S0-BSC-653

RHEUMATOLOGY

SECOND EDITION

JOHN H KLIPPEL
PAUL A DIEPPE

VOLUME ONE

RHEUMATOLOGY

SECOND EDITION

JOHN H KLIPPEL
National Institute of Arthritis and Musculoskeletal and Skin Diseases
National Institutes of Health
Bethesda, USA

PAUL A DIEPPE
Faculty of Medicine
University of Bristol
Bristol, UK

Frank C Arnett
Division of Rheumatology
Department of Internal Medicine
University of Texas Health Science Center
Houston, USA

Peter M Brooks
Department of Medicine
The University of New South Wales
St. Vincent's Hospital
Sydney, Australia

Juan J Canoso
American British
Cowdray Hospital
Mexico City, Mexico

Simon Carette
Département de Rheumatologie
Le Centre Hospitalier de l'Université Laval
Québec, Canada

Jan Dequeker
Division of Rheumatology
Department of Internal Medicine
University Hospitals KU Leuven
Belgium

Rodney Grahame
Department of Rheumatology
UMDS Guy's Hospital
London, UK

Andrew CS Keat
Department of Rheumatology
Northwick Park Hospital
Harrow, UK

Robert P Kimberly
Division of Clinical Immunology and Rheumatology
Department of Medicine
University of Alabama at Birmingham
Birmingham, USA

Matthew H Liang
Department of Rheumatology, Immunology and Allergy
Brigham & Women's Hospital
Boston, USA

Ravinder N Maini
Kennedy Institute of Rheumatology
London, UK

Leo BA van de Putte
Department of Rheumatology
University Hospital Nijmegen
Nijmegen, The Netherlands

John S Sergent
Vanderbilt University Medical Center
The Vanderbilt Clinic
Nashville, USA

Nathan J Zvaifler
Division of Rheumatology
School of Medicine
University of California at San Diego
San Diego, USA

Theme editors

Joseph A Buckwalter
Department of Orthopedic Surgery
University of Iowa
Iowa City, USA

Charles G Peterfy
Department of Radiology
University of California at San Francisco
San Francisco, USA

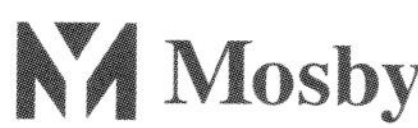

Mosby

London Philadelphia St. Louis Sydney Tokyo

Cataloging-in-Publications Data:
Cataloging records for this book are available from the US Library of Congress and the British Library

ISBN: 0 7234 2405 5

For full details of Mosby International titles please write to:
Mosby International
Lynton House
7–12 Tavistock Square
London WC1H 9LB
UK

Typeset in Times, legends set in Univers.
Produced by Reeds Reprographics, Ipswich, UK.
Printed and bound by Grafos, SA Arte sobre papel, Barcelona, Spain.

Published in 1998 by Mosby, an imprint of Mosby International, a division of Times Mirror International Publishers Limited.
First edition published in 1994 by Mosby-Year Book Europe Limited.

SECOND EDITION

Publisher	Fiona Foley
Development Editors	Sue Hodgson
	Jeremy Gross
Managing Editor	Alison Whitehouse
Project Managers	Katie Pattullo
	Sarah Edwards
	Elaine Graham
	Nigel Wetters
Designer	Pete Wilder
Design and Illustration	The EDI Partnership: Mark Willey, Lee Smith, Zak Knowles
	Lynda Payne
	Danny Pyne
	Mike Saiz
Proofreader/Editor	John Ormiston
Copyeditor	Ellen Sarewitz
Editorial Assistant	Susan Rana
Production	Siobhan Egan
	Susan Walby
	Adam Phillips
Index	Janine Ross

FIRST EDITION

Publisher	Fiona Foley
Project Managers	David Cooke
	Michael Smith
	Lucy Hamilton
	Alison Whitehouse
Design and Illustration	Judith Gauge
	Richard Prime
	Jenni Miller
	Mark Willey
	Chris Read
	Tim Read
	Anne-Marie Woodruff
	Dereck Johnson
Linework	Lee Smith
Editorial Assistant	Chris Downs
Production	Adam Phillips
	Jane Tozer
	Susan Bishop
Index	Nina Boyd

DRUG NOTICE

The contributors, the editors, and the publishers have made every effort to ensure the accuracy and appropriateness of the drug dosages presented in this textbook. The medications described do not necessarily have specific approval by the Food and Drug Administration for use in the diseases and dosages for which they are recommended. The package insert for each drug should be consulted for use and dosage as approved by the FDA. Because standards for usage change, it is advisable to keep abreast of revised recommendations, particularly those concerning new drugs.

COPYRIGHT

PREFACE

Jack Klippel and Paul Dieppe

The second edition of *Rheumatology* is:

- A comprehensive, authoritative text reference book, designed to meet the complete needs of all practicing clinical and academic rheumatologists as well as all health care professionals and scientists interested in disorders of the musculoskeletal system.
- Based firmly on modern medical science, integrating the relevant basic biology with current clinical practice.
- Of immediate bedside value through its innovative use of 'practical problems' and other clinical material.
- An easily accessible, user-friendly, beautifully illustrated color publication.
- Consistent in style and format, each chapter being written to a strict template and rigorously edited.
- A genuinely international book, with editors, authors and material drawn from all over the world.
- Fully up-to-date, with carefully selected references to original work and key reviews up to and including 1997 publications.

THE SECOND EDITION OF *RHEUMATOLOGY* IS A TOTALLY NEW AND VERY EXCITING BOOK

Although the first edition was an unqualified success – being voted 1994 Book of the Year by Doody's *Health Sciences Book Review Journal*, for example – the editorial team and publishers both knew that they could do even better. We therefore commissioned independent, critical reviews of the first edition from clinicians and scientists worldwide, analyzed their comments and embraced the exciting challenge of re-structuring the format and contents of the book in a way that would retain all the best features of the first edition of *Rheumatology*, while also striving to make a great book even better. We believe that we have succeeded and that the second edition of *Rheumatology* will become the first choice authoritative text reference for all practicing rheumatologists and their trainees.

As noted by the reviewers, ("a model for other textbooks" – *NEJM*; "a departure from everything that has preceded it" – *JAMA*) the success of the first edition owed much to our consistency of style and content, innovative use of color illustration, many 'practical problems' and user-friendly format. We have retained all these features of the book. We have continued to use tightly controlled templates for each chapter, and have pursued a rigorous editorial policy in order to ensure that the content and format of the book remain both consistent and of the highest possible standard. The different sections remain color coded (although users of the first edition should note that the colors have changed!).

Whilst much of what made the first edition so successful has therefore been retained, we have also made many major changes to the contents. We have increased the number of practical problems by 30%, with new information on disease assessment, management and rehabilitation, and completely rewritten over 50% of the original contributions. We have included even more full-color illustrations.

The introductory section, as well as that on principles of therapy, has been extensively restructured, and many new editors and contributors have joined the team. Every chapter has either been carefully revised (15%) or updated (50%), or, in many cases, completely rewritten (25% of chapters). Much new information has been added, but we have also cut out some of the material found in the first edition, so that the total extent of the book is only some 80 pages longer. We have also worked hard on the index, in order to make it even easier for the reader to find the material that he or she wants. Another major change that will come as a relief to many, and may well reduce the incidence of upper limb, soft tissue lesions, is that the book is now in two, much lighter volumes.

Contributions from the crucial allied sub-specialities of imaging and orthopedics have been greatly strengthened by the addition of 'theme editors' in these areas (Charles Peterfy and Joseph Buckwalter, respectively). They have both responded to the difficult tasks that we gave them magnificently, keeping a watching brief on their areas of interest throughout the book, as well as contributing a lot of new material themselves.

A modern textbook must respond to the fast pace of change in the science and practice of medicine. Since publication of the first edition of *Rheumatology*, there have been many important advances in rheumatology, which we have addressed by the inclusion of new contributions in the second edition (see Table below).

The production of the second edition of *Rheumatology* has been a greatly enjoyable team effort. We would like to thank every one of the editors and authors who have contributed to either the first or second editions of the book, as well as the excellent team at Mosby, led by Fiona Foley: Sue Hodgson, Katie Pattullo, Alison Whitehouse, Sarah Edwards, Elaine Graham, Jeremy Gross, Andrea Ford, Lynda Payne, Susan Rana and Pete Wilder. However, above all, *Rheumatology* is a tribute to the vision, leadership and hard work of Fiona Foley, to whom we are proud to dedicate this book.

RECENT KEY ADVANCES IN THE SCIENCE AND PRACTICE OF RHEUMATOLOGY

- New understanding of endothelial cell biology (Chapters 5.12 and 7.18) and mediator systems in inflammatory arthritis – such as nitric oxide and the neuroendocrine system (Chapter 5.11).
- Significant advances in our understanding of pain and pain management (Chapter 3.4).
- Developments in procedural rheumatology (Chapter 2.13).
- Advances in the molecular genetics of rheumatoid arthritis (Chapter 5.7), osteoarthritis (Chapter 8.7), and SLE (Chapter 7.3).
- Advances in evidence-based medicine, health services research (Chapters 1.2 and 1.5) and outcome assessment (Chapter 3.14 and the Appendix).
- New understanding of the risk factors and control of osteoporosis (Chapters 8.38 and 8.40).
- The cause of conditions such as Whipple's disease (Chapter 6.24) and Marfan's syndrome (Chapter 1.6) have been discovered.
- The impact of magnetic resonance imaging on rheumatology (Chapter 2.14).
- The molecular understanding of connective tissue turnover and the discovery of new enzymes, such as aggrecanase (Chapters 1.8 and 8.6).
- The potential development of structure-modifying drugs for osteoarthritis (Chapter 8.9).
- The development of new immunotherapeutic approaches, based on the advances in molecular biology (Chapter 3.10).

USER GUIDE

VOLUMES, SECTIONS AND COLOR-CODING

Rheumatology Second Edition is divided into two volumes. The book is organized into eight sections, which are color-coded as follows for quick and easy reference:

VOLUME ONE

SECTION 1 — Rheumatic diseases

SECTION 2 — Evaluation, signs and symptoms

SECTION 3 — Principles of management

SECTION 4 — Regional pain problems

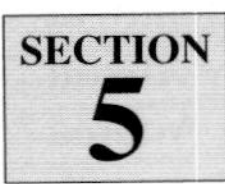

Rheumatoid arthritis and other synovial disorders

VOLUME TWO

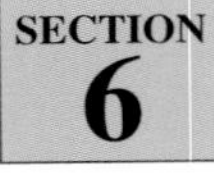

Infection-related rheumatic diseases and spondyloarthropathies

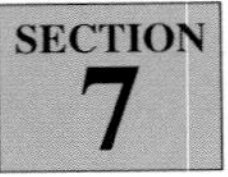

Connective tissue disorders

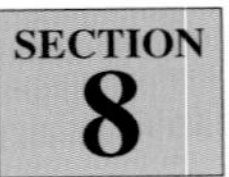

Disorders of bone, cartilage and connective tissue

Sections 1–5 appear in Volume One, and Sections 6–8 appear in Volume Two.

Rheumatology Second Edition has a total extent of 1920 pages. Volume One has 888 pages, and Volume Two has 1032 pages.

FINDING CHAPTERS AND PAGES

Within each section the chapters are numbered consecutively, with each chapter paginated and beginning on page 1. Each page gives the section, chapter and page number. An example is shown below. This example is page 4 of chapter 3 in Section 5, page 5.3.4.

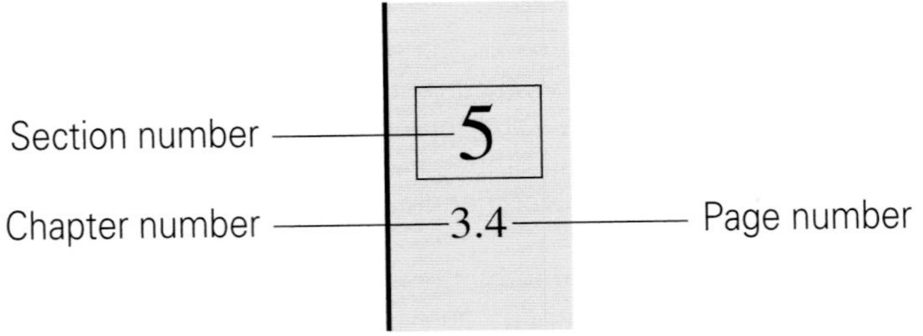

To find this chapter, turn to the yellow section (Section 5), find chapter 3 and then turn to page 4.

A comprehensive subject index, covering the entire book, appears in the back of both volumes of *Rheumatology Second Edition*.

FINDING PRACTICAL PROBLEMS

A Classification Guide to the Practical Problems, which categorizes the titles of the Practical Problems under 12 different subject headings, appears after the Contents list at the front of both volumes. Practical Problems are also colored in a gray tint in the Contents list.

ACKNOWLEDGEMENTS

This book would not exist without the huge contribution made by previous Section Editors and contributors to the first edition.

Lynn H Gerber
Brian L Hazelman
Roger D Sturrock
Murray B Urowitz
Frank A Wollheim

Adewale O Adebajo
M H Arnold
Roger M Atkins
Howard A Austin III
Colin G Barnes
Maurice A Barry
Edward J Bieber
Anders Bjelle
Scott D Boden
Henry H Bohlman
Dimitrios T Boumpas
Giles Campion
Ramon M Carbotte
Joseph M Cash
James T Cassidy
Hereward S Cattell
David E Caughey
Leo M Cooney Jr
Leslie J Crofford
Pierre D Delmas
François Delrieu
Judah A Denburg
Susan D Denburg
Anthony S Fauci
Gilbert C Faure
Mark P Figgie
Darragh Foley-Nolan
Paul R Fortin
Eric P Gall
Marc T Galloway
Kevin L Garvin
Charles Goldsmith
Eva Hedfors
Pascal Hilliquin
David W L Hukins
Michael H Huo
Robert Inman
Lawrence J Kagen
Joachim R Kalden
Ronald L Kirby
Reva Lawrence
Ron Laxer
Timothy JK Leonard
Randall J Lewis
Stephen Lipson
Sverre Maehlum
John A Mathews
Charles-Jöel Menkes
Colin D Merrick
John Moll
Kenneth D Muirden
Michael S Mulligan
Andrew K Palmer
Ross E Petty
Kevin D Pile
David S Pisetsky
David N Podell
Andrew J Porges
Carlos D Rosé
James T Rosenbaum
Robert T Schoen
James R Seibold
Nancy A Shadick
Walter H Short
Lola Sicard-Rosenbaum
Bernard H Singsen
Ezra Sohar
Louis Solomon
Richard D Sontheimer
David E Trentham
Peter Tugwell
Anthony S Unger
Robert PS van den Berg
Martin H van Rijswijk
James A Varani
Peter A Ward
B Paul Wordsworth
David Yocum

CONTENTS

VOLUME ONE

VOLUME 1 SECTION 1

RHEUMATIC DISEASES

Matthew H Liang & Leo BA van de Putte

VOLUME 1 SECTION 2

EVALUATION, SIGNS AND SYMPTOMS

Rodney Grahame & John S Sergent

VOLUME 1 SECTION 3

PRINCIPLES OF MANAGEMENT

Peter M Brooks

VOLUME 1 SECTION 4

REGIONAL PAIN PROBLEMS

Juan J Canoso & Simon Carette

SECTION 4

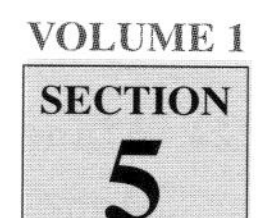

VOLUME 1
SECTION 5

RHEUMATOID ARTHRITIS AND OTHER SYNOVIAL DISORDERS

Ravinder N Maini & Nathan J Zvaifler

RHEUMATOID ARTHRITIS

SECTION 5

JUVENILE CHRONIC ARTHRITIS

UNCOMMON ARTHROPATHIES

VOLUME TWO

VOLUME 2

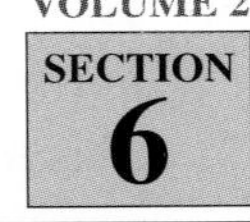

SECTION 6

INFECTION-RELATED RHEUMATIC DISEASES AND SPONDYLOARTHROPATHIES

Frank C Arnett & Andrew CS Keat

INFECTION

SPONDYLOARTHROPATHIES

VOLUME 2 SECTION 7

CONNECTIVE TISSUE DISORDERS

John H Klippel & Robert P Kimberly

SYSTEMIC LUPUS ERYTHEMATOSUS

VOLUME 2
SECTION 8

DISORDERS OF BONE, CARTILAGE AND CONNECTIVE TISSUE

Jan Dequeker & Paul Dieppe

OSTEOARTHRITIS AND RELATED DISORDERS

CRYSTAL-RELATED ARTHROPATHIES

ENDOCRINE AND HEMOGLOBIN-RELATED ARTHRITIS AND STORAGE DISEASES

SECTION
8

SECTION
8

CLASSIFICATION GUIDE TO PRACTICAL PROBLEMS

This guide classifies the 148 Practical Problems in *Rheumatology Second Edition* under nine different subject categories, to help the reader find the information they need quickly and easily. Many of the Practical Problems appear under more than one category. The categories are as follows:

1. Patient outcome and rehabilitation
2. Drug and surgical interventions
3. Spinal problems
4. Upper limb problems
5. Lower limb problems
6. Generalized musculoskeletal pain
7. Inflammatory joint disease, divided into rheumatoid arthritis and others
8. Connective tissue disease, divided into systemic lupus erythematosus and others
9. Bone, cartilage and metabolic disorders, divided into bone and others

This guide is not an index. The index to both volumes of *Rheumatology Second Edition* can be found at the back of this book.

1. PATIENT OUTCOME AND REHABILITATION

2. DRUG AND SURGICAL INTERVENTIONS

3. SPINAL PROBLEMS

4. UPPER LIMB PROBLEMS

5. LOWER LIMB PROBLEMS Page

6. GENERALIZED MUSCULOSKELETAL PAIN Page

7. INFLAMMATORY JOINT DISEASE Page

RHEUMATOID ARTHRITIS

OTHERS

8. CONNECTIVE TISSUE DISEASE Page

SYSTEMIC LUPUS ERYTHEMATOSUS

OTHERS

9. BONE, CARTILAGE AND METABOLIC DISORDERS Page

BONE

OTHERS

CONTRIBUTING AUTHORS

MICHA ABELES **7.08**
Associate Professor of Medicine, Department of Medicine, Division of Rheumatology, University of Connecticut Health Center; Associate Director, Multipurpose Arthritis Center, Farmington, Connecticut, USA

BRIAN D ADAMS **5.16**
Professor, Department of Orthopedic Surgery, University of Iowa College of Medicine, Iowa City, Iowa, USA

DAVID M ADLAM **4.13**
Consultant Oral & Maxillofacial Surgeon, Addenbrookes Hospital, Cambridge, UK

SALVATORE ALBANI **5.20**
Assistant Professor of Pediatrics; Director, Center for Pediatric Rheumatology, Department of Pediatrics, University of California at San Diego School of Medicine, La Jolla, California, USA

JEFF A ALLOWAY **7.23**
Assistant Professor of Medicine, Uniformed Services University of the Health Sciences; Staff Rheumatologist, Wilford Hall Medical Center, Lackland Airforce Base, San Antonio, Texas, USA

MARY-CARMEN AMIGO **7.08, 7.36**
Associate Professor of Rheumatology, Instituto Nacional de Cardiologìa I. Chàvez, Universidad Nacional Autònoma de México, Mexico City, Mexico

BERNARD AMOR **6.25**
Professor of Rheumatology, Clinique de Rhumatologie, Hôpital Cochin, Paris, France

BARBARA M ANSELL **5.19, 5.24**
Dumgoyne, Stoke Poges, Berkshire, UK

FRANK C ARNETT **6.10**
Professor and Director, Division of Rheumatology and Clinical Immunogenetics, Department of Internal Medicine, University of Texas-Houston, Health Science Center, Houston, Texas, USA

ELIZABETH M BADLEY **3.02**
Director, Arthritis Community Research and Evaluation Unit, The Wellesley Hospital Research Institute; Associate Professor, Department of Preventive Medicine & Biostatistics, Faculty of Medicine, University of Toronto, Toronto, Ontario, Canada

W TIMOTHY BALLARD **3.12**
Director, Chattanooga Orthopedic Group Foundation for Research, Chattanooga, Tennessee, USA

JAMES E BALOW **7.08**
Clinical Director, NIDDK, National Institutes of Health, Bethesda, Maryland, USA

THOMAS BARDIN **8.28, 8.29, 8.30, 8.31**
Professor of Rheumatology, Clinique de Rhumatologie, Centre Viggo Pertersen, Hôpital Lariboisière, Paris, France

LES BARNSLEY **4.04, 4.06**
Consultant Rheumatologist, Concord Hospital, Sydney, Australia; Senior Lecturer in Rheumatology, Sydney University, Australia

WERNER F BARTH **6.25**
Chairman, Section of Rheumatology, Washington Hospital Center; Professor of Medicine, George Washington University Medical Center, Washington DC, USA

ADRIAN E BAUMAN **3.03**
Associate Professor (Public Health); Head, Epidemiology Unit, The Liverpool Hospital Liverpool, New South Wales, Australia

NICHOLAS BELLAMY **3.14** **8.12**
Professor of Medicine, Epidemiology and Biostatistics, University of Western Ontario; Director, Division of Rheumatology LHSC - Victoria Campus, London, Ontario, Canada

J SYBIL BIERMANN **8.53**
Assistant Professor, Department of Surgery; Director of Orthopedic Oncology, The University of Michigan, Ann Arbor, Michigan, USA

JOHANNES WJ BIJLSMA **8.43**
Professor of Rheumatology, Department of Rheumatology and Immunology, University Hospital, Utrecht, The Netherlands

HOWARD A BIRD **3.07**
Professor of Pharmacological Rheumatology, Clinical Pharmacology Unit (Rheumatism Research), University of Leeds, Research School of Medicine, Chapel Allertown Hospital, Leeds, West Yorkshire, UK

CAROL M BLACK **7.11**
Director, Royal Free Academic Unit of Rheumatology & Connective Tissue Diseases; Professor of Rheumatology, Royal Free Hospital School of Medicine, London, UK

TOMÁS S BOCANEGRA **6.04**
Senior Director, Clinical Research GD Searle & Co, Skokie, Illinois, USA

NIKOLAI BOGDUK **4.02, 4.06**
Professor of Anatomy; Director, Cervical Spine Research Unit, Faculty of Medicine and Health Sciences, Discipline of Anatomy, University of Newcastle, Callaghan, Newcastle, Australia

STEFANO BOMBARDIERI **7.31**
Associate Professor; Chief, Clinical Immunology Unit, University of Pisa, Pisa, Italy

DAVID G BORENSTEIN **4.03, 4.06**
Clinical Professor of Medicine, The George Washington University Medical Center, Washington DC, USA

JOANNE BORG-STEIN **4.18**
Chief, Physical Medicine and Rehabilitation; Assistant Professor, Tufts University; Medical Director, Spaulding and Newton-Wellesley Hospital Rehabilitation Center, Newton-Wellesley Hospital, Newton, Massachusetts, USA

STEPHEN M BREATHNACH **6.22**
Consultant Dermatologist and Senior Lecturer, St John's Institute of Dermatology, St Thomas' Hospital, London, UK

BARRY BRESNIHAN **2.04**
Professor of Rheumatology, University College; Consultant Rheumatologist, St Vincent's Hospital, Dublin, Ireland

ANTHONY J BRON **5.16**
Professor of Ophthalmology and Head of Department, Nuffield Laboratory of Ophthalmology, University of Oxford, Oxford, UK

PETER M BROOKS **3.01, 3.05, 3.12** **5.16** **6.09** **8.12**
St. Vincent's Hospital, Sydney, New South Wales, Australia

ANNE C BROWER **5.05** **6.17**
Professor and Chair, Department of Radiology, Eastern Virginia Medical School, Hofheimer Hall Norfolk, Virginia, USA

STUART I BROWN **5.16**
Director, The Shiley Eye Center; Professor and Chair of Ophthalmology, University of California, San Diego, La Jolla, California, USA

W WATSON BUCHANAN **1.01**
Director, Rheumatic Diseases Unit, McMaster University Hospital, Hamilton, Ontario, Canada

JOSEPH A BUCKWALTER **3.01, 3.12** **4.14** **8.09, 8.12, 8.43**
Professor of Orthopedic Surgery, Department of Orthopedic Surgery, University of Iowa, Iowa City, Iowa, USA

PETER G BULLOUGH **8.08**
Director of Laboratory Medicine, The Hospital for Special Surgery; Professor of Pathology, Cornell University Medical College, New York, New York, USA

ADOLF BURSSENS **8.49**
Lecturer, University of Louvain, Wilsele-Leuven, Belgium

JOEL BUXBAUM **8.27**
Chief, Rheumatology Section, New York Department of VA Medical Center; Professor of Medicine, New York University School of Medicine, Research Service, New York VA Medical Center, New York, New York, USA

Numbers in colored boxes refer to contributors' chapters

JILL P BUYON **7.08**
Director, Lupus Clinic, Hospital for Joint Diseases; Associate Professor of Medicine, New York University School of Medicine, New York, New York, USA

MARGARET A BYRON **5.16**
Consultant and Honorary Senior Lecturer, Rheumatology Unit, Bristol Royal Infirmary, Bristol, UK

ERIC GL BYWATERS **5.17**
Former Director MRC Rheumatism Unit, Taplow, Emeritus Professor of Medicine (Rheumatology), Royal Postgraduate Medical School of London, London, UK

LEONARD H CALABRESE **6.07**
Vice Chairman, Department of Rheumatic and Immunologic Disease, Cleveland Clinic Foundation, Cleveland, Ohio, USA

JOHN J CALLAGHAN **8.12**
Professor, Department of Orthopedics, University of Iowa College of Medicine, Iowa City, Iowa, USA

JEFFREY P CALLEN **7.29, 7.30**
Professor of Medicine (Dermatology); Chief, Division of Dermatology, University of Louisville School of Medicine, Louisville, Kentucky, USA

JOHN STEWART CAMERON **2.09**
Emeritus Professor of Renal Medicine, UMDS, London, Clinical Science Labs, Guy's Hospital, London, UK

JUAN J CANOSO **2.12** **4.01**
Adjunct Professor of Medicine, Tufts University, Boston, Massachusetts, USA; Rheumatologist, American British Cowdray Hospital, Mexico City, Mexico

SIMON CARETTE **4.01, 4.10**
Professor of Medicine, Division of Rheumatology, Centre Hospitalier, Universitaire de Quebec, Quebec, Canada

LUIS J CATOGGIO **7.15**
Head, Rheumatology Section, Medical Services, Hospital Italiano de Buenos Aires and Fundacion Dr Pedro M Catoggio para el Progreso de la Reumatologia, Buenos Aires, Argentina

ARNOLD CATS **5.15, 5.16**
Emeritus Professor of Rheumatology, Department of Rheumatology, Leiden University Hospital, Leiden, The Netherlands

TIM E CAWSTON **1.08**
Professor of Rheumatology, Department of Rheumatology, The Medicine School, University of Newcastle, Newcastle, UK

KUNTAL CHAKRAVARTY **6.20**
Consultant Rheumatologist, Old Church and Haroldwood Hospital, Havering Hospital NHS Trust, Romford, Essex, UK

M ANNE CHAMBERLAIN **5.16**
Professor of Rheumatological Rehabilitation, Rheumatology & Rehabilitation Research Unit, University of Leeds School of Medicine, Leeds, UK

G DAVID CHAMPION **3.13**
Rheumatologist, St Vincent's Hospital and Sydney Children's Hospital, Sydney, New South Wales, Australia

MICHAEL D CHARD **4.08**
Consultant Rheumatologist, Worthing Hospital, Worthing, West Sussex, UK

ERNEST HS CHOY **3.10**
Lecturer, Rheumatology Units, Guy's and King's College Hospitals, London, UK

FLAVIA M CICUTTINI **8.07**
Senior Lecturer, Department of Epidemiology and Preventive Medicine, Monash University, Australia

ANTHONY CLARKE **8.12**
Consultant in Rheumatology and Rehabilitation, Royal National Hospital for Rheumatic Diseases, Bath, UK

DANIEL J CLAUW **7.34**
Assistant Professor of Medicine, Chief, Division of Rheumatology, Immunology and Allergy, Georgetown University Medical Center, Washington DC, USA

PHILIP J CLEMENTS **3.09**
Professor of Medicine, Department of Medicine, Center for Health Sciences, University of California at Los Angeles, Los Angeles, California, USA

MARC D COHEN **5.04**
Director, Division of Rheumatology; Associate Professor of Medicine, Mayo Clinic, Jacksonville, Florida, USA

MILTON COHEN **3.04**
Chairman, Department of Rheumatology and Pain Clinic, St Vincent's Hospital, Sydney, New South Wales, Australia

MICHAEL G COHEN **8.14**
Consultant Rheumatologist, Gordon, Sydney, New South Wales, Australia

DOYT L CONN **5.04** **7.20**
Senior Vice President for Medical Affairs, Arthritis Foundation: Clinical Professor of Medicine, Emory University School of Medicine, Atlanta, Georgia, USA

F RICHARD CONVERY **5.29**
Professor of Orthopedic Surgery, University of California at San Diego, San Diego, California, USA

CYRUS COOPER **4.06** **8.02**
Reader in Rheumatology, University of Southampton, MRC Senior Clinical Scientist, MRC Environmental Epidemiology Unit; Consultant Rheumatologist, Southampton General Hospital, Southampton, UK

BRETT G COURTENAY **6.09**
Consultant Orthopaedic Surgeon, St. Vincent's Campus, Sydney, New South Wales, Australia

EDWARD V CRAIG **4.14**
Attending Surgeon, Hospital for Special Surgery; Clinical Professor of Orthopedics Surgery, Cornell University Medical School; Attending Surgeon: Orthopedics, New York Hospital, New York, New York, USA

MICHAEL H CRAWFORD **2.07**
Robert S Flinn Professor and Chief of Cardiology, University of New Mexico Health Sciences Center, Albuquerque, New Mexico, USA

PAUL CREAMER **1.06** **8.11, 8.12**
Visiting Assistant Professor, Department of Rheumatology and Clinical Immunology, University of Maryland Medical School, Baltimore, Maryland, USA

ADRIAN J CRISP **4.14**
Consultant Rheumatologist, Department of Rheumatology, Addenbrooke's NHS Trust, Cambridge, UK

MARY K CROW **7.06**
Professor of Medicine, Department of Medicine, Hospital for Special Surgery, New York, New York, USA

MARTA L CUÉLLAR **6.23**
Research Instructor, Department of Medicine, Section of Rheumatology, Louisiana State University School of Medicine, New Orleans, Louisiana, USA

THOMAS R CUPPS **7.23**
Associate Professor of Medicine, Georgetown University Hospital, Washington DC, USA

JANET CUSHNAGHAN **8.12**
Rheumatology Clinical Specialist, The County Hospital, Hereford, UK

SEAMUS E DALTON **4.07** **8.53**
Consultant in Rehabilitation and Sports Medicine, Director of Sports Medicine, North Sydney Orthopaedic and Sports Medicine Center, Crows Nest, Sydney, Australia

LAWREN H DALTROY **3.03**
Associate Director, RBB Multipurpose Arthritis and Musculoskeletal Diseases Center, Brigham & Womens Hospital; Assistant Professor in Medicine, Harvard Medical School; Assistant Professor of Health & Social Behavior, Harvard School of Public Health, Brigham Women's Hospital Boston, Massachusetts, USA

JOHN C DAVIS, JR **7.08**
Clinical Associate, Clinical Investigation Unit, National Institute of Arthritis, Musculoskeletal and Skin Diseases, National Institutes of Health, Bethesda, Maryland, USA

DAVID M DAWSON **7.16**
Professor of Neurology, Harvard Medical School, Neurology Service, Brockton/West Roxbury Department of Veteran Affairs Medical Center, West Roxbury, Massachusetts, USA

RICHARD O DAY **3.08** **5.16**
Professor of Clinical Pharmacology, St Vincent's Hospital, Darlinghurst, Sydney, Australia

KAREL DE CEULAER **8.25**
Consultant Rheumatologist, Department of Medicine, University of the West Indies, Kingston, Jamaica, West Indies

JAN DEQUEKER **1.01** **8.34, 8.36, 8.39, 8.44, 8.49**
Professor of Rheumatology, Faculty of Medicine, Katholieke Universiteit Leuven; Director Arthritis and Metabolic Bone Research Unit, Division of Rheumatology, University Hospitals Leuven, Belgium

JEAN-PIERRE DEVOGELAER **8.45**
Professor of Rheumatology, Saint-Luc University Hospital; Medical Director, the Arthritis Unit, Louvain University in Brussels, Brussels, Belgium

Numbers in colored boxes refer to contributors' chapters

PAUL DIEPPE 2.01
8.01, 8.03, 8.04, 8.09, 8.12, 8.13, 8.19, 8.33, 8.53
Director, MRC Health Services Research Initiative; Professor of Rheumatology, University of Bristol, Bristol, UK

JOSH J DIXEY 5.25
Consultant Rheumatologist and Medical Director, The Robert Jones and Agnes Hunt Orthopaedic and District NHS Trust Hospital, Oswestry, Shropshire, UK

ALLAN ST J DIXON 5.16
Helston, Cornwall, UK

MICHAEL DOHERTY 8.12, 8.13, 8.16, 8.19
Professor of Rheumatology, Nottingham University Medical School; Consultant in Rheumatology, City Hospital, Nottingham, UK

MAXIME DOUGADOS 6.20
Professor of Rheumatology, Service de Rhumatologie B, Université René Descartes, Hôpital Cochin, Paris, France

PAUL DOURY 8.44
Professeur du Val De Grâce, Spécialiste de Rhumatologie, Rhumatologie Service Polyclinique, Institution Nationale des Invalides, Paris, France

ROBERT B DUTHIE 8.33
Emeritus Professor, Oxford University; Honorary Consultant, Nuffield Orthopaedic Centre, Oxford, UK

JOHN B EASTWOOD 8.42
Senior Lecturer in Medicine & Consultant Renal Physician, Department of Renal Medicine, St George's Hospital and Medical School, London, UK

JEFFREY C EDBERG 7.02
Assistant Professor of Medicine, Department of Medicine, The University of Alabama at Birmingham, Birmingham, Alabama, USA

JO CW EDWARDS 5.06
Professor of Connective Tissue Medicine, University College London Rheumatology Unit, Arthur Stanley House, London, UK

N LAWRENCE EDWARDS 8.19
Chief, Section of Rheumatology, Professor of Medicine, Veterans Administration Medical Center, University of Florida, Gainesville, Florida, USA

JOHN A EISMAN 8.37
Professor of Medicine and Director, Bone and Mineral Research Program, The Garvan Institute of Medical Research, St Vincent's Hospital, Sydney, New South Wales, Australia

KEITH B ELKON 7.05
Professor of Medicine, Department of Medicine, The Hospital for Special Surgery, New York, New York, USA

BRYAN T EMMERSON 8.14, 8.15, 8.19
Professor Emeritus and Honorary Research Consultant, University of Queensland; Consultant Emeritus, Princess Alexandra Hospital, Brisbane, Queensland, Australia

JOHN M ESDAILE 1.02 5.22
Research Director, Mary Pack Arthritis Centre; Head, Division of Rheumatology, Professor of Medicine, University of British Columbia, Vancouver, British Columbia, Canada

LUIS R ESPINOZA 6.23
Professor and Chief, Section of Rheumatology, Department of Medicine, Louisiana State School of Medicine, New Orleans, Louisiana, USA

JOHN A FAIRCLOUGH 4.11
Consultant in Trauma and Orthopaedics, Cardiff Royal Infirmary, Cardiff, Wales, UK

ADEL G FAM 4.09, 4.12
Professor of Medicine and Head, Division of Rheumatology, Sunnybrook Health Science Centre, University of Toronto, Toronto, Ontario, Canada

BARRI J FESSLER 7.08
Senior Staff Physician, Department of Rheumatic and Immunologic Diseases, The Cleveland Clinic Foundation, Cleveland, Ohio, USA

GARY S FIRESTEIN 5.13
Professor of Medicine, Division of Rheumatology, UCSD School of Medicine, La Jolla, California, USA

JAMES L FLECKENSTEIN 7.16
Medical Director Algur H Meadows Diagnostic Imaging Center; Associate Professor of Radiology, Department of Radiology, University of Texas Southwestern Medical Center at Dallas, Dallas, Texas, USA

SÁNDOR S FORGÁCS 8.20, 8.23
Professor of Radiology, Head of Department of Diagnostic Radiology, Uzsoki Hospital, Budapest, Hungary

JOHN V FORRESTER 2.06
Professor of Ophthalmology, Cockburn Chair in Ophthalmology, Department of Ophthalmology, University of Aberdeen, Medical School, Aberdeen, Scotland

VICTOR H FRANKEL 1.11
President, Hospital for Joint Diseases Orthopedic Institute; Professor of Orthopedic Surgery, New York University School of Medicine, New York, New York, USA

ANTHONY J FREEMONT 2.11
Professor of Osteoarticular Pathology, Department of Rheumatology, University of Manchester, Manchester, UK

STEVEN M FRIEDMAN 7.06
Professor of Medicine, Department of Medicine, Hospital for Special Surgery, Cornell University Medical College, New York, New York, USA

BEATRICE E FRUEH 5.16
Assistant Professor, Department of Ophthalmology, Inselspital Bern, Switzerland

DANIEL E FURST 3.09 5.16
Director of the Arthritis Clinical Research Unit and Medical Director, Virginia Mason Research Center; Clinical Professor of Medicine and Rheumatology, University of Washington, Seattle, Washington, USA

SHERINE E GABRIEL 1.03
Associate Professor of Medicine and Epidemiology, Department of Health Sciences Research and Department of Internal Medicine, Division of Rheumatology, Mayo Clinic, Rochester, Minnesota, USA

JS HILL GASTON 5.10
Professor of Rheumatology, Department of Medicine, University of Cambridge School of Clinical Medicine, Addenbrooke's Hospital, Cambridge, UK

HARRY K GENANT 8.43
Professor of Radiology, Medicine & Orthopedic Surgery; Chief, Musculoskeletal Radiology; Executive Director, Osteoporosis Research Group, University of California Medical Center, San Francisco, California, USA

DAVID L GEORGE 2.05
Associate Director of Medicine, Department of Medicine, Reading Hospital and Medical Center; Clinical Professor of Medicine, Pennsylvania State University, West Reading, Pennsylvania, USA

EMMANUEL GEORGE 4.14
Consultant Rheumatologist, Arrowe Park Hospital, Upton, Wirral, Merseyside, UK

PIET PMM GEUSENS 8.35, 8.43
Professor, Clinical Research Center for Bone and Joint Diseases, Dr L Willems-Instituut, Limburgs Universitair Centrum, Diepenbeek, Belgium

DAFNA D GLADMAN 7.01
Deputy Director, Centre for Prognosis Studies in the Rheumatic Diseases; Program Director, Division of Rheumatology; Professor of Medicine, University of Toronto, Toronto, Ontario, Canada

DON L GOLDENBERG 4.15. 4.18
Chief of Rheumatology, Newton-Wellesley Hospital; Professor of Medicine, Rheumatology Department, Tufts University School of Medicine, Newton, Massachusetts, USA

DUNCAN A GORDON 5.03
Senior Rheumatologist, Toronto Hospital Arthritis Centre; Professor of Medicine, University of Toronto, Toronto, Ontario, Canada

GEOFFREY P GRAHAM 4.11
Consultant Orthopaedic Surgeon, Cardiff Royal Infirmary and BUPA Hospital, Cardiff, UK

RODNEY GRAHAME 2.02 8.51
Emeritus Professor of Clinical Rheumatology, UMDS Guy's Hospital, London, UK

JAN T GRAN 6.15
Head of Department of Rheumatology, Regional Hospital of Tromsø; Professor of Rheumatology, University of Tromsø, Tromsø, Norway

JERRY M GREENE 7.16
Chief, Rheumatology Section, Medical Service Brockton/West Roxbury Department of Veteran Affairs Medical Center; Instructor in Medicine, Harvard Medical School, West Roxbury, Massachusetts, USA

GERALD D GROFF 4.14
Associate Professor Clinical Medicine, College of Physicians and Surgeons, Columbia University, Bassett Healthcare, Cooperstown, New York, USA

Numbers in colored boxes refer to contributors' chapters

CHARLOTTE GRONDIN **5.24**
Professeur de Clinique, Service de Rhumatologie, Centre Hospitalier Universitaire de Québec, Pavillon Chul, Sainte-Foy, Québec, Canada

WOLFGANG L GROSS **7.19**
Professor of Internal Medicine, Department of Rheumatology, Medical University of Luebeck and Rheumaklinik Bad Bramstedt GmbH, Luebeck/ Bad Bramstedt, Germany

LOÏC P GUILLEVIN **7.24, 7.31**
Professor of Medicine, Head of Department of Internal Medicine, Hôpital Avicenne, Faculté de Médecine Paris-Nord, Bobigny Cedex, France

NORTIN M HADLER **5.16**
Professor of Medicine and Microbiology/Immunology, University of North Carolina at Chapel Hill; Attending Rheumatologist, University of North Carolina Hospitals, Chapel Hill, North Carolina, USA

POUL HALBERG **5.01**
Physician-in-Chief, Department of Rheumatology, Hvidovre Hospital, University of Copenhagen, Hvidovre, Denmark

STEPHEN HALL **4.05**
Associate Professor of Rheumatology, Department of Medicine, Monash University, Box Hill Campus, Melbourne, Victoria, Australia

VEDAT HAMURYUDAN **7.26**
Associate Professor of Medicine, Division of Rheumatology, Department of Medicine, Cerrahpasa Medical Faculty, University of Istanbul, Aksaray, Istanbul, Turkey

JOHN G HANLY **7.08**
Head, Division of Rheumatology, Department of Medicine, Dalhousie University, Halifax, Nova Scotia, Canada

JOHN L HARKNESS **6.09**
Head, Division of Microbiology, St Vincent's Hospital, Darlinghurst, Sydney, Australia

JOHN B HARLEY **7.03**
Professor of Medicine, Department of Medicine, Oklahoma Medical Research Foundation, University of Oklahoma, Oklahoma City, Oklahoma, USA

E NIGEL HARRIS **7.35**
Dean and Senior Vice President for Academic Affairs; Professor of Medicine, Morehouse School of Medicine, Atlanta, Georgia, USA

IAN HASLOCK **6.19**
Consultant Rheumatologist, Visiting Professor in Clinical Bioengineering, University of Durham, Department of Rheumatology, South Cleveland Hospital, Middlesborough, UK

PETER HASSELBACHER **1.10**
Professor of Medicine, University of Louisville, Louisville, Kentucky, USA

DAVID E HASTINGS **5.03**
Professor of Surgery, University of Toronto, The Wellesley Hospital, Toronto, Ontario, Canada

JOHANNA MW HAZES **5.15**
Head of the Outpatient Rheumatology Department, Associate Professor of Rheumatology, Department of Rheumatology, University Hospital, Leiden, The Netherlands

BRIAN L HAZLEMAN **7.21**
Consultant Rheumatologist, Addenbrooke's Hospital; Director, Rheumatology Research Unit; Fellow, Corpus Christi College, Cambridge, UK

SVEN ÅKE HEDSTRÖM **6.02**
Director, Associate Professor, Department of Infectious Diseases, Halmstad Hospital, Halmstad, Sweden

PHILIP S HELLIWELL **6.21**
Consultant Rheumatologist; Senior Lecturer in Rheumatology, Rheumatology and Rehabilitation Research Unit, University of Leeds School of Medicine, Leeds, UK

DAVID B HELLMANN **7.31**
Executive Vice Chairman, Department of Medicine, Mary Betty Stevens Professor of Medicine, The Johns Hopkins Hospital, Baltimore, Maryland, USA

JEANNE E HICKS **7.16**
Associate Professor of Internal Medicine, George Washington University Hospital, Washington DC; Associate Professor of Rehabilitation Medicine in the Department of Orthopedics; Deputy Chief, Rehabilitation Medicine, National Institutes of Health, Bethesda, Maryland, USA

GARY S HOFFMAN **7.22**
Chairman, Department of Rheumatic & Immunologic Diseases, The Cleveland Clinic Foundation, Cleveland, Ohio, USA

V MICHAEL HOLERS **7.04, 7.08**
Associate Professor of Medicine and Immunology, Department of Medicine, University of Colorado Health Sciences Center, Denver, Colorado, USA

PETER HOLLINGWORTH **5.24**
Consultant Rheumatologist, Department of Rheumatology, Southmead General Hospital, Bristol, Avon, UK

OSVALDO HÜBSCHER **2.03**
Head, Rheumatology Unit, Department of Internal Medicine, CEMIC, Buenos Aires, Argentina

RODNEY A HUGHES **4.14**
Consultant Physician, Rheumatology Department, St Peter's Hospital, Chertsey, Surrey, UK

SHEPARD R HURWITZ **4.14**
Associate Professor, Department of Orthopedic Surgery, University of Virginia, Health Sciences Center, Charlottesville, Virginia, USA

GUNNAR HUSBY **6.15**
Professor of Medicine (Rheumatology), Rikshospitalet, Oslo Sanitetsforening Rheumatism Hospital, Oslo, Norway

ROBERT IGWE **8.21, 8.22**
Endocrinology Fellow, Division of Endocrinology, Wayne State University, Detroit, Michigan, USA

ROBERT W IKE **2.13**
Associate Professor of Internal Medicine, Department of Internal Medicine, Division of Rheumatology, University of Michigan Medical Center, Rackham Arthritis Research Unit, Ann Arbor, Michigan, USA

CHRISTOPHER J JACKSON **5.12**
Henry Langley Research Fellow, University of Sydney at the Sutton Rheumatism Research Laboratories, Royal North Shore Hospital, St Leonards, New South Wales, Australia

DAVID RW JAYNE **7.31**
Senior Lecturer in Renal Medicine, Division of Renal Medicine, St George's Hospital Medical School, London, UK

SERGIO A JIMENEZ **7.12**
Professor of Medicine; Professor of Biochemistry & Molecular Biology; Director, Division of Rheumatology, Thomas Jefferson University, Philadelphia, USA

JEREMY G JONES **5.16**
Specialist in Rheumatology and Rehabilitation Medicine, Queen Elizabeth Hospital, Rotorua, New Zealand

JACQUELYN JOSEPH-SILVERSTEIN **7.18**
Associate Professor of Biological Science, Associate Provost, St. John's University, New York, New York, USA

ROBERT A KALISH **7.08**
Assistant Professor of Medicine, Division of Rheumatology, Tufts University School of Medicine, New England Medical Center, Boston, Massachusetts, USA

CEES GM KALLENBERG **7.31**
Professor of Clinical Immunology, Department of Clinical Immunology, University Hospital, Groningen, The Netherlands

DIMITRIOS G KASSIMOS **8.11**
Consultant Rheumatologist, Rheumatology Unit, 401 Military Hospital of Athens, Athens, Greece

DANIEL L KASTNER **5.23**
Chief, Genetics Section, Arthritis and Rheumatism Branch, National Institute of Arthritis and Muscoskeletal and Skin Diseases, National Institutes of Health, Bethesda, Maryland, USA

TOMISAKU KAWASAKI **7.27**
Director, Kawasaki Disease Research Center, Tokyo, Japan

ANDREW CS KEAT **6.10, 6.25**
Consultant Rheumatologist, Department of Rheumatology, Northwick Park Hospital, Harrow, UK

EDWARD C KEYSTONE **7.25, 7.31**
Professor of Medicine, University of Toronto; Chief, Rheumatology Disease Unit; Director, Division of Advanced Therapeutic Studies in Rheumatic Disease, Arthritis & Autoimmunity Research Center, Wellesley Hospital, Toronto, Ontario, Canada

MUHAMMAD ASIM KHAN **6.16**
Professor of Medicine, Case Western Reserve University, Cleveland, Ohio, USA

ROBERT P KIMBERLY **7.02**
Director, UAB Arthritis and Musculoskeletal Diseases Center; Director, Division of Clinical Immunology and Rheumatology; Howard L Holley Professor of Medicine, University of Alabama School of Medicine, Birmingham, Alabama, USA

GABRIELLE H KINGSLEY **3.10**
Consultant Senior Lecturer, Lewisham Hospital, Rheumatology Unit, UMDS, Guy's Hospital, London, UK

Numbers in colored boxes refer to contributors' chapters

JOHN R KIRWAN **3.06**
Consultant & Reader in Rheumatology, Division of Medicine, Rheumatology Unit, University of Bristol, Bristol, UK

RODANTHI C KITRIDOU **7.12**
Professor of Medicine, Directress of Clinical Rheumatology, Los Angeles County University & Southern California Medical Center, Los Angeles, California, USA

MICHAEL KLEEREKOPER **8.21, 8.22**
Division of Endocrinology, Wayne State University School of Medicine, Detroit, Michigan, USA

JOHN H KLIPPEL **7.07**
Clinical Director, National Institute of Arthritis & Musculoskeletal & Skin Diseases, Bethesda, Maryland, USA

ARNOLDO S KRAUS **7.08**
Assistant Professor of Medicine (Rheumatology), Department of Immunology and Rheumatology, Instituto Nacional de la Nutricion Salvador Zubiran, Mexico City, Mexico

BARRY S KRAUSHAAR **4.14**
Former fellow, Nirschl Orthopedic Sportsmedicine Clinic, Arlington, Virginia, USA

KLAUS E KUETTNER **8.06**
Professor and Chairman, Department of Biochemistry, Rush Medical College, Rush-Presbytarian - St Luke's Medical Centre, Chicago, Illinois, USA

DANIEL KUNTZ **8.28, 8.29, 8.30, 8.31**
Professor of Rheumatology, Clinique de Rhumatologie, Centre Viggo Petersen, Hôpital Lariboisière, Paris, France

NANCY E LANE **8.38, 8.40**
Associate Professor of Medicine and Rheumatology, Division of Rheumatology, University of California at San Francisco, San Francisco, California, USA

LUC M LATEUR **8.52**
Clinical Head, Department of Radiology, University Hospital Gasthuisberg, Leuven, Belgium

CARLOS LAVERNIA **5.29**
Assistant Professor of Orthopedics and Bioengineering, University of Miami, Miami, Florida, USA

MARJATTA LEIRISALO-REPO **6.20**
Consultant in Rheumatology, Department of Medicine, University of Helsinki, Helsinki, Finland

E CARWILE LEROY **7.10**
Professor and Chairman, Department of Microbiology and Immunology; Professor of Medicine, College of Medicine, Medical University of South Carolina, Charleston, South Carolina, USA

FRANÇOIS LHOTE **7.24, 7.31**
Praticien Hospitalier - Medécine des Hôpitaux, Service de Medécine Interne, Hôpital Delafontaine, Saint-Denis, France

MATTHEW H LIANG **1.02**
Professor of Medicine, Harvard Medical School; Professor of Health Policy and Management, Harvard School of Public Health; Director, Robert B Brigham Multipurpose Arthritis and Musculoskeletal Diseases Center, Boston, Massachusetts, USA

LARS LIDGREN **6.02**
Chairman and Professor, Department of Orthopedic Surgery, University Hospital of Lund, Lund, Sweden

ROBERT W LIGHTFOOT, JR **7.17**
Division of Rheumatology, University of Kentucky Medical Centre, Lexington, Kentucky, USA

KEITH KT LIM **8.03, 8.33**
Consultant Rheumatologist, University Hospital, Kuala Lumpur; Honorary Lecturer in Medicine, Bristol University, England; Consultant Rheumatologist and General Physician, Subang Jaya Medical Centre, Petaling Jaya, Selangor, Malaysia

YLVA LINDROTH **3.03**
Rheumatology Department, University Hospital of Malmö, Malmö, Sweden

PETER E LIPSKY **6.12**
Professor of Internal Medicine and Microbiology, Department of Internal Medicine, Rheumatic Diseases Division, University of Texas Southwestern Medical Centre at Dallas; Director, Harold C Simmons Arthritis Research Center, Dallas, Texas, USA

GEOFFREY LITTLEJOHN **4.18** **8.10**
Director Rheumatology and Associate Professor, Department of Medicine, Monash University at Monash Medical Centre, Melbourne, Victoria, Australia

MICHAEL D LOCKSHIN **7.08**
Director, Barbara Volcker Center for Women and Rheumatic Disease, Hospital for Special Surgery, New York, New York, USA

C MARTIN LOCKWOOD **7.31**
University Reader in Therapeutic Immunology and Consultant Physician, Department of Medicine, University of Cambridge School of Clinical Medicine, Addenbrooke's Hospital Cambridge, UK

MARTIN K LOTZ **5.11**
Member MEM/Division of Arthritis Research, The Scripps Research Institute, La Jolla, California, USA

JOHN LOUGHLIN **1.06**
ARC Postdoctoral Research Fellow, Institute of Molecular Medicine, John Radcliffe Hospital, Oxford, UK

PETER J LOWTHIAN **4.05**
Director of Clinical Services, Cedar Court Rehabilitation Hospital, Melbourne, Australia

HARVINDER S LUTHRA **5.27**
John F Finn Minnesota Arthritis Foundation Professor of Medicine; Chair, Division of Rheumatology, Department of Internal Medicine, Mayo Medical School, Rochester, Minnesota, USA

ROGER LYON **5.29**
Assistant Professor of Orthopedics, Medical College of Wisconsin, Milwaukee, Wisconsin, USA

ALEX J MACGREGOR **5.02**
Honorary Senior Lecturer, Department of Rheumatology, St Thomas' Hospital, London, UK

MAREN LAWSON MAHOWALD **6.03**
Professor of Medicine, University of Minnesota; Rheumatology Section Chief Minneapolis VAMC, Rheumatology Office, Department of Veterans Affairs Medical Center, Minneapolis, Minnesota, USA

JOAN C MARINI **8.50**
Chief, Section on Connective Tissue Disorders, Heritable Disorders Branch, National Institute of Child Health & Human Development, Bethesda, Maryland, USA

PIERRE MAROTEAUX **8.32**
Directeur de Recherches Émèrite au CNRS, Hôpital des Enfants Malades, Paris, France

CLAYTON MARSH **6.20**
Consultant Orthopaedic Surgeon, Taunton and Somerset Hospital, Taunton, Somerset, UK

MANUEL MARTÍNEZ-LAVÍN **8.46**
Chief, Rheumatology Department, Insitituto Nacional de Cardiologìa Ignacio Chàvez; Professor of Rheumatology, Universida de Nacional Autònoma de México, Mexico

ERIC L MATTESON **5.04**
Associate Professor of Medicine, Consultant in Rheumatology, Department of Rheumatology and Internal Medicine, Mayo Clinic, Rochester, Minnesota, USA

BERNARD MAZIÈRES **4.10** **8.47**
Chef de Service, Service de Rhumatologie, University Hospital of Rangueil, Toulouse Cedex, France

GERALDINE M MCCARTHY **8.17**
Associate Professor of Medicine, Department of Medicine (Rheumatology), Medical College of Wisconsin, Milwaukee, Wisconsin, USA

CONOR MCCARTHY **8.12**
Consultant Rheumatologist, Mater Hospital, Dublin, Ireland

NEIL W MCGILL **8.19**
Consultant Rheumatologist, Department of Rheumatology, Royal Prince Alfred and Rachel Forster Hospitals, Sydney, Australia

THOMAS A MEDSGER, JR **7.13**
Department of Medicine/Rheumatology, University of Pittsburgh, Pittsburgh, Pennsylvania, USA

HERMAN MIELANTS **2.08** **6.24**
Professor of Rheumatology; Head of Rheumatology Department, University Hospital, Gent, Belgium

FREDERICK W MILLER **7.14**
Senior Investigator, Laboratory of Molecular and Developmental Immunology, Center for Biologics Evaluation and Research, Food and Drug Administration, Bethesda, Maryland, USA

Numbers in colored boxes refer to contributors' chapters

DONALD N MITCHELL **5.26**
Honorary Consultant Physician, Royal Brompton Hospital, London, UK

KATHY L MOSER **7.03**
Senior Research Scientist, Oklahoma Medical Research Foundation, Oklahoma City, Oklahoma, USA

HARALAMPOS M MOUTSOPOULOS **7.32**
Professor and Head, Department of Pathophysiology, National University of Athens, Athens, Greece

GREGORY R MUNDY **8.34, 8.39, 8.40**
JC & Irene H Heyser Professor of Bone and Mineral Metabolism, Professor and Head, Division of Endocrinology, Department of Medicine, University of Texas Health Science Center at San Antonio, Texas, USA

CHARLES NAGANT DE DEUXCHAISNES **8.45**
Professor, Saint-Luc University Hospital, The Arthritis Unit, Louvain University in Brussels, Brussels, Belgium

STANLEY J NAIDES **6.06**
Associate Professor of Internal Medicine, Division of Rheumatology, Department of Internal Medicine, University of Iowa, Iowa City, Iowa, USA

DAVID J NASHEL **4.16, 4.18**
Chief, Rheumatology Section, Veterans Affairs Medical Center; Professor of Medicine, Georgetown University, Washington DC, USA

CHRISTOPHER NEEDS **5.16**
Consultant Rheumatologist, Eastwood, Sydney, Australia

GERALD T NEPOM **5.07**
Director, Virginia Mason Research Center & Affiliate Professor, University Washington School of Medicine, Seattle, Washington, USA

BARBARA NEPOM **5.07**
Research Associate Member, Virginia Mason Research Center, Seattle, Washington, USA

ROBERT P NIRSCHL **4.14**
Chairman, Founding Director Orthopedic Surgery/Sportsmedicine, Nirschl Orthopedic & Sportsmedicine Clinic; Director, Orthopedic Sportsmedicine Fellowship Program, Arlington Hospital, Georgetown University, Arlington, Virginia, USA

CHESTER V ODDIS **7.13**
Associate Professor of Medicine, Division of Rheumatology and Clinical Immunology, Department of Medicine, University of Pittsburgh, Pittsburgh, Pennsylvania, USA

NANCY J OLSEN **7.16**
Associate Professor of Medicine, Division of Rheumatology and Immunology, Vanderbilt University, Nashville, Tennessee, USA

K SIGVARD OLSSON **8.26, 8.33**
Senior Medical Officer, Department of Medicine, Sahlgren's University Hospital, Mölndal; Associate Professor, University of Göleborg, Sweden

PHILIPPE ORCEL **8.31**
Professor of Rheumatology, Service de Rhumatologie, Hôpital Pitie-Salpetrière and INSERM U349, Centre Viggo Petersen, Hôpital Lariboisiére, Paris, France

MICHAEL T OTTE **8.12, 8.53**
Clinical Instructor, Department of Musculoskeletal Radiology, University of California at San Francisco, San Francisco, California, USA

STEPHEN A PAGET **5.16**
Physician-in-Chief, Chairman, Division of Rheumatology; Professor of Medicine, Department of Rheumatoid Medicine, Hospital for Special Surgery, New York, New York, USA

GABRIEL S PANAYI **3.10**
ARC Professor of Rheumatology, Division of Medicine, Rheumatology Unit, UMDS Guy's and St Thomas's Medical and Dental School, London, UK

MICHAEL PAZIANAS **8.42**
Associate Professor of Medicine, Department of Medicine, University of Pennsylvania, Philadelphia, Pennsylvania, USA

J DAVID PERRY **4.17**
Consultant Rheumatologist, Royal London Hospital, Mile End; Medical Officer, Crystal Palace National Sports Centre, London, UK

CHARLES G PETERFY **2.14** **4.18**
Assistant Professor of **8.04, 8.12, 8.33, 8.43, 8.53**
Radiology; Medical Director of MRI Research, Osteoporosis and Arthritis Research Group, Department of Radiology, University of California at San Francisco, San Francisco, California, USA

INGEMAR F PETERSSON **8.05**
Director, Spenshult's Hospital for Rheumatic Diseases, Halmstad, Sweden

MICHELLE A PETRI **7.08**
Director, Lupus Center; Associate Professor of Medicine, Division of Rheumatology, Johns Hopkins University School of Medicine, Baltimore, Maryland, USA

JACQUES G PEYRON **8.12**
Centre de Rhumatologie Hopital de la Pitié, Paris, France

THEODORE PINCUS **2.10**
Professor of Medicine and Microbiology, Division of Rheumatology and Immunology, Department of Medicine,Vanderbilt University Medical Center, Nashville, Tennessee, USA

PAUL H PLOTZ **7.14**
Chief, Arthritis and Rheumatism Branch, National Institute of Arthritis and Musculoskeletal and Skin Diseases, National Institutes of Health, Bethesda, Maryland, USA

SOLOMON POSEN **8.35**
Emeritus Professor of Medicine, University of Sydney; Consultant Physician, Royal North Shore Hospital, North Shore Medical Center, St Leonards, New South Wales, Australia

MORDECHAI PRAS **5.23**
Professor of Medicine; Director of Heller Institute of Medical Research and Department of Medicine F, Heller Institute of Medical Research, Sheba Medical Center, Tel-Hashomer, Israel

ELON PRAS **7.36**
Department of Medicine, Chaim Sheba Medical Center, Institute of Human Genetics, Tel-Hashomer, Israel

ANNE-MARIE F PRIEUR **5.21**
Médecin des Hôpitaux, Unité d'Immunologie et d'Hómatologie, Département de Pédiatrie, Hôpital Necker-Enfants Malades, Université Paris V Paris, France

WALDEMAR PRUZANSKI **7.31**
Professor of Medicine, Department of Medicine, The Wellesley Hospital, Toronto, Ontario, Canada

BRIAN QUILTY **8.53**
Clinical Research Fellow, Rheumatology Unit, Bristol Royal Infirmary, Bristol, UK

DANIEL W RAHN **6.05, 6.09**
Professor of Medicine, Vice Dean for Clinical Affairs, Medical College of Georgia, Augusta, Georgia, USA

ELIZABETH RANKIN **6.09**
Senior Registrar in Rheumatology, Bristol Royal Infirmary, Bristol, UK

HEINER RASPE **8.36**
Professor of Social Medicine; Director, Institute for Social Medicine, Medical University, Lübeck, Germany

DONALD RESNICK **6.13**
Professor of Radiology, UCSD; Chief, Osteoradiology, Veterans Affairs Medical Center, San Diego, California, USA

BRUCE C RICHARDSON **7.36**
Associate Professor of Internal Medicine, Division of Rheumatology, University of Michigan Medical Center, Ann Arbor, Michigan, USA

DWIGHT R ROBINSON **1.07**
Professor of Medicine, Harvard Medical School; Physician, Arthritis Unit, Massachusetts General Hospital, Boston, Massachusetts, USA

IAN F ROWE **6.09**
Consultant Rheumatologist, Worcester Centre for Rheumatic Disease, Worcester Royal Infirmary, Worcester, UK

MICHAEL K RUHOY **6.13**
Genesis Community Imaging Center, Phoenix, Arizona, USA

ANTHONY S RUSSELL **6.14, 6.20**
Professor of Medicine, Rheumatology/Clinical Immunology, University of Alberta, Edmonton, Alberta, Canada

JANE E SALMON **7.02**
Professor of Medicine, Hospital for Special Surgery, Cornell University Medical College, New York, New York, USA

PHILIP N SAMBROOK **8.36, 8.43**
Professor of Rheumatology, Florance & Cope, Department of Rheumatology, Royal North Shore Hospital, Sydney, New South Wales, Australia

OLIVER SANGHA **3.11**
Harvard Medical School, Brigham & Women's Hospital, Multipurpose Arthritis & Musculoskeletal Diseases Center, Boston, Massachusetts, USA

ELLIOT SAVDIE **5.16**
Nephrologist, St Vincent's Hospital, Sydney, New South Wales, Australia

Numbers in colored boxes refer to contributors' chapters

ALLEN DALE SAWITZKE 5.16
Assistant Professor of Medicine, Salt Lake, Utah, USA

LESLIE SCHRIEBER 5.12
Associate Professor of Medicine, Department of Rheumatology, Royal North Shore Hospital, Department of Medicine, University of Sydney, St Leonards, New South Wales, Australia

H RALPH SCHUMACHER, JR 8.18
Professor of Medicine, University of Pennsylvania School of Medicine; Director, Arthritis Immunology Center, Veterans Affairs, Philadelphia, Pennsylvania, USA

MARK E SCHWEITZER 6.13
Associate Professor of Radiology and Orthopedic Surgery, Department of Radiology, Thomas Jefferson University Hospital, Philadelphia, Pennsylvania, USA

DAVID L SCOTT 5.16
Reader in Rheumatology & Consultant Rheumatologist, Department of Rheumatology, Kings College Hospital, London, UK

J THOMAS SCOTT 5.16
Winters Lodge, Taunton, Somerset, UK

STEPHEN L SEAGREN 6.20
Professor of Radiation Oncology, School of Medicine, University of California at San Diego, San Diego, California, USA

JOHN S SERGENT 2.01, 2.07
Chief Medical Officer, Vanderbilt University Medical Centre, Nashville, Tennessee, USA

ALAN SILMAN 5.02
Director/Professor of Rheumatic Disease Epidemiology, ARC Epidemiology Research Unit, University of Manchester, Manchester, UK

ROY L SILVERSTEIN 7.18
Chief, Division of Hematology and Medical Oncology; Mark W Pasmantier Professor of Medicine, Cornell University Medical College, New York, New York, USA

PETER A SIMKIN 1.09
Professor of Medicine; Adjunct Professor of Orthopedics, Division of Rheumatology, Department of Medicine, University of Washington, Seattle, Washington, USA

EDWIN A SMITH 7.10
Associate Professor of Medicine, Division of Rheumatology and Immunology, Medical University of South Carolina, Charleston, South Carolina, USA

HUGH A SMYTHE 8.10
Professor, Department of Medicine, Rheumatic Diseases Unit, University of Toronto, The Wellesley Hospital, Toronto, Ontario, Canada

DAVID H SONNABEND 8.12
Associate Professor and Chairman, Department of Orthopaedic Surgery, Prince of Wales Hospital, Sydney, New South Wales, Australia

TIM D SPECTOR 8.07
Consultant Rheumatologist, Department of Rheumatology, St Thomas' Hospital, London, UK

HARRY SPIERA 7.36
Chief, Division of Rheumatology, Clinical Professor of Medicine, Division of Rheumatology, Mount Sinai Medical Center, New York, New York, USA

TREVOR C B STAMP 8.41
Consultant Physician & Senior Lecturer, Royal National Orthopaedic Hospital NHS Trust, Stanmore, Middlesex, UK

VIRGINIA D STEEN 7.12
Professor of Medicine, Department of Medicine, Georgetown University, Washington DC, USA

LYNNE S STEINBACH 7.16
Associate Professor of Radiology, University of California, San Francisco, California, USA

CHRISTINA H STENSTRÖM 5.16
RPT, Research Assistant, Department of Physical Therapy, Karolinska Institutet, Huddinge, Sweden

GEROLD STUCKI 3.11
Medical Director, Institute of Physical Medicine, Department of Rheumatology and Physical Medicine; Associate Professor of Physical Medicine and Rheumatology, University Hospital Zurich, Zurich, Switzerland

BERNARD N STULBERG 6.09
Director, Cleveland Center for Joint Reconstruction, Cleveland, Ohio, USA

ANGELA SWAN 8.19
Department of Medicine, Rheumatology Unit, Bristol Royal Infirmary, University of Bristol, Bristol, UK

DEBORAH P M SYMMONS 1.04
Consultant Senior Lecturer, ARC Epidemiology Research Unit, University of Manchester, Manchester, UK

ILONA S SZER 7.28
Director, Division of Pediatric Rheumatology, Children's Hospital San Diego; Associate Professor of Pediatrics, Department of Pediatrics, UCSD School of Medicine, University of California at San Diego School of Medicine, San Diego, California, USA

ANTONIO TAVONI 7.31
Clinical Assistant, Clinical Immunology Unit, University of Pisa, Pisa, Italy

DAVID S TEARSE 4.14
Associate Professor, Department of Orthopaedic Surgery, University of Iowa Hospitals, Iowa City, Iowa, USA

EUGENE J-M.A. THONAR 8.06
Professor and Associate Chairman, Department of Biochemistry, Rush Medical College, Rush-Presbyterian-St Luke's Medical Centre, Chicago, Illinois, USA

PHILLIP F J TIRMAN 8.12
Medical Director, San Francisco Magnetic Resonance Center; Assistant Clinical Professor, University of California at San Francisco, San Francisco, California, USA

PAAVO TOIVANEN 6.01
Professor of Bacteriology and Serology, Department of Medical Microbiology, Turku University, Turku, Finland

AULI TOIVANEN 6.11
Professor of Medicine, Department of Medicine, Turku University, Turku, Finland

ALAN G TYNDALL 6.09
Professor and Head, University Department of Rheumatology, Felix Platter Spital and Kantonsspital, Basle, Switzerland

ATHANASIOS G TZIOUFAS 7.32
Consultant Rheumatologist, Department of Pathophysiology, National University of Athens, Athens, Greece

MURRAY B UROWITZ 7.01
Director, Centre for Prognosis Studies in the Rheumatic Diseases; Associate Dean, Postgraduate Medical Education, Faculty of Medicine and Professor of Medicine, University of Toronto, Toronto, Ontario, Canada

ROBERT M VALENTE 7.20
Assistant Professor of Medicine, Mayo Medical School; Consultant in Internal Medicine and Rheumatology, Department of Internal Medicine, Division of Rheumatology, Mayo Clinic, Rochester, Minnesota, USA

LEO BA VAN DE PUTTE 5.14 8.33
Professor and Chairman, Department of Rheumatology, University Hospital Nijmegen, Nijmegen, The Netherlands

DÉSIRÉE VAN DER HEIJDE 8.33
Assistant Professor of Rheumatology, Department of Rheumatology, University Hospital Maastricht, Maastricht, The Netherlands

PIET LCM VAN RIEL 5.14
Professor, Director Clinical Research Unit, Department of Rheumatology, University Hospital Nijmegen, The Netherlands

JOHN VARGA 7.12
Chief, Section of Rheumatology; Professor of Medicine, Department of Medicine, University of Illinois, Chicago College of Medicine, Chicago, Illinois, USA

PATRICK J W VENABLES 7.33
Kennedy Institute of Rheumatology, London, UK

BARRIE VERNON-ROBERTS 6.18
George Richard Marks Professor and Head of Department, Department of Pathology, University of Adelaide; Head, Division of Tissue Pathology, Institute of Medical and Veterinary Science, Adelaide, Australia

ERIC M VEYS 2.08 6.24
Professor of Rheumatology, Department of Rheumatology, University Hospital, Gent, Belgium

EDUARDO R WAINSTEIN 7.31
Instructor in Medicine, University of Chile School of Medicine, Santiago, Chile

ANTHONY B WARD 5.16
Consultant Physician in Rehabilitation Medicine, North Staffordshire Rehabilitation Centre, Haywood Hospital, Stoke-on-Trent, Staffordshire, UK

JOHN R WARD 5.16
Professor Emeritus, Rheumatology Division, University of Utah Medical Center, Salt Lake City, Utah, USA

Numbers in colored boxes refer to contributors' chapters

IAIN WATT **8.04**
Consultant Clinical Radiologist, Bristol Royal Infirmary, Bristol, UK

JAMES N WEINSTEIN **4.06**
Center for the Evaluative Clinical Sciences, Dartmouth Medical School, Hanover, New Hampshire, USA

MICHAEL H WEISMAN **5.16**
Director, Arthritis Center; Professor of Medicine, Division of Rheumatology, Department of Medicine, University of California San Diego School of Medicine, San Diego, California, USA

DENNIS R WENGER **8.48**
Director, Pediatric Orthopedics; Clinical Professor of Orthopedic Surgery, Children's Hospital, San Diego, California, USA

PATIENCE H WHITE **5.18**
Chairman, Division of Adult and Pediatric Rheumatology; Professor of Medicine and Pediatrics, Children's National Medical Center, George Washington University Medical Center, Washington DC, USA

STEPHEN G WIENER **2.05**
Chairman, Section of Dermatology, The Reading Hospital and Medical Center, West Reading, Pennsylvania, USA

FREDRICK M WIGLEY **7.09, 7.12**
Professor of Medicine & Director, Rheumatology Division, Department of Medicine, The Johns Hopkins University, The Richard Starr Ross Research Building, Baltimore, Maryland, USA

MATH J H WIJNANDS **5.14**
Rheumatologist, Tweesteden Ziekenhuis Tilburg, The Netherlands

DANIEL M WILEN **8.53**
Department of Orthopaedic Surgery, Hospital for Joint Diseases, New York, New York, USA

DAVID G WILLIAMS **5.09**
Senior Scientist, The Mathilda and Terence Kennedy Institute of Rheumatology, London, UK

RALPH C WILLIAMS, JR **6.08**
Eminent Scholar, Marcia Whitney Schott Chair in Rheumatoid Arthritis Research, Division of Rheumatology and Clinical Immunology, Department of Medicine, University of Florida, Gainesville, Florida, USA

ROBERT A WISE **7.12**
Associate Professor of Medicine, Department of Medicine, Johns Hopkins University, School of Medicine, Baltimore, Maryland, USA

FRANK A WOLLHEIM **6.09**
Professor and Chairman, Department of Rheumatology, Lund University Hospital, University of Lund, Lund, Sweden

PATRICIA WOO **6.25**
Professor of Paediatric Rheumatology, Department of Molecular Pathology, Molecular & Paediatric Rheumatology Unit, UCL Medical School, London, UK

PAUL H WOOLEY **5.08**
Associate Professor of Medicine, Immunology and Orthopaedic Surgery, Division of Rheumatology, Hutzel Hospital, Wayne State University, Detroit, Michigan, USA

ANTHONY D WOOLF **8.43**
Consultant Rheumatologist, Duke of Cornwall Rheumatology Unit, Royal Cornwall Hospital Trust, Truro, Cornwall, UK

ROBERT L WORTMANN **7.16**
Professor and Chairman, Department of Medicine, East Carolina University School of Medicine, Greenville, North Carolina, USA

CHRISTOPHER WRAY **4.06**
Orthopaedic Consultant, Orthopaedics Department, Airedale General Hospital, Steeton, W Yorks, UK

VERNA WRIGHT **6.21, 6.25**
Professor of Rheumatology, Rheumatology and Rehabilitation Research Unit, University of Leeds, Leeds, UK

HASAN YAZICI **7.26**
Professor and Chief, Division of Rheumatology, Department of Medicine, University of Istanbul, Aksaray, Istanbul, Turkey

ARTHUR M F YEE **7.08**
Instructor in Medicine, Department of Medicine and Division of Rheumatic Diseases, Cornell University Medical College, Hospital for Special Surgery, New York, New York, USA

EDWARD YELIN **1.05**
Professor of Medicine and Health Policy, Department of Medicine, University of California at San Francisco, San Francisco, California, USA

NEVILLE YEOMANS **5.16**
Professor of Medicine, Department of Medicine, The University of Melbourne, Western Hospital, Footscray, Melbourne, Victoria, Australia

JOHN R YORK **8.24, 8.33**
Clinical Associate Professor, Department of Rheumatology, Royal Prince Alfred and Rachel Forster Hospitals, Redfern, Australia

RAYMOND L YUNG **7.36**
Assistant Professor of Internal Medicine, Divisions of Rheumatology and Geriatric Medicine, University of Michigan Medical Center, Ann Arbor, Michigan, USA

SEBAHATTIN YURDAKUL **7.26**
Professor of Medicine, Division of Rheumatology, Department of Medicine, Cerrahpasa Medical Faculty, University of Istanbul , Aksaray, Istanbul, Turkey

JOSEPH D ZUCKERMAN **8.53**
Chairman, Department of Orthopedic Surgery, Hospital for Joint Diseases, New York, New York, USA

NATHAN J ZVAIFLER **5.28, 5.30** **6.20**
Professor of Medicine, Division of Rheumatology, School of Medicine, University of California San Diego, California, USA

Numbers in colored boxes refer to contributors' chapters

1

RHEUMATIC DISEASES

Matthew H Liang & Leo BA van de Putte

1

HISTORY OF RHEUMATIC DISEASES

W Watson Buchanan
& Jan Dequeker

Summary
- The reasons why the past is relevant to both the present and future are outlined.
- Methods available to the historian studying rheumatoid disease are summarized.
- Difficulties arising in interpreting data from such methods are discussed – in particular the changes in ancient bones and joints that may resemble disease.

Who controls the past controls the future.
Who controls the present controls the past.
George Orwell, 1949

HISTORICAL PERSPECTIVE

In the face of the rapid advance of medical knowledge, both medical students and their teachers have little time to study medical history. Many universities do have departments of medical history, but courses for undergraduates are often elective and the subject does not have a regular place in the curriculum. As a consequence only a few medical students are aware that medicine has a past as well as a future. Indeed, most teachers in medical schools, apart from a few elderly eccentric professors who still teach by anecdote, conduct their tuition as if only what is happening today is important, and the past totally irrelevant and better discarded.

Implicit in this neglect of the history of medicine is the belief that only what is new is relevant for the present and the future, be it new insights into pathogenesis or treatment[1]. It has been said that of all the information learned today, approximately one-half will be obsolete after 5 years: hence, the catchy phrase 'the half-life of medical knowledge is a scant 5 years'[2]. The past is thus simply destroyed and has no relevance to either the present or the future. But if this is so, can the present likewise not be discarded for not having relevance for the future[1]? If present knowledge is to become obsolete as it passes into the forgotten past, why then should such emphasis be placed on learning what is known at present? Logically, if we deny the existence of history we deny the existence of the present, an assertion of the futility of human endeavor.

The problems facing modern medicine differ little from those of the past: the answers change, but the questions and problems remain much the same. The current debate on the value of plasmapheresis in connective tissue disease differs little from that on blood-letting a century or so ago[2]. The nature/nurture controversy in the pathogenesis of tuberculosis is not so different from that today in rheumatoid arthritis (RA). The major infectious diseases have been conquered, but humans must still live with their microbes, and today's students of medicine have similar if not identical problems to those of their predecessors a century ago. The recent epidemic of acquired immune deficiency syndrome (AIDS) is not so dissimilar in its problems to syphilis when it first occurred in Europe. *Plus ça change, plus c'est la même chose.*

As King has emphasized, the timeless problem in medicine is the disease[2]. If today's doctor needs reminding of the limitations of medicine then it is useful for today's doctor to know that predecessors faced similar problems. Change implies something constant, and in medicine today it is salutary to keep this Aristotelian doctrine in mind and be aware of the factors that remain unaltered. There is a body of knowledge in Western medicine that remains unaltered, although the doctrines are always in a state of flux. The modern doctor would be ill advised to ignore this wisdom of history.

We believe that the importance of a study of the history of rheumatic diseases is essentially that of understanding the changing concepts of pathogenesis and treatment. The study of history highlights 'fashions' in medical thinking, which in turn promotes caution in drawing conclusions. This chapter will deal with the various methods available for study of the history of rheumatic disease.

PALEOPATHOLOGY

Paleopathology, a term popularized by Sir Marc Armand Ruffer (1859–1917), Professor of Bacteriology at the Cairo Medical School at the turn of the century[3], consists of the study of disease in human populations as revealed by their mummified and skeletal remains. Dieppe and Rogers[4] have commented that paleopathology provides the addition of a time dimension to the study of disease, which they aptly described as 'two-dimensional epidemiology'. There are a number of pitfalls in interpreting ancient skeletal remains which have been admirably summarized by Wells[5]. These include the circumstances of burial, which are often unknown, and the nature of the soil, since burial in chalk will result in chemical changes so that the bones become light and pliable. Fossilized specimens undergo chemical changes, known as pyrites disintegration, which can lead to changes simulating periostitis. Roots encircling bones can also produce lesions on the surface of bones which may be interpreted as periosteal reactions. Erosions of joints may occur as a result of soil erosion[6,7], as well as a number of conditions, including frostbite, syringomyelia, leprosy and peripheral gangrene. Artefacts are innumerable, and precipitate judgments and hasty conclusions are best avoided. As Wells commented: 'the best opinions are usually tentative opinions'[5].

Dieppe and colleagues have advocated a multidisciplinary approach to the study of paleopathology, the team consisting of an archeologist, paleopathologist, radiologist, and rheumatologist[8]. These workers have also suggested a system of classification of common rheumatic diseases for use by archeologists and others[9]. These suggestions, if put into practice, should avoid diagnostic 'howlers', such as femoral shaft changes in a young girl from an Anglo-Saxon cemetery ascribed to the forcible abduction of the thighs during rape[10].

A thorough knowledge of pathology of bones and joints is indispensible in interpreting changes in ancient skeletons. This is most apparent in the interpretation of changes in the spine being due to ankylosing spondylitis. Although this disease undoubtably is present in several speciments[11–14], earlier descriptions were confused with osteophytosis and diffuse idiopathic skeletal hyperostosis (DISH) (see Fig. 1.1)[15–23]. From earlier studies it is clear that many of the authors were unaware of other diseases, such as psoriatic arthritis, Reiter's disease and fluorosis, which can involve the spine. Several studies have failed to identify ankylosing spondylitis[24–26]. This may have been due to the low prevalence of HLA-B27 in the subjects studied, since spondyloarthropathies and ankylosing spondylitis are relatively uncommon in the absence of HLA-B27. Some authors have found spinal osteophytes useful in defining age[27].

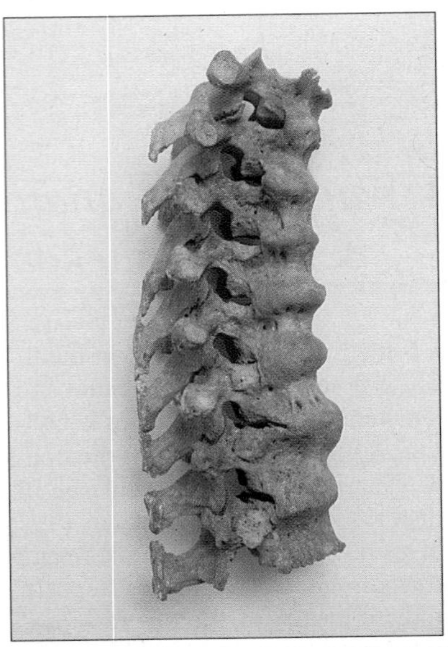

Fig. 1.1 Spine of a medieval bishop from Wells, UK. This shows evidence of idiopathic skeletal hyperostosis (Forestier's disease). Spines with this condition have sometimes been confused with ankylosing spondylitis. Courtesy of Dr J Rogers.

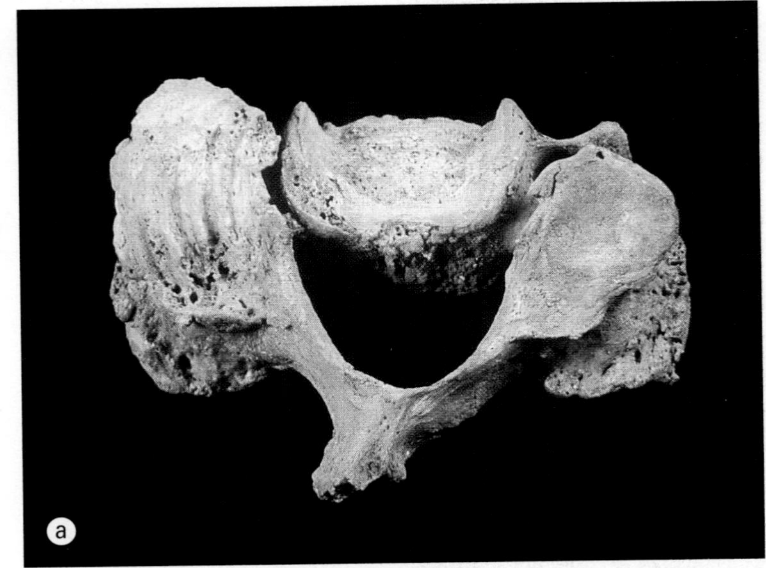

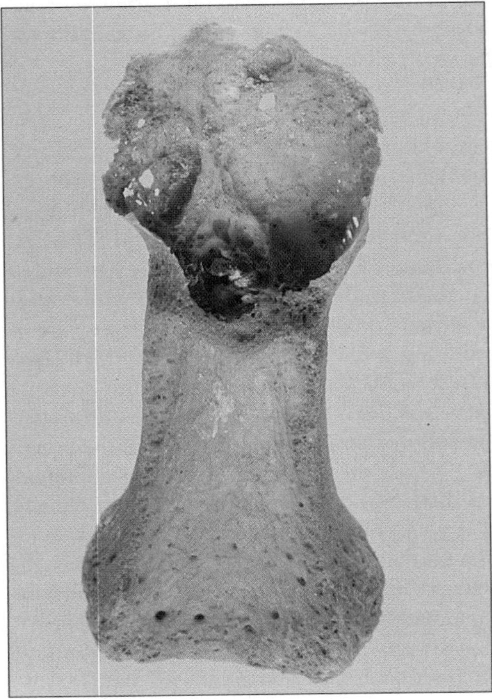

Fig. 1.2 Metatarsal bone from a Saxon skeleton. This shows a large erosion with a bony 'hook', suggesting chronic gouty arthritis. Courtesy of Dr J Rogers.

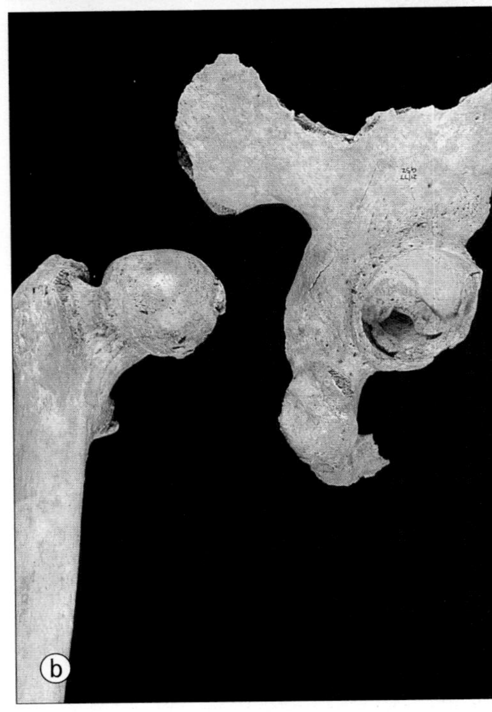

Fig. 1.3 Romano–British skeletal material: advanced OA of a spinal vertebra (a) and hip joint (b). Note the osteophytes, bony sclerosis and remodeling of the articular surfaces.

Intervertebral disc calcification is an extremely common finding in Egyptian mummies[11,28]. This might lead the unwary to a diagnosis of ochronosis. The calcification has been shown to be the result of the dehydrating agent natron (a mixture of sodium carbonate and sodium bicarbonate) used in the embalming process[29]. Ochronosis has, however, been described in an Egyptian mummy[30]. Chondrocalcinosis has been observed in several ancient skeletal remains[31,32], but X-ray crystallography has not been performed to confirm the presence of calcium pyrophosphate crystals. Urate crystals have been identified in gouty tophi in ancient remains[33]. Although lead poisoning has long been recognized as a cause of gout[34,35], and the content of lead in ancient bones has been extensively studied[36], no such study has been performed on ancient remains with gouty arthritis (Fig. 1.2).

There is little difficulty in diagnosing osteoarthritis (OA) in ancient remains (Fig. 1.3) and the disease appears little different in both prevalence and distribution than it is today[37]. Difficulty has arisen, however, in the interpretation of erosive arthritis, especially as environmental factors such as burial in chalky soil can lead to articular erosions[8,9]. Whether RA has been demonstrated in ancient skeletons has been the subject of debate[7,8,26,38–42]. Undoubtedly, lack of knowledge of rheumatic diseases led some workers at the turn of the century to report mummies with RA when it is clear that they had generalized OA[43]. However, in their defense one has to recall that the differentiation between OA and RA had not clearly been established[44]. Because of the absence of RA in paleopathologic material and of convincing descriptions in older medical texts, speculation arose as to whether the disease might be a relatively recent affliction of humankind[39,42]. However, paleopathologic material is sporadic and selective, and suffers from a lack of clinical information[45]; it is also difficult to prove a negative association[46]. Sir James Paget (1814–1894), in discussing whether osteitis deformans and Charcot's arthropathy could be 'new' diseases, provided a word of caution. He is reported as commenting: 'In speaking of a new disease, the great difficulty lay in the fact that one had to establish not a positive conclusion but a negative one; for, when proving a thing was new, the real thing to prove was that it was not old, and to do that was a much greater difficulty in regard to most diseases than at first sight appeared'[47]. Furthermore, speculation has been fueled by the demonstration of erosive polyarthritis in ancient Indian remains in North America[48–50], although this has been disputed on the grounds that a number of joint diseases, including the seronegative arthropathies[51], can cause an erosive polyarthritis. Speculation has now arisen as to whether RA had its origins in the New World[52].

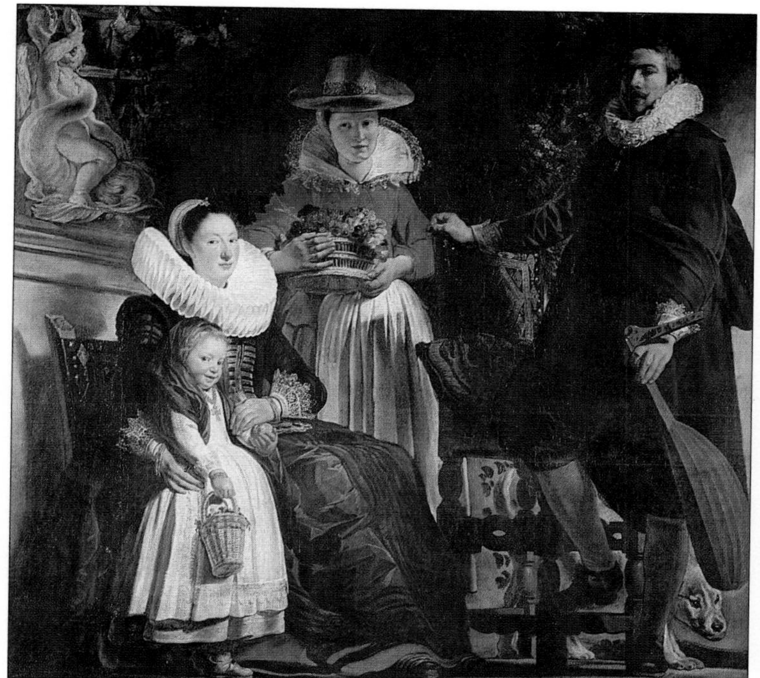

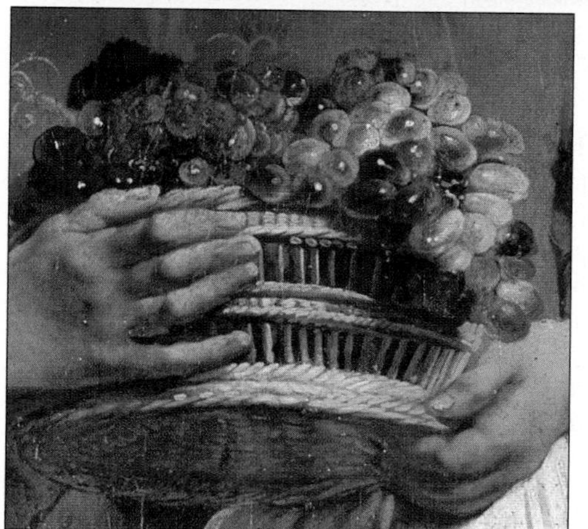

Fig. 1.4 Evidence of rheumatoid arthritis. Painting by Jacob Jordaens (1593–1678), entitled *The Painter's Family*, which now hangs in the Prado Museum. The hands of the serving maid, seen holding the basket of fruit (and in the detail), are suggestive of RA. Reproduced by kind permission of the Museo del Prado, Madrid, Spain.

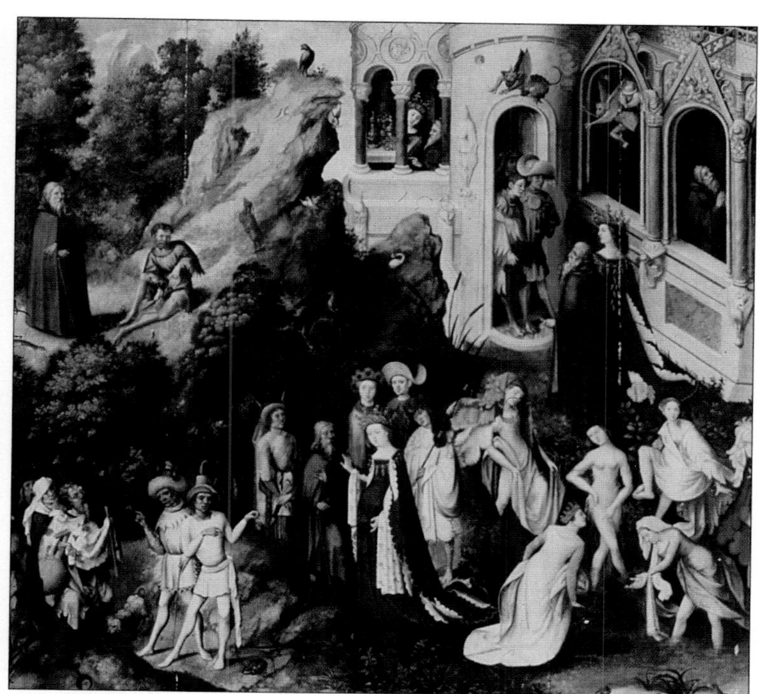

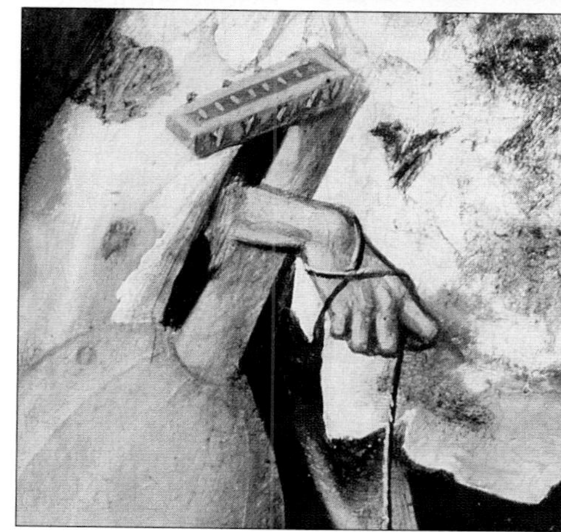

Fig. 1.5 Evidence of rheumatoid arthritis. *The Temptation of St Anthony:* painting by an anonymous artist of the Flemish–Dutch School, mid-15th to early 16th century, now in the Escorial Museum. Hand and wrist deformities of the beggar in the left corner (and in the detail) are very suggestive of RA. By kind permission of the Spanish Art Heritage, Madrid, Spain.

A number of new techniques, both radiologic[53,54] and biochemical[55–57], have become available for the study of ancient skeletal remains but have yet to be evaluated. Visual assessment of bones is still, however, regarded to be just as important as radiography[58].

VISUAL ARTS AND LITERATURE

If humankind does not leave clues to its illnesses in its mortal remains, then perhaps it might do so in its works of art. The problem is that the essence of art is not mimesis, but expression[59], and artistic style often precludes accurate diagnosis[60]. In an extensive study of Flemish paintings between 1400 and 1700, only five showed possible RA[61], the most convincing being that of the serving maid in Jacob Jordaens' *The Painter's Family* (Fig. 1.4). Another example is the beggar in the painting *The Temptation of St Anthony* (Fig. 1.5). Other paintings that have been claimed to illustrate RA are not entirely convincing[62].

Perhaps the most impressive identification of a rheumatic disease in a painting is that of temporal arteritis in Canon Van der Paele by Jan Van Eyck (c. 1385–1440) (see Fig. 1.6). According to minutes of the cathedral, the Canon began to have difficulty in performing his duties in 1431, as a result of morning stiffness, weakness and general ill health, which lasted some 12 years[63]. The painting shows scar formation over the temporal artery with loss of hair of the eyebrow and in front of the left ear. Another example of temporal arteritis has been suggested in the portrait of Francesco Gambetti by Piero di Cosimo in 1505[64].

Although certain deformities such as achondroplasia and Pott's disease of the spine can be readily identified in sculptures[65], OA and other rheumatic diseases are not so clearly defined[66, 67]. Appleboom *et al.*[62,68] suggested that Peter Paul Rubens (1577–1640) may have suffered from RA, which may have influenced his art. If this were so then it might be expected that the works of Pierre Auguste Renoir (1841–1919) would show evidence of his severe rheumatoid disease, but this is not found[69,70]. A better case can be made, however, for the effects of corticosteroid therapy on the arthritis of Raoul Dufy (1877–1953) in making his art more lively[71]. Bywaters[72] has suggested that the 'happy and joyous style' of the paintings of Paul Klee (1879–1940) 'gave way to heavy lines, dark colours and foreboding titles reflecting his imprisonment in the flesh' as a result of developing progressive systemic sclerosis in 1935. However, Klee, a Jew, fled Germany in 1933 and the change in artistic style could as easily have been caused by depression as to what was happening to his people. Arthritis and rheumatic disease, and their treatment, may influence but never create artistic genius[73]. A convincing case has been made for scleroderma in a painting of Bishop Francisco Domonte by Murillo[74].

There is no reference to joint disease in the Bible. Ehrlich[75] has reviewed the works of Shakespeare and noted sciatica and gout to be the most commonly cited diseases. Surprisingly, there is no mention of polyarthritis. Authors, even those who were doctors, seldom refer to arthritic and rheumatoid disorders in their works[76], perhaps due to the

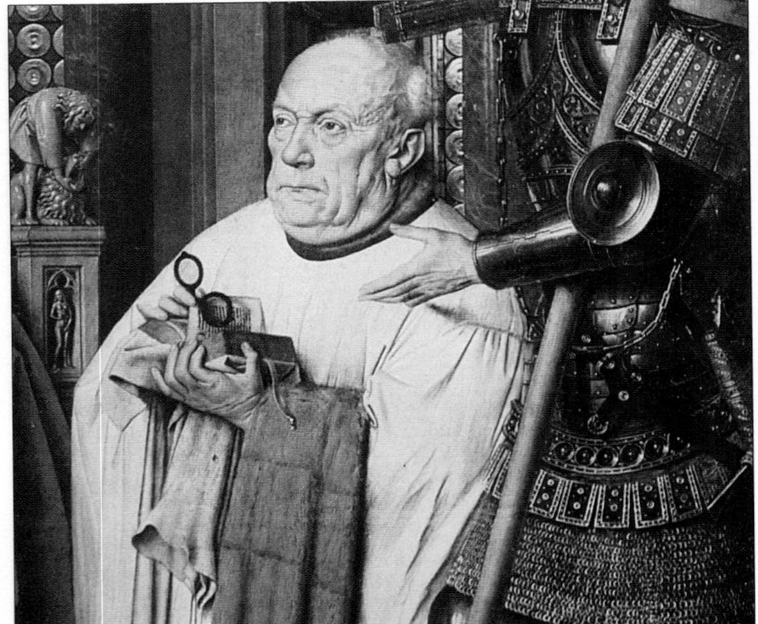

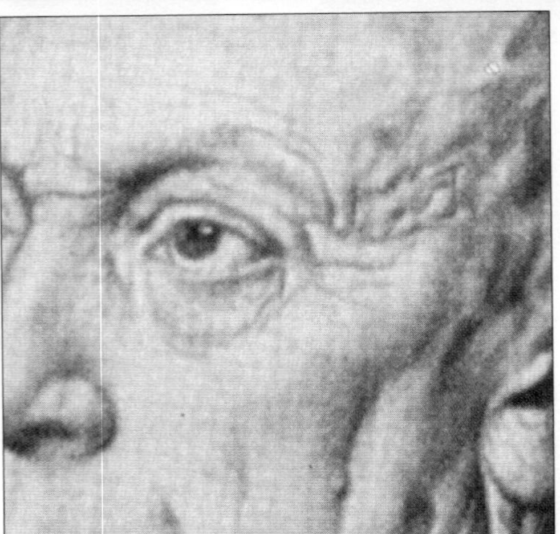

Fig. 1.6 Evidence of temporal arteritis: painting by Jan Van Eyck (c. 1385–1440), entitled *The Virgin with Canon Van der Paele,* 1436. By kind permission of Groeeningemuseum, Bruges, Belgium.

SOME POSSIBLE RHEUMATIC ILLNESSES AMONG SIGNIFICANT HISTORIC FIGURES	
Constantine IX Monomachus (980–1055)	RA?
Peter il Giottosa (1414–1469)	Ankylosing spondylitis?
Christopher Columbus (1451–1506)	Reiter's disease
Mary Queen of Scots (1542–1587)	Marfan's syndrome
Siebrandus Sixtius (1568–1631)	RA?
Benjamin Franklin (1706–1790)	Gout
Nicolo Paganini (1782–1840)	Ehlers–Danlos syndrome
Renoir (1841–1919)	RA?

Fig. 1.7 Some possible rheumatic illnesses among significant historic figures. Students of the history of medicine have sometimes suggested that illness has been the basis of creative activity or greatness, the so-called 'creative malady'. Nothing can, of course, be further from the truth.

fact that these diseases lack drama. However, Sir Arthur Conan Doyle in the story *Missing Three-Quarters* describes the opulent Lord Mount-James, 'one of the richest men in England', as being able to 'chalk his billiard cue with his knuckles'. Chronic tophaceous gout was the subject of a contribution by Conan Doyle to the *Lancet* in 1884[77]. Kahn and colleagues[78] reviewed rheumatic disease in nonmedical French literature and reported that Hervé Bazin introduced systemic lupus erythematosus (SLE) in his novel *Que J'ose Aimer* in 1956. The descriptions of gout given by Gourevitch[79] in Greco–Roman nonmedical literature are difficult to interpret.

EARLY MEDICAL LITERATURE

Study of early medical literature is seldom of particular value in view of the vagueness of the descriptions[38]. For example, Soranus of Ephesus (98–138AD) in his treatise *On Chronic Disease* describes polyarthritis affecting middle-aged men, causing the joints to 'become twisted, with the toes and fingers either turned sideways, or bent over backwards, or rest immovable upon their neighbours'. This might not unreasonably be interpreted as RA, unless it is appreciated that the description includes an acute attack of gout with discharging tophi[38]. Translators of early medical writings are often nonmedical. Usually, it is not possible to verify the accuracy of the translation so that diagnosis can only be tentative[80].

It is only in the 17th or 18th century that literature becomes more reliable, although RA is still not clearly defined[81–83]. Berk and Cowan have made a plea for the inclusion of classic descriptions in the modern curriculum[84]. Certainly, the description of clinical gout by Sydenham cannot be bettered[81]. However, these early medical writers have also much clinical wisdom to teach today's student of medicine. For example, the observation by John Hunter (1728–1793)[82] that inflammation was a reparative process should not go unnoticed by those practising sports medicine who would prescribe nonsteroidal anti-inflammatory analgesics for traumatic inflammation. This might be better treated conservatively along the lines suggested by John Hilton (1807–1876) in his famous treatise *Rest and Pain*[83]. Clinical rheumatologists might consider the therapy advised by William Heberden (1710–1801) for pulmonary tuberculosis: 'the best remedies seem to be a cool air; quiet; a very sparing mild nourishment, administered in small quantities of time'. Considering that Heberden lived in an era of ferocious blood-letting and violent purges it is understandable that Dr Samuel Johnson (1709–1784), whom Heberden attended during his last illness, should have described him as 'timidorum timidissimus'. Would that modern clinical rheumatologists could be referred to as such!

HISTORICAL FIGURES

In 1989 Appelboom reviewed a 'gallery' of famous people who suffered from arthritis or rheumatic disease[85]. These make fascinating reading and are particularly useful for biographers (Fig. 1.7). Little, however, is added to the serious study of the history of rheumatic disease. However, there are several exceptions, such as the crippling polyarthritis which affected Constantine IX Monomachus (980–1055)[86] and Siebrandus Sixtius[87] but which may have been RA, thus supporting the view that RA is not a recent disease of humankind. Illnesses in notable historic figures can, however, be useful in teaching medical students, both in terms of diagnosis[88] and in highlighting the misery of the affliction suffered by patients (for example, the torment of Eramus's pustulotic arthro-osteitis[89] and of Renoir's RA).

MUSEUMS

There has been a sad decline in interest in medical museums, despite the fact that many of the older museums contain much of current interest[90]. For example, there is a remarkable collection of pathologic specimens in William Hunter's collection in the University of Glasgow[91]. This collection is of particular value because clinical histories, including details of surgical operations and postmortem findings, are available. Thus, one can appreciate which diseases were common in the 18th century. As might be expected, there are numerous examples of injuries and infections of all sorts, as well as a variety of arthritic disorders, with the single exception of RA. The museum includes a classic case of osteitis fibrosa cystica[92]. Diseases affecting the ancient Egyptians, as evidenced in museum collections, have been well described and, perhaps more importantly, properly catalogued[93].

Surely it is time for a careful and unhurried appraisal of the material held in medical museums. Perhaps the most interesting could be published as is currently done with art galleries. This will probably add little to our understanding of arthritic and rheumatic diseases, but might prove of inestimable value in medical education.

SUMMARY

This section has reviewed the methods which a student of rheumatic disease history may pursue. The weaknesses and strengths of each approach are discussed. The comments of the late Sir William Osler (1849–1919), in his introductory lecture at the 45th Session of the Medical Faculty, McGill University in Montreal, should be noted[94]:

> Remember you enter upon a glorious heritage; you will reap where you have not sown and gotten where you have not strained and the knowledge which is your privilege today to acquire so early has cost others. We are, all of us, debtors to our profession.

REFERENCES

1. Wilson LG. Medicine without its history. Editorial. J Hist Med Allied Sci. 1978;33:467–8.
2. King LS. Medical thinking: An historical preface. Princeton: Princeton University Press; 1982:227–44.
3. Ruffer MA. Studies in palaeopathology in Egypt. J Path Bact. 1913;18:149–62.
4. Dieppe PA, Rogers J. Two-dimensional epidemiology. Br J Rheumatol. 1985;24:310–2.
5. Wells C. Pseudopathology. In: Brothwell D, Sandison AT, eds. Diseases of antiquity. Springfield, Illinois: Charles C Thomas; 1967:5–19.
6. Molleson TI. The role of environment in the acquisition of rheumatic diseases. In: Appleboom T, ed. Art, history and antiquity of rheumatic diseases. Brussels: Elsevier; 1987:100–8.
7. Rogers JM, Dieppe PA. Symmetrical erosive arthritis in Ohio woodland Indians (Letter). J Rheumatol. 1989;16:1012.
8. Dieppe P, Heywood A, Rogers J, Waldron T, Watt J. The paleopathology of rheumatic diseases. In: T. Appelboom, ed. Art, history and antiquity of rheumatic diseases. Brussels: Elsevier; 1987:109–12.
9. Rogers JM, Waldron T, Dieppe P, Watt J. Arthropathies in paleopathology: the basis of classification according to most probable cause. J Archaeol Sci. 1987;14:179–93.
10. Hawkes SC, Wells C. Crime and punishment in an Anglo-Saxon cemetery. Antiquity. 1975;49:118–22.
11. Zorab PA. The historical and prehistorical background to ankylosing spondylitis. Proc R Soc Med. 1961;54:415–20.
12. Steinbock RT. Paleopathological diagnosis and interpretation. Springfield, Illinois: Charles C Thomas; 1976:306–8.
13. Spencer DG, Sturrock RD, Buchanan WW. Ankylosing spondylitis: yesterday and today. Med Hist. 1980;24:60–9.
14. Kramar C. A case of ankylosing spondylitis in mediaeval Geneva. OSSA. 1982;8:115–29.
15. Smith GE, Wood Jones F. Archaelogical survey of Nubia. Report for 1907–1908. Cairo: National Print Department;. 1910;2:273.
16. Ruffer MA, Rietti A. On osseous lesions in ancient Egyptians. J Path Bact. 1912;16:439–65.
17. Shore LR. Some examples of disease of the vertebral column found in skeletons in ancient Egypt. A contribution to paleopathology. Br J Surg. 1936;24:256–71.
18. Roche MB. Incidence of osteophytosis and osteoarthritis in 419 skeletonized vertebral columns. Am J Phys Anthrop. 1957;15:433–4.
19. Salib P. Orthopaedic and traumatic skeletal lesions in ancient Egyptians. J Bone Joint Surg. 1962;44B:944–7.
20. Chapman FH. The incidence and age distribution of osteoarthritis in an archaic American Indian population. Proc Indiana Acad Sci. 1964;72:64–6.
21. Bourke JB. The paleopathology of the vertebral column in ancient Egypt and Nubia. Med Hist. 1971;15:363–75.
22. Wells C. Joint pathology in ancient Anglo-Saxons. J Bone Joint Surg. 1962;44B:948–9.
23. Rogers J, Watt J, Dieppe P. Paleopathology of spinal osteophytosis, vertebral ankylosis, ankylosing spondylitis, and vertebral hyperostosis. Ann Rheum Dis. 1985;44:113–20.
24. Clarke GA, Delmond JA. Vertebral osteophytosis in Dickson Mound populations: a biomechanical interpretation. Henry Ford Hosp Med J. 1979;27:54–8.
25. Rogers J, Watt I, Dieppe P. Arthritis in Saxon and mediaeval skeletons. Br Med J. 1981;283:1668–71.
26. Rothschild BM, Turner KR, DeLuca MA. Symmetrical erosive peripheral polyarthritis in the late archaic period of Alabama. Science. 1988;241:1488–501.
27. Stewart TD. The rate of development of vertebral hypertrophic arthritis and its utility in age estimation. Am J Phys Anthropol. 1957;15:433–49.
28. Gray PHK. Calcinosis intervertebralis, with special reference to similar changes in mummies of ancient Egyptians. In: Brothwell D, Sandison AT. Diseases of antiquity. Springfield, Illinois: Charles C Thomas; 1967:5–19.
29. Sandison AT. The use of natron in mummification in ancient Egypt. J Near East Stud. 1963;22:259–61.
30. Milgram JW. Osteoarthritic changes at the severely degenerated disc in humans. J Soc Orthop Med. 1984;1:8–11.
31. Rothschild BM, Thillaud PL. Oldest bone disease. Nature. 1991;349:288.
32. Braunstein EM, White SJ, Russell W, Harris JE. Paleoradiologic evaluation of the Egyptian royal mummies. Skeletal Radiol. 1988;17:348–52.
33. Elliot Smith G, Dawson WR. Egyptian mummies. London: Allen and Unwin; 1924.
34. Wells C. A paleopathological rarity in a skeleton of Roman date. Med Hist. 1973;17:399–400.
35. Ball GV. Two epidemics of gout. Bull Hist Med. 1971;45:401–8.
36. Waldron HA. Lead poisoning in the ancient world. Med Hist. 1973;17:391–9.
37. Berato J, Dutour O, Williams J, Zakarian H, Acquaviva PC. Epidémiologie des affections rheumatismales dans une population antique. Etude de la Nécropole du Haut Empire de Saint-Lambert (Fréjus, Van). Rev Rheumat. 1990;57:397–400.
38. Short CL. The antiquity of rheumatoid arthritis. Arthritis Rheum. 1974;17:193–205.
39. Buchanan WW, Murdoch RM. Hypothesis: that rheumatoid arthritis will disappear. J Rheumatol. 1979;6:324–9.
40. Rogers J, Dieppe P. The Alabama findings and the New World pathogen theory in antiquity of erosive arthritis In: Rogers J, Dieppe P, eds. The antiquity of erosive arthropathies. (Conference Proceedings No 5) London: Arthritis and Rheumatism Council; 1989.
41. Rogers J, Dieppe P. Skeletal paleopathology and the rheumatic diseases: where are we now? Leader. Ann Rheum Dis. 1990;49:885–6.
42. Buchanan WW, Laurent RM. Rheumatoid arthritis: an example of ecological succession? Canad Bull Med Hist. 1990;7:77–91.
43. May WP. Rheumatoid arthritis (osteitis deformans) affecting bones 5500 years old. Br Med J. 1897;2:1631–2.

44. Balint GP, Rooney PJ, Buchanan WW. A legacy for rheumatology from Sir William Osler. Clin Rheumatol. 1987;6:423–35.
45. Kirwan J. The antiquity of erosive arthropathies: the way forward. In: Rogers J, Dieppe P, eds. Antiquity of erosive arthropathies (Conference Proceedings No. 5). London: Arthritis and Rheumatism Council; 1989:66–9.
46. Wood PHN. Is rheumatoid arthritis a recent disease? In: Dumonde DC, ed. Infection of immunology in the rheumatic diseases. Oxford: Blackwell; 1976:619–22.
47. Buchanan WW. The contribution of Sir James Paget (1814–1894) to the study of rheumatic disease. Clin Rheumatol. 1996;15(in press).
48. Rothschild BM, Woods RJ. Symmetrical erosive peripheral polyarthritis in the late archaic period of Alabama. Science. 1988;241:1498–501.
49. Woods RJ, Rothschild BM. Population analysis of symmetrical arthritis in Ohio Woodland Indians (1200 years ago). J Rheumatol. 1988;15:1258–63.
50. Rothschild BM, Woods RJ. Symmetrical erosive disease in archaic Indians: the origin of rheumatoid arthritis in the new world? Semin Arthritis Rheum. 1990;19:278–84.
51. Ledem J, Peisson E, Peisson O. Aspects of the history of rheumatoid arthritis in the light of recent osteoarchaeological finds. Scand J Rheumatol. 1988;17:341–52.
52. Buchanan WW. Rheumatoid arthritis: another New World disease. Semin Arthritis Rheumat. 1994;23:289–94.
53. Leisen JC, Duncan H, Riddle JM. Scanning electron miscroscopy of the rheumatoid erosion in macerated bone specimens. In: Rogers J, Dieppe P, eds. Antiquity of erosive arthropathies (Conference Proceedings No. 5). London: Arthritis and Rheumatism Council; 1989:21–4.
54. Pickering RB, Conces DJ Jr, Braunstein EM, Yurco F. Three-dimensional computed tomography of the mummy Wenuhotep. Am J Phys Anthropol. 1990;83:49–55.
55. Hagelberg E, Sykes B. Ancient bone DNA amplified. Nature. 1989;342:485.
56. Cattaneo C, Gelsthorpe K, Phillips P, Sokol RJ. Blood in ancient human bone. Nature. 1990:347–39.
57. Marshall E. Paleoanthropology gets physical. Science. 1990;247:798–801.
58. Rogers J, Watt I, Dieppe P. Comparison of visual and radiographic detection of bony changes at the knee joint. Br Med J. 1990;300:367–8.
59. Dequeker J, Rico H. Rheumatoid arthritis-like deformities in an early 16th century painting of the Flemish–Dutch school. JAMA. 1992;268:249–251.
60. Bridgman GB. The book of a hundred hands. New York: Dover; 1971.
61. Dequeker J. Arthritis in Flemish paintings. Br Med J. 1977;1:1196–7.
62. Appelboom T, deBoelpaepe C, Ehrlich GE, Famaey J-P. Rubens and the question of antiquity of rheumatoid arthritis. JAMA. 1981;245:483–6.
63. Dequeker J. Polymyalgia rheumatica with temporal arteritis, as painted by Jan Van Eyck in 1436. Can Med Assoc J. 1981;124:1597–8.
64. Roth WG. Arteriitis temporalis, dargestellt an einem Gemälde des Reichmuseums in Amsterdam. Hautartz. 1969;20:330–2.
65. Buchanan WW. Ancient Egyptian dwarfs. Proc Roy Coll Phys Edin. 1990;9:358–61.
66. Alarcon-Segovia D, Ramon de la Fuente J. Pre-Columbian representation of rheumatic diseases in Mesoamerica. In: Appelboom T, ed. Art, history and antiquity of rheumatic diseases. Brussels: Elsevier; 1987:27–30.
67. Jobba G. Locomotor diseases in sculpture. J Rheumatol. 1990;17:1684–5.
68. Appelboom T, Preaux C. Rubens' rheumatism approached by his correspondence and painting. In: Appelboom T, ed. Art, history and antiquity of rheumatic diseases. Brussels: Elsevier; 1987:41–2.
69. Saudan Y. Did Renoir's arthritis have a repercussion on his work? In: Appelboom T, ed. Art, history and antiquity of rheumatic diseases. Brussels: Elsevier; 1987:46–8.
70. Louie JS. Renoir his art and his arthritis. In: Appelboom T, ed. Art, history and antiquity of rheumatic diseases. Brussels: Elsevier; 1987:43–5.
71. Hamburger E, Donner CD. The treatment of Raoul Dufy's arthritis. N Engl J Med. 1979;301:669–72.
72. Bywaters EGL. Paul Klee: the effect of scleroderma on his painting. In: Appelboom T, ed. Art, history and antiquity of rheumatic diseases. Brussels: Elsevier; 1987:49–50
73. Pickering GG. Creative malady. London: Allen and Unwin; 1974.
74 Dequeker J, Vanopdenbosch L, Castillo Ojugas A. Early evidence of scleroderma. Br Med J. 1995;311:1714–5.
75. Ehrlich GE. Shakespeare's rheumatology. Ann Rheum Dis. 1967;26:562–3.
76. Smithers DW. The idle trade. Tunbridge Wells: Dragonfly Press; 1989.
77. Doyle A. The remote effects of gout. Lancet. 1884;ii:978–9.
78. Kahn MF, Beraner L, Daudin M. Rheumatic diseases in nonmedical French literature. In: Appleboom T, ed. Art, history and antiquity of rheumatic diseases. Brussels: Elsevier; 1987:56–61.
79. Gourevitch D. Gout in Greco-Roman nonmedical literature. In: Appelboom T, ed. Art, history and antiquity of rheumatic diseases. Brussels: Elsevier; 1987:66–8,
80. Lopez Ferez JA. Rheumatism, arthritis and gout in Galen. In: Appelboom T, ed. Art, history and antiquity of rheumatic diseases. Brussels: Elsevier; 1987:84–6.
81. Latham RG. The works of Thomas Sydenham, MD. Translation of Latin Edition of Dr Greenhill, Vols 1 & 2. London: The Sydenham Society; 1848. (Reprinted by the Classics of Medicine Library, Birmingham: AL; 1979.)
82. Palmer JF, ed. The works of John Hunter. Vols I–IV. London: Langman; 1835–7.
83. Hilton J. Rest and pain. London: G. Bell and Sons; 1863.
84. Berk SL, Cowan J. Classic disease descriptions in the modern curriculum. JAMA. 1989;86:693–5
85. Appleboom T. The past: a gallery of arthritis. Clin Rheumatol. 1989;8:442–52.
86. Caughey DE. The arthritis of Constantine IX. Ann Rheum Dis. 1974;33:77–80.
87. Dequeker J. Siebrandus Sixtius: evidence of rheumatoid arthritis of the robust reaction type in a seventeenth-century Dutch priest. Ann Rheum Dis. 1992;51:561–2.
88. Balint GP, Buchanan WW. Historical perspective in undergraduate education of rheumatology: a lost cause? Eular Bull. 1986;3:107–10.
89. Dequeker J. Art history and rheumatism: the case of Erasmus of Rotterdam (1466–1536), suffering from pustulotic arthro-osteitis. Ann Rheum Dis. 1991;50:517–21.
90. Waugh D. The decline and fall of our medical museums. Can Med Assoc J. 1990;142:236.
91. Palmer DG, Marshall AJ, Buchanan WW. Eighteenth century bone and joint disease: William Hunter's Collection, Pathology Department, Royal Infirmary, Glasgow. Rheumatology. 1977;4:34–38.
92. Buchanan WW, Kraag GR, Palmer DG, Cockshott WP. The first recorded case of osteitis fibrosa cystica. Can Med Assoc J. 1981;124:812–15.
93. Ghalioungui P, El Dawakhly Z. Health and healing in Ancient Egypt. A pictorial essay. Cairo: The Egyptian Organisation for Authorship and Translation; 1965.
94. Osler W. At the opening of the Forty-Fifth Session of the Medical Faculty, McGill University, Introductory Lecture: Why history matters. Can Med Surg J. 1877–78;VI:193–210.

2

IMPACT AND COST EFFECTIVENESS OF RHEUMATOLOGIC CARE

Matthew H Liang & John M Esdaile

- Rheumatology is the medical specialty that deals with the prevention, treatment and rehabilitation of over 100 diverse arthritis and musculoskeletal disorders, which are the most important cause of disability in society.
- The treatment repertoire of rheumatology is diverse and, by necessity, multidisciplinary.
- Early recognition, early treatment and managed or coordinated care are essential for the best outcomes and cost effectiveness.
- Rheumatic disease care is a model for how health care should be delivered and organized and, from a number of views, it is richly satisfying and stimulating for its students.

Rheumatology is the medical specialty that deals with the prevention, treatment and rehabilitation of individuals with arthritis and musculoskeletal diseases. Since the early 1950s, it has matured as a subspeciality of internal medicine. This chapter introduces the specialty and reviews its impact on rheumatic disease care and the health and welfare of individuals and the population.

THE BURDEN OF RHEUMATIC AND MUSCULOSKELETAL DISEASES

Arthritis and musculoskeletal disorders are more prevalent and a more frequent cause of disability than either heart disease or cancer[1,2]. In the USA, they are the most common illnesses evaluated in ambulatory care (accounting for an estimated 315 million physician visits per year), the second most common reason for visits to surgeons, the third most common reason for visits to family doctors and the fourth most common reason for visits to specialists[3,4]. Studies show that new musculoskeletal complaints are the most time consuming for physicians to evaluate and manage[5].

Despite the enormous prevalence and significant individual and societal burden imposed by these disorders, few countries have an integrated health care system in place for their management. This gap between what is known and what is practised is explained in part by the misperception of the public and its leaders that the disorders are one condition and/or an inevitable part of aging and/or incurable, and in part by the nature of the disorders themselves and their epidemiology.

Rheumatic and musculoskeletal diseases encompass over 100 discrete acute and chronic disorders, some with multisystem involvement and others affecting musculoskeletal regions (see Fig. 2.1). No age or racial group is spared and the clinical manifestations are diverse. Although many of the disorders are chronic or remitting, significant advances have been made in their management: once fatal or major debilitating diseases are now curable and others are managed successfully. Osteoarthritis (OA) is the most common arthritis disorder but it is overdiagnosed and poorly treated. In contrast, the systemic rheumatic conditions (connective tissue diseases and vasculitis) are uncommon but potentially fatal, and the incidence of many diseases is so low that most physicians will not have had much experience with their diagnoses and/or management.

The gap between what is known and what is practised represents a failing of medical education. Despite the high prevalence and impact of arthritis and musculoskeletal conditions, medical school, postgraduate and continuing medical education programs have provided little curriculum time to them[6–9]. Studies worldwide show that primary care physicians are less likely to make correct or timely diagnoses of arthritis and musculoskeletal disease, to manage musculoskeletal disease appropriately, and to do it in a cost-effective manner[10–17].

THE SCOPE OF RHEUMATOLOGY

Because of the nature of rheumatologic and musculoskeletal disorders, the cognitive span required for their diagnosis draws on the entire field of medicine. Understanding their pathogenesis, interpreting the specialized laboratory tests used for diagnosis and following the clinical status of the patient draws on knowledge of cellular and humoral immunology, immunogenetics, muscle biology, bone and cartilage biochemistry and biomechanics, to name just a few.

Laboratory studies, diagnostic imaging and synovial fluid analysis are important, but they require interpretation. For example, immunologic testing has played a critical role in the diagnosis and evaluation of systemic rheumatic diseases such as rheumatoid arthritis (RA), systemic lupus erythematosus (SLE), poly- and dermatomyositis and Wegener's granulomatosis, but it requires expertise to use the results wisely. Standardization of the assays is not consistent and their performance characteristics – sensitivity, specificity and predictive value – depend on the test and the clinical setting. A false-positive immunochemical test such as an antinuclear antibody can cause unnecessary anguish for the patient and prompt inappropriate, potentially dangerous treatment. Although radiodiagnostic imaging studies are valuable, they need to be selectively ordered in situations where the information is likely to make a diagnosis or prompt a change in management. For example, an expert history and musculoskeletal examination and explanation to the patient with low back pain costs far less than a magnetic resonance image study and is probably far more cost-effective, more appropriate and addresses the patient's concerns. Conversely, for early diagnosis and treatment of septic arthritis and crystalline disease, accurate interpretation of synovial fluid chemistry and microscopy is essential, but studies show disturbing variation in the accuracy of synovial fluid interpretation, further underscoring the need for expert consultation[18,19].

For those with chronic arthritis and musculoskeletal diseases, the need for health services, unlike that for more publicized conditions such as cancer and heart disease, unfolds and undulates over the person's life and presents unique problems for coordinated care. Providers must distinguish the consequences of the disease from its treatment and from comorbid illness, and advise patients on multiple therapeutic, rehabilitative and surgical options. In acute disease, the patient is a passive recipient of health care and relies upon the physician to resolve the problem[20]. In chronic illness, the patient is 'experienced' and is the most important source of information about his/her well being and functioning. Here, in contrast to acute disease, ambulatory and community services are much more important than hospital care. Central to chronic disease management is a consistent provider–patient relationship which establishes the trust and understanding that are essential to a long-term dialogue as the patient faces a maze of medical choices and the vicissitudes of his/her disease.

A rheumatologist directs and coordinates a team of health professionals and draws on a host of diagnostic, therapeutic, and rehabilitation services. The members of the team vary, depending on the patient's

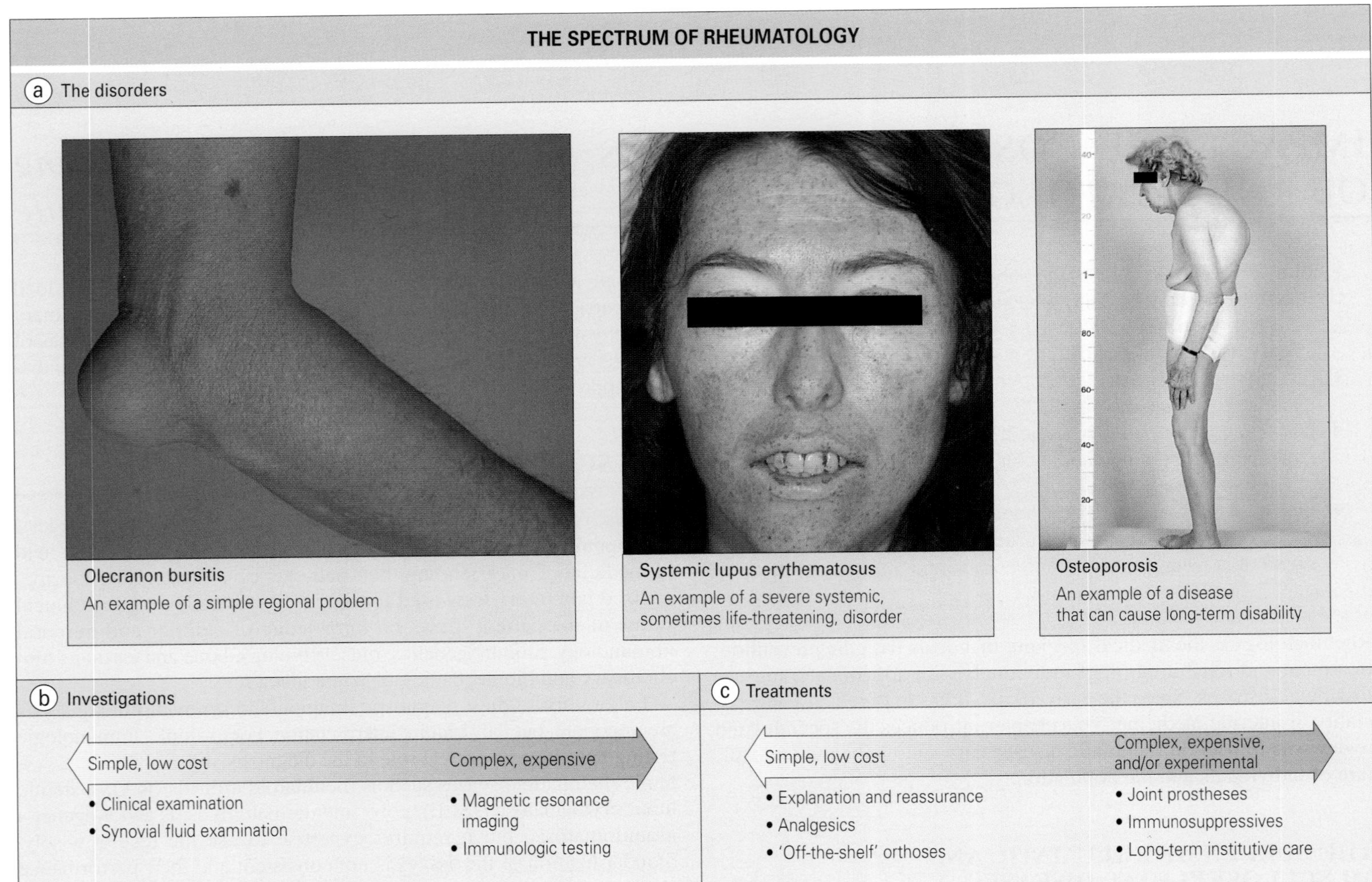

Fig. 2.1 The spectrum of rheumatology. Musculoskeletal disorders range from regional conditions to severe life-threatening or disabling diseases. In addition, investigations range from physical examination to expensive high technology investigations. Finally, therapeutic options range from simple low-cost interventions to complex, expensive and occasionally experimental options.

problems at a given time (Fig. 2.2). Depending on the health care system, the team may be physically proximate, as on an inpatient or outpatient rheumatic disease unit; or it may be in a center 'without walls', where the services of other health professionals knowledgeable in the special problems of rheumatic disease patients (particularly in systemic rheumatic disorders) are available. The essential features, irrespective of site or constituent members, is that the approach is comprehensive, coordinated and problem-oriented over the life of the patient. The division of responsibility should be explicit and consensual, and repeated assessment should be lifelong. If the team approach is managed well, the patient and family are secure in the support and expertise made available to them, and the results are frequently more effective than the sum of the results of the individual components.

ELEMENTS OF RHEUMATIC DISEASE MANAGEMENT
Rheumatology
Primary care
Physical therapy
Occupational therapy
Orthopedic surgery
Podiatry
Rehabilitation medicine
Clinical psychology
Vocational counseling
Dermatology
Neurology
Ophthalmology
Social work

Fig. 2.2 Elements of rheumatic disease management.

THE IMPACT OF RHEUMATOLOGIC CARE

Early, appropriate rheumatologic intervention reduces morbidity, maintains function and prolongs life. Timely treatment improves outcome and/or reduces health care costs in such diverse diseases as septic arthritis, rheumatoid arthritis, lupus nephritis[21,22], polymyalgia rheumatica and giant cell arteritis[23], Lyme disease[24], polymyositis and dermatomyositis[25], familial Mediterranean fever[26], gout and tophaceous gout, scleroderma renal crisis[27], Wegener's granulomatosis[28], systemic necrotizing vasculitis[29] and Kawasaki syndrome[30]. Furthermore, in end-stage arthritis from all causes, total joint arthroplasty is dramatically effective, reduces pain, improves function and prevents dependency[31,32].

Many rheumatic diseases are chronic and symptoms fluctuate, thus patients commonly require repeated evaluation and modifications in therapy. More frequent specialty consultation and follow-up care is associated with better outcomes in patients with musculoskeletal complaints, and regular care by a rheumatologist (as opposed to intermittent care) is associated with better function in patients with RA[33].

Continuity of care also provides patients with security in the face of an uncertain future[34] and we believe that in chronic illnesses, health care systems have an ethical obligation to preserve doctor–patient relationships.

Rheumatologic care encompasses the expertise of rheumatology, orthopedics, nursing, physical therapy, occupational therapy, social work, podiatry, vocational counseling and clinical psychology. As single-dimension interventions, these are effective. For example, prescribed exercise programs reduce pain and improve function for patients with OA of the knee[35,36], RA[37], fibromyalgia[38], ankylosing spondylitis[39–41] and SLE[42]. Patient education programs and psychoeducational interventions improve function and quality of life in patients with arthritis[43–52], reduce physician visits by 40% and decrease health care costs[47]. However, not all services may be used for all patients and, even if they are, they are not all used at once or in the same intensity over the lifetime of a patient. They are most effectively coordinated by a knowledgeable and experienced clinician, and the data show that *coordinated* managed care improves the function and quality of life of patients with arthritis[53–59].

All economically developed countries are facing a crisis in health care financing. Reduced utilization of services for patients with arthritis has been observed in health care systems with restricted access to rheumatology specialists, and these patients have poorer outcomes than those who do have access[53]. In systems of care funded by global budgets, referrals for critical pain therapies, medications used in rheumatic disease, assistive devices and other durable medical equipment, and referral to physical therapy and orthopedic surgery are often restricted, but the effects on patients have been little studied. Even more troubling is the ethical dilemma presented when economic incentives are provided to physicians for doing less. In this environment of fiscal pressure, making choices over which medical services are provided for patients becomes a major issue for physicians: making choices wisely and humanely is paramount.

Rheumatology, a relatively small specialty, has demonstrated what expert, comprehensive and cost effective care can do for a group of disorders with enormous public health impact. Given the prevalence of rheumatic and musculoskeletal disorders, physicians trained in these conditions bring added value to integrated delivery systems. As the lead physicians in the management of multidisciplinary care for patients with systemic rheumatic diseases, they provide direct care for the more complicated cases or confirmation or reassurance when diagnostic uncertainty exists, provide advice and education for those with less severe disease and guide the use of scarce resources.

The appeal of rheumatology is diverse. It may be the fascination with rare potentially fatal systemic diseases or the equally mysterious common disabling disorders; the lack of procedures; the links to basic immunology; or the ability to help, no matter how bleak the prognosis or incurable or rare the underlying disorder. In the end, it is stimulating, challenging and personally satisfying to learn, and it takes a lifetime to master.

REFERENCES

1. Decker JL. American Rheumatism Association nomenclature and classification of arthritis and rheumatism. Arthritis Rheum. 1983;26:1029–32.
2. Lawrence RC, Hochberg MC, Kelsey JL, *et al.* Estimates of the prevalence of selected arthritic and musculoskeletal diseases in the United States. J Rheumatol. 1989;16:427–41.
3. Yelin EH, Felts WR. A summary of the impact of musculoskeletal conditions in the United States. Arthritis Rheum. 1990;33:750–5.
4. Communicable Diseases Center. Arthritis prevalence and activity limitations – United States. MMWR. 1990;43:433–4.
5. Lion J, Henderson MG, Malbon A, Wiley MM, Noble S. Ambulatory visit groups: a prospective payment system for outpatient care. J Ambulatory Care Manage. 1984;7:30–45.
6. Goldenberg DL, DeHoratius RJ, Kaplan SR, *et al.* Rheumatology training at internal medicine and family practice residency programs. Arthritis Rheum. 1985;28:471–6.
7. Goldenberg DL, Meenan RF, Allaire S, Cohen AS. The educational impact of rheumatology elective. Arhtritis Rheum. 1983;26:658–63.
8. Meenan RF, Goldenberg DL, Allaire SH, Anderson JJ. The rheumatology knowledge and skills of trainees in internal medicine and family practice. J Rheumatol. 1988;5:1693–700.
9. Strosberg MA, Strosberg JM. Do family practice residents in the United States learn clinical rheumatology? An important question. J Rheumatol. 1980;7:923–6.
10. Bellamy N, Gilbert JR, Brooks PM, Emmerson BT, Campbell J. A survey of current prescribing practices of antiinflammatory and urate lowering drugs in gouty arthritis in the province of Ontario. J Rheumatol. 1988;15:1841–7.
11. Chan KW, Felson DT, Yood RA, Walker AM. The lag time between onset of symptoms and diagnosis of rheumatoid arthritis. Arthritis Rheum. 1994;37:814–20.
12. Hanly JG, McGregor A, Black C, Bresnihan B. Late referral of patients with rheumatoid arthritis to rheumatologists. Ir J Med Sci. 1984;153:316–18.
13. Mazzuca SA, Brandt KD, Katz BP. Improved training of house officers in a rheumatology consult service. Arthritis Care Res. 1993;6:59–63.
14. Panush RS, Carias K, Kramer N, Rosenstein ED. Acute arthritis in the hospital. Comparison of rheumatologic with non-rheumatologic care. J Clin Rheumatol. 1995;1:74–80.
15. Bjelle A, Magi M. Rheumatic disorders in primary care. A study of two primary care centres and a review of previous Swedish reports on primary care. Scand J Rheumatol. 1981;10:331–41.
16. Kidd BL, Cawley MI. Delay in diagnosis of spondarthritis. Br J Rheumatol. 1988;27:230–2.
17. Stross JK, Bole GG. The impact of a new rheumatologist on the management of rheumatic disease patients in community hospitals. Arthritis Rheum. 1983;26:1033–6.
18. Schumacher HR Jr, Sieck MS, Rothfuss S, *et al.* Reproducibility of synovial fluid analyses. A study among four laboratories. Arthritis Rheum. 1986;29:770–4.
19. Hasselbacher P. Variation in synovial fluid analysis by hospital laboratories. Arthritis Rheum. 1987;30:637–42.
20. Holman HR. Thought barriers to understanding rheumatic diseases. Arthritis Rheum. 1994;37:1565–72.
21. Ward MM, Leigh JP, Fries JF. Progression of functional disability in patients with rheumatoid arthritis. Associations with rheumatology subspecialty care. Arch Intern Med. 1993;153:2229–37.
22. McInnes PM, Schuttinga J, Sanslone WR, Stark SP, Klippel JH. The economic impact of treatment of severe lupus nephritis with prednisone and intravenous cyclophosphamide. Arthritis Rheum. 1994;37:1000–6.
23. Hazleman BL. Polymyalgia rheumatica and giant cell arthritis. In: Klippel JH, Dieppe PA,eds. Rheumatology, 2 Ed. London: Mosby, 1997. [Chapter 7.21].
24. Steere AC. Lyme disease. N Engl J Med. 1989;321:586–96.
25. Fafalak RG, Peterson MG, Kagen LJ. Strength in polymyositis and dermatomyositis. Best outcome in patients treated early. J Rheumatol. 1994;21:643–8.
26. Zemer D, Revach M, Pras M, *et al.* A controlled trial of colchicine in preventing attacks of familial Mediterranean fever. N Engl J Med. 1994;291:932–4.
27. Lopez-Ovejero JA, Saal SD, D'Angelo WA, Cheigh JS, Stenzel KH, Laragh JH. Reversal of vascular and renal crises of scleroderma by oral angiotensin-converting-enzyme blockade. N Engl J Med. 1979;300:1417–19.
28. Hoffman GS, Kerr GS, Leavitt RY, *et al.* Wegener granulomatosis: an analysis of 158 patients. Ann Intern Med. 1992;116:488–98.
29. Cohen RD, Conn DL, Ilstrup DM. Clinical features, prognosis, and response to treatment in polyarteritis. Mayo Clin Proc. 1980;55:146–55.
30. Newburger JW, Takahashi M, Beiser AS, *et al.* A single intravenous infusion of gamma globulin as compared with four infusions in the treatment of acute Kawasaki syndrome. N Engl J Med. 1991;324:1633–9.
31. Liang MH, Cullen KE, Larson MG, *et al.* Cost-effectiveness of total joint arthroplasty in osteoarthritis. Arthritis Rheum. 1986;29:937–943.
32. Chang RW, Pellissler JM, Hazen GB. A cost effectiveness analysis of total hip arthroplasty for osteoarthritis of the hip. JAMA. 1996;275:858–65.
33. Esdaile JM, Joseph L, MacKenzie T, Kashgarian M, Hayslett JP. The benefit of early treatment with immunosuppressive agents in lupus nephritis. J Rheumatol. 1994;21:2046–51.
34. Quill TE, Cassel CK. Nonabandonment: a central obligation for physicians. Ann Intern Med. 1995;122:368–74.
35. Kovar PA, Allegrante JP, MacKenzie CR, Peterson MG, Gutin B, Charlson ME. Supervised fitness walking in patients with osteoarthritis of the knee. A randomized, controlled trial. Ann Intern Med. 1992;116:529–34.
36. Puett DW, Griffin MR. Published trials of nonmedicinal and noninvasive therapies for hip and knee osteoarthritis. Ann Intern Med. 1994;121:133–40.
37. Semble EL, Loeser RF, Wise CM. Therapeutic exercise for rheumatoid arthritis and osteoarthritis. Semin Arthritis Rheum. 1990;20:32–40.

38. McCain GA. Role of physical fitness training in the fibrositis/fibromyalgia syndrome. Am J Med. 1986;81:73–77.
39. Bakker C, Hidding A, van der Linden S, van Doorslaer E. Cost effectiveness of group physical therapy compared to individualized therapy for ankylosing spondylitis. A randomized controlled trial. J Rheumatol. 1994;21:264–68.
40. Bulstrode SJ, Barefoot J, Harrison RA, Clarke AK. The role of passive stretching in the treatment of ankylosing spondylitis. Br J Rheumatol. 1987;26:40–2.
41. Kraag G, Stokes B, Groh J, Helewa A, Goldsmith CH. The effects of comprehensive home physiotherapy and supervision on patients with ankylosing spondylitis: an 8-month followup. J Rheumatol. 1994;21:261–63.
42. Robb-Nicholson LC, Daltroy L, Eaton H, *et al.* Effects of aerobic conditioning in lupus fatigue: a pilot study. Br J Rheumatol. 1989;28:500–5.
43. Burckhardt CS, Mannerkorpi K, Hedenberg L, Bjelle A. A randomized, controlled clinical trial of education and physical training for women with fibromyalgia. J Rheumatol. 1994;21:714–20.
44. Daltroy LH, Liang MH. Arthritis education: opportunities and state of the art. Health Educ Q. 1993;20:3–16.
45. deVellis RF, Blalock SJ. Psychological and educational interventions to reduce arthritis disability. Bailliere's Clin Rheumatol. 1993;7:397–416.
46. Holman H, Mazonson P, Lorig K. Health education for self-management has significant early and sustained benefits in chronic arthritis. Trans Assoc Am Physicians. 1989;102:204–8.
47. Lorig KR, Mazonson PD, Holman HR. Evidence suggesting that health education for self-management in patients with chronic arthritis has sustained health benefits while reducing health care costs. Arthritis Rheum. 1993;36:439–46.
48. Mullen PD, Laville EA, Biddle AK, Lorig K. Efficacy of psychoeducational interventions on pain, depression, and disability in people with arthritis: a meta-analysis. J Rheumatol. 1987;14(suppl 15):33–9.
49. Parker JC, Singsen BH, Hewett JE, *et al.* Educating patients with rheumatoid arthritis: a prospective analysis. Arch Phys Med Rehabil. 1984;65:771–4.
50. Rene J, Weinberger M, Mazzuca SA, Brandt KD, Katz BP. Reduction of joint pain in patients with knee osteoarthritis who have received monthly telephone calls from lay personnel and whose medical treatment regimens have remained stable. Arthritis Rheum. 1992;35:511–15.
51. Strauss GD, Spiegel JS, Daniels M, *et al.* Group therapies for rheumatoid arthritis. A controlled study of two approaches. Arthritis Rheum. 1986;29:1203–9.
52. Winfield JB. Arthritis patient education. Efficacy, implementation, and financing. ACR/AHPA/AF/NAAB Task Force on Arthritis Patient Education. Arthritis Rheum. 1989;32:1330–3.
53. Clement DG, Retchin SM, Brown RS, Stegall MH. Access and outcomes of elderly patients enrolled in managed care. JAMA. 1994;271:1487–92.
54. Clarke AE, Esdaile JM, Hawkins D. Inpatient rheumatic disease units: are they worth it? [editorial]. Arthritis Rheum. 1993;36:1337–40.
55. Helewa A, Bombardier C, Goldsmith CH, Menchions B, Smythe HA. Cost-effectiveness of inpatient and intensive outpatient treatment of rheumatoid arthritis. A randomized, controlled trial. Arthritis Rheum. 1989;32:1505–14.
56. Helewa A, Goldsmith CH, Lee P, *et al.* Effects of occupational therapy home service on patients with rheumatoid arthritis. Lancet. 1991;337:1453–56.
57. Helewa A, Smythe HA, Goldsmith CH. Can specially trained physiotherapists improve the care of patients with rheumatoid arthritis? A randomized health care trial. J Rheumatol. 1994;21:70–9.
58. Raspe HH, Deck R, Mattussek S. The outcome of traditional or comprehensive outpatient care for rheumatoid arthritis (RA). Results of an open, non-randomized, 2-year prospective study. Z Rheumatol. 1992;51(suppl 1):61–6.
59. Spiegel JS, Spiegel TM, Ward NB, Paulus HE, Leake B, Kane RL. Rehabilitation for rheumatoid arthritis patients. A controlled trial. Arthritis Rheum. 1986;29:628–37.

CLASSIFICATION OF RHEUMATIC DISEASES

Sherine E Gabriel

- Classification criteria are a powerful tool for identifying and distinguishing patients with a target disease from those without the condition.
- Classification criteria in the rheumatic diseases have made a substantial contribution to advancing both the art and the science of rheumatology.
- Like any other diagnostic tool, classification criteria must be appropriately designed and interpreted.
- The current environment of economic constraints dictates that we evaluate the cost-effectiveness of our approaches to developing classification criteria.
- Classification criteria are most useful when they pertain to clinically recognizable disease entities rather than vague, nonspecific syndromes.

INTRODUCTION

Standardized nomenclature and classification are necessary in order to distinguish patients with a specific rheumatic disease from those without the disease. This is especially problematic in rheumatology because the rheumatic diseases are syndromes with overlapping and variable clinical features that lack diagnostic laboratory tests. Moreover, many of these conditions have an unknown or incompletely understood etiology and pathogenesis. Because of this, classification schemes often combine various types of information including clinical and laboratory features, tests of suspected pathogenic mechanisms (e.g. autoantibodies), anatomic abnormalities, organ system involvement, genetic factors (e.g. HLA B-27), and etiologic agents (e.g. L-tryptophan), among others.

Classification criteria for the rheumatic diseases serve many important functions. Criteria are necessary for the proper conduct and interpretation of clinical trials, epidemiologic studies, and clinical research. Without clear, standardized definitions, epidemiologic studies estimating the prevalence and incidence of diseases in a population would be meaningless since they would vary due to the use of different definitions of disease. In clinical studies, standard classification criteria ensure that study subjects all have the same disease, facilitating comparison and interpretation of results. Classification criteria are also useful in health services research. For example, when physician practice patterns are studied, standardized classification criteria allow the separation of variation due to differences in disease characteristics from variation due to physician practice style[1–5]. Classification criteria encourage international collaboration by ensuring that patients studied from widely divergent locations have the same disease entity. Finally, while classification criteria are explicitly proscribed for diagnosis[6], they are useful for teaching purposes and as diagnostic guides. In summary, classification criteria provide a uniform language which is fundamental to accurate communication, thus facilitating our understanding of the rheumatic diseases[7].

TYPES OF CRITERIA

Classification criteria are only one of the numerous types of criteria used in describing disease processes. Criteria have also been developed for measuring or classifying disease severity, disease activity, organ damage, function, outcome and prognosis[7,8]. This chapter focuses on classification criteria.

Classification criteria have two purposes: first to separate patients with the target disease from patients with similar conditions which might be confused with the disease and second to separate patients with the target disease from normal subjects. Occasionally, subclassification criteria are needed when disease subsets have been identified which have different clinical, laboratory, serologic, immunologic or prognostic features. These criteria delineate subgroups within a disease cluster; for example, the subtypes of juvenile rheumatoid arthritis[9] or the CREST syndrome, which is a subtype of scleroderma[10,11].

DIAGNOSTIC TOOLS

Although classification criteria are imperfect measures of the presence of disease, they are often used as diagnostic tools in the clinical setting. A critical consideration in determining the usefulness of any diagnostic tool is the disease prevalence in the population in which the tool will be applied. Most classification criteria used in rheumatology have been created by comparing groups of patients with the disease in question with patient groups who have similar conditions which could be confused with the disease. Although this may be the most clinically relevant comparison, when such criteria are applied to a population setting where the frequency of the target disease is likely to be much lower, the positive predictive value of the criteria or the probability that the subject having the criteria indeed has the disease in question decreases substantially. For example, assume classification criteria have been developed in 1000 patients where the target disease is present in 50% (Fig. 3.1) such as might occur in a rheumatology practice. Now assume that these criteria perform nearly perfectly, with a sensitivity, specificity and positive predictive value of 98%. When the same criteria are applied to a general population of 10,000 where the target disease is present in only 1% of the population, the positive predictive value falls to only 33% (Fig. 3.1).

As with any other diagnostic tool, studies proposing classification criteria must demonstrate:

- validity (i.e. they must accurately define the disease),
- appropriate selection of cases and controls,
- comprehensiveness in selection of potential criteria (i.e., the list of attributes which will be tested to determine if they distinguish cases from controls),

PREVALENCE OF TARGET DISEASE

	Target disease		
Classification criteria	Present	Absent	Total
Prevalence = 50%*			
Positive	490	10	500
Negative	10	490	500
Total	500	500	1000
Prevalence = 1%†			
Positive	98	198	296
Negative	2	9702	9704
Total	100	9900	10,000

*Sensitivity = specificity = positive predictive value = 98%;
†Sensitivity = 98%; specificity = 98%; positive predictive value = 33%

Fig. 3.1 Prevalence of target disease: 50%; 1%.

- absence of circular reasoning (where the identified criteria are identical to those used to select cases),
- independent validation (criteria should be developed in one sample and tested in another), and
- proper application of statistical techniques[8].

Many of the classification criteria currently in use in rheumatology do not adhere to these standards. Because of these limitations, classification criteria should never be the only means by which a diagnosis is made. The fact that a particular individual does not meet all the classification criteria for a disease does not necessarily imply an incorrect diagnosis. Conversely, not all individuals who fulfill classification criteria actually have the disease in question.

CLASSIFICATION CRITERIA RELEVANT TO RHEUMATIC DISEASES

A major purpose for gathering data on the prevalence of diagnostic entities is to allow comparisons over time and among different places. The World Health Organization International Classification of Diseases (ICD) classification criteria have made such comparisons possible. Without a standard classification system which remains fixed over time and is applied uniformly from place to place, meaningful comparative analyses would not be possible. The ICD is, by far, the most widely used of such tools.

The ICD has been developing for more than two centuries[12]. Its roots date back to 18th century works by Francois de Lacroix, William Cullen and Linnaeus[12], the father of biological classification systems. The importance of an international, standardized statistical classification of diseases was widely recognized at the first International Statistical Congress in Brussels in 1853. Today, the ICD classification has been accepted by most countries of the world. It is a statistical classification of diseases, complications of pregnancy, childbirth, and puerperium, congenital abnormalities, causes of perinatal morbidity and mortality, accidents, poisoning and violence, as well as symptoms and ill-defined conditions. 'Nondisease' states can also be coded using a special section on 'special conditions and examinations without sickness'[13]. The ICD classification as it pertains to the rheumatic diseases is summarized in Figure 3.2.

Disease-specific classification criteria have also been developed and evaluated for most of the rheumatic diseases, including all the major vasculitides (polyarteritis nodosa, Churg–Strauss vasculitis, Wegener's granulomatosus, Henoch-Schönlein purpura, giant cell arteritis and Takayasu's arteritis)[6], the spondyloarthropathies[14–17], rheumatoid arthritis[18–21], Sjögren's syndrome[22], Behçet's disease[23], systemic lupus

NOMENCLATURE AND CLASSIFICATION OF RHEUMATIC DISEASES

Code	Description
Diffuse diseases of connective tissue	
710.0	Systemic lupus eryth. (SLE) and
581.81	Nephrotic syndrome (SLE)
583.81	Nephritis (SLE)
710.1	Systemic sclerosis
710.2	Keratoconjunctivitis sicca/ Sjögren's syndrome
710.3	Dermatomyositis
710.4	Polymyositis
710.9	CTD – unspecified diffuse
443.0	Raynaud's
Rheumatoid arthritis and inflammatory polyarthritis	
714.0	Rheumatoid arthritis
714.1	Felty's
714.2	Other/Visceral or syst. involv.
714.30	JRA – chronic or unspecified
714.31	JRA – acute
714.32	JRA – pauci
714.33	JRA – monoarticular
714.9	Inflammatory arth., seronegative
Osteoarthritis	
715.91	Osteoarthritis – shoulder
715.92	Osteoarthritis – upper arm
715.93	Osteoarthritis – forearm
715.94	Osteoarthritis – hand
715.95	Osteoarthritis – pelvic region and thigh
715.96	Osteoarthritis – lower leg
715.97	Osteoarthritis – ankle and foot
715.98	Osteoarthritis – other spec. site
715.09	Osteoarthritis – mult. sites/gen.
715.2_	Osteoarthritis – local., second., site__
721.0	Osteoarthritis – cervical spine
721.3	Osteoarthritis – lumbosacral spine
721.42	Osteoarthritis – lumbar spine
Spine disorders	
720.0	Ankylosing spondylitis
722.0	Displac. of cervical inter. disc
722.10	Displac. of lumbar inter. disc
722.11	Displac. of thoracic inter. disc
722.2	Displac. of inter. disc, unspec., incl. herniation
722.4	Degener. of cerv. inter. disc
722.51	Degener. of thoracic inter. disc
722.52	Degener. of lumbar inter. disc
722.6	Degenerative disc Disease (NOS)
723.1	Neck pain
723.4	Cervical neuritis
724.00	Spinal stenosis, unspecific region
724.02	Lumbar stenosis
724.3	Sciatica
724.4	Lumbar radiculopathy
724.5	Backache – NOS (also MBP)
733.00	Osteoporosis – unspecified
733.1	Compression fracture
733.6	Tietze's disease
733.99	DISH syndrome
737.30	Scoliosis
756.12	Spondylolisthesis
Arthropathy	
716.9	Arthropathy, unspecified site__
719.4	Pain in joint, site__
Internal derangement of knee	
717.7_	Chrondromalacia patellae (CMP)
717.9_	Internal derangement knee, unspec.
Joint disorders	
719.0_	Joint effusion, site__
719.30	Palindromic rheumatism, site unspecified
719.44	Pain, hand
719.45	Pain, hip or thigh
719.46	Pain, lower leg or knee
729.5	Pain in limb
725	Polymyalgia rheumatica
Symptoms involving skin and other integumentary tissue	
782.0	Paresthesia
447.6	Vasculitis
446.0	Polyarteritis nodosa
446.1	Kawasaki disease
446.2	Hypersensitivity vasculitis/ Goodpasture's syndrome
446.4	Wegener's
446.5	Giant cell arteritis/temporal arteritis
446.6	Thrombocytopenic purpura
446.7	Takayasu arteritis
287.0	Henoch–Schönlein purpura
Tendinitis and bursitis	
726.0	Adhesive capsulitis/ Frozen shoulder
726.10	Bursae/tendons Disorder – shoulder
726.11	Tendinitis, calcific, shoulder
726.12	Tenosynovitis, bicipital
726.2	Periarthritis, left and/or right shoulder
726.32	Lateral epicondylitis
726.33	Olecranon bursitis
726.5	Trochanteric bursitis (TBS)
726.60	Knee bursitis
726.61	Pes Anserine bursitis
726.65	Bursitis, prepatellar
726.70	Metatarsalgia
726.90	Tendinitis, unspecified
727.3	Heel bursitis
Disorders of synovium, tendon, bursitis	
727.04	De Quervain's tenosynovitis
727.51	Baker's cyst
Disorders of muscle, ligament, fascia	
728.71	Plantar fasciitis
Disorders of soft tissue	
333.99	Restless leg syndrome
353.0	Thoracic outlet syndrome
354.0	Carpal tunnel syndrome
729.0	Fibrositis/fibromyalgia
729.1	Myalgia and myositis, unspecified
729.2	Radiculopathy, unspecified
729.4	Fasciitis, unspecified
729.82	Nocturnal leg cramps
Crystal arthropathies	
274.0	Gouty arthritis
274.81	Tophaceous gout–ear only
274.82	Tophaceous gout
275.4	Disorders of calcium Metabolism and
712.1_	Chondrocalcinosis due to dicalcium phosphate, site__
712.2_	Pseudogout, site__
712.3_	Chondrocalcinosis, unspecified , site__
712.8_	Other specified crystal arthropathies, site__
712.9_	Unspecified crystal arthropathy, site__
Disorders of plasma protein metabolism	
273.9	Unspecified disorder plasma protein metabolism
Other inflammatory diseases	
696.0	Psoriatic arthritis
099.3	Reiter's disease and
711.1_	Arthropathy assoc. with Reiter's disease, site__
555.9	Regional enteritis, unspecified
556	Ulcerative colitis and
713.1	Arthropathy assoc. with GI (not infections)
695.2	Erythema nodosum and
713.3	Arthropathy assoc. with dermatologic disorders
088.81	Lyme disease

Fig. 3.2 Nomenclature and classification of rheumatic diseases. (The following fifth-digit subclassification is for use with categories 711–712, 715–16, 718–19 and 730: 0 – site unspecified; 1 – shoulder region; 2 – upper arm; 3 – forearm; 4 – hand; 5 – pelvic region and thigh; 6 – lower leg; 7 – ankle and foot; 8 – other specified sites; 9 – multiple sites.)

erythematosus[24–26], dermatomyositis/polymyositis[27], rheumatic fever[28], primary gout[29], Reiter's syndrome[30], juvenile rheumatoid arthritis[9,31], systemic sclerosis (scleroderma)[10], fibromyalgia[32] and osteoarthritis[33,34].

METHODOLOGICAL AND STATISTICAL CONSIDERATIONS

While there is no doubt that classification criteria have played a critical role in our understanding of disease, there is little agreement as to the optimal, or the most cost-effective, approach to developing such criteria[8,35]. Historically, classification criteria have been developed by means of consensus of a panel of expert clinicians, who generate the candidate criteria and identify cases and comparison subjects. Statistical approaches are often used to reduce the set of potential diagnostic features to a manageable number; for example, by examining each variable's ability to distinguish cases from controls and eliminating redundant variables. Statistical techniques, such as receiver-operating characteristic (ROC) curves, discriminant analysis and logistic regression analysis, may be used to create classification criteria from a series of diagnostic measures. In recent years, classification and regression trees (CART), based on the work of Breiman *et al.*[36–38], has been used for a number of classification exercises. Advantages of this method include the graphic display of results, the ability to use attributes multiple times in different parts of the tree and the ability to perform internal cross-validation.

The newest technique applied to disease classification in rheumatology is artificial neural networks[12,39–44]. In this technique, sequences of cases and controls are fed into the network and a function to predict cases from the clinical data is built empirically. The neural network 'learns', just as a physician learns, to distinguish disease from nondisease by seeing one patient after another and categorizing their clinical information. However, because the function is quite complex, wide application of neural networks is not likely.

Obviously, resource utilization and cost vary greatly depending on the methods used. Historic, empirically derived classification criteria developed *ad hoc* have proven extremely useful. Statistically derived and validated criteria provide added confidence in the final criteria set – however, at a substantial added cost. There is no 'correct' approach to classification criteria development. However, it is necessary to keep in mind that the main goal of classification criteria is simply to facilitate communication.

A WORD OF CAUTION

While classification criteria provide a guide to diagnosis, criteria do not necessarily describe real pathologic entities. Rather, classification criteria are evolving representations of disease which permit convenient communication and allow some insight into the nature of a disorder[45]. In rheumatology, there are several examples of evolving classification criteria which have provided better and more exact information about the disease under consideration (e.g. the 1958 American Rheumatology Association criteria for rheumatoid arthritis; 1987 American College of Rheumatology criteria for rheumatoid arthritis). By contrast, some entities have been defined which are not really 'diseases.' A definition of disease has been given by Scadding[46] – 'A disease is the sum of the abnormal phenomenon displayed by a group of living organisms in association with a specific common characteristic or set of characteristics by which they differ from the norm of their species in such a way as to place them at a biological disadvantage'[46]. The use of classification criteria for labeling certain conditions that do not meet this definition of disease (e.g. post-traumatic syndrome, post-traumatic stress disorder, chronic fatigue syndrome and repetitive strain injury[45]) has been severely criticized. Such diagnostic labels may, in themselves, induce illness behavior, particularly if these entities are being contested in the courtroom. Similarly, Cohen and Quinter have challenged the usefulness of diagnostic criteria for fibromyalgia and suggest that they 'convey no pathophysiologic insight and that they have been validated via a circular argument in which the evidence on which the construct is based is taken as proof of its veracity'[47].

REFERENCES

1. Yelin EH, Henke CJ, Kramer JS, Nevitt MC, Shearn M, Epstein WV. A comparison of the treatment of rheumatoid arthritis in health maintenance organizations and fee-for-service practices. N Engl J Med. 1985;312:962–7.
2. Henke CJ, Epstein WV. Practice variation in rheumatologists' encounters with their patients who have rheumatoid arthritis. Med Care. 1991;29(8):799–812.
3. Nevitt MC, Yelin EH, Henke CJ, Epstein WV. Risk factors for hospitalization and surgery in patients with rheumatoid arthritis: implications for capitated medical payment. Ann Intern Med. 1986;105:421–8.
4. Cherkin DC, Deyo RA, Wheeler K, Ciol MA. Physician variation in diagnostic testing for low back pain. Who you see is what you get. Arthritis Rheum. 1994;37:15–22.
5. Criswell LA, Redfearn WJ. Variation among rheumatologists in the use of prednisone and second-line agents for the treatment of rheumatoid arthritis. Arthritis Rheum. 1994;37:476–80.
6. Hunder GG, Arend WP, Bloch DA, *et al.* The American College of Rheumatology 1990 criteria for the classification of vasculitis. Arthritis Rheum. 1990;33(8):1065–1144.
7. Fries JF, Hochberg MC, Medsger TA,Jr, Hunder GG, Bombardier C, American College of Rheumatology Diagnostic and Therapeutic Criteria Committee. Criteria for rheumatic disease. Arthritis Rheum. 1994;37:454–62.
8. Felson DT, Anderson JJ. Methodological and statistical approaches to criteria development in rheumatic diseases. Baillière's Clin Rheumatol. 1995;9:253–66.
9. Brewer EJ,Jr., Bass J, Baum J et al. Current proposed revision of JRA criteria. Arthritis Rheum. 1977;20:195–9.
10. Subcommittee for Scleroderma Criteria of the American Rheumatism Association Diagnostic and Therapeutic Criteria Committee: Preliminary criteria for the classification of systemic sclerosis (scleroderma). Arthritis Rheum. 1980;23:581–90.
11. Masi AT, Rodnan GP, Medsger TA Jr, *et al.* Preliminary criteria for the classification of systemic sclerosis (scleroderma). Bull Rheum Dis. 1981;31:1–6.
12. Israel RA. The history of the international classification of diseases. Health Trends. 1991;22:43–4.
13. Sartorius N. Conference working papers: Methodologic problems of common terminology, measurement, and classification. 11. Modifications and new approaches to taxonomy in long-term care: advantages and limitations of the ICD. Med Care. 1976;14:109–15.
14. Dougados M, van der Linden S, Juhlin R, *et al.* The European Spondylarthropathy Study Group preliminary criteria for the classification of spondylarthropathy. Arthritis Rheum. 1991;34:1218–27.
15. Moll JMH, Wright V. New York clinical criteria for ankylosing spondylitis. A statistical evaluation. Ann Rheum Dis. 1973;32:354–63.
16. Boyer GS, Templin DW, Goring WP. Evaluation of the European Spondylarthopathy Study Group preliminary classification criteria in Alaskan Eskimo populations. Arthritis Rheum. 1993;36:534–8.
17. Collantes-Estevez E, Cisnal Del Mazo A, Munoz-Gomariz E. Assessment of 2 systems of spondyloarthropathy diagnostic and classification criteria (Amor and ESSG) by a Spanish multicenter study. J Rheumatol. 1995;22:246–51.
18. Arnett FC, Edworthy SM, Bloch DA, *et al.* The American Rheumatism Association 1987 revised criteria for the classification of rheumatoid arthritis. Arthritis Rheum. 1988;31(3):315–24.
19. Erickson AR, Reddy V, Vogelgesang SA, West SG. Usefulness of the American College of Rheumatology recommendations for liver biopsy in methotrexate-treated rheumatoid arthritis patients. Arthritis Rheum. 1995;38:1115–9.
20. Paimela L. The radiographic criterion in the 1987 revised criteria for rheumatoid arthritis. Reassessment in a prospective study of early disease. Arthritis Rheum. 1992;35:255–8.
21. Hochberg MC, Chang RW, Dwosh I, Lindsey S, Pincus T, Wolfe F. The American College of Rheumatology 1991 revised criteria for the classification of global functional status in rheumatoid arthritis. Arthritis Rheum. 1992;35:498–502.
22. Vitali C, Bombardieri S, Moutsopoulos HM, *et al.* Preliminary criteria for the classification of Sjogren's

syndrome. Arthritis Rheum. 1993;36:340–7.
23. The International Study Group for Behçet's Disease. Evaluation of diagnostic ('classification') criteria in Behçet's disease – towards internationally agreed criteria. Br J Rheumatol. 1992;31:299–308.
24. Tan EM, Cohen AS, Fries JF, *et al.* The 1982 revised criteria for the classification of systemic lupus erythematosus. Arthritis Rheum. 1982;25:1271–7.
25. Somogyi L, Cikes N, Marusic M. Evaluation of criteria contributions for the classification of systemic lupus erythematosus. Scand J Rheumatol. 1993;22:58–62.
26. Clough JD, Elrazak M, Calabrese LH, Valenzuela R, Braun WB, Williams GW. Weighted criteria for the diagnosis of systemic lupus erythematosus. Arch Intern Med. 1984;144:281–5.
27. Bohan A, Peter JB, Bowman RL, Pearson CM. A computer-assisted analysis of 153 patients with polymyositis and dermatomyositis. Medicine. 1977;56:255–86.
28. Stollerman GH, Markowitz M, Taranta A, Wannamaker LW, Whittemore R. Jones criteria (revised) for guidance in the diagnosis of rheumatic fever. Circulation. 1965;32:664–8.
29. Wallace SL, Robinson H, Masi AT, Decker JL, McCarty DJ, Yu T-F. Preliminary criteria for the classification of the acute arthritis of primary gout. Arthritis Rheum. 1977;20:895–900.
30. Willkens RF, Arnett FC, Bitter T, *et al.* Reiter's syndrome. Evaluation of preliminary criteria for definite disease. Arthritis Rheum. 1981;24:844–9.
31. Cassidy JT, Levinson JE, Bass JC, *et al.* A study of classification criteria for a diagnosis of juvenile rheumatoid arthritis. Arthritis Rheum. 1986;29:274–81.
32. Wolfe F, Smythe HA, Yunus MB, *et al.* The American College of Rheumatology 1990 criteria for the classification of fibromyalgia. Report of the multicenter criteria committee. Arthritis Rheum. 1990;33(2):160–72.
33. Altman R, Asch E, Bloch D, *et al.* Development of criteria for the classification and reporting of osteoarthritis. Classification of osteoarthritis of the knee. Arthritis Rheum. 1986;29(8):1039–49.
34. Altman R, Alarcon G, Appelrouth D, *et al.* The American College of Rheumatology criteria for the classification and reporting of osteoarthritis of the hip. Arthritis Rheum. 1991;34:505–14.
35. Katz JN, Liang MH. Classification criteria revisited. Arthritis Rheum. 1991;34:1228–30.
36. Breiman L, Friedman J, Olshen RA, Stone D. Classification and regression trees. Belmont, CA: Wadsworth; 1984.
37. Bloch DA, Moses LE, Michel BA. Statistical approaches to classification. Arthritis Rheum. 1990;33:1137–44.
38. Taylor RM, Gabriel SE, O'Fallon WM, Bowles CA, Duffy J. A diagnostic algorithm for distinguishing eosinophilia-myalgia-syndrome from fibromyalgia and chronic myofascial pain. J Rheumatol. 1996 (in press).
39. Astion ML, Wener MH, Thomas RG, Hunder GG, Bloch DA. Application of neural networks to the classification of giant cell arteritis. Arthritis Rheum. 1994;37:760–70.
40. Baxt WG. Use of an artificial neural network for the diagnosis of myocardial infarction. Ann Intern Med. 1991;115:843–8.
41. Guerriere MRJ, Detsky AS. Neural networks: what are they? Ann Intern Med. 1991;115:906–7.
42. Astion ML, Wilding P. The application of backpropagation neural networks to problems in pathology and laboratory medicine. Arch Pathol Lab Med. 1992;116:995–1001.
43. Mulsant BH. A neural network as an approach to clinical diagnosis. MD Comput. 1990;7:25–36.
44. Zelicoff AP, Browner WS, Carter JH, Baxt WG. Myocardial infarction prediction by artificial neural networks. Ann Intern Med. 1992;116:701–2.
45. Pearce JMS. New diagnoses for old diseases: dangers and distractions. Q J Med. 1994;87:253–8.
46. Scadding JG. Diagnosis: the clinician and the computer. Lancet. 1967;ii:877–82.
47. Cohen ML, Quintner JL. Fibromyalgia syndrome, a problem of tautology. Lancet. 1993;342:906–9.

4

EPIDEMIOLOGIC CONCEPTS AND RHEUMATOLOGY

Deborah Symmons

- Rheumatic disease epidemiology is concerned with determinants and distribution of rheumatic diseases in different populations.
- Frequency of disease in a population can be expressed in terms of incidence (the number of new cases) and prevalence (the proportion of the population with the disease).
- Rheumatic disease frequency and severity vary with age, gender, ethnic origin and country.
- Differences in disease or outcome frequency can be explored to yield hypotheses about demographic, genetic, hormonal, environmental and psychosocial risk factors for development or severity of disease.
- These hypotheses can be tested in case control or cohort studies which involve the use of a comparison group.

INTRODUCTION

Epidemiology is the clinical science which studies the distribution and determinants of disease in populations. It involves describing the frequency of diseases and their consequences (including morbidity and mortality), and understanding the risk factors for developing a disease or its complications. There are two basic types of epidemiologic studies (Fig. 4.1). Descriptive epidemiology 'describes' the number of people who develop the disease in a particular time period or who currently have the disease, what type of people are susceptible (in terms, for example, of age, gender or ethnic background) and where and when the disease occurs (geographic variations on a large or small scale, secular trends)[1]. Put more succinctly, descriptive studies investigate the distribution of disease in relation to person, place and time.

Analytic epidemiology tests hypotheses of causation and involves using a comparison group (Fig. 4.2). By comparing people with and without a particular disease or outcome, or people who have particular factors (such as drugs, pregnancy or certain genotypes), it is possible to identify risk factors for developing disease or attributes which affect outcome or disease severity. Such studies may select subjects on the basis of their exposure status or being disease-free and follow them to see how many develop the disease. This basic design is known as a cohort study. Cohort studies may be prospective, if the outcome has not occurred when the study begins, or retrospective if the outcome has already happened. Alternatively, two groups may be selected on the basis of their disease status, those with the disease being the 'cases' and those without being the 'controls'. All the subjects are then studied to see how many in each group have been exposed to the risk factor(s) of interest. This design is called a case-control study. Each design has its advantages and disadvantages, and the choice is often dictated by the relative prevalence of the disease and the exposure[2].

This chapter introduces the fundamental concepts of epidemiology and describes how these have been used to study the frequency of rheumatic disorders and their burden worldwide. It also discusses how hypotheses concerning risk factors for developing rheumatic diseases or particular outcomes can be generated and tested.

QUESTIONS ADDRESSED BY EPIDEMIOLOGIC STUDIES

Question	Methodology
How many? Who? Where? When?	Descriptive epidemiology
Why? How does it happen?	Analytic epidemiology

Fig. 4.1 Questions addressed by epidemiologic studies.

HOW MANY PEOPLE HAVE THE DISEASE?

The two most common measures of disease frequency are prevalence and incidence (Fig. 4.3)[1]. Prevalence relates to existing cases of disease. The term point prevalence is used to describe the proportion of the population that has the disorder at a particular point in time (sometimes called 'prevalence day'). This measure is useful for chronic disorders such as rheumatoid arthritis (RA) and osteoarthritis (OA). For intermittent conditions such as back pain and gout it is more appropriate to measure period prevalence – the proportion of the population that has the disorder at some time during a given time period (usually one year). The one-year period prevalence of back pain includes all those who had back pain at the beginning of the year plus all those who develop back pain during the year regardless of how long any individual episode of back pain lasts. Finally, cumulative prevalence is the proportion of the population who have had, or who now have, the disorder up to a specified time point, for example by age 60 years or up to the time of the study.

Prevalence in the population setting is commonly determined by

COMPARISON OF CASE-CONTROL AND COHORT STUDY DESIGNS

Study design	Past	Present	Future
Prospective cohort study		Exposed Not exposed	Disease / No disease Disease / No disease
Retrospective case-control study	Exposed / Not exposed Exposed / Not exposed	Disease Controls	
Retrospective cohort study	Exposed Not exposed	Disease / No disease Disease / No disease	

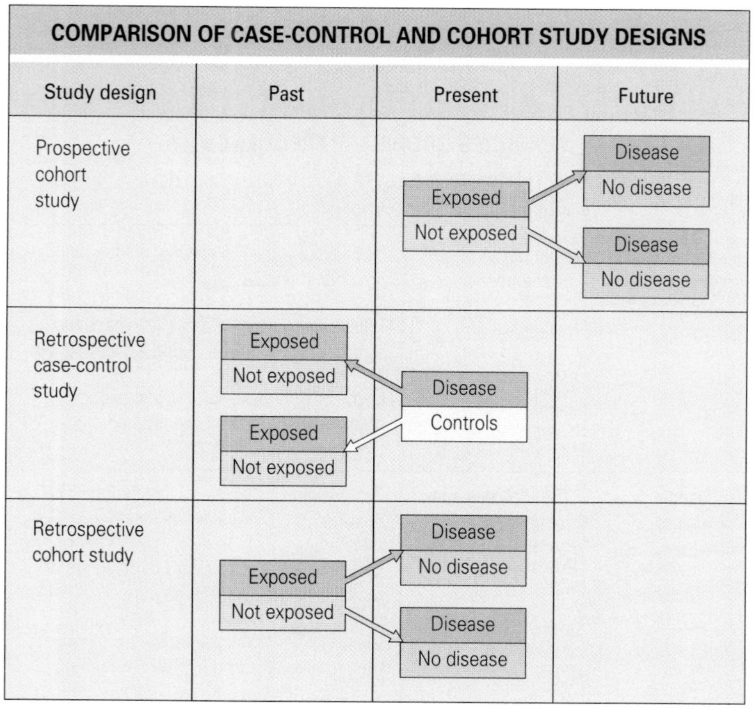

Fig. 4.2 Comparison of case-control and cohort study designs.

questionnaire, by clinical evaluation or by using a combination of both. In the hospital or primary care setting prevalence is often assessed by identifying diagnosed cases. Although this may be a practical way of measuring prevalence for uncommon conditions[3], the cases identified in this way are often skewed towards the more severe end of the clinical spectrum because mild cases may not be under current medical review.

While the term prevalence relates to existing disease, the term incidence relates to new cases of disease. Investigators of disease etiology will want to know the number of individuals in a defined population who first develop the disorder in a given time period, usually one year. This figure is known as the incidence rate or, more accurately, the first incidence rate. However, planners and providers of health care services may be more interested in the total number of episodes of a disorder, which is known as the episode incidence, than in the number of individuals affected. The episode incidence of back pain is usually higher than the first incidence rate since it includes people who have second or subsequent episodes of back pain and counts more than once those who have repeated episodes during the time frame of interest. Those who are studying outcome may want to consider cumulative incidence up to a particular time. This measure can be used, for example, to compare the frequency of certain side effects in patients exposed to antirheumatic drugs.

Incidence is measured either by monitoring for new cases as they are diagnosed, or by conducting two cross-sectional studies some time apart and identifying new cases which have occurred between the two surveys.

MORTALITY

Disease incidence and prevalence are related by the formula:

$$\text{incidence} \times \text{mean duration} = \text{prevalence}.$$

Individuals may leave the prevalent pool of cases either through recovery or through death. The mean disease duration is determined by the average length of time to recovery or death. Rheumatoid arthritis has a relatively low incidence but a long duration so the prevalence is relatively high. The rate of death may be expressed as the mortality rate (the number of deaths from a disease in a given time period divided by the total population) or the case-fatality rate (the number of deaths from a disease in a given time period divided by the number of cases of the disease).

MEASURES OF DISEASE FREQUENCY

Term	Denominator	Numerator
Prevalence (relates to existing disease)	Number of people in the population	Point prevalence (number who have the disorder at a given time point)
		Period prevalence (number who have the disorder at some time during a given period)
		Cumulative prevalence (number who have the disorder at some time up to a given time point)
Incidence (relates to disease onset)	Total person–time of observation	First incidence (number who have their first onset of the disorder in a given time period)
		Episode incidence (number of episodes of the disorder in a given time period)
		Cumulative incidence (number who have their first onset up to a given time point)

Fig. 4.3 Measures of disease frequency.

PRACTICAL ISSUES IN MEASURING DISEASE FREQUENCY

Issues relating to the numerator

Accurate estimation of incidence and prevalence depends on reliable case definition and case ascertainment. Most rheumatic diseases do not have a specific diagnostic test. Sets of classification criteria (see Chapter 1.3) have therefore been developed in order to identify homogeneous patient populations for epidemiologic studies and clinical trials. There are many problems in interpreting and applying these criteria. The construction of nearly all the classification criteria is such that early or mild cases may not meet the criteria. In addition some criteria sets require expensive, invasive or nonstandard investigations, such as radiography or immunochemical tests, which are not routinely obtained or are not suitable for use in a population setting. This makes it difficult to apply the criteria retrospectively using patients' medical records or to use them unaltered in population surveys.

In inflammatory conditions such as RA or systemic lupus erythematosus (SLE) the criteria were developed using patients with active disease. A population survey of RA prevalence will therefore identify those individuals who currently have active disease plus those people who in the past have had disease was sufficiently severe to leave stigmata such as joint deformities. People who had mild disease that is now in natural or drug-induced remission will not be detected. Thus the resultant figure is a cross between point prevalence and cumulative prevalence.

Determining the time of disease onset is problematic for some rheumatic diseases. If OA is defined in terms of radiologic change then it is usually impossible to say when this first appeared. The classification criteria for SLE require an individual to satisfy four out of 11 criteria[4], which may be accumulated over several years. The disease is 'diagnosed' on the day the fourth criterion is met, and yet the onset was presumably on the day that the first feature appeared. It is, therefore, important to define precisely how the time of onset was determined and to recognize the consequences of this definition when interpreting studies.

Finally all cases of the disease within the population should be identified. Disease in the population has a continuum of severity (Fig. 4.4) and ascertainment may not be complete depending on where it is carried out. Clinic-based studies rely on the patient having sought medical care, being (more or less) correctly diagnosed and being referred to the appropriate specialist. With severe life-threatening diseases one might reasonably assume all cases are referred, but this is not the situation with most rheumatic diseases. To overcome this problem several approaches may be used simultaneously (for example, ascertaining SLE cases from hospital clinics, self-help groups and laboratory records of ANA results) to try to 'capture' those with the disorder concerned. Studies that use different case definitions or methods of case ascertainment will not yield comparable results. For example, a study of the prevalence of knee OA which begins by screening the population by radiography and then evaluates those with abnormal radiographs will not yield the same number of cases as one which screens the population for knee symptoms and then radiographs those who are symptomatic.

Issues relating to the denominator

To calculate rates it is necessary to know the size of population from which the cases have been identified. This is difficult when cases are identified only from hospital or clinic attenders because many medical facilities do not have defined catchment populations. There are many factors that determine whether an individual case is referred to a particular center (referral bias). The denominator population should comprise only those individuals at risk of developing the disease. Thus the incidence of juvenile arthritis should be expressed per 100,000 children aged under 16, not per 100,000 of the total population.

SOURCES OF DATA FOR ESTIMATING DISEASE OCCURRENCE

Routinely collected data may prove useful in building up a picture of the epidemiology of a rheumatic disease. Researchers using

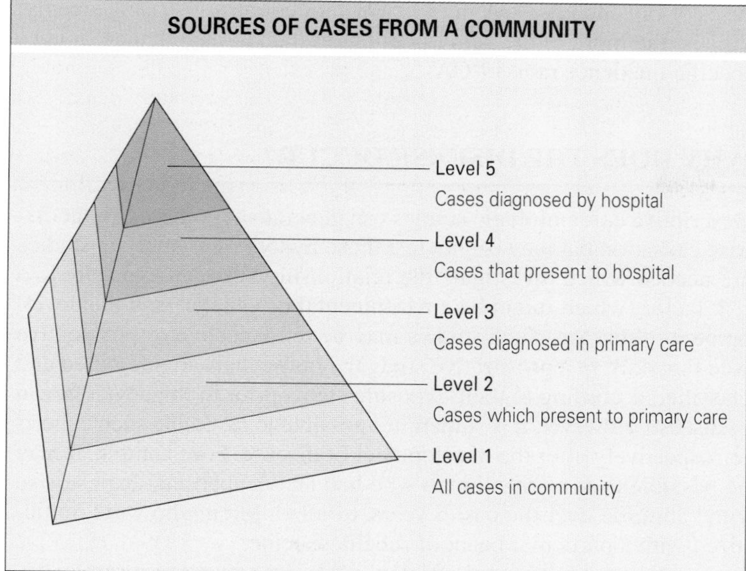

Fig. 4.4 Sources of cases from a community.

routinely collected data need to assess the diagnostic accuracy and level of completeness. A variety of sources have been used in rheumatic disease epidemiology.

Death certificates

Mortality records have, with a few exceptions, been of little use in rheumatic disease epidemiology because the rheumatologic disorder is often not recorded on the death certificate. Therefore it is not possible to tell, for example, how many people with RA die each year in a particular country. However, if a cohort of RA patients has already been identified, death certificates will provide valuable information on the number of the cohort who have died and their attributed causes of death. Because most countries code the cause of death using the International Classification of Diseases it is possible to make comparisons of the attributed causes of death between RA cohorts in different locations, and between RA cohorts and the general populations from which they were drawn.

Morbidity registers

While many countries have cancer registers, the same is not true for the rheumatic diseases. Some Scandinavian countries have registers of people who are disabled or who can claim reimbursable medication and, using a unique personal identity number, they are able to link information on these registers with, for example, mortality data. The Mayo Clinic in Rochester, Minnesota, USA, has developed a record linkage system whereby the health care records of all residents in Olmsted County are maintained on a central database. Information from this database, which dates back to 1910, has been used to generate incidence estimates of a number of rheumatic diseases. However the population of Olmsted County is only about 100,000 and the majority of the population is of Scandinavian descent. This limits the reliability of estimates for rare diseases and the generalizability of all estimates. In the UK, during the 10-yearly census years, a large group of primary care physicians code the reason for every patient consultation and whether it is the first consultation for the particular diagnosis. Standard disease definitions are not used. Nevertheless, these Royal College of General Practitioner (RCGP) morbidity surveys provide unique national primary care based data on the incidence and prevalence of musculoskeletal diseases. In all these situations information about the denominator, that is the number of people covered by the registers, is known.

Health insurance databases

In some countries, healthcare which is reimbursed by the government is linked to diagnostic codes on large computerised databases. These have provided a rich source of data on the frequency of rare events such as drug toxicity or major complications of orthopaedic surgery. They enable the identification of individuals for detailed study. Examples include the data on medicare patients in the USA or on Canadians covered by their national healthcare system.

Population surveys

In many countries there are regular population surveys which examine social and demographic trends. These may include health-related information such as number of visits to a physician, self-reported illness and disability. Examples include the General Household Survey in the UK and the National Health and Nutrition Examination Surveys in the USA.

Work absenteeism records

In some countries information on the reason for absence from work for sickness is recorded and can be used to examine the profile of rheumatologic complaints in an occupational cohort.

WHO IS SUSCEPTIBLE TO THE DISEASE?

Differences in disease occurrence provide useful starting points for the investigation of disease causation. Striking differences in age- and sex-specific rates are seen in many rheumatic diseases. For example, RA is three times more common in females than males[5]; and the onset of ankylosing spondylitis is rare after the age of 55 years[6]. Apparent differences in overall or crude (that is all age and sex combined) incidence and prevalence between populations may simply reflect differences in the proportions of men and women or in the age structures of the populations. It is therefore important, whenever possible, to see epidemiologic data broken down into age (for example 10-year age bands) and sex-specific groups before making inferences. It is then possible to apply the age- and sex-specific incidence rates from one population to the age–sex distribution of another population in order to calculate the 'expected' number of incident cases in the second population – a process known as standardization. This is the principle underlying the calculation of standardized mortality ratios (SMRs). The number of observed deaths in a population (for example of patients with RA) is compared with the number of deaths which would be expected in a sample of the general population with the same age and sex distribution.

Differences in disease frequency or adverse outcomes may also be found between racial groups (for example, SLE is more common in people of Afro-American and Afro-Caribbean origin than in Caucasians)[7], occupations (for example, hip OA is more common in farmers)[8] and social classes (for example, back pain is more common in the lower social classes)[9]. It can be difficult, however, to determine the relative contributions of race, occupation and socioeconomic factors to disease etiology because these factors are often interrelated.

WHERE DOES THE DISEASE OCCUR?

Differences in disease rates between countries or regions may be due to genetic (including racial) and/or environmental factors. Possible environmental factors include diet and socioeconomic factors. In rheumatology there are hints of geographic patterns which are still being unraveled (Fig. 4.5). For example, RA occurs with similar frequency in most white Caucasian populations. However, it has a higher prevalence among some native American peoples, such as the Pima, and a lower prevalence in rural southern Africa, China and Indonesia[10]. Migration studies suggest whether geographic differences in disease frequency are predominantly due to genetic or environmental factors.

If a migrating people have the same frequency of disease in their native and newly adopted countries, this suggests that genetic factors are more important. If the disease frequency changes, especially if it changes within one or two generations, this suggests a change in environment or lifestyle as being important. Most of the geographic variation in the frequency of ankylosing spondylitis can be explained by the varying prevalence of HLA-B27 in different racial groups. Further investigation of the frequency and clinical characteristics of SLE in people of African origin may yield important etiologic clues. There is a high frequency of SLE in Afro-Americans and Afro-Caribbeans but a low frequency in West Africa[7]. Although this suggests an environmental cause for SLE, it is possible that genetic admixture may play a part in the changing incidence of SLE in this group of people.

WHEN DOES THE DISEASE OCCUR?

Time trends in disease occurrence may also provide important etiologic clues. Clusters of incident cases in a particular season of the year or sporadic time–space clusters suggest that all or most of the cases in the cluster may have been exposed to an etiologic agent from a common source. In rheumatology, Lyme disease provides a good example of a disease identified because of clustering of cases of juvenile and adult inflammatory arthritis in place and time[11]. A rise or fall in disease incidence year-on-year may suggest a change in the level of exposure to risk factors. Between around 1970 and 1985 there was a marked fall in the incidence of RA in women in the USA and the UK. This coincided with the increasing use of the oral contraceptive pill and there is evidence to suggest that the two phenomena are linked[12]. Changes in disease prevalence with time are more difficult to interpret because they may be caused by alterations in disease incidence, recovery rates or survival – or a combination of all three. When considering future health service provision, health care planners have to take account of trends in incidence and prevalence, both of which may be affected by increasing life expectancy. For instance, the number of new cases of hip and knee OA in most Western countries is rising steeply. This is due more to the aging population than to any change in age-specific incidence rates of OA.

VARIATIONS IN RHEUMATIC DISEASE FREQUENCY COMPARED TO EUROPEAN WHITES		
	Increased frequency	**Decreased frequency**
RA	Native American (Pima, Chippewa, Yakima)	Rural African Chinese Indonesian
Juvenile chronic arthritis	Canadian Inuit	Afro-Americans
Ankylosing spondylitis	Haida people	Australian aboriginals
Gout	Polynesians Filipinos	Africans
SLE	Afro-Americans Afro-Caribbeans Chinese	West Africans
Scleroderma	Southern US	Australian aboriginals
Polymyalgia rheumatic	Northern Europeans	Afro-Americans
OA knee	Afro-American women	
OA hip		Chinese Asian Indians Africans
Osteoporosis	Northern Europeans	Africans

Fig. 4.5 Some geographic and racial variations in rheumatic disease.

WHY DOES THE DISEASE OCCUR?

Descriptive epidemiologic studies can generate hypotheses about disease causation but they cannot test those hypotheses. Analytic studies are needed which investigate the relationship between exposure to a risk factor (which might be environmental or genetic) and the development of disease. Such studies may be retrospective or prospective (see Fig. 4.2). In a prospective study the individuals are identified and classified according to their exposure status prior to the development of disease. However, it is sometimes possible to assemble such cohorts retrospectively after the development of disease. For example, it may be possible to identify all men who had an occupational exposure to vinyl chloride over the past 5 years, or all children who were immunized with a particular batch of rubella vaccine.

A cohort study is more efficient when investigating a rare exposure, while a case-control design is more efficient when investigating a rare disease (Fig. 4.6). The case-control study is best for investigating multiple risk factors simultaneously. Although either incident or prevalent cases can be used for a case-control study, incident cases are usually preferred because it is then clear that any risk factors identified are markers for disease susceptibility rather than severity. For example, clinic attenders with RA have a high frequency of HLA-DR4 compared with the general population. However, in studies which were confined to incident cases of RA, no association with HLA-DR4 was found. This means that people who are HLA-DR4 positive do not have an increased risk of developing RA, but if they do develop RA they are more likely to develop complications such as Felty's syndrome. The most difficult aspect of a case-control study is the selection of appropriate controls. Controls should be individuals who, if they had developed the disease, would have been included among the cases. Thus the cases and controls should be selected from the same catchment population. It is not ideal to conduct a study where, for example, the cases are elderly people with knee OA and the controls are healthy blood donors from another area.

The results in longitudinal studies are usually expressed as a relative risk, that is the risk (or incidence) of the disease in the exposed

ADVANTAGES AND DISADVANTAGES OF EPIDEMIOLOGIC STUDY DESIGNS		
Study design	**Advantages**	**Disadvantages**
Prospective cohort	Good exposure data Accurate timing of exposure and disease onset Little recall bias	Expensive May be long delay before disease onset Large numbers needed Only suitable for frequent outcomes
Case control	Relatively inexpensive Quick to perform Useful for rare diseases	Subject to recall bias Cases may not be representative Controls difficult to select and ascertain Exposure data may be unreliable Time of exposure and disease onset may be imprecise
Descriptive prevalence study	Quick to perform Generalizable	Difficult to distinguish cause and effect Biased towards inclusion of chronic cases

Fig. 4.6 Advantages and disadvantages of epidemiologic study designs.

ASSESSING THE ASSOCIATION BETWEEN EXPOSURE AND DISEASE				
		Disease		
		+	–	
Exposure	+	a	b	a+b
	–	c	d	c+d
		a+c	b+d	a+b+c+d

Relative risk = $\frac{a}{a+b} \div \frac{c}{c+d} = \frac{a(c+d)}{c(a+b)}$ (Cohort)

Odds ratio = $\frac{a}{b} \div \frac{c}{d} = \frac{ad}{bc}$ (Case-control)

Fig. 4.7 Assessing the association between exposure and disease.

ASSESSING CAUSALITY BETWEEN A RISK FACTOR AND A DISEASE OR OUTCOME
An association between an exposure and an outcome may be due to:
Direct causation
Chance
Bias
Confounding
Causality is more likely if:
Exposure precedes the outcome of interest
Association is biologically plausible
Association is strong (high relative risk)
Association is consistent between studies
Association is supported by experimental evidence

Fig. 4.8 Assessing causality between a risk factor and a disease or outcome.

INCIDENT CASES PER 100,000 MALES (MUSCULOSKELETAL DISEASES TEMPLATE)

Condition	0–14 years	15–24 years	25–44 years	45–64 years	65–74 years	75+ years	All ages
Inflammatory arthritis[a]	=JCA	12	25	45	49	64	32
Juvenile chronic arthritis[b]	12	1	0	0	0	0	—
Ankylosing spondylitis[c]	1	15	23	8	4	4	12
Gout[d]	0	0	170	450	470	760	210
SLE[e]	0	0	1	5	2	0	1
Scleroderma[f]	—	—	—	—	—	—	0.2
OA[g]	0	120	250	1500	2500	2900	—
Back pain[h]	NA	3800	6300	6300	4900	4500	5500
Soft tissue rheumatism[i]	100	1800	3360	4830	4370	2920	3530
Osteoporosis [j]:							
Hip fracture	NA	8	15	26	116	721	—
Fractured vertebra	0	3	19	61	148	466	—

a Data from the Norfolk Arthritis Register, UK[15]. All cases of inflammatory polyarthritis of >4 weeks' duration that present to primary care are notified to the register which covers a population of around 500,000. About half the cases satisfy the 1987 American Rheumatism Association criteria for RA at presentation.

b Data from Helsinki, Finland[16]. These figures are based on children who satisfied the ARA criteria for juvenile chronic arthritis, 37% of whom were male.

c Data from the Mayo Clinic, USA, over a 50-year period.

d Third RCGP Morbidity Survey[17].

e Cases ascertained from multiple sources (predominantly hospital-based) in Nottingham, UK (1988–1989)[18].

f Scleroderma is a rare disease and no studies have been large enough to provide reliable age- and sex-specific data. Data from the Mayo Clinic, USA[19].

g Third RCGP Morbidity Survey[17]; data include OA of all sites.

h Third RCGP Morbidity Survey[17].

i Third RCGP Morbidity Survey[17]; data include shoulder pain, bursitis, tendinitis, tenosynovitis and other nonarticular rheumatism.

j Hospital admissions in the Trent region, UK (1989–1990), for fractured neck of femur[20]; data for fractured vertebrae are from the Mayo Clinic, USA (1950–1982)[21].

Fig. 4.9 Incident cases per 100,000 males (musculoskeletal diseases template). JCA = juvenile chronic arthritis (inflammatory arthritis at <15 years is classified here as JCA).

cohort (a/a+b) divided by the risk of disease in the unexposed cohort (c/c+d) (Fig. 4.7). In a case-control study the relative frequency of risk factors is determined by the number of cases and controls and so, in this situation, the odds ratio is calculated; that is, the odds of disease in the exposed (a/b) divided by the odds of disease in the unexposed (c/d). The relative risk or odds ratio indicates the strength of the association between the risk factor and the disease. In a case-control study causality cannot be assumed because information about disease state and exposure status are collected cross-sectionally. It is therefore impossible to be sure which came first. In a longitudinal study the higher the relative risk, the more likely the exposure and the outcome are to be linked in a causal chain. Figure 4.8 shows the other factors which should be considered when examining causality.

WHAT HAPPENS TO PEOPLE WITH THE DISEASE?

The investigation of prognosis is analogous to investigating the development of disease and can be assessed with either cohort or case-control studies. In prognosis studies all the individuals studied have the disease in question. In longitudinal studies patients are selected on the basis of exposure to a predictor variable (for example being HLA-DR4 positive in RA, or having a particular radiographic grading in OA) and then followed for the incidence of the outcome of interest (for example death or the development of disability). In a case-control study patients are selected on the basis of whether or not they have developed a particular complication of their disease (for example vasculitis in RA, or vertebral fracture in osteoporosis) and then compared with patients without this outcome for predictors such as corticosteroid use.

APPLICATIONS OF EPIDEMIOLOGIC DATA

PLANNING RHEUMATOLOGY HEALTH CARE SERVICES

The ability of a population to benefit from rheumatology health care depends on three things:

- the incidence and prevalence of rheumatic disease in that community,
- the effectiveness of the regimens available to treat or prevent rheumatic disease, and
- the proportion of those affected or potentially affected who might benefit from such interventions[13].

The first step in planning rheumatology services is to compile a profile of the community's musculoskeletal health. Ideally, this would involve conducting a detailed interview with each resident. A reasonable substitute is to perform a survey using a stratified sample of the population. However, even when this is done, it is not possible to cover every aspect

INCIDENT CASES PER 100,000 FEMALES (MUSCULOSKELETAL DISEASES TEMPLATE)

Condition	0–14 years	15–24 years	25–44 years	45–64 years	65–74 years	75+ years	All ages
Inflammatory arthritis[a]	=JCA	31	53	93	97	49	71
Juvenile chronic arthritis[b]	24	2	0	0	0	0	—
Ankylosing spondylitis[c]	1	4	5	3	1	0	3
Gout[d]	0	0	40	120	170	250	70
SLE[e]	3	4	7	13	5	3	6
Scleroderma[f]	—	—	—	—	—	—	1.6
OA[g]	0	130	490	2500	4500	5000	—
Back pain[h]	NK	3900	6000	6800	5300	5000	—
Soft tissue rheumatism[i]	160	2200	4030	5220	4290	3350	3950
Osteoporosis[j]:							
Hip fracture	0	3	5	76	216	1935	—
Fractured vertebra	0	1	12	218	549	1081	—

a Data from the Norfolk Arthritis Register, UK[15]. All cases of inflammatory polyarthritis of >4 weeks' duration that present to primary care are notified to the register which covers a population of around 500,000. About half the cases satisfy the 1987 American Rheumatism Association criteria for RA at presentation.
b Data from Helsinki, Finland[16]. These figures are based on children who satisfied the ARA criteria for juvenile chronic arthritis, 37% of whom were male.
c Data from the Mayo Clinic, USA, over a 50-year period.
d Third RCGP Morbidity Survey[17].
e Cases ascertained from multiple sources (predominantly hospital-based) in Nottingham, UK (1988–1989)[18].
f Scleroderma is a rare disease and no studies have been large enough to provide reliable age- and sex-specific data. Data from the Mayo Clinic, USA[19].
g Third RCGP Morbidity Survey[17]; data include OA of all sites.
h Third RCGP Morbidity Survey[17].
i Third RCGP Morbidity Survey[17]; data include shoulder pain, bursitis, tendinitis, tenosynovitis and other nonarticular rheumatism.
j Hospital admissions in the Trent region, UK (1989–1990), for fractured neck of femur[20]; data for fractured vertebrae are from the Mayo Clinic, USA (1950–1982)[21].

Fig. 4.10 Incident cases per 100,000 females (musculoskeletal diseases template).

PREVALENT CASES PER 100,000 MALES (MUSCULOSKELETAL DISEASES TEMPLATE)

Condition	0–14 years	15–24 years	25–44 years	45–64 years	65–74 years	75+ years	All ages
RA[a]	0	100	200	1100	2000	2500	—
JCA[b]	15	6	5	4	3	3	—
Ankylosing spondylitis[c]	—	90	207	720	97	142	197
Gout[d]	0	170	170	1060	1220	1220	610
SLE[e]	0	13	13	10	8	8	12
Scleroderma[f]	0	0	1	3	3	2	—
OA[g]	0	270	500	2890	5750	7000	—
Back pain[h]	—	4900	8400	6700	6100	6100	7500
Soft tissue rheumatism[i]	125	450	820	1207	1092	730	885
Osteoporosis[j]	—	—	—	—	—	—	No data
Disablement	—	—	—	—	—	—	5120

a Data from the Mayo Clinic, USA,1974, based on attendance in primary and secondary care[5].
b Figures frim the Mayo Clinic, USA, 1990, based on cases of active disease[22]. It has been assumed that two thirds of cases remit by adult life and that 2% die per annum thereafter.
c Mayo Clinic, USA[6].
d Figures from a study based on attendance at primary care in the UK[23].
e Southern Sweden, 1982[24].
f Cases ascertained from multiple sources (predominantly hospital-based) in the West Midlands region, UK[25].
g Third RCGP Morbidity Survey[17].
h Third RCGP Morbidity Survey[17].
i Third RCGP Morbidity Survey[17] The survey provides information on new episodes of soft tissue problems in 1 year. For the template it has been assumed that each episode lasts 3 months.
j Data from the Mayo Clinic, USA, based on noninvasive bone density measurement at the spine, neck of femur and distal radius[21].

Fig. 4.11 Prevalent cases per 100,000 males (musculoskeletal diseases template).

of musculoskeletal health in a single survey. Therefore a picture of the community's burden of illness has to be built up piecemeal using all available sources of data, including published incidence and prevalence data, allowing for modifiers such as socioeconomic group, ethnicity and cultural factors, which may affect the applicability of external data.

The templates shown in Figures 4.9–4.12 give estimates of the incidence and prevalence of the principal rheumatic disorders for white Caucasian populations. Each sex is shown separately and the age format is based on the life cycle framework proposed by Pickin and St Leger[14]. The framework is based on the fact that each stage of life is associated with particular risks of ill health and particular opportunities for health promotion. Because there are relatively few data on the epidemiology of rheumatic disease in childhood, the first four stages of the life cycle – late pregnancy to 1 week after birth, 1 week to 1 year, 1–4 years, and 5–14 years – have been combined.

Wherever possible the sources of the estimates have been based at primary care level. This template therefore represents health care demands rather than health care needs. The main conditions for which there is likely to be a discrepancy between need and demand are OA and osteoporosis. A similar exercise was conducted by the National Arthritis Data Workgroup, whose remit was to estimate the number of prevalent cases of the various rheumatic diseases in the USA using national data[26]. Figures 4.9–4.12 present the data from published studies from North America and Europe, with some rounding, smoothing and adjustment of age groupings in a format that can be applied to a population with a known age and sex structure in order to estimate roughly the number of incident and prevalent cases that will present to primary care.

The next stage in health care planning is an evaluation of available interventions (see Chapter 1.2). One approach, being adopted by the musculoskeletal group of the international Cochrane Collaboration, is to conduct systematic reviews of the efficacy and effectiveness of various interventions for rheumatic diseases. The final, and most difficult, step is deciding what proportion of sufferers could or should benefit from an effective intervention considering comorbidity, cost, ability to improve and many other factors. In the absence of data some countries have attempted empirically to estimate the proportion of sufferers who should be referred to hospital or remain under specialist care[27] (see Chapter 3.2).

DETERMINING ATTRIBUTABLE RISK AND POPULATION ATTRIBUTABLE RISK FRACTION

The size of the relative risk indicates the strength of association between an exposure and outcome, but it does not indicate the relative importance of the exposure in accounting, for example, for the prevalence of the disease in the population. Patients with Sjögren's syndrome have a relative risk of 44 of developing non-Hodgkin's lymphoma (NHL) compared with the general population[28]. However, NHL is a rare disease in the general population, and even when the incidence is increased 44-fold the actual occurrence is still uncommon. Thus, despite this high relative risk few patients with Sjögren's syndrome develop NHL.

From a public health perspective two other measures are more important. The attributable risk, which is the difference between the

PREVALENT CASES PER 100,000 FEMALES (MUSCULOSKELETAL DISEASES TEMPLATE)							
Condition	0–14 years	15–24 years	25–44 years	45–64 years	65–74 years	75+ years	All ages
RA[(a)]	3	200	625	2025	3750	4700	—
JCA[(b)]	100	43	35	29	23	19	—
Ankylosing spondylitis[(c)]	—	35	125	165	55	65	73
Gout[(d)]	0	10	10	300	130	—	100
SLE[(e)]	3	59	99	99	38	38	65
Scleroderma[(f)]	0	1	1	9	5	5	—
OA[(g)]	0	250	750	4750	10,520	13,400	—
Back pain[(h)]	NA	4400	7500	9000	7500	7000	7200
Soft tissue rheumatism[(i)]	135	550	1008	1305	1073	838	988
Osteoporosis[(j)]	—	—	420	21,210	47,500	75,000	—
Disablement	—	—	—	—	—	—	10,870

(a) Data from the Mayo Clinic, USA,1974, based on attendance in primary and secondary care[5].

(b) Figures frim the Mayo Clinic, USA, 1990, based on cases of active disease[22]. It has been assumed that two thirds of cases remit by adult life and that 2% die per annum thereafter.

(c) Mayo Clinic, USA.

(d) Figures from a study based on attendance at primary care in the UK[23].

(e) Southern Sweden, 1982[24].

(f) Cases ascertained from multiple sources (predominantly hospital-based) in the West Midlands region, UK[25].

(g) Third RCGP Morbidity Survey[17].

(h) Third RCGP Morbidity Survey[17].

(i) Third RCGP Morbidity Survey[17]. The survey provides information on new episodes of soft tissue problems in 1 year. For the template it has been assumed that each episode lasts 3 months.

(j) Data from the Mayo Clinic, USA, based on noninvasive bone density measurement at the spine, neck of femur and distal radius[21].

Fig. 4.12 Prevalent cases per 100,000 females (musculoskeletal diseases template).

SOME ETIOLOGIC, PROTECTIVE AND PROGNOSTIC FACTORS IN RHEUMATOLOGY			
	Etiologic	Protective	Risk factors for poor prognosis
RA	Nulliparity Breast feeding Female gender	Oral contraceptive use	HLA-DR4 Rheumatoid factor
Ankylosing spondylitis	HLA-B27 Male gender		
Gout	Hyperuricemia Obesity Hypertension Lead exposure		
SLE	Complement deficiency Some drugs, e.g. hydralazine Female gender		Lower socio-economic status
Scleroderma	Silica Organic solvents Some drugs, e.g. bleomycin Female gender		
OA knee	Obesity Certain occupations, e.g. mining		Obesity
OA hip	Acetabular dysplasia Certain occupations, e.g. farming	?Squatting	
Back pain	Obesity Certain occupations Driving		Previous back pain Psychological factors
Osteoporosis	Early menopause Low body mass index Corticosteroid use	Obesity African Thiazide diuretics Exercise	Falls

Fig. 4.13 A summary of some of the etiologic, protective and prognostic factors in rheumatology.

risk of the outcome in the exposed and in the unexposed, gives an estimate of the number of cases among an exposed population that can be attributed to the exposure. The population attributable risk fraction is the proportion of the disease in the population which can be attributed to the risk factor. An example is found in the association between nonsteroidal anti-inflammatory drug (NSAID) ingestion and gastrointestinal (GI) bleeding and ulceration. Individuals taking NSAIDs have a relative risk of 2.25 of having a GI bleed compared to those not taking NSAIDs[29], that is, they are 2.25 times more likely to have a GI bleed than the general population. However, GI bleeds do occur in those not taking NSAIDs and some of the observed bleeds in NSAID users would have occurred by chance. It is estimated that NSAIDs have an attributable risk of 13/1000 per year for admission to hospital with a GI problem in patients with RA[30]. That is, for every 1000 RA patients who take an NSAID for a year, 13 more will be admitted to hospital each year for a GI problem than in a comparable group of RA patients not taking NSAIDs. It is also estimated that NSAIDs are responsible for 60% of all ulcer-related deaths[31].

A summary of some of the etiologic, protective and prognostic factors for selected rheumatic diseases is shown in Figure 4.13. Some of these factors are more definitive than others, and further study is required.

REFERENCES

1. Hennekens CH, Buring JE. Measures of disease frequency and association. In: Mayrent SL, ed. Epidemiology in medicine. Boston: Little, Brown; 1987:54–98.
2. Silman AJ. Epidemiologic studies: a practical guide. Cambridge: Cambridge University Press; 1995:16–25.
3. Safavi KH, Heyse SP, Hochberg MC. Estimating the incidence and prevalence of rare rheumatologic diseases: a review of methodology and available data sources. J Rheumatol. 1990;17:990–3.
4. Tan E, Cohen A, Fries J, *et al.* The 1982 revised criteria for the classification of systemic lupus erythematosus. Arthritis Rheum. 1982;25:1271–7.
5. Linos A, Worthington JW, O'Fallon WM, Kurland LT. The epidemiology of rheumatoid arthritis in Rochester, Minnesota: a study of the incidence, prevalence and mortality. Am J Epidemiol. 1980;111:97–8.
6. Carbone LD, Cooper C, Michet CJ, *et al.* Ankylosing spondylitis in Rochester, Minnesota 1935–89. Arthritis Rheum. 1992;35:1476–82.
7. Symmons DPM. Lupus around the world. Frequency of lupus in people of African origin. Lupus. 1995;4:176–8.
8. Croft P, Coggon D, Cruddas M, Cooper C. Osteoarthritis of the hip; an occupational disease in farmers. Br Med J. 1992;304:1269–72.
9. Mason V. The prevalence of back pain in Great Britain. London: Her Majesty's Stationery Office; 1994.
10. Silman AJ, Hochberg MC. Rheumatoid arthritis. In: Epidemiology of the rheumatic diseases.

Oxford: Oxford University Press; 1993:7–68.
11. Steere AC, Malwista SE, Snydman DR, Shope RE, Andiman WA. An epidemic of oligoarticular arthritis in children and adults in three Connecticut counties. Arthritis Rheum. 1977;20:7–37.
12. Spector TD, Hochberg MC. The protective effect of the oral contraceptive pill on rheumatoid arthritis. Clin Epidemiol. 1990;43:1221–30.
13. Frankel S. Health needs, health-care requirements, and the myth of infinite demand. Lancet. 1991;337:1588–90.
14. Pickin C, St Leger S. Assessing health needs using the life cycle framework. Buckingham: Open University Press; 1993.
15. Symmons DPM, Barrett EM, Bankhead C, *et al.* The incidence of rheumatoid arthritis in the United Kingdom: Results from the Norfolk Arthritis Register. Br J Rheumatol. 1994;33:735–9.
16. Kunnamo I, Kallio P, Pelkonen P. Incidence of arthritis in urban Finnish children: a prospective study. Arthritis Rheum. 1986;29:1232–8.
17. Royal College of General Practitioners, OPCS, Department of Health and Social Security. Morbidity statistics from general practice. 3rd National Morbidity Survey 1981–2. London: Her Majesty's Stationery Office; 1988.
18. Hopkinson ND, Doherty M, Powell RJ. The prevalence and incidence of systemic lupus erythematosus in Nottingham, UK, 1989–1990. Br J Rheumatol. 1993;32:110–15.
19. Michet CJ, McKenna CH, Elveback LR, Kaslow RA, Kurland LT. Epidemiology of systemic lupus erythematosus and other connective tissue diseases in Rochester, Minnesota, 1950 through 1979. Mayo Clin Proc. 1985;60:105–13.
20. Kanis JA. The incidence of hip fracture in Europe. Osteoporos Int. 1993;3(Suppl 1):10–15.
21. Melton LJ, Chrischilles EA, Cooper C, Lane AW, Riggs BL. How many women have osteoporosis? J Bone Miner Res. 1992;7:1005–10.
22. Towner SR, Michet CJ, O'Fallon WM, Nelson AM. The epidemiology of juvenile arthritis in Rochester, Minnesota 1960–1979. Arthritis Rheum. 1983;26:1208–13.
23. Currie WJC. Prevalence and incidence of the diagnosis of gout in Great Britain. Ann Rheum Dis. 1979;38:101–6.
24. Nived O, Sturfelt G, Wollheim F. Systemic lupus erythematosus in an adult population in southern Sweden – incidence, prevalence and validity of ARA revised classification criteria. Br J Rheumatol. 1985;24:147–54.
25. Silman A, Jannini S, Symmons D, Bacon P. An epidemiological study of scleroderma in the West Midlands. Br J Rheumatol. 1988;27:286–90.
26. Lawrence RC, Hochberg MC, Kelsey JL, *et al.* Estimates of the prevalence of selected arthritic and musculoskeletal diseases in the United States. J Rheumatol. 1989;16:427–41.
27. Marder WD, Meenan RF, Felson DT, *et al.* The present and future adequacy of rheumatology manpower. Arthritis Rheum. 1991;34:1209–17.
28. Kassan SS, Thomas TL, Moutsopoulos HM, *et al.* Increased risk of of lymphoma in sicca syndrome. Ann Intern Med. 1978;89:888–92.
29. Bloom BS. Risk and cost of gastrointestinal side-effects associated with non-steroidal anti-inflammatory drugs. Arch Intern Med. 1989;149:1019–22.
30. Fries J. NSAID gastropathy: the second most deadly rheumatic disease? Epidemiology and risk appraisal. J Rheumatol. 1991;18(suppl 28):6–10.
31. Zeidler H. Epidemiology of NSAID induced gastropathy. J Rheumatol. 1991;18(suppl 28):2–5.

5

THE ECONOMIC AND FUNCTIONAL IMPACT OF RHEUMATIC DISEASE IN THE US

Edward H Yelin

- The cost of musculoskeletal conditions may be as high as 2.5% of the US gross national product.
- In the US, musculoskeletal conditions account for 315 million physician visits, 8.26 million hospital admissions and more than 1.5 billion restricted activity days each year.
- About half the absolute cost of musculoskeletal conditions is due to medical care and the rest is due to the indirect costs of lost wages.
- Most of the increment in costs for people who have musculoskeletal conditions, relative to costs for those who don't, is due to indirect costs.
- About 40% of people with musculoskeletal conditions report some form of disability.
- The average total annual cost of RA and SLE for an individual patient is about 80% of US per capita income.

INTRODUCTION

Studies of the economic and social burden of the rheumatic diseases provide prognostic information for individuals about their ability to function and the extent to which family income will be affected. They also provide an indication of the impact of the condition on the nation's economy.

Most studies of the economic and social burdens of individual conditions have been conducted on patients sampled in clinical environments (usually the practices of rheumatologists), most concern rheumatoid arthritis (RA), and, until very recently, most have been conducted in North America. In contrast, most studies of the economic impact of rheumatic diseases on the population as a whole have been conducted on national, community-based samples, with the information collected by self-report in a survey format[1–3]. Indeed, in the latter, because diagnoses are self-reported, costs are usually presented for the overall category 'musculoskeletal conditions' rather than for specific rheumatic diseases. The clinical samples offer greater diagnostic precision and greater specificity with respect to the impact of the conditions studied, ensuring that the information relevant to the condition in question is collected and that all those included in the studies actually have the condition; the community-based samples ensure that the information is more representative.

The costs of illness typically are divided into those due to direct expenditures for medical care services and those due to the indirect impact of illness on function. Usually costs are defined in economic terms by the wages lost from reduced employment, but sometimes they are defined as the amount an individual is willing to pay to avoid losses in all kinds of activities[4–5].

In studies using either clinical or community-based samples, the proportion of total costs of rheumatic conditions attributed to indirect costs is relatively higher than in most other chronic conditions[1]. The high proportion of indirect costs reflects the great impact of musculoskeletal conditions on function, but also the relatively low cost of most medical interventions for these conditions. Thus, even though some individuals experience very high medical costs, especially for procedures such as total joint replacement, for the vast majority the medical interventions involve only ambulatory care, physical modalities and drugs.

Because the most detailed studies of the economic and functional impact of musculoskeletal conditions have been done in the US, this chapter concentrates on the results of US studies rather than international data.

NATIONAL ECONOMIC IMPACT OF MUSCULOSKELETAL CONDITIONS

In the US, there have been four systematic studies of the costs of major diagnostic condition groups since the early 1960s. Figure 5.1 summarizes the results of these studies for musculoskeletal conditions. In the studies conducted in 1963, 1972 and 1980, the total costs of musculoskeletal conditions were just under 1% of gross national product (GNP)[4,6–8]. Using the National Bureau of Economic Research definition of a recession as three consecutive quarters of a year in which GNP declines by 1% or more, musculoskeletal conditions may be said to have had an impact on the national economy roughly equivalent to a permanent recession.

In 1963 and 1972, direct medical care costs attributed to musculoskeletal conditions accounted for about half the total costs of these conditions. In 1980, however, the medical care portion exceeded the indirect costs by a wide margin. This reflects the high rate of inflation in medical care costs that occurred in the US during the 1970s and the stagnant wages among the working population.

In the most recent nationwide US study of the costs of illness conducted in 1988, the total costs of musculoskeletal conditions consumed the equivalent of 2.5% of GNP, with roughly equal portions attributed to direct medical care costs and indirect costs due to wage losses. The 1988 study reported that total costs of musculoskeletal conditions were three times as great as in 1980. The National Arthritis Data Work Group in the US concluded that about half the increase was due to improvement in the ability to document the costs of illness and the remainder was due to the increased prevalence of musculoskeletal conditions in an aging population[2]. The 1988 estimate for the US is consistent with an estimate that the total costs of musculoskeletal conditions in Canada represented 2.0% of GNP in 1986[3]. Thus, overall, musculoskeletal conditions would appear to have an impact equivalent to a severe permanent recession, not just a mild one.

COSTS OF MUSCULOSKELETAL CONDITIONS AS PERCENTAGE OF US GNP

Year	Direct costs (%)	Indirect costs (%)	Total costs (%)
1963	0.3	0.3	0.7
1972	0.3	0.4	0.7
1980	0.5	0.3	0.8
1988	1.2	1.3	2.5

Fig. 5.1 Costs of musculoskeletal conditions as a percentage of US GNP in 1963, 1972, 1980 and 1988. With permission from Yelin and Callahan[2].

HEALTH CARE USE BY 41.18 MILLION PERSONS WITH MUSCULOSKELETAL CONDITIONS			
Type of health care	Total (million)	Mean per person	% with ≥1 visit/admission
Physician visits	315.22	7.69	90.8
Hospital admissions	8.26	0.20	16.8
Hospital days	60.30	1.46	
Length of stay days		6.88	

Fig. 5.2 Health care use by 41.18 million persons with musculoskeletal conditions over a 1-year period (US, 1990–1992). Adapted from Yelin and Callahan[2].

NATIONAL ECONOMIC IMPACT OF ALL FORMS OF ARTHRITIS

The US studies summarized in Figure 5.1 present results for the absolute costs of the conditions; that is, all the costs incurred by those who have the conditions, without comparison with the costs incurred by similar people who do not have the conditions. For RA and all forms of arthritis, 55 and 51% of total costs, respectively, are attributable to direct costs of medical care (Fig. 5.2)[9,10]. However, when evaluating the incremental costs of RA and all forms of arthritis, indirect costs constitute a much larger part of the total: 80% in the former and 64% in the latter. Thus, as expensive as the medical care for these conditions may appear to be, indirect costs due to wage losses account for most of the increment in costs, an indication that the unique feature of musculoskeletal conditions is their impact on functioning, particularly on functioning in employment.

NATIONAL ESTIMATES OF MEDICAL CARE USE

Using the data from the 1990–1992 National Health Interview Survey (HIS), the National Arthritis Data Work Group[2] calculated the amount of health care attributable to musculoskeletal conditions; the results are summarized in Figure 5.2. All told, 41.18 million individuals reported having one or more musculoskeletal conditions and made in excess of 315 million physician visits each year, or just under 8 per person. Most of these visits were probably attributable to their musculoskeletal condition[11]. In addition, about 90% of these individuals reported making at least one physician visit a year.

In a smaller scale study focusing on access to care among individuals with musculoskeletal conditions in one California county, close to 90% of those with one or more of these conditions reported ever having seen a physician for the condition and just under 60% had seen one in the year prior to study[12]. Comparable figures were reported in a study in Yorkshire, in the UK[13]. People with musculoskeletal conditions also use hospital-based care with great frequency. Among the HIS respondents with musculoskeletal conditions, more than 16% reported one or more hospital admissions; the total number of admissions for these conditions was in excess of 8 million.

IMPACT ON ACUTE AND CHRONIC DISABILITY

Musculoskeletal conditions have a major impact on the population in terms of acute disability, defined as the number of days with restricted activity, days spent in bed and days lost to work. Among the 41.18 million individuals with musculoskeletal conditions, 10.87 million (26.4%) reported one or more restricted activity days (Fig. 5.3). However, those with one or more such days actually averaged more than 38 days each year, or more than a month. These individuals experienced in excess of 1.5 billion restricted activity days a year. Work loss days were far less common, averaging 3.53 per person; nevertheless, in excess of 145 million days were lost to work among this group. This number is relatively low because so many individuals with musculoskeletal conditions completely stop working (see Prevalence of Work Disability, below) and thus do not respond to the question in the HIS about work loss days. Verbrugge and Patrick compared major chronic conditions for prevalence, disability (defined as activity limitation in their study) and medical care contact for six strata defined by gender and age[14]. They reported that arthritis was the most common cause of disability in four of the six strata.

Musculoskeletal conditions are an important cause of long-term disability, defined in the HIS by the ability to perform the major activities appropriate to one's age for example, among those aged 18–69 years, the ability to work; or, for those over 70 years, the ability to perform personal care activities. Among all 41.18 million reporting a musculoskeletal condition, 5.65 million (13.7%) state that they are unable to

CHRONIC AND ACUTE DISABILITY AMONG 41.18 MILLION PEOPLE WITH MUSCULOSKELETAL CONDITIONS				
Type of disability	Number (million)	% of total	No. per person	Total days (millions)
Chronic				
Activity limitation: general				
Unable to do major activity	5.65	13.7		
Limited in amount/type of major activity	6.12	14.9		
Limited in non-major activities	5.55	13.5		
Not limited	23.86	57.9		
Activity limitation: specific to work				
Unable to do major work activity	5.48	18.4		
Limited in amount/type of major work activity	3.56	12.0		
Limited in non-major work activities	2.75	9.2		
Not limited	17.99	60.4		
Activity limitation: personal care activities				
Unable to perform personal care needs	0.79	4.8		
Limited in other routine needs	1.56	9.4		
Not limited	14.16	85.6		
Acute				
Restricted activity (days)	10.87	26.4	38.21	1574
Bed days	22.85	55.5	15.92	649
Work days lost	1.73	4.2	3.53	145

Fig. 5.3 Chronic and acute disability among 41.18 million persons with musculoskeletal conditions over a 1-year period (US, 1990–1992). Adapted from Yelin and Callahan[2].

WORK DISABILITY RATES ASSESSED IN COMMUNITY STUDIES	
Study group	Work disability rate (%)
Arthritis symptoms, arthritis diagnosis	54
Arthritis symptoms, no diagnosis	36
Arthritis diagnosis, no symptoms	44
RA defined by symptoms and diagnosis	72
OA defined by symptoms and diagnosis	53

Fig. 5.4 Work disability rate among people with musculoskeletal conditions sampled in community environments. Adapted from Pincus, Mitchell and Burkhauser[19].

ESTIMATES OF THE ABSOLUTE NATIONAL COSTS OF RA AND ALL FORMS OF ARTHRITIS IN 1994 (US$)

	Direct costs							Indirect costs			Grand total
	Physician visits			Hospital admissions			Total				
Disease entity	Number (million)	Unit price	Total	Number (million)	Unit price	Total		Number (million)	Unit price	Total	
RA	19.65	$75	$1.47 bn (0.02% GNP)	0.54	$6136	$3.29 bn (0.05% GNP)	$4.76 bn (0.07% GNP) (55%)	1.05	$24,076	$3.98 bn (0.06% GNP) (46%)	$8.74 bn (0.13% GNP)
Arthritis, all forms	226.3	$75	$16.97 bn (0.3% GNP)	6.90	$6136	$42.33 bn (0.6% GNP)	$59.30 bn (0.9% GNP) (51%)	2.34	$24,076	$56.34 bn (0.8% GNP) (49%)	$115.64 bn (1.7% GNP)

Fig. 5.5 Estimates of the absolute national costs of RA and all forms of arthritis in 1994 (US$). Adapted from Pincus *et al.*[19] and Jonsson *et al.*[23]

do their major activity, 6.12 million (14.9%) that they are limited in the amount or type of their major activity and 5.55 million (13.5%) that they are limited in activities other than their major one (Fig. 5.3). All told, more than 42% are limited in some way in their activities. Similarly, about 40% of those of working age report limitation specific to working, with 18.4% stating that they are unable to work at all and another 12.0% stating that they are limited in the amount or kind of work they can do. Despite the relative frequency of disability in musculoskeletal conditions, inability to care for oneself is relatively rare, with 0.79 million individuals stating they are unable to perform their personal care needs and another 1.56 million stating they are limited in the amount or particular type of personal care activities.

In a recent Canadian survey, people with musculoskeletal conditions also reported high rates of disability. Almost 90% of Canadians with self-reported arthritis had some trouble with mobility and almost 70% were physically dependent. The overall prevalence rate of activity limitation associated with musculoskeletal conditions would appear to be relatively similar among nations where comparable data exist, affecting between 3 and 8% of the entire adult population[15–17]. All economically advanced nations face a pandemic of musculoskeletal-related disability in the years to come, however, due to the rapid aging of the population[15].

PREVALENCE OF WORK DISABILITY

Musculoskeletal conditions are among the most common causes of work disability because of their overall prevalence and their severity. In the US, the number of persons making claims on Social Security Disability Insurance (the public program of disability compensation) as a result of musculoskeletal conditions is increasing rapidly, suggesting that this serious problem may be worsening with the passage of time[18].

Unfortunately, few studies of the prevalence of work disability use community-based samples of the population. In the most systematic study (Fig. 5.4), out of all respondents who had symptoms consistent with any form of arthritis and a diagnosis of an arthritic condition, 54% ceased work[19]. Among those with symptoms of arthritis, but no specific diagnosis, the work disability rate was 36%. People who reported symptoms consistent with RA and had an RA diagnosis experienced the highest work disability rate (72%); among those who had symptoms of osteoarthritis (OA) and had an OA diagnosis, the work disability rate was 53%. Clearly, work loss from musculoskeletal conditions is a major problem.

THE ECONOMIC BURDEN OF SPECIFIC RHEUMATIC DISORDERS

Several detailed studies on the economic costs of RA were conducted between 1976 and 1984[1]. Despite different methods, and sampling in different kinds of clinical settings, the results of the studies were consistent (Fig. 5.5). Direct medical care costs were substantial, averaging (for each patient) the equivalent of 20% of US per capita income[20]. Indirect costs were far larger, constituting between two thirds and three fourths of the total cost of RA. Stated in relative terms, indirect costs were equivalent to 60% of US per capita income and 45% of the median salary and wages of all US full-time workers[20].

Over time, the relatively high medical care costs experienced by individuals with RA continue (Fig. 5.6), with total medical care costs still averaging the equivalent of about 20% of US per capita income[9,21–23]. However, this average masks tremendous variability. Persons in the tenth percentile incurred medical care costs of about $300 a year, or the equivalent of less than 2% of US per capita income. However, the 90th percentile incurred costs more than 40% higher than per capita income, and the 99th percentile incurred costs almost four

ESTIMATES OF THE INCREMENTAL NATIONAL COSTS OF RA AND ALL FORMS OF ARTHRITIS IN 1994 (US$)

	Direct costs							Indirect costs			Grand total
	Physician visits			Hospital admissions			Total				
Disease entity	Incremental number	Unit price	Total	Incremental number	Unit price	Total		Incremental number	Unit price	Total	
RA	1.07	$75	$0.14 bn (0.002% GNP)	0.45	$6136	$0.48 bn (0.007% GNP)	$0.62 bn (0.009% GNP) (20%)	0.102	$24,076	$2.45 bn (0.036% GNP) (80%)	$3.07 bn (0.045% GNP)
Arthritis, all forms	0.98	$75	$2.28 bn (0.03% GNP)	0.06	$6136	$11.41 bn (0.17% GNP)	$13.69 bn (0.20% GNP) (36%)	1.000	$24,076	$24.08 bn (0.36% GNP) (64%)	$37.77 bn (0.56% GNP)

Fig. 5.6 Estimates of the incremental national costs of RA and all forms of arthritis in 1994 (US$). Adapted from Thompson *et al.*[5] and Jonsson *et al.*[23]

times as large as per capita income. The latter two groups typically had surgical admissions and were using multiple disease-modifying agents during the year. When hospital admissions did not occur and when only one such agent was reported, costs were about $2000 a year, or less than 10% of per capita income.

The high indirect costs of RA are a function of the prevalence of work disability, with the rate varying from a low of 34% in one study to a high of 59% in another[1]. One study reported on the duration of time from onset of the condition until work disability occurred: of persons with RA, 10% stopped working in the first year after onset, about half had stopped working in the first decade, and close to 90% left work prior to the normal age of retirement[24]. However, the impact of RA on functioning extends far beyond work to encompass all domains of activity. Compared with people of the same age and gender, those with RA experienced a significant reduction in the number of household chores, shopping and errands, social relationships, leisure and recreation pursuits, public service and voluntary activities, and in the ways they could move around the community[1]. In addition to the impact of RA on function, psychologic disturbance, especially depression, is frequently associated with RA[2].

With respect to OA, direct medical care costs averaged $1884 (US) in 1994 terms in the three studies which assessed this parameter, or about 9% of US per capita income (versus 20% among persons with RA)[1,2]. Indirect costs have been assessed in only one study and amounted to $10,705 (US) in 1994 terms, or roughly half the US per capita income and a third of the median salary and wages of full-time workers (versus 60 and 45%, respectively, among persons with RA)[1].

In every domain, people with OA reported more activity losses than did matched controls without OA, though the difference between their activity mix and that of the controls was smaller than the difference between that of controls and people with RA[1].

The economic impact of systemic lupus erythematosus (SLE) has only recently been studied[25]. Using a sample from a Canadian tertiary care clinic, it was shown that 54% of the total costs of SLE were due to the indirect costs of lost wages. Overall, the total cost of SLE averaged $13,094 (Canadian) in 1990, which is equivalent to 80% of per capita income in Canada for that year[20]. The one published study of the economics of juvenile chronic arthritis (JCA) was conducted among a panel of patients attending a hospital clinic[26] and indicated that total costs amounted to about 40% of per capita income in the US for that year[20]. However, because children do not incur wage losses, almost all the costs of JCA were due to direct medical expenditure.

CONCLUSIONS

In the US, the cost of all forms of musculoskeletal disease is about 2.5% of GNP, with much of the increment in costs relative to other conditions being due to lost wages and reduced functional capacity. Studies of RA indicate that medical care costs of this condition may average as much as 20 and indirect costs as much as 60% of per capita income. Average costs of SLE may be comparable to those of RA; average costs of OA and JCA would appear to be lower, in the former because of lesser severity, and in the latter because children do not incur lost wages.

REFERENCES

1. Felts W, Yelin E. The economic impact of the rheumatic diseases in the United States. J Rheum. 1989;16:867–84.
2. Yelin E, Callahan L. The economic cost and social and psychological impact of musculoskeletal conditions. Arthritis Rheum. 1995;38:1351–62.
3. Badley E. The economic burden of musculoskeletal disorders in Canada is similar to that for cancer and may be higher. J Rheumatol. 1995;22:204–6.
4. Rice D. Estimating the cost of illness. Rockville, MD: National Center for Health Statistics Health Economics Series No. 6; 1966.
5. Thompson M, Read J, Liang M. Feasibility of willingness to pay measurements in chronic arthritis. Med Decis Making. 1984;4:195–212.
6. Cooper B, Rice D. The economic cost of illness revisited. Soc Secur Bull. 1979;39:21–35.
7. Rice D, Hodgson T, Kopstein A. The economic costs of illness: a replication and update. Health Care Fin Rev. 1985;7:61–80.
8. Rice D. Cost of musculoskeletal conditions. In: Praemer A, Furner S, Rice D, eds. Musculoskeletal conditions in the US. Chicago: American Academy of Orthopedic Surgeons; 1992.
9. Yelin E. The costs of rheumatoid arthritis: absolute, incremental, and marginal estimates. J Rheumatol. 1996;23(suppl. 44):47–51.
10. Yelin E. The economics of osteoarthritis. In: Brandt K, Lohmander S, Doherty M, eds. Osteoarthritis. Oxford: Oxford University Press; in press.
11. National Center for Health Statistics. The National Ambulatory Care Survey, U.S., 1975–1981 and 1985 Trends. Rockville, MD: National Center for Health Statistics Publication No. 88–1754; 1988.
12. Yelin E, Bernhard G, Pflugrad D. Access to medical care among persons with musculoskeletal conditions: a study using a random sample of households in San Mateo County, California. Arthritis Rheum. 1995;38:1128–33.
13. Badley E, Tennant A. Impact of disablement due to rheumatic disorders in a British population: estimates of severity and prevalence from the Calderdale Rheumatic Disablement Survey. Ann Rheum Dis. 1993;52:6–13.
14. Verbrugge L, Patrick D. Seven chronic conditions: their impact on U.S. adults' activity levels and use of medical services. Am J Public Health. 1995;85:173–82.
15. Badley E. The impact of disabling arthritis. Arth Care Res. 1995;8:221–8.
16. Centers for Disease Control and Prevention. Arthritis prevalence and activity limitations, United States, 1990. MMWR. 1994;43:433–8.
17. Reynolds D, Chambers L, Badley E, *et al.* Physical disability among Canadians reporting musculoskeletal diseases. J Rheum. 1992;19:1020–30.
18. Chirikos T. An analysis of compositional trends in Social Security Disability Awards, 1960–1991. J Dis Policy Stud. 1995;6:2–22.
19. Pincus T, Mitchell J, Burkhauser R. Substantial work disability and earnings losses in individuals less than 65 with osteoarthritis: comparisons with rheumatoid arthritis. J Clin Epidemiol. 1989;42:449–57.
20. US Bureau of the Census. Statistical abstract of the US, 1995. Washington, DC: USGPO; 1995:431, 461, 856.
21. Lambert C, Hurst N. Health economics as an aspect of health outcome: basic principles and application in rheumatoid arthritis. Br J Rheumatol. 1995;34:774–80.
22. Eberhardt K, Larsson B-M, Nived K. Early rheumatoid arthritis: some social, economical, and psychological aspects. Scand J Rheumatol. 1993;22:119–23.
23. Jonsson B, Rehnberg C, Borgquist L, Larsson S. Locomotion status and costs in destructive rheumatoid arthritis. Acta Orthop Scand. 1992;63:207–12.
24. Yelin E, Henke C, Epstein W. The work dynamics of the person with rheumatoid arthritis. Arthritis Rheum. 1987;30:507–12.
25. Clarke A, Esdaile J, Bloch D, *et al.* Canadian study of the total medical costs for patients with systemic lupus erythematosus and the predictors of costs. Arthritis Rheum. 1993;36:1548–59.
26. Allaire S, DeNardo B, Szer I, Meenan R, Schaller J. The economic impacts of juvenile rheumatoid arthritis. J Rheumatol. 1992;19:952–5.

6

GENETIC FACTORS IN RHEUMATIC DISEASE

Paul Creamer
& John Loughlin

- Genes code for proteins which are produced by a process of transcription, translation and post-translational modification.
- Mutations in genes result in production of abnormal proteins which may also be functionally deficient.
- Molecular biology techniques used to elucidate the genetic basis of connective tissue disorders include restriction fragment length polymorphisms, polymerase chain reaction, tandem repeat sequences, single-stranded conformational polymorphisms, heteroduplex analysis, *in situ* hybridization and cloning.

Rheumatic diseases and genetics

- Most rheumatic diseases have an element of genetic susceptibility in their etiology.
- The genetic component of many rheumatic diseases is by association with certain major histocompatibility complex (MHC) antigens.
- Collagen gene defects are the basis of osteogenesis imperfecta (type I collagen), type VII Ehlers–Danlos syndrome (type I collagen), premature osteoarthritis (OA) (type II collagen) and Marfan syndrome (fibrillin).
- Defects in processing enzymes are involved in many diseases and one of the best characterized is the HPRT gene defect that results in hyperuricemia (e.g. Lesch–Nyhan syndrome).
- Defects in genes for cytokines, hormones and their receptors may contribute to chronic rheumatic disease, for example vitamin D receptor polymorphisms in osteoporosis.

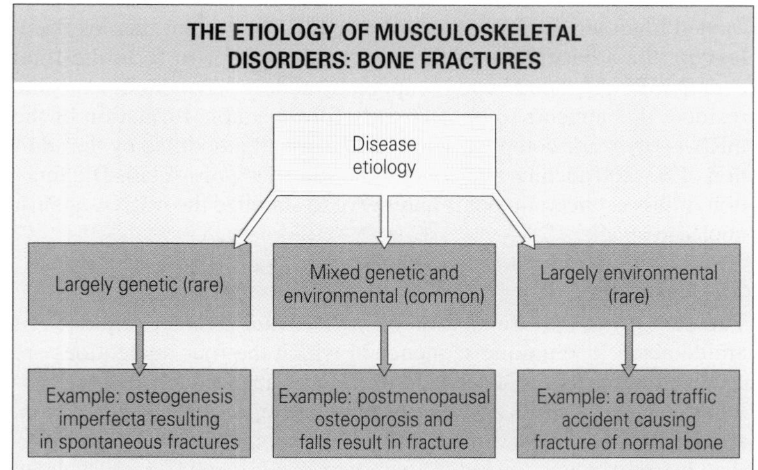

Fig. 6.1 The etiology of rheumatic diseases is usually a mixture of genetic and environmental factors. Bone fractures are an example.

INTRODUCTION

Rheumatic disease, like all diseases, may be purely genetic, purely environmental or, more commonly, a mixture of the two. Hip fracture, for example, is mostly genetic if it arises as a result of osteogenesis imperfecta and mostly environmental if it results from a car crash. The commonest type of hip fracture (osteoporotic fracture) is the result of a complex interaction between genetic and environmental influences (Fig. 6.1).

While for some conditions the genetic component is confined to a single gene ('monogenic') as, for example, in some cases of multiple epiphyseal dysplasia (MED) or the Lesch–Nyhan syndrome, the majority are multifactorial and polygenic. The use of modern molecular genetics to identify the genetic predisposition to such common conditions as OA and osteoporosis is one of the challenges facing rheumatology today.

The genetic component of many rheumatic diseases is by association with certain MHC antigens. This is covered in detail in Chapters 5.7, 6.12 and 7.3. For other conditions, the linkage is with non-MHC gene products including connective tissue matrix components and enzymes such as those involved in the metabolism of uric acid.

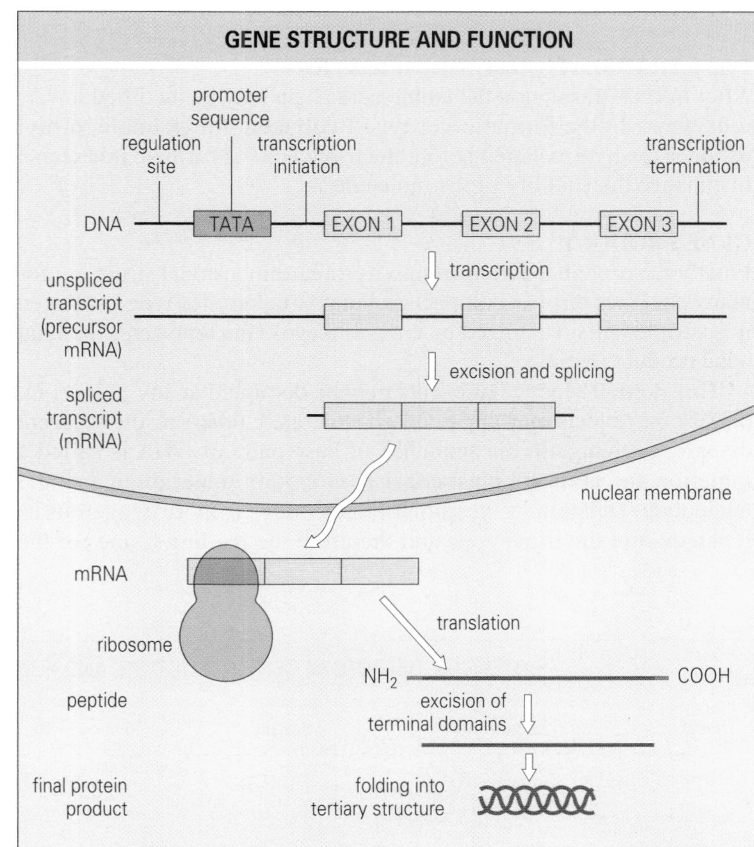

Fig. 6.2 Gene structure and function.

GENE STRUCTURE AND FUNCTION

The human genome contains all the information for the structure and function of the organism, though not all the genes are active at any one time. Genes consist of functional units of deoxyribonucleic acid (DNA) ('exons') separated by noncoding regions or 'introns' (Fig. 6.2). Genomic DNA exists primarily to specify the amino acid sequence of proteins. The DNA sequences that flank both ends of the gene have important regulatory functions. Genes are separated by large stretches of DNA with no obvious function, termed 'intergenic' DNA.

TRANSCRIPTION

DNA itself is not a template for protein synthesis; rather the information coded by DNA must first be transferred to messenger ribonucleic acid (mRNA). This process is known as 'transcription' and is controlled by promoter sequences located 30–40 base pairs upstream from the gene: an example of such a sequence is the consensus sequence TATAAAA, or 'TATA box'. Transcription begins with uncoiling of the tightly packed DNA molecule to allow RNA polymerase enzymes access to the relevant gene. The primary RNA transcript is an exact copy of the gene containing both introns and exons. Introns are first looped together – a process involving U1 RNA – and then excised, leaving the adjacent exons to be spliced together to form the final coding mRNA[1]. The 5′ end is capped by adding a 7-methylguanosine residue; this appears to be necessary for the stable formation of the mRNA–ribosome complex. The 3′ end is usually modified by the addition of 50–200 adenine nucleotides, the so-called poly-A tail. The function of this is uncertain but it may serve to stabilize the mRNA against nuclease attack.

TRANSLATION

The next process is translation of mRNA into a linear sequence of amino acids. The unique sequence in which the four nucleotides are arranged in nucleic acids encodes the amino acid sequence of the protein to be synthesized. A group of three nucleic acids forms a codon, specifying a particular amino acid. Uncommon amino acids are specified by only one codon but frequently occurring amino acids have up to six codons. This 'degeneracy' of the code may represent a built in fail-safe mechanism which allows correct amino acid synthesis even if one nucleotide in the codon is altered. Other codons specify 'start' or 'stop' protein synthesis. The chain is synthesized from N-terminal to C-terminal using the three nucleotide reading frame.

POST-TRANSLATIONAL MODIFICATION

After mRNA translation the amino acid chain may be modified in various ways. In the formation of type I collagen, for example, prolyl residues are hydroxylated before the triple helix is formed: this seems to enhance the stability of the molecule.

GENE PRODUCT

Finally the protein is arranged into its three-dimensional structure: for many enzymes this is a compact globular structure; for type I collagen it is a triple helix, stabilized by cross-linkage. This represents the final gene product.

This normal seqence of events may be disrupted at any point (Fig. 6.3). Some defects may apparently be tolerated; others result in severe disease. A change in the sequence of base pairs of DNA is called a mutation and at its simplest consists of a point mutation in a single nucleotide. Deletion or insertion of nucleotides is more dangerous as it can disrupt the triple code and therefore the reading frame for the whole gene. Translocation is a more drastic defect: whole chromosomal segments are moved from the original site to a new one either within the same chromosome or on a different one. Gene conversion is a special example in which a pair of homologous genes interact so that part of the nucleotide sequence of one is incorporated into the other. An example is the rearranging of genes coding for the T-cell receptor. This is important in generating diversity from a limited genetic repertoire.

Errors may occur at other points including transcription, splicing, translation and post-translational modification. It is of interest that many of the defined antigens to which autoantibodies are directed in rheumatic diseases such as systemic lupus erythematosus are structures that have vital roles in DNA replication and protein synthesis (see Chapter 7.5). The Scl-70 antigen, for example, is an enzyme (topoisomerase I) that unwinds the supercoiled DNA so that transcription can take place[2]. Both Sm and RNP are small ribonucleic proteins which play a part in removing introns from the primary RNA transcript and splicing exons to make mRNA[3]. Finally, Jo-1, an antibody found in myositis, represents aminoacyl-tRNA synthetase, an enzyme required for amino acid addition at the ribosome[4].

DETECTION METHODS

The development of methods to detect genes and their products has been fundamental to our current understanding of the genetic basis of connective tissue diseases. Of crucial importance to these techniques is the ability of DNA and RNA to 'hybridize'. If a solution of DNA is heated, the two strands separate giving rise to single-stranded or denatured DNA. If allowed to cool, the two strands come together again or 'hybridize' resulting in exactly the same double-stranded structure as the original. A radiolabeled strand of DNA will also hybridize to its exact complementary form and can be detected by autoradiography.

Because genetic material normally exists in very small quantities, the ability to amplify DNA sequences using plasmid or viral cloning vehicles has been essential. A 'complementary' or cDNA copy of mRNA is made using the enzyme reverse transcriptase and converted into double-stranded DNA by DNA polymerase. This fragment is then inserted into a cloning vehicle and the resulting chimeric molecule used to transform a bacterial cell (usually *Escherichia coli*). Reproduction of the *E coli* results in replication ('cloning') of the recombinant DNA molecule, producing multiple copies for analysis.

RESTRICTION ENZYMES AND BLOT TESTS

'Restriction enzymes (endonucleases)' (Fig. 6.4) are bacterial cell products which recognize particular DNA nucleotide sequences and cut the molecule at that point. Different enzymes recognize different sequences, usually 4–6 nucleotides long. Using these 'molecular scissors', a solution of native DNA isolated from millions of cells can

POTENTIAL DEFECTS IN GENE STRUCTURE AND FUNCTION

Defect	Example	Result	Gene	Disease
Missense mutation	TGC→TGT	Arg→Cys	*COL2A1*	Premature OA/dysplasia
Frameshift insertion or deletion	CCTTGA→CCTTTGA	Insertion of STOP	*HPRT*	HPRT Chicago (HPRT deficiency)
Major deletions	Deletion of exon 8	Loss of phe_{178}–asn_{203}	*HPRT*	HPRT Connersville (HPRT deficiency)
Splicing defects	Skipping of exon 6	Loss of N-propeptide cleavage site	*COL1A2*	Ehlers–Danlos type VII
Post-translational modification	Reduced galactosyl transferase activity	Reduced post-translational glycosylation of IgG		RA (increased agalactosyl IgG)

Fig. 6.3 Types of genetic abnormality which can cause rheumatic disease. (HPRT, hypoxanthine phoshorylribotransferase.)

Name	Source	Cutting site
BamH I	*Bacillus amyloliquefaciens*	5'↓ 3' G GATCC
EcoR I	*Escherichia coli* RY13	↓ G AATTC
Hae III	*Haemophilus aegyptius*	↓ GG CC
Taq I	*Thermus aquaticus*	↓ T CGA
Hind III	*Haemophilus influenzae*	↓ A AGCTT

Fig. 6.4 Some examples of restriction enzymes.

be cut so that the DNA from each cell is cleaved into an identical set of fragments. These fragments can be separated by agarose gel electrophoresis on the basis of size. The DNA is transferred and fixed to nitrocellulose paper and subsequently hybridized with a specific radiolabeled DNA probe (Southern blot tests)[5]. In this way, the gene can be mapped relative to enzyme cutting sites. Occasionally a gene mutation may inactivate a cutting site, resulting in the appearence of a single large fragment instead of two smaller fragments on gel electrophoresis (Fig. 6.5).

Identification of a gene does not neccessarily give information on its expression *in vivo*: for this reason it is sometimes more useful to look at the mRNA product. The same technique of hybridization using radiolabeled gene probes is used. Such 'Northern' blot tests differs fom Southern blot tests in that there is no need to denature the RNA (being naturally single stranded) and restriction enzymes are not required.

In order to establish the precise cellular expression of a gene, RNA probes may be hybridized directly to paraffin tissue sections, using a technique analagous to immunocytochemistry[6]. Such '*in situ* hybridization' permits *in vivo* mRNA expression studies and avoids the possibility of artefactual gene activation which may result from *in vitro* tissue culture techniques. Several mRNA species can be visualized simultaneously and, when combined with conventional phenotyping using monoclonal antibodies, the cells producing the mRNA can be positively identified.

RESTRICTION FRAGMENT LENGTH POLYMORPHISMS

The noncoding region of DNA is relatively unconserved: point mutations in the introns appear to be well tolerated and may become established. The intragenic regions of a pair of homologous genes are therefore more variable than the coding regions of the genes and may differ on average once every 100 or 200 nucleotide bases. On digestion by restriction enzymes, therefore, different sized fragments will result if these nucleotide changes affect restriction enzyme sites. These are termed restriction fragment length polymorphisms (RFLPs). An RFLP is therefore a change in the DNA sequence that either destroys or creates a restriction enzyme recognition site or alters the distance between two sites (Fig. 6.6). Such restriction patterns are allelic and the haplotype can be followed through generations of a specific family. The presence or absence of a restriction site is denoted + or – : thus an individual may be +/+, +/– or –/–. When the restriction site is close to the gene responsible for a dominant trait, the disease gene is linked to the restriction site and can be followed. Cosegregation of disease with a specific polymorphism haplotype thus provides strong evidence that the gene located near the restriction site is responsible for the disease. Though it cannot identify the exact mutation, RFLP analysis is a relatively simple way to establish (or refute) linkage of disease to a particular gene. To perform RFLP studies requires large families spanning at least

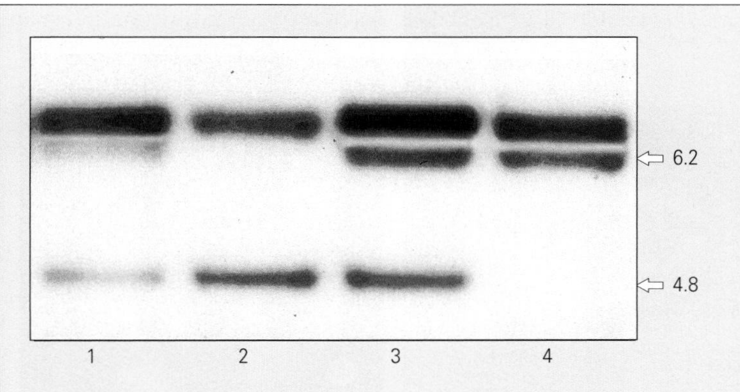

Fig. 6.5 An example of gel electrophoresis. This gel shows the restriction pattern obtained in four individuals. A RFLP exists, which, if present, cuts a 6.2kb fragment into 4.8kb and 1.4kb fragments (the 1.4kb fragment is too small to appear on the gel). Lanes 1 and 3 show subjects heterozygous for the RFLP (1/2). Lane 2 is homozygous for the presence of the site (1/1), while lane 4 is homozygous for its absence (2/2). An invariable band appears at about 7.0kb (unlabeled).

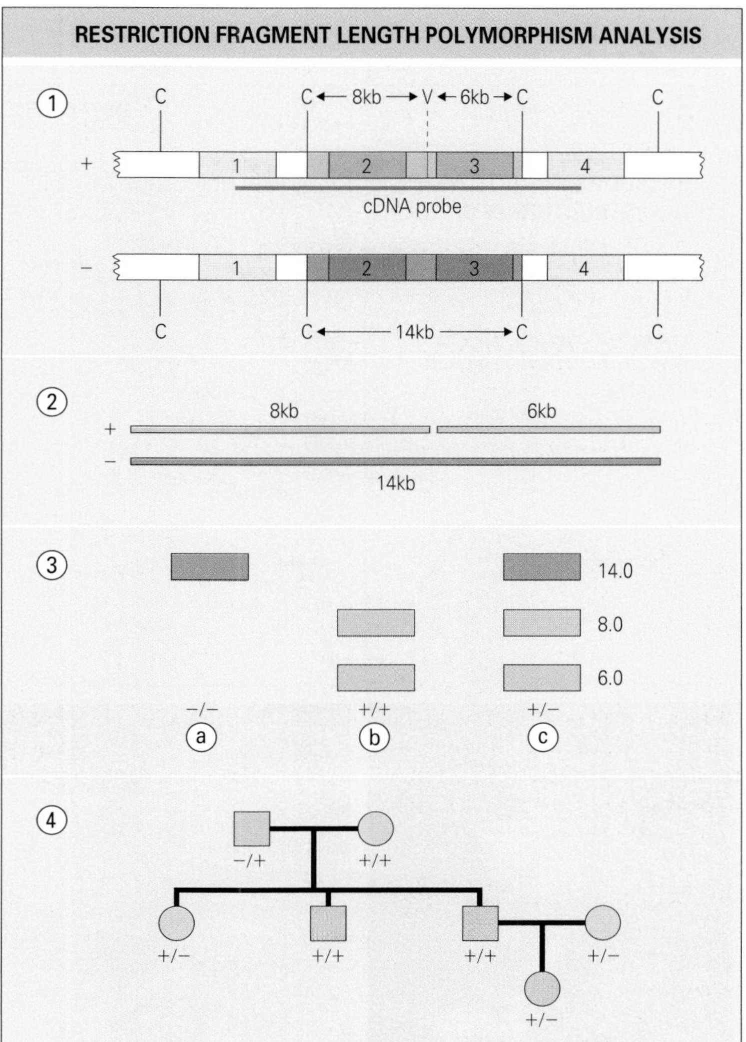

Fig. 6.6 Restriction fragment length polymorphism analysis. Consider a hypothetical gene consisting of four exons. A particular restriction enzyme invariably cuts the gene at two points (C). A polymorphism exists in the site at V. Polymorphisms are detected by a cDNA probe to part of the gene (1). The (–) allele which lacks the cutting site results in a 14kb fragment on digestion with the enzyme. The presence of V splits the (+) allele into two smaller fragments of 8 and 6kb (2). On Southern blot tests characteristic patterns are seen. Lane (a) represents the pattern in a subject homozygous for the (–) allele, (b) is homozygous for the (+) allele and (c) is the heterozygous state (3). The pedigree of an informative family is indicated (4). The disease always segregates with the (+) allele, indicating linkage at or near the gene of interest.

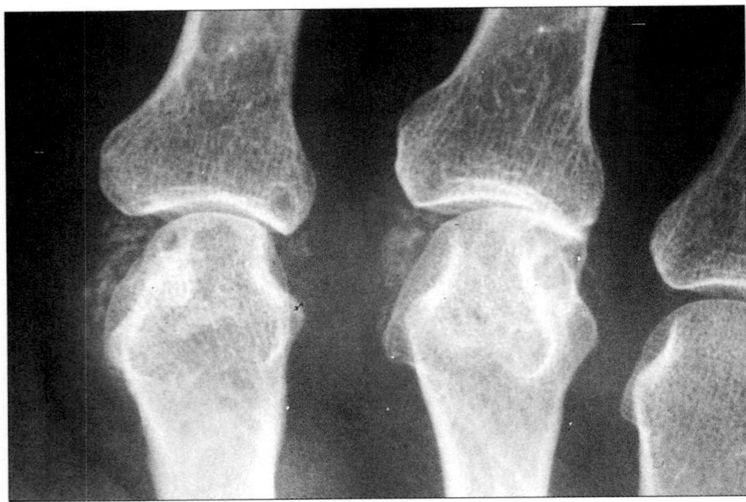

Fig. 6.7 Calcification affecting metacarpophalangeal joints.

three generations to provide sufficient meioses to confirm that the segregation pattern observed has not arisen by chance alone. They depend for success on the presence of key members who are 'informative' or heterozygous for the polymorphism, allowing the two chromosomes to be distinguished.

POLYMERASE CHAIN REACTION

Genetic studies on small amounts of genetic material have been greatly facilitated by the development of the polymerase chain reaction (PCR)[7]. This is a serial reaction involving the use of a heat-stable DNA polymerase to amplify a DNA sequence millions of times. The technique involves the use of two single-stranded oligonucleotide probes complementary to DNA sequences flanking the region to be amplified. First the DNA is heat denatured; the primers are then annealed to their complementary sequences and extended using DNA polymerase. Heat denaturing releases the newly manufactured segment and the process can begin again. Up to 30 or 40 cycles can be performed, each one doubling the amount of DNA present. Enough DNA can thus be generated to allow direct sequencing of the gene.

The PCR can be used in other ways. The genome contains many copies of short DNA sequences that are composed of tandemly repeating units. The function of these 'tandem repeat sequences' is unknown.

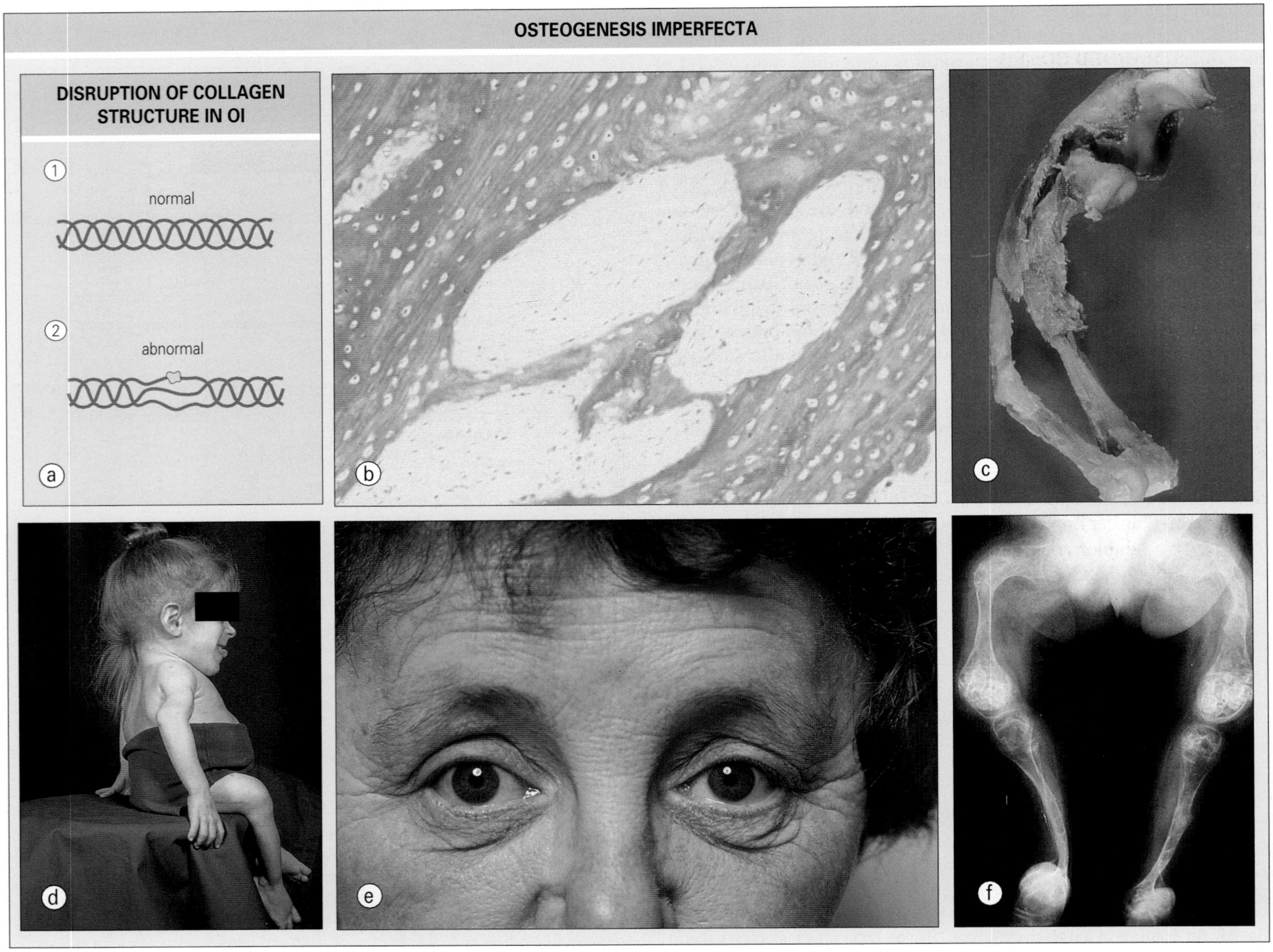

OSTEOGENESIS IMPERFECTA

DISRUPTION OF COLLAGEN STRUCTURE IN OI

1 normal

2 abnormal

Fig. 6.8 Osteogenesis imperfecta. Triple helical structure of normal collagen: a single amino acid substitution in OI can disrupt the helical structure resulting in abnormal collagen (a). Bone biopsy from a patient with OI showing marked hypercellularity of the bone with a fine lamellar pattern and extensively eroded surfaces (hematoxylin & eosin stain) (b). Dissected specimen of forearm bones showing multiple fractures, including a fracture dislocation of the radial head (c). A patient with OI congenita showing defects in all four limbs, an increased anteroposterior diameter of the chest and spinal deformity (d). The characteristic blue sclerae of OI (e). Radiograph showing characteristic deformity in OI (f).

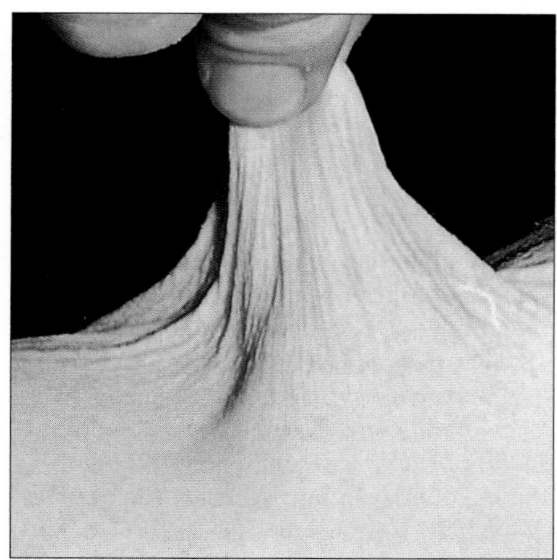

Fig. 6.9 Ehlers-Danlos syndrome. Excessive skin laxity. The skin can be pulled away from the sybcutaneous tissue and will snap back when released (Courtesy of Dr H. Bird).

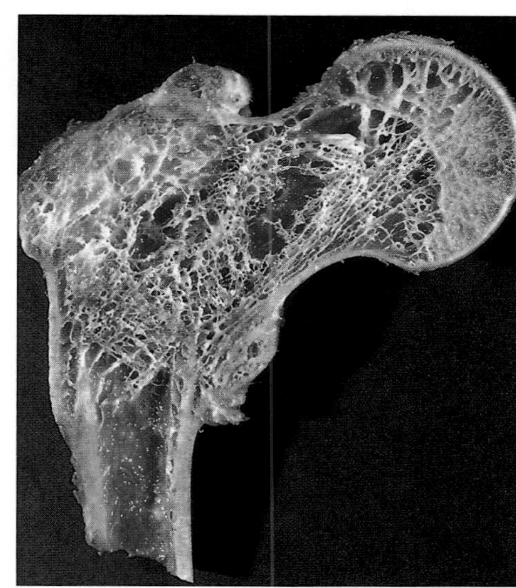

Fig. 6.10 Photograph of an autopsy section through the femur of a young man with Ehlers–Danlos syndrome shows a healed pathologic fracture and sever osteoporosis.

Using PCR the pattern of tandem repeats can be determined and, since each person's pattern of tandem repeats is likely to be unique, they can be used to follow allele cosegregation. Tandem repeat sequences are often more informative than RFLPs in linkage studies due to their greater number of potential alleles and therefore higher heterozygosity.

SINGLE-STRANDED CONFORMATIONAL POLYMORPHISMS

A commonly used PCR-based method for detecting DNA sequence changes is single-stranded conformational polymorphisms (SSCP). This technique relies on the fact that primary sequence differences will alter the secondary structure of single-stranded DNA, which affects its rate of migration through a polyacrylamide gel. Thus a section of DNA that contains a mutation and has been heat denatured and allowed to form single-stranded secondary structures will have a different mobility to the normal sequence. Clearly this technique works best when the mutation to be detected results in a large difference in mobility. Also, PCR can be used simply and quickly to detect mismatches between double-stranded DNA containing one wild-type strand and one strand from a mutant gene – 'heteroduplex analysis'. The PCR product for the test sample and the control are mixed, heated and allowed to reanneal. If the test and control differ in sequence, half the reannealed DNA will be heteroduplex. Such complexes migrate at different rates through a gel due to a 'kink' in the DNA at the region of the mismatch. Use of bacteriophage enzymes that cleave DNA at mismatched nucleotides ('resolvases') further improves the efficiency of this technique[8]. Unlike standard heteroduplex analysis, in which not all mismatches cause the heteroduplex molecules to have a different mobility to that of the normal sequence, resolvases will cut at nearly all mismatches.

GENETIC DEFECTS AND RHEUMATIC DISEASES

Most rheumatic diseases have an element of genetic susceptibility in their etiology. In addition to the MHC-related associations, examples include structural defects of connective tissue elements, abnormalities of enzymes involved in key metabolic pathways and cytokines, hormones and their receptors.

STRUCTURAL ABNORMALITIES IN CONNECTIVE TISSUES

Genetic defects in collagen genes

Collagen is a major constituent of all connective tissue and mutations in collagen genes have now been described in association with a large number of musculoskeletal disorders[9]. It is becoming increasingly clear that mutations in distinct but related genes can result in the same apparent disease; conversely, mutations in the same gene can produce different clinical phenotypes. Linkage of disease expression to a single genetic locus is therefore the exception rather than the rule. At least two loci, for example, have been described in multiple epiphyseal dysplasia, including type IX collagen[10] and cartilage oligomeric matrix protein (COMP)[11,12]. Calcium pyrophosphate disease, characterized by deposition of calcium-containing crystals in joint tissue (Fig. 6.7) and development of a form of OA, appears to be familial and early onset in some cases. Linkage has been established to two loci located on chromosome 8q[13] and chromosome 5p[14].

Type I collagen consists of three α chains folded into a triple helix. Two major mechanisms exist to ensure correct three-dimensional structure. First, chains are synthesized as precursor pro-α chains containing globular terminal extensions called N- and C-propeptides. These are cleaved from the loosely associated chains to form insoluble collagen. Second, post-translational glycosylation and hydroxylation ensure correct alignment of residues[9].

Osteogenesis imperfecta (OI) is an inherited disorder of connective tissue that results in abnormally brittle bones (see Chapter 8.50). Most patients have defects in other connective tissue, resulting in blue sclera, teeth deformities and fragile skin (Fig. 6.8). There is wide heterogeneity in expression of disease. The genetic basis for OI is now established as residing in the two genes encoding type I procollagen, *COL1A1* and *COL1A2*[15,16]. Many of the mutations in the *COL1A1* and *COL1A2* genes involve substitutions of invariant glycine residues located in the major helix of the protein with larger amino acids. Larger deletions of three exons have also been reported[17]. Generally these mutations do not prevent transcription into mRNA but rather result in production of an abnormal chain, which profoundly affects three-dimensional structure and stability. For example, substitution of cysteine for glycine at position 748 disrupts or kinks the triple helix, resulting in abnormally branched fibrils and a weaker overall bone structure.

Mutations in the type I procollagen gene *COL1A2* have also been found in the type VII variant of the Ehlers–Danlos syndrome (EDS), (Figs 6.9 & 6.10) which is associated with extreme joint laxity. Interestingly, all five mutations so far described result in skipping of exon 6 in RNA splicing[18]. This exon codes for the cleavage site of N-propeptide. Without it, the precursor cannot be cleaved, resulting in abnormally long chains which disrupt fibril formation. Type IV EDS, associated with arterial rupture and catastrophic hemorrhage, has been linked to mutations in the type III collagen gene, including a single substitution of aspartate for glycine at position 883. The type III collagen that is produced is both quantitatively and qualitatively abnormal[19]. Other mutations result in aberrant splicing of RNA[9]. Also, EDS type II has been linked to the *COL5A1* gene[20].

Osteoarthritis and the type II procollagen gene

The predominant collagen in articular cartilage is type II collagen coded by the *COL2A1* gene on chromosome 12. Mutations of this gene have been implicated in several conditions that share as common features cartilage loss and premature joint failure. Some cases of chondrodysplasias[21] and spondyloepiphyseal dysplasias[22] are linked to *COL2A1* mutations though in other dysplasia families type II collagen has been specifically excluded[23]. Stickler syndrome (hereditary arthro-ophthalmopathy) is clearly linked to *COL2A1*: all mutations so far reported introduce a premature stop codon[24].

The contribution of *COL2A1* mutations to generalized OA remains uncertain. Three families were originally described in whom inheritance of OA as a dominant trait appeared to be linked to a polymorphism in the type II procollagen gene[25,26]. For one family the defect was identified as a single base mutation converting arginine at position 519 of the α_1(II) chain to a codon for cysteine[27]. This mutation has been sought in a further seven families with familial OA and found in two[28]. It seems to define a distinctive pattern of early-onset aggressive generalized OA with mild spinal chondrodysplasia and autosomal dominant inheritance. The gene product has been analyzed by obtaining articular cartilage from one family member at the time of joint replacement[29]. About a quarter of the α_1(II) chains present in the collagen of this cartilage contained the arginine to cysteine substitution. Such abnormal collagen might be expected to reduce the durability of cartilage and predispose to OA. There should be caution, however, in extrapolating these results to OA as whole. Sibling pair analysis of subjects with more typical generalized OA excluded *COL2A1* as a major susceptibility locus[30]. Neverthless these findings are of enormous potential significance, in terms of prediction of at-risk individuals and even genetic therapy. It also confirms the impact that a single nucleotide mutation can have in causing widespread articular cartilage damage. Recent twin studies[31] have indicated that the overall genetic component in OA may be as high as 70% though currently the genes responsible remain unknown.

Fibrillin and the gene for Marfan syndrome

Fibrillins are the most prominent proteins in the extracellular microfibril. Fibrillin-1 is encoded by gene *FBN1* on chromosome 15q. It is now clear that mutations of this gene result in Marfan syndrome: a heterogeneous autosomal dominant condition characterized by ocular, skeletal and cardiovascular abnormalities (Fig. 6.11)[32]. One described mutation results in substitution of proline for arginine at position 716[33]. This is a nonconservative change, and is likely to disrupt the secondary structure of the molecule. A related condition – congenital contractural arachnodactyly – is due to mutations in *FBN2*, the gene on chromosome 5q coding for fibrillin-2[34].

ENZYME DEFECTS

Processing enzymes are involved in many diseases. The concept of 'inborn errors of metabolism' was initiated by Sir Archibald Garrod's studies on alkaptonuria in the early 20th century[35]. Garrod realized that the familial nature of such conditions could be explained in terms of the laws of Mendelian inheritance, implying an underlying genetic cause. Such defects are not confined to rheumatologic disorders, but one of the best characterized results is in a severe form of gout. Hypoxanthine phosphoribosyl transferase is an enzyme concerned with purine metabolism. Deficiency of HPRT results in a clinical condition characterized by overproduction of uric acid and hyperuricemia (see Practical Problem 8.19, Gout in young people). Almost complete deficiency is found in the Lesch–Nyhan syndrome, a disorder further characterized by choreoathetosis, mental retardation, spasticity and self-mutilation (Fig. 6.12), whereas partial deficiencies result in urate calculi and gouty arthritis but not the severe neurologic complications[36]. Levels of HPRT activity vary from 0.01 to 70% of normal. Studies of purified enzyme from unrelated patients with deficiency showed that the enzyme differed in kinetic and electrophoretic properties, suggesting that different mutations may be responsible in different patients. This is indeed the case as has been confirmed by amino acid sequencing, cDNA cloning and direct sequencing of PCR-amplified mRNA transcripts[37]. A large number of mutations have been described comprising, in order of frequency, point mutations, deletions and insertions. The finding of the same mutation in unrelated individuals is extremely rare. Mutations are not randomly dispersed throughout the molecule but are clustered into regions, some of which are highly conserved in evolutionary terms and are predicted to be involved in substrate binding. Single amino acid changes may have large structural consequences; for example, in the variety known as HPRT (Banbury) substitution of proline for arginine at position 51 breaks the α helical structure, while in HPRT (Milwaukee) conversion of alanine at 161 to serine causes a loss in the β turn structure. All mutations have in common a reduction in enzyme activity[38].

Another example is homocystinuria, an autosomal recessive disorder that resembles Marfan syndrome. The defect lies in the enzyme cystathionine β-synthetase, though the genetic basis remains to be established. Alkaptonuria is another autosomal recessive enzyme

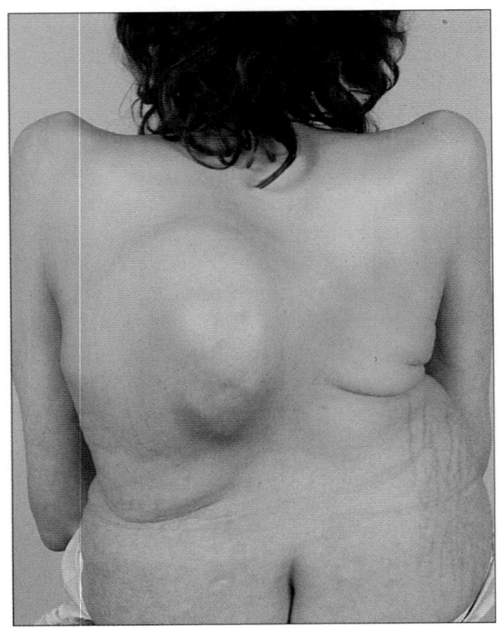

Fig. 6.11 Marfan syndrome.

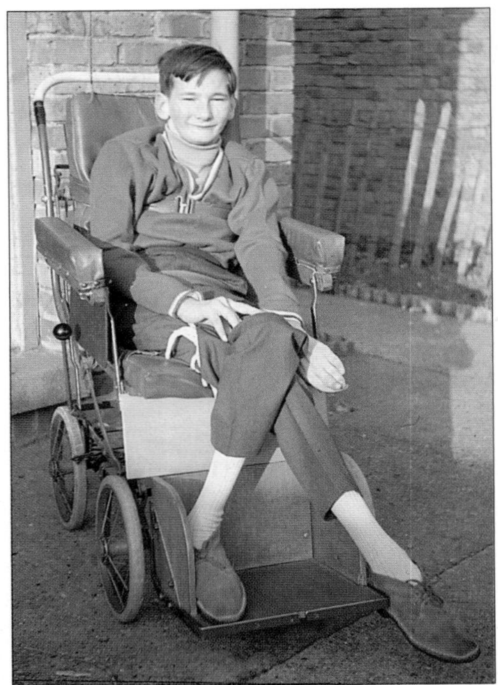

Fig. 6.12 Lesch–Nyhan syndrome. A boy suffering from Lesch–Nyhan syndrome. He is confined to a wheelchair because of mental retardation and tendency to self-mutilation as well as problems arising from gout.

defect, due to reduction in activity of an enzyme concerned with tyrosine metabolism, homogentisic acid oxidase. Deposition of pigment derived from polymerized metabolites of homogentisic acid in cartilage, skin and sclera results in the clinical condition ochronosis (see Chapter 8.28). Rheumatologic manifestations include calcification and ossification of intervertebral disks and peripheral OA affecting knees, shoulders and hips.

CYTOKINES, HORMONES AND THEIR RECEPTORS

Cytokines mediate acute inflammation, chronic inflammation and tissue destruction in diseases such as rheumatoid arthritis (RA). Like hormones, they mediate their effect via receptors on the cell surface. Naturally occurring inhibitors exist to limit their activity.

Allelic polymorphism in the promoter and controlling regions of genes for tumor necrosis factor (TNF-α) and interleukin-1 (IL-1) exist and may be related to differences in cytokine production rates between individuals. Such cytokine gene polymorphisms may contribute to genetic susceptibility to chronic inflammatory diseases

An example of hormone receptor polymorphisms is provided by the vitamin D receptor in osteoporosis. Genetically determined factors are known to contribute strongly to bone mass in healthy individuals. Certain alleles of the gene encoding the vitamin D receptor appear to be associated with differences in bone mineral density[39].

GENE THERAPY

As the genetic basis of diseases is established, the possibility emerges of manipulating the genome[40]. Two major areas can be considered. Monogenic diseases, for example cystic fibrosis, osteogenesis imperfecta or the Lesch–Nyhan syndrome, are in theory amenable to correction by inserting a normal gene into the host organism. Polygenic diseases or those with a mixture of genetic and environmental influences such as RA might be treatable by adding a gene which produces a beneficial or protective product. Such genes might include those for the naturally occurring inhibitors of proinflammatory cytokines, such as IL-1 or TNF-α, or the adhesion molecules that allow invasion of inflammatory cells in the rheumatoid synovium[41]. Other cytokines, such as insulin-like growth factor (IGF-1) or transforming growth factor (TGF-β), are capable of repairing cartilage and may be useful in OA.

Two major approaches have been used to introduce DNA into host cells. In the first, cells are removed from the host, cultured and infected with a retrovirus into which has been inserted the human gene of interest. The modified cell population is then reinserted into the host. The second method involves direct infection of the host with recombinant virus carrying the gene of interest. Such an approach has successfully been used to insert the human gene for HPRT into mice, using a neurotropic DNA virus as vector. The gene product was shown to be produced in the brains of infected animals[42]. Physical methods such as the use of liposomes have also been used and have the advantage of low toxicity and ease of delivery.

The IL-1 receptor antagonist protein (IRAP) has received most interest in rheumatic disease. In rabbits, synovial cells modified to express IRAP and then reinjected migrate back to synovium, produce IRAP and can protect the joint against certain experimental arthritis[43]. Using retroviral transduction of hemopoietic stem cells, prolonged secretion of IRAP is possible in mice[44].

Though considerable progress has been made in gene therapy, there are several reasons for caution. First, considerable technical problems will have to be overcome before the techniques can be widely applied to human disease. Second, most diseases are the result of both genetic and environmental factors, both of which need to be clearly established before gene therapy can be contemplated. Third, for many genetic diseases the detrimental effects of a mutant gene have already manifested themselves in the phenotype before any corrective gene therapy can be applied. It is therefore too late to correct the damage. Fourth, treatment is directed at somatic cells, rather than germ cells, so the condition can still be transmitted to offspring. Finally, ethical considerations[45] and financial constraints may limit progress.

Since 1990, when the first approved gene therapy experiment was conducted on a girl with adenosine deaminase deficiency, gene therapy has been used in molecular deficiency diseases such as severe combined immunodeficiency, familial hypercholesterolemia and cystic fibrosis. Preliminary results appear promising. Gene therapy trials are also under way using antisense oligonucleotides, adoptive immunotherapy with genetically modified T-cells and delivery vectors containing IL-1 receptor inhibitor for arthritis (see Chapter 3.10). Over the past 5 years gene therapy has become a reality with every likelihood of further advances in the years to come. Rheumatic disorders with a genetic basis may, for the first time, become curable diseases.

REFERENCES

1. Rogers J, Wall R. A mechanism for RNA splicing. Proc Natl Acad Sci USA. 1980;77:1877–9.
2. Shero JH, Bordwell B, Rothfield NF, Earnshaw WC. High titres of autoantibodies to topoisomerase 1 (Scl-70) in sera from scleroderma patients. Science. 1986;231:737–40.
3. Lerner MR, Boyle JA, Mount SM, *et al.* Are sn RNPs involved in splicing? Nature. 1980;283:220–4.
4. Mathews MB, Bernstein RM. Myositis autoantibody inhibits histidyl-tRNA synthetase: a model for autoimmunity. Nature. 1983:304:177–9.
5. Southern EM. Detection of specific sequences among DNA fragments separated by gel electrophoresis. J Mol Biol. 1975;98:503–17.
6. Ogilvie AD, Wood NC, Dickens E, Wojtacha D, Duff GW. *In situ* hybridisation. Ann Rheum Dis. 1990;49:434–9.
7. Saiki RK, Gelfand DH, Stoffel S, *et al.* Primer directed enzymatic amplification of DNA with a thermostable DNA polymerase. Science 1988;239:487–91.
8. Mashal RD, Koontz J, Sklar J. Detection of mutations by cleavage of DNA heteroduplexes with bacteriophage resolvases. Nature Genet. 1995;9:177–83.
9. Kuivaniemi H, Tromp G, Prockop DJ. Mutations in collagen genes: causes of rare and some common diseases in humans. FASEB. 1991;5:2052–60.
10. Muragaki Y, Mariman E, van Beersum S, *et al.* A muation in the gene encoding the α_2 chain of the fibril associated collagen IX, *COL9A2*, causes multiple epiphyseal dysplasia (MED2). Nature Genet. 1996;12:103–5.
11. Briggs MD, Hoffman S, King LM, *et al.* Pseudoachondroplasia and multiple epiphyseal dysplasia due to mutations in the cartilage oligomeric matrix protein gene. Nature Genet. 1995;10:330–6.
12. Hecht JT, Nelson LD, Crowder E, *et al.* Mutations in exon 17B of cartilage oligomeric matrix protein (COMP) cause pseudoachondroplasia. Nature Genet. 1995;10:325–9.
13. Baldwin CT, Farrer LA, Adair R, Dharmavaram R, Jimenez S, Anderson L. Linkage of early onset osteoarthritis and chondrocalcinosis to human chromosome 8q. Am J Hum Genet. 1995;56:692–7.

14. Hughes AE, McGibbon D, Woodward E, Dixey J, Doherty M. Localisation of a gene for chondrocalcinosis to chromosome 5p. Hum Molecular Genet. 1995;4:1225–8.
15. Prockop DJ, Constantinou CD, Dombrowski KE, *et al.* Type I procollagen: the gene protein system that harbors most of the mutations causing osteogenesis imperfecta and probably more common heritable disorders of connective tissue. Am J Med Genet. 1989;34:60–7.
16. Sykes B, Ogilvie D, Wordsworth B, *et al.* Consistent linkage of dominantly inherited osteogenesis imperfecta to the type I collagen loci: COL1A1 and COL1A2. Am J Hum Genet. 1990;46:293–307.
17. Chu ML, Gargiulo V, Williams SC, Ramirez F. Multiexon deletion in an osteogenesis imperfecta variant with increased type III collagen mRNA. J Biol Chem. 1985;260:691–4.
18. Vasan NS, Kuivaniemi H, Vogel BE, *et al.* A mutation in the pro alpha$_2$(1) gene (*COL1A2*) for type I procollagen in Ehlers–Danlos syndrome type VII: evidence suggesting that skipping of exon 6 in RNA splicing may be a common cause of the phenotype. Am J Hum Genet. 1991;48:305–17.
19. Tromp G, Kuivaniemi H, Stolle C, Pope FM, Prockop DJ. Single base mutation in the type III procollagen gene that converts the codon for glycine 883 to aspartate in a mild variety of Ehlers–Danlos syndrome IV. J Biol Chem. 1989;264:19313–17.
20. Loughlin J, Irven C, Hardwick LJ, *et al.* Linkage of the gene that encodes the α_1 chain of type V collagen (COL5A1) to type II Ehlers-Danlos syndrome (EDS II). Hum Mol Genet. 1995;4:1649–51.
21. Bogaert R, Tiller GE, Weiss MA, *et al.* An amino acid substitution (Gly 853-Glu) in the collagen α_1 (II) chain produces hypochondrogenesis. J Biol Chem. 1992;267:22522–6.
22. Murray LW, Bautista J, James PL, Rimoin DL. Type II collagen defects in the chondrodysplasias: spondyloepiphyseal dysplasias. Am J Hum Genet. 1989;45:5–15.
23. Weaver EJ, Summerville GP, Yeh G, *et al.* Exclusion of type II and type VI procollagen gene mutations in a five generation family with multiple epiphyseal dysplasia. Am J Med Genet. 1993;45:345–52.
24. Ahmad NN, Ala-Kokko L, Knowlton RG, *et al.* Stop codon in the procollagen II gene (*COL2A1*) in a family with the Stickler syndrome (arthro-ophthalmopathy). Proc Natl Acad Sci USA. 1991;88:6624–7.
25. Palotie A, Vaisanen P, Ott J, *et al.* Predisposition to familial osteoarthritis linked to type II collagen gene. Lancet. 1989;i:924–7.
26. Knowlton RG, Katzenstein PL Moskowitz RW, *et al.* Genetic linkage of a polymorphism in the type II procollagen gene (*COL2A1*) to primary osteoarthritis associated with mild chondrodysplasia. N Eng J Med. 1990;322:526–30.
27. Ala-Kokko L, Baldwin CT, Moskowitz RW, Prockop DJ. Single base mutation in the type II procollagen gene (*COL2A1*) as a cause of primary osteoarthritis associated with a mild chondrodysplasia. Proc Natl Acad Sci USA. 1990;87:6565–8.
28. Pun YL, Moskowitz RW, Lie S, *et al.* Clinical correlations of osteoarthritis assocaited with a single-base mutation (arginine 519 to cysteine) in type II procollagen gene. Arthritis Rheum. 1994;37:264–9.
29. Eyre DR, Weis MA, Moskowitz RW. Cartilage expression of a type II collagen mutation in an inherited form of osteoarthritis associated with a mild chondrodysplasia. J Clin Invest. 1991;87:357–61.
30. Loughlin J, Irven C, Fergusson C, Sykes B. Sibling pair analysis shows no linkage of generalized osteoarthritis to the loci encoding type II collagen, cartilage link protein or cartilage matrix protein. Br J Rheumatol. 1994;33:1103–6.
31. Spector TD, Cicuttini F, Baker J, Loughlin J, Hart D. Genetic influences on osteoarthritis in women: a twin study. Br Med J. 1996;312:940–4.
32. Dietz HC, Pyeritz RE. Mutations in the human gene for fibrillin-1 (*FBN1*) in the Marfan syndrome and related disorders. Hum Mol Genet. 1995;4:1799–809.
33. Dietz HC, Cutting GR, Pyeritz RE, *et al.* Marfan syndrome caused by a recurrent *de novo* missense mutation in the fibrillin gene. Nature. 1991;352:337–9.
34. Putnam EA, Zhang H, Ramirez F, Milewicz DM. Fibrillin-2 (*FBN2*) mutations result in the Marfan-like disorder, congenital contractural arachnodactyly. Nature Genet. 1995;11:456–8.
35. Garrod AE. Inborn errors of metabolism (Croonian Lectures). Lancet. 1908;ii:1,73,142,214.
36. Kelley WN, Rosenbloom FM, Henderson JF, *et al.* A specific enzyme defect in gout associated with overproduction of uric acid. Proc Natl Acad Sci. USA. 1967;57:1735–9.
37. Davidson BL, Tarle SA, Palella TD, Kelley WN. Molecular basis of hypoxanthine-guanine phosphoribosyltransferase deficiency in ten subjects determined by direct sequencing of amplified transcripts. J Clin Invest. 1989;84:342–6.
38. Davidson BL, Tarle SA, van Antwerp, *et al.* Identification of 17 independent mutations responsible for human hypoxanthine-guanine phosphoribosyltransferase (HPRT) deficiency. Am J Hum Genet. 1991;41:951–8.
39. Morrison NA, Qi JC, Tokita A, *et al.* Prediction of bone density from vitamin D receptor alleles. Nature. 1994;367:284–7.
40. Doherty PJ. Gene therapy and arthritis [editorial]. J Rheum. 1995;22:1220–2.
41. Chernajovsky Y, Feldmann M, Maini RN. Gene therapy of rheumatoid arthritis via cytokine regulation: future perspectives. Br Med Bull. 1995;51:503–16.
42. Palella TD, Hidaka Y, Silverman LJ, Levine M, Glorioso J, Kelley WN. Expression of human HPRT mRNA in brains of mice infected with a recombinant herpes simplex virus-1 vector. Gene. 1989;80:137–44.
43. Bandara G, Mueller GM, Galea-Lauri J, *et al.* Intra-articular expression of biologically active interleukin 1 receptor antagonist protein by *ex vivo* gene transfer. Proc Natl Acad Sci USA. 1993;90:10764–8.
44. Boggs SS, Patrene KD, Mueller GM, Evans CH, Doughty LA, Robbins PD. Prolonged expression of human IL-1 receptor antagonist (hIL-1ra) in mice reconstituted with haematopoietic cells transduced with a retrovirus carrying the hIL-1ra cDNA. Gene Ther. 1995;2:632–8.
45. Krimsky S. Human gene therapy: must we know where to stop before we start? Hum Gene Ther. 1990;1:171–3.

7

INFLAMMATION

Dwight R Robinson

- Inflammation is an essential defense mechanism, as well as an important pathologic process. It is responsible for symptoms and tissue injury in a number of rheumatic and other diseases. The control of inflammatory processes is a major aim in therapy, but achieving this goal is often difficult in practice.
- Currently, a large number of biological agents are known or suspected to be involved in the pathogenesis of inflammation.
- Inflammation is highly complex and probably involves many mediators and cell types in any disease state. Mediators appear to coordinate cellular infiltration and proliferation, the chemical modification of tissues and even tissue destruction.
- Knowledge of the important biochemical mediators in any specific inflammatory process may lead to the rational development of new and more effective therapeutic agents.

INTRODUCTION

Inflammation is a complex process which may be defined as the response of living tissues to injury[1]. The response only occurs in vascularized tissues, delivering essential molecules and cells to sites of inflammation in extravascular tissues. Inflammation is essential to protect the host from pathogenic microorganisms and to repair wounds from physical or chemical injury. The repair of injured tissues is an integral part of inflammation, after elimination of injurious organisms or matter.

In some forms of tissue injury, repair is the major beneficial result of inflammation, such as in the repair of 'clean' lacerations. In other cases, such as acute bacterial infections, the invaders may be removed and inflammation resolved with little tissue damage. However, in other infections, elimination of the invading microorganisms may be accompanied by significant tissue destruction. For example, in a bacterial abscess, extensive repair of tissues may be necessary, possibly with some degree of permanent functional impairment. This can occur with articular cartilage destruction in septic arthritis or with the formation of scar tissue in vital organs. In some cases, commonly in rheumatic disease, such tissue destruction and attempted repair may occur in the presence of chronic inflammation in which the cause is uncertain, and no apparent microorganism or foreign material is present.

Here we review some of the mediators and cells which are currently thought to be important in the genesis of inflammatory reactions. It should be noted at the outset that in spite of extensive research in this area, inflammation is still not well understood. It seems likely that many different mediators and several cell types are required for any inflammatory reaction to occur. However, there is no inflammatory reaction for which a list of mediators and cells comprising all important components could be provided, much less determine the relative importance of each mediator and cell type. It should also be noted that establishing this kind of detailed information about inflammatory reactions is not just a theoretic academic exercise, since this information would serve as a basis for the rational design of therapeutic agents.

ACUTE AND CHRONIC INFLAMMATION

Inflammation may be either acute or chronic, although this division is arbitrary and elements of both are usually present at some time during the process[1]. The initial inflammatory response is usually acute, involving vascular responses, neutrophils and/or mast cells as the most prominent elements. Acute inflammation usually evolves into chronic forms, with or without a repair phase. Chronic inflammation is usually of longer duration and characterized by the presence of the mononuclear cell series, macrophages, lymphocytes and plasma cells, as well as the proliferation of connective tissue fibroblasts. Chronic inflammation may either follow the acute form or it may characterize the reaction from the beginning. Examples of chronic inflammatory reactions are those associated with persistent intracellular organisms, such as *Mycobacterium tuberculosis*, certain viruses, physical agents with low-grade toxicity such as in silicosis, and various autoimmune reactions. Acute inflammation is usually seen with highly virulent organisms, such as pyogenic bacteria, which may result in extensive neutrophil accumulation and tissue necrosis to form abcesses.

THE VASCULAR AND CELLULAR PHASES OF INFLAMMATION

The heat, redness and swelling of inflammatory reactions are a result of the vascular response to injury[1]. A transient period of vasoconstriction typically follows injury, after which vasodilatation of the arterioles occurs. Subsequently, there is increased permeability of the microvasculature, through gaps in the junctions between endothelial cells, resulting in exudation of plasma into the extravascular spaces. The plasma loss leads to increased blood viscosity and stasis of erythrocytes. Leukocytes then adhere to endothelium, a process called margination, migrate through the widened gap junctions and then through the basement membrane into the extravascular space (Fig. 7.1).

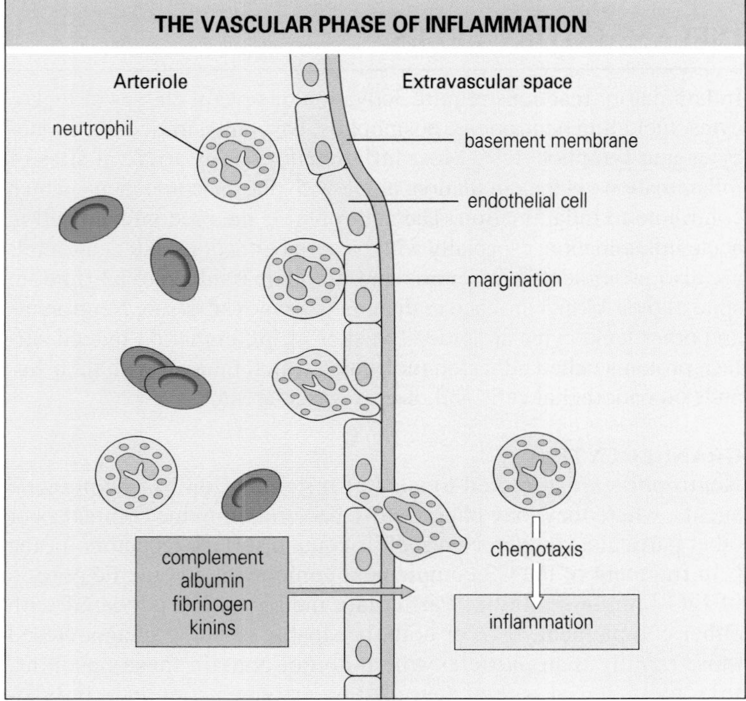

Fig. 7.1 The vascular phase of inflammation.

PHAGOCYTOSIS

Neutrophils and monocytes identify noxious particles, such as bacteria, cell debris, crystals or foreign particles, and engulf these materials through phagocytosis. Most microorganisms must be coated with serum components called opsonins in order to be recognized by phagocytes. Opsonins include IgG antibodies to antigens on the surface of microorganisms or the C3b fragment of the C3 complement component. These are recognized by specific receptors on the surfaces of phagocytes which surround the invading particle with pseudopodia, eventually encasing it in a phagocytic vacuole. The vacuole fuses with lysosomes to form phagolysosomes, followed by discharge of the contents of the lysosome, usually resulting in degradation of the ingested particle. The phagocytosed particle is exposed to a variety of degradative enzymes, such as proteases, and chemical agents, such as oxygen free radicals. At the same time, however, some of these potent degrading agents escape from the phagocytic cell into the extracellular space, contributing to tissue injury.

CELLS AND MEDIATORS OF INFLAMMATION

The vascular and cellular events in inflammation briefly outlined above, as well as other events in inflammation, are induced and modulated by a large number of biochemical agents. These agents include low molecular weight materials of a variety of chemical classes, and larger molecules including enzymes. These agents are produced by infiltrating inflammatory cells and by resident cells in the inflamed tissues. The synthesis and release of these agents is often a result of specific signaling mechanisms, usually as a consequence of interactions with specific cell receptors. Several dozens of mediators can be identified in any inflammatory exudate, and the complexity of the process is increased by synergistic or antagonistic effects which exist between different mediators. The number of candidate compounds for important roles in inflammation increases with new research, and it is a major challenge to determine the functionally significant mediators in any given inflammatory reaction. We attempt to briefly review here the cells and mediators which have generally been considered to play important roles in inflammation, although important omissions are undoubtedly made. However, future research may almost certainly indicate new compounds which should be added to those which we discuss here.

INFLAMMATORY CELLS

Inflammatory reactions require activation of several classes of leukocytes, including neutrophils, eosinophils, basophils, mast cells, monocytes and lymphocytes[2]. Most inflammatory cells arrive at sites of inflammation via the circulation, along with plasma components which contribute to inflammation. The neutrophil is the predominant cell in acute inflammation, especially with bacterial infections, but neutrophils are also prominent in vasculitis and in rheumatoid synovial fluid, in spite of their virtual absence in rheumatoid synovial tissue. Neutrophils and other leukocytes are guided to sites of inflammation by cell surface proteins called adhesion molecules which interact with their ligands on endothelial cells and on extravascular sites.

GRANULOCYTES

Neutrophils are attracted to sites of inflammation by chemotactic agents, where they may phagocytose bacteria, immune complexes or other particulate matter. Neutrophils contain surface receptors for the C3b fragment of the C3 complement component and the Fc portion of IgG immunoglobulin. Particulate matter which is coated with either complement, IgG, or both, is capable of being phagocytosed more rapidly than particles which do not contain these opsonins. Ingested material is then degraded by enzymes contained in lysosomes within the neutrophil.

Neutrophils contain two major types of lysosomes, or granules, the azurophil granule and the specific granules (Fig. 7.2). The azurophil granules contain elastase, cathepsin G, glycosidases and lysozyme. The specific granules contain collagenase, lysozyme and lactoferrin. During phagocytosis, lysosomes fuse with the phagocytic vacuole and discharge their component enzymes into the vacuole. However, neutrophils may also discharge their lysosomal contents into tissues, which can lead to tissue injury or cell death. This may occur either during phagocytosis or when the cell encounters substances such as immune complexes fixed to surfaces which cannot be phagocytosed. In addition to degradative enzymes, phagocytosis or activating agents can elicit the production of oxygen free radicals, hydrogen peroxide and hypochlorous acid from neutrophils, all of which may further contribute to tissue injury.

Other granulocytes which are important elements in inflammatory responses are eosinophils, mast cells and basophils. These cells release a variety of lipid and peptide mediators, as do neutrophils. The eosinophil appears to be particularly involved in host defense against parasitic infections, whereas mast cells and basophils are involved in the inflammatory response generated by allergic or immediate hypersensitivity reactions.

MACROPHAGES

Macrophages are one of the most important cells in inflammatory reactions. They are especially important in chronic inflammation and play crucial roles in chronic inflammatory rheumatic diseaseas, such as rheumatoid arthritis (RA)[1]. Macrophages are produced as monocytes in the bone marrow and travel to various tissue sites via the circulation where they take up residence in peripheral tissues. Monocytes are long-lived and survive in tissues for periods of months or even years. Monocytes can then differentiate into active macrophages, which become capable of a variety of phagocytic and secretory functions in response to environmental stimuli.

Macrophages have several functions and produce a large number of biologically active substances. Among their most important functions are phagocytosis and the digestion of ingested material. In addition, soluble molecules, such as soluble immune complexes, are internalized by macrophages following attachment to surface receptors by a process termed pinocytosis. The ingested material is either transported to the interior of the cell by phagocytosis or pinocytosis in endocytotic vesicles, which then fuse with lysosomes initiating degradation of the material. A large number of substances are produced and often secreted from macrophages, and these materials may contribute to inflammation and its consequences.

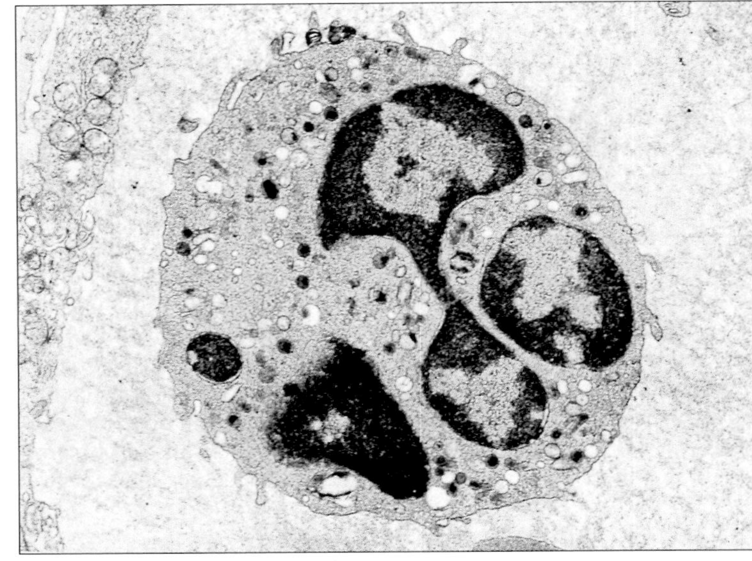

Fig. 7.2 The ultrastructure of a neutrophil. Note the presence of granules in the cytoplasm.

Enzymes capable of degrading proteins and other macromolecules include lysozyme, which degrades bacterial cell walls, and neutral proteinases, including plasminogen activator, elastase and collagenase. Other important proteins include interleukin-l (IL-l), tumor necrosis factor-α (TNF-α) and complement components. Activated macrophages produce active oxygen molecules, including free radicals and a number of eicosanoids are produced, including prostaglandin E_2 (PG E_2), prostacyclin, thromboxane A_2 and leukotrienes B_4 and C_4 (LTB_4, LTC_4). Some proteins which are produced may counteract the actions of other products, such as the protease inhibitor, α_2-macroglobulin. The majority of the macrophage products serve to augment inflammation and destroy invading microorganisms, but tissue injury may clearly result.

Finally, macrophages play a key role in the immune response by functioning as antigen presenting cells. Antigenic material is ingested, degraded into low molecular weight fragments and presented on the cell surface bound to class II major histocompatibility complex (MHC) antigens. Here, the antigenic fragments are recognized by T-cells in the context of the MHC antigens, leading to clonal expansion and activation of antigen-specific T-cells.

LYMPHOCYTES

Lymphocytes are important in identifying foreign (and auto) antigens as well as in participating in the responses which lead to elimination of those antigens[1]. B cells recognize antigenic epitopes, proliferate and differentiate into antibody-forming plasma cells. T-cells recognize antigens through their T-cell receptors which also leads to their proliferation.

The expanded T-cell population contributes to inflammation in several ways. The CD4 T-cell subset facilitates immune reactions by amplifying the B cell population through secretion of lymphokines, including IL-2, IL-4 and IL-5. CD4 cells also augment delayed hypersensitivity reactions based on the enhancement of antigen-specific cytotoxic T-cells, which respond to viral antigens and other antigens. The lymphokines secreted by CD4 cells also include interferon-γ (IFN-γ), which activates macrophages and induces the expression of MHC antigens, IL-3 and granulocyte–macrophage colony stimulating factor (GM-CSF), which promote the growth and differentiation of bone marrow stem cells participating in inflammation and repair.

The CD8 cells, the other major T-cell subset, carry out two important functions. These cells are cytolytic to cells bearing certain antigens in combination with class I MHC antigens, and are important in host defense against virus infected cells, as well as in rejection of alloantigens. The second important function of this T-cell subset is the general suppression of immune responses.

Other T-cells, which belong to neither the CD4 nor CD8 subsets, exist and carry out important functions. One of these classes of T-cells is the natural killer (NK) cells, which recognize and eliminate neoplastic cells and are therefore important in immune surveillance of cancerous cells. Another T-cell subset comprises cells expressing a different class of T-cell receptor, containing γ–δ receptor chains instead of the α–β chains found on most T-cells. The exact function of these cells is uncertain, but they are known to recognize antigens of *Mycoplasma* organisms, and thus may be important in host defense against this class of organism.

MEDIATORS OF INFLAMMATION

The coordination of vascular and cellular responses, and other events which are required for inflammation to take place, is dependent on a number of active mediators. These are derived either from the plasma, from migrating inflammatory cells or from cells comprising the local vasculature or other tissues at sites of inflammation. Several of the more important groups of inflammatory mediators are discussed below.

COMPLEMENT

The ability of the immune system to function properly in host defense depends on a group of proteins called the complement system (see Chapter 7.4)[1,2]. This system comprises over 20 proteins which circulate in the plasma in inactive forms. Many complement components are converted into their active forms through selective proteolytic cleavage. The complement system is activated by a series of sequential proteolytic steps which are carried out by the complement components themselves, each of which become active proteases, following their own activation by proteolytic cleavage. The complement system has three important functions: the activation of inflammatory cells, the cytolysis of cells infected with invading microorganisms and the opsonization of foreign matter to facilitate phagocytosis.

Complement facilitates the elimination of harmful microorganisms as part of the system of innate immunity[2]. Immunity may be divided into two distinct systems which cooperate to provide host defense, and differ primarily in the mechanism by which they recognize foreign organisms. Phylogenetically, the oldest of these is the system of innate, or natural immunity, recognizes organisms by identifying them as harmful through their surface carbohydrate molecules, through the mannose receptors on macrophages, NK cells and complement. Thus the innate immune system distinguishes between foreign bacteria and the host through surface carbohydrates, resulting in recognition with a broad specificity. The system of acquired, or specific immunity, on the other hand, is highly specific and recognizes foreign peptide antigens that are processed from proteins from microorganisms and bound to class I and class II antigens of the MHC on the surface of antigen presenting cells. The recognition of protein fragments, as opposed to carbohydrates that are recognized by the system of innate immunity, enables recognition of an almost infinite number of structures, and allows recognition of the genetically variable microorganisms. Cellular and soluble components (complement) of the innate immune system also may direct the specific immune system to assist in eliminating harmful organisms and distinguish them from autoantigens, to prevent autoimmune disease[2].

In order to carry out these functions, activation of the complement pathway takes place by two mechanisms, outlined in Figure 7.3. These two activation pathways each culminate in the activation of C3, which may either function as an opsonin or activate the remainder of the complement pathway by cleavage of C5 leading to formation of the membrane attack complex.

Classic complement cascade

The classic complement activation pathway is initiated when antigen–antibody complexes activate Cl. Active Cl cleaves both C4 and C2 to form the active C4bC2b complex, which is a C3 convertase, cleaving C3 into C3a and C3b. The C3b component binds to receptors on the surfaces of neutrophils, eosinophils and macrophages facilitating adherence and phagocytosis of bacteria and other particles. The second function of C3b is to continue the activation of the complement sequence. The C3b component forms a complex with the C3 convertase, C4b2b, to form a specific protease which cleaves C5 into C5a and C5b. The larger fragment, C5b, becomes bound to cell membranes where it is responsible for initiating assembly of the membrane attack complex, C5–C9, by the sequential addition of C6, C7, C8 and C9. This complex is inserted into cell membranes, perturbing them sufficiently to produce cell lysis. Two of the products of the activation of the complement pathway, C3a and C5a, are termed anaphylatoxins, small peptides which cause histamine release from mast cells and cause smooth muscle contraction, therefore mimicking anaphylactic reactions. The C5a component is also a potent chemotactic factor for neutrophils; it triggers the neutrophil oxidative burst, and stimulates LTB_4 synthesis.

KININS AND RELATED PROTEINS

The so-called contact system consists of a group of four proteins which circulate in the plasma in inactive forms, and are activated to provide a host defense system[1,3]. The contact system consists of Hageman factor (also called coagulation factor XII), prekallikrein, high molecular weight kininogen (HMWK) and coagulation factor XI (plasma thromboplastin antecedent). Thus, the contact system is closely related to the coagulation system.

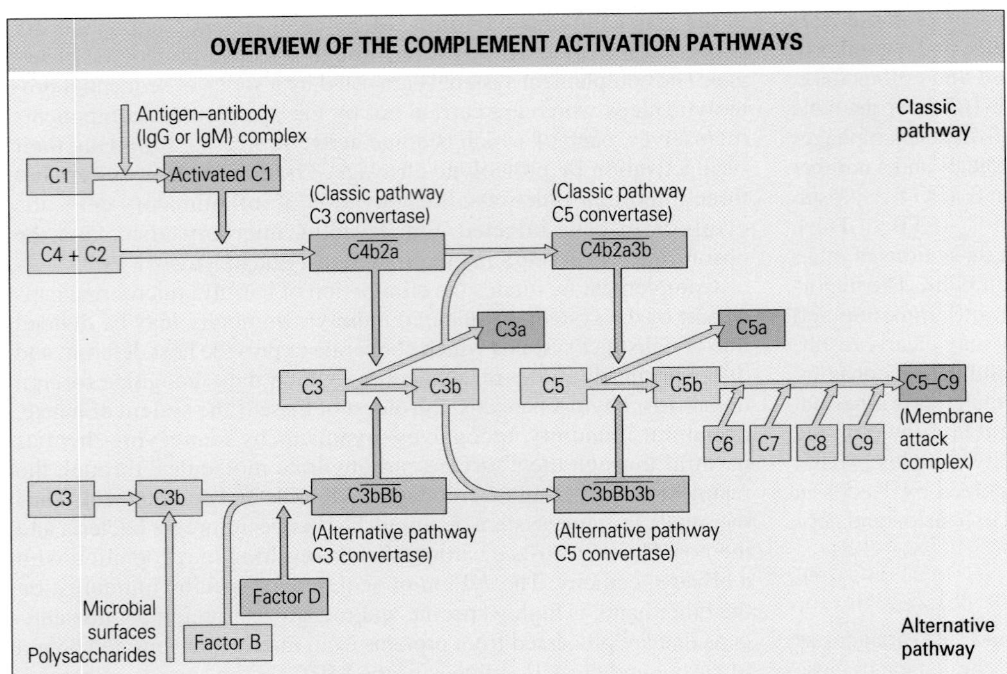

Fig. 7.3 Overview of the complement activation pathways. Activation of the classic pathway follows antigen–antibody complex binding to C1, and activation of the alternative pathway follows C3b binding to microbial agents or other surfaces. Both pathways act on C3 and C5 to generate the inflammatory components, C3, C5a, and the C5–C9 attack complex. Adapted from Abbas AK *et al.* Cellular and molecular immunology, 2E. Philadelphia: WB Saunders Co; 1994.

The contact system is activated by contact with negatively charged surfaces, which may be found in a variety of substances, including monosodium urate and calcium pyrophosphate dihydrate crystals, collagen, vascular basement membranes, glycosaminoglycans and immune complexes. Activation is initiated by Hageman factor binding to negatively charged surfaces through positively charged amino acids near its amino-terminal end. Binding may be accompanied by a low level of activation by limited cleavage of Hageman factor to form active Hageman factor. The activation is accelerated by binding in the vicinity of bimolecular complexes of both prekallikrein and HMWK, and factor XI and HMWK. The active fragment of Hageman factor, HFa, then cleaves prekallikrein to release the active enzyme, kallikrein, and factor XI to produce active factor XIa. Factor XIa and kallikrein are capable of cleaving HMWK to release bradykinin (Fig. 7.4). A kallikrein–kinin system also exists in the vascular wall, where it contributes to vasodilatation. Vascular tissues contribute substances that mediate vasodilatation including endothelium-derived relaxing factor, now known to be nitric oxide (NO), endothelium-derived hyperpolarizing factor (EDHF), which causes vasodilatation by opening vascular smooth muscle K^+ channels, and prostacyclin.

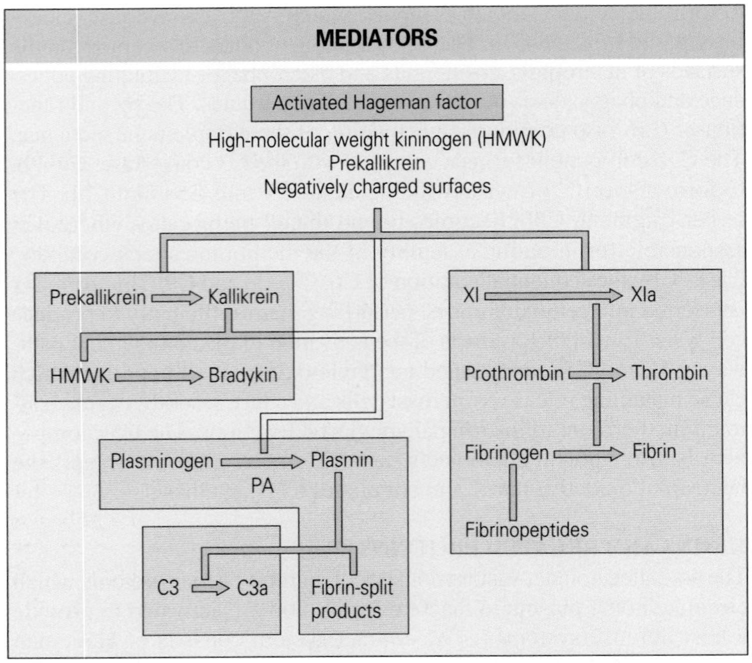

Components of the contact system may function in several ways as mediators of inflammation. Active Hageman factor may increase vascular permeability, and when active Hageman factor is infused it causes hypotension. Bradykinin is a peptide consisting of nine amino acids which causes vasodilatation, increases vascular permeability and also produces hypotension. In addition, it produces pain and causes leukocyte margination in blood vessels. It is inactivated by kininases, one of which (kininase II) is a dipeptidase, cleaving the two carboxy-terminal amino acids, and is identical to angiotensin-converting enzyme (ACE). Therefore ACE inhibitors not only promote vasodilatation by inhibiting the conversion of angiotensin I to the more potent angiotensin II by ACE, but ACE inhibitors potentiate the vasodilatating effects of bradykinin by inhibiting bradykinin breakdown by kininase II[3].

MEDIATORS

Activated Hageman factor
High-molecular weight kininogen (HMWK)
Prekallikrein
Negatively charged surfaces

Prekallikrein ⟹ Kallikrein
HMWK ⟹ Bradykin
XI ⟹ XIa
Prothrombin ⟹ Thrombin
Fibrinogen ⟹ Fibrin
Fibrinopeptides
Plasminogen ⟹ Plasmin
PA
C3 ⟹ C3a
Fibrin-split products

Fig. 7.4 Interrelations between the four plasma mediator systems. Interrupted lines indicate that the pathway may not be physiologically important.
PA = plasminogen activator. Adapted from Cotran RS, Kumar V, Robbins SL, Schoen FJ[1].

VASOACTIVE AMINES AND NITRIC OXIDE

There are three low molecular weight amines which are potentially important inflammatory mediators: histamine, serotonin, and adenosine[1].

Histamine

Histamine is the decarboxylation product of the amino acid, histidine, and is stored in mast cell granules. It is released on mast cell activation by substances such as IgE immunoglobulin, which promote immediate hypersensitivity reactions. The biological effects of histamine are mediated through its interactions with specific receptors. Histamine produces vasodilatation and enhanced permeability of postcapillary venules in addition to bronchoconstriction and the enhanced flow of bronchial mucous.

Serotonin

Serotonin (5-hydroxytryptamine) is stored in the dense body granules of platelets. It is a vasoconstrictor, but also enhances microvascular permeability. Serotonin also promotes fibrosis by enhancing the synthesis of collagen by fibroblasts.

Adenosine

Adenosine is a nucleotide generated during mast cell activation from the breakdown of adenosine triphosphate (ATP)[4]. Adenosine inhibits platelet aggregation and modulates the activation of inflammatory cells through interaction with two different surface receptors. Studies of neutrophils have demonstrated that at low adenosine concentrations, occupancy of the A_1 receptor enhances phagocytosis of immune complexes through Fc receptors and superoxide formation, whereas at high adenosine concentrations, these effects are inhibited by occupancy of the A_2 receptor.

Nitric oxide

The discovery in 1987 that endothelial-derived relaxing factor was NO began an important new area of research with implications for inflammation and several other fields (see Chapter 5.11)[5]. The synthesis of NO in endothelial cells is stimulated by bradykinin, thrombin and serotonin and adenosine derived from platelets. The enzyme that catalyzes the release of NO from arginine is NO synthase, which exists in two forms. One form of NO synthase is a constitutive, cytosolic enzyme, dependent on Ca^{2+} and calmodulin, and releases NO for short periods in response to various stimuli. The other form of NO synthase is induced by interactions of cytokines and other stimuli, including NO, with macrophages and endothelial cells. The inducible NO synthase is cytosolic, Ca^{2+} independent and synthesizes NO for longer periods of time than the constitutive enzyme. It requires tetrahydrobiopterin and other cofactors. The induction of NO synthase is inhibited by glucocorticoids. The constitutive enzyme activates guanylate cyclase and causes vasodilatation and other physiologic responses. The inducible NO synthase acts as a cytotoxic molecule for invading microorganisms and tumor cells, and may have other consequences including the vascular changes in inflammation[5].

THE CLOTTING SYSTEM

As noted above, the contact and clotting systems are intimately related[1]. Activation of Hageman factor is the initial step in both of these systems and the end product of the clotting pathway, fibrin, is a component of many inflammatory reactions. The fibrinolytic system may also be considered to be a component of the clotting system, which also has an important role in inflammation. Fibrinopeptides, which are cleaved from fibrin by the fibrinolytic system, primarily plasmin, possess chemotactic activity and increase vascular permeability. Plasmin, in addition to lysing fibrin clots, is capable of activating Hageman factor and cleaving the C3 component of complement. Thus, components of the complement, kinin and clotting pathways each interact to facilitate inflammation.

ACTIVATED FORMS OF OXYGEN

Molecular oxygen is activated to form free radicals and other species which are important in host defense against microorganisms[1]. However, active oxygen may react with several components of tissues including lipids, proteins and other compounds resulting in tissue injury during inflammatory reactions.

Molecular oxygen has a unique electron structure which is responsible for many of its biological properties. However, unlike most stable molecules, molecular oxygen has two unpaired electrons in its outer orbitals. In its fully reduced state with a two valence, as it exists in water and most stable organic molecules, each oxygen molecule may be considered to have gained four electrons. Reactive oxygen species are formed by partial reduction. Addition of a single electron to molecular oxygen yields the superoxide anion, and reduction by two electrons yields the peroxide anion. Other reactive species are derived from superoxide and hydrogen peroxide; oxygen may also undergo electron rearrangement to form singlet oxygen, as described below.

Phagocytosis of bacteria, crystals or other particulate matter by neutrophils and macrophages is accompanied by a burst of oxygen consumption and by the production of several reactive oxygen species. The first reduction is due to a pyridine nucleotide linked oxidase, which reduces oxygen to the superoxide anion free radical. Superoxide is converted into hydrogen peroxide (H_2O_2) by the enzyme superoxide dismutase (equations 7.1 & 7.2)

$$2O_2 + NAD(P)H \text{— oxidaze} \rightarrow 2O_2^- + NAD(P)^+ + H^+ \qquad (7.1)$$

$$2O_2^- + 2H^+ \text{— superoxide dismutase} \rightarrow H_2O + O_2 \qquad (7.2)$$

Formation of H_2O_2 in neutrophils, however, probably cannot account for the bactericidal activity of these cells. The most important bactericidal agent in neutrophils appears to be hypochlorous acid, HOCl, formed from H_2O_2 by the enzyme myeloperoxidase. Macrophages lack this enzyme, probably utilizing other reactive oxygen species for bacterial killing.

The superoxide anion (O_2^-) and hydrogen peroxide (H_2O_2) form the reactive hydroxyl radical ($OH^·$) in the Haber–Weiss reaction (equation 7.3).

$$O_2^- + H_2O_2 \rightarrow O_2 + OH^0 + OH^- \qquad (7.3)$$

The reactive hydroxyl radical may actually result from two reactions catalyzed by ionic iron. First, the superoxide ion reduces ferric iron to ferrous iron, following which hydrogen peroxide is reduced to form a hydroxyl radical by ferrous iron (equations 7.5 & 7.6).

$$O_2 + Fe^{3+} \rightarrow O_2 + Fe^{2+} \qquad (7.5)$$

$$Fe^{2+} + H_2O_2 \rightarrow Fe^{3+} + OH^0 + OH^- \qquad (7.6)$$

The hydroxyl radical and singlet oxygen are highly reactive oxygen species and are able to induce lipid peroxidation and polypeptide chain cleavage, in addition to other reactions.

In its stable ground state with two unpaired electrons in the outer orbital, oxygen is referred to as a triplet state due to its electromagnetic behavior[6]. This triplet structure stabilizes oxygen, since in order to be reduced by a two-electron donor, the donor electrons must also have parallel spins, or in molecular orbital terms, each electron must have the same spin quantum number. The electronic structure of singlet oxygen differs from that of the triplet state by having all electrons paired, leaving vacant the antibonding orbital which has a single unpaired electron within the triplet molecule.

Singlet oxygen is formed in many reactions, such as enzymatic degradation of lipid peroxides, including the formation of PGH_2 from PGG_2 (Fig. 7.5), and by the one-electron oxidation of the superoxide anion by heavy metal anion-containing catalysts. The anti-inflammatory activity of gold compounds and carotenoids has been postulated to be due in part to quenching singlet oxygen or converting it into its ground state, triplet oxygen[7].

ARACHIDONIC ACID METABOLITES

A large number of biologically active metabolites are derived from the reactions of oxygen with arachidonic acid. These include the cyclooxygenase (COX) products (prostaglandins and thromboxanes) and lipoxygenase products, which include leukotrienes[8,9].

Arachidonic acid is a polyunsaturated fatty acid abundant in nearly all tissues. It is primarily found in ester linkage in the (see Fig. 7.5) *sn*-2 or middle carbon position of the glycerol portion of phospholipids. Before arachidonic acid can be metabolized, it must be released by phospholipases. There are two classes of phospholipases which account for most of the arachidonic acid that is hydrolyzed. Phospholipase A_2 hydrolyzes arachidonic acid from the ester group at the *sn*-2 position, producing arachidonic acid and lysophospholipids. The second route for arachidonic acid release is the hydrolysis of the glycerophosphate bond at the *sn*-3 carbon position by phospholipase C. This reaction produces the phosphoryl-base and diacylglycerols. Subsequently, lipases cleave arachidonic acid and other fatty acids from diacylglycerol.

Prostaglandins and thromboxane A_2

Cyclooxygenases, also called PGG/H synthases, are lipoxygenases which catalyze the addition of molecular oxygen to arachidonic acid to form, initially, the endoperoxide intermediate PG_2. The same

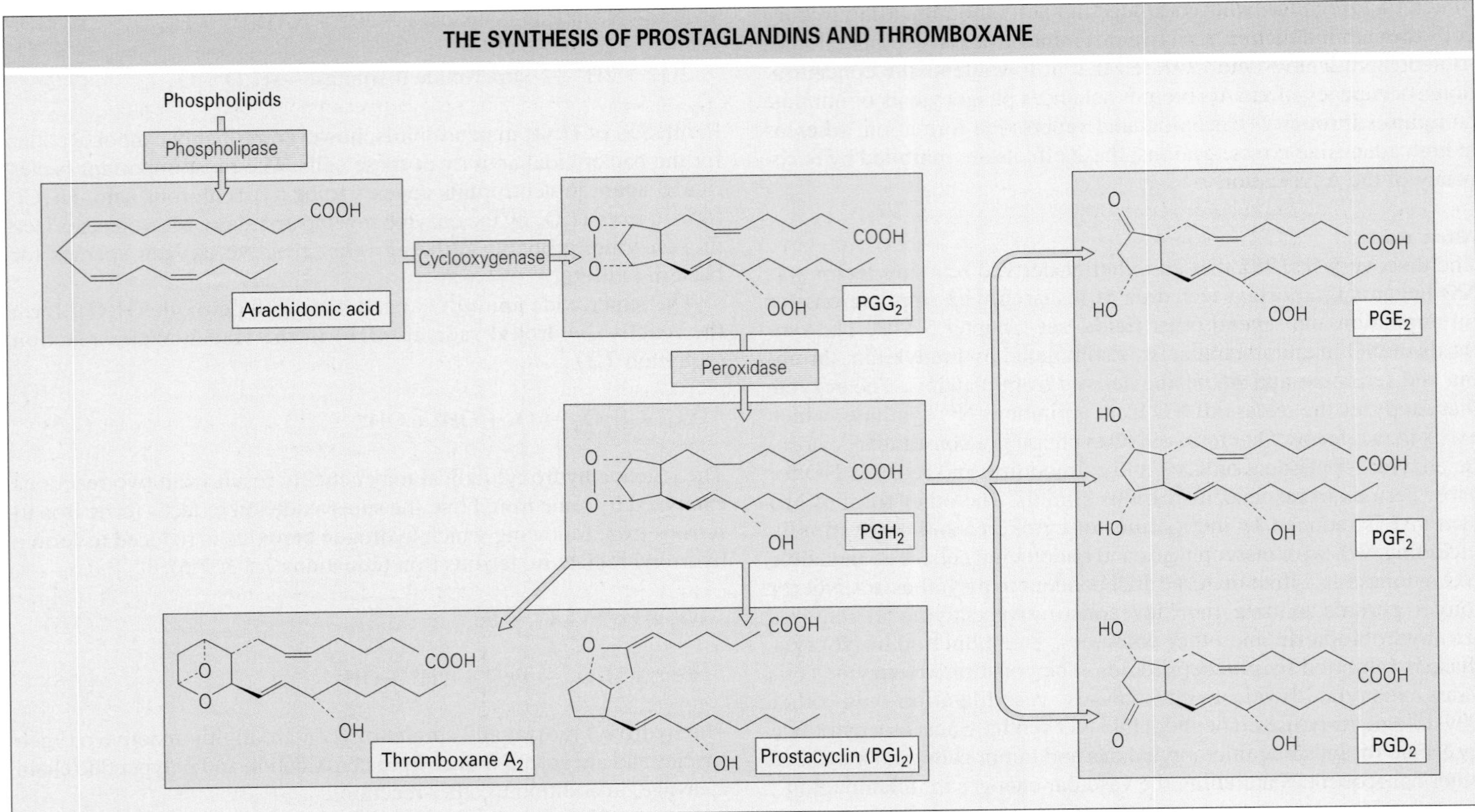

Fig. 7.5 The synthesis of prostaglandins and thromboxane A_2. Adapted from Robinson DR[8].

enzyme also possesses peroxidase activity and catalyzes reduction of the 15-hydroperoxy group of PGG_2 to form the 15-hydroxy compound, PGH_2. This endoperoxide (PGH_2) may then react with a number of enzymes, sometimes called isomerases, to become one of the prostaglandins or thromboxanes (see Fig. 7.5).

The prostaglandins are characterized by a 5-membered ring, which determines the type of prostaglandin. In addition, PGH_2 can be converted into a 6-membered ring, thromboxane A_2. These compounds differ markedly in spite of the similarities in structure. For example, thromboxane A_2 is a powerful vasoconstrictor and causes platelet aggregation, whereas prostacyclin, or PGI_2, causes vasodilatation and opposes platelet aggregation.

Two prostaglandins, PGE_2 and PGI_2, are mediators of the vascular phases of inflammation and are both potent vasodilators. In addition, they act synergistically with certain other vasoactive mediators, such as histamine and kinins, to increase vascular permeability. Prostaglandins E_2 and I_2 also stimulate osteoclastic bone resorption, suggesting that bone erosion in chronic inflammatory diseases such as RA may be mediated, at least in part, by prostaglandins produced by inflamed tissues. In addition to their vascular effects, PGE_2 and PGI_2 elevate levels of cyclic 3′, 5′-adenosine monophosphate (cAMP) in cells; many of their biological effects may be related to this elevation of cAMP.

It is widely recognized that in addition to proinflammatory effects, PGE_2 (and probably PGI_2 as well) may have anti-inflammatory effects. One of the most prominent is their immunosuppressive effects in which both T-cell activation and IL-2 formation, as well as the proliferation and maturation of B cells, may be inhibited by exposure to PGE_2. In addition, several investigators have documented that PGE_2 may inhibit the secretion of inflammatory mediators by cells. This is especially prominent in the case of the synthesis of leukotrienes, which may be actively inhibited both *in vitro* and *in vivo*. Finally, it has been shown that administration of the E prostaglandins, or their derivatives, suppresses experimental inflammation in several model systems, although pharmacologic doses are often required. It is not well established whether endogenous production of PGE_2 acts as a suppressing agent in these pathologic models.

Two cyclooxygenase gene products

An important advance in prostaglandin biochemistry in recent years has been the discovery that PGH synthase exists in two isoforms, PGHS-1 and PGHS-2, also called COX-1 and COX-2, respectively[10]. These enzymes are the products of different genes but they have a large degree of amino acid homology and identity. Their kinetic parameters are similar and both enzymes are inhibited by nonsteroidal anti-inflammatory drugs (NSAIDs). A major difference between the two enzymes is the regulation of their levels in cells. The levels of COX-1 are constitutive in most tissues; it is considered a ‘housekeeping’ enzyme, maintaining stable capacity for prostaglandin and thromboxane synthesis in tissues such as stomach, kidney, endothelial cells and blood platelets. In contrast, COX-2 is less widely distributed, but it is an inducible enzyme and may be stimulated up to 80-fold by growth factors, cytokines or other agents. It may be considered a part of the inflammatory response and is produced in stimulated monocytes, synovial cells and fibroblasts.

The presence of two isoforms of PGH synthase raises the important possibility that the enzymes may differ in their response to inhibitory drugs. That is, selective drugs might inhibit COX-2 in inflamed tissues while sparing COX-1 in the gastrointestinal tract, kidney and vasculature. While currently available drugs lack the desirable degree of selectivity towards COX-2, some investigational compounds are highly selective for COX-2 *in vitro*[9].

Evidence for the roles of cyclooxygenases from gene deletion experiments.

The genes for both COX-1 and COX-2 were deleted in separate experiments utilizing stem cell technology, providing evidence for the roles of each of these enzymes in murine health and development and in inflammatory reactions[11–14]. Knockout mice for COX-2 had a shortened life span due to failure of normal kidney development. Myocardial fibrosis also occurred, but the explanation for this finding is unknown. Female mice were infertile, indicating that COX-2 is required for ovulation. The results of experimental inflammatory reactions were somewhat unexpected, in that inflammations induced by either carrageenan or tetradecanoyl phorbol acetate (TPA) were similar in mice lacking the COX-2 gene and in the controls, and these agents were expected to be at least in part dependent on COX-2. Arachidonic acid-induced swelling was also similar in mice lacking COX-2 and in controls, but since this reaction occurs within 30 minutes of the application of arachidonic acid, any requirement for prostaglandins would be expected to be dependent on COX-1, since the induction of COX-2 requires longer time periods. In an additional model of inflammation, TNF-α-induced hepatotoxicity generated by the endotoxin, lipopolysaccharide, was reduced in mice lacking COX-2, suggesting that macrophage prostaglandin production contributes to this inflammatory reaction. In addition, the absence of COX-2 was associated with suppurative peritonitis, suggesting that COX-2 may confer protection from this bacterial infection[11,13].

Similar methods were used to delete the murine COX-1 gene[12]. Even though these mice have gastric PGE levels that are only about 1% of normals, they had no gastric pathology. The mice lacking COX-1 have reduced platelet aggregation as expected, since platelet thromboxane synthesis is essentially all from COX-1. Mice lacking COX-1 have a reduced inflammatory response to arachidonic acid applied to the skin, demonstrating that this response is dependent on COX-1. On the other hand, the inflammatory response to TPA in skin is normal, and thus these experiments and those described above demonstrate that this reaction is dependent on neither COX-1 nor COX-2. Although the fertility of mice lacking COX-1 is normal, few live births result from matings in which both males and females are homozygous for the COX-1 deletion. The lack of live births appeared to be based on impaired parturition in these animals, indicating that prostaglandin production by COX-1 is required for normal parturition. These models should be valuable in further determining the functions of COX-1 and COX-2 in health and in disease[12].

Evidence for a role of cyclooxygenase products in neoplasia.

Several lines of evidence indicates that cyclooxygenase products may play a role in neoplasia. Epidemiologic observations have shown that aspirin ingestion is associated with a reduction in the incidence of colon cancer by 40–50%[15]. In experimental studies in rodents, NSAIDs inhibit carcinogen-induced colon tumors[16]. In humans, NSAIDs inhibit formation of adenomas in the colon, and these drugs induce apoptosis of intestinal epithelium in patients with familial adenomatous polyposis[17,18]. In addition, COX-2 mRNA and enzyme levels are increased in human adenocarcinomas of the colon[19,20]. Finally, rat intestinal epithelial cells that were transfected with the COX-2 gene expressed enhanced levels of COX-2, and were resistant to apoptosis. This enhanced proliferative response in the transfected cells was reduced by the NSAID, sulindac sulfide. Thus *in vitro* studies demonstrate that enhanced expression of the COX-2 gene is associated with a change in cell phenotype resembling neoplasia[21]. Evidence is thus accumulating that cyclooxygenase products may contribute to the development of cancer, and that at least some of this effect may be modified by NSAIDs.

Leukotrienes

Lipoxygenases, other than PGG/H synthase, also catalyze the addition of molecular oxygen to specific double bonds in polyunsaturated fatty acids, again primarily arachidonic acid[10]. The most important lipoxygenases are named for the position in the arachidonic acid molecule to which oxygen is added. The 5-lipoxygenase leads to the formation of leukotrienes, as illustrated in Figure 7.6. The addition of oxygen to

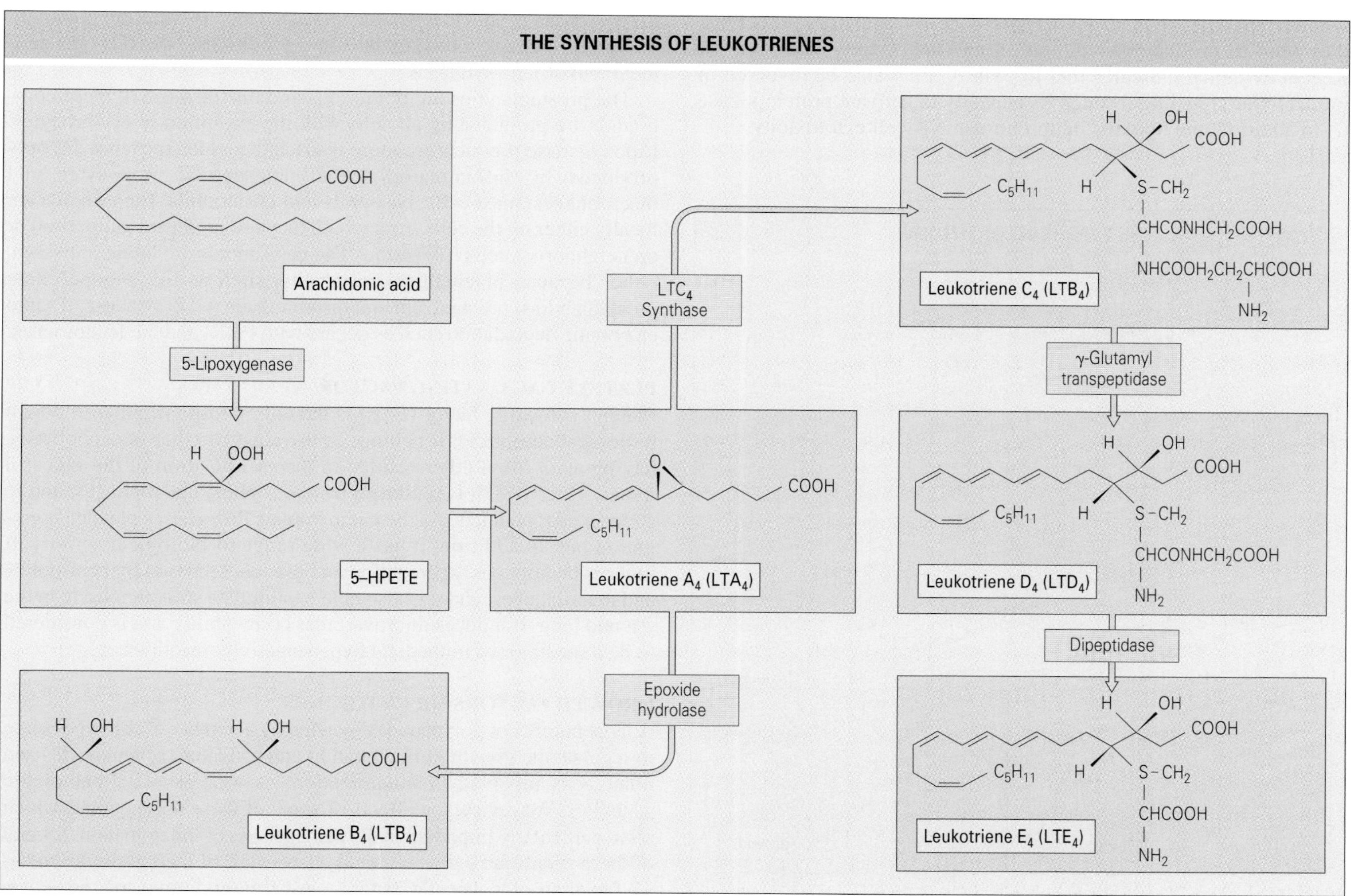

Fig. 7.6 The synthesis of leukotrienes. Adapted from Robinson[8].

the 5 position of arachidonic acid forms 5-hydroperoxyeicosatetraenoic acid (5-HPETE). The same molecule catalyzes the cyclization of the hydroperoxy compound to form cyclic 5,6-epoxide (LTA_4). The LTA_4 intermediate undergoes two important reactions to form two different classes of leukotrienes. In the first, the LTA_4 hydrolase reaction converts LTA_4 into the stereospecific dihydroxy derivative LTB_4. Alternatively, LTA_4 may react with glutathione to form LTC_4, which is further metabolized to LTD_4 and LTE_4 by elimination of a gammaglutamyl residue and, subsequently, a glycine residue. The three compounds LTC_4, LTD_4 and LTE_4 are collectively called the sulfidopeptide leukotrienes, compounds which account for the activity of the previously recognized slow reacting substance of anaphylaxis, an important mediator of immediate hypersensitivity reactions.

Products of the 5-lipoxygenase pathway are important mediators of inflammation. For example, LTB_4 is a chemoattractant for leukocytes and promotes the adherence of leukocytes to endothelial cells. It also activates secretion of active oxygen species and degradative enzymes from neutrophils. In contrast, the sulfidopeptide leukotrienes LTC_4, LTD_4 and LTE_4 contract smooth muscle in vascular, respiratory and intestinal tissues. In addition, they cause vasoconstriction, but increase microvascular permeability. They are important mediators of bronchial asthma because of their ability to cause bronchoconstriction and their ability to increase the flow of bronchial mucus. Other organs may also be affected by these compounds. For example, the sulfidopeptide leukotrienes stimulate mesangial cell contraction and exert a negative inotropic and an arrhythmogenic effect on the heart. In addition to the leukotrienes, the lipoxygenases can also produce hydroperoxy derivatives of arachidonic acid, many of which have biological activity but have not been characterized in detail. Finally, the combined action of the 5- and 15-lipoxygenases produces triple lipoxygenation of the lipoxins (Fig. 7.7). These compounds are produced by neutrophils and by neutrophils interacting with certain other cells. Lipoxins have counter-regulatory properties; they tend to produce vasodilatation and are weakly chemotactic. Recent evidence indicates that lipoxin A_4 may also be involved in intracellular signaling through its capacity to activate protein kinase C. In addition, the lipoxins inhibit human NK cell cytotoxicity.

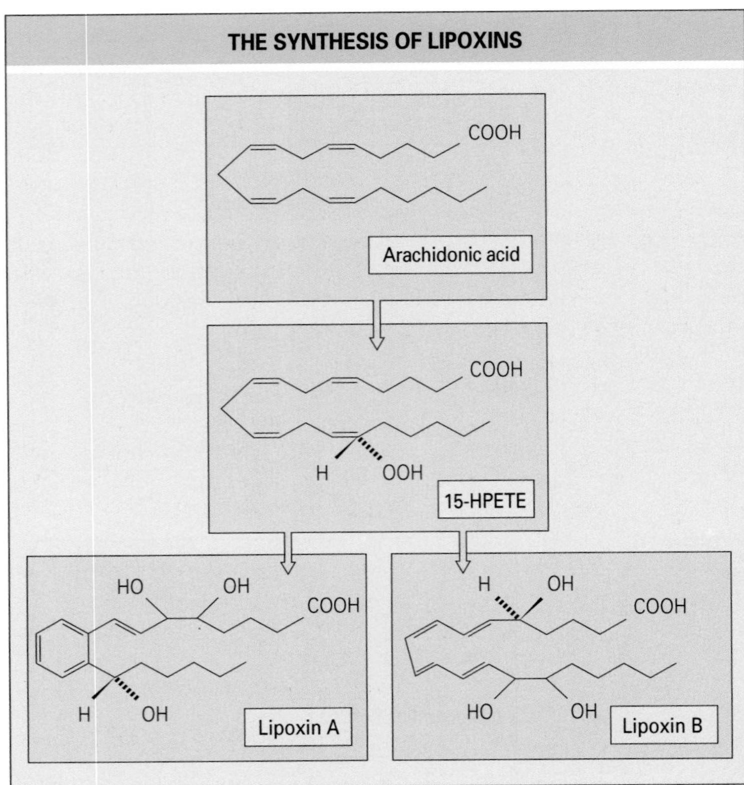

Fig. 7.7 The synthesis of lipoxins. Adapted from Robinson DR[8].

Regulation of eicosanoid synthesis

A large number of factors are capable of stimulating the synthesis of eicosanoids. However, the mechanism by which these factors augment eicosanoid synthesis is not well understood. It is generally accepted that stimulation of eicosanoid synthesis requires stimulation of phospholipase activity. This is necessary to provide adequate quantities of free arachidonic acid for cyclooxygenase and lipoxygenase, since quantities of free arachidonic acid existing in resting cells are low.

The mechanism of inhibition of cyclooxygenase activity most familiar to physicians is inhibition by NSAIDs[8,9]. Vane and Botting proposed that the major therapeutic action of aspirin and other NSAIDs may be accounted for by the inhibition of the enzyme cyclooxygenase[9]. In part, this is based on reasonably good correlations between the relative anti-inflammatory potencies of the different NSAIDs and their potencies as cyclooxygenase inhibitors. In addition, many toxic effects of NSAIDs can also be accounted for by cyclooxygenase inhibition. For example, the tendency for NSAIDs to cause erosive gastritis may be related to elimination of the cytoprotective effects of PGE_2 in the gastric mucosa. While other pharmacologic effects of NSAIDs may also be important for their activity, cyclooxygenase inhibition appears to be a prominent mechanism of action of these agents.

Glucocorticoids also inhibit the synthesis of prostaglandins and leukotrienes, but the mechanism of action differs from that of NSAIDs. Glucocorticoids appear to inhibit release of free arachidonic acid from phospholipids[8,9]. Several laboratories have provided evidence that glucocorticoids induce the synthesis of proteins called lipocortins, which in turn inhibit the hydrolysis of arachidonic acid from phospholipids. At least one of the lipocortins is similar to cytoskeletal proteins called calpactins, which inhibit phospholipases by complexing phospholipids, effectively making phospholipids ineffective substrates for phospholipases. Other lipocortins apparently inhibit phospholipases directly. Glucocorticoids inhibit the formation of both cyclooxygenase and lipoxygenase products whereas NSAIDs lack any important activity on lipoxygenases. In fact, under some conditions, NSAIDs may augment leukotriene synthesis.

The prostaglandins are ubiquitous and one or more of these compounds are produced by all cells with the exception of erythrocytes. Lipoxygenase products are more restricted, and leukotrienes are only produced by inflammatory cells, neutrophils, monocytes and macrophages, mast cells, basophils and eosinophils. Eicosanoids act locally either on the cells from which they are produced (autocrine) or on neighboring cells (paracrine) The eicosanoids are labile in tissues, either because of chemical instability, such as the endoperoxide prostaglandins, prostacyclin and thromboxane A_2, or because of rapid enzymatic degradation such as occurs with PGE_2 and the leukotrienes.

PLATELET ACTIVATING FACTOR

Platelet activating factor (PAF) is the only phospholipid with potent biological activities[1]. It belongs to the class of ether phospholipids, having an O-alkyl ether residue in the *sn*-l position of the glycerol moiety (Fig. 7.8). It is produced by neutrophils, macrophages, and to some extent, platelets. As the name implies PAF causes platelet aggregation but, in addition, it has a wide range of biological activity. It induces chemotaxis, aggregation and granule secretion by neutrophils and macrophages, and it is also able to stimulate smooth muscle in the gut and lung. It induces microvascular permeability and is considered to be a mediator of immediate hypersensitivity reactions.

GROWTH FACTORS OR CYTOKINES

A large number of polypeptides secreted by a number of cell types serve to regulate the growth, differentiation and activation of leukocytes and other cells involved in inflammation, as well as other pathologic states[22,23]. We review the effects of some of these polypeptides which seem particularly important in the pathogenesis of inflammation. Several of these agents are called interleukins because of their ability to mediate functions of leukocytes, but it is clear that this term is too restrictive, since interleukins affect many cells other than leukocytes.

PLATELET ACTIVATING FACTOR

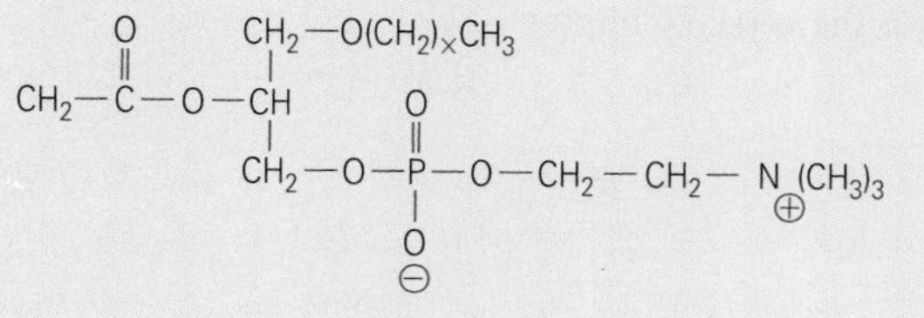

Fig. 7.8 The chemical structure of platelet activating factor.

The actions of IL-l, TNF and IL-6 are sometimes considered together because of their overlapping functions. These cytokines are produced in large quantities by monocytes. The numerous effects of IL-l illustrate the pleiotropic activity of cytokines. It is an endogenous pyrogen, stimulating the synthesis of acute phase proteins by the liver, augments the growth of T-cells and facilitates B cell proliferation and immunoglobulin secretion. Also, IL-1 induces IL-6 secretion and potentiates the responses of immature hematopoietic cells to macrophage-colony stimulating factor (M-CSF) and IL-3. It stimulates production of PGE_2 and collagenase, and augments the expression of adhesion molecules on endothelial cells, therefore increasing the adherence of leukocytes. Like IL-l, TNF-α is pyrogenic and promotes an acute phase reaction, stimulates PGE_2 and collagenase synthesis, and promotes osteoclast activation. It has also been called cachectin because it may mediate the wasting accompanying inflammatory and neoplastic states. The activation of synthesis of IL-l and TNF-α in macrophages by bacterial endotoxin may account for tissue injury and shock produced by endotoxin. TNF-α acts synergistically with IFN-γ to enhance antiproliferative effects. The actions of IL-6 include growth stimulation of a variety of cell types, including stem cells for neutrophils and monocytes, B cells and T-cells. Also, IL-6 stimulates the synthesis of acute phase proteins by the liver.

Several interleukins augment the growth and activation of lymphoid cells, and therefore are of primary importance in immune reactions. IL-2 is produced by T-helper cells and stimulates the proliferation of T-cells and the expression of IL-2 receptors on T-cells. IL-4 also promotes the growth of T-lymphocytes, and modifies the function of B cells, including the induction of immunoglobulin class switching and enhancement of IgE production. In addition to these effects, IL-4 increases the expression of class II MHC antigens on B cells and macrophages. It also stimulates the fusion of macrophages to form multinucleated giant cells, and augments macrophage aggregation. IL-4 may thus participate in the development of the granulomatous response. Other interleukins are also pleiotropic growth factors including IL-3, IL-5 and IL-7. IL-3 promotes the growth and differentiation of hematopoietic stem cells leading to the production of all blood cell types. IL-5 facilitates the growth and function of B cells, and the growth of eosinophils. IL-7 is a growth factor for B cells and T-cells. Granulocyte-macrophage colony stimulating factor promotes the growth of neutrophils, macrophages, eosinophils, fibroblasts and endothelial cells. Another polypeptide, granulocyte-colony stimulating factor (G-CSF), is a more specific growth factor for neutrophils. IL-8 is a member of a family of low molecular weight, basic heparin-binding polypeptides. It causes chemotaxis and activation of neutrophils and produces inflammation on injection, as does IL-l and TNF-α. A slightly larger form of IL-8 has been reported to have antichemotactic and anti-inflammatory effects.

The interferons were identified, on the basis of their antiviral activity, in three major forms, α, β, and δ, based on their cells of origin[14]. Interferon-γ, or immune interferon, is produced by activated T-cells. It induces the expression of class II MHC antigens on several cell types, including connective tissue cells, monocytes, and epithelial and endothelial cells. Interferon-δ also activates macrophages for antigen presentation and for killing of intracellular parasites and tumor cells. It also acts synergistically with TNF-α in the lysis of tumor cells.

PROTEINASES AND TISSUE INJURY

Proteinases are among the most important mediators of tissue injury and degradation[24]. Many proteinases are stored within the lysosomes of leukocytes, while others are synthesized and secreted in response to inflammatory stimuli. Proteinases may be divided into two classes, those active at acid pH and those active at neutral pH. The former enzymes probably function to degrade bacteria and cell debris at low pH within phagolysosomes, and it is doubtful that they have significant extracellular activity where the pH is near neutrality. Degradation of extracellular proteins in connective tissues is carried out by several neutral proteinases derived from neutrophils, monocyte–macrophages, fibroblasts and other cells.

Neutral proteinases include important enzymes[24]. They may be divided into two groups, the metalloenzymes, which require metal ions such as Zn^{2+} as a cofactor, and the serine proteinases, which have a serine hydroxyl group in their catalytically active sites. Collagenase initiates the degradation of extracellular or interstitial collagens. It is highly specific and cleaves five types of collagen, including type I, the most abundant type, and type II collagen which is the major form of collagen in articular cartilage. Collagenase cleaves a single specific peptide bond between the glycine–isoleucine residues 775–776, in each of the three polypeptide α-chains. Collagen must be in its native, triple-helical form to be cleaved by collagenase. The products of collagen cleavage by collagenase are two fragments, the larger consisting of three quarters of the original collagen molecule from the amino terminal end, and a quarter length fragment containing the carboxyl terminal end. The triple helices of each of these two products are more susceptible to thermal denaturation than is the native collagen molecule, and on denaturation become susceptible to proteolytic degradation by gelatinase and other proteinases. One form of collagenase is produced by fibroblasts, macrophages, synovial cells and endothelial cells, and a different form of collagenase is produced by neutrophils.

Gelatinases are enzymes which specifically degrade gelatin, which is denatured collagen. Their synthesis is regulated by many of the same factors which regulate collagenase synthesis. Gelatinases are produced by both macrophages and neutrophils. These enzymes cleave native collagens, types V and XI, as well as gelatin.

Proteoglycanase is an enzyme which is capable of degrading proteoglycans by cleaving the proteoglycan core protein. It has been found in articular cartilage and also may be produced by rheumatoid synovial tissue.

Several serine proteinases arise from the activation of inactive precursors in host defense systems which were discussed above. These include complement components, the coagulation cascade and the fibrinolytic system. Plasma kallikrein and plasmin both may activate collagenase, but the roles of other enzymes in these systems in degradation of connective tissue proteins remain unclear. Neutrophils produce elastase and cathepsin G, both of which are probably important in proteoglycan degradation. Elastase degrades elastin and may participate in collagen degradation by cleaving the telopeptide, nonhelical portion containing collagen cross-links. Many serine proteinases are capable of degrading a variety of tissue proteins.

REGULATION OF PROTEOLYTIC ENZYME ACTIVITY

It is clear that proteolytic enzymes are tightly regulated in order to avoid uncontrolled tissue degradation. Some metalloproteinases are stored preformed in granules or lysosomes, such as both the specific granules and the azurophilic granules of neutrophils. Release of stored enzymes can be stimulated by many substances which activate neutrophils, such as C5a and LTB_4. Other proteolytic enzymes are synthesized in response to various stimuli. For example, IL-l markedly augments synthesis of collagenase and gelatinase and secretion from synovial cells, chondrocytes and macrophages.

Metalloproteinases are often secreted as inactive precursors or proenzymes, which are activated by other proteolytic enzymes and certain chemical agents. For example, procollagenase is activated by plasmin, trypsin or by a specific enzyme called procollagenase activator. Reactive oxygen species may activate human neutrophil collagenase.

Proteinase inhibitors

Inhibitors of proteolysis are normally abundant in plasma and tissues and are essential to prevent unwanted tissue degradation. Both metalloproteases and serine proteases are inhibited by a 720kDa α-macroglobulin, a large protein abundant in plasma. Another important inhibitor is called tissue inhibitor of metalloproteinases TIMP, a 28kDa molecular weight protein which inhibits proteases by complexing with them (see Chapter 1.8).

REFERENCES

1. Cotran RS, Kumar V, Robbins SL, Schoen FJ, eds. Robbins SL. Pathologic Basis of Disease, 5E. Ch 3. 1994;51–92.
2. Fearon DT, Locksley RM. The instructive role of innate immunity in the acquired immune response. Science. 1996;272:50–4.
3. Vanhoutte PM, Boulanger CM, Illiano SC, Nagao. T, Vidal M, Mombouli J-V. Endothelium-dependent effects of converting-enzyme inhibitors. J Cardiovasc Pharm. 1993;22:S10–S16.
4. Salmon JE, Cronstein BN. Fc receptor-mediated functions in neutrophils are modulated by adenosine receptor occupancy. Al receptors are stimulatory and A2 receptors are inhibitory. J Immunol. 1990;145:2235–40.
5. Moncada S, Palmer RMJ, Higgs EA. Nitric oxide: physiology, pathophysiology, and pharmacology. Pharmacol Rev 1991;43:109–142.
6. Naqui A, Chance B. Reactive oxygen intermediates in biochemistry. Annu Rev Biochem. 1986;55:137–66.
7. Corey EJ, Mehrotra MM, Rhan AU. Antiarthritic gold compounds effectively quench electronically excited singlet oxygen. Science. 1987;236:68.
8. Robinson DR. Eicosanoids and related agents. In Arthritis and Allied Conditions, 13E. Koopman WJ, ed. Williams & Wilkins: Baltimore; 1997:515–28.
9. Vane JR, Botting RM. New insights into the mode of action of anti-inflammatory drugs. Inflamm Res. 1995;44:1–10.
10. Smith WL, Meade EA, DeWitt DL. Interactions of PGH synthase isozymes-1 and -2 with NSAIDs. Ann NY Acad Sci. 1994;744:50–7.
11. Dinchuk JE, Car BD, Focht RJ, *et al.* Renal abnormalities and an altered inflammatory response in mice lacking cyclooxygenase II. Nature. 1995;378:406–9.
12. Langenbach R, Morham SG, Tiano HF, *et al.* Prostaglandin synthase 1 gene disruption in mice reduces arachidonic acid-induced inflammation and indomethacin-induced gastric ulceration. Cell. 1995;83:483–92.
13. Morham SG, Langenbach R, Loftin CD, *et al.* Prostaglandin synthase 2 gene disruption causes severe renal pathology in the mouse. Cell. 1995;83:473–82.
14. DeWitt D, Smith WL. Yes, but do they still get headaches? Cell. 1995;83:345–8.
15. Giovannucci E, Rimm EB, Stampfer MJ, Colditz GA, Ascherio A, Willett WC. Aspirin use and the risk for colorectal cancer and adenoma in male health professionals. Ann Intern Med. 1994;121:241–6.
16. Reddy BS, Rao CV, Rivenson A, Kelloff G. Inhibitory effects of aspirin on azoxymethane-induced colon carcinogenesis in F344 rats. Carcinogenesis. 1993;14:1493–7.
17. Giardiello FM, Hamilton SR, Krush AJ, *et al.* Treatment of colonic and rectal adenomas with sulindac in familial adenomatous polyposis. N Engl J Med. 1993;328:1313–16.
18. Pasricha PJ, Bedi A, O'Connor K, *et al.* The effects of sulindac on colorectal proliferation and apoptosis in familial adenomatous polyposis. Gastroenterology. 1995;109:994–8.
19. Eberhart CE, Coffey RJ, Radhika A, Giardiello FM, Ferrenbach S, DuBois RN. Up regulationof cyclooxygenase 2 gene expression in human colorectal adenomas and adenocarcinomas. Gastroenterology. 1994;107:1183–8.
20. Kargman S, O'Neill G, Vickers P, Evans J, Mancini J, Jothy S. Expression of prostaglandin G/H synthase-1 and -2 protein in human colon cancer. Cancer Res. 1995;55:2556–9.
21. Tsujii M, DuBois RN. Alterations in cellular adhesion and apoptosis in epithelial cells overexpressing prostaglandin endoperoxide synthase 2. Cell. 1995;83:493–501.
22. Arai S-I, Lee F, Miyasima A, Miyatake S, Arai N, Yokota T. Cytokines: Coordinators of immune and inflammatory responses. Annu Rev Biochem. 1990;59:783–836.
23. Feldmann M, Brennan FM, Maini RN. Role of cytokines in rheumatoid arthritis. Annu Rev Immunol. 1996;14:397–440.
24. Nagase H, Okada Y. Proteinases and matrix degradation. In: Textbook of Rheumatology, 5E. Kelley WN, Ruddy S, Harris ED, Sledge CB, eds. WB Saunders: Philadelphia; 1997:323–41.

8

TISSUE DESTRUCTION AND REPAIR

Tim Cawston

- Cartilage is made up of collagens and proteoglycans which can be degraded by active proteases.
- All classes of proteases play a part in connective tissue turnover. The pathway that predominates varies with the resorptive status.
- MMPs are potent enzymes that degrade connective tissue and are inhibited by TIMPs; the balance between active MMPs and TIMPs determines the extent of degradation.
- Various cytokines and growth factors stimulate the production of proteases and inhibitors while inhibiting matrix synthesis, which leads to matrix destruction.
- Growth factors can increase the synthesis of matrix. Mixtures of growth factors can be used in conjunction with artificial matrix to promote the repair of cartilage defects in large joints.

INTRODUCTION

The breakdown of cartilage and bone in the arthritides prevents joints from functioning normally. In severe cases both cartilage and the underlying bone can be destroyed. Cartilage contains collagens. These long rod-shaped molecules aggregate to form cross-linked collagen fibers giving connective tissues their strength and rigidity[1]. Trapped between the collagen fibers are the proteoglycans. These large molecules consist of three globular domains interspersed with heavily glycosylated and sulfated polypeptide that form highly charged aggregates[2]. These attract water into the tissue and allow cartilage to resist compression. Chondrocytes maintain a steady state in normal adult cartilage where the rate of matrix synthesis equals the rate of degradation. Any change in this steady state will rapidly affect the functional integrity of the cartilage. Thus, during growth and development synthesis of matrix components exceeds the rate of degradation and a net increase in tissue mass results. Where resorption of tissue is required then the rate of matrix synthesis is reduced and the rate of degradation increases. In some pathologies a net loss of matrix results.

The primary cause of cartilage and bone destruction in the arthritides involves the elevated levels of active proteases, secreted from a variety of cells, that degrade collagen and proteoglycan. The sources of these proteases will depend on the type of disease. In osteoarthritis (OA) the proteases produced by chondrocytes are likely to play a major role. In contrast, in a highly inflamed rheumatoid joint the proteases produced by chondrocytes, synovial cells and inflammatory cells all play a part in the destruction that is found.

The tissues of the joint are capable of repair. While proteoglycan can be readily resynthesized, the replacement of collagen, after its destruction, is rare[3]. Various growth factors and cytokines present in the joint are able to upregulate matrix synthesis. These factors have been studied to determine if cartilage and bone defects can be repaired *in vivo*.

PROTEOLYTIC PATHWAYS OF CONNECTIVE TISSUE BREAKDOWN

Extracellular matrix proteins are broken down by different proteolytic pathways. The four main classes of protease[4] are classified according to the amino acid or chemical group at the active center of the enzyme which participates in the hydrolysis of peptide bonds. Cysteine and aspartate proteases are predominantly active at acid pH and so act intracellularly; the serine and metalloproteinases are active at neutral pH and are responsible for extracellular digestion. Examples of these enzymes and the different matrix proteins cleaved are shown in Figure 8.1. Enzymes, such as elastase, are stored within neutrophils and can be instantly released in certain situations. Some enzymes may not participate in the cleavage of matrix proteins but are able to activate other proteases that can then degrade the matrix. There is increasing interest in proteases that are membrane-bound rather than released from

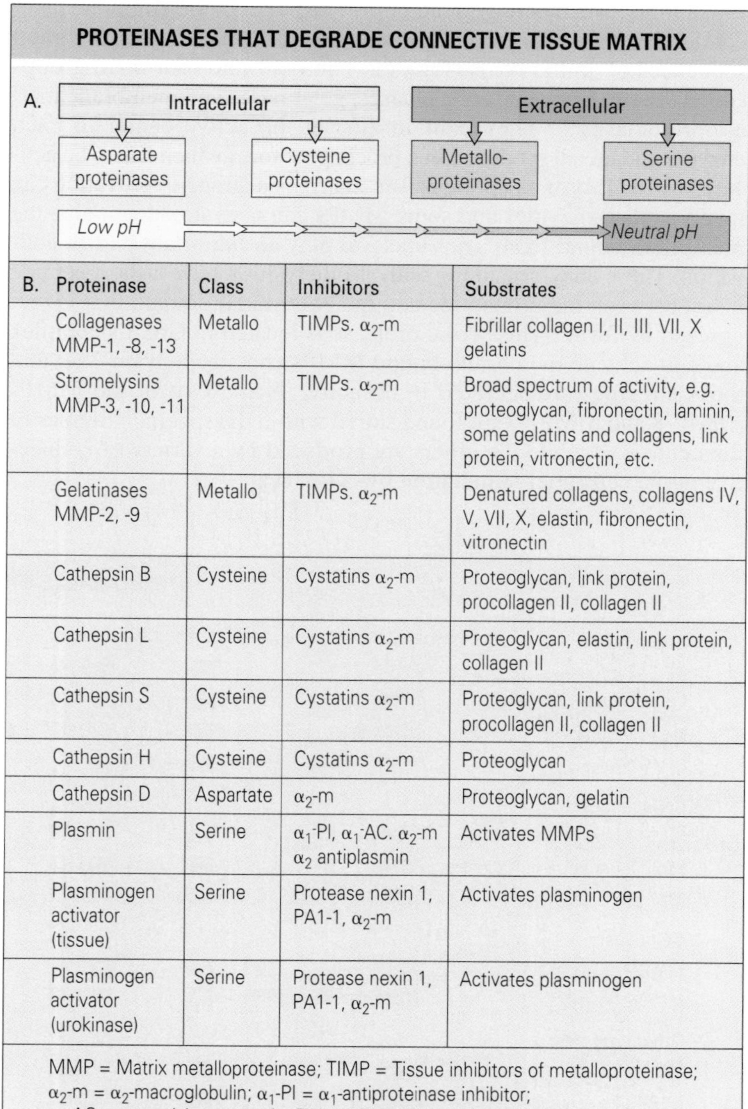

PROTEINASES THAT DEGRADE CONNECTIVE TISSUE MATRIX

B. Proteinase	Class	Inhibitors	Substrates
Collagenases MMP-1, -8, -13	Metallo	TIMPs. α_2-m	Fibrillar collagen I, II, III, VII, X gelatins
Stromelysins MMP-3, -10, -11	Metallo	TIMPs. α_2-m	Broad spectrum of activity, e.g. proteoglycan, fibronectin, laminin, some gelatins and collagens, link protein, vitronectin, etc.
Gelatinases MMP-2, -9	Metallo	TIMPs. α_2-m	Denatured collagens, collagens IV, V, VII, X, elastin, fibronectin, vitronectin
Cathepsin B	Cysteine	Cystatins α_2-m	Proteoglycan, link protein, procollagen II, collagen II
Cathepsin L	Cysteine	Cystatins α_2-m	Proteoglycan, elastin, link protein, collagen II
Cathepsin S	Cysteine	Cystatins α_2-m	Proteoglycan, link protein, procollagen II, collagen II
Cathepsin H	Cysteine	Cystatins α_2-m	Proteoglycan
Cathepsin D	Aspartate	α_2-m	Proteoglycan, gelatin
Plasmin	Serine	α_1-PI, α_1-AC. α_2-m α_2 antiplasmin	Activates MMPs
Plasminogen activator (tissue)	Serine	Protease nexin 1, PA1-1, α_2-m	Activates plasminogen
Plasminogen activator (urokinase)	Serine	Protease nexin 1, PA1-1, α_2-m	Activates plasminogen

MMP = Matrix metalloproteinase; TIMP = Tissue inhibitors of metalloproteinase; α_2-m = α_2-macroglobulin; α_1-PI = α_1-antiproteinase inhibitor; α_1-AC = α_1- antichymotrypsin; PAI-1 = Plasminogen activator-1.

Fig. 8.1 Proteases that degrade connective tissue matrix. The four main classes of proteinases are named according to the chemical group involved in catalysis. The aspartate and cysteine proteases act at low pH and are thought to act within the lysosomal system where they degrade protein intracellularly. These enzymes can also be released in small pockets near the cell membrane to degrade extracellularly. Secreted serine and metalloproteases act extracellularly at neutral pH. Some enzymes are membrane bound, ensuring that they act locally to the cell (a). Each enzyme is listed with its protease class, inhibitors and major matrix proteins degraded (b).

the cell in a free form. These enzymes are known to be associated with various processes such as cytokine processing, receptor shedding and the removal of proteins that are associated with cell–cell or cell–matrix interactions.

All classes of protease play a part in the turnover of the connective tissues. The pathway that predominates will vary with different resorptive situations. One protease pathway may precede another. The osteoid layer in bone is removed by osteoblast metalloproteinases prior to the attachment of osteoclasts which secrete predominantly cysteine proteases. These in turn strip bone matrix. In septic arthritis neutrophils release both serine and metalloproteases that exceed the local concentration of inhibitors, resulting in a rapid stripping of the cartilage matrix from the fluid phase.

EXTRACELLULAR PROTEOLYSIS–NEUTRAL PROTEASES

MATRIX METALLOPROTEINASES

Collagenase, the first member of the matrix metalloproteinase family (MMPs) to be discovered, specifically cleaves triple helical collagen. This family, when acting together, can degrade all the components of connective tissue matrix. These enzymes are made up of common sequences of amino acids (Fig. 8.2a) and fall into four main groups called the stromelysins, collagenases, gelatinases and membrane metalloproteinases[5,6]. They contain zinc at the active center of each enzyme and are all produced in a proenzyme form which has to be activated by the loss of a peptide before matrix is degraded. Activation can involve other enzymes and some MMPs can activate others; also the membrane-bound MMPs are likely to play an important part in activation. These enzymes, along with stromelysin-3, have a short peptide insert between the propeptide and the N-terminal domain that is recognized by furin[7]. This serine protease is located in Golgi's complex and can activate membrane-bound MMPs and stromelysin-3 so that these enzymes are secreted in an active form. Two of the MMPs (MMP-8 and MMP-9) are found stored within the specific granules of the neutrophil while the others are produced by a variety of connective tissue cells after stimulation by cytokines.

The stromelysins have a broad substrate specificity (see Fig. 8.1). The natural substrates of these enzymes are probably the proteoglycans fibronectin and laminin. Stromelysin-1 is not normally widely expressed but can be readily induced by growth factors and cytokines such as interleukin (IL)-1. The expression pattern of these enzymes is often distinct. This may explain why there are different enzymes with very similar substrate specificity[8].

There are four collagenases: collagenase-1 (MMP-1), collagenase-3 (MMP-13), neutrophil collagenase (MMP-8) and collagenase-4 (MMP-18). These enzymes cleave fibrillar collagens at a single site, producing three-quarter- and one-quarter-sized fragments. The enzymes differ in their specificity for different collagens. Both MMP-1 and MMP-13 are synthesized by fibroblasts and macrophages when these cells are stimulated with inflammatory mediators. Neutrophil collagenase is predominantly synthesized by neutrophils and released upon stimulation of the cell. The way in which collagenase-3 is controlled is not yet known although retinoic acid, which downregulates MMP-1, is known to upregulate MMP-13. However, MMP-13 has a much broader substrate specificity than the other collagenases[9]. It was originally described as rat collagenase; it is now known that rodents do not appear to have an equivalent enzyme to MMP-1.

The structure of porcine collagenase was solved by X-ray crystallography and is shown in Figure 8.2b. The active site zinc is found within the N-terminal domain and a second zinc ion is also present, along with three calcium ions. An exposed linking peptide joins this domain to the C-terminal domain which has a unique structure with four units of repeating β-sheet held together by a disulfide bond and forming a four-bladed propellor[10].

The two gelatinases cleave denatured collagens, type IV and V collagen and elastin. Expression of the 72kDa gelatinase (MMP-2) is the most widespread of all the MMPs; 92kDa gelatinase (MMP-9) is expressed in a wide variety of transformed and tumor-derived cells[11]. The main substrates of the MMPs are summarized in Figure 8.1.

These proteases are involved in the normal turnover of connective tissue matrix that takes place during growth and development, and are implicated in the pathologic destruction of joint tissue. Also, there is an increase in levels of different MMPs in rheumatoid synovial fluid, in conditioned culture media from rheumatoid synovial tissues and

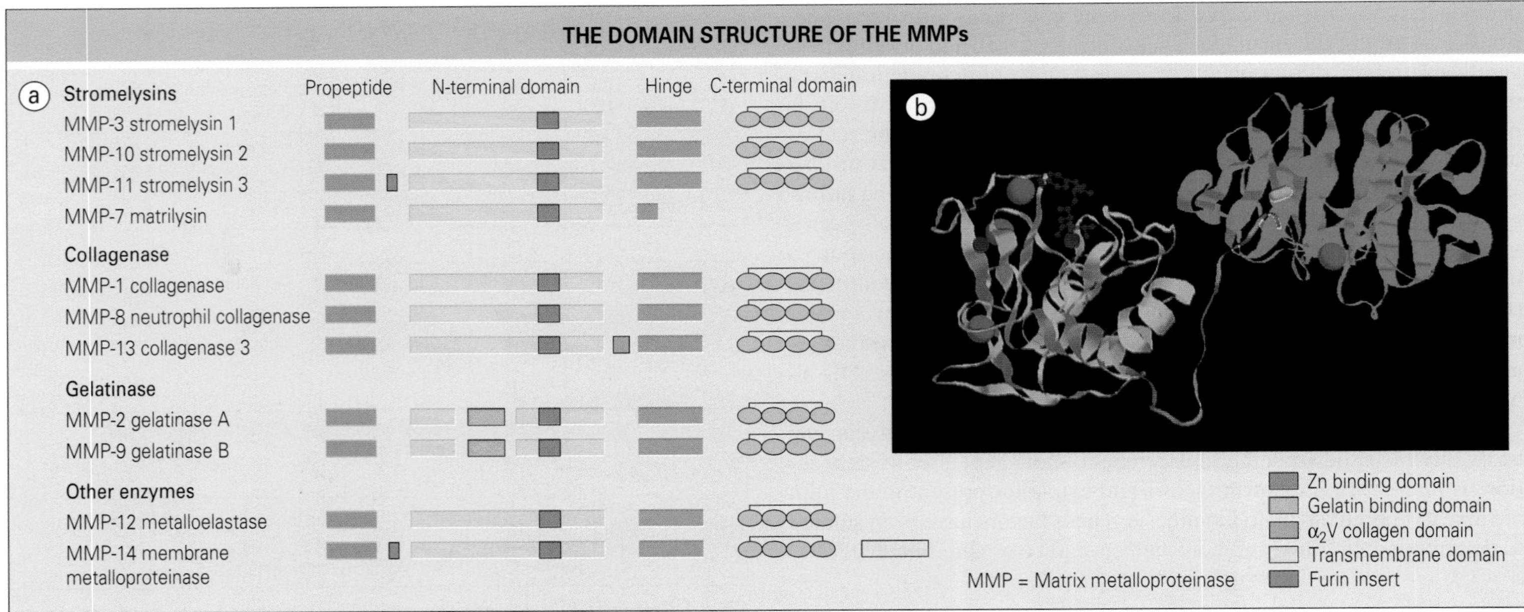

Fig. 8.2 The domain structure of the matrix metalloproteinases (MMPs) (a). The groups of enzymes among the MMPs differ in the matrix components that they cleave. Some enzymes contain inserts of amino acid that change the enzyme's ability to cleave its substrate or bind to other proteins. The structure of porcine MMP-1. The N-terminal domain (yellow) and C-terminal domain (blue) are joined by a highly exposed linking peptide (orange) that is susceptible to cleavage. In the N-terminal domain, two zinc ions (purple) and three calcium ions (green), held tightly into the protein, are essential for either maintaining structure or for catalysis. A synthetic inhibitor (dark blue) of enzyme activity binds to the active site zinc. Similar inhibitors are effective at blocking collagen breakdown *in vitro* and in animal models. The C-terminal domain of the molecule is important for binding to collagen and also increases the binding to tissue inhibitor metalloproteinase (TIMP). A further calcium is found at the center of the so-called four-bladed β propellor, four units of β-sheet which are held together by a disulfide bond (yellow) (b).

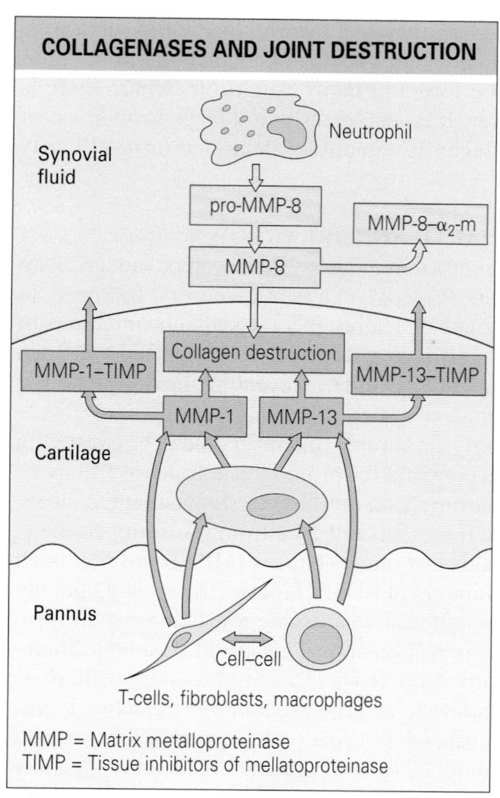

Fig. 8.3 Collagenases and joint destruction. Cell–cell interactions between T-cells, fibroblasts and macrophages within the pannus tissue give rise to a mixture of cytokines and growth factors that act on these cells and on the chondrocytes to increase collagenase-1 (MMP-1) or collagenase-3 (MMP-13). After activation, if local levels exceed the available TIMPs, collagen destruction ensues. Within the joint cavity neutrophils can release neutrophil collagenase (MMP-8) at or close to the cartilage surface where degradation will occur unless α_2-macroglobulin is available.

cells, in synovial tissue at the cartilage–pannus junction from rheumatoid joints and in animal models of arthritis[6].

The MMPs are carefully controlled at a number of different points that include:

- synthesis and secretion,
- activation of the proenzymes and
- inhibition of the active enzymes.

Synthesis and secretion

Both IL-1 and tumour necrosis factor (TNF) have similar properties and affect numerous cell types to produce proinflammatory and degradative effects. The synthesis and secretion of collagenase-1 and stromelysin-1 are stimulated by IL-1 and TNF[12]. Within the arthritic joint there are large numbers of different cell types. Specific cytokines and growth factors differ in their action on individual cell types. Agents may suppress the release of one enzyme while promoting that of another and have different effects in different cells. It is therefore difficult to predict the outcome of blocking the action of individual cytokines to prevent cartilage destruction. These interactions are illustrated in Figure 8.3.

Activation of the proenzymes

Activation of MMP is an important control point in connective tissue breakdown. All MMPs are produced in a proenzyme form[13]. The propeptide is removed proteolytically and this allows the enzyme to hydrolyze peptide bonds. Active stromelysin activates procollagenase, suggesting that, *in vivo*, a cascade mechanism occurs. Plasminogen activators are able to generate plasmin and this enzyme and the membrane MMPs activate some members of the MMPs. Activation is likely to be achieved in a tightly controlled environment close to the cell surface.

Inhibition of the active enzymes

All active MMPs are inhibited by tissue inhibitors of metalloproteinases (TIMPs)[6,14], stable proteins that bind tightly to active MMPs in a 1:1 ratio. After secretion, TIMP-3 is bound by the extracellular matrix; TIMP-4 is predominantly localized in heart tissue. These TIMPs play an important role in controlling connective tissue breakdown by blocking the action of the activated MMPs and preventing activation[15]. If TIMP levels exceed those of active enzyme then connective tissue turnover is prevented. The

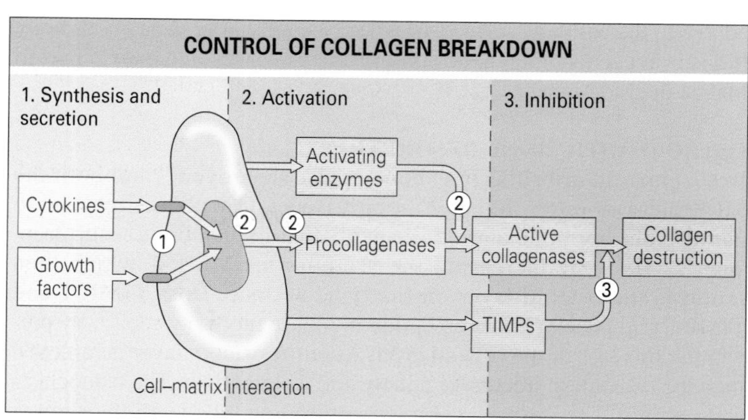

Fig. 8.4 Control of collagen breakdown. The matrix metalloproteinases (MMPs) are controlled by mechanisms that include upregulation by combinations of cytokines and growth factors, activation of the secreted enzymes and the inhibition by tissue inhibitors of metalloproteinases (TIMPs).

mechanisms that control the extracellular activity of the MMPs are illustrated in Figure 8.4 using collagenase as an example.

ENDOGENOUS SERINE PROTEASES

Low levels of endogenous serine proteases are found in cartilage and are likely to be derived from neutrophils[16]. Cartilage contains plasminogen activators, plasmin activity and other serine proteases that may also activate metalloproteinases. It is not known if chondrocytes are able to synthesize and secrete serine proteases but no such enzyme has been purified and characterized from cartilage tissue[17].

PLASMINOGEN-DEPENDENT PATHWAYS

The plasminogen-dependent pathway is implicated in a wide variety of situations where connective tissue matrix is remodeled. Both tissue plasminogen activator and urokinase plasminogen activator are found in cartilage and cleave plasminogen to plasmin. Inhibitors and protease nexins can bind and inactivate the released enzymes. The activity of plasminogen and the activating enzymes is maximized when bound to fibrin or to the cell surface; this localizes the degradation and protects proteases from inhibitors. Many experiments *in vitro* with tissue or cells point to a role for the plasminogen–plasmin system in the activation of pro-MMPs in some situations of matrix turnover[17].

NEUTROPHIL-DEPENDENT PATHWAYS

A large influx of polymorphonuclear leukocytes are often found in joint diseases. Neutrophils contain both serine (elastase and cathepsin G) and metalloproteinases (MMP-2 and MMP-9). Discharge of enzyme-containing granules close to or while attached to the cartilage surface can lead to binding of elastase and damage to the cartilage[18]. Enzymes released into the synovial fluid cannot avoid the inhibitors present such as α_2-macroglobulin (which can inhibit all the classes of proteases), α_1-antiproteinase inhibitor, TIMP-1 and TIMP-2. Once enzymes are complexed they are thought to be cleared from the joint. An excess of inhibitory activity is found in most synovial fluids and so it is unlikely that neutrophil proteases are able to cause damage to the matrix from the fluid phase. In septic arthritis the normal inhibitory capacity of the synovial fluid is exceeded and neutrophil proteases rapidly degrade cartilage from the fluid phase. Large amounts of protease–inhibitor complexes are present in these fluids[6].

Neutrophil serine proteases have a limited role in matrix turnover within the joint and in cartilage matrix. The release of degraded matrix components does not correlate with markers of neutrophil granules. Antigen-induced arthritis in beige mice produce severe cartilage loss, although elastase and cathepsin G are absent and the same loss is also seen if the animals are first depleted of neutrophils[19]. However, these enzymes are capable of degrading cartilage matrix. Where there are neutrophils in inflammatory cellular infiltrates that abut cartilage or adhere to the cartilage surface, or where the inhibitory capacity of body fluids is exceeded, then neutrophil serine proteases may play a part in matrix degradation.

OSTEOCLASTIC BONE RESORPTION

In rheumatoid arthritis (RA) bone is also destroyed[20] and both the MMPs and cysteine proteases are involved[21]. Osteoblasts respond to parathyroid hormone and other agents that induce bone resorption, such as IL-1, by increasing the secretion of MMP-1 which then removes the osteoid layer on the bone surface. Both TIMP-1 and TIMP-2 can prevent bone resorption in mouse model systems[22] by preventing this loss of the osteoid layer. After the osteoid layer is removed then the osteoclast precursors adhere and differentiate. The osteoclasts form a tightly sealed low pH microenvironment beneath their lower surface, which removes mineral and lysosomal proteases, then resorb the exposed decalcified matrix. Cathepsin B-like enzymes are capable of destroying cross-linked collagen matrix at low pH[23].

INTRACELLULAR PATHWAYS – ACID PROTEASES

LYSOSOMAL PROTEASES

The involvement of an intracellular route for the breakdown of cartilage was suggested as cathepsin D (an aspartate protease), and cathepsin B (cysteine) are raised in OA tissue. Cathepsins B, L and H (all cysteine proteases) are found in raised levels in cartilage in antigen-induced rat arthritis. Incubation of resorbing cartilage with specific cathepsin B inhibitors that are designed to cross cell membranes, and so enter the cell, blocked the release of proteoglycan fragments[24].

Lysosomal enzymes probably play a role in connective tissue turnover where fragments of cleaved matrix are engulfed and digested intracellularly. Most of the evidence that points to the existence of an intracellular pathway comes from ultrastructural studies where fragments of material containing the characteristic banding pattern of collagen have been seen within the cell and, in some cases, associated with lysosomal enzymes. Inhibition studies suggest that aspartate and cysteine proteases are involved and possibly MMPs[25]. There is considerable controversy concerning the normal mechanisms of collagen turnover with opinion divided as to the relevant contribution of both intracellular and extracellular pathways. A large number of studies (reviewed by Everts *et al.*[25]) have shown that collagen-containing vacuoles have been found within connective tissue fibroblasts. Some workers consider that these vacuoles contain recently synthesized collagen rather than collagen that was first secreted and then subsequently phagocytozed. However, tissues in which a rapid resorption of connective tissue is taking place, or which have been stimulated to resorb, appear to have an increased number of collagen-containing vacuoles, which suggests that these may be linked to resorption. It is possible that tissue such as the periodontal ligament, in which there is a very high turnover of collagen, predominantly resorb collagen via this route in preference to the extracellular route. Everts *et al.*[25] have suggested that this pathway is the predominant normal pathway in connective tissues and that the extracellular route only predominates in pathologic conditions.

As far as cartilage is concerned, it is known that cathepsin B inhibitors targeted to enter the cell can block resorption induced by IL-1 but not by retinoic acid[24]. It may be the case that MMP inhibitors completely block cartilage breakdown induced by either pathway. However, Buttle *et al.*[24] only looked at proteoglycan degradation and not at collagen turnover. Some authors do not think that there is much normal turnover of the collagen fibrillar network in adult cartilage. Everts *et al.*[25] have proposed the following sequence of events:

1. formation of contacts between the cell and the collagen fibril,
2. segregation of the fibril by cellular processes,
3. partial digestion of the fibril by membrane-bound MMPs and probably gelatinase,
4. intracellular digestion within the lysosomal system by cathepsin B or L.

It should be noted that this sequence of events closely links extracellular events with intracellular events, so it is likely that this close apposition of pathways will be found in many conditions where there is connective tissue turnover. It is also clear that a large proportion of recently synthesized collagen is sometimes degraded intracellularly before secretion.

MODEL SYSTEMS OF CARTILAGE BREAKDOWN

Initiation of cartilage breakdown in model systems can be induced with either IL-1 or retinoic acid. Proteoglycan is released first followed, in some circumstances, by collagen. Highly specific synthetic inhibitors of MMPs completely block cartilage resorption. It is expected that such inhibitors may be of therapeutic benefit in preventing the destruction of cartilage seen in the arthritides[26].

The turnover of proteoglycan is rapid and reversible in contrast with collagen. The enzyme responsible for proteoglycan release from cartilage was thought to be stromelysin until it was shown that the cleavage point in proteoglycan fragments released from resorbing cartilage could not be cleaved by this enzyme[27]. Thus, TIMPs could not block the cleavage, although inhibitors of MMPs blocked the release but only at very high concentration[6]. These results suggest that a metalloproteinase, but not an MMP, is responsible. This could be a membrane-bound protease on the chondrocyte surface. Studies suggest that, as both metalloproteinase and cysteine protease inhibitors can block proteoglycan release from cartilage, multiple pathways could be involved and cartilage resorption induced by different agents could proceed by different pathways or include different activation mechanisms.

The loss of collagen from cartilage is irreversible as any attempt at repair does not lead to restoration of normal cartilage. Whereas IL-1 is sometimes able to initiate cartilage collagen resorption alone, when this cytokine is combined with oncostatin M a rapid and reproducible release of collagen is found in bovine and porcine cartilage[28]. Synthetic inhibitors of MMPs and TIMP-1 and TIMP-2 are able to prevent the release of collagen fragments from the cartilage[29]. This firmly implicates the collagenolytic MMPs in this process. It is known that both collagenase-1 and -3 can be made by chondrocytes. Interestingly, retinoic acid is known to downregulate MMP-1 but increases production of TIMP and of collagenase-3. The breakdown of cartilage in response to retinoic acid may be caused by increased levels of collagenase-3 exceeding the local TIMP concentrations even though the levels of collagenase-1 are reduced.

The future prospects for the prevention of connective tissue breakdown using synthetic protease inhibitors look promising. Compounds that inhibit the MMPs are the most advanced[30]. It is likely that treatment with such agents will shift the balance away from degradation of matrix to preventing the loss of connective tissue matrix without leading to excess synthesis. There were early problems with the oral availability of these compounds. Some inhibitors are active in animal models and initial clinical trials should soon begin. It will be interesting to see if blocking one MMP with some inhibition of others is sufficient to halt the progressive and chronic destruction of connective tissue seen in the arthritides. If the release of connective tissue fragments drives joint inflammation leading to a chronic cycle of damage then these compounds could be effective on their own. It may be necessary to combine different protease inhibitors, either in sequence or with other agents that hit different specific steps in the pathogenesis before the chronic cycle of joint destruction found in these diseases can be broken[6] (Fig. 8.5).

REPAIR OF CONNECTIVE TISSUE MATRIX

Within arthritic tissues there are areas of cartilage where synthesis of new matrix takes place and areas where net loss of the extracellular matrix occurs. The chondrocytes are intimately involved in both these processes. Polypeptide growth factors have a profound effect on chondrocytes and it is apparent that these factors play a major role in the regulation of the synthesis of normal matrix as well as in the processes that are involved in the destruction of cartilage in disease. These agents

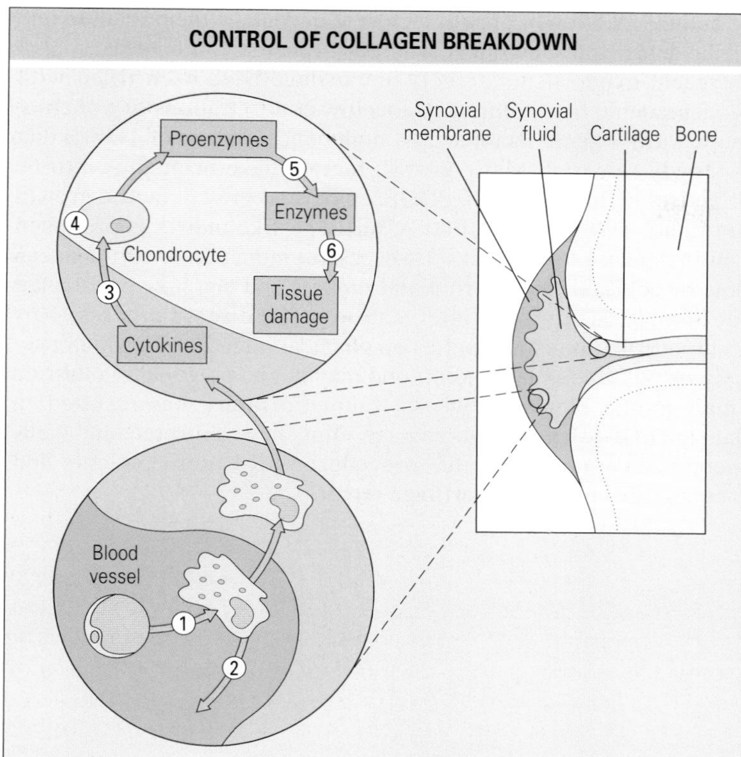

Fig. 8.5 Therapeutic intervention points for preventing connective tissue destruction. The destructive cycle of events can be broken in a number of ways, including: (1) blocking entry of harmful cells; (2) removal of harmful cells from the joint; (3) blocking or mimicking cytokine or growth factor action; (4) blocking intracellular signaling pathways; (5) preventing activation of proteases; (6) direct inhibition of destructive protease.

act on chondrocytes via cell surface receptors coupled to intracellular signaling pathways. Other factors, such as hormones, corticosteroids, prostaglandins, peptides or retinoids, may also influence the response of any particular cell type to these growth factors.

Cartilage metabolism may be influenced by effects on cellular proliferation, migration or differentiation or the control of individual genes (Fig. 8.6). The effect of any particular growth factor will also depend on the state of differentiation of the cell. Various types of cells in tissues may well respond differently to particular cytokines and growth factors. Other local conditions will affect the response of individual tissues such as mechanical loading, oxygen tension and the presence of other factors (Fig. 8.6).

Transforming growth factor (TGF)-β and insulin-like growth factor (IGF)-1 are acknowledged as having profound effects on the synthesis of matrix components by chondrocytes. Details of these growth factors have been well reviewed[31,32]. Transforming growth factor-β can also downregulate the production of matrix-degrading proteases and upregulate protease inhibitors such as TIMP or plasminogen activator inhibitor, suggesting that TGF-β may prevent cartilage destruction by both stimulating synthesis and blocking breakdown pathways. It can also generally affect protein synthesis by chondrocytes and has been found to potentiate the stimulation of DNA synthesis achieved with other growth factors, rather that initiating this itself[33]. Although TGF-β is locally synthesized by chondrocytes, IGF-1 mimics many of the actions of TGF-β, but it does not have the mitogenic properties of, or generally affect protein synthesis to the extent found for TGF-β.

These growth factors are recognized as having a generally protective effect on cartilage, stimulating matrix resorption and blocking the effects of the proinflammatory cytokines. Other factors also show similar protective effects in some circumstances. Interferon (IFN)-γ inhibits cytokine-stimulated bone resorption and IL-1- or TNF-stimulated collagenase production by chondrocytes as well as reducing IL-1-stimulated prostaglandin release from cartilage. Interleukin-4, -13 and -10 have recently been shown similarly to oppose the effects of the proinflammatory cytokines by blocking protease secretion, and increasing inhibitor production and matrix synthesis. Also, IL-4 and -13 can protect cartilage by blocking matrix resorption induced by IL-1.

Other growth factors can affect cartilage homeostasis by inducing cells to migrate, differentiate or proliferate. Platelet-derived growth factor (PDGF) has a mitogenic effect on chondrocytes and can stimulate collagenase production in some connective tissue fibroblasts. Fibroblast growth factor (bFGF) stimulates DNA synthesis in chondrocytes in culture and can also stimulate plasminogen activator inhibitors and TIMP in fibroblasts and endothelial cells.

All these factors are likely to stimulate repair within cartilage. However, growth factors do not act alone and many are known to act synergistically in promoting matrix synthesis. Within the cartilage, TGF-β and IGF are synthesized by the chondrocytes and are stored in considerable quantity within the matrix, bound to different matrix

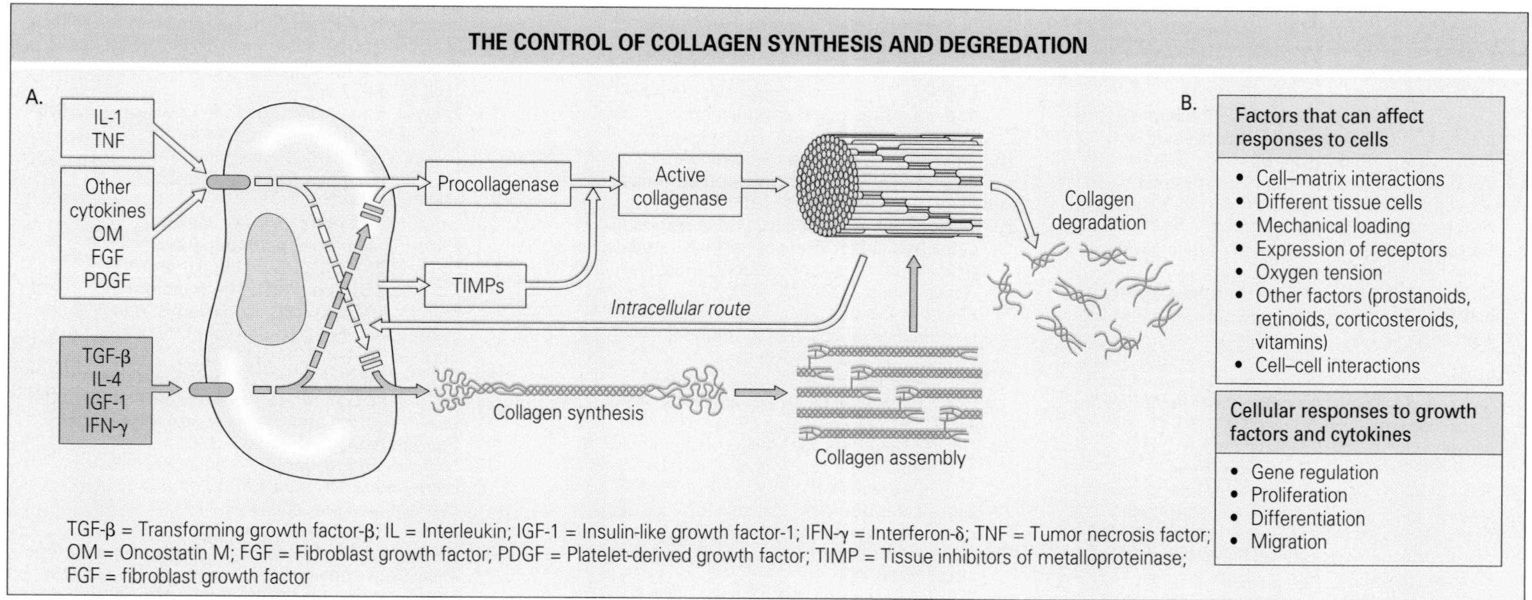

Fig. 8.6 The control of collagen synthesis and degradation. Increased synthesis of collagen or protease inhibitors, often linked to reduced production of proteases, is found after treatment with a variety of growth factors which include transforming growth factor-β, interferon-γ, insulin-like growth factor-1 and interleukin (IL)-4. IL-1 and tumor necrosis factor-β increase the production of proteases and reduce collagen synthesis. Other agents, such as oncostatin M, fibroblast growth factor and platelet-derived growth factor can also influence this process. Pathways that increase synthesis and reduce degradation are shown in red; pathways that increase degradation and reduce synthesis are shown in yellow (a). Other factors can alter the cellular response to these stimuli, and cells can respond to growth factors in a number of ways (b).

components. Thus the source of these growth factors will vary. They can be produced by cells outside the cartilage and diffuse in, or they can be produced locally by the chondrocytes or released from the matrix as it is degraded. The control mechanisms are thus complex and growth factors often exist in a latent form. Other proteins may also be present that sequester the factors and prevent them from binding to cellular receptors.

MODELS OF MATRIX REPAIR

Increasing interest is being shown in the possibility that defects found in diseased or damaged cartilage can be repaired after the delivery of agents that will stimulate chondrocytes to synthesize new matrix[34]. Different approaches have been used, including:

- the isolation of chondrocytes, which are grown in culture and then implanted into defects at high density;
- grafting of cartilage into large defects;
- filling of defects with various natural or synthetic polymers;
- and the addition of growth factors to encourage the migration into the defect and subsequent synthesis of matrix components.

In recent experiments defects in cartilage have been filled with biodegradable matrix that contains low concentrations of a chemotactic or mitogenic factor with a high concentration of TGF-β that is slowly released. Many growth factors have been shown to be effective, including bFGF, PDGF, epidermal growth factor, growth hormone, TGF-β and IGF-1. A cartilage-like matrix is produced within defects after 6 weeks[35]. Successful induction of cartilage can now be achieved in experimental models and can now be adapted for clinical use to allow intervention in the disease process. This technique is limited as it relies on physical intervention which may only be possible in large joints and may not be practical in multiple small joints. However, where traumatic injury has resulted in damage to cartilage, or where large joints have a discrete and well-recognized injury, then this procedure will benefit patients and increase the chances of cartilage repair.

REFERENCES

1. Prockop DJ, Kivirikko KI. Collagens; molecular biology, diseases, and potentials for therapy. Annu Rev Biochem. 1995;64:403–34.
2. Hardingham TE, Fosang AJ. Proteoglycans: many forms and many functions. FASEB. 1992;6:861–70.
3. Jubb RW, Fell HB. The breakdown of collagen by chondrocytes. J Pathol. 1980;130:159–62.
4. Barrett AJ. Introduction to the history and classification of proteases. In: Barrett AJ, ed. Proteases in mammalian cells and tissues. Amsterdam: Elsevier NH, 1977:1–55.
5. Woessner JF. Matrix metalloproteinases and their inhibitors in connective tissue remodeling. FASEB. 1992;5:2145–54.
6. Cawston TE. Metalloproteinase inhibitors and the prevention of connective tissue breakdown. Pharm Ther. 1996;3:163–82.
7. Pei D, Weiss SJ. Furin-dependent intracellular activation of the human stromelysin-3 zymogen. Nature. 1995;375:244–7.
8. Nagase H. Human stromelysin 1 & 2. Methods Enzymol. 1995;248:449–70.
9. Dioszegi M, Cannon P, Van Wart HE. Vertebrate collagenases. Methods Enzymol. 1995;248:413–31.
10. Li J, Brick P, O'Hare MC, *et al.* Structure of full length porcine synovial collagenase reveals a C-terminal domain containing a calcium-linked four-bladed propeller. Structure. 1995;3:541–9.
11. Murphy G, Crabbe T. Gelatinases A and B. Methods Enzymol. 1995;248:470–84.
12. Goldring MB. Degradation of articular cartilage in culture: regulatory factors in joint cartilage degradation. In: Woessner JF, Howell DS, eds. Joint cartilage degradation. New York: Marcel Dekker; 1993:281–345.
13. Kleiner DE Jr, Stetler-Stevenson G. Structural biochemistry and activation of matrix metalloproteinases. Curr Biol. 1993;5:891–7.
14. Murphy G, Willenbrock F. Tissue inhibitors of matrix metalloendopeptidases. Methods Enzymol. 1995;248:496–510.
15. Denhardt DT, Feng B, Edwards DR, Cocuzzi ET, Malyankar UM. Tissue inhibitor of metalloproteinases (TIMP, aka EPA): structure, control of expression and biological functions. Pharmacol Ther. 1993;59:329–41.
16. Birkedal-Hansen H, Moore WGI, Bodden MK, *et al.* Matrix metalloproteinases – a review. Crit Rev Oral Biol Med. 1993;4:197–250.
17. Nagase H, Woessner JF. Role of endogenous proteases in the degradation of cartilage matrix. In: Woessner JF, Howell DS, eds. Joint cartilage degradation. New York: Marcel Dekker, 1993:159–85.
18. Sandy JD, Sriratana A, Brown HLG, Lowther DA. Evidence for polymorphonuclear leukocyte derived proteases in arthritic cartilage. Biochem J. 1981;193:193–202.
19. Schalkwijk J, Joosten LAB, Van den Berg WB, Van de Putte LBA. Antigen induced arthritis in beige mice. Ann Rheum Dis. 1990;49:607–10.
20. Oyajobi BO, Russell RGG. Bone remodelling, cytokines, and joint disease. In: Kuettner K, *et al.* Articular cartilage and osteoarthritis. New York: Raven Press; 1992:333–48.
21. Everts V, Delaiss J-M., Korper W, *et al.* Degradation of collagen in the bone-resorbing compartment underlying the osteoclast involves both cysteine-proteinases and matrix metalloproteinases. J. Cell Physiol. 1992;150:221–31.
22. Hill PA, Reynolds JJ, Meikle MC. Inhibition of stimulated bone resorption *in vitro* by TIMP-1 and TIMP-2. Biochim Biophys Acta. 1993;1177:71–4.
23. Barrett AJ, Buttle DJ, Mason RW. Lysosomal cysteine proteases. Institute for Scientific Information, Atlas of Science. Biochemistry. 1988;1:256–60.
24. Buttle DJ, Bramwell H, Hollander AP. Proteolytic mechanisms of cartilage breakdown: a target for arthritis therapy? Clin Pathol: Mol Pathol. 1995;48:167–77M.
25. Everts V, Van Der Zee E, Creemers L, Beertsen W. Phagocytosis and intracellular digestion of collagen, its role in turnover and remodelling. Histochem J. 1996;28:229–45.
26. Vincenti MP, Clark IM, Brinkerhoff CE. Using inhibitors of metalloproteinases to treat arthritis. Easier said than done? Arthritis Rheum. 1994;37:1115–26.
27. Sandy JD, Flannery CR, Neame PJ, Lohmander LS. The structure of aggrecan fragments in human synovial fluid: evidence for the involvment in osteoarthritis of a novel protease. J Clin Invest. 1992;89:1512–16.
28. Cawston TE, Ellis AJ, Humm G, *et al.* IL-1 and oncostatin M in combination promote the release of collagen fragments from bovine nasal cartilage in culture. Biochem Biophys Res Commun. 1995;215:377–85.
29. Ellis AJ, Powell LK, Curry VA, Cawston TE. TIMP and TIMP-2 prevent the release of collagen fragments in cartilage stimulated with IL-1. Biochem Biophys Res Commun. 1994;201:94–101.
30. Gordon JL, Drummond AH, Galloway WA. Metalloproteinases as therapeutics. Clin Exp Rhematol. 1993;11(Suppl 8):91–4.
31. Roberts AB, Sporn MB. The transforming growth factors. In: Sporn MB, Roberts AB, eds. Peptide growth factors and their receptors. Heidelberg: Springer-Verlag; 1990:419–72.
32. Rechler MM, Nissley PS. Insulin like growth factors. In: Sporn MB, Roberts AB, eds. Peptide growth factors and their receptors. Heidelberg: Springer-Verlag; 1990:263–336.
33. Morales TI. Polypeptide regulators of matrix homeostasis. In: Kuettner K, *et al.* Articular cartilage and osteoarthritis. New York: Raven Press; 1992:265–80.
34. Hamerman D. Prospects for medical intervention in cartilage repair. In: Woessner JF, Howell DS, eds. Joint cartilage degradation. New York: Marcel Dekker; 1993:529–46.
35. Tyler JA, Hunzinker E. Articular cartilage regeneration. In: Brandt K, Lohmander S, Doherty M. Osteoarthritis. Oxford: Oxford University Press; 1996 (in press).

9

THE MUSCULOSKELETAL SYSTEM

Peter A Simkin

Summary
- Malfunctions of the musculoskeletal system are the principle focus of rheumatology.
- The major tissues that constitute the musculoskeletal system include bones, cartilage, ligaments and tendons, synovium, bursae, and skeletal muscle.
- Pathologies of these tissues compromise the supportive and mechanical functions of the musculoskeletal system.

INTRODUCTION

All multicellular organisms require a skeletal structure to provide support and to facilitate mechanical function. So fundamental is this role that terms such as 'skeletal' and 'bare bones' are regularly used to denote the most basic elements of any plan. Just as an architect's plans vary in response to the proposed use of a building, musculoskeletal designs vary in accordance with the needs of each species. Among mammals, for instance, specific plans have evolved to meet the unique activities of the tree shrew, the hippopotamus, the giraffe, the blue whale, the cheetah and the human being. In each of these examples, the musculoskeletal system comprises the same fundamental building materials and it serves the same basic needs. Among these are requirements for stable support, for facilitation of work, for protection of vital organs and for growth and renewal over the lifetime of the individual.

Stable support is perhaps the most fundamental role of organized structure in any living thing. When one is as stationary as a tree, a coral, or an oyster the supporting structure may be relatively simple while still providing both a framework for other systems and positioning for subsistence in a competitive world. The issue becomes greatly complicated when mobility is also required. Then the animal must have the characteristics of a living machine with the biological analogs of engines, bearings and levers arranged in a manner that enable it to perform work.

Malfunctions of this machine provide the principal focus of clinical rheumatology. It is the afflictions and vulnerabilities of the musculoskeletal system that form the core of rheumatologic practice and the primary content of this book. This chapter introduces the components of this system and provides a brief overview of their integrated function in normal people.

The relative preponderance of musculoskeletal tissues provides one indication of the importance of this system to total body function. In elderly cadavers, muscle and bone respectively account for 50% and 21% of fat free mass, and these values would surely be higher in young, normal subjects[1–5]. Other critical musculoskeletal components include the tensile connectors represented by tendons and ligaments, the flexible interfaces provided by cartilage and the unique synovial tissue that lines and supports most mammalian joints (see Fig. 9.1). All musculoskeletal tissues are of course supplied by the circulation and guided and protected by their innervation, but the components of those systems are not reviewed here.

MUSCULOSKELETAL TISSUES

STRIATED MUSCLE

Skeletal muscle provides the engine or driving force for musculoskeletal activity. It is here that the chemical energy derived from foodstuffs is ultimately converted to the mechanical energy required to do work.

Individual striated fibers are bundled in perimysial tissue that transmits the force of muscle contraction through tendons to attachments on bone (Fig. 9.2). Each fiber can do work only in the direction of its long axis. It is the great variety of arrangements within muscles and the cooperation between muscles that permits the full range of human activities.

From the raw power of a well-trained weight lifter to the digital dexterity of an accomplished musician, all musculoskeletal motion is driven by the same basic contractile units. To achieve simple motions more than one muscle may act together by adding forces, as do the biceps and the brachialis in elbow flexion. The work of these agonists is closely coordinated with opposing antagonists – in this case the triceps. Often gravity contributes a significant additional force. Thus, in the upright individual, elbow extension may be driven by gravity and controlled by relaxing flexor muscles while the triceps extensor plays a largely passive role. Similarly, the tibialis anterior muscle, an ankle extensor, plays its most important role in controlling ankle flexion after heel strike in the normal gait cycle. This active 'relaxation' which is also known as 'eccentric contraction', has been likened to the gradual 'playing out' of rope as a suspended load is safely brought to earth.

Synergism is the remaining major form of muscle interaction. Synergistic muscles work together to drive motions that no one of them could produce alone. At the wrist, for instance, muscles at the 'four corners' (radial and ulnar sides, dorsal and volar aspects) interact to produce adduction, abduction, flexion, extension and circumduction. Each of these actions requires a different combination of muscles. A somewhat different example of synergism occurs when one muscle, or set of muscles, positions a joint to facilitate or enhance the mechanical advantage of other muscles. Again, using the wrist as an example, the extensor muscles 'cock' the wrist to increase the power of the finger flexors when one 'makes a fist'. In the intact person, not only the wrist but also the arm and the rest of the body must be coordinated to put that fist in position to perform its intended role. Thus, the mechanics of human activities are never simple but require the complex interactions of many synergistic muscle groups.

BONE

Essentially no muscle contraction would be effective unless it could produce directed motion through a skeletal lever. Each effective motion comes about as muscles act on bones to move the limbs, head or torso. In some cases, such as the transverse and spinous processes of vertebrae, the lever function is obvious and the mechanical advantage is relatively good. In many others, however, the mechanical advantage is poor and muscles must exert substantial transarticular compressive forces in order to generate the desired moment. To initiate flexion of phalangeal joints for instance, there must be many pounds of articular compression for each pound of flexor force exerted. The bones of the skeleton have evolved in a way that withstands and distributes these normal forces as well as the minor impacts involved in everyday trauma. Only in the case of a marked overload does the normal skeletal support fail with resultant fracture of bone.

Bone is characterized by the deposition of hydroxyapatite crystals in a well-organized collagenous matrix. When bone is newly formed, as in a child or in a healing fracture, this matrix is relatively loose and the bone is described as 'woven'. With full maturation, however, the bone becomes denser and better adapted to load bearing, especially under compressive forces.

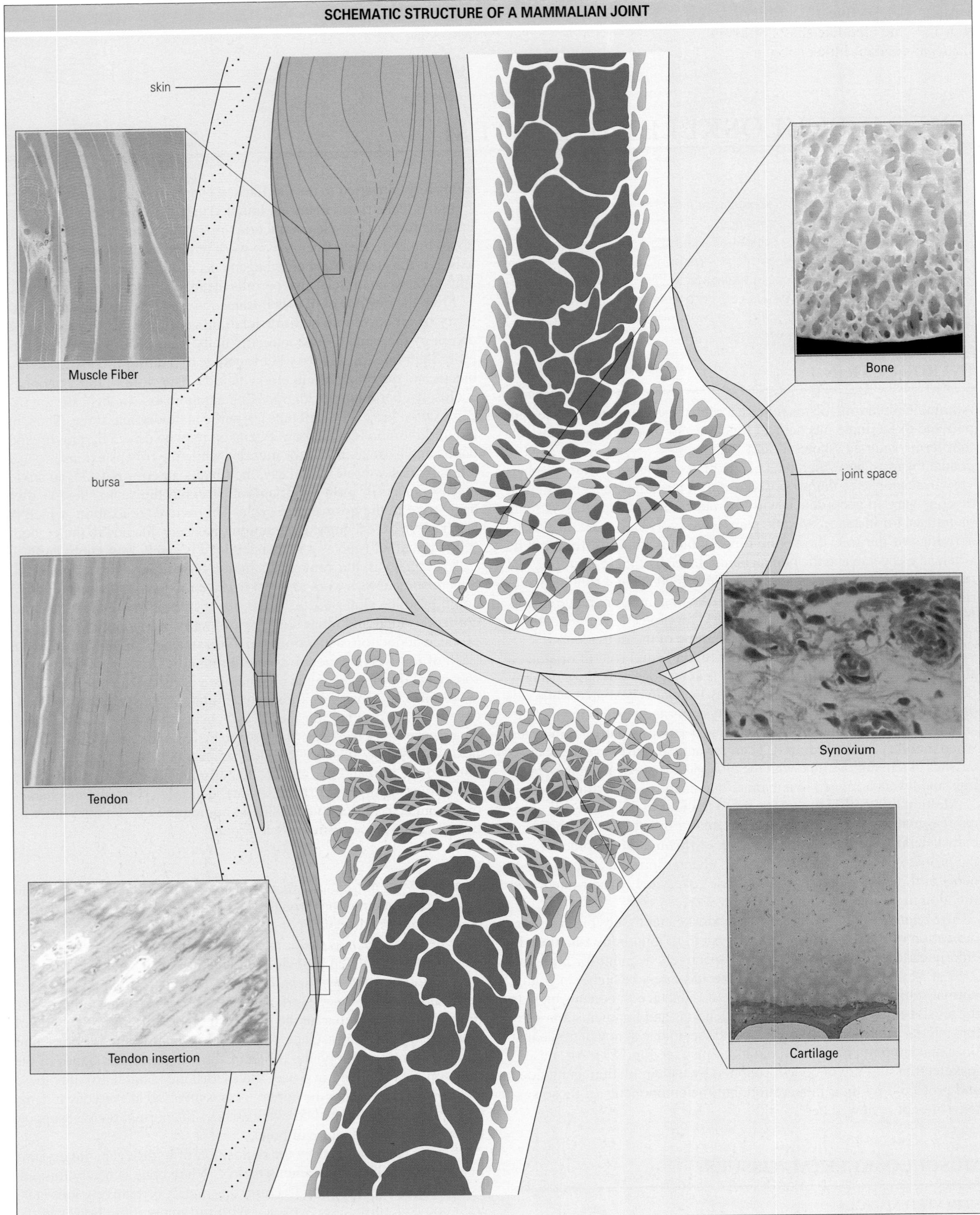

Fig. 9.1 Schematic structure of a mammalian joint. The histologic appearances of the main tissues are highlighted. The thin layers of synovial fluid in the joint and in the bursa are exaggerated for clarity.

Mature bone is histologically described as compact (dense) or trabecular (spongy) (Fig. 9.3). Compact bone is predominant, and most typical, in the pipe-like shafts of long bones. There, the mid-shaft or diaphysis contains little or no internal osseous structure, but a marrow cavity largely filled with fat and loose interstitial tissue. The bone itself undergoes regular haversian remodeling and is covered by a sensitive periosteum that is capable of new bone formation. Compact bone is also found in the subchondral plate of concave joint members such as

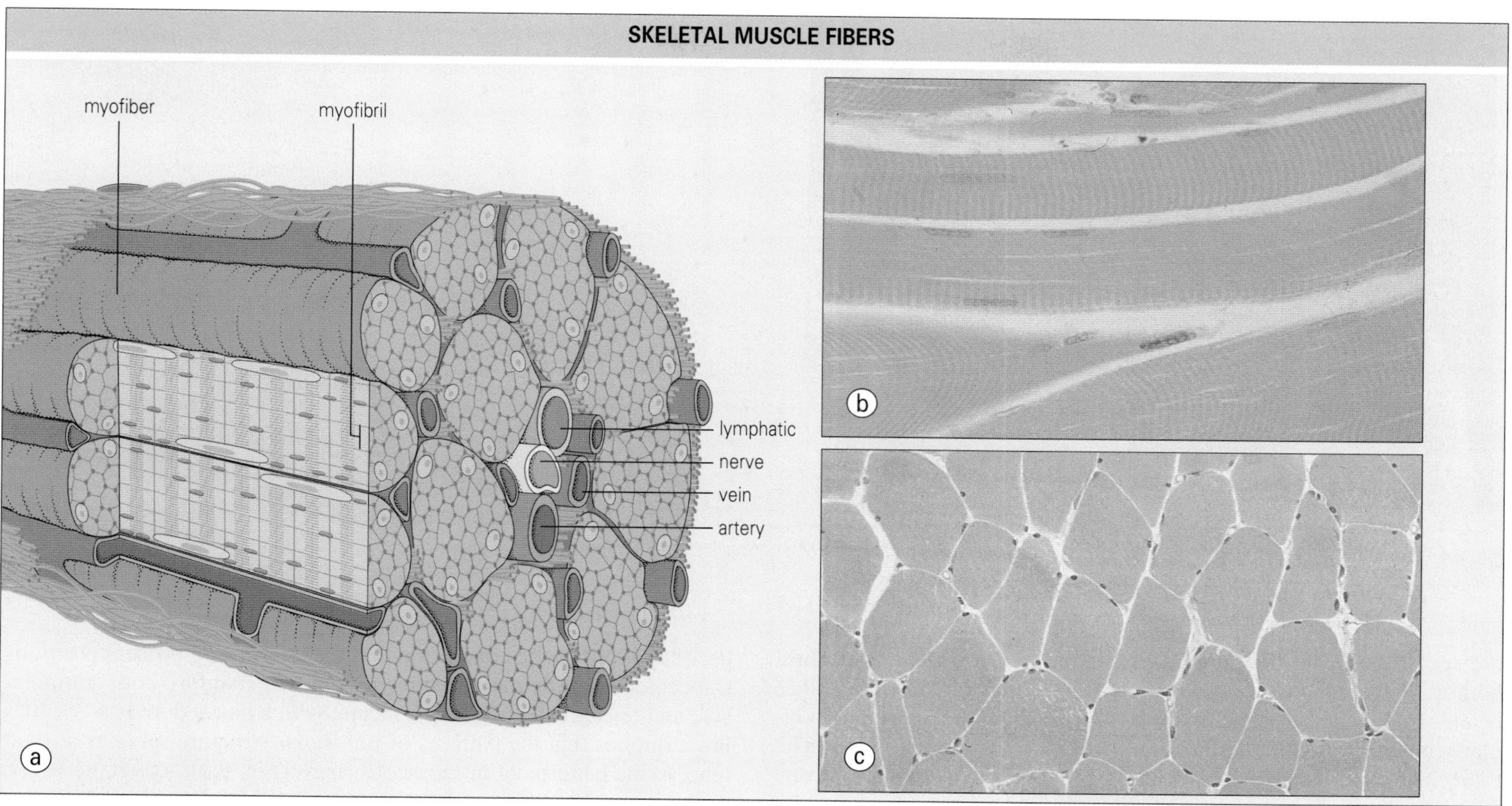

Fig. 9.2 Skeletal muscle. Schematic diagram of a muscle bundle (a). Micrograph of skeletal muscle fibers in a longitudinal section show prominent cross striations (b). Micrograph of skeletal muscle fibers in a transverse frozen section illustrating the roughly hexagonal profiles (c). Reproduced with permission from Stevens A, Lowe J. Histology, 2E. London: Mosby, 1992.

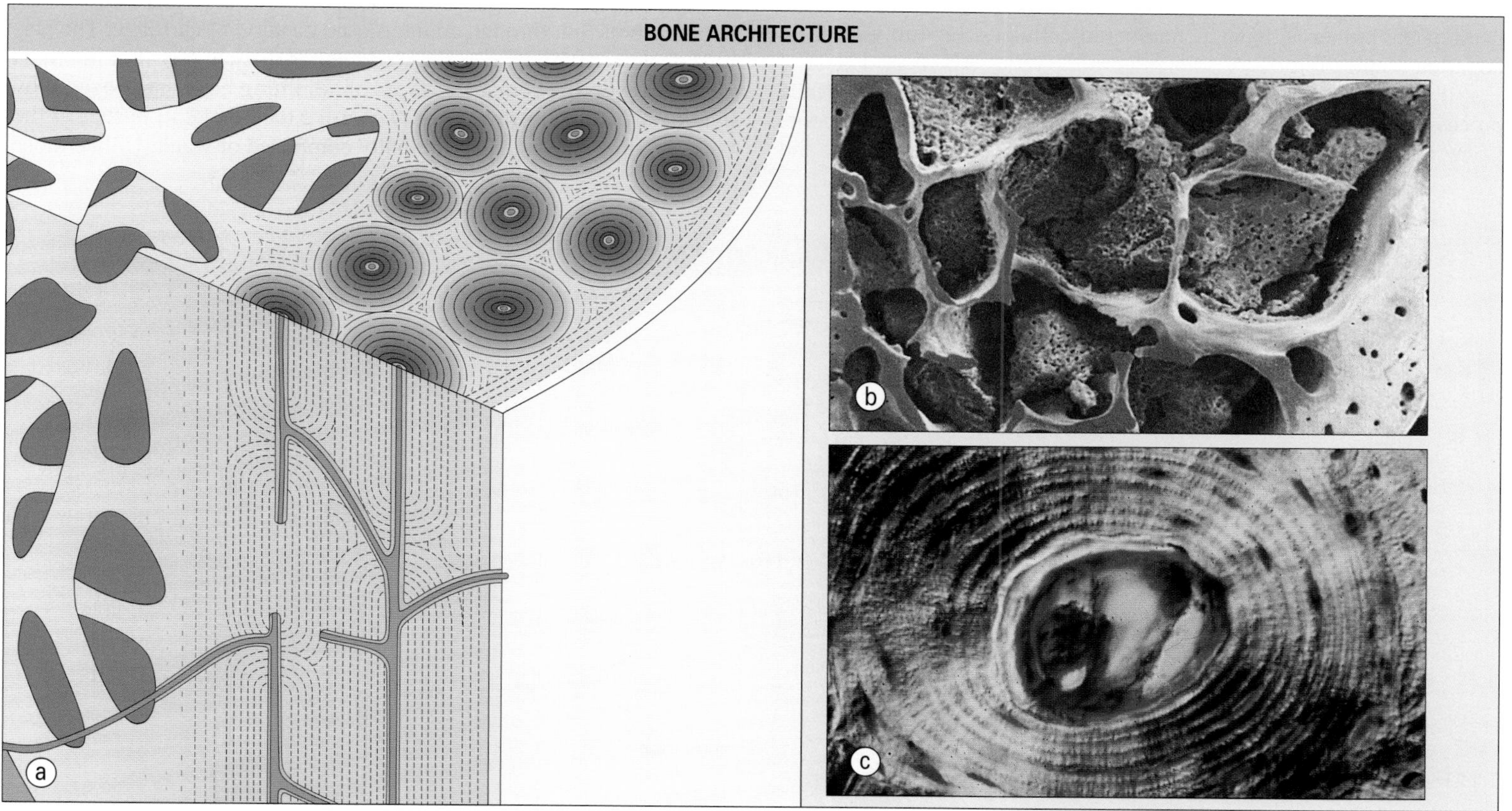

Fig. 9.3 Bone architecture. Schematic diagram showing transverse and longitudinal cuts through the shaft of a long bone. The cortical shell (foreground) is haversian bone while the more central trabeculae are lamellar bone (a). Low power scanning electron microscopy showing the cortical and trabecular architecture of bone (b). Polarizing micrograph of a single osteon (haversian system) showing concentric pattern of bone deposition (c). Reproduced with permission from Stevens A, Lowe J. Histology, 2E. London: Mosby, 1992.

TRABECULAR PATTERNS IN THE HIP

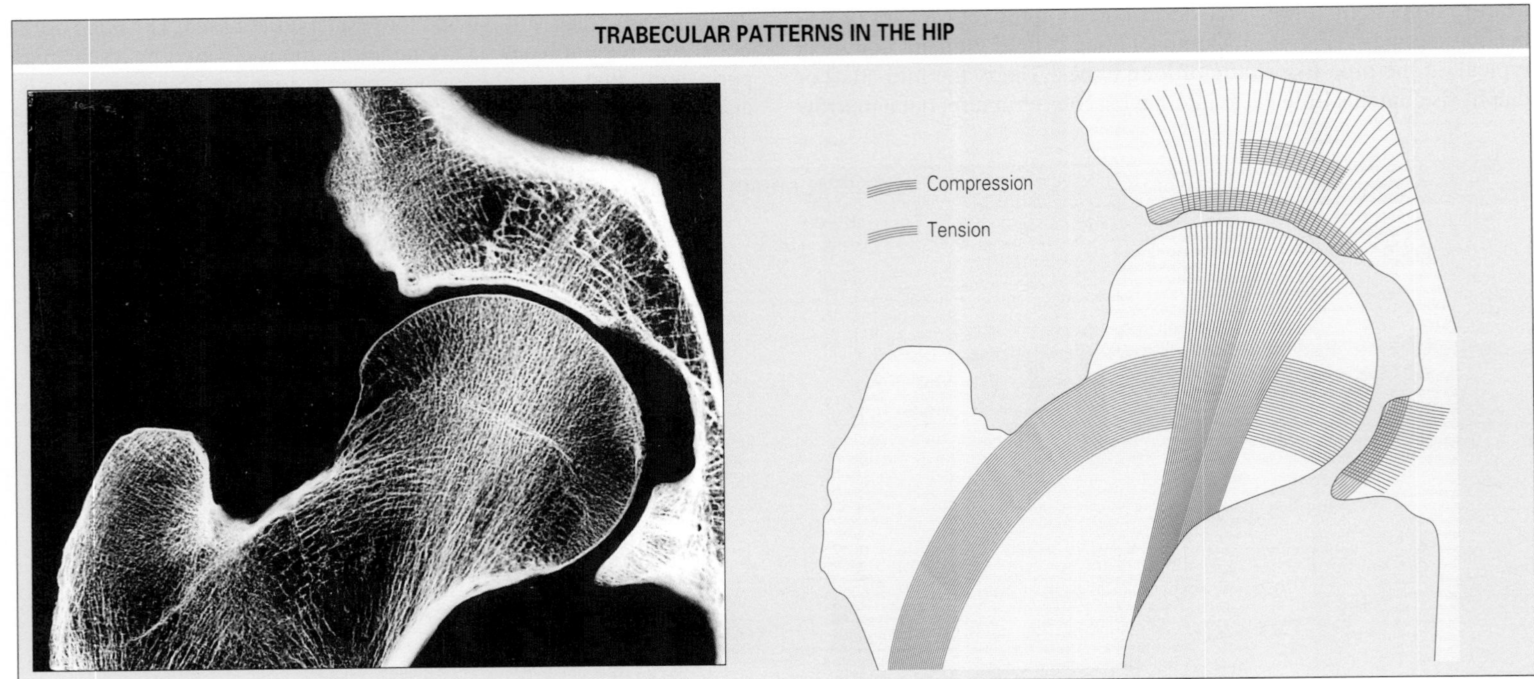

Fig. 9.4 Trabecular patterns. Radiograph of a 3mm slab cut through both bones of a normal hip. The compressive and tensile trabecular patterns are shown schematically on the right.

the acetabulum and the glenoid fossa, and in the walls of vertebral bodies. Trabecula is a term derived from Latin roots meaning 'little beam'. In bone it is applied to the cross-braced architecture found regularly beneath articular surfaces and within the vertebral bodies. The trabecular pattern varies considerably from one site to another. In vertebral bodies it characteristically forms vertical 'plates' connected by horizontal 'struts'. In low stress areas it may form a lace-like three-dimensional filigree which maximizes the continuum throughout adjacent marrow spaces. In contrast, areas subjected to substantial compressive stress, such as the subchondral bone of the patella or the head of the humerus, have a chambered cellular structure with little apparent connectivity.

All trabeculae undergo remodeling through ongoing surface processes of osteoclastic resorption and osteoblastic formation of bone. Long ago observations of trabecular patterns in the femoral neck and head led Wolff to the conclusion that the remodeling process positions trabeculae for maximal effectiveness in withstanding both compressive and tensile stresses. This concept, which has endured as 'Wolff's law', implies that the patterns of trabecular structure serve as a 'road map' to the patterns of intraosseous stress (Fig. 9.4). As yet, however, we have not been able to read the messages inherent in the varying trabecular designs described above.

CARTILAGE

When one bone articulates with another the contact is not directly bone-on-bone but through an interposed cushion of cartilage. The various designs of joints are reviewed later in this chapter. For the most part, however, the contact surfaces of adjoining bones are covered by hyaline articular cartilage (Fig. 9.5). Like the other soft tissues of the body, hyaline cartilage is principally composed of water. Unlike those

ARTICULAR CARTILAGE

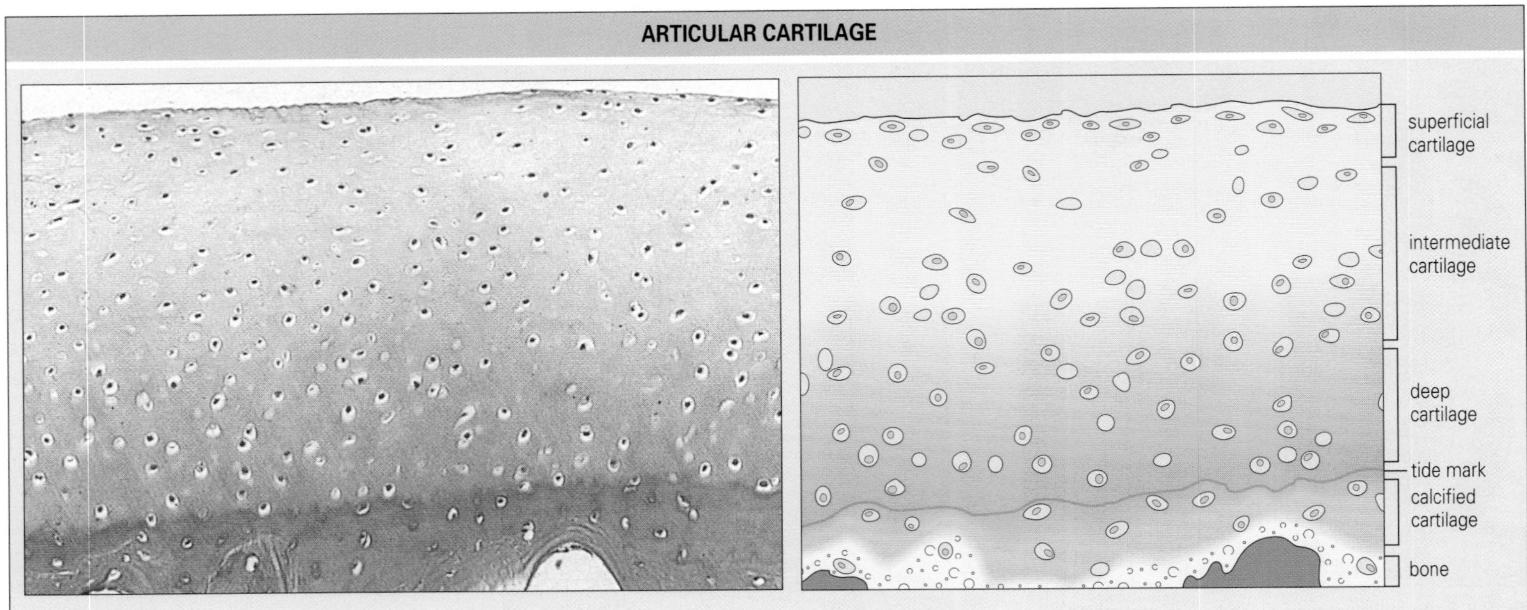

Fig. 9.5 Cartilage. Photomicrograph of articular cartilage over the subchondral bone. On the right is a schematic drawing illustrating the different zones within the cartilage.

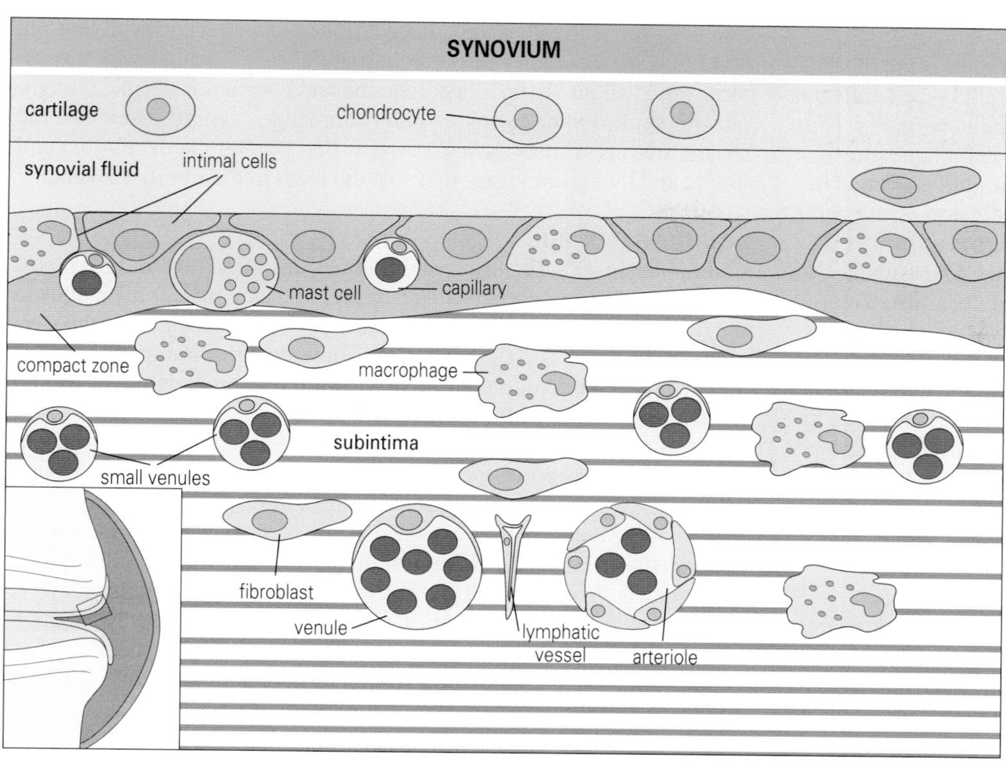

Fig. 9.6 Synovium. Schematic illustration of synovium showing the delicate synovial lining resting on a fibroadipose subintimal layer rich in capillaries, lymphatics and nerve endings.

other tissues, however, normal hyaline cartilage is remarkably firm and resilient. The reason for its striking consistency lies in a unique system of pressurization that makes this tissue a turgid gel. Proteoglycan aggregates, restrained within an arching framework of type II collagen fibers, provide the basis for a tissue pressure that may be as great as three or more atmospheres. Such aggregates are largely made up of chondroitin sulfate and keratan sulfate. The high density of fixed negative charge within these moieties gives each the expansile properties of a coiled spring. It is the net outward thrust of these electrostatic forces that renders articular cartilage firm and resilient. When the proteoglycans are lost, as they are in a variety of articular diseases, the cartilage softens and loses its resilience. Chondromalacia, a term derived from the Greek roots for 'cartilage' and 'soft', describes this stage in the progress of joint diseases. Normal articular cartilage is not static but undergoes continuing turnover and renewal akin to that in other tissues. The principal players in this process are the chondrocytes that are individually quite active but are sufficiently sparse in their distribution that the overall metabolic activity of cartilage is relatively low. The biochemistry of proteoglycan turnover, and of chondromalacia, is developed in detail in the chapter on osteoarthritis (Chapter 8.6).

Perhaps in part because of its turgor, normal hyaline cartilage lacks both blood vessels and nerves. This means that the nutritional needs of chondrocytes must be met by the vasculature of adjacent tissues. For the most part, this is thought to be a function of synovial microvessels. Synovial fluid then becomes the vehicle that carries nutrients to chondrocytes and returns their metabolic wastes to the blood stream. The concomitant absence of nerves may be a blessing to patients with arthritis. Damage to cartilage alone cannot be painful. Thus the pain of arthritis always indicates involvement of adjacent soft tissues or of subjacent bone.

Not all cartilage is hyaline. Fibrocartilage is an alternative design often found at sites subjected to shearing forces under tensile stress. Examples include the crescentic menisci over each tibial plateau and the principal load-bearing region in the roof of the acetabulum. Histologically similar fibrocartilage also joins the ribs to the sternum and unites the anterior pelvis at the pubic symphysis. This tissue actually fills an intermediate place between hyaline cartilage and the dense connective tissue of ligaments and tendons. Its cells are still recognizable as chondrocytes in characteristic lacunae, but they are found within a surrounding matrix that is more notable for its fibrous component (in this case mainly type I collagen) than for its proteoglycan composition.

SYNOVIUM

Although it is the least substantial in bulk, the synovium is among the most important articular tissues. This is clearly true for clinicians since this tissue is the seat of the many inflammatory conditions known collectively as 'synovitis'. Fundamentally a living lining, the synovium covers all intra-articular surfaces other than the articulating areas of cartilage. The synovium itself is shallow with a normal depth of 25–35μm. Perhaps its most characteristic feature is a seemingly well-organized matrix composed of numerous microfibrils and abundant proteoglycan aggregates. Within this matrix lie the synovial cells[6]. These have traditionally been classified morphologically as macrophage-like type A cells and fibroblast-like type B cells. The precise origins and interrelations of these cell types are uncertain and it now seems more important to remember the respective protective and synthetic capabilities of the synovium than to allocate these roles to specific cell populations[7].

All synovial cells loosely interdigitate without tight intercellular junctions. The lining is sometimes described as 'one to three cell layers deep'. This phrase accurately reflects the paper-thin quality of the tissue but implies a laminar arrangement of cells that is not obvious on inspection (Fig. 9.6). Among the normal synovial cells are occasional resident mast cells as well as rare leukocytes that are presumably in transit between plasma and synovial fluid.

The synovial lining is sometimes classified in terms of its subjacent connective tissue. Thus, areas of 'areolar', 'fibrous' and 'adipose' synovium respectively overlie regions of loose, dense and fatty connective tissue. These in turn reflect both the overall design of each joint and the physical stresses upon its lining. Areolar areas often withstand substantial tensile stress as the tissue expands or contracts with joint motion. The cartilaginous surfaces that comprise the knuckles, for instance, are covered by a thin layer of synovium that then 'accordions' out of the way as extension of the fingers brings the phalangeal bases back from the volar to the distal aspects of the metacarpal heads. This stretching and contracting presumably leads to corresponding changes in the thickness of the synovium and in the depth of its supporting vascular and neurologic elements. The structure and the functions of these critical components of normal synovium as well as their relationship to synovial fluid are reviewed in Chapter 1.10 on joint physiology.

LIGAMENTS AND TENDONS

Dense connective tissue plays a number of important roles in the machinery of the body. Ligaments are strong bundles of parallel type I collagen fibers that serve as 'check reins' to prevent inappropriate motions. Thus each 'hinge' joint, for instance, is bordered by collateral ligaments that largely limit its motion to flexion and extension. Similarly, a broad ligament across the flexor surface prevents hyperextension of the same joints. Every ligament runs from bone to bone. For the most part they cross joints and connect one bone with its neighbors. Occasionally, as in the transverse ligament of the atlas, they run between insertions on different parts of the same bone. Ligaments resemble tendons histologically (Fig. 9.7). Tendons, however, serve as active drivers of joint motion whereas ligaments are passive restraints. Both tendons and ligaments insert into bone at anatomic sites known as entheses. At these loci, the collagenous extraosseous fibers are continuous with the 'Sharpey's fibers' of the bone itself. Entheses are of interest to clinicians primarily because of their vulnerability to the inflammatory disease, ankylosing spondylitis and its related 'spondyloarthropathies' (see Chapter 6.13).

TENDON SHEATHS AND BURSAE

As they connect muscle bodies to sometimes distant insertion sites, tendons often run through sheaths that preclude adherence to adjacent tissues along their paths. Similarly, points of potential friction such as those between ligaments, bony prominences and overlying skin are often protected by lubricating bursae. These flimsy structures are little more than flattened sacks whose opposing inner surfaces slide freely against each other as the less forgiving, overlying tissues move. Both tendon sheaths and bursae are lined by a tissue that is histologically indistinguishable from synovium, and they contain a film of fluid that also appears synovial. It is perhaps not surprising then that tendon sheaths and bursae are often targets of the same inflammatory diseases that affect synovial joints.

CLASSIFICATION OF JOINTS

SYNARTHROSIS

Articulations permit motion between adjoining bones. This primary role is met by various designs depending on the respective requirements for motion and stability. These demands are unique between the adjoining plates of the skull and it is not surprising that they are met by a singular design. Here the rate of motion is the glacial pace of growth as the skull slowly enlarges to accommodate the maturing brain. Here, too, the need for stability is great as the bones unite to form a sturdy helmet that protects the soft and vulnerable brain. The solution is an interlocking suture line that 'sews' together the adjacent bones in an exceptionally strong bond that grows readily throughout maturation. When growth is complete, articulations are no longer required and bony union occurs throughout the skull. Other forms of barely movable 'synarthroses' are the strong, fibrous 'syndesmoses', such as that joining the distal tibia and fibula, and the 'gomphoses' that seat the teeth in their bony sockets.

AMPHIARTHROSIS

In amphiarthroses, the articulating bones are joined by an interposed segment of flexible fibrocartilage. Such joints are most conspicuous in the rib cage where costal cartilage joins the ends of each rib to the sternum. These tissues easily bend to accommodate respiratory excursions and also provide a tough but flexible union that protects the heart and lungs during chest wall trauma.

Similar bonds provide an element of flexibility to the pelvic ring. At the pubic symphysis, fibrocartilage forms a sturdy union that may bend more readily than bone during acute trauma. In response to the hormone, relaxin, these bonds normally loosen in late pregnancy to provide a more generous birth canal. At the rear of the pelvic ring, the sacroiliac joints are somewhat more mobile and are synovial in design. In older subjects of either sex the range of sacroiliac motion diminishes markedly although bony ankylosis (fusion across the joint) does not usually occur[8].

Intervertebral discs provide a special form of amphiarthrosis between adjoining vertebral bodies. Here a thin plate of fibrocartilage, the vertebral end plate, forms a boundary between the trabecular bone within each vertebral body and the proteoglycan-rich nucleus pulposus. The latter forms the bulk of the disc material. It is bounded and restrained by the circumferential annulus fibrosus that ties each vertebra to the next. The interposed nucleus provides a unique hydraulic system that distributes loading forces broadly across the vertebral end plates and stores loading energy within the surrounding annulus fibrosus.

DIARTHROSIS

The diarthroses, or synovial joints, are by far the most common type of articulation and they are clearly the most important joints in clinical rheumatology. These are the joints that are actively driven by muscles and tendons, are stabilized by ligaments, are cushioned by hyaline cartilage and are both nourished and lubricated by synovial tissue (Fig. 9.8).

In mechanical terms, synovial joints are 'journal bearings'. In each of them the normal design consists of two well-lubricated contact surfaces that slide across, against or around each other. A film of synovial fluid lubricates both the bearing itself (cartilage-on-cartilage) and the adjacent interfaces of synovium-on-cartilage and synovium-on-synovium. These additional contact areas reflect the surface redundancy required to facilitate the full range of motion of each synovial joint.

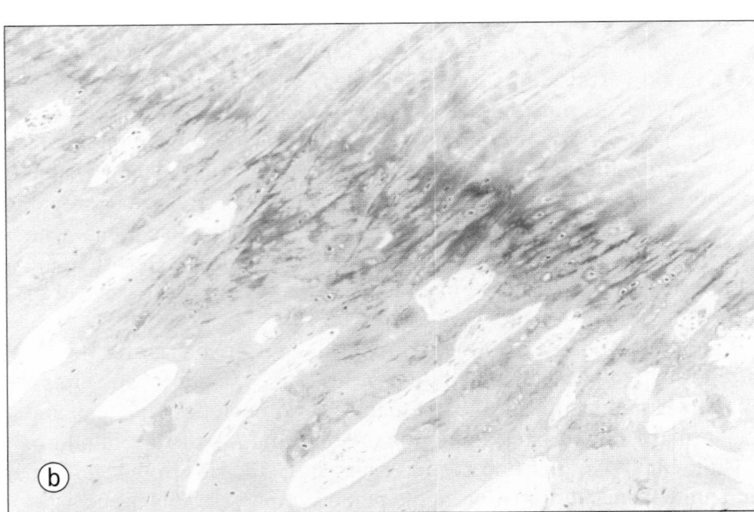

Fig. 9.7 Tendon. Micrograph of tendon showing the organized bundles of collagen (a). Tendon insertion showing a population of chondrocytes at the bone–tendon interface and the collagen fibers crossing the interface (b). Courtesy of Dr John Clark.

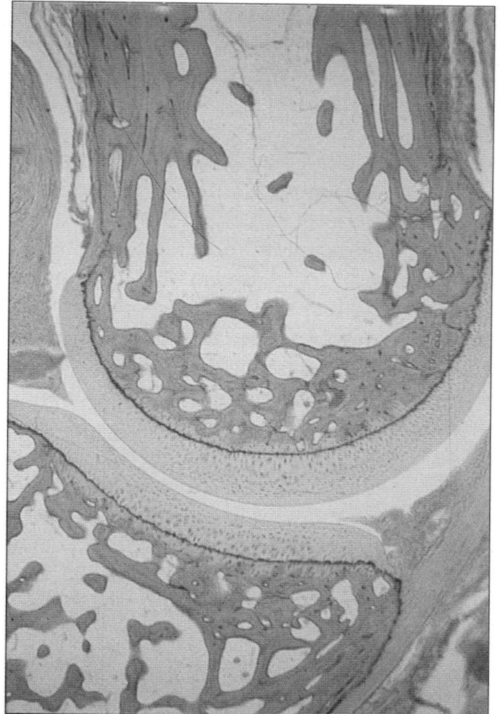

Fig. 9.8 The diarthrodial joint. Reproduced with permission from the Clinical Slide Collection on the Rheumatic Diseases, copyright 1991. Used by permission of the American College of Rheumatology.

As a finger extends, for instance, the dorsal synovial surface will contract and the volar surface will expand, while these roles then reverse during flexion. Both tissue elasticity and accordian-like folding and unfolding are involved. Not surprisingly, these functions can be compromised by the tissue hyperplasia and edema of chronic synovitis with resultant stiffness and loss of full joint motion.

FORM AND FUNCTION OF SYNOVIAL JOINTS

UNIAXIAL

Joints move along one or more axes of motion. Among uniaxial joints, the 'hinge' provides a classic model exemplified by the elbow joint (Fig. 9.9). Here, the distal ulna flexes and extends around the proximal humerus. As this occurs, the contact surfaces of cartilage slide against each other with a concave member to some extent enclosing its opposing convex mate. Essentially all of the former is a contact surface throughout flexion and extension. In contrast, the convex member has a much larger surface, only part of which articulates at any time. This disparity of surface areas largely defines the range of each hinge joint. Other articulations such as the knees and metacarpophalangeals, also mainly flex and extend, but they have subtle, but important, additional motions.

The only significant joint motion that does not require disparate surface areas is the pivot action best exemplified by the head of the radius and the humeral capitellum during pronation and supination of the forearm. Here, one surface simply spins against the other. Opposing contact areas are also comparable at many plane joints where normal motion is minimal. Examples include the sacroiliac and many intertarsal and intercarpal articulations.

POLYAXIAL JOINTS

Just as the 'hinge' is the classic uniaxial joint, the 'ball and socket' is the classic polyaxial joint exemplified both by the hip and the shoulder (Fig. 9.10). The basic motions permitted are not only flexion and extension but also abduction (away from the midline), adduction (towards the midline), rotation and any combination of these. Other configurations of polyaxial joints include ellipsoid joints, such as the wrist, that may flex, extend, abduct and adduct but cannot rotate. They can, however, combine their primary motions sequentially in a motion known as circumduction. Similar motions are also achievable through the 'saddle' configuration found at the base of the thumb. In each of these examples a configuration has evolved that meets the needed range of motion while preserving maximal stability.

STABILITY

To achieve directed motion, articular surfaces must slide upon each other yet that sliding must track along precise paths. For most activities, the joints serve as fulcrums and the adjoining bones as lever arms. An unstable, sloppy fulcrum compromises the lever's work just as a sliding ladder base imperils the workman who has climbed it. The

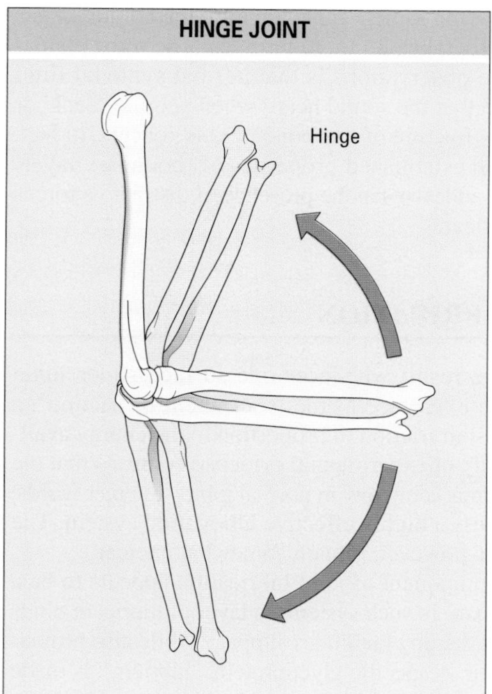

Fig. 9.9 The elbow joint between the humerus and ulna is a hinge joint and is capable only of flexion and extension.

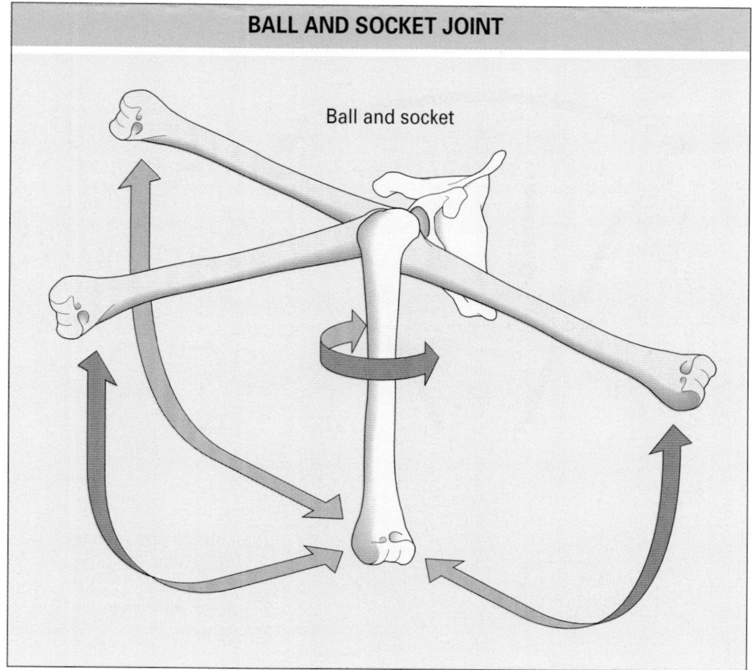

Fig. 9.10 The shoulder is a polyaxial, ball and socket joint.

requisite stability is brought about by four principal mechanisms:

- the shape of the joint components,
- the 'check rein' role of ligaments and capsule,
- the active guidance of muscles and tendons crossing the joint, and
- the adhesive properties of synovial fluid reinforced by atmospheric pressure.

SHAPE

Most limb motions are arc-like and arise from opposing nearly congruent convex and concave surfaces of articular cartilage (Fig. 9.11). In this configuration, the concave member forms a 'socket' that serves to restrain the opposing 'ball'.

Only two human joints really fit this classic 'ball in socket' model. In the hip, a relatively deep acetabulum retains the femoral head throughout its normal range of motion. In the shoulder, the glenoid fossa is much shallower and additional mechanisms are needed to stabilize this most mobile of human joints. In both the hip and the shoulder, the hemispherical shape of the contact surface facilitates rotation as well as flexion, extension, abduction and adduction. Most joint surfaces, however, are oblate rather than hemispherical, with long and short radii of curvature resembling the surface of an American football or rugby ball. This configuration facilitates motion in the direction of the short axis and prevents rotation just as an egg cannot be spun along its long axis if it is constrained within a spoon. In almost all joints, the fit of opposing surfaces confers at least a measure of stability.

LIGAMENTS

Ligaments usually run from one bone to its partner and form a tough but flexible limit to inappropriate joint motions. The collateral ligaments of interphalangeal joints, for instance, remain taut throughout flexion and extension and thereby prevent abduction and adduction. In the same joint a thickened portion of joint capsule, the 'volar plate', overlies the flexor aspect and provides a ligamentous check against hyperextension.

Since ligaments are purely passive restraints, they do their jobs without an energy cost. This economy is particularly important in the hips and knees which 'lock' in extension during simple standing. The strong ligaments that provide this support thus permit relaxation of the major muscles that drive these joints. In contrast, there is no comparable ligamentous check at the ankle and the leg muscles therefore must continue to expend energy during otherwise relaxed standing.

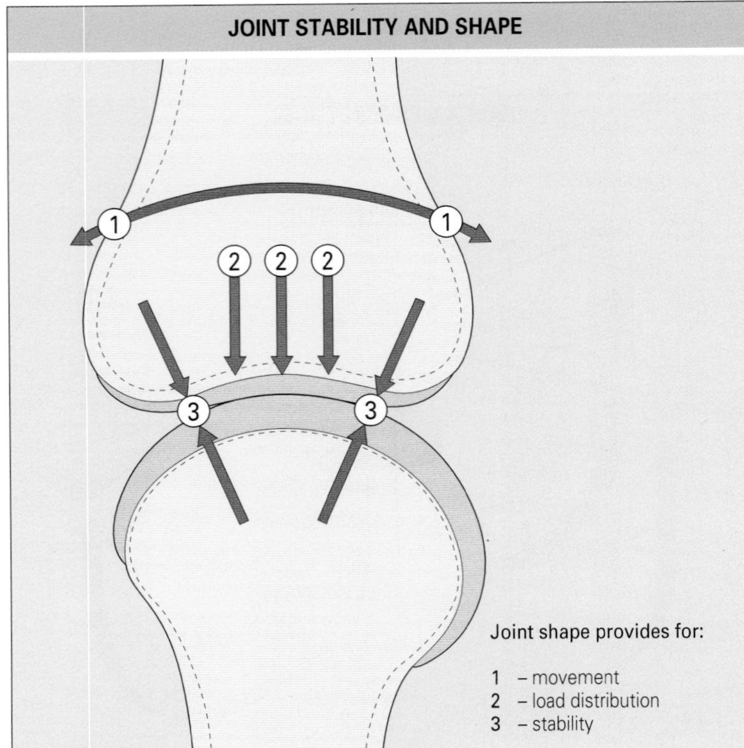

Fig. 9.11 Joint stability and shape.

MUSCLES AND TENDONS

When muscles act, the force of their contraction drives the joint members together. In fact, the mechanical advantage of most muscles is so poor that much more energy goes into joint compression than is spent on useful work. The 'up side' of this expenditure lies in the stability conferred when interlocking joint members are driven together. Unlike ligaments, muscles change their length as they contract or relax and thus their tendons provide a stabilizing factor even in the direction of joint motion. Since all tendons are strong ties that cross joints, they may all be considered to be factors promoting joint stability. Some, however, are obviously more involved as stabilizers than are others. Perhaps the best example of this role is that provided by the 'rotator cuff' muscles of the shoulder. This inner layer of muscles arises on the scapula and forms a vault around the humeral head beyond which it inserts in an inverted 'U'. These small muscles serve to seat the humeral head in the glenoid fossa throughout all shoulder motions and to resist the distracting vectors of the more powerful outer muscles that act across this joint[9].

THE SYNOVIAL FLUID BOND

As important as the rotator cuff is, its muscles need not contract to maintain shoulder contiguity when a relaxed arm hangs at the side. The joint does not sublux under the force of gravity because its members are in effect 'glued' together. Part of this property is simple atmospheric pressure. At sea level, a force of fifteen pounds per square inch weighs on all exterior surfaces and acts against distraction of adjacent tissues. Thus, if the surface area of the glenoid fossa was one square inch, a force of fifteen pounds would be required to induce distraction even though all shoulder muscles were completely relaxed.

Evidence from studies of normal human third metacarpophalangeal joints indicates that an additional adhesive factor is involved. If the contact surface of this small joint is roughly one square centimeter, a force of about one kilogram should overcome the stabilizing force of atmospheric pressure. In fact, however, it takes a pull of ten kilograms to distract this joint[10]. At the instant of distraction, there is an audible 'knuckle crack', a gas bubble appears within the joint, and both the bubble and significant distraction become recognizable radiographically. This phenomenon is readily distinguished from audible crepitus and other mechanically induced articular or periarticular sounds by the subject's inability to crack the same joint again until the bubble of gas has dissolved. This usually takes 20 to 30 minutes. The most plausible explanation for these observations is that normal synovial fluid serves as an adhesive and that the sound heard when people 'crack' or 'pop' their knuckles is the fracture of this bond[11]. This concept, in fact, is entirely consistent with established properties of 'boundary layer' lubricants which serve as adhesives in the presence of distractive forces but as lubricants under shear.

FRICTION AND LUBRICATION

Friction is the inevitable result whenever one surface slides upon another. Its extent is best expressed as the 'coefficient of friction', a measure of the energy cost in friction in proportion to the energy available for work. A large body of experimental evidence confirms that the coefficient of friction is remarkably low in normal joints. In other words, this means that they possess a highly effective lubrication system. The mechanics of that system, however, remain somewhat unclear.

The most important component of joint lubrication appears to be a 'boundary layer' mechanism. In such systems, a layer of lubricant binds to the bearing surface and thereby facilitates slippage while also providing protection against wear. A specific glycoprotein, 'lubricin', is made within synovial joints and appears to be the principal binding substance.

On the surface of cartilage, lubricin may then bind water which through its cohesion with bound water on the opposing cartilage provides the bond described in the preceding section on joint stability. This simple picture has been made more complex by evidence that not only lubricin but also phospholipids may play an important boundary layer role.

Hydrodynamic lubrication is a second process that appears to contribute to the low friction found in synovial joints. In this mechanism, motion of the joint generates a layer of fluid that then serves to cushion and separate the bearing surfaces. As we have seen, articular cartilage is a hydrated gel backed by a continuous layer of subchondral bone.

When a region of cartilage is compressed under load, a portion of its fluid content may flow laterally and exude from the adjacent, unloaded surface. As joint motion proceeds to load that area in turn, the exuded fluid provides a cushion. In this fashion, as in related examples of hydrodynamic lubrication, motion of the loaded joint plays the principal role in sustaining a fluid layer between opposing faces of cartilage.

When a loaded convex cartilage slides across its concave mate, their interface experiences a high degree of shearing stress. In contrast, shear is low when the same convex cartilage opposes unloaded synovium. The lessened shear forces comparably diminishes the potential friction and therefore ameliorates the lubrication problem. It is in the low shear setting that the hyaluronan of synovial fluid is thought to play a role. Hyaluronan makes the fluid viscid like the white of an egg. This resemblance reportedly led Paracelsus to coin the term 'synovia' (like egg) in the early 16th century. It is hyaluronan that allows the synovial surfaces to slide easily against each other and over the exposed articular cartilage. The effectiveness of this system is best attested to by the rarity of synovial pinching during the normal use of joints.

DISTRIBUTION OF LOADING FORCE

Although shear stresses across joints can be minimized by an effective lubrication system, there is no comparable mechanism to reduce the compressive stress of articular loading. Instead, the various tissues of the joint share this burden through an impressive system of energy distribution. When this system fails, the overloaded tissue fractures or ruptures with resultant pain and disability. A number of different tissues participate in the normal system.

SKELETAL MUSCLE

Skeletal muscle offers by far the most important means of distributing loading energy. It often does so by subtly giving way as it accepts the load, just as a hard-thrown ball is caught best by 'soft hands' that yield as they accept the ball's energy. Thus at heel strike in normal walking, the ankle, knee and hip are all in flexion. The extensor muscles of these joints then accept much of the impact of the stride. When the energy level is greater, as in a jump from a height, the role of extensor muscles is more obvious as each joint flexes farther while their extensor muscles 'play out rope' by actively lengthening under load. To appreciate the extent of this contribution, imagine simply jumping down from the height of a chair and landing with fully extended hips and knees, The jolt of that impact would jar every organ system, including the brain, and could easily lead to fractures as the energy of the drop was distributed not through the adjacent muscles but directly through the bones and joints.

CARTILAGE

Of that loading energy that does reach the joint, it long seemed obvious that the highly resilient articular cartilage must be an important biological 'shock absorber'. Indeed, the physical properties of cartilage are quite appropriate for this role. Its extent, however, is not. There is simply not enough thickness of cartilage in the load-bearing line to accept a major portion of impact energy[12].

SUBCHONDRAL BONE

In contrast to the shallow layers of articular cartilage, a deep region of trabecular bone adjoins essentially all synovial joints (Fig. 9.12). This structure is both flexible and elastic. It thus is able to store impact energy while bending, just as the springs on a bed or an automobile do. The energy is then recovered as elastic recoil when the joint is unloaded. In contrast to the shock absorption of skeletal muscle, the elastic behavior of trabecular bone does not require energy to absorb energy and thus is, in this respect, a more attractive mechanism. There are limits, however, on the load-accepting capacity of juxta-articular bone. This is particularly true of concave articular members. If such a surface flexes, its constituent parts are driven away from each other and a fracture failure may ensue. On the opposite side of the joint, however, the convex member behaves like a 'Roman arch' in that its constituent parts are driven together or compacted under load. It thus can flex and still remain strong. It is because of these principles that the 'subchondral plate' of a concave joint member must be significantly thicker and less compliant than that of the opposing convex mate[13].

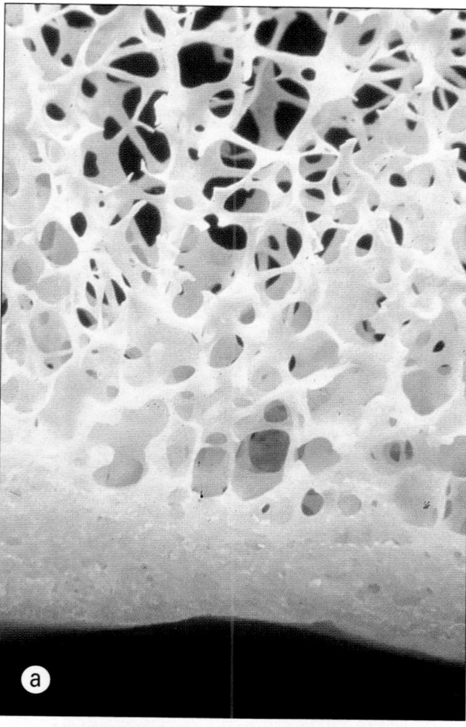

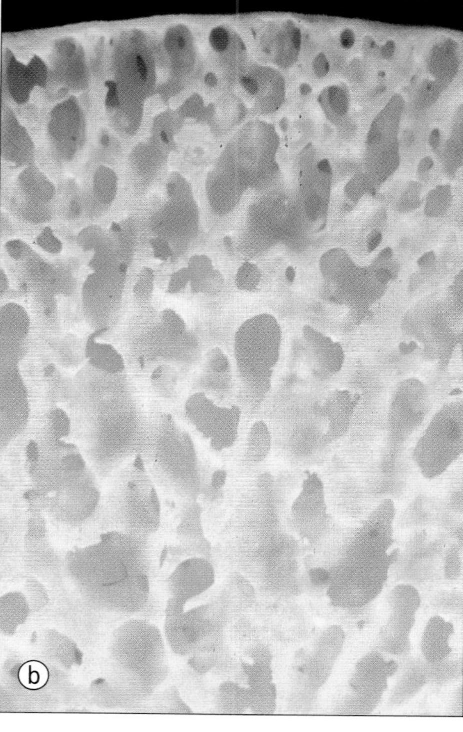

Fig. 9.12 Subchondral bone. A 3mm slab from the acetabulum (a) appears above another from the femoral head of a normal human hip (b). Both have had soft tissues, including cartilage, removed and are seen at low magnification. The acetabulum has a much thicker subchondral plate and a more open trabecular structure.

MUSCULOSKELETAL DEVELOPMENT

Musculoskeletal development begins early in embryonic life with the appearance of limb buds for each of the four extremities. Within these growing blastemic structures, cellular condensations form and define the primordial skeletal components (Fig. 9.13). These condensations chondrify with dense cellular interzones, indicating the future sites of synovial joints. Articulations then arise as the interzones cavitate to form a complete model of cartilaginous bones and synovial joints well before the end of the embryonal period (Fig. 9.14). These rapid-fire events have been the subject of extensive embryologic study intensified by the clinical problem of teratogenesis. Physical malformation may occur without known antecedents or after a viral infection in early pregnancy. Its most marked association, however, is with embryonal exposure to the teratogenic drug thalidomide. Early exposure to this agent may result in complete or partial absence of long bones and or hand and foot components, but the patterns are highly variable and the precise mechanism remains uncertain. This lack of predictability underscores the continuing need for a better understanding of fetal development.

By the end of the embryonal period (approximately 60 days) the bones and synovial joints have all appeared and the course from there on is essentially one of growth and development (Fig. 9.15). Use of the joints appears to be essential during fetal growth to permit development of the normal muscular and skeletal configuration and to prevent fibrous ankylosis of joints that have initially cavitated in a normal fashion.

By the time of birth, the primary growth centers of most bones have completed the transition from the earliest, avascular anlage, through a purely cartilaginous model, past the early vascularization and calcification of that model, to the presence of true bone. Most of the secondary growth centers in the epiphyses remain in the vascularized cartilage stage at birth and begin to form bone during infancy.

As development progresses through childhood and adolescence these growth centers account for most of the length gained. This process involves a cartilaginous proliferation at the growth site so that from the earliest ossification of the cartilaginous prototype to the ultimate physeal closure in full-sized young people, most new bone formation can be described as endochondral. From the time of birth, the lifelong process of bony remodeling is also underway, however, and both apposition and resorption occur on trabecular, endosteal and periosteal surfaces.

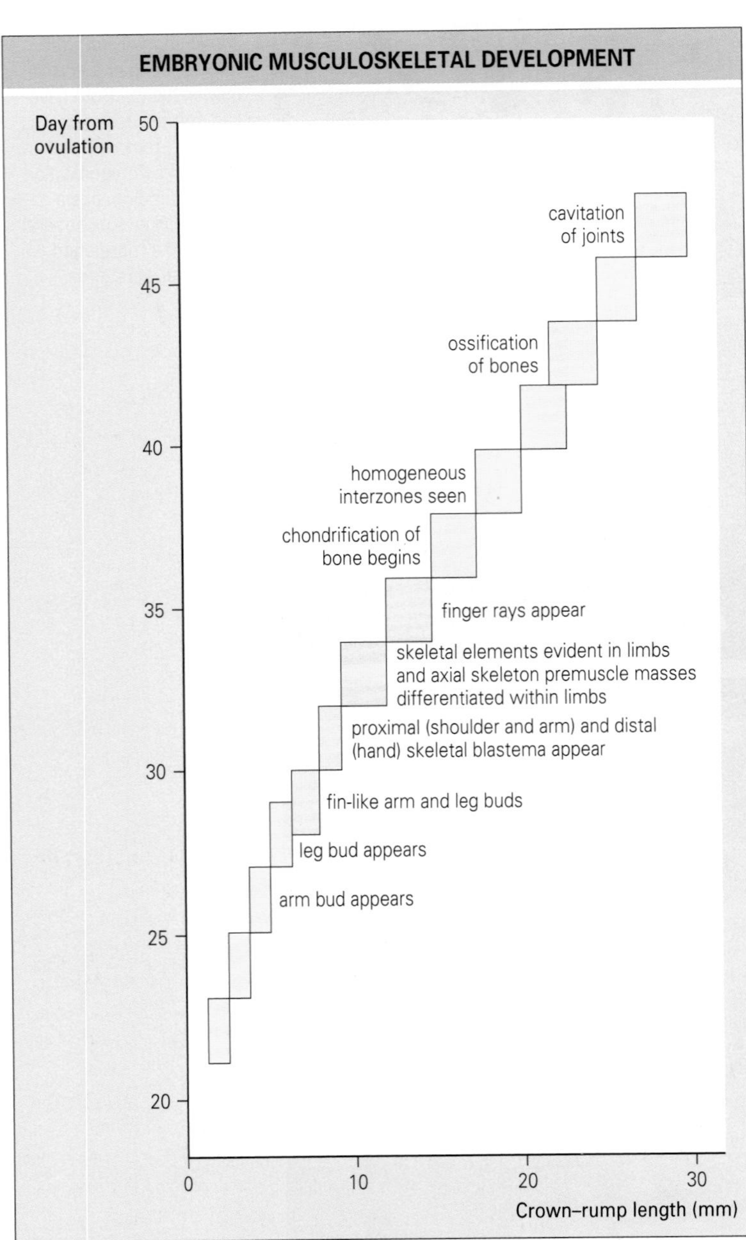

Fig. 9.13 Events of musculoskeletal development. Measures of crown–rump length and estimates of days from ovulation show variation for stages of observed development.

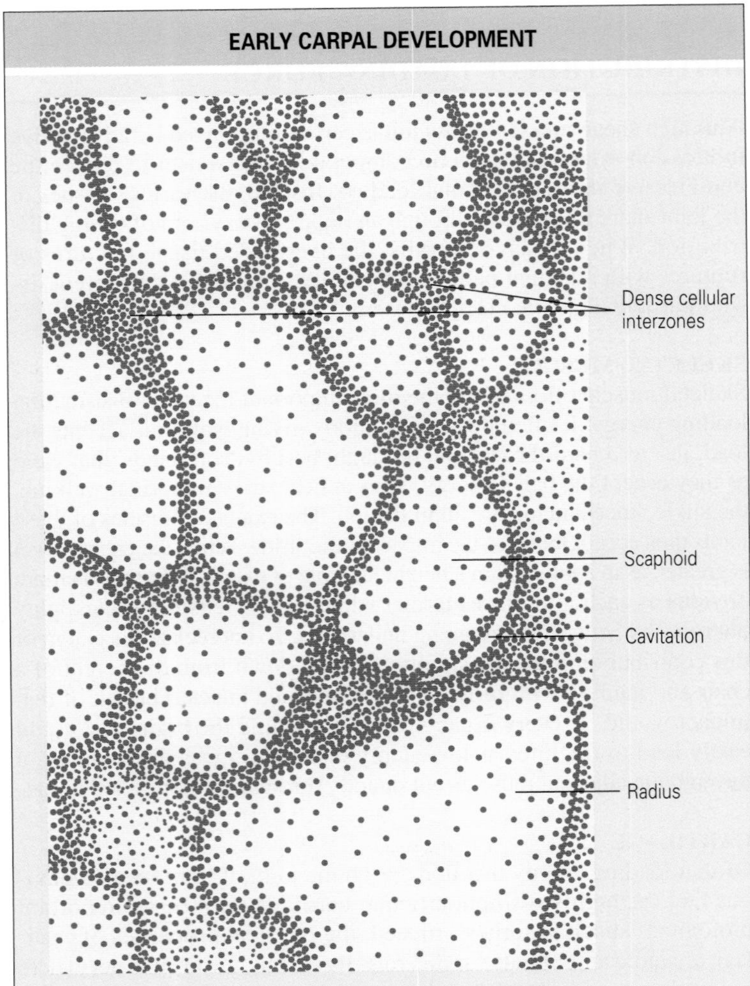

Fig. 9.14 In the early fetus, the radius and ulna appear at the bottom with metacarpal bases above and carpals in the middle. Each of these structures is cartiagenous at this stage. Dense cellular interzones are obvious and 'cavitation' has occurred in the one between the radius and scaphoid to intiate the articular cavity of this joint. From O'Rahilly R, Gardner E. The.embryology of movable joints. In: Sokoloff L, ed. The joints and synovial fluid, Vol I. New York: Academic Press; 1978.

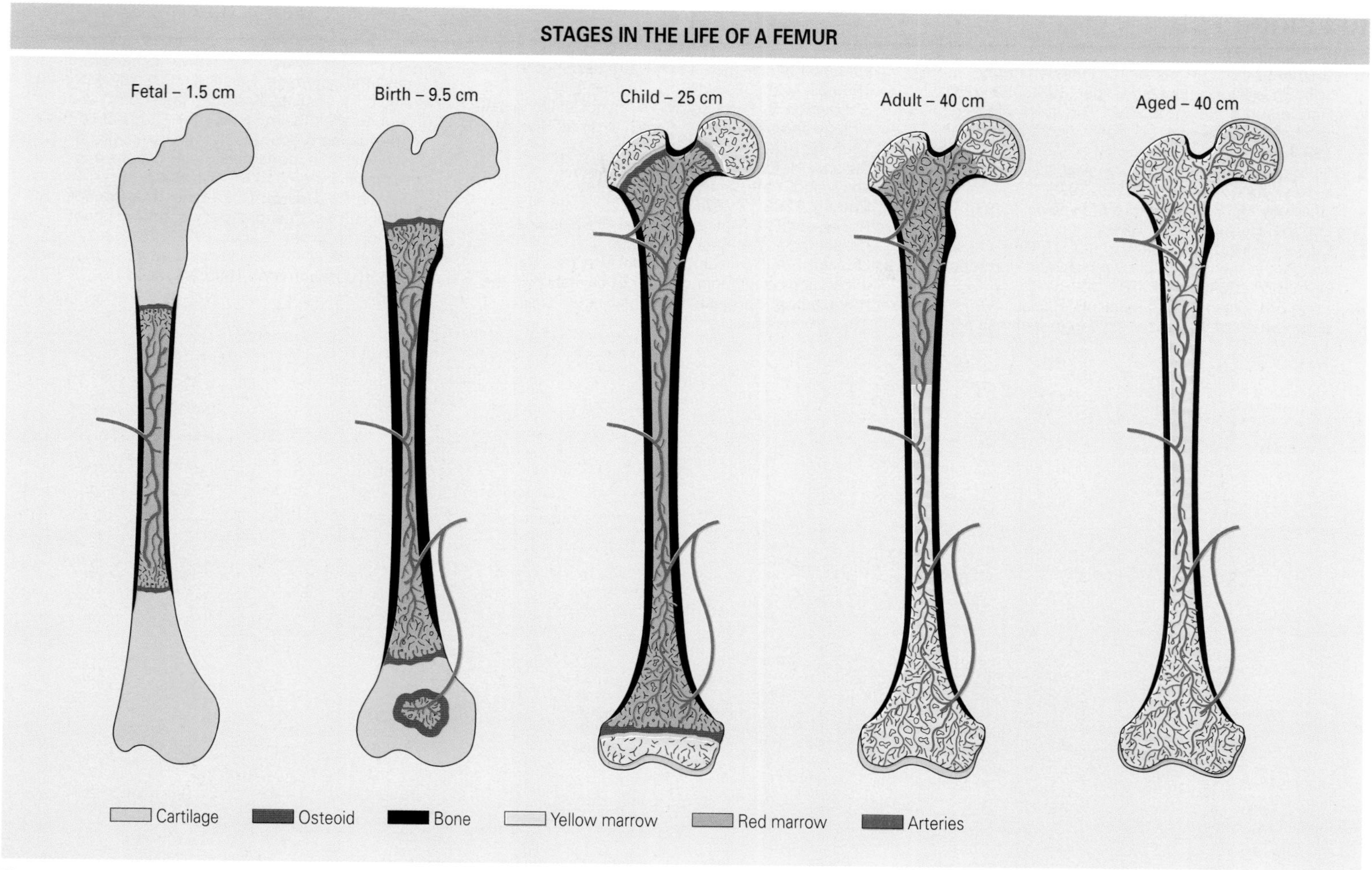

STAGES IN THE LIFE OF A FEMUR

Fig. 9.15 Appearance and length of the femur as a representative long bone at five different ages. Appearance and length of the femur as a representative long bone in black, un-calcified osteoid in purple, arteries in red, 'red marrow' in pink, and 'yellow marrow' in light yellow. In the fetal femur at approximately 10 weeks, the mesenchymal model hass fully chodrified, a perichondrial 'collar' of new bone has formed, and a nutrient vessel is supplying the primary growth center of the shaft. By the time of birth, a secondary growth center has begun in the distal epiphysis and fully formed epiphyseal 'plates' are present in the child at approximately age 7. Most femoral growth in length takes place in the distal epiphysis. Proximal growth centers are present in the head, greater trochanter, and lesser trochanter (latter not shown). Cortical thickness diminishes as the 'woven' bone of childhood becomes denser in the adult and then begins to atrophy with advancing age. As adult stature is attained, the epiphyseal 'plates' close sequentially and the marrow cavity becomes continuous. The transition from 'red' to 'yellow' marrow is well underway in the long bones of young adults and complete in the elderly.
Note that all five femurs are shown at the same length but the true length increases by almost 30-fold. Marked remodeling occurs throughout the period of growth to accommodate the progressive changes in both length and breadth.

Bone plays another essential role as the housing for the blood-forming marrow. Early in fetal life most blood is made in the liver, but by the time of birth this responsibility has passed to the bone marrow. Virtually all long bones as well as the axial skeleton are initially involved in this process. As the individual grows, however, there is a progressive transformation of red (blood forming) marrow to yellow (fatty) marrow (Fig. 9.15). For the most part, this process begins with the digits and moves steadily in a central direction. Some interesting work suggests that low temperature is in some way inhospitable to red marrow and the transition is driven by the cooler temperatures in normal extremities. Exceptions exist, however, such as the early and complete transition to fatty marrow in the femoral and humeral heads. The explanation for this distribution seems likely to be interesting if and when it can be found.

As we have seen, all musculoskeletal tissues undergo a continuous remodeling process. It should not be surprising, then, that the musculoskeletal framework does not remain static, but continues to evolve throughout adulthood into old age. Thus, for instance, progressive changes in the nucleus pulposus may make disc herniation less likely but contribute significantly to progressive loss of height. Corresponding changes in the biochemistry of articular cartilage are well recognized although their import in progressive joint diseases remains unclear. The skeleton reaches its peak mass in early adulthood and begins to decline thereafter in both sexes. Women appear to be more susceptible to the manifestations of osteoporosis not because they lose bone more rapidly, but because they start from a lower peak. These and other aspects of aging are reviewed in Chapter 8.37.

Our perceptions of rheumatic diseases depend in large measure on their patterns of presentation. These conditions vary greatly from each other in the specific joints most likely to be affected and in those which are likely to be spared. With relatively few exceptions, these patterns are not understood[14]. It seems reasonable to suspect, however, that the local pathophysiology of each condition may in part depend upon the unique structural or functional characteristics of its preferred target tissues. Thus, the comparative study of specific articulations, of tissue changes over time and of sex-related variations in musculoskeletal structures will continue to be important areas of rheumatologic investigation.

REFERENCES

1. Clemente CD. The joints. In: Gray's Anatomy, 30E. Philadelphia: Lea & Febiger; 1980:329–428.
2. Henderson B, Edwards JCW. The synovial lining in health and disease. London: Chapman and Hall; 1987.
3. Sokoloff L. The joints and synovial fluid, Vols I & II. New York: Academic Press; 1978.
4. Ghadially FN. Fine structure of synovial joints. London: Butterworths; 1983.
5. Clarys JP, Martin AD, Drinkwater DT. Gross tissue weights in the human body by cadaver dissection. Hum Biol. 1984;56:459–73.
6. Price FM, Mason RM, Levick JR. Radial organization of interstitial exchange pathway and influence of collagen in synovium. Biophys J. 1995;69:1429–39.
7. Henderson B, Pettipher R. The synovial lining cell: biology and pathbiology. Semin Arthritis Rheum. 1985;15:1–32.
8. Bellamy N, Park W, Rooney PJ. What do we know about the sacroiliac joint? Semin Arthritis Rheum. 1983;12:282–313.
9. Rockwood CA, Matsen FA, eds. The shoulder. Philadelphia: WB Saunders; 1990.
10. Unsworth A, Dowson D, Wright V. 'Cracking joints': a bioengineering study of cavitation in the metacarpophalangeal joint. Ann Rheum Dis. 1971;30:348–58.
11. Chen YL, Israelachvili J. New mechanism of cavitation damage. Science. 1991;252:1157–60.
12. Radin EL, Paul IL. Does cartilage compliance reduce skeletal impact loads? The relative force-attenuating properties of articular cartilages, synovial fluid, periarticular soft tissues and bone. Arthritis Rheum. 1970;13:139–44.
13. Simkin PA, Heston TF, Downey DJ, Benedict RS, Choi HS. Subchondral architecture in bones of the canine shoulder. J Anat. 1991;175:213–27.
14. Simkin PA. Why this joint and why not that joint? Scand J Rheumatol. 1995;24:13–16.

10

JOINT PHYSIOLOGY

Peter Hasselbacher

Summary

- Articular structures are supported by physiologic systems that allow for efficient movement.
- Changes in intraarticular pressure and temperature, in particular, have profound influences on normal joint physiology.
- Joint pathology may result from disturbances of circulation, lymphatic drainage, innervation, and processes that alter diffusion of macromolecules across the synovial membrane.

INTRODUCTION

Physiology seeks to teach how living things work, and the use of this word in this textbook reminds us that joints are indeed made of living tissues. The body of knowledge of the physiology of joints is not as old, voluminous, nor quantitative as the physiology of other organ systems, but the application of new investigational technology and molecular biological techniques is rapidly expanding the body of information[1–4]. Such knowledge provides a framework within which we can conceptualize normal joint biology or pathophysiology, and which can be used to rationally interpret symptoms and physical findings in patients with rheumatic diseases.

The principal function of almost all joints is movement. Other processes necessarily support that function but, in turn, movement alters these other physiologic activities. Microscopic examination of synovium and cartilage shows them to be composed of metabolically active, healthy-appearing cells. This implies that they have the same nutritional requirements as other tissues, produce similar waste products and respond to hormonal and other metabolic stimuli in ways analogous to other tissues. It therefore is no surprise that joints are vulnerable to ischemia[5], or suffer along with the rest of the body in systemic diseases such as acromegaly, hemochromatosis, hyperparathyroidism or a multitude of genetic, metabolic, endocrinologic, toxic, immunologic or other toxic or immunologic disorders. Joints age as well, with subsequent effects on function[6].

A reasonable initial hypothesis is that joint tissues follow basic physiologic principles that hold true for other tissues. Some of these principles can be demonstrated particularly well in joint tissues; some may even be unique. Joint fluid is easily sampled and offers a special opportunity to study processes of extravascular compartments[7]. Many of the traditional aspects of physiology can and have been studied in the diarthrodial joint: circulation, lymphatics, pressure, diffusion, innervation, temperature, etc. Not surprisingly, changes in one physiologic 'system' within the joint can have important effects on other systems. Furthermore, all are uniquely modified by physical movement. New information suggests that, far from being sequestered from the rest of the body, processes within the joint interact with and alter the physiology of the whole body.

CIRCULATION

Joints require a blood supply to ensure the health of hyaline articular cartilage, which lacks blood vessels of its own and which is at the far end of the blood delivery system[8]. The nearest available blood vessels are the capillaries of the synovium. In the adult there is little if any diffusion of nutrients across the tidemark of calcified and metabolically inactive-appearing tissue that separates bone from articular cartilage. Chondrocytes are among the cells most remote from their blood supply. Transport across the final few millimeters of synovial intima, joint fluid and cartilage matrix is entirely dependent on diffusion. Even in osteonecrosis, when subchondral bone is dead and disorganized, overlying cartilage can be viable. The presence of freely mobile, living intra-articular cartilaginous joint 'mice' is additional evidence that cartilage nutrition occurs solely through synovial fluid. Thus the synovium and synovial cavity have a major role in facilitating metabolic exchange, and in maintaining a normal joint space environment.

Large blood vessels of the limbs pass the articular regions, and feeder vessels enter and leave the joint capsule at positions protected from mechanical pressure during movement. The arterial, venous and lymphatic systems of the synovium anastomose extensively with the corresponding vessels of the joint capsule, attached ligaments and tendons, periosteum and adjacent bone. These interconnections imply that hydrostatic changes in one anatomic region have effects elsewhere. Certainly when there is increased central venous pressure, as from congestive heart failure, the venous pressure in the synovium is also increased and a true transudate in the joint space may result. This is particularly likely to occur in the presence of hypoalbuminemia[9]. In conditions such as osteonecrosis, sickle cell crisis or osteoarthritis in which intraosseous pressure is elevated, the joint effusions and synovial changes seen clinically may well be due in part to increased venous and lymphatic pressures.

The microscopic structure of the synovium is well suited to facilitate nutrition of the cartilage and the synovium. The capillary network is particularly rich, with individual loops numerous at the juxtacavitary or intimal surface of the synovial membrane. Unlike the deeper subintimal capillaries, these surface capillaries are fenestrated, a property thought to allow rapid exchange of small solutes and water. The capillary system and its postcapillary venules do more than just deliver to and remove plasma from the joint. Mediator cells of inflammation and immunity arrive at and exit the vascular compartment through these vessels. Synovial intimal macrophages derived from the bone marrow arrive by this route[10]. It appears that specific targeting of subpopulations of lymphocytes and other cells occurs through cell surface recognition at the endothelium of the capillary and small venules.

LYMPHATICS

There is an easily demonstrated and typical lymphatic system in the synovium, but not in the cartilage[11]. The blind end-pouches and collecting vessels lie somewhat deeper than do the surface capillaries; the main trunks follow arteries and veins. As elsewhere, synovial lymphatics carry excess fluid, high molecular weight solutes and protein, tiny particulates and some cells (but not erythrocytes) out of the joint. This bulk transfer is powered by normal movement of the joint, and is presumably impeded by synovial disorganization or excessive intra-articular pressure. The lymphatics provide a removal mechanism for macromolecules that is relatively insensitive to molecular weight. Proteins and proteoglycans from the joint enter the systemic circulation through this route. Very little is known about the effects of lymphatic dysfunction during disease, but it may be fair to extrapolate from the effects of lymphatic obstruction elsewhere.

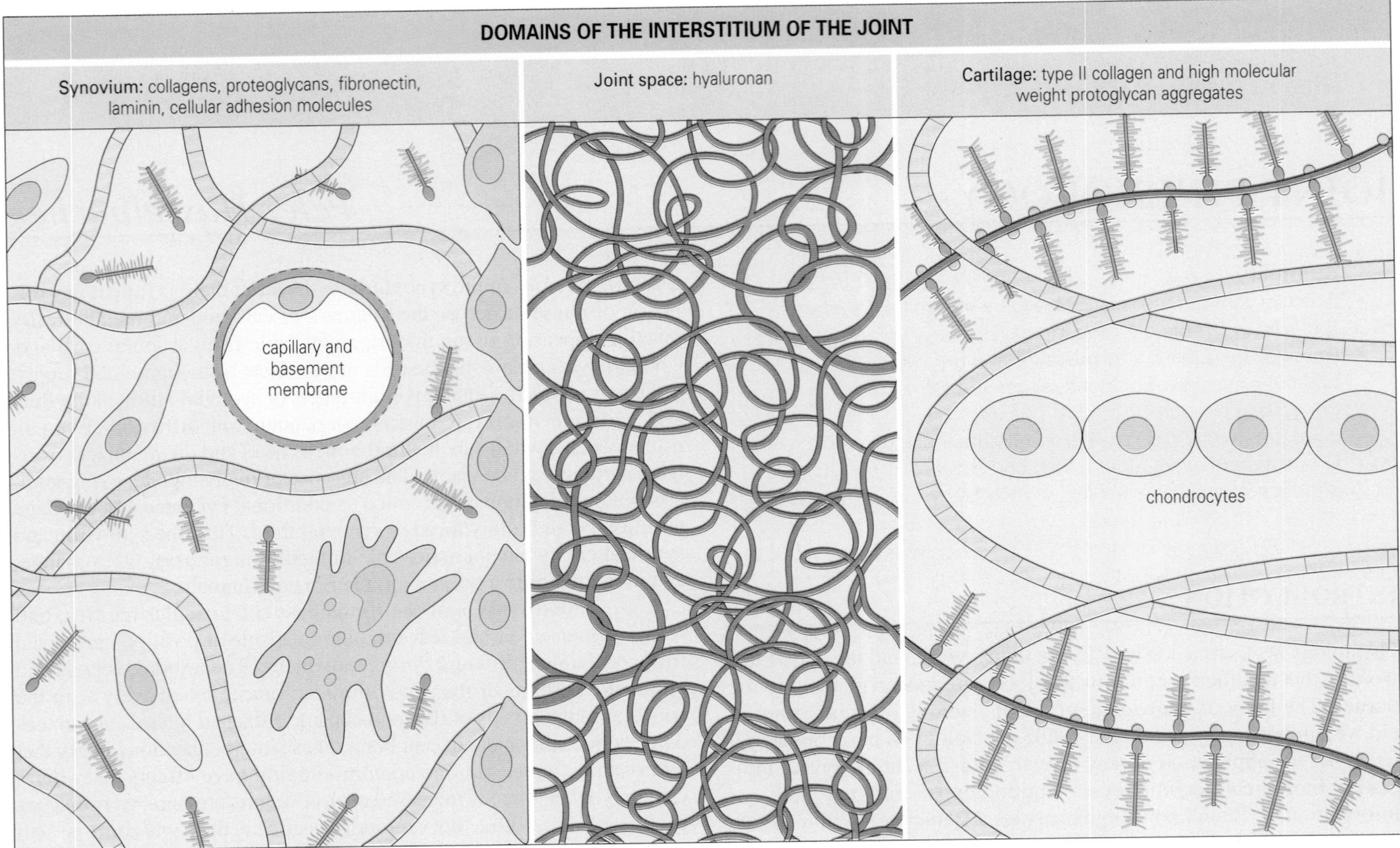

Fig. 10.1 Schematic representation of the domains of the interstitium of the joint space. The thin basement membrane of the synovial capillary may be the most concrete barrier to diffusion of large molecules.

INTERSTITIAL DOMAINS WITHIN THE JOINT

It has been traditional to consider the joint space, extracellular synovium and hyaline articular cartilage as one continuous, extravascular, interstitial space[12] (Fig. 10.1). Certainly the discrete mechanical barriers between plasma and tissue spaces are small compared to other tissues. There is no basement membrane underlying the synovial intima as there is beneath the lining cells of the pleura or of the gut. Intimal cells lack appreciable tight junctions. Thus, the only basement membrane separating the chondrocyte from the intravascular space is the fragile capillary basement membrane. In simple terms, a small molecule leaving the capillary and diffusing towards a chondrocyte must traverse a host of connective tissue macromolecules[13,14]. These include those of the basement membrane of the capillary, the collagens and lower molecular weight proteoglycans of synovial tissue, matrix molecules associated with intimal cell membranes, the high molecular weight hyaluronate of synovial fluid, the organized surface structure (lamina splendens) of cartilage, the dense, highly structured matrix of type II collagen and the uniquely high molecular weight proteoglycan aggregates of hyaline articular cartilage itself. Although discrete traditional anatomic barriers are not present, the substantial influence of these macromolecules on diffusion and cellular interactions is increasingly being appreciated. The joint has proven to be a good place to study these new concepts.

The extracellular matrix is synthesized and maintained by the cells of the synovium and cartilage. Even in the normal state, this ‘obstacle course’ of cells and macromolecules offers differing resistance to the passage of molecules and cells across the joint. In the presence of disease, the alterations of relative barriers to ingress and egress afforded by the different layers, compartments and macromolecules are profound and deleterious. The sequences of the genes that encode the protein portion of these connective tissue components are becoming known. Mutations that cause abnormal gene products are associated with an increasing number of hereditary disorders that were previously unknown, including some forms of premature osteoarthritis[15]. Such experiments of nature will give additional and insight into the physiologic significance of matrix macromolecules.

DIFFUSION

Early physiologic studies of the joint focused on measurement of substances in the excess synovial fluid present in diseased joints, or in saline instilled into normal joints. Such studies have been informative and clinically useful, yet such static snapshots of a dynamic process cannot fully describe the magnitude or direction of the fluxes that occur[16].

Properties of molecules that predict how well they enter and traverse the various joint ‘compartments’ include: molecular weight, effective molecular radius, electrical charge at physiologic conditions, lipid solubility, protein binding and degree of interaction with other structural and nonstructural molecules or cells of the joint. An instructive clinical example of these effects is that large molecular weight proteins such as IgM or fibrinogen are largely excluded from synovial fluid when compared to lower molecular weight albumin[17]. This exclusion occurs at the normal capillary basement membrane and as a result of exclusion of large proteins from the molecular domain of synovial fluid hyaluronan and joint proteoglycans. The albumin–globulin ratio (r) of normal synovial fluid is 20.4 compared to the usual 1.0–2.1 in plasma. This ratio falls dramatically, even in noninflammatory arthritis such as osteoarthritis (r=5.4), and falls even further in rheumatoid arthritis (r=2.2) or infectious arthritis (P. Hasselbacher, unpublished data). The normal superficial layers of cartilage also provide a barrier to diffusion of protein into the matrix of cartilage. Not surprisingly, pathologic disruption of joint tissues interferes markedly with the physical diffusion of molecules in to and out of joints. Compared to the ingress of molecules, which is highly dependent on molecular size, the rate of egress through the lymphatic system is much less sensitive; albumin leaves as easily as IgM.

In steady-state conditions, small molecules such as synovial fluid gases, electrolytes or urea are generally found in joint fluid in concentrations similar to those in plasma and other interstitial fluid (which is the more proper comparison). Glucose concentrations may be lower, but glucose is utilized locally by cells on the way in. Small molecules can re-enter the distal vascular capillary network just as they do in other capillary beds. Although, in the normal state, diffusion of small molecules is not limiting to the tissues, in disease states, they can be, for both physiologic molecules as well as drugs. In infectious arthritis or other severely inflammatory disease states, the local metabolic conditions are quite harsh. Anoxia, acidosis and low glucose are clinically observed as the joint switches to anaerobic metabolism and metabolic demands outstrip availability[18]. This results from physical disruption of normal pathways for diffusion, added layers of fibrin on the synovial lining cells, compromise of blood supply by thrombosis or increased intra-articular pressure and increased local consumption of necessary metabolites by inflammatory cells. Such conditions are not compatible with life, even that of a chondrocyte. Clinical consequences can be devastating. Even a successful bacterial cure of an infected joint cannot bring dead cartilage back to life. Postinfectious degenerative arthritis is therefore an important complication of this disease and why early diagnosis and treatment are so important.

Not all small or large molecules in the synovial fluid derive from plasma. Many cell types of the synovium contribute to synovial interstitial fluid. Mast cells, fibroblasts, tissue macrophages, immunocompetent cells, nerve endings and other resident or pathologic cells of the synovium presumably affect what substances eventually reach the joint space and cartilage. A number of serum proteins, such as immunoglobulin or complement, can be synthesized within the confines of the capsule. Just as systemic hormones have an effect on chondrocytes and cartilage, it must be assumed that local cell products or cytokines also influence chondrocyte expression and joint function. It is tempting to speculate that some cellular messenger produced by chondrocytes signals in turn to synovial intimal cells. There is increasing realization that intracapsular events can affect the rest of the body. If acute gout or pseudogout can cause an increase in acute phase reactants in blood, it is certainly possible that some of the systemic features of rheumatoid arthritis are initiated or maintained by factors produced within the joints.

INTRA-ARTICULAR PRESSURE

The joint space is really more of a potential one, empty and collapsed. Even the normal knee, the largest joint space, contains 2ml or less of synovial fluid. Normal intra-articular pressure in a resting joint is actually subatmospheric, presumably due to Starling forces and perhaps some lymphatic pumping[19]. The redundant synovial cavity wall, with its folds and recesses, is necessary for normal excursions of motion to occur. Joint immobility permits the potential volume of the joint to decrease. In adhesive capsulitis of the shoulder, decreased potential articular volume from fibrosis and lack of compliance of the synovial space restrict movement. The presence of a chronic effusion under pressure can stretch the capsule and increase the maximal intrasynovial volume. The manifestations of increased intra-articular volumes and pressures can be extraordinary and have practical consequences in the management of joint disease as discussed below[20,21].

The walls of the synovial cavity are elastic and as the volume of fluid increases, pressure increases nonlinearly (Fig. 10.2). The resulting pressure–volume curves define the compliance of the synovial membrane and its surrounding connective tissue. In diseases such as rheumatoid arthritis, in which there is thickening and fibrosis of the synovium and capsule, the pressure rises more rapidly and with smaller volumes than does a normal joint, i.e. the rheumatoid joint has reduced compliance. The mechanical strength of the thickened tissues is greater and the pressures attained can be truly colossal. Flimsy normal joint structures will rupture at their weakest point long before such pressures are attained.

When a normal joint (without effusion) is carried through its range of motion, intra-articular pressure does not increase and, in fact, may substantially decrease, such as occurs during active extension of the knee. This decrease is due presumably to the effect of muscular action on the shape of the potential cavity. When excess fluid is present, the effect of motion and position is very different. For each joint, there is a position in which intra-articular pressure for a given volume is minimal[22]. Movement in any direction away from this position

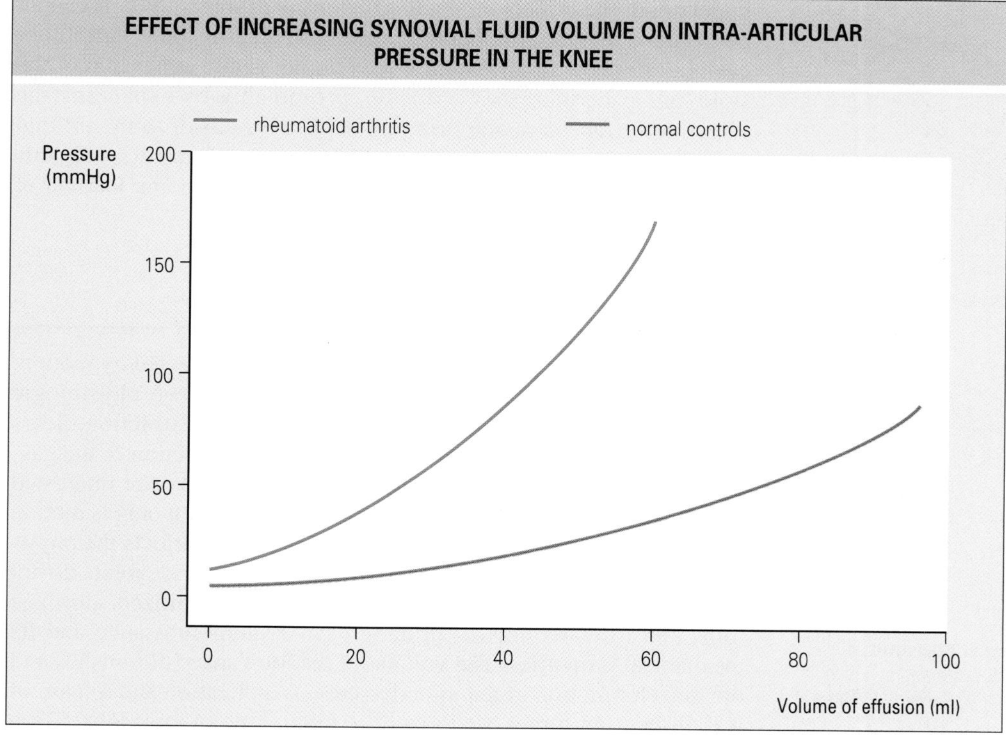

Fig. 10.2 Effect of increasing synovial fluid volume on intra-articular pressure in the knee. Pressure rises much more rapidly for a given volume in the rheumatoid joint. Substantial pressures can be present clinically. (Adapted with permission from Dieppe PA, Bacon PA, Bamji AN, Watt I. Atlas of Clinical Rheumatology. London: Gower; 1986.)

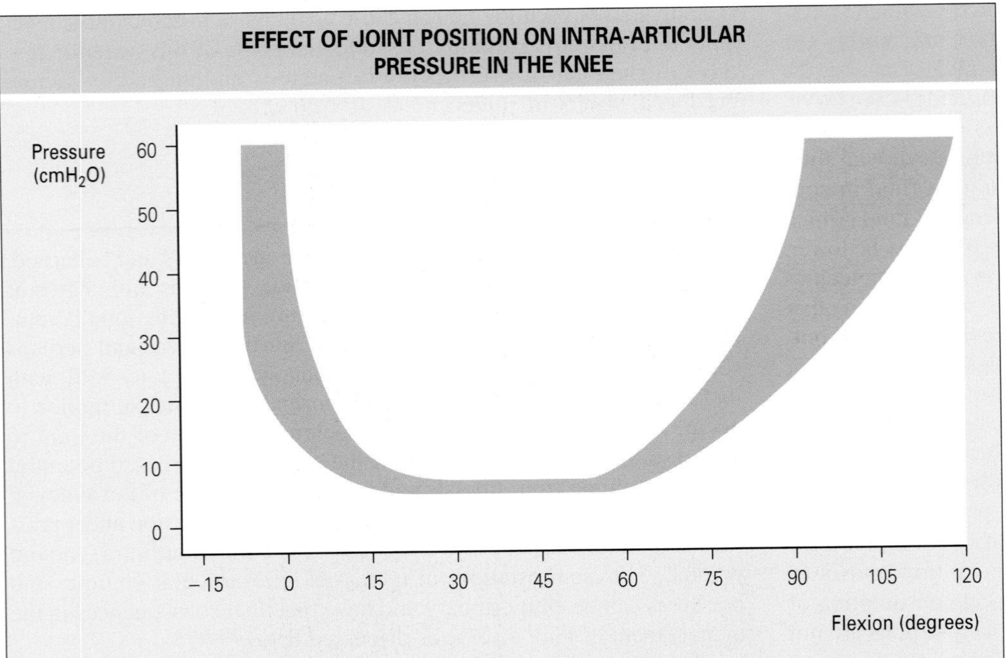

Fig. 10.3 Effect of joint position on intra-articular pressure in the knee. When the knee has an effusion, intra-articular pressure is minimal in partial flexion and rises rapidly as the joint is straightened (0°) or flexed further. (Reproduced with permission from Eyring and Murray[22]).

increases pressure (Fig. 10.3). For example, the position of minimal pressure in the elbow is one of intermediate flexion. Thus, the ability to extend the elbow fully is a physical finding which rules against a significant inflammatory intra-articular process. Because minimum pressure usually equates to minimum pain, such positions are spontaneously assumed when disease is present. Unfortunately, these positions are not usually those of maximum function, which is why prevention of contractures is an important goal for the clinician.

On weight bearing or the application of muscular force around the effused joint, or at extremes of passive motion, intra-articular pressure may easily achieve several hundred millimeters of mercury. In addition to causing pain, this energy has great destructive potential (Fig. 10.4). It is not surprising that diseased joints will develop herniations of the cavity through weak points in the capsule (which become synovial cysts) or through the subchondral bony plate (which causes bone cysts or geodes). The capsule and synovium may stretch to accommodate greater equilibrium volumes but do so at the expense of their stabilizing function.

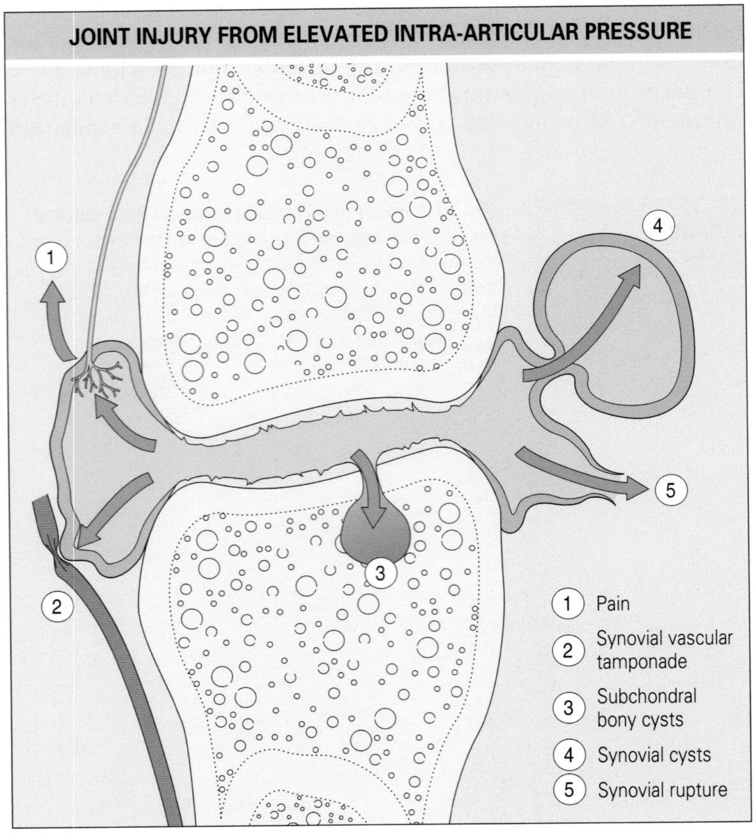

JOINT INJURY FROM ELEVATED INTRA-ARTICULAR PRESSURE

1 Pain
2 Synovial vascular tamponade
3 Subchondral bony cysts
4 Synovial cysts
5 Synovial rupture

Fig. 10.4 Examples of joint injury from elevated intra-articular pressure: pain, synovial vascular tamponade, subchondral bony cysts, synovial cysts and synovial rupture. (Reproduced with permission from Dieppe PA, Bacon PA, Bamji AN, Watt I. Atlas of Clinical Rheumatology. London: Gower; 1986.)

An effect of pressure on blood flow is easily demonstrated. Pressures within diseased joints that are greater than systolic blood pressure are easily attained during routine activities. Experimentally it has been shown that increased intra-articular pressure can cause tamponade of the capillary bed. Intra-articular pressure >45mmHg has been associated with acidosis in joints, suggesting that this physiologic effect has clinical significance[23]. The effect of such intra-articular pressure on synovial lymphatics is unknown but potentially they are similarly vulnerable.

Although the deleterious effects of extremes of pressure are easily understood, the effects of small effusions are more subtle. It cannot be assumed that the simple presence of a small effusion is harmful or even interferes with diffusion. For example, gentle expansion of the synovial space increases diffusion, presumably by expanding the effective surface area and bringing capillaries closer to the intimal surface. There are a variety of new techniques available to study diffusion in humans and animal models and much is being learned of practical use.

MOTION

The joint is not the only organ or body part that is affected by motion. The rhythmic expansion of the chest has well-known physiologic effects on cardiopulmonary function. Muscular contraction clears peripheral edema. Peristalsis of bowel is a major function of the gastrointestinal system. Physiologists and clinicians alike are interested in a variety of sphincter and intraluminal pressures. Not only is motion in diarthrodial joints, but motion itself affects the physiology and health of the joint[24]. Without motion *in utero*, joints do not develop normally. If a mature joint is strictly immobilized, cartilage thins and loses its normal proteoglycan ground substance and its mechanical properties. The volume of the joint space diminishes and the range of motion of the joint decreases. Application and release of weight-bearing forces are thought to play a role in joint lubrication and in the diffusion of substances in and out of cartilage[25]. There are other reasons why continued use is required for joint health, including the maintenance of normal strength and coordination of muscles, the preservation of bone mass, the maintenance of desired weight and preservation of normal range of joint motion. Exercise increases blood flow to synovial tissues. Joint motion permits, and may be required for, the lymphatic system to clear the joint of particulates, macromolecules and excess fluid. In inflamed joints, the lack of movement allows fibrosis and rapid shortening of ligaments and capsule so that range of motion is lost.

INNERVATION

There is much new information about the innervation of the joint[26]. The one observation that has not changed is that there are no nerve endings in hyaline articular cartilage. This explains why osteoarthritis is asymptomatic until it is already well advanced. Traditionally it was thought that there were no nerve endings in the synovium either. This was shown to be untrue with a bold self-experiment involving cutaneous anesthesia[27]. Although most of the synovium is relatively insensitive to mechanical stimulation, there are some areas (such as at the superior pole of the patella) that are painful when pinched. Histologic and more sophisticated histochemical and immunologic staining methods demonstrate small-diameter nerve fibers within the confines of the capsule. These generally follow the course of the arterioles and it was assumed that these are related to vasomotor function. However, some sensory or chemoreceptor function has to be present as the intra-articular injection of bradykinin or intrasynovial injection of hypertonic saline causes pain. That the vasculature of the synovium is responsive to autonomic and other chemical stimulus is now well established. Concepts of antidromic conduction and proinflammatory mediators released from nerve endings open new areas of understanding how the neurologic system modulates inflammatory joint disease[28]. No doubt as a result of this improved understanding of articular neurology, use of physical modalities and other nonmedicinal therapies will become more rational and effective.

Whereas cartilage has none, and synovium has limited innervation the capsule, intra-articular fat pads, attached ligaments, periosteum, muscles and adjacent bone are abundantly innervated. Certainly at arthrocentesis, penetration of the capsule penetration of the capsule by the needle, or touching the periosteum adjacent to the joint is painful. Such pain sensation may have a normal function in preventing joint overload. It has been thought that a major function of such articular innervation is proprioception – the perception of joint position, and the direction and velocity of movement. Although joints are excellent low-friction bearings, the cartilage and subchondral bone unit make a poor shock absorber. The presence of a normally functioning proprioceptive mechanism and intact sensorimotor reflexes prevents and dissipates potentially destructive forces of gravity and movement. The magnitude of such potential and kinetic energy is evident from the frequency of fractures from simple falls and is suggested by the force felt in the everyday phenomenon of descending stairs in the dark and expecting there to be one more step than there is.

The paradigm of failure of these protective mechanisms is Charcot's joint (Fig. 10.5), in which loss of normal sensory function can lead to gross mechanical disruption within days[29]. Exactly which sensory components are most critical is uncertain, but the usual clinical correlates of Charcot's joints appear to be loss of deep pain or position sense. Lack of pain sensation from needle contact with juxta-articular bone appears to be a reliable correlate of Charcot's joint, even when more superficial sensation is relatively normal. Such mechanisms of joint destruction are most often seen in individuals with diabetic neuropathy.

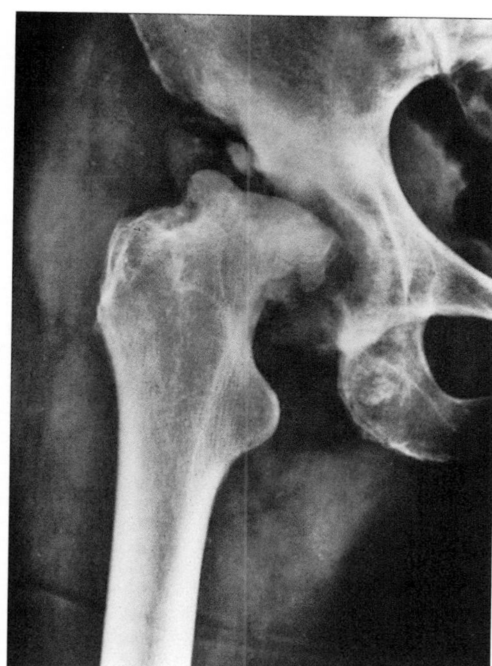

Fig. 10.5 Charcot's joint. Anteroposterior view of the right hip of a 57-year-old woman with neurosyphilis (tabes dorsalis) shows the typical features of Charcot's joint. (Reproduced with permission from Greenspan A. Orthopedic Radiology: A Practical Approach. New York: Gower; 1988.)

TEMPERATURE

The temperature of the skin overlying joints is a cardinal item of physical examination. Although there may be a few joints close enough and deep enough to the body's center to share its core temperature, the normal intra-articular temperature of peripheral joints is far less than 37°C. The temperature of the resting knee for example is around 32°C, the ankle 29°C. The distal joints of fingers and toes may approach ambient temperature. Even the most inflamed knee in a patient with rheumatoid arthritis rarely rises above 37°C. Since temperature is largely a function of blood flow, it is not surprising that manipulations that change blood flow, such as the smoking of a cigarette or the application of external heat or cold will effect intra-articular temperature[30]. Joint movement itself increases joint temperature. Although the friction of movement may produce some heat, it is likely that the substantial heat of muscular contraction and a generalized increase in blood flow to the limb is more important.

Biochemical, cellular and physiologic studies of tissues are usually performed at the standard 37°C. We must remain wary of the possible effects of lower temperatures on metabolic, biochemical, biophysical, and immunologic processes that we know participate in the pathophysiology of joint disease. Is lower temperature the simple explanation of why urate deposition and gout are more frequent in distal joints and unheard of in the shoulder and hip? Why is there no such apparent relationship in chondrocalcinosis, the other major crystal-induced form of arthritis? Does temperature have any effect on precipitation of immune complexes? A potential list of similar questions is vast.

CONCLUSION

This chapter has offered an introductory overview of the physiology of the joint. The intention has been to emphasize the dynamic interaction of different physiologic processes involved in normal and abnormal articular function. All physicians are practical physiologists with the unique opportunity to study the human subject. It has been gratifying to see the broad proliferation of new knowledge in this area. Questions that were unanswered in reviews two decades ago are solved. Because of the wonderful self-perpetuating nature of scientific inquiry, for every question that is answered, two more are posed. It will always be true that there remains a great deal to be learned and all can make a contribution.

REFERENCES

1. Edwards JCW, ed. Second International Meeting on Synovium; Cell Biology and Physiology. Ann Rheum Dis. 1995; 54:389–436.
2. Sokoloff L. The joints and synovial fluid. Vol 1. New York: Academic Press; 1978.
3. Sokoloff L. The joints and synovial fluid. Vol 2. New York: Academic Press; 1980.
4. Hasselbacher P. The biology of the joint. Clinics in Rheumatic Diseases. Vol 7(1). London: WB Saunders; 1981.
5. Edmonds SE, Ellis G, Gaffney K, Archer J, Blake DR. Hypoxia and the rheumatoid joint: immunological and therapeutic implications. Scand J Rheumatol, Suppl. 1995;101:163–8.
6. Karvonen RL, Negendank WG, Teitge RA, Reed AH, Miller PR; Fernandez-Madrid F. Factors affecting articular cartilage thickness in osteoarthritis and aging. J Rheumatol. 1994;21:1310–18.
7. Hasselbacher P. Arthrocentesis, synovial fluid analysis, and synovial biopsy. In: Primer on the rheumatic diseases, 10E, Atlanta: Arthritis Foundation; 1993, 67–72.
8. Simkin PA. Synovial perfusion and synovial fluid solutes. Ann Rheum Dis. 1995;54:424–8.
9. McDonald JN, Levick JR. Effect of extravascular plasma protein on pressure–flow relations across synovium in anaesthetized rabbits. J Physiol. 1993;465:539–59.
10. Edwards JC. The nature and origins of synovium: experimental approaches to the study of synoviocyte differentiation. J Anat. 1994;184:493–501.
11. Davies DV. The lymphatics of the synovial membrane. J Anat. 1946;80:21–3.
12. Hadler NM. The biology of the extracellular space. Clin Rheum Dis. 1981;7(1):71–97.
13. Levick JR, McDonald JN. Fluid movement across synovium in healthy joints: role of synovial fluid macromolecules. Ann Rheum Dis. 1995;54:417–23.
14. Laurent TC, Laurent UB, Fraser JR. Functions of hyaluronan. Ann Rheum Dis. 1995;54:429–32.
15. Williams CJ, Jimenez SA. Heritable diseases of cartilage caused by mutations in collagen genes. J Rheumatol Suppl. 1995;43:28–33.
16. Levick JR. An analysis of the interaction between interstitial plasma protein, interstitial flow, and fenestral filtration and its application to synovium. Microvasc Res. 1994;47:90–125.
17. Weinberger A, Simkin PA. Plasma proteins in synovial fluids of normal human joints. Semin Arthritis Rheum. 1989;19:66–76.
18. Najafipour H, Ferrell WR. Comparison of synovial PO_2 and sympathetic vasoconstrictor responses in normal and acutely inflamed rabbit knee joints. Exp Physiol. 1995;80:209–20.
19. Levick JR. An investigation into the validity of subatmospheric pressure recordings from synovial fluid and their dependence on joint angle. J Physiol. 1979;289:55–67.
20. Jayson MIV. Intra-articular pressure. Clin Rheum Dis. 1981;7(1):149–66.
21. Ahlqvist J, Harilainen A, Aalto K, Sarna S, Lalla M, Osterlund K. High hydrostatic pressures in traumatic joints require elevated synovial capillary pressure probably associated with arteriolar vasodilatation. Clin Physiol. 1994;14:671–9.
22. Eyring EJ, Murray WR. The effect of joint position on the pressure of intra-articular effusion. J Bone Joint Surg. 1964;46A:1235–41.
23. James MJ, Cleland LG, Rofe AM, Leslie AL. Intra-articular pressure and the relationship between synovial perfusion and metabolic demand. J Rheumatol. 1990;17:521–7.
24. Schollmeier G, Uhthoff HK, Sarkar K, Fukuhara K. Effects of immobilization on the capsule of the canine glenohumeral joint. A structural functional study. Clin Orthop. 1994;304:37–42.
25. Mow VC, Ateshian GA, Spilker RL. Biomechanics of diarthrodial joints: a review of twenty years of progress. J Biomech Eng. 1993;115:460–7.
26. Mapp PI. Innervation of the synovium. Ann Rheum Dis. 1995;54:398–403.
27. Kellgren JH, Samuel EP. The sensitivity and innervation of the articular capsule. J Bone Joint Surg. 1950;32B:84–92.
28. Scott DT, Lam FY, Ferrell WR. Acute joint inflammation – mechanisms and mediators. Gen Pharmacol. 1994;25:1285–96.
29. Sequeira W. The neuropathic joint. Clin Exp Rheumatol. 1994;12:325–37.
30. Oosterveld FG, Rasker JJ. Effects of local heat and cold treatment on surface and articular temperature of arthritic knees. Arthritis Rheum. 1994;37:1578–82.

11

BIOMECHANICS

Victor H Frankel

- Kinematics is the branch of mechanics describing motion. It is concerned with gait, joint surface movement and activities of daily living.
- Joint surfaces slide either over each other in a tangential fashion or roll. The motion is controlled by the axis or center of rotation of the joint. If the center of rotation is displaced, compression or tension at the joint surfaces can result in articulate damage and osteoarthritis.
- The lower extremity joint forces during activities such as walking or running are high and are multiples of body weight.
- Bone tissue is viscoelastic and demonstrates anisotropic behavior.
- Collagenous tissues such as tendon, ligament and joint capsule have a characteristic stress–strain curve with a toe portion followed by a very steep stiff portion prior to rupture.
- Synovial fluid is thixotropic. The viscosity changes with the velocity gradient.
- Joint lubrication is a combination of boundary lubrication, hydrodynamic lubrication and boundary film lubrication.

RANGE OF TIBIOFEMORAL JOINT MOTION IN THE SAGITTAL PLANE DURING COMMON ACTIVITIES

Activity	Range of motion from knee extension to knee flexion (degrees)
Walking	0–67
Climbing stairs	0–83
Descending stairs	0–90
Sitting down	0–93
Tying a shoe	0–106
Lifting an object	0–117

Fig. 11.1 Range of tibiofemoral joint motion in the sagittal plane during common activities.

INTRODUCTION

Purposeful motion is a requirement for life. Loss of motion results in deterioration of function, disability and, ultimately, an inability to perform the activities necessary for daily living. Biomechanics is the study of biological systems, utilizing engineering science and methodology[1]. It involves the study of body motion and the forces that produce that motion. The rheumatologist, like the orthopedic surgeon, is concerned with motion of the human body. The first specialty is concerned with joint function from a medical standpoint; the other, from a surgical reconstructive view. The basic biomechanical science is the same for both.

Kinematics is the branch of mechanics concerned with motion of a body without reference to force or mass. It can be assessed at several different levels: gross motion of joints, motion during activities, motion necessary for the activities of daily living and, finally, joint surface motion.

The recording of joint motion, and deviation from normal joint motion, is an important element of the physical examination, well known to all who treat the locomotor system. It is necessary to understand the range of motion needed for activities of daily living (Figs 11.1 & 11.2).

GAIT

A common reason for seeking care for the musculoskeletal system is difficulty with gait, and the study of normal gait serves as an entrance point to the study of biomechanics. Motion in gait is so rapid that special techniques are necessary to study the angular and linear displacements that occur. Linear progression of the body is produced by angular motion of the joint. Utilizing high speed cinematography, stroboscopic photography, television sampling or electronic goniometry, these angular displacements can be registered. Gait laboratories are utilized to perform such studies and consist of a walkway, a method of recording motion, a force plate to record the ground reaction forces and electromyographic systems to study phasic muscle contraction. Through computer acquisition and processing of data the displacements of the limbs during gait can be recorded.

Specific portions of the gait cycle may be analyzed. Linear and angular displacements are recorded and, by studying successive displacements, the velocity of a limb segment may be determined as the time during which the displacement occurred. Successive velocities are studied to determine the accelerations which produced the velocity changes. Knowledge of the accelerations aide in understanding joint loading.

Gait has been classified into several distinct phases with reference to the limbs. These are the stance phase, the swing phase and the period of double support when both feet are on the ground (Fig. 11.3). The period of double support occurs at about 60% of the gait cycle. The range of motion used in the sagittal plane for normal gait for the hip, knee and ankle joints is given in Figure 11.4.

MEAN VALUES FOR MAXIMUM HIP MOTION IN THREE PLANES DURING COMMON ACTIVITIES

Activity	Plane of motion	Recorded value (degrees)
Tying shoe with foot on the floor	Sagittal Frontal Transverse	124 19 15
Tying shoe with feet across opposite thigh	Sagittal Frontal Transverse	110 23 33
Sitting down on chair and rising from sitting	Sagittal Frontal Tranverse	104 20 17
Stooping to obtain object on floor	Sagittal Frontal Transverse	117 21 18
Squatting	Sagittal Frontal Transverse	122 28 26
Ascending stairs	Sagittal Frontal Transverse	67 16 18
Descending stairs	Sagittal	36

Fig. 11.2 Mean values for maximum hip motion in three planes during common activities.

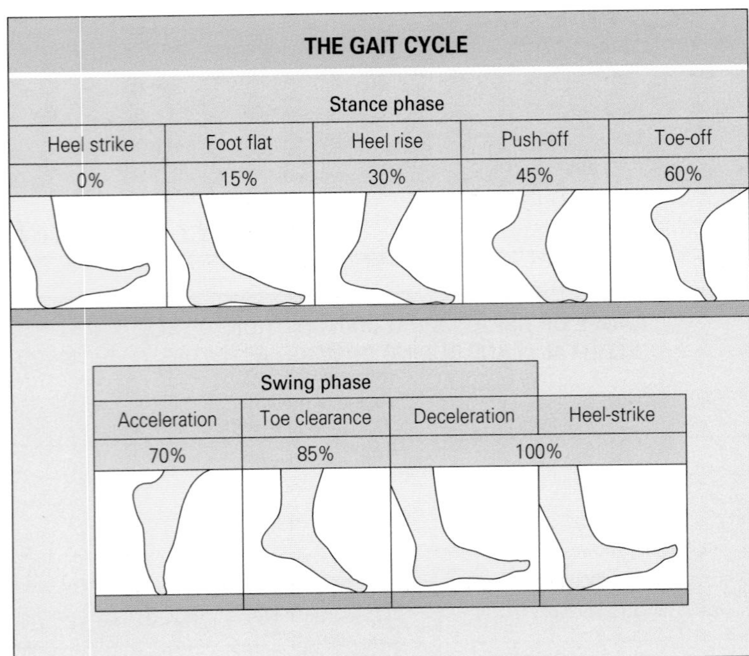

Fig. 11.3 The gait cycle. About 60% of the normal gait cycle is spent in stance phase and about 40% in swing phase. After heel strike the center of the load progresses forward rapidly to the great toe, where toe-off occurs at about 60% of the gait cycle.

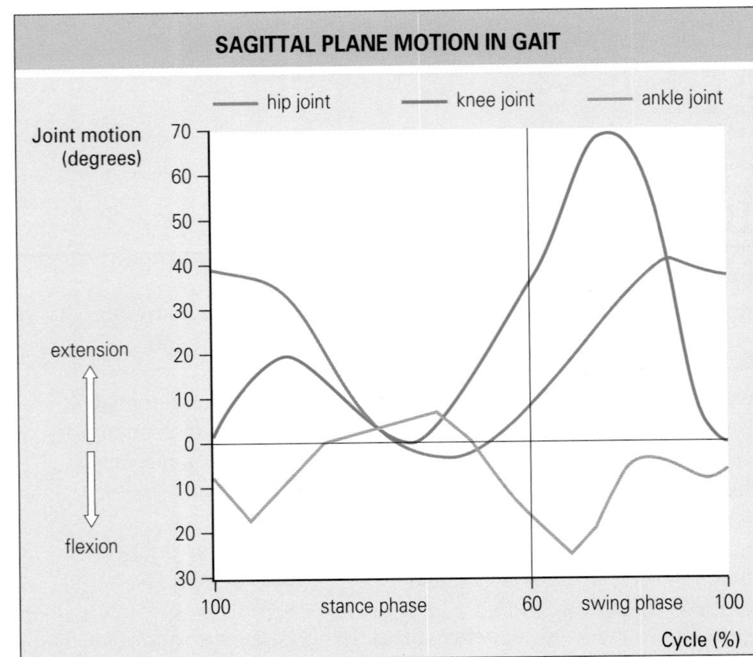

Fig. 11.4 Sagittal plane motion in gait. Range of motion in the sagittal plane of the hip, knee and ankle for one gait cycle.

Motions also occur in the frontal and transverse planes. In the knee joint, transverse rotations are important in stance phase flexion and extension. In the hip joint, too, small degrees of rotation are necessary for smooth gait (Fig. 11.5).

Progression in gait requires the displacement of the center of gravity of the body, which in turn requires energy expenditure. There are three types of energy. Potential energy is the energy stored in a body through its elevation above a base; strain energy is the energy stored in the body under deformation; and kinetic energy is the energy possessed by a moving mass and is equal to one half the mass times its velocity squared. The energy level is constant if no work is done, as in the example of a simple pendulum where the loss of potential energy as it swings down is exactly compensated for by the gain in kinetic energy. If the energy level is not constant, work must be done to produce the change in energy level. This situation occurs during gait. The energy level in the different segments of the lower extremity is not constant. The difference in energy is made up by the work done by the muscles at the joints; forward displacement of the body results, but a large part of the energy is dissipated in the rotations of the segments. In pathologic gait situations, or situations in which external supports are used, more energy is expended in gait. This is an important consideration where gait is desired but general health conditions mean that excess energy requirements will have a deleterious effect. Energy expenditure during gait with arthritic joints can rise easily by 50%.

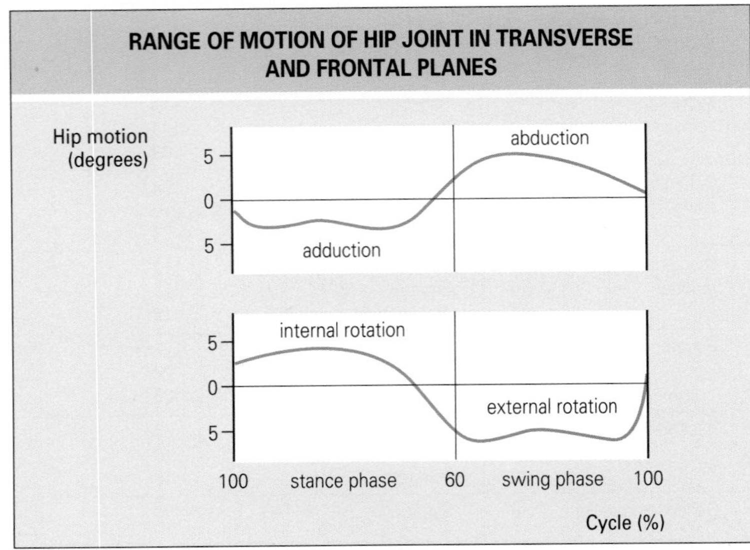

Fig. 11.5 Hip joint motion in the transverse and frontal planes during level walking. One gait cycle.

The energy required for changing the center of gravity of the body during gait progression has five determinants[2]:

- Pelvic rotation. The pelvis rotates alternately to the right and to the left during normal level walking. This rotation is approximately 4° from the central axis for a total of 8°.
- Pelvic tilt. The pelvis tilts downwards relative to the horizontal on the opposite side to that of the weight-bearing limb. The angular displacement averages 5°. This lateral list helps decrease the amount of vertical displacement of the center of gravity required, thus saving energy.
- Knee flexion in the stance phase. As the body weight passes over the supporting leg, the knee undergoes flexion during midstance. The knee flexes approximately 15° and displacement of the center of gravity of the body is minimized. A knee that is stiff or weak will not permit midstance knee flexion, producing an increased energy expenditure. Pelvic rotation, pelvic tilt and knee flexion all act to flatten the arc through which the center of gravity of the body is translated. This minimizes the energy expended during gait.
- Foot and ankle mechanisms. Motions of the foot and ankle are closely interrelated during the gait cycle to avoid abrupt changes in the center of gravity and produce a smooth sinusoidal motion with a consequent large reduction in energy cost.
- Lateral displacement of the pelvis. The center of gravity of the body is displaced laterally over the weight-bearing extremity twice during the cycle of motion. This is achieved by a horizontal shift of the pelvis or by a relative abduction of the hip. The presence of the normal tibiofemoral angle obviates the need for excessive lateral displacement of the pelvis, which would require more energy. The net result of this is to keep the center of gravity of the body close to the line of projection, thus minimizing the energy expenditure.

Disorders of the hip, knee and ankle prevent some or all of these energy-saving mechanisms from operating so that more effort is required for gait. For the rheumatologist managing a patient with both joint and systemic problems, minimizing energy expenditure during gait is an important biomechanical goal.

JOINT SURFACE MOTION

During motion, the surfaces of the joint accelerate over each other in a reciprocal manner as the joint goes from flexion to extension. A technique for studying surface joint motion is to study the center of rotation of the joint[3]. The distal humerus forms an almost perfect cylinder and, as the olecranon rotates about the distal humerus, in effect it does so about a simple axis of rotation (Fig. 11.6). The surface motion at any particular point on the surface is perpendicular to the line which connects that point to the center of rotation. In the case of the distal humerus, the joint motion is always tangential to the joint surface. However, in the case of the knee joint with its changing curvature of radius, the instant center of rotation must move as the joint goes from flexion to extension in order to keep the joint surfaces moving parallel to each other (Fig. 11.7). If the center of rotation for a particular range of motion is displaced due to an arthritic process or to an interarticular injury, the normal gliding will be altered and the joint may be distracted or compressed (Fig. 11.8). If the center of rotation is on the surface there is no sliding friction because only rolling occurs. Rotating a joint about an abnormally located instant center can cause joint surface damage and begin a degenerative arthritic process (see page 11.6).

ACCELERATIONS

Accelerations are necessary for motion, which the body generates through the forces produced by muscle contraction. In a model of a limb, the muscle is attached distal to the limb's axis of rotation (Fig. 11.9), and its contraction produces a torque about that axis. A torque, or moment, is the product of a force and a distance. The torque (T) is related to the acceleration (A) by the expression $T = I \times A$. The mass moment of inertia (I) is an expression not only of the mass but of the distribution of the mass about an axis.

Muscle forces have both an external and an internal effect. The external effect of the force produces a joint torque which results in an acceleration with concomitant motions: force; torque; acceleration; motion. The internal effect of the force produces both deformation of the joint surfaces and internal stresses: force; deformation; strain.

STATICS AND DYNAMICS

When all of the forces acting on a body sum to zero, the body is said to be in equilibrium – the so-called static state. When the forces are not in equilibrium, the dynamic state may exist and accelerations are produced, resulting in motion.

A study of statics is useful in determining the loads on joints. In the hip joint in single leg stance, the force is produced from two sources:

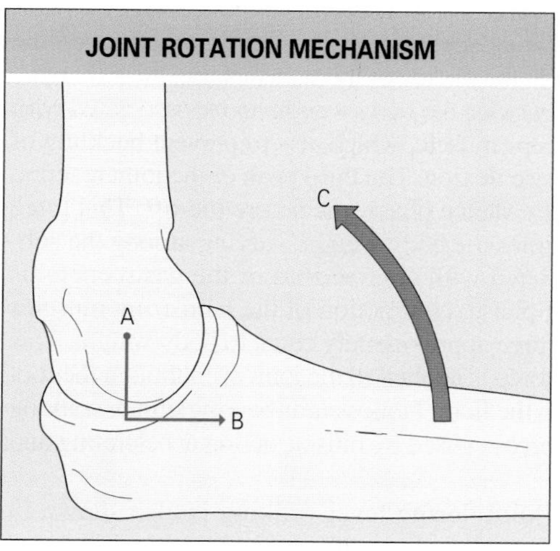

Fig. 11.6 Joint rotation mechanism. This illustrates surface motion at the humeroulnar joint.

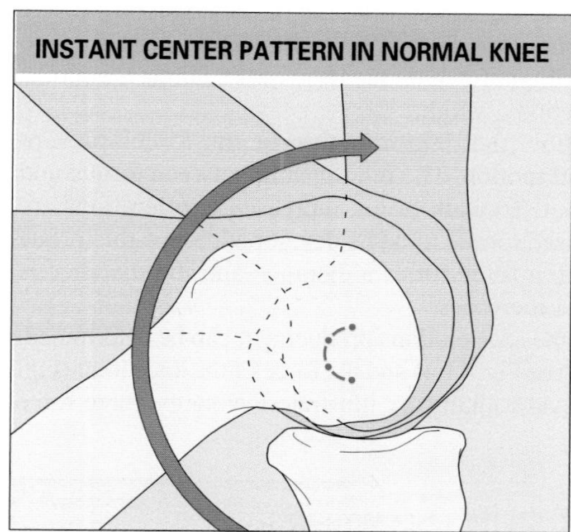

Fig. 11.7 Instant center pattern in the normal knee. Semicircular instant center pathway for the tibiofemoral joint in a normal knee. Each point is the instant center for a particular range of motion.

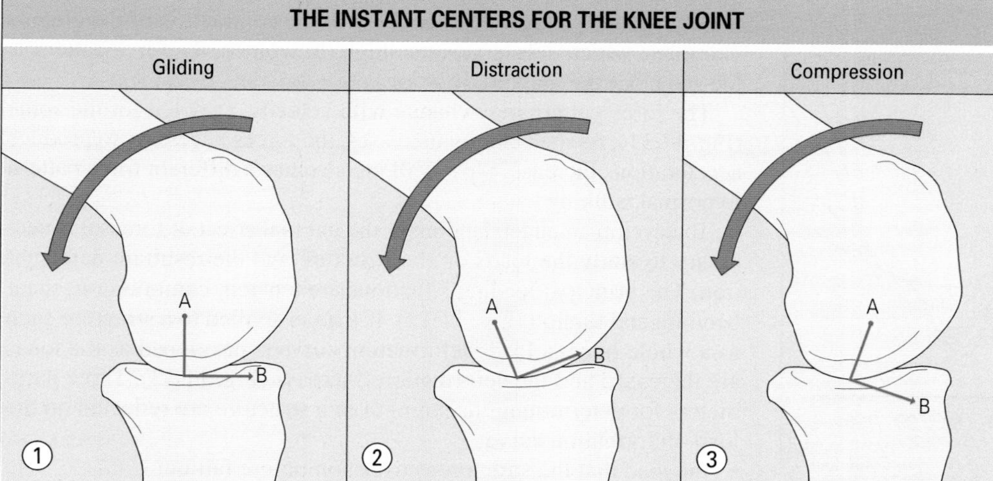

Fig. 11.8 The instant centers for the knee joint. (1) In a normal knee, a line drawn from the instant center of the tibiofemoral joint to the tibio-femoral contact point (line A) forms a right angle with a line tangential to the tibial surface (line B). The arrow indicates the direction of displacement of the contact points. Line B is tangential to the tibial surface, indicating that the femur glides on the tibial condyles during the measured interval of motion. (2,3) Where the center of rotation is displaced, the joint may be distracted or compressed.

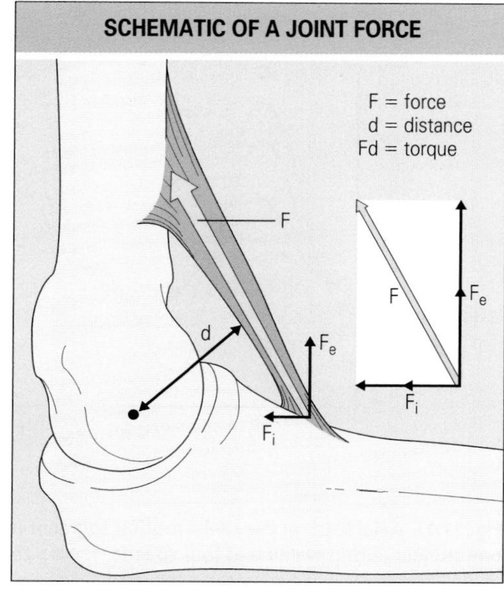

Fig. 11.9 Schematic of a joint force. (F_e: Force vector producing angular acceleration; F_i: Force vector producing joint compression).

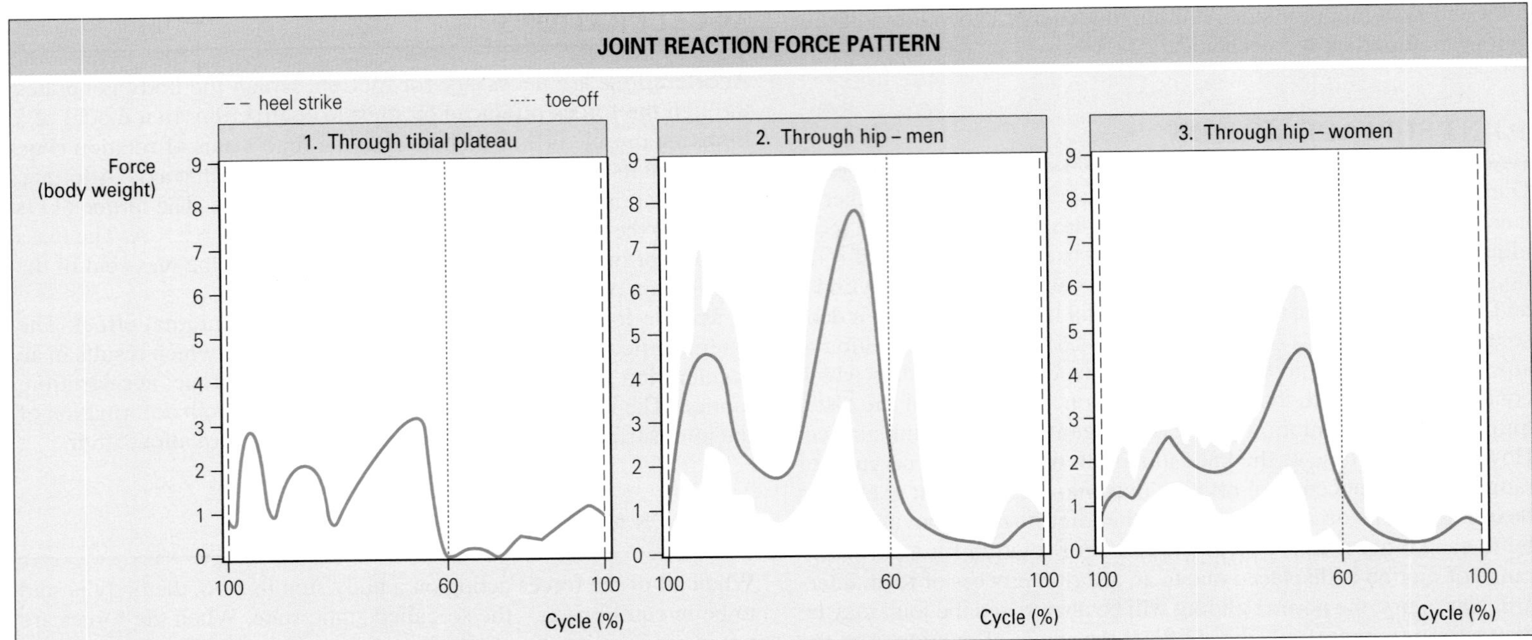

Fig. 11.10 Joint reaction force. (1) Knee joint reation force in terms of body weight transmitted through tibial plateau during walking (one gait cycle: 12 subjects). (2,3) Hip joint reaction force in units of body weight during walking (one gait cycle). The shaded area indicates variations among subjects.

the superincumbent body weight, which is equivalent to approximately 85% of the total body weight, and the abductor muscle, which contracts to keep the pelvis level. The contraction of the abductor muscle produces a force of about twice the body weight, so that when the two forces are added, the resultant force on the head of the femur is approximately three times the body weight.

Dynamic studies allow the determination of the forces present during accelerations and motion. The relationship between torque and acceleration is important. To walk faster, increased accelerations are required, thus an increased torque must be developed. Since the torque about a joint is equal to a force times a distance and the distance is constant, the force must increase.

By studying motion, the accelerations producing it can be determined. The motion of the knee (see Fig. 11.4) and the force of the knee joint (Fig. 11.10) during normal level walking are illustrated. Note the three force peaks present during the stance phase. They are due to normal muscle activity. Just after heel strike, the joint reaction force ranges from two to three times the body weight and is associated with contraction of the hamstring muscles, which have a decelerating and stabilizing effect on the knee. During knee flexion in the middle of the stance phase, the joint reaction force is approximately twice the body weight and is associated with contraction of the quadriceps muscle, which acts to prevent buckling of the knee during stance-phase flexion. The third peak of the joint reaction force occurs during the late stance phase just before toe-off. This force ranges from two to four times the body weight, varying among the subjects tested, and is associated with contractions of the gastrocnemius muscle. In the late swing phase, contraction of the hamstring muscles results in a joint reaction force approximately equal to body weight. This demonstrates that a large force is applied to the joint even though the foot may not be in contact with the floor. Non-weight-bearing crutch walking does not eliminate joint forces caused by muscle action accelerating and decelerating the limb.

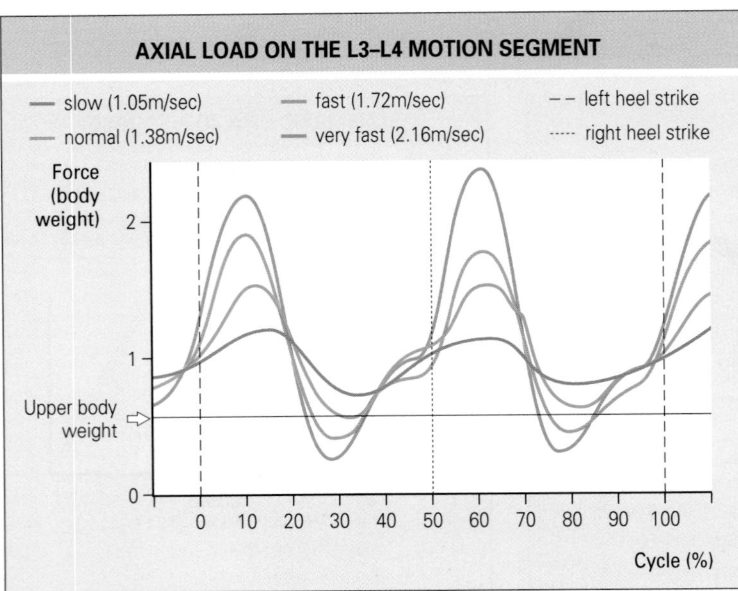

Fig. 11.11 Axial load on the L3–L4 motion segment in terms of body weight for one subject during walking at four speeds. The horizontal line denotes the weight of the upper body, which represents the gravitational component of this load. Loads were predicted using experimental data from photogrammetric measurements along with a biomechanical model of the trunk.

The force on the hip joint during level walking is also shown in Figure 11.10. In men, two peak forces are produced during the stance phase. During the swing phase, the joint reaction force is approximately equal to body weight because of the contraction of the gluteus maximus, which decelerates the thigh. In women, the force pattern is the same but the magnitude is lower.

The force pattern may change with velocity, as noted for the spine (Fig. 11.11). As the velocity increases, the forces necessary to produce accelerations increase. Slow walking also has a different force pattern to normal walking.

To develop an understanding of the internal effect of forces it is necessary to study the loads on the structure and the resultant deformation. The principal loading situations are tension, compression, shear bending and torsion (Fig. 11.12). If load is applied to a structure such as a whole bone, a load–deformation curve is developed as the loads are increased and the deformations increase (Fig. 11.13). Three parameters for determining the strength of a structure are reflected on the load–deformation curve:

- the load that the structure can sustain before failing;
- the deformation that it can sustain before failing;
- the energy that it can store before failing.

The strength in terms of load and deformation, or ultimate strength, is indicated on the curve by the ultimate failure point. The strength in terms of energy storage is indicated by the size of the area under the entire

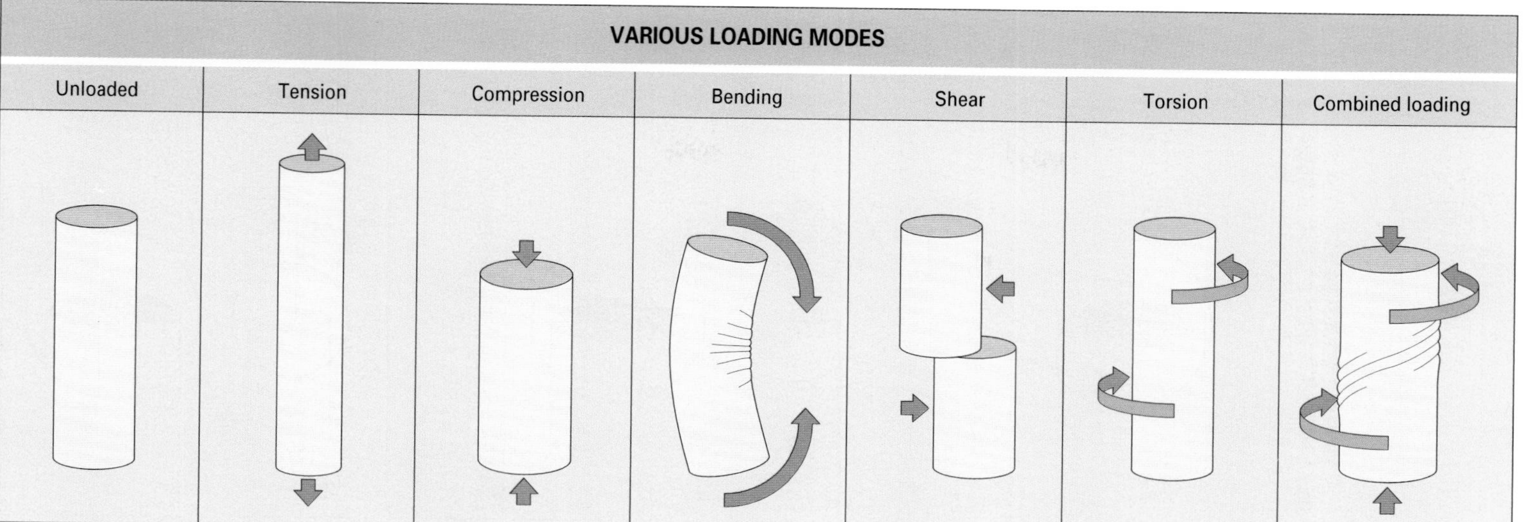

Fig. 11.12 Schematic representation of various loading modes.

curve. The larger the area, the greater is the energy stored in the structure as the load is applied. The stiffness of the structure is indicated by the slope of the curve in the elastic region. The steeper the slope, the stiffer the material. The load–deformation curve is useful for determining the mechanical properties of whole structures such as a whole bone, an entire ligament or tendon, or a surgical implant. This knowledge is helpful in the study of fracture behavior and repair, the response of a structure to physical stress or the effect of various treatment programs.

Characterizing a bone or other structure in terms of the material that composes it, independent of its geometry, requires standardization of the testing conditions and the size and shape of the test specimens. Such standardized testing is useful for comparing the mechanical properties of two or more materials, such as the relative strength of bone and tendon tissue or the relative stiffness of various materials used in prosthetic implants. More precise units of measurement can be used when standardized samples are tested, i.e. the load per unit of area of the sample (stress), and the amount of deformation in terms of the percentage of change in the sample's dimensions (strain). The curve generated is a stress–strain curve (Fig. 11.14).

Stress is the load, or force, per unit area that develops on a plane surface within a structure in response to externally applied loads. The three units most commonly used for measuring stress in standardized samples of bone are newtons per centimeter squared (N/cm^2); newtons per meter squared, or pascals (N/m^2, Pa); and meganewtons per meter squared, or megapascals (MN/m^2, MPa). Figure 11.15 illustrates the stress in a perpendicular plane of a cylinder under tension and compression, and the stress in a shear plane.

Strain is the deformation (change in dimension) that develops within a structure in response to externally applied loads. The two basic types of strain are linear strain, which causes a change in the length of the specimen, and shear strain, which causes a change in the angular relationships within the structure. Linear strain is measured as the amount of linear deformation (lengthening or shortening) of the sample divided by the sample's original length. It is a nondimensional parameter expressed as a percentage (for example, centimeter per centimeter). Shear strain is measured as the amount of angular change in a right angle lying in the plane of interest in the sample.

Biological tissues have different stress–strain relationships

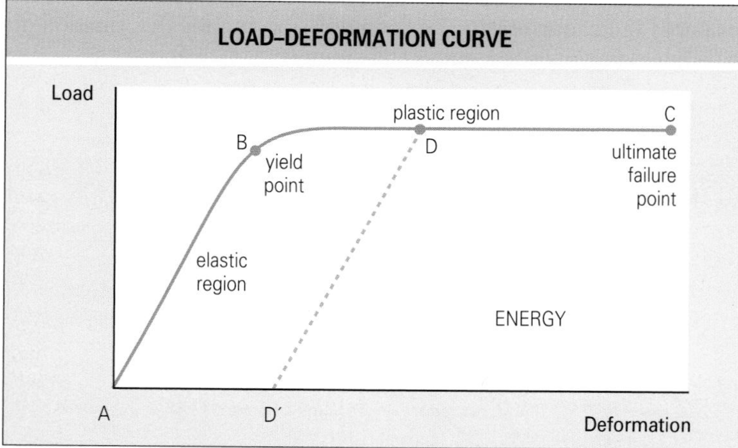

Fig. 11.13 Load–deformation curve for a structure composed of a pliable material. If a load is applied within the elastic range of the structure (A to B on the curve) and is then released, no permanent deformation occurs. If loading is continued past the yield point (B) and into the plastic range of the structure (B to C on the curve) and then released, permanent deformation results. The amount of permanent deformation that occurs if the structure is loaded to point D in the plastic region and then unloaded is represented by the distance between A and D′. If loading continues within the plastic range the ultimate failure point (C) is reached.

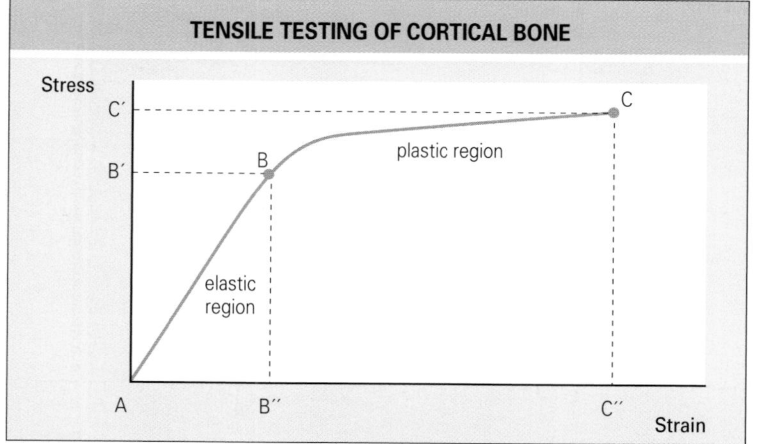

Fig. 11.14 Stress–strain curve for a cortical bone sample tested in tension. Yield point (B): point past which some permanent deformation of the bone sample occurs. Yield stress (B′): load per unit area sustained by the bone sample before plastic deformation takes place. Yield strain (B′′): amount of deformation withstood by the sample before plastic deformation occurs. The strain at any point in the elastic region of the curve is proportional to the stress at that point. Ultimate failure point (C): the point past which failure of the sample occurs. Ultimate stress (C′): load per unit area sustained by the sample before failure. Ultimate strain (C′′): amount of deformation sustained by the sample before failure.

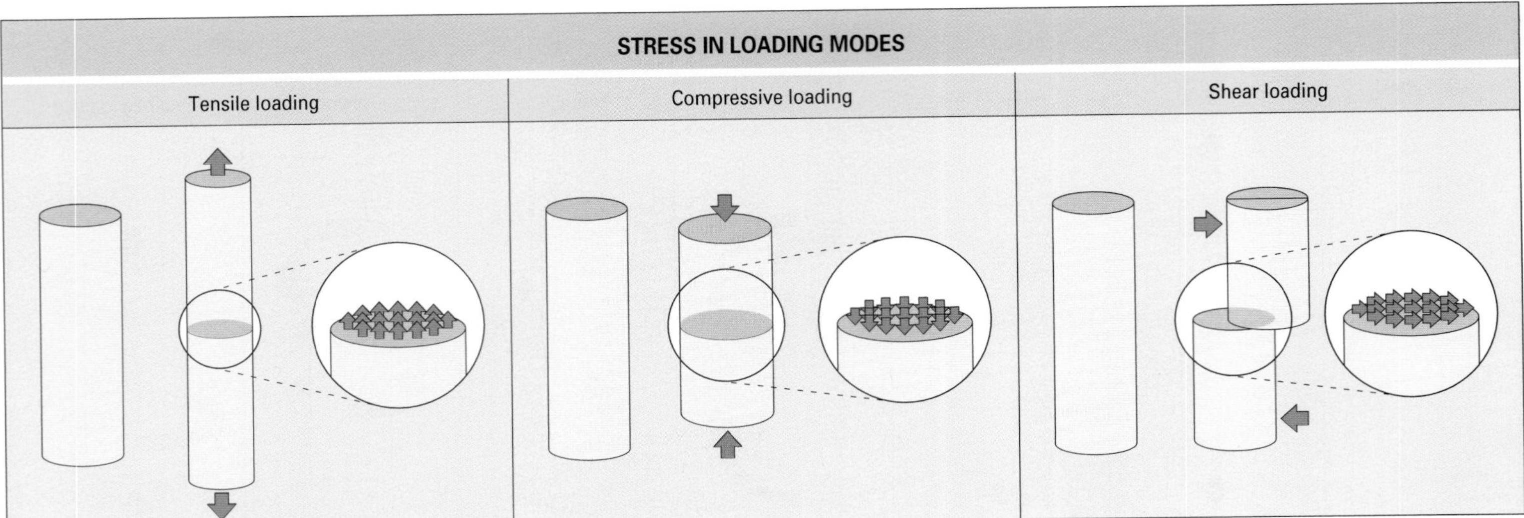

Fig. 11.15 Stress produced in loading modes.

depending upon their composition. In the case of the soft tissues, made up of collagen and elastin fibers, the curve has a characteristic 'toe' portion and, as the force increases, becomes much stiffer (see Fig. 11.16). Cartilage under tension loading exhibits a similar type of stress–strain relationship. Biological tissues also exhibit properties that are not found in structural material, such as stainless steel; they are anisotropic so that the stress–strain relationships of, for instance, a bone sample depends upon the direction in relation to the long axis of the bone from which the sample is taken (Fig 11.17).

Another property which tissue may exhibit is viscoelastic time-dependent behavior under load. Cartilage under a constant compressive stress shows a creep response due to exudation of fluid from the sample until an equilibrium is reached (Fig. 11.18). If a constant compression rate is applied to the cartilage, the phenomenon of stress relaxation occurs.

The collagenous tissues also demonstrate viscoelasticity. It is evident that the duration of the contact pressure is of great importance.

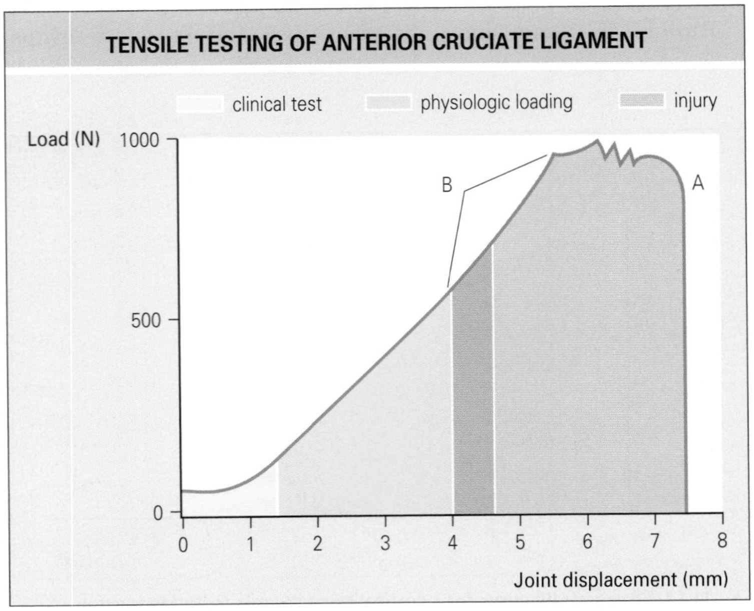

TENSILE TESTING OF ANTERIOR CRUCIATE LIGAMENT

clinical test
physiologic loading
injury
Load (N)
1000
500
0
B
A
0 1 2 3 4 5 6 7 8
Joint displacement (mm)

Fig. 11.16 Tensile testing of a human anterior cruciate ligament *in vitro*. The curve produced has been converted into a load–displacement curve and divided into three regions correlating with clinical findings: the load imposed on the anterior cruciate ligament during the anterior drawer test; that placed on the ligament during physiologic activity; and that imposed on the ligament from partial injury to complete rupture (A). It should be noted that the divisions shown here represent a generalization. Microfailure (B) is shown to begin towards the end of the physiologic loading region, but it may take place well before this point in any given ligament.

For example, it has been demonstrated that earlobe tissue under tension loading exhibits a time-dependent stretch, i.e. the material will continue to stretch as a constant load is left on for measureable periods of time. This reaction to the load comprises four well-defined regions. As the load is applied there is an area of immediate elastic deformation; if the load is taken off immediately the material recoils elastically back to its original size. If, however, the load is left on, the material continues to stretch. This stretching tends to reach a limiting or steady-state value. If the load is allowed to remain for an appreciable period of time and is then removed, there is an immediate elastic recoil towards the material's original dimension.

This response to prolonged loading is typical of the response shown by materials classified as viscoelastic. Load relaxation and creep phenomena are found in ligaments and tendons – knowledge of this time-dependent behavior is useful in overcoming contractures. Bone also exhibits viscoelastic, time-dependent behavior. As the loading or strain rate increases, the stress–strain curve also changes, becoming steeper in the elastic region to level off at higher values of stress. This effect is present in bone tissue or whole bone. A complex state of stress and strain can result from simple loading conditions, tension, compression and shear. If a joint structure is placed under compressive loading, compressive stresses and strains will result in certain planes, while tension and shear stresses and strains occur in other directions. Note the change in shapes indicating tension and compression and the deformation of the angles showing shear stress and strain (Fig. 11.19).

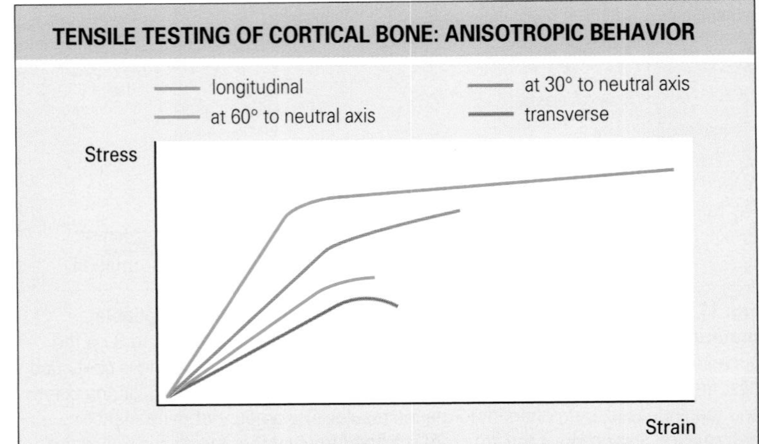

Fig. 11.17 Anisotropic behavior of cortical bone specimens from a human femoral shaft: tested in tension in four directions: longitudinal, tilted 30° with respect to the neutral axis of the bone, tilted 60°, and transverse.

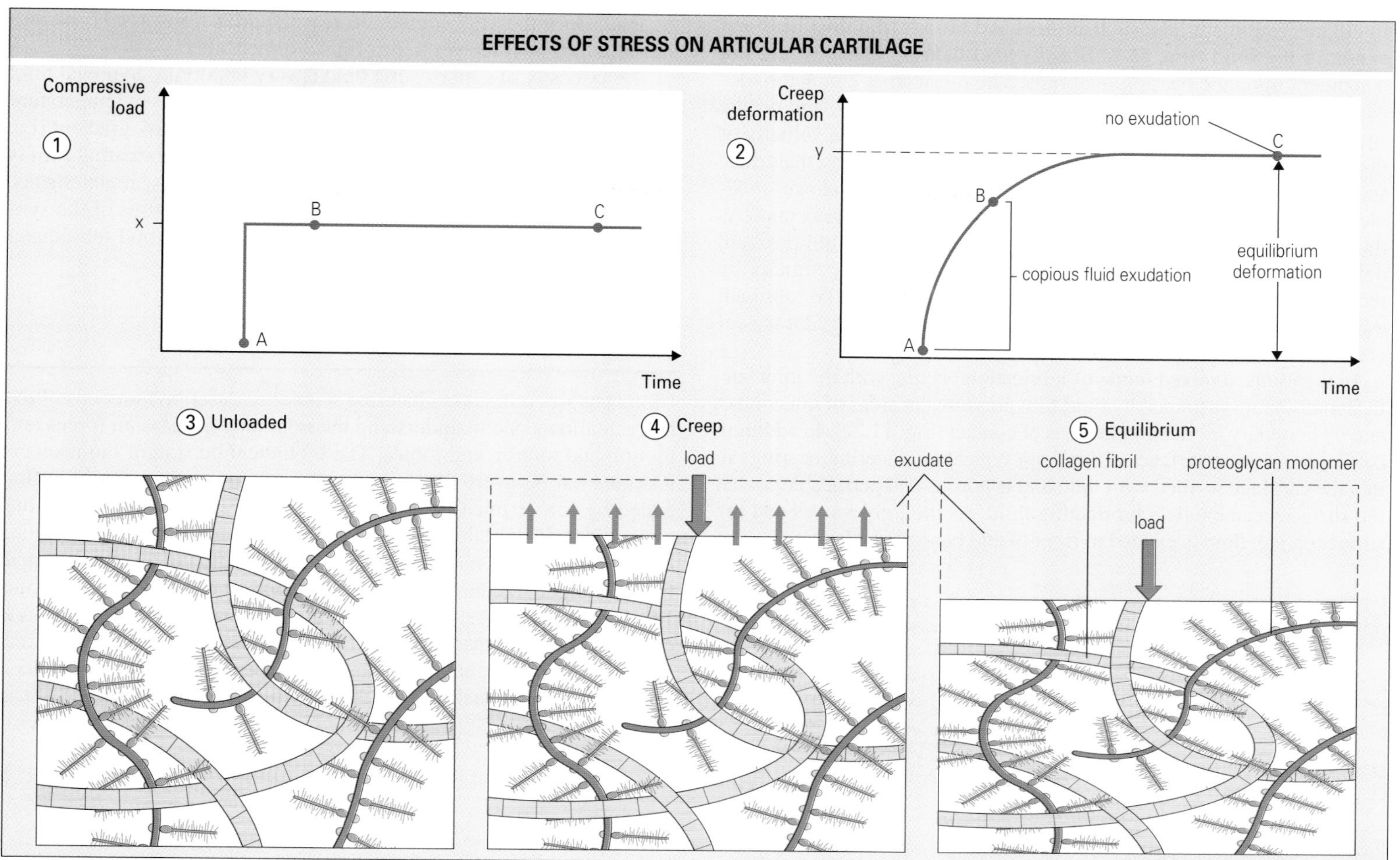

Fig. 11.18 Effects of stress. A constant stress (x) applied to a sample of articular cartilage (1) and creep response of the sample under the constant applied stress (2). The drawings of a block of tissue (3–5) illustrate that creep is accompanied by copious exudation of fluid from the sample and that the rate of exudation decreases over time from point A to B to C. At equilibrium (y), fluid flow ceases and the load is borne entirely by the solid matrix (point C).

A change in normal kinematics resulting in an altered state of stress or strain in a joint is one of the mechanisms leading to degenerative arthritis. For example, a bucket handle tear converts the knee joint from a three-dimensional joint to a planar joint by blocking normal tibial rotation. As a result of this restriction to motion, the instant center is displaced from its normal position. Forcing the joint to rotate about an abnormal instant center is similar to forcing a door to rotate about a bent hinge; the door jamb or the door will be worn down. This same process occurs in any joint that is forced to revolve about an abnormal instant center. Distraction may cause stretching of the ligaments. Compression will cause articular surface wear and an abnormal stress distribution in the articulating surfaces. This altered stress distribution may occur not only in the contact areas of the cartilage, but also adjacent to this area. The synovial reaction will occur in the region of altered stress and strain, followed by osteophyte formation. Small mechanical changes can induce biological processes that result in degenerative arthritis. Caution should be exerted in exercising joints that display kinematic abnormalities on physical examination.

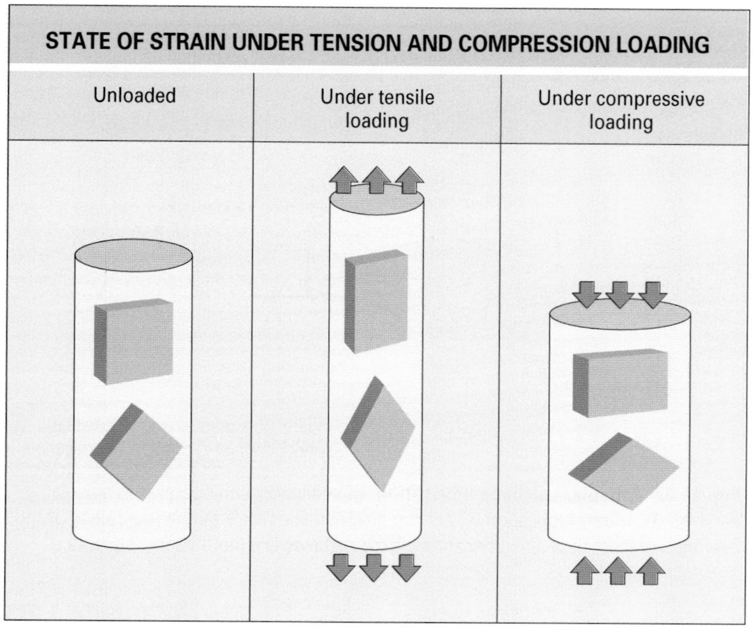

Fig. 11.19 State of strain under tension and compressive loading. Tension and compression strain are indicated by an increase or decrease in the length of a line. The presence of shear strain in a structure loaded in tension and in compression is indicated by angular deformation.

LUBRICATION

The human joints are exposed to a great variation of loading conditions. There can be high impact, short duration loads such as in running, moderately low loads with a prolonged loading time such as in standing, and low loads with rapid motion in the swing phase of walking. Over a lifetime there is relatively little wear in the joints, indicating a very superior lubricating system.

There are two types of lubrication. One is boundary lubrication, which is due to a single layer (monolayer) of lubricant adsorbed on each bearing surface. In the case of a joint, boundary lubrication is achieved by a macromolecular monolayer attached to each articular surface. These layers carry loads and are effective in reducing friction. The second type of lubrication, fluid film lubrication, produces a greater bearing surface separation and is due to a thin film of lubricant. The pressure developed in the lubricating fluid carries the loads (Fig. 11.20).

In engineering materials, such as steel and bronze, the thickness and extent of the fluid film, as well as its load-bearing capacity, are not dependent upon the bearing materials. The lubricating characteristics depend upon the lubricant properties, such as viscosity, and on the shape of the gap between the two bearing surfaces and the velocity of the relative surface motion. In the human joint, the bearing materials, such as the articular cartilage, are not rigid and have much lower modules of elasticity. Elastohydrodynamic lubrication therefore occurs. As the joint surfaces move and pressure is developed, the fluid pressure deforms the surfaces (Fig. 11.21). This changes the film geometry by increasing the surface area, thus there is less chance of the lubricant escaping between the bearing surfaces and a longer lasting film is generated. This results in a lower stress.

In the joints, a mixed mode of lubrication occurs, with the joint surface loads being sustained by fluid film pressures in areas of noncontact and by boundary lubrication in areas of contact (Fig. 11.22). In addition, cartilaginous joint surfaces differ from typical engineering bearings in that the cartilage is filled with fluid and is porous and permeable so that the surfaces can exude a lubricating fluid. As the joint moves and the surfaces slide, fluid is exuded in front of and beneath the leading half of the load. Once the peak stresses decrease, fluid is reabsorbed back into the cartilage and it returns to its original dimensions.

The viscosity of a lubricating fluid is very important. Synovial fluid undergoes large changes in viscosity, both with changes in temperature (i.e. it is a Newtonian fluid) and with changes in velocity gradient (i.e. it is thixotropic). For very low velocities, a thinner lubricating film is desirable. Being thixotropic, synovial fluid can meet these requirements.

If a joint effusion is present, the thixotropic properties of the synovial fluid may be lost, resulting in reduced lubrication and subsequent wear of the joint surfaces.

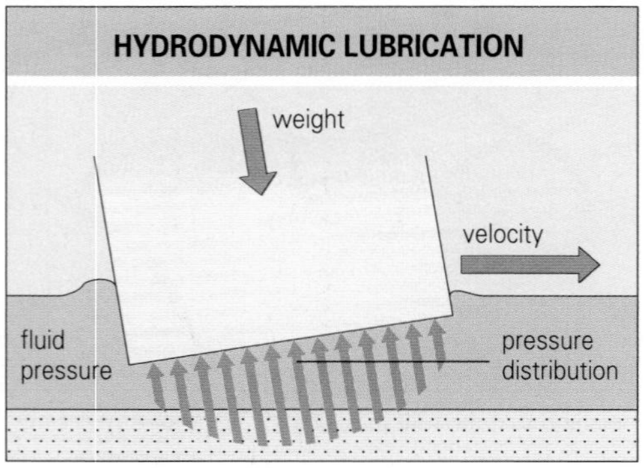

Fig. 11.20 Hydrodynamic lubrication. During motion at sufficiently high velocities the weight tilts and forms a wedge shape. Because of the viscous properties of the fluid, a pressure will be created within the fluid to support the weight.

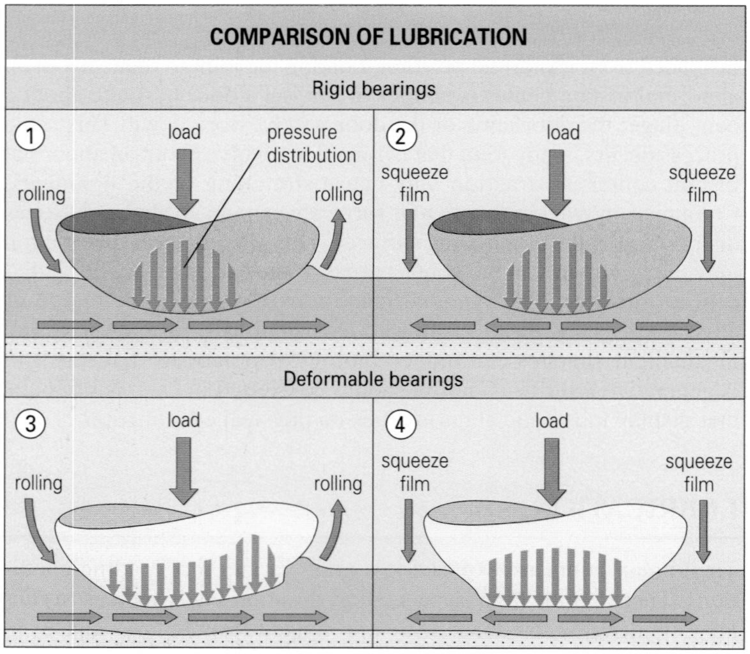

Fig. 11.21 Load-carrying by lubricated bearing. A comparison of hydrodynamic lubrication (1) and squeeze film lubrication (2) of rigid surfaces, and elastohydrodynamic lubrication of deformable bearing surfaces under a hydrodynamic (sliding) action (3) and a squeeze film action (4). Surface deformation of elastohydrodynamically lubricated bearings increases the contact area, thus increasing the load-carrying capacity of these bearings.

SUMMARY

Biomechanics utilizes engineering science to describe functions of the body. It allows one to understand the relationship between forces and motion and motion and forces. The biological portion of biomechanics must not be overlooked. Biological processes that may be influenced by forces must be studied with a knowledge of not only the magnitude and direction of the forces but also their rate of application. Disuse osteoporosis may result from the application of less than normal forces. Fatigue fractures result from the application of increased forces. Joint wear and subsequent degenerative arthritis may result from a change of both the magnitude and direction of the forces on an injured joint. An understanding of the basic concepts of biomechanics is necessary for anyone dealing with the musculoskeletal system.

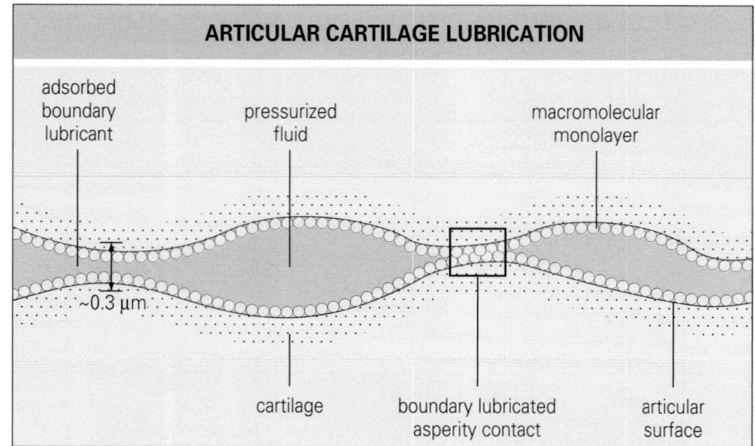

Fig. 11.22 Articular cartilage lubrication. Mixed lubrication operates in articular cartilage: boundary lubrication where the fluid film is as thick as the roughness of the bearing surfaces; fluid film lubrication where surfaces are more widely separated.

REFERENCES

1. Nordin M, Frankel VH. Basic biomechanics of the musculoskeletal system, 2E. Philadelphia: Lea & Febiger; 1989.
2. Saunders JB DeC M, Inman VT, Eberhardt HD. The major determinants in normal and pathological gait. J Bone Joint Surg. 1953;35A:543–58.
3. Frankel VH, Burstein AH, Brooks DB. Biomechanics of internal derangement of the knee. Pathomedics as determined by analysis of the instant centers of motion. J Bone Joint Surg. 1971;53A:945.

2

EVALUATION, SIGNS AND SYMPTOMS

Rodney Grahame & John S Sergent

1

HISTORY

Paul Dieppe & John Sergent

- History taking is the most important skill needed in rheumatology.
- A good history ('the story') can be a powerful therapeutic experience for the patient, as well as provide the physician with some 80% of the diagnostic information required.
- History taking involves an initial (patient-centred) listening phase and a second (physician-centred) interrogative phase.
- The physician needs to learn about the major presenting symptoms, the chronology of the disorder and its impact on the patient and people around the patient, as well as ancillary information such as past and family history and involvement of other systems.
- Patients must have the opportunity to voice the problems that matter most to them.

INTRODUCTION – THE MEDICAL CONSULTATION

The consultation between physician and patient is at the core of all rheumatologic practice. The process is often divided into three overlapping phases: history taking, examination and analysis of the data obtained. History taking is by far the most important part of the process.

The division of the medical consultation into distinct phases is artificial, as in practice all three components take place together. From the moment of first meeting a patient, the physician is simultaneously observing and examining the way in which the patient walks and the manner of introduction, hand shaking and responses to the consultation process, for example, as well as listening to what is being said and trying to piece together what the nature of the problem might be.

The purpose of the medical consultation is twofold: first it allows the patient to present the problem to the physician, a therapeutic process in itself; and second it can enable the physician to sort out the nature of the problem (diagnosis) and decide on any further course of action that might need to be taken. In this context, the physician must always ask what has brought the patient to the consultation and what the expectations of the patient are. In some cases a patient visits the physician because of referral by or on the advice of a third party, in which case both the patient's perception of the problem and the expectations of the referring party must be considered. The diagnostic process is also complex, as the physician needs to establish the physical or psychosocial issues that are of most importance to the patient and that are most disrupting to normal life, as well as try to diagnose the anatomic and pathologic aspects of any disease that might be present.

ESTABLISHING THE HISTORY

One of the great advantages of rheumatology over many other medical subspecialties is that the history and examination provide most of the key information required for diagnosis, assessment and treatment. In most cases special investigations are either unnecessary or add relatively little more than confirmatory evidence of the conclusions drawn from the history and physical examination. One of the key aspects of a rheumatic disease that the physician needs to understand, the history provides much information about the pathologic processes involved and the impact of the condition on the patient, whereas the examination is essential to sort out the anatomic structures involved; together they allow differentiation of the rheumatic disorders into different categories (Fig. 1.1).

Obtaining a good rheumatology history involves the art of medicine as much as its science. However, it is very difficult both to teach or to learn the central art of history taking, which probably depends more on experience than does any other aspect of medical practice. When junior physicians complain that patients do not tell them the same crucial facts as they reveal to the senior consultants, they are exposing their inability to take a good history. Most physicians think that they are good at communicating with their patients, but surveys of the patients themselves disagree; all physicians should be prepared to be critical of their technique when interviewing patients and to spend more time learning the key skills involved in communication.

The history can be established at different levels, depending on the nature of the consultation and time available. If the only need is to establish quickly the presence or absence of major musculoskeletal problems, then the screening questions (and examination) described in the 'GALS' (gait, arms, legs, spine) regime will suffice – this includes questions such as 'Do you suffer from any pain or stiffness in your arms or legs, neck or back?' and 'Do you have any difficulty with washing and dressing or with stairs and steps?' At the second level, it may be appropriate to concentrate relatively quickly and exclusively on a specific regional problem, such as the elbow pain with which the patient presented. However, in the majority of cases it is both necessary and rewarding to take a full history, particularly as an apparently simple regional problem may be the manifestation of a more generalized condition and may be associated with a large amount of physical and psychosocial overlay that is all too easy to miss or ignore.

Full history taking can be divided into two phases, an initial 'open' phase in which the physician listens, followed by a second 'specific' phase in which direct questioning elicits ancillary information.

DIAGNOSIS OF MUSCULOSKELETAL DISORDERS
1. The history provides information on the pathologic process, including: Inflammatory rheumatic disorders Mechanical rheumatic disorders Systemic diseases affecting the musculoskeletal system Functional disorders
2. The **examination** defines the **anatomic site** of the problem, including: Articular disorders Periarticular disorders Myalgias or muscle disease
3. Both **history and examination** help determine **disability**, as in the pneumonic 'PILS': P Preventable causes of disability (falls, pressure sores, etc.) I Independent living (washing, dressing, toileting, etc.) L Lifestyle (role, goals and soul) S Social support (housing, family, friends, money, etc.)

Fig. 1.1 The diagnosis of musculoskeletal disorders.

THE INITIAL PATIENT-CENTRED 'OPEN' PHASE OF HISTORY TAKING

The history is the patient's story. The physician's first job is to listen to what the patient has to say. After the initial introductions have been made, through which the physician should create a relaxed atmosphere, the history can begin with an open question, such as 'Tell me about it' – allowing the patient to start wherever he or she wishes ('it' should not be defined). The physician needs to be prepared to wait, to encourage the patient with nonverbal signals and to avoid talking him- or herself; the physician should not use any closed question which can be answered with a 'yes' or 'no' or simple factual statement. This should help the patient bring the problems that really bother him or her out into the open and also avoid that all too common complaint that 'the physician didn't listen to me' – which often means that the patient was not given the chance to say what he or she wanted to say. The stoic, macho, monosyllabic patient may need a lot of coaxing and encouragement, whereas the garrulous, flighty, anxious and distracted patient may need help and direction to get to the point, but all should be given the opportunity to open up before the physician risks closing the interview down with specific questions. During this phase a few remarks will often help steer the conversation along the lines required, but nonverbal communication is often the key; for example the physician can lean forward, establish eye contact and look more interested as the patient begins to focus on the issues that matter, and lean back when it seems that less relevant information is being proffered. However, the value judgment as to what is and is not relevant is in itself one of the crucial analytic skills employed during this first phase of the interview.

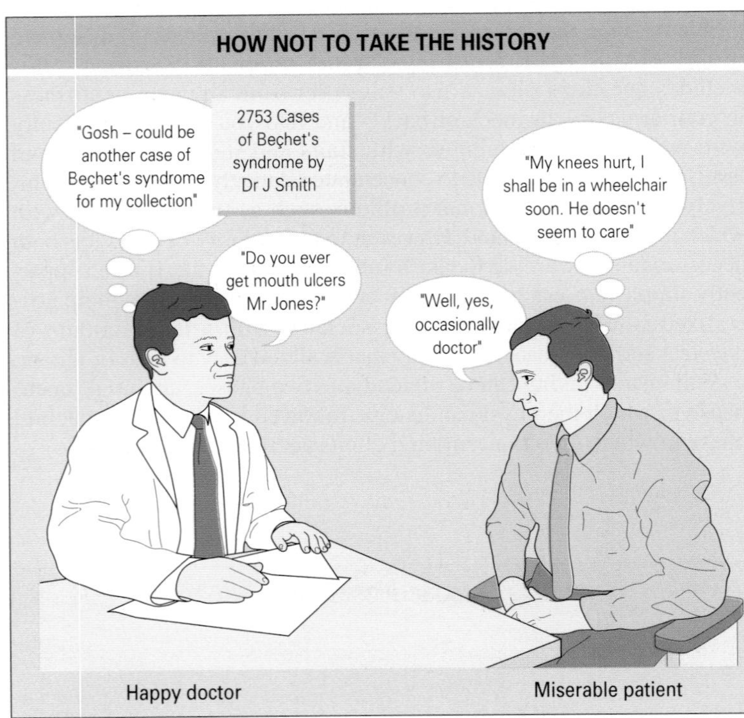
HOW NOT TO TAKE THE HISTORY
"Gosh – could be another case of Beçhet's syndrome for my collection"
2753 Cases of Beçhet's syndrome by Dr J Smith
"My knees hurt, I shall be in a wheelchair soon. He doesn't seem to care"
"Do you ever get mouth ulcers Mr Jones?"
"Well, yes, occasionally doctor"
Happy doctor
Miserable patient

Fig. 1.2a How not to take the history. The physician is obsessed with the diagnosis and with the discovery of more cases of a disorder that particularly interests him; the patient is aware of this, but is intimidated and unable to voice his fears that he is going to be in a wheelchair within a few months.

FOUR KEY SKILLS OF GOOD HISTORY TAKING
Active listening
Soliciting attribution
Providing support
Establishing agreement

Fig. 1.2b The four key skills of good history taking.

CATEGORIES FOR TAKING A CHRONIC RHEUMATIC DISEASE HISTORY
Demographic data (age, sex, occupation, etc.)
Presenting symptoms (pain, stiffness, swelling, weakness, fatigue, anxiety, etc.)
Chronology of the disorder (how it started, course and effect of interventions)
Impact (impairment, disability and handicap)
Past medical history and family history
Drug (and other interventions), occupational history, social history
Review of other systems

Fig. 1.3 Categories of information that need to be obtained when taking a history from someone with a chronic rheumatic disease.

THE SECOND, PHYSICIAN-CENTRED 'INTERROGATIVE' PHASE OF HISTORY TAKING

Only when the first phase has been completed should the physician turn to the second phase, to learn more about what they still wish to know. As soon as a physician starts to ask highly specific questions, such as the dose of a drug that is being taken, the whole nature of the interview changes and many people immediately stop being able to say what is really troubling them. All too often physicians begin with specific questions, so their patients never have the chance to express the real problem. This helps explain why physicians are sometimes accused of investigating and treating something of interest to themselves rather than the item of real importance to the patient (Fig. 1.2).

It is generally taught that during the specific phase of history taking the information obtained should be split into demographic data (age, sex, occupation, etc.), the presenting problems and history of presenting complaint, past history, family and psychosocial history, past and current therapy, and review of systems. In patients with chronic rheumatic diseases it is often useful to order the information in a slightly different way to emphasize three issues – the current symptoms, the chronology of the condition (including the influence of any therapy) and the impact of the disorder in both physical and psychologic terms – before reviewing the other features, including the past and family history, occupational, sexual and psychosocial issues, and other systems (Fig. 1.3).

SYMPTOMS

The most important presenting symptoms in rheumatologic practice include pain, stiffness or locking, swelling, weakness or difficulty moving, fatigue and emotional lability such as anxiety or depression. Of these pain is most common.

Analysis of these symptoms helps the physician to differentiate a rheumatic complaint into five main types:

- inflammatory musculoskeletal disease,
- mechanical joint or periarticular disorder,
- nonrheumatic disease causing musculoskeletal symptoms,
- a functional disorder,
- or another of unknown cause.

PAIN

Many rheumatic diseases are characterized by specific patterns of pain and stiffness. For example, gout usually begins in the middle of the night with a pricking sensation in the great toe, which quickly builds up into an intolerable burning pain; whereas osteoarthritis is characterized by use-related pain and inactivity stiffness of the affected joints. The many different patterns of pain can be distinguished by finding out 'when, why, where and what'.

When and why?

The time and mode of onset, diurnal pattern and factors that affect pain are all important. Pain caused by inflammation is usually worse at the

COMMON PERIARTICULAR PROBLEMS AND PRECIPITATING ACTIVITIES	
Periarticular syndromes	**Precipitating events**
Subachromial bursitis	Carpentry, painting, sports
Rotator cuff tendinitis	Throwing, repetitive work
Bicipital tendinitis	Repetitive lifting
Olecranon bursitis	Trauma
Lateral epicondylitis (tennis elbow)	Tennis, housework
Medial epicondylitis (golfer's elbow)	Tennis, housework
Tendinitis of abductor pollicis longus and extensor pollicis brevis (de Quervain's disease)	Repetitive lifting
Ilipsoas bursitis	Running, climbing
Trochanteric bursitis	Running, climbing
Prepatellar bursitis	Gardening, carpet laying
Achilles tendinitis	Running on hills, climbing steps
Plantar fasciitis	Walking, sports (especially if obese)

Fig. 1.4 Common periarticular problems and activities that may precipitate them.

ends of the day and associated with stiffness, whereas mechanical pain is generally use-related. The factors that bring on a mechanical pain may provide clues as to the precise diagnosis, it is useful to ask specific questions about what kinds of activities induce pain – repetitive motion, climbing stairs, arising from a low chair, and so on. Periarticular problems are often induced by a specific type of activity (Fig. 1.4). Other disorders may also present with pain that has a specific relationship to activity; for example, when a twisting movement produces sharp pain and locking of the knee joint, it is likely that an internal derangement (such as a torn meniscus) is the problem; similarly it may be an easy task to diagnose spinal stenosis from the pain history when it is apparent that buttock and leg pain is activity related and that walking downhill (which extends the spine) causes more pain than walking uphill or cycling. Constant severe pain, present throughout the day and night and not affected by or linked to anything might be due to a bone disorder, but can also be functional.

Where?

It is obviously important to establish the site of pain. Regional disorders, associated with pain in one area, must be differentiated from systemic conditions in which there is generalized pain. However, it is often difficult to obtain any precise localization of musculoskeletal pain as it is mostly visceral, and therefore poorly localized, rather than somatic in origin. Furthermore, pain is often referred to areas of the body distal to the lesion. Classic examples of this include the referral of neck or shoulder pain to the upper arm and the presentation of hip disease with knee pain (Fig. 1.5). Generalized pain all over can be due to fibromyalgia or polymyalgia rheumatica, whereas pain in multiple joints (arthralgia) can be due to a number of other possible causes, such as viral infections and many arthropathies. However, the full differentiation of the anatomic site of origin of both generalized or regional pain usually requires examination of the patient in addition to history taking (see Fig. 1.1).

COMMON PATTERNS OF REFERRED PAIN	
Source of pain	**Pattern of referral**
Cervical spine	Occipital, shoulders
Shoulder	Lateral aspect of arm
Lateral epicondyle	Mid forearm
Carpal tunnel	Radial fingers, occasionally forearm or arm
Lumbar spine	Sacroiliac joints, buttocks, posterior thigh, lower leg, foot
Hip joint	Groin, medial thigh, medial knee, greater trochanteric, buttock above gluteal fold
Trochanteric bursa	Lateral thigh, buttock

Fig. 1.5 Common patterns of referred pain.

What and so what?

The quality of musculoskeletal pain sometimes provides important diagnostic clues. For example, a nerve entrapment may produce pain that is described as being like an electric shock and of a shooting type. In contrast, vascular pain may be throbbing and joint pains are often described as a severe aching sensation. However, neither the adjectives that people use to describe their pain nor their assessment of its severity is generally of great diagnostic value. Of much greater importance than 'what quality' in diagnosis is the 'so what' value of these descriptions; they provide important insights into the person, their response to the pain and the degree to which it disrupts their lives. Pain is a subjective sensation that cannot be felt by others, cannot be remembered exactly and brings with it a great deal of psychologic baggage, interpretation and fear; also, it has quite different effects on different individuals.

STIFFNESS

Rheumatologists and their patients often give great value to the symptom of stiffness with neither knowing quite what they mean. Stiffness (or 'gelling') of joints is important because an inflammatory joint disorder is generally associated with severe and prolonged morning and evening stiffness, whereas osteoarthritis is associated with short-lived but severe stiffness after inactivity. However, 'stiffness' can be used to describe many different sensations and phenomena; it is also difficult to describe. Inactivity gelling of the osteoarthritic joint appears to be largely due to difficulty in the initiation of movement, whereas morning stiffness in rheumatoid arthritis (RA) may describe a more constant difficulty in moving the joints through any part of their range. Stiffness can also be used to describe pain or aching in joints with movement, or to mean a reduced or limited range of movement. One of the disorders most characterized by stiffness is polymyalgia rheumatica, in which morning stiffness can be so severe that it even becomes impossible to move enough to role out of bed, although a few hours after getting up the patient may be virtually asymptomatic. The duration of morning stiffness can also indicate the activity of RA; simple questions such as 'What time do you wake?' followed by 'When are you as loose as you are going to get?' help pin down its duration.

Locking of the joints, limbs or spine is a less common, but associated, symptom. Locking may be used to describe very severe stiffness, but more commonly describes a specific mechanical event in which some internal derangement of a joint actually causes it to lock in one position until a trick movement or help from someone else frees it up. This is a classic symptom of meniscal injury of the knee joint, but it also occurs in the neck and spine when there is disk or apophyseal joint disease, and it can affect other joint sites.

SWELLING

Swelling is an important symptom and sign of joint disease; true swelling implies inflammation of a joint or periarticular structure. However, while patients should always be asked if they have joint swelling, one must beware of interpreting their positive answer to mean that there will be evidence of inflammation on examination. Pain and stiffness of joints may be accompanied by the feeling that they are swollen, and patients may genuinely believe that their hands or feet look swollen even when there is no objective sign of this to the examiner.

WEAKNESS AND DIFFICULTY MOVING

Patients often describe weakness of limbs or of the whole body. This can be an important clue to an uncommon rheumatic disorder such as polymyositis or a neuropathy; the pattern of asymmetric or symmetric muscle weakness and its central or peripheral distribution may give vital clues to the diagnosis. However, as with symptoms such as stiffness and swelling, weakness may mean different things. It may describe the difficulty that the patient has with movement because of joint disease, or the feeling of insecurity that is associated with a loss of proprioception that accompanies many forms of joint disease. It may also be used to describe the regional weakness of a joint or limb caused by the local muscle-wasting that can accompany joint damage. Finally, the term 'weakness' may be used by a patient to describe general fatigue rather than loss of muscle power.

Difficulty with movement and specific impairments of function can also be the presenting complaint of a musculoskeletal disease. This can occur in regional or systemic disorders (either of which can prevent someone reaching or dressing, for example) and may present as difficulty in climbing in and out of the bath or performing some other crucial activity of daily living (ADL). However, it is uncommon for these problems to arise in the absence of a complaint of pain and/or stiffness.

FATIGUE

Fatigue is an important manifestation of most generalized rheumatic disorders, including RA and most notably systemic lupus erythematosus (SLE). It may be severely disabling, with a general sense of overwhelming tiredness and fatigue making it impossible for the patient to do anything. It is a symptom that is often ignored by physicians and which is sometimes inappropriately passed off as being functional in origin. Although fatigue is sometimes functional, and can be prominent in noninflammatory conditions such as fibromyalgia, the fatigue of RA or SLE is a good indicator of the systemic activity of the disease; the time at which fatigue becomes a problem is sometimes used, along with the duration of morning stiffness, as one of the monitors of disease activity.

People with inflammatory arthritis are often able to function well for several hours, only to suffer overwhelming fatigue in mid or late afternoon. It is useful to ask specifically if the patient needs to lie down before completing a day's work, or if he or she needs a nap immediately after arriving home in the evening, for example. (It is also useful to advise people with inflammatory arthritis to take regular midday rests to prevent the later onset of severe fatigue.)

EMOTIONAL LABILITY

Fear and anxiety accompany most patient contacts with a rheumatologist, particularly first or 'new patient' consultations. Patients are usually anxious that they may have some severe disease which will cause them to become crippled. Pain is a potent cause of anxiety, as it tends to signal damage to the body. Someone who is good at taking the history will be particularly skilled at allaying anxiety at an early stage and at creating a relaxed 'timeless' environment, to ensure that anxiety does not prevent the patient from telling 'his or her story' properly. It is important that the physician responds to patient fears and tries to address them specifically and honestly, rather than concentrating too much on the physical diagnosis (see Fig. 1.2).

Emotional lability, depression and other psychiatric disturbances can also be the direct result of a rheumatic disease, as in the common development of depression and less common onset of psychoses in SLE, for example.

OTHER PRESENTING SYMPTOMS

Patients with a rheumatic disorder occasionally present with a variety of other symptoms, including cracking or clicking of joints, deformity or general malaise. Joint cracking is usually of no pathologic significance and patients should be reassured that it does not damage joints.

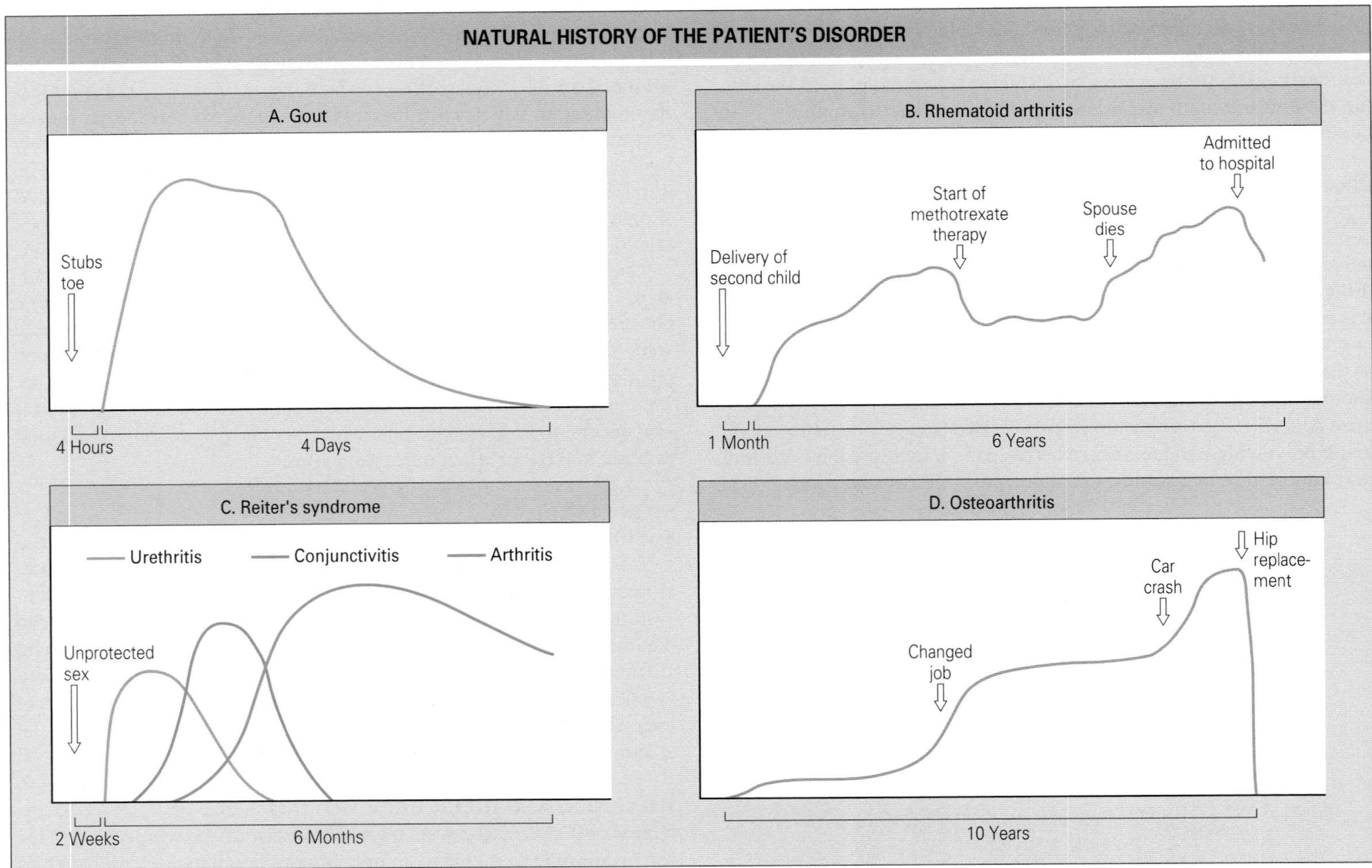

Fig. 1.6 At the end of the history-taking process, the physician should be able to draw a graph that outlines the natural history of the patient's disorder. Shown is a graphic representation of the typical chronologic pattern of four common rheumatic diseases: (a) gout, (b) rheumatoid arthritis, (c) Reiter's syndrome, (d) osteoarthritis.

Malaise may be functional, but it is important to ask for the presence of any other symptoms, such as fever, night sweats or weight loss, which may indicate the presence of a serious systemic disorder such as a malignancy or active inflammatory disease.

THE CHRONOLOGY OF THE DISORDER

A good history taker will be able to draw a clear graphic representation of the chronology of the patient's illness by the end of the consultation (Fig. 1.6).

Nothing in the history is as important as the first symptom. Even if the condition has been present for months or years, the physician nearly always gains great insight by asking the simple question 'Exactly how did this begin?' The subsequent course is also important; the rate of development of the disorder, the influence of any drug therapy or other interventions and the relationship of the condition to life events should be investigated. Disease chronology is particularly important in understanding the likely pathologic process involved. For example, a traumatic condition obviously relates to a specific event, whereas a degenerative pathology usually presents in a slow insidious fashion. Crystal-related inflammation is particularly rapid in onset and severe, but self-limiting, whereas untreated sepsis causes a steadily worsening situation over a few days. Many of the idiopathic inflammatory or immunologic rheumatic diseases have a variable course with spontaneous remissions and exacerbations, whereas others, such as reactive arthritis, follow a more predictable course with the sequential development of mucocutaneous and joint inflammation over a period of a few weeks after the initiating event, which gradually subsides over a period of months. Other specific patterns include that of palindromic rheumatism which, as the word implies, involves symmetric attacks of arthritis that come and go spontaneously over a few days.

The influence of treatment and life events on the course of a disease can also be of great relevance to the understanding of its nature and impact. Response to anti-inflammatory therapy is an important feature of many disorders and a sudden and almost miraculous response to corticosteroids is characteristic of polymyalgia rheumatica.

THE IMPACT OF THE CONDITION ON THE PATIENT

The 'GALS' system asks two screening questions, one of which searches for key symptoms of rheumatic disease (pain and stiffness) and the other for common disabilities (difficulty with washing, dressing, stairs or steps). However, a more complete history of the physical and psychosocial impact of the condition – or disability – is usually called for.

Several different frameworks or paradigms of disability have been described. For example, the World Health Organization (WHO) adopted the definition of impairment, disability and handicap shown in Figure 1.7. However, many disabled persons' groups regard this as a medical model of dubious value; they prefer a psychosocial description of handicap, which they regard as being due to society's inability to cope with people who have varying functional abilities. It is helpful to have some model in mind when thinking about disability, and to remember that the patient's perception of their problem will be molded by adaptation as well as aspirations. The WHO or medical model of disability has the advantage of differentiating a disability, such as difficulty moving a limb, from the handicap that this may produce, which can vary from virtually none in someone of a sedentary occupation and nature to disastrous in the aspiring athlete or musician (Fig. 1.7).

THE WHO MODEL OF IMPAIRMENT, DISABILITY AND HANDICAP	
Pain and a disease process can lead to: **Impairment**	Loss of function (such as inability to flex left index finger due to tendon rupture, for example)
This can result in: **Disability**	Inability to perform a task (e.g. difficulty playing the violin and minor problems with other tasks)
This may result in: **Handicap**	Psychosocial disadvantage (e.g. loss of earnings of concert violinist; others with this impairment may have little or no handicap)

Fig. 1.7 The WHO model of impairment, disability and handicap.

It is often helpful to ask the patient to talk the physician through a typical day – what time the patient wakes, whether he or she can get to the toilet easily, any problems with washing and dressing, does the patient go out of the house much, do his or her own shopping and so forth. Potentially embarrassing or frustrating problems such as those associated with toilet difficulties or sexual dysfunction should be approached openly and frankly with simple direct questions. Some people will not answer at first, but many will return to the topic later, having been given 'permission' to talk about it through the open, direct approach of the physician.

The patient's needs and aspirations are a critical part of the impact of the condition, and will interact with their ability to adapt to a rheumatic condition. Questions such as 'What things do you find difficult that you would like to be able to do?', 'Are there things that you cannot do now that you could do a year ago?', 'What is it about your arthritis that you find most frustrating?' and 'What do you most enjoy doing?' may be helpful in bringing out critical issues. It is important to look for the positive things as well as the negative ones. When you do discuss one of the more emotionally charged problems, patients will sometimes falter and show signs of emotion; it is often best to say nothing but continue with sympathetic eye contact, which may result in a helpful, tearful catharsis. The psychosocial issues are just as important as the physical ones when considering the impact of a rheumatic disease on a person.

A further *aide memoir* to some of the more important aspects of disability is the 'PILS' pneumonic, which reminds the physician to think about four issues:

- preventable causes of disability (P), such as falls or pressure sores;
- independence (I), including issues such as ability to wash and toilet without aid;
- lifestyle (L), including roles and goals;
- social factors (S), such as family, friends and housing (see Fig. 1.1).

OTHER ASPECTS OF THE HISTORY

The full patient interview should always include direct questions on the topics covered included in all medical history taking.

PREVIOUS MEDICAL HISTORY

The previous medical history may include past events which give clues to the present problem, such as an attack of unexplained epilepsy in someone with lupus, now presenting with painful swollen hands, or a story of a swollen ankle in childhood in a young man with back pain who has now developed ankylosing spondylitis. In other cases, relevant previous medical events may relate to the associations between disorders, such as bronchiectasis preceding RA, or hypermobility in childhood as a risk factor for osteoarthritis.

FAMILY HISTORY

In most individual cases of rheumatic disease the family history is of marginal benefit, although it is easy to place too much emphasis on it (everyone has a relative with arthritis!). However, there are notable exceptions, such as the solid family history of ankylosing spondylitis in a young man presenting with back pain, or a history of gout in the family.

SOCIAL HISTORY AND OCCUPATION

Much of the most important information on the social history should be obtained when thinking about the impact of the condition – factors such as housing, spouse and so forth covered in the PILS checklist. Other issues, such as smoking and alcohol intake, can be important in a few cases: smoking may be of great relevance in someone with RA who develops fibrosing alveolitis, for example, and alcohol can be an important factor in the pathogenesis of gout. In addition, occupation can be important, so a full occupational history is sometimes informative. For example, certain jobs, such as farming, appear to increase the risk of osteoarthritis of the hip, whereas others, such as carpet laying, are associated with knee disease.

THE DRUG HISTORY

It is always valuable to take a clear history of current drug intake; remember that patients often take 'alternative', 'complimentary' or other over-the-counter medicines in addition to prescribed drugs, and that they may be loath to admit this. The efficacy of a drug may be a valuable diagnostic clue – as in the value of night-time anti-inflammatory drugs in cases of inflammatory back pain – and drugs themselves may be the cause of the problem, as in drug-induced lupus.

THE REVIEW OF SYSTEMS

The general review of other systems is very helpful in the differentiation of the many forms of inflammatory joint disease. Specific patterns of association are common; for example, mucocutaneous problems in the seronegative spondyloarthritides, dry eyes and mouth in sicca syndrome (although a 'dry mouth' is a common complaint), and a variety of systemic features in the connective tissue disorders, including rashes, mouth ulcers, Raynaud's phenomenon, neuropsychiatric disturbances and many others. In practice it is often helpful to have a mental checklist of specific questions (such as 'Have you ever had to see a physician or optician about your eyes for anything other than glasses?') for each of the common associations of a disorder which you consider likely when taking the history (Fig. 1.8).

In this general context it is also vital to be able to sort out the local, relatively minor disorders from the systemic, severe problems. Fever, night sweats, anorexia, weight loss and other systemic symptoms may provide the clue to the generalized, severe illness. In addition, it may be useful to ask questions such as 'If you had no joint pain, would you feel well?' in order to gauge the relative importance of general or other system-related problems to that of joint disease.

PATIENT SELF-ASSESSMENT

A large number of self-assessment forms and instruments are used in rheumatology (see Appendix: selected measures for outcome assessment of rheumatic diseases – volume 2). These can be given to patients in waiting rooms and are sometimes used to assist the interview. In some cases it can be helpful to go over the forms with a patient – to discuss responses to treatment, for example. However, the forms must not be used to replace the important skill of open history taking, as outlined earlier.

SOME OF THE SYSTEMIC FEATURES OF RHEUMATIC DISORDERS

- General features of active inflammation in the musculoskeletal system: Fever, night sweats, anorexia, weight loss
- Organ specific features, examples include:

Organ system	Rheumatoid arthritis and connective tissue diseases	The seronegative spondyloarthritides
Skin	Photosensitivity, alopecia, various rashes	Psoriasis, palmar and solar pustules
Eyes	Red eye, dryness, visual loss	Red or painful eye
Mouth	Oral ulcers, dryness	Ulcers
Chest	Pleuritic pain, dyspnea	Dyspnea, cough
Gastrointestinal	History of peptic ulcer	Diarrhea
Genitourinary		Penile/vaginal discharge Sexually transmitted disease
Neurologic/ psychologic	Stroke, neuropathies	Seizures, psychiatric change
Hematologic	Thromboembolic disease, anemia, bleeding disorders	

Fig. 1.8 Rheumatic diseases systems review: some of the symptoms that can arise from other systems as a result of inflammatory disorders of the musculoskeletal system.

CONCLUSION – SORTING OUT THE INFORMATION OBTAINED

Finally, it is important to remember that the medical consultation is a major part of the therapeutic opportunity that a rheumatologist has to offer. With this in mind, the consultation should always end on a positive note. It may be appropriate to make sure that the patient has had the chance to say what he or she wants to with a question such as 'Is there anything else that you want to tell me?' (it is helpful to ask this at the end of the formal history taking, before examining the patient, thus allowing the opportunity for something else to be brought up during the examination). It is also important to make sure that the patient feels positive about the consultation; it may be useful, for example, to congratulate and thank the patient for sharing their problems and opening up about their illness. This can be particularly important if a patient has shown emotion, such as crying, during the interview – unless such patients are reassured that they have done well and that the consultation was helpful for both you and them, they may leave with a feeling that they have let themselves down.

It has been said that 80–90% of diagnoses are made from the history alone. It is both challenging and rewarding to listen to a new patient with a rheumatic complaint with this knowledge, and the understanding that the correct diagnosis, as well as your ability to address the issues that matter most to the patient, will depend on your skills in the all important art of history taking.

FURTHER READING

1. Doherty M, Dacre J, Dieppe P, Snaith M. The 'GALS' locomotor screen. Ann Rheum Dis. 1992;51:1165–9.
2. Matthews DA, Suchman AL, Branch WT. Making 'connexions': enhancing the therapeutic potential of patient-clinician relationships. Ann Intern Med. 1993;118:973–7.
3. Smith RC, Hoppe RB. The patient's story: integrating the patient and physician centred approaches to interviewing. Ann Intern Med. 1991;115:470–7.
4. Lipkin M. The medical interview. In: Branch WT, ed. Office Practice of Medicine. Philadelphia: WB Saunders, 1987:1287–1306.
5. Bechman HB, Frankel RM. The effect of physicians' behavious on the collection of data. Ann Intern Med. 1984;101:692–6.
6. Billings JA, Stoeckle JD. The Clinical Encounter: a Guide to the Medical Interview and Case Presentation. Chicago Year Book Publishers, 1989.
7. Bechman H, Markakis K, Suchman A, Frankel R. Getting the most from a 20 minute visit. Am J Gastroenterol. 1994;89:662–4.
8. Nardone DA, Johnson GK, Faryona A, Coulehan JL, Parnno TA. A model for the diagnostic medical interview: nonverbal, verbal and cognitive assessments. J Gen Intern Med. 1992;7:437–42.

2

EXAMINATION OF THE PATIENT

Rodney Grahame

- The clinical examination is pivotal in the assessment of the rheumatic patient.
- The techniques of the examination process are the time-honored ones, suitably adapted to the specific needs of the locomotor system, namely, inspection, palpation and observing movement (look, feel, move).
- To facilitate the maximum yield of clinical information the patient is examined with the limbs and spine exposed. Because of the complexity of the locomotor system, part of the examination is conducted with the patient sitting on the side of the examination table, part standing, part lying prone and part lying supine.
- Since the affected part may be painful, it is imperative that maximum attention is paid to the avoidance of inflicting unnecessary discomfort on the patient. It behoves the examiner to give the patient every consideration in this respect.
- The patient is more than the sum of his or her joints. No rheumatological assessment is complete without a complete clinical examination, to include the patient's general physical and psychological state of health.

INTRODUCTION

The system of examination proposed in this chapter assumes that the reader has received a general grounding in clinical medicine, but has had little or no previous specialist exposure to locomotor medicine (including rheumatology and orthopedics). It aims, however, to pave the way to enabling the rheumatologic novice to pursue logically and with a degree of confidence the diagnosis of any condition that falls within the purview of this book.

As the generalist edges towards the specialty, so our quest commences with a generalist approach to the patient as a whole, before focusing in on the locomotor system in depth. After a sweep of the 'other' major systems (to detect multisytem involvement), the process concludes its holistic circuit by exploring the patient's functional capacity and psychosocial adjustment.

The clinical examination complements the history and with it completes the clinical assessment. The clinician should now be in a position to establish a clinical diagnosis (or, at least, profer a differential diagnosis), make an estimate of the severity and extent of the rheumatological disorder, the impact that it has had on the patient's life, his/her mobility, his/her emotional state, capacity for self-care, his/her ability to work and enjoy leisure activities.

Only then is it appropriate to select those special investigations which the clinician considers necessary to confirm his clinical suspicions regarding diagnosis, gauging disease activity, prognosis and choice of treatment. In this way the performance of unnecessary, expensive, unpleasant (even dangerous) investigations may be avoided.

GENERAL EXAMINATION

The first impressions – observations made while taking history – are often the most revealing and careful observation is worthwhile:

- *What is the overall appearance* of the patient? Estimate the approximate age. Note the gender. Note the body height and shape for evidence of body disproportion such as obesity, tallness (marfanoid habitus?), restricted growth, obvious skeletal deformity or increased head size. Does the appearance of the face 'spell' illness or health, anemia or polycythemia, depression or emotional distress? Is there evidence of cushingoid features, alopecia, emaciation or self-neglect?
- *Are the patient's movements* hesitant, labored, inhibited, painful or restricted? Is the gait abnormally slow? Is there an obvious limp? Is a walking aid being used, or is the patient wheel-chair-bound?
- *How is the patient's manner?* Does it appear resentful, aggressive, unduly demanding, manipulative, argumentative or self-contradictory? What about the affect? Is there a suggestion of hypomania, depression or *la belle indifférence*, or of an obsessional, compulsive or anxiety neurosis?

THE LOCOMOTOR SYSTEM

A useful approach in examination of the locomotor system is to seek answers to five Key Questions, with the aim of proceeding in a logical manner. Once all five have been answered, it should be possible to establish a differential diagnosis (Fig. 2.1).

PERIPHERAL JOINTS

The initial joint screen

An efficient strategy for elucidating the cause of a symptomatic joint complaint is firstly to ask:

Key Question 1
'Are any of the joints abnormal?'

The answer is obtained by undertaking a rapid joint screening examination, the initial joint screen (Fig. 2.2). Abnormal joint(s) thus identified are then subjected to a more rigorous examination.

Re-examination

Any joint(s) found to be abnormal on rapid screening is(are) then submitted to a careful re-examination. The key elements of the 're-examination examination' are:

- *inspection* – swelling, redness, deformity;
- *palpation* – warmth, crepitus, tenderness;
- *movement* – active, passive and against resistance.

LOCOMOTOR SYSTEM EXAMINATION: QUESTIONS TO BE ANSWERED
1. Are any of the joints abnormal?
2. What is the nature of the joint abnormality?
3. What is the extent (distribution) of the joint involvement?
4. Are other features of diagnostic importance present?
5. Do the answers to questions 1–4 provide sufficient clues to enable one to establish a differential diagnosis? (They should!)

Fig. 2.1 Locomotor system examination: questions to be answered.

THE INITIAL JOINT SCREEN

Upper extremity

Finger flexion (MCPs, PIPs, DIPs)

Maneuver	Make a fist
Assessment	Ability/inability to embed finger tips into palm
Normal angle	–
Active/passive	Active

The patient is asked to make a fist and to try to bury the fingers in the palm.With the volar aspect uppermost the observer can immediately see if one or more fingers fail to reach the palm, indicating that a reduced range of flexion exists in one or more small finger joints (MCP, PIP of DIPs) of the respective digit(s). There is simultaneous assessment of joint swelling, redness, tenderness on palpation and whether movement elicits pain.

Finger extension (MCPs, PIPs, DIPs)

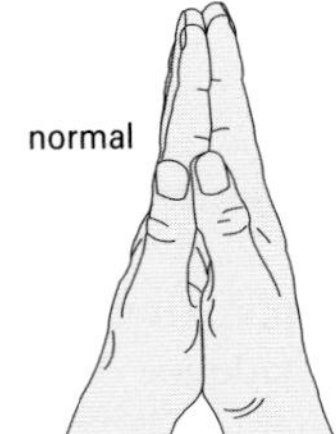

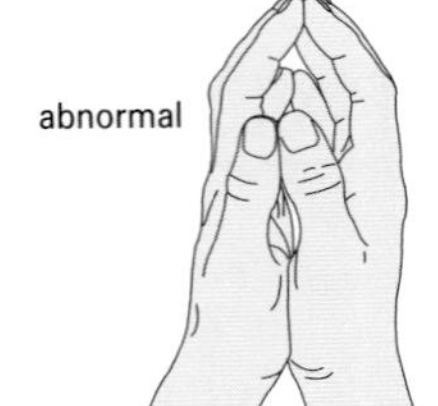

Maneuver	Prayer sign
Assessment	Contact of digits
Normal angle	–
Active/passive	Active

The patient is asked to place the palms of both hands together in the position of prayer.Full small finger joint extension is denoted by complete contact of all digits along their whole length. When a gap remains between the fingers, this indicates the presence of fixed flexion, affecting one or more small finger joints in the affected finger(s).

Finger hyperextension 5th MCP >90∞

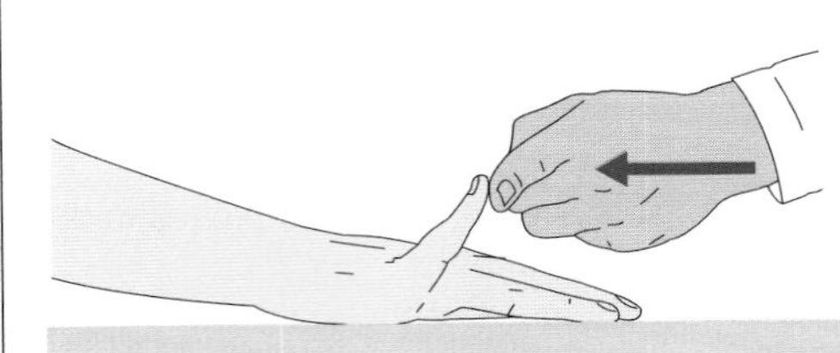

Maneuver	–
Assessment	On each side, ads 1 to Beighton score
Normal angle	< 90°
Active/passive	Passive

With the hand placed flat on a table, the little finger is gently extended as far as it will go, short of causing pain. If an angle of 90° of extension or more is achieved, the 5th MCP is deemed to be hypermobile.

Wrist flexion

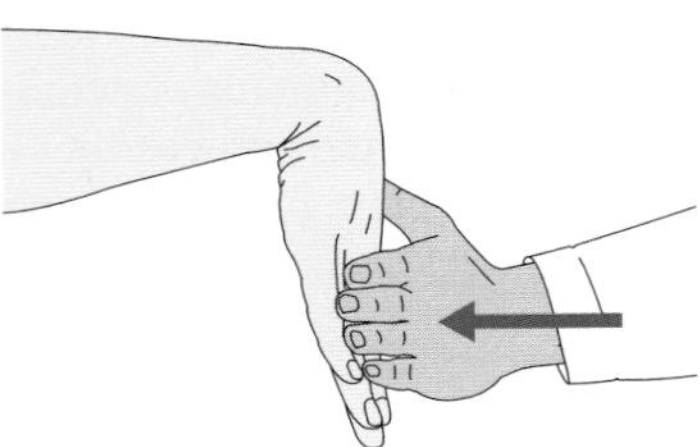

Maneuver	Bend wrist palmarly
Assessment	Estimate angle
Normal angle	60 – 90°
Active/passive	Passive

With the forearm outstretched, the hand is gently coaxed downwards until the maximal range of wrist flexion is achieved, short of causing pain.The angle achieved is estimated by 'eye-balling'. There is simultaneous assessment of joint swelling, redness, tenderness on palpation and whether the movement elicits pain.

Wrist extension

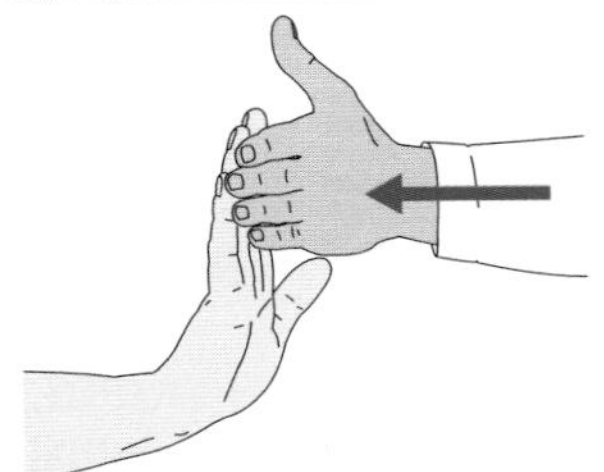

Maneuver	Bend wrist dorsally
Assessment	Estimate angle
Normal angle	60 – 90°
Active/passive	Passive

With the forearm outstretched, the hand is gently coaxed upwards until the maximal range of wrist extension is achieved, short of causing pain. The angle achieved is estimated by 'eye-balling'.

Thumb apposition to volar aspect of wrist

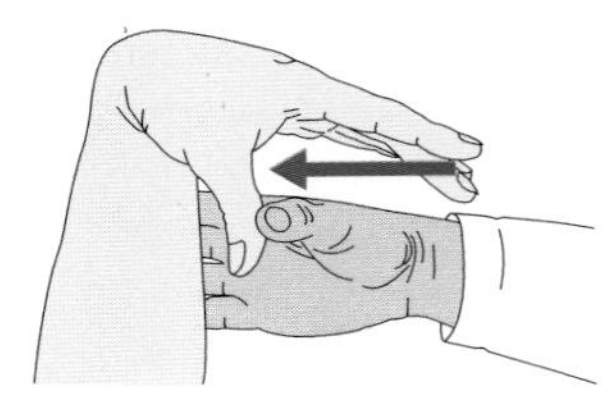

Maneuver	–
Assessment	On each side, adds 1 to Beighton score
Normal angle	–
Active/passive	Passive

The thumb is passively moved towards the volar aspect of the forearm. Where contact is made the thumb/wrist complex is deemed to demonstrate hypermobility.

Elbow flexion

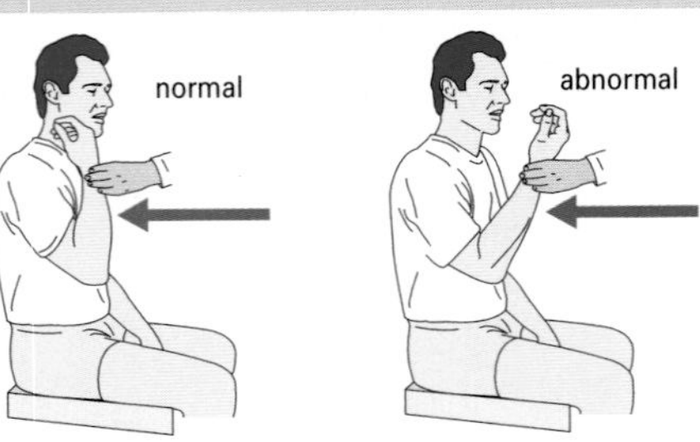

Maneuver	Flex elbow
Assessment	Estimate angle
Normal angle	145°
Active/passive	Passive

The forearm is gently moved as close as possible to the upper arm and the maximum angle of passive elbow flexion is estimated by eye.

Elbow extension

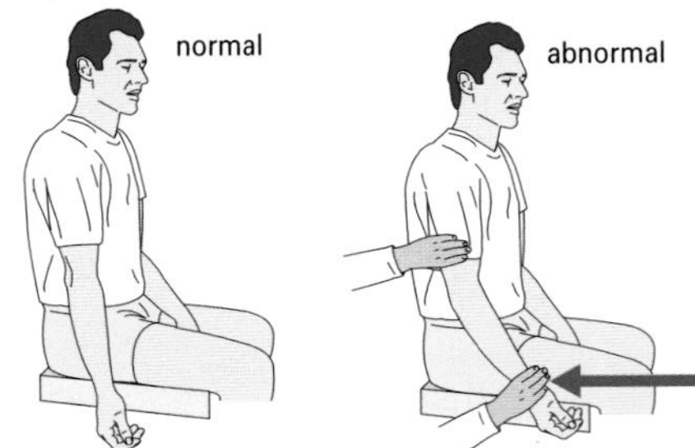

Maneuver	Extend elbow
Assessment	Estimate angle
Normal angle	0°
Active/passive	Passive

The upper limb is straightened at the elbow to achieve maximal elbow extension. When it is not possible to straighten the elbow completely, the maximum angle achieved subtracted from 180° is referred to as the angle of 'fixed flexion' of the elbow. There is simultaneous assessment of joint swelling, redness, tenderness on palpation and whether movement elicits pain.

Elbow hyperextension

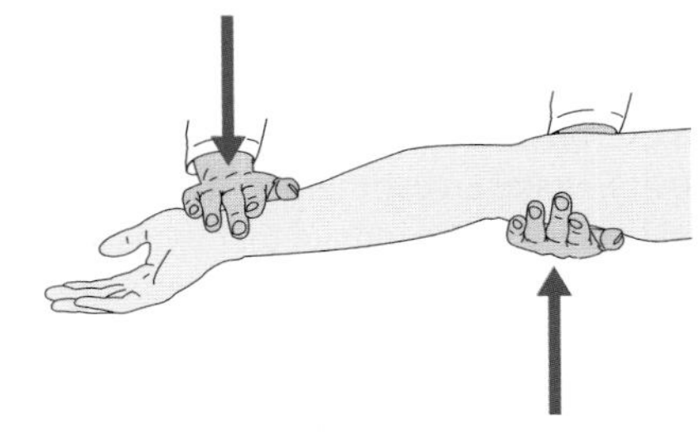

Maneuver	–
Assessment	On each side, adds 1 to Beighton score
Normal angle	< 10° hyperextension
Active/passive	Passive

Where elbow extension proceeds to beyond 180°, elbow hyperextension is deemed to exist. More than 10° from the 180° position is considered to be a significant degree of hyperextension.

Fig. 2.2 The initial joint screen: how to inspect, palpate and assess the range of movement in the joints in the most efficient and expeditious manner.

THE INITIAL JOINT SCREEN

Shoulder

Active elevation

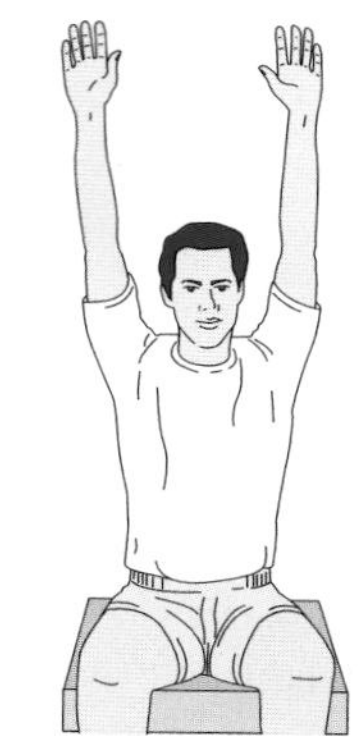

Maneuver	Arms in air
Assessment	Degree of elevation
Normal angle	–
Active/passive	Active

The patient is asked to place each arm together or in turn in the air as high as he/she can. Failure to achieve total elevation (in the absence of muscle paralysis) indicates limitation of gleno-humeral joint motion. Where the failure appears to be the result of pain (such as a painful arc), a tendonitis may be present.

Abduction/lateral rotation

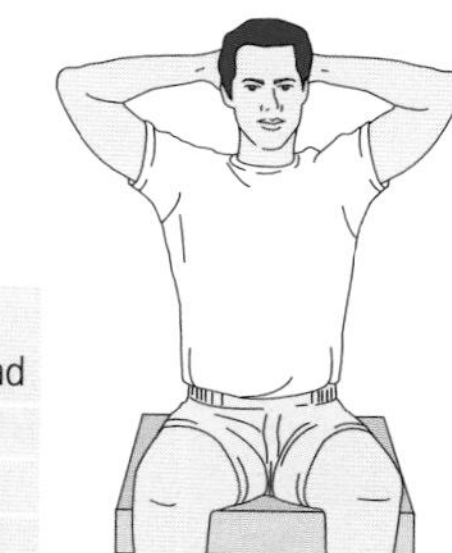

Maneuver	Hands behind head
Assessment	–
Normal angle	–
Active/passive	Active

The patient is asked to place both hands on the back of his/her neck. If they cannot reach it, then there is limitation of gleno-humeral abduction and/or lateral rotation. If failure appears to be due to pain, consider a painful arc due to a supraspinatus/infraspinatus tendonitis.

Extension/internal rotation

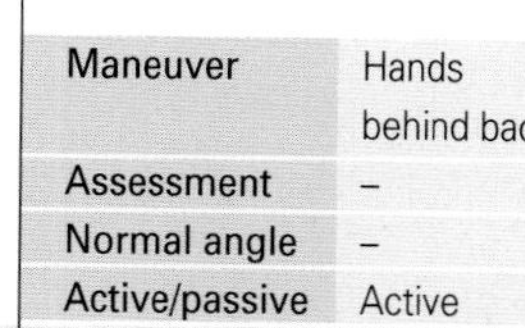

Maneuver	Hands behind back
Assessment	–
Normal angle	–
Active/passive	Active

The patient is asked to place both hands behind his/her lower back region. If they cannot reach it, then there is limitation of gleno-humeral extension and/or medial rotation. If failure appears to be due to pain, consider a painful arc due to a subscapularis tendonitis.

If any of these three shoulder maneuvers appears restricted, a more detailed shoulder examination is required

Glenohumeral external rotation

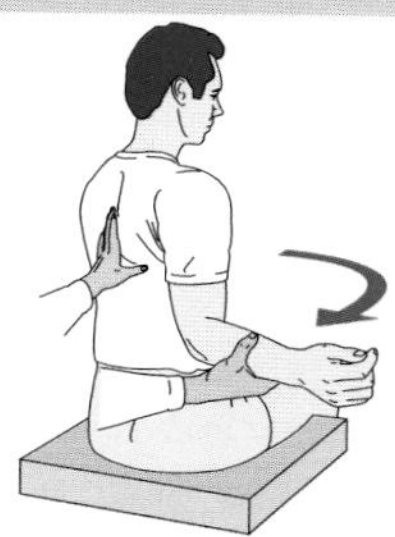

Maneuver	Angle estimated by examiner fixing scapula with one hand, while moving upper arm passively with other
Assessment	Estimate angle
Normal angle	30–60°
Active/passive	Passive

The examiner gently steadies the patient's left scapula with his right hand, while he passively rotates the patient's left shoulder laterally with his left hand, using the humerus held vertically as the axis of rotation. The angle of lateral rotation achieved is estimated by eye. He then gently steadies the patient's right scapula with his left hand, while he passively rotates the patient's right shoulder laterally with his right hand, again using the humerus held vertically as the axis of rotation. The angle of lateral rotation achieved is estimated by eye. A range greater than 70° indicates shoulder hypermobility.

Glenohumeral abduction

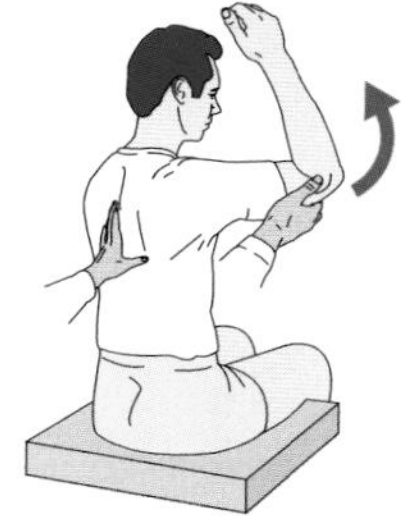

Maneuver	Angle estimated by examiner fixing scapula with one hand, while moving upper arm passively with other
Assessment	Estimate angle
Normal angle	about 90°
Active/passive	Passive

The examiner gently steadies the patient's left scapula with his right hand, while he passively flexes the patient's left shoulder with his left, measuring by eye the angle of flexion achieved. He then gently steadies the patient's right scapula with his left hand, while he passively flexes the patient's right shoulder with his right hand, again measuring by eye the angle of flexion achieved.

Glenohumeral flexion

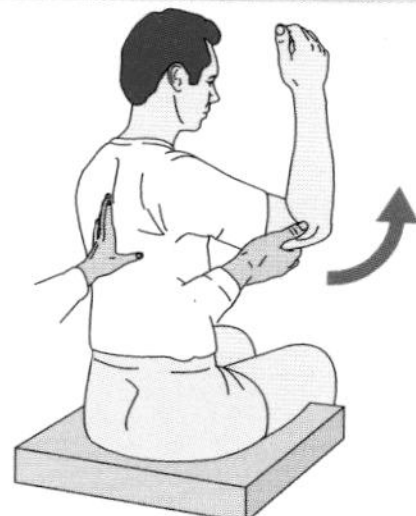

Maneuver	Angle estimated by examiner fixing scapula with one hand, while moving upper arm passively with other
Assessment	Estimate angle
Normal angle	about 90°
Active/passive	Passive

The examiner gently steadies the patient's left scapula with his right hand, while he passively abducts the patient's left shoulder with his left, measuring by eye the angle of abduction achieved. He then gently steadies the patient's right scapula with his left hand, while he passively abducts the patient's right shoulder with his right hand, again measuring by eye the angle of abduction achieved.

Palpation

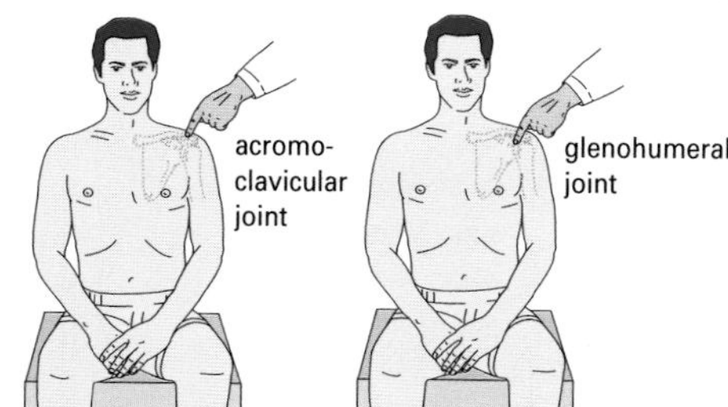

Maneuver	Eliciting tenderness in gap between coracoid and humeral head
Assessment	–
Normal angle	–
Active/passive	Passive

The shoulder examination is completed by palpation. Tenderness in the groove between the coracoid process and the humeral head (the site of the gleno-humeral joint) (right) and between the clavicle and acromion is indicative of acromioclavicular arthritis (left).

Temporomandibular joints

Mouth opening

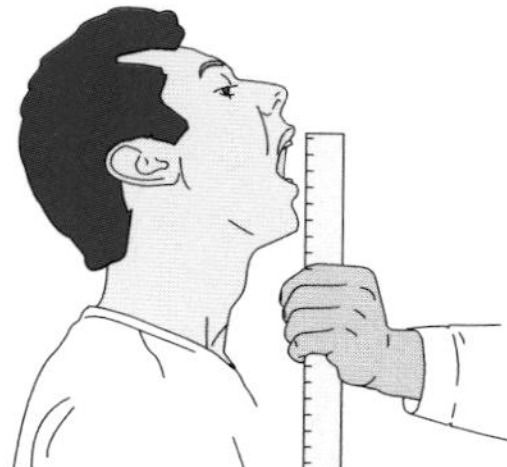

Maneuver	Distance between tips of upper and lower incisor teeth using ruler
Assessment	–
Normal angle	–
Active/passive	Active

The TMJ is tested by asking the patient to open his/her mouth as wide as possible. The distance between the tips of the upper and lower incisor teeth may be measured serially to gauge progress.

Side–to–side movement of jaw

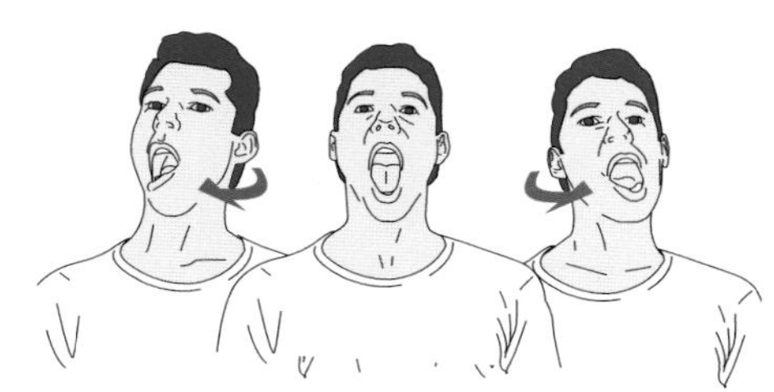

	Deviate lower jaw
	–
	–
	Active

Another movement is to ask the patient to move his/her jaw from side to side. Such movement may not be possible in the presence of significant TMJ damage or dysfunction.

Fig. 2.2 continued

THE INITIAL JOINT SCREEN

Cervical spine

Right rotation

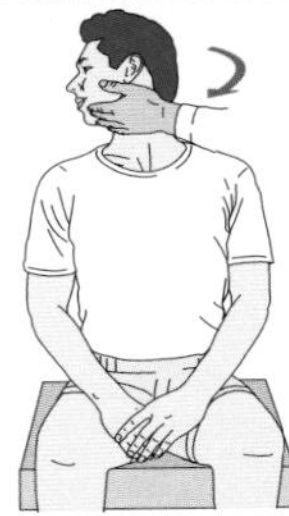

Maneuver	Turn head to right
Assessment	Estimate angle
Normal angle	60–90° diminishing with age
Active/passive	Active

The patient sits comfortably on the edge of the examining table with the legs hanging free, facing the examiner. The patient is asked to turn his/her head to the right as far as they can. The examiner gently guides the patient's jaw with his hand to ensure that the maximum range is achieved, and then estimates the angle.

Left rotation

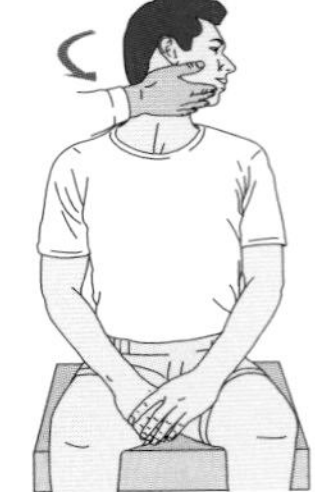

Maneuver	Turn head to left
Assessment	Estimate angle
Normal angle	60–90° diminishing with age
Active/passive	Active

The patient sits comfortably on the edge of the examining table with the legs hanging free, facing the examiner. The patient is asked to turn his/her head to the left as far as he/she can. The examiner gently guides the patient's jaw with his hand to ensure that maximum range is achieved, and then estimates the angle.

Flexion

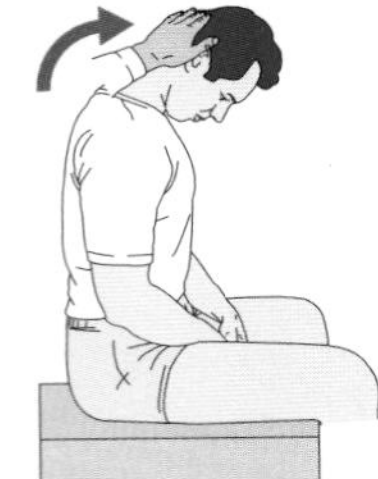

Maneuver	Flex neck forward
Assessment	Estimate angle
Normal angle	60–90° diminishing with age
Active/passive	Active

The patient sits comfortably on the edge of the examining table with the legs hanging free, facing the examiner. The patient is asked to bend their head forward as far as they can. The examiner gently guides the patient's head with his hand to ensure that the maximum range is achieved, and then estimates the angle.

Extension

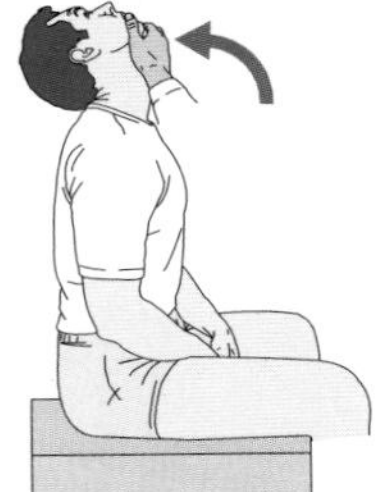

Maneuver	–
Assessment	Estimate angle
Normal angle	60–90° diminishing with age
Active/passive	Active

The patient sits comfortably on the edge of the examining table with the legs hanging free, facing the examiner. The patient is asked to look up as far as he/she can. The examiner gently guides the patient's jaw with his hand to ensure that the maximum range is achieved, and then estimates the angle.

Right lateral flexion

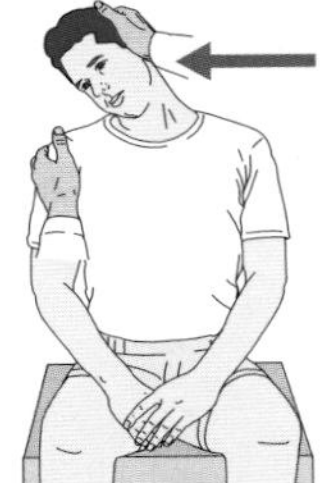

Maneuver	Flex neck to right
Assessment	Estimate angle
Normal angle	30–60° diminishing with age
Active/passive	Active

The patient sits comfortably on the edge of the examining table with the legs hanging free, facing the examiner. The patient is asked to angle their head to the right to try to touch his/her ear with his/her shoulder. The examiner gently guides the patient's head with his hand to ensure that maximum range is achieved, and then estimates the angle. The normal range, which diminishes with age, is 30–60°.

Left lateral flexion

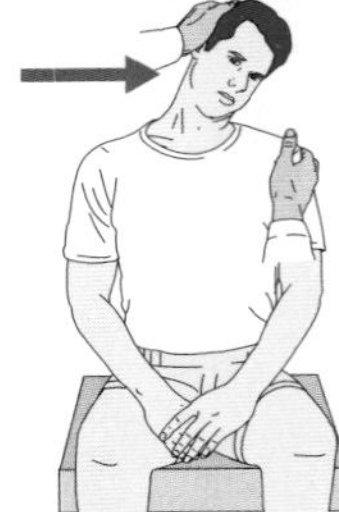

Maneuver	Flex neck to left
Assessment	Estimate angle
Normal angle	30–60° diminishing with age
Active/passive	Active

The patient sits comfortably on the edge of the examining table with the legs hanging free, facing the examiner. The patient is asked to angle his/her head to the left to try to touch his/her ear with his/her shoulder. The examiner gently guides the patient's head with his hand to ensure that maximum range is achieved, and then estimates the angle.The normal range, which diminishes with age, is 30–60°.

Dorsal spine

Right rotation

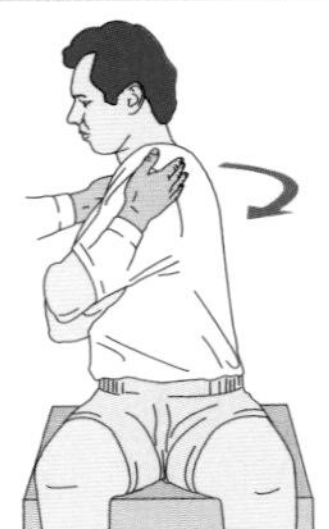

Maneuver	Turn upper body to right
Assessment	Measurement of rotation angle between the plane of the shoulder and the pelvis
Normal angle	45–75°
Active/passive	Passive

The patient sits comfortably on the edge of the examining table with the legs hanging free, facing the examiner. The patient is asked to turn the upper trunk to the right as far as he/she can. The examiner gently guides the patient's shoulders with his hands to ensure that the maximum range has been achieved, and then estimates the angle.

Left rotation

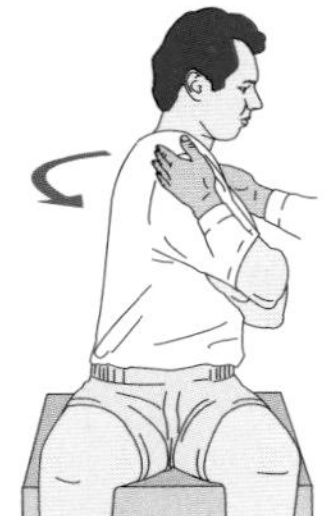

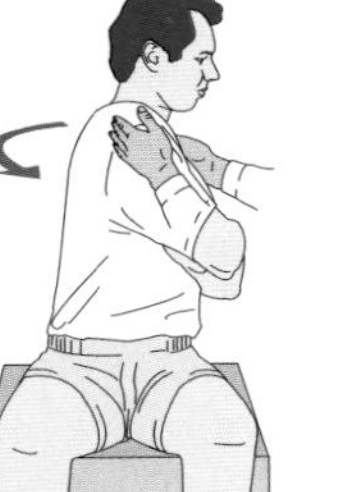

Maneuver	Turn upper body to left
Assessment	Measurement of rotation angle between the plane of the shoulder and the pelvis
Normal angle	45–75°
Active/passive	Passive

The patient sits comfortably on the edge of the examining table with the legs hanging free, facing the examiner. The patient is asked to turn the upper trunk to the left as far as he/she can. The examiner gently guides the patient's shoulders with his hands to ensure that the maximum range has been achieved, and then estimates the angle.

Occiput–wall distance

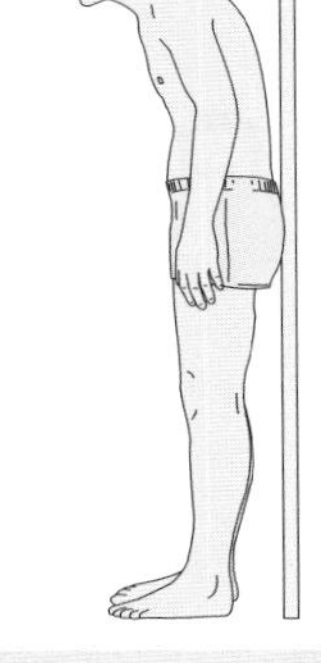

Maneuver	(In ankylosing spondylitis)
Assessment	Measurement of distance
Normal angle	–
Active/passive	Active

The patient is asked to stand with his back to a wall, at the same time trying to touch the wall with the back of his/her head. A person with normal cervical spine mobility would have no difficulty with this. A patient with advanced ankylosing spondylitis with cervical spine involvement would be unable to close the gap. Serial measurement of the distance between the occiput and the wall by means of tape measure is a useful index of progress in ankylosing spondylitis.

Fig. 2.2 continued

THE INITIAL JOINT SCREEN

Lumbar spine

Lumbar flexion

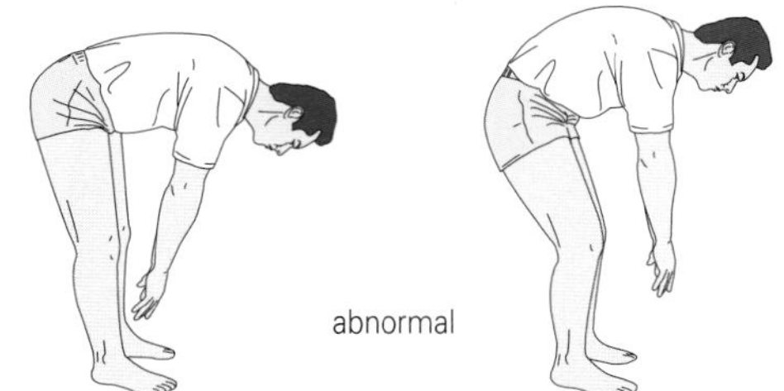

Maneuver	For ankylosing spondylitis, also include overall spinal movement (C7 to line between dimples of venus), Schober index and finger–floor distance
Assessment	Note the distance between the fingertips and the floor
Normal angle	–
Active/passive	Active

The patient stands in the erect posture, with his/her back to the examiner. The patient is asked to bend forward as if trying to touch his/her toes. Note is made of the range of movement, the presence of spasm of the erector spinae muscles, pain on movement, deviation to one or other side (sciatic scoliosis) or the induction of sciatica (indicating nerve root compression). The last two conditions listed are found in herniated intervertebral disc (Chapter 4.3).

Hypermobility

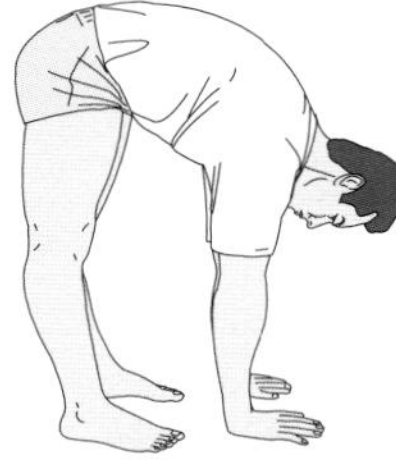

Maneuver	Try to place flat on floor while knees are extended
Assessment	Adds 1 to Beighton score if hands are placed flat on floor
Normal angle	–
Active/passive	–

The patient stands in the erect posture, with their back to the examiner. The patient is then asked to bend forward and try to place his/her hands flat on the floor without bending his/her knees. If they succeed, the patient is deemed to have a hypermobile spine.

Right/left lateral flexion

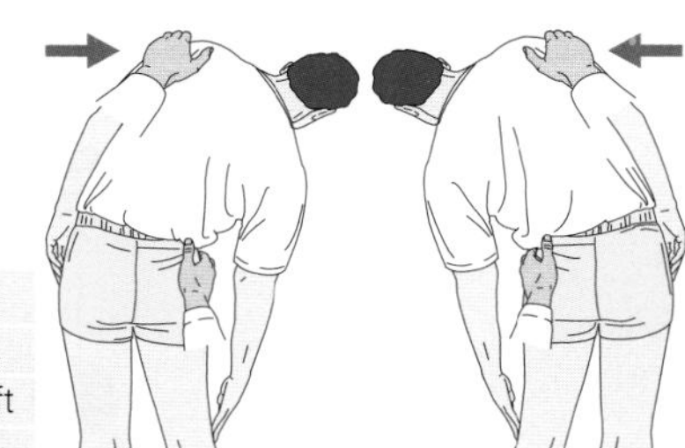

Maneuver	Bend to sides
Assessment	Estimate angle
Normal angle	30° to right – 30° to left
Active/passive	Active

The patient stands in the erect posture with his/her back to the examiner. The patient is asked to bend to the right, then to the left, as if trying to edge his/her fingers as far as the knee. Note is made of the range of movement. Reduction of lateral flexion is typically seen in ankylosing spondylitis, while in disc prolapse it is characteristically relatively well preserved.

Lumbar extension

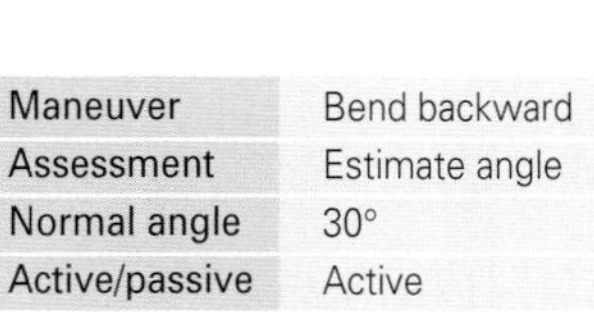

Maneuver	Bend backward
Assessment	Estimate angle
Normal angle	30°
Active/passive	Active

The patient stands in the erect posture, with their back to the examiner. The patient is then asked to bend backwards as if trying to arch his/her back as much as possible. Note is made of restricted range. Pain on extension is encountered in facet joint syndrome but may also be seen in herniated intervertebral disc (Chapter 4.3).

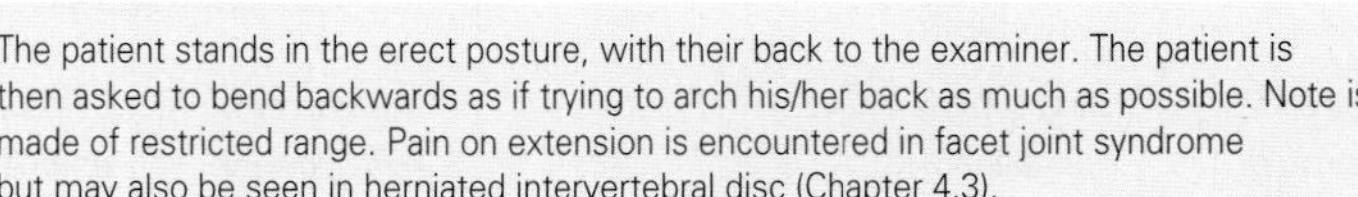

The spinal examination is completed by careful palpation of each individual spinous process in order to detect tenderness, thereby indicating the site of a lesion (but not, of course, its nature). This may be most effectively achieved with the patient in a prone position. A similar process is adopted for the facet joints (in facet joint syndrome) by palpating 3cm from the midline on both sides at each vertebral level.

The lumbar spine houses the lumbar spinal nerve roots and the cauda equina. These nerve roots and their sheathes are thus liable to come under tension or by compression disease, affecting adjacent spinal structures. The examination of the lumbar spine is completed by a complete neurological examination of the lower limbs and the performance of tests to detect the presence of tension affecting the nerve roots in either the femoral or sciatic nerves.

Test for cruralgia

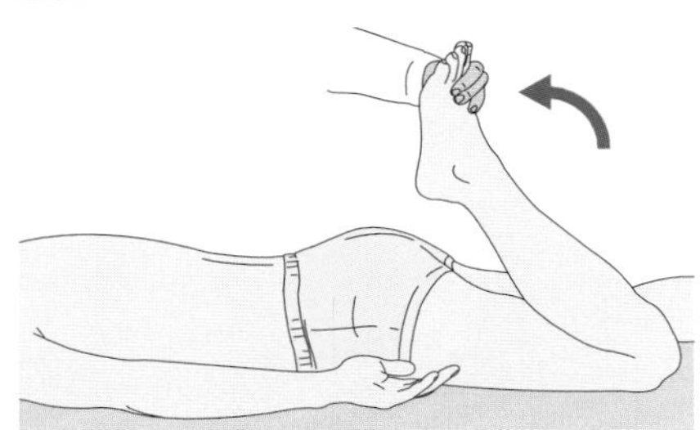

Maneuver	Femoral nerve stretch test
Assessment	Pain in the ipsilateral anterior thigh
Normal angle	–
Active/passive	Passive

The patient lies prone and as relaxed as possible. The examiner takes hold of the patient's ankle and gently passively flexes the knee as far as it will go, carefully ensuring that the procedure is not causing distess. In a positive test the patient feels pain in the isolateral anterior thigh, i.e. in the distribution of the femoral nerve which has been put on stretch (cruralgia), indicating that there is a compressive lesion affecting the femoral roots on that side. The test is then repeated on the other side. Pain felt in the back does not constitute a positive test. Caution is advised in interpreting a test which appears symmetrically positive, which is commonly the case in healthy subjects in old age.

Test for sciatica

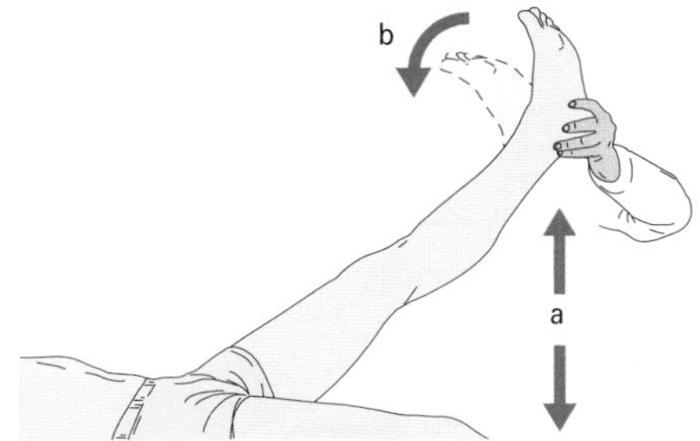

Maneuver	Straight leg raise (Lasègue) test
Assessment	Estimate angle
Normal angle	60 – 90°
Active/passive	Passive

The patient lies supine, while the examiner gently raises the patient's leg from the bed, at the same time observing the patient's face for signs of distress. The maximum angle achievable without causing pain is recorded as the SLR (straight leg raise) (a). The normal varies between 60 and 90°. Below 60° suggests sciatic nerve root tension (sciatic nerve roots L5, S1). Tight hamstring muscles, which may limit SLR and cause pain behind the knees, must be distinguished from true sciatica.The ankle is dorsiflexed (extended) at the point of maximal SLR (b). Any increase in pain confirms the presence of sciatic nerve root tension.

Fig. 2.2 continued

THE INITIAL JOINT SCREEN

Lower extremity – Hip

Flexion

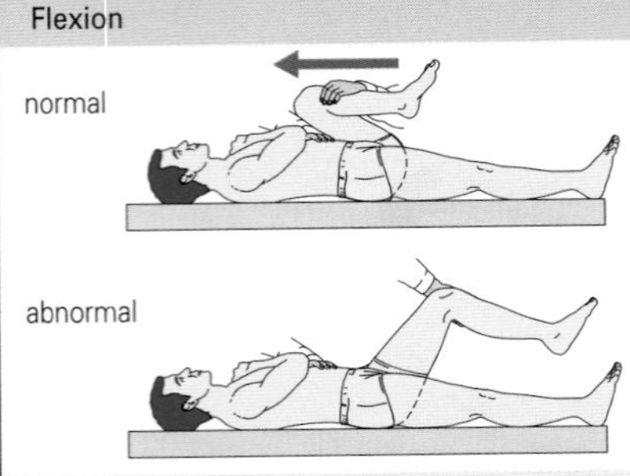

Maneuver	Lying supine, patient bends knee
Assessment	Estimate angle
Normal angle	120° diminishing with age
Active/passive	Passive

The patient lies supine, while the fully extended limb is passively flexed at the hip and knee as far as it will go. The angle formed by the flexed thigh and the extended contralateral limb is estimated.

Medial rotation

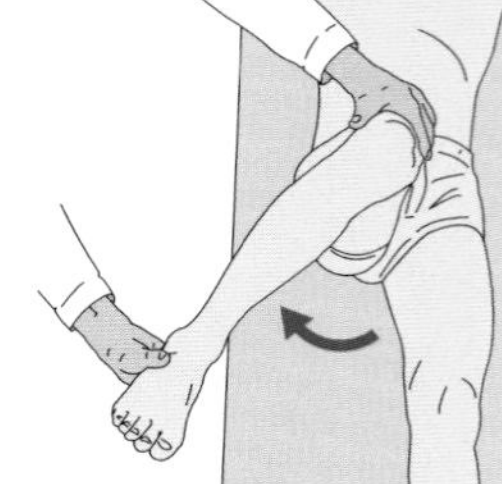

Maneuver	With hip/knee flexed 90°
Assessment	Estimate angle
Normal angle	Medial rotation 30°
Active/passive	Passive

Medial: the patient lies supine, while the hip is passively flexed and held at 90°. Holding the patient's foot with his right hand and steadying the patient's thigh (held vertical) with his left hand, the examiner rotates the lower limb outwards, noting the angles of hip medial rotation achieved in the process, and at the same time, guarding against inflicting pain.

Lateral rotation

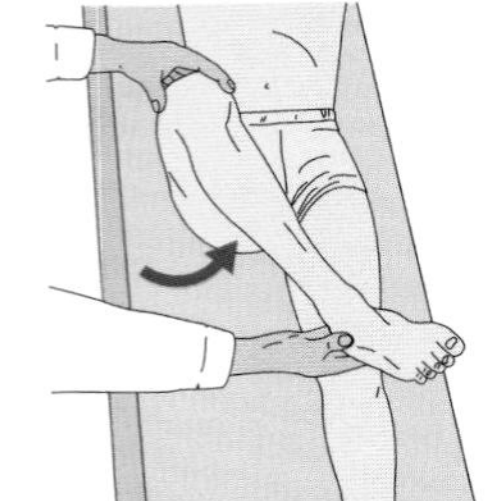

Maneuver	With hip/knee flexed 90°
Assessment	Estimate angle
Normal angle	Lateral rotation 60°
Active/passive	Passive

Lateral: the patient lies supine, while the hip is passively flexed and held at 90°. Holding the patient's foot with his right hand and steadying the patient's thigh (held vertical) with his left hand, the examiner rotates the lower limb inwards, noting the angle of hip lateral rotation achieved in the process, and at the same time, guarding against inflicting pain.

Adduction

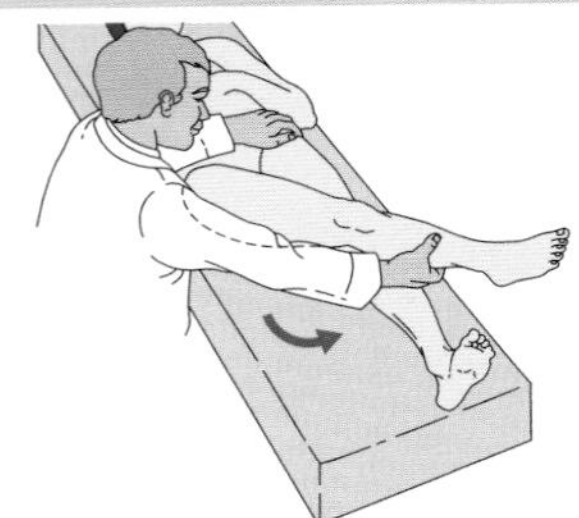

Maneuver	Lying supine
Assessment	Estimate angle
Normal angle	40°
Active/passive	Passive

The patient lies supine, while the fully extended limb is passively abducted as far as it will go. Steadying the patient's contralateral anterior superior iliac spine to prevent pelvic movement, the examiner notes the angles subtended by the fully adducted hip and the midline.

Abduction

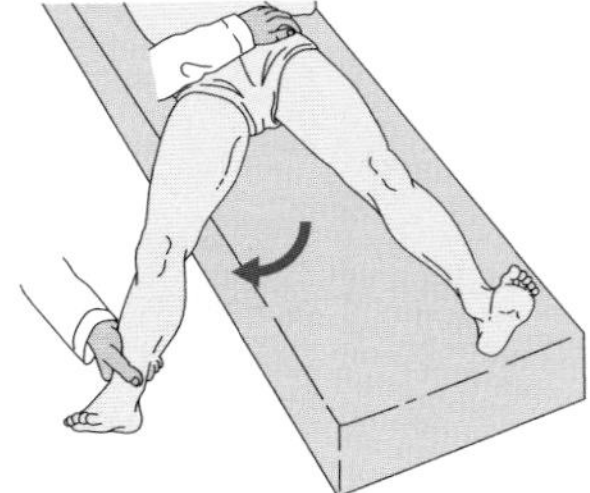

Maneuver	Lying supine
Assessment	Estimate angle
Normal angle	25°
Active/passive	Passive

To estimate adduction the fully extended limb is passively swung towards and beyond the midline as far as it will go. The angle subtended with the starting position then represents the angle of hip abduction.

Extension

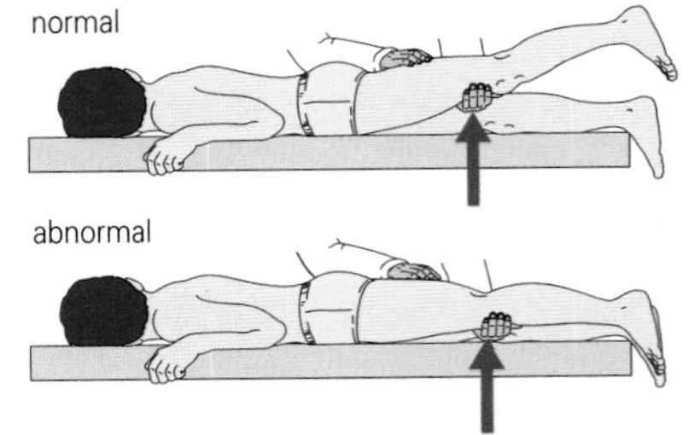

Maneuver	Lying controlateral side
Assessment	Estimate angle
Normal angle	5–20°
Active/passive	Passive

The patient lies on his/her side with their body in a straight line. The uppermost limb, couched in the examiner's right arm, is passively extended as far as it will go short of causing pain, while the patient's trunk is steadied with the examiner's left hand. The angle subtended with the starting position is the angle of hip extension. The patient then turns on his/her other side and extension of the other hip is measured.

Knee

Flexion

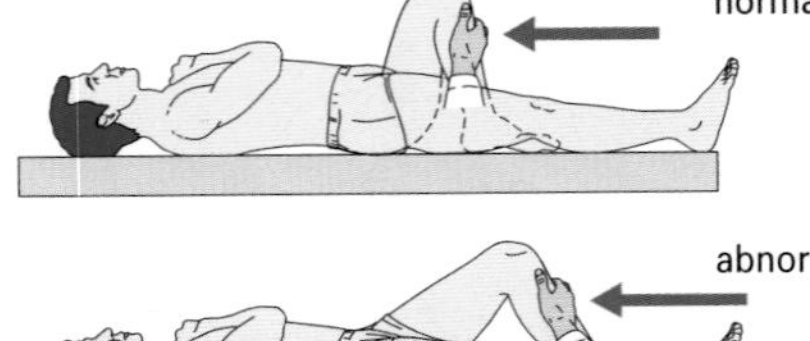

Maneuver	Lying supine
Assessment	Estimate angle
Normal angle	about 135°
Active/passive	Passive

This has already been partly covered in hip flexion. Note will also be made of the presence of crepitus or an effusion (see text). There is simultaneous assessment of joint swelling, redness, tenderness on palpation and whether movement elicits pain.

Extension

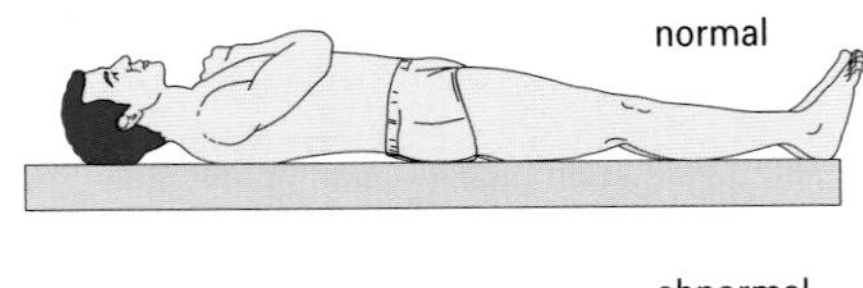

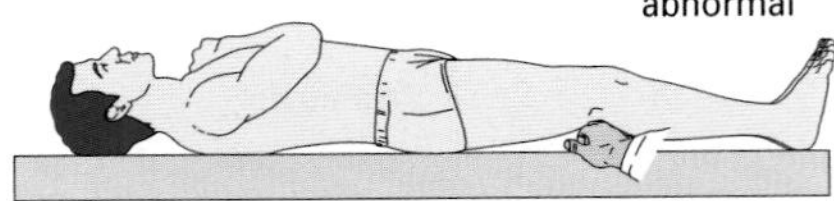

Maneuver	Lying supine, leg flat, no gap
Assessment	Estimate angle
Normal angle	0°
Active/passive	Passive

With the patient sitting on a couch with legs outstretched, there should be no gap between the knees and the couch. The presence of such a gap denotes incomplete knee (or hip) extension.

Hyperextension >10°

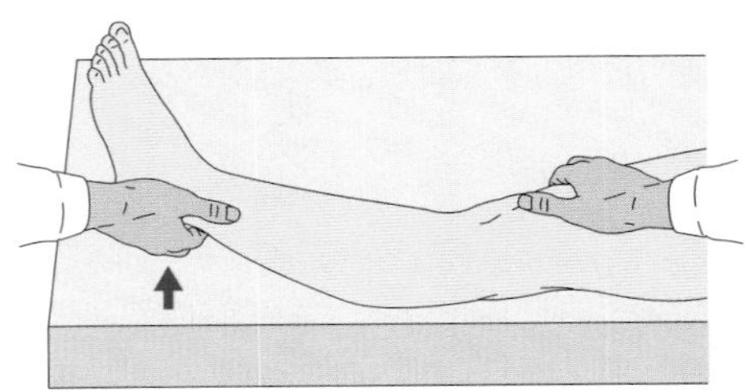

Maneuver	Lying supine, heel raised
Assessment	On each side adds 1 to Beighton score
Normal angle	–
Active/passive	Passive

This is best demonstrated with the patient sitting on a couch with knees outstretched. The examiner takes the patient's heel in his right hand and lifts it off the couch, at the same time placing his left hand firmly on the patient's knee to prevent it from rising off the couch. In the presence of joint laxity the knee will go into hyperextension. An angle of greater than 10° denotes hypermobility.

Fig. 2.2 continued

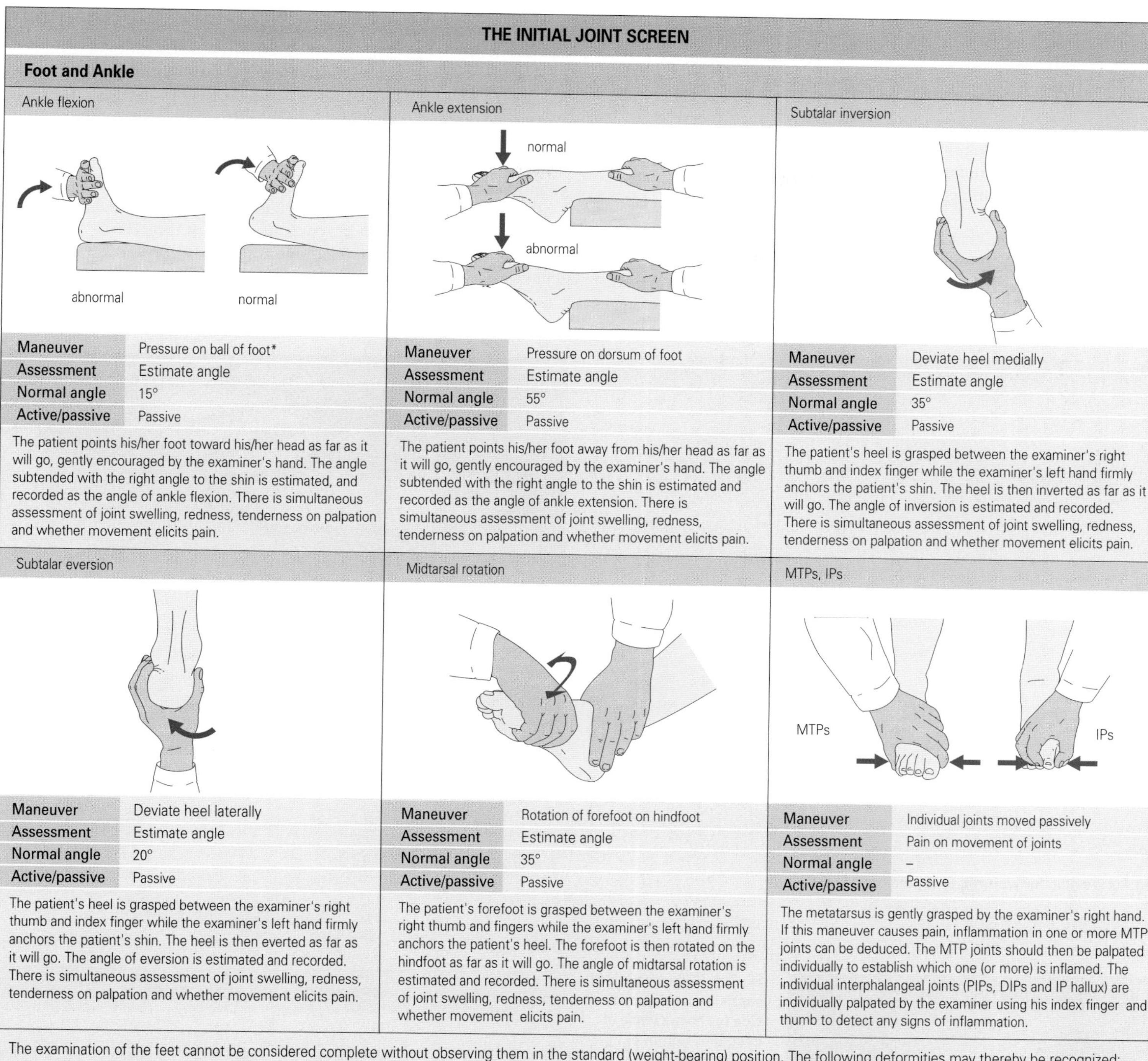

THE INITIAL JOINT SCREEN

Foot and Ankle

Ankle flexion

Maneuver	Pressure on ball of foot*
Assessment	Estimate angle
Normal angle	15°
Active/passive	Passive

The patient points his/her foot toward his/her head as far as it will go, gently encouraged by the examiner's hand. The angle subtended with the right angle to the shin is estimated, and recorded as the angle of ankle flexion. There is simultaneous assessment of joint swelling, redness, tenderness on palpation and whether movement elicits pain.

Ankle extension

Maneuver	Pressure on dorsum of foot
Assessment	Estimate angle
Normal angle	55°
Active/passive	Passive

The patient points his/her foot away from his/her head as far as it will go, gently encouraged by the examiner's hand. The angle subtended with the right angle to the shin is estimated and recorded as the angle of ankle extension. There is simultaneous assessment of joint swelling, redness, tenderness on palpation and whether movement elicits pain.

Subtalar inversion

Maneuver	Deviate heel medially
Assessment	Estimate angle
Normal angle	35°
Active/passive	Passive

The patient's heel is grasped between the examiner's right thumb and index finger while the examiner's left hand firmly anchors the patient's shin. The heel is then inverted as far as it will go. The angle of inversion is estimated and recorded. There is simultaneous assessment of joint swelling, redness, tenderness on palpation and whether movement elicits pain.

Subtalar eversion

Maneuver	Deviate heel laterally
Assessment	Estimate angle
Normal angle	20°
Active/passive	Passive

The patient's heel is grasped between the examiner's right thumb and index finger while the examiner's left hand firmly anchors the patient's shin. The heel is then everted as far as it will go. The angle of eversion is estimated and recorded. There is simultaneous assessment of joint swelling, redness, tenderness on palpation and whether movement elicits pain.

Midtarsal rotation

Maneuver	Rotation of forefoot on hindfoot
Assessment	Estimate angle
Normal angle	35°
Active/passive	Passive

The patient's forefoot is grasped between the examiner's right thumb and fingers while the examiner's left hand firmly anchors the patient's heel. The forefoot is then rotated on the hindfoot as far as it will go. The angle of midtarsal rotation is estimated and recorded. There is simultaneous assessment of joint swelling, redness, tenderness on palpation and whether movement elicits pain.

MTPs, IPs

Maneuver	Individual joints moved passively
Assessment	Pain on movement of joints
Normal angle	–
Active/passive	Passive

The metatarsus is gently grasped by the examiner's right hand. If this maneuver causes pain, inflammation in one or more MTP joints can be deduced. The MTP joints should then be palpated individually to establish which one (or more) is inflamed. The individual interphalangeal joints (PIPs, DIPs and IP hallux) are individually palpated by the examiner using his index finger and thumb to detect any signs of inflammation.

The examination of the feet cannot be considered complete without observing them in the standard (weight-bearing) position. The following deformities may thereby be recognized:

- Flat feet (pes planus) – flattening of the longitudinal arch of the foot.
- Pronation of the foot (often associated with pes planus).
- Valgus deformity of the hindfoot (eversion of sub-talar joint).
- Pes cavus – an exceptionally high longitudinal arch.
- Talipes equinovarus – the heel is raised to produce an 'equine' posture.
- Hallux valgus – great toe pointing away from the midline.
- Subluxation of MTPs – toes deviated upwards proximally and curled distally.

Fig. 2.2 continued

Remember that the examination of these three cardinal elements is integrated on a regional basis – joint set by joint set. The purpose of each stage of the examination and the techniques to be used should be explained to the patient as it progresses around the locomotor system. Great gentleness should be observed at all times in order to avoid inflicting unnecessary pain or discomfort: joints or other sensitive structures may indeed be very sensitive. To facilitate this, the examiner's eyes should study the patient's in order to anticipate discomfort before it happens.

ARTICULAR AND PERIARTICULAR SWELLING

Site of swelling	Tissue involved	Indicative of
Articular soft tissue	Joint synovium/effusion	Inflammatory joint disease
Periarticular soft tissue	Subcutaneous tissue	Inflammatory joint disease
Non-articular synovial	Bursa/tendon sheath	Inflammation of structure
Bony areas	Articular ends of bone	Osteoarthritis

Fig. 2.3 Articular and periarticular swelling.

Key Question 2
'What is the nature of the joint abnormality?'

Here, what is being sought are signs of:

- active current inflammation? (see Key Question 5),
- irreversible joint damage from past inflammation, and
- mechanical defect.

It is important to note that these are not mutually exclusive; a combination of them may be found.

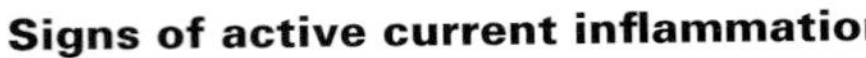

Signs of active current inflammation

These are crucial in distinguishing arthritis from arthragia of noninflammatory origin, such as mechanical defects, hypermobility, and so on.

Warmth is elicited by using the back of the fingers as a 'thermocouple'. Because its value depends on the amount of heat generated within the joint, it is mainly suitable for medium and large-sized joints, for example the knee, ankle and wrist joints (Fig. 2.4).

Redness is uncommon but is encountered in gout, especially around the big toe (Fig. 2.5), and in sepsis in any joint (Fig. 2.6).

Swelling is variable, depending on its cause; Figure 2.3 describes what to look out for. There are a number of specific techniques for

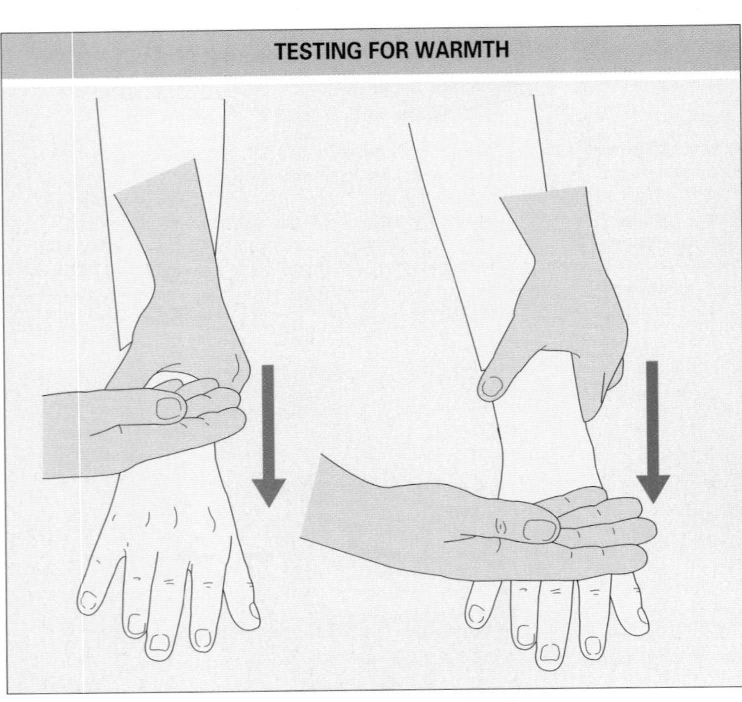

Fig. 2.4 Testing for warmth, using the back of the hand.

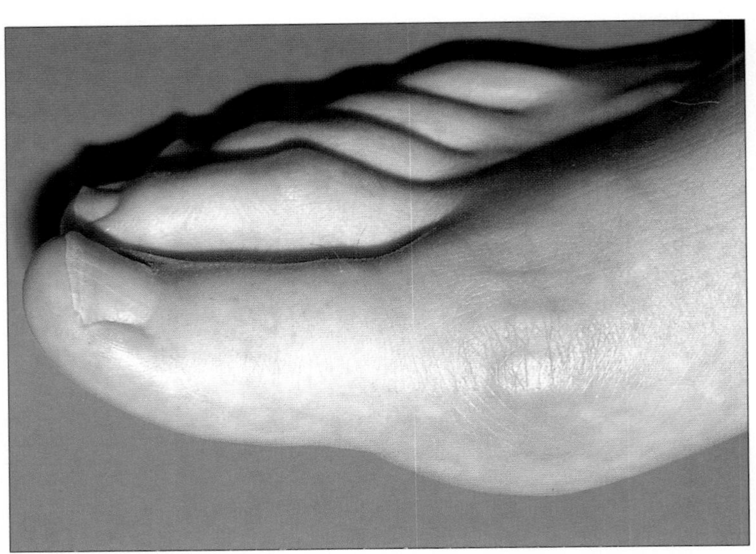

Fig. 2.5 Redness as seen in gout – a valuable indicator of the intensity of underlying joint inflammation.

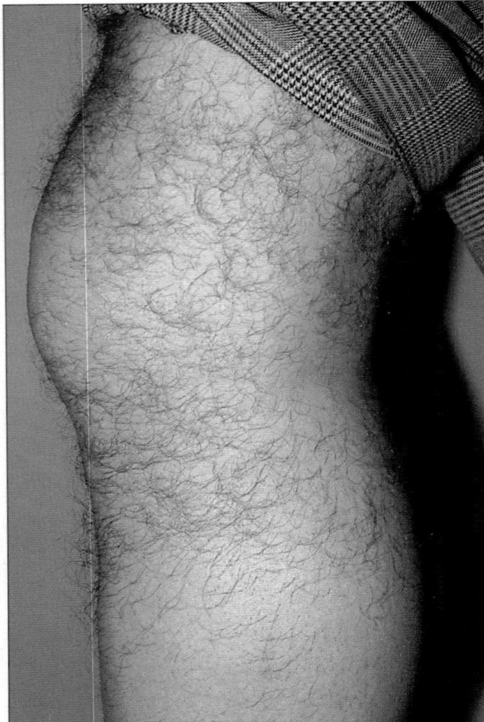

Fig. 2.6 Redness seen in sepsis is an additional clue to the presence of infections within or around the joint.

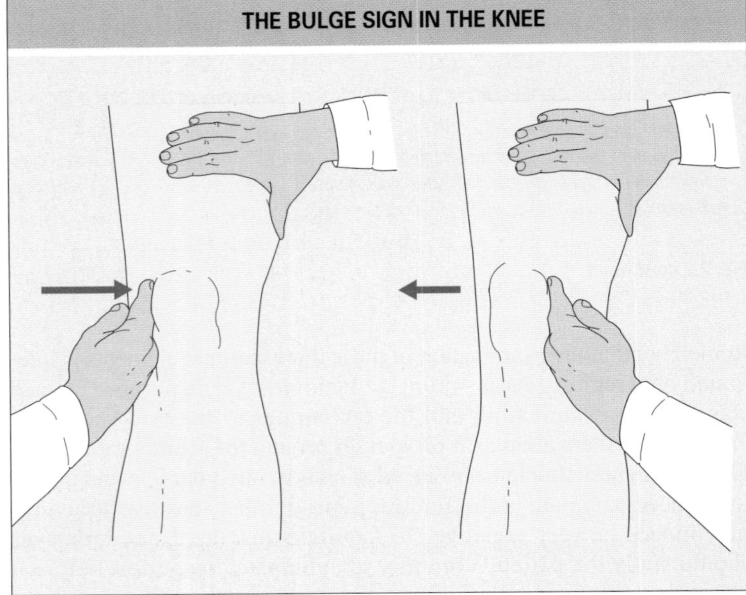

Fig. 2.7 The bulge sign in the knee. The back of the hand gently wafts the fluid from one side of the knee to the other. This is most helpful in detecting small knee effusions.

detection of effusion. Various signs are used in the knee (Fig. 2.7) and elbow (Fig. 2.8), wrist, ankle, small finger (Fig. 2.9) and toe joints to establish the presence of a joint effusion (by fluctuation using the index finger against the contralateral thumb/index in combination). Baker's cyst should not be forgotten – a tense fluctuating swelling in the popliteal fossa (best palpated with patient lying prone) (see Chapter 5.16).

Tenderness is elicited by gentle palpation (squeezing). The 'composite compression' test is particularly suitable for a group of adjacent small joints in a group, for example the MCPs (Fig. 2.10), PIPs and MTPs. This is followed by gentle palpation (squeezing) of individual joints to establish which within the group are the tender, and therefore the inflamed, ones.

Crepitus is an audible and palpable sensation resulting from the movement of one roughened surface on another. In osteoarthritis the crepitus has a fine quality. This should be distinguished from the coarser, clicking sensation encountered in normal joints, with which it may be confused.

Loss of function, effectively loss of range of movement or motion, can be assessed based on motions described in Figure 2.11.

Irreversible joint damage from past inflammation

Essentially this is recognized by the presence of deformity, crepitus, and loss of joint range (or abnormal plane) of motion *in the absence* of features of current inflammation.

Mechanical defects

Examples of these include a knee with an impacted meniscus tear or fragment of bone with osteochondritis dissecans; or 'locking' of the spine in cervical spondylosis or lumbar intervertebral disc prolapse. Mechanical defects are identified by finding a painful restriction of motion favoring a certain plane(s) *in the absence* of features of present, or the sequellae of past, inflammation.

Planes of joint motion

To determine whether the plane of joint motion is abnormal, it is necessary to be familiar with the normal planes of movement relevant to that particular joint (Fig. 2.11). For example, the elbow is a simple hinge joint; hence its normal range is flexion/extension only. Any other movement, such as elbow abduction, is therefore abnormal elbow movement, which is likely to indicate gross joint disruption. Where appropriate, the affected side should always be compared with the unaffected side. Problems may arise when the contralateral joint is, itself, abnormal.

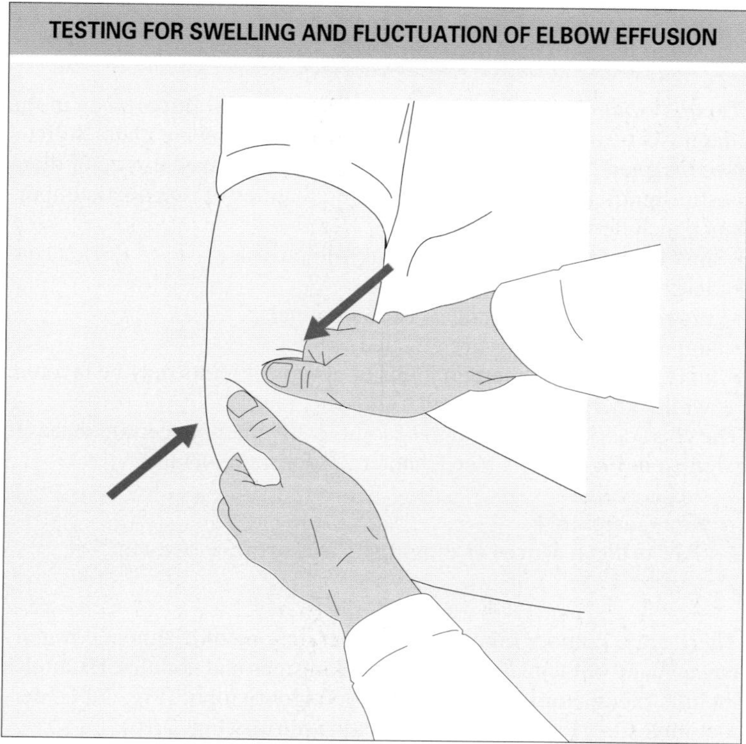

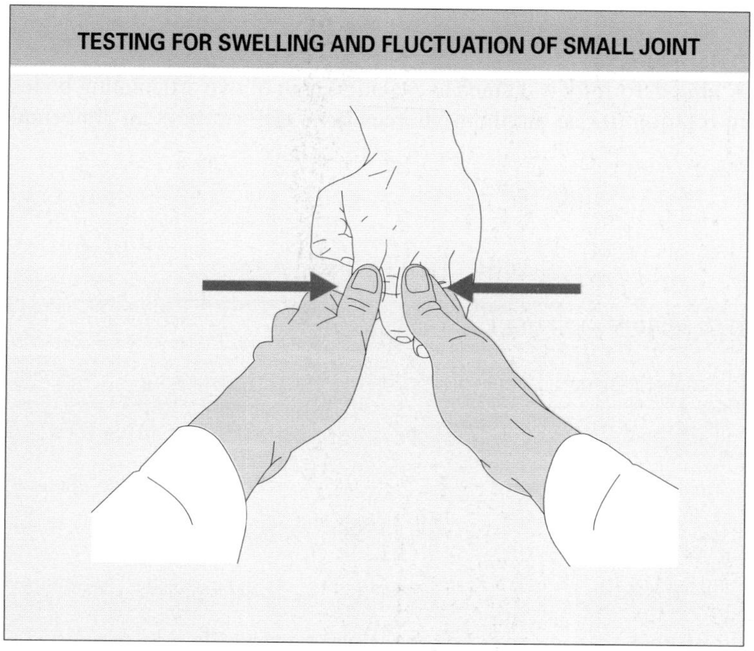

Fig. 2.8 The bulge sign in the elbow. Normally there is a dimple (concavity) seen between the olecranon and the lateral epicondyle. In the presence of an elbow joint effusion the dimple becomes a bulge, which is itself fluctuable.

TESTING FOR SWELLING AND FLUCTUATION OF SMALL JOINT

Fig. 2.9 Testing small joints for fluctuation. The index finger and contralateral thumb/index finger are used to detect cross-fluctuation.

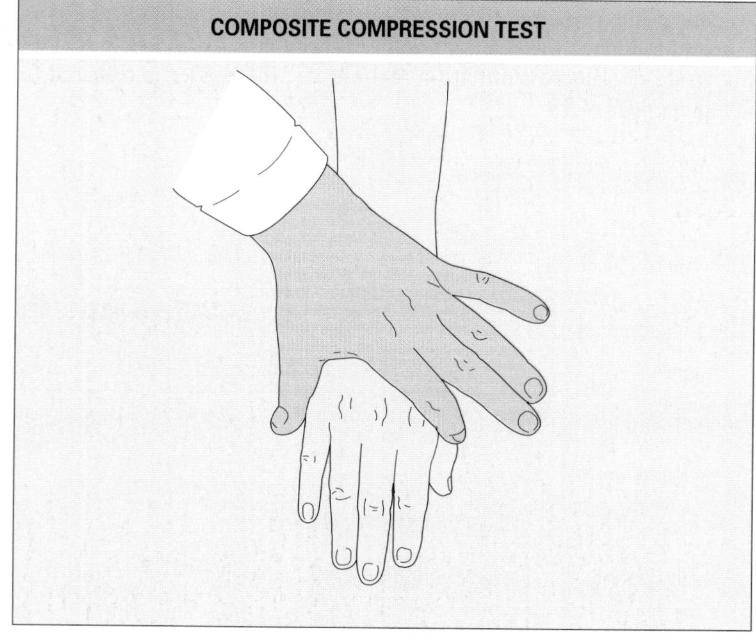

Fig. 2.10 The 'composite compression' test to elicit tenderness in a group of small joints. A gentle squeeze is applied across the knuckles (for MCPs) or forefoot (MTPs). If pain is ellicited this indicates that one or more of the groups of joints encompassed is inflamed. Each one is then palpated individually to determine the culprit.

EXAMPLES OF DIFFERENT JOINT PLANE CHARACTERISTICS		
Joint type	No. of planes	Examples
Hinge	1	Elbow, knee, ankle, MCP, PIP, DIP, MTP
Two-way hinge	2 (circumduction)	Wrist, trapeziometacarpal
Ball and socket	All planes	Shoulder, hip

Fig. 2.11 Examples of different joint plane characteristics.

Range of joint motion

For every joint there is a spectrum of normal range of joint motion, which is genetically determined. It varies with age, gender and ethnic origin. A range that is considered to be outside the upper limit is deemed to be hypermobile, and that below the lower limit, hypomobile. It is therefore necessary to familiarize oneself with 'normal' ranges of motion for all peripheral joints (see Fig. 2.2).

The normal inherent joint range is diminished by joint inflammation (the bulk of inflamed synovium and the effusion) or by irreversible damage to the joint structures (articular cartilage) as a result of disease. Movement is first lost from the extremes of the range. Increasing joint damage results in a narrower and narrower range of motion about the neutral position. Ultimately, movement is lost completely, a situation know as ankylosis.

Hypermobility is recognized by a series of passive maneuvers collectively known as the Beighton scale (see Chapter 8.51). Each hypermobile joint scores a single point; if the sum is greater than three, the patient can be classed as hypermobile.

Assessing joint movement

There are three methods of assessing joint movement. All three are valuable, each has primacy in particular situations:

- *In examination of joints* a combination of active and passive is recommended.
- *In detecting lesions in tendons* or at tendino-osseous junctions, the against-resistance method is principally of use (see tendon inflammation, below).
- *For measuring muscle power*, the against-resistance method is, of course, the principal technique (see under Power below).

General guidance for assessing joint movement is given in Figure 2.2. For more detailed examination techniques, the reader is referred to Chapters 4.07–4.13.

Power

Assessing power is an essential feature of the neurological examination. It impinges on the rheumatological examination in two main areas. Firstly, at the interface of rheumatology and neurology (see Chapter 2.04), where rheumatic disease manifests as neurological complications, for example rheumatoid neuropathy, cervical myelopathy and radiculopathy, and lumbar nerve root compression resulting in foot drop. Secondly, muscle power is lost as a result of inhibition due to pain arising in adjacent inflamed joints. This effect forms the basis of the grip-strength test for assessing progress in rheumatoid arthritis.

Key Question 3
'What is the extent (distribution) of the joint involvement?'

The *distribution* of joint involvement is of crucial importance in the diagnosis of rheumatic disease, as certain patterns are characteristic (see Chapter 2.3). The *number* of involved joints may also be of diagnostic significance. Other characteristic features of diagnostic importance include whether:

- involvement is symmetrical or asymmetrical,
- large or small joints are affected,
- distribution is peripheral or central(spinal),
- upper or lower limbs are affected,
- in certain diseases certain joints or groups of joints may be favored, while others may be spared.

The characteristic distribution of joint involvement in certain diseases is given in Figure 2.12 (see Chapter 2.3 for more detail).

Key Question 4
'Are other features of diagnostic importance present?'

There are a number other features that may be of diagnostic importance, many of them easily visible as skin signs and nodules. Examples include rheumatoid nodules (Fig. 2.13), gouty tophi (Fig. 2.14), dermatomyositis (Fig. 2.15) and psoriatic arthritis (Fig. 2.16).

Key Question 5
'Do the answers to questions 1–4 provide sufficient clues to enable one to establish a differential diagnosis?' (They should!)

Deformities

A *joint* deformity is defined as malalignment of two articulating bones in relation to one another, whereas *bone* deformity is an abnormal

CHARACTERISTIC DISTRIBUTION OF JOINT INVOLVEMENT						
Diagnosis	Symmetry	Number of joints involved*	Large/small joints	Peripheral/central distribution	Upper/lower limb	Predilection
Rheumatoid arthritis	Symmetrical	Mono/oligo/polyarthritis	Large/small	Peripheral	Upper/lower	MCPs, PIPs, MTPs, DIPs
Ankylosing spondylitis				Central		Sacroiliac joints, hip, shoulder
Psoriatic arthritis	Asymmetrical	Polyarthritis	Large/small	Peripheral	Upper/lower	DIPs, sacroiliac joints
Reactive arthritis	Asymmetrical	Oligo/polyarthritis	Large	Peripheral	Lower	Sacroiliac joints, DIPs (toes)
Gout	Asymmetrical	Mono/oligoarthritis	Large/small	Peripheral	Lower > upper	1st MTP, knee, hip
*Monoarthritis denotes inflammation in a single joint, oligoarthritis denotes 2–4 joints, polyarthritis denotes 5 or more joints						

Fig. 2.12 Characteristic distribution of joint involvement in the most common rheumatic diseases.

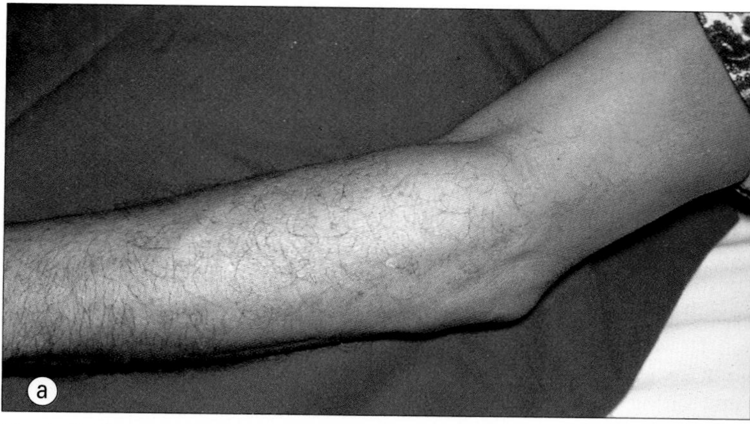

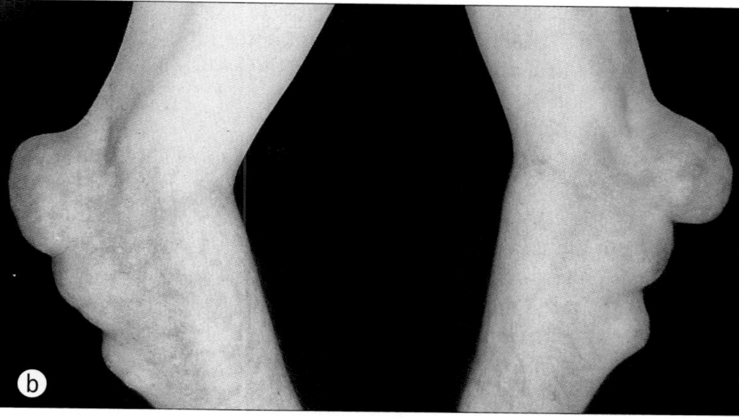

Fig. 2.13 Rheumatoid nodules seen most commonly on the extensor surfaces on the forearms. Early small nodules (a) are best detected by the examiner running their fingers along the border of the ulna. Large nodules (b) may develop in the olecrenon bursa as well as the subcutaneous tissue. The presence of rheumatoid nodules is a strong indicator of rheumatoid arthritis.

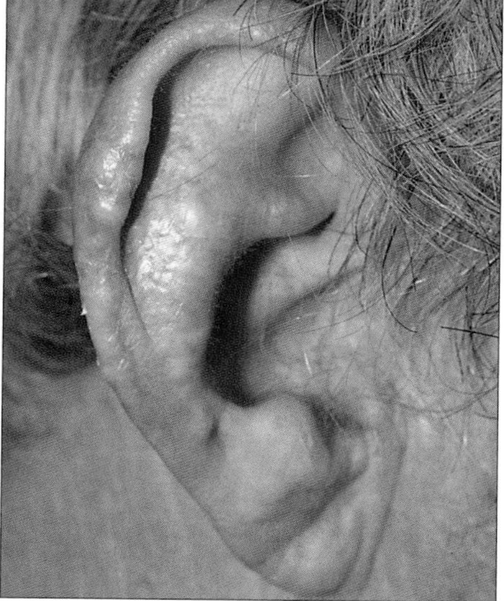

Fig. 2.14 Gouty tophi, seen on the ear pinna (as shown here), over affected joints of the toes, and so on. They represent deposits of urate crystals.

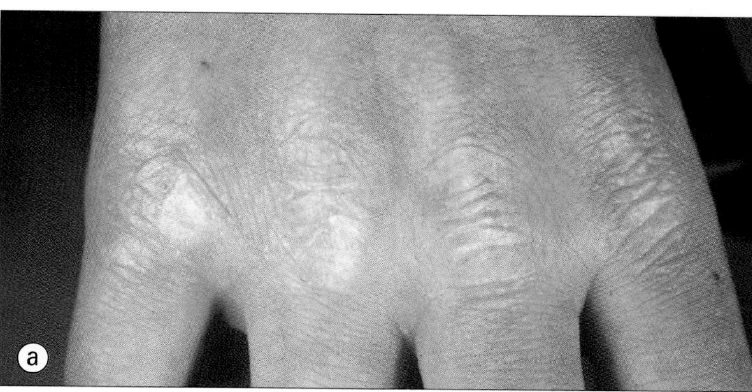

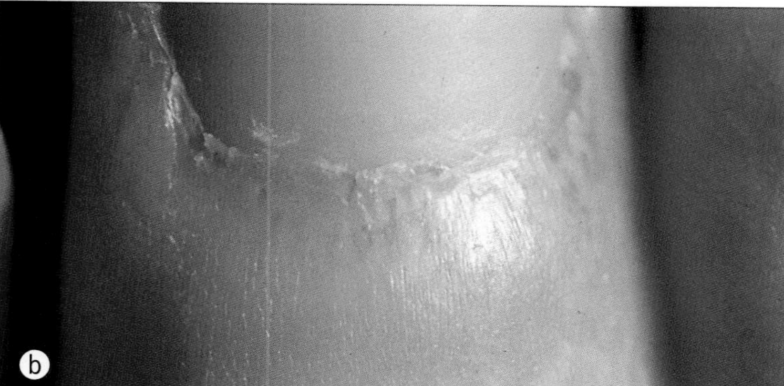

Fig. 2.15 Skin and nailfold lesions in dermatomyositis. These show characteristic erythematosus dermatis (Goddron's patches) (a) and periungual edema and nailfold capillary changes that often occur in this and other connective tissue diseases (b).

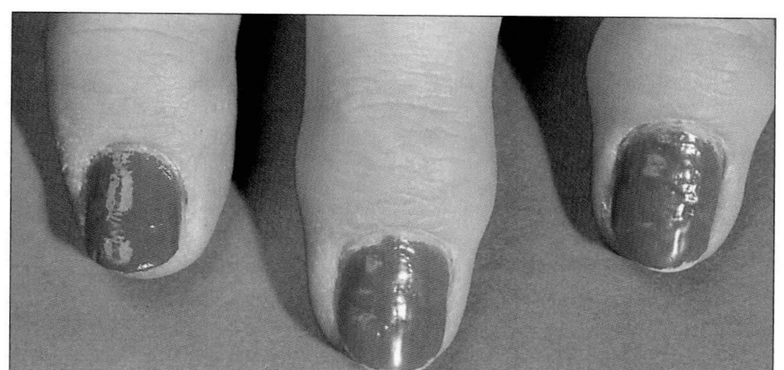

Fig. 2.16 Psoriatic arthritis. Swelling of the distal IP joints is characteristic of psoriatic arthritis. Note the pitting in the adjacent finger nails.

shape of the bone(s) itself (themselves). There are a number of terms in common use to describe peripheral joint deformities:

- *Dislocation*: articulating surfaces are displaced so that they are no longer in contact with one another.
- *Subluxation:* partial dislocation.
- *Fixed flexion*: loss of extension, so that the joint is permanently flexed.
- *Valgus:* a lower limb deformity whereby the distal part is directed away from the midline (e.g. hallux valgus).
- *Varus:* a lower limb deformity whereby the distal part is directed towards the midline (e.g. genu varum).

Commonly encountered specific deformities are given in Figure 2.17.

Instability

It is a fair statement that a joint that provides movement without stability is functionally useless. Weight-bearing joints are particularly (but not exclusively) vulnerable to instability. Joint stability is impaired when:

- *ligaments* are stretched or torn through injury, weakened by disease (RA) or when inherently lax;
- *articular bony surfaces* are congenitally deformed (dysplastic) or damaged by disease (e.g. RA, OA, neuropathic arthropathy);
- *muscle power* is reduced as a result of myopathy, myositis, paralysis (multiple sclerosis, cerebral palsy, stroke, motor neuron disease, poliomyelitis, etc.) or cachexia.

Common examples of observable joint instability in clinical practice are given in Fig. 2.18.

THE SPINE

The spinal structures, including the joints, are relatively inaccessible to clinical examination. Much clinically useful information is therefore derived by indirect means. Examination of the spine is covered in more detail in Chapters 4.2–4.5, but the overall approach is described here.

To achieve the maximum yield, a complete examination requires that the patient is examined in erect posture, lying prone, lying supine and sitting.

Erect posture

As in the re-examination of peripheral joints, the key elements are:

- inspection,
- palaption,
- movement.

Inspection will reveal a postural defect such as a scoliosis, kyphosis

COMMONLY ENCOUNTERED SPECIFIC DEFORMITIES	
Deformity	Description
Lower limb	
Hallux abductovalgus	Great toe diverted outwards
Genu varum	Tibia directed medially on femur
Genu valgum	Tibia directed laterally on femur
Dislocation of the patella	Displacement of patella laterally or medially on the femur
Valgus deformity of the heel	Heel angulated laterally in respect of the ankle
Coxa vara	Reduced angle between femoral neck and shaft
Pes planovalgus	Flattening of the longitudinal arch of the foot (+ valgus heel)
Fixed flexion of the knee	Loss of extension, so that knee joint is permanently flexed
Fixed flexion of the hip	Loss of extension, so that the hip is permanently flexed
Upper limb	
Fixed flexion of DIPs/PIPs/MCPs ('prayer sign')	Inability to straighten fingers
Ulnar deviation	Lateral deviation of fingers with partial subluxation of MCPs
Swan neck deformity of finger	Hyperextension of PIPs with fixed flexion of DIPs
Boutonnière deformity	Permanent fixed flexion of PIPs
Z-shaped thumb	Hyperextension of 1st IP joint with palmar subluxation of 1st MCP
Volar subluxation of wrist	Back displacement of carpus in relation to distal radius
Dorsal subluxation of inferior radioulnar joint	Prominent ulnar styloid
Fixed flexion of elbow	Inability to straighten elbow fully
Cubitus valgus	Angular displacement of forearm in relation to upper arm
Upward subluxation of shoulder	Humerus rides up vertically on account of atrophy/rupture of rotator cuff
Anterior dislocation of shoulder	Forward displacement of humeral head from glenoid
Posterior dislocation of shoulder	Backward displacement of humeral head from glenoid

Fig. 2.17 Specific deformities of the locomotor system.

or hyperlordosis (Fig. 2.19). It may even be possible to see a 'step' indicating a spondylolisthesis. Careful palpation will reveal an asymmetrical spasm of erector spini muscles. Loss (or increase) of range of spinal movement is an important feature in the process of identifying spinal disease (see Fig. 2.2).

Lying prone

Palpation may uncover an area of localized tenderness over a spinous process suggesting the presence of a localized lesion at that site. However, palpation will not determine the nature of the lesion. Diffuse lumbar tenderness is of doubtful significance.

In the femoral nerve stretch test (see Fig. 2.2), pain felt in the anterior thigh region of the ipsilateral leg denotes compression of the femoral nerve roots (L2,3,4) on that side. The test is of dubious significance if positive bilaterally (as is commonly seen in the elderly).

Lying supine

Inspection will reveal wasting, limb shortening, swelling or deformity.

The straight leg raising and sciatic nerve stretch test (see Fig. 2.2) are important tests for sciatica (compression of the sciatic nerve roots L5 and S1). Sacroiliac joint stress tests, including compression, distraction and sacral pressure tests, will help to confirm the presence of a uni- or bilateral sacroiliitis (see Chapter 6.16).

Sensory loss is assessed when the patient is lying supine, checking the dermatomal distribution of any sensory loss (Fig. 2.20), for example the sock/stocking distribution. Global and myotomal motor weakness and reflex changes (i.e. knee, ankle, gluteal and cremasteric reflexes) should also be sought using the normal methods for the detection of neurologic deficits.

Sitting

The 'slump' test is a subtle test for the detection of minor degrees of, or dubiously 'true' sciatic nerve root entrapment. With the patient sitting on edge of table, the knee is gently extended while the trunk slumps forward. If this increases sciatic pain, the test is positive. Neck flexion and/or ankle extension will increase the sciatica further, while neck extension and/or ankle flexion will obviously have the opposite effect in genuine cases.

THE SOFT TISSUES

Soft tissue swelling

Be it articular, periarticular, bursal or tenosynovial (see Fig. 2.3), soft tissue swelling as a physical sign is pathognomic of inflammation.

COMMONLY ENCOUNTERED EXAMPLES OF JOINT INSTABILITY

Instability	Example
Passive side-to-side movement of the tibia on the femur (collateral knee ligaments)	Ruptured collateral knee ligaments
Passive anteroposterior movement of the tibia on the femur (cruciate ligaments)	Ruptured cruciate knee ligaments
Gross genu recurvatum	Polio Hypermobility/Ehlers–Danlos syndrome
Positive Trendelenburg sign (see Fig. 14.10.7)	Unstable hip
'Arthritis mutilans' – flail interphalangeal joints	Psoriatic arthritis RA
Spontaneous dislocation of the shoulder or patella	Hypermobility/Ehlers–Danlos syndrome
Pes planus (collapse of the longitudinal arch)	Obesity/laxity

Fig. 2.18 Commonly encountered examples of joint instability.

SPINAL DEFORMATION

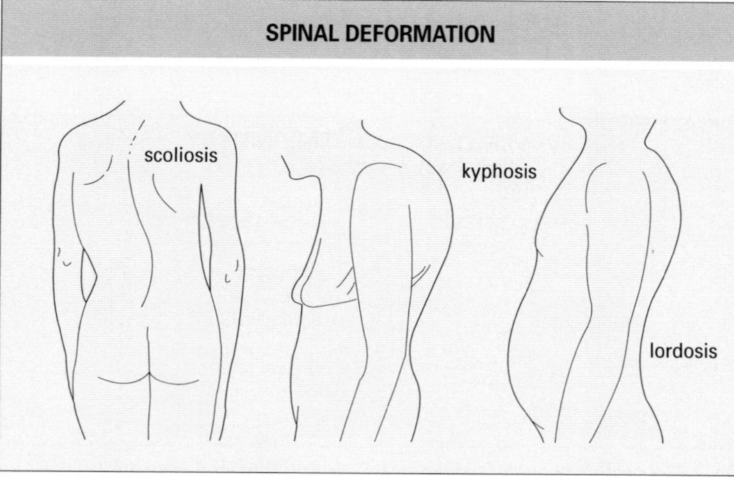

Fig. 2.19 Spinal deformities. These are best observed from behind and from the side, with the patient in the erect posture.

IDENTIFICATION OF NEUROLOGIC DEFICITS IN THE LOWER BACK

Root level	Sensory loss	Motor loss	Reflex
L3	Anterior thigh	Quadriceps	Knee
L4	Medial shin	Quadriceps	
	Invertors of foot	Knee	
L5	Lateral shin	Evertors of foot	None
		Extensors of ankles/toes	
S1	Lateral foot	Flexors of ankle/toe	Ankle
S2,3,4	Saddle area	External sphincters	Gluteal

Fig. 2.20 Identification of neurologic deficits in the lower limbs.

A subjective feeling of joint swelling that is not accompanied by swelling apparent to the observer carries no such significance. It is detected by careful observation and, where appropriate, by comparison with the contralateral side. Since joint, bursal or tenosynovial (Fig 2.21) inflammation is almost invariably accompanied by the presence of an inflammatory exudate, termed an effusion, an important step in confirming inflammation is the detection of an effusion. In gross cases where a joint, for example, is distended with fluid, inspection will leave the examiner in no doubt. However, it is important in all cases to confirm the presence or (otherwise) of an effusion by palpation. In small joints, such as in the fingers, cross-fluctuation is applied between the examiner's index finger pressing dorsally, while at the same time the joint is gently squeezed from the sides between the examiner's index and thumb (Fig. 2.9). A similar technique may also be applied to larger joints. However, this may not be sufficiently sensitive to detect a small knee effusion. To detect such an effusion, fluid is gently massaged into either the lateral or medial side of the joint thereby forming a bulge, which is then stroked across to the other side of the joint. The formation of this bulge is known as the 'bulge sign'.

Ligament injuries

These are detected by eliciting tenderness over the damaged portion of the affected tendon, and by eliciting pain on attempting to distract the bony structures held together by the ligament.

Tendon rupture

When the tendon is subject to disease or is subjected to excessive load, it may rupture. An example of the former is the rupture of the extensor tendons of the little and ring finger tendons, which occurs in RA when synovitis of the wrist begins to erode the tendons directly. An example of the latter is the rupture of the Achilles tendon in sports injuries. Such cases are recognized when attempted movement is nullified, because the muscle is no longer in continuity with the tendon. In extensor tendon rupture, the fingers can be flexed normally but cannot be actively extended. In Achilles tendon rupture, if the patient kneels and the soleus muscle is tapped, the expected flexion of the ankle is not elicited.

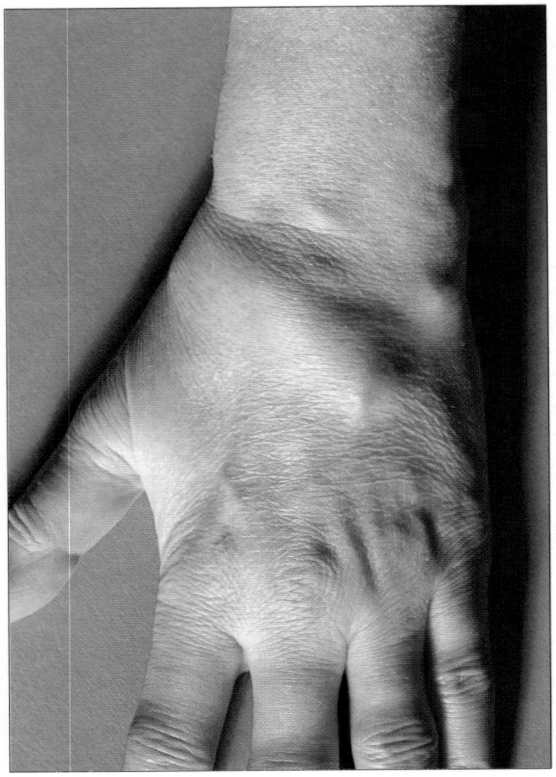

Fig. 2.21 Dorsal sheath effusion in RA. This is often painless. It may also show fluctuation on palpation.

Tendon inflammation (tendonitis)

In shoulder rotator cuff injuries, tendinitis is detected by eliciting a 'painful arc' of *active* movement in the plane of action of the affected tendon, whereas *passive* movement in the same plane is almost pain free. The 'painful arc' effect is enhanced when the active movement is performed against resistance. The relevant tendons and their principal plane of shoulder motion are shown in Figure 2.22). Localized tenderness is elicited over the course of the affected tendon.

Paratenon inflammation

This is seen around the Achilles tendon. Pain and tenderness are detected along the course of the lower soleus and adjacent Achilles tendon.

Tendon sheath

Findings on physical examination will allow recognition of the type of damage to the tendon sheath:

- mechanical obstruction causing triggering (flexor pollicis longus/flexor digitorum longus) (see Chapter 4.9),
- overuse injury, as in De Quervain's tenosynovitis (abductor pollicis longus) (see Chapter 4.9),
- synovial inflammation, for example dorsal sheath effusion in RA (Fig. 2.20) (see Chapter 4.9).

Bursal inflammation (bursitis)

This occurs in inflammatory synovial diseases (gout, rheumatoid arthritis or infection) or arises from unaccustomed friction in overuse injuries or chronic trauma. Common sites include the olecranon, prepatellar, infrapatellar, Achilles insertion, subacromial, ischial and semimembranosus bursae. It is recognized by the detection of a tender, warm fluctuant swelling at the site of a bursa. The overlying skin may be reddened. See Chapter 4.14 – Olecranon bursitis.

Nerve entrapment

It is important to recognize the symptoms and signs of:- carpal tunnel syndrome (Chapter 5.16), ulnar neuritis (Chapter 4.16), common peroneal nerve lesion, meralgia paresthetica (Chapter 4.16) and tarsal tunnel syndrome (Chapter 4.16). These peripheral nerve entrapment lesions are common, and may be provoked by overuse injury. Careful attention to detection of neurological deficit in the territory of the trapped nerve will point to the correct diagnosis, which may be confirmed by a provocative sign such as tapping over the course of the median nerve (Tinel's sign) in the carpal tunnel syndrome (Chapter 4.16).

LOCATING SHOULDER TENDONITIS BY ELICITING A 'PAINFUL ARC'

Muscle/tendon affected	Plane of motion (arc)
Supraspinatus	Abduction
Infraspinatus	Lateral rotation
Subscapularis	Medial rotation
Biceps	Flexion

Fig. 2.22 Locating shoulder tendonitis by eliciting a 'painful arc': the plane of motion in which there is pain on active but not passive motion identifies the tendon affected.

OTHER SYSTEMS: THE 'POLYARTHRITIS PLUS' CONCEPT

The chronic rheumatic diseases (including the inflammatory disorders of connective tissue) constitute a group of multisystem conditions in which a symmetrical peripheral polyarthritis without distinctive characteristics is likely to be a common presenting feature. It follows that detecting a clinical association with an abnormality in another system is more likely to prompt the correct diagnosis than pondering the results of a battery of antibody tests, which can at best only offer a list of relative probabilities.

'POLYARTHRITIS PLUS': ASSOCIATIONS OF OTHER DISORDERS WITH ARTHRITIS	
Polyarthritis +	Potential diagnosis
Abdominal pain	Polyarteritis nodosa
Abortions	Primary antiphospholipid syndrome
Alopecia	SLE
Butterfly rash	SLE
Calcinosis	Dermatomyositis, scleroderma
Cardiac failure	Too nonspecific
Clubbing	Hypertrophic osteoarthropathy
Coma	SLE
Confusional state	SLE
Diarrhea	Reactive arthritis
Digital vasculitis	RA
Deep vein thrombosis	Primary antiphospholipid syndrome
Dysphagia	Scleroderma
Fits	SLE
Headaches	Temporal arteritis
Hemolysis	SLE
Hypertension	SLE, PAN
Malabsorption	Scleroderma
Mononeuritis multiplex	PAN, RA
Neuropathy	RA, PAN
Neutropenia	Drugs, Felty's syndrome, SLE
Pericarditis	RA, SLE, JCA
Pleural effusion	RA, SLE
Pneumonitis	SLE
Proteinuria	SLE, drugs
Pulmonary fibrosis	RA, scleroderma, methotrexate
Purpura	SLE, drugs
Raynaud's phenomenon	Scleroderma, SLE, RA
Renal failure	SLE, drugs
Thrombocytopenia	SLE, drugs
Urethritis	Reactive arthritis

Fig. 2.23 Polyarthritis plus: associations of other disorders with arthritis.

The concept of *'polyathritis plus'* is thus a useful guide to solving such clinical diagnostic problems. Only a full examination of all systems can exhaust the totality of diagnostic clues that may be brought to light and marshaled. Caution is urged in assuming that an observed clinical association necessarily has diagnosic significance. Two alternative explanations should always also be born in mind: the possibility either that the associated feature may be iatrogenic (i.e. the result of treatment) or that it may have arisen entirely by coincidence.

The most important *'polyarthritis plus'* features together with their likely diagnoses are listed in Figure 2.23. It is outside the scope of this chapter to document in detail the significance of all possible interpretations of the associations listed. Many, however, are covered in other chapters in this section, in other sections and in the index.

PSYCHOSOCIAL STATUS

An integral part of the examination will concern the patient's state of mind. In no other branch of medicine does *psyche–soma* interaction play a more important role. This is because:

- Pain is such a prominent symptom;
- Disability and loss of mobility cause such frustration and dismay;
- Inability to work and dependence on others causes loss of self-esteem; it is hardly surprising that such patients become clinically depressed.

In a condition referred to as somatization or amplification syndrome, somatic symptoms (including pain and loss of function) may become elaborated or even generated subconsciously in order, apparently, to achieve secondary gain, for example after an accident when compensation is pending. Although such problems may be difficult to distinguish from organic syndromes, an astute and experienced clinician will often be able to recognize the spurious symptoms and signs for what they are.

Although a formal psychological examination lies outside the scope of the clinical assessment (indeed, few rheumatologists will be appropriately skilled to perform it), it should nevertheless be possible during the course of history taking and examination to glean sufficient information to draw the appropriate conclusions as to the patient's mental status, and advise psychiatric intervention where necessary.

FUNCTIONAL IMPAIRMENT

No assessment of a disorder affecting the locomotor system, either local or generalized, can be considered complete without consideration of the patient's functional status and quality of life. This covers the impact of the condition on the ability to self-care in daily living and on the capacity to carry out normal daily routine, including work, leisure, sporting and other social activities. A complete functional assessment will include aspects of:

- self-care – ability to wash, bath, attend to toilet needs, dress, cook and feed oneself;
- mobility – including standing, transferring, walking, negotiating stairs, driving and using public transport;
- nature of occupation, work capacity and social security benefits.

A recommended approach is to obtain the services of trained health care professionals (rheumatology nurse practitioner, occupational therapist and/or physiotherapist, medical social worker), who are specially trained for these tasks. Much of this important information can be gleaned by the physician during the clinical evaluation either from the history, during the examination or from questionnaires such as the Heath Assessment Questionnaire (HAQ) and the AIMS2, which the patients can be asked to complete prior to the consultation (see the Appendix: selected measures for outcome assessment).

FURTHER READING

Gross J, Fetto J, Rosen E. Musculoskeletal Examination. Cambridge: Blackwell Science, 1996.

Little AH. The Rheumatological Physical Examination. Orlando: Grune and Stratton, 1986.

Polley HF, Hunder GG. Rheumatologic Interviewing and Physical Examination of Joints, 2E. Phliadelphia: WB Saunders, 1978.

Doherty M, Dacre J, Dieppe P, Snaith M. The 'GALS' locomotor screen. Annals of the Rheumatic Diseases 1992;51:1165–9.

Doherty M. An Introduction to the Musculoskeletal System. Chesterfield: The Arthritis and Rheumatism Council, 1991.

Doherty M, Hazleman BL, Hutton CW, Maddison PJ, Perry JD. Rheumatology Examination and Injection Techniques. London: WB Saunders Co Ltd, 1992.

PATTERN RECOGNITION IN ARTHRITIS

Osvaldo Hübscher

Pattern recognition is the key to diagnosis of the rheumatic disorders; the central questions that need to be asked are:

- Is there a locomotor problem or a disease of another system?
- Is the condition articular or periarticular?
- Is the condition mechanical (arthrosis) or inflammatory?
- Does it affect appendicular or axial structures or both?

These questions can be answered from a synthesis of data from the history and examination, in particular:

- From the *history* – the mode of onset, sequence of development of different features, and the duration and pattern of the symptoms.
- From the *examination* – the number, distribution and pattern of the affected joints or periarticular structures, and the nature of any systemic involvement.

INTRODUCTION

The history and physical examination are the two most important components of the diagnostic process for patients complaining of musculoskeletal pain, stiffness or other rheumatic symptoms[1]. Clinical judgment in interpreting findings elicited from the history and physical examination should allow the physician to answer several key questions:

- Do the symptoms originate in the locomotor system or do they reflect diseases primarily affecting other systems (e.g. neurologic disorders, vascular disease)?
- Is it an articular or nonarticular process?
- Does the patient have arthralgias or arthritis?
- Is there evidence of other organ involvement (e.g. systemic connective tissue disorders) or does it appear to be a disorder restricted to the musculoskeletal system (e.g. osteoarthritis)?
- Is the articular problem inflammatory, degenerative or something else?
- Does the disease affect axial or appendicular structures, or both?

A substantial number of patients will have localized mechanical problems or nonspecific soft tissue conditions. Muscular syndromes or pain originating in periarticular foci can often mimic an articular origin (sometimes affecting more than one site). Examples are uni- or bilateral anserine bursitis resembling an intra-articular knee joint disorder and extensor tendinitis of the thumb (de Quervain's tenosynovitis)mimicking wrist involvement. Bone lesions (e.g. Paget's disease, osteoid osteoma) may also provoke pain referred to a joint. Arthralgia is used to refer to pain localized in a joint whereas arthritis refers to the objective evidence of an inflammatory or degenerative change of the joint. Arthritis is a much more specific sign of an articular disorder.

Once the physician establishes that the disorder originates in the joints, several other aspects of the history and physical examination should be considered in order to delineate a diagnostic pattern of arthropathy (Fig. 3.1). The attributes of joint involvement which will be considered in this section focus on those dominating the clinical picture during the early phases of rheumatic disorders, when treatment could be of greater benefit. Moreover, the diagnostic value of pattern recognition will be considered without taking into account other characteristics of the patient (e.g. gender, age, family history) or the presence or absence of extra-articular features of disease normally contributing to diagnostic certainty.

MAJOR DIAGNOSTIC FEATURES OF JOINT DISORDERS

Mode of onset
- Acute
- Insidious

Duration of symptoms
- Self-limiting
- Chronic

Number of affected joints
- Monoarthritis
- Oligoarthritis (2–4 joints)
- Polyarthritis

Distribution of joint involvement
- Symmetric
- Asymmetric

Localization of affected joints
- Axial
- Appendicular
- Both

Sequence of involvement
- Additive
- Migratory
- Intermittent

Local pattern of involvement (in individual joints)

Fig. 3.1 Major diagnostic features of joint disorders.

MODE OF ONSET AND DURATION OF SYMPTOMS

Some arthropathies typically present with an acute onset of pain with the peak intensity reached within hours or a few days[2], whereas in others maximum severity is reached gradually (over several weeks or months). Variations may occur and the same disorder may have a sudden onset in some patients and be gradual in others. Rheumatoid arthritis (RA), for instance, may present as an acute polyarthritis (especially in the elderly) and psoriatic arthropathy as an acute monoarthritis resembling gout, whereas in most cases both disorders begin insidiously. Examples of an acute onset also include bacterial and viral arthritis (e.g. parvovirus B19 and rubella), rheumatic fever, reactive arthritis, palindromic rheumatism and crystal-induced arthritis (the best example being nocturnal attacks of gout). An insidious pattern is common in early onset pauciarticular juvenile chronic arthritis (EOPA-JCA) as well as in the polyarticular onset type and in osteoarthritis (OA), hypertrophic osteoarthropathy, mycobacterial and fungal arthritis and most cases of neuropathic arthropathy (Charcot's joints).

Arthritic disorders lasting less than 4–6 weeks are considered self-limiting in practical terms, while those lasting longer are considered chronic. In self-limiting arthritic disorders the duration of symptoms and signs may be a valuable discriminating feature. Early episodes of monoarticular gout tend to subside spontaneously after 3–10 days and resolution is complete; acute or subacute pseudogout attacks of calcium pyrophosphate dihydrate crystal deposition disease (CPPD) may last from 2 or 3 days to 3–4 weeks; most articular or periarticular episodes of palindromic rheumatism disappear within hours to several days with no articular sequelae. A steady inflammation in an individual joint for more than a few days or a week in children is highly unlikely to be due to rheumatic fever.

THE RED HOT JOINT
Infectious Bacterial Neisserial (may be preceeded by transient polyarticular disease) Mycobacterial Virus Lyme disease
Crystal induced Gout CPPD (pseudogout type) Hydroxyapatite (acute calcific periarthritis)
Traumatic
Palindromic rheumatism
Psoriatic arthropathy
Reactive arthritis
Bacterial endocarditis

Fig. 3.2 Acute monoarthritis: important diagnostic possibilities.

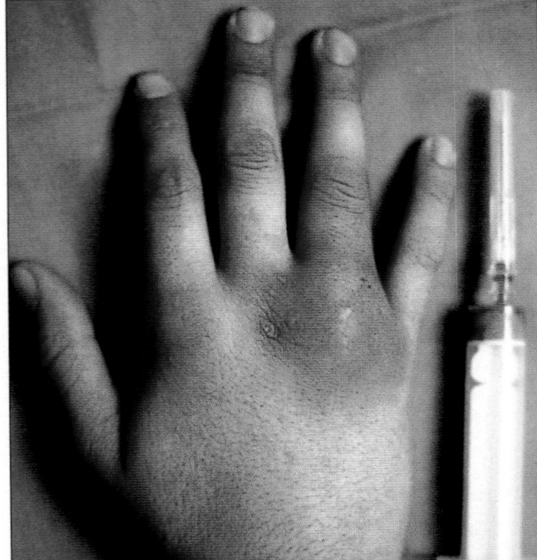

Fig. 3.3 The red hot joint. Septic arthritis of the ring finger MCP showing swelling and intense redness of the skin.

THE NUMBER OF AFFECTED JOINTS

The clinical pattern may be monoarticular or polyarticular. Although almost any individual arthropathy may begin as monoarthritis, the initial pattern of some disorders is characteristically monoarticular regardless of the subsequent course. In particular, patients with an acute painful synovitis of a single joint and varying degrees of overlying redness represent a challenging subset in clinical rheumatology[3,4]. Although redness may occur in any acute arthritis regardless of the etiology, its presence usually evokes a restricted list of possible diagnoses (Fig. 3.2). The most common diagnoses are crystal-induced synovitis (including acute calcific periarthritis[5]), bacterial infectious arthritis (Fig. 3.3), traumatic conditions, psoriatic arthritis and palindromic rheumatism (in which the joint may reach a dark bluish redness). Very occasionally rheumatologists are confronted with rare causes of acute monoarthritis such as synovitis associated with pancreatic disease or with unusual findings in the synovial fluid examination (e.g. lipid microspherulites).

Owing to the frequency of the underlying disease it should be remembered that the uncommon occurrence of a red hot joint in the context of RA may be due to superimposed infectious synovitis and not to the disease process itself[6]. Nonetheless, a syndrome of acute sterile arthritis mimicking articular infection may occur in RA patients and respond to anti-inflammatory therapy[7]. Although systemic lupus erythematosus (SLE) causes a number of articular problems, the occurrence of monoarthritis suggests infection or osteonecrosis.

Chronic monoarthritis is often the presenting manifestation of a variety of joint disorders (Fig. 3.4); histologic elucidation may be necessary to make the correct diagnosis[8]. In a substantial number of patients the cause remains undetermined[9].

Involvement of two to four separate joints is referred to as oligoarthritis. In general, rheumatic disorders manifesting as monoarthritis may also be oligoarticular. Despite this overlap there are examples in which involvement of two or three joints (rather than one) may significantly narrow the diagnostic spectrum. As an example, lower limb oligoarthritis (especially of the knees and ankles) in an asymmetric fashion is reminiscent of reactive arthritis[10]. An asymmetric oligoarthritis affecting scattered distal interphalangeal (DIP) and proximal interphalangeal (PIP) finger joints and metacarpophalangeal (MCP) joints characterizes a common subgroup of patients with psoriatic arthropathy.

The third articular pattern is the one in which polyarticular involvement dominates the clinical picture. A wide variety of inflammatory and noninflammatory disorders, both common and uncommon, may present as polyarthritis[11] (Fig. 3.5).

SELECTED CAUSES OF CHRONIC MONOARTHRITIS
Infectious arthritis Mycobacterial, fungal, bacterial, viral, Lyme disease
Inflammatory arthritis Crystal induced Monoarticular RA EOPA-JCA Seronegative spondyloarthropathies (ankylosing spondylitis, reactive arthritis, inflammatory bowel disease arthritis, undifferentiated) Psoriatic arthropathy Foreign body synovitis (e.g. plant thorn synovitis) Sarcoidosis
Noninflammatory arthritis Osteoarthritis Internal derangement Osteonecrosis Synovial osteochondromatosis Reflex sympathetic dystrophy Hemarthrosis (e.g. coagulopathy, anticoagulants) Neuropathic (Charcot's joint) Stress fracture Transient regional osteoporosis Juvenile osteochondroses
Tumors Pigmented villonodular synovitis Lipoma arborescens Synovial metastasis from solid tumors Synovial sarcoma
Undiagnosed
EOPA-JCA = Early onset pauciarticular juvenile chronic arthritis

Fig. 3.4 Selected causes of chronic monoarthritis.

IS IT A SYMMETRIC OR AN ASYMMETRIC DISORDER?

This distinction is very helpful in the differential diagnosis of oligo- and polyarticular conditions, with RA being the classic example of symmetric arthritis. Symmetry is not necessarily strict in the hands; the same MCP or PIP joint may not be equally affected in both extremities of RA patients. Erosive inflammatory OA, parvovirus arthritis and many cases of SLE may resemble RA, whereas reactive arthritis, psoriatic arthropathy and polyarticular gout usually present with asymmetric involvement of appendicular joints.

This feature of the articular pattern has obvious limitations; every patient with a symmetric disorder may have an initial asymmetric phase. Figure 3.5 lists a number of conditions classified according to the most characteristic pattern.

DISTRIBUTION OF OLIGO- AND POLYARTHRITIS		
	Symmetric	**Asymmetric***
Inflammatory	RA; JCA (systemic and polyarticular types) Adult onset Still's disease SLE Mixed connective tissue disease Polymyalgia rheumatica Rheumatic fever (adult onset) Jaccoud's arthritis	Ankylosing spondylitis Reactive arthritis Psoriatic arthropathy (oligoarticular type) Enteropathic arthritis Undifferentiated spondyloarthropathy JCA (pauciarticular types) Palindromic rheumatism
Degenerative/ crystal induced	OA (primary generalized, erosive and nodal types) CPPD(pseudo-RA type) 'Milwaukee shoulder' Hemochromatosis arthropathy	Gout (especially oligoarthritis) CPPD (pseudogout type)
Infectious	Viral arthritis Lyme disease	Bacterial arthritis Bacterial endocarditis
Miscellaneous	Hypertrophic osteoarthropathy Amyloid arthropathy Myxedematous arthropathy Sarcoid arthritis (acute type)	

*Most asymmetric arthritides may be or are characteristically initially monoarticular
JCA = Juvenile chronic arthritis; CPPD = Calcium pyrophosphate dihydrate crystal deposition disease

Fig. 3.5 Distribution of selected oligo- and polyarthritis.

CHRONIC ARTHROPATHIES WITH PERIPHERAL AND AXIAL INVOLVEMENT
Inflammatory
Spondyloarthropathies Ankylosing spondylitis Reactive arthritis Psoriatic arthropathy (a subset of patients) Enteropathic arthritis Undifferentiated
Juvenile chronic arthritis Systemic and polyarticular onset
Adult onset Still's disease
Syndrome of SAPHO (synovitis, acne, pustulosis, hyperostosis and osteitis)
Noninflammatory
OA
Diffuse idiopathic skeletal hyperostosis
Acromegaly
Ochronosis
Spondyloepiphyseal dysplasia

Fig. 3.6 Chronic arthropathies with peripheral and axial involvement.

LOCALIZATION OF AFFECTED JOINTS

AXIAL INVOLVEMENT

Axial structures include, apart from the spine, centrally located joints such as the sacroiliac, sternoclavicular, manubriosternal and the rest of the chest wall and sometimes shoulders and hips.

In the presence of peripheral arthritis one of the most helpful clues in the differential diagnosis is to determine the presence of concomitant axial involvement. While some rheumatic conditions rarely affect the axial segments (e.g. gout, SLE, systemic vasculitis), a combined pattern is often seen in others (Fig. 3.6). Osteoarthritis of the spine often coexists with appendicular involvement. Patients with ankylosing spondylitis (AS), psoriatic arthropathy, reactive arthritis (both following enteric and sexually transmitted infection) and arthritis accompanying inflammatory bowel disease may also exhibit varying degrees of combined axial and peripheral involvement. Polyarticular and systemic onset JCA as well as adult onset Still's disease commonly affect the apophyseal joints of the cervical spine in addition to peripheral joints. The SAPHO syndrome (synovitis, acne, pustulosis, hyperostosis and osteitis) is a further example among the much less frequent arthritides[12].

Involvement of the cervical spine structures is frequent in RA patients whereas the dorsal and lumbar segments are spared. Persistent pain in these areas should lead to other diagnoses (e.g. insufficiency fractures of the spine, sacrum or iliac bones)[13].

PERIPHERAL INVOLVEMENT

Individual joints (as well as tendon sheaths and bursae) may eventually be affected by a large number of rheumatic disorders. Some joints, however, are closely associated with the early phases of a selected group of diseases. Consequently, their involvement often facilitates the diagnostic process. Common examples seen in clinical rheumatology include the following:

- bilateral and symmetric involvement of small and large joints, typical of RA;
- exclusive inflammatory DIP joint involvement of the fingers, a relatively infrequent, although important clue in the diagnosis of psoriatic arthropathy (Fig. 3.7);
- bilateral bony enlargement of the second and third MCP joints with restricted motion, characteristic of hemochromatosis arthropathy[14];
- the metatarsophalangeal (MTP) joint of the big toe, typically affected in acute gouty attacks (see Fig. 3.8);

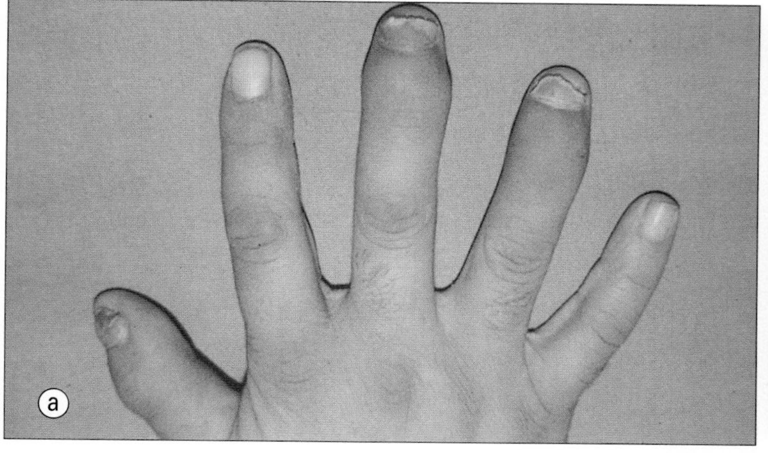

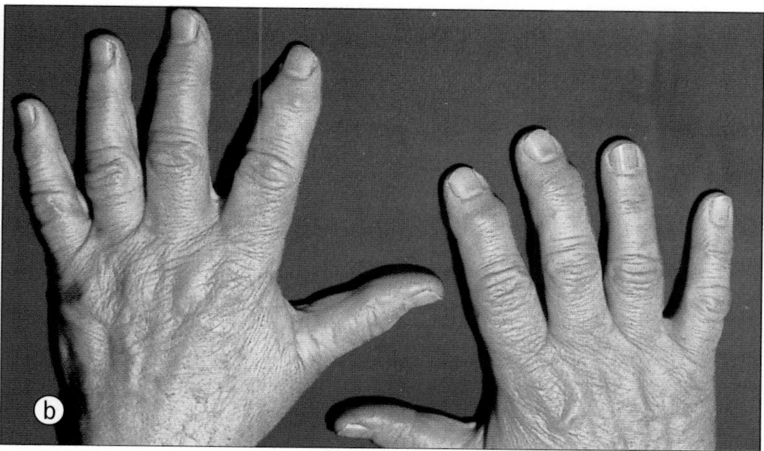

Fig. 3.7 Rheumatic disorders affecting the DIP joints. Psoriatic arthropathy of two DIP joints and of the interphalangeal joint of the thumb together with nail dystrophy (a). Osteoarthritis is the commonest disorder affecting this segment (Heberden's nodes) (b).

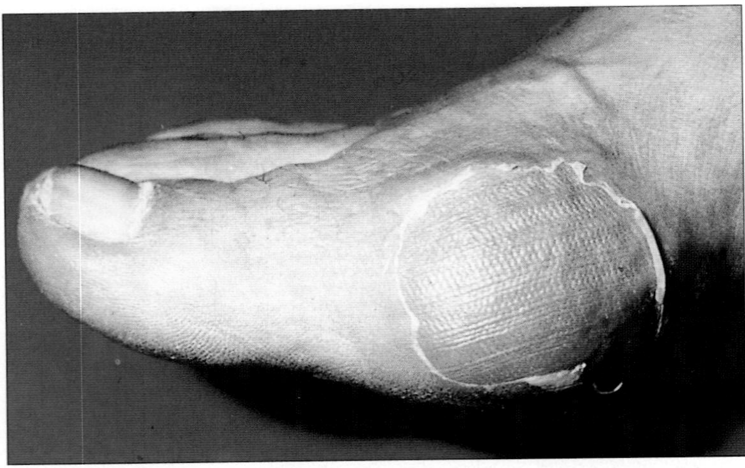

Fig. 3.8 Acute gout. The first MTP joint is involved at some time in approximately 75% of patients. Desquamation of the skin often occurs.

- pain in the muscle girdles (neck, shoulders, lower back, buttocks) in an appropriate clinical setting is highly indicative of polymyalgia rheumatica although the onset of RA in the elderly may be difficult to differentiate from this entity[15];
- juxta-articular pain and tenderness (symptoms of inflammatory enthesopathies may dominate the clinical picture in some patients with seronegative spondyloarthropathies;
- acute involvement of a sternoclavicular joint (one of the less frequently involved joints), suggests septic arthritis in intravenous drug abusers[16];
- bilateral and symmetric bony enlargment of the DIP and PIP joints (Heberden's and Bouchard's nodes).

The MCP and PIP joints of the fingers, wrists, knees and MTP joints are commonly affected bilaterally or symmetrically, with a striking absence of DIP joint disease. Patients with SLE or other systemic rheumatic diseases may occasionally present with a 'rheumatoid' pattern of disease. Nodal osteoarthritis (Heberden's nodes) is by far the most frequently encountered poly-articular disorder affecting the DIP joint (Fig. 3.7). Crystalline disorders[17], such as CPPD, as well as OA, psoriatic arthropathy and a wide variety of conditions, may mimic the podagra of gout[18]. The occurrence of 'pseudopodagra' is one of the best examples of how the specific site of the index joint, although helpful, can only suggest the diagnosis.

An enthesopathy is a pathologic process at the sites of tendinous, ligamentous or articular capsule attachment to bone and can be inflammatory, degenerative, crystalline or metabolic[19]. Achilles tendon and plantar fascia insertions into the calcaneum (heel pain) are principally involved. The costosternal areas, iliac crests, ischial tuberosities, greater trochanters and manubriosternal joint may be also affected. The presence of inflammatory tarsal involvement and enthesopathy in pediatric patients (<16 years of age) may be a discriminating feature in distinguishing between AS and JCA (except late onset pauciarticular JCA) in the absence of axial disease[20]. The finding of an enthesopathic digit or dactylitis (sausage finger) strongly suggests psoriatic arthropathy (more common in the hands) or reactive arthritis (more common in the feet) (Fig. 3.9).

SEQUENCE OF JOINT INVOLVEMENT

Clinical involvement of joints may follow three major patterns: additive, migratory and intermittent. An additive pattern refers to the involvement of more joints while the previous joints remain symptomatic. Polyarticular OA, reactive arthritis and RA are typical examples of this progressive sequence.

A migratory pattern means that the process ceases or abates in one joint while simultaneously or immediately after starts in a previously normal joint. Neisserial arthritis may present as a migratory arthritis and tenosynovitis while the fleeting arthritis of rheumatic fever in children is a classic example.

In the intermittent rheumatic disorders there is complete remission of symptoms and signs until the next recurrence in the same or other joints. No evidence of active disease or residual signs can be detected during intervals. Crystal-induced arthritis, familial Mediterranean fever and palindromic rheumatism usually follow this pattern for years with asymptomatic periods that vary in length. Patients with SLE often show complete resolution of synovitis (commonly polyarthritis) and follow a discontinuous pattern of arthropathy. Adult onset Still's disease may also run a polycyclic clinical course[21].

LOCAL PATTERN OF JOINT DISEASE

Local signs may be of great diagnostic help. In the same manner as the presence of redness often suggests a particular group of diagnoses (see above), the occurrence of skin desquamation when inflammation declines is suggestive of acute gouty monoarthritis. Additional findings which may be of diagnostic value include:

- symmetric or asymmetric enlargement of individual joints;

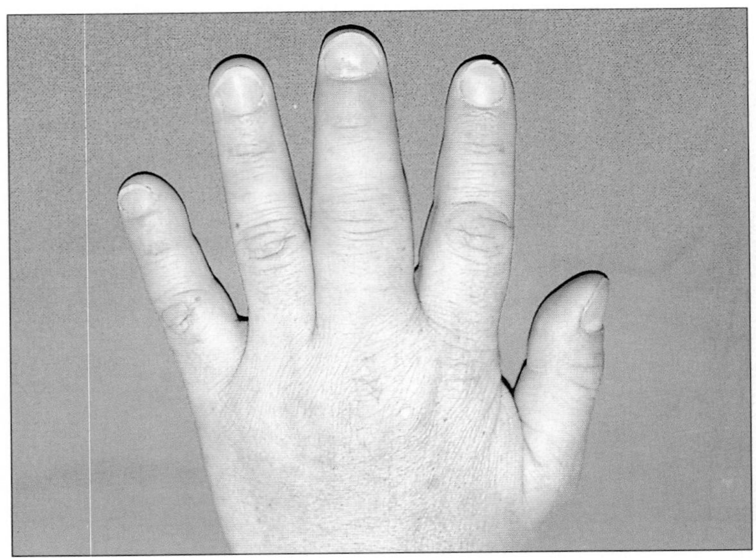

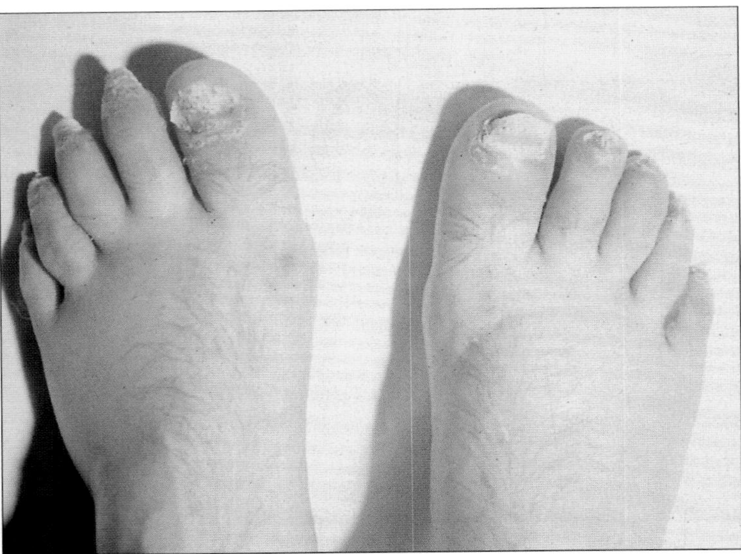

Fig. 3.9 Sausage fingers and toes. Psoriatic arthropathy; dorsal and volar aspects of dactylitis at the 3rd finger (a). Reactive arthritis: dactylitis more evident at the 2nd and 3rd left toes and nail dystrophy (b)l

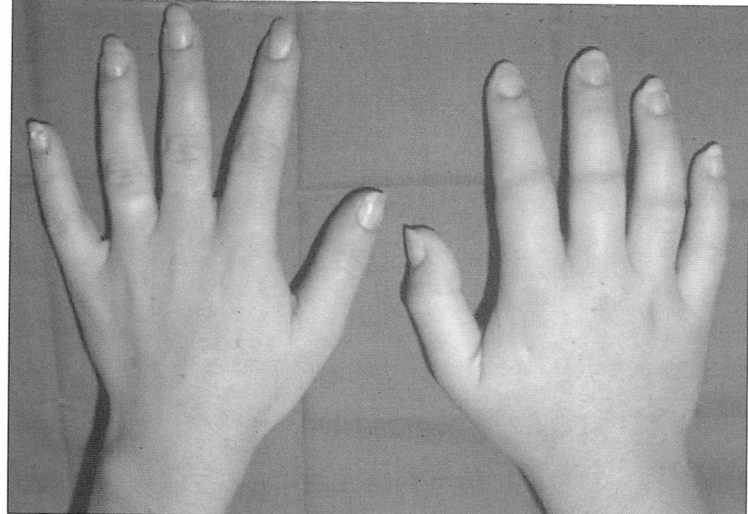

Fig. 3.10 Reflex sympathetic dystrophy syndrome. There is diffuse, edematous swelling of the entire right hand.

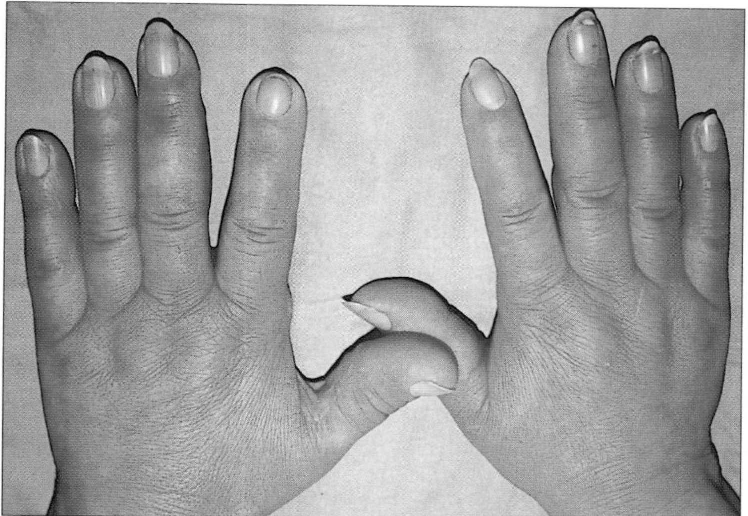

Fig. 3.11 Swollen hands in mixed connective tissue disease. The presence of symmetric puffy hands is a common early finding. Similar changes are often seen in the early stages of scleroderma.

- in some forms of arthritis, local signs of inflammation extending beyond the anatomic limits of the joint.

The physical sign of joint enlargement is more obvious in the finger joints. Fusiform swelling of PIP joints in RA is the best example of symmetric involvement as opposed to Heberden's nodes, erosive OA, chronic sarcoidosis and tophaceous gout which often produce asymmetric enlargement of the affected joint.

Inflammation extending beyond the joint may be a major diagnostic contribution as illustrated by the presence of dactylitis, a characteristic sign of an enthesopathic process (see above). A diffusely painful swollen hand or foot may indicate reflex sympathetic dystrophy syndrome in that extremity (Fig. 3.10). Bilateral symmetric puffy swelling of hands and fingers (and sometimes the feet) may be seen in the early phases of systemic sclerosis and mixed connective tissue disease (Fig. 3.11). Indurative edema of hands and feet is also a characteristic early feature of Kawasaki disease.

Diffuse swelling of both hands with pitting is a conspicuous feature of the syndrome of remitting seronegative symmetric synovitis with pitting edema (RS^{3}PE syndrome)[22] (Fig. 3.12). These findings have occasionally been noted in the hands and feet of patients with polymyalgia rheumatica[23]. Unilateral painless swelling of the dorsum of one hand (extending to a variable degree to the elbow) with pitting edema due to lymphatic obstruction is an infrequent finding in RA patients[24]:

Flexion contractures of the fingers with a striking painful thickening of the palmar fascia and marked decreased active and passive mobility (Fig. 3.13) may be seen. The first of these may be seen in association with neoplastic conditions (especially ovarian carcinoma)[25]. Diabetic patients may also develop painless contractures of the finger joints[26].

From time to time rheumatologists see patients who complain of variable pain in the hands and feet. Digital clubbing and local signs of inflammation may or may not be prominent. Hypertrophic osteoarthropathy, acquired pachydermoperiostosis, acromegaly and thyroid acropachy should be considered when encountering these cases.

THE CLINICAL VALUE OF PATTERNS OF ARTHROPATHY

Evidence of some distinct articular patterns focuses the spectrum of diagnostic options and reduces unnecessary diagnostic testing[27]. These patterns are not diagnostic *per se* and they must always be viewed as a rough guide only for various reasons. First, unrelated arthropathies may share one or more clinical patterns. As an example, EOPA-JCA, tuberculous arthritis and foreign body arthritis (e.g. plant thorn synovitis)[28] may all present as a gradual onset chronic monoarthritis of the knee in

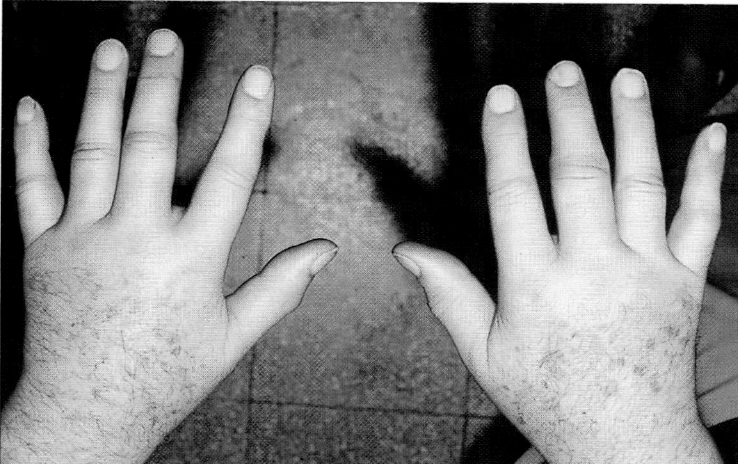

Fig. 3.12 Remitting seronegative symmetric synovitis with pitting edema. Massive acute painful edema of both hands in an 80-year-old man.

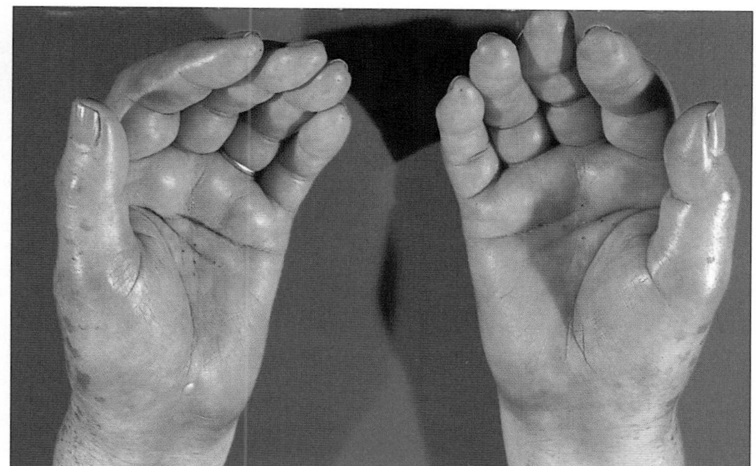

Fig. 3.13 Flexion contractures of all fingers in carcinoma-associated fasciitis. A 50-year-old woman developed painful swelling and contractures of both hands secondary to marked hardening and thickening of the palmar fascia. Palmar erythema is also present. Investigations revealed an ovarian carcinoma, the most commonly associated neoplasm in these patients.

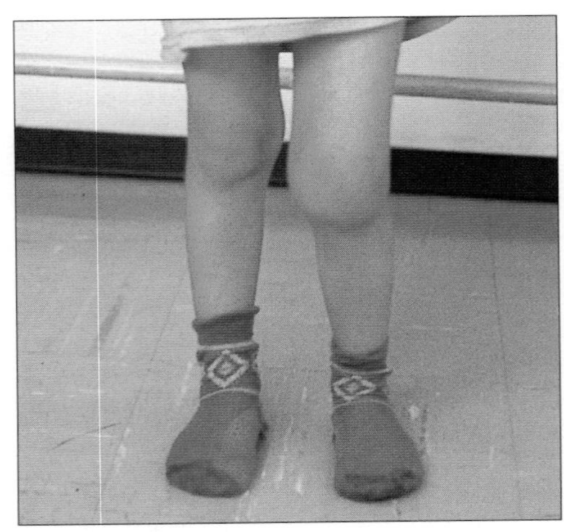

Fig. 3.14 EOPA-JCA in a young girl with monoarthritis. This patient had associated asymptomatic iridocyclitis. In some cases a synovial biopsy is mandatory to exclude other disorders.

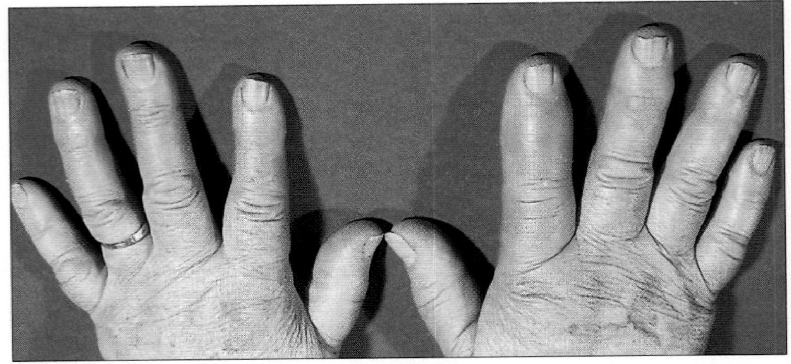

Fig. 3.15 Gouty attack superimposed on a Heberden's node. The clinical combination may be found in elderly patients treated with diuretics as seen in the distal interphalangeal joint of the right index finger in this 78-year-old woman. Note mild desquamation of the overlying skin.

a young girl before the age of 6 years (Fig. 3.14). Both gout and pseudogout can mimic septic arthritis in the setting of febrile acute mono- or polyarthritis[29]. Second, some major arthritides have more than one mode of onset. It should be remembered, for example, that chronic or intermittent mono- and oligoarthritis (with no involvement of the small joints of the hands) may occasionally dominate the early course of RA before a symmetric poly-arthritis evolves. The same presentation may also precede the appearance of typical inflammatory low back pain in patients with AS. Moreover, CPPD has many clinical patterns with pseudogout and pseudo-osteoarthritis being the most frequent[30]. Third, the articular pattern may change with time in the course of a single disorder. In these cases the correct diagnosis is facilitated when the patient is seen during the 'typical' phase of the disease or may be hampered during the 'atypical'phases. Early gout, for instance, is an acute, intermittent, monoarticular arthropathy; as the disease progresses, however, the patient may present with a chronic additive, relatively symmetric, polyarticular disease leading to confusion with RA on physical examination[31]. Finally, a single clinical pattern of joint disease may correspond to more than one diagnosis. Chronic gout superimposed on Heberden's nodes[32] and the coexistence of crystals and infection in cases of subacute monoarthritis[33] are examples of this clinical situation (Fig. 3.15).

The combination of features analyzed above can often contribute to the accurate diagnosis of an arthropathy. A deeper knowledge of each of the individual disorders is necessary to enhance the specificity of the diagnostic process. However, this may require the addition of laboratory studies, joint fluid examination, imaging techniques and other tests to refine the analysis. The more varied the articular patterns possible in a given arthropathy, the more necessary complementary studies become. Systemic vasculitis, SLE, bacterial endocarditis, HIV infection, solid tumors and leukemia, Behçet's syndrome, sickle cell disease and relapsing polychondritis are examples of disorders in which several patterns of arthropathy have been described and which may require a panoply of investigations in addition to the physical findings. However, the careful history and physical examination remains the cornerstone of a diagnostic evaluation for all patients who present with rheumatic complaints.

REFERENCES

1. American College of Rheumatology Ad Hoc Committee on Clinical Guidelines. Guidelines for the initial evaluation of the adult patient with acute musculoskeletal symptoms. Arthritis Rheum. 1996;39:1–8.
2. Carias K, Panush R. Acute arthritis. Bull Rheum Dis. 1994;43:1–4.
3. Rogachefsky RA, Carneiro R, Altman RD, Burkhalter W. Gout presenting as infectious arthritis. J Bone J Surg. 1994;76A:269–73.
4. Baker DG, Schumacher HR. Acute monoarthritis. N Engl J Med. 1993;329:1013–20.
5. McCarthy GM, Carrera G, Ryan L. Acute calcific periarthritis of the finger joints. A syndrome of women. J Rheumatol. 1993;20:1077–80.
6. Goldenberg DL. Infectious arthritis complicating RA and other chronic rheumatic disorders. Arthritis Rheum. 1989;32:496–502.
7. Singleton JD, West S, Nordstrom D. 'Pseudoseptic'arthritis complicating RA. J Rheumatol. 1991;18:1319–22.
8. Fletcher M, Scott JT. Chronic monarticular synovitis. Ann Rheum Dis. 1975;34:171–6.
9. Blocka K, Sibley JT. Undiagnosed chronic monarthritis. Clinical and evolutionary profile. Arthritis Rheum. 1987;30:1357–61.
10. Keat A. Reiter's syndrome and reactive arthritis in perspective. N Engl J Med. 1983;309:1606–15.
11. Pinals RS. Polyarthritis and fever. N Engl J Med. 1994;330:769–74.
12. Kahn MF. Why the 'SAPHO' syndrome? J Rheumatol. 1995;22:2017–19.
13. Stroebel R, Ginsburg W, McLeod R. Sacral insufficiency fractures: an often unsuspected cause of low back pain. J Rheumatol. 1991;18:117–9.
14. Faraawi R, Hart M, Kertesz A, Bell D. Arthritis in hemochromatosis. J Rheumatol. 1993; 20:448–52.
15. Healey LA. Polymyalgia rheumatica and seronegative RA may be the same entity. J Rheumatol. 1992;19:270–2.
16. Rosenthal J, Bole GG, Robinson WD. Acute nongonococcal infectious arthritis. Arthritis Rheum. 1980;23:889–97.
17. Fam A, Stein J. Hydroxyapatite pseudopodagra in young women. J Rheumatol. 1992,19:662–4.
18. Bomalaski JS, Schumacher HR. Podagra is more than gout. Bull Rheum Dis. 1984;34:77–84.
19. Resnik D, Niwayama G. Enthesis and enthesopathy: anatomic, pathological and radiological correlation. Radiology. 1983;146:1–9.
20. Burgos Vargas R, Vazquez Mellado J. The early clinical recognition of juvenile-onset ankylosis spondylitis and its differentiation from juvenile RA. Arthritis Rheum. 1995;38:835–44.
21. Cush J, Medsger T, Christy W, Herbert D, Cooperstein L. Adult-onset Still's disease. Arthritis Rheum. 1987;30:186–94.
22. Russell E, Hunter JB, Pearson L, McCarty DJ. Remitting seronegative, symmetrical synovitis with pitting edema. J Rheumatol. 1990;17:633–9.
23. Salvarani C, Gabriel S, Hunder G. Distal extremity swelling with pitting edema in polymyalgia rheumatica. Arthritis Rheum. 1996;39:73–80.
24. Sant S, Tormey V, Freyne P, Casey E. Lymphatic obstruction in rheumatoid arthritis. Clin Rheumatol. 1995;14:445–50.
25. Shiel WC, Prete PE, Jason M, Andrews BS. Palmar fasciitis and arthritis with ovarian and non-ovarian carcinomas. Am J Med. 1985;79:640–4.
26. Kapoor A, Sibbitt WL. Contractures in diabetes mellitus: the syndrome of limited joint mobility. Semin Arthritis Rheum. 1989;18:168–80.
27. Fries JF, Mitchell DM. Joint pain or arthritis. JAMA. 1976;235:199–204.
28. Reginato A, Ferreiro JL, Riester O'Connor C, *et al.* Clinical and pathologic studies of 26 patients with penetrating foreign body injury to the joints, bursae and tendon sheaths. Arthritis Rheum. 1990;33:1753–62.
29. Ho G, DeNuccio M. Gout and pseudogout in hospitalized patients. Arch Intern Med. 1993;153:2787–90.
30. Chuzhin Y, Panush RS. CPPDDD: what is it and why is it underrecognized? Bull Rheum Dis. 1995;44:3–5.
31. Talbott J, Altman RD, Yu T. Gout arthritis masquerading as rheumatoid arthritis or vice versa. Semin Arthritis Rheum. 1978;8:77–114.
32. Lally E, Zimmermann B, Ho G, Kaplan S. Urate-mediated inflammation in nodal osteoarthritis: clinical and roentgenographic correlations. Arthritis Rheum. 1989;32:86–90.
33. Zyskowski L, Silverfield J, O'Duffy JD. Pseudogout masking other arthritides. J Rheumatol. 1983;10:449–53.

4

ARTHRITIS AND MUSCLE WEAKNESS OR NEUROPATHY

Barry Bresnihan

Definition

- Muscle weakness and neuropathy occur frequently in rheumatic diseases.
- Muscle weakness may be primary or secondary to other factors.
- Neuropathy is usually caused by ischemia secondary to vasculitis or localized nerve entrapment.
- Detailed evaluation may be required to determine the cause and extent of muscle disease or neuropathy in rheumatic diseases.

CLINICAL ASSESSMENT

A systematic approach is essential when assessing muscle weakness or neuropathic features in a patient with a primary rheumatic disease. Many patients with chronic arthritis complain of lethargy or fatigue, muscle wasting or weakness, loss of fine function or coordination and paresthesia or numbness. These symptoms may represent the constitutional effects of chronic inflammatory disease or indicate specific myopathic or neuropathic complications.

HISTORY OF SYMPTOMS

The most frequent symptoms of neuromuscular disease are weakness and pain, but limpness, heaviness or stiffness, fatigue, wasting, spontaneous movements, palpable tenderness, local or diffuse swelling of nerves or muscles and contractures are other features of importance. Patients with chronic rheumatic disease may have associated anemia, cardiac or pulmonary disease, loss of physical fitness or even malnutrition, depression or anxiety, which may account for fatigue or subjective weakness. Appropriate questioning by the physician should elicit evidence of these background factors.

Weakness

Muscle weakness may be proximal, distal or local (Fig. 4.1). The impact of early muscle weakness depends on the individual's lifestyle. Proximal limb girdle weakness usually presents with lower limb symptoms such as difficulty with walking, running, climbing steps or rising from a low seat. Sudden falls may occur due to instability of the knee. Shoulder girdle weakness may be equally prominent, but may not have a great impact unless individuals are required to use upper limb girdle muscles vigorously. Eventually, performing simple tasks above head level will produce symptomatic weakness.

Distal weakness leads to tripping over carpets, steps and footpaths. Weakness of the hands is usually first noted as clumsiness, before progressing to impairment of grip strength. Patients with a compressive myelopathy, as in cervical spondylosis, or cerebellar ataxia may present with lower limb weakness. They often complain of particular difficulty walking down stairs. Patients with neuromuscular disease may present with localized muscle weakness, such as wristdrop or footdrop in peripheral neuropathy. Cranial nerve lesions may cause ptosis or ophthalmoplegias. Inflammatory muscle diseases involving the muscles of respiration, the pharyngeal laryngeal muscles or those of the upper esophagus may cause dyspnea, dysphonia or dysphagia.

The mode of onset and progression of weakness are of great importance in assessment. The weakness of peripheral neuropathy induced by vasculitis may be sudden in onset, reaching maximal severity over hours or days. The weakness of an entrapment neuropathy or a compressive myelopathy is usually more gradual, progressing over months or years. Weakness associated with inflammatory muscle disease may present acutely over a number of days, but patients would more usually notice weakness over a period of weeks or months. Other causes of acute onset muscle weakness include Guillain–Barré syndrome, myasthenia gravis and poliomyelitis. Inflammatory muscle disease may also progress more insidiously over months or even years. Similarly, myasthenia gravis, the muscular dystrophies and motor neuron disease may follow a more chronic progressive course.

Neuromuscular pain, numbness and paresthesia

Persistent muscle contraction at rest is a common cause of chronic musculoskeletal pain including low back pain, neck pain and perhaps fibromyalgia. Stress, depression or anxiety may be responsible in some cases. Painful muscle spasms may accompany inflammatory or degenerative joint disease. It may be difficult to distinguish true muscle pain from articular pain in a patient with arthritis. Muscle pain at rest may also occur in infectious myopathy. Inflammatory myopathy is rarely painful except in very severe cases, but many patients will have night cramps and pain with fatigue after significant exertion.

Muscle pain on exertion is usually attributable to ischemia, as in intermittent claudication. Some metabolic muscle disorders may cause muscular pain after exertion. Other rare causes of muscular pain and cramp include myoglobinuria and lipid storage diseases. Occasionally muscular dystrophy, motor neuron disease and early spasticity present with exertional pain.

Peripheral neuropathy, dorsal nerve root compression, as in intervertebral disc prolapse, and spinal cord lesions may cause neurogenic pain at rest. In these situations, numbness and paresthesia may also be

EXAMPLES OF NEUROMUSCULAR WEAKNESS IN RHEUMATIC DISORDERS
Proximal
Subjective Anemia, chronic illness, malignancy, chronic infection, endocrine disorder, depression
Apparent Proximal upper and lower limb arthropathy
True Inflammatory myopathy, drug-induced myopathy, eosinophilia–myalgia syndrome, cervical myelopathy, osteomalacia
Distal
Apparent Peripheral arthropathy
True Peripheral neuropathy
Local
Apparent Monoarthritis
True Isolated neuropathy, localized myopathy

Fig. 4.1 Examples of neuromuscular weakness in rheumatic disorders.

present. Spinal cord lesions may be accompanied by painful flexor spasms. Disorders of anterior horn cells, the motor segments of spinal roots and neuromuscular junctions are not painful. Spinal stenosis may also present with lower limb neuropathic pain, numbness, and weakness on exertion. It is often relieved by rest.

FAMILY HISTORY

Familial occurrence is a feature of several primary neuromuscular diseases[1]. Seeking a positive family history requires careful and detailed enquiry. Mild cases and variants of congenital neuromuscular diseases may have been unrecognized. It may be necessary to examine other family members in detail if a suspicion of congenital neuromuscular disease exists. It is important to know that considerable intersibling variation may be observed in some disease categories. Thus, for example, in glycogen storage disease of muscle slowly progressive proximal weakness in one sibling may bear little resemblance to severe and rapidly fatal disease in another. In sex-linked and dominant conditions a family history can be most helpful: the early diagnosis of Duchenne, facioscapulohumeral and myotonic muscular dystrophy and the periodic paralyses is greatly facilitated if other family members are known to be affected.

DRUGS AND TOXINS

Many drugs have been implicated as causes of neuromuscular disease and a detailed drug history is essential. Several medications commonly prescribed by rheumatologists have been associated with neuromuscular complications (Fig. 4.2). In all instances neuromuscular side-effects are rare complications of therapy. Individual case reports of reversible peripheral neuropathy associated with therapeutic doses of various nonsteroidal anti-inflammatory drugs have been described. A severe neuropathy and myopathy has been described following excessive intake of colchicine. Chloroquine therapy has been associated with reversible polyneuropathy and myopathy involving both skeletal and cardiac muscle. Administration of gold salts has also been complicated by the development of peripheral polyneuropathy and myokymia. Myokymia is a rhythmic and sometimes painful rippling of muscles. All extremities and the tongue may be involved. Myokymia gradually resolves after cessation of gold salt administration. D-Penicillamine has been associated with several neuromuscular side-effects including the development of polymyositis, dermatomyositis and myasthenia gravis. These complications resolve after discontinuation of D-penicillamine. Corticosteroid therapy is the most common drug-induced cause of muscle weakness encountered in patients with rheumatic diseases. Corticosteroid myopathy is usually dose related and is uncommon in patients receiving less than the equivalent of prednisone 20mg daily. It is also important to determine if exposure to compounds such as organophosphates or heavy metals which are toxic to neuromuscular tissues has occurred.

PHYSICAL EXAMINATION

General

When examining a patient with arthritis who may have neuromuscular complications it is necessary to complete a preliminary general examination to seek evidence of anemia, cardiopulmonary disease, an endocrine disorder, malignancy, chronic infectious disease or depression. Each of these may cause weakness, wasting, pain, stiffness, fatigue or other symptoms suggestive of neuromuscular disease. Where the cause of arthritis has not been established, it is necessary to search for clues such as rash, vasculitis, calcinosis, lymphadenopathy and sicca manifestations, which might facilitate making the primary diagnosis. It is necessary to search for nonmuscular signs of primary muscle disease, such as premature baldness or cataracts in myotonic dystrophy.

Joints

When assessing neuromuscular features in a patient with arthritis it is necessary to establish the pattern, extent and severity of joint involvement. Articular pain and limitation may contribute to adjacent muscle wasting and weakness. Similarly, joint deformity or contracture complicates assessment of muscle tone and power, tendon reflexes and plantar responses. It may not be possible to measure muscle power accurately in actively inflamed joints. Apparent muscle weakness may recover when joint inflammation resolves. Involvement of lower limb joints may interfere with normal gait and erroneously suggest a neuromuscular disease.

Muscles

Muscles should be examined for evidence of wasting or hypertrophy, abnormal movement, flaccidity or spasticity, weakness and tenderness. In the inflammatory myopathies muscle bulk is usually normal. Wasting is seen only in unresponsive or advanced cases. Proximal limb girdle weakness may be profound and tenderness is common during active inflammatory stages. Proximal limb girdle weakness is also encountered in metabolic and endocrine myopathies, corticosteroid myopathy and some forms of muscular dystrophy. Weakness is usually most profound in the deltoids and hip flexors. Proximal weakness can also be demonstrated in the neck flexors and abdominal muscles. Thus, the patient has difficulty raising the head from the supine position against resistance and may be unable to sit upright without using the arms. Localized wasting suggests a regional nerve lesion. Predominantly distal muscle wasting and weakness suggests peripheral neuropathy or motor neuron disease. Increased muscle tone suggests an upper motor neuron lesion. Hypertrophy of calf muscles appears early in the course of Duchenne's dystrophy. This is followed by pseudohypertrophy as the muscles are replaced by fat. Atrophy occurs in the later stages. Fasciculation is an important clue in the diagnosis of motor neuron disease. Tenderness may be present in infectious myopathies. Tenderness, but without weakness, may be present in fibromyalgia, muscle strain and spasm. Progressive muscle weakness with continued use, or fatiguability, is characteristic of myasthenia gravis. The muscle weakness may be reversed within one minute of giving an intravenous injection of edrophonium chloride. In addition to the limb and trunk muscles it is important to examine facial muscles and expression. Facial asymmetry, ptosis and muscle weakness and the appearance of the tongue may give important clues to diagnosis.

A standard semiquantitative scale of muscle strength is the Medical Research Council's grading system: 0, no contraction; 1, flicker; 2, muscle contraction possible only after elimination of gravity; 3, muscle contraction against gravity; 4, decreased power, but muscle contraction against resistance possible; 5, normal.

Peripheral nervous system

A systematic examination of the peripheral nervous system requires a thorough knowledge of the anatomy of the cranial and peripheral nerves and of the autonomic nervous system. Disorders of the cranial nerves, particularly ophthalmoplegias and involvement of V and VII, are well recognized complications of SLE, systemic sclerosis, mixed connective tissue disease and Sjögren's syndrome. Disorders of the peripheral motor and sensory nerves will cause muscle wasting, flaccidity and weakness, reduction or absence of deep tendon reflexes and impaired sensation which will depend on the extent and distribution of nerve involvement. Excellent guidelines for the examination of the peripheral nerves have been published by the Medical Research Council[2].

The autonomic nervous system may be selectively involved in some peripheral neuropathies such as familial amyloid neuropathy. Sympathetic vasomotor function is usually tested by studying changes in heart rate and blood flow that occur when the autonomic nervous system is stimulated either directly or indirectly. The Valsalva maneuver with monitoring of blood pressure and heart rate is particularly useful. Monitoring blood presure following other stimuli such as cold water immersion of a limb, emotion and sustained hand grip also provide a means of measuring sympathetic outflow.

LABORATORY ASSESSMENT

Screening tests

The approach to the laboratory investigation of patients with neuromuscular symptoms depends on what physical signs have been demonstrated and on whether the patient has a known or suspected primary rheumatic

DRUGS THAT MAY CAUSE NEUROMUSCULAR COMPLICATIONS
Affecting peripheral nerves
Nonsteroidal anti-inflammatory drugs
Colchicine
Chloroquine, hydroxychloroquine
Gold salts
D-Penicillamine
Affecting muscle
Nonsteroidal anti-inflammatory drugs
Colchicine
Chloroquine, hydroxychloroquine
Gold salts
D-Penicillamine
Cyclosporin
Corticosteroids
Affecting neuromuscular junctions
D-Penicillamine

Fig. 4.2 Drugs prescribed by rheumatologists that may cause neuromuscular complications.

CAUSES OF ELEVATED SERUM CREATINE PHOSPHOKINASE LEVEL
Inflammatory myopathy
Muscular dystrophy
Motor neuron disease
Metabolic myopathies
Hypokalemic periodic paralysis
Parasitic infestations
Drug-induced myopathy
Alcoholic myopathy
Hypothyroidism
Intramuscular injection
Crush injury
Myocardial infarction
Strenuous exercise

Fig. 4.3 Causes of elevated serum creatine phosphokinase level.

or connective tissue disease. A direct explanation for neuromuscular symptoms may be immediately evident. Thus, screening tests of neuromuscular manifestations are directed towards assessing the activity and extent of the primary disease. Where neuromuscular features cannot be attributed directly to a primary rheumatologic disorder, the choice of screening test is dependent on the presence or absence of objective weakness. In the absence of objective weakness, screening tests should include full blood count and eosinophil count, erythrocyte sedimentation rate or C-reactive protein, liver function tests, electrolytes, renal function tests, chest radiographs, pulmonary function tests, electrocardiograph and thyroid function tests, in order to identify evidence of anemia, chronic liver, renal, hepatic or cardiopulmonary disease, malignancy, chronic inflammation, infection or thyroid disease. If abnormal results cannot be easily explained, a more systematic search for the precise diagnosis is necessary. Occasionally, an inflammatory myopathy may present in the absence of objective muscle weakness. Thus, serum creatine phosphokinase (CPK) measurement should be included among the screening tests.

If objective weakness, or elevated muscle enzymes, is demonstrated, more specific tests of neuromuscular function are usually indicated.

Specific tests

Elevated serum levels of CPK and other muscle enzymes such as aldolase, lactic dehydrogenase and aspartate aminotransferase are suggestive of, but not specific for, an inflammatory myopathy. Elevated levels may also be found in other disorders, listed in Figure 4.3. Serial measurements of muscle enzyme levels are important in assessing the response to treatment in inflammatory myopathy.

In the presence of an inflammatory myopathy, serologic tests such as those for various antinuclear antibodies and complement levels provide evidence of an associated connective tissue disease. Measurements of cryoglobulins, antineutrophil cytoplasmic antibodies (ANCA) and hepatitis surface B antigen are required in patients with suggested vasculitis. Positive antiacetylcholine receptor antibody tests are usually present in myasthenia gravis. Serum calcium, phosphate, vitamin D and parathyroid hormone levels are necessary when osteomalacia or hyperparathyroidism are the suspected causes of weakness.

Electromyography and nerve conduction studies

Electrophysiologic assessment of neuromuscular function has become highly sophisticated and requires considerable expertise and experience. Electrophysiologic studies can confirm the presence of and more precisely localize a neuromuscular lesion. Neuropathic and myopathic patterns can be identified. Peripheral nerve and spinal root lesions can be distinguished and entrapment neuropathies localized.The classic electromyographic appearance of an inflammatory myopathy includes a marked increase in electrical activity as the needle is inserted into resting muscle. Weak muscle contraction elicits a motor unit action potential that is more polyphasic and of lower amplitude and shorter duration than normal (Fig. 4.4). The electromyographic appearance of a neuropathic disorder includes characteristic positive sharp waves or fibrillation potentials at rest (Fig. 4.5). Weak muscle contraction elicits motor unit action potentials which are polyphasic and of larger amplitude and longer duration than normal.

Nerve conduction studies include tests of both motor and sensory function. When testing motor function a stimulus is applied to the relevant peripheral nerve. The velocity of conduction from the application of the stimulus to the initiation of the evoked muscle action potential is measured. The amplitude and duration of the muscle action potential are also measured. Sensory nerve conduction can be measured by applying a stimulus to a digital sensory nerve and measuring the latency and conduction velocity of the sensory nerve action potential. Using these techniques, the characteristics of ischemic or entrapment neuropathies, segmental demyelination, hypertrophic neuropathies and reinnervation may be determined.

Muscle biopsy

Muscle biopsy is the definitive diagnostic test in the evaluation of myopathy[3]. The muscle selected for biopsy should be clinically involved, but not excessively weak. In muscle diseases with a patchy distribution, CT, MR imaging or ultrasonography may facilitate the selection of biopsy material. Muscle samples may be examined after routine staining with hematoxylin and eosin (see Fig. 4.6), or after specific staining to demonstrate the presence or absence of specific muscle enzymes or the abnormal accumulation of lipid or glycogen. Thus, details of muscle fiber necrosis, inflammatory cell infiltration, necrotizing vasculitis and granuloma formation may be characterized and inflammatory metabolic or drug-induced myopathies and other muscle disorders may be identified[4].

Nerve biopsy

A decision to obtain a nerve biopsy should be carefully considered, as this is not a routine procedure. Prior consultation with the neuropathologist is recommended. A sensory nerve biopsy is preferable. The sural nerve in the calf is the most frequently selected. Considerable care is required and crushing the nerve fibers must be avoided. For detailed analysis a portion of the nerve must be prepared in frozen sections and other portions fixed in glutaraldehyde for embedding in epoxy resin and fixed in Susa fixative for paraffin embedding[5]. Nerve biopsy is diagnostic in a few conditions, such as vasculitis, amyloidosis or leprosy. Usually these conditions may be identified by alternative diagnostic methods.

DISEASES ASSOCIATED WITH ARTHRITIS AND MUSCLE WEAKNESS

RHEUMATOID ARTHRITIS

Muscle stiffness and weakness are common in RA. This is usually secondary to articular disease, peripheral or entrapment neuropathy or may be a constitutional effect of systemic chronic inflammatory disease. Wasting of interosseous muscles in the hands, the quadriceps and muscles of the shoulder and pelvic girdle is frequently observed and is usually caused by disuse secondary to local joint disease.

Several patterns of muscle pathology have been described, including type II fiber atrophy and necrosis, vasculitis and perivascular mononuclear cell accumulations[6]. Rheumatoid myositis, characterized by patchy muscle fiber necrosis and mononuclear cell infiltration, has

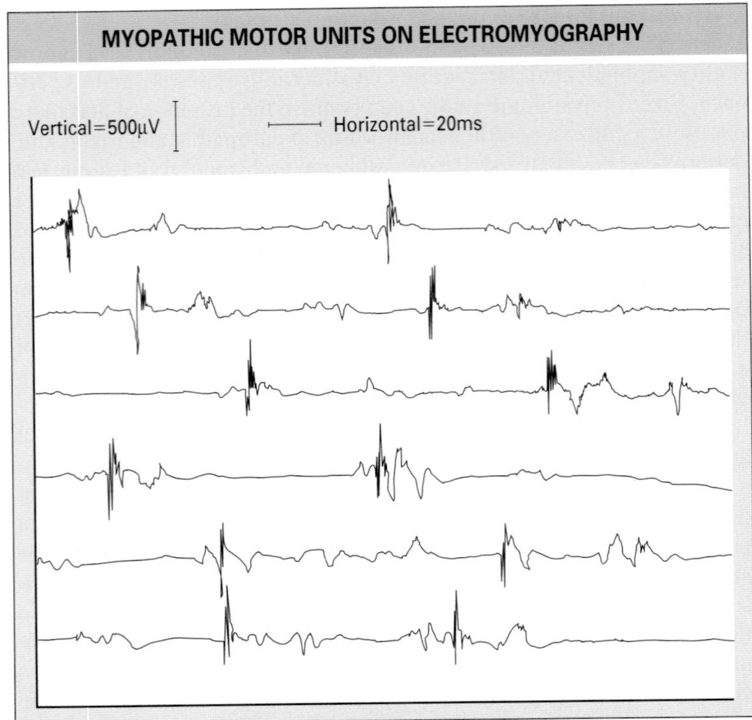

Fig. 4.4 Myopathic motor units on electromyography (EMG). Units are of short duration and low amplitude and are polyphasic. Courtesy of Dr Michael Hutchinson, St Vincent's Hospital, Dublin.

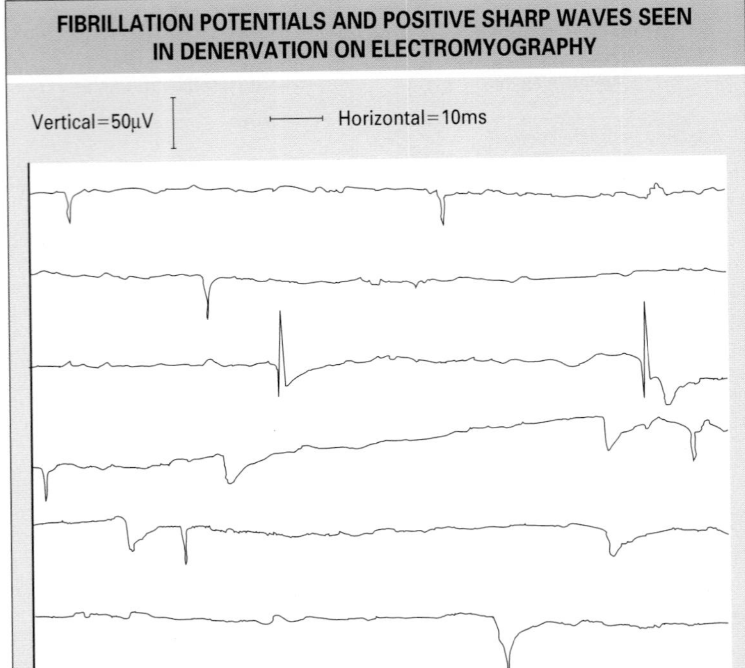

Fig. 4.5 Fibrillation potentials and positive sharp waves seen in denervation on electromyography. Courtesy of Dr Michael Hutchinson, St Vincent's Hospital, Dublin.

been described as a distinct entity occurring in patients with systemic disease or an elevated CPK level[7]. It was noted that muscle tissue samples from patients with rheumatoid myositis exhibited spontaneous synthesis of rheumatoid factor and immunoglobulin, suggesting that local immune events may be important in the pathogenesis.

OTHER CHRONIC ARTHROPATHIES

As in RA, muscle stiffness and weakness may occur in other forms of arthropathy such as the spondyloarthropathies and osteoarthritis. No specific muscle pathology has been described and features of muscle disease are secondary to articular disease or entrapment neuropathy. In ankylosing spondylitis involvement of the cauda equina may occur in the later stages and account for radicular features in the lower limbs[8] (see Chapter 6.20).

POLYMYOSITIS, DERMATOMYOSITIS AND INCLUSION-BODY MYOSITIS

Polymyositis, dermatomyositis and inclusion-body myositis are a heterogeneous group of acquired inflammatory muscle disorders. They have been extensively reviewed recently[9,10] and are considered in Chapters 7.13–7.15. Arthralgia or low-grade arthritis may occur, particularly when there is an associated connective tissue disease such as scleroderma or mixed connective tissue disease. Diagnostic confusion between an inflammatory myopathy and a connective tissue disease should not arise with detailed clinical and serologic assessment.

MYOSITIS IN CONNECTIVE TISSUE DISEASES

Variable myalgia, muscle tenderness and weakness are relatively common in scleroderma, mixed connective tissue disease, SLE and Sjögren's syndrome. In scleroderma, muscle weakness may be caused by diffuse atrophy secondary to progressive cutaneous disease. In some patients with scleroderma proximal muscle weakness is associated with mild elevation of muscle enzymes, polyphasic motor unit potentials of normal amplitude and duration on EMG, and interstitial fibrosis and variation in diameter of muscle fibers, but without inflammation on biopsy. Others present with features resembling polymyositis including very high muscle enzyme concentrations, inflammatory changes on biopsy and polyphasic motor unit potentials of short duration and small amplitude on EMG[11]. Clinical, biochemical and histologic features identical to those of polymyositis have also been well described in mixed connective tissue disease[12]. In SLE and Sjögren's syndrome clinical features of inflammatory myopathy are quite uncommon. In a prospective study of 55 patients with SLE an inflammatory myopathy was noted in 13%, though histologic abnormalities were noted in 87%[13]. Of 104 patients with primary Sjögren's syndrome, only three were found to have biopsy proven myositis[14].

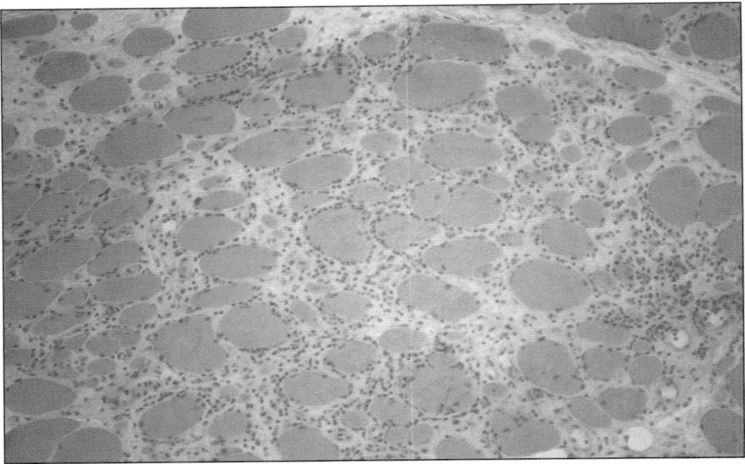

Fig. 4.6 Histologic features. Histologic features of inflammatory muscle disease. Infiltrating mononuclear cells are interspersed between atrophic muscle fibers. By courtesy of Dr Michael Farrell, Beaumont Hospital, Dublin.

BEHÇET'S DISEASE

Mild muscle pain is relatively frequent, but a clinical myopathy is unusual. Subclinical myopathology is purported to be quite common[15]. Focal or diffuse necrotizing myositis with muscle pain and weakness and elevated muscle enzymes has been described[16].

THE EOSINOPHILIA–MYALGIA SYNDROME

A syndrome characterized by marked eosinophilia and severe incapacitating myalgia following ingestion of L-tryptophan was first reported in the USA in 1989[17] (see Chapter 7.34). L-Tryptophan, an essential amino acid, available without prescription, was often recommended in individuals suffering from anxiety, premenstrual tension, fibromyalgia or depression. The severe myalgia usually affects proximal muscles. Muscle weakness, which also involves the proximal muscles predominantly, may be profound.

POLYMYALGIA RHEUMATICA AND GIANT CELL ARTERITIS

Muscle pain and stiffness in proximal limb girdle muscles is characteristic of polymyalgia rheumatica[18] (see Chapter 7.21). In the majority the shoulder girdle is the first to become symptomatic. Muscle strength is usually maintained, but the pain may impede vigorous contraction. In the later stages muscle atrophy may develop and restriction of shoulder movement may be noted. Prominent muscle symptoms may occur in patients with giant cell arteritis. Many complain of profound constitutional fatigue and weakness. Ischemia secondary to arteritis may cause claudication symptoms in the muscles of mastication and swallowing, the tongue or the limbs[19].

SARCOIDOSIS

Sarcoid myopathy is usually asymptomatic (see Chapter 5.26). In acute sarcoidosis with erythema nodosum asymptomatic granulomatous myopathy is common and random muscle biopsy may contribute to establishing the diagnosis. Sarcoid myopathy may also be symptomatic in acute disease and presents with fever, severe muscle pain and tenderness involving proximal limb girdle muscles[20]. The histologic appearances of both asymptomatic and symptomatic sarcoid myopathy, which include noncaseating granulomata, are identical. The immunohistologic features are characteristic with macrophages and $CD4^+$ T-cells diffusely distributed throughout the cellular exudate. $CD8^+$ T-cells are interspersed irregularly within the granulomatous infiltrate during the early phase of granuloma maturation and confined to a lymphocytic mantle surrounding the granuloma in the later stages[21]. A chronic insidious myopathy with muscle wasting and weakness may be associated with chronic persistent multisystem sarcoidosis.

OSTEOMALACIA

Muscle weakness is frequently encountered in patients with osteomalacia. Weakness is predominantly proximal and is occasionally asymmetric. Patients may develop a characteristic waddling gait. Muscle wasting may occur without fasciculation or reflex change. Bone pain and tenderness may be present.

HYPOTHYROIDISM

Patients with hypothyroidism may present with proximal muscle weakness and marked elevation of CPK levels (see Chapter 8.21). However, EMG and muscle biopsy are normal. Muscle weakness resolves after successful treatment with thyroid hormone replacement.

LYME DISEASE

Lyme disease has been associated with polymyositis and dermatomyositis[22]. Lyme myositis may occur early or late in the course of disease and usually resolves after appropriate antibiotic therapy, with or without corticosteroids.

HUMAN IMMUNODEFICIENCY VIRUS (HIV)

HIV-associated myopathies meet the criteria for polymyositis in most patients and resemble HIV-negative polymyositis both clinically and histologically[23].

DISEASES ASSOCIATED WITH ARTHRITIS AND NEUROPATHY

RHEUMATOID ARTHRITIS

A number of distinct forms of neuoropathy occur in RA: entrapment neuropathy, peripheral neuropathy due to vasculitis, amyloid neuropathy and neuropathy due to drugs or coincidental diseases.

Entrapment neuropathy

The two most frequently observed entrapment neuropathies in RA are the carpal and tarsal tunnel syndromes[24] (see Chapter 4.16). Both are the result of synovial thickening occurring in a location where the peripheral nerve passes through a confined anatomic space. Carpal tunnel syndrome may occur early in the course of the disease. The median nerve becomes compressed where it is contained between the carpal bones and the transverse carpal ligament. The median nerve in the hand innervates the thenar muscles and supplies palmar digital nerves to the thumb, index and middle fingers and half the ring finger. The motor fibers innervate the abductor pollicis brevis, the opponens pollicis and the first two lumbricals. Carpal tunnel syndrome usually presents as pain and paresthesia in the wrist and hand, waking the patient at night. Pain frequently extends to the forearm. Paresthesia is usually localized to the median nerve area of the hand, though poor localization of sensory symptoms is not uncommon. Corresponding neurologic deficit may be elicited as weakness of abductor pollicis brevis or opponens pollicis, or as impaired pin-prick or light touch sensation, or as hyperesthesia in the median nerve distribution in the hand. Wasting of the thenar eminence is a late feature. Median nerve irritability may be demonstrated by 1) Tinel's sign, which involves tapping over the palmar aspect of the carpal tunnel, or 2) Phalen's maneuver, which requires flexion of the wrist causing increased pressure within the carpal tunnel (see Chapter 5.16).

The tarsal tunnel along the medial aspect of the ankle and foot contains the tibial nerve; it is formed by the medial mallelous and the flexor retinaculum. As it leaves the tarsal tunnel the tibial nerve divides into medial plantar, lateral plantar and medial calcaneal branches. The medial plantar nerve supplies sensation to the medial surface of the sole of the foot, the medial aspect of the first 3.5 toes and motor supply to abductor hallucis, flexor digitorum brevis, flexor hallucis brevis and the first lumbrical. The lateral plantar provides sensation to the lateral 1.5 toes and sole of the foot and motor supply to the remaining intrinsic muscles of the foot, except for the short extensors. The calcaneal branches innervate the median surface of the calcaneus and the plantar aspect of the heel. The tarsal tunnel syndrome is characterized by burning pain and paresthesia in the toes and sole of the foot, which is usually worse at night. Physical signs include diminished sensation corresponding to the distribution of the nerves, a positive Tinel's sign and pain on pronation of the foot. In advanced cases weakness and atrophy of the intrinsic muscles of the foot may be observed.

Peripheral nerve compression secondary to synovial proliferation may occur very occasionally at other locations such as the elbow joint[25].

Peripheral neuropathy due to vasculitis

A mild distal sensory symmetric polyneuropathy may occur in RA, especially in patients who have long-standing erosive disease, nodules and high titer IgM rheumatoid factor (see Chapter 5.04). The patient usually complains of numbness and burning paresthesia affecting the feet. Upper limb symptoms are less frequent. All sensory modalities may be impaired with diminished pin-prick and light touch sensation observed in a patchy distribution. Sensory impairment may progress gradually in lower and upper limbs, giving a typical glove and stocking distribution. Ocasionally clinically demonstrable peripheral motor loss is also encountered in this form of neuropathy. A less common but potentially more severe form of neuropathy is mononeuritis multiplex. This usually occurs in patients who may be quite ill with more severe rheumatoid disease manifestations and results from asymmetric involvement of multiple individual peripheral nerves. Symptoms of motor impairment usually accompany sensory symptoms. Footdrop is frequently present in mononeuritis multiplex. In some patients neuropathic features appear in the presence of relatively mild joint disease.

Amyloid neuropathy

Peripheral neuropathy due to secondary amyloidosis occurs in a minority of patients (see Chapter 8.27). Patients usually develop a painful polyneuropathy which is predominantly sensory. There may be an associated autonomic neuropathy. Motor loss usually occurs as a late manifestation.

Autonomic neuropathy

Autonomic neuropathy is characterized by an impaired heart-rate response to standing and occurs in up to one-third of patients. Patients with autonomic neuropathy often have coexisting neuropathy suggesting that vasculitis is the underlying pathogenic mechanism. Antonomic neuropathy is usually asymptomatic in RA.

SYSTEMIC LUPUS ERYTHEMATOSUS

Clinical features of peripheral neuropathy occur in less than 10% of SLE patients (see Chapter 7.1). In most, the symptoms are mild, usually affecting the sensory more than the motor nerves. Occasionally mononeuritis multiplex may occur. Cranial neuropathy is probably more common than peripheral neuropathy. Diplopia and facial numbness are the most frequent symptoms. Signs of intermittent ptosis or ophthalmoplegia may accompany other acute manifestations of disease. Additional features of cranial neuropathy encountered in lupus include visual field defects, dysarthria, facial weakness and vertigo.

SCLERODERMA

Cranial neuropathy has been well described in scleroderma, though it occurs uncommonly[26]. An insidious trigeminal sensory neuropathy which may occur bilaterally is the most frequently observed lesion. Unilateral or bilateral facial weakness may also occur. Other cranial nerve disorders are less common. Signs and symptoms of peripheral nerve involvement are rare, although subclinical peripheral neuropathy has been demonstrated in a considerable proportion of patients[27]. Entrapment neuropathy such as carpal tunnel syndrome may rarely occur.

POLYARTERITIS NODOSA AND OTHER FORMS OF VASCULITIS

Peripheral neuropathy occurs in most patients with classic polyarteritis nodosa and the Churg–Strauss syndrome[28] (see Chapter 7.20). Neuropathic features are frequently present as initial manifestations. The onset of symptoms may be sudden, involving a single peripheral nerve and progressing to a mononeuritis multiplex pattern within hours or days. The distribution of pain, paresthesia and sensory and motor deficit depends on the peripheral nerves involved by the vasculitic process. If peripheral nerve involvement progresses, a generalized symmetric polyneuropathy involving all sensory and motor functions may evolve. A slowly progressive distal sensorimotor neuropathy is less common. Cranial neuropathy occurs occasionally. Other forms of systemic vasculitis may also cause peripheral neuropathy. In patients with hypersensitivity vasculitis, including Henoch-Schönlein purpura, mixed cryoglobulinemia, Wegener's granulomatosis and giant cell arteritis, peripheral neuropathy is not frequent.

SARCOIDOSIS

Cranial nerve lesions are the most frequently encountered neuropathic manifestations of sarcoidosis. Cranial nerves II and VII are the most often affected, and bilateral involvement is common.

INFECTIONS

Lyme disease

Lyme disease is caused by the spirochete, *Borrelia burgdorferi*. The clinical presentation and cause of Lyme disease has been fully described[29] (see Chapter 6.5). Migratory musculoskeletal pain is a frequent early manifestation. Articular features, ranging from arthralgia and intermittent arthritis to chronic erosive arthritis, may develop within a few weeks of the onset of the illness. Frank neurologic abnormalities, including facial palsies, motor and sensory radiculopathies and mononeuritis multiplex develop in approximately 15% of patients within several weeks to months. These features are usually associated with a lymphocytic pleocytosis in the cerebrospinal fluid. Typically, neurologic abnormalities persist for months, but may recur or become chronic.

Acquired immune deficiency syndrome (AIDS)

A number of rheumatological disorders have been described in patients with AIDS[30] (see Chapter 6.7). Peripheral neuropathy may also occur and is usually a distal, symmetric, predominantly sensory neuropathy with a glove and stocking distribution. Painful dysesthesia and distal weakness occur.

REFERENCES

1. Walton JN. Clinical examination of the neuromuscular system. In: Watson JN, ed. Disorders of voluntary muscle. Edinburgh: Churchill Livingstone; 1981:448–80.
2. Medical Research Council. Aids to the examination of the peripheral nervous system. Memorandum No. 45. London: Her Majesty's Stationery Office; 1981.
3. O'Rourke KS, Blaivas M, Ike RW. Utility of needle muscle biopsy in a university rheumatology practice. J Rheumatol. 1994;21:413–24.
4. Dubowitz V. Muscle biopsy. A modern approach. London, Ballière Tindall, 1985.
5. Dyck PJ, Thomas PK, Lambert EH, Bunge T, eds. Peripheral neuropathy: Philadelphia, W.B. Saunders; 1984.
6. Reza M, Verity M. Neuromuscular manifestations of rheumatoid arthritis: a clinical and histomorphological analysis. Clin Rheum Dis. 1977;3:565–88.
7. Halla JT, Koopman WJ, Fallahi S, Oh SJ, Gay RE, Schrohenloher RE. Rheumatoid myositis. Clinical and histologic features and possible pathogenesis. Arthritis Rheum. 1984;27:737–43.
8. Russell ML, Gordon DA, Ogryzlo MA. The cauda equina syndrome of ankylosing spondylitis. Ann Int Med. 1973;78:551–4.
9. Dalakas MC. Polymyositis, dermatomyositis and inclusion-body myositis. N Eng J Med. 1991;325:1487–98.
10. Askannas V, Engel WK, Mirabella M. Idiopathic inflammatory myopathies: inclusion-body myositis, polymyositis and dermatomyositis. Curr Opin Rheumatol. 1994;7:448–56.
11. Clements PJ, Furst DE, Campion DS, *et al.* Muscle disease in progressive systemic sclerosis. Diagnostic and therapeutic considerations. Arthritis Rheum. 1978;21:62–71.
12. Oxenhandler R, Hart M, Corman L, Sharp G, Adelstein E. Pathology of skeletal muscle in mixed connective tissue disease. Arthritis Rheum. 1977; 20:985–8.
13. Lim KL, Abdul-Wahab R, Lowe J, Powell RJ. Muscle biopsy abnormalities in systemic lupus erythematosus: correlation with clinical and laboratory parameters. Ann Rheum Dis. 1994;53:178–82.
14. Kraus A, Cifuentes M. Villa AR, Jakez J, Reyes E, Alancon-Segovia D. Myositis in primary Sjögren's syndrome: report of 3 cases. J Rheumatol. 1994;21:649–53.
15. Afifi AK, Frayha RA, Bahuth NB, Tekian A. The myopathology of Behçet's disease. A histochemical, light-, and electron-microscopic study. J Neurol Sci. 1980;48:333–42.
16. Arkin CR, Rothschild BM, Florendo NT, Popoff N. Behçet syndrome with myositis. A case report with pathologic findings. Arthritis Rheum. 1980;23:600–4.
17. Shulman LE. The eosinophilia-myalgia syndrome associated with ingestion of L-tryptophan. Arthritis Rheum. 1991;33:913–7.
18. Cohen M, Ginsburg WW. Polymyalgia rheumatica. Rheum Dis Clin North Am. 1990;16:325–39.
19. Calamia KT, Hunder GG. Clinical manifestations of giant cell arteritis. Clin Rheum Dis. 1980;6:389–403.
20. Douglas AC, Macleod JG, Matthews JD. Symptomatic sarcoidosis of skeletal muscle. J Neurol Neurosurg Psychiatr. 1973;36:1034–40.
21. Tews DS, Pongratz DE. Immunohistological analysis of sarcoid myopathy. J Neurol Neurosurg Psychiatr. 1995;59:322–5.
22. Horowitz HW, Sanghera K, Goldberg N, *et al.* Dermatomyositis associated with lyme disease: case report and review of lyme myositis. Clin Infect Dis. 1994;18:166–71.
23. Illa I, Nath A, Dalakas M. Immunocytochemical and virological characteristics of HIV-associated inflammatory myopathies: similarities with seronegative polymyositis. Ann Neurol. 1991;29:474–81.
24. Nakano KK. The entrapment neuropathies of rheumatoid arthritis. Orthop Clin North Am 1975;6:837–60.
25. Fernandes L, Goodwill CJ, Grivatsa SR. Synovial rupture of rheumatoid elbow causing radial nerve compression. Br Med J. 1979;2:17–18.
26. Teasdall RD, Frayha RA, Shulman LE. Cranial nerve involvement in systemic sclerosis (scleroderma): a report of 10 cases. Medicine (Baltimore). 1980;59:149–59.
27. Schady W, Sheard A, Hassell A, Holt L, Jayson MIV, Klimiuk P. Peripheral nerve dysfunction in scleroderma. Quart J Med. 1991;292:661–5.
28. Moore PM, Fauci AS. Neurologic manifestations of systemic vasculitis. A retrospective and prospective study of the clinicopathologic features and responses to therapy in 25 patients. Am J Med. 1981;71:517–24.
29. Reik L, Steere AC, Bartenhagen NH, Shope RE, Malawista S. Neurologic abnormalities of Lyme disease. Medicine (Baltimore). 1979;58:281–94.
30. Snider WD, Simpson DM, Nielsen S, Gold JWM, Metroka CE, Posner JB. Neurological complications of acquired immune deficiency syndrome. Analysis of 50 patients. Ann Neurol. 1983;14:403–18.

5

SKIN AND RHEUMATIC DISEASE

David L George
& Stephen G Wiener

- Skin lesions often provide valuable diagnostic clues for a number of rheumatic diseases
- The spectrum of dermatoarthropathies ranges from primary immunologic syndromes to infectious, metabolic and neoplastic disorders.
- The principal types of skin lesions seen in patients with arthritis are exanthems papulosquamos rashes, nodules, vesicles and bullae, ulcers, and pupura.

INTRODUCTION

The diagnosis of rheumatic diseases is commonly based on pattern recognition. The skin is the most accessible organ and often provides valuable diagnostic clues that may lead to a specific diagnosis or limit the list of possibilities[1–3]. For example, a diagnosis of psoriatic arthritis might be based upon the presence of distal interphalangeal (DIP) joint synovitis, erythematous scaling plaques over extensor surfaces and nail pitting. Conversely, unrelated skin lesions may occasionally mislead the clinician. For example, incorrect diagnosis of systemic lupus erythematosus (SLE) might be made in a patient with a symmetric polyarthritis who manifests the facial rash of acne rosacea.

Pattern recognition of skin lesions is based upon the type (Fig. 5.1), configuration, distribution and evolution of the lesions. Selective laboratory techniques may further assist diagnosis. This chapter focuses on the cutaneous diseases most relevant in patients with rheumatic complaints (Fig. 5.2) and emphasizes characteristic features that will allow the physician to distinguish those cutaneous lesions commonly associated with musculoskeletal syndromes from entities with which they are often confused.

IMPORTANT DERMATOLOGIC TERMS	
Macule	Flat lesion differentiated from surrounding skin by its color
Papule/nodule	Raised solid lesion less than/greater than 1cm in diameter, respectively
Vesicle/bulla	Raised fluid filled lesion less than/greater than 0.5cm, respectively
Pustule	Vesicle filled with purulent exudate
Wheal (urticaria)	Pale erythematous papule or plaque resulting from upper dermal edema.
Ulcer	Lesion resulting from destruction of the epidermis and at least the upper dermis
Petechia/purpura	Intradermal hemorrhage less than/greater than 3mm in diameter, respectively
Desquamation (scaling)	Abnormal shedding or accumulation of the stratum corneum
Sclerosis	Hardening or induration of the skin
Pathergy (Koebnerization)	Induction of skin lesion in location of minor trauma

Fig. 5.1 Important dermatologic terms.

EXANTHEMS

An exanthem is a diffuse rash with fever and systemic symptoms which is usually due to a viral, allergic or primary immunologic illness, but certain bacterial infections must be considered.

TYPES OF CUTANEOUS LESIONS OBSERVED IN RHEUMATIC DISORDERS

Disorder	Lesion type: Macules/ papules	Papulonodular	Vesicular/bullous	Pustular	Ulcerating	Petechia/purpura
Primary immune disease						
Systemic lupus erythematosus	•	•	•		•	•
Scleroderma		•			•	
Dermatomyositis	•	•			•	•
Rheumatoid arthritis		•			•	•
Still's disease	•					
Sjögren's syndrome					•	•
Erythema nodosum		•				
Pyoderma gangrenosum		•		•	•	
Sarcoid	•	•				
Inflammatory bowel disease	•	•	•	•	•	•
Psoriatic arthritis	•			•		
Reiter's syndrome	•			•		
Behçet's syndrome	•	•	•	•	•	•
Multicentric reticulohistiocytosis		•				
Serum sickness	•					•
Neutrophilic dermatoses	•	•	•	•	•	
Kawasaki disease	•		•	•		
Necrotizing venulitis	•	•	•		•	•
Polyarteritis nodosa	•	•			•	•
Wegener's granulomatosus	•	•	•		•	•
Lymphomatoid granulomatosis	•	•			•	
Infections						
Neisserial infections	•	•	•	•		•
Rheumatic fever	•	•				
Subacute bacterial endocarditis		•				•
Hydradenitis suppurativa/ acne conglobata		•		•		
Syphilis	•	•		•	•	
Lyme disease	•		•			
Rickettsial infections	•					•
Viral infections	•		•	•		•
Fungal infections		•			•	
Mycobacterial infections		•			•	
Other conditions						
Diabetes mellitus		•	•		•	
Thyroid disease	•	•				
Hyperlipidema (Type II)		•				
Crystal disease		•				
Neoplasms	•	•			•	•

Fig. 5.2 Types of lesions observed in diseases with rheumatic expression [1–3].

Dermatomyositis, SLE, Lyme disease and rheumatic fever may have characteristic cutaneous lesions in association with acute systemic disease and are discussed later in this chapter. Characteristic exanthems are also seen in Still's disease and Kawasaki disease (Fig. 5.3).

The patient with Still's disease develops discrete pink to salmon colored macules or slightly elevated papules several millimeters in size on the trunk and extremities, although lesions may occur on the face and rarely on the palms and soles[4,5]. The lesions are maximal during episodes of fever and are prominent in areas of minor skin trauma (Koebner's phenomenon). Still's lesions are irregular in shape and have no associated purpura or vesicles. They are asymptomatic or only mildly pruritic. The lesions do not spread, and last only minutes to hours. When the rash recurs, lesions are in new locations. No oral lesions accompany the rash. Such a rash in the presence of quotidian fever, diffuse palpable lymphadenopathy and polyarthritis is diagnostic of Still's disease.

Kawasaki disease presents with a polymorphous rash (morbilliform, scarlatiniform, pustular or erythema-multiforme-like rash), which is notable for early erythema of the palms and soles with desquamation days later, along with scarlet-fever-like oral mucosal changes, including strawberry tongue, dry red fissured lips and conjunctival congestion[6]. The rash is often prominent in the diaper area. Such a rash in the setting of prolonged fever, pronounced lymphadenopathy and polyarthralgias or arthritis in a child would strongly favor the diagnosis of Kawasaki disease.

Bacterial infections with exanthems include acute and chronic meningococcemia. A nonspecific measles-like eruption may antedate the petechial and purpuric lesions of acute meningococcemia. This diagnosis should be considered in a child or young adult who presents with prostration, fever and morbilliform rash. Early polyarthralgia or polyarthritis during the bacteremic phase has been observed, and reactive pauciarthritis may occur days later[7]. Periodic fever, maculopapular skin rash and arthritis may occur with chronic meningococcemia[8]. Lesions are often distributed near involved joints or over areas of pressure. They are variable in appearance but are most often macules or papules that later develop central hemorrhage. Petechiae, pustules and erythema-nodosum-like lesions may also be seen.

Rocky Mountain spotted fever, a rickettsial disease, may have a maculopapular eruption before becoming purpuric. Diagnosis is aided by a characteristic evolution that begins in the distal parts of extremities and spreads centrally. This infection is often associated with arthralgias and myalgias, and rarely with severe muscle weakness, but not generally with arthritis[9,10]. Secondary syphilis should be considered in the sexually active patient with fever and diffuse maculopapular eruption, especially that involving palms and soles[11]. Toxic shock syndrome may express a scarlatiniform eruption similar to that of Kawasaki disease, and also a reactive arthropathy accompanied by fever and hypotension secondary to toxin-producing staphylococcal infection[12]. *Streptobacillus moniliformis* infection manifests a nonspecific diffuse maculopapular eruption with arthritis of large joints that occurs within a few days to 1 week after a bite from an infected rat or ingestion of contaminated rat excretions[13]. Where endemic, leptospirosis should be considered in the patient with unexplained fever, arthralgia and myalgia. Erythematous macules over the tibia are an important diagnostic clue[14].

Viral infections[15] and drug reactions are the illnesses most commonly confused with exanthem-associated primary rheumatic disorders. Some viral rashes have a characteristic pattern and course. Rubella rash classically begins on the face and spreads rapidly to the neck, arms, trunk and legs, and resolves in the same order. The rash is of short duration, only 2–3 days, and arthritis usually develops as the rash fades. Human parvovirus B19 infection (erythema infectiosum) may be associated with a similar rash; the slapped cheek appearance and a lace-like body rash are more common in children than in adults[16]. Hepatitis B virus may commonly be associated with polyarthritis and rash but, in addition to erythematous papules, urticarial lesions are commonly observed. The presence of an enanthema, petechiae or vesicles and localized lymphadenopathy may also suggest a viral illness, although mononucleosis, cytomegalovirus infection and acute human immunodeficiency virus infection[17] may be associated with diffuse lymphadenopathy and diffuse maculopapular rash. Arthralgias rather than frank arthritis are usually seen with these illnesses.

Drug eruptions usually develop almost simultaneously over the entire body, although the intensity may increase with time. The initial appearance may be in the flexure creases before becoming generalized[18]. Fever generally resolves within 3 days of stopping the drug. Erythema multiforme[19] may result from drug allergy or infection. The skin findings are characterized by round erythematous lesions which are symmetrically distributed, involving the palms, soles and oral mucosa. The presence of target lesions is helpful diagnostically (Fig. 5.4). The milder form of the disease, erythema multiforme minor, may be associated with fever and polyarthralgias. High fever and polyarthritis are common in erythema multiforme major (Stevens–Johnson syndrome), and this illness must be distinguished from Kawasaki syndrome. Inspection of the oral mucosa may help in this clinical differential diagnosis[20] (see *Oral Lesions*).

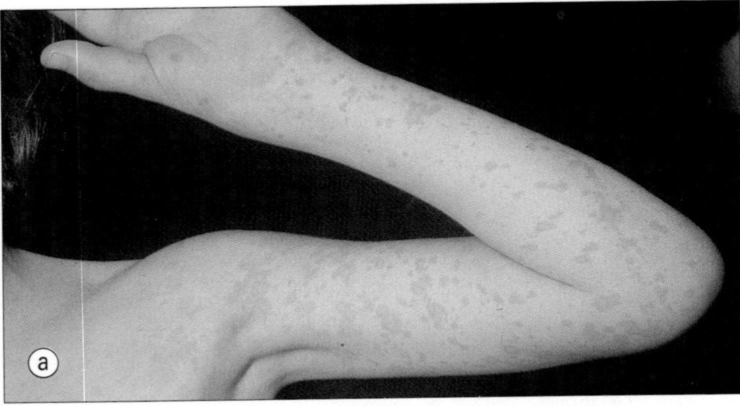

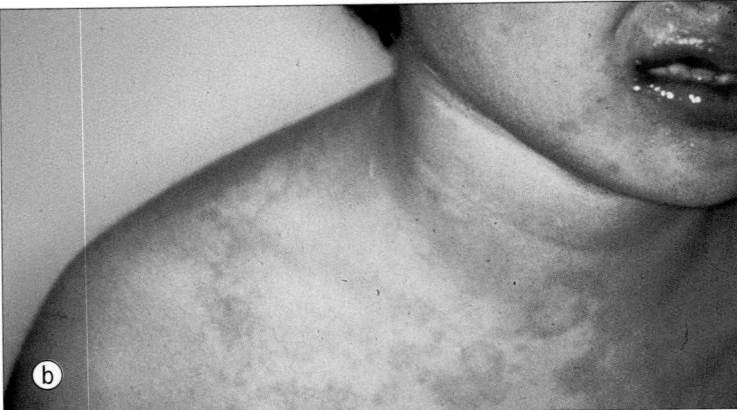

Fig. 5.3 Exanthems: Still's rash (a); Kawasaki syndrome (b). Reproduced from the Revised Clinical Slide Collection on the Rheumatic Diseases, copyright 1981. Used by permission of the American College of Rheumatology.

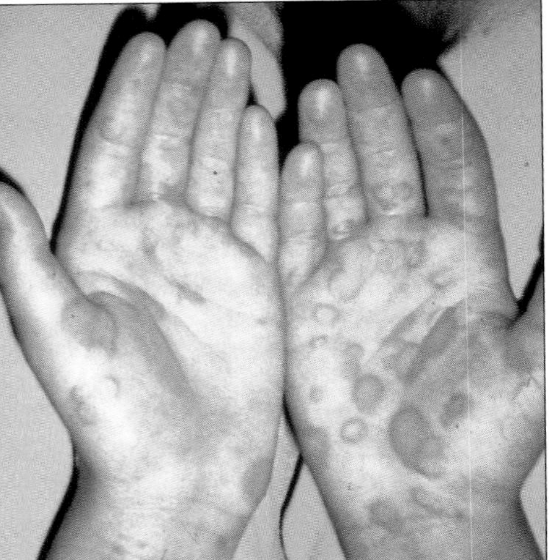

Fig. 5.4 Erythema multiforme.

Other potentially serious drug reactions associated with joint symptoms include hypersensitivity and serum sickness-like reactions[21].

Rare disorders with rash, fever and arthritis include familial Mediterranean fever[22], in which a characteristic erysipelas-like rash may exist on the lower extremity in conjunction with an acute monoarthritis and fever. Angioimmunoblastic lymphadenopathy[23] should be considered in the adult with fever, generalized morbilliform rash, polyarthritis and diffuse lymphadenopathy.

PAPULOSQUAMOUS LESIONS

Rheumatic diseases notable for papulosquamous lesions include psoriatic arthritis, Reiter's syndrome and lupus erythematosus (subacute and discoid). Scale formation in patients with inflammatory cutaneous papules or plaques results from accumulation of the stratum corneum.

The characteristic lesions of psoriasis are sharply demarcated inflammatory plaques with a silvery scale most commonly present on extensor surfaces of the elbows and knees as well as the scalp, ears and presacral area (Fig. 5.5). Nail abnormalities are common. Pustular psoriasis results from a greater collection of neutrophils and therefore differs histologically from usual psoriasis only in a quantitative way[24]. The lesions of keratoderma blennorrhagicum and pustular psoriasis are histologically identical, but Reiter's patients usually have lesions restricted to the palms and soles (Fig. 5.6) and are identified by other clinical characteristics, such as conjunctivitis and urethritis.

Scale formation is also a prominent feature of discoid lupus (Fig. 5.7) and the papulosquamous variety of subacute cutaneous lupus erythematosus (SCLE). In addition to an adherent scale, characteristic features of discoid lesions include follicular plugging, hyper- or hypopigmentation, atrophy (loss of skin markings), sclerosis and telangiectasia. Lesions are most common on the face (but sparing the nasolabial folds), scalp, neck and ears. Lesions may occur elsewhere on the body only if also present above the neck[25]. Lesions of SCLE do not reveal signs of follicular plugging, pigmentary change or scarring and are distributed primarily on the shoulders, the extensor surface of the forearm and the upper back and upper chest. The face and scalp are generally spared and lesions below the waist are very rare. In the papulosquamous form of SCLE, papules may commonly enlarge and coalesce, leading to a reticulate pattern. Histopathologic studies are diagnostic, although immunofluorescence is not routinely positive in SCLE[25].

Lichen planus and pityriasis rosea may be confused with papulosquamous rashes due to rheumatic disease but have features which allow their differentiation. Lichen planus is a pruritic eruption with violet colored, polygonal, flat-topped lesions with thin white scales often present on flexor aspects of the wrists and ankles, the presacral area, glans penis and mucous membranes. Pityriasis rosea is manifested by erythematous papules with thin scaly borders following truncal lines of cleavage (Christmas tree pattern). The initial lesion, or herald spot, is larger than subsequent lesions. Lichen planus may occur secondary to gold or D-penicillamine therapy, and pityriasis rosea may be seen secondary to gold or antimalarial drug therapy[26]. Diffuse papulosquamous lesions and arthralgias may occur in T-cell lymphoma[27] or secondary syphyllis[11].

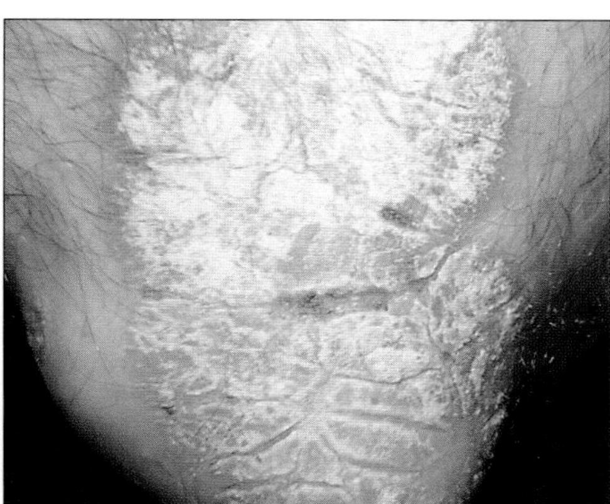

Fig. 5.5 Psoriatic plaque on elbow with characteristic silver scale.

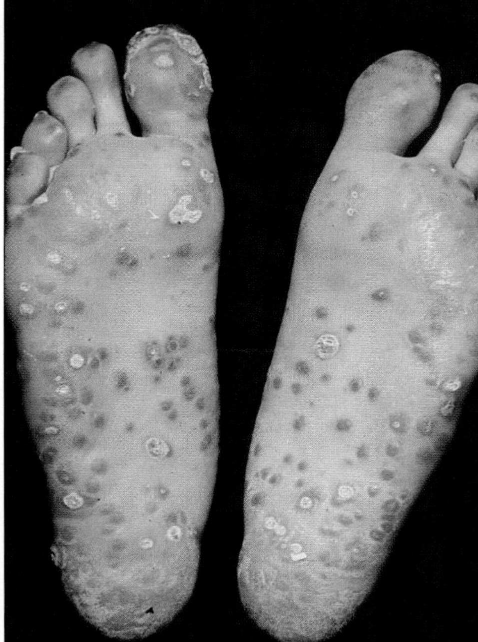

Fig. 5.6 Keratodermia blennorrhagicum on the soles of a patient with Reiter's syndrome.

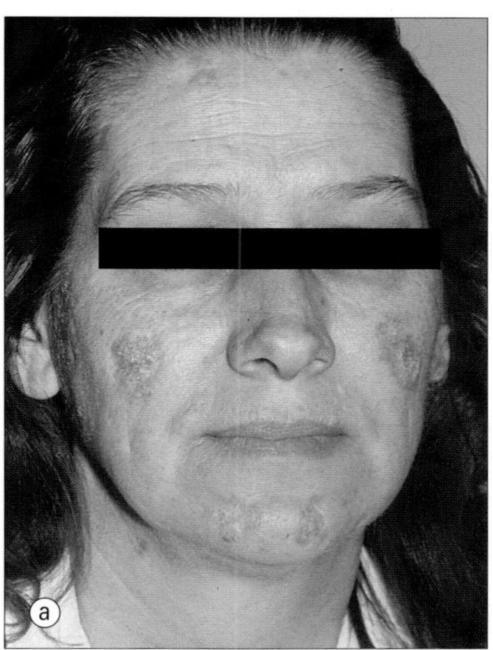

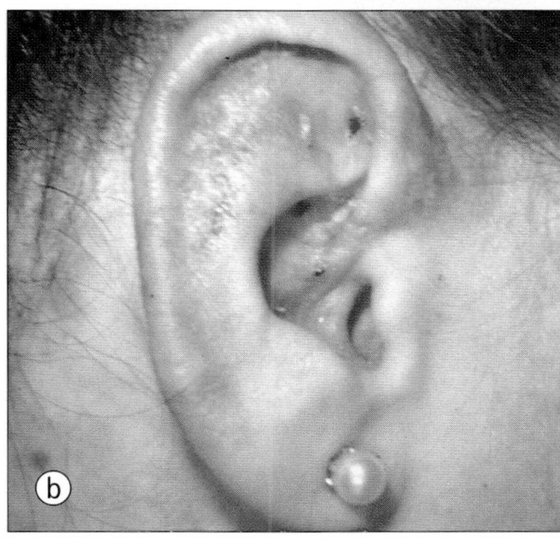

Fig. 5.7 Discoid lupus involving the face (a) and ear (b).

ANNULAR LESIONS

Three rheumatic illnesses, rheumatic fever, SCLE and Lyme disease, are suggested by characteristic annular or arciform skin lesions in which the central portion has a distinctive appearance compared with the border.

In rheumatic fever, migratory polyarthritis may be accompanied by erythema marginatum, an annular eruption with a round or serpiginous border which may be flat or slightly raised and is usually present on the trunk or proximal extremities (Fig. 5.8). Lesions migrate rapidly over a period of hours. The rash typically develops in crops lasting hours to several days[28].

The annular variety of SCLE (Fig. 5.9) is nonmigratory and has the same distribution as the papulosquamous variety. A form of primary cutaneous annular erythema, erythema annulare centrifigum, may occur in association with chloroquine therapy[20].

The primary lesion of erythema migrans (EM), which is nearly pathognomonic of acute Lyme disease[29], is at the site of the tick bite, most often the axillae, groin, thigh or buttocks (Fig. 5.10). The primary lesion migrates outward, much more slowly than that of erythema marginatum, and reaches an average size of 15cm. The central area may reveal blue discoloration, vesicles, purpura, necrosis or ulceration. A target lesion may form. Secondary lesions are smaller, migrate less and have less indurated centers. Erythema migrans spares the palms, soles and oral mucosa and commonly accompanies constitutional symptoms, headache and arthralgias. Recurrent EM may be coincident with pauciarthritis.

Other distinctive annular lesions include elastosis perforans serpiginosa, which is seen as a side effect of D-penicillamine therapy. Annular rashes may be observed in cutaneous granuloma annulare, cutaneous T-cell lymphoma, secondary syphilis, sarcoid, erythema multiforme and psoriasis[30], and the clinical picture and histopathology are distinctive.

FACIAL LESIONS AND PHOTOSENSITIVE SKIN RASH

In a patient with polyarthritis, photosensitive dermatitis involving the face prompts consideration of a diagnosis of SLE and, less commonly, dermatomyositis.

As described above, discoid lupus has a virtually diagnostic appearance and distribution. Facial lesions that mimic discoid lesions[25,31,32,33] are described in Figure 5.11. In addition to the clinical features which may help discriminate these lesions, histopathology and immunofluorescence studies may be required[34]. It should be noted that some immunofluorescent deposits may be found at the dermal–epidermal junction in polymorphous light eruption, Jessner's lymphocytic eruption, seborrheic dermatitis, and acne rosacea (Fig. 5.12), and that early

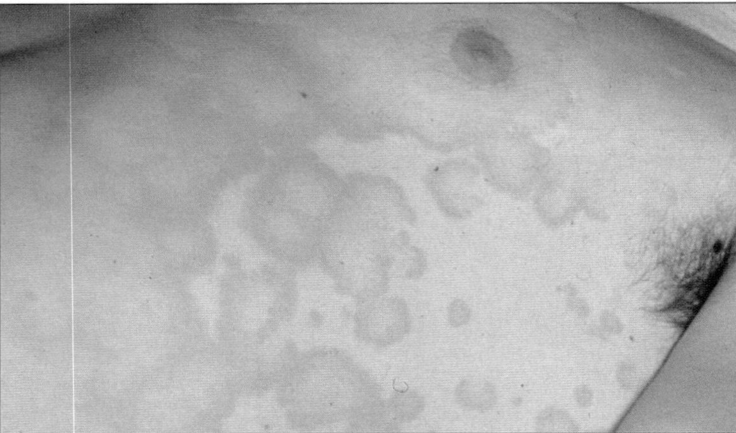

Fig. 5.8 Erythema marginatum. Reproduced from the Revised Clinical Slide Collection on the Rheumatic Diseases, 1981. Used by permission of the American College of Rheumatology.

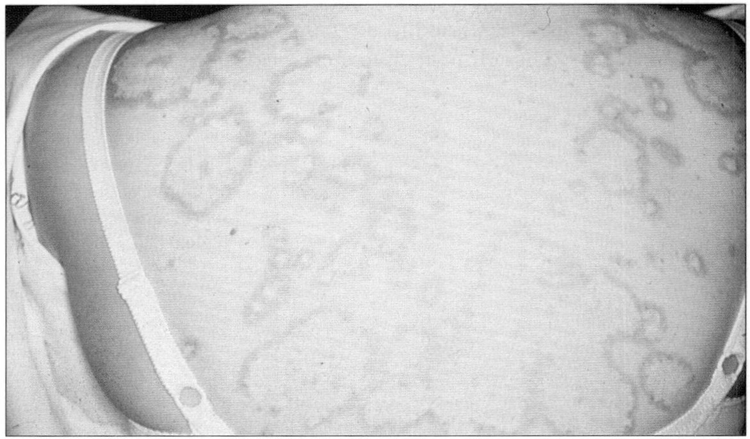

Fig. 5.9 Annular variety of subacute cutaneous lupus. Reproduced, with permission, from Sontheimer RD, *et al.* Ann Int Med. 1982;96:664–71.

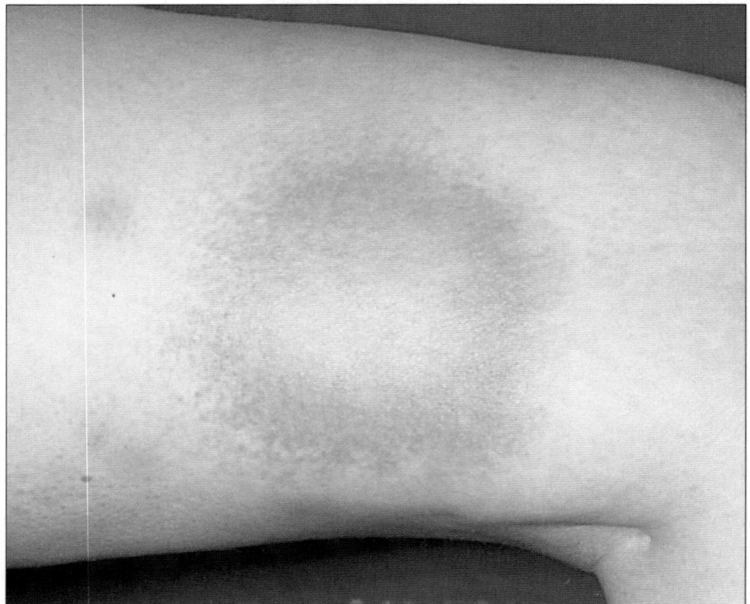

Fig. 5.10 Erythema migrans. This annular, erythematous lesion developed over a preiod of 3 weeks around the site of a tick bite. Reproduced, with permission, from: Pathology of the Skin, 2E McKee PH, London: Mosby Wolfe; 1996.

FACIAL LESIONS – MIMICS OF DISCOID LUPUS	
Diagnosis	Discriminating features
Polymorphous light eruption (occasional)	Large papule/edematous plaque without follicular plugging, scar, or telangiecstases following early season sun exposure
Benign lymphocytic infiltration of Jessner (rare)	Red, slightly raised discoid appearance without follicular plugging or scar
Seborrheic dermatitis (common)	Erythema with yellow greasy scale, involving nasolabial fold, eyebrows and hairline
Acne rosacea (common)	Erythematous papules and plaques involving nasolabial folds; the presence of pustules
Tinea faciei (occasional)	Localized dermatophyte infection; scale present but no follicular plugging; positive fungal scraping; may coexist with discoid lupus lesion
Lupus vulgaris tuberculous (rare)	Solitary papule/nodule slowly extends leaving atrophy and scar but not follicular plugging; smooth yellow–brown (apple jelly) nodules at periphery by diascopy
Lupus pernio sarcoida (rare)	Small nodules on the nose, or nodules/plaques on cheeks and ears; associated with upper respiratory involvement and pulmonary fibrosis

Fig. 5.11 Facial lesions – mimics of discoid lupus.

discoid lesions may lack this finding.

The malar rash of acute lupus is a photosensitive dermatitis which may be flat (malar blush) or raised (butterfly eruption)[35]. There is no atrophy or sclerosis and little scale. Nasolabial folds are not involved. This rash may resolve over hours or it may persist for days. The facial rash of acute lupus may be more widespread than the malar area. The chin is often involved but the area below the chin is spared. A heliotrope eruption similar to that of dermatomyositis may be observed. Features of dermatomyositis rash (Fig. 5.13) that might allow discrimination from lupus include occasional nasolabial fold involvement, prominent heliotrope and extrafacial involvement including erythema over the interphalangeal joints rather than the extensor surface of skin between phalangeal joints (Fig. 5.14), erythema following the course of extensor tendons and scaling and fissuring of lateral aspects of the fingers (mechanic's hands). The presence of papules with erythema over the interphalangeal joints, Gottron's papules, is pathognomonic for dermatomyositis[36].

Misdiagnosis of acute lupus may occur in patients expressing other photosensitive eruptions[37–41] and in those with conditions that produce vascular dilation (Fig. 5.15). Facial lesions of erysipelas (Fig. 5.16) and porphyria cutanea tarda (Fig. 5.17) human parvovirus infection[42] have rarely been confused with the malar rash of lupus. Clinical history and examination are usually sufficient to discriminate these processes, but rarely histopathology and immunofluorescence are indicated.

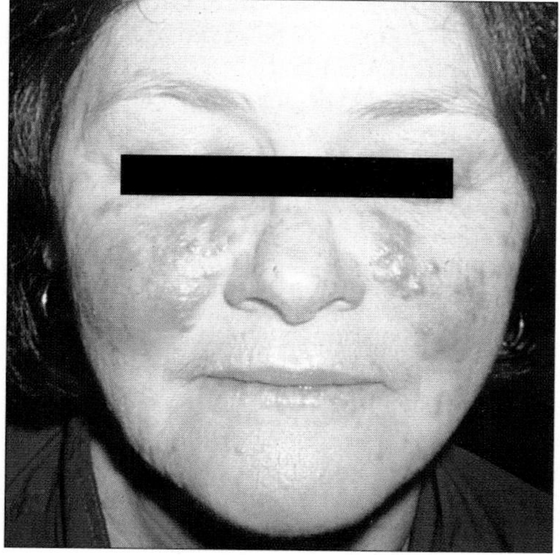

Fig. 5.12 Acne rosacea.

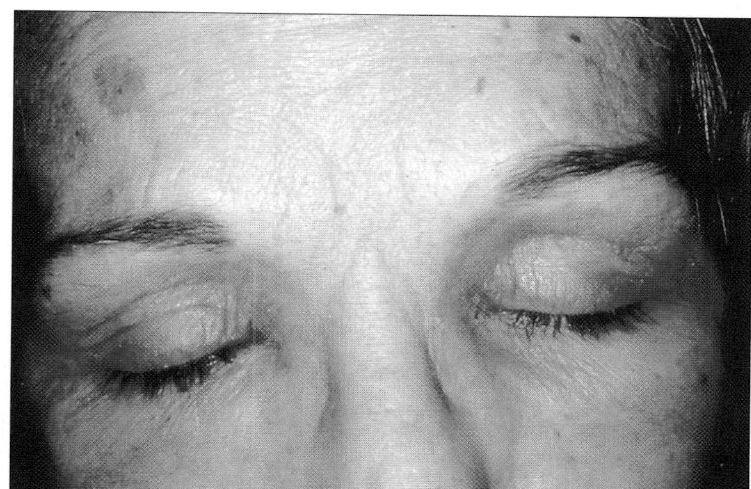

Fig. 5.13 Dermatomyositis. Reproduced, with permission, from the American Academy of Dermatology.

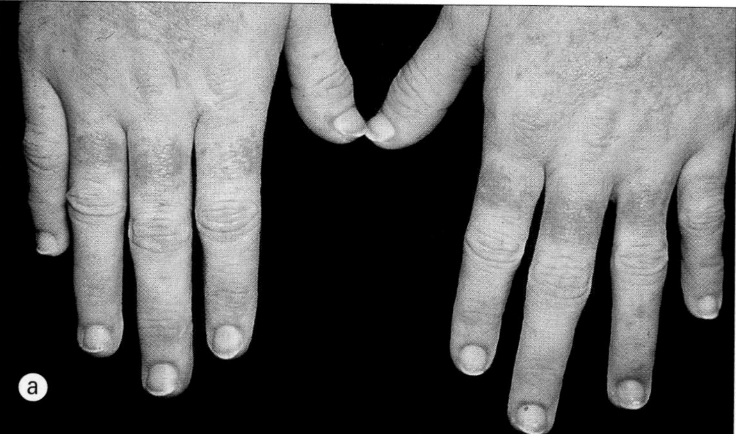

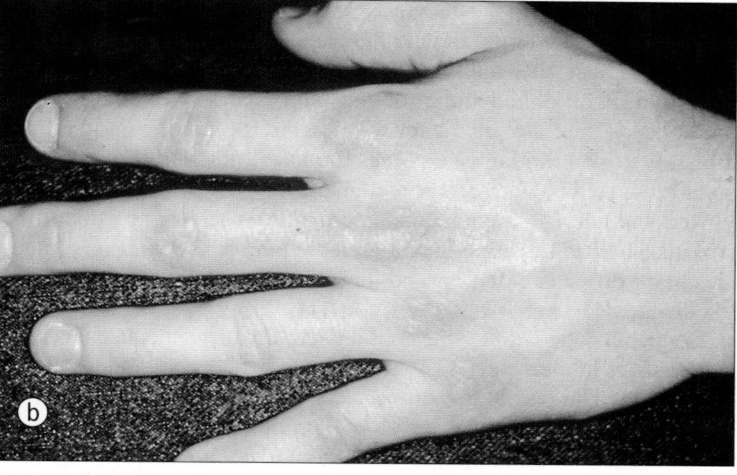

Fig. 5.14 Acute lupus (hand) (a) Reproduced from the Revised Clinical Slide Collection on the Rheumatic Diseases, 1981. Used by permission of the American College of Rheumatology.; **Dermatomyositis (b)** Reproduced, with permission, from the American Academy of Dermatology. All rights reserved.

FACIAL LESIONS – MIMICS OF ACUTE LUPUS	
Diagnosis	Discriminating features
Dermatomyositis• (occasional)	Heliotrope version more common; the rash often involves nasolabial folds; the rash has a distinctive pattern at other body locations
Photoallergic/phototoxic drug reactions• (common)	Clinical history of exposure to drugs including sulfa, thiazides, phenothiazines, tetracycline, piroxicam (phototoxic within days of first exposure), naproxen (porphyria-like)
Polymorphous light eruption• (common)	Small papule/papulovesicle variety; occasionally on face and commonly on forearms, chest or thighs, very pruritic, fewer recurrences with further sun exposure over the season
Porphyria• (rare)	Vesicular/bullous lesions and skin fragility in photosensitive distribution; may coexist with SLE
Pellagra• (rare)	Mucosal erythematous patches and ulcers antedate rash; associated gastrointestinal and psychological disturbances
Early acne rosacea (common)	Malar erythema involving nasolabial folds
Carcinoid (rare)	Episodic flushing, associated with other systemic symptoms including diarrhea
Erysipelas (rare)	Bridge of nose and one or both cheeks involved with raised, rapidly spreading, warm erythematous rash which may later vesiculate and crust in the febrile patient
Parvovirus infections (occasional)	Slapped cheek rash (rare in adults)

Fig. 5.15 Facial lesions – mimics of acute lupus. * Photosensitive processes

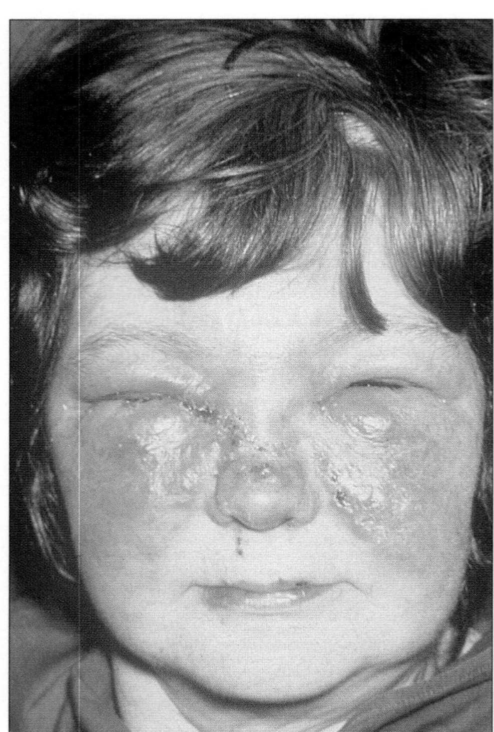

Fig. 5.16 Erysipelas. Reproduced, with permission, from Farrar WE *et al.* Infectious Diseases, 2E. London: Gower; 1991.

URTICARIA

Diseases that might be considered in the setting of urticaria and arthritis include hepatitis B infection[43], serum sickness[44], primary urticarial vasculitis, mononucleosis and C1q complement deficiency[45].

Leukocytoclastic vasculitis is the pathologic process in a small number of patients with urticaria (urticarial vasculitis). Such urticaria is more likely to be associated with symptoms of burning or pain rather than pruritus, tends to resolve more slowly (generally in not less than 4 hours and up to about 72 hours) and may have a purpuric component. Secondary skin changes of pigmentation, scaling or purpura may be found after resolution of the urticaria.

Arthralgias may be observed in chronic urticaria resulting from processes other than leukocytoclastic vasculitis, but arthritis generally suggests underlying vasculitis[46]. The erythrocyte sedimentation rate is nearly always elevated in patients with urticarial vasculitis, and early components of complement are depressed in about 50% of cases of primary urticarial vasculitis[47].

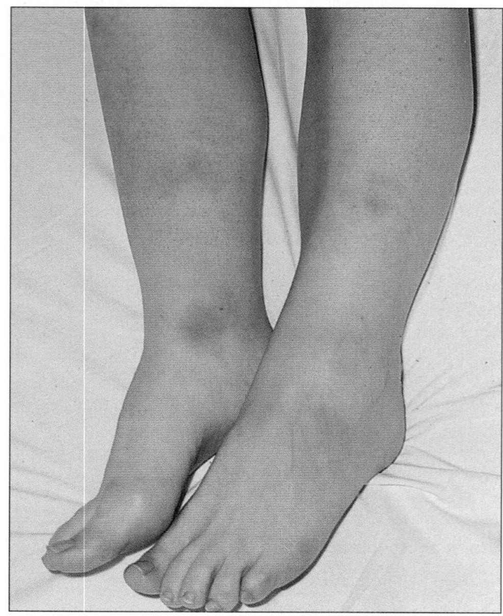

Fig. 5.17 Erythema nodosum – tender subcutaneous nodules on the lower legs. By permission of St Mary's Hospital Medical School, London.

NODULAR LESIONS

The character and distribution of cutaneous and subcutaneous nodules are critical in the evaluation of patients with diseases such as rheumatoid arthritis (RA), rheumatic fever, crystal deposition diseases, atypical infections, panniculitis, vasculitis and malignancy. Rheumatoid nodules[48] are firm, nontender, flesh colored subcutaneous lesions about 0.5–4cm in diameter which may be movable or fixed to periosteum or deep fascia. They are observed most commonly over areas of pressure and are found in about 20% of patients with RA and a small fraction of lupus patients[49]. Nearly all of these patients are observed to be serologically positive for rheumatoid factor.

Rheumatoid nodules may be pathologically indistinguishable from necrobiosis lipoidica diabeticorum (NLD) or granuloma annulare (GA), but these disorders do not present a problem of clinical differential diagnosis since NLD is most commonly observed as a pretibial subcutaneous nodule in the diabetic patient and GA is usually intracutaneous rather than subcutaneous. However, generalized GA is more commonly seen in patients with RA and lupus[50].

Rheumatic-fever-associated nodules are also firm, nontender lesions in areas of pressure but tend to be smaller, usually less than 1cm[49], and shorter-lived (the average duration is 4–6 days, and the lesions rarely last longer than 1 month). Rheumatic nodules at the elbow tend to occur at the point of the olecranon, rather than several centimeters distal as with rheumatoid nodules. Rheumatic nodules are rare. When they occur the nodules tend to form in crops late in the course of the illness in patients who also manifest signs of carditis.

Tophi secondary to uric acid deposits may produce subcutaneous nodules with a distribution similar to those of rheumatoid nodules. Helpful discriminating features include asymmetry, DIP joint involvement, involvement of the helix of the ear, origin at the joint margin rather than adjacent tissue, yellow appearance, overlying erythema, history of recurrent monoarthritis, asymmetric joint involvement and absence of a positive rheumatoid factor. Such signs should prompt joint aspiration and possible nodule biopsy to define the histopathology. A portion of the pathologic specimen should be placed in ethanol rather than formaldehyde to prevent dissolution of monosodium urate crystals.

Periarticular deposits of calcium crystals (pyrophosphate dihydrate, hydroxyapatite and oxalate) may rarely produce subcutaneous nodules and inflammatory or mechanical joint symptoms[51–53]. In oxalosis, miliary intradermal papules of calcium are more characteristic than nodule formation.

Achilles tendonitis in association with subcutaneous nodules of cholesterol at the tendon may be observed in the homozygous and heterozygous forms of type II hyperlipoproteinemia. In the homozygous state patients may also develop subcutaneous nodules over extensor surfaces of the knees and elbows and a migratory polyarthritis of large joints[49].

Multicentric reticulohistiocytosis[54] is a rare disorder associated with a destructive polyarthritis and multiple nodules. These nodules are usually cutaneous rather than subcutaneous, light copper to red–brown and often involve the hands, forearm and face. Periungual lesions, 'coral beads', are also characteristic. Unlike RA, multicentric reticulohistiocytosis commonly involves the DIP joint. This entity is frequently associated with occult malignancy.

Red and tender subcutaneous nodules may occur in panniculitis, arteritis, atypical infections and metastatic tumor. The location of nodules, their propensity to scar and their histopathology assist differential diagnosis[3,55,56].

Erythema nodosum (EN) lesions are red or violet subcutaneous nodules, 1–5cm in diameter, without associated epidermal abnormalities (Fig. 5.18). The pathology shows a septal panniculitis without vasculitis. Usually EN nodules develop in pretibial locations and resolve spontaneously over several weeks without ulceration or scarring. The lesions may develop less frequently on the thighs, arms, face, neck and trunk[56]. Whether idiopathic or associated with a known precipitant, EN lesions are often accompanied by acute polyarthralgias or arthritis

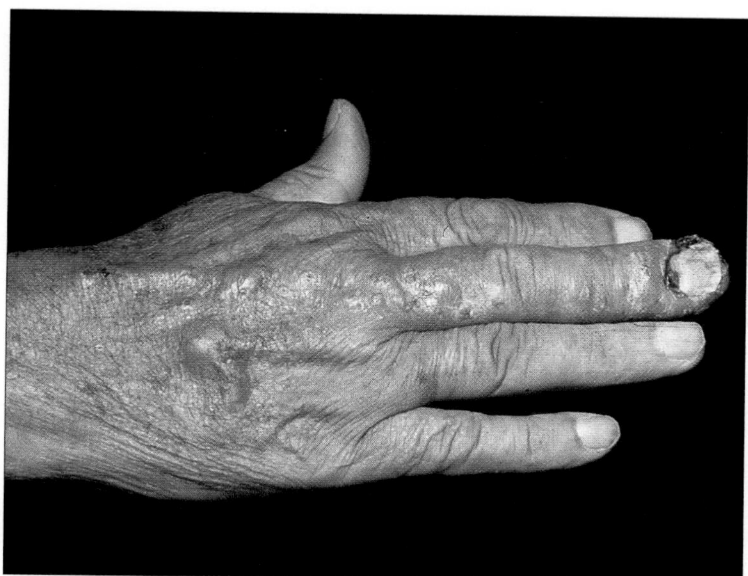

Fig. 5.18 Sporotrichosis. Several secondary nodules are apparent along lymphatic channels. Courtesy of Dr TF Sellers Jr.

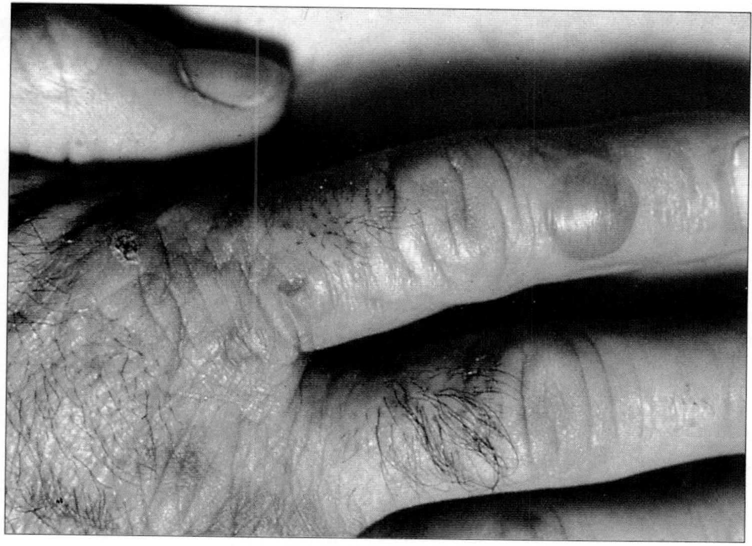

Fig. 5.19 Porphyria cutanea tarda.

predominantly in large joints of the lower extremities. A diagnosis of EN should prompt consideration of primary immune processes, for example sarcoidosis (Lofgren's syndrome), or inflammatory bowel disease, Behçet's syndrome, the effects of drugs (sulfa, birth control pills), pregnancy and infections (post-β hemolytic streptococcus, *Mycobacterium tuberculosis or M. leprae*, fungus, *Yersinia, Chlamydia*, etc.)

Erythematous subcutaneous nodules that are unusually painful, develop in locations other than the pretibial region, ulcerate or scar, persist for more than several weeks, or are not in association with the above diseases, may be expressions of a different pathologic entity. Weber–Christian disease is an idiopathic lobular panniculitis with fever, polyarthralgias and painful subcutaneous nodules more widespread than in EN and which often ulcerate or scar (secondary to fat necrosis). Panniculitis with pancreatitis or pancreatic carcinoma may manifest similar skin lesions and polyarthritis. Serum lipase levels are often elevated. Excisional biopsy will reveal a lobular panniculitis often with characteristic 'ghost-like' fat cells, presumed to be due to the enzyme effects upon the adipose cell.

Lupus profundus is a lobular panniculitis found on the face, upper arms or buttocks. Overlying cutaneous involvement with discoid lesions is common. The lupus band test in the overlying skin is positive in about 70% of cases[56]. This entity usually follows a chronic course associated with local scarring.

Diffuse granulomas in the subcutaneous tissue may also produce lobular panniculitis in sarcoidosis, although the septal panniculitis of EN is a much more common expression[57].

Erythema induratum (nodular panniculitis) is a lobular panniculitis with local vasculitis which may be idiopathic or associated with tuberculosis. Unlike EN nodules, the nodules of erythema induratum are commonly on the calf and tend to ulcerate[56]. Erythema nodosum leprosum lesions tend to be more widespread, and upper extremity joint involvement is seen more often than in primary EN[58].

Necrotizing arteritis such as polyarteritis nodosa and Wegener's granulomatosis may be associated with painful cutaneous and subcutaneous nodules. These lesions tend to be smaller than those of EN. They develop in crops and are found most commonly on the lower legs and feet, especially along the course of arteries, although they may have a widespread distribution. Other skin lesions, such as purpura and livedo reticularis, may also be present[3,59].

Polyarthralgias may accompany erythema elevatum diutinum, nodular skin lesions secondary to leukocytoclastic vasculitis. These vasculitic lesions have a predilection for extensor surfaces of joints as well as skin overlying the buttocks and Achilles' tendons[60].

Nodules adjacent to an inflammatory joint or tendon sheath should prompt consideration of local infections, such as sporotrichosis (Fig. 5.18), atypical mycobacterial infection and treponemal infections[49,61]. Ulceration develops frequently.

Cutaneous and subcutaneous nodules may also result from infiltration of metastatic tumor cells. When there are multiple nodules, hematologic malignancies are most common[27].

VESICLES AND BULLAE

Vesicles and bullae result from a disturbance of intraepidermal coherence or dermal–epidermal adherence[59]. A host of pathologic mechanisms may lead to blistering of the skin. Two blistering eruptions are seen in SLE. First, a generalized bullous eruption may develop in normal appearing or erythematous skin (bullous eruption of SLE). This eruption is bullous pemphigoid like and has histologic similarities to dermatitis herpetiformis: it may be dapsone responsive. Unlike dermatitis herpetiformis, it is not pruritic and is more widespread. Immunofluorescence and electron microscopic studies may be helpful diagnostically[62,63]. Second, blistering may be seen in areas of photosensitive dermatitis. Such lesions must be distinguished from the rash of porphyria cutanea tarda, which is seen occasionally in the lupus patient (Fig 5.19)[64].

Some primary immune skin disorders have been described at increased frequency in a number of rheumatic diseases[64]. Bullous pemphigoid is significantly more common in the rheumatoid patient and has been described in SLE, polymyositis and primary biliary cirrhosis. Dermatitis herpetiformis is commonly associated with autoimmune thyroid disease and has been reported in RA, Sjögren's syndrome, dermatomyositis and ulcerative colitis. Pemphigus has been described in patients with SLE, RA, Sjögren's syndrome and lymphomatoid granulomatosis. Pemphigus foliaceous may result from a D-penicillamine reaction.

Vesicles and bullae may accompany more characteristic lesions in patients with necrotizing vasculitis, ecthyma gangrenosum and disseminated intravascular coagulation (DIC). Blistering may also be a prominent feature in erythema multiforme major, and short-lived bullae may be seen in staphylococcal scalded skin syndrome. Musculoskeletal symptoms may accompany each of these entities.

Localized or generalized vesicles may also be seen in varicella or herpes viral infections. Tzanck test or culture may be helpful[65]. Lesions of EM may vesiculate centrally.

PUSTULAR LESIONS

Pustular skin lesions in patients with rheumatic disease include pustular vasculitis associated with several bowel-associated processes, Sweet's syndrome, Behçet's syndrome, disorders with palmar and plantar pustular skin lesions and disorders associated with severe forms of acne. In addition, disseminated gonococcemia (Fig. 5.20), chronic meningococcemia, disseminated viral infections, such as varicella and disseminated herpes simplex, and reactions to drugs (especially sulfa drugs, hydantoins and halogen compounds) may produce disseminated pustular lesions[65].

A syndrome of cutaneous pustules, fever and polyarthritis is seen in patients with inflammatory bowel disease and those having undergone Billroth II surgery, thus prompting the descriptive term bowel-associated dermatosis–arthritis syndrome[66]. Episodic painful cutaneous pustules on a purpuric base are seen primarily on the upper extremities and upper trunk.

Patients with Sweet's syndrome (acute febrile neutrophilic dermatosis) may also present with painful papulonodules or pustules[67] (Fig. 5.21). Although painful oral and genital ulcers are most characteristic of Behçet's syndrome, pustular skin lesions, especially at sites of minor trauma (e.g. needlestick pathergy), should also lead to its consideration. The arthritis is frequently pauciarticular in these disorders. Histology of pustular skin lesions may be similar in Behçet's syndrome, Sweet's syndrome and bowel-associated dermatitis–arthritis[66].

Isolated palmar and plantar pustulosis, pustular psoriasis and keratoderma blennorrhagicum are identical pathologically. Patients with psoriasis and keratoderma blennorrhagicum may have symptoms of spondyloarthropathy. An association of palmar pustulosis with sternal clavicular hyperostosis and chronic recurrent multifocal osteomyelitis (CRMO) has been described[68].

Severe forms of acne have also been associated with rheumatic illnesses[69]. Acne fulminans has also been associated with sternal clavicular hyperostosis and CRMO. The patients described have usually been young, white males who become acutely ill with fever, weight loss, arthralgias, myalgias and multiple inflammatory skin lesions with ulceration on the back and chest. Acne conglobata and related illnesses exhibit extensive cystic and nodular acne on the buttocks, thighs and upper arms as well as the conventional locations of acne vulgaris. Some of these patients, most notably young black males, have a higher frequency of spondyloarthropathy and sternal clavicular hyperostosis. Isotretinoin, a vitamin A derivative used for severe acne, has been associated with mild myalgias and arthralgias which often resolve spontaneously without cessation of therapy, and with axial skeletal hyperostoses.

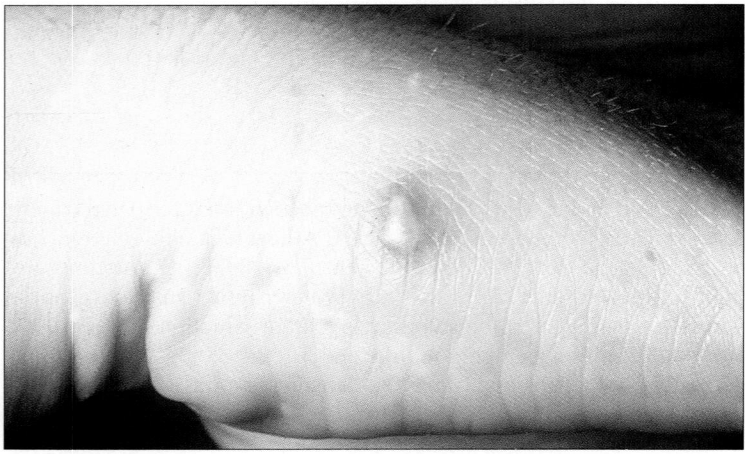

Fig. 5.20 Gonococcemia. Pustules are commonly found on the hands and feet. Reprinted with permission from *Pathology of the Skin 2E*, McKee PH, Mosby-Wolfe 1996 and by courtesy of Dr RN Thin, St Thomas' Hospital, London, UK.

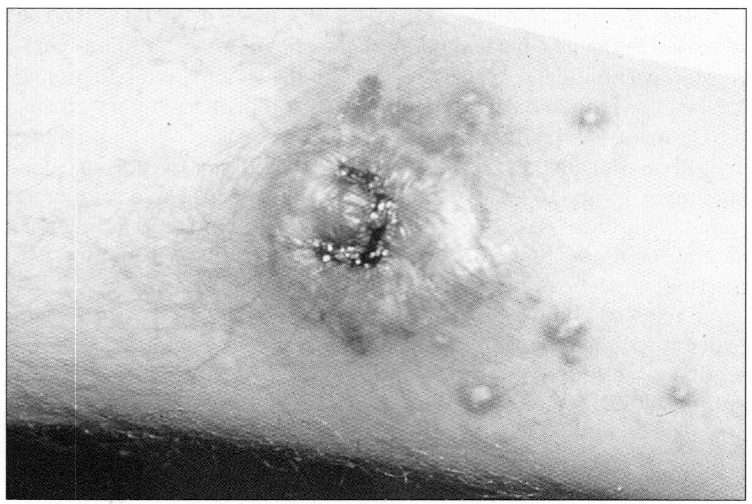

Fig. 5.21 Sweet's syndrome. Erythematous plaque with pustulation and ulceration. Courtesy of Dr Kenneth DeBenedictus.

PURPURA

Purpura, nonblanching erythematous lesions, should be evaluated by size and palpability[70]. Petechiae are characteristic of platelet disorders. They result from leakage of erythrocytes from dermal capillaries where platelet plugs serve as the major source of coagulation. Larger collections of blood form ecchymoses that are due to leakage from arterioles or venules at sites of minor trauma; ecchymoses are also common in platelet and other bleeding disorders. These lesions are not usually palpable unless bleeding occurs into an unrelated inflammatory lesion.

Nonpalpable purpura result from extravasation of erythrocytes in the absence of inflammation. Causes of nonpalpable purpura in the patient with rheumatic complaints include: platelet deficiency states such as immune thrombocytopenia; vascular fragility as observed in primary amyloid, scurvy and genetic disorders of collagen formation; reduced integrity of supportive connective tissue as observed in corticosteroid therapy; and vessel thrombosis or nonseptic emboli such as thrombotic thrombocytopenic purpura, antiphospholipid syndrome, cholesterol emboli and merantic endocarditis[30].

In primary amyloid, vascular fragility results from infiltration of the vessel with amyloid light chain protein. Purpura is most common in the periorbital region, at skin folds and in areas of minor trauma (pinch purpura). Patients may manifest polyarthritis secondary to amyloid infiltration of synovium. In scurvy, altered collagen formation probably contributes to vascular fragility[71] and the lesions are rarely palpable. Perifollicular hemorrhage with central corkscrew hairs on the lower extremities is characteristic. Hemorrhage into muscle or joints may occur. Cholesterol emboli, a consequence of severe atherosclerotic vessel disease, may mimic vasculitis and characteristically involves the lower extremity with purpura, livedo reticularis, nodules and ischemic ulcers[30,72]. Rickettsial and certain viral illnesses (echovirus and coxsackie viral infections) may show petechial lesions in the course of the illness.

PALPABLE PURPURA

Petechiae and flat purpuric lesions are rarely observed in necrotizing angiitis[73] because vascular inflammation leads to increased permeability. Palpable hemorrhage of lesions of the dermis should suggest vasculitis or embolus associated with an infectious agent.

Palpable purpura in dependent locations (areas with increased orthostatic pressure, such as the buttocks or lower extremities) is the most common presentation of necrotizing venulitis (Fig. 5.22). Lesions are round or oval secondary to radial diffusion of erythrocytes from the postcapillary venules of the upper vascular plexus of the dermis[73]. The differential diagnosis includes chronic bacterial infection, acute hepatitis B infection, drug reaction, associated lymphoproliferative disorder, associated rheumatic disease and Henoch–Schönlein purpura (HSP). Biopsy within 24–48 hours helps define the inflammatory nature of the

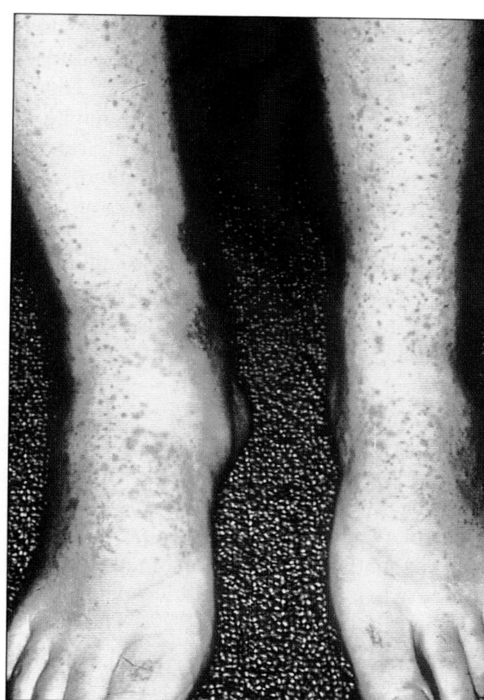

Fig. 5.22 Palpable purpura of necrotizing venulitis.

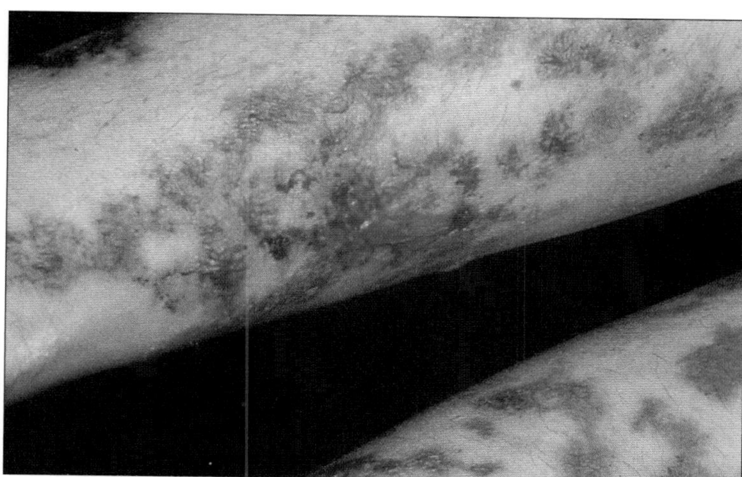

Fig. 5.23 Polyarteritis nodosa with irregular purpura, livedo reticularis and necrosis. Reproduced, with permission from the American Academy of Dermatology.

lesion. The presence of IgA immunofluorescent deposits at the dermal–epidermal junction supports the presence of HSP. In isolated leukocytoclastic vasculitis the prognosis is generally good; nevertheless, necrotizing venulitis may be associated with larger vessel vascultitis and should prompt a careful search for systemic necrotizing arteritis[59,74]. Signs of necrotizing arteritis include irregularly outlined purpura, since inflammation and thrombosis of deep dermal and subcutaneous vessels result in areas of hemorrhage and infarction[73]. Cutaneous nodules, livedo reticularis, digital infarcts and deep cutaneous ulcers (Fig. 5.23) are also seen.

Acute onset of purpuric lesions in the febrile patient is sepsis until otherwise proven[75]. Acute meningococcemia begins as small, irregular, often palpable purpura which are more widely distributed and less symmetric than leukocyclastic vasculitis. The lesions may progress rapidly over hours to extensive bullous and irregular hemorrhagic lesions with central necrotic gunmetal gray patches (Fig. 5.24). The vascular lesions result from direct invasion of the organism as well as being secondary to DIC.

Gram-negative infection may embolize to the skin (ecthyma gangrenosum) and also seed the joint. The skin lesions are erythematous wheals or papules with irregular areas of purpura followed by necrosis and ulceration. The morphology of wheal or papule containing an irregular purpuric area is a specific sign of septicemia with gram-negative organisms including gonococcus, meningococcus, *Klebsiella* spp., *Pseudomonas* spp. and *Escherichia coli*[76].

ULCERS

Vascular, infectious and tumor-associated causes must be considered in the patient with cutaneous ulceration and musculoskeletal symptoms. Ulcerations secondary to ischemia may result from vasospasm in Raynaud's phenomenon, vascular thrombosis in antiphospholipid syndrome or paraproteinemia and vascular necrosis in necrotizing venulitis or arteritis. Other skin findings and associated systemic signs and symptoms differentiate among these causes.

Lower extremity ulcers in the debilitated rheumatoid patient[77–80] present a common diagnostic dilemma. The differential diagnosis includes vasculitis, pyoderma gangrenosum, pressure sores, infection and vascular insufficiency. Pyoderma gangrenosum (Fig. 2.25) is observed more commonly in patients with RA, inflammatory bowel disease, Behçet's syndrome, Wegener's granulomatosis, paraproteinemias or chronic active hepatitis[81].

Pyoderma gangrenosum is a rare ulcerating lesion of unknown cause which begins as a nodule or hemorrhagic pustule that breaks down to form a painful ulcer with an irregular, undermined, raised violaceous border. The lesion is usually single and is most commonly observed in the lower extremities, buttock or abdomen. Such lesions often develop at sites of previous minor trauma. Pathologic specimens may be suggestive of this entity but are not diagnostic. Differential diagnosis of the lesion includes necrotizing arteritis and infectious causes, including atypical mycobacterial or fungal infection, amoebiasis, tropical ulcer and anaerobic bacterial synergistic gangrene (Meleney's ulcer)[30,81].

Rheumatoid vasculitic ulcers classically develop suddenly on the calves or dorsum of the foot[82]. They are multiple, painful, have a 'punched out' appearance and an indurated base, and may enlarge

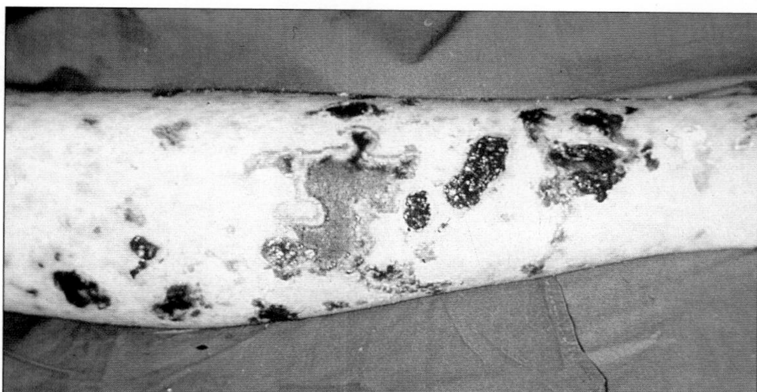

Fig. 5.24 Purpura fulminans with secondary skin necrosis. Reproduced, with permission, from Farrar WE *et al.* Infectious Diseases, 2E, London: Gower; 1991.

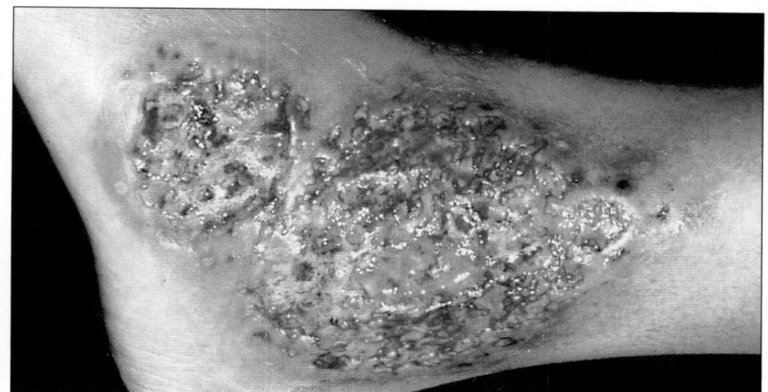

Fig. 5.25 Pyoderma gangrenosum.

rapidly (Fig. 5.26). They are most often seen in patients with long-standing erosive nodular RA, especially those with Felty's syndrome or other signs of vasculitis. Chronic superficial leg or sacral ulcers are also observed in rheumatoid patients with other signs of vasculitis, but these lesions are less specific[82]. Venous stasis ulcers are most common in the ankle area, especially near the medial malleolus, and are painless unless there is secondary infection. These ulcers are shallow and wide and have an irregular outline. They are often surrounded by thick and hyperpigmented skin secondary to the chronic venous insufficiency.

Venous insufficiency ulcers are common in the rheumatoid patient because of reduced skin integrity, increased venous stasis due to inactivity and possibly reduced venous muscle pump activity secondary to reduced ankle mobility[83].

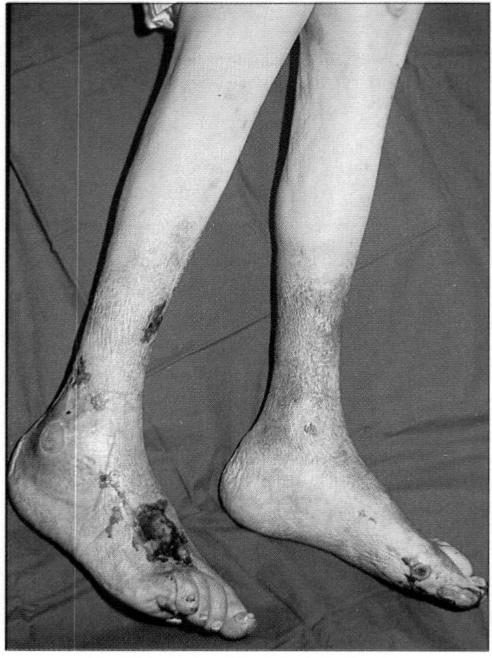

Fig. 5.26 Rheumatoid vasculitic ulceration in various stages of evolution. Reproduced from the Revised Clinical Slide Collection on the Rheumatic Diseases, 1981. Used by permission of the American College of Rheumatology.

MIMICS OF SCLERODERMA	
Disease	Cutaneous expression
Eosinophilic fasciitis	Cutaneous sclerosis of extremities sparing hands and feet often lack Raynaud's phenomenon, nailfold abnormalities and body telangiectases, fascial inflammation on biopsy
Diabetes mellitus	Bound-down skin over hands with joint contractures in the chronic diabetic
Scleredema	Benign skin tightening developing rapidly over the neck and upper back in the noninsulin dependent diabetic
Monoclonal gammopathy POEMS syndrome	Polyneuropathy, organomegaly, endocrinopathy, M protein, and skin changes (POEMS)– skin is thickened and may be hyperpigmented but is not bound down
Primary amyloid	Scleroderma-like skin changes are rare, waxy cutaneous papules are more characteristic
Scleromyxedema	Induration of hands, face, arms (trunk and lower extremities to a lesser degree) with multiple fine waxy papules (may be associated with monoclonal gammopathy)
Carcinoid	Scleroderma-like lesions of lower extremities in association with other carcinoid symptoms
Palmar fasciitis/polyarthritis paraneoplastic syndrome	Bound-down palmar or plantar fascia associated with internal malignancy
Reflex sympathetic dystrophy (late phase)	Tight dystrophic skin of extremity following period of vasomotor instability, altered sympathetic nerve function

Fig. 5.27 Mimics of scleroderma.

Ulcers occur over bony prominences associated with undue pressure. They can become quite deep and are frequently infected in patients with severe peripheral neuropathies. Painful ulceration with pale edges on the toes and dorsum of the foot, or the heel, and poor granulation tissue in a leg with trophic changes and reduced peripheral arterial pulse pressures suggest arterial insufficiency ulcers on an atherosclerotic basis. Vasculitis may reduce the threshold of pressure or atherosclerotic disease that will produce ischemia and ulceration.

Other ulcerating lesions may be of assistance in differentiating various immune diseases. For example, perianal ulcers secondary to cutaneous granulomatous disease may be seen in Crohn's disease[84]. Genital ulcers are often a sign of Behçet's syndrome.

DERMAL SCLEROSIS

Fibrosis of the skin producing visible and palpable thickening is a characteristic feature of scleroderma (see Chapter 7.9). Attention to the appearance, distribution and histopathology of the involved skin can be helpful in distinguishing between patients with scleroderma and those with scleroderma-like abnormalities[85–92] (Fig. 5.27). The distribution of involvement helps to distinguish the limited form of scleroderma [formerly the CREST (calcinosis cutis, Raynaud's phenomenon, esophegeal dysfunction, sclerodactyly and telangiectasai) syndrome] variant from progressive systemic sclerosis. The CREST variant does not generally produce scleroderma of the proximal extremities or of the trunk and has a more benign prognosis.

TELANGIECTASES

Telangiectases result from dilated venules, capillaries and arterioles. Periungual telangiectases and broad lesions called mat telangiectases are important types to identify because of their specificity for scleroderma (Fig. 5.28). Mat telangiectases are broad, oval or polygonal macules 2–7mm in diameter and found on the face, mucous membranes and hands. These lesions are clinically distinguishable from the broad often palpable telangiectases of hereditary hemorrhagic telangiectasia. In this latter disease, telangiectases are actually arteriovenous malformations and are associated with epistaxis and gastrointestinal bleeding (Osler–Rendu–Weber disease)[93].

Linear telangiectases are nonspecific and may be seen in sun damage, acne rosacea, venous hypertension (lower extremities), carcinoid and hypercorticism. When linear telangiectases are present on the face, malar erythema may result which can be confused with a non-raised malar rash of lupus.

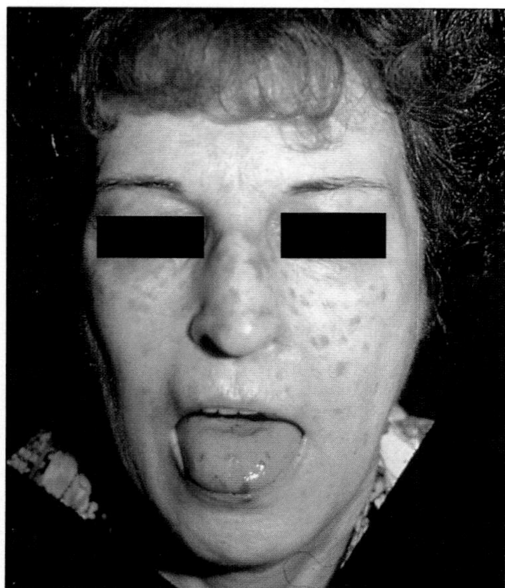

Fig. 5.28 Mat telangiectases in a patient with CREST syndrome. Reprinted from the Clinical Slide Collection on the Rheumatic Diseases, copyright 1991, 1995. Used by permission of the American College of Rheumatology.

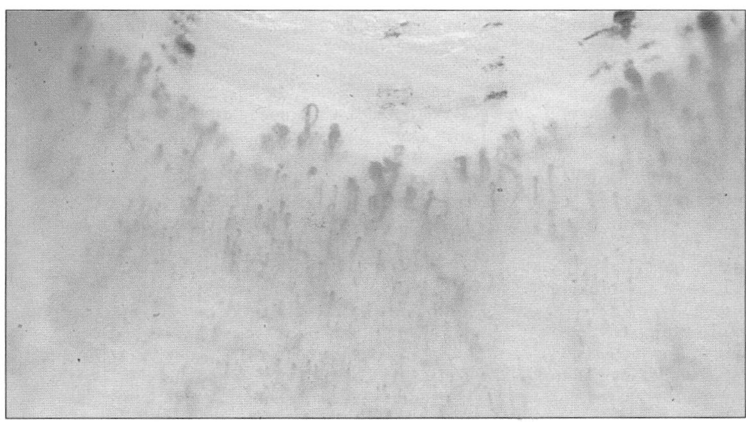

Fig. 5.29 Nailfold capillary pattern in a patient with scleroderma. Notice the avascular areas. Courtesy of Dr Hildegard Maricq.

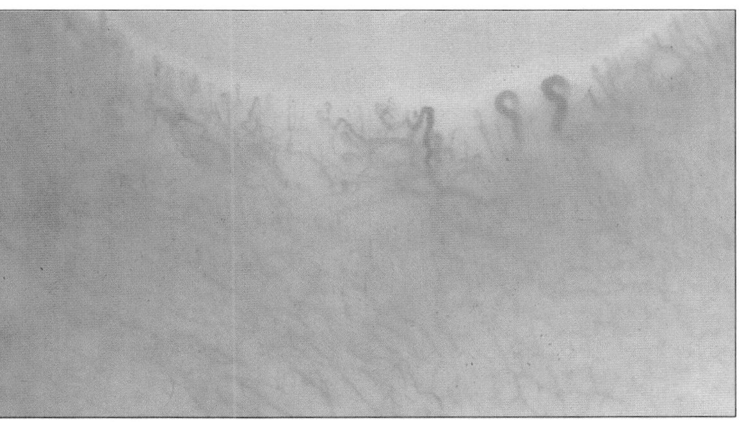

Fig. 5.30 Nailfold capillary pattern in a patient with discoid lupus erythematosus. Courtesy of Dr Hildegard Maricq.

Nailfold telangiectases observed by the naked eye or, preferably, by capillary microscopy are quite specific for the presence of systemic rheumatic disease, especially scleroderma (Fig. 5.29), dermatomyositis and occasionally lupus (Fig. 5.30), and may occur in as many as two thirds of patients with such conditions. They may be helpful as early markers of these diseases[93,94]. The characteristic pattern of scleroderma and dermatomyositis is dilated capillaries frequently bordered by avascular areas. In SLE a tortuous pattern of capillaries without avascular areas is characteristic. In dermatomyositis and lupus, periungual erythema is commonly present as well.

HYPERPIGMENTATION

Pigmentary changes of the skin may be a clue to diagnosis in patients with rheumatic complaints[30]. Joint pain and diffuse hyperpigmentation may be seen in primary biliary cirrhosis, hemochromatosis and Whipple's disease. Rarely, diffuse hyperpigmentation may antedate the more characteristic skin changes of scleroderma[33]. Generalized hyperpigmentation has also been reported rarely in SLE[33]. Hyperpigmentation may also be present without dermal sclerosis in patients with POEMS syndrome, but arthritis occurs infrequently.

Brown to blue–gray discoloration of the skin secondary to drug deposition may occur in rheumatoid patients treated with gold (chrysiasis). Diffuse yellow discoloration is observed frequently with quinacrine therapy, and bluish–black pigmentation of the pretibial area, face and nailbeds is associated with the use of antimalarial drugs[94]. A diagnosis of ochronosis should be considered in the osteoarthritic patient with pigmentary changes overlying cartilage and tendons.

ORAL LESIONS

A careful evaluation of the mouth and pharynx is helpful in the evaluation of rheumatic disease. Findings of ulceration, xerostomia and gingivitis, and an assessment of tongue size and color, may all be of diagnostic importance.

Oral ulcers are common findings in Behçet's syndrome, Crohn's disease, Reiter's syndrome and SLE. Oral ulcerations of Behçet's syndrome and Crohn's disease may be indistinguishable from those of recurrent aphthous stomatitis. Patients with Behçets syndrome or Crohn's disease may experience painful, shallow, round to oval ulcers with discrete borders, which often occur in crops. These lesions tend to occur on mucosa not bound to periosteum as opposed to the lesions of recurrent intraoral herpes which tend to be present upon the hard palate and gingiva. Histopathology of the lesions of Behçet's syndrome or Crohn's disease is not helpful for differential diagnosis, and other clinical signs and symptoms are required to distinguish between these illnesses. In contrast, the lesions of Reiter's syndrome are painless, have an irregular border and are commonly located upon the palate or dorsum of the tongue[96].

Oral ulcers are common in patients with active lupus and may herald a disease flare. Lesions are usually painless, but may occasionally be painful, and are most common on the hard palate[35]. Discoid lesions may produce irregularly shaped white scars upon the mucosa that may be confused with lichen planus or leukoplakia. Histopathology and immunofluorescence studies are diagnostic of these discoid lesions. Nonspecific oral ulcers frequently develop in patients receiving nonsteroidal anti-inflammatory drugs or disease modifying drugs such as gold, D-penicillamine, methotrexate and azathioprine.

Gingivitis secondary to immune disease has been described rarely in lupus[35] and may also be seen as an early manifestation of Wegener's granulomatosis[3].

Kawasaki disease and erythema multiforme major may both reveal signs of fever, conjunctivitis and oral mucosa lesions as well as a polymorphic skin eruption. In Kawasaki disease diffuse erythema of the oral cavity is seen, as well as erythema of the lips followed by dryness, fissuring and surface erosions which contrast to the bloody, crusting lips of a patient with erythema multiforme major. Erythema of the tongue with prominent ungual papillae leads to the strawberry tongue of Kawasaki disease which can be seen in scarlet fever but not in erythema multiforme major.

REFERENCES

1. Braverman IM. Skin signs of systemic disease, 2E. Philadelphia: WB Saunders; 1981.
2. Fitzpatrick TB, Eisen AZ, Wolff K, Freedberg IM, Austen KF, eds. Dermatology in General Medicine, 4E. New York: McGraw-Hill; 1993:27–55.
3. Cupps TR, Fauci AS. The Vasculitides. Philadelphia: WB Saunders; 1981.
4. Ansell BM. Rheumatic Disorders in Childhood. London: Butterworths; 1980:50–51.
5. Case records of the Massachusetts General Hospital. N Engl J Med. 1989; 321:34–43.
6. Burns JC, Mason WH, Glode MP, Shulman ST *et al.* Clinical and epidemiologic characteristics of patients referred for evaluation of Kawasaki disease. J Pediatr. 1991;118:680–6.
7. Kidd BG, Hart HH, Gregor RR. Clinical features of meningococcal arthritis: a report of four cases. Ann Rheum Dis. 1985;44:790–2.
8. Weinberg AN, Schwartz MN. Gram-negative coccal and bacillary infections. In: Fitzpatrick TB, Eisen AZ, Wolff K, Freedberg IM, Austen KF, eds. Dermatology in General Medicine, 4E. New York: McGraw-Hill; 1993:2334–51.
9. Krober MS. Skeletal muscle involvement in Rocky Mountain spotted fever. South Med J. 1978;71:1575–6.
10. Case records of the Massachusetts General Hospital. N Engl J Med. 1971;288:1400–4.
11. Gerster JC, Weintraub A, Vischer TL, Fallet GH. Secondary syphilis revealed by rheumatic complaints. J Rheumatol. 1977;4:197–200.
12. Gertner E, Inman RD. Aseptic arthritis in a man with toxic shock syndrome. Arthritis Rheum. 1986;29:910–16.
13. Schwartz MN, Weinberg AN. Miscellaneous bacterial infections with cutaneous manifestations.

In: Fitzpatrick TB, Eisen AZ, Wolff K, Freedberg IM, Austen KF, eds. Dermatology in General Medicine, 4E. New York: McGraw-Hill; 1987:2354–70.
14. Kreisberg RA. Clinical problem solving. An abundance of options. N Engl J M. 1993;281–3.
15. Mangi RJ. Viral arthritis – the great masquerader. Bulletin Rheum Dis. 1994;43:5–6.
16. Woolf AD, Campion GV, Chishick A, *et al.* Clinical manifestations of human Parvovirus B19 in adults. Arch Intern Med. 1989;149:1153–6.
17. Hulsebosch HJ, Claesson FA, van Ginkel CJ, Kuiters GR, Goudsmit J, Lange JM. Human immunodeficiency exanthem. J Am Acad Dermatol. 1990;23:483–6.
18. Braverman IM. Skin Signs of Systemic Disease, 2E. Philadelphia: WB Saunders; 1981:825.
19. Huff JC, Weston WL, Tonneson MG. Erythema multiforme: a critical review of characteristics, diagnositic criteria and causes. J Am Acad Dermatol. 1983;8:763–75.
20. Braverman IM. Skin signs of systemic disease, 2E. Philadelphia: WB Saunders; 1981:453–516.
21. Roujeau JC, Stern RS. Severe adverse cutaneous reactions to drugs. N Engl J Med. 1994;331:1272–85.
22. Majeed HA, Quabazard Z, Hijazi Z, Farwana S, Harshani. The cutaneous manifestations in children with familial Mediterranean fever (recurrent hereditary polyserositis). A six-year study. Q J Med. 1990;278:607–16.
23. Helfgott SM. Polyarthritis in a 78 year old woman. Clinicopathologic conference. Arthritis Rheum. 1994;37:1087–95.
24. Braverman IM. Skin Signs of Systemic Disease, 2E. Philadelphia: WB Saunders; 1981:740–60.
25. Rothfield N. Lupus erythematosus. In: Fitzpatrick TB, Eisen AZ, Wolff K, Freedberg IM, Austen KF, eds. Dermatology in General Medicine, 4E. New York: McGraw-Hill; 1993:2137–48.
26. Wintroub BU, Stern R. Cutaneous drug reactions: Pathogenesis and clinical classification. J Am Acad Dermatol. 1985;13:167–79.
27. Piette WW. An approach to cutaneous changes caused by hematologic malignancies. Dermatol Clin. 1987;7(3):467–79.
28. Ansell BM. Rheumatic Disorders in Childhood. London: Butterworths; 1980:155–6.
29. Malone MS, Grant-Kels JM, Feder HM, Luger SW. Diagnosis of Lyme disease based on dermatologic manifestations. Ann Intern Med. 1991;114:490–8.
30. Bolognia J, Braverman I. Skin manifestations of internal disease. In: Wilson JD, Braunwald E, Isselbacher KJ, *et al.*, eds. Harrison's Principles of Internal Medicine. New York: McGraw-Hill; 1994:290–307.
31. Almeida L, Grossman M. Widespread dermatophyte infections that mimic collagen vascular disease. J Am Acad Dermatol. 1990;23:855–7.
32. Braverman IM. Skin Signs of Systemic Disease, 2E. Philadelphia: WB Saunders; 1981:255–377.
33. Zax RH, Callen JP. Sarcoidosis. Dermatol Clin. 1989;7(3):505–14.
34. Weigard DA. Cutaneous immunofluorescence. In: Callen JP, ed. Med Clin North Am. 1989;73(5):1263–74.
35. Wallace DJ. Cutaneous manifestations of SLE. In: Wallace DJ, Hahn BH, eds. Dubois' Lupus Erythematosus, 4E. Philadelphia: Lea and Febiger; 1993:356–69.
36. Plotz PH. Current concepts in the idiopathic inflammatory myopathies: polymyositis, dermatomyositis, and related disorders. Ann Intern Med. 1989;111:143–57.
37. Taylor CR, Hawk JLM. Recognizing photosensitivity. Ann Rheum Dis 1994;53:705–707.
38. Harber LC. Abnormal responses to ultraviolet radiation: drug induced photosensitivity. In: Fitzpatrick TB, Eisen AZ, Wolff K, Freedberg IM, Austen KF, eds. Dermatology in General Medicine, 4E. New York: McGraw-Hill; 1993:1677–89.
39. Epstein JH. Polymorphous light eruption. In: Beare JM, Ruiz Maldonaudo R, Parish LC, eds. Textbook of Pediatric Dermatology. Philadelphia: Grune and Stratton; 1989:706–10.
40. Bickers DR, Patrick MA, Lim HW. The porphyrias. In: Fitzpatrick TB, Eisen AZ, Wolff K, Freedberg IM, Austen KF, eds. Dermatology in General Medicine, 4E. New York: McGraw-Hill; 1993:1854–94.
41. Barthelmy H, Chouvet B, Cambazard F. Skin and mucosal manifestations in vitamin deficiency. J Am Acad Dermatol. 1986;15:1263–74.
42. Nesher G, Osborn TG, Moore TL. Parvovirus infection mimicking systemic lupus erythematosus. Semin Arthritis Rheum. 1995;24:297–303.
43. McElgunn PS. Dermatologic manifestations of hepatitis B virus infection. J Am Acad Dermatol. 1983;8:539–48.
44. Bielory L, Gascon P, Lawley TJ, Young NS, Frank MM. Human serum sicknes: A prospective analysis of 35 patients treated with equine anti-thymocyte globulin for bone marrow failure. Medicine. 1988;67:40–57.
45. Burrall BA, Halpern GM, Huntley AC. Chronic urticaria. West J Med. 1990;152:268–76.
46. Pasero G, Oliveri I, Gemignani G, Vitali C. Urticaria/ arthritis syndrome: report of four B51 positive patients. Ann Rheum Dis. 1989;48:508–11.
47. Monroe EW. Urticarial vasculitis: An updated review. J Am Acad Dermatol. 1981;5:88–95.
48. Kaye B, Kaye D, Bobrove A. Rheumatoid nodules. Am J Med. 1984;76:279–92.
49. Moore CP, Willkens RF. The subcutaneous nodule: Its significance in the diagnosis of rheumatic disease. Semin Arthritis Rheum. 1977;7:63–79.
50. Dabski K, Winkelman RK. Generalized granuloma annulare: Clinical and laboratory findings in 100 patients. J Am Acad Dermatol. 1989;20:39–47.
51. Reginato AJ, Kurnik B. Calcium oxalate and other crystals associated with kidney diseases and arthritis. Semin Arthritis Rheum. 1989;18:198–224.
52. Resnick C. Tumoral calcinosis. Arthritis Rheum. 1989;32:1484–6.
53. Leisen JC, Austard ED, Bluhm GB, Sigler JW. The tophus in calcium pyrophosphate deposition disease. JAMA. 1980;244:1711–12.
54. Rapini RP. Multirentric reticulohistocytosis. Clin Dermatol. 1993;11:107–11.
55. Bondi EE, Lazarus GA. Panniculitis. In: Fitzpatrick TB, Eisen AZ, Wolff K, Freedberg IM, Austen KF, eds. Dermatology in General Medicine, 3E. New York: McGraw-Hill; 1993:1330–44.
56. Braverman IM. Skin Signs of Systemic Disease, 2E. Philadelphia: WB Saunders; 1981:710–40.
57. Kalb RE. Sarcoidosis with subcutaneous nodules. Am J Med. 1988; 85:731–6.
58. Albert DA, Weisman MH, Kaplan R. The rheumatic manifestations of leprosy. Medicine. 1980;59:442–8.
59. Francis C, Huong LT, Piehe J *et al.* Wegener's granulomatosis. Dermatological manifestations in 75 cases with clinicopathologic correlation. Arch Derm. 1994;130:861–7.
60. Katz SI. Erythema elevation diutinum. In: Fitzpatrick TB, Eisen AZ, Wolff K. Freedberg IM, Austen KF, eds. Dermatology in General Medicine, 3E. New York: McGraw-Hill; 1993:1167–71.
61. Fritch PO, Elias PM. Mechanisms of vesicle formation and classification. In: Fitzpatrick TB, Eisen AZ, Wolf K, Freedberg IM, Austen KF, eds. Dermatology in General Medicine, 3E. New York: McGraw-Hill; 1987:546–54.
62. Hall RP, Lawley TJ, Katz SI. Bullous eruption of systemic lupus erythematosus (editorial). J Am Acad Dermatol. 1982;7:797–9.
63. Kutz DC, Bridges AJ. Bullous rash and brown urine in a systemic lupus erythematosus patient treated with hydroxychloroquine. Arthritis Rheum. 1995;38:440–3.
64. Callen J. Internal disorders associated with bullous disease of the skin. J Am Acad Dermatol. 1980;3:107–19.
65. Fitzpatrick TB, Bernhard JD. The structure of skin lesions and fundamentals of diagnosis. In: Fitzpatrick TB, Eisen AZ, Wolff K, Freedberg IM, Austen KF, eds. Dermatology in General Medicine, 4E. New York: McGraw-Hill; 1993:27–55.
66. McNeely MC, Jorizzo JL, Solomon AR, Schmalstieg FC, Cavallo T. Primary idiopathic cutaneous pustular vasculitis. J Am Acad Dermatol. 1986;14:939–44.
67. Daniel SU, Fett DL, Gibson LE, Pittelkow MR. Sweet syndrome: acute febrile neutrophilic dermatosis. Sem Dermatol. 1995;14:173–8.
68. Laxer RM, Shore AD, King S, Silverman ED, Wilmot DM. Chronic recurrent multifocal osteomyelitis and psoriasis: A report of a new association and review of related disorders. Semin Arthritis Rheum. 1988;17:260–70.
69. Knitzer RH, Needleman BW. Musculoskeletal syndromes associated with acne. Semin Arthritis Rheum. 1991;20:247–55.
70. Schreiner DT. Purpura. Dermatol Clin. 1989;7:481–9.
71. Reuler JB, Broudy VC, Cooney TG. Adult scurvy. JAMA. 1985;253:803–7.
72. Cappiello RA, Espinoza LR, Adelman H, Aquilar J, Vassey FB, German BF. Cholesterol embolism: A pseudo-vasculitis syndrome. Semin Arthritis Rheumatol. 1989;18:240–6.
73. Braverman IM. Skin Signs of Systemic Disease, 2E. Philadelphia: WB Saunders; 1981:378–452.
74. Gibson LE, Daniel SU. Cutaneous vasculitis. Rheum Dis Clin North Am. 1990;16:309–24.
75. Spencer LV, Callen JP. Cutaneous manifestations of bacterial infections. Dermatol Clin. 1989;7:579–89.
76. Braverman IM. Skin Signs of Systemic Disease, 2E. Philadelphia: WB Saunders; 1981:809–922.
77. Cawley MI. Vasculitis and ulceration in rheumatic disease of the foot. Baillière's Clin Rheumatol. 1987;1:315–33.
78. Vollersten RS, Conn DL. Vasculitis with rheumatoid arthritis. Rheumatol Dis Clin North Am. 1990;16:445–61.
79. Jorizzo JL, Daniels JC. Dermatologic conditions reported in patients with rheumatoid arthritis. J Am Acad Dermatol. 1983;8:439–57.
80. Levine JM. Leg ulcers: Differential diagnosis in the elderly. Geriatrics. 1990;45:32–42.
81. Wolff K, Stingl G. Pyoderma gangrenosum. In: Fitzpatrick TB, Eisen AZ, Wolff K, Freedberg IM, Austen KF, eds. Dermatology in General Medicine, 4E. New York: McGraw-Hill; 1993:1171–1183.
82. Bacon DG, Tribe CR. Systemic rheumatoid vasculitis: A clinical and laboratory study of 50 cases. Medicine. 1981;60:288–97.
83. Gaylarde PM, Dodd HJ, Sarlcony I. Venous leg ulcers and arthropathy. Br J Rheumatol. 1990;29:142–4.
84. Burgdorf W. Cutaneous manifestations of Crohn's disease. J Am Acad Dermatol. 1981;5:689–95.
85. Rocco VK, Hurd ER. Scleroderma and scleroderma-like disorders. Semin Arthritis Rheum. 1986;16:22–69.
86. Lakhanapal S, Ginsburg WW, Michet CJ, Doyle JA, Moore SB. Eosinophilic fasciitis: Clinical spectrum and therapeutic response in 52 cases. Semin Arthritis Rheum. 1988;17:221–31.
87. Varga J, Peltonen J, Vitto J, Jimenez S. Development of diffuse fasciitis with eosinophilia during L-tryptophen: Demonstration of elevated type I collagen gene expression in affected tissues. Ann Intern Med. 1990;112:344–51.
88. Feingold KR, Elias P. Endocrine skin interactions. J Am Acad Dermatol. 1987;17:921–40.
89. Feingold KR, Elias P. Endocrine skin interactions. J Am Acad Dermatol. 1988;19:1–20.
90. Viard J, Lasavre P, Boitard C, *et al.* POEMS syndrome presenting as systemic sclerosis. Am J Med. 1988;84;524–7.
91. Gabriel SE, Perry HO, Oleson GB, Bowles CA. Scleromyxedema: A scleroderma-like disorder with systemic manifestations. Medicine. 1988;67:58–65.
92. Pfinsgraff J, Buckingham RB, Killian PJ, *et al.* Palmar fasciitis and arthritis with malignant neoplasms: A paraneoplastic syndrome. Semin Arthritis Rheum. 1986;16:118–25
93. Braverman IM. Skin Signs of Systemic Disease, 2E. Philadelphia: WB Saunders; 1981:532–65.
94. Minkin W, Rabhan NB. Office nail fold microscopy using ophtalmoscope. J Am Acad Dermatol. 1982;7:191–3.
95. Bailin PL, Matkaluk. Cutaneous reactions to rheumatologic drugs. Clin Rheumatol Dis. 1982;8:493–516.
96. Winchester R. Reiter's syndrome. In: Fitzpatrick TB, Eisen AZ, Wolff K, Freedberg IM, Austen KF, eds. Dermatology in General Medicine, 4E. New York: McGraw-Hill; 1993;2199–211.

6

THE EYE AND RHEUMATIC DISEASES

John Forrester

Ocular and periocular involvement in rheumatic disease
- Uveitis and uveoretinitis.
- Keratitis and keratoconjunctivitis sicca.
- Scleritis.

Uveitis

Definition
- Inflammation of the uveal tract (iris, ciliary body or choroid).

Types
- Anterior (iridocyclitis), posterior (retinochoroiditis) or both (panuveitis).
- Acute (e.g. acute anterior uveitis or iritis) or chronic (most posterior uveitides).
- Recurrent.

Presentation
- Anterior uveitis presents with pericorneal redness (injection), flare and cells in the anterior chamber of the eye as seen on slit-lamp examination. Cellular deposits (keratic precipitates) form on the posterior surface of the cornea. In juvenile seronegative arthritis uveitis may present with loss of vision in the absence of redness of the eye (white eye uveitis).
- Posterior uveitis presents with 'floaters' and blurring or loss of vision; in rheumatic disease it is more commonly a retinal vasculitis as in Behçet's disease or polyarteritis nodosa

Corneal involvement in rheumatologic disease
- Rheumatoid corneal ulcers normally present as marginal or peripheral areas of corneal thinning leading eventually to perforation. Staining with fluorescein dye will reveal the extent.
- They may be relatively painless compared to idiopathic marginal ulcers (Mooren's ulcer).
- Sudden loss of vision is a prominent feature, particularly if perforation has occurred.
- Corneal opacification is known as sclerosing keratitis.
- Keratoconjunctivitis sicca can promote corneal ulceration and opacification.

INTRODUCTION

The eye may be involved in many ways as part of multisystem connective tissue diseases. Usually one or more of the ocular coats are affected by an inflammatory process, but on occasion the clinical evidence of inflammation may not be immediately apparent, as in the melting corneal ulcer of rheumatoid arthritis (RA). Ocular involvement in arthritic disease may be linked to infectious diseases, as seen in the triad of Yersinia enterocolitis, ankylosing spondylitis (AS) and uveitis. Indeed, the possible association between such disease clusters and pathogenetic mechanisms involving infectious agents, autoimmunity and molecular mimicry is a field of active investigation, particularly with regard to the role of major histocompatibility (MHC) class I antigens in susceptibility to disease.

Other ocular disorders associated with connective tissue diseases include the several forms of dry eye syndrome (keratoconjunctivitis sicca, KCS) in which the clinical manifestations are secondary to low-grade lymphocytic infiltration of the lacrimal and accessory lacrimal glands. However, this produces a disturbance of tear film physiology with potentially serious sight-threatening complications.

The major manifestations of ocular involvement in rheumatologic disease are uveitis, corneal disease and dry eye syndromes, and scleritis. This chapter deals with each of these disease entities separately.

UVEITIS

Uveitis denotes inflammation of the middle coats of the eye (Fig. 6.1), i.e. the iris (iritis), the ciliary body (cyclitis) or the choroid (choroiditis). Certain forms of uveitis may affect only a small part of the eye and are thus described according to their anatomic location, for example, inflammation of the pars plana of the ciliary body is known as pars planitis. The types of uveitis were originally subdivided into granulomatous and nongranulomatous on the basis of their appearance by slit lamp microscopy, and this partly assisted in providing an explanation for a presumptive pathology. While this was valuable in assisting our understanding of the mechanism of induction of uveitis, it has become outdated with the development of newer experimental models.

Probably the clearest pathogenetic distinction we can make in uveitis depends on whether the disease is restricted to the anterior segment or whether it is predominantly a posterior segment disease with variable 'spill over' into the anterior segment[1]. Anterior uveitis is most frequently an acute, recurrent illness involving the iris and ciliary body and may occur as an HLA-B27+ or an HLA-B27– disease[2]. Chronic forms of anterior uveitis also occur, as with juvenile seronegative arthritis, but are much less common. Posterior uveitis, by contrast, presents with a bewildering variety of clinical syndromes of markedly different

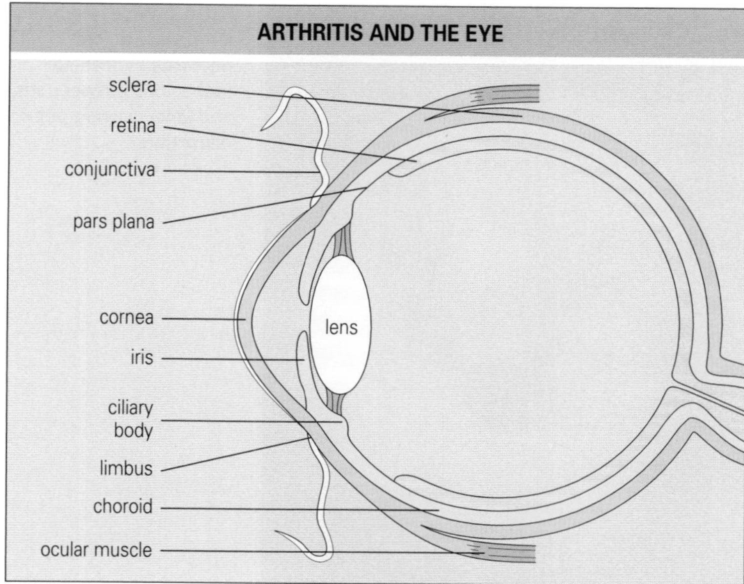

Fig. 6.1 The structural elements of the eye which may be primarily involved in rheumatic disease processes.

severity and visual consequences. Despite this heterogeneity, many forms of this disease are increasingly recognized as representing part of a spectrum of uveoretinal inflammatory disease[3].

The association of uveitis with rheumatologic disease, in which autoimmune mechanisms are considered to play a major part, has led to the notion that many forms of uveitis are also 'autoimmune' in nature. However, autoimmune disease may also be initiated through infectious agents, as demonstrated in the link between microbial heat-shock proteins and rheumatoid disease[4]; uveitis may serve as an excellent paradigm for such diseases.

CLINICAL PRESENTATION

Anterior uveitis

Acute anterior uveitis (AAU) is restricted to the iris and ciliary body (iridocyclitis). Typically, the patient presents with a moderately injected eye, variable pain and discomfort, depending on the degree of ciliary muscle spasm and/or rise in intraocular pressure, and some degree of reduced vision. External examination may show some corneal clouding, which depends on the intraocular pressure and the inflammatory cell infiltrate in the anterior chamber. Slit-lamp examination reveals cells in the anterior chamber which may be fine (single cells) or discrete (aggregates of cells). These tend to deposit on the posterior corneal endothelium (keratic precipitates). Protein exudation in the anterior chamber is best seen with a small narrow slit-lamp beam and may be so marked that a fibrin clot forms in the anterior chamber. Iris vessel engorgement is present during the acute stage and adhesions form between the posterior iris and the lens surface (posterior synechiae); synechiae frequently persist long after the inflammation has settled (Fig. 6.2). Anterior synechiae also form between the peripheral iris and the posterior cornea and may be so dense as to occlude the drainage angle of the eye, causing secondary glaucoma.

Inflammation of the ciliary body (cyclitis) causes difficulty in accommodation, affecting reading ability in the acute phase; if cyclitis becomes chronic, a retrolental fibrous membrane may form (cyclitic membrane) which may traverse the visual axis and also reduce vision. Chronic cyclitis may also affect aqueous production by the ciliary body and lead to ocular hypotension, which is an important sign of persistent intraocular inflammation.

The annual incidence of AAU is 8.2 new cases per 100,000 population and it is the commonest form of uveitis[5]. The severity of the inflammation depends on the HLA-B27 allotype[5]. Approximately half of the cases are HLA-B27+ and have AS or some similar joint disease. Initial studies suggested that clinically HLA-B27+ AAU could be distinguished by the unilaterality and high protein exudation in such patients, while HLA-B27– AAU patients were more likely to have mutton-fat keratic precipitates[6]. Rothova *et al.*[7] have confirmed these findings in a study of 144 AAU patients in whom 50 clinical variables were analyzed using statistical methods. Significantly different findings in HLA-B27+ patients were: younger age at onset; male predominance; unilaterality with alternating recurrences; plastic and/or fibrinoid aqueous; absence of mutton-fat keratic precipitates; high ocular complication rate; and frequent association with spondyloarthropathies. In both groups of patients, persistent posterior synechiae occurred (36% and 15% in the HLA-B27+ and HLA-B27– cases, respectively) and it may therefore be difficult to exclude pars planitis from some of these cases. Despite this caveat, it appears from this comprehensive study that HLA-B27$^+$ AAU is a separate entity from HLA-B27$^-$ AAU and that the former has a worse visual prognosis.

Genetic heterogeneity in AAU and its association with arthritis has recently been further demonstrated in the phenotypic association with polymorphisms in the HLA-linked proteasome subunit gene, *LMP2*[8]. These novel findings strongly implicate MHC Class I associated mechanisms in the induction of AAU (see below).

Chronic anterior uveitis is much less frequent than AAU and most commonly occurs in association with seronegative juvenile chronic arthritis (JCA) (see Chapter 5.18)[7]. Due to the insidious nature of this inflammatory disorder (the 'white eye' uveitis) (Fig. 6.3), the visual consequences of this disease can be severe. The inflammation occurs predominantly as a low-grade cellular infiltrate, with marked flare and relative hypotonia oculi. Extensive posterior synechiae, with cataract formation and secondary cystoid macular edema, account for the visual loss. The etiology is obscure.

Various types of juvenile arthropathy may be associated with this form of uveitis including the spondyloarthropathies and all forms of JCA (systemic, pauciarticular and polyarticular)[9]. The 5-year incidence of uveitis in seronegative JCA is 20% and the disease is more frequently bilateral. In 6–20%, the uveitis precedes the arthritis by an average of 5 years and this may be as long as 20 years. Unlike most forms of uveitis, in which serologic testing is of little value, a search for antinuclear antibody can be informative[10].

A recent extensive study of children with various forms of arthropathy found that factors significantly associated with sight threatening complications of uveitis were (1) a chronic course of uveitis, (2) juvenile psoriatic arthropathy, (3) diagnosis of uveitis prior to, or at the time

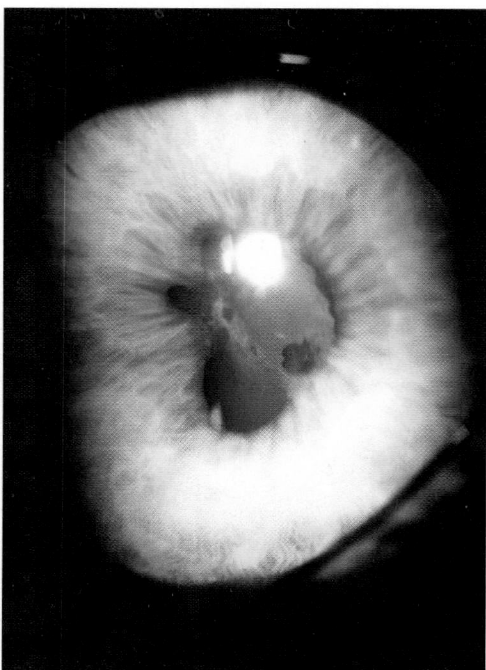

Fig. 6.2 Wide beam slit lamp view of 'old' posterior synechiae (adhesions between iris and lens) causing pupil distortion.

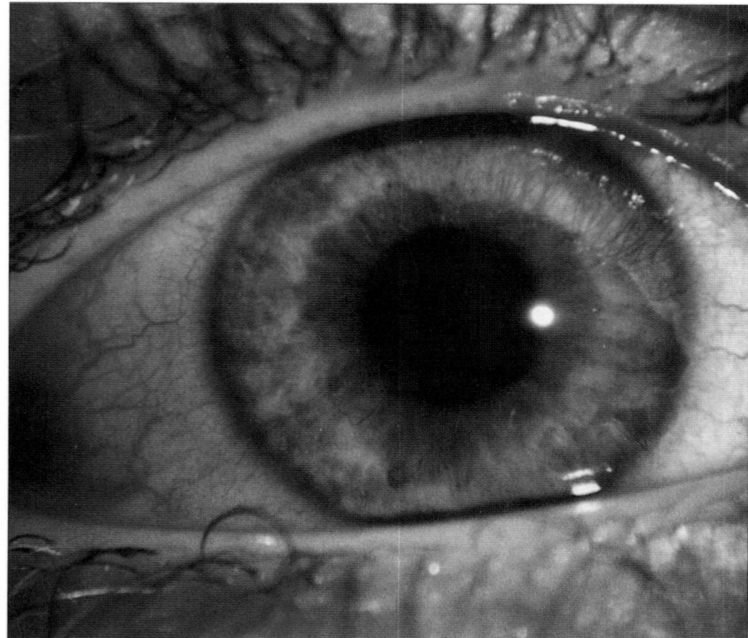

Fig. 6.3 Chronic uveitis in seronegative juvenile arthitis — 'white eye' uveitis.

of, arthritis onset and (4) symptomatic onset[11]. The risk of developing uveitis late (5 years) after the onset of arthritis is small. In addition, while ocular complications are common (33%), sight-threatening complications affect a minority of patients. However, this group requires close ophthalmological follow-up. In summary, AAU is the more common manifestation in most juvenile arthropathies but the chronic form is the more serious, if only because it is easily missed.

Posterior uveitis

Posterior uveitis occurs in association with many rheumatic diseases. However, in a major prospective study of systemic disease linkage with uveitis, only 26% of cases of posterior uveitis were found to have an association with systemic disease, of which the most common was sarcoidosis[12]. In most cases of posterior uveitis, an etiology cannot be found and the disease is considered to be 'endogenous'. However, pathologic and other studies have shown that there is little difference in the mechanism of tissue destruction that occurs, for example, in the retinal vasculitis of Beçhet's disease compared to retinal vasculitis in isolation. It may be that, in isolated retinal vasculitis, a systemic 'event' has taken place, but thus far tests are unable to determine the cause. Perhaps with ultrasensitive techniques, such as the polymerase chain reaction, it will be possible to identify causative (possibly infectious) agents in tissues or cells from patients who were presumed to have 'endogenous' autoimmune uveitis, such as retinal vasculitis. The same probably applies to other autoimmune diseases. Endogenous posterior uveitis includes several discrete clinical entities, which at first sight might seem to be unrelated. Pars planitis (intermediate uveitis), for instance, involves predominantly the peripheral retina and vitreous base, and characteristically is associated with vitreous inflammatory cell infiltrates (snowballs) and extensive subretinal chorioretinal infiltrates. However, careful examination and fluorescein angiography will show that many of these cases also have signs of peripheral retinal vasculitis while visual loss is most frequently due to macular edema, itself usually a manifestation of increased perifoveal capillary leakiness.

Sympathetic ophthalmia is characterized by focal chorioretinal nodules or microgranulomas – the Dalen–Fuchs nodule – which typically accumulate as healed scars within the fundus after a short self-limiting period of active inflammation. Similar micrograulomas are observed in sarcoid uveoretinitis (Fig. 6.4), in Vogt–Koyanagi–Harada's syndrome, a systemic inflammatory disease common in Asian races, and in the less well-defined disorder of multifocal, diffuse choroiditis. They are also frequently the cause of exacerbations of vitritis in cases of 'intermediate' uveitis or pars planitis where one or two small, round, white foci in the equatorial or pre-equatorial fundus may be sufficient to cause symptoms of floaters. They often escape detection, however, because they are short-lived and self-limiting and may disappear leaving virtually no trace. When they occur in large numbers as in sympathetic ophthalmia, less so in sarcoidosis, they have a characteristic appearance on fluorescein angiography during the active phase: hypofluorescent choroidal 'spots' in the early sequence with late hyperfluorescence[13]. Healed, inactive lesions are overlaid by depigmented retinal pigment epithelium and appear as pigment epithelial defects on fluorescein angiography. The similarity both clinically and pathogenetically has recently been reviewed[14].

Retinal vasculitis involving the posterior pole may present as an 'idiopathic' disorder or as part of a disease entity such as sarcoidosis, Behçet's disease, multiple sclerosis or systemic lupus erythematosus (SLE) (Fig. 6.5). The vasculitis may affect small or large vessels, and occurs usually as a phlebitis with retinal hemorrhages. Less frequently, an arteritis and phlebitis occur with widespread retinal infiltrates and ischemia even to the point of retinal necrosis. Retinal vasculitis rarely occurs in isolation. Careful examination will reveal that chorioretinal infiltrates similar to those in sympathetic ophthalmia are present. In addition, vitreous inflammatory cells are almost a prerequisite for the differentiation of retinal vasculitis from other retinal vascular thrombotic disorders.

Pars planitis or intermediate uveitis is assuming increasing importance as a clinical entity due to its increasing frequency in audit studies of patients attending uveitis clinics. This disorder commonly affects young males who present with symptoms of floaters and gradually decreasing vision due to secondary cystoid macular edema. Clinically, examination of the peripheral retina reveals inflammatory cell aggregates in the vitreous (snowballs), pre- and subretinal exudative material with fibrogliosis (snow banking), and peripheral retinal vasculitis. Cases have been described in association with a variety of systemic diseases such as sarcoidosis, multiple sclerosis and Lyme borreliosis. However, in most cases no etiological agent can be found. Recently, an association between intermediate uveitis and HLA-A28 has been identified. In addition HLA-A28+ patients were significantly more likely to suffer arthralgia and to have evidence of hypocomplementemia[15].

It is important to differentiate uveitis associated with systemic disease from those forms of uveitis which have a clear infectious etiology, such as *herpes simplex*-induced acute retinal necrosis, cytomegalovirus

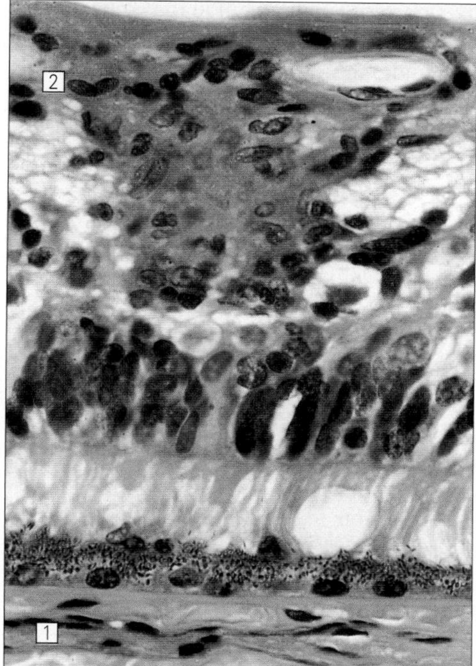

Fig. 6.4 Microgranuloma in sarcoid uveoretinitis. Choroid (1); retina (2). Note the large numbers of epithelioid giant cells.

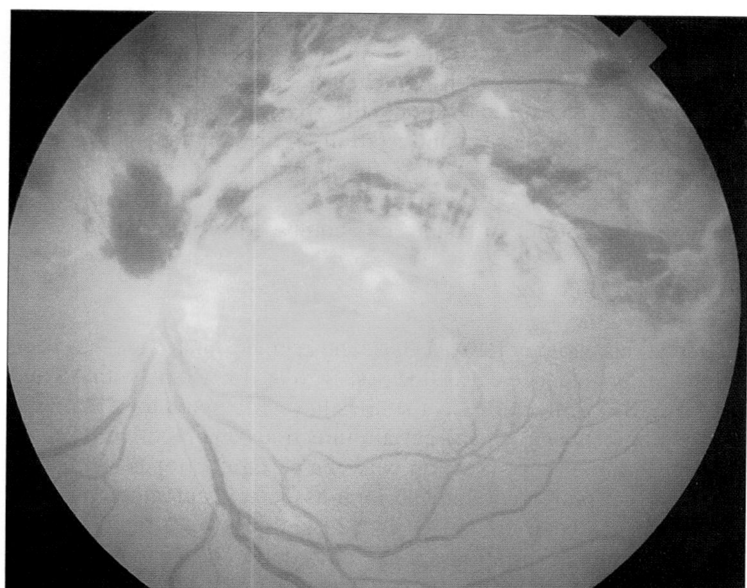
Fig. 6.5 Acute, severe, retinal vasculitis affecting the upper temporal retinal vessels. Note the large number of hemorrhages and white choroidal and retinal infiltrates.

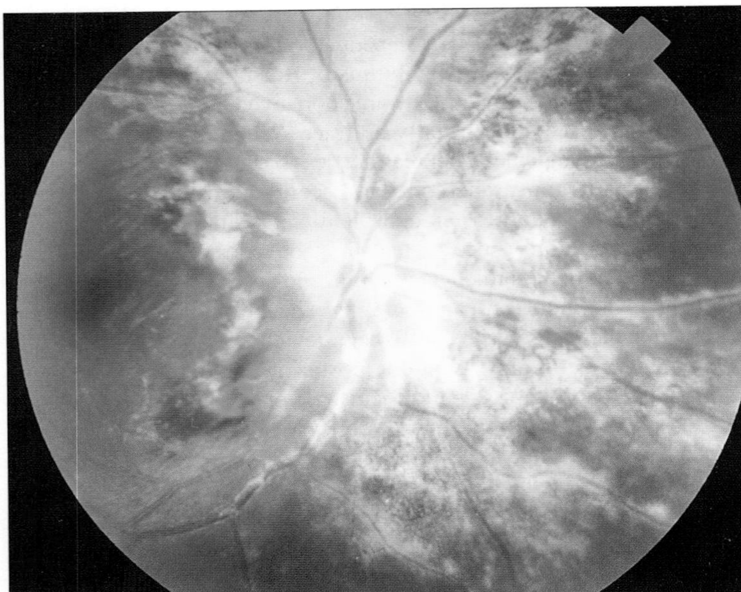

Fig. 6.6 Massive retinal infiltration and necrosis in a case of cytomegalovirus retinitis.

retinitis (Fig. 6.6) and toxoplasmosis retinochoroiditis, although the evidence for the last has become less compelling in the light of recent data showing no clear serologic difference between clinically 'toxoplasma' patients and healthy controls[16]. Most uveitis syndromes, however, are of unknown etiology and much of the reported histopathology has been concerned with end-stage disease. Immunohistopathologic studies have shown that T-cells, particularly T-helper ($CD4^+$) cells, and monocytes predominate in many lesions such as the Dalen–Fuchs nodule in sarcoidosis and in sympathetic ophthalmia[17]. In general, the available histologic data have supported the concept of an immunologically mediated process in most forms of posterior uveitis. In addition, despite the differences in clinical presentation, most forms of posterior uveitis have four cardinal features:

- vitreous inflammatory cells and exudate (vitreous haze);
- focal chorioretinal infiltrates;
- retinal vasculitis;
- macular edema.

In some forms, there may be a greater emphasis on one or more of these features, for example retinal vasculitis, or, in birdshot choroidoretinopathy, focal chorioretinal infiltrates. In other forms, additional features may be present, for example retinal necrosis, exudative retinal detachment (in Vogt–Koyanagi–Harada syndrome), or subretinal and preretinal neovascularization. However, as will be seen from the discussion below, these manifestations represent the spectrum of choroidoretinal responses to an inflammatory stimulus and this limited set of responses is essentially the same whether the stimulus is immunologic, chronic infectious or a combination of both.

PATHOGENESIS

Anterior uveitis

An infectious etiology for AAU has long been postulated and has been given greater credence during the past 10 years by its link with AS and the HLA-B27 antigen. Recent studies have attempted to explain the association between AS and certain infectious enterocolitic diseases by suggesting a cross-reaction between certain epitopes (antigenic sites) on the foreign antigen and joint-associated autoantigen which bind specifically to certain HLA-B27 antigens on articular lining cells[2,18]. Protein crystallographic studies have shown that the HLA class I antigen contains an antigenic peptide-binding region in a cleft between two α helical regions on the external domains of the α_1 and α_2 chains on its extracytoplasmic surface[19]. Single amino acid point mutations within the variable region of this binding cleft account for the different allotypes of HLA-B27 (there are seven), and each of these types has variable binding affinity for antigenic peptide and/or the T-cell receptor (see Chapter 6.12). It has been suggested that the binding cleft of the HLA antigen is normally occupied by (nonimmunogenic) autoantigen but, if this site were occupied by cross-reacting or competing foreign peptide, then an immune response might be elicited by presentation of the peptide to the appropriate sensitized cytotoxic lymphocytes which recognize the peptide–MHC antigen complex.

In the case of AS, associations have been detected with various infectious diseases, including *Klebsiella* and *Yersinia* enterocolitis, and with Reiter's syndrome. Similarly, in AAU association with fecal carriage of *Klebsiella* and with recent *Yersinia* infection have been reported, although there is still considerable controversy concerning these results[20,21].

However, there is abundant documented and undocumented clinical evidence for an association of enteric and similar infections with AAU and AS. The increasingly convincing laboratory data and the incontrovertible association with HLA-B27 generally support a pathogenetic mechanism in AAU requiring an infectious agent, plus a genetically susceptible host. Autosensitized cross-reactive cytotoxic lymphocytes target the appropriate peptide–MHC class I antigen complex on the host cells in both the eye and the joint, and induce inflammation by damaging these cells. A simpler mechanism for the induction of AAU during infectious states has been proposed which involves release of endotoxin by the invading microorganisms. This is based on the experimental model of endotoxic uveitis induced in rats by intradermal injections of *Shigella* toxin[22]. However, this fails to account for the genetic susceptibility of AAU patients and for the delay between development of enteric disease and the later onset of uveitis.

The mechanisms proposed above for HLA-B27+ AAU does not explain the inflammatory response in the AAU patient who is HLA-B27–, or the chronic uveitis in seronegative patients with connective tissue disease. From the clinical presentation it is clear that these patients have a different type of disease, possibly involving different cell types (mutton-fat keratic precipitates are more likely to be aggregates of macrophages, while fine keratic precipitates are probably T lymphocytes)[7]. In some of these patients, autoimmunity to connective tissue matrix components, such as cartilage and vitreous type II collagen or proteoglycan, has been proposed. In a model of adjuvant arthritis, in which subcutaneous injections of Freund's complete adjuvant induce an RA-like condition, 60% of the animals develop an acute anterior uveitis[23]. However, even in this form of disease, infectious agents have been implicated via a molecular mimicry model whereby cross reaction between a mycobacterial component in the adjuvant and a component in the cartilage proteoglycan has been proposed[24].

Therefore, the emerging understanding of AAU is that, while microorganisms, autoimmune or immune-mediated responses and inflammatory destructive disease are inextricably entwined via processes such as molecular mimicry, the precise mechanisms involved vary significantly between HLA-B27+ disease and HLA-B27– connective-tissue-associated disease: this distinction probably has important implications for the sequelae of the disease[7]. Our understanding of these mechanisms may be assisted by the recent description of experimental models of autoimmune anterior uveitis using ocular melanin-associated autoantigen[25,26].

Posterior uveitis

Despite the marked clinical heterogeneity of posterior uveitis syndromes, information derived from experimental models has greatly assisted us in defining these disorders. Experimental autoimmune uveoretinitis (EAU) is a disorder similar to experimental autoimmune encephalomyelitis (a model for multiple sclerosis) or to collagen- or adjuvant-induced arthritis in which a presumed autoantigen is used to induce organ-specific inflammation. Several retinal antigens, each with the ability to induce EAU, have been described, including retinal

S-antigen, interphotoreceptor retinol binding protein (IRBP) and even rhodopsin itself[27–29]. Considerable information is now available concerning the amino acid sequence and secondary structure of these proteins, and more recently immunodominant epitopes on these antigens have been described, at least for retinal S-antigen[30] and IRBP[31]. However, the list of potential retinal autoantigens has continued to increase[25,28,32] such that there are now at least 30 possible autoantigenic epitopes which have been identified for uveoretinitis. Despite the lack of sequence homology between these proteins, they all induce a spectrum of uveitis severity which can be modified not so much by the nature of the antigen, but by the dose of antigen, the species and strain of experimental animal, and the state of immunosuppression of the animal[3]. Thus, low-dose antigen in a low responder rat strain may produce a few focal microgranulomata (similar to Dalen–Fuchs nodules) and minimal evidence of retinal vasculitis (Fig. 6.7), while high-dose antigen will produce extensive destruction of the photoreceptor layer, severe thrombotic retinal vasculitis, exudative retinal detachment and even retinal necrosis[3]. Clinically, these two extremes might be represented by intermediate uveitis (pars planitis) and severe Behçet's-associated retinal vasculitis.

The mechanism of the inflammatory response in EAU is currently under intensive investigation. The similarities with other experimental models of autoimmune disease are further supported by the fact that they can all be induced by transfer of $CD4^+$ activated T-cells to naïve recipients. In addition, as in human uveitis, there is considerable genetic variability in susceptibility to the disease, which further emphasizes the importance of the MHC antigen in disease induction. For instance, one of the white dot syndromes (known as bird-shot retinochoroiditis due to the clinical appearance of the fundus 'peppered' with small white lesions) has a very high association with -HLA-A29[33]. In addition Behçet's disease has an association with HLA-B5101/02 but also shows a link with cell-mediated immune responses to retinal autoantigens even when there are no ocular signs[34].

Generation of an immune response requires processing of antigen (proteolysis) by antigen presenting cells (APCs) and presentation of an antigenic fragment(s) (immunogenic peptide) bound to cell surface MHC antigens to the responding T-cell. $CD4^+$ (T-helper) cells are activated by antigenic peptide bound to MHC class II molecules on the APC while $CD8^+$ (T-cytotoxic) cells are activated by antigen–MHC class I complexes. Considerable information is now available concerning the sequences of peptides likely to be involved in these mechanisms in uveitis, including Behçet's disease[35].

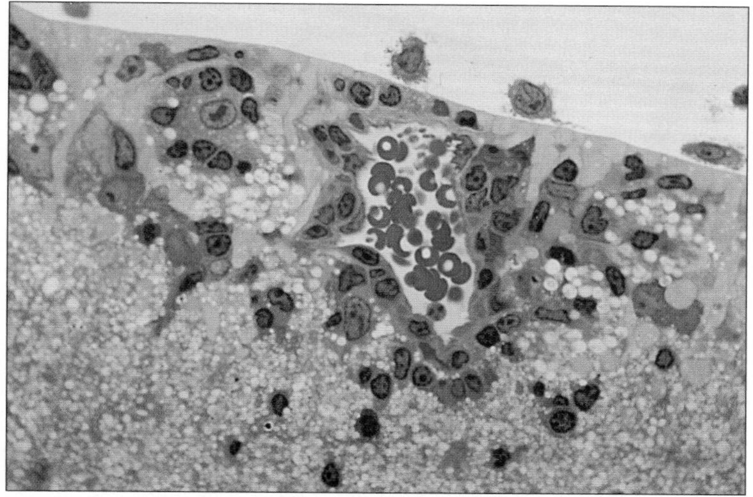

Fig. 6.7 Retinal vasculitis in an experimental model of uveitis. Note the predominantly mononuclear cell inflitrate with relative absence of neutrophils.

Many questions arise from such data. For instance, is there a minimum size of peptide required to induce an immune response? Why are some peptides good inducers while others are not? Is the relative affinity of the peptide for the MHC antigen important, and is this reflected in genetic susceptibility to disease? Recent studies on peptides from retinal S-antigen have suggested that there is a 'core sequence' within the protein which is essential for disease induction and that this sequence has considerable homology for certain sequences from viral and fungal proteins[36]. Indeed, immunization of animals with peptide sequences from baker's yeast fungi has induced an ocular inflammation similar to EAU[37]. If these results are confirmed, they would provide the strongest evidence yet for the molecular mimicry hypothesis involving cross-reactive antigens in the mechanism of induction of uveitis. Parallel studies in Behçet's disease have shown that T-cell epitopes are shared between the heat shock protein hsp65 and mycobacterial antigen, providing circumstantial evidence that these mechanisms are operative in human disease also[38].

Pathogenetic mechanisms in uveitis are slowly being unraveled and involve several different cellular and molecular pathways. For each type of uveitis, however, it is likely that the mechanisms are qualitatively similar and that quantitative differences are reflected in the clinical severity and/or pattern of uveitic disease. This offers hope for a logical and uniform approach to immuno-intervention.

MANAGEMENT

Anterior uveitis usually responds to topically applied corticosteroids, which reduce the inflammatory response, and mydriatics, which prevent the sequelae of the disease such as synechiae. It is important to give adequate treatment since the inflammation can escape control and lead to hypopyon uveitis and secondary glaucoma. Corticosteroid drops may be required on an hourly regime, and on occasion subconjunctival corticosteroid may be necessary. Very rarely, systemic corticosteroids may be necessary to treat severe AAU. Chronic anterior uveitis is more difficult to treat and, while it is usually responsive to systemic corticosteroids, clearly their long-term use is ill-advised, particularly since many patients are children. Exceptionally, resort has been made to treating such cases with alternative immunosuppression, including methotrexate, azathioprine and cyclosporin A, as for posterior uveitis.

Posterior uveitis may not require therapy when vision is not affected and the symptoms are restricted to floaters, as occurs in milder forms of pars planitis. However, if vision is threatened, treatment with systemic immunosuppressants is usually indicated, provided that all infectious causes of uveitis have been excluded. It is current practice to start treatment with systemic corticosteroids at a high dose and to reduce this rapidly to a level at which the inflammation can be adequately controlled. If this controlling dose is unacceptably high, or if the inflammation is reactivated during dose reduction, alternative therapies may be necessary. Recently, cyclosporin A has been shown to be effective in chronic sight-threatening posterior uveitis, but the initial studies reported a significant level of renal toxicity among other side effects[39]. Low-dose cyclosporin A therefore has been used with less but still appreciable renal toxicity[40]. It has been shown that close monitoring of renal glomerular and tubular function together with early detection of signs of hypertension minimize the risks of renal damage.

Other immunosuppressants, such as azathioprine, cyclophosphamide and chlorambucil, are within the armamentarium of therapy but each has significant side effects restricting its use. In addition some value has been obtained from the use of low-dose methotrexate.

Despite these new approaches, treatment of severe refractory uveitis can be unsatisfactory in some cases. Accordingly, new therapies are currently under evaluation such as the immunosuppressants FK506 and mycophenolic acid; monoclonal antibody therapy such as antibodies to CD4 lymphocytes[41]; and protocols such as tolerance induction via mucosal immunization[42,43]. However, these are mostly within the experimental realm at present.

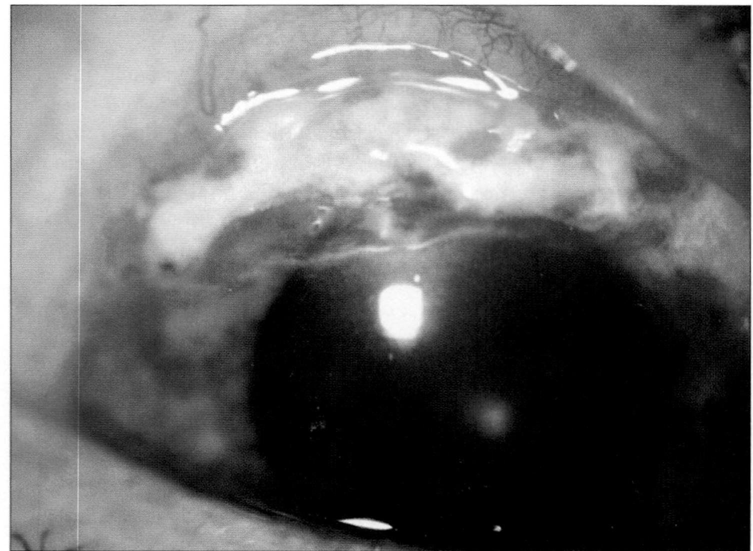

Fig. 6.8 Marginal ulceration of cornea in a patient with systemic vasculitis and nephropathy.

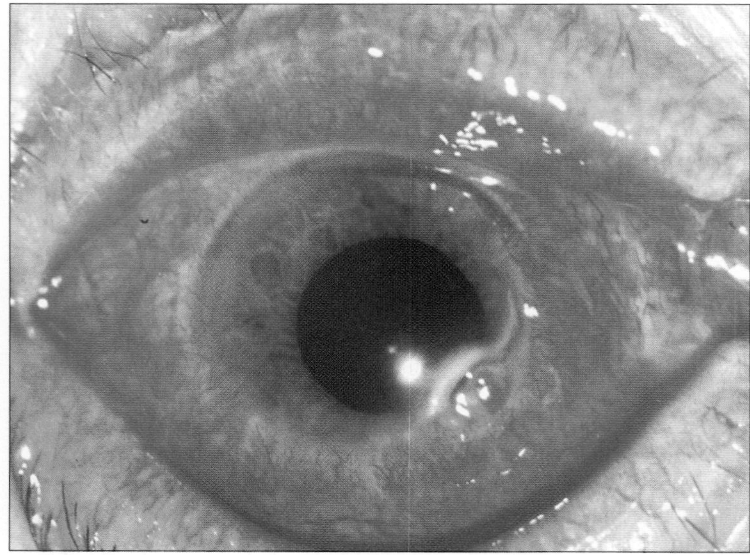

Fig. 6.9 Active corneal ulceration with corneal infiltrates at the 'leading edge' of an ulcer, and considerable associated conjunctival injection.

CORNEAL DISEASE

Corneal manifestations of rheumatologic disease include marginal ulceration, marginal thinning, keratolysis and sclerosing keratitis. Limbal vasculitis may also be seen as a rare manifestation. The cornea is also involved in dry eye disease, which is dealt with separately.

MARGINAL ULCERATION AND MARGINAL THINNING

Both of these conditions are relatively common in RA and may even occur in the elderly in the absence of arthritis as part of the aging process. Usually the lower half of the cornea is involved in a painless furrowing of the corneal periphery (Fig. 6.8) which normally remains epithelialized. The etiology is unknown and it has been linked to immunologically mediated vasculitis of the pericorneal vessels. In the absence of systemic disease, however, it is assumed to be due to impaired vascular supply at the limbus. Marginal thinning with descemetocele and corneal perforation may also occur in other connective tissue disorders, such as Wegener's granulomatosis, relapsing polychondritis, SLE and progressive systemic sclerosis. No treatment is necessary unless there is an associated inflammation or there is breakdown of the corneal epithelium with development of corneal ulceration, as shown in Figure 6.9.

KERATOLYSIS

Keratolysis may occur as a primary disorder related to the underlying connective tissue disease but more commonly occurs secondary to some other pathology, such as dry eye disease leading to corneal ulceration and perforation. Frequently, this sequence of events is precipitated by intercurrent infection producing, for example, a corneal abscess which causes loss of central corneal stromal tissue. In a number of series, RA accounted for 8–15% of all cases of corneal perforation[44].

Treatment of corneal ulceration and incipient perforation can be difficult. Topical antibiotics and mydriatics are required to clear any secondary infection and prevent complications of intraocular inflammation. A corneal abscess or hypopyon (Fig. 6.10) mandates a thorough search for causative organisms, sometimes requiring sampling of aqueous fluid or corneal biopsy material. The latter may be particularly necessary in antibiotic-resistant cases in which mycotic infection is suspected.

In sterile corneal ulcers and perforations the management is aimed more towards a presumed immunologically mediated cause. Local and systemic immunosuppression is indicated, initially with corticosteroids. In cases of Wegener's granulomatosis the drug of choice is cyclophosphamide; recently, in some cases of incipient perforation, systemic cyclosporin A has proved valuable. Recent attempts to introduce topical cyclosporin as a treatment for severe marginal corneal ulceration (Mooren's ulcer, see below)[45] have been reported but this drug awaits the introduction of a suitable vehicle for topical use due to its high lipophilicity.

In many cases, surgical intervention is necessary. Very small central corneal perforations (<1.5mm in diameter) may be sealed with a tissue adhesive such as cyanoacrylate glue. Frank perforation usually requires emergency keratoplasty if any useful vision is to be salvaged. In certain disorders that have a significant vasculitic component, recession of the limbal conjunctiva has been attempted in order to reduce the level of inflammatory cytokines draining towards the site of damage, but no study has shown clear benefit using this approach.

In patients who are systemically unwell and unfit for major surgery, a temporary conjunctival hood may be used but this consigns the eye to the development of a dense corneal leukoma. Ultimately, a planned penetrating keratoplasty will be required if vision is to be restored.

In cases of fulminant infection with endophthalmitis, it may be impossible to salvage the eye itself, even with major anterior segment reconstruction, including lensectomy and vitrectomy. In these cases, evisceration of the globe may be necessary to control the infection.

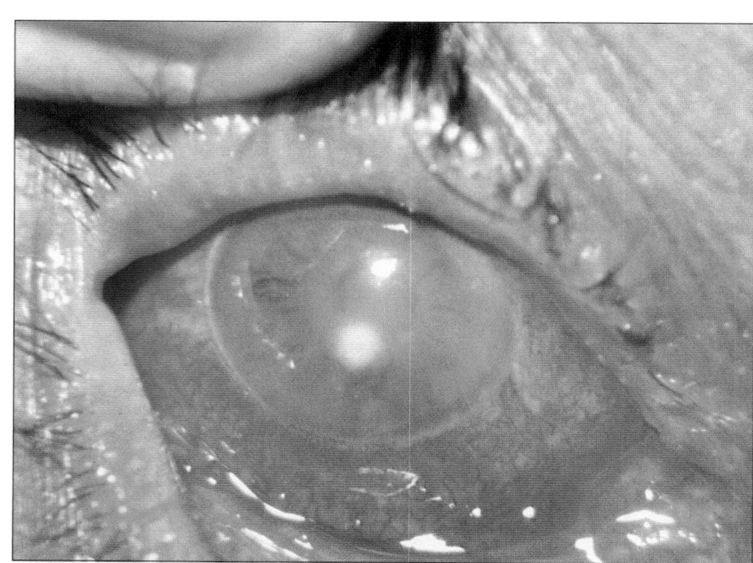

Fig. 6.10 Paracentral corneal abscess with diffuse corneal edema and conjunctival infection.

As indicated above, the etiology of many of these melting disorders of the cornea is unclear. Since they occur predominantly in severe RA, often with a vasculitic component, it is assumed that the same autoimmune processes are at work, but the precise nature of the antigen in the cornea is not known. In some cases, differentiation from Mooren's ulcer, a painful melting disorder of the peripheral cornea characterized by an overhanging edge to the ulcer, can be difficult and is based merely on the absence of systemic connective tissue disease. Recent studies have suggested that the cornea contains pathogenic autoantigens which can induce disease in patients with Mooren's ulcer[46]. Corneal stromal dissolution due to collagenase secretion by infiltrating inflammatory cells, and even by the corneal epithelium, has long been suggested as a mechanism, but the nature of the stimulus for this process is also not known. If this group of disorders is autoimmune in nature, then animal studies indicate that they are likely to be T-cell mediated and tissue damage is probably induced by activated cytolytic T-cells or macrophages. The latter cell is a major source of collagenase.

SCLEROSING KERATITIS

Sclerosing keratitis is the most common corneal complication of scleritis (see below)[47]. In this disorder, pericorneal or limbal inflammation is accompanied by peripheral corneal vessels which advance across the central cornea preceded by superficial stromal opacities, which probably represent inflammatory lymphocytes. In nodular scleritis the corneal involvement may be restricted to one segment (Fig. 6.11), but in diffuse scleritis the entire cornea may be involved, producing a dense corneal leukoma. Perforation of the cornea may occur even when it is sclerosed and is associated with corneal epithelial breakdown. Treatment of the disease is the same as that for the underlying condition (scleritis, see below).

SCLERAL DISEASE

SCLERITIS AND EPISCLERITIS

Scleritis is a relatively common extra-articular manifestation of RA but is also a feature of other connective tissue diseases, particularly those with a vasculitic component. Such conditions include SLE, AS, psoriatic arthritis, Behçet's disease, relapsing polychondritis and Wegener's granulomatosis. However, approximately 50% of the cases of scleritis present in the absence of systemic disease.

Clinical presentation of episcleritis

The clinical presentation depends on whether only the episclera is involved or whether there is deeper tissue destruction. Episcleritis may be nodular or diffuse and is usually a benign recurrent condition, easily controlled by topical steroid therapy. The disease occurs twice as frequently in women as in men and has a sudden onset of moderate pain and redness of the eye. Sometimes there is minimal pain or only slight discomfort and the redness is noticed by an observer. The redness is often intense and may involve the entire anterior sclera, but more frequently the redness is segmental. The lack of discharge and the good preservation of vision serve to differentiate this condition from other causes of the 'red eye', such as conjunctivitis and iritis.

Nodular episcleritis has a similar presentation but a much more protracted course. The initial segmental redness remains localized over 2–3 days but increases in size and becomes swollen, forming a tender nodule. Slit-lamp examination with a red-free light shows that the underlying deep episcleral and scleral vessels remain normal in contour. Visualization of the deep episcleral vessel system can be assisted by decongesting the superficial vascular bed with a drop of either 1/1000 epinephrine (adrenaline) or 10% phenylephrine. In RA, most of the episcleritis is of the diffuse type, and nodular episcleritis occurs more commonly in nonarthritic or rheumatologic conditions. However, this is not the case with scleritis (see below).

Episcleritis is a self-limiting condition, in the majority of cases resolving spontaneously within 3 weeks. Resolution of the inflammation may be expedited with the use of local corticosteroids; nonsteroidal anti-inflammatory agents such as flurbiprofen have also been used. In severe or recurrent cases, and especially in those where there is a risk of corneal involvement, systemic therapy may be necessary to control the disease.

Clinical presentation of scleritis

Scleritis may be anterior or posterior. Anterior scleritis occurs in three forms: diffuse, nodular and necrotizing with or without inflammation. Scleromalacia perforans is the end stage of severe necrotizing scleritis and is very rare. Perforation may be associated with accompanying malnutrition. Although posterior scleritis is relatively underdiagnosed, anterior scleritis still occurs with greater frequency but the reason for this is not known.

The main feature differentiating episcleritis from scleritis is pain, which in the latter is usually severe and deep-seated. Pain is frequently transmitted to the orbit and face. Scleritis also has an insidious onset and tends to recurrences which can be minimized if the initial attack is adequately treated. Awareness of the condition is therefore probably the most important factor in successfully managing the disease. The course of diffuse and nodular scleritis (Fig. 6.12) is one of eventual resolution, perhaps with some degree of scleral thinning; the course of necrotizing scleritis, however, is usually progressive (see Fig. 6.13).

Clinical signs differentiating episcleritis from diffuse scleritis may be difficult to detect, but a careful examination of the deep scleral vessels

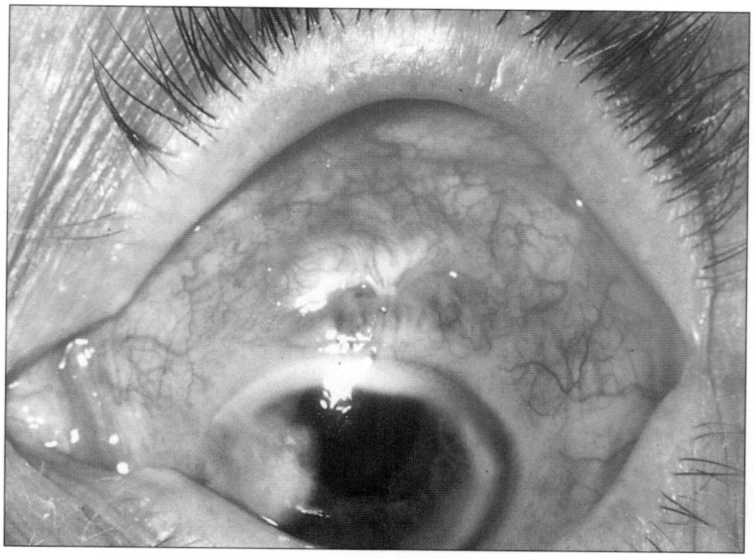

Fig. 6.11 Sclerosing keratitis (white corneal lesion) associated with active necrotizing scleritis (upper quadrant).

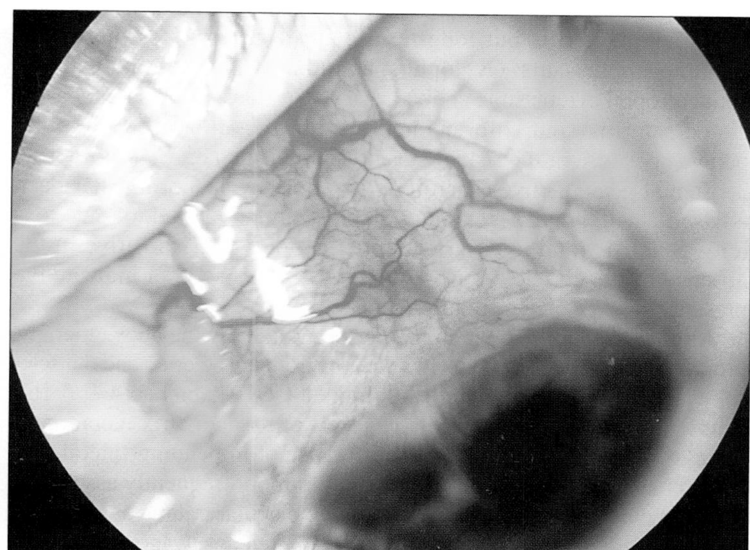

Fig. 6.12 Diffuse and nodular scleritis involving predominantly the upper temporal quadrant of the globe.

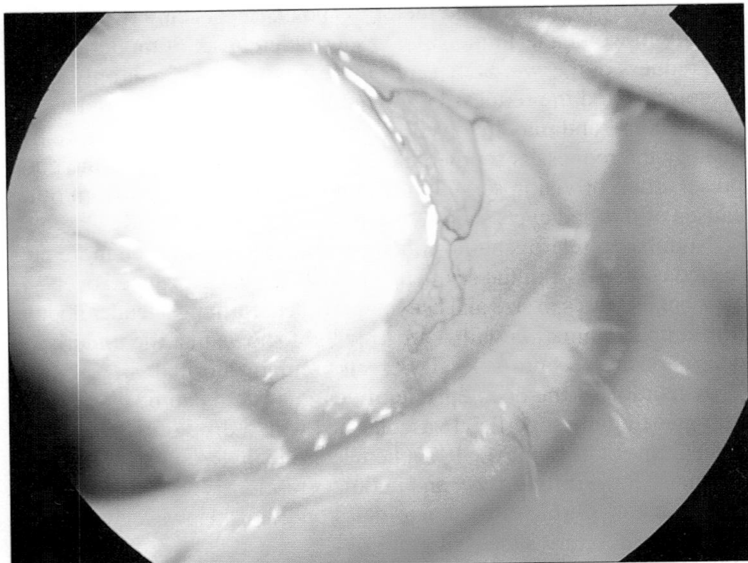

Fig. 6.13 Necrotizing scleritis in severe RA. The area of involved sclera is completely avascular, at risk of perforation, and unresponsive to a range of immunosuppressants.

(see above) will show their involvement in the latter condition. In nodular scleritis, the nodule has a deep red or violaceous color with a consistently abnormal vascular pattern. Recent studies using low-dose anterior segment fluorescein angiography have proved of considerable value in determining the vascular pattern and in estimating the degree of vasculitis-related anterior scleral ischemia[48].

The pathogenesis of scleritis remains poorly understood mainly due to the lack of suitable material for study. A recent large retrospective study of 290 patients with scleritis indicated that patients generally remained within the same category of disease activity through their course. In terms of severity, diffuse scleritis was least progressive while visual loss was 74% in necrotizing disease[49]. In a study of conjunctival and scleral biopsies from 25 patients with scleritis, immune-complex deposition and neutrophil invasion were observed in the vessels, suggesting a role for immune complexes in this aspect of the disease. However, there was also a marked T-cell and macrophage infiltration, with widespread expression of MHC class II antigen on many cell types[50].

The treatment of scleritis requires attention to relief of pain and to halting the progression of the disease. Nonsteroidal anti-inflammatory drugs are useful in controlling non-necrotizing forms of scleritis. Some patients require low-dose systemic corticosteroids for disease control. High-dose corticosteroids are required for initial control of severe necrotizing scleritis but long-term control necessitates the use of immunosuppressants. Cyclophosphamide, particularly indicated in antineutrophil cytoplasmic antibodies (ANCA)-positive vasculitis-associated scleritis, and chlorambucil are not recommended in young patients because of the risk of sterility, and in such cases azathioprine is often also ineffective. Therefore, low-dose cyclosporin A has been advised[51] with good effect, but with close attention paid to renal toxicity. Scleritis (and uveitis) patients may be ANCA positive in the absence of the classic c- or p-antigen and thus need not indicate the presence of Wegener's granulomatosis[52].

Although the inflammation may be controlled by the above therapy, progressive destruction occurs in severe necrotizing scleritis and the scleral wall may become dangerously thinned (see Chapters 5.4 & 5.16). This appears to be due to excessive levels of tissue matrix metalloproteinases[53]. However, despite the appearance of impending scleral rupture in many cases, this rarely occurs and is more frequently associated with some additional pathology, such as mild ocular trauma or infection. When rupture occurs, scleral patching is required to salvage the eye, and fixed donor sclera provides a good support. The graft should cover the entire area of necrosis plus some of the surrounding 'normal' sclera. In addition, a wide conjunctival flap should be fashioned to provide as much vascularization as possible. Corneoscleral perforations are more common in patients with severe RA in whom peripheral corneal ulceration is associated with limbal and scleral inflammation. In these patients, a combined corneoscleral graft may be required to patch the defect.

KERATOCONJUNCTIVITIS SICCA

The classic ocular complication of rheumatologic disease is KCS (dry eye syndrome), and if this is associated with a reduction in salivary secretion, the triad constitutes one form of Sjögren's syndrome (see Chapter 7.32). Pathologically, there is chronic lymphocytic infiltration of the lacrimal and salivary glands as well as involvement of the accessory lacrimal glands and the conjunctival and epithelial layers[54,55]. As a result, conjunctival and corneal punctate erosions occur not only because of the failure of aqueous tear secretion but also because chronic damage to the oil-secreting glands of the palpebral conjunctiva induces more rapid evaporation of tears from the ocular surface and a greater tendency to tear spill-over at the lid margin, due to loss of surface tension. Punctate erosions on the conjunctiva probably occur at sites of focal lymphocytic infiltrate.

CLINICAL MANIFESTATIONS OF KCS

Symptoms of KCS include dryness, ocular irritation, foreign body sensation, photophobia and pain. Sometimes patients complain of excessive tearing which may merely describe a sensation or may in fact be real, due to tear spill-over as described above. The patient is more vulnerable to bouts of recurrent infectious conjunctivitis, perhaps as a result of reduced antibacterial tear lysozyme and lactoferrin. As a result patients are more likely to develop corneal ulcer and perforation.

Clinically the eyes appear minimally affected with loss of surface lustre and perhaps some accumulation of matter at the medial canthus (Fig. 6.14). There is mild pericorneal redness (injection) reflecting the degree of corneal punctate erosions or other keratopathy, but more commonly there is interpalpebral injection and/or inferior bulbar injection, evidence of mild corneal exposure due to nocturnal lagophthalmos and associated with increased evaporation of tears. In severe cases discrete corneal filaments may be macroscopically visible (filamentary keratitis) and these represent tags of exfoliated epithelium, still attached at one end and intermixed with surface mucin.

TESTING FOR KCS

Commonly used tests for dry eye disease include the Schirmer filter paper test in which a strip of absorbent filter paper is placed in the lower fornix and the flow of tears measured in millimeters with time. This test is unreliable, especially when performed in the resting state since there are many variables which regulate normal tear flow[56]. The augmented tear test, in which tear flow is stimulated using agents such as concentrated ammonia or oil of cloves, is more informative but is unpleasant and not frequently used. Decreased flow can be simply observed by determining the

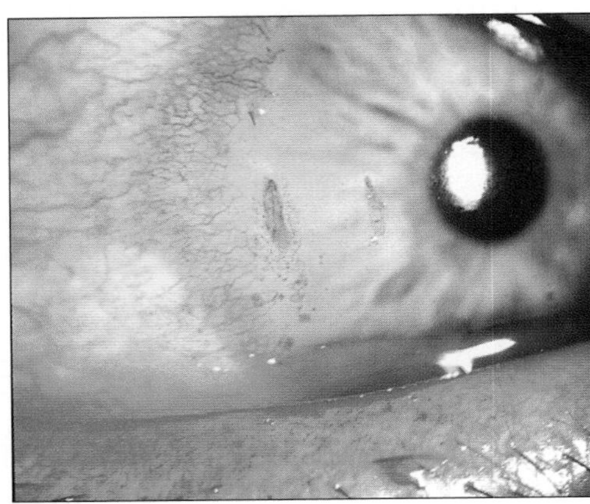

Fig. 6.14 Keratoconjunctivitis sicca.

height of the tear meniscus, since this is a measure of tear volume. Only 7% of normal individuals have a tear meniscus <0.1mm. Interestingly the height of the meniscus does not correlate with the Schirmer test in normal subjects. Reduced aqueous tear component can be confirmed by an increase in tear osmolality, but this test is limited by the difficulties of obtaining a sufficiently large sample for measurement.

Dry spots on the conjunctiva and cornea can readily be made apparent by instilling a drop of fluorescein or Rose Bengal dye, and this is the most reliable method of establishing the diagnosis. Examination using a yellow filter on the slit-lamp microscope will reveal the extent of disease. However, the test with Rose Bengal dye may be acutely irritating due to the dye's low pH, and it should be used with caution. A useful test of disturbed tear film dynamics is the tear film break-up time (BUT) which is determined by examining the tear film with the slit lamp after the instillation of fluorescein drops. More recently a non-invasive test using a grid projected onto the surface of the preocular tear film has been described. In addition the blink rate and the degree of blepharospasm will reflect the extent of corneal erosive disease.

LABORATORY TESTS FOR KCS

There are no specific tests for KCS. Biochemical studies have shown that certain proteins, such as lysozyme and lactoferrin[56], may be reduced in concentration in tears, but these tests are not sensitive enough for clinical use. Other proteins derived from the circulation appear to be increased in concentration. Tear viscosity in KCS is reduced, suggesting a decrease in tear mucin content.

Pathologically, in addition to the chronic round cell infiltration and progressive atrophy of the lacrimal glands, there is goblet cell loss, increased cellular stratification and keratinization of the conjunctiva, and loss of surface microvilli which may reduce mucin adherence and thus wettability of the ocular surface. Impression cytology of the conjunctival epithelium has shown increasingly marked changes in epithelial morphology with severity of KCS. Most of these tests are of research value only and the simple clinical tests described above usually provide the diagnosis. The treatment of KCS is essentially tear replacement therapy. In severe cases this can become extremely difficult and even procedures such as punctal occlusion may be insufficient to control the disease. Recent attempts to control the progressive immunologic destruction of the lacrimal glands have been made using topical cyclosporin but the problem of drug solubility remains[57]. Progressive and repeated corneal ulceration leads to loss of vision due to corneal opacification. However, this extremely rare condition occurs in patients who have KCS in addition to other vasculitis-related disease of the anterior segment of the eye.

REFERENCES

1. Forrester JV. Uveitis. Br J Ophthalmol. 1990;74:620–2.
2. Feltkamp TEW, BreurVriesendorp BS, Derhaag PJFM. HLA-B27 subtypes and acute anterior uveitis: a review. Reg Immunol. 1994;6:8–11.
3. Forrester JV, Liversidge JM, Dua HS, Towler HM, McMenamin PG. Comparison of clinical and experimental uveitis. Curr Eye Res. 1990;9(suppl):75–84.
4. Acha-Orbea H, Palmer E. Mls-a retrovirus exploits the immune system. Immunol Today. 1991;12:356–61.
5. Smit RLMJ, Baarsma GS. Epidemiology of uveitis [editorial review]. Curr Opin Ophthalmol. 1995;6:57–61.
6. Miettinen R, Sari M. Clinical characteristics of familial acute anterior uveitis. Can J Ophthalmol. 1977;12:1–8.
7. Rothova A, van Veenendal WG, Linssen A, Glasius E, Kijlstra A, de Jong P. Clinical features of acute anterior uveitis. Am J Ophthalmol. 1987;103:137–45.
8. Machsymowych WP, Russell AS. Polymorphism in the *LMP2* gene influences the relative risk for acute anterior uveitis in unselected patients with ankylosing spondylitis. Clin Invest Med. 1995;18:42–6.
9. Kanski JJ. Juvenile arthritis and uveitis. Survey Ophthalmol. 1990;34:253–67.
10. Murray P. Serum autoantibodies and uveitis. Br J Ophthalmol. 1986;70:266–8.
11. Cabral DA, Petty RE, Malleson PN, Ensworth S, McCormack AQ, Shroeder ML. Visual prognosis in children with chronic anterior uveitis and arthritis. J Rheumatol. 1994;21:2370–5.
12. Rothova A, Buitenhuis HJ, Meenken C, *et al.* Uveitis and systemic disease. Br J Ophthalmol. 1991;76:137–41.
13. Sharp DC, Bell RA, Patterson E, Pinkerton RMH. Sympathetic ophthalmia: histopathologic and fluorescein angiographic correlation. Arch Ophthalmol. 1984;102:232–5.
14. BenEzra D, Forrester JV. Fundal white dots: the spectrum of a similar pathological process. Br J Ophthalmol. 1995;79:856–60.
15. Martin T, Weber M, Schmitt C, Weber JC, Tongio MM, Flament J. Association of intermediate uveitis with HLA-A28: definition of a new syndrome? Albrect von Graefe's Arch Klin Exp Ophthalmol. 1995;233:269–74.
16. Kijlstra A. The value of laboratory testing in uveitis. Eye. 1991;4:732–6.
17. Jakobiec F, Marboe C, Knowles D, *et al.* Human sympathetic ophthalmia. Ophthalmology. 1983;90:76–95.
18. Feltkamp TEJ. Are gram-negative bacteria involved in HLA-B27 associated uveitis? Br J Ophthalmol. 1995;79:718.
19. Bjorkman PJ, Sayer MA, Samraoui B, Bennett WS, Strominger JL, Wiley DC. The foreign antigen binding site and T cell recognition regions of Class 1 histocompatibility antigens. Nature. 1987;329:566–72.
20. Careless DJ, Inman RD. Acute anterior uveitis: clinical and experimental aspects. Semin Arthritis Rheum. 1995;24:432–41.
21. LeirisaloRepo M. Enteropathic arthritis, Whipple's disease, juvenile spondyloarthropathy and uveitis. Curr Opin Rheum. 1994;6:385–90.
22. Rosenbaum JT, McDevitt HO, Guss RB, Egber PR. Endotoxin-induced uveitis in rats as a model for human disease. Nature. 1980;286:611–13.
23. Waksman BH, Bullington SJ. Studies of arthritis and other lesions induced in rats by injection of mycobacterial adjuvant. Arch Ophthalmol. 1960;64:751–61.
24. Cohen IR. The self, the world and autoimmunity. Sci Am. 1988;258:834–40.
25. Broekhuyse RM, Kuhlmann ED, Winkens HJ. Experimental autoimmune anterior uveitis. 1. Induction by a detergent-insoluble, intrinsic protein fraction of the retinal pigment epithelium. Exp Eye Res. 1991;52:465–11.
26. Chan CC, Hikita N, Dastgheib K, Whitcup SM, Nussenblatt RB. Experimental melanin-protein induced uveitis (EMIU,formerly EAAU): immunopathologic processes. Ophthalmology. 1994;101:1275–81.
27. Gery I. Retinal antigens and the immunopathologic process they provoke. Prog Retinal Res. 1986;5:75–109.
28. Gery I, Chanaud NP, Anglade E. Recoverin is highly uveitogenic in Lewis rats. Invest Ophthalmol Vis Sci. 1994;35:3342–5.
29. McMenamin PG, Broekhuyse RM, Forrester JV. Ultrastructural pathology of experimental autoimmune uveitis: a review. Micron. 1992;24:521–46.
30. Borst DF, Donoso L, Merryman C, *et al.* S antigen: Characterisation of a pathogenic epitope which mediates experimental autoimmune uveitis and pinealitis in Lewis rats. Curr Eye Res. 1987;6:1151–9.
31. Sanui H, Redmond TM, Kotake S, *et al.* Identification of an immunodominant and highly immunopathogenic determinant in the retinal interphotoreceptor retinoid-binding protein (IRBP). J Exp Med. 1989;169:1947–60.
32. Dua HS, Lee RH, Lolley RN, *et al.* Induction of experimental autoimmune uveitis by the retinal photoreceptor cell protein, phosducin. Curr Eye Res. 1992;11(suppl):107–12.
33. Priem HA, Oosterhuis JA. Birdshot retinochoroidopathy. Am J Ophthalmol. 1988;105:182–5.
34. Yamamoto JH, Minami M, Inaba G, Masuda K, Mochizuki M. Cellular immunity to retinal specific antigens in patients with Behçet's disease. Br J Ophthalmol. 1993;77:584–9.
35. Falk K, Rotzschke O, Takiguchi M, *et al.* Peptide motifs of HLA-B51, -B52 and -B78 molecules, and implications for Behçet's disease. Int Immunol. 1995;7:223–8.
36. Singh VK, Hanspreet KK, Kumihiko Y, Tohru A, Donoso LA, Shinohara T. Molecular mimicry between a uveitopathogenic site of S-antigen and viral peptide. J Immunol. 1990;144:1282–7.
37. Singh VK, Yamaki K, Donoso LA, Shinohara T. Yeast histone H3-induced experimental autoimmune uveoretinitis. J Immunol. 1989;142:1512–7.
38. Pervin K, Childerstone A, Shinnick T, *et al.* T cell epitope expression of mycobacterial and hohmologous human 65-kiladalton heat shock protein peptides in short term cell lines from patients with Behçet's disease. J Immunol. 1993;151:2273–82.

39. Nussenblatt RB, Palestine AG, Chan CC. Cyclosporin A therapy in the treatment of intraocular inflammatory disease resistant to systemic corticosteroids and cytotoxic agents. Am J Ophthalmol. 1983;96:275–82.
40. Towler HM, Cliffe AM, Whiting PH, Forrester JV. Low dose cyclosporin A therapy in chronic posterior uveitis. Eye. 1989;3:282–7.
41. Isaacs JD, Hale G, Waldmann H, *et al.* Monoclonal antibody therapy of chronic intraocular inflammation using campath-1H. Br J Ophthalmol. 1995;79:1054–5.
42. Dick AD, Cheng YF, Liversidge J, Forrester JV. Intranasal administration of retinal antigens suppresses retinal antigen-induced experimental autoimmune uveoretinitis. Immunology. 1994;82:625–31.
43. Nussenblatt RB, Caspi RR, Mahdi R, *et al.* Inhibition of S-antigen induced EAU by oral induction of tolerance with S-antigen. J Immunol. 1990;144:1689–95.
44. Portnoy SL, Insler MS, Kaufman HE. Surgical management of corneal ulceration and perforation. Survey Ophthalmol. 1989;34:47–58.
45. Zhao JC, Jin XY. Immunological analysis and treatment of Mooren's ulcer with cyclosporin A applied topically. Cornea. 1993;12:481–8.
46. Gottsch JD, Liu SH, Minkovitz JB, Goodman DF, Srinivasan M, Strak WJ. Autoimmunity to a corneal-associated stromal antigen in patients with Mooren's ulcer. Invest Ophthalmol Vis Sci. 1995;36:1541–7.
47. De la Maza MS, Jabbur NS, Foster CS. Severity of scleritis and episcleritis. Ophthalmology. 1994;101:389–396.
48. Watson PG, Booth-Mason S. Fluorescein angiography in the differential diagnosis of sclerokeratitis. Br J Ophthalmol. 1987;71:145–51.
49. Tuft SJ, Watson PG. Progression of scleral disease. Ophthalmology. 1991;98:467–71.
50. Fong LP, de la Maza MS, Rice B, Kupperman AE, Foster CS. Immunopathology of scleritis. Ophthalmology. 1991;98:472–9.
51. Hakin KN, Ham J, Lightman SL. Use of cyclosporin in the management of steroid-dependent non-necrotising scleritis. Br J Ophthalmol. 1991;75:340–1.
52. Hagen EC, van de VijverReenalda H, de Keizer RJW, *et al.* Uveitis and anti-neutrophil cytoplasmic antibodies. Clin Exp Immunol. 1994;95:56–9.
53. Di Girolamo N, McLuskey PJ, Lloyd A, Wakefield D. Stromelysin (matrix metalloproteinase-3) and tissue inhibitor of metalloproteinas (TIMP-1) mRNA expression in scleritis. Ocular Immunol Inflamm. 1995;3:181–5.
54. Williamson J, Gibson AAM, Wilson T, Whaley K, Forrester JV. The histology of the lacrimal gland in keratoconjunctivitis sicca. Br J Ophthalmol. 1973;57:852–8.
55. Damato B, Allan D, Murray SB, Lee WR. Senile atrophy of the human lacrimal gland: the contribution of chronic inflammatory disease. Br J Ophthalmol. 1984;68:674–8.
56. Bron AJ, Mengher LS. The ocular surface in keratoconjunctivitis sicca. Eye. 1989;3:428–37.
57. Laibovitz RA, Solch S, Andriano K, O'Connell M, Silverman MH. Pilot trial of cyclosporine 1% ophthalmic ointment in the treatment of keratoconjunctivitis sicca. Cornea. 1993;12:315–23.

7

CARDIOPULMONARY SYMPTOMS IN RHEUMATIC DISEASE

Michael H Crawford & John Sergent

- Cardiopulmonary symptoms are a common clinical feature of most systemic rheumatic disorders.
- Cardiac and pulmonary pathologies may develop in virtually all of the connective tissue disorders as well as in RA and the seronegative spondyloarthropathies.
- Rheumatologic symptoms, including arthritis and myositis, may be a complication of drugs used to treat cardiopulmonary disorders.

SYMPTOMS OF CARDIOPULMONARY DISEASE

Cardiopulmonary symptoms may develop in virtually all of the systemic inflammatory rheumatic diseases. However, with the exception of systemic lupus erythematosus (SLE), they are usually not among the presenting features of rheumatic disorders. For the most part, rheumatic disease patients with cardiopulmonary symptoms have a well established diagnosis at the time of their chest symptoms. The most important chest symptoms indicative of cardiopulmonary pathology are chest pain, dyspnea, cough, hemoptysis and edema.

PLEURITIC CHEST PAIN

Pericarditis

Patients with acute pericarditis in association with a rheumatic disease have a presentation which is usually identical to idiopathic pericarditis, with sharp, pleuritic substernal pain exacerbated by lying flat and occasionally by swallowing. The pain is typically relieved by sitting up or assuming an upright posture. Tamponade or constrictive pericarditis are uncommon, and the diagnosis is relatively easy once it is suspected. Elevated jugular venous pressure and a pulsus paradoxus are present in nearly all patients, and many patients with constrictive pericarditis will have a paradoxic increase in the jugular venous pressure during inspiration (Kussmaul's sign).

Clinical pericarditis occurs at some time during the course of at least 25% of patients with SLE (see Chapter 7.1). It is also common in systemic juvenile rheumatoid arthritis (Still's disease) and occurs less frequently in rheumatoid arthritis (RA) and scleroderma. Large pericardial effusions and tamponade, with or without prior symptoms of pericarditis, may develop in SLE[1].

Patients with RA are at risk of developing chronic constrictive pericarditis[2]. While uncommon, it is important to recognize and treat this syndrome early. Patients are most likely to be seropositive men with rheumatoid nodules and other nonarticular manifestations[3]. The presentation is typically insidious, with the gradual development of edema, exertional fatigue, some dyspnea and general failure to thrive[4].

Clinical pericarditis, with or without significant effusion, may be seen rarely in patients with dermatomyositis, systemic sclerosis and several forms of vasculitis. In systemic sclerosis the development of an often asymptomatic pericardial effusion has been noted as an occasional forerunner of scleroderma renal crisis and a poor prognosis[5].

Pleurisy

The pain of pleurisy is usually moderate and intermittent, but occasional patients have severe, constant pain, requiring narcotics for relief. The pain may be localized or migratory, and splinting may be so severe that patients may complain of dyspnea as well as pain. The combination of dyspnea and pleuritic pain raises the possibility of a pulmonary embolus, especially in patients with antiphospholipid antibodies.

The majority of patients with systemic lupus will have episodes of pleuritic pain during their course, usually in association with general flares of the disease (see Chapter 7.1). Any pleural effusions which develop are usually small and resolve with either corticosteroid treatment or the passage of time.

Rheumatoid arthritis is associated with symptomatic pleural disease in up to 20% of cases. In most patients this consists of mild pleuritic pain which is intermittent and relatively easily managed, and usually occurs early in the course. About 1% will have an associated rheumatoid pleural effusion of variable size. On occasion these can be large enough to impair lung function, with associated dyspnea or exertion. These large effusions often have the characteristics of an empyema, and can fibrose, causing restrictive lung disease[6].

Pleuritic chest pain is an occasional feature of systemic sclerosis, but it is rarely an important clinical problem. Still's disease may be frequently associated with pleural pain during the acute, toxic phase of the disease. Various forms of vasculitis, especially Wegener's granulomatosis, may also be associated with pleural chest pain. Pleurisy, in association with connective tissue disease or vasculitis, obligates the clinician to search for other causes of pleural disease, in particular infection.

DYSPNEA

Dyspnea in the rheumatic diseases may be due to a variety of causes including lung disease, heart disease, severe anemia, diseases of the chest wall, generalized or focal muscle weakness or severe deconditioning.

Dyspnea in patients with RA is nearly always an indication of serious underlying disease. In addition to the large pleural effusions mentioned above, rheumatoid lung disease occurs in over 10% of patients with seropositive RA[7]. It consists of an inflammatory interstitial infiltrate, associated with progressive pulmonary fibrosis.

Cardiac involvement due to RA can also present with dyspnea. Patients with constrictive pericarditis (see above) often have mild dyspnea, although their major complaint is usually marked fatigue and weakness. Involvement of the heart itself due to RA is rare, but can present as a catastrophic emergency. Rheumatoid nodules can occur anywhere in the heart, but tend to concentrate along the heart skeleton. For this reason, involvement of the heart with rheumatoid nodules can present with complete heart block or acute aortic insufficiency. Finally, there have been a few cases reported of valvular heart disease due to rheumatoid nodules forming on the valve leaflets[8].

Systemic lupus erythematosus

The most common cause of dyspnea in SLE is probably diaphragmatic weakness. In most cases this is a rather mild problem, and can only be detected by sophisticated methodologies. However, in severe cases patients with lupus may actually present with 'vanishing lung disease', due to the virtual total paralysis of the diaphragm. Patients with lupus may also develop interstitial pneumonitis and pulmonary fibrosis identical to that seen in RA and in some of the other rheumatic diseases.

Cardiac disease due to Libman–Sacks endocarditis is usually asymptomatic for many years after the murmurs are first audible. However, this disorder can eventually cause either aortic or mitral insufficiency, or both, and present with dyspnea as a manifestation of cardiac failure.

A small subset of lupus patients will develop pulmonary hypertension. These can be broken down into two groups. First of all, some patients develop a pulmonary hypertension that resembles idiopathic pulmonary hypertension, with onion-skin changing of the small arterioles in the lung. This is relatively uncommon in lupus, and more frequently seen in systemic sclerosis (see below). In addition, patients with lupus who have antiphospholipid antibodies are at risk for thrombogenic pulmonary hypertension (see below).

Finally, patients with lupus may develop severe anemia, due to autoimmune hemolytic anemia, the anemia of end-stage renal disease or occasionally due to bone marrow failure. These patients typically have dyspnea as one of their major clinical manifestations.

Systemic sclerosis

Systemic sclerosis may cause dyspnea through a number of different mechanisms, but lung disease is a major cause of morbidity and mortality in the disease (see Chapters 7.9 and Practical Problem 7.12, Pulmonary evaluation and management). Occasional patients have severe involvement of the chest wall to the point that they develop restrictive lung disease. These patients are usually nearly at end-stage, and have marked restriction of their exercise capacity. Restrictive lung disease usually presents as an inflammatory interstitial pneumonitis with cough and dyspnea, and often progresses to severe pulmonary fibrosis.

Pulmonary hypertension in scleroderma, as in lupus, may resemble idiopathic pulmonary hypertension. The pulmonary hypertension is usually progressive and severe, leading to death in virtually all patients.

Finally, patients with scleroderma and dyspnea should always be evaluated for the possibility of chronic aspiration. Many of these patients complain of heartburn and nocturnal and early morning cough, but symptoms are by no means present in all. It is the practice of many physicians to assume that virtually all patients with scleroderma have nocturnal aspiration, and to prophylax accordingly, since virtually all have esophageal dysfunction.

Polymyositis and dermatomyositis

Polymyositis and dermatomyositis are both associated with dyspnea due to weakness of the chest wall and diaphragm (see Chapter 7.13). They present as restrictive lung disease and, especially in children, can be quite severe and the occasional cause of death. In addition, these disorders are associated with a pulmonary fibrosis which resembles that seen in RA patients. The vast majority of these individuals will have antisynthetase autoantibodies, most commonly antihistidyl tRNA synthetase (Jo-1).

Antiphospholipid antibody syndrome

Patients with antiphospholipid antibodies, with or without systemic lupus, may present with insidious worsening of dyspnea (see Chapter 7.35). These patients are very likely to have thrombogenic hypertension, and may have never had acute pulmonary embolus symptoms. The etiology is presumed to be a combination of small emboli plus *in situ* pulmonary thrombosis.

Sjögren's syndrome

Sjögren's syndrome patients are at extremely high risk of recurrent pulmonary infections (see Chapter 7.32). These infections are due to dryness of the tracheobronchial tree, leading to abnormal ciliary function and the inability to clear bacteria. Many of these patients have a chronic productive cough and other symptoms of infection, but many do not. Patients with Sjögren's syndrome who are developing these symptoms should be treated with appropriate antibiotics and good pulmonary toilet. Sjögren's syndrome is also occasionally associated with an inflammatory pulmonary fibrosis similar to that seen in RA.

Ankylosing spondylitis and other spondyloarthropathies

Ankylosing spondylitis (AS) and, less frequently, the other spondyloarthropathies may cause dyspnea for a number of different reasons. The most frequent is restrictive lung disease due to involvement of the costovertebral joints, with restriction of thoracic cage movement. This is rarely a major problem in people who do not have another lung disease but, especially in smokers, a combination of chronic bronchitis and/or emphysema plus AS may lead to severe pulmonary dysfunction.

Patients with AS may also develop aortic insufficiency. Involvement of the aorta in this disease occurs in patients after many years of disease and is more or less proportional to the severity of the AS. The aortitis causes a gradual dilation of the aorta, with the slow progression of aortic insufficiency[9]. The murmur is typically audible for several years before dyspnea develops.

Finally, patients with AS may develop apical pulmonary fibrosis. This generally presents with dyspnea and cough, but rarely causes severe pulmonary dysfunction unless it is also accompanied by another lung disease.

OTHER CARDIOPULMONARY SYMPTOMS

Cough and hemoptysis may be the initial or late presentation of Wegener's granulomatosis (see Chapter 7.22). On rare occasions, when a granulomatous region within the lungs sloughs, the hemoptysis may be life threatening. Alveolar hemorrhage with hemoptysis is a rare but also life-threatening manifestation of SLE.

Systemic lupus patients, especially when hypocomplementemic or immunosuppressed, have an increased susceptibility to a variety of community-acquired and nosocomial pneumonias.

In addition lupus patients, and to a lesser extent other rheumatic disease patients treated with corticosteroids, are at increased risk for coronary artery disease. Lupus mortality has a bimodal distribution, with an increased death rate in the first 5 years of disease, usually due to complications of the disease or its treatment, and a second period of increased death at 15–20 years, primarily due to early coronary artery disease. The etiology of this coronary artery disease is thought to be multifactorial, and includes hypertension, small vessel coronary arteritis, and hyperlipidemia due to nephrotic syndrome and/or corticosteroids[10].

Fever

Subjective fever can be caused by pericarditis or myocarditis, but should also raise the possibility of endocarditis. Fever is a major symptom of endocarditis, and patients with rheumatic diseases such as SLE or the antiphospholipid antibody syndrome may have underlying valvular abnormalities that can serve as a nidus for infectious endocarditis. Fever can also be a manifestation of opportunistic infections in the lungs, hypersensitivity pneumonitis or pleurisy.

Palpitations

Palpitations may represent cardiac arrhythmias due to myocarditis or pericarditis. Pericarditis more often irritates the atria, causing atrial tachyarrhythmias such as fibrillation or flutter. Myocarditis usually causes premature contractions of the ventricles or ventricular tachycardia. Heart failure can be a complication of myocarditis or severe valvular involvement in the rheumatologic diseases. Heart failure can also result in atrial and ventricular tachyarrhythmias. Finally, hypoxia from lung involvement in rheumatic diseases may result in cardiac arrhythmias, especially ventricular arrhythmias.

Syncope

Syncope may be caused by atrial or, more commonly, by ventricular tachyarrhythmias. Syncope can also be caused by atrioventricular block, which can occur as a manifestation of the rheumatologic involvement of the myocardium. In addition, syncope can be due to pulmonary hypertension secondary to rheumatologic involvement of the lungs. Severe pulmonary hypertension fixes the cardiac output, and so any exertion or other demand for increased blood supply may result in reduced cerebral blood flow and syncope.

Edema

Edema may be due to right, left or biventricular heart failure, caused by rheumatologic involvement of the heart or lungs. In addition, chronic constrictive pericarditis due to rheumatologic involvement of the pericardium, or chronic restrictive cardiomyopathy due to amyloidosis of the heart secondary to rheumatologic diseases, can lead to significant peripheral edema.

TESTING FOR CARDIOPULMONARY DISEASE

ELECTROCARDIOGRAM

The electrocardiogram (ECG) is extremely useful for confirming the diagnosis of pericarditis. The classic pattern of diffuse ST segment elevation is almost pathognomonic of this entity (Fig. 7.1). Unfortunately, not all patients with pericarditis display this classic ECG pattern. Some have more nonspecific ST T-wave changes, which could suggest the diagnosis of myocarditis. There are no specific ECG findings for myocarditis, and the typical ECG pattern of acute myocardial infarction is rarely seen. Conduction abnormalities are readily detected by the ECG, the most serious being complete atrioventricular (AV) block. The ECG may show right ventricular hypertrophy in patients with severe pulmonary hypertension. Patients with marked valvular disease of the left heart can show left ventricular hypertrophy and left atrial enlargement. Systemic hypertension can result in the pattern of left ventricular hypertrophy and left atrial enlargement as well. Continuous ECG recordings (using a Holter monitor) or event recorders can be useful in patients with palpitations and syncope to record any rhythm disturbances during their symptoms.

RADIOGRAPHIC TECHNIQUES

A plain radiograph of the chest is extremely useful for detecting cardiac enlargement, pleural effusion and parenchymal lung disease. With severe pulmonary hypertension there may be peripheral pruning of the pulmonary vasculature and selective right heart enlargement. Computed tomography (CT) or magnetic resonance imaging (MRI) are particularly useful for confirming thickened pericardium in cases of suspected constrictive pericarditis or chronic symptomatic pericarditis. It is important to confirm that the pericardium is diseased before attempting pericardiectomy for patients with chronic chest pain syndromes.

LABORATORY TESTS

In patients with cardiac symptoms, routine blood work may reveal anemia. This can either cause or aggravate cardiac symptomatology, especially in patients with underlying rheumatologic involvement of the heart. Pulmonary manifestations of rheumatologic diseases may be shown by the presence of hypoxia, which can be detected by arterial blood gases or the measurement of oxygen saturation by finger oximeter. Rheumatologic tests are usually of little value in the evaluation of patients with cardiopulmonary symptomatology, since there is no defined relationship between abnormal rheumatologic tests and cardiopulmonary manifestations of disease.

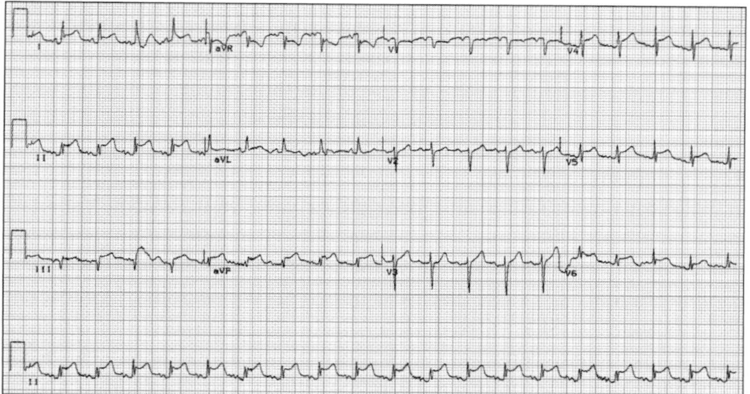

Fig. 7.1 12-lead ECG exhibiting changes consistent with acute pericarditis in a 23-year-old woman with SLE. Note ST elevation in all but leads AVL and V1, which are isoelectric, and AVR, which shows reciprocal ST depression. This pattern is practically diagnostic for pericarditis in the appropriate clinical setting.

EXERCISE TESTS

Exercise or pharmacologic stress tests are occasionally of value in diagnosing chest pain syndromes in patients with rheumatologic diseases. Because rheumatologic involvement of the heart may result in nonspecific ST T-wave changes on the electrocardiogram, standard exercise ECG testing has a lower sensitivity and specificity in patients with rheumatologic disease. Thus, in most patients an imaging stress test should be performed by utilizing either nuclear perfusion scanning or echocardiography (see below).

PULMONARY FUNCTION TESTS

In patients with pulmonary symptoms, pulmonary function testing can confirm the presence of restrictive or obstructive lung disease due to the rheumatologic involvement of the chest wall, pulmonary parenchyma and bronchial system. The most common abnormalities on pulmonary function testing are those of restrictive lung disease due to fibrosing alveolitis: reduced vital capacity and static lung volumes, reduced carbon dioxide diffusing capacity, increased lung stiffness and occasionally hypoxia (see Fig. 7.2).

FLUID ANALYSIS

Pericardial or pleural fluid can be valuable in establishing the etiology of a suspected rheumatic disease process. Pericardial fluid is rarely obtained solely for diagnostic purposes because of the dangers of this technique, but diagnostic pleural taps are frequently done when there are pleural effusions of unknown etiology. Usually, SLE fluids are exudative with lymphocytosis, normal glucose and a low C3. A positive ANA in pleural fluid is considered diagnostic. Rheumatoid arthritis fluid is exudative and serosanguineous with high neutrophil counts (> 200/mm^3), high lactic dehydrogenase (LDH) levels, and low glucose and C3 levels.

BIOPSY

It may be useful to perform a myocardial biopsy in selected patients to confirm the diagnosis of myocarditis. Such a decision may dictate the aggressiveness of anti-inflammatory treatment. Pericardial biopsy can be done if surgical drainage of fluid is required, and shows deposits of IgG, IgM, C3 and C1q by immunofluorescence. Pleural biopsy can also be useful in patients with RA if nodules are seen. Usually rheumatologic involvement of the pleura produces a chronic inflammatory histologic picture without vasculitis. Diagnostic heart or lung biopsies are rarely indicated.

RADIONUCLIDE STUDIES

Radionuclide tagging of red blood cells with technetium-99m is a useful technique for determining right and left ventricular performance[11]. Myocardial perfusion scanning with thallium-201 or technetium-99m-labeled sestimibi is useful for determining vascular problems with the myocardium. A lack of myocardial perfusion may be seen segmentally during stress testing in patients with myocarditis or significant coronary vasculitis. If such defects then resolve at rest, this suggests inducible myocardial ischemia due to large-vessel coronary artery disease. Finally, ventilation perfusion scans of the lung are useful for detecting pulmonary emboli, hemorrhage or primary ventilatory problems.

ANGIOGRAPHY

In patients with suspected venous thrombotic problems associated with the antiphospholipid antibody syndrome, systemic venograms are often useful for confirming the diagnosis. In patients with suspected coronary vasculitis or coronary atherosclerosis, coronary angiography is frequently indicated. Finally, pulmonary angiography may be required to differentiate pulmonary emboli from other types of pulmonary vascular disease.

ECHOCARDIOGRAPHY

Echocardiography is the most useful current technique for making the diagnosis of pericarditis, since it is highly sensitive for detecting small amounts of pericardial fluid (Fig. 7.3). Almost all cases of significant

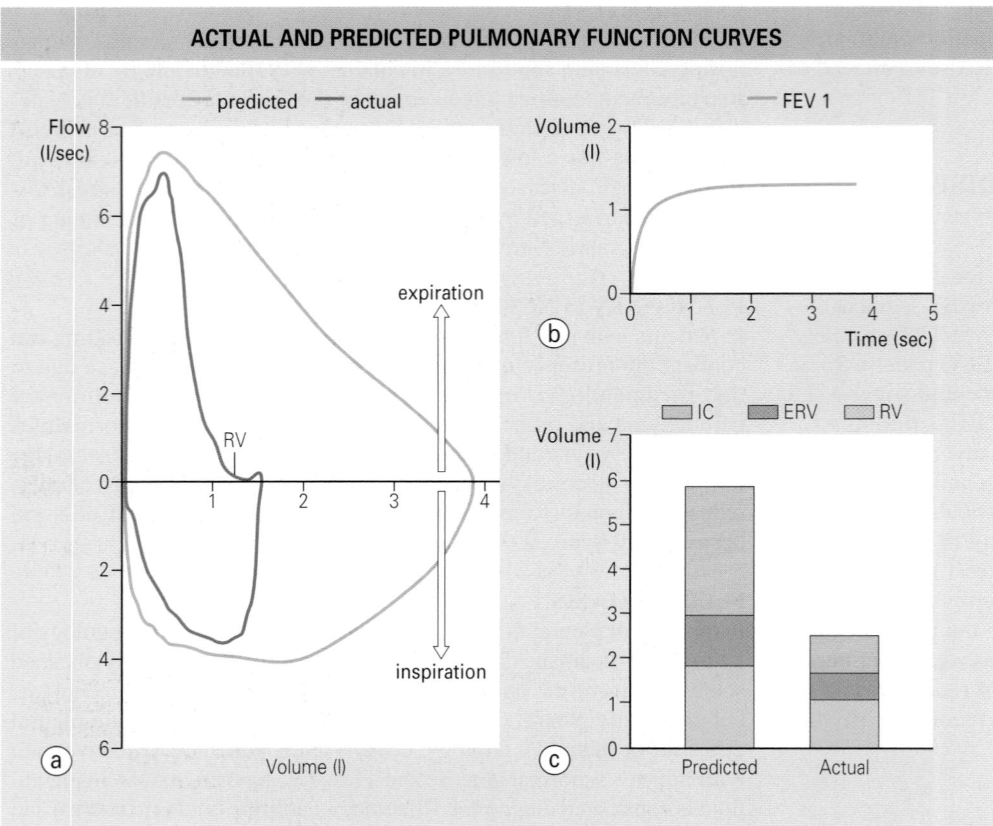

Fig. 7.2 Results of pulmonary function testing in a 55-year-old man with scleroderma and pulmonary fibrosis. Actual and predicted flow volume curves during inspiration and expiration are shown. Note that the peak flow rate is relatively unaffected, demonstrating a lack of airway obstruction, but the residual volume (RV) is markedly reduced compared to the predicted value (a). Spirometry tracing of expiration shows a low forced expiratory volume at one second (FEV1), but when corrected for the reduced forced vital capacity (FEV1/FVC × 100%) it is normal at 93% (predicted 81%) (b). A bar graph of lung volumes exhibits substantial reductions in inspiratory capacity (IC), expiratory reserve volume (ERV), RV and total lung capacity (height of bar) compared to predicted values. The diffusing capacity for carbon dioxide is one quarter of the predicted value, reflecting alveolar fibrosis (c).

pericarditis are associated with pericardial fluid accumulation. Echocardiography is not as useful for determining the thickness of the pericardium if chronic pericarditis or chronic constrictive pericarditis is suspected. Usually, MRI is the best technique for defining pericardial thickness, but a CT scan can also be helpful. Echocardiography is highly accurate for detecting abnormalities of the valve leaflets which are frequently involved in rheumatologic diseases. Readily detectable abnormalities include Libman–Sacks vegetations in patients with SLE, leaflet fibrosis and valve granulomas (Fig. 7.4)[12]. Doppler echocardiography can detect and assess the severity of valvular regurgitation, and imaging of the left ventricle can determine the impact of the valvular regurgitation on ventricular size and function (Fig. 7.5)[13]. Involvement of the ventricle or the atria with myocarditis can also be demonstrated on echo by evidence of ventricular dilatation, thinning, reduced contractility and segmental wall motion abnormalities (Fig. 7.6). In patients with left ventricular hypertrophy or amyloidosis, diastolic dysfunction of the ventricle can be detected by Doppler echocardiography[14]. Finally, pulmonary artery pressures can be estimated by the Doppler echocardiography assessment of trivial or greater tricuspid regurgitant jets. Thus, Doppler echo can be used to estimate the degree of pulmonary hypertension. Also useful in this regard is the assessment of the size of the right ventricle and atrium and the size and dynamics of the inferior vena cava (Fig. 7.6). Finally, duplex Doppler of the peripheral veins can be useful for detecting venous thrombosis in patients with hypercoaguable states.

RHEUMATIC DISEASES INVOLVING THE JOINTS AND THE HEART AND LUNGS

Cardiac and pulmonary complications are a feature of most of the systemic rheumatic disorders (see Figs 7.7 & 7.8).

SYSTEMIC LUPUS ERYTHEMATOSUS

SLE is associated with widespread cardiopulmonary involvement of the pericardium, myocardium, endocardium, conduction system and valve leaflets. The underlying pathology is believed to be due to immune complex deposition and complement activation on the vascular endothelial surfaces, leading to an inflammatory reaction (see Chapter 7.2). In addition, antiphospholipid antibodies may be associated with venous and arterial thrombosis, but their primary pathogenetic role in SLE-associated heart and lung disease has not been defined[15–18].

As with other rheumatic diseases, involvement of the heart and lungs at pathologic examination is much more frequent than clinical disease[19, 20]. Clinically evident pericarditis is perhaps the most common clinical manifestation of SLE heart disease, and concomitant pleural effusion is frequent. Both commonly accompany increases in SLE disease activity. Acute pericarditis is usually uncomplicated and tamponade and chronic constrictive pericarditis occur rarely. It must also be remembered that pericardial effusion may occur in SLE patients because of uremia. Treatment with nonsteroidal anti-inflammatory drugs (NSAIDs) usually causes resolution of the pericarditis, although low-dose corticosteroids may be needed in treatment-resistant patients. Large pericardial effusions unresponsive to medical therapy or cardiac tamponade should be treated with pericardiocentesis. Rare cases of chronic constrictive pericarditis may require pericardiectomy.

Valvular heart disease is probably the most important clinical manifestation of SLE heart disease. The classic feature is small vegetations (Libman–Sacks) seen almost exclusively on the mitral and aortic valves, either on the atrial or great vessel side rather than on the ventricular side (see Fig. 7.9). Larger valve masses can also be seen and leaflet thickening is frequent and may result in valve regurgitation, but rarely stenosis. Regurgitation is usually mild, but may be moderately severe and can result in congestive heart failure and the need for valve replacement. Valvular involvement in SLE is unrelated to other clinical manifestations and may spontaneously remit, irrespective of anti-inflammatory therapy[21]. Another complication of SLE valve disease is infectious endocarditis. Because of the prevalence of SLE valve disease, antibiotic prophylaxis for all SLE patients undergoing dental and other forms of nonsterile surgery has been recommended[22]. This practice has little risk and is probably less expensive than performing echocardiograms on all patients with SLE to detect subclinical valvular disease regardless of their symptoms.

Infrequently, SLE acute myocarditis is diagnosed clinically, but can be seen in up to 80% of autopsy patients. Myocarditis is usually

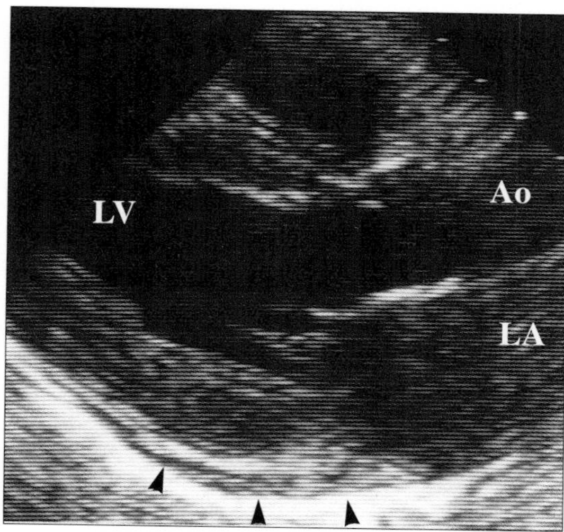

Fig. 7.3 Transthoracic echocardiogram in a patient with SLE, showing a small pericardial effusion (arrows) posterior to the left ventricle (LV). Aorta (AO), left atrium (LA). Courtesy of CA Roldan.

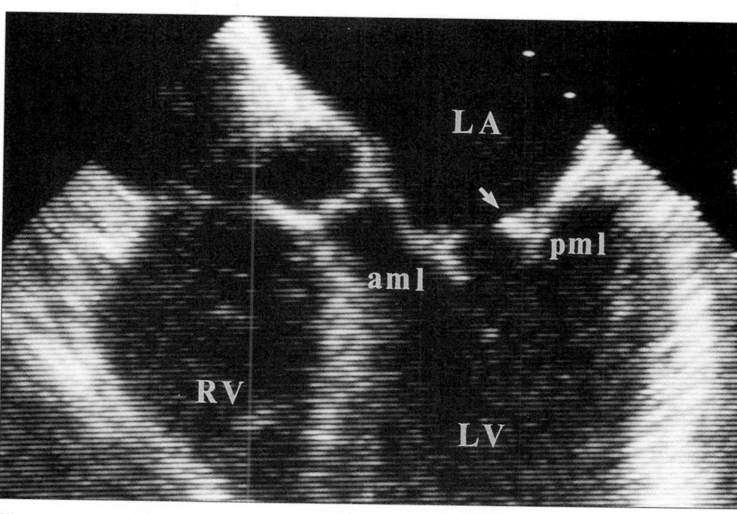

Fig. 7.4 Transesophageal echocardiogram from a patient with SLE demonstrating thickening of the anterior (aml) and posterior (pml) mitral leaflets and a Libman–Sacks vegetation (arrow) on the pml. Left atrium (LA), left ventricle (LV), right ventricle (RV). Courtesy of CA Roldan.

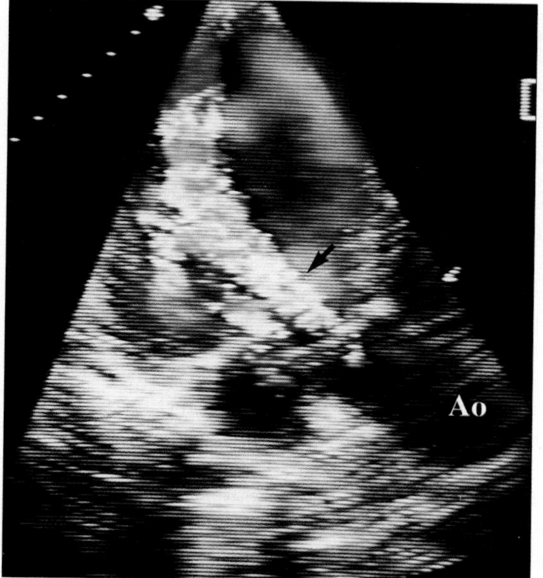

Fig. 7.5 Transthoracic color-flow Doppler echocardiogram, apical view, showing a moderately severe aortic regurgitation jet (arrow) into the left ventricle in a patient with AS. Courtesy of CA Roldan.

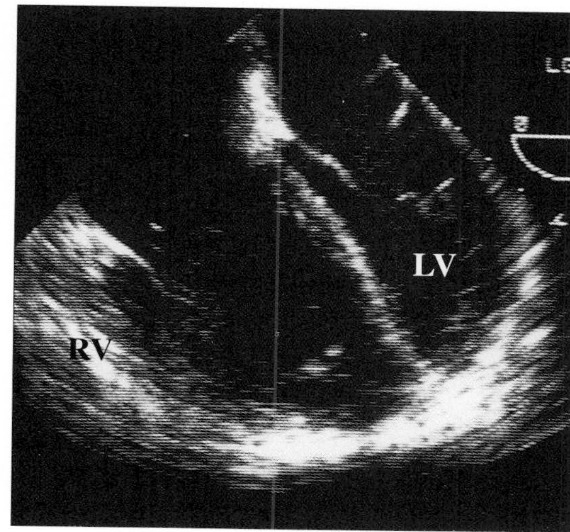

Fig. 7.6 Transesophageal echocardiogram in a patient with SLE and pulmonary hypertension due to chronic pulmonary emboli. Note the dilated right ventricle (RV) compared to the left ventricle (LV). Courtesy of CA Roldan.

mild and does not cause significant left ventricular dysfunction. Less than 10% of patients with SLE are found to have coronary vasculitis. Coronary vasculitis is more common in older patients with SLE, perhaps because of acceleration of underlying atherosclerosis. It may be difficult to differentiate SLE coronary vasculitis from myocarditis on clinical grounds. Although anti-inflammatory therapy is recommended for coronary vasculitis, it must be remembered that in the presence of frank myocardial infarction, corticosteroids are contraindicated because of wound-healing retardation and the potential for ventricular rupture.

Venous thromboemboli are a frequent complication in SLE patients. Both arterial and venous thrombotic events have been described in patients with antiphospholipid antibodies. In some patients arterial embolism may be due to embolization of valve masses or Libman–Sacks or infectious vegetations. Thromboembolic disease in SLE patients is treated in the standard fashion. No specific role for anti-inflammatory therapy has been documented.

Patients with SLE may present with arrhythmias and conduction disturbances in association with myopericarditis, or as isolated clinical events. Chronic inflammation of the conduction system can lead to a high degree heart block, which may resolve with the use of corticosteroid therapy. Patients who are unresponsive to corticosteroids may require a pacemaker.

RHEUMATOID ARTHRITIS

Cardiovascular disease in RA is caused by immune-mediated inflammation, vasculitis or granulomatous deposition in the various parts of the heart and great vessels. Clinical recognition of cardiac disease occurs in approximately one third of patients with chronic RA, but is more common in autopsy series. Pericarditis and pleural effusion are quite frequent in hospitalized patients with active disease. They are also more common in patients with positive rheumatoid factor and nodular disease. Cardiac tamponade or chronic restrictive pericarditis are less common than acute pericarditis. If pericardial or pleural fluid is removed, analysis of its characteristics can be useful if the diagnosis is in question. Ordinarily the fluid is serosanguinous with a high protein and high LDH content, but with a low glucose level. The cellular content is high and consists mainly of neutrophils. Pleuropericarditis is generally treated with anti-inflammatory drugs; pericardiectomy is occasionally required for chronic pericardial constriction.

Rheumatoid involvement of the mitral and aortic valves is usually mild, asymptomatic and rarely progresses. Some patients may develop aortitis, leading to root dilatation and aortic regurgitation (Fig. 7.10). This is more common in patients with long-standing disease, erosive polyarticular and nodular disease, systemic vasculitis and high rheumatoid factors. The value of anti-inflammatory treatment for rheumatoid valvular disease is unclear, but if necessary surgical valve treatment can be successfully accomplished.

FREQUENCY OF CARDIAC COMPLICATIONS OF RHEUMATOLOGIC DISEASES

Disease	Complication	Frequency
Systemic lupus erythematosus	Pericarditis	++++
	Leaflet fibrosis	++++
	Libman–Sacks vegetations	+++
	Mild valve regurgitation	+++
	Coronary occlusion	+++
	Myocarditis, cardiomyopathy	++
	Pulmonary hypertension	++
Rheumatoid arthritis	Leaflet fibrosis	++++
	Pericardial effusion	++++
	Coronary occlusion	++++
	Myocarditis/cardiomyopathy	++
	Valve granulomas	+
	Mild valve disease	+
Ankylosing spondylitis	Aortic valve disease	++++
	Subaortic bump	+++
	Conduction system disease	+++
	Coronary occlusion	+++
	Pericarditis	++
	Myocarditis/cardiomyopathy	++
	Mild aortic regurgitation	++
Systemic sclerosis	Myocarditis/cardiomyopathy	+++
	Pulmonary hypertension	+++
	Pericarditis	++
	Coronary occlusion	++
	Valve disease	++
Polymyositis/dermatomyositis	Myocarditis/cardiomyopathy	+++
	Pericarditis	+++
	Pulmonary hypertension	+

Fig. 7.7 Frequency of cardiac complication of rheumatologic diseases.

Rheumatoid myocarditis is rarely observed clinically. Coronary arteritis is also rare in patients with RA and is usually seen in patients with severe disease. Patients with arrhythmias and conduction disturbances are often elderly and differentiating a rheumatoid etiology from other forms of heart disease may be difficult. Finally, pulmonary vasculitis and interstitial fibrosis leading to pulmonary hypertension are rare in RA, but can produce cor pulmonale[23]. Such patients have a poor prognosis, despite anti-inflammatory therapy[24].

SYSTEMIC SCLEROSIS

The most common primary cardiac disease in patients with systemic sclerosis is coronary artery disease of the intramural coronary arteries and arterioles[25]. How much of the clinical findings are due to intramyocardial Raynaud's phenomenon is unclear, but most patients with evidence of coronary artery disease have peripheral Raynaud's phenomenon (see Chapter 7.9). Patients with systemic sclerosis may also develop myocarditis, but pericarditis is very uncommon. Interestingly, conduction defects are not uncommon and are caused by fibrosis of the conduction system. Conduction system disease can lead to atrial and ventricular arrhythmias and high degrees of heart block. There is no known specific treatment for conduction system involvement and so patients are treated in the standard fashion with antiarrhythmic drugs and pacemakers as appropriate. Valvular heart disease is rare in patients with systemic sclerosis, but echocardiography may reveal mitral regurgitation in a high proportion of patients due to nonspecific thickening of the mitral valve[26]. Pulmonary vasculopathy and primary interstitial lung disease occur in systemic sclerosis and can

FREQUENCY OF PULMONARY COMPLICATIONS OF RHEUMATOLOGIC DISEASES

Disease	Complication	Frequency
Systemic lupus erythematosus	Pleural effusion	++++
	Fibrosing alveolitis	+++
	Acute alveolitis	+
	Pulmonary hemorrhage	+
	Pulmonary vasculitis	+
Rheumatoid arthritis	Pleural effusion	+++
	Fibrosing alveolitis	+++
	Necrobiotic nodules	+
	Obliterative bronchiolitis	+
	Pulmonary vasculitis	+
Ankylosing spondylitis	Fibrosing alveolitis	++
Systemic sclerosis	Fibrosing alveolitis	++++
Polymyositis/dermatomyositis	Fibrosing alveolitis	++

Fig. 7.8 Frequency of pulmonary complications of rheumatologic diseases.

cause considerable disability due to dyspnea. Pulmonary hypertension and cor pulmonale may result from these lung diseases[27].

ANKYLOSING SPONDYLITIS

Cardiovascular complications of AS usually occur in patients who have had the disease for a decade or more (see Chapter 6.16). The most important cardiovascular manifestation of AS is aortitis, which frequently results in aortic regurgitation because of aortic root dilatation (Fig. 7.11). The regurgitation is generally mild and does not commonly progress in severity. Valvular surgery has been successfully carried out in these patients.

The second most common cardiac diseases in AS are conduction disturbances, caused by a subaortic fibrotic process extending into the base of the septum and resulting in high degree atrioventricular block[28]. There is no specific therapy for conduction disturbances, but pacemakers usually take care of the problem.

Patients may develop granulomatous root fibrosis in the subaortic basilar portion of the anterior mitral leaflet (subaortic bump), leading to mitral regurgitation as a result of decreased anterior leaflet mobility[29]. Left ventricular dilation from aortic regurgitation may also cause mitral regurgitation in some patients. This form of mitral regurgitation is not often progressive and rarely results in the need for valve surgery. However, as with all valvular regurgitation, endocarditis prophylaxis is indicated[30]. Myocardial and pericardial disease are rare in AS.

POLYMYOSITIS AND DERMATOMYOSITIS

The most common cardiac manifestations of polymyositis and dermatomyositis are myocarditis, arrhythmias and conduction disturbances (see Chapter 7.13)[31]. Other forms of cardiac disease are much less common[32,33]. ECG changes are frequently seen and are probably due to myocarditis. Severe myocarditis can result in congestive heart failure. Pulmonary vasculopathy and primary interstitial lung disease also occur in patients with polymyositis and dermatomyositis. Anti-inflammatory therapy rarely helps any of the cardiopulmonary manifestations of this disease, and a poor prognosis is indicated.

RHEUMATIC FEVER

Arthritis is one of the five major Jones criteria for the diagnosis of rheumatic fever (see Chapter 6.8). It frequently involves the large joints bilaterally, and is associated with heat and swelling in addition to discomfort. A chronic form of arthritic deformity of the fingers, known as Jaccoud's arthritis, can occur in rheumatic fever. It is characterized by a lateral deviation of the second to fifth digits of the hands. It can

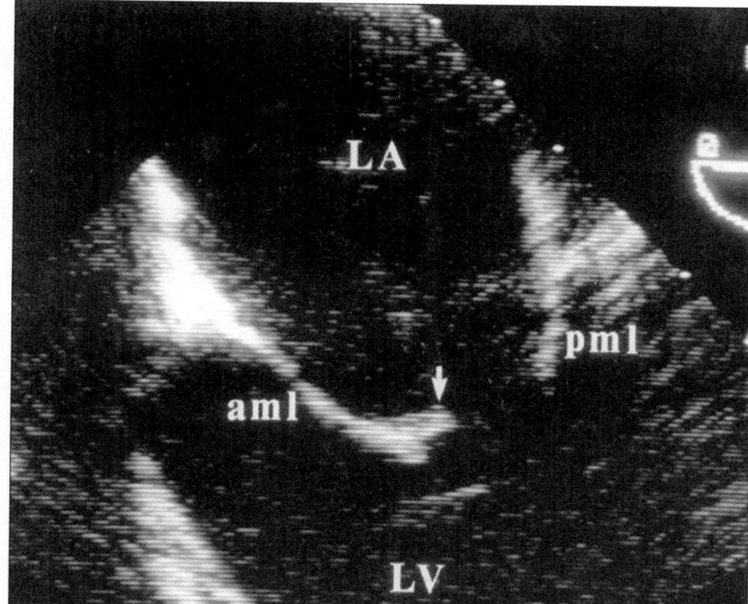

Fig. 7.9 Libman–Sacks vegetation (arrow) at the tip of the anterior mitral leaflet (aml) as seen on a transesophageal echocardiography in a patient with SLE. Courtesy of CA Roldan.

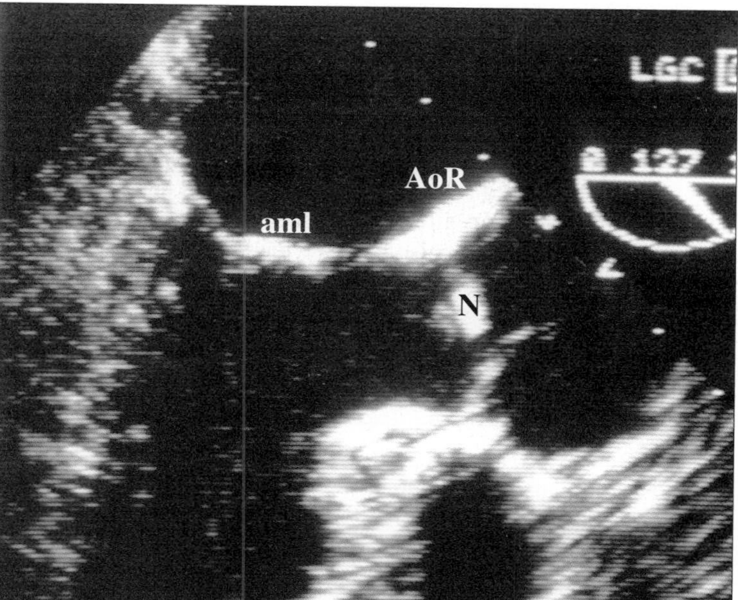

Fig. 7.10 A transesophageal echocardiogram in a patient with RA, showing a nodule (N) on the noncoronary cusp of the aortic valve and thickening of the aortic root (AoR) and anterior mitral valve leaflet (aml). Courtesy of CA Roldan.

be differentiated from the deformity of RA since the patient can voluntarily straighten the fingers in Jaccoud's arthritis, but not in RA, and there are nor erosions on hand radiographs in Jaccoud's arthritis.

CARDIOPULMONARY COMPLICATIONS OF RHEUMATOLOGIC CONDITIONS

PULMONARY HYPERTENSION

Vascular or interstitial lung disease leading to pulmonary hypertension and cor pulmonale is most frequently seen in systemic sclerosis, RA, and polymyositis and dermatomyositis. Valvular heart disease due to SLE or other rheumatologic diseases can also result in secondary pulmonary hypertension due to left heart failure. In patients with SLE, consideration must be given to pulmonary emboli since there may be venous thromboembolic disease in those with high antiphospholipid antibody levels.

SYSTEMIC HYPERTENSION

Many rheumatologic diseases can be associated with systemic hypertension, especially if there is any significant renal involvement. Hypertension is often severe and can lead to hypertensive heart disease. Systemic hypertension is perhaps the most common cardiopulmonary manifestation of systemic sclerosis, due principally to renal involvement (see Practical Problem 7.12, Scleroderma renal crisis). It is unclear if specific anti-inflammatory therapy helps this form of hypertension, and treatment is usually directed at the high blood pressure *per se*.

INFECTIOUS ENDOCARDITIS

The incidence of infectious endocarditis is higher in patients with SLE than in age-matched controls, suggesting that subclinical Libman–Sacks endocarditis has a propensity to become infected during periods of bacteremia. For this reason, it is recommended that patients with SLE have antibiotic prophylaxis for dental or other non-sterile surgery. An alternative would be to carry out echocardiograms on all patients with lupus planning such surgery, and only prophylax those with significant valvular lesions or regurgitation[34,35]. However, this approach may be more costly and less effective than routine antibiotics as long as the patient is not allergic. Infectious endocarditis can also be seen in patients with AS and RA who have involvement of the aorta and aortic valve or mitral regurgitation. Right-sided endocarditis is rare in patients with rheumatologic disease because of the rarity of involvement of the right-sided valves. However, in patients presenting with pulmonary symptomatology, right-heart endocarditis with septic embolization must be considered.

HYPERKINETIC HEART SYNDROME

Abnormally increased left ventricular performance has been demonstrated in up to one third of patients with polymyositis and dermatomyositis. The cause of this usually asymptomatic form of heart disease is unknown. Some believe that hyperkinetic heart syndrome can lead to systemic hypertension or hypertrophic cardiomyopathy, but documented cases in patients with polymyositis and dermatomyositis have not been reported. Anti-inflammatory therapy does not seem to help the hyperkinetic heart syndrome and treatment is usually directed at suppressing the heart with beta blockers.

AMYLOIDOSIS

In patients with chronic RA, amyloid deposits in the heart may lead to restrictive cardiomyopathy (see Chapter 8.27). This may manifest clinically as diastolic heart failure. Echocardiography usually shows a

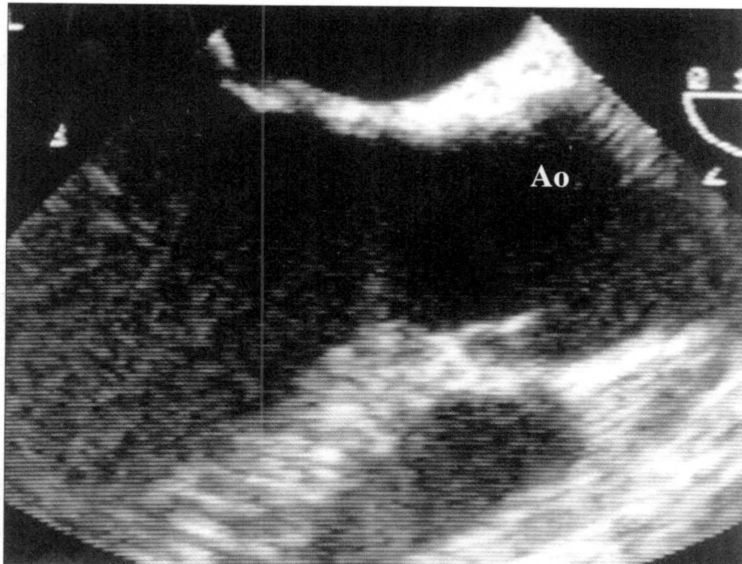

Fig. 7.11 A Transesophageal echocardiogram in a patient with ankylosing spondylitis, showing aortic root dilatation and thickening indicative of aortitis. The patient also had severe aortic regurgitation (not shown). Courtesy of CA Roldan.

thickened, shiny or speckled myocardium with normal systolic function. The atria are frequently large and the cavity of the ventricles small. Another clue that the thickened ventricles are due to amyloid is that the ECG does not show left ventricular hypertrophy, since there is no increase in the muscle mass of the ventricles.

Amyloidosis can also lead to conduction abnormalities and arrhythmias. There is no specific treatment for amyloidosis and it is unclear whether treatment of RA affects the rate of progression of amyloid heart disease. Amyloid can also infiltrate the lung, leading to restrictive pulmonary disease.

CARDIOPULMONARY COMPLICATIONS OF DRUGS USED IN RHEUMATOLOGY

NONSTEROIDAL ANTIINFLAMMATORY DRUGS

The most common cardiopulmonary complications of NSAIDs result from salt and water retention. Although this does not usually cause any problems, patients with significant valvular heart disease or myocardial disease may go into congestive heart failure on NSAID treatment.

CORTICOSTEROIDS

Corticosteroids also cause salt and water retention and can lead to heart failure in susceptible individuals. In addition, corticosteroids may lead to release of encapsulated *Mycobacterium tuberculosis* organisms in the lungs or in the other parts of the body, resulting in secondary tuberculosis. It is recommended that all patients receive a chest radiograph and a purified protein derivative (PPD) skin test prior to starting corticosteroid therapy.

Patients who have their long-term corticosteroid therapy stopped abruptly may develop acute Addison's disease due to suppression of the adrenal gland during the corticosteroid therapy. Addison's disease is manifest as symptoms of orthostatic hypotension, reduced blood pressure, low serum sodium and high potassium levels. The heart size is often small on chest radiographs and the ECG may document sinus tachycardia. Treatment after fluid replacement is by maintenance doses of corticosteroids, which are then slowly tapered to allow adrenal function to return.

IMMUNOSUPPRESSIVE DRUGS

The most common complication of immunosuppressive drugs is the potentiation of infections in the lung and occasionally the heart. Infection with opportunistic organisms, particularly of the lungs, is a complication associated with most immunosuppressive agents. Patients on methotrexate may develop 'methotrexate lung', which may be a hypersensitivity pneumonitis and can be seen in up to 6% of patients taking the drug (see Practical Problem Chapter 5.16: Methotrexate in rheumatoid arthritis). Cyclosporin A may be associated with hyperuricemia and gouty arthritis.

SLOW ACTING ANTIRHEUMATIC DRUGS

Several of the slow acting antirheumatic drugs (SAARDs) may be associated with pulmonary complications including hypersensitivity pneumonitis, bronchiolitis obliterans and fibrosing alveolitis (see Chapter 3.8).

REFERENCES

1. Kahl LE. The spectrum of pericardial tamponade in systemic lupus erythematosus: Report of ten patients. Arthritis Rheum. 1992;35:1343–9.
2. Escalante A, Kaufman RL, Quismorio FP, Beardmore TD. Cardiac compression in rheumatoid pericarditis. Semin Arthritis Rheum. 1990;20:148–63.
3. Hara KS, Ballard DJ, Ilstrup DM, Connally DC, Vollersten RS. Rheumatoid pericarditis: Clinical features and survival. Medicine. 1990;69:81–91.
4. Kelly CA, Bourke JP, Malcom A, Griffiths ID. Chronic pericardial disease in patients with rheumatoid arthritis: a longitudinal study. Q J Med. 1990;75:461–70.
5. Lee P, Langevitz P, Alderdice CA, *et al.* Mortality in systemic sclerosis (scleroderma). Q J Med. 1992;82;139–48.
6. Dieppe PA. Empyema in RA. Ann Rheum Dis. 1975;34:181–5.
7. Saag KG, Kolluri S, Koehnke RK, *et al.* Rheumatoid arthritis lung disease. Determinants of radiographic and physiologic abnormalities. Arthritis Rheum. 1996; 39:1711–19.
8. Mullins PA, Grace AA, Stewart SC, Shapiro LM. Rheumatoid heart disease presenting as acute mitral regurgitation. Am Heart J. 1991;122:242–5.
9. O'Neill TW, Bresnihan B. The heart in ankylosing spondylitis. Ann Rheum Dis. 1992;51:705–6.
10. Petri M, Perez-Gutthann S, Spence D, Hochberg MC. Risk factors for coronary artery disease in patients with systemic lupus erythematosus. Am J Med. 1992;93:513–9.
11. Bahl VK, Aradhye S, Vasar RS, Malhotra A, Reddy KS, Malaviya A. Myocardial systolic function in systemic lupus erythematosus: A study based on radionuclide ventriculography. Clin Cardiol. 1992;15:433–5.
12. Crozier IG, Li E, Milne MJ, Nicholls MG. Cardiac involvement in systemic lupus erythematosus detected by echocardiography. Am J Cardiol. 1990;65:1145–8.
13. Enomoto K, Kaji Y, Mayumi T, *et al.* Frequency of valvular regurgitation by color Doppler echocardiography in systemic lupus erythematosus. Am J Cardiol. 1991;67:209–11.
14. Sasson Z, Rasooly Y, Wai Chow C, Marshall S, Urowitz MB. Impairment of left ventricular diastolic function in systemic lupus erythematosus. Am J Cardiol. 1992;69: 1629–34.
15. Gleason CB, Stoddard MF, Wagner SG, Longaker RA, Pierangeli S, Harris EN. A comparison of cardiac valvular involvement in the primary antiphospholipid syndrome versus anticardiolipin-negative systemic lupus erythematosus. Am Heart J. 1993;125:1123–9.
16. Khamashta MA, Cervera R, Asherson RA, *et al.* Association of antibodies against phospholipids with heart valve disease in systemic lupus erythematosus. Lancet. 1990;335:1541–4.
17. Logar D, Kveder T, Rozman B, Dobovisek J. Possible association between anti-Ro antibodies and myocarditis or cardiac conduction defects in adults with systemic lupus erythematosus. Ann Rheum Dis. 1990;49:627–9.
18. Roldan CA, Shively BK, Lau CC, Gurule FT, Smith EA, Crawford MH. Systemic lupus erythematosus valve disease by transesophageal echocardiography and the role of antiphospholipid antibodies. J Am Coll Cardiol. 1992;20:1127–34.
19. Bahl VK, Vasan RS, Aradhye S, Malaviya AN. Prevalence of cardiac abnormalities early in the course of systemic lupus erythematosus. Am J Cardiol. 1991;68:1540–1.
20. Nihoyannopoulos P, Gomez PM, Joshi J, Loizou S, Walport MJ, Oakley CM. Cardiac abnormalities in systemic lupus erythematosus. Association with raised anticardiolipin antibodies. Circulation 1990;82:369–75.
21. Roldan CA, Shively BK, Crawford MH. An echocardiographic study of valvular heart disease associated with systemic lupus erythematosus. N Engl J Med. 1996;335:1424–30.
22. Lehman TJA, Palmeri ST, Hastings C, Klippel JH, Plotz PH. Bacterial endocarditis complicating systemic lupus erythematosus. J Rheumatol. 1983;10:655–8.
23. Young ID, Ford SE, Ford PM. The association of pulmonary hypertension with rheumatoid arthritis. J Rheumatol. 1989;16:1266–9.
24. Mutru O, Laakso M, Isomäki H, Koota K. Cardiovascular mortality in patients with rheumatoid arthritis. Cardiology. 1989;76:71–7.
25. Anvari A, Graninger W, Schneider B, Sochor H, Weber H, Schmidinger H. Cardiac involvement in systemic sclerosis. Arthritis Rheum. 1992;35;1356–61.
26. Maione S, Yalentini G, Giunta A, *et al.* Evaluation of cardiac structures and function in systemic sclerosis by Doppler echocardiography. Cardiology. 1991;79:165–71.
27. Silver RM. Clinical aspects of systemic sclerosis (scleroderma). Ann Rheum Dis. 1991;50:854–61.
28. Peeters AJ, ten Wolde S, Sedney MI, de Vries RRP, Dijkmans BAC. Heart conduction disturbance: An HLA-B27 associated disease. Ann Rheum Dis. 1991;50:348–50.
29. O'Neill TW, King G, Graham IM, Molony J, Bresnihan B. Echocardiographic abnormalities in ankylosing spondylitis. Ann Rheum Dis. 1992;51:652–4.
30. Hoppman RA, Wise CM, Challa VR, Peacock JE. Subacute bacterial endocarditis and ankylosing spondylitis. Ann Rheum Dis. 1988;47:423–7.
31. Schwartz MI. Pulmonary and cardiac manifestations of polymyositis–dermatomyositis. J Thorac Imaging. 1992;7:46–54.
32. Buchpiguel CA, Roizenblatt S, Lucena-Fernandes MF, *et al.* Radioisotopic assessment of peripheral and cardiac muscle involvement and dysfunction in polymyositis/dermatomyositis. J Rheumatol. 1991;18:1359–63.
33. Byrnes TJ, Baethge BA, Wolf RE. Noninvasive cardiovascular studies in patients with inflammatory myopathy. Angiology. 1991;42:843–8.
34. Comens SM, Alpert MA, Sharp GC, *et al.* Frequency of mitral valve prolapse in systemic lupus erythematosus, progressive systemic sclerosis and mixed connective tissue disease. Am J Cardiol. 1989;63:369–70.
35. Leung WH, Wong KL, Lau CP, Wong CK, Cheng CH, Tai YT. Echocardiographic identification of mitral valvular abnormalities in patients with mixed connective tissue disease. J Rheumatol. 1990;17:485–8.

8

GASTROINTESTINAL TRACT AND RHEUMATIC DISEASE

Herman Mielants & Eric M Veys

- Abdominal symptoms in a patient with arthritis may reflect several different etiologies.
- Inflammatory bowel disorders, particularly Crohn's disease and ulcerative colitis, are often complicated by the development of peripheral or axial arthritis.
- Most systemic rheumatic diseases can be associated with intermittent inflammation involving the peritoneum or gastrointestinal tract.
- A number of anti-rheumatic drugs can produce bowel symptoms; NSAID-induced gastropathy is by far the most common.

INTRODUCTION

An association between pathology of the gut and imflammatory arthritis has long been recognized. As early as 1922[1] colectomy was advocated a treatment for rheumatoid arthritis (RA) and the development of peripheral arthritis in occational patients with chronic ulcerative colitis and inflammatory bowel disease was noted. In recent years inflammatory joint disease has been established following intestinal bypass surgery and in celiac disease and Whipple's disease. The gut could play a role in the pathogenesis of the arthritis in these diseases. In other inflammatory joint diseases, abdominal manifestations can be a symptom of a complication of rheumatic diseases such as systemic vasculitis, scleroderma, or amyloidosis. Finally, nonsteroidal anti-inflammatory drugs (NSAIDs) can cause damage of the gastrointestinal tract, especially in the stomach and duodenum, but probably also in the small intestine and colon.

Major abdominal symptoms are diarrhea, abdominal pain and intestinal blood loss (Fig. 8.1):

- diarrhea is mainly a symptom of intestinal inflammation and/or of hypermotility;
- abdominal pain can be associated with diarrhea, but can also exist as an independent abdominal manifestation;
- intestinal blood loss is predominantly a symptom of a major gut lesion.

THE GUT AND ARTHRITIS
Arthritis associated with diarrhea
Crohn's disease Ulcerative colitis Enterogenic (bacterial) reactive arthritis (Reiter's) Undifferentiated spondyloarthropathies Whipple's disease Blind loop syndrome Celiac disease Behçet's disease Collagenous colitis
Arthritis associated with abdominal pain
Ulcerative colitis Crohn's disease Vasculitic syndromes Henoch–Schönlein (leukocytoclastic vasculitis) Rheumatoid arthritis Systemic lupus erythematosus Polyarteritis nodosa Scleroderma Amyloidosis Familial Mediterranean fever Behçet's disease Whipple's disease
Arthritis associated with intestinal blood loss
Ulcerative colitis Vasculitic syndromes Henoch–Schönlein Whipple's disease

Fig. 8.1 The gut and arthritis.

DIFFERENTIAL DIAGNOSIS

The differential diagnosis of inflammatory locomotor diseases associated with abdominal symptoms is aided by determining the distribution of the joint inflammation. Inflammatory symptoms of the locomotor system can be subdivided into peripheral joint involvement, with or without tendinitis, and axial inflammation (of the spine and sacroiliac joints).

Peripheral arthritis can be subdivided into mono- or pauciarticular and polyarticular joint involvement.

PAUCIARTICULAR OR MONOARTICULAR INVOLVEMENT

This clinical presentation is typical of the spondyloarthropathies (see Chapters 6.11 and 6.24). Pauciarticular joint involvement is usually asymmetric, involving large and small joints, predominantly of the lower limbs, and frequently associated with tendinitis (Fig. 8.2). Enthesitis (inflammation of the insertion of the tendon into the bone) is the hallmark of these diseases, and usually involves the feet (Achilles tendon, insertion of plantar fascia) or knee (insertion of patellar ligament) (Fig. 8.2) (see Chapter 6.13). Sacroiliitis and spondylitis (which is also an enthesitis) can be associated. Other features include clinical overlap of the different diseases, familial aggregation among members of the group and the frequent association with HLA-B27[2].

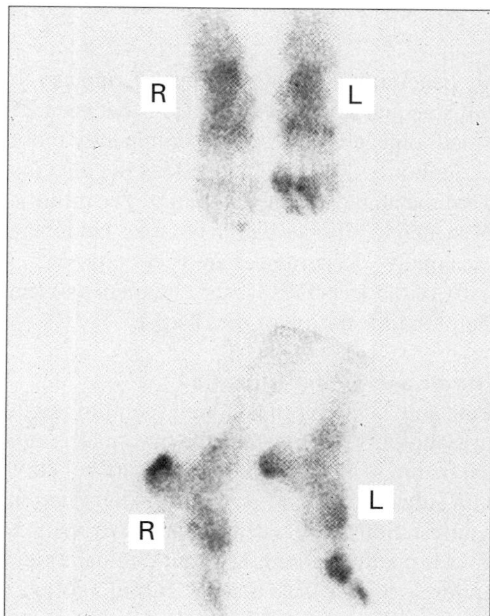

Fig. 8.2 ^{99m}Technetium methylene diphosphonate (MDP) scans of pauciarticular asymmetric joint involvement and enthesopathies in spondyloarthropathies.

Diagnosis	Abdominal symptoms	General symptoms	Extra-articular features	Relationship between abdominal symptoms and arthritis: Onset	Course
Crohn's disease	Diarrhea Abdominal pain Fistulae	Weight loss Ill-being Fever	Erythema nodosum Clubbing Uveitis, conjunctivitis	Usually before arthritis, sometimes coincident or postdated	Flares rarely coincide
Ulcerative colitis	Diarrhea Blood loss	Rare	Erythema nodosum Uveitis	Before arthritis, frequently coincident	Flares directly related
Enterogenic reactive arthritis	Diarrhea Vomiting	Spiking fever Ill-being Dehydration	Uveitis Urethritis	1–4 weeks before arthritis	Longer arthritis duration
Undifferentiated spondyloarthropathies	Rare diarrhea	None	Uveitis Erythema nodosum Urethritis	Arthritis before abdominal symptoms 'subclinical' gut inflammation	Related

DISORDERS WITH MONOARTICULAR OR PAUCIARTICULAR JOINT INVOLVEMENT AND ABDOMINAL SYMPTOMS

Fig. 8.3 Disorders with monoarticular or pauciarticular joint involvement and abdominal symptoms.

Diseases belonging to this group in which abdominal symptoms are present are Crohn's disease, ulcerative colitis, enterogenic reactive arthritis and undifferentiated spondyloarthropathies (see Fig. 8.3).

CROHN'S DISEASE

The prevalence of Crohn's disease has increased during the past three decades to about 75/100,000 population. A screening study for colorectal cancer in an asymptomatic population detected 21 cases of inflammatory bowel disease (IBD), suggesting that the true prevalence may be underestimated by 30%[3]. This study also suggests the existence of patients with subclinical IBD and Crohn's disease.

Abdominal symptoms

Crohn's disease is characterized by the classic triad of diarrhea, abdominal pain and weight loss. Disease onset may be insidious and progression subclinical. Diarrhea consists mainly of frequent watery bowel movements and typically follows meals. The stool volume depends on the anatomic location of the disease. Intestinal bleeding is uncommon. Abdominal pain is present in the majority of patients and described as cramping, predominantly in the right lower quadrant of the abdomen. Pain is usually not reported as severe[4].

Weight loss is a common feature and is in the range of 10–20% of body weight. General debility is a common complaint together with low grade fever.

In the later stages of Crohn's disease perianal involvement appears, with fistulae and abscesses. The finding of a tender abdominal mass may be a sign of an intra-abdominal abscess or fistulae.

Peripheral arthritis

Peripheral arthritis, mainly pauciarticular and asymmetric, appears in about 20% of patients, with an equal sex ratio. Peak age is between 25 and 44 years. Large and small joints are involved, predominantly those of the lower limbs (most commonly the knees and ankles but also the metacarpophalangeal and the metatarsophalangeal joints). The arthritis is mainly migratory and transient and subsides within 6 weeks, but it may also become chronic and destructive. Recurrences are very common.

Enthesopathies, especially of the feet (Fig. 8.2) are frequent and can be considered as a peripheral manifestation of the disease.

Relationship between arthritis and gut inflammation

In most cases gut symptoms antedate or coincide with the joint manifestations, but the articular symptoms may precede the intestinal symptoms by years[5]. It is argued that in some cases of spondyloarthropathy, Crohn's disease can remain subclinical, joint or tendon inflammation being the only clinical manifestation[6]. In a recent prospective study, 8 out of 129 (6%) spondyloarthropathy patients without clinical manifestations of IBD at onset developed Crohn's disease during a follow-up period of up to 9 years[7]. Colonic involvement increases the susceptibility to peripheral arthritis. Attacks of arthritis can be related temporally to flares of bowel disease although this is less pronounced than in ulcerative colitis.

Extra-articular features

Skin lesions, specifically erythema nodosum and pyoderma gangrenosum, are frequently associated and occur in 10–21% of patients. Erythema nodosum parallels the activity of the bowel disease and tends to occur in patients with active peripheral arthritis; it is probably a manifestation of Crohn's disease. Pyoderma gangrenosum is less common and more severe. It is not related to bowel and joint diseases and is probably an associated disorder[8]. Clubbing is also reported in this disease.

Acute anterior uveitis is the ocular manifestation most commonly associated with Crohn's disease, occurring in 3–11% of patients. It is acute in onset, unilateral and transient, but recurrences are common. It generally spares choroid and retina, but a chronic progressive form with lesions in the posterior part has been described. Mutton-fat keratic precipitates are a sign of granulomatous uveitis and can be present. Acute anterior uveitis is more related to those spondyloarthropathies showing axial involvement and associated with HLA-B27. Inflammatory gut lesions were found on ileocolonoscopy in 66% of patients with acute anterior uveitis associated with spondyloarthropathies[9]. Conjunctivitis and episcleritis are also described: in these cases a red eye without photophobia or pain is typically seen.

Secondary amyloidosis with involvement of major organs is not uncommon, and is usually lethal.

Laboratory and radiographic features

Raised inflammatory serum parameters (especially C-reactive protein), marked thrombocytosis and a hypochromic anemia due to chronic inflammation are common findings. The synovial fluid analysis is nonspecific and consistent with inflammatory arthritis, with a cell count varying from 1500–50,000/mm^3 (1.5–50 $\times$ 10^9/l). Cultures are negative.

As a rule, radiographs of the peripheral joints show no erosive lesions. However, erosive lesions of MCP and MTP joints have been described (Fig. 8.4), and these only differ from the arthritis seen in RA by their pauciarticular and asymmetric distribution. Adjacent bone proliferation is frequently present. The radiographic appearance of the enthesopathies is similar to that found in other spondyloarthropathies.

Genetics

There is substantial evidence favoring a genetic cause for Crohn's disease. Familial aggregation of Crohn's disease and ulcerative colitis has been frequently described[10]. Both diseases are believed to be genetically linked, since both occur within the same families. No significant associations with HLA antigens have been demonstrated, in particular the peripheral arthritis is not associated with HLA-B27. HLA-Bw16 and HLA-Bw18 have been found elevated in Crohn's disease, while

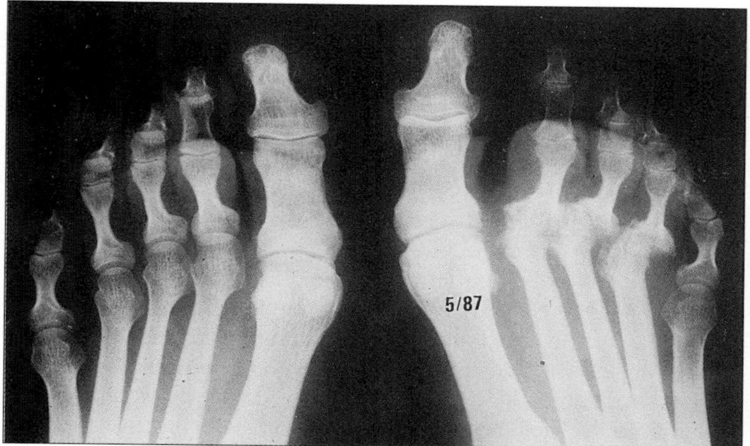

Fig. 8.4 Erosive metatarsophalangeal joint lesions in a patient with Crohn's disease (asymmetric joint involvement).

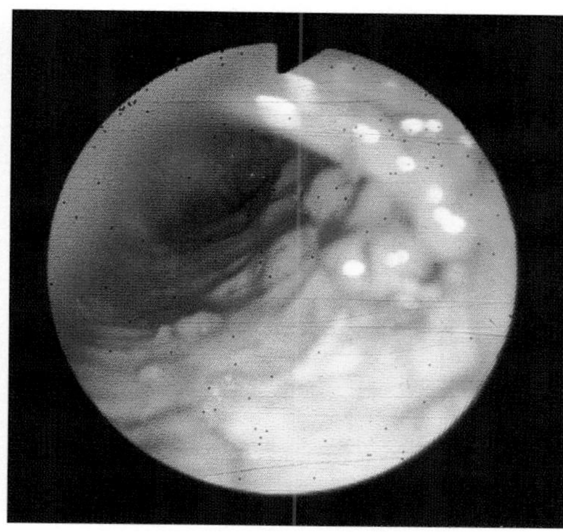

Fig. 8.5 Endoscopy revealing cobblestone formation in a patient with Crohn's disease.

HLA-Bw62 has been described in spondyloarthritic patients presenting Crohn's-disease-like lesions on gut biopsy[11]. HLA-Bw62 could be a predisposing factor to the development of arthritis and tendinitis in HLA-B27-patients with chronic inflammatory gut lesions.

Diagnosis

The laboratory and radiographic findings are also identical to those of Crohn's disease.Histologic evidence of Crohn's disease is essential and can be obtained at colonoscopy (in cases of colonic involvement) or ileocolonoscopy. Macroscopically, the presence of patchy aphthous ulcers, and of cobblestones (Fig. 8.5) will raise suspicions and point to the diagnosis. Although the differential diagnosis with ulcerative colitis can be difficult, some histologic features of Crohn's disease, such as the patchy distribution of the lesions, the involvement of different layers of the bowel wall and the presence of aphthous ulcers, pseudopyloric metaplasia and granulomas (Fig. 8.6) are pathognomonic.

ULCERATIVE COLITIS

The prevalence of ulcerative colitis is 50–100/100,000 population; the disease seems to be more frequent in whites than in non-whites.

Abdominal symptoms

The most frequent abdominal manifestations of ulcerative colitis are diarrhea and blood loss. In distal locations, there can be passage of blood with each bowel movement. With more extensive colon involvement, the blood will be mixed with a soft, liquid and sometimes mucopurulent stool.

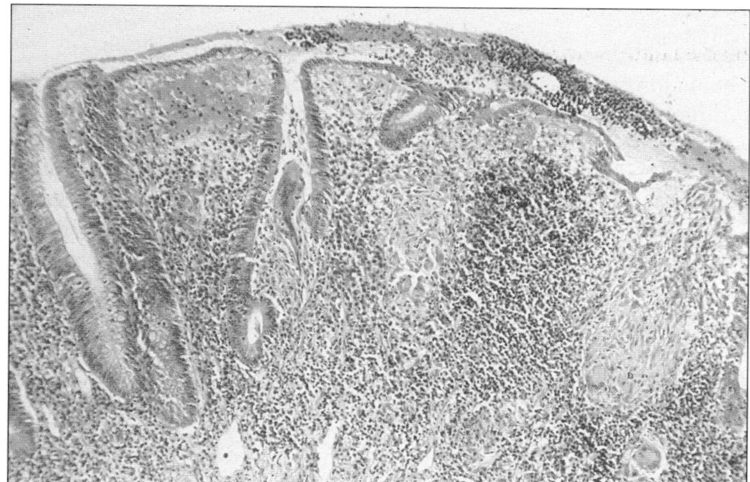

Fig. 8.6 Crohn's disease of colon. Microscopic aspect of colon biopsy showing irregular distorted crypts which are interrupted by infiltrations of inflammatory cells. The lamina propria contains sarcoid granulomas and a mononuclear infiltrate. (H&E stain, × 120.)

Diarrhea is practically always present. Defecation is frequent, sometimes every few minutes, and usually in small amounts. Abdominal pain, rectal cramps and fever are less frequent than in Crohn's disease, and considerable weight loss is distinctly uncommon.

Peripheral arthritis

The patterns of peripheral arthritis and enthesopathy associated with ulcerative colitis are identical to those seen in Crohn's disease, but their prevalence is much lower (5–10%).

Relationship between arthritis and gut inflammation

Disease onset usually precedes the joint symptoms but a coincidental onset of joint and abdominal symptoms is not uncommon. In the course of the disease the temporal relationship between attacks of arthritis and flares of the bowel disease is more marked than in Crohn's disease. Joint symptoms are more common in total than in partial colonic involvement. Surgical removal of the inflamed colon has a therapeutic effect on the joint symptoms[12].

Extra-articular features

The dermatologic and ocular manifestations of ulcerative colitis are comparable to those seen in Crohn's disease, but they are less common. Clubbing and amyloidosis are absent.

Genetics

A genetic predisposition to ulcerative colitis has been substantiated; familial aggregation for Crohn's disease and ulcerative colitis has been amply documented[10] and both diseases seem to be genetically linked. No association with HLA-antigens, especially HLA-B27, has been demonstrated in relation to the peripheral arthritis.

Diagnosis

The endoscopic appearance is different from that seen in Crohn's disease: the mucosa is extensively involved, with edema, friability and bleeding on minor trauma. Subsequently, ulcerations and strictures may appear. The histologic picture differs from Crohn's disease by the continuous involvement of only the mucosa, with no damage to the deeper layers (see Fig. 8.7).

ENTEROGENIC REACTIVE ARTHRITIS

Different enterogenic bacteria are capable of initiating peripheral arthritis (see Chapter 6.24). *Shigella flexneri*, *Salmonella typhimurium*, *Yersinia enterocolitica* (especially serotype 3), *Y. pseudotuberculosis* and *Campylobacter jejuni* are the most common species[13], although arthritis has frequently been reported in outbreaks of diarrhea in which no pathogens were identified.

The disease has been termed reactive arthritis, since the causative organisms cannot be isolated from the joint[14]. The sterile arthritis develops as a reaction to a distant infection.

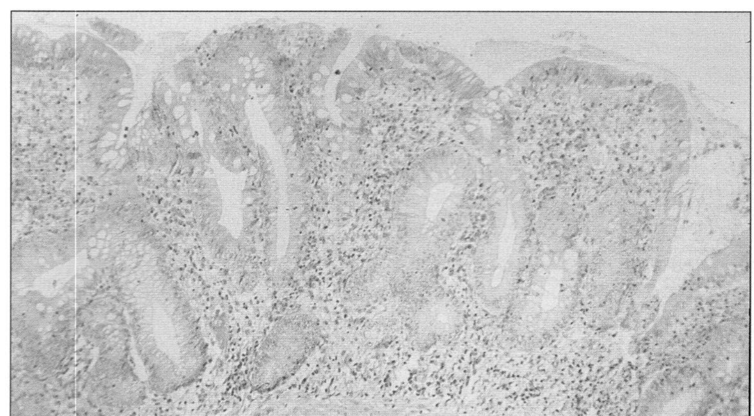

Fig. 8.7 Ulcerative colitis. Microscopic aspect of colon biopsy showing irregular villous surface with distorted and branching crypts. There is mucin depletion. The lamina propria contains infiltrates with mononuclear cells and granulocytes. The bottom of the crypts does not reach the muscularis mucosa. (H&E stain, × 120.)

Abdominal symptoms

The clinical picture mainly consists of very profuse diarrhea, accompanied by spiking fever, general malaise, abdominal cramps, vomiting and progressive dehydration. In some cases blood loss in stools may be present. The interval between infection and the onset of intestinal symptoms is very short.

In salmonella epidemics the frequency of those reporting gastrointestinal distress is between 1% and 10% depending on the antimicrobial resistance pattern. Most patients recover within 1 month although a fatal outcome is not uncommon.

Peripheral arthritis

The peripheral arthritis related to intestinal bacterial infections resembles that seen in the spondyloarthropathies: an asymmetric oligoarticular pattern of joint involvement, predominantly of the lower limbs, accompanied by tendinitis (10%). Monoarthritis is a common finding, as well as dactylitis (sausage-like toes and fingers). Men are more frequently affected than women (1.5:1).

The duration of the joint symptoms is usually restricted and in more than 70% of cases the patient is symptom-free after about 19 weeks. Nevertheless, about 20% of patients experience multiple episodes of flare-up of joint disease and in about 10–30% of cases (depending on the causative organism) the joint inflammation becomes chronic. In the majority of cases antibiotic treatment has no effect on the joint manifestations.

Relationship between arthritis and gut inflammation

Arthritis develops generally 6–14 days after the diarrhea. The interval is less than 30 days in 80% of patients, although it may amount to 3 months. The joint symptoms usually take longer to subside than the abdominal symptoms. In some cases, mainly of Yersinia arthritis, diarrhea can be absent.

There is no relationship between the severity of gut symptoms and the severity of joint symptoms.

Extra-articular features

The most common extra-articular lesions are ocular manifestations. Acute anterior uveitis and conjunctivitis occur in about 5–30% of cases and are usually self-limited. The uveitis is frequently associated with attacks of arthritis, but can subsequently follow an independent course.

Urogenital inflammation (urethritis, balanitis, vaginitis) occurs in about 12–20% of cases, although the infectious organism is usually absent from the urogenital tract.

Oral ulcers and erythema nodosum (especially in Yersinia enteritides) are not uncommon, while keratoderma blennorrhagicum is never seen in enterogenic reactive arthritis. Neurologic, cardiac and renal complications are rare.

Laboratory and radiographic features

During the initial stage of reactive arthritis patients develop the specific laboratory features of an acute bacterial infection. The causative organisms can be cultured from the stools during the active stage of intestinal manifestations.

Increased levels of immunoglobulins can be detected in the serum. The IgM increase is very short-lived, but the increases in IgG and IgA levels may be persistent. It appears, however, that these immunoglobulins are not organism-specific.

The joint fluid is inflammatory and contains 4000–120,000 cells/mm^3 (4–120 $\times$ 10^9/l), mainly polymorphonuclear cells. A characteristic of reactive arthritis is that the causative organism cannot be cultured in the joint fluid or synovium. However, specific bacterial antigenic material (lipopolysaccharide) has been demonstrated in the synovial fluid cells[15] and the synovium of patients with reactive arthritis. Other work suggests the persistence of the causative organism in the gut submucosa of patients with chronic joint disease due to defective local defense mechanisms[16].

Erosive lesions of the involved joint are uncommon but may be present. Typical aspects are the combined presence of bone proliferation and bone erosions, and the asymmetric pattern of involvement.

Genetics

Predisposition to arthritis associated with gut infection is strongly linked with the HLA-B27 antigen, which is present in 60–80% of patients. There is also a striking association with sacroiliitis, spondylitis and acute anterior uveitis.

In epidemics of enteric bacteria the relative risk of developing reactive arthritis in HLA-B27 positive patients is about 20%, while in HLA-B27 negative patients the risk is lower than 1%.

Carriage of HLA-B27 antigen influences not only the development of the disease, but also the severity, extent and duration of symptoms.

Diagnosis

The diagnosis is made by stool cultures obtained during the active episode of intestinal symptoms, or by determining specific immunoglobulins in the serum (although the specificity of these tests is questionable).

Endoscopic confirmation can be obtained. The histology mainly demonstrates an infiltrate with polymorphonuclear cells, mucosal ulceration and crypt abscesses. The architecture of crypts and villi is usually preserved.

UNDIFFERENTIATED SPONDYLOARTHROPATHIES

A large number of patients presenting the clinical, biological, radiographic and genetic features of the spondyloarthropathies cannot be classified into one of the known clinical entities. These patients are classified under 'undifferentiated spondyloarthropathies'.

Abdominal symptoms

The majority of these patients do not present pronounced abdominal symptoms. However, about 20–30% regularly experience short episodes of diarrhea or regularly have more than two stools per day[17].

Peripheral arthritis

The clinical picture is identical to that seen in other forms of spondyloarthropathy. There is asymmetric involvement of the small and large joints, predominantly of the lower limbs. Enthesopathies, mainly of the feet, and dactylitis are frequently associated.

Relationship between arthritis and gut inflammation

The gut inflammation in undifferentiated spondyloarthropathies is mainly subclinical and can only be demonstrated by ileocolonoscopy[6]. In about 60% of patients inflammatory gut lesions can be detected on biopsy. These lesions either resemble acute bacterial enteritis and are then classified as 'acute', or resemble idiopathic inflammatory bowel disease and are then classified as 'chronic'[18].

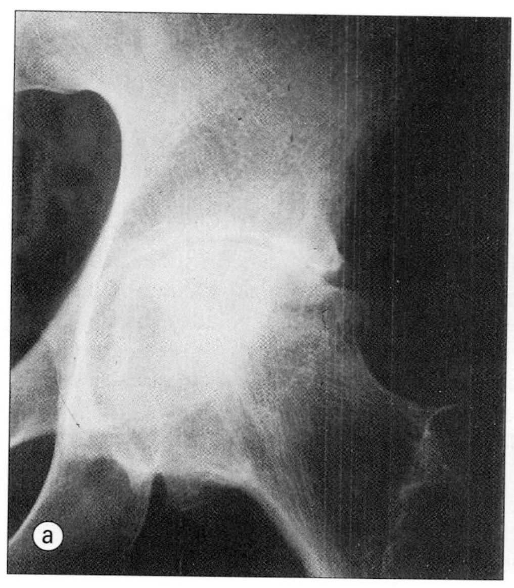

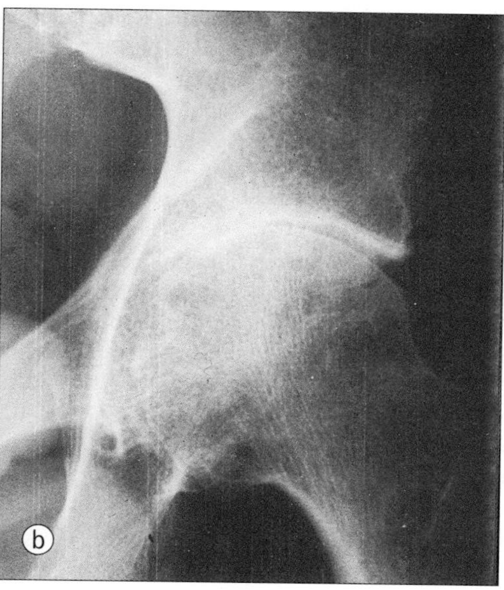

Fig. 8.8 Hip involvement in spondyloarthropathies. The concentric type with concentric joint-space narrowing and ruff-like osteophytosis (a). The destructive type with eccentric joint-space narrowing, osteolysis and destruction of femoral head (b).

Repeat ileocolonoscopy has demonstrated a strong relationship between the persistence of intestinal inflammation and that of joint inflammation[19]. In a recent study[7] it was demonstrated that the remission of rheumatic disease was always associated with the disappearance of gut inflammation, whereas half of the patients with persistent locomotor inflammation still presented chronic gut inflammation; 20% of the latter developed IBD. This finding supports the hypothesis that the gut triggers the joint disease in the majority of spondyloarthritis patients. This close relationship was confirmed in the animal model of HLA-B27 transgenic rats in which most animals developed gut and joint inflammation[20]; in germ-free conditions, however, there was no development of either form of inflammation[21].

Extra-articular features

Acute anterior uveitis, erythema nodosum and urogenital symptoms are the most frequent extra-articular features.

Laboratory and radiographic features

Most patients have elevations of acute phase reactants with an increased erythrocyte sedimentation rate (ESR) and C-reactive protein (CRP). Inflammatory reactants are significantly more raised in patients with 'chronic' inflammatory gut lesions than in those presenting acute lesions or a normal histology. Erosive joint lesions, particularly of the small joints of hands and feet, are not uncommon. They resemble the lesions seen in RA, but differ by their asymmetric and pauciarticular pattern. Destructive lesions of the hip joint, mimicking RA hip involvement and different from the concentric hip involvement in ankylosing spondylitis (AS), have been described[22] (Fig. 8.8). Like the erosive joint lesions they are related to the presence of subclinical gut inflammation.

Genetics

The prevalence of HLA-B27 is similar to that found in the reactive arthritis, while HLA-Bw62 positivity has been reported to be increased in relation to gut inflammation[11]. Family studies have also revealed familial aggregation of the subclinical gut inflammation in undifferentiated spondyloarthropathies and Crohn's disease.

Diagnosis

The diagnosis is made by the clinical picture and by excluding proven enteric infections. Ileocolonoscopy can confirm the presence of subclinical gut inflammation.

POLYARTICULAR INVOLVEMENT

As a rule, abdominal symptoms are not prominent in those forms of joint disease characterized by polyarticular involvement (Fig. 8.9), and they frequently appear as a complication. There is no specific relationship between these different diseases.

DISORDERS WITH POLYARTICULAR JOINT INVOLVEMENT AND ABDOMINAL SYMPTOMS

Diagnosis	Abdominal symptoms	General symptoms	Extra-articular features	Relationship between abdominal symptoms to arthritis
Whipple's disease	Diarrhea (steatorrhea) Abdominal pain	Fever Weight loss Lymphadenopathy	Neurologic Dermatologic	Onset Different Course No relationship
Blind loop syndrome	Abdominal pain Diarrhea	Fever Weight loss	Erythema nodosum Vesicopustulae Urticaria	Onset 2–30 months after surgery Course No relation
Celiac disease	Absent in 50% Abdominal pain Steatorrhea	Malaise Weight loss	Osteomalacia	Relationship unknown
Vasculitic syndromes Henoch–Schönlein Rheumatoid arthritis Systemic lupus erythematosus Polyarteritis nodosa	Abdominal pain Intestinal bleeding Perforation	Disease-related	Purpura Disease-related	No direct relationship
Scleroderma	Obstipation Abdominal cramps	Disease-related	Disease-related	No direct relationship

Fig. 8.9 Disorders with polyarticular joint involvement and abdominal symptoms.

WHIPPLE'S DISEASE

Whipple's disease is probably a form of enterogenic reactive arthritis caused by an infection of the gut. Characteristic periodic acid Schiff (PAS)-staining deposits are found in macrophages of the small intestine and in the mesenteric nodes; these cells contain rod-shaped free bacilli[23]. These bacilliform bodies are considered to be the etiologic agent since they disappear when a patient is successfully treated with antibiotics[24]. Recently, using polymerase chain reaction, a bacterial 16S RNA sequence was amplified from duodenal tissue, and shown to be a gram-positive actinomycete, designated as *Tropheryma whipplii*[25]. The clinical picture is characterized by weight loss, pyrexia, lymphadenopathy, abdominal pain and migratory polyarthritis. Diarrhea with steatorrhea is usually the chief complaint and is observed in 75% of the cases.

The peripheral arthritis may be transient or chronic, it involves larger joints more often than small ones, and is predominantly polyarticular and symmetric. The arthritis may antedate the intestinal complaints. Flares of arthritis are not related to exacerbations of intestinal symptoms. The synovial fluid usually contains a high number of cells (4000–100,000/mm^3; 4–100 $\times$ 10^9/l), predominantly polymorphonuclear cells (up to 100%).

Erosive lesions on radiographs are absent, although destructive lesions have been reported. The incidence of sacroiliitis and spondylitis is controversial and ranges between 8% and 20%. The relationship with HLA-B27 has also been described.

The disease responds very well to antibiotic treatment, usually with tetracyclines, which have to be continued for more than one year.

BLIND LOOP SYNDROME

Intestinal bypass surgery can cause a syndrome associated with arthritis and dermatitis. The pathogenesis involves bacterial overgrowth and mucosal alterations in the blind loop and is probably immune-mediated[26].

Polyarthritis develops in 20–50% of patients with the blind loop syndrome, 2–30 months following surgery. The arthritis is polyarticular, symmetric and migratory, and may become chronic. The most frequently affected joints are the knees, wrists, metacarpophalangeal and metatarsophalangeal joints. The duration of the arthritis is unpredictable. Radiographic deformities or erosions are not seen. There is no relationship between joint symptoms and gut symptoms. Erythema nodosum, vesicopustular eruptions and urticaria may be associated. Surgical reanastomosis gives complete resolution of all symptoms.

Acute symmetric polyarthritis involving the peripheral and axial skeleton was described 1 week to 2 years after a restorative proctocolectomy with an ileal pouch and anastomosis for ulcerative colitis[27].

CELIAC DISEASE

Celiac disease (gluten-sensitivity enteropathy) is known to be associated with abnormal intestinal permeability. Bowel symptoms, however, are absent in 50% of patients. Many disorders, such as dermatitis herpetiformis, hyposplenism and autoimmune disorders, have been associated with the disease.

Celiac disease can be divided into three types:

- one in which diarrhea (usually steatorrhea) is the main feature;
- one with constitutional disturbances such as lassitude, weight loss and malaise;
- one with varied symptoms such as neuropathy and osteomalacia.

The distribution of the arthritis varies widely but is mainly polyarticular and symmetric, involving predominantly the large joints, hips, knees and shoulders. Radiographic changes are rare. A higher frequency of HLA-B8, DR3 has been described. There is a striking response of joint manifestations to a gluten-free diet28, although rechallenge generally does not provoke arthritis.

VASCULITIC SYNDROMES

This entity includes a number of autoimmune diseases in which the gut is not primarily involved, although inflammation of the abdominal (usually mesenteric) arteries and secondary vasculitic lesions in gut mucosal and submucosal layers may arise.

Henoch-Schönlein purpura

This disease, which mainly occurs in children, is a form of hypersensitivity vasculitis. It is characterized by the triad of nonthrombocytopenic purpura, arthritis and abdominal pain.

The characteristic skin lesions are manifested as palpable purpura and represent leukoclastic venulitis. Arthritis, predominantly involving the lower limbs, is transient.

Gastrointestinal symptoms are characterized by severe cramping and colicky abdominal pain sometimes associated with gastrointestinal hemorrhage. Rarely, protein-losing enteropathy and even perforation may occur. There is no direct temporal relationship between articular and intestinal symptoms. Mild renal involvement, consisting of glomerulitis with microscopic hematuria, occurs in 50% of cases.

The disease usually remits spontaneously within a week, but recurrences are frequent before complete remission is achieved.

Rheumatoid arthritis

The initial pathologic change in RA is believed to occur in small blood vessels. The most important extra-articular complications of RA are due to an inflammatory vascular disease giving rise to digital arteritis, peripheral neuropathy and arteritis of viscera.

Intestinal involvement, due to a partial infarction of intestinal arteries, causes abdominal pain, at first intermittent and later continuous. This can lead to intestinal bleeding or perforation. There is no direct relation with the joint manifestations, but most RA patients with this complication have high rheumatoid factor titers and usually present subcutaneous nodules. The prognosis is very poor, and a fatal outcome is frequent.

Systemic lupus erythematosus (SLE)

The most common intestinal manifestation of SLE is abdominal pain, which may be accompanied by nausea and less often by diarrhea (see Chapter 7.1). In most patients abdominal pain occurs in association with evidence of disease activity in other systems. Abdominal pain is usually colicky and not related to joint manifestations. The symptoms are mainly caused by mesenteric arteritis, and colonic perforations may occur.

Polyarteritis nodosa

This disease is characterized by panmural necrotizing inflammatory lesions in small and medium-sized muscular arteries (see Chapter 7.20).

On angiography of the truncus coeliacus and the abdominal arteries, characteristic saccular or fusiform aneurysms and narrowing of arteries can be found (Fig. 8.10) which are of diagnostic importance.

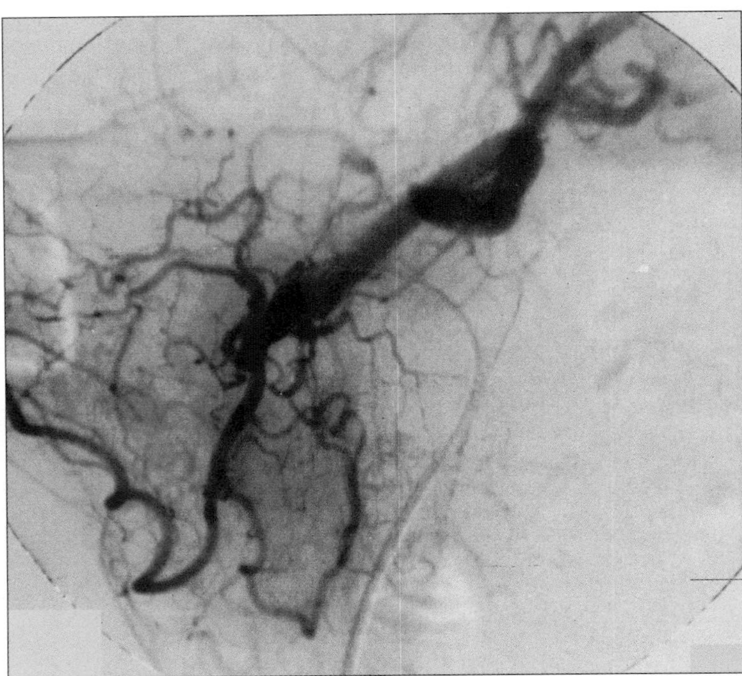

Fig. 8.10 Aneurysms on the mesenteric artery in polyarteritis.

Gastrointestinal involvement, mainly abdominal pain, is seen in 50% of patients. Nausea, vomiting, diarrhea, jaundice, ulceration with bleeding, infarction or perforation are other possible manifestations. Infarction and perforation are usually fatal.

SCLERODERMA

Scleroderma is a systemic disease characterized by excessive deposition of collagen and other connective tissue components in the skin and multiple internal organs (see Chapter 7.9). Gastrointestinal involvement is very frequent in this disease and is mainly characterized by a motility dysfunction of the entire gastrointestinal tract[29].

Reduced oral aperture, loss of lamina dura with loosening of the teeth and a severe esophageal dysfunction with dysphagia are features of upper gastrointestinal tract involvement.

Characteristically, hypomotility with atony, marked dilatation and functional ileus are present in the small intestine and the colon. Abdominal cramps, malabsorption and mainly constipation, sometimes alternating with diarrhea, are the clinical manifestations. The disturbed intestinal motility leads to stasis and secondary bacterial overgrowth.

The pathology consists of a normal mucosa with mild villous atrophy, infiltrations of the lamina propria by lymphocytes and plasma cells, fibrous thickening of the submucosa and thickening of the walls of small arteries and arterioles. Almost unique to systemic sclerosis is the development of wide-mouthed, often square-shaped pseudodiverticula along the anti-mesenteric border of the transverse and descending colon.

MISCELLANEOUS RHEUMATIC DISEASES

Behçet's syndrome

Behçet's syndrome is characterized by the presence of buccal, ocular, genital and skin ulcerations accompanied by arthritis (see Chapter 7.26). It has been related to the spondyloarthropathies (since sacroiliitis and spondylitis may be present) and to inflammatory bowel disease. Virtually all features of Behçets syndrome can be seen in Crohn's disease of the colon. Diarrhea, abdominal pain, ulceration of the colon and more rarely perforation are possible clinical manifestations. Controversy exists as to whether these cases represent true involvement of the colon by Behçet's syndrome, or merely coincidental inflammatory bowel disease.

Amyloidosis

Primary amyloidosis, or amyloidosis secondary to chronic inflammatory diseases, may cause gastrointestinal manifestations, including obstruction, ulceration, malabsorption, hemorrhage, protein loss and diarrhea (see Chapter 8.27). At a later stage, gastrointestinal bleeding may occur, which can be fatal. These manifestations may occur through direct infiltration with amyloid or through infiltration of the autonomic nervous system.

Familial Mediterranean fever

Familial Mediterranean fever is a genetic disorder, inherited as an autosomal recessive disorder with complete penetrance (see Chapter 5.23). The characteristic symptoms include intermittent fever, recurrent abdominal pain and joint inflammation.

The abdominal crises resemble acute peritonitis, lasting from 12–24 hours. Serous fluid in the abdominal cavity may be found. Intestinal obstruction may occur. The arthritis occurs together with, or independent of, the other manifestations. The arthritis is mainly asymmetric, predominantly involving the lower limbs. Attacks can persist for 2–3 weeks. Amyloidosis is a frequent complication.

AXIAL INVOLVEMENT

The axial involvement related to intestinal inflammation consists of sacroiliitis and syndesmophytes. Both lesions can be regarded as forms of enthesopathy. Sacroiliitis can be present without vertebral lesions; in cases of spondylitis, sacroiliitis is practically always associated.

INFLAMMATORY BOWEL DISEASE (CROHN'S DISEASE AND ULCERATIVE COLITIS)

There is no significant difference between the axial involvement in these two diseases. The true prevalence of sacroiliitis is difficult to estimate since the onset frequently is insidious. Prevalence rates of 10–15% for sacroiliitis and of 7–12% for spondylitis have been described, although the real figures are probably higher. The male to female ratio is 3:1, which is comparable to uncomplicated AS[30].

The clinical picture is indistinguishable from uncomplicated AS. The patient complains of inflammatory low back pain, thoracic or cervical pain, alternate buttock pain or chest pain. Limitation of motion in the lumbar or cervical region and reduced chest expansion are classic clinical signs.

The onset of axial involvement does not parallel that of bowel disease and frequently precedes it. Its course is also totally independent of the course of the gut disease; neither colectomy in ulcerative colitis nor surgery in Crohn's disease alter the course of any associated sacroiliitis or spondylitis.

Radiographically, the axial involvement is indistinguishable from uncomplicated AS. The frequency of asymmetric sacroiliitis could be higher (Fig. 8.11).

Sacroiliitis and spondylitis, as opposed to the peripheral arthritis, are associated with HLA-B27, but to a lesser degree than in uncomplicated AS. HLA-B27 positivity is found in 66% of ulcerative colitis patients and in 53% of Crohn's disease patients with spondylitis. The prevalence of HLA-B27 is lower in patients with inflammatory bowel disease and sacroiliitis alone. AS patients not carrying the HLA-B27 antigen are at a higher risk of developing IBD than are HLA-B27 positive AS patients. This has been confirmed in a prospective study on the evolution of spondyloarthropathies in which only 2 out of 6 ankylosing spondylitis patients evolving to IBD were found to be HLA-B27 positive[7]. In first degree relatives of patients with IBD, there is an increased prevalence of IBD and of AS. The HLA-B27-B44 phenotype has been found to place patients at a higher risk of developing the common manifestations of Crohn's disease and AS[31].

It has been postulated that axial involvement in inflammatory bowel disease is not a manifestation of this disease but an associated disorder[8].

ENTEROGENIC REACTIVE ARTHRITIS

Axial involvement in patients with reactive arthritis caused by enterogenic bacteria is relatively rare. Radiographic evidence of sacroiliitis has been found in 6–9% of patients and is more likely in chronic and recurrent disease. Ankylosing spondylitis is relatively rare.

The presence of sacroiliitis and spondylitis may be accounted for by a common genetic basis rather than by a predisposition to one as a result of the other.

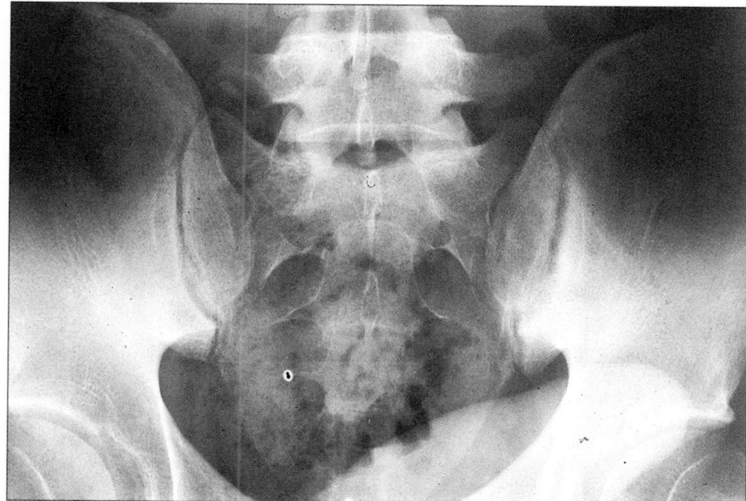

Fig. 8.11 Asymmetric sacroiliitis in a patient with inflammatory bowel disease.

OTHER SPONDYLOARTHROPATHIES

During evolution 7.5% of AS patients will develop IBD[7]. Sacroiliitis and spondylitis have also been described in Whipple's disease and in Behçet's syndrome but the relation of these diseases to the spondyloarthropathies remains speculative. Axial involvement in these diseases is rare and the association with HLA-B27 is questionable.

(NSAIDS) AND THE GASTROINTESTINAL TRACT

Long-term NSAID use increases the relative risk for gastric ulcer to 5 and for duodenal ulcer to 1.1[32], with a combined prevalence of 10–20% (see Chapter 3.5 and Practical Problem 5.16)[33]. These lesions can cause dangerous complications such as bleeding and perforation, and sometimes death. These drugs, however, are not only toxic for the upper gastrointestinal tract, but can induce subclinical intestinal abnormalities manifested by an increased intestinal loss of protein and blood[34], sometimes causing bowel ulcerations and small intestinal strictures[35].

Sulfasalazine can reduce intestinal inflammation and blood loss caused by NSAIDs[36]. NSAID-induced enteropathy is more common in the proximal parts of the jejunum and ileum than in the terminal ileum and colon.

There is no association found between the use of NSAIDs and the presence of inflammatory gut lesions in the terminal ileum and colon found during ileocolonoscopy in the spondyloarthropathies.

REFERENCES

1. Smith R. Treatment of rheumatoid arthritis by colectomy. Ann Surg. 1922;76:515–78.
2. Wright V, Moll JHD. Seronegative polyarthritis. Amsterdam: North–Holland; 1976.
3. Mayberry JF, Ballantyne KC, Hardcastle JD, Maugham C, Pye C. Epidemiological study of asymptomatic inflammatory bowel disease: the identification of cases during a screening programme for colorectal cancer. Gut. 1989;30:481–83.
4. Kirsner JB, Shorter RG. Inflammatory bowel disease. Philadelphia: Lea & Febiger; 1988.
5. Haslock I. Arthritis and Crohn's disease. Ann Rheum Dis. 1973;32:479–86.
6. Mielants H, Veys EM. The gut in the spondyloarthropathies. J Rheumatol. 1990;17:7–10.
7. Mielants H, Veys EM, Cuvelier C, *et al.* The evolution of spondylarthropathies in relation to gut histology. J Rheumatol.1995;22:2266–84.
8. Schorr–Lesnick B, Brandt LJ. Selected rheumatologic and dermatologic manifestations of inflammatory bowel disease. Am J Gastroenterol. 1988;83:216–23.
9. Banares AA, Jover JA, Fernandez-Gutierrez B, *et al.* Bowel inflammation in anterior uveitis and spondyloarthropathy. J Rheumatol. 1995;22:1112–17.
10. Kirsner JB. Genetic aspects of inflammatory bowel disease. Clin Gastroenterol. 1973;2:557–62.
11. Mielants H, Veys EM, Joos R, Noens L, Cuvelier C, De Vos M. HLA-antigens in seronegative spondyloarthropathies, reactive arthritis and arthritis in ankylosing spondylitis. Relation to gut inflammation. J Rheumatol. 1987;14:466–71.
12. Wright V, Watkinson G. The arthritis of ulcerative colitis. Br Med J. 1965;2:670–5.
13. Keat AE. Reiter's syndrome and reactive arthritis in perspective. N Engl J Med. 1983;309:1606–15.
14. Ahvonen P, Sievers K, Aho K. Arthritis associated with *Yersinia enterocolitica* infection. Acta Rheum Scand. 1969;15:323–32.
15. Granfors K, Jalkanen S, Von Essen R, *et al.* Yersinia antigens in synovial fluid cells from patients with reactive arthritis. N Engl J Med. 1989;320:216–21.
16. De Koning J, Heeseman J, Hoogkamp–Korstanje JAA, *et al.* Yersinia in intestinal biopsy specimens from patients with seronegative spondylarthropathies: correlation with specific serum IgA antibodies. J Infect Dis. 1989;159:109–12.
17. Mielants H, Veys EM, Goemaere S, Goethals K, Cuvelier C, De Vos M. Gut inflammation in the spondylarthropathies: clinical, radiological, biological and genetic features in relation to the type of histology. A prospective study. J Rheumatol. 1991;18:1542–51.
18. Cuvelier C, Barbatis C, Mielants H, De Vos M, Roels H, Veys EM. The histopathology of intestinal inflammation related to reactive arthritis. Gut. 1987;2:394–401.
19. Mielants H, Veys EM, Joos R, Cuvelier C, De Vos M. Repeat ileocolonoscopy in reactive arthritis. J Rheumatol. 1987;14:456–8.
20. Hammer RE, Maika SD, Richardson JA, Tang JP, Taurog JD. Spontaneous inflammatory disease in transgenic rats expressing HLA-B27 and Human b2M : an animal model of HLA-B27 associated human disorders. Cell 1990;63:109–12.
21. Taurog J, Richardson JA, Croft JAT, Simmons A, Ming Zhou S, Hammer E. The germfree state prevents development of gut and joint inflammatory disease in HLA-B27 transgenic rats. J Exp Med. 1994;180:2359–64.
22. Mielants H, Veys EM, Goethals K, Van Der Straeten C, Ackerman C, Goemaere S. Destructive hip lesions in seronegative spondylarthropathies. Relation to gut inflammation. J Rheumatol. 1990;17:315–40.
23. Fleminc JL, Wiesner RH, Shorter RG. Whipple's disease: clinical, biochemical and histopathologic features and assessment of treatment in 29 patients. Mayo Clin Proc. 1988;63:539–52.
24. Dobbins WO. Whipple's disease: an historical perspective. Q J Med. 1985;56:523–31.
25. Relman DA, Schmidt TM, Mac Dermott RP, *et al.* Identification of the uncultured bacillus of Whipple's disease. N Eng J Med. 1992;327:293–301.
26. Wands JA, Le Mont JT, Mann E, Isselbachter K. Arthritis associated with intestinal bypass procedure for morbid obesity. Complement activities and characterization of circulatory cryoproteins. N Engl J Med. 1976;294:121–4.
27. Axon JMC, Hawley PR, Huskisson EC. Ileal pouch arthritis. Br J Rheumatol. 1993;32:586–8.
28. Bourne JT, Kumar P, Huskisson E. Arthritis and coeliac disease. Ann Rheum Dis. 1985;44:592–8.
29. Battle WM, Shape WJ, Scott–Weight, *et al.* Abnormal colonic mobility in progressive systemic sclerosis. Ann Intern Med. 1981;94:749–52.
30. Isdale A, Wright V. Seronegative arthritis and the bowel. In: Baillières Clinical Rheumatology: The gut and rheumatic diseases. 1989;3:285–301.
31. Purmann J, Zeidler H, Bertram S, *et al.* HLA-antigens in ankylosing spondylitis associated with Crohn's disease. Increased frequency of the HLA phenotype B27–B44. J Rheumatol. 1988;15:1659–61.
32. Duggan JM, Dobson AJ, Johnson H, *et al.* Peptic ulcer and non-steroidal antiinflammatory agents. Gut. 1986;27:929–33.
33. Larkam EN, Smith JL, Lidsky MD, Gramad DY. Gastroduodenal mucosa and dyspeptic symptoms in arthritic patients during chronic nonsteroidal anti-inflammatory drug use. Am J Gastroenterol. 1987;82:1153–1158.
34. Bjarnason I, Hayllar J, MacPherson AT, Russell A. Side-effects on non-steroidal antiinflammatory drugs in the small and large intestine in man. Gastroenterology 1993;104:1832–47.
35. Morek AJ, Madhock R, Sturrock RD, Capell HA, Mac Kenzie JF. Enteroscopic diagnosis of small bowel ulceration in patients receiving nonsteroidal antiinflammatory drugs. Lancet 1991;337:520.
36. Hayllar T, Smith T, MacPherson A, Price AB, Gumpel M, Bjarnason I. Nonsteroidal anti-inflammatory drug-induced small intestinal inflammation and blood loss. Arthritis Rheum. 1994;37:1146–50.

9

THE KIDNEY AND RHEUMATIC DISEASE

J Stewart Cameron

- Renal manifestations of rheumatic diseases occur commonly.
- Rheumatologic conditions may occur in patients with renal diseases.
- Antirheumatic drugs may have adverse effects on the kidneys.
- There is a group of disorders which manifest themselves in the kidney as well as in soft tissues and in joints.
- The kidney and kidney function are important in rheumatologic practice.

SYMPTOMS OF KIDNEY DISEASE

Kidney disease is unlike rheumatic disease in that there are few syndromes in which renal involvement comes to attention – renal disease is characterized more by its silence than its symptoms[1]. Occasionally, if proteinuria is profuse, the nephrotic syndrome (edema, hypoalbuminemia and profuse proteinuria) will appear. However, blood and protein in the urine go unnoticed unless tests are performed, and macroscopically visible hematuria is unusual. Uremia, with all its complications, creeps up insidiously and causes feelings of general ill-health and debility that may not be attributed to renal dysfunction unless urine is tested. Polyuria and nocturia may give a clue to reduced renal function, but in men with normal renal function may also be the result of prostatic enlargement. Pain is not a feature of renal disease, although it does of course occur with renal and (above all) ureteric stones. Thus, to detect early changes in renal function, the clinician is particularly dependent upon laboratory tests of urine and blood.

TESTING FOR KIDNEY DISEASE

PROTEINURIA

There are no outward signs of proteinuria unless a large amount of protein is excreted, in which case the urine may be frothy and edema may appear as part of a nephrotic syndrome. The glomerular filter is complex, permitting a high flux of solvent (water) and of molecules up to an Einstein–Stokes radius of 1.5nm, above which there is a gradual cutoff with increasing molecular size[2]. A practical consequence of this selectivity is that glomerular proteinuria is overwhelmingly albumin, reinforced by the fact that the concentration of albumin in plasma is higher than that of any other protein.

Ordinarily less than 150mg of protein are excreted in the urine per 24 hours (80 ± 24mg) so that 128mg/24h represents the upper limit of normal[3]. More than half of these are low molecular weight proteins or protein fragments, although albumin is the largest single component. Proteinuria in excess of this arises if the glomerular filter is damaged and becomes more permeable ('glomerular' proteinuria). However, if the proximal renal tubules are damaged, proteins of low molecular weight, normally almost completely reabsorbed, pass into the urine ('tubular' proteinuria). This usually occurs as part of Fanconi's syndrome of multiple proximal tubular damage and dysfunction[4].

Testing for proteinuria

Heating the urine to test for albuminuria is rare today, having been replaced by various 'stick' tests[5] (Fig. 9.1). These are based on the principle that the titration curve of certain dyes is shifted in the presence of protein, especially albumin. However, it must be remembered that immunoglobulin light chains and some low molecular weight proteins are not detected by stick tests. The sticks are buffered to keep the pH

DIFFERENT METHODS OF DETECTING AND MEASURING URINE PROTEIN

Method	Description	Detection limit (mg/l)	Comments
Kjeldahl	Remove nonprotein nitrogen, digest protein, measure protein nitrogen	10–20	Reference and research method
Biuret	Copper reagent, measures peptide bonds	50	Requires precipitation of proteins, used for 24h measurement in some labs
Turbidimetric	Addition of trichloracetic or sulfosalicylic acids alters colloid properties and produces turbidity read in densitometer; benzethomecin also used	50–100	Imprecise, different readings from albumin and globulin
Dye binding	Indicator changes colour in presence of protein (e.g. Coomassie brilliant blue)	50–100	Different proteins bind differently; used in many labs for 24h excretion
Stick tests	Impregnated with indicator dye (bromcresol green) which changes colour in presence of protein	100	Reacts poorly with globulins; Usual clinical screening test

Fig. 9.1 Different test methods of detecting and measuring urine protein. The commonest today are 'stick' tests (bottom) using paper strips impregnated with indicator dye which are dipped into the urine.

constant and should be read immediately: leaving them in the urine will wash out the buffer and give a false reading. Commercial sticks such as Albustix are very sensitive, giving a trace or positive reading in many normal urine samples containing protein at only about 100mg/l. An alternative test is sulfosalicylic acid precipitation (0.5ml of 3% solution to 0.5ml urine), which can be read in a densitometer to give a rough quantitative reading. Again, this is insensitive to immunoglobulin light chains.

If proteinuria is found, it is usual to quantitate it over 24 hours. Alternatively, the protein:creatinine ratio can be determined on 'spot' urine samples. Upper limits of normal are 0.2 by weight (21mg/mmol); more than 3.5 (360mg/mmol) represents nephrotic range proteinuria[6]. Many individuals without renal disease will show a positive stick test for proteinuria, often only in 'trace' or '+' quantities. Thus 2–5% of children, 5% of young adults and up to 16% of the elderly will show detectable proteinuria[7]. Proteinuria in excess of normal is often found incidentally in daytime specimens taken from adolescent boys, but levels return to normal during recumbency ('postural' or 'orthostatic' proteinuria), with a benign prognosis in almost all cases[8]. Strenuous exercise will lead to the appearance of protein, red cells and even casts in the urine[9,10], and a resting sample may need to be checked.

Quantities of protein in excess of normal but insufficent to register on stick testing, termed microalbuminuria, have been studied extensively in diabetics. Microalbuminuria is present in the majority of patients with systemic lupus erythematosus (SLE), even in those with apparently normal urine and renal function[11]: biopsy may reveal histologic changes, and some of these patients subsequently develop obvious clinical proteinuria and nephritis.

Cellulose acetate electrophoresis is the easiest way of assessing the pattern of proteinuria, and is particularly valuable in the diagnosis and assessment of tubular proteinuria, where it rarely exceeds 1.5–2g/24h in the urine. In glomerular proteinuria, in contrast, up to 100g/24h proteinuria may be found. In myeloma, however, there may be concomitant glomerular damage, and thus albuminuria as well. Specific radioimmunoassays and enzyme-linked immunosorbent assays (ELISAs) are available for β_2-microglobulin, one of the many microglobulins which form the major part of tubular proteinuria (see later). Patients with primary amyloidosis and light-chain nephropathy, as well as those with myeloma, may have κ and λ light chains in their urine. The most accurate and sensitive method to detect this is immunofixation using specific antisera to probe blots of electrophoresed urines. The concentration in the plasma may be negligible, while high in the urine.

HEMATURIA

This is a cardinal symptom of renal disease. Visible blood in the urine may be bright red but more often, after a delay, is brownish and like tea or cola in appearance, especially in acid urine. Usually the blood loss is trivial but in some patients (generally, those with bleeding lesions of the urinary tract) there is major bleeding with clot colic. This is not common but occurs from tumors, after trauma and, occasionally, from polycystic kidneys and in sickle cell trait, all of which can appear in rheumatologic patients. Invisible blood or hemoglobin in the urine may be detected by the appropriate test – microscopy and stick tests, respectively.

Unlike proteinuria, which almost invariably arises from the kidneys, hematuria may arise from anywhere in the urinary tract[7]. Urinary tract infections and prostatic disease are common causes of hematuria (Fig. 9.2). In all cases, the test should be repeated several times over 1–2 weeks and urinary infection sought. In any individual over 45–50 years of age the possibility of a tumor must be investigated[12]; the likelihood of significant lesions in an otherwise well young patient with hematuria unaccompanied by proteinuria is very small[13]. The presence of red cell casts confirms glomerular hematuria[14], as does concomitant proteinuria in higher than trace amounts. In the presence of either, cystourethroscopy is unnecessary, although still often performed in practice. The side effects of warfarin and other anticogulants should not be overlooked, but in most such cases there will be an identifiable lesion or lesions within the urinary tract[15].

CAUSES OF HEMATURIA	
Disorders of coagulation	**Infections**
Anticoagulants Bleeding disorders (hemophilia, etc.)	Acute pyelonephritis/cystitis Schistosomiasis Urethritis Prostatitis
Glomerular diseases	**Stones**
IgA nephropathy Endocapillary nephritis Alport's syndrome Thin membrane nephropathy Mesangiocapillary glomerulonephritis Crescentic glomerulonephritis Fabry's disease Vasculitis/lupus, etc.	Anywhere in urinary tract Calcium oxalate crystalluria Urate crystalluria
	Obstruction
	Release of obstruction
Interstitial diseases	**Trauma**
Interstitial nephritis Polycystic disease	To kidney, bladder, ureter
Medullary diseases	**Miscellaneous**
Papillary necrosis from: Analgesic nephropathy Sickle cell disease Diabetes mellitus Sponge kidney Tuberculosis	Hypertension Loin pain hematuria syndrome Familial telangectasia Atrioventricular malformations Endometriosis Chemical cystitis Meatal ulcers Urethral caruncle Foreign body Trapped renal vein Factitious (added blood)
Renal and urinary tract tumous	
Wilms' tumor Renal cell carcinoma Transitional cell lesions Carcinoma of the prostate Carcinoma of the urethra	

Fig. 9.2 Causes of hematuria.

Testing for blood in the urine

Blood is only visible in urine to a concentration of 5ml/l (25,000 cells/μl). In health, fewer than 10^7 red blood cells (RBCs)are excreted per day in 2 liters of urine. In normal urine, the upper limit of the number of RBCs is less clearly defined than that of normal proteinuria, perhaps because some normal individuals have thin glomerular capillary basement membranes: 90% of normal individuals will have <1 cell/ml (10^5 cells/h), but a few will show up to 10 cells/ml without having any renal dysfunction. A number of drugs and foods that give a pinky red color to the urine – phenindione, phenolphthalein, rifampin (rifampicin), beets, etc. – may be confused with hematuria. Hemoglobin and myoglobin may be excreted as free compounds when intravascular hemolysis or rhabdomyolysis occurs, and will need to be differentiated from hematuria. Porphyrins may also discolor urine and be mistaken for hematuria.

Stick tests detect the hemoglobin from lysed RBCs, which break up more quickly in dilute alkaline urine. The reaction is between the hemoglobin and *O*-toluidine, and the sensitivity of the tests is close to the normal range – about 1–5 cells/μl. Some individuals without kidney disease will show positive reactions from time to time, for example after vigorous exercise – 'jogger's nephritis'[9]. Negative results may be obtained using stick testing in urine samples when they contain ascorbic acid because the patient has been taking 'mega' doses of vitamin C[16].

Microscopy of unspun normal urine usually shows about 1 RBC/μl, and should be performed on fresh concentrated acid urine to avoid breakup of the cells. Hemoglobinuria or myoglobinuria can only be distinguished by doing both tests. A Fuchs–Rosenthal counting chamber should be used for unspun, unstained urine, preferably using phase-contrast rather than bright-field illumination. Concentration of the urine by centrifugation is useful for qualitative analysis only, to look for casts or white cells.

It is obviously valuable to be able to distinguish the site of origin of the RBCs if possible; for example, concomitant proteinuria and red cell casts have already been noted as indicators of hematuria that is glomerular in origin. Birch *et al.* reintroduced the idea of using red cell morphology for this purpose[17].

Normal hematuria shows less than 1% of dysmorphic erythrocytes[18], while glomerular hematuria usually contains a high proportion of bizarre-shaped RBCs with knobs protruding from them (acanthocytes)[19] and considerable anisocytosis (see Fig. 9.3). Smooth disks are usually observed with bleeding from lesions in the urinary tract. Both phase-contrast microscopy of unspun urine, which is strongly observer-dependent, and red cell analysers have been used to make the distinction; however, the latter, although convenient, do not provide accurate information at low red cell excretion rates.

Urine microscopy and casts

In renal diseases, particularly glomerulonephritis, the urine may contain 'casts' of the renal tubules. These casts are made up principally of a unique polymeric glycoprotein of high molecular weight (Tamm–Horsfall protein[20,21]) and various plasma proteins (principally albumin)[22], with formed elements of the renal tubular epithelium, white or red blood cells trapped in them[23] (Fig. 9.3c). A skilled observer examining fresh urine in the clinic can learn a great deal about what is going on in the kidney, but casts dissolve rapidly, especially in dilute alkaline urines, so that delayed observation is relatively useless. Nevertheless, the presence of casts containing red cells in particular is a valuable clue to the presence of glomerular inflammation, and it suggests immediately that the associated hematuria is of glomerular origin. Granular casts contain disintegrating renal tubular cells, and they too indicate significant disease. In renal failure, the dilated atrophic tubules give rise to broad casts ('renal failure casts'). Bland 'hyaline' casts made only of the protein matrix may be seen in simple proteinuric states or even in healthy individuals.

ENZYMURIA AND BRUSH BORDER ANTIGENS IN THE URINE

Small amounts of enzymes from renal tubular cells are found in normal urine[24]. Increased excretion of these enzymes has been shown to be a sensitive index of renal tubular damage because they are too large to pass the normal glomerular filter. These measurements have the advantage that they can be made easily and with great sensitivity, but they are unfortunately nonspecific. Their main value lies in screening populations at risk for renal damage, such as those taking potentially nephrotoxic agents or exposed to environmental hazards. Various enzymes have been studied, the most common being *N*-acetyl-β-D-glucosaminidase (NAG).

TESTS OF RENAL FUNCTION

These nearly always involve testing of glomerular function. Tubular function is rarely tested[4], although enzymuria and β_2-microglobulin excretion can be used as indicators of tubulointerstitial damage, as mentioned earlier. Some measure of glomerular filtration rate (GFR) is needed to assess glomerular function and allow safe prescription of renally excreted drugs. Unfortunately there is no single simple measurement that gives high-quality data from which GFR can be derived. It is important to realise, too, that renal function, along with almost every body function, declines with age.

Plasma creatinine measurement

Because of its convenience and low cost, this is the test most frequently used to assess glomerular function: no injections or infusions are required, and the technique is available in all clinical laboratories. However, it does have a number of disadvantages.

First, the chemistry of the reaction on which the test is based is only partially understood[25] and many substances interfere with the reaction (see Fig. 9.4), often resulting in false elevations of the measured concentration[25]. With improving technology and greater specificity (e.g. high-performance liquid chromatography), the 'normal levels' for plasma creatinine have been set lower and lower.

Second, the profound reduction in GFR with age is offset by

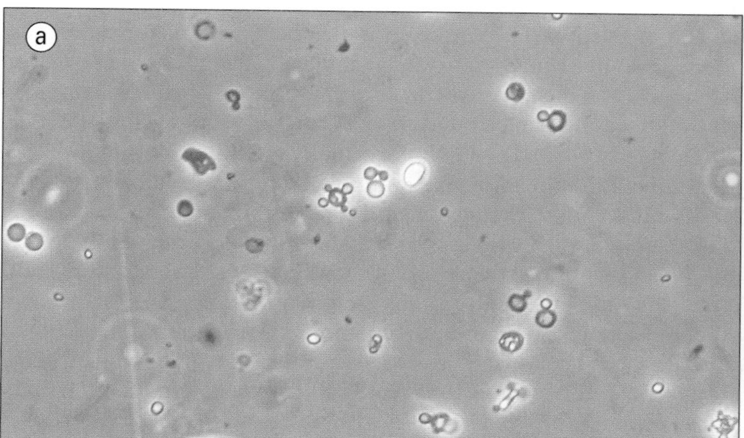

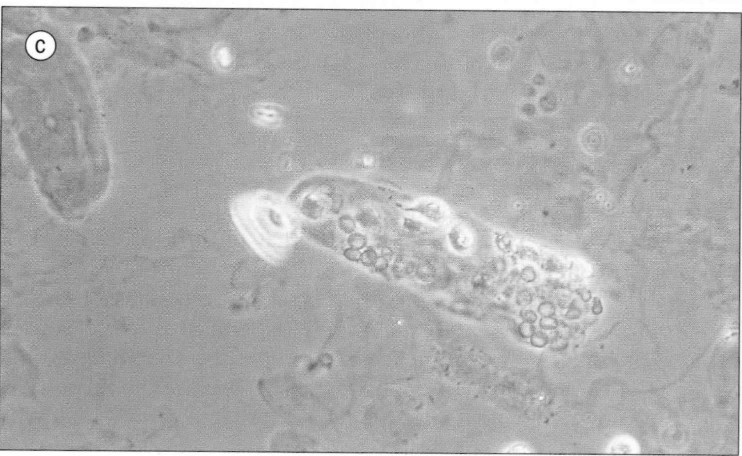

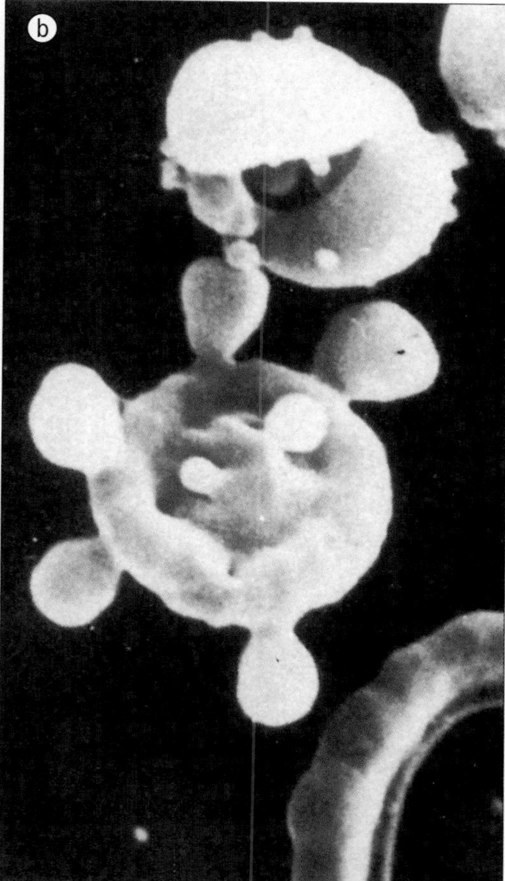

Fig. 9.3 Microscopy of urine. (a) Acanthocytes seen through the microscope which indicate a renal (probably glomerular) origin for the hematuria (×640, phase contrast). Courtesy of Dr GB Fogazzi. (b) Acanthocytes seen by scanning elecron microscope: details of the 'knobs' and protrusions can be seen. Reprinted by permission of Blackwell Science, Inc.[9] (c) A tubular cast containing red cells, which usually indicates a glomerular origin for concomitant hematuria (Rath *et al.*[14]) and in general an active proliferative/infiltrative glomerular disease (×400, phase contrast). Courtesy of Dr GB Fogazzi.

reduced creatinine production as muscle mass also decreases with age; thus the plasma creatinine at 100 years of age is the same as at 25, despite a reduction in GFR by two-thirds or more (Fig. 9.5). This holds as well for any other state in which muscle mass is lost (such as starvation).

Third, the increase in plasma creatinine concentration is not related linearly to a falling GFR. About half of renal function – even more in aged and wasting patients – can be lost before the plasma creatinine exceeds the upper limit of normal (Fig. 9.6).

Fourth, as renal function declines, creatinine is secreted increasingly by the renal tubules. Several drugs in common use interfere with this (e.g. cimetidine and trimethoprim) and raise the plasma creatinine concentration without a concomitant fall in GFR.

Finally, diet contributes to plasma creatinine in the form of creatine in meat, especially stewed meat. Blood urea is almost useless as an estimate of GFR because it depends to a greater degree both on dietary intake of protein and on body mass.

To derive GFR from the plasma creatinine, various formulae have been described which take account of some of these variables. The best validated and most reproducible is that of Cockroft and Gault (see [27]), which nevertheless remains an approximation:

$$GFR = \frac{1.2(140 - A)W}{P_{creat}}$$

where GFR is the glomerular filtration rate, measured in milliliters per minute; A is age of the patient, measured in years; W is weight of the patient, measured in kilograms; and P_{creat} is plasma concentration of creatinine, measured in micromoles per liter. If P_{creat} is expressed as milligrams per deciliter, then the factor 1.2 in the numerator must be replaced by a factor 72 in the denominator.

Creatinine clearance

While a number of exogenous substances such as inulin satisfy the criteria for an ideal substance capable of measuring the GFR[4], the many techniques used require infusions, catheterization, etc., and so are impractical for clinical use. However, creatinine comes near to being ideal: creatinine clearance approximates to inulin clearance, and in many centers it is measured instead of plasma creatinine. Having said this, the weakness of any clearance measurement is the need for accurate urine collection, usually over 24 hours, which despite its apparent simplicity proves almost impossible on a regular basis. Furthermore, creatinine secretion by the renal tubules increases as the plasma concentration rises. In some patients this also occurs in the presence of proteinuria. Thus there is probably no point in measuring creatinine clearance unless the measurement can be repeated many times to obtain an average figure or a trend.

Clinical measurement of GFR by other methods

The difficulties in measuring GFR have led to a search for other methods more suitable for routine clinical use. The methods used are more accurate than plasma creatinine measurement, especially at normal or near normal renal function. Most involve the injection of an easily measured exogenous substance by a single injection, usually intravenously, and the derivation of the GFR from the rate of reduction in plasma concentration in a variable number of blood samples taken during the hours following the injection[4]. Iohexol measured by fluorescent excitation[28,29] has become widely used, as has ^{131}I-iothalamate in the USA[30] and ^{51}Cr-EDTA (ethylenediaminetetra-acetic acid)[31] in Europe. The former can also be given by subcutaneous injection so that an approximately stable concentration is present in the blood and a quantity excreted per unit time (UV) and plasma concentration (P) clearance measured[32]. Finally, ^{99}Sn^{m}-DTPA (diethylene penta acetic acid), which is normally used for imaging, can be used to measure the GFR too[33], although the short radioactive half-life (6 hours) of the chelate makes it inconvenient to use.

A search has been made for substances that occur naturally in the plasma and whose concentrations rise linearly with the fall in GFR, rather than hyperbolically as does creatinine (Fig. 9.6). β_2-Microglobulin satisfies some of these conditions[34] but is not easy to measure. Recently, the serine protease inhibitor cystatin C[29,35] has been proposed as a substitute for creatinine and seems to have distinct advantages. It may be that its use will increase.

INTERFERENCE WITH THE MEASUREMENT AND RENAL HANDLING OF CREATININE

Substances that interfere with the measurement of plasma creatinine or creatinine clearance	
Endogenous	
Protein	Deproteination is essential; note the influence of hyperproteinemia in some kinetic methods
Ketones and ketoacids	Actetoacetate and acetone elevate levels (red complex); this depends on the timing of rate analysis, temperature, ascorbic acid
Glucose and other sugars	Picrate to picramate (red); effect on levels is with temperature, rate and method
Bilirubin	Reduces kinetic levels by increasing blank (biliverdin)
Fatty acids	Elevates levels; especially palmitic
Urate	Elevates levels; Jaffé reactive on heating
Urea	Elevates levels; weakly Jaffé reactive
Exogenous	
Cephalosporins	Strongly elevates levels to as high as 500μmol/l (5.7mg/dl); varies with drug and method of analysis; cefoxitin, cephalothin, cephamandole, cephaloridine, cefotaxime react, but the rate of reaction varies
5-Fluorocytosine	Only with methods using creatinine deaminase – chromogen strongly elevates levels
Phenylacetylurea	Elevates levels, picrate reactive
Methanol metabolites	Elevates levels; metabolites not identified
Substances that block tubular secretion of creatinine and induce true elevation of plasma creatinine (reducing calculated creatinine clearance)	
Triamterene	Probenecid
Spironolactone	Cimetidine (not ranitidine)
Amiloride	Trimethoprim

Fig. 9.4 Interference with the measurement and renal handling of creatinine. See Spencer [25] for discussion and further references.

MULTISYSTEM DISEASES PRESENTING BOTH IN JOINTS AND IN KIDNEYS

SYSTEMIC LUPUS ERYTHEMATOSUS

Only about one-third of patients with lupus nephropathy first present directly in a renal clinic (see Chapters 7.3–7.8)[36]. In one study of 1000 lupus patients seen in rheumatologic practice, renal involvement was present in 16% at presentation, and in half during follow up[37]. Review shows a variation of 25–65% in different series – greater in younger and less in older patients. Because patients with SLE may develop nephropathy later, microscopic examination of the urine and testing for protein need to be performed at every visit to the rheumatology clinic, and not merely at the first attendance. A regular check on renal function is also useful (see earlier).

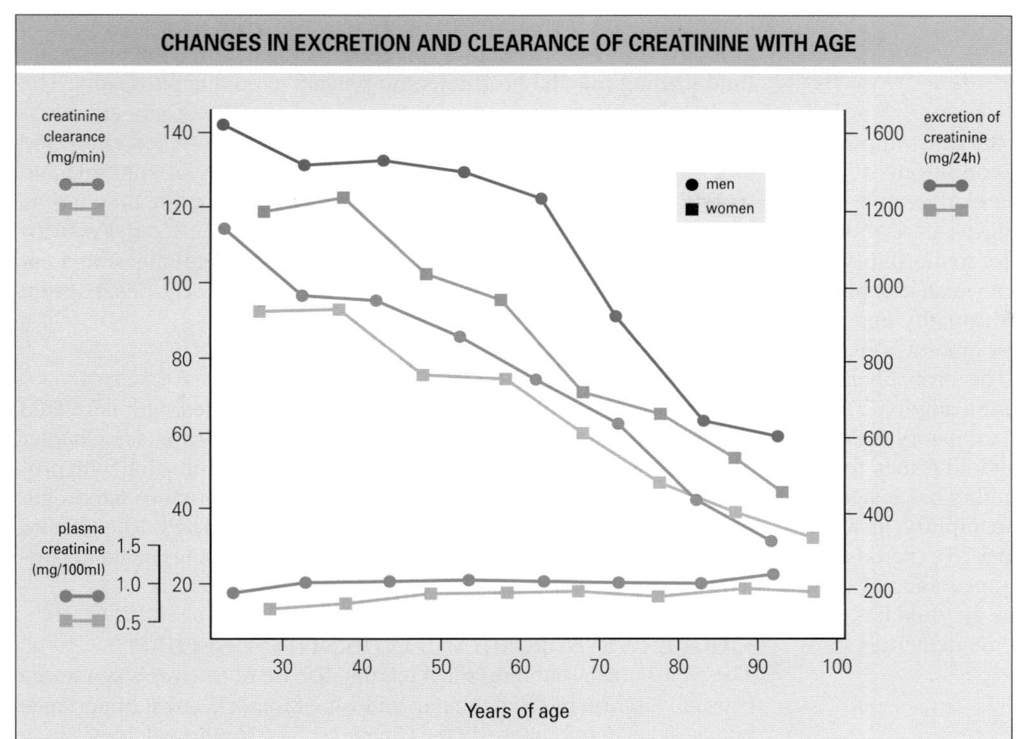

Fig. 9.5 The 'hidden' reduction in renal function with age. Although the normal creatinine clearance decreases dramatically with age to a mean of only 40ml/min in the very elderly, the plasma creatinine remains constant up to 100 years of age because of a concomitant reduction in excretion (and by inference, production) of creatinine due to reduction in muscle mass (data from Kampmann *et al.*[26]).

About 10% of patients with lupus nephritis develop distal renal tubular acidosis with hyperchloremia and hyperkalemia. Usually this is of little importance, except that the hyperkalemia may be worsened by drug therapy, especially by the use of mixed diuretics containing a potassium-sparing diuretic such as amiloride or triamterene. Thus plasma electrolytes should be checked periodically. In patients with hyperkalemia resistant to dietary manipulation, 9α-fludrocortisone may be of value[38]. The role of renal biopsy in patients with lupus is considered in Chapter 7.8.

THE VASCULITIDES (WEGENER'S GRANULOMATOSIS, MICROSCOPIC POLYANGIITIS, ETC.)

Although a polyarthropathy is common in the early stages of various forms of vasculitis (Chapters 7.17–7.31), the arthralgias are not often the dominant long-term problem. As with SLE, an important point in patients with vasculitis is that they may develop renal manifestations later in the course of their disease, and urine assessment at every visit should be the rule, with plasma creatinine, or better GFR, measurements at intervals.

Children with Henoch–Schönlein purpura (Chapter 7.28) have by definition a polyarthralgia which may precede the rash and usually precedes the renal manifestations. About 50% of patients develop nephritis, but only in a minority is it severe. Nevertheless, nephritis is a source of major morbidity and an important cause of end-stage renal failure in children[1,39].

Renal disease is an inconstant feature of relapsing polychondritis (Chapter 5.27) and often takes the form of a crescentic glomerulonephritis, although other histologic patterns, including focal segmental glomerulosclerosis, are found. Treatments of both the primary condition and the renal disease are controversial, and the role of immunosuppressive therapy is unclear.

SYSTEMIC SCLEROSIS

It is important to remember that renal vasoconstriction with diminished renal blood flow and increased filtration fraction is a very early manifestation of scleroderma (see Chapters 7.9–7.12), appearing long before hypertension, urinary changes or renal failure[40]. A close watch needs to be kept on renal function and above all blood pressure in every patient.

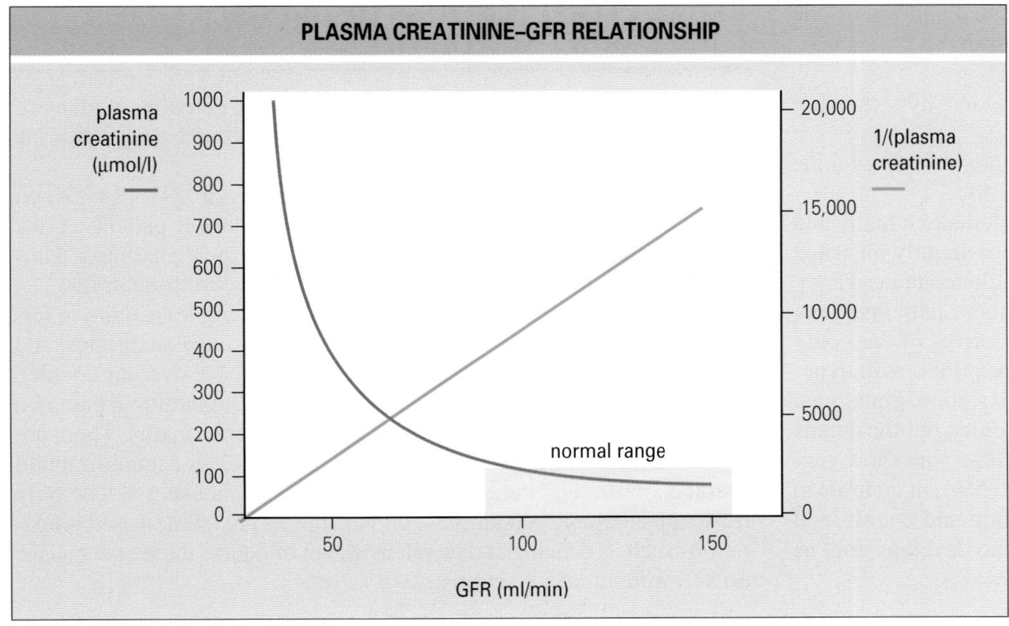

Fig. 9.6 The relationship of plasma creatinine to GFR. As the GFR decreases, plasma creatinine rises but in a hyperbolic fashion, so that plasma creatinine levels only become abnormal (normal range shaded) after a considerable loss of renal function. One way of compensating for this hidden information is to use the reciprocal of the plasma creatinine, which is approximately linear.

RENAL COMPLICATIONS OF RHEUMATOLOGIC CONDITIONS

AMYLOIDOSIS

Reactive amyloid A (see Chapter 8.27) is by far the most important renal complication arising from rheumatologic conditions. It may follow any inflammatory condition except SLE (and ulcerative colitis), but is particularly common in rheumatoid arthritis (RA), both in adults and in children, when it is a major contributor to morbidity and a common cause of death (see Chapter 5.24). It may also complicate ankylosing spondylitis, more rarely psoriatic arthropathy and very rarely Behçet's syndrome[41]. However, it is almost unknown in SLE and only a handful of cases have been recorded[42]. This probably arises from the fact that in lupus there is no increase in serum amyloid A protein concentrations during the acute or chronic inflammatory episodes that is found in all the other conditions listed[43]. Amyloid A may follow prolonged joint or bone sepsis, particularly when this has lasted for several years, although it may appear early and rapidly in a few patients. In familial Mediterranean fever (Chapter 5.23), there is evidence that colchicine prophylaxis prevents the appearance of renal damage and proteinuria. However, in general, once amyloid has been deposited within the kidney it does not regress, although there is some evidence for partial resolution in a few cases[44].

GOUTY NEPHROPATHY

The common form of gout (Chapters 8.14 & 8.15) is a disorder of renal function in the form of relative underexcretion of filtered urate (fractional excretion of urate, FE_{urate}, 5.4% versus 10–12%) in the face of a normal or increased purine load of dietary origin. Glomerular renal function of gouty patients attending rheumatology clinics is almost always normal when corrected for age (see Fig. 9.6) and chronic renal impairment is now rare; conversely, gout is rare as a cause of chronic renal insufficiency (0.5–1.0%). Renal biopsies from these patients, even when appropriately processed into alcohol to prevent washout of uric acid/urate from the sections, usually show few or absent intratubular or interstitial deposits of urate/uric acid, while vascular and tubulointerstitial lesions are prominent.

If gouty patients with impaired renal function have been treated with allopurinol, appropriate adjustment for age and renal function must be made to achieve plasma oxypurinol concentrations of between 60μmol/l and 100μmol/l[45]. Most cases of allopurinol 'sensitivity' result from absolute or relative overdosing in relation to diminished renal function. Uricosuric agents such as benzbromarone and probenecid become relatively less effective as renal function decreases, losing their effect altogether when the plasma creatinine reaches about 250–300μmol/l.

If gout and renal failure are present together, the diagnosis of one of three possible subgroups of gout should be considered[46]:

- familial juvenile hyperuricemia (Chapter 8.19)[47];
- chronic lead intoxication, gout, renal failure and hypertension (Chapter 8.14);
- gout from complete or partial deficiency of hypoxanthine guanine phosphoribosyl transferase (HPRT) (Chapter 8.14).

Familial juvenile hyperuricemia affects males and females equally and is frequently associated with renal failure. It is a dominantly inherited disorder characterized by severe underexcretion of filtered urate (FE_{urate} 3–4%). The cause of the interstitial nephritis in these patients is not clear. An important point is that symptom-free relatives of the gouty patient, even children, may also be severe underexcretors, with hyperuricemia and reduction in GFR. Chronic lead intoxication, gout, renal failure and hypertension are associated with each other, but the details of the association are not clear. Subjects with saturnine gout show very low fractional excretions of filtered urate (FE_{urate} 3–5%). In contrast to classic gout, renal failure is common in this group and occult lead intoxication should be suspected in any patient who develops gout as renal failure progresses[48,49].

Gout from complete or partial deficiency of HPRT may show such gross overproduction of urate that even treatment with allopurinol and fluid loading may be insufficient to prevent crystal nephropathy. The crystals in patients treated with allopurinol may be of any combination of uric acid, xanthine and oxypurinol, infiltrating the kidney and clogging the urine[47]. Because of the poor solubility of xanthine and oxypurinol, even in alkaline urine, alkalinizing the urine may not be effective in preventing crystal nephropathy and acute renal insufficiency; increasing the urine flow rate is the most useful measure. Less severe forms of HPRT deficiency may present as early-onset severe gout, sometimes with a family history.

RHEUMATOID ARTHRITIS

The existence of a specific glomerulopathy associated with untreated RA has been the subject of controversy for some years (see Chapter 5.4)[50]. However, it now seems established that in association with proteinuria, minor degrees of hypercellularity or membranous nephropathy may be found. IgA nephropathy has also been noted[51]. Rheumatoid vasculitis is not usually complicated by nephritis, but crescentic nephritis has been recorded[52].

SJÖGREN'S SYNDROME AND INTERSTITIAL NEPHRITIS

The well-known (but rare) renal tubular disease of Sjögren's syndrome is usually a form of renal tubular acidosis of minor clinical importance but great academic interest (see Chapter 7.32). Nephrocalcinosis may be seen occasionally. The glomerulopathy associated with Sjögren's syndrome is less common, and usually of a membranous pattern.

OTHER RHEUMATOLOGIC DISORDERS

Relapsing polychondritis (Chapter 5.27) has been mentioned above. Other glomerulopathies seen in association with rheumatic conditions include IgA nephropathy in ankylosing spondylitis (Chapters 6.15–6.20)[51,53,54], membranous nephropathy[55] and various forms of nephritis in association with either psoriasis or psoriatic spondyloarthropathy[54] (Chapters 6.21–6.23). Because skin lesions are common (2% of the Caucasian population), some reports probably represent coincidence rather than a causal relationship. IgA nephropathy has also been reported in association with Reiter's syndrome[54] (Chapter 6.12). The glomerulopathy of mixed connective tissue disease is discussed in Chapter 7.33. It is now recognized to be more common than initially supposed, but it is still much less commonly found than in patients with lupus and is not usually severe. There is an infrequent association of Behçet's syndrome (Chapter 7.26) with a nephritis; it may be crescentic and severe[56], with or without evident glomerular immune aggregates.

RENAL COMPLICATIONS OF DRUGS USED IN RHEUMATOLOGY

All rheumatologists are aware of the nephrotoxic potential of many of the drugs they prescribe[50], and it goes without saying that regular urine and renal funtion tests are necessary.

The toxicity of nonsteroidal anti-inflammatory drugs (NSAIDs) on the kidney is discussed in Chapters 3.5 and 5.16. Many patients at risk purchase ibuprofen or naproxen direct from their local pharmacy. Thus it is important to question patients about their use of these drugs.

Analgesic nephropathy (Chapter 3.4) is becoming less common following educational programs on the dangers of mixed analgesics, and the removal of phenacetin from preparations available over the counter. One practical problem is how to treat chronic rheumatologic pain in a patient who has previously suffered analgesic nephropathy. There are few hard data in this field, but many clinicians use acetaminophen (paracetamol), despite its close relationship to phenacetin. The only truly safe analgesics under these circumstances are opiate-based preparations such as codeine and its relatives, but of course these agents have no anti-inflammatory actions.

The induction of membranous nephropathy by penicillamine and sodium aurothiomalate[50] (Chapter 5.16) is also seen with other sulfydryl-containing drugs. It seems likely that, in the case of gold, it is the thiol group which is responsible, especially since forms of gold which do not contain a thiol group do not induce proteinuria. If significant proteinuria or a nephrotic syndrome develops, there is some evidence that the proteinuria will diminish or even disappear despite continued drug ingestion. The rare syndrome of pulmonary hemorrhage and crescentic nephritis induced by penicillamine[57,58] may be fatal. The use of either penicillamine or aurothiomalate has been rarely associated with a minimal change nephrotic syndrome rather than the more common membranous nephropathy (see Chapter 5.16).

The experimental drug Tenidap[59] which has several effects, including those of a cyclo-oxygenase inhibitor, induces a minor degree of mostly tubular proteinuria. In one study β_2-microglobulin was observed in 40% of patients given the drug, but only 1.5% had the drug withdrawn because proteinuria exceeded 1.5g/24h. In almost all patients this proteinuria disappeared within 3–12 months; its mechanism is not clear but presumably represents reversible proximal tubular damage.

RHEUMATOLOGIC COMPLICATIONS OF RENAL DISEASE[60–62]

ACUTE MONOARTHROPATHY

An acute hot single joint in renal patients has the usual differential diagnosis and management, but the proportion of the different diagnoses may vary widely[62].

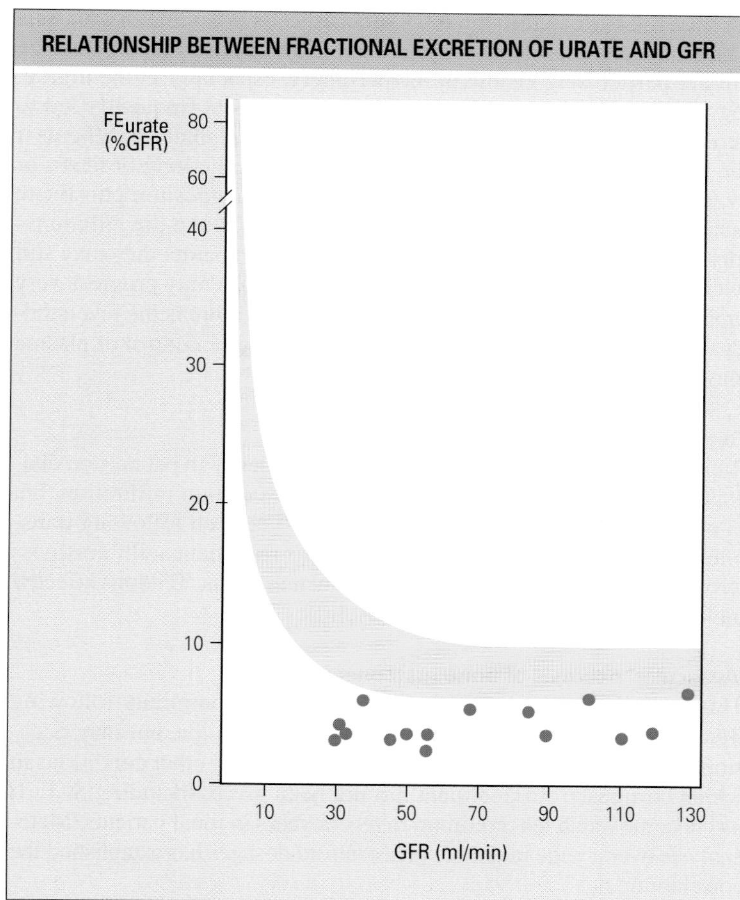

Fig. 9.7 The relationship between fractional excretion of urate (FE_{urate}) and GFR[63]. As the GFR falls below half of normal, the fractional excretion rises also, so that the rise in plasma urate is limited and its solubility limit is not exceeded. This accounts in part for the rarity of gout in uncomplicated renal failure. The points are data from patients with familial juvenile hyperuricemic nephropathy (FJHN) who have a low FE_{urate} at all levels of function; data from patients with lead-induced gout and renal failure are similar.

Gout

Gout is paradoxically rare in association with chronic renal failure, despite hyperuricemia, in part because the fractional excretion of urate rises steadily to as much as 80%[63] (Fig. 9.7) as GFR falls. Nevertheless, hyperuricemia does appear, and it has been suggested that the uremic milieu suppresses acute inflammation, although evidence for this is poor. When a diagnosis of gout is confirmed by the presence of the characteristic negatively birefringent crystals in joint fluid from patients already in uremia, in end-stage renal failure or on dialysis, lead-induced disease should be suspected[49] and excluded using a versenate test, although this is difficult to interpret in those with advanced renal failure.

In transplant recipients gout is common[64] and is usually precipitated by therapy with diuretics, cyclosporin or both, and may present even in young women. The volume contraction caused by diuretic use increases the net reabsorption of filtered urate and is probably the predominant factor. Cyclosporin diminishes the GFR, probably the main effect that leads to retention of urate and to gout.

In terms of treatment, an acute attack of gout can be conventionally managed in renal patients with intra-articular corticosteroids, colchicine or NSAIDs, although the potential risks of volume contraction in the diuretic-treated transplant recipient and the increased risk of gastrointestinal hemorrhage in the uremic (Chapter 5.16) must not be forgotten. Colchicine is retained in renal failure and the required dosage (usually 0.6mg every 2h until relief or diarrhea appears) may be lower than usual.

In the long-term management of chronic gout in patients with renal disease the most important points are:

- the dosage of allopurinol must be adjusted to the degree of renal function, to maintain an effective but safe plasma oxypurinol concentration of 60–100μmol/l [65];
- in transplant recipients a reduction in either diuretic or cyclosporin dosage, or both, will often solve the problem and avoid the need for chronic drug treatment;
- many transplant recipients receive treatment with azathioprine.

Even with reduction in dosage, allopurinol and azathioprine together usually produce severe marrow depression, from inhibition of conversion of 6-mercaptopurine (derived from the azathioprine) to 6-thiouric acid. The choice then is between using a uricosuric drug such as probenecid or benzbromarone, rather than allopurinol, or stopping the azathioprine so that allopurinol can be used.

Pseudogout

Pseudogout, in which weakly birefringent crystals of calcium pyrophosphate can be identified in the aspirated joint fluid (Chapter 8.16), is appreciably more common in patients with chronic or end-stage renal failure than in those with true gout, and is often found in association with secondary hyperparathyroidism. Articular calcification (chondrocalcinosis) is often present as well. In the acute attack, intra-articular corticosteroids are useful, followed by oral NSAIDs (remembering the caveats made above). Management of chronic pseudogout centers around controlling the phosphate concentration and alleviating the hyperparathyroidism, by parathyroidectomy if necessary.

Arthritis associated with articular and periarticular deposits of calcium oxalate crystals has also been reported in uremic patients[66,67] (see Chapter 8.17).

Septic arthritis

Uremic patients on dialysis are immunosuppressed by their uremia and are subject to repeated bacteremias, either from the needling procedures required for hemodialysis, or in association with episodes of peritoneal contamination or frank peritonitis in those on continuous ambulatory peritoneal dialysis (CAPD). Septic arthritis (Chapter 6.2) is therefore common in patients with end-stage renal disease[60], and may occur in almost any site – from spinal (with psoas abscess on occasion) through to phalangeal joints.

The most common infecting organism is *Staphylococcus aureus*, but, as always in the immunosuppressed, many other organisms may be seen, particularly gram-negative bacteria, but even fungi and *Mycobacterium tuberculosis* must not be forgotten[68]. Sometimes osteomyelitis of adjacent bone will complicate the course, especially if treatment is delayed.

All of the above also holds true for transplant recipients, except that their mechanism of immunosuppression is drug induced. Septic arthritis is seen less often in transplant recipients than in dialysed patients and may occur in almost any joint.

Hemarthrosis

The anticoagulated uremic patient may bleed into a large joint, resulting in hemarthrosis[69] (see Chapter 8.24). In some patients this is associated with β_2-microglobulin amyloid infiltration of periarticular structures (see Chapter 8.29).

JOINT EFFUSIONS

In association with transplant rejection

Painful effusions into joints, especially the knees, are sometimes seen in association with rejection episodes in transplant recipients. The pathogenesis is not known and the condition rapidly subsides during treatment of the rejection.

In association with β_2-microglobulin arthropathy

Effusions are common in joints affected by periarticular deposits of β_2-microglobulin (see below and Chapter 8.29), but these are usually noninflammatory. Under polarizing microscopy, fibrils of β_2-microglobulin amyloid may be seen in the joint fluid.

CHRONIC POLYARTHROPATHY AND SPONDYLOARTHROPATHY

This group of complaints (Chapter 6.10) in patients in chronic renal failure and on dialysis is a major cause of morbidity in patients who have had uremia for 5 years or more. Apart from the familiar conditions, a number of apparently new syndromes have been partially delineated in dialysed uremics, although the area remains confused and confusing.

Erosive osteoarthritis

The first group of patients shows an otherwise typical erosive osteoarthritis, mainly of the phalangeal and metacarpal joints, but also of major joints or in the spine. This does not differ radiologically or clinically from that seen in nondialysed patients, with an increasing incidence with age and a predominance of women. However, it appears to be much commoner than in the nondialysed population[70], and appears at sites other than the hand. Whether this raised incidence relates to the frequency of hyperparathyroidism in the dialysed population is not clear. It has been suggested that iron overload and deposition may be the central feature of pathogenesis[71].

Destructive cervical spondylarthropathy

In the second group of patients a destructive cervical spondyloarthropathy develops in older patients during the first years after starting hemodialysis or CAPD, or even in those who have never been dialysed, with the appearance of severe chondrocalcinosis. This may be another associated feature of hyperparathyroidism. It may be a spinal manifestation of the erosive joint changes in peripheral joints, discussed above.

β_2-Microglobulin-related amyloidosis

The third group of patients suffers from clinical syndromes associated strongly but not exclusively with β_2-microglobulin amyloidosis, and which overlap to some extent; they have received much attention (see Chapter 8.29)[72]. These conditions appear to arise in association with local deposition of an amyloid derived from β_2-microglobulin which accumulates in uremia.

Carpal tunnel syndrome in dialysed patients

A major associated feature of β_2-microglobulin accumulation in uremia is the frequency of carpal tunnel symptoms (Chapters 4.16 and 8.29) associated with local deposition of this compound. Only transient relief is gained from local injections of corticosteroids or local anesthetic agents, or by using splints; decompression is the only effective treatment for these symptoms, which are frequently severe and do not differ from those in patients with carpal tunnel symptoms in other settings. One or more decompressions may be needed.

Carpal tunnel syndromes may also be seen early in uremic patients in whom creation of arteriovenous fistulas at the wrist for dialysis has resulted in an edematous hand. Symptoms generally improve if blood flow to the hand can be reduced by surgical intervention on the fistula, but a decompression may be required later, when the hyperperfusion is seen merely to have precipitated the onset of symptoms.

UREMIC OSTEODYSTROPHY

This includes osteitis fibrosa, osteomalacia, fracturing aluminum-induced renal bone disease and 'adynamic' bone (Chapter 8.42). Bone diseases, particularly rickets, may also complicate renal tubular disorders that lead to excessive urinary losses of phosphate[73].

Soft tissue calcification

Ectopic deposition of calcium (Chapter 8.29) is common in uremic patients, especially those who have been untreated or inadequately dialysed for long periods. The crucial factor is a high calcium–phosphate product arising from secondary hyperparathyroidism, plus failure to control the plasma phosphate by diet or by phosphate binders. Eventually the only treatment is parathyroidectomy (see Chapter 8.42).

Periarticular inflammatory deposits of microcrystalline hydroxyapatite may mimic arthritis, affect tendon sheaths, or occur in the eye (uremic red eye), in the skin or as subcutaneous inflammatory masses. They may also present as vascular calcification of vessels of any size but are particularly visible in the periphery, especially in the digital, leg and forearm vessels. In the past these deposits frequently led to actual digital gangrene[60]. They may make transplantation difficult if the iliac vessels are involved. In organs such as the lung or heart, or even muscle, amorphous deposits of calcium magnesium phosphate occur and spread rapidly; although they do not evoke the inflammatory reaction associated with crystalline hydroxyapatite, they may still lead to organ dysfunction. Metastatic calcification may progress very rapidly (calciphylaxis), but an equally striking feature is the reversibility of such calcification after parathyroidectomy or control of plasma phosphate.

Tendon rupture

Rupture of tendons is seen with moderate frequency in patients on dialysis, in some in association with amyloid or calcium infiltration, but in others without apparent cause. It can also be seen following transplantation, when it presumably relates to treatment with corticosteroids[74], as occurs in other conditions such as lupus. Tendons affected include the biceps, quadriceps and Achilles.

'Avascular' necrosis of bone (osteonecrosis)

This complication (Chapter 8.47) is seen most commonly following transplantation during treatment with corticosteroids, but may occasionally appear in dialysis patients[75,76] or in certain other conditions in which corticosteroid treatment has not been given, including SLE. It has become much less common in recent years in renal patients. Meta-analysis over a wide range of corticosteroid dosages has established the correlation[77].

Osteopenia following transplantation

Osteoporosis is dealt with in Chapters 8.36–8.40. It has become apparent that, following renal transplantation, there is a rapid loss of some 8–10% of cancellous vertebral bone, but not of cortical bone[78], even in patients treated with low-dose corticosteroids as part of triple drug regimens. The most likely explanation is that this is an effect of glucocorticoid administration. This has been observed in other patients given these drugs[79], and there is some evidence that bone loss may be prevented by the use of corticosteroid-free or ultra-low-dose corticosteroid regimens[80]. This early phase after transplantation seems to be crucial since it appears that after 2 years the bone losses are normal for the patient's age and sex[81]. Fracturing osteopenia does not yet appear to be a major problem in transplant clinics.

REFERENCES

1. Bacon P, Hadler N. The kidney in rheumatic disease. London: Butterworth; 1982.
2. Myers BD, Guasch A. Mechanisms of proteinuria in nephrotic humans. Nephrol Dial Transplant. 1994;8:107–12.
3. Berggård I. Plasma proteins in normal urine. In: Manuel H, Bétuel H, Revillard J-P, eds. Proteins in normal and pathological urine. Basel: Karger; 1970:719.
4. Cameron JS, Greger R. Renal function testing and its physiological basis. In: Cameron JS, Davison AM, Grünfeld J-P, Kerr DNS, Ritz E, eds. Oxford Textbook of Clinical Nephrology, 2E. London: Oxford University Press; 1997 (in press).
5. McElderry LA, Tarbit IF, Cassells-Smith AJ. Six methods for urinary protein compared. Clin Chem. 1982;28:356–60.
6. Ginsberg JM, Chang BS, Matarese RA, Garella S. Use of single voided urine samples to estimate quantitative proteinuria. N Engl J Med. 1983;309:1543–6.
7. Cameron JS. The patient with proteinuria or haematuria. In: Cameron JS, Davison AM, Grünfeld J-P, Kerr DNS, Ritz E, eds. Oxford Textbook of Clinical Nephrology, 2E. London: Oxford University Press; 1997 (in press).
8. Springberg PD, Garrett LE, Thompson AL *et al.* Fixed and reproducible orthostatic proteinuria: results of a 20 year follow-up study. Ann Intern Med. 1982;97:516–9.
9. Fassett RG, Owen JE, Fairley J, Birch DF, Fairley KF. Urinary red cell morphology during exercise. Br Med J. 1982;285:1455–7.
10. Kallmeyer G, Miller NM. Urinary changes in ultra-long distance marathon runners. Nephron. 1993;64:119–21.
11. Terai C, Nojima Y, Takano K, Yamada A, Takaku F. Determination of urinary albumin excretion by radioimmunoassay in patients with subclinical lupus nephritis. Clin Nephrol. 1987;27:79–83.
12. Britton JP, Dowell AC, Whelan PO. Dipstick haematuria and bladder cancer in men over 60: results of a community study. Br Med J. 1989;299:1010–12.
13. Froom P, Ribak J, Benbassat J. Significance of microhaematuria in young adults. Br Med J. 1984;288:20–21.
14. Rath B, Turner C, Hartley B, Chantler C. Evaluation of light microscopy to localise the site of haematuria. Arch Dis Child. 1991;65:338–40.
15. Culclasure TF, Brady VJ, Hasbargen JA. The significance of hematuria in the anticoagulated patient. Arch Intern Med. 1994;154:649–52.
16. Brigden ML. High incidence of significant urinary ascorbic acid in a West coast population. Implication for routine analysis. Clin Chem. 1992;38:426–31.
17. Birch DF, Fairley KF, Whitworth JA *et al.* Urinary erythrocyte morphology in the diagnosis of glomerular hematuria. Clin Nephrol. 1983;20:78–84.
18. Loh EH, Keng VW, Ward PB. Blood cells and red cell morphology in the urine of healthy children. Nephron. 1990;34:185–7.
19. Köhler H, Wandel E, Brunck B. Acanthocyturia – a characteristic marker for glomerular bleeding. Kidney Int. 1991;40:115–20.
20. McQueen EG. Composition of urinary casts. Lancet. 1966;i:397–8.
21. Hoyer J, Seiler MW. Pathophysiology of Tamm–Horsfall protein. Kidney Int. 1979;16:279–89.
22. Rustecki GJ, Goldsmith C, Schreiner GE. Characterization of proteins in urinary casts. Fluorescent antibody identification of Tamm–Horsfall protein in matrix and serum proteins in granules. N Engl J Med. 1971;284:1049–52.
23. Fogazzi GB, Passerini P, Ponticelli C, Ritz E. The urinary sediment. An integrated view. Milan: Masson; 1993.
24. Mondorf AW. Urinary enzymatic markers of renal damage. In: Whelton A, Neu H, eds. The aminoglycosides. New York: Marcel Dekker; 281–301.
25. Spencer K. Analytical reviews in clinical chemistry: the estimation of creatinine. Ann Clin Biochem. 1986;23:1–25.
26. Kampmann J, Siersbaek-Nielsen K, Kristensen K, Moholm-Hamnsen J. Rapid evaluation of creatinine clearance. Acta Med Scand. 1974;196:517–20.
27. Gault MH, Longereich LL, Harnett JD, Wesolowski C. Predicting glomerular function from adjusted serum creatinine. Nephron. 1992;62:249–56.
28. Brown SCW, O'Reilly PH. Iohexol clearance for the determination of glomerular filtration rate in clinical practice: evidence for a new gold standard. J Urol. 1991;146:675–9.
29. Nilsson-Ehle P, Grubb A. New markers for the determination of GFR: iohexol clearance and cystatin C concentration. Kidney Int. 1994;46(suppl 47):s17–s19.
30. Hall JE, Guyton AC, Farr BM. A single injection method for measuring glomerular filtration rate. Am J Physiol. 1976;233:F72–6.
31. Brochner-Mortensen J. A simple method for the determination of glomerular filtration rate. Scand J Clin Lab Invest. 1972;30:271–4.
32. Levey AS, Greene T, Schluchter PA *et al.* Glomerular filtration rate measurements in clinical trials. J Am Soc Nephrol. 1993;4:1159–71.
33. Shemesh O, Golbetz H, Kriss JP, Myers BD. Limitations of creatinine as a filtration marker in glomerulopathic patients. Kidney Int. 1985;28:830–8.
34. Schardijn GHC, Statius van Eps LW. β_2-Microglobulin: its significance in the evaluation of renal function. Kidney Int. 1987;32:635–41.
35. Newman DJ, Thakkar H, Edwards RG *et al.* Serum cystatin C measured by automated immunoassay: a more sensitive marker of changes in GFR than serum creatinine. Kidney Int. 1995;47:312–8.
36. Lewis EJ. Lupus Nephritis. London: Oxford University Press; 1997 (in press).
37. Cervera R, Khamashta M, Font J *et al.* Systemic lupus erythematosus: clinical and immunologic patterns of disease expresssion in a cohort of 1000 patients. Medicine. 1993;72:113–24.
38. Dreyling KW, Wanner C, Schollmeyer P. Control of hyperkalaemia with fludrocortisone in a patient with systemic lupus erythematosus. Clin Nephrol. 1990;33:179–83.
39. Haycock GR. Henoch–Schönlein purpura. In: Cameron JS, Davison AM, Grünfeld J-P, Kerr DNS, Ritz E, eds. Oxford Textbook of Clinical Nephrology, 2E. London: Oxford University Press; 1997 (in press).
40. Urai L, Nagy Z, Szinay G, Waltner W. Renal function in scleroderma. Br Med J. 1958;ii:1264–6.
41. Peces R, Riesgo I, Ortega F, Velasco J, Alvarez

Grande J. Amyloidosis in Behçet's disease. Nephron. 1984;36:114–7.
42. Orellana C, Collado A, Hernandez MV, *et al.* When does amyloidosis complicate systemic lupus erythematosus? Lupus. 1995;4:415–7.
43. De Beer FC, Mallya RK, Fagan EA, *et al.* Serum amyloid A protein concentration in inflammatory diseases and its relationship to the incidence of reactive amyloidosis. Lancet;1982;ii:231–7.
44. Tang AL, Davies DR, Wing AJ. Remission of nephrotic syndrome in amyloidosis associated with a hypernephroma. Clin Nephrol. 1989;32:225–8.
45. Cameron JS, Simmonds HA. Use and abuse of allopurinol. Br Med J. 1987;294:1504–5.
46. Cameron JS, Moro F, Simmonds HA. Inherited disorders of uric acid metabolism and transport. In: Cameron JS, Davison AM, Grünfeld, J-P, Kerr DNS, Ritz E, eds. Oxford Textbook of Clinical Nephrology, 2E. London: Oxford University Press; 1997 (in press).
47. Cameron JS, Simmonds HA, Moro F. Gout uric acid and purine metabolism in pediatric nephrology. Pediatr Nephrol. 1993;7:105–18.
48. Batuman V, Landy E, Maesaka JK, Wedeen RP. Contribution of lead to hypertension with renal impairment. N Engl J Med. 1983;309:17–21.
49. Colleoni N, D'Amico G. Chronic lead accumulation as a possible cause of renal failure in gouty patients. Nephron. 1986;44:32–5.
50. Emery P, Adu, D. Rheumatoid arthritis and related conditions. In: Cameron JS, Davison AM, Grünfeld J-P, Kerr DNS, Ritz E, eds. Oxford Textbook of Clinical Nephrology, 2E. London: Oxford University Press; 1997 (in press).
51. Sato M, Kojima H, Koshikawa, S. IgA nephropathy in rheumatoid arthritis. Nephron. 1988;48:169–70.
52. Breedeveld FC, Valentijn RM, Westedt M-L, Weening JJ. Rapidly progressive glomerulonephritis with glomerular crescent formation in rheumatoid arthritis. Clin Rheumatol. 1985;4:353–9.
53. Bailey KR, Burry AF, McGiven AR, *et al.* A renal lesion in ankylosing spondylitis. Nephron. 1980;26:171–3.
54. Jennette JC, Ferguson AL, Moore MA, Freeman DG. IgA nephropathy associated with seronegative spondylarthropathies. ArthritisRheum. 1982;25:144–9.
55. Botey A, Torras A, Revert L. Membranous nephropathy in ankylosing spondylitis. Nephron. 1981;29:203.
56. Tietjen DP, Moore WJ. Treatment of rapidly progressive glomerulonephritis due to Behçet's syndrome with intravenous cyclophosphamide. Nephron. 1990;55:69–73.
57. Sternlieb I, Bennett B, Scheinberg IH. D-Penicillamine-induced Goodpasture's syndrome in Wilson's disease. Ann Intern Med. 1975;82:673–6.
58. Swainson CP, Thomson D, Short AIK, Winney RJ. Plasma exchange in the successful treatment of drug-induced renal disease. Nephron. 1982;30:244–9.
59. Madhok R. Tenidap. Lancet. 1995;346:481–5.
60. Massry S, Bluestone R, Klinenberg J, Coburn, J. Abnormalities of the musculoskeletal system in hemodialysis patients. Semin Arthritis Rheum. 1975;4:321–49.
61. CT, Wasserstein A, Schumacher HR Jr, Fernandez P. Musculoskeletal manifestations in hemodialysis patients. J Rheumatol. 1985;12:1149–53.
62. Julian BA. Complications of the musculoskeletal system in renal transplant recipients. J Nephrol. 1995;8:231–7.
63. Danovitch GM, Weinberger J, Berlyne GM. Uric acid in advanced renal failure. Clin Sci. 1972;43:331–41.
64. Li H-Y, Rocher LL, McQillan MA, *et al.* Cyclosporin-induced hyperuricemia and gout. N Engl J Med. 1989;321:287–92.
65. Simmonds HA, Cameron JS, Morris GS, Davies PM. Allopurinol in renal failure and the tumour lysis syndrome. Clin Chim Acta. 1986;160:189–95.
66. Hoffman GS, Schumacher HR, Paul H, *et al.* Calcium oxalate microcrystalline-associated arthritis in end-stage renal disease. Ann Intern Med. 1982;97:36–42.
67. Rosenthal A, Ryan LM, McCarty DJ. Arthritis associated with calcium oxalate crystals in an anephric patient treated with peritoneal dialysis. JAMA. 1981;260:1280–1.
68. Ascher NL, Simmons RL, Marker S, Klugman J, Najarian JS. Tuberculous joint disease in transplant patients. Am J Surg. 1978;135:835–6.
69. Brown EA, Gower PE. Joint problems in patients on maintenance haemodialysis. Adv Nephrol. 1982;18:247–50.
70. Duncan IJS, Hurst NP, Disney A, Sebben R, Milazzo SC. Is chronic renal failure a risk factor for the development of erosive osteoarthritis? Ann Rheum Dis. 1989;48:183–7.
71. Cary NRB, Sethi D, Brown EA, Erhardt CC, Gower PE. Dialysis arthropathy: amyloid or iron? Br Med J. 1986;293:1392–5.
72. Van Ypersele C, Drüecke TB. Dialysis amyloid. London: Oxford University Press; 1996.
73. Amiel C, Bailly C, Escoubet B, Friedlander G. Hypo- and hyperphosphataemia. In: Cameron JS, Davison AM, Grünfeld J-P, Kerr DNS, Ritz E, eds. Oxford textbook of clinical nephrology. London: Oxford University Press, 1992:1783–1801.
74. Khan MA, Ballou SP. Tendon rupture in systemic lupus erythematosus. J Rheumatol. 1981;8:308–10.
75. Bailey GL, Griffiths HI, Mocelin AJ, Gundy DH, Hampers CL, Merrill JP. Avascular necrosis of the femoral head in patients on maintenance hemodialysis. Trans Am Soc Artif Int Org. 1972;18:401–3.
76. Langevitz P, Busilka D, Stewart J, Sherrard DJ, Hercz G. Osteonecrosis in patients receiving dialysis: report of two cases and review of the literature. J Rheumatol. 1990;17:402–6.
77. Felson DT, Anderson JJ. A cross-study evaluation of association between steroid dose and bolus steroids and avascular necrosis of bone. Lancet. 1987;i:902–6.
78. Julian BA, Laskow DA, Dubovsky J, *et al.* Rapid loss of vertebral mineral density after renal transplantation. N Engl J Med. 1992;325:544–50.
79. Lukert BP, Raisz LG. Glucocorticoid-induced osteoporosis: pathogenesis and management. Ann Intern Med. 1990;112:352–64.
80. Briner VA, Thiel G, Monier-Faugere MC *et al.* Prevention of cancellous bone loss but persistence of renal bone disease despite normal 1,25-vitamin D levels two years after kidney transplantation. Transplantation. 1995;59:1393–1400.
81. Grotz WH, Mundinger FA, Gugel B, Exner VM, Kirste G, Schollmeyer PJ. Bone mineral density after kidney transplantation. Transplantation. 1995;59:982–6.

10 LABORATORY TESTS IN RHEUMATIC DISORDERS

Theodore Pincus

- Laboratory studies are useful for the diagnosis and monitoring of many of the rheumatic diseases.
- Interpretation of laboratory studies is confounded by problems of false positive results, false negative results, and measurement error.
- Rheumatology and screening laboratory panels are not cost effective and introduce a major source of false–positive findings.

INTRODUCTION

Four major sources of data are used to arrive at a diagnosis of a rheumatic disease:

- history and physical examination,
- laboratory tests,
- radiographs and imaging procedures and
- synovial fluid.

For many, or perhaps even most, rheumatic diseases laboratory testing has limited utility for diagnosis (in contrast to disease monitoring). Relevant diagnostic information for the major rheumatic diseases is summarized in Figure 10.1, with the most important single contributing factor highlighted. For example, in rheumatoid arthritis (RA), the diagnosis may be best established from the history and physical examination; for systemic lupus erythematosus (SLE), from a laboratory test, the antinuclear antibody (ANA) – albeit with a requirement for multisystem disease; for gout, from a synovial fluid examination; and for ankylosing spondylitis (AS) from a radiograph. For common diseases like osteoarthritis (OA) or fibromyalgia, there is essentially no diagnostic role for laboratory tests except to exclude other possible diagnoses. The common practice of ordering a battery of laboratory tests rarely leads to a definitive diagnosis, and often introduces considerable 'false–positive' information and unnecessary costs into the diagnosis of rheumatic disease.

PROBLEMS OF INTERPRETING LABORATORY TESTS IN RHEUMATOLOGY

The problems of interpreting the results of laboratory testing generally involve one of four major areas:

- false-positive results,
- false-negative results,
- measurement error and
- differences in groups of patients compared with individual patients.

FALSE-POSITIVE RESULTS

Inflammatory musculoskeletal diseases, for which patients are often 'screened' with laboratory tests, are seen in about 1% of the population, perhaps 2% if gout is included[1]. However, even a 1% false-positive rate of serologic tests for lupus or Lyme disease, for example, will result in many people being 'labeled' as having SLE or Lyme disease

DIAGNOSIS OF RHEUMATIC DISEASES

Diagnosis	History & physical examination	Blood tests	Radiographs	Synovial fluid
RA	**Symmetric polyarthritis** **Morning stiffness**	RF+ in ~80% Elevated ESR in 50–60%	Demineralization Erosions Joint space narrowing	Inflammation WBC >10,000
SLE	Multisystem disease	**ANA+ in >99%** **DNA antibodies in 60–75%**	Generally nondestructive	Mild inflammation
AS	Back pain Axial involvement	HLA-B27 in ~90%	**Sacroiliitis** **Vertebral squaring**	Inflammation WBC 5–20,000
Gout	Recurrent attacks	Uric acid elevated in 75–90%	Erosions, cysts	**Negatively birefringent crystals**
OA	Pain ± swelling ± limited motion	Nonspecific abnormalities	**Joint space narrowing** **Osteophytes**	Noninflammatory WBC <10,000
Fibromyalgia	**Chronic pain 'all over'** **No swollen joints** **Muscle spasm**	No abnormalities ANA+ in 2–5% Uric acid >8.0 in 2–5%	No severe abnormalities (may have cervical OA)	None
Scleroderma	**Skin tightness dorsum of hand** **Facial skin tightening**	ANA+ in >90% with Hep-2 cells	± Pulmonary fibrosis ± Esophageal dysmotility ± Calcinosis	Not specific
Polymyositis	Muscle weakness ± pain	**CPK elevated in 80%** **ANA+ in 33%**	Not helpful	Not specific

Fig. 10.1 Diagnosis of rheumatic diseases. The clinical data is from different sources, with source of most valuable data in bold.

on the basis of laboratory findings alone without clinical evidence of disease. The problem of false-positive interpretations of laboratory data in rheumatic diseases extends beyond serologic tests. For example, gout is often misdiagnosed on the basis of an elevated serum uric acid, rather than on the finding of urate crystals in synovial fluid. Most people with elevated uric acid do not have gout, and need not be treated for hyperuricemia. In all likelihood, many more people are diagnosed as having SLE, Lyme disease and gout who do not have these diseases than who have them.

Antinuclear antibodies are a good example of problems caused by false-positive laboratory testing in rheumatology. False-positive results of ANA testing constitute one of the primary reasons for rheumatology consultations. However, whereas SLE occurs in 1 in 2000 of the population, positive ANA tests occur in 1–5% of normal individuals, and musculoskeletal symptoms are seen in about 15% of the population (Fig. 10.2). Because of the prevalence of musculoskeletal symptoms and the practice of using laboratory testing rather than a history and physical examination to 'screen' for SLE, ANA tests may be ordered for up to 1 in 6 women in their lifetime, whereas only 1 in 2000 will have SLE. Therefore, even if ANA tests are restricted to people with musculoskeletal symptoms, 1 in 600 women will have a positive ANA test, only 1 in 3.3 of whom will have SLE. However, the actual rate of positive ANA tests in normal individuals is generally at least 5%, particularly with the use of more sensitive human Hep-2 cells[2], suggesting that the prevalence of individuals with musculoskeletal symptoms and a positive ANA who have SLE is probably more in the region of 1 in 15 (at most). Therefore, most people with a positive ANA test do not have SLE or any other inflammatory disease.

Similar considerations pertain to tests for other autoantibodies, which may be positive in 1–5% of the normal population, only a small fraction of whom have an inflammatory rheumatic disease (Fig. 10. 3). Furthermore, positive tests for Lyme borreliosis[3] and elevated uric acid are seen in about 3–5% of the normal population, only a small fraction of whom have Lyme disease or gout. Therefore, many patients with noninflammatory rheumatic conditions may be labeled with the diagnosis of rheumatic disease on the basis of a false-positive laboratory test, despite the absence of supporting clinical findings.

FALSE-NEGATIVE RESULTS

False-negative problems are more unusual but may have serious consequences. Patients with RA who have a negative rheumatoid factor (RF) test and/or normal erythrocyte sedimentation rate (ESR) may suffer joint destruction while treatment is deferred on the basis of 'normal' laboratory values. Similarly, patients with vasculitis and other life-threatening rheumatic diseases may develop irreversible end-organ renal failure or stroke, or even die, while undergoing extensive laboratory evaluation (and elaborate imaging studies), despite classic physical

ANALYSIS OF A POSITIVE TEST FOR ANA

Assumption	1% of normals ANA$^+$	5% of normals ANA$^+$
Prevalence of ANA$^+$ in SLE	99%	99%
Prevalence of ANA$^+$ in normal population	1%	5%
Prevalence of SLE	1:2000	1:2000
If 2000 people have ANA tests:		
Number who have SLE	1	1
Number who do not have SLE	20	100
Likelihood of SLE in ANA$^+$ group	1/20	1/100
If 15% of population has musculoskeletal symptoms, likelihood of individual with ANA$^+$ and musculoskeletal symptoms having SLE	1/3	1/15

Fig. 10.2 Analysis of a positive test for ANA.

PREVALENCE OF AUTOANTIBODIES IN NONDISEASED POPULATIONS

Autoantibody	Population	Prevalence	Reference
RF	Normal subjects age >65	16%	Cammarata, 1967[4]
Titer >1:32	Normal males	3.6%	Ball & Lawrence, 1961[5]
	Normal females	4.8%	
ANA	2500 blood donors		Fritzler, 1985[6]
	female 20–50 years	45% > 1:40	
	male 45–50 years	58% > 1:160	
ANA	63 blood donors	3.2%	Burnham *et al*, 1966[7]
ANA	255 >65 years	36%	Camarata, 1967[4]
ANA	71 elderly (?)	22%	
	<65 years	6%	
Antimitochondrial antibody	2500 blood donors 20–50 years	3.6%	Fritzler, 1985[6]
SS-A/Ro	2500 blood donors 20–50 years	0.44%	Fritzler, 1985[6]
SS-B/La	32?? normal subjects	3%	
	52–72 years	9%	
ANA	Relatives of children with SLE	29/94	Lehman, 1984[8]
	Relatives of adults with SLE	7/33	Lehman, 1984[8]
Anti-SS-A	Relatives of children with SLE	4/94	Lehman, 1984[8]
	Relatives of adults with SLE	1/33	Lehman, 1984[8]
Anti-DNA	Relatives of children with SLE	26/94	
	Relatives of adults with SLE	13/33	
SS-A	Normal pregnant women	2/445	Taylor, 1988[9]
SS-B	Normal pregnant women	3/445	Taylor, 1988[9]

Fig. 10.3 Prevalence of autoantibodies in nondisease populations.

findings such as palpable purpura and foot drop, which, to an experienced rheumatologist, make a clear diagnosis at presentation.

MEASUREMENT ERROR

Another important factor to take into consideration is measurement error. Although laboratories perform extensive procedures to minimize measurement error, it is an intrinsic component of any measurement – even precise measurements in the physical sciences, much less serologic testing. Although measurement error outside a normal range is uncommon, the inevitable consequence of testing large numbers of people who present with musculoskeletal symptoms is incorrect results in a significant number of individuals.

An interesting analysis of measurement error in rheumatology testing was conducted in two university laboratories. The sera of 667 patients with connective tissue diseases were tested for C3 complement component and anti-DNA antibodies[10] (Fig. 10.4). Agreement was essentially linear for the C3 tests and most DNA antibody measures. However, based on the measurement of DNA antibodies, two patients who were classified as having SLE in Laboratory B were normal according to Laboratory A, and more were found with the reciprocal pattern. The differences in measurement of anti-DNA antibodies may be explained in part on the basis of denaturation of double-stranded DNA (dsDNA) into single-stranded DNA in many preparations, but unrecognized sources of variation are also seen in the application of any laboratory test.

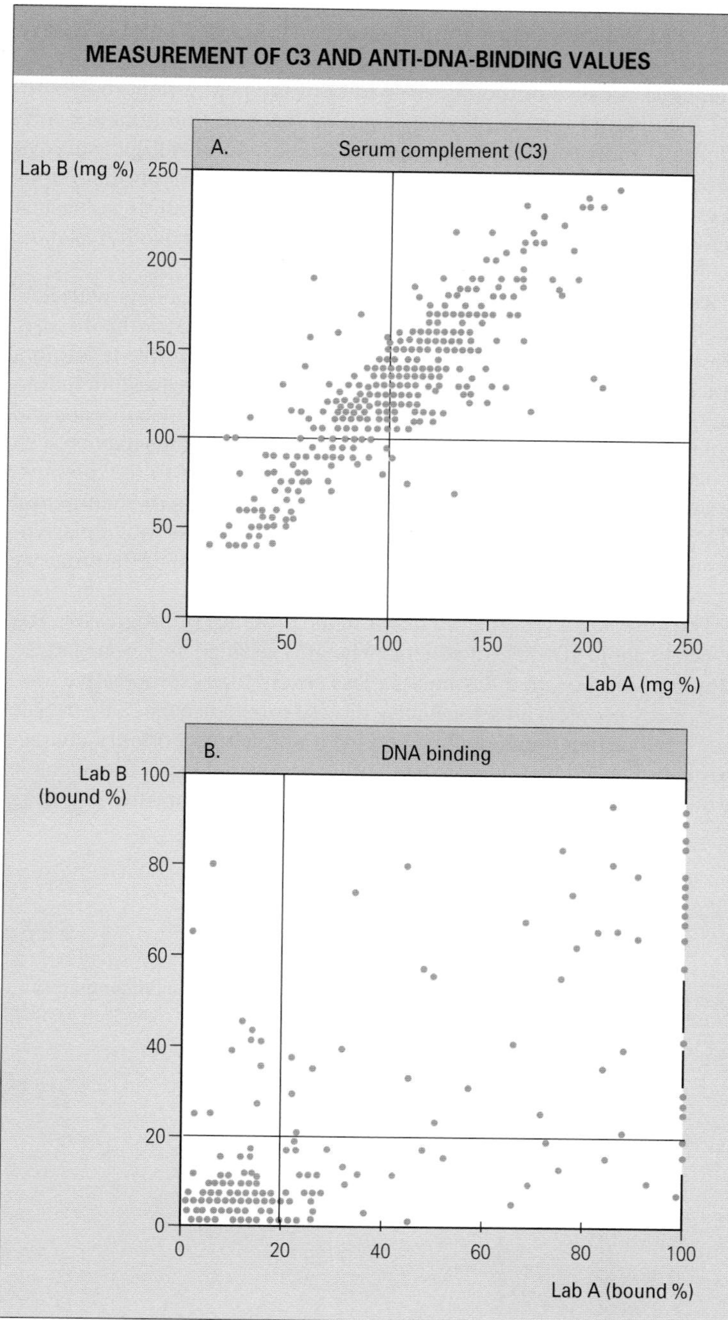

Fig. 10.4 Measurement of C3 and anti-DNA binding values in two reference laboratories (normal value for DNA binding – <20%). With permission from Feigenbaum *et al.*[10].

Whenever a laboratory value does not agree with clinical observation, the clinician should always include consideration of laboratory error in an explanation of the findings. Measurement error is considerably more common than is generally acknowledged.

DIFFERENCES IN GROUPS OF PATIENTS COMPARED WITH INDIVIDUALS

Evidence of statistically significant differences in the proportion of individuals with certain autoantibodies who have particular clinical features may provide clues to pathogenesis for groups of patients analogous to data obtained from epidemiologic studies. However, these data often are of limited value in an individual patient, and their collection may add considerable expense without meaningful value for diagnosis and management. Clinical decisions in individual patients must be based primarily on clinical findings rather than laboratory values.

Many studies have found that specific autoantibodies have a much higher prevalence in patients with particular clinical features. For example, patients with the CREST (calcinosis, Raynaud's phenomenon, esophageal hypomotility, sclerodactyly, telangeictasia) syndrome typically have anticentromere antibody (ACA). Although this observation may provide powerful clues to pathogenesis, the value of testing for ACA in the management of patients with obvious clinical signs of the disease is far less certain (see Chapter 7.9). Another example involves the observation that the HLA haplotype B27 is found in 90% of patients with AS compared with 8% of the normal population. This observation may be interpreted to suggest that HLA typing has a clinical role in helping identify patients who have AS. However, 10% of patients with AS are HLA-B27 negative. This group may experience disease of equal severity to those who are HLA-B27-positive. Further, only about 1 in 20 people who have HLA-B27 have AS, and only 1 in 3 people who have back pain and HLA-B27 have AS. Therefore, HLA typing is rarely indicated in the diagnosis or management of patients with AS (see Chapter 6.16).

ACUTE PHASE REACTANTS

Nonspecific indicators of the presence of inflammation, including ESR and C-reactive protein (CRP), are often valuable in patients suspected of having inflammatory rheumatic diseases and in monitoring clinical status[11,12]. The ESR may be elevated on the basis of large increases in serum fibrinogen levels or smaller increases in serum immunoglobulins. It is measured in a vertical cylindrical tube, either 200mm (Westergren) or 100mm (Wintrobe). The Westergren method is preferred as it has a greater capacity to differentiate normal from abnormal and to monitor disease. The upper limit of normal may increase with age; values up to 40mm/h Westergren ESR are not uncommon in elderly people.

Initially, CRP was identified as a precipitin from the serum of patients with pneumococcal pneumonia, rheumatic fever or streptococcal infection, which reacted with the 'C' or somatic polysaccharide of the pneumococcus. An association of elevated CRP levels with inflammatory rheumatic diseases was first described in 1951[13]. C-reactive protein is composed of nonglycosylated polypeptide subunits, each 27,000Da, encoded on a single gene on chromosome 1 with no polymorphism. The concentration may rise more than 500-fold in acute inflammation, doubling in up to every 6 hours. Radioimmunodiffusion, solid phase radioimmunoassay and nephelometry can be used to detect CRP.

Most patients with inflammatory rheumatic diseases have elevated ESR and/or CRP; persistently high levels are usually associated with disease progression in patients with RA[14–16]. Nonetheless, up to 40% of patients with active RA have a normal ESR despite radiographic progression and progressive disability[17]. According to Pereira *et al.*, CRP is not elevated in active SLE, and elevated levels in a patient with SLE are an indicator of infection rather than inflammation[18].

Elevated ESR may be seen in normal individuals, and in patients with noninflammatory rheumatic diseases, including OA and fibromyalgia[15]. In addition, a number of factors may influence ESR (Fig. 10.5). Although there is a tendency for ESR to rise with age, one study found ESR levels higher than 40mm/h in eight female patients aged 30–40 years with non-inflammatory rheumatic conditions. Overall, about 10% of men and women with OA had elevated ESR[17]. Therefore, while an abnormal ESR increases the likelihood of an inflammatory rheumatic disease, it does not exclude a noninflammatory condition. Conversely, a normal ESR does not exclude an inflammatory rheumatic disease.

AUTOANTIBODIES

The modern era of rheumatology began in the 1940s with the discovery of rheumatoid factor[19] and the lupus erythematosus (LE) cell[20], which revealed the presence of immune dysfunction in inflammatory rheumatic diseases. It was originally hoped that laboratory tests for autoantibodies would provide sensitive and specific markers in rheumatic diseases, analogous to cultures in infectious diseases or serum glucose in diabetes.

Over the past few decades, however, it has been recognized that autoantibodies are not qualitatively abnormal proteins but immunoglobulins which can be produced by most normal individuals to quantitatively detectable levels under conditions of immune dysregulation. Most autoantibodies are not specific for a clinical syndrome, but may be detected in people with markedly different clinical features as well as in some normal individuals. Furthermore, autoantibodies may not be detected in many individuals who have clinical findings similar to patients in whom serum autoantibodies are detected, and treatment is similar for both groups. Therefore, while research into autoantibodies has yielded considerable information about pathogenetic mechanisms, serologic testing for autoantibodies in clinical practice remains generally more an adjunct to diagnosis and management rather than a precise clinical guide.

RHEUMATOID FACTOR

Rheumatoid factors are immunoglobulin molecules which bind to the Fc portion of immunoglobulin G (IgG) (see Chapter 5.9). Rheumatoid factors of the immunoglobulin classes IgM, IgA, IgG and IgE have been described, although IgM rheumatoid factor is the most easily detectable because of the higher avidity of the pentavalent molecule. IgG rheumatoid factors may be found in synovial fluid, but are considerably more difficult to detect in serum. In serologic surveys rheumatoid factor has been found in at least 1% of the normal population. Thus, since RA occurs in 0.5–1% of the population, at least as many individuals who have rheumatoid factor do not have RA as have the disease (Fig. 10.6).

Rheumatoid factor is found in about 70–90% of patients with RA, and has often been misinterpreted as being diagnostic for the disease. However, a false-positive rheumatoid factor, i.e. a positive result in a patient who does not have RA, is found in many diseases, including sarcoidosis, leprosy, tuberculosis, pulmonary fibrosis, liver disease and syphilis (Fig. 10.7). Moreover, musculoskeletal symptoms may be seen in patients with many of these diseases to add further to the diagnostic confusion with RA. Conversely, the highest titers of rheumatoid factor are often seen in patients with conditions such as Sjögren's syndrome or macroglobulinemia who have no signs of inflammatory arthritis.

The absence of rheumatoid factor in the presence of progressive RA is seen in about 10–30% of patients who are classified as 'seronegative'. Although seronegative RA may be less severe than 'seropositive' disease, many people with seronegative disease experience the radiographic progression, functional decline and even premature mortality characteristic of RA. Perhaps most importantly, rheumatoid factor is detectable in only 33% of patients who ultimately become 'seropositive' during

FACTORS THAT INFLUENCE THE ERYTHROCYTE SEDIMENTATION RATE

Increase	Decrease
Anemia	Sickle cell disease
Hypercholesterolemia	Anisocytosis
Female sex	Spherocytosis
Pregnancy	Acanthocytosis
High room temperature	Microcytosis
Inflammatory disease	Polycythemia
Chronic renal failure	Bile salts
Obesity	Clotting of blood samples
Heparin	Greater than 2h delay in running test
Tissue damage (myocardial infarction, stroke)	Low room temperature
	Hypofibrinogenemia
	Congestive heart failure
	Cachexia

Fig. 10.5 Factors that influence ESR. With permission from Sox HC Jr, Liang MH. The erythrocyte sedimentation rate: guidelines for rational use. Ann Intern Med. 1986;104:515–23.

LABORATORY TESTS USED IN INFLAMMATORY RHEUMATIC DISEASES – LIKELIHOOD OF DISEASE IN A PATIENT WITH A POSITIVE TEST

	RF	ANA	HLA-B27	Elevated uric acid
Suspected disease	RA	SLE	AS	Gout
Patients with positive test (%)	80	99	90	80
Prevalence of positive test in normals	2/100	1/100	6/100	5/100
Disease prevalence	1/100	1/2000	1/300	1/200
Likelihood of disease if positive test	1/2	1/20	1/18	1/10
Likelihood of disease if positive test and joint pain	1/1.5	1/5	1/4.8 (1/3 for back pain)	1/2.5

Fig. 10.6 Laboratory tests used in inflammatory rheumatic diseases. Likelihood of disease in a patient with a positive test.

the first 3 months of disease, and in only 60% during the first 6 months[21]. Therefore, a test for rheumatoid factor is least likely to be positive in early disease when it might be most helpful to the clinician. This is particularly important in view of mounting evidence that patients with RA should be treated early, prior to end-organ damage, when rheumatoid factor is as likely to be negative as positive.

ANTINUCLEAR ANTIBODIES

The lupus erythematosus cell

The LE cell, a polymorphonuclear leukocyte (PMN) which contains the phagocytosed nuclear material of a second cell[20], has been identified in 50–75% of patients with SLE, as well as in patients with other rheumatic diseases. The LE cell test is readily available as it can be performed in a physician's office using only a conventional microscope. However, the test has many drawbacks, for example it:

- is tedious to perform,
- is less sensitive in screening for SLE than is ANA,
- is less specific in the diagnosis of SLE than anti-DNA antibodies,
- can be seen in other inflammatory rheumatic diseases and
- does not provide quantitative data for monitoring the course of SLE.

Therefore, the LE cell test is of historic interest and is rarely, if ever, used in the clinical setting for patients with suspected autoimmunity.

Fluorescent antinuclear antibody test

The fluorescent ANA test is performed by overlaying a patient's serum on fixed cells on a microscope slide. It is a sensitive and simple screen for SLE[22]. Clinicians are rightly concerned to attempt to identify SLE in patients who have musculoskeletal symptoms. However, many disorders may be associated with a positive ANA and all clinicians have under their care patients with a positive ANA who do not have SLE (Fig. 10.8).

DNA antibodies

A test for DNA antibodies is less sensitive than that for ANA, but is more specific for SLE, particularly as these antibodies are rarely seen in normal individuals. Antibodies to dsDNA may be measured using immunodiffusion, complement fixation, radioimmunoassay, a fluorescent assay for a DNA-containing organelle in the parasite *Crithidia lucillae* and enzyme-linked immunosorbant assays (ELISA). These antibodies are found in 50–80% of untreated patients with SLE and, apart from some cases of Sjögren's syndrome and chronic active hepatitis, are virtually diagnostic for the disease.

In addition, DNA antibodies also appear significant in the pathogenesis of lupus nephritis (see Chapter 7.2). High titers of DNA antibodies are usually associated with renal disease and are often accompanied by low levels of serum complement activity, indicating the presence of circulating immune complexes[22,23]. Clinical improvement in SLE is usually associated with a significant decline in or complete disappearance of DNA antibodies, accompanied by normalization of serum complement levels[24] (Fig. 10.9). Conversely, a rise in DNA antibodies in the presence of a decline in serum complement generally is associated with a high frequency of exacerbation of SLE nephritis. In clinical practice, a test for DNA antibodies is useful to establish a diagnosis of SLE, and to monitor patients with SLE nephritis.

Antiribonucleoprotein and anti-Sm

An antibody reactive with soluble saline extracts from calf or rabbit thymus, termed extractable nuclear antigen (ENA), includes a ribonuclease-sensitive fraction, known as ribonucleoprotein (RNP), and a ribonuclease-resistant fraction known as Sm[25]. High titers of antibodies to the RNP component of ENA, at levels of 1:10 000 or higher, have been described in a clinical syndrome known as mixed connective tissue disease (MCTD), characterized by arthritis, Raynaud's phenomenon, hand swelling, myositis and esophageal hypomotility (see Chapter 7.33). Long-term follow up of patients with MCTD has revealed that many of these patients go on to develop RA, scleroderma or other conditions[26]. Thus, ENA antibodies are clinically not as specific as previously suggested to identify a specific syndrome.

RHEUMATOID FACTORS IN DISEASE STATES AND NORMALS	
Disease	Percentage positive for rheumatoid factor
Rheumatoid arthritis Sjögren's syndrome	50–85
Subacute bacterial endocarditis Systemic lupus erythematosus Leprosy Liver disease	25–50
Juvenile chronic arthritis Pulmonary diseases Tuberculosis	10–25
Ankylosing spondylitis Rheumatic fever Osteoarthritis Psoriatic arthritis Gout	5–10
Normals	<5

Fig. 10.7 Rheumatoid factors in disease states and normals.

CONDITIONS ASSOCIATED WITH ANA
1. Rheumatic diseases
Systemic lupus erythematosus Polymyositis Sjögren's syndrome Scleroderma Vasculitis Rheumatoid arthritis
2. Normal, healthy individuals
Females > males, prevalence increases with age Relatives of patients with rheumatic diseases ? Pregnant females
3. Drug-induced
4. Hepatic diseases
Chronic active hepatitis Primary biliary cirrhosis Alcoholic liver disease
5. Pulmonary diseases
Idiopathic pulmonary fibrosis Asbestos-induced fibrosis Primary pulmonary hypertension
6. Chronic infections
7. Malignancies
Lymphoma Leukemia Melanoma Solid tumors (ovary, breast, lung, kidney)
8. Hematologic disorders
Idiopathic thrombocytopenic purpura Autoimmune hemolytic anemia
9. Miscellaneous
Endocrine disorders (type I diabetes mellitus, Graves' disease) Neurologic diseases (multiple sclerosis) End-stage renal failure After organ transplantation

Fig. 10.8 Conditions associated with ANA.

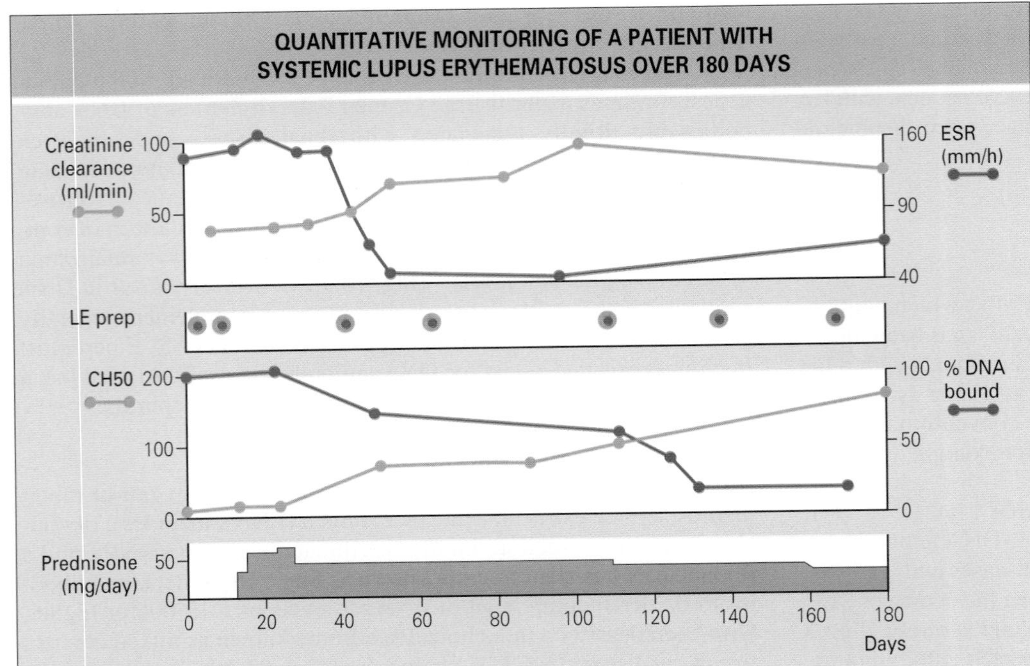

Fig. 10.9 Disease course of SLE in 14-year-old boy over 6 months, showing the relation of anti-DNA binding and CH50 levels to other clinical and laboratory measures. With permission from Pincus *et al.*[23]. Copyright (1969), Massachusetts Medical Society. All rights reserved.

Antibodies to Sm, the ribonuclease-resistant component of ENA, have been considered specific for SLE, as in the case of DNA antibodies, but these antibodies are seen in only about 30% of SLE cases.

Antibodies to Ro (SS-A) and La (SS-B)

The autoantibodies anti-Ro, which is identical to anti-SS-A, and anti-La, which is identical to anti-SS-B, have been found in patients with SLE, Sjögren's syndrome and other autoimmune diseases[27]. In addition, these antibodies have been found in mothers who had infants with congenital complete heart block, including some with SLE or Sjogren's syndrome as well as in mothers with no evidence of connective tissue disease. It has been suggested that anti-Ro and anti-La antibodies should be measured in pregnant patients with SLE to raise an index of suspicion of congenital heart block in the fetus. However, the absence of anti-Ro does not exclude the possibility of congenital heart block, which is diagnosed through a physical examination and electrocardiogram. Furthermore, most mothers with anti-Ro antibodies who have infants with congenital heart block show no signs of connective tissue disease (see Chapter 7.8). The anti-Ro test may have some utility for screening pregnant women with SLE, but does not add clinically useful information in the majority of patients.

Antibodies to histones

Antibodies to histones have been described in about 50% of patients with SLE and about 75% of patients with drug-induced lupus[28] (see Chapter 7.36). Some observers have suggested that these antibodies may be regarded as a marker for drug-induced lupus. However, 25% of people with drug-induced lupus have a negative test for antibodies to histones, and the diagnosis of drug-induced lupus can be made effectively without this test.

Antiproliferating cell nuclear antigen

An interesting antinuclear antibody reacting with proliferating tissue culture cells has been identified in fewer than 5% of SLE patients[22,28]. The antigenic moiety, termed proliferating cell nuclear antigen (PCNA), provides a valuable marker for cell proliferation but is not clinically useful in the diagnosis or management of SLE.

Anticentromere and anti-Scl-70

Anticentromere antibodies directed to restricted regions of chromosomes are found in 80–90% of patients with the CREST variant of scleroderma. Another antibody, anti-Scl-70, is found in 40% of patients with systemic sclerosis (see Chapter 7.9). However, ACAs are seen in some patients with systemic sclerosis and anti-Scl-70 in some patients with the CREST syndrome. The scleroderma variants are diagnosed on the basis of clinical features, so these tests are primarily of research interest.

Antibodies to nuclear enzymes

Autoantibodies with specificity for enzymes involved in nuclear functions, including antibodies to RNA polymerase-1 and antibodies to enzymes involved in the synthesis of transfer RNA, have been identified in patients with rheumatic diseases. An antibody termed Jo-1 has been reported in approximately 30% of patients with polymyositis and in 70% of patients with polymyositis who have interstitial lung disease (see Chapter 7.13). Studies of these antibodies appear likely to result in a better understanding of nuclear structure and function, but are not of current value in clinical care.

Antinuclear antibodies in polymyositis

Another type of ANA, PM-1, is reported in approximately 50% of patients with polymyositis and in 10% with dermatomyositis[28]. Routine measurement of PM-1 has not proved clinically useful to date, but further studies may contribute to the understanding of pathogenetic mechanisms in polymyositis.

Antiphospholipid antibodies

The antiphospholipid antibody syndrome is characterized by clinical features of thrombosis, recurrent fetal loss and thrombocytopenia (see Chapter 7.35). This syndrome can be seen in patients who have features of SLE and other connective tissue diseases, but can also be seen without these features as 'primary' antiphospholipid antibody syndrome.

Three types of tests are used in diagnosis of the antiphospholipid syndrome:

- a standard test for syphilis, such as the venereal disease research laboratory (VDRL) and Wasserman tests;
- lupus anticoagulant tests, in which the capacity of a serum to inhibit *in vitro* clot formation is tested; and
- a specific ELISA to detect antiphospholipid antibodies.

Similar phenomena may be measured in all three types of tests: it is not clear whether more than one type of test is needed.

In a patient who has recurrent fetal loss or unexplained thrombosis, a search for antiphospholipid antibodies is of value. However, many individuals with antiphospholipid antibodies have no clinical abnormalities.

Antineutrophil cytoplasmic antibodies

Antineutrophil cytoplasmic antibodies (ANCA) have been described in patients with vasculitis, primarily in Wegener's granulomatosis (WG) (see Chapters 7.22 and 7.31). Clinical observations suggest that the test for ANCA may not be as specific for WG as previously thought[29]. Furthermore, the diagnosis of WG is based on clinical criteria, not laboratory tests. Some authors have suggested that ANCA may be useful in monitoring the clinical course of WG; further studies are required to confirm this.

OTHER IMMUNOLOGIC TESTS

ANTISTREPTOLYSIN O TITER

In patients with acute rheumatic fever, the antistreptolysin O titer (ASOT) shows an acute rise, reflecting the presence of an active streptococcal infection (see Chapters 6.8 and 6.9). An increase in the incidence of acute rheumatic fever has been recorded over the past decade, although the disease remains relatively unusual, and a simple elevated ASOT in itself is not diagnostic.

In clinical practice, if a history of antecedent 'strep throat' plus clinical features suggest acute rheumatic fever, paired sera drawn acutely and after 10–14 days should be tested to determine ASOT. Nonetheless, most individuals have been exposed to streptococci and many normal people have elevated ASOT. Patients with musculoskeletal pain need an ASOT test only rarely.

LYME BORRELIOSIS TITERS

In view of the low prevalence of Lyme disease versus the high prevalence of positive Lyme titers, probably fewer than 1 in 100 people with a positive test have Lyme disease. Therefore, it is recommended that a Lyme titer only be obtained in patients with clinical evidence of Lyme disease, most notably the erythema chronicum migrans rash. The presence of musculoskeletal pain with a history of a tick bite is not an indication for a Lyme antibody test (see Practical Problem 6.9, Positive Lyme serology with nonspecific symptoms).

SERUM COMPLEMENT

The complement cascade involves a series of proteins which may be activated by immune complexes, as well as other mechanisms (see Chapter 7.4). A low serum complement level may indicate the presence of circulating complexes, a complement component deficiency or a problem with protein synthesis, e.g. in liver failure.

In practice, serum complement has proved valuable in one clinical setting: the management of SLE nephritis. Low levels of serum complement are associated with persistent nephritis, and normalization is associated with a better long-term outcome[23,24].

Three measures of serum complement are available in routine clinical practice: total complement activity, termed a CH50, and the C3 and C4 complement components. In more than 99% of clinical situations, only one of these measures is needed. The CH50 has the advantage of measuring biological activity. A normal value excludes any type of disorder that would lower serum complement, including circulating immune complexes. The disadvantage of the CH50 is that it requires serum to be frozen within an hour after collection to preserve biological activity. The C3 and C4 assays measure serum levels of these proteins, and do not depend on biological activity, so that careful handling is not required. In usual clinical practice, the only indication for a serum complement assay is in monitoring SLE nephritis, and only one measure is needed.

ASSAYS FOR CIRCULATING IMMUNE COMPLEXES

A number of assays have been described to detect circulating immune complexes in serum, including the Raji cell assay, in which immune complexes bind to the Raji cell line, and the C1q binding assay, in which immune complexes are bound to the first component of complement. These were originally proposed as possible techniques to monitor autoimmune diseases. However, they are not infrequently found to be positive in normal individuals, and their use is as research tools rather than as clinical tests.

HLA HAPLOTYPE TYPING

The association of several rheumatic diseases with the major histocompatibility complex, HLA, may provide important advances in our understanding of the pathogenesis of rheumatic diseases (see Chapter 5.7). For example, HLA-B27 is found in 90% of patients with AS (versus 8% in the normal population), and HLA-DR4, now termed D0401, in 67% of Caucasian people with RA (versus 30% in the normal population). These findings confer a relative risk of about 80–100 for AS in individuals who have HLA-B27, and of 5–7 for RA in individuals who have HLA-DR4, compared with the general population.

These observations have been interpreted to suggest that HLA typing may be useful clinically in helping identify disease. However, this is not the case, for several reasons. A significant proportion of patients with HLA-associated diseases do not bear the HLA marker, i.e. 10% of patients with AS are HLA-B27-negative and 33% of patients with RA are HLA-DR4-negative. Disease in these patients may have equally severe consequences, and requires a diagnosis based on other criteria. Conversely, most people with HLA-B27 or -DR4 do not have AS or RA. A calculation of the number of individuals in the population with back pain who have HLA-B27 indicates that only 1 in 3 would be expected to have AS. These considerations render HLA typing inappropriate in routine clinical settings, although its importance as a research procedure remains unquestioned.

URIC ACID

Uric acid measurement is included in the evaluation of patients with musculoskeletal symptoms, as elevated uric acid is seen in 90% of people with gout, either through overproduction or underexcretion. However, elevated uric acid levels are common in the general population, particularly in patients who take diuretics for hypertension and other conditions, as well as in 3–5% of normal individuals[1]. Overdiagnosis of gout is associated with at least one potentially disastrous complication – allopurinol vasculitis (see Chapter 8.19).

The diagnosis of gout is established definitively in the laboratory through identification of urate crystals in synovial fluid (see Chapter 8.14). Identification is most specific using a polarizing microscope, although a thin needle-like crystal penetrating a PMN through its entire depth, indicating a urate crystal, may be seen using a regular microscope.

RHEUMATOLOGY SCREENING PANELS

Recognition of the potential severity of rheumatic diseases has led to widespread use of 'rheumatology screeining panels' in an effort to 'rule out' or 'not miss' inflammatory rheumatic diseases. These screens are available in all national laboratories in the US. The simplest screen includes rheumatoid factor, ANA, and uric acid, although more elaborate screens are available, which may include erythrocyte sedimentation rate, C-reactive protein, anti-streptolysin O titer, protein electrophoresis, quantitative immunoglobulins, and ANA subsets such as anti-Ro and anti-LA, anti Sm, and anticentromere antibodies[1].

Although well–meaning in attempts to screen thoroughly for disease, 'rheumatology screens' introduce a major source of potential 'flase–positive' information to patient evaluations. As noted above, a positive ANA or elevated uric acid may be seen in up to 5% of the normal population, while the diseases associated with these tests are seen in fewer than 1% of the population. Therefore, most individuals with positive tests will not have these diseases. As musculoskeletal symptoms are quite common in thepopulation, even when screens are restricted to people with musculoskeletal diseases, a large number of 'false–positive' results will nonetheless be seen[1]. Therefore, rheumatology screens should not be performed, not only because they are intellectually in appropriate, but also because much 'false–positive' information will result.

REFERENCES

1. Lichtenstein MJ, Pincus T. How useful are combinations of blood tests in 'rheumatic panels' in diagnosis of rheumatic diseases? J Gen Intern Med. 1988;3:435–42.
2. Miller MH, Littlejohn GO, Jones BW, Strnad H. Clinical comparison of cultured human epithelial cells and rat liver as substrates for the fluuorescent antinuclear antibody test. J Rheumatol. 1985;12:265–9.
3. Cammarata RJ, Rodnan GP, Fennell RH. Serum anti-γ-globulin and antinuclear factors in the aged. JAMA. 1967;199:115–8.
4. Ball J, Lawrence JS. Epidemiology of the sheep cell agglutination test. Ann Rheum Dis. 1961;20:235–43.
5. Fritzler MJ, Pauls JD, Kinsella TD. Antinuclear, anticytoplasmic, and anti-Sjogren's syndrome antigen A (SSA/Ro) antibodies in female blood donors. Clin Immunol Immunopathol. 1985;36:120–8.
6. Burnham TK, Fine G, Neblett TR. The immunofluorescent tumor imprint technique: II. The frequency of antinuclear factors in connective tissue diseases and dermatoses. Ann Intern Med. 1966;65:9–19.
7. Lehman TJA, Hanson V, Zvaifler N, Sharp G, Alspaugh M. Antibodies to nonistone nuclear antigens and antilymphocyte autobodies among children and adults with systemic lupus erythematosus and their relatives. J Rheumatol. 1984;11:644–7.
8. Taylor PV, Taylor KF, Norman A, Griffiths S, Scott JS. Prevalence of maternal Ro (SS-A) and La (SS-B) autoantibodies in relation to congenital heart block. Br J Rheumatol. 1988;27:128–32.
9. Magnarelli LA. Quality of lyme disease tests (editorial). JAMA. 1989;262:3464–5.
10. Feigenbaum PA, Medsger TA, Jr, Kraines RG, Fries JF. The variability of immunologic laboratory tests. J Rheumatol. 1982;9:408–14.
11. Ballou SP, Kushner I. C-reactive protein and the acute phase response. Adv Intern Med. 1992;37:313.
12. Weinstein A, Del Giudice J. The erythrocyte sedimentation rate – time honored and tradition bound (editorial). J Rheumatol. 1994;21:1177–8.
13. Hill AGS. C-reactive protein in the chronic rheumatic diseases. Lancet 1951;ii:807–11.
14. Emery P, Luqmani R. The validity of surrogate markers in rheumatic disease. Br J Rheumatol. 1993;32:3–8.
15. van Leeuwen MA, van Rijswijk MH, van der Heijde DMFM, *et al.* The acute-phase response in relation to radiographic progression in early rheumatoid arthritis: a prospective study during the first three years of the disease. Br J Rheumatol. 1993;32:9–13.
16. Hassell AB, Davis MJ, Fowler PD, *et al.* The relationship between serial measures of disease activity and outcome in rheumatoid arthritis. Q J Med. 1995;86:601–7.
17. Wolfe F, Michaud K. The clinical and research significance of the erythocyte sedimentation rate. J Rheumatol. 1994;21:1227–37.
18. Pereira DA, Silva JA, Elkon KB, Hughes GRV. C-reactive protein levels in systemic lupus erythematosus: a classification criterion? Arthritis Rheum. 1980;23:770.
19. Rose HM, Ragan C, Pearce E, Lipman MO. Differential agglutination of normal and sensitized sheep erythrocytes by sera of patients with rheumatoid arthritis. Proc Soc Exp Biol Med. 1948;68:1–6.
20. Hargraves MM, Richmond H, Morton R. Presentation of two bone marrow elements: the 'tart' cell and 'LE' cell. Proc Staff Meet Mayo Clin. 1948;23–5.
21. Jacoby RK, Jayson MIV, Cosh JA. Onset, early stages, and prognosis of rheumatoid arthritis: a clinical study of 100 patients with 11–year follow–up. Br Med J. 1973;2:96–100.
22. von Muhlen CA, Tan EM. Autoantibodies in the diagnosis of systemic rheumatic diseases. Semin Arthritis Rheum. 1995;24:323–58.
23. Pincus T, Schur PH, Rose JA, Decker JL, Talal N. Measurement of serum DNA-binding activity in systemic lupus erythematosus. N Engl J Med. 1969;281:701–5.
24. Lightfoot RW Jr, Highes GRV. Significance of persisting serologic abnormalities in SLE. Arthritis Rheum. 1976;19:837–43.
25. Sharp GC, Irvin WS, May CM, et al. Association of antibodies to ribonucleoprotein and Sm antigens with mixed connective–tissue disease, systemic lupus erythematosus and other rheumatic disease. N Engl J Med. 1976;295:1149–54.
26. Nimelstein SH, Brody S, McShane D, Holman HR. Mixed connective tissue disease: a subsequent evaluation of the original 25 patients. Medicine. 1980;59:239–48.
27. Reichlin M. Autoantibodies to the RoRNP particles. Clin Exp Immunol. 1995;99:7–9.
28. Pisetsky DS. Antinuclear antibodies. Rheum Dis Clin North Am. 1992;18:283–505.
29. Rao JK, Weinberger M, Oddone EZ, *et al.* The role of antineutrophil cytoplasmic antibody (c-ANCA) testing in the diagnosis of Wegener granulomatosis. Ann Intern Med. 1995;123:925–32.

11

SYNOVIAL FLUID ANALYSIS

Anthony J Freemont

- Normal synovial fluid is a hypocellular, avascular connective tissue.
- In disease the synovial fluid increases in volume and can be aspirated.
- Changes in the composition of synovial fluid reflect the pathogenesis of the arthropathy.
- Elements that change can be either visualized with the light microscope or measured biochemically.
- Synovial fluid microscopy is a simple, cheap and accurate test that yields information of diagnostic and prognostic significance.
- Synovial fluid biochemical analysis is less well studied, from the perspective of its use as a diagnostic test, although it has a great deal to offer as a research tool.

INTRODUCTION

NORMAL SYNOVIAL FLUID

Synovial fluid (SF) is a transudate of plasma supplemented with high-molecular weight, saccharide-rich molecules, notably hyaluronans, produced by fibroblast-derived type B synoviocytes. The fluid is kept free of debris by macrophage-derived type A synoviocytes. Formation of SF is balanced by its removal via synovial lymphatics.

The surface of synovium and cartilage are not covered by an intact cell layer seated on a basement membrane, but by an incomplete layer of cells. Thus the matrix of cartilage and synovium are in contact with the SF, allowing a relatively homogeneous chemical environment to develop within the joint. Because of this unusual arrangement, it is perhaps better to regard the synovial fluid as a tissue rather than a true body fluid. As such it contains few cells[1], mainly chondrocytes and synoviocytes shed from the tissues lining the joint, together with migratory defense cells. The chemical composition of SF is poorly understood and complex (Fig 11.1).

THE CHEMICAL COMPOSITION OF NORMAL SYNOVIAL FLUID			
Osmolarity	296mOsm/l	Total protein	~25g/l
pH	7.44	Albumin	~8g/l
P_{CO_2}	6.0kPa (range 4.7–7.3)	α_1-antitrypsin	0.78μg/l
P_{O_2}	<4.0kPa	Ceruloplasmin	~43mg/l
Potassium	4.0mmol/l	Haptoglobin	~90mg/l
Sodium	136mmol/l	α_2-macroglobin	0.31g/l
Calcium	1.8mmol/l	Lactoferrin	0.44mg/l
Urea	2.5mmol/l	IgG	2.62g/l
Uric acid	0.23mmol/l	IgA	0.85g/l
		IgM	0.14g/l
Glucose	100mmol/l	IL-1β	20pg/ml
Chondroitin sulfate	40mg/l	IL-2	15.1U/ml
Hyaluronate	2.14g/l	TNF-α	1.38ng/ml
Cholesterol	Small amounts	INF-α	350U/ml
		INF-δ	13.7U/ml

IL = Interleukin; TNF = Tumor necrosis factor; INF = Interferon.

Fig. 11.1 The chemical composition of normal synovial fluid[2].

SYNOVIAL FLUID IN DISEASED JOINTS

Variation in the volume and composition of synovial fluid reflects pathologic processes within the joint. Because of the unusual relationship between the tissues within the joint, chemically mediated events such as inflammation and enzyme-mediated degradation within the synovium and cartilage are reflected in changes in the chemical composition of SF. These changes include the production of factors responsible for the accumulation of different cell types within the fluid. In terms of their diagnostic utility, both chemical and cytologic changes in the synovial fluid have been studied. These data will be summarized here.

SYNOVIAL FLUID MICROSCOPY

Analysis of synovial fluid differs in three important respects from that of other body fluids:

- synovial joints are rarely affected by neoplastic processes;
- recognition of noncellular particulate material, such as crystals and cartilage fragments, as well as microorganisms, is essential for understanding the disease process within the joint; and
- the greatest diagnostic information comes not only from recognition of cell types but also from their quantification[3,4].

THE BASIC APPROACH TO SYNOVIAL FLUID MICROSCOPY

Examination of synovial fluid is in four parts[5]:

- gross analysis,
- nucleated cell count,
- 'wet preparation' and
- cytocentrifuge preparation.

Gross analysis

Since SF from inflamed joints has a tendency to clot it should be anticoagulated. The best anticoagulant is lithium heparin. It is not possible to fix SF, which is therefore fresh tissue. Even with refrigeration, optimal cytologic information can be extracted from the sample only if it reaches the laboratory within 24 hours (preferably as soon as possible) of aspiration.

Upon arrival, SF is examined for color, clarity and viscosity and by a long-established piece of bench chemistry called the mucin clot test.

Color

Normally, SF is pale yellow. In hemarthroses it will be red or orange and in inflammatory arthropathies cream or white. In septic arthritis it may be colored by bacterial chromogens.

Clarity

Normal SF is clear, but with increasing numbers of particles and/or cells it becomes cloudier.

Viscosity

Synovial fluid is viscid because of the complex saccharides it contains. In inflammatory joint disease the viscosity of the fluid falls due to enzymic digestion and altered saccharide synthesis. This is easily demonstrated at the bedside by simply dripping the fluid from the end of the syringe immediately after aspiration. In cases of inflammatory joint disease the low-viscosity SF will form individual droplets whereas, in noninflammatory arthropathies with more viscid fluid, a 'stringing' effect is seen (Fig. 11.2).

Nucleated cell count

The nucleated cell count may be performed manually or automatically. For convenience, the nucleated cell count of SF is expressed as cells/mm^3. Normal SF contains <200 cells/mm^3 (<0.2 $\times$ 10^9/l). In inflammatory joint disease the cell count is greater than 1000 cells/mm^3 (1 $\times$ 10^9/l) and in noninflammatory arthropathies it is lower. Cell counts in excess of 25, 000 cells/mm^3 (25 $\times$ 10^9/l) are found in three clinical conditions: rheumatoid arthritis (RA), septic arthritis and reactive arthritis.

'Wet preparation'

Synovial fluid aspirates often contain visible particles. In making the 'wet preparation', the specimen is agitated and a small aliquot, containing as many of these particles as possible, is placed on a microscope slide. It is then gently squeezed flat beneath a cover slip and viewed unstained with a conventional microscope. For optimal results the condenser diaphragm is closed to produce diffuse light in which the unstained cells and particles are more clearly seen. This preparation is examined for one cell type, the ragocyte, and several different classes of noncellular particulate material.

Classes of crystalline material

Several classes of crystalline materials are found in the joints[6]. Monosodium urate monohydrate crystals are needle-shaped – 5–30µm in length – and highly birefringent (see Chapter 8.13, Fig. 13.3). They can be distinguished from other crystals as they are negatively birefringent when viewed in polarized light with an interposed quarter wave plate. These crystals, especially when intraleukocytic, are diagnostic of gout. If found within the background of a high cell count SF, their presence usually signifies acute gout, but even if the cell count is low the diagnosis is confirmed.

Calcium pyrophosphate dihydrate crystals accumulate normally within joints with advancing age. In elderly patients, they can therefore be regarded as a normal finding, a condition known as chondrocalcinosis. Sometimes the crystals are associated with a high nucleated cell count in an acute monoarthritis. This is the typical presentation of pseudogout. The presence of calcium pyrophosphate crystals in association with otherwise typical features of osteoarthritis (OA) characterizes hypertrophic OA[6].

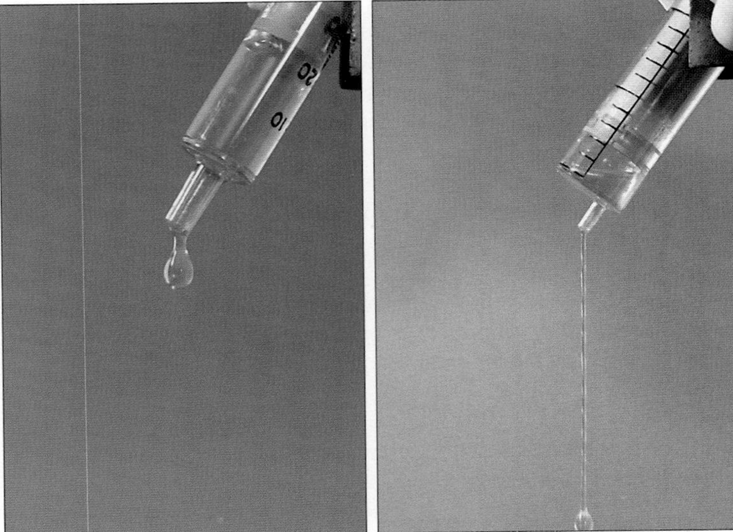

Fig. 11.2 The synovial fluid 'drip' test.
On the left, in a case of inflammatory joint disease, the low-viscosity SF falls as individual droplets. On the right, in a non-inflammatory arthropathy with more normally viscid fluid, a 'stringing' effect is seen. Courtesy of Professor Rodney Grahame.

Hydroxyapatite within SF indicates damage to calcified cartilage or underlying subarticular bone. Loss of cartilage, sufficient to expose these structures, is seen most commonly in OA and RA. The crystals are too small and amorphous to be seen with the light microscope, but staining with alizarin red stain[7] produces a birefringent red product which is easily visualized. A specific arthropathy, 'Milwaukee shoulder', is associated with larger apatite microspherules[8].

Lipids enter SF in inflammatory joint disease, in fracture of juxta-articular bone and in hemarthrosis. They can be distinguished from one another by their shape and differential solubility in hydrocarbon solvents[5]. Following intra-articular injection of depot corticosteroids, the crystalloid remains within the joint for up to 10 weeks and may mislead the unwary if they are not recognized[9].

Other crystals are found within SF, but are too numerous and rare to describe here. For a further description see Freemont and Denton[5].

Noncrystalline particles

Synovial joints are lined by cartilage and synovium and may be crossed by ligaments and bands of fibrocartilage. Alteration to the physical structure of any of these components by primary disease or trauma may lead to small fragments appearing free within the SF. Most common are fragments of articular cartilage or, depending on the joint, internal ligament and fibrocartilage[5].

Articular cartilage has a silken sheen in polarized light. In OA, the most common disorder in which cartilage is found free in the joint, fragments typically show the crimping of early fibrillation and clustered chondrocytes.

Fragments of fibrocartilage can be recognized by the curved arrays of collagen fibers and flattened chondrocytes they contain. They are typically found within traumatized knee joints.

Both in traumatized joints and in RA small fragments of ligament may be found within SF. They consist of long, thin twisted fibrils of no more than a dozen collagen fibers.

With the advent of prosthetic surgery, and particularly as the number of aging prostheses increases, wear of implanted material leads to foreign material within the joint. Many modern plastics, such as high-density polyethylene, used in prostheses, methylmethacrylate cement and composites such as Dacron and carbon fiber, mimic crystals if they fragment and can cause diagnostic problems. Metal debris from metal-based prostheses appear as tiny black particles. Although difficult to recognize these may be important harbingers of imminent prosthetic failure.

Occasionally, peculiar extraneous material such as plant fibres or other foreign bodies introduced accidentally (see Chapter 5.30) is found within SF.

Ragocytes are cells of various lineages characterized by the presence of cytoplasmic refractile granules which are larger than conventional granulocyte granules (Fig. 11.3). Ragocytes were first described in RA[10], in which they have been shown to contain immune complexes. They are not restricted to RA, being a constant feature of all inflammatory arthropathies, so that their diagnostic value is somewhat limited. However, with the exception of RA, septic arthritis, gout and pseudogout, ragocytes rarely account for more than 50% of all nucleated cells. If a crystal arthropathy is excluded, ragocyte counts above 70% are diagnostic of RA, and above 95% diagnostic of septic arthritis. The latter is diagnostic even in the absence of detectable organisms.

Cytocentrifuge preparation

Synovial fluid cytoanalysis can only be conducted on cytocentrifuge preparations. Optimal preparations are made by diluting the fluid to 400 cells/mm^3 (0.4 $\times$ 10^9/l) with isotonic saline and staining with Jenner–Giemsa stain. The one exception is when septic arthritis is suspected, when the greatest likelihood of identifying organisms is afforded by diluting the fluid to 1200 cells/mm^3 (1.2 $\times$ 10^9/l).

Careful microscopic examination of synovial fluid allows microorganisms to be identified in approximately 85% of instances of clinical infectious arthritis[5]. Most infective arthritis is caused by gram-positive cocci. The greatest problems in diagnosing septic arthritis are the

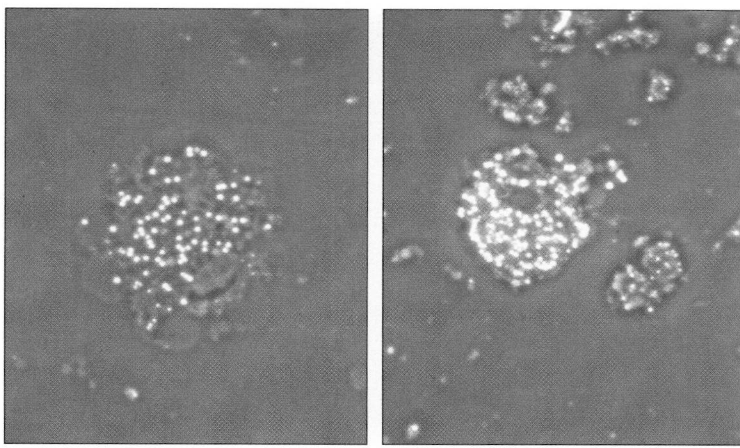

Fig. 11.3 Ragocytes from a patient with RA, showing the typical granules. Phase microscopy. (× 300)

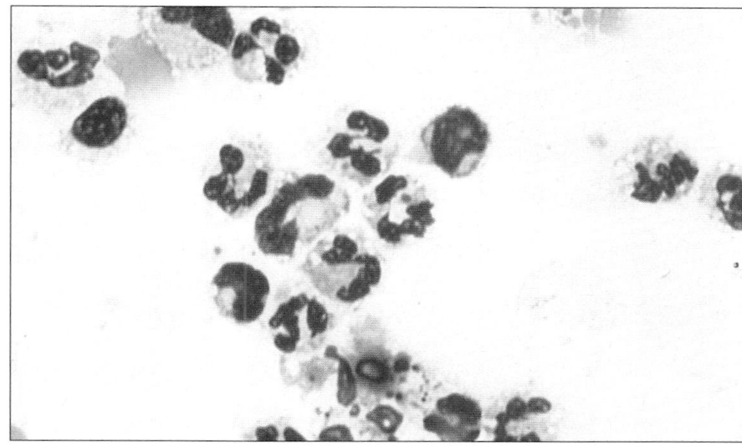

Fig. 11.4 A Jenner–Giemsa-stained cytocentrifuge preparation from an SF specimen with a cell count of 8500 cells/mm³ diluted to 400 cells/mm³. It shows neutrophils and small lymphocytes. (× 150)

recognition of gram-negative organisms and organisms rendered gram-negative by incomplete antibiotic therapy, and distinguishing contaminating organisms from true pathogens.

Immunosuppressed patients have an increasing incidence of nonsuppurative infectious arthritis, particularly caused by *Mycobacteria* and fungi. Although it is often possible to see the organism in these cases, the closest cooperation between clinician and cytopathologist is necessary to achieve the optimal detection rate, particularly in patients with a pre-existing arthritis.

Many different cell types are found within SF, reflecting the pathogenesis of the various joint diseases. Generally, in inflammatory arthropathies, polymorphs dominate the cytologic picture (Fig. 11.4). In noninflammatory arthropathies, macrophages, lymphocytes and synoviocytes are the most commonly encountered cells. There is a number of diagnostically useful cells commonly encountered in Jenner–Giemsa-stained cytocentrifuge preparations.

Neutrophils predominate in inflammatory arthropathies and in intra-articular hemorrhage where they commonly represent 60–80% of cells. Septic arthritis is the only disorder in which neutrophils regularly account for more than 95% of nucleated cells. The presence of small lymphocytes, the major SF cell in 10% of inflammatory arthropathies, is indicative of a better long-term prognosis in RA[11]. Plasma cells, rare in synovial fluid, are usually indicative of RA.

Reider cells have lobed nuclei, the lobes of which show symmetry about a pale attenuated center. Their singular morphology is caused by cytoskeletal abnormalities induced by the cellular environment. Other cells exhibiting morphologic changes secondary to altered internal membrane and microfilament or microtubule dysfunction include Mott cells and Döhle's body cells. All these cells are restricted to RA fluids[5].

Macrophages are the predominant cell in viral arthritis, acute monocytic arthritis and, with appropriate intracytoplasmic inclusions, pigmented villonodular synovitis (PVNS) and prosthetic debris-induced arthropathy. Cytophagocytic mononuclear cells (CPM) are mononuclear cells that have phagocytosed apoptotic polymorphs (Fig. 11.5). These cells are seen wherever apoptosis is taking place and, as this is the usual way in which polymorphs are removed from joints; they are common. They are abundant in the seronegative spondyloarthropathies[12]. If more than 5% of all macrophages are CPM a confident diagnosis of a seronegative spondyloarthropathy can be made. In RA, apoptosis occurs in the absence of CPM formation, a feature of such universal occurrence that it can be used diagnostically.

Synoviocytes, a morphologically distinct subgroup of large cells with a low nuclear–cytoplastic ratio, have a round, eccentrically situated nucleus and 'pericellular frill'. They are found most commonly in noninflammatory arthropathies in which multinucleate forms may occur. Eosinophils are seen following intra-articular hemorrhage and arthrography, as well as in the rare joint infestations. Mast cells, although found in most arthropathies, are seen most commonly in the seronegative spondyloarthropathies and in traumatic arthritis[12]. Lupus erythematosus cells are common in many arthritides.

THE CLINICAL VALUE OF SYNOVIAL FLUID MICROSCOPY

By retrospective analysis of proved cases using the criteria listed above, and others, it is possible to recognize patterns of microscopic features specific for certain arthropathies. These have been used to derive a diagnostic algorithm[5] which provides valuable diagnostic and prognostic data.

Tested blind it gives an accurate diagnosis in approximately 40% of cases[13] and a short differential diagnosis in a further 25%. In all but 4% it proves possible to say whether the patient has an inflammatory or noninflammatory arthropathy. The overall diagnostic rate in synovial fluid cytoanalysis is therefore 96%, although in half the diagnoses it is not precise. The false-positive rate is almost zero. Synovial fluid cytoanalysis is a highly selective and specific rheumatologic and orthopedic investigation.

THE PLACE OF SYNOVIAL FLUID MICROSCOPY IN DIAGNOSIS

The tissue pathologist has limited access to tissue from diseased joints. The articular surfaces are rarely biopsied except in end-stage disease, when they are removed, usually at joint replacement surgery. These specimens offer little of diagnostic value.

Synovium is not infrequently biopsied. Synovial biopsy is the investigation of choice in diseases with specific appearances, such as granulomatous inflammation and PVNS. However, even experienced histopathologists can find difficulty distinguishing inflammatory from noninflammatory arthropathies on a synovial biopsy, and even then it is usually impossible to be more specific as there are few histologic features that differentiate disorders in the same broad group.

Synovial fluid microscopy is of greatest value in differentiating inflammatory and noninflammatory arthropathies, in identifying specific disorders within these two groups, in diagnosis of early inflammatory disease, where it is often possible to identify a specific arthropathy before the clinical syndrome develops, in the diagnosis of mono- and oligoarthropathies and in the rapid diagnosis of joint disease, in particular suspected cases of septic arthritis where prognosis is inversely related to the delay in diagnosis.

BACTERIOLOGIC AND VIROLOGIC CULTURE

An essential part in the investigation of any arthropathy is the submission of specimens of SF to culture for microorganisms. As well as in cases of suspected infective arthritis, unsuspected infections may also be identified by this means. In addition to common bacterial joint pathogens (*Staphylococcus*, *Steptococcus*, etc.), *Neisseria*, *Salmonella*, *M. tuberculosis*, fungi and viruses requiring special culture methods should also be considered. For further details, see the relevant chapter(s) in Section 6.

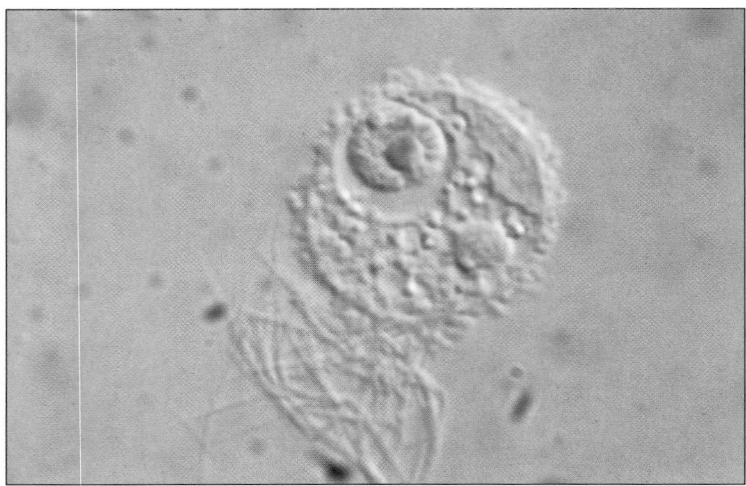

Fig. 11.5 A cytophagocytic mononuclear cell in which an apoptotic polymorph has been phagocytosed by a macrophage. Unstained 'wet prep' viewed in Nomarski phase optics. (× 500)

SOME OF THE POTENTIAL SF 'BIOCHEMICAL MARKERS' OF DISEASE PROCESSES UNDER INVESTIGATION

Process	SF markers
Inflammation	Eicosanoids, other small molecular weight mediators, breakdown products of complement cytokines, proteases
Matrix turnover	
Synovium/capsule	Hyaluronate, type III collagen propeptides
Cartilage degradation	Keratin sulfate, cartilage oligomeric matrix protein, other proteoglycan epitopes, type II collagen products
Cartilage synthesis	'Neo-epitopes' on proteoglycans, collagen type II propeptides
Bone	Osteocalcin, bone sialoprotein, other bone proteins and growth factors

Fig. 11.6 Some of the potential SF 'biochemical markers' of disease processes that are being investigated.

CHEMICAL CHANGES IN THE SYNOVIAL FLUID IN DISEASE

The chemistry of normal SF is outlined in Figure 11.1. Biochemical changes in the SF in disease may reflect abnormalities in the blood, or result from the production of excess or abnormal products in the synovium or cartilage. In general, products of normal or abnormal joint metabolism will be in a dynamic equilibrium with the serum, and dependent on a complex set of variables such as the hydrostatic and osmotic gradients across the joint, so that isolated single estimations of a product are not easy to interpret. Additional problems include the lack of availability of normal SF for comparison with disease samples, and the variable volumes of fluid aspirated and variable dilution of chemicals within the joint. It may be for these reasons that, in general, biochemical changes in SF have not proved to be disease specific or of great value as a diagnostic tool. However, recent work has shown that some changes may help pinpoint a specific disease process within a joint.

PRODUCTS OF INFLAMMATION

Levels of inflammatory mediators, such as eicosanoids[14], proteases and cytokines[15], are elevated in the SF of patients with a variety of arthropathies, reflecting the level of inflammation. Several antibodies, such as rheumatoid factor, have been described in SF, reflecting local production[16]. Similarly, SF complement levels change with local joint inflammation, and in RA complement breakdown products correlate with the severity of the synovitis[17]. However, most of these findings lack either consistency or specificity.

BIOCHEMICAL 'MARKERS' OF TISSUE BREAKDOWN AND REPAIR

Recent research has highlighted the potential value of assaying a number of products of matrix degradation and repair in body fluids, including SF. Local production of several tissue-specific peptides occurs as part of the disease process of both inflammatory arthropathies and osteoarthropathies, and these products can be identified by immunologic or other assay systems[18].

For example, degradation of cartilage proteoglycans by specific enzymes results in cleavage at specific sites within the peptide chain. The peptide sequences which are exposed at the ends of the fragments can then be identified[19]. Similarly, synthesis of new proteoglycan molecules may result in the expression of sugar motives that are not usually found in adult cartilage[20]. Assays of potential markers of synthesis and breakdown of collagens, proteoglycans and a variety of noncollagenous proteins with connective tissue matrices are now being developed and used as research tools to investigate disease processes (Fig. 11.6).

REFERENCES

1. Cohen AS, Brandt KD, Krey PR. Synovial fluid analysis. In: Cohen AS, ed. Laboratory diagnostic procedures in the rheumatic diseases, 2E. Boston: Little Brown; 1975:105–36.
2. Gardner DL. Pathological basis of the connective tissue diseases. London; Edward Arnold. 1992:90.
3. Revell PA. The value of synovial fluid analysis. Curr Top Pathol. 1982;71:1–24.
4. Currey HLF, Vernon-Roberts B. Examination of synovial fluid. Clin Rheum Dis. 1976;2:149–77.
5. Freemont AJ, Denton J. Atlas of synovial fluid cytopathology, vol 18. Current histopathology. Dordrecht, Boston, London: Kluwer Academic Publishers; 1991.
6. Dieppe PA, Calvert P. Crystals and joint disease. London: Chapman and Hall; 1983.
7. Paul H, Reginato AJ, Schumacher HR. Alizarin red-S staining as a screening test to detect calcium compounds in synovial fluid. Arthritis Rheum. 1983;26:191–200.
8. McCarty DJ, Halverson PB, Carrera GF, Brewer BJ, Kozin F. Milwaukee shoulder: association of microspheroids containing hydroxyapatite crystals, active collagenase, and neutral protease with rotator cuff defects. II; Synovial fluid studies. Arthritis Rheum. 1981;24:474–83.
9. Kahn CB, Hollander JL, Schumacher HR. Corticosteroid crystals in synovial fluid. JAMA. 1970;211:807–9.
10. Rawson AJ, Abelson NM, Hollander JL. Studies of the pathogenesis of rheumatoid joint inflammation. II; Intracytoplasmic particulate complexes in rheumatoid synovial fluids. Ann Int Med. 1965;62:281–4.
11. Davies MJ, Denton J, Freemont AJ, Holt PJL. Comparison of serial fluid cytology in rheumatoid arthritis; delineation of the subgroups with prognostic implications. Ann Rheum Dis. 1988;47:559–62.
12. Freemont AJ, Denton J. The disease distribution of synovial fluid mast cells and cytophagocytic mononuclear cells in inflammatory arthritis. Ann Rheum Dis. 1985;44:312–15.
13. Freemont AJ, Denton J, Chuck A, Davies MJ, Holt PJL. The diagnostic value of synovial fluid cytoanalysis; a reassessment. Ann Rheum Dis. 1991;50:101–7.
14. Bombardieri S, Cattani P, Ciabottoni R, *et al.* The synovial prostaglandin system in chronic inflammatory arthritis: differential effects of steroidal and non-steroidal anti-inflammatory drugs. Br J Pharmacol. 1981;73:891–901.
15. Di Giovine FS, Nuki G, Duff GW. Tumour necrosis factor in synovial exudates. Ann Rheum Dis. 1988;47:768–72.
16. Mimms CA, Stokes A, Grahame R. Synthesis of antibodies including antiviral antibodies in the knee joints of patients with arthritis. Ann Rheum Dis. 1985;44:734–41.
17. Doherty M, Richards N, Hornby J, Powell R. Relation between synovial fluid C3 degradation products and local joint inflammation in rheumatoid arthritis, osteoarthritis and crystal associated arthropathy. Ann Rheum Dis. 1988;47:190–7.
18. Heinegaard D, Lohmander S, Sasene T. Acta Orthop Scand. 1995;66(suppl 266):1–212.
19. Sandy JD, Flannery CR, Neame PJ, Lohamander LS. The structure of aggrecan freagments in human synovial fluid: evidence for the involvement in osteoarthritis of a novel protease. J Clin Invest. 1992;215:377–85.
20. Poole AR, Ionescu M, Swan A, Dieppe P. Changes in cartilage metabolism in arthritis are reflected by altered serum and synovial fluid levels of the cartilage proteoglycan aggrecan. J Clin Invest. 1994;94:25–33.

12

ASPIRATION AND INJECTION OF JOINTS AND PERIARTICULAR TISSUES

Juan J Canoso

- Synovial aspiration is the basic diagnostic tool in rheumatology.
- Synovial fluid analysis allows distinction between inflammatory and noninflammatory conditions and provides direct proof of crystal arthropathy, infection and hemarthrosis.
- Major diagnostic errors can be made by simply assuming the nature of an effusion.
- Corticosteroid injections and infiltrations are basic treatment tools in rheumatology, orthopedics and general medicine.
- Synovial aspiration and corticosteroid injections and infiltrations carry minimal risk to the patient when properly indicated and performed.
- Technical difficulties vary; some of these procedures require specialized knowledge for optimal results.

Joints and periarticular structures such as bursae and tendon sheaths may need aspiration for diagnostic or therapeutic purposes. In addition, corticosteroids and other drugs are often injected in and around soft tissue periarticular lesions to treat regional pain syndromes (Fig. 12.1). The principles and practice of inserting a needle into either a joint cavity or periarticular lesion are very similar.

INDICATIONS FOR ASPIRATING OR INJECTING MUSCULOSKELETAL TISSUES

ASPIRATING FLUID FOR DIAGNOSTIC OR THERAPEUTIC PURPOSES

In patients in whom sepsis, crystal synovitis or bleeding is the suspected cause of a joint, bursal or tendon sheath lesion, aspiration and analysis of the fluid is essential for diagnosis[1–3]. In addition, in patients who have poorly defined forms of arthritis, knowledge of the nature of the synovial fluid, particularly the inflammatory cell content, will complement findings from the history and physical examination and help provide the basic framework for diagnosis and treatment. In patients with tense joint or bursal effusions, aspiration of synovial fluid provides prompt relief of pain and permits the patient to move or bear weight on the affected joint. Finally, in hemarthrosis or septic arthritis, the blood and pus within a synovial cavity may be toxic to the joint cartilage and synovial membrane, so evacuation of the fluid is necessary to avoid permanent joint damage. Large articular effusions should be drained as fully as possible to decrease pressure, improve synovial circulation and prevent muscle atrophy.

Synovial fluid should be aspirated into sterile syringes, which are either capped or immediately aliquoted into sterile containers. Anticoagulants can help avoid the formation of fibrin clots, making the fluid easier to handle and assisting in analyses of the cellular content. If unusual or chronic infections are suspected it may be prudent to inoculate some of the fluid into appropriate growth media (such as chocolate agar for gonococcal infections) immediately after aspiration. The fluid should be inspected for the presence of blood and to see how opaque it is, which is a rough guide to cell content. Three laboratory investigations should then be carried out on all fluids aspirated for diagnostic purposes:

- the total and differential cell count,
- examination for organisms (gram stain, culture, etc.),
- polarized light microscopy for the presence of urate or pyrophosphate crystals.

As crystal synovitis and infections can coexist it is never wise to rely on one of these investigations alone. The cellular content is indicative of the type of arthritis (Fig. 12.2). Other special investigations that can be of value include cytology and the assay of a variety of biochemical markers of connective tissue turnover, such as products of the synthesis and degradation of cartilage aggrecan.

PRACTICAL PROCEDURE AND AFTERCARE

Technical considerations

Some joints are easier to enter than others. There is a rank order of technical difficulty in which knee aspiration stands as the easiest procedure and sacroiliac joint injection [4,5] as the most difficult. Because sacroiliac joint injection, facet joint injection[6] and epidural block[7] fall in the specialism of interventional radiology they are not discussed further in this chapter.

The procedure

Aspiration or injection of joints or soft tissues is an outpatient procedure that does not require specialized equipment (see Fig. 12.3).

INDICATIONS FOR ASPIRATING OR INJECTING JOINTS	
Diagnosis	Mandatory if septic arthritis suspected Strongly advised if crystal arthritis or hemarthrosis suspected Differentiation of inflammatory from noninflammatory arthritis Imaging studies – arthroscopy and arthrography Synovial biopsy
Therapy	To remove tense effusions to relieve pain and improve function To remove blood or pus from a joint For injection of corticosteroids and other intra-articular therapies For tidal lavage of joints

Fig. 12.1 Indications for aspirating or injecting joints.

SYNOVIAL FLUID FINDINGS				
	Normal	Osteoarthritis	Rheumatoid and other inflammatory arthritis	Septic arthritis
Gross apperance	Clear	Clear	Opaque	Opaque
Volume (ml)	0–1	1–10	5–50	5–50
Viscosity	High	High	Low	Low
Total white cell count/mm^3	<200	200–10,000	5000–75,000	>50,000
% Polymorphonuclear cells	<25%	<50%	>50%	>75%

Fig. 12.2 Knee joint synovial fluid findings in common forms of arthritis.

EQUIPMENT REQUIRED FOR JOINT AND SOFT TISSUE INJECTIONS	
Skin preparation	Antiseptic solution (povidone-iodine), alcohol swabs, 4 × 4 gauze pads
Local anesthetics	1% lidocaine
Needles	23–27 gauge needles for local anesthetic; 18 gauge for large to moderate size joints (knees, shoulders, ankles, etc.); 23–25 gauge for small joints (wrists, MCP's, etc.)
Syringes	3 or 5ml syringe for anesthetic–steroid injection and 10–50ml syringe for fluid aspiration
Miscellaneous	Gloves; forceps for removing needles from syringe; specimen tubes/plates for cultures and fluid studies

Fig. 12.3 Equipment required for joint and soft tissue injections. All of the required supplies should be assembled in advance. Very importantly, the needle should be long enough to reach the intended place and have a caliber adequate to the nature of the fluid. While standard needle lengths work well in thin patients, longer needles and even a spinal needle may be required in obese patients. Purulent effusions require #18 or #16 needles. A failure to fully drain a septic joint indicates large debris or loculation and calls for tidal lavage (*vide infra*), arthroscopy or arthrotomy.

Universal precautions must be followed during the procedure; gloves are recommended and required by medical practice regulations in many countries.

The patient should be placed in a comfortable supine or recumbent position (in case of possible fainting, as well as to aid relaxation), and the procedure must be fully explained. Prior to cleaning the skin, bony and other landmarks need to be identified by palpation and the needle site marked in some way, such as with a thumbnail imprint in the skin. The skin must then be carefully cleaned with antiseptic agents. For local anesthesia, the skin and subcutaneous tissues can be infiltrated down to the level of the periarticular lesion or joint capsule using 1% lidocaine (lignocaine) without epinephrine (adrenaline) and a small-bore needle. However, physicians experienced with the procedure often prefer to use topical ethyl chloride or no anesthetic at all. This is often appropriate for joint aspiration, as it is difficult to anesthetize the capsule, so a single, simple, quick needle thrust may be much less painful than the local anesthesia. With the proper technique, the needle passes freely through the extra-articular tissues and a 'pop' is felt as the needle enters the joint. The ease with which fluid can be withdrawn depends on the needle size used, viscosity of the fluid, extent of synovitis and presence of any fibrin clots or 'rice bodies' in the joint fluid. Free flow of fluid is often suddenly interrupted due to clogging of the needle end by the synovial membrane or debris. Rotating the needle, withdrawing it slightly or even re-injecting a little of the fluid will often help unclog the needle and allow additional fluid to be withdrawn. If corticosteroids or other substances are to be injected, this can be done through the same needle, but removing the aspirating syringe from the needle hub may be difficult and require forceps.

At the end of any procedure, the needle should be swiftly withdrawn, and light pressure put on the needle site of the skin. The application of a simple adhesive plaster for a few hours afterwards is all that is usually required thereafter.

Aftercare

There is a great deal of variation in the advice given to patients after aspiration or therapeutic injection of joints or soft tissues. Some doctors give no specific instructions, others recommend a prolonged period of rest to help facilitate the best possible therapeutic response. In most cases, it is sensible for patients to rest the affected joint for 24–48 hours after a therapeutic injection, to minimize leakage of the therapeutic agent and improve the anti-inflammatory response. However, this advice must depend on the patient's circumstances.

CONTRAINDICATIONS AND COMPLICATIONS

CONTRAINDICATIONS

There are few absolute contraindications to joint or soft tissue aspirations and injections; if infection is suspected then fluid should always be aspirated from a joint. In other indications, the procedures should probably be avoided if there is infection of the overlying skin or subcutaneous tissues or if bacteremia is suspected. The presence of a significant bleeding disorder or diathesis, such as a patient receiving anticoagulant therapy or with severe thrombocytopenia, may also preclude joint aspiration. However, if it is deemed necessary for diagnosis or therapy, the procedure may be carried out after an injection of factor VIII in a hemophiliac for example, or with other appropriate cover for the bleeding disorder. Aspiration of a joint with a prosthesis in it carries a particularly high risk of infection, and is often best left to surgeons using full aseptic techniques.

Lack of response to previous injections may be a relative contraindication to therapeutic injections and, if there is any suspicion of infection being the underlying cause of the musculoskeletal problem, corticosteroids must not be injected, for fear of exacerbating the infection.

COMPLICATIONS

There are surprisingly few complications of these procedures. The most significant issue is the risk of infection, and care must always be taken to use sterile 'no-touch' techniques, as well as avoiding corticosteroids in those who could have existing sepsis. It is estimated that the risk of a septic arthritis following aspiration or corticosteroid injection is in the order of 1 per 15,000 procedures[8]. Patients who have severe immunodeficiency problems, as well as those with implants, may be at greater risk.

Other complications can arise from misplaced injections. The best described problem is tendon rupture following corticosteroid injections for tendinitis. The risk can be minimized by avoiding injection into the tendon itself, and no therapeutic agent should be injected against any unexpected resistance. Occasionally nerve damage can also result from a misplaced injection, for example median nerve atrophy following attempted injections for a carpal tunnel syndrome.

CORTICOSTEROID INJECTIONS

Corticosteroid injections are frequently used to achieve local anti-inflammatory activity. The indications for their use include the presence of persistent inflammation at a single site in the absence of a contraindication, such as suspicion of infection (see below). Synovial joints and other cavities should generally be injected with a long-acting, crystalline form of corticosteroid such as triamcinolone hexacetonide or acetonide. These agents are taken up by the synovial lining cells, allowing continued local release into the targeted area. Only a relatively small proportion escapes into the general circulation but, during the first 24 hours after injection, patients may experience flushing or other evidence of a corticosteroid 'pulse'. For periarticular injections, particularly subcutaneous bursae and de Quervain's tenosynovitis, methylprednisolone acetate should be used, as the more potent triamcinolone hexacetonide is likely to induce skin atrophy. Local anesthetic is sometimes mixed with corticosteroids for such injections. In the case of some periarticular lesions, for example rotator cuff lesions around the shoulder, this can have the advantage of confirming the correct placement of the injection, as the local anesthetic should result in almost immediate relief of the problem if the injection is correctly placed.

Corticocosteroid doses vary with the structure injected. For each of the described procedures below a dose range is shown based on the use of methylprednisolone acetate 40mg/ml. If the more potent triamcinolone hexacetonide 20mg/ml is used, the lower figure of the range should be chosen.

Corticosteroid injections are used in joints, bursae, tendon sheaths and entheses[9]. Some of these procedures are easy to perform while others are technically demanding or have dubious results. The simple procedures include infiltrations for trigger finger[10,11], carpal tunnel syndrome[12,13], ganglia, olecranon bursitis[14,15], rotator cuff tendinitis, trochanteric bursitis, anserine[16] bursitis and 'trigger points'. The technically demanding group includes injections for de Quervain's tenosynovitis[17,18], lateral epicondylitis (tennis elbow)[19], medial epicondylitis (golfer's elbow), suprascapular nerve block[20] (see Chapter 2.13), iliopsoas bursitis[21], ischial 'bursitis', Achilles tendinitis, retrocalcaneal bursitis[22], plantar fasciitis, posterior tibialis tenosynovitis and Morton's neuroma[23]. Intracavitary position of the needle can be ascertained by withdrawing some articular fluid or checking to see if the cavity distends as fluid is injected. In the soft tissues, correct positioning may be ascertained by elimination of pain by a preceding lidocaine infiltration. Rest of the injected site for 48 hours following the procedure is generally recommended. Additional rest may lead to better results and should be considered under special circumstances.

COMPLICATIONS OF CORTICOSTEROID INJECTIONS AND INFILTRATIONS

Facial flushing. Very common, occurring in perhaps 40% of cases. Transient and inconsequential, it may nevertheless worry patients who have not been warned.

Postinjection flare. Corticosteroid crystal-induced synovitis occurs in about 5% of intra-articular injections. Pain appears several hours following the procedure and may last from a few hours to 1 day. Persisting pain and mounting swelling may indicate missed or iatrogenic infection; these joints should be re-aspirated for gram stain and aerobic and anaerobic cultures. Tennis elbow infiltrations are often followed by protracted pain, which may last several weeks. Repeated tennis elbow infiltrations are believed to contribute to the development of chronic pain.

Skin atrophy. This is a frequent complication of superficial infiltrations and olecranon bursa injections. The condition is characterized by cigarette paper-like skin, recurrent ecchymosis and chronic pressure pain. Post-injection atrophy is more likely to develop in elderly individuals.

Skin hypopigmentation. Superficial corticosteroid infiltrations such as those used in de Quervain's tenosynovitis often cause a hypopigmented patch which may be quite disfiguring in people with dark skin. The condition resolves in a few months to 2 years.

Infection. This is an extremely rare complication of corticosteroid injections, except for injections in the olecranon bursa. Postinjection septic bursitis may occur from exacerbation of a missed infection (infections of superficial bursae may be quite subdued) or may be caused by contamination of a sterile bursa through the needle track. The skin at the elbow tip has little recoil. Taps made at the bursal apex, where the skin is maximally stretched, often create a leaking point that may act as a portal of entry.

Tendon rupture. A ruptured tendon following a corticosteroid injection may indicate abuse of the procedure, intratendinous injection or coincidental rupture caused by the very condition that lead to the injection. Athletes who have received multiple infiltrations around the Achilles' tendon are at a high risk of tendon rupture. Conditions that lead to spontaneous tendon rupture include dorsal wrist tenosynovitis and posterior tibialis tenosynovitis in rheumatoid arthritis (RA), chronic subacromial impingement damaging the rotator cuff and the long biceps tendon, senile changes in the supraspinatus or long biceps tendon, chronic corticosteroid use, fluoroquinolone-induced tendinitis, uremia, hyperparathyroidism and systemic lupus erythematosus.

Corticosteroid arthropathy. Abuse of intra-articular injections may result in a Charcot's-like arthropathy similar to the one described in calcium pyrophosphate crystal deposition disease (see Chapter 8.16).

Osteonecrosis. This is a reported complication of abused articular or soft tissue corticosteroid infiltrations.

Corticosteroid-induced osteoporosis. Patients who have been serially injected, for recurrent tendinitis, for example, are at an enhanced risk of osteoporosis during the injection period, particularly if additional factors are present such as prolonged bed rest or a low calcium intake. Intra-articular corticosteroids are said to have less effect on bone than do oral corticosteroids[24]. However, the relative safety of the intra-articular route has not been shown in clinical trials.

Other systemic complications. Corticosteroid injections cause transient pituitary inhibition, lasting up to several days. Serial infiltrations may cause adrenal suppression.

ASSOCIATED PROCEDURES

A number of other agents apart from corticosteroids have been used for intra-articular or periarticular therapy via injection. Examples include the radioactive colloids such as yttrium-90, which can irradiate the synovium to achieve a form of chemical synovectomy, other sclerosing agents and long-acting local anesthetics, sometimes used alone to help sort out the origin of musculoskeletal pain.

There are a number of other procedures outlined in Chapters 2.13 and 2.14 that may require joint puncture, which include:

- Imaging joints with contrast agents: injection of contrast agents with or without air can help image soft tissue and cartilage lesions in joints using radiography (arthrography).
- Joint lavage: tidal lavage of joints with saline, through a simple percutaneous cannula, or during arthroscopy can result in lasting relief of pain and inflammation in chronic arthritis.
- Synovial biopsy: synovial biopsy can be of diagnostic value, and is essential for the diagnosis of pigmented villonodular synovitis and other neoplastic lesions, as well as sometimes being necessary to diagnose chronic infections such as tuberculosis and foreign body synovitis. This can be done percutaneously, using a 'Parker Pearson' needle, or through arthroscopy.
- Needle arthroscopy and 'chondroscopy': full arthroscopic examination and surgery is largely the province of the orthopedic surgeon. However, arthroscopic examination of some joints, especially the knee, can be carried out under local anesthesia, particularly if modern small-bore arthroscopes (needlescopes) are used. This can be of value in examining the synovium and cartilage (chondroscopy) and in joint lavage, as well as allowing biopsy under direct vision.

THE WRIST AND HAND

FINGER AND METACARPOPHALANGEAL JOINTS

Indications. Injection in RA, psoriatic arthritis, active Bouchard's nodes.

Corticosteroid dose. 10–15mg methylprednisone (no. 25 or no. 27 needle).

Approach. Dorsolateral with the digit in semiflexion (see Figs 12.4 & 12.5). Corticosteroid injection produces circumferential distention of the joint. Multiple joints may be injected in one session.

Precautions. Do not overdistend joint(s). Fluid has a tendency to back up; keep firm pressure with a sterile gauze for at least 5 minutes following the procedure.

Complications. Joint hyperlaxity, capsular calcification (frequent but inconsequential).

FLEXOR TENDON SHEATHS

Indications. Injection in trigger finger; flexor tenosynovitis in RA, psoriatic arthritis.

Corticosteroid dose. 15–20mg methylprednisone mixed with 1–2ml lidocaine (no. 25 or no. 27 needle or no. 23 butterfly).

Approach. Just distal to palmar crease of thumb, proximal palmar crease (index), distal palmar crease (long, ring and little fingers) with needle held at a 45° distal inclination (Fig. 12.6).

Precautions. Avoid intratendinous injection. Reciprocal needle movements upon gentle finger motion indicate tendon engagement; back up by the millimeter, free the needle and inject. Up to three injections given 3 weeks apart are allowed.

Complications. Superficial extravasation may produce asymptomatic

INJECTION OF THE METACARPOPHALANGEAL JOINT

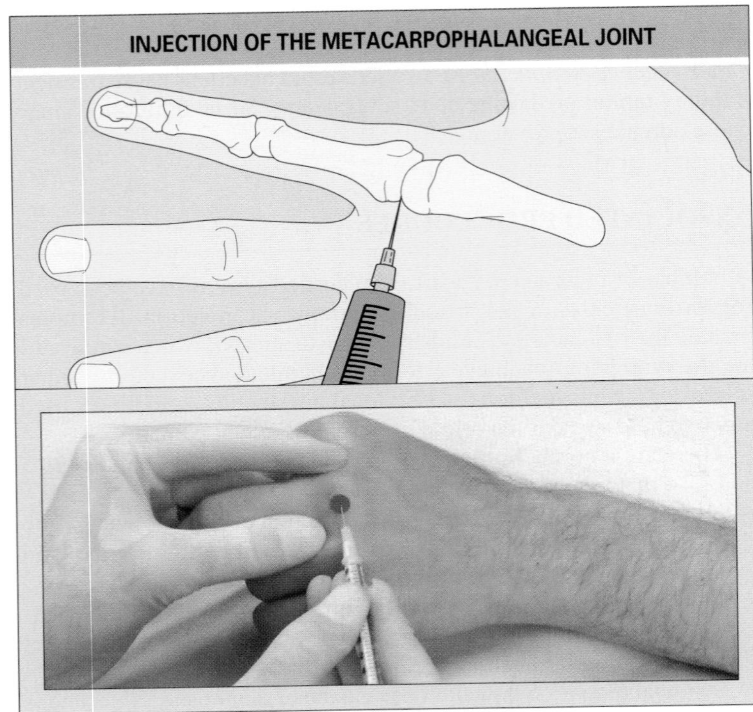

Fig. 12.4 Injection of the metacarpophalangeal joint.

INJECTION OF THE INTERPHALANGEAL JOINT

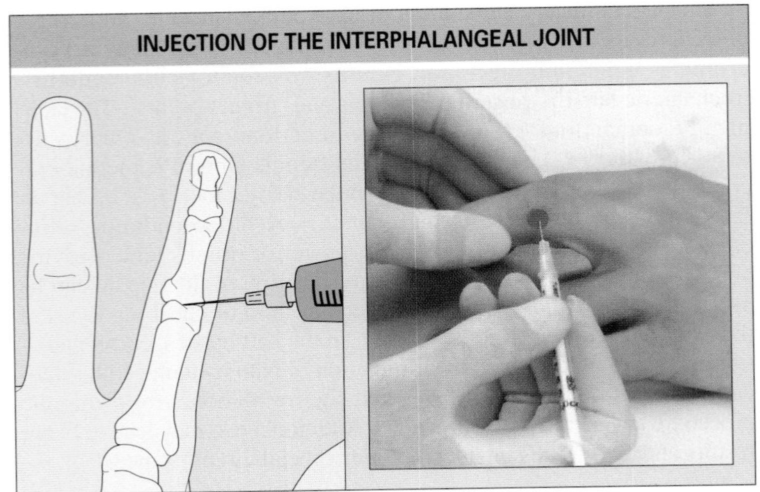

Fig. 12.5 Injection of the proximal interphalangeal joint.

focal palmar fat atrophy. Large published series comment on a lack of tendon rupture and iatrogenic infection.

DE QUERVAIN'S TENOSYNOVITIS

Indications. Most instances of inflammation of the common sheath of the abductor pollicis longus and extensor pollicis brevis result from hand overuse. Corticosteroid injections are highly successful in these cases.
Corticosteroid dose. 20–30mg methylprednisolone acetate (no. 25 needle).
Approach. The needle is aimed towards the radial styloid, which underlies the sheath. The needle is then pulled back by the millimeter and injection is attempted. Successful injection distends the sheath distally to the metacarpal base.
Precautions. Make sure that the corticosteroid remains within the sheath. Do not infiltrate grossly thickened sheaths, as mycobacterial infection may be present.
Complications. As mentioned previously, skin hypopigmentation frequently complicates this procedure. Skin atrophy, leading to recurring ecchymosis, is particularly prevalent in elderly patients.

CARPAL TUNNEL SYNDROME

Indications. Injection treatment is indicated in all etiologies of carpal tunnel syndrome (CTS) except acute cases due to fracture, hemorrhage, infection and CTS of late pregnancy.
Corticosteroid dose. 30–40mg methlyprednisone mixed with 2–3ml lidocaine (no. 22 or no. 25 needle or no. 23 butterfly).
Approach. Just distal to the distal wrist crease and just medial to palmaris longus (PL) tendon (Fig. 12.7). If the PL tendon is absent (25% of people lack the PL tendon), use the midline. The needle is inserted to a depth of 1cm with a 45° distal inclination and a 45° lateral inclination.
Precautions. Paresthesias indicate median nerve engagement; if they occur, reposition the needle. Reciprocal needle motion upon gentle finger motion (which should be rehearsed beforehand) indicates tendon engagement; again, reposition the needle.
Complications. Transient increase of paresthesias.

Note: A properly made resting splint to hold the wrist in the neutral position provides the lowest pressures within the carpal tunnel.

FIRST CARPOMETACARPAL JOINT

Indications. Painful osteoarthritis (OA). The patient presents with a 'square hand' with grating and tenderness at the prominence.
Corticosteroid dose. 15–30mg methlyprednisone (no. 23 or no. 25 needle).
Approach. Within the anatomic snuffbox. After localizing the joint line at the base of the first metacarpal, the joint is entered at the anatomic snuffbox between the common sheath of the abductor pollicis longus and extensor pollicis brevis anteriorly and the extensor pollicis longus posteriorly. To optimally expose the joint the thumb is flexed across the palm towards the little finger.

INJECTION OF THE FLEXOR DIGITAL TENDON SHEATH IN TRIGGER FINGER

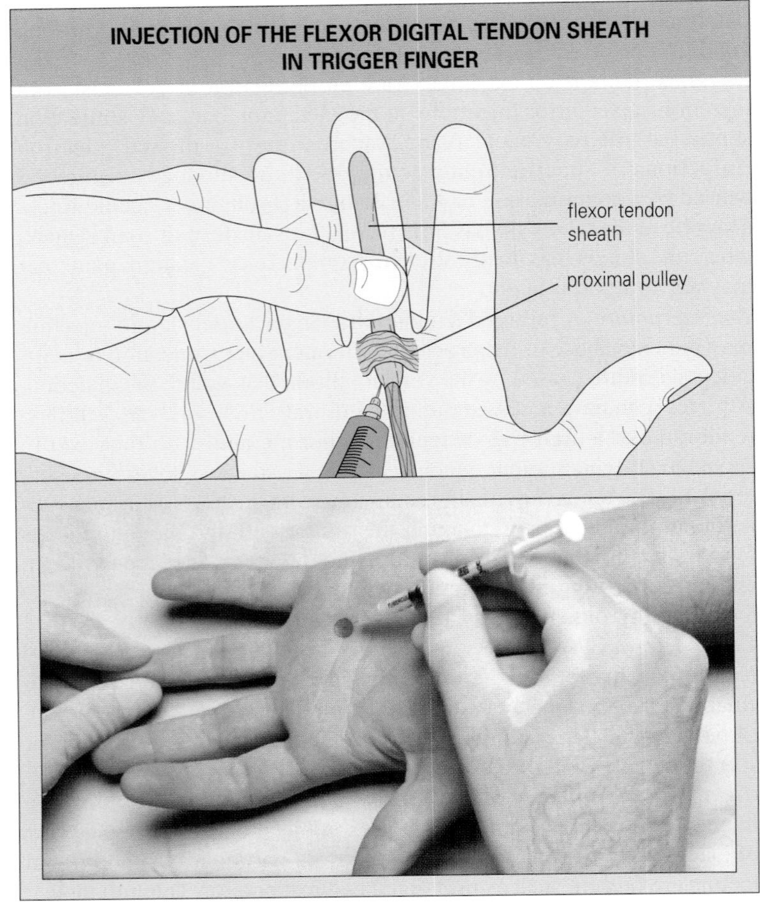

Fig. 12.6 Injection of the flexor digital tendon sheath in trigger finger.

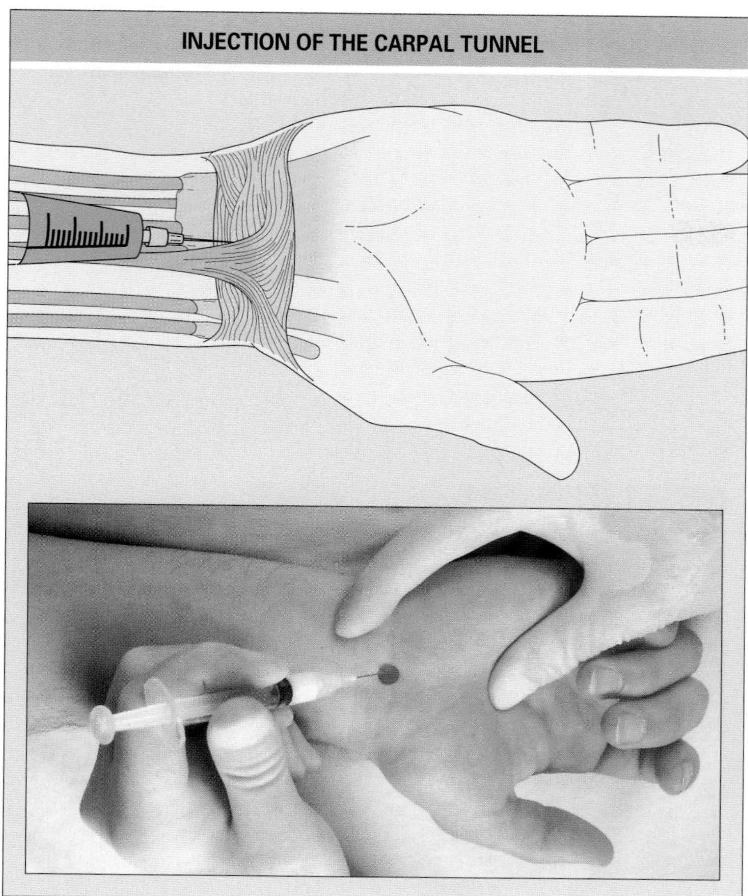

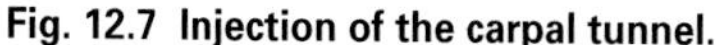
Fig. 12.7 Injection of the carpal tunnel.

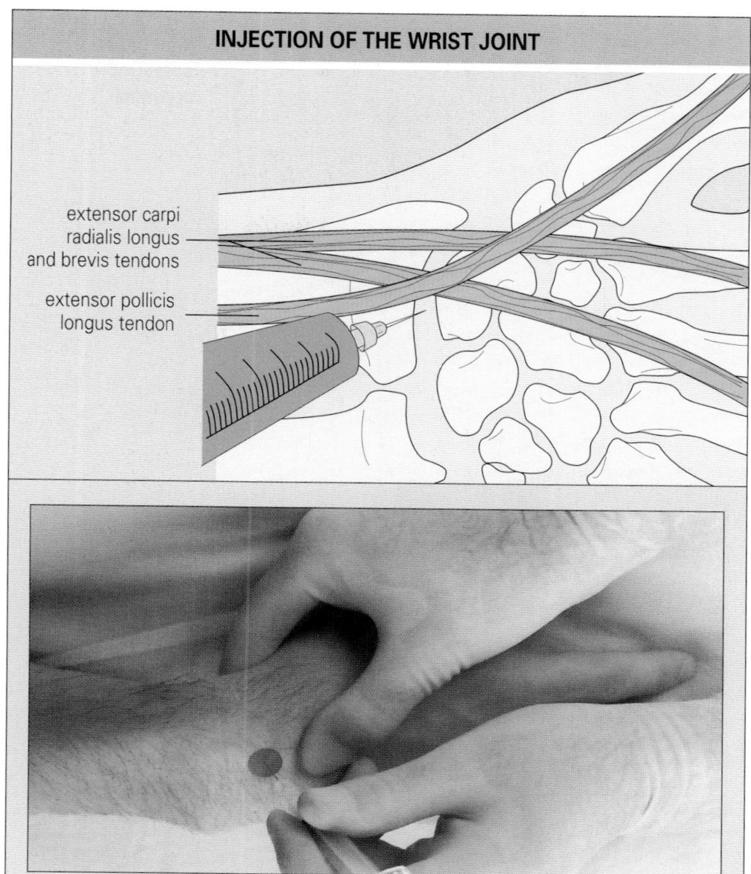

Fig. 12.8 Injection of the wrist joint.

Precautions. Avoid the radial artery. The course of this vessel varies and may encircle the joint line.
Complications. None, as long as the radial artery is avoided.

WRIST

Indications. For diagnosis in acute arthritis. Most cases of acute wrist arthritis are due to calcium pyrophosphate dihydrate pseudogout, gout and septic arthritis. For injection in RA, other sterile synovitides and OA such as associated with chondrocalcinosis and hemochromatosis.
Corticosteroid dose. 30–40mg methylprednisone (no. 23 needle). Aspiration should be attempted before injection. For aspiration alone use a no. 20 or no. 18 needle.
Approach. Dorsal, just distal to Lister's tubercule (a bone prominence in the dorsal distal radius where the extensor pollicis longus bends radially to reach the thumb), just ulnar to the extensor pollicis longus tendon (Fig. 12.8). The wrist should be slightly palmar flexed to facilitate the procedure.
Precautions. There are no important neurovascular structures of concern at this site.
Complications. None.

GANGLIA

Indications. Local corticosteroids are highly effective in the treatment of routine dorsal ganglia. Ganglia within the carpal tunnel, which impinge on neurovascular structures, or that are larger than 3cm in diameter, should be treated surgically.
Corticosteroid dose. Depends on the lesion; usually 15–20mg methylprednisone (no. 20 or no. 18 needle; thinner needles may be clogged).
Approach. The needle is aimed to the center of the lesion, which is aspirated prior to injection. Ganglia contain a very viscous, translucent fluid. Fluids with other characteristics indicate that the lesion is not a ganglion; they should therefore be cultured and inspected for crystals.
Precautions. In wrist ganglia, rule out radial artery aneurysm, which mimicks a ganglion. These lesions are expansile with the pulse, as opposed to the focal pulsation caused by a normal adjacent radial artery.
Complications. None.

THE ELBOW REGION

ELBOW

Indications. Aspiration in acute arthritis, injection in RA and psoriatic arthritis.
Corticosteroid dose. 30–40mg methylprednisone (no. 22 needle). Aspiration should be attempted before injection. For aspiration alone use a no. 20 or no. 18 needle, depending on the suspected diagnosis.
Approach. There are three commonly used entries. For all entries the elbow is held flexed at 90°.

- Posterior approach. The depression in the midline between the two halves of the triceps tendon is palpated at the back of the elbow. The needle is then passed perpendicular to the skin into the olecranon fossa (see Fig. 12.9).
- Inferolateral approach. The midpoint cleft between the olecranon tip and the lateral epicondyle is palpated. The needle is then inserted perpendicularly, aiming at the center of the joint.
- Lateral approach. The radiocapitular joint may be entered from the side, just proximal to the radial head. The needle is passed tangentially between the two bones, rather than directly (see Fig. 12.10).

Precautions. There are no neurovascular structures in the vicinity.
Complications. None.

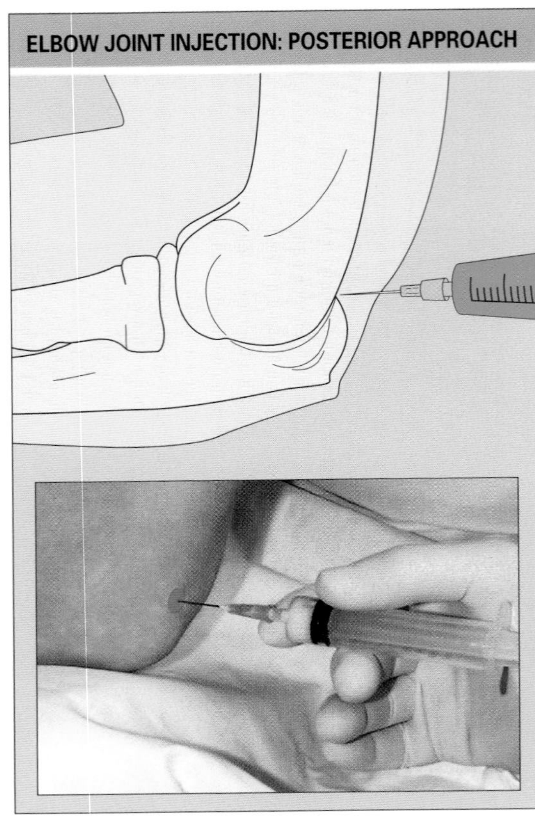

Fig. 12.9 Elbow joint injection: posterior approach.

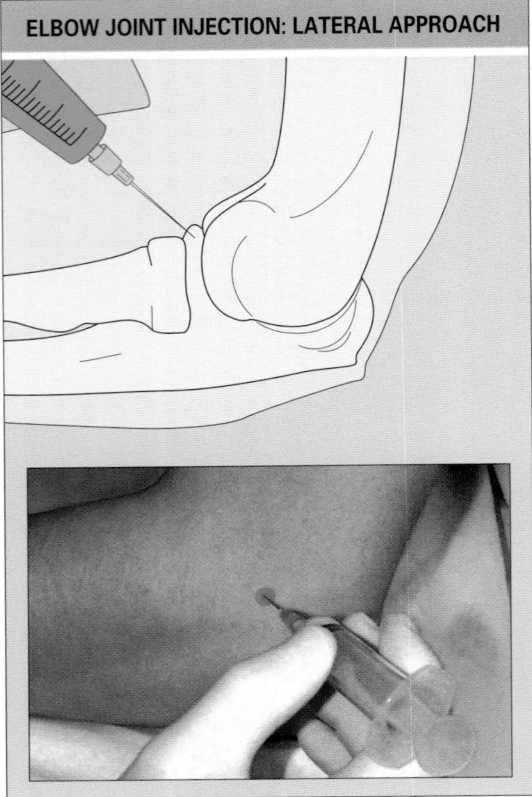

Fig. 12.10 Elbow joint injection: lateral approach.

OLECRANON BURSA

Indications. For diagnosis of effusion and for treatment of aseptic bursitis (traumatic or idiopathic) in cases that are refractory to conservative treatment. A negative bursal fluid culture is required for the procedure to be performed.

Corticosteroid dose. 20mg of methylprednisolone acetate (no. 22 needle). Aspiration should be attempted before injection. For aspiration alone use a no. 20 needle.

Approach. Lateral through normal skin, aiming at the center of the bursa.

Precautions. Taps at the tip of the bursa may create a chronic leak. Medial entries may damage the ulnar nerve.

Complications. Skin atrophy, pain on leaning and septic bursitis are recognized complications of the intrabursal administration of 20mg of triamcinolone hexacetonide[13]. The injection of 20mg of methylprednisolone acetate has not caused complications[14].

Note: In traumatic or idiopathic olecranon bursitis conservative treatment is recommended, namely avoiding leaning on the elbow, for 3 months. Intrabursal corticosteroids may be tried in cases that fail to resolve.

TENNIS ELBOW

Indications. Failure of conservative treatment. To speed up recovery in high performance athletes, although this is a controversial procedure.

Corticosteroid dose. 10–20mg methylprednisone (no. 22 needle).

Approach. At the most tender point (Fig. 12.11). Pass the needle to periosteal contact and infiltrate with 2–3ml lidocaine. Failure to eradicate pain on resisted wrist dorsiflexion indicates the wrong injection site; reposition needle and reinfiltrate with lidocaine. The corticosteroid should be infiltrated deeply, at the tenoperiosteal junction.

Precautions. Avoid injecting too superficially.

Complications. Transient increase in pain in 40% of patients. Repeated corticosteroid infiltrations may result in chronic pain.

Note: The current trend is to be conservative, avoiding infiltrations. Lack of improvement with lidocaine infiltration suggests an alternative diagnosis such as compressive neuropathy of the deep branch of the radial nerve or cervical radiculopathy.

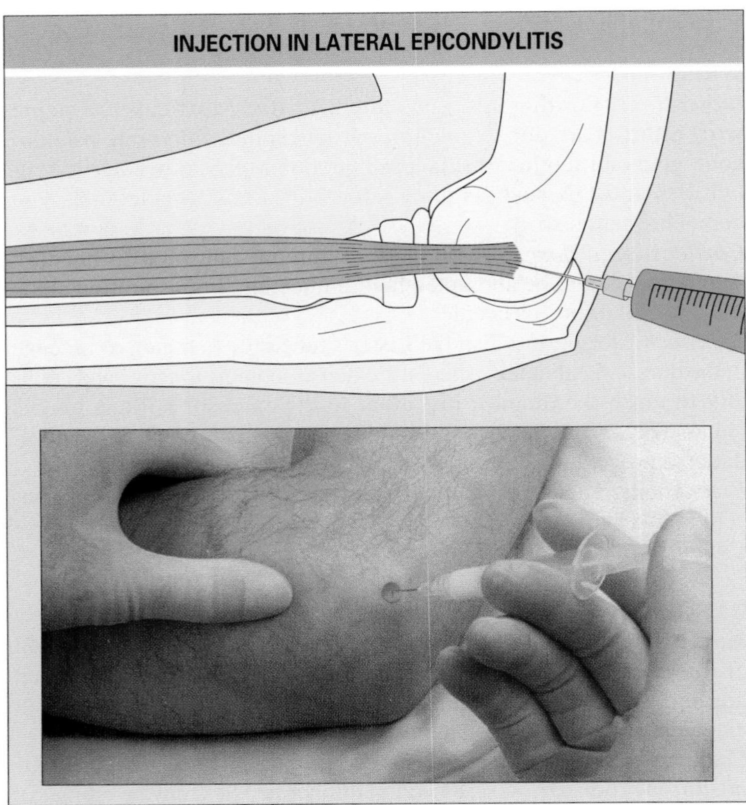

Fig. 12.11 Injection of corticosteroid and local anesthetic into the common extensor tendon origin at the lateral humeral epicondyle.

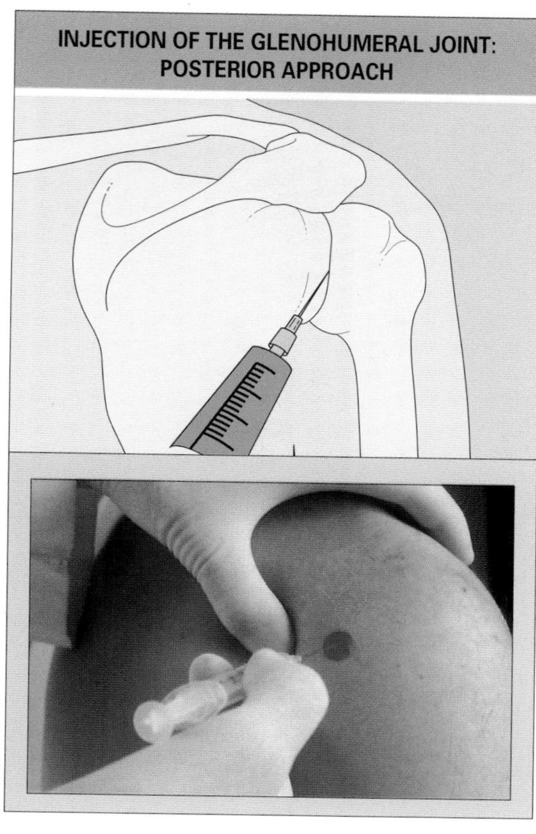

Fig. 12.12 Injection of the glenohumeral joint: posterior approach.

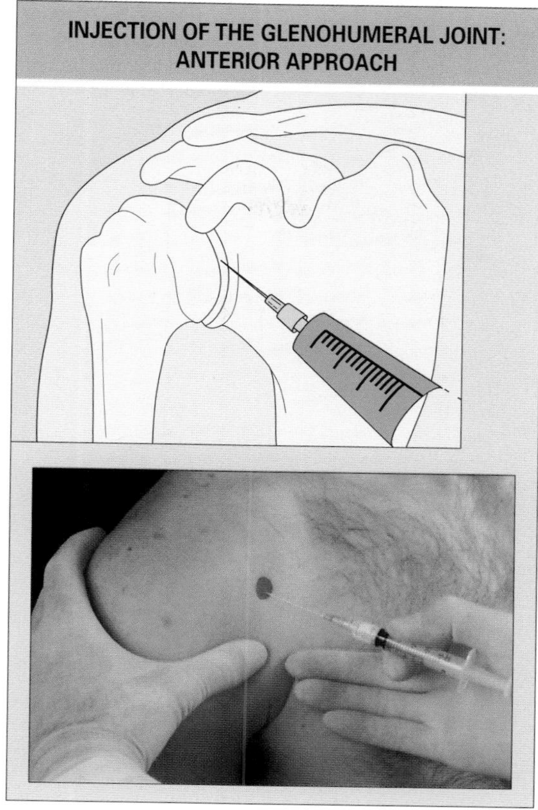

Fig. 12.13 Injection of the glenohumeral joint: anterior approach.

THE SHOULDER REGION

SHOULDER (GLENOHUMERAL JOINT)

Indications. Aspiration in acute arthritis; injection in RA, spondyloarthropathy, the initial stages of frozen shoulder; OA.

Corticosteroid dose. 40–60mg methlyprednisone (no. 22 needle). Aspiration should be attempted before injection. In the frozen shoulder, injection into the joint may be difficult on account of the capsular restriction. For aspiration alone use a no. 20 or larger needle.

Approach. Two entries are described, the posterior approach, which is often preferred because it causes less apprehension and pain, and the needle is farther away from neurovascular structures, and the anterior approach.

- Posterior approach. The patient should be sitting. The posterior margin of the acromion is palpated. The needle is then inserted posteroanteriorly 1cm below and 1cm medial to posterior corner of the acromion, aiming towards the coracoid process until bone is touched at the articular space (Fig.12.12).
- Anterior approach: Again, the patient should be sitting (landmarks are lost in the recumbent position) with the arm hanging at the side of the body, elbow flexed 90°, and forearm in the sagittal plane. The needle is entered anteroposteriorly 1cm distal and 1cm lateral to the coracoid process (Fig. 12.13). Prior to each advancement of the needle some lidocaine is injected, so the needle is moving through an anesthetized front. Once the bone is touched (which happens soon after the capsular toughness is felt) the forearm is very gently and passively brought into internal rotation as the needle is pushed into the articular space.

Precautions. Use a chair with armrests, have an assistant present, watch for fainting.

Complications. Vasovagal syndrome. Prior to the procedure patients should be asked about previous fainting upon venipuncture or other minor procedures. Any such experience dictates a posterior approach. Misplaced anterior injections may encounter neurovascular structures.

Note: Glenohumeral joint aspiration may be difficult. In cases of acute arthritis in which a 'dry tap' results, the procedure should be repeated under fluoroscopic or echo control.

SUBACROMIAL BURSA

Indications. Injection may be indicated in subacromial impingement and some cases of calcific tendinitis.

Corticosteroid dose. 30–40mg methylprednisone (no. 22 or no. 25 needle).

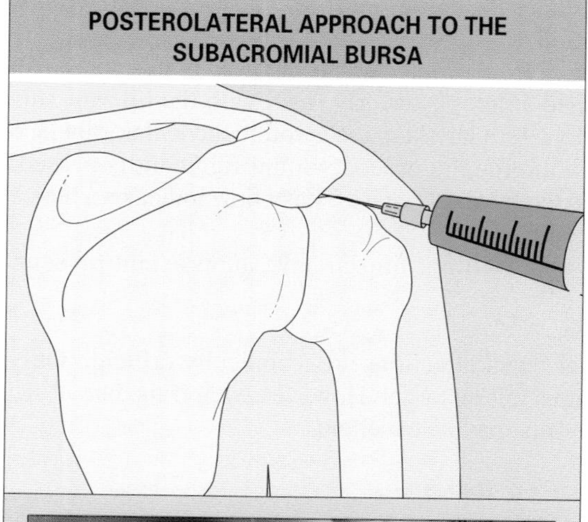

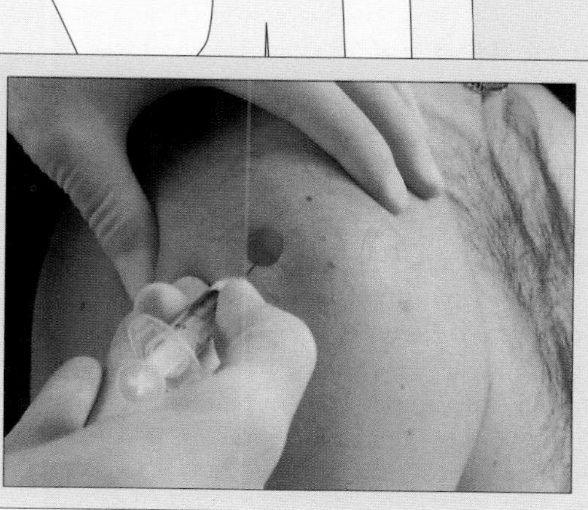

Fig. 12.14 Posterolateral approach to the subacromial bursa.

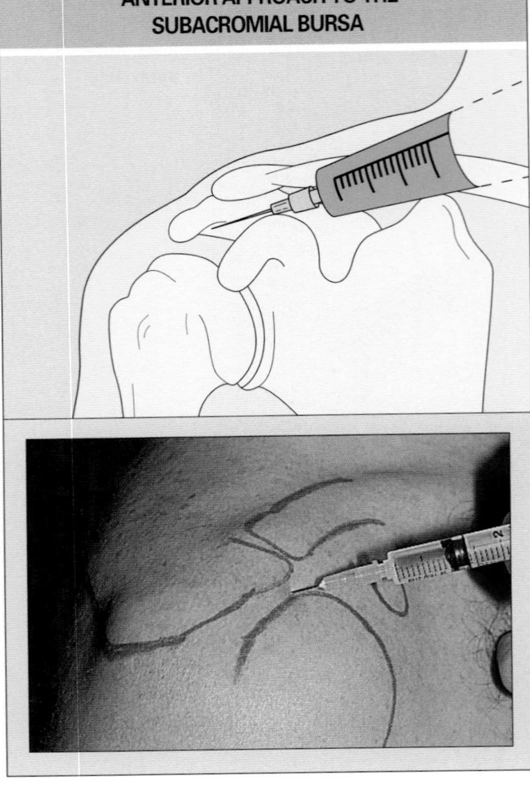

Fig. 12.15 Anterior approach to the subacromial bursa.

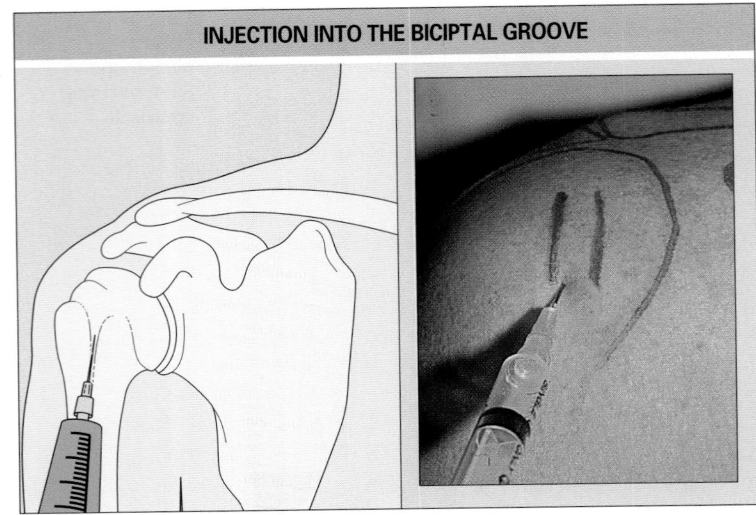

Fig. 12.16 Injection into the bicipital groove.

Approach. There are several possible entries. Two are described here, the posterolateral approach and the anterior approach. Adequate muscle relaxation is important, as it allows a better palpation of the gap between the acromion and humeral head.

- Posterolateral approach. The needle is aimed anteromedially ensuring that it passes under the acromion (Fig. 12.14). Easy flow indicates bursal injection.
- Anterior approach. A front of lidocaine is required in this approach. The needle is aimed anteroposteriorly flush with the inferior surface of the acromion, 1cm lateral to the acromioclavicular joint (see Fig. 12.15). Once the tough coracoacromial ligament is passed, tissue resistance to the lidocaine ceases. Easy flow indicates a bursal location of the needle.

Precautions. Use a chair with armrests, have an assistant present, watch for fainting.
Complications. None.

Note: Subacromial bursa injections are technically difficult. Only about 50% of injections fall on target. However, even if the bursal sac is not entered, the results may be excellent.

ACROMIOCLAVICULAR JOINT
Indications. Aspiration in acute arthritis, injection in OA, RA and spondyloarthropathy.
Corticosteroid dose. 10–20mg methylprednisone (no. 23 butterfly or no. 22 needle). Aspiration should be attempted before injection. For aspiration alone use a no. 20 needle.
Approach. Aim the needle perpendicular to the articular cleft; advance it by 0.5cm; aspirate or inject to distend joint.
Precautions. The procedure is difficult because the acromioclavicular (AC) joint is very narrow and has a partial meniscus. Septic AC arthritis should be suspected in drug addicts and in patients who have, or have recently had, an indwelling subclavian catheter. If sepsis is suspected, corticosteroids should not be injected.
Complications. None.

BICIPITAL TENDINITIS
Indications. Bicipital tenosynovitis. This is a tenuous indication, as most cases of bicipital tendinitis are caused by subacromial impingement, which is best treated by subacromial bursa injection.
Corticosteroid dose. 15–20mg methylprednisone (no. 22 or no. 25 needle).
Approach. The bicipital tendon should be palpated and a mark made on the skin. The needle is then directed somewhat superiorly, tangentially to the tendon (Fig. 12.16). A deeper injection is also possible if easy flow of fluid is obtained.
Precautions. Inject under low pressure.
Complications. The integrity of the biceps tendon may be already compromised by the usual underlying condition, subacromial impingement. Thus, the relatively common postinjection ruptures may reflect this underlying damage as much as a direct effect of the corticosteroid on the tendon. This is the reason why the author does not favor direct injection of the bicipital tendon sheath.

THE SPINE

INTERSPINOUS LIGAMENTS
Indications. Reactive arthritis, ankylosing spondylitis with interspinous ligament enthesopathy.
Corticosteroid dose. 15–20mg methylprednisone (no. 22 needle).
Approach. Posteroanterior at the midline between the vertebral spinous processes; infiltrate ligament and its attachments. Several levels may have to be treated.
Precautions. This is an intraligamentous infiltration and a fair amount of pressure is required. There is no need to infiltrate deeper than 1.5cm; this precaution should keep the needle away from the dural sac.
Complications. None.

THE HIP REGION

HIP
Indications. Diagnosis of septic arthritis of the hip, including the differential diagnosis of septic arthritis versus aseptic loosening in a prosthetic hip.
Corticosteroid dose. None: the procedure is performed strictly for diagnosis.
Approach. Hip aspiration is performed with the patient lying supine and the affected leg in external rotation. The femoral neck projection

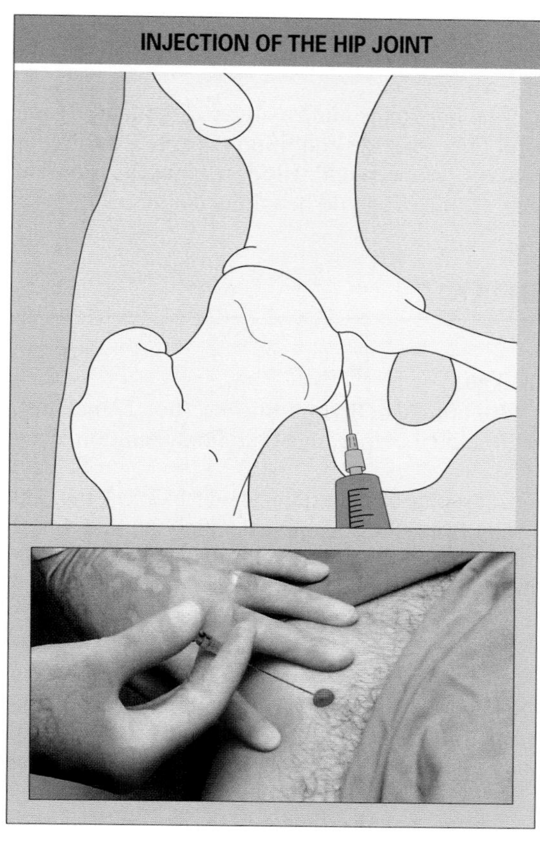

Fig. 12.17 Injection of the hip joint.

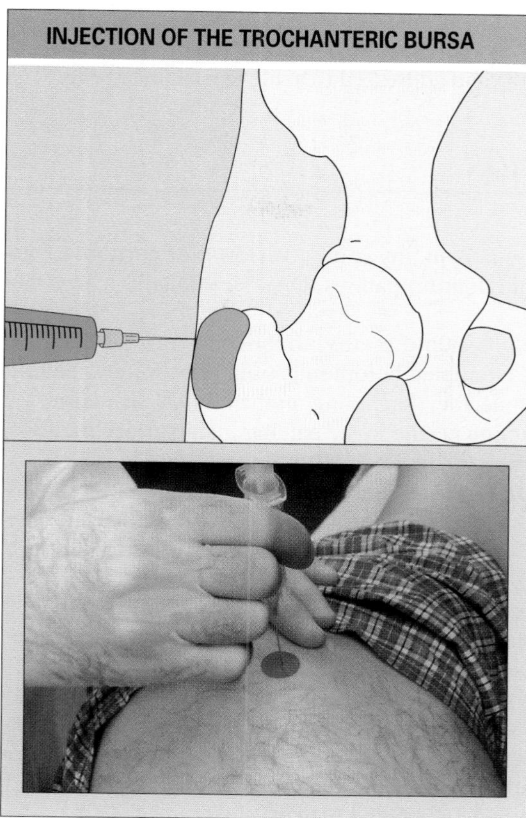

Fig. 12.18 Injection of the trochanteric bursa.

follows a line bisecting the angle between the inguinal ligament and the femoral artery. The needle is inserted cephalad medially, one finger breadth lateral to the femoral artery and two finger breadths distal to the inguinal ligament (Fig. 12.17).
Precautions. The danger of injuring the femoral neurovascular bundle is averted by using an imaging procedure as control.
Complications. None.

Note: Hip aspiration belongs in the realm of orthopedics and radiology. The yield of the procedure can be maximized by using fluoroscopic, ultrasound or computed tomography (CT) guidance.

ILIOPSOAS BURSA
Indications. Painful iliopsoas bursitis.
Corticosteroid dose. 30–40mg methylprednisone mixed with 3ml of 1% lidocaine (no. 22 needle). Aspiration should be attempted before injection.
Approach. As for hip aspiration. Once the femoral head is contacted, the needle is withdrawn by the millimeter and small amounts of a contrast medium are injected until the iliopsoas bursa is outlined. At this time the corticosteroid is injected.
Precautions. The use of a contrast medium is essential for injecting intrabursally, rather than within the joint or in more supeficial planes.
Complications. None.

TROCHANTERIC 'BURSA'
Indications. Trochanteric 'bursitis' syndrome.
Corticosteroid dose. 30–40mg mixed with 3ml of 1% lidocaine (no. 22 1.5 inch needle; a spinal needle may be required in obese patients).
Approach. With the patient lying on his or her opposite side, the greater trochanter is identified by distal to proximal palpation along the femur. The point of maximal tenderness is usually located at the posterior corner of the greater trochanter. The needle is inserted vertically to make periosteal contact (Fig. 12.18).

- Step 1. Lidocaine should then be infiltrated radially to cover the base of a cone 3cm in diameter, half on bone and half in the proximal soft tissues.
- Step 2. If pain is relieved, the mixture of corticosteroid and lidocaine is infiltrated in the same area. Experienced physicians may skip Step 1.

Precautions. The needle should be of sufficient length to reach the bone.
Complications. None.

Note: Rather than bursitis, this process represents a stress enthe-

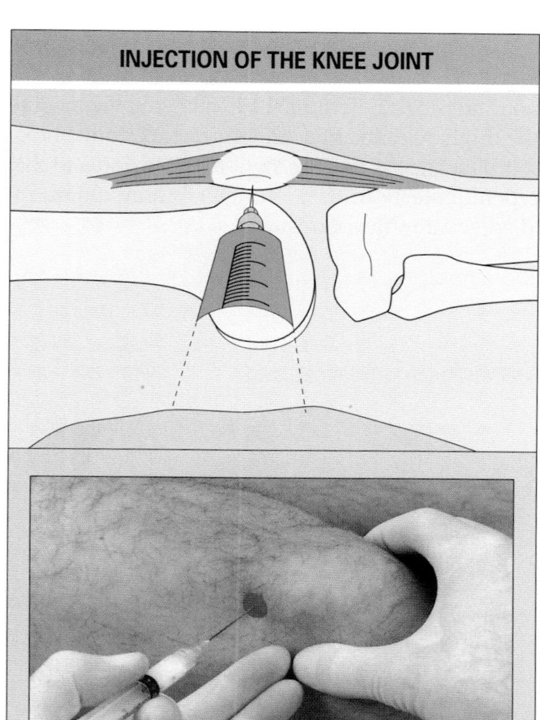

Fig. 12.19 Injection of the knee joint.

sopathy at the gluteus medium and minimus insertion. The cause of the excessive pull should be sought (foot, knee, hip or back disorder, a discrepant leg length) and addressed to achieve sustained relief.

THE KNEE REGION

KNEE

Indications. For diagnosis in any joint effusion. For corticosteroid injection in RA, spondyloarthropathies, OA, occasionally in crystal-induced synovitis.
Corticosteroid dose. 40–60mg methylprednisone (no. 22 needle). Aspiration should be attempted before injection. For aspiration alone use a no. 20 or no. 18 needle, depending on the clinical suspicion.
Approach. Medial, aiming needle to the patellar undersurface mid-distance between the upper and lower poles of the patella (Fig. 12.19). A medial approach is preferred because the lateral patellofemoral cleft is narrower than the medial and the joint capsule is tougher laterally than medially. There are, however, many possible entries to the knee and the choice is very personal.
Precautions. Beware of superimposed septic arthritis in RA patients. Postpone the injection of an acutely inflamed joint until a negative synovial fluid culture result becomes available.

Note: If SF analysis has not been performed any fluid removed during the procedure should be studied for cell count, differential, crystals, and culture. Because corticosteroid crystals remain in joints for weeks and even months an erroneous diagnosis of gout or pseudogout can be made in a previously injected patient.
Complications. None.

BAKER'S CYST

Aspiration or injection of the cyst is unnecessary. In adults, Baker's cysts develop in connecting gastrocnemius–semimembranosus bursae and depend for their persistence and growth on excessive SF produced in the knee. Baker's cysts are best treated by correcting the causative knee disorder with systemic treatment, corticosteroid injection or surgery such as arthroscopic meniscectomy or synovectomy.

ANSERINE 'BURSITIS'

Indications. The syndrome of anserine bursitis.
Corticosteroid dose. 20–30mg methylprednisone mixed with 2–3ml of lidocaine (no. 22 needle).
Approach. The injection site is best determined by following the medial tendinous border of the thigh, with the knee in semiflexion, to the tibia where a mark is placed. The knee is then brought to extension and the needle is entered perpendicularly to tibial contact. An area 3cm in diameter is infiltrated adjacent to the periosteum.
Precautions. Paresthesias extending along the medial leg indicate engagement of the saphenous nerve; reposition needle.
Complications. None.

Note: Because anserine bursitis is almost always secondary (genu valgum, patellofemoral OA, etc.) the condition is expected to recur unless the primary process has been addressed. A vigorous program of isometric quadriceps exercises should be initiated at once.

THE ANKLE AND FOOT

ANKLE

Indications. As for the knee.
Corticosteroid dose. 40–60mg methylprednisone (no. 22 needle). Aspiration should be attempted before injection. For aspiration alone use a no. 20 needle.
Approach. With the patient supine on the examination table, seek the cleft between tibia and talus by gently flexing and extending the foot. Insert the needle vertically medial to the anterior tibialis tendon (Fig. 12.20).
Precautions. Avoid the dorsalis pedis artery.
Complications. None.

SUBTALAR JOINT

Indications. As for the knee.
Corticosteroid dose: 20–30mg methylprednisone (no. 22 needle). Aspiration should be attempted before injection. For aspiration alone use a no. 20 needle.
Approach. By gently inverting and everting the foot find the soft cleft (sinus tarsi) anterior to the lateral malleolus. Insert the needle perpendicularly towards the tip of the medial malleolus (Fig. 12.21). Aspiration of fluid proves an articular insertion. Inject under low pressure.
Precautions. None.
Complications. None.

POSTERIOR TIBIALIS TENDON SHEATH

Indications. Posterior tibialis tenosynovitis in RA and spondyloarthropathies; tarsal tunnel syndrome.
Corticosteroid dose. 20–30mg methlyprednisone (no. 22 needle).
Approach. Patient lies supine with the injected leg resting on the contralateral knee. The needle is inserted perpendicularly, three finger breadths proximal to the tip of the medial malleolus and flush with the posterior surface of tibia to a depth of about 1.5cm. Inject under low pressure. Fluid may be felt distending the sheath.
Precautions. Aspirate first to make sure that the posterior tibial artery has not been punctured. Plantar paresthesias indicate engagement of the posterior tibial nerve. Avoid intratendinous injection by assuring free flow of the corticosteroid. *This procedure should only be*

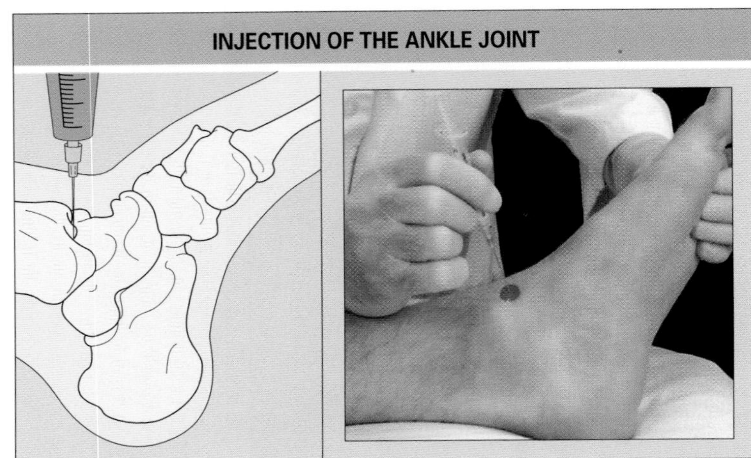

Fig. 12.20 Injection of the ankle joint.

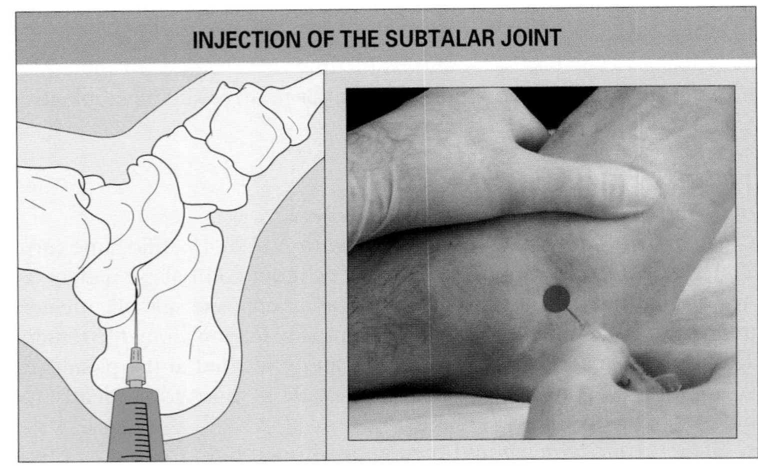

Fig. 12.21 Injection of the subtalar joint.

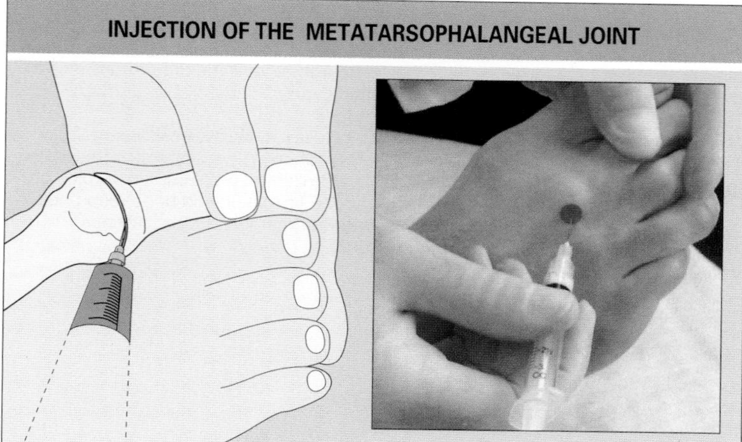

Fig. 12.22 Injection of the MTP joint.

performed by rheumatologists, orthopedists or other health professionals with a thorough knowledge of anatomy.
Complications. The posterior tibialis tendon is prone to spontaneous rupture in RA. A misplaced (intratendinous) injection enhances this tendency.

RETROCALCANEAL BURSA

Indications. Refractory Achilles' tendon enthesitis in the spondyloarthropathies; RA.
Corticosteroid dose. 15–20mg methylprednisone (no. 22 needle or butterfly). Aspiration should be attempted before injection. Presence of fluid (usually a trace) proves intrabursal location. *Do not inject if the intrabursal position of the needle cannot be shown.*
Approach. Patient lies prone on examination table with foot outside mattress. Allow calf relaxation.

- Posterior approach. The needle is advanced vertically, transtendinous, aiming at the posterior superior calcaneal angle. Touch the bone and back up 1mm.
- Lateral approach. An alternative is a lateral approach. Bursal pressures may be decreased by keeping the foot in a slight plantar flexion.

Precautions. Do not inject large volumes; high pressures produce back flow as the needle is removed. The distal leg and foot should be placed in a cast for 10 days to achieve maximal anti-inflammatory effect. *This procedure should only be performed by rheumatologists, orthopedists, or other health professionals with a thorough knowledge of anatomy.*
*Complications.*Tendon rupture is possible and more than one reinjection is discouraged. A period of 2–3 weeks should elapse between the initial injection and the first (and last) reinjection.

PLANTAR FASCIA ATTACHMENT

Indications. Refractory plantar fasciitis in the spondyloarthropathies.
Corticosteroid dose. 20–30mg methylprednisone diluted with 2ml of lidocaine (no. 22 needle).
Approach. Medial, needle parallel to the plantar skin 2cm deep to plantar surface. Aim the needle into the medial plantar tubercle of the calcaneus. Resilience indicates fascial location. Relocate the needle and inject deeply and superficially to the fibrous fascia.
Precautions. This procedure should only be performed by rheumatologists, orthopedists or other health professionals with a thorough knowledge of anatomy.
Complications. Repeated infiltrations result in fat atrophy and pressure plantar heel pain. Discourage more than one reinjection (2–3 weeks after the initial injection).

MORTON'S NEUROMA

Indications. Morton's neuroma.
Corticosteroid dose. 20–30mg mixed with 1ml lidocaine (no. 22 needle).
Approach. Dorsal between metatarsal heads. The needle must be advanced plantarly about 2cm and pass through the intermetatarsal ligament, which is indicated by tough fibrous resistance.
Precautions. Inject under low pressure. *This procedure should only be performed by rheumatologists, orthopedists or other health professionals with a thorough knowledge of anatomy.*
Complications. None are expected; up to two reinjections 2–3 weeks apart are allowed.

METATARSOPHALANGEAL JOINTS

Indications. Aspiration for the diagnosis of gout (usually the first metatarsophalangeal). Injection in hallux rigidus, RA and the spondyloarthropathies.
Corticosteroid dose. 10–20mg (no. 22 needle). Attempt aspiration before injection. For aspiration alone use a no. 22 needle.
Approach. Dorsal, lateral or medial to extensor tendon. Slight passive plantar flexion facilitates the procedure (Fig. 12.22).
Precautions. None.
Complications. None.

TRIGGER POINTS IN THE MYOFASCIAL SYNDROMES

Indications. Acute cases if pressure on a point or nodule consistently reproduces pain.
Corticosteroid dose. 3–5ml of lidocaine or bupivacaine (no. 22 needle). Do not use corticosteroids.
Approach. Aim at a tender point or the center of a nodule, which should be infiltrated radially throughout the indurated area.
Precautions. None.
Complications. None.

REFERENCES

1. Cohen AS, Goldenberg D. Synovial fluid. In Cohen AS. (ed.) Laboratory diagnostic procedures in the rheumatic diseases 3E. Orlando: Grune & Stratton; 1985:1–54.
2. Schumacher HR Jr, Reginato AJ. Atlas of synovial fluid analysis and crystal identification. Philadelphia: Lea & Febiger; 1991:1–257.
3. Canoso JJ, Yood RA. Reaction of superficial bursae in response to specific disease stimuli. Arthritis Rheum. 1979;22:1361–4.
4. Schwarzer AC, Aprill CN, Bogduk N. The sacroiliac joint in chronic low back pain. Spine. 1995;20:31–7.
5. Braun J, Bollow M, Seyrekbasan F, *et al.* Computed tomography guided corticosteroid injection of the sacroiliac joint in patients with spondyloarthropathy with sacroiliitis: Clinical outcome and followup by dynamic magnetic resonance imaging. J Rheumatol. 1996;23:659–64.
6. Carette S, Marcoux S, Truchon R, *et al.* Facet joint injection of corticosteroids in chronic low back pain: A randomized double-blind placebo controlled trial. N Engl J Med. 1991;325:1002–7.
7. Bogduk N. Spine update: Epidural steroids. Spine. 1995;20:845–8.
8. Hollander JL. Intrasynovial steroid injections. In: Hollander JL, McCarty DL Jr, eds. Arthritis and allied conditions. Philadelphia: Lea & Febiger; 1972;517–34.
9. Neustadt DH. Local corticosteroid injection therapy in soft tisssue rheumatic conditions of the hand and wrist. Arthritis Rheum. 1991;34:923–6.
10. Murphy D, Failla JM, Koniuch MP. Steroid versus placebo injection for trigger finger. J Hand Surg. 1995;20A:628–31.
11. Lambert MA, Morton RJ, Sloan JP. Controlled study of the use of local steroid injection in the treatment of trigger finger and thumb. J Hand Surg. 1992;17B:69–70.
12. Kay NRM. A safe, reliable method of carpal tunnel injection. J Hand Surg. 1992;17A:1160–1.
13. Weiss A-PC, Sachar K, Gendreau M. Conservative management of carpal tunnel syndrome: A

reexamination of steroid injection and splinting. J Hand Surg. 1994;19A:410–15.
14. Weinstein PS, Canoso JJ, Wohlgethan JR. Long-term follow-up of corticosteroid injection for traumatic olecranon bursitis. Ann Rheum Dis. 1984;43:44–6.
15. Smith DL, McAfee JH, Lucas LM, Kumar KL, Romney DM. Treatment of nonspecific olecranon bursitis. A controlled, blinded prospective trial. Arch Intern Med. 1989;149:2527–30.
16. Larsson L-G, Baum J. The syndrome of anserina bursitis: An overlooked diagnosis. Arthritis Rheum. 1985;28:1062–5.
17. Anderson BC, Manthey R, Brouns MC. Treatment of de Quervain's tenosynovitis with corticosteroids. Arthritis Rheum. 1991;34:793–8.
18. Weiss A-PC, Akelman E, Tabatabai M. Treatment of de Quervain's disease. J Hand Surg. 1994;19A:595–8.
19. Price R, Sinclair H, Heinrich I, Gibson T. Local injection of tennis elbow. Hydrocortisone, triamcinolone and lignocaine compared. Br J Rheumatol. 1991;30:39–44.
20. Vecchio PC, Adebajo AO, Hazleman BL. Suprascapular nerve block for persistent rotator cuff lesions. J Rheumatol. 1993;20:453–5.
21. Fortin L, Bélanger R. Bursitis of the iliopsoas: Four cases with pain as the only clinical indicator. J Rheumatol. 1995;22:1971–3.
22. Canoso JJ, Wohlgethan JR, Newberg AH, Goldsmith MR. Aspiration of the retrocalcaneal bursa. Ann Rheum Dis. 1984;43:308–12.
23. Greenfield J, Rea J Jr, Ilfeld FW. Morton's interdigital neuroma. Indications for treatment by local injections versus surgery. Clin Orthop. 1984;185:142–4.
24. Emkey RD, Lindsay R, Lyssy J, Weisberg JS, Dempster DW, Shen V. The systemic effect of intraarticular administration of corticosteroids on markers of bone formation and bone resorption in patients with rheumatoid arthritis. Arthritis Rheum. 1996;39:277–82.

13

MINIMALLY INVASIVE PROCEDURES

Robert W Ike

- Invasive procedures applicable to diagnosis or management in rheumatology include:
  - biopsies (skin, muscle, salivary gland, synovium),
  - arthroscopy,
  - joint lavage,
  - regional perineural injections.
- The use and sequence of each procedure depends, in practice, on the focus of the individual rheumatologist, but can include independent work by a procedure-oriented rheumatologist who has acquired the appropriate training and equipment.

INTRODUCTION

This chapter reviews applications and technique for several minimally invasive procedures for the diagnosis or management of a patient with a rheumatic disorder. These procedures are often handled via referral to a specialist. However, some rheumatologists have found it useful to learn and practice at least some of these procedures themselves.

BIOPSIES

The histology of structures that can be sampled with minimally invasive techniques can sometimes be sufficiently characteristic to suggest a specific diagnosis when coupled with the appropriate clinical information. Tissue findings can influence the management of patients with an established diagnosis when these demonstrate the accelerated end-organ involvement by a process related to the underlying disease, the effects of supervening conditions or an unexpected process. Interaction between pathologist and clinician guides the clinician to select and handle the sample correctly and helps the pathologist choose appropriate methods of analysis to answer the clinical questions being asked[1].

SKIN AND SUBCUTANEOUS TISSUE

Many abnormalities of the integument can provide clues to rheumatic disease diagnosis (see Chapter 2.5). Tissue confirmation is sometimes helpful. Biopsy of a suspicious lesion can confirm the diagnosis of lupus in a patient with other suggestive clinical manifestations[1]. Immunofluorescence shows immunoglobulin and complement deposition at the dermal–epidermal junction of lesional skin in 90% of cases, and of normal sun-protected skin in about 50% of cases. This latter feature is specific for systemic lupus, and justifies biopsy of normal skin for the 'lupus band test'[2]. Scleroderma involves skin and subcutaneous structures in a characteristic manner, although similar findings can occur as a localized process (e.g. morphea) or deeper pathology, as in the fasciitis syndromes. Vasculitis seen on skin biopsy often prompts a search for systemic involvement, but seldom stands alone as a diagnostic finding[3]. IgA deposition indicates Henoch–Schönlein purpura or one of its variants. Not all palpable purpura are due to vasculitis; biopsy can show other responsible processes, including microthrombi, cholesterol emboli and hemorrhage.

Tender soft nodular lesions in the patient with systemic rheumatic features can be due to inflammation of fat lobules, or panniculitis. Biopsy can refine the diagnosis according to the distribution of inflammation through the fat lobule, or by showing granulomata or vasculitis[4]. Subcutaneous nodules that accompany polyarthritis usually show features of the characteristic rheumatoid granuloma, which can also occur in rheumatoid-like polyarthritis accompanying scleroderma or lupus, rheumatic fever or juvenile chronic polyarthritis. However, nodules composed of other material – monosodium urate, calcium pyrophosphate dihydrate, cholesterol, amyloid – can be defined by biopsy, which sometimes provides an alternative diagnosis for a perplexing arthritis[5].

A relatively recent skin lesion should be sampled and the specimen should contain the lesion's edge along with some normal skin. Biopsy can be obtained with a disposable dermal punch or by excision with scalpel and forceps. The latter technique obtains larger and deeper samples, and is required when features such as fasciitis or vasculitis of small muscular arteries are being sought. While excision of a subcutaneous nodule allows study of its architecture, percutaneous needle sampling is simple and usually adequate to demonstrate the material of which the nodule is composed.

MUSCLE

Information from muscle biopsy can influence the diagnosis and therapy in several rheumatic disorders. For suspected inflammatory myopathy, muscle biopsy may be required when the diagnosis cannot be established with certainty from the clinical evidence available. If inflammatory myopathy diagnosis is reasonably certain, tissue confirmation of myositis might be desired when toxic, expensive or experimental therapies are being considered. For the patient with inflammatory myopathy who becomes weaker on treatment, muscle biopsy can differentiate persistent disease from the effects of corticosteroids or disuse, and sometimes disproves the original diagnosis[6]. Myopathies can accompany other rheumatic diseases. In the scleroderma patient with myopathy, tissue confirmation should be sought before initiating treatment as inflammatory corticosteroid-responsive myopathy is but one of several possibilities[7]. Predominant or progressive weakness and myalgia that arise in patients with other common rheumatic diseases may prompt a search for myopathy; muscle biopsy can disclose the occasional myositis or vasculitis case and often identifies treatment-related myopathy[8].

Occult or subclinical muscle involvement disclosed on biopsy can help confirm the diagnosis of certain multisystem disorders. Polyarteritis and other systemic necrotizing vasculitides are confirmed by finding necrotizing vasculitis that involves medium-sized arteries. The yield of 'blind' muscle biopsy is about 40% and rises to 80% in patients with muscle pain[9]. Sarcoidosis is diagnosed when noncaseating granulomata are found in at least two organ systems. Muscle biopsy yields diagnostic granulomata in 50%, rising to 90% if the erythema nodosum lesions overlie the muscle to be biopsied[10].

In patients with primary noninflammatory disorders of muscle, the wider availability of molecular diagnostic techniques is increasing the yield and specificity of muscle biopsy. For the metabolic and genetic disorders that can be thus identified, specific remedies are rare[6,11].

The muscle for biopsy should be clinically abnormal, but not grossly wasted or fibrotic. An electromyographic needle can cause focal traumatic myositis; hence muscle should come from the side opposite any recent electromyographic evaluation. Magnetic resonance imaging (MRI) may be helpful in identifying affected muscle groups and thus increase the likelihood of finding pathology on the muscle biopsy. If the biopsy is required to seek vasculitis, a distal muscle group should be selected. Biopsy is performed after infiltrating local anesthetic into the skin and subcutaneous tissue in the region of interest, avoiding muscle. Pain fibers occupy the perimysial areas and fascia, but are not found in muscle itself. Hence, pain from the procedure can be minimized, if not completely eliminated. Conscious sedation using short-acting benzodiazepines and narcotics further reduces patient discomfort. An open or percutaneous technique can be used.

Open biopsy is more commonly performed; it permits direct inspection of the muscle while obtaining an easily processed specimen that is more likely to contain larger blood vessels than percutaneous samples[11,12]. A longitudinal incision of at least 5cm, with dissection carried out through subcutaneous tissue and fat to reach the muscle, should permit excision of a sample measuring approximately 2 × 1 × 1cm. The two ends of the sample should be lightly affixed to an object that holds the muscle at resting length, using formal muscle clamps or by stitching or pinning each end to a stiff object, such as cork, swab stick, tongue blade or stiff card. The sample should be kept moist for 1–2h before being placed in fixative to avoid contraction artifact. Snap freezing a portion of the sample is required for histochemical studies, and permits storage of unprocessed muscle for later specialized tests.

Percutaneous sampling of muscle using specially designed instruments yields adequate material for light and electron microscopy, histochemistry and chemical analysis[11]. Skin overlying an area anesthetized as for open biopsy is incised with a scalpel to enable penetration of deeper tissues by the biopsy instrument; the cutting window is opened to admit tissue, which is cut free and contained by the encircling blade. The suction-assisted University College Hospital instrument can collect several samples with each penetration, held in the barrel of the cutting blade after each bite (Fig. 13.1). The technique can be performed at the bedside or in an outpatient room and is relatively atraumatic as it avoids the occasional infection or wound-healing problems that can complicate open biopsy. The small size of the samples obtained mandate special care in processing; concern that focal lesions might be missed in these small pieces may be unwarranted, as a wide area of muscle can be sampled by the percutaneous biopsy instrument oriented in several different directions through the same skin puncture, thus encompassing a much larger region than that obtained by an open biopsy[13]. Collected samples are kept moist, oriented under a dissecting microscope and then snap frozen. Routine histopathology and histochemistry are carried out on the frozen section, with processing for additional studies as indicated by the clinical situation and frozen section findings.

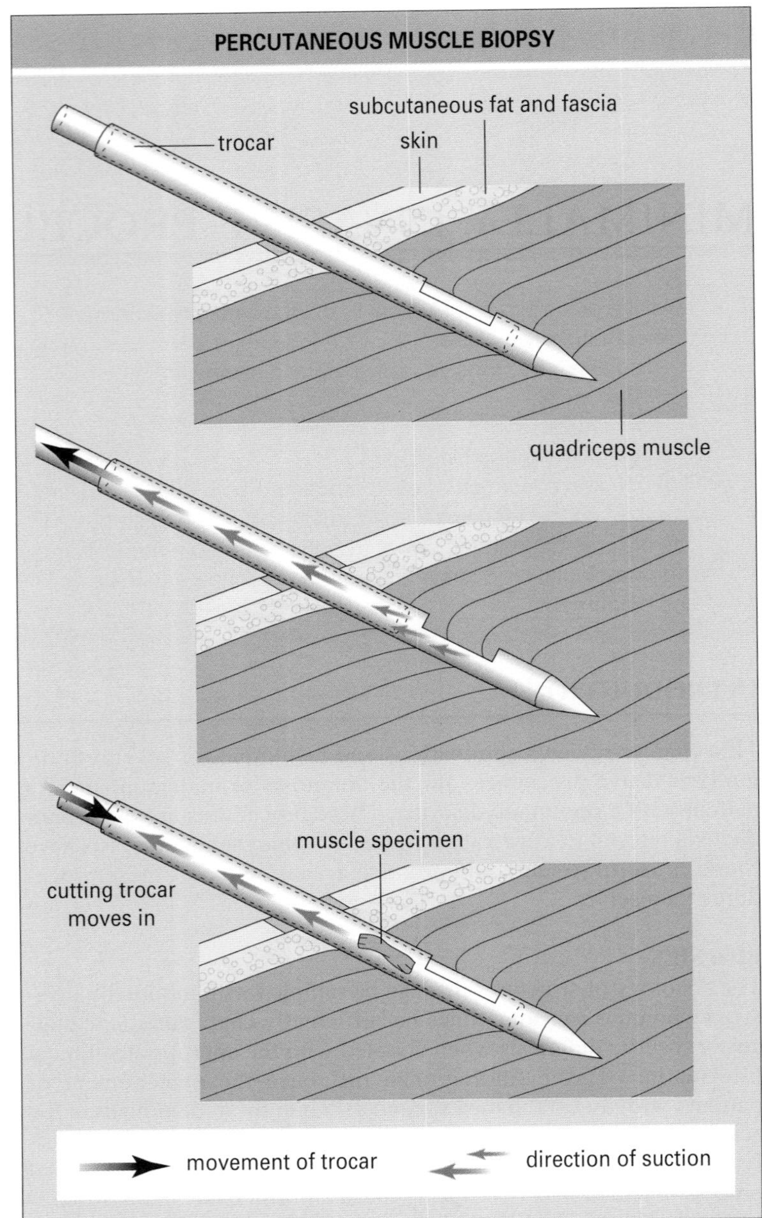

Fig. 13.1 Percutaneous muscle biopsy using suction-assisted instrument.

SALIVARY GLAND

Salivary gland histology provides one technique by which Sjögren's syndrome is diagnosed. Characteristic findings of focal lymphocytic infiltrates in the parotid and submandibular glands are also found in the minor salivary glands, which can be retrieved from their submucosal location inferior to the lower lip[14]. Subclinical involvement of these glands is common in amyloidosis[15], sarcoidosis[16] and hemochromatosis[14], and so biopsy can substitute for more extensive organ sampling in a diagnostic search for these multisystem processes.

Labial salivary gland biopsy is a simple outpatient procedure. Lidocaine (lignocaine) with epinephrine (adrenaline) is injected into the area that contains the densest collection of glands, determined by palpation. The overlying mucosa is incised with a horizontally oriented scalpel after vasoconstriction has been confirmed by pallor, care being taken to avoid damaging the small nerves and blood vessels that lie at the same depth as the salivary glands. Glands are isolated by blunt dissection with the closed forceps, then removed with the same forceps until at least six pieces have been retrieved (Fig. 13.2). The tissue defect is closed with an absorbable suture. Local discomfort is not uncommon, but usually subsides in a day or two.

The clinician should clearly state the features to be sought by the pathologist. All sets of clinical criteria for the diagnosis of Sjögren's syndrome require that minor salivary glands meet a certain focus score, defined by number of clusters of 50 or more lymphocytes seen in 4mm^2 of gland tissue.

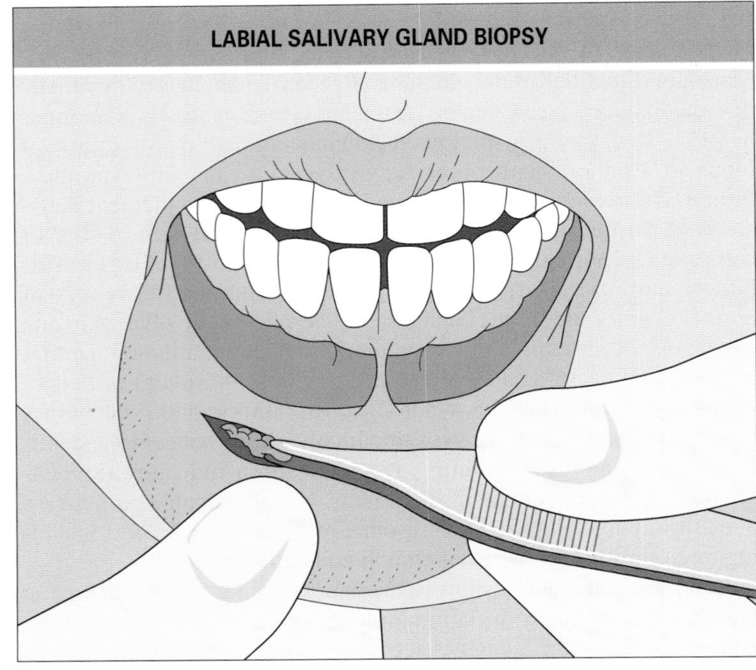

Fig. 13.2 Labial salivary gland biopsy.

SYNOVIUM

Of the many disease processes that can involve joints, only a few exhibit characteristic synovial pathology (Fig. 13.3). Some of these entities are quite rare, while some can usually be diagnosed by inference from other clinical data. For patients with arthritis that remains unclassifiable, biopsy is clinically indicated when the differential diagnosis includes processes that can be confirmed by synovial features. Reaching a tissue diagnosis is particularly relevant when the disorder revealed might disseminate or cause joint destruction if untreated, as with infectious or invasive processes.

Several clinical situations present diagnostic problems that sometimes require synovial tissue to resolve[18]. Otherwise unexplained chronic or subacute cases of monoarthritis or oligoarthritis should be biopsied when indolent infection is considered a possibility, however remote. Other unexpected diagnoses may include tumors, foreign bodies and crystal deposits. Joint infection nearly always involves synovium before the agent enters synovial fluid, so cultures of synovial tissue can yield the agent when fluid does not[19]. Hence, cases of acute monoarthritis or oligoarthritis with systemic features that suggest infection should be considered for synovial biopsy when other cultures are negative. Unexplained inflammatory arthropathy involving multiple joints should be considered for biopsy when there is some reason to suspect less common diseases with distinctive features, such as sarcoidosis, leukemia, Crohn's disease or Whipple's disease. However, most cases

CHARACTERISTIC FEATURES OF SYNOVIUM IN SELECTED RHEUMATIC DISEASES		
Diagnosis	**Macroscopic features**	**Microscopic features**
Crystalline diseases		
Calcium pyrophosphate disease	Calcific deposits	Calcium pyrophosphate crystals
Gout	Refractile urate deposits	Monosodium urate crystals
Hydroxyapatite arthropathy	Calcific deposits	Hydroxyapatite crystals (electron microscopy); globular calcium-containing deposits (Von Kossa, Alizarin S stains)
Infectious arthritis		
Bacterial and fungal	Adhesions, necrotic synovium, cartilage discoloration	Organisms; intense polymorphonuclear infiltrate
Chronic borreliosis (Lyme disease)	Hypertrophic synovium	*Borrelia burgdorferi* spirochete (silver stain)
Filariasis	Guinea worm	
Tuberculosis		Caseating granulomata with acid-fast bacilli
Infiltrative diseases		
Amyloidosis		Amyloid deposition (Congo red stain)
Fabry's disease		Foam cells in vessel walls
Inflammatory arthropathies		
Behçet's disease	Synovial 'slough'	
Postvenereal reactive (Reiter's syndrome)		Chlamydial bodies, *Yersinia* antigens (with special immunofluorescent agents)
Systemic lupus erythematosus		Hematoxylin bodies
Malignancy		
Primary (e.g. synovioma) or metastatic, leukemia, lymphoma		Malignant cells
Metabolic arthropathies		
Hemochromatosis		Blue hue predominantly of synovial lining cells (due to iron deposition)
Ochronosis	Black pigment, shards	Fragments of pigmented cartilage
Synovial disorders		
Pigmented villonodular synovitis	(As name describes)	Villous hypertrophy with hemosiderin and giant cells
Synovial chondromatosis	Cartilage in synovium	Islands of metaplastic cartilage
Other		
Hemangioma		Excessive (often irregular or cavernous) blood vessels
Foreign body (e.g. plant thorn)		Birefringent plant material; granulomatous reaction
Multicentric reticulohistiocytosis		Histiocytes and multinucleated giant cells
Sarcoidosis		Noncaseating granulomata
Whipple's disease		Periodic acid Schiff-positive, diastase resistant macrophages

Fig. 13.3 Characteristic features of synovium in selected rheumatic diseases. (Modified from O'Rourke and Ike[17], with permission.)

of polyarthritis will not have diagnostic findings. Unexplained non-inflammatory arthropathy can occasionally be due to some important and readily diagnosed systemic disease, including hemochromatosis, amyloidosis, multicentric reticulohistiocytosis and ochronosis. Hemarthrosis not due to obvious trauma can be the presenting feature of pigmented villonodular synovitis, osteochondromatosis and metastatic tumors. For the patient with totally unexplained subtle joint findings, biopsy can help determine whether there is any pathologic process in the synovium and can help guide symptomatic treatment.

Synovial tissue can be obtained blindly from the joint using a needle instrument. Of the several tools applicable to this task, the Parker–Pearson instrument – comprising a cutting hook, stylet and 14 gauge needle through which both can be passed – is the most popular specialized tool[18]; the Tru-Cut biopsy needle, used for a variety of soft issue biopsies, is an inexpensive, disposable item which can retrieve synovial tissue through an action similar to that of the Parker–Pearson instrument[20]. Of the joints accessible to blind biopsy, the knee is the most commonly approached, followed by the wrist, ankle, elbow and olecranon bursa. Smaller joints and tendon sheaths can be biopsied if sufficiently swollen to discern synovium from adjacent structures. With radiographic guidance, the shoulder, hip and sacroiliac joint can be entered[20]. The procedure can be performed at the hospital bedside or in the clinic (Fig. 13.4). Aseptic technique is mandatory, with local anesthesia usually sufficient to assure patient comfort. Conscious sedation is reserved for the anxious patient or anticipated difficult joint. The joint should be aspirated, then reinstilled with saline or dilute local anesthetic. The tip of the biopsy instrument is directed to an area of palpable synovial thickening. With the cutting window open, the operator or an assistant presses the skin overlying the instrument to fill the cutting window with tissue; sliding the sharp-edged outer cylinder of the instrument over the cutting window frees the sample, which can then be removed from the joint. The process is repeated, directing the instrument to other areas if possible, until sufficient tissue for the planned studies is obtained. The operator should become familiar with the gross appearance of synovial tissue (pink) so that necrotic tissue, fibrin or cartilage is not submitted instead. Once collected, tissue samples should distributed into appropriate vials for the planned studies as soon as possible, including absolute alcohol for crystal analysis, and into appropriate media for microbiological studies.

Patients are instructed to rest biopsied joints for at least 24 hours, and then to resume normal activities if no increased pain or swelling is noted. Complications of the procedure such as hemarthrosis and infection are theoretically possible but extremely rare. Tips of reusable biopsy instruments have been reported to break off into the joint on occasion; hence, such instruments should be carefully inspected for wear or distortion before each procedure[18].

Larger amounts of synovial tissue can be obtained with arthroscopic guidance (discussed below) or through open arthrotomy. The latter method may be the procedure of choice for small joints that would not easily admit a biopsy needle or arthroscope. Arthrotomy of a larger joint made for the sole purpose of sampling tissue need not be as large as that for full exploration of the joint. Analyzable synovial tissue can sometimes be obtained serendipitously, as when discovered in a tissue specimen removed from the patient in a previous procedure or found at arthrocentesis, either floating in synovial fluid or embedded in the aspirating needle.

ARTHROSCOPY

The endoscopy of joints (or arthroscopy) permits direct inspection of intra-articular structures, magnified 10–15 times and shown without grossly perturbing their spatial relationships (Fig. 13.5). The visualized tissues can be probed, sampled, grasped, cut and otherwise modified using instruments inserted through other small incisions. These generic capabilities of arthroscopy – visualization, guided sampling and tissue modification – have been applied to a variety of joint disorders, with an explosive rate of expansion over the past two decades.

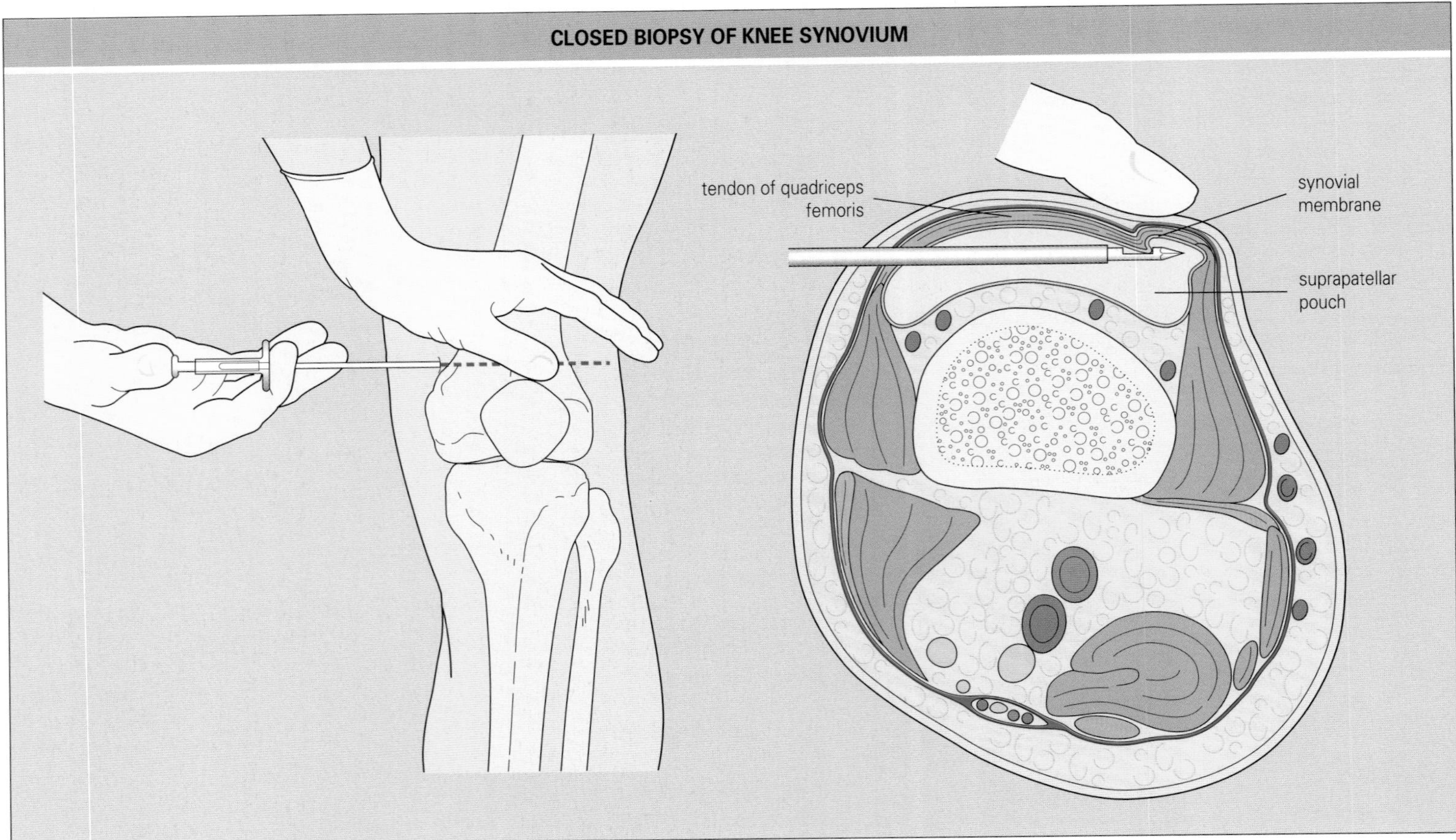

Fig. 13.4 Closed biopsy of knee synovium.

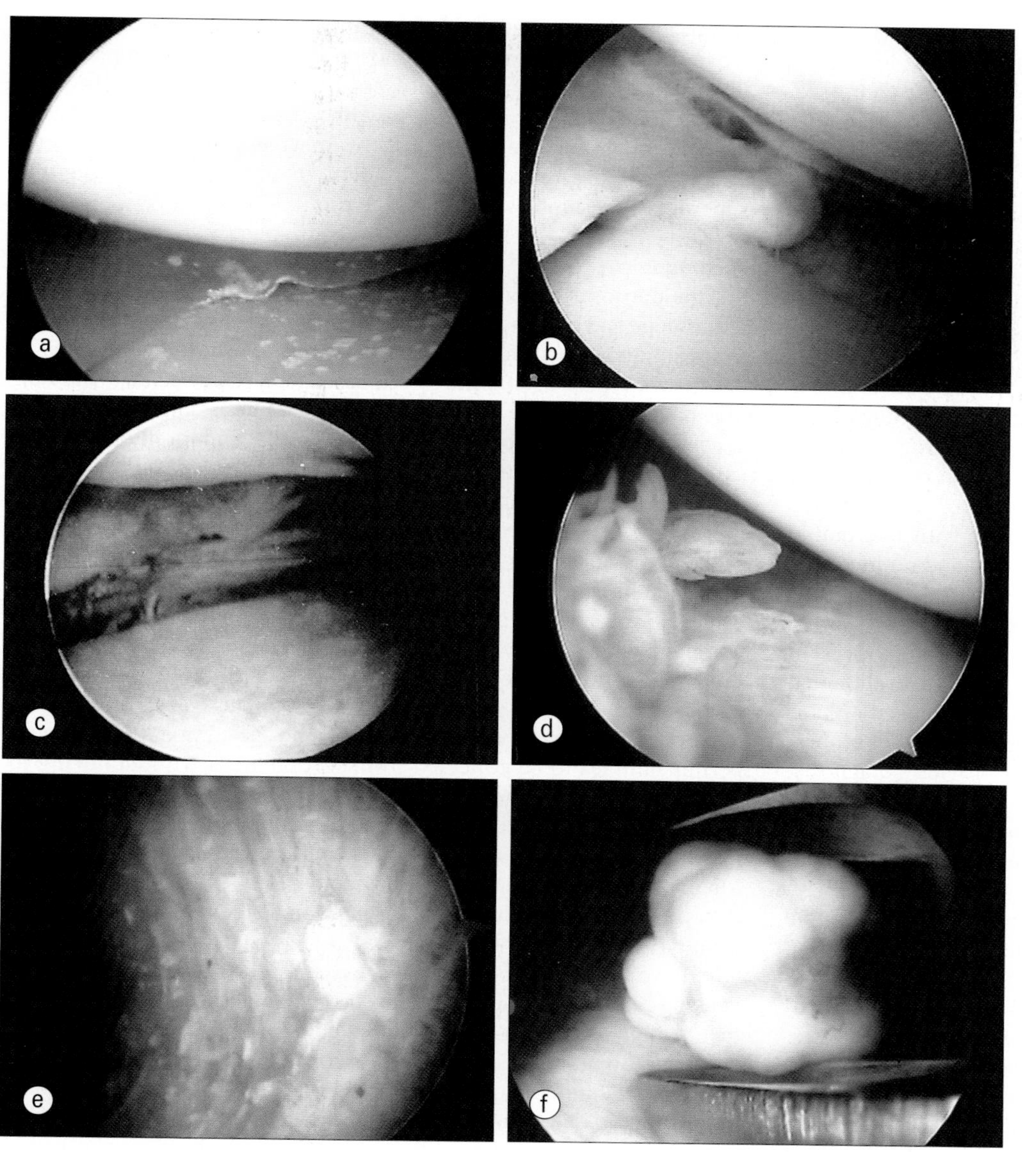

Fig. 13.5 Examples of intra-articular pathology seen at arthroscopy. Refractile white deposits of monosodium urate on the otherwise normal femoral condyle, medial meniscus and tibial plateau in a patient with gout (a); flap tear of the medial meniscus with ulceration of adjacent tibial plateau cartilage (b); complex (degenerative) tear of the medial meniscus, posterior horn, in a patient with OA (c); villous synovitis overlying the outer rim of the medial meniscus in a patient with psoriatic arthritis and knee effusion following minor trauma (d); hyperemic synovium embedded with cartilage fragments in a patient with OA and persistent effusion (e); osteocartilaginous loose body being removed from the knee of a patient with OA and locking symptoms (f).

Arthroscopically guided techniques developed by orthopedic surgeons to supplant an array of interventions once done through arthrotomy account for most of this growth. However, a role for arthroscopy is also emerging for certain subacute and chronic joint conditions that present to the rheumatologist. Refinement in techniques and equipment have made it feasible to perform arthroscopy in an office or procedure-room setting. Some rheumatologists have taken advantage of such developments to begin performing arthroscopy themselves, a trend that should help further define the utility of arthroscopy in rheumatology[23].

ARTHROSCOPIC SURGERY FOR ARTHRITIS

The consequent reduction in postoperative morbidity afforded by arthroscopic performance has made certain surgical interventions for patients with arthritis more widely applicable.

Synovectomy, the physical removal of accumulated inflamed synovium, can palliate otherwise refractory knee symptoms for several years – despite radiographic progression – in patients with an inflammatory arthropathy and minimal secondary joint destruction. Arthroscopic synovectomy is more tedious and time consuming than open synovectomy, but can guide removal of tissue from areas not reached in the open process, thus effecting a more thorough resection. In addition, undamaged structures can be spared instead of being removed as a matter of course, such as for menisci handled at open synovectomy[24]. Finally, arthroscopy avoids the large arthrotomy required for open synovectomy, which mandated additional leg immobilization and hospitalization, and often left a stiff joint only partly remediable by vigorous physical therapy or manipulation under anesthesia. However, the long-term advantages of arthroscopic synovectomy over open methods have yet to be demonstrated in a controlled trial; a retrospective review of long-term outcomes in patients with rheumatoid arthritis (RA) and refractory knee synovitis randomly allocated to undergo either arthroscopic or open synovectomy demonstrated a less frequent recurrence and a longer-lived benefit for those who underwent open synovectomy[25].

'Joint debridement', performed through open arthrotomy as a palliative operation for knee osteoarthritis (OA) in the era before total joint replacement became feasible, has been resurrected as an arthroscopic procedure. For the open procedure, all 'impediments to smooth joint motion' were identified and removed, including osteophytes and chondrophytes, areas of fibrillated cartilage, damaged menisci, loose bodies and clumps of synovium; some proponents advocated the drilling of bare bone to promote fibrocartilaginous ingrowth. 'Abrasion arthroplasty' is an adaptation of this latter intervention to arthroscopy, in which curettage of exposed bone using a motorized burr replaces the drilling, but this component has since been abandoned due to lack of reproducible efficacy[26]. Of the remaining aspects of joint debridement, all are feasible under arthroscopic guidance. The procedure is widely practiced, partly because of the prevalence of knee OA, the paucity of management options short of total joint replacement and the perception of arthroscopy as a minor procedure. Although open series report high rates of satisfactory outcomes[27], controlled trials have failed to show additional benefits beyond those achieved with arthroscopic lavage[28] or closed lavage[29]. Knee OA is a heterogeneous condition when defined by features of intra-articular anatomy[30]. It is possible that some subsets of this condition could be quite effectively addressed by specific arthroscopic resections. However, the concept of 'debridement' masks these differences; it conveys the notion of knee OA as a collection of rough bits that need to be cleaned up. With this concept clouding our understanding and the intervention being of dubious value, perhaps the term 'debridement' should be used with caution when arthroscopic approaches to OA are discussed.

Other chronic joint conditions have been addressed with arthroscopic versions of older open interventions. The painful shoulder with signs of impingement is amenable to curettage of the common inferior subacromial spur, trimming of the partial rotator cuff tear and cleaning of the subacromial bursa; however, debate continues as to whether this procedure is comparable to the older, more extensive interventions[31]. Other joints less commonly affected by OA – such as the ankle[32], elbow[33] and wrist[34] – have been submitted to 'debridement' with reported successes. Hip arthroscopy is feasible, with a favorable outcome when collections of loose bodies are found and removed[35].

ARTHROSCOPY IN CLINICAL RHEUMATOLOGY

Several broadly defined clinical situations in rheumatology present combinations of diagnostic uncertainty and therapeutic frustration that the arthroscope can sometimes untangle[17]. In an undiagnosed inflammatory arthropathy with the knee involved alone or as part of a polyarticular process, synovial biopsy can occasionally provide a diagnosis; arthroscopic guidance assures that abnormal tissue is obtained from a variably distributed process and sometimes demonstrates diagnostic or highly suggestive macroscopic features (such as the 'synovial slough' of Behçet's syndrome). Acute intense joint inflammation with systemic features – acute pyarthrosis – requires arthroscopy to sample synovium for culture to settle any suspicion of infection not confirmed by synovial fluid findings; arthroscopy can help treat established infectious arthritis by providing large-volume joint lavage, removing impediments to drainage and resecting synovitis that sometimes persists after eradication of infection. Arthroscopy has reawakened interest in synovectomy for 'refractory' knee synovitis in patients with a diagnosed inflammatory arthropathy, such as RA (discussed above); for many such patients, the arthroscope shows features in addition to synovitis, particularly the consequences of long-standing synovitis such as 'rice bodies', synovial scarring, damaged intra-articular structures (menisci, ligaments) and pannus. In patients with diagnosed inflammatory arthropathy who have troublesome symptoms but no overt signs of synovitis, such consequences of synovitis can be at fault. For patients with knee pain, normal radiographs and noninflammatory fluid, arthroscopy can identify the offending 'internal derangement', which often involves only hyaline cartilage ('preradiographic' OA) or synovium (in an early synovitis that has not yet produced fluid-phase inflammation). Refractory knee pain in OA for which radiographs do not dictate total knee arthroplasty has become a popular, if controversial, focus of arthroscopic surgery, as discussed above. Using magnetic resonance imaging (MRI) to detect deranged structures before proceeding to arthroscopy assigns undue weight to abnormal meniscal signals, which can be found in asymptomatic knees[36], while ignoring pathologies that might be missed by MRI.

ARTHROSCOPIC ASSESSMENT OF TREATMENT EFFECTS

Tissue effects of rheumatic disease treatments are seldom directly documented. Arthroscopy provides the means by which this might be accomplished for interventions directed at joint tissues. Besides the directed biopsy of target tissues, arthroscopy can serve to provide quantitative scores of the global effect on joint tissues[37].

OFFICE-BASED ARTHROSCOPY

Arthroscopy requires a conventional operating room environment when concomitant open arthrotomy might be performed. This applies to complex procedures such as cruciate ligament allografting, meniscal repair and transplantation, and combined arthroscopic and/or open repair procedures, but not to diagnostic procedures and simple resections. The development of arthroscopes small enough to be inserted into the joint under local anesthesia with needle puncture has reopened the concept of office-based arthroscopy, in which the procedure is done on an awake (or lightly sedated) patient in an outpatient setting that superficially resembles the operating room, if at all.

Technique

For the purposes of joint inspection, lavage and tissue sampling, the arthroscope and other necessary instruments can be comfortably inserted following delivery of local anesthesia to the sites of joint entry and to the synovial space itself. Mild systemic sedation can be given to the anxious patient, or when a more extensive procedure is anticipated. These preparations are delivered by the arthroscopist and monitored by the assisting nurse, obviating the need for a formal anesthetist. Principles of asepsis are followed for all items that might touch the patient. The clarity of the video image delivered depends in part on the type of arthroscope used – glass-lens systems produce a sharper image than that from fiberoptic instruments, which transmit optical data in pixels through a cable. However, adequate visualization also depends on clear intra-articular fluid, which is provided by the lavage accompanying the procedure. Fiberoptic systems have proved adequate to locate and characterize areas of gross intra-articular pathology[21]. Tissue samples can be removed by hand-operated forceps with scoop-tipped ends; suction-assisted devices permit samples to be collected from several areas without having to remove and reinsert the instrument. Motorized shavers remove tissue drawn by suction into the cutting end of a rotating blade, and can collect large amounts of tissue, sometimes blurring the distinction between 'diagnostic' and 'therapeutic' arthroscopy[38]. Following the procedure, patients can return to full activities as soon as their symptoms permit, usually within 2 days. Assist devices are recommended only for those who have undergone considerable tissue resection or those who find walking painful afterwards. Since the procedure requires no general anesthetic, thigh tourniquet or leg-holding device the risk of complications associated with conventional arthroscopy (deep venous thrombosis, thrombophlebitis, joint effusion or quadriceps atrophy) is quite low[39]. Since office-based arthroscopy is usually performed to settle diagnostic issues, patient expectations of the procedure tend to be more reasonable than those of the arthritis patient facing conventional arthroscopy in the operating room.

Arthroscopy in the office setting can also be used for joints other than the knee, including the ankle, wrist, shoulder, elbow and bursae of the olecranon and prepatellar regions. A number of orthopedic surgeons have made this transition from the operating room for some interventions that involve these joints (as well as the knee), a trend that is likely to be perpetuated by the cost savings. Rheumatologists are beginning to explore the utility of inspecting these medium-sized joints, as well as the small joints of the hand, in early disease state[40].

JOINT LAVAGE

Passing a volume of physiologic fluid through a joint can sometimes confer temporary benefit in several different disorders, including OA, RA, crystal-associated arthritides and infection of joints and bursae[41]. For most of these conditions, this phenomenon was first observed in joints that had undergone arthroscopy in the era before arthroscopic surgery became feasible. Methods devised to lavage joints without using an arthroscope employ a large bore needle to instill physiologic fluid (usually normal saline), and then remove the fluid and associated joint contents through various routes. The volume of fluid used can vary from 50ml to several liters, with smaller amounts for a single injection. Installation and removal of a small volume can be performed as an adjunct to arthrocentesis in the clinic, and larger volumes are delivered in repeated cycles of joint distention and lavage in dedicated procedures.

For most conditions approached with lavage, the therapeutic effect is presumably achieved by removing material that is somehow perpetuating adverse features of the observed clinical situation. In OA several components derived from articular cartilage have phlogistic properties *in vitro* and in animal models, including macroscopic 'wear particles', proteoglycan aggregates and crystals; lavage of these free-floating materials from the joint can reduce the synovial burden and thereby ameliorate the synovitis that is so common in clinical flares of OA[42]. Physical alteration of the joint milieu in RA is less likely to have a lasting effect on inflammatory mediators, which are mainly cellular or molecular species that arise from the synovium. However, remnants of past inflammatory events – fibrin, sloughed synovial villi, clumped inflammatory cells – can coalesce and persist as rice bodies, which can cause persistent joint swelling if abundant and can clog arthrocentesis needles[43]. Lavage through a large bore needle (to remove rice bodies and material that might derive from the accompanying secondary OA) can ameliorate signs of local inflammation and perpetuate the effects of an intra-articular glucocorticoid given at the same setting[44]; a single exchange of 50ml can be effective, although larger volumes have also been used. The phlogistic agents in crystal-associated arthropathies are well identified and as readily recognized as the crystals themselves. However, conventional treatments are usually adequate to ameliorate clinical flares, so lavage is rarely used. Joint lavage can occasionally trigger a flare in a joint that harbors crystals, usually when encountered at arthroscopy performed for other indications[39]. Nevertheless, the anti-inflammatory effects of lavage on crystal-associated arthropathies are sufficiently well documented to warrant consideration of this intervention in a patient for whom more conventional therapy may be contraindicated[41,42]. Thorough evacuation of purulent synovial fluid and other debris that impedes joint drainage is an important component of septic arthritis management. When joint drainage can no longer be accomplished with bedside arthrocentesis, closed lavage through a large bore needle using a liter or more of fluid can sometimes provide sufficient additional drainage to obviate the further consideration of surgery[45]. This intervention has been described for the knee joint and for olecranon and peripatellar bursae, but could be applied to other large joints if correct placement of the lavage needle within the capsule can be assured.

Joint lavage can be undertaken in the same setting as arthrocentesis, but requires additional preparation. Aseptic conditions apply to all items that might touch the patient. Local anesthetic should be delivered along tracks to be used for joint entry, and to the joint space if repeated distention and lavage are anticipated. To minimize infection risk, a closed system should be used to traffic fluid from reservoir [usually an intravenous (i.v.) bag] to effluent container (suction canister or empty evacuated bottle); an adequate system can be fashioned from three-way stopcocks, plastic tubing and other connectors available as standard i.v. supplies. A large bore needle (14 gauge or larger) should be used; several reusable needles manufactured to penetrate and evacuate body cavities – mainly the peritoneum (for laparoscopy) and joints (for arthroscopy) – serve very well for joint lavage. Complications are rare; they include vasovagal reactions, extracapsular fluid extravasation, persistent pain at the puncture site and cellulitis. Patients should refrain from driving for several hours afterwards if a weight-bearing joint has been given intra-articular anesthesia, as this can impair joint proprioception.

REGIONAL PERINEURAL INJECTIONS

Principles of nerve block for regional anesthesia have been adapted for pain management. Symptoms due to focal nerve entrapment by soft tissue often respond to corticosteroids placed at the site of tissue hypertrophy, frequently obviating the need for surgical release. Techniques for injection treatment of the common entrapment neuropathies consequent to periarticular soft tissue impingement (e.g. carpal, cubital and tarsal tunnel syndromes) are an established part of many rheumatologists' practice, and are described elsewhere in this volume (see Chapter 4.16). The two procedures described in this section – while applicable to several clinical situations encountered by rheumatologists – are not yet widely utilized, either by referral or by direct performance. However, each is within the capabilities of the rheumatologist who is already assured with other procedures and able to master the relevant regional anatomy (see Chapter 2.12).

SUPRASCAPULAR NERVE BLOCK

The suprascapular nerve arises from the upper trunk of the brachial plexus and contains afferent, efferent and sympathetic components. It courses down and laterally from the brachial plexus deep to the trapezius muscle, then passes downwards to the upper border of the scapula through the suprascapular notch, reaching the posterior aspect of the scapula in the supraspinatus fossa where it supplies the supraspinatus muscle and gives off articular branches to the glenohumeral and acromioclavicular joints. The suprascapular nerve thus provides sensory fibers to approximately 70% of the shoulder region, mainly the superior and posterior aspects.

Placement of local anesthetic (with or without corticosteroids) near the suprascapular notch and in the supraspinous fossa interrupts afferent nerve fibers, usually without a concomitant motor effect. This intervention has been used to palliate shoulder pain from several conditions, including adhesive capsulitis, glenohumeral degenerative arthritis, chronic rotator cuff tears, reflex sympathetic dystrophy, humeral metastases and recent surgery[46,47]. In RA, where shoulder pain can arise from several combinations of anatomic damage and focal inflammation, suprascapular nerve block has provided relief superior to that attained with intra-articular injections in controlled studies, and the effect is not dependent on corticosteroids[48]. Mechanisms for prolonged pain relief are obscure, but could relate to the relative immobility of the nerve at the suprascapular notch (rendering it susceptible to trauma with scapular movement) or to an effect on C fibers, interrupting the cycle of feedback amplification that can occur with chronic pain.

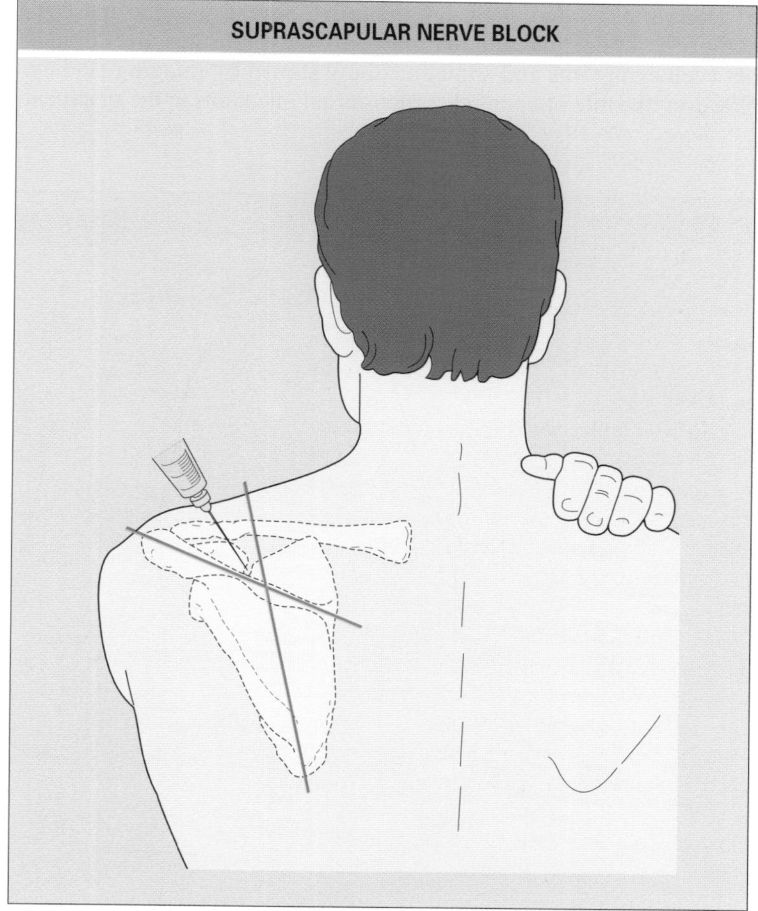

Fig. 13.6 Suprascapular nerve block.

With the seated patient grasping the unaffected shoulder, suprascapular nerve block begins by locating a point 2–3cm above and lateral to the intersection of two lines (one drawn on the scapular spine and the other drawn superiorly from the inferior angle of the scapula, bisecting it); local anesthetic is infiltrated down to bone through a needle directed inwards, forwards and down (see Fig. 13.6). The needle is then 'walked' along the floor of the supraspinous fossa while delivering small amounts of anesthetic, moving cephalad and laterally, until the suprascapular notch is entered. The patient may feel mild pain at the shoulder tip and radiating down the arm. After aspirating to assure that no vascular structure has been entered, the desired mix of long-acting anesthetic and corticosteroid is delivered. Entering the suprascapular notch may not be imperative, since anesthetic delivered along the floor of the supraspinous fossa should reach the suprascapular nerve as it lies between the scapular periosteum and adjacent fascia of the supraspinatus muscle.

Suprascapular nerve blocks are not entirely without risks. Pleural space violation may result in pneumothorax. Great caution must therefore be employed in carrying out the procedure.

EPIDURAL CORTICOSTEROID INJECTION

The space between the periosteum of the vertebral canal and the spinal dura mater runs from the tip of the sacrum to the foramen magnum. Spinal nerve roots exit the dural sac to occupy this space before blending with the periosteum as they pass through the vertebral foramina. Epidural injection of local anesthetic agents can predictably block spinal sensory input below the level at which the agent is placed. Used mainly as an alternative to general anesthesia, such injections have also been employed in the management of sciatica. Corticosteroids have been included in therapeutic epidural injections to treat soft-tissue inflammation and edema that might account for nerve root compression that is not directly caused by pressure from a herniated disk. Findings that support this concept include the chronic inflammation and fibrosis commonly shown in perineural tissue examined at laminectomy as well as the phlogistic properties of intervertebral disk material, including potent phospholipase A_2 activity[48]. These phenomena may partly explain the discordance between symptoms and spinal anatomy shown by imaging studies. However, the role of epidural corticosteroid injections in the treatment of various back syndromes remains uncertain.

The few controlled studies of epidural corticosteroids indicate that they hasten recovery from lower-extremity radicular pain, with a therapeutic effect persisting at intermediate term follow-up (2 weeks to 3 months). The difference between injected and control groups becomes negligible after a year or more, consistent with the tendency for most low back syndromes to remit with time[48]. Beneficial effects from epidural corticosteroids in lumbar spinal stenosis have been described, with neurogenic claudication symptoms often palliated for several months or more by a series of 2–3 epidural injections spaced several days apart[49]. Axial pain is seldom affected by epidural corticosteroids. Radicular pain is less likely to respond if chronic or associated with previous back surgery[48].

The technique for lumbar epidural injection (Fig. 13.7) resembles that for lumbar puncture. The interspace at or above the clinically affected nerve root is marked, then anesthetized after the skin has been cleansed. The anesthetizing needle can often locate the depth of the ligamentum flavum, thus defining the track for the epidural needle. Specifically designed blunt tipped needles with side-directed openings minimize the chance for dural puncture and assure delivery of medication to the epidural space. Entry of the epidural space is suggested by a 'pop' as the fibers of the ligamentum flavum are breached, and confirmed by immediate loss of resistance in an attached glass syringe. A mixture of depot corticosteroid and lidocaine (lignocaine) is then instilled unless cerebrospinal fluid flows from the hub, which indicates a dural puncture. A volume of 10ml that contains 80–160mg of methylprednisolone or triamcinolone is sufficient to infiltrate several levels. Immediately after injection, the patient may transiently experience increased discomfort in the region served by the irritated nerve root, a useful sign that indicates the successful placement of corticosteroid. The patient then rests, laying on the side of greater symptoms, and is discharged after any regional hypoesthesia has worn off (see Chapter 2.12).

The epidural space can also be approached via a caudal route, using a needle inserted through the sacral hiatus. A larger volume must be used to traverse the caudal canal and reach the affected lumbar region. Compared to the lumbar approach, this method is usually easier to perform in patients operated on previously, minimizes the risk of dural puncture and delivers medication closer to the sacral roots.

The potential for infection and hematoma formation following epidural injection contraindicates the procedure in patients with local

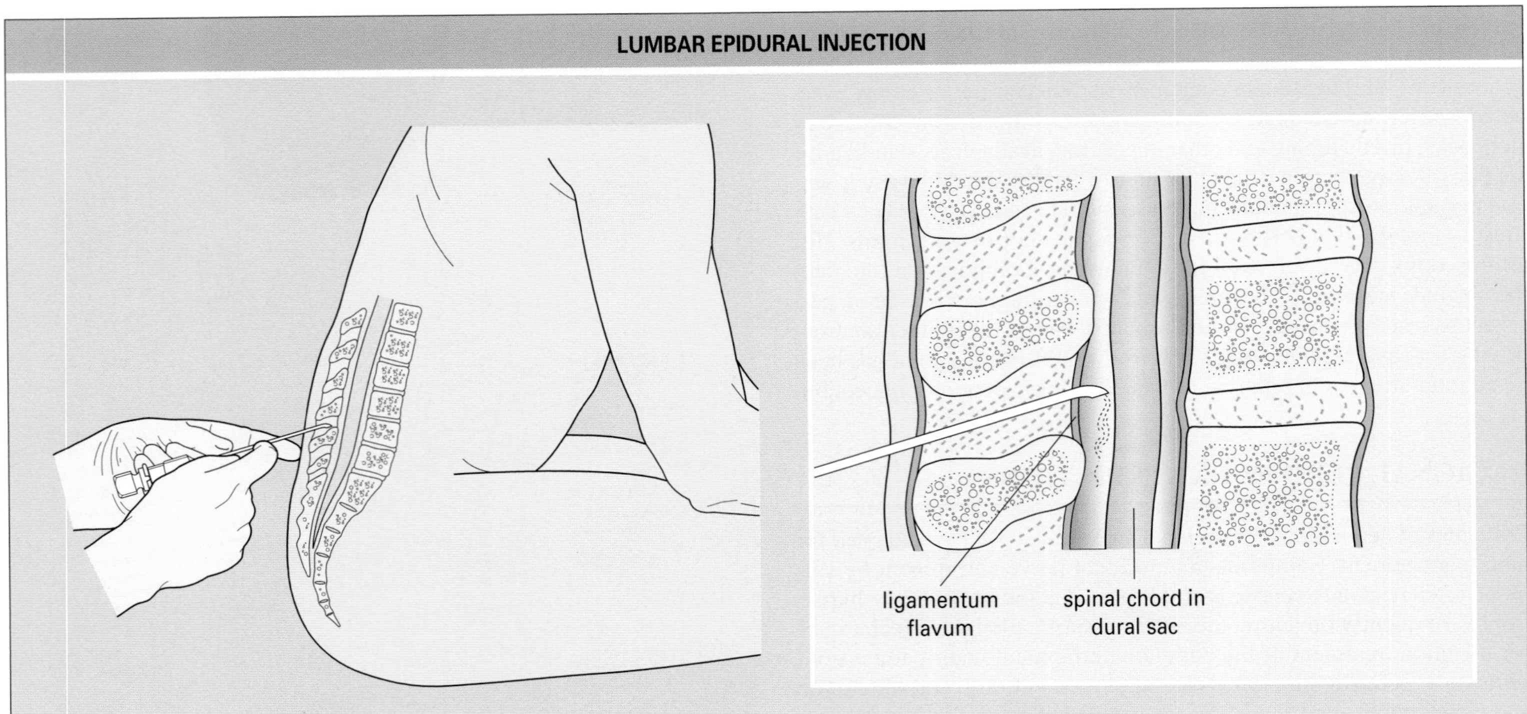

Fig. 13.7 Lumbar epidural injection.

and systemic infections or an established bleeding diathesis; fortunately, such complications are extremely rare[49]. Minor complications include unintentional dural puncture (with occasional associated headache), vasovagal reaction and the systemic effects of injected corticosteroids, including salt and water retention, exacerbation of diabetes and hypothalamic–pituitary–adrenal (HPA) axis suppression. This latter effect can persist for 1–3 months following a series of three weekly injections[50]. Thus, it would be prudent to administer supplemental corticosteroids or test the HPA axis in patients who face major physiologic stress and have recently undergone a series of epidural injections.

REFERENCES

1. Bywaters EGL, Edmonds JP. Biopsies and tissue diagnosis in the rheumatic diseases. Clin Rheum Dis. 1976;2:179–208.
2. Harrist TJ, Mihm MC Jr. Specificity and clinical usefulness of the lupus band test. Arthritis Rheum. 1980;23:479–90.
3. Gibson LE. Cutaneous vasculitis: approach to diagnosis and systemic associations. Mayo Clin Proc. 1990;65:221–9.
4. Bondi EE, Lazarus GS. Panniculitis. In: Fitzpatrick TB, Eisen AZ, Wolff K, Freedberg IM, Austen KF, eds. Dermatology in general medicine, 4E. New York: McGraw-Hill, Inc.; 1993:1329–44.
5. Moore GP, Wilkens RF. The subcutaneous nodule: its significance in the diagnosis of rheumatic disease. Semin Arthritis Rheum. 1977;7:63–78.
6. Mastaglia FL, Laing NG. Investigation of muscle disease. J Neurol Neurosurg Psych. 1996;60:256–74.
7. Clements PJ, Furst DE, Campion DS, *et al.* Muscle disease in progressive systemic sclerosis: diagnostic and therapeutic considerations. Arthritis Rheum. 1978;21:62–71.
8. Zucker J. Drug-induced myopathies. Semin Arthritis Rheum. 1990;19:259–68.
9. Dahlberg PJ, Lockhart JM, Overholt EL. Diagnostic studies for systemic necrotizing vasculitis. Arch Int Med. 1989;149:161–5.
10. Stjernberg N, Cajander S, Truedsson H, Uddenfeldt P. Muscle involvement in sarcoidosis. Acta Med Scand. 1981;209:213–16.
11. O'Rourke KS, Ike RW. Muscle biopsy. Curr Opin Rheumatol. 1995;7:462–8.
12. Dubowitz V. Muscle biopsy: a practical approach, 2E. London: Ballière-Tindall; 1985.
13. Haddad MG, West RL, Treadwell EL, Fraser DD. Diagnosis of inflammatory myopathy by percutaneous needle biopsy with demonstration of the focal nature of myositis. Am J Clin Pathol. 1994,101:661–4.
14. Daniels TE. Labial salivary gland biopsy in Sjögren's syndrome. Assessment as a diagnostic criterion in 362 suspected cases. Arthritis Rheum. 1984;27:147–56.
15. Delgado WA, Mosqueda A. A highly sensitive method for diagnosis of secondary amyloidosis by labial salivary gland biopsy. J Oral Pathol Med. 1989;18:310–14.
16. Nessan VJ, Jacoway JR. Biopsy of minor salivary glands in the diagnosis of sarcoidosis. N Engl J Med. 1979;301:922–4.
17. O'Rourke KS, Ike RW. Diagnostic arthroscopy in the arthritis patient. Rheum Dis Clin North Am. 1994;20(2):321–42.
18. Saaibi DL, Schumacher HR Jr. Percutaneous needle biopsy and synovial histology. Baillière's Clin Rheumatol. 1996;10(3):535–54.
19. Wofsy D. Culture-negative septic arthritis and bacterial endocarditis. Diagnosis by synovial biopsy. Arthritis Rheum. 1980;23:605–7.
20. Beaule V, Laredo JD, Cywiner C, Bard M, Tubiana JM. Synovial membrane: percutaneous biopsy. Radiology. 1990;177:581–5.
21. Ike RW, O'Rourke KS. Detection of intra-articular abnormalities in osteoarthritis of the knee: a pilot study comparing needle arthroscopy with standard arthroscopy. Arthritis Rheum. 1993;36:1353–63.
22. Ike RW. Diagnostic arthroscopy. Baillière's Clin Rheumatol. 1996;10:495–517.
23. Wei N, Delauter SK and Erlichman MS. Office based arthroscopy. Evolution of the procedure: the next 100 cases. J Clin Rheumatol. 1995;1:219–27.

24. Fiocco U, Cozzi L, Rigon C, *et al.* Arthroscopic synovectomy in rheumatoid and psoriatic knee joint synovitis: long-term outcome. Br J Rheumatol. 1996;35:463–70.
25. Ryu J, Saito S, Honda T, Sano S. Comparison between arthroscopic and open synovectomy for the rheumatoid knee: a retrospective study on the results of the two methods. J Orthop Rheumatol. 1996;9:28–32.
26. Bert JM, Maschka K. The arthroscopic treatment of unicompartmental gonarthrosis: a five year follow-up study of abrasion arthroplasty plus arthroscopic debridement and arthroscopic debridement alone. Arthroscopy. 1989:5:25–32.
27. Novak PJ, Bach BR Jr. Selection criteria for knee arthroscopy in the osteoarthritic patient. Orthop Rev. 1993;22:798–804.
28. Moseley JB Jr, Wray NP, Kuykendall D, Willis K, Landon G. Arthroscopic treatment of osteoarthritis of the knee: a prospective, randomized, placebo controlled trial. Results of a pilot study. Am J Sports Med. 1996;24:28–34.
29. Chang RW, Falconer J, Stulberg SD, Arnold WJ, Mannheim LM, Dyer AR. A randomized controlled trial of arthroscopic surgery versus closed-needle joint lavage for patients with osteoarthritis of the knee. Arthritis Rheum. 1993;36:289–96.
30. Ike RW. The role of arthroscopy in the differential diagnosis of osteoarthritis of the knee. Rheum Dis Clin North Am. 1993;19:673–96.
31. Van Holsbeeck E, DeRycke J, Declercq G, Martens M, Verstreken J, Fabry G. Subacromial impingement: open versus arthroscopic decompression. Arthroscopy. 1992;8:173–8.
32. Ogilvie-Harris DJ, Sekyi-Otu A. Arthroscopic debridement for the osteoarthritic ankle. Arthroscopy. 1995;11:433–6.
33. O'Driscoll SW. Operative treatment of elbow arthritis. Curr Opin Rheumatol. 1995;7:103–6.
34. Bain GI, Roth JH. The role of arthroscopy in arthritis. 'Ectomy' procedures. Hand Clin. 1995;11:51–8.
35. McCarthy JC, Busconi B. The role of hip arthroscopy in the diagnosis and treatment of hip disease. Orthopedics. 1995;18:753–6.
36. Fernandez-Madrid F, Karvonen RL, Teitge RA, Miller PR, Negendank WG. MR features of osteoarthritis of the knee. Magn Reson Imaging. 1994;12:703–9.
37. Ayral X. Quantitative arthroscopy. Baillière's Clin Rheumatol. 1996;10:477–94.
38. Moreland LW, Calvo-Alén J, Koopman WJ. Synovial biopsy of the knee joint under direct visualization by needle arthroscopy. J Clin Rheumatol. 1995;1:103–8.
39. Szachnowski P, Wei N, Arnold WJ, Cohen LM. Complications of office based arthroscopy of the knee. J Rheumatol. 1995;22:1722–5.
40. Arayssi TK, Schumacher R. Closed needle biopsy of small joints in patients with synovitis: development and testing of a new biopsy needle. Arthritis Rheum. 1996;39:S157.
41. Ayral X, Dougados M. Joint lavage. Rev Rhumatisme [Engl Ed]. 1995;62:281–7.
42. Ike RW. Joint lavage. In: Brandt KD, Doherty M, Lohmander S (eds). Textbook on osteoarthritis.Oxford:Oxford University Press (in press).
43. Popert AJ, Scott DL, Wainwright AC, Walton KW, Williamson N, Chapman JH. Frequency of occurrence, mode of development, and significance of rice bodies in rheumatoid joints. Ann Rheum Dis. 1982;41:109–17.
44. Srinivasan A, Amos M, Webley M. The effects of joint washout and steroid injection compared with either joint washout or steroid injection alone in rheumatoid knee effusion. Br J Rheumatol. 1995;34:771–3.
45. Ike RW. Tidal irrigation in septic arthritis of the knee: a potential alternative to surgical drainage. J Rheumatol. 1993;20:2104–11.
46. Brown DE, James DC, Roy S. Pain relief by suprascapular nerve block in gleno-humeral arthritis. Scand J Rheumatol. 1988;17:411–15.
47. Vecchio PC, Adebajo AO, Hazleman BL. Suprascapular nerve block for persistent rotator cuff lesions. J Rheumatol. 1993;20:453–5.
48. Gado K, Emery P. Modified suprascapular nerve block with bupivacaine alone effectively controls chronic shoulder pain in patients with rheumatoid arthritis. Ann Rheum Dis. 1993;52:215–18.
49. Spaccarelli KC. Lumbar and caudal epidural corticosteroid injections. Mayo Clin Proc. 1996;71:169–78.
50. Ciocon JO, Galindo-Ciocon D, Amaranath L, Galindo D. Caudal epidural blocks for elderly patients with lumbar canal stenosis. J Am Geriatr Soc. 1994;42:593–6.

14

IMAGING TECHNIQUES

Charles G Peterfy

- Imaging plays a valuable clinical role in defining pathologies which affect the musculoskeletal system.
- The most commonly used procedures include conventional radiography, CT, scintigraphy, ultrasonography and MRI.
- The procedures differ in their abilities to image soft tissue pathologies, bone and cartilage and the choice of procedures depends on the question being asked.
- Communication between a radiologist familiar with the procedures and the clinician caring for the patient is essential to optimize information obtained with imaging.

INTRODUCTION

The discovery of the X-ray by Wilhelm Konrad Roentgen in 1895 marked a turning point in the history of medicine. That the study of electrical discharges in a vacuum would one day yield a method for 'seeing' through the flesh of living humans could not have been anticipated by the physicians of the time. This is evident from the statements of another visionary scientist of that period, Berkeley George Moynihan of Leeds, one of the forefathers of modern surgery, who at about the same time felt that with the advent of anesthesia and sterile technique there was little room for further discovery in the field of surgery. It was not long, however, before the implications of Roentgen's discovery were recognized, and in 1901 he was awarded the first Nobel Prize.

For most of the following century, radiography remained the principal imaging modality used to evaluate arthritis and related disorders. More recently, other advances in medical imaging have profoundly enhanced the ability to diagnose disease. Chief of these was computed tomography (CT), developed in the 1970s by GN Hounsfield who also received a Nobel Prize for his work. The approach to cross-sectional imaging introduced by CT formed the basis for two additional modalities: real-time ultrasonography and magnetic resonance imaging (MRI). The latter, in particular, has brought unprecedented soft-tissue imaging capabilities to routine clinical use. In addition to these techniques for delineating structural detail, radionuclide scintigraphy has enabled functional imaging of a variety of organs and tissues.

Although this explosion of technological development has advanced the ability to image arthritic joints, the increased technical sophistication coupled with the rapid pace of development has hindered the ability of some physicians to understand and properly utilize them. Familiarity with the strengths and limitations of these modalities should enable rheumatologists and other clinicians dealing with arthritis to take full advantage of the growing armamentarium, as well as to help direct further development to serve the needs of their patients better.

GENERAL APPROACHES TO MEDICAL IMAGING

There are three basic approaches to medical imaging: transmission imaging, reflection imaging and emission imaging (Fig. 14.1). Each involves three fundamental components: a source of radiation, a patient and an image receptor. Transmission imaging (radiography, fluoroscopy, CT and photon or X-ray absorptiometry) and reflection imaging (ultrasonography) utilize an external energy source, whereas in emission imaging (scintigraphy, MRI and thermography) the patient serves as the energy source. A variety of different radiation types can be used to generate medical images. These include electromagnetic radiation in the form of high-frequency X-ray and γ radiation (radiography, fluoroscopy, CT, scintigraphy, and photon or X-ray absorptiometry), radiofrequency radiation (MRI) or infrared radiation (thermography), and sound (ultrasonography). The image receptor can be light-sensitive film (radiography) or an X-ray image intensifier (fluoroscopy), an array of ionization chambers or scintillation detectors (CT), a scintillation crystal coupled to photomultiplier tubes (scintigraphy), a piezoelectric crystal (ultrasonography) or simply a wire coil (MRI).

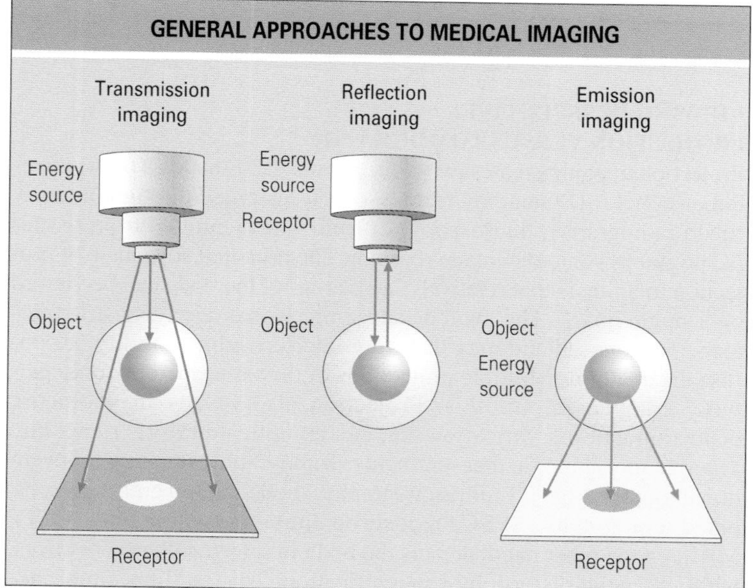

Fig. 14.1 General approaches to medical imaging. In transmission imaging (e.g. radiography, CT), X-ray radiation is transmitted through the object to the receptor. In reflection imaging (ultrasonography), the transducer serves as both the energy source and the receptor for sound waves reflected by the body. In emission imaging (scintigraphy), the body serves as both the object and the energy source for γ-radiation absorbed by the receptor.

CHARACTERISTICS AND QUALITY OF THE RADIOLOGIC IMAGE

The performance of imaging tools can be described in terms of:
- technical parameters such as signal-to-noise ratio, contrast-to-noise ratio, image blurring or spectral separation, acquisition speed, etc., or
- diagnostic parameters, such as sensitivity, specificity and the area under the receiver–operator–characteristic (ROC) curve (see Fig. 14.2).

Both of these perspectives are important, although the former will be emphasized in the following discussion. The amount of useful information in a radiologic image depends not only on the particular modality, but also on the viewing perspective and the image clarity. Viewing perspective can be either projectional or tomographic (see Figs 14.3 & 14.4). Image clarity, or quality, is a function of four factors: contrast, blurring, noise and the presence of distortion and artifacts.

IMAGE QUALITY	
Technical parameters	Diagnostic parameters
Contrast	Sensitivity
Blur	Specificity
Noise	Area under ROC curve
Artifacts/distortion	
ROC = Receiver–operator–characteristic.	

Fig. 14.2 Image quality.

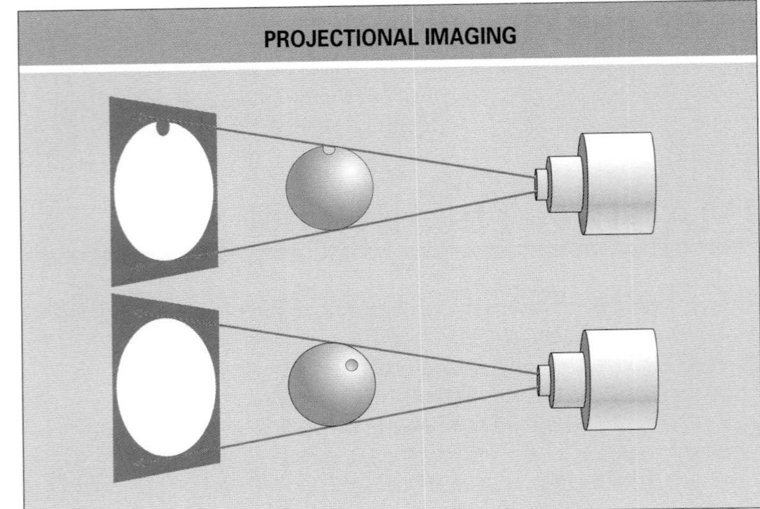

Fig. 14.3 Projectional imaging. Conventional radiography and scintigraphy cast 2D shadows of 3D objects onto the receptor. This results in morphologic distortion, magnification and superimposition that may obscure anatomic features.

VIEWING PERSPECTIVE: PROJECTION VERSUS TOMOGRAPHY

Projection imaging creates two-dimensional (2D) shadows of the three-dimensional (3D) anatomy from X-rays transmitted through the body (plain radiography, fluoroscopy) or from γ-rays emitted from tissues (scintigraphy) onto the image receptor. The principal advantage of projection imaging is that relatively large areas of the body can be viewed on a single image. The main disadvantage is that overlying structures are superimposed and may therefore interfere with visibility or confuse the anatomy. Multiple projections of the same anatomy only partially compensate for this. Projection also results in geometric distortion and magnification that can complicate efforts to acquire accurate morphologic measurements. Tomographic imaging [conventional tomography, CT, ultrasonography, single photon emission computed tomography (SPECT), positron emission tomography (PET), MRI], on the other hand, depicts the body in selected planes, or slices, without spatial distortion or magnification. This facilitates morphologic measurements and eliminates superimposition. However, only a small area of the body is depicted on each image, so that a large number of images must be evaluated to cover a region of the anatomy.

CONTRAST

Contrast is the most fundamental image characteristic. An anatomic structure is visible only if there is sufficient contrast with its background or surrounding tissues (Fig. 14.5). Contrast depends on differential tissue properties, the particular imaging modality used and the specific settings employed to acquire the image. It is measured as the difference in attenuation or signal between two regions of interest (ROIs), divided by the sum of their values. Contrast-to-noise ratio is calculated as $ROI_1 - ROI_2$ divided by the background noise (standard deviation of background values). Radiography offers high contrast between noncalcified soft tissues and bone and between fatty and nonfatty tissues, but discriminates poorly among different nonfatty, noncalcified tissues.

BLURRING

Some degree of blurring is present in all imaging techniques. Blurring reduces the contrast and visibility of small anatomic structures (i.e. detail) and results in a variable degree of image 'unsharpness'. The spatial resolution of an image depends on the amount of image blur. Three basic sources of blurring are: geometric blurring, motion blurring and receptor blurring.

Geometric blurring relates to the geometry of the imaging system and is affected by the size of the radiation source and the distances

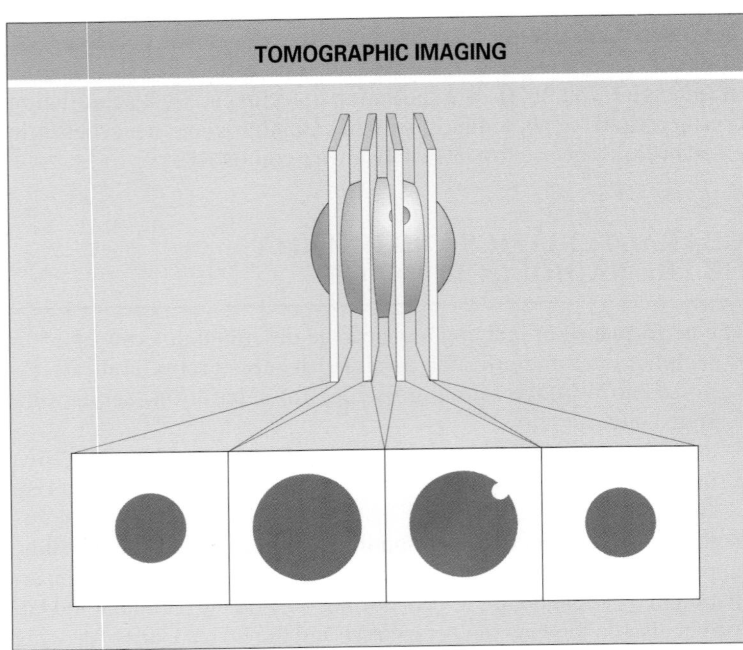

Fig. 14.4 Tomographic imaging. Tomographic techniques, such as CT, ultrasonography and MRI, produce cross-sectional images without morphologic distortion, magnification or superimposition.

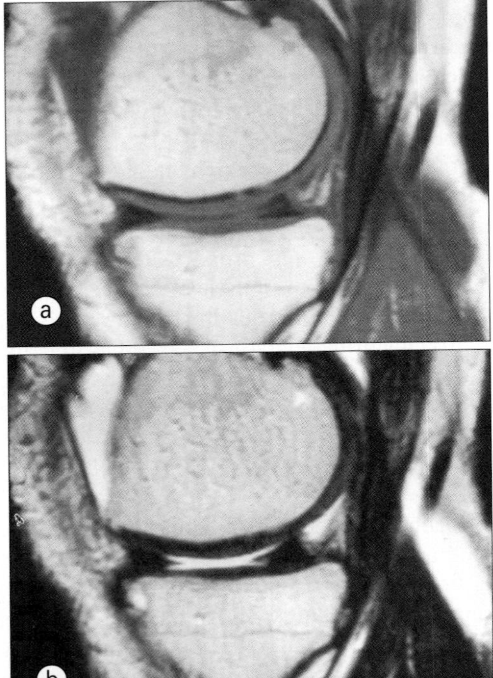

Fig. 14.5 Image contrast. Articular cartilage is difficult to differentiate from adjacent synovial fluid on a T1-weighted MRI image of the knee (a) because both structures have similar signal intensity and therefore show poor contrast. Contrast between cartilage and synovial fluid is increased on T2-weighted MRI image (b), which shows thinning of the articular cartilage over the posterior horn of the meniscus.

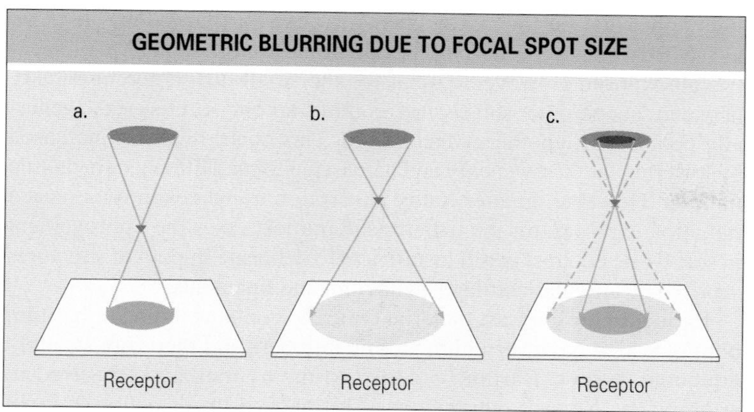

Fig. 14.6 Geometric blurring due to focal spot size. As an object (in this case a point) is moved closer to the source, or focal spot, from (a) to (b) blurring of the projected image is increased. This blurring can be decreased by reducing the size of the focal spot (c).

between the source and the patient and between the patient and the image receptor (Fig. 14.6). Moving the patient closer to the energy source or farther from the receptor magnifies the projected image (magnification radiography) but also increases blurring. A very small X-ray source, or focal spot (microfocal radiography), is therefore used to offset blurring. Geometric blurring, particularly severe in scintigraphy because of the large size of the energy source (i.e. the patient), can be mitigated by placing a grid, or collimator, over the camera to filter out obliquely oriented γ-rays (see below), and by increasing the distance between the patient and the receptor (Fig. 14.7). In CT, the distances between the focal spot, patient and receptor are more or less fixed, so that geometric blurring is governed primarily by the size of the focal spot. Geometric blurring in ultrasonography is determined by the size of the transducer and the depth of the reflective interface.

Motion blurring – caused by nonsynchronized movements of the energy source, patient or receptor during image acquisition – results in a loss of image sharpness and the development of artifacts. The energy source and imaging receptor can be stabilized, but it is more difficult to suppress voluntary movements by the patient. Restraints or sedation may be necessary for disoriented patients or children, but acquisition times are generally short for radiography or CT and most patients can keep still enough for satisfactory images to be obtained. Even with the more time-consuming MRI, reasonable-quality scans of the extremities can usually be obtained. Involuntary movements such as cardiac contractions, vascular pulsations and gastrointestinal peristalsis, and semivoluntary movements, such as breathing and swallowing, are, however, more problematic. Gating techniques can be used to synchronize image acquisition with periodic movements but tend to prolong the examination time. Motion blur is not affected by magnification.

The imaging receptor contributes to image unsharpness. In plain radiography, receptor blurring is determined primarily by the thickness of the intensifying screen over the film (see below). Thicker screens improve receptor sensitivity, allowing reduced patient exposure and faster imaging, but also increase image blurring. High-speed film–screen combinations typically show two to three times the degree of blurring observed with high-detail film–screen combinations. Geometric magnification reduces receptor blur relative to the image size, but it must be remembered that magnification also increases focal spot blur.

NOISE

Noise in imaging comes from a variety of sources. In radiography, noise typically manifests as a grainy background that reduces the visibility of small, low-contrast detail. Higher contrast thus lessens the impact of noise. In conventional radiography the major cause is scatter radiation. Radiation scattered by Compton interactions exits the body in random directions and therefore carries little usable spatial information. Scatter radiation must therefore be removed by placing a grid in front of the receptor, or allowed to miss the receptor by moving the body farther away (air gap). In scintigraphy, both scattered and primary γ-rays emitted from the body lack directionality. The scatter radiation, however, tends to be less energetic, and therefore can be filtered out electronically. Scatter radiation is usually less pronounced in tomographic imaging (e.g. CT and SPECT). In ultrasonography, refraction, or bending, of sound waves as they cross tissue interfaces in the body causes spatial distortions in the image rather than background noise.

Under certain circumstances, statistical fluctuations in the number of photons that reach the receptor become a significant source of image noise. This effect, known as quantum mottle, is most problematic in digital subtraction angiography (DSA), fluoroscopy, CT and scintigraphy, but can also be significant in radiography using highly sensitive intensifying screens and fast film. Quantum mottle can be reduced by increasing the exposure (i.e. the number of photons striking the receptor).

Nonuniformity of the receptor itself can also be a source of image

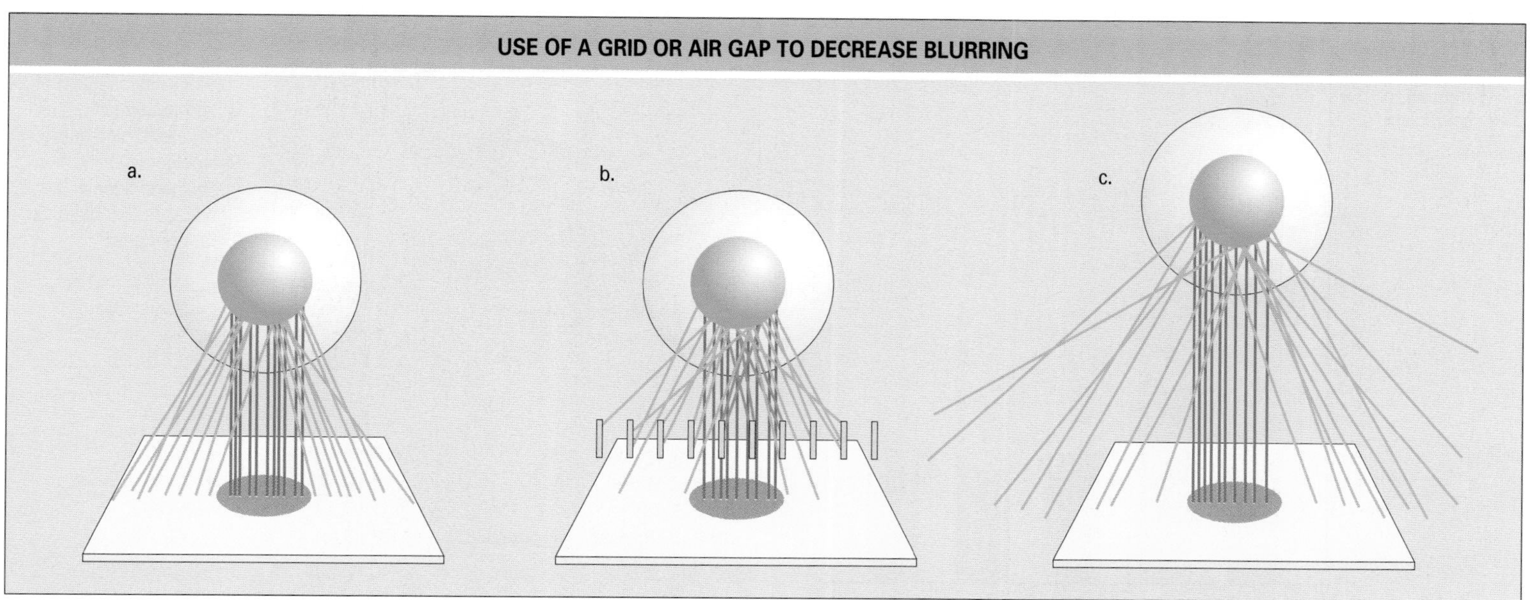

Fig. 14.7 Use of a grid or air gap to decrease blurring. Obliquely oriented scatter radiation adds noise to an image (a). A grid placed between the patient and the receptor filters out the scatter radiation, thus decreasing image noise (b). Moving the receptor away from the patient (i.e. introducing an air gap) allows oblique scatter radiation to miss the receptor and thus also reduces image noise (c).

noise. This can be significant with some scintigraphy cameras. However, modern radiographic film–screen combinations are so uniform that receptor noise is rarely a problem.

RADIOGRAPHY (X-RAY TRANSMISSION IMAGING)

BASIC PRINCIPLES

Radiography is a generic term for any imaging technique based on the transmission of X-rays through the body, including fluoroscopy and CT. However, the term is generally used for plain radiography. X-rays are a form of electromagnetic radiation similar to visible light but of sufficiently high energy to penetrate tissue. The higher the energy of the X-ray (measured in keV), the greater its tissue penetration. As X-rays pass through the body, they are variably attenuated by the different tissues depending on a number of factors: the thickness of the tissues, the physical characteristics (density, atomic number) of the tissues and the energy of the X-ray photons. Radiographic images are created by the transmitted X-rays that reach the imaging receptor. In plain radiography, the receptor is the film–screen combination. In fluoroscopy, the receptor is the X-ray image intensifier; in CT, it is an array of ionization chambers or scintillation detectors.

Differential attenuation of X-ray photons by different tissues is the basis for contrast on the radiographic image. As X-rays pass through tissue they are attenuated by two principal mechanisms: photoelectric absorption and Compton scattering. Photoelectric absorption completely removes photons from the X-ray beam, whereas Compton scattering deflects photons into a random course. This scattered radiation carries no useful information and is a cause of noise (e.g. film 'fog'). Scattered photons must therefore be filtered out before reaching the receptor either by placing a grid or a collimator in front of the receptor or by introducing an air gap large enough to allow most of the scattered photons simply to miss the receptor (Fig. 14.7).

Photoelectric absorption is most pronounced with low-energy X-ray imaging (Fig. 14.8) and in tissues with high atomic number and physical density. At moderate to high X-ray energies (>60keV) – and for most clinical applications – Compton scattering is the chief mechanism of X-ray attenuation and increases with the physical density of tissue. Since bone is around twice as dense as most other tissues, contrast between bone and adjacent soft tissue is relatively high on radiographs obtained with either high or low X-ray energy. Contrast is particularly high on low-energy images because of the additional contribution of photoelectric absorption. However, except for the small difference in density between fat and other soft tissues, contrast among soft tissues is generally poor with high-energy techniques. This contrast can be increased by lowering the X-ray energy and harnessing tissue differences in atomic number. However, greater X-ray absorption translates into increased radiation exposure for the patient, and in most cases the improvement in soft-tissue contrast is still insufficient to delineate important structures such as the articular cartilage, synovium and ligaments.

Radiographic contrast material typically contains iodine or barium, both of which have very high atomic numbers and therefore strongly attenuate X-rays. Barium is added to methylmethacrylate used in arthroplasty to opacify this cement. This permits the detection of small radiolucent separations that form between the opaque cement and adjacent bone or metal during biomechanical loosening. Iodine-containing contrast material injected into a joint during arthrography opacifies the synovial cavity to delineate the surface of articular structures, such as the hyaline cartilage, menisci and cruciate ligaments. Intravascular administration of iodinated contrast material opacifies vessel lumens and is the basis for angiography. However, tissue opacification is generally too mild to be detected by conventional radiography. It must be remembered that iodinated contrast material can be toxic to certain organs, particularly the kidneys, and carries a mild risk of systemic reaction, which on rare occasions can be life threatening. The risk is lower with intra-articular administration, but is still present.

Radiographic film is composed of a thin emulsion composed of a gelatin matrix impregnated with silver halide crystals and layered over a polyester backing (Fig. 14.9). Exposure of the silver halide crystals to appropriate wavelengths of X-ray and/or visible light creates a latent image in the emulsion that is then amplified with the developer. Excess unexposed silver halide crystals are subsequently washed away and the film is fixed. To maintain image sharpness, the emulsion layer needs to be as thin as possible and to cover only one side of the film (single-emulsion film). To minimize patient exposure, it is also important that the film be highly sensitive or 'fast'. Film speed (sensitivity) can be improved by flattening the halide crystals and aligning them parallel to the surface of the film. Even with this, however, relatively high exposures are necessary to achieve sufficient image quality. Additional sensitivity is gained by adding an intensifying screen to the receptor system.

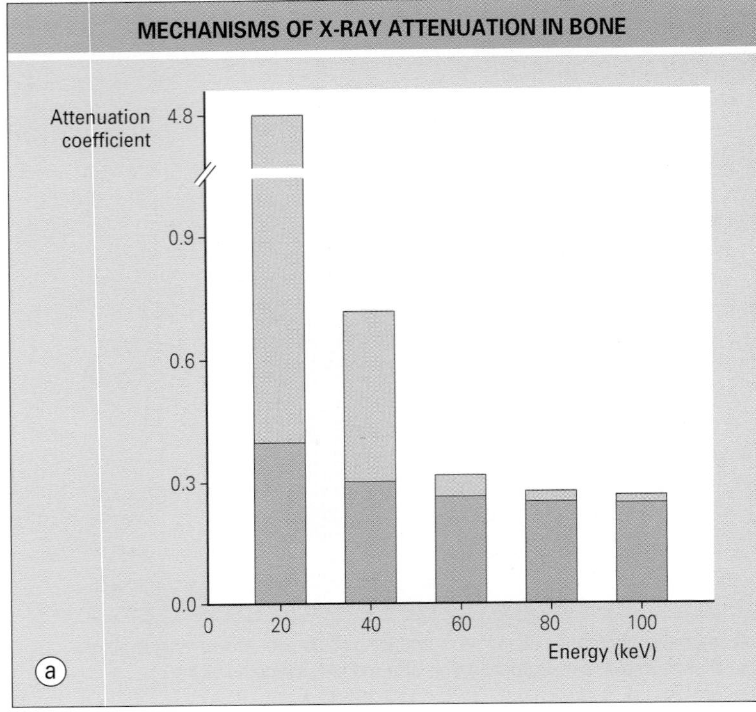

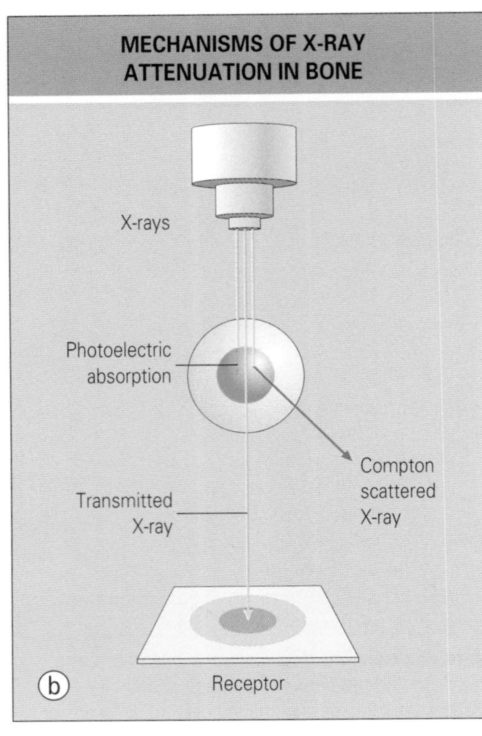

Fig. 14.8 Mechanisms of X-ray attenuation in bone. Compton scatter (purple bars) is the dominant mechanism of X-ray attenuation at moderate to high energies. Photoelectric absorption (green bars) adds a significant contribution at lower energies.

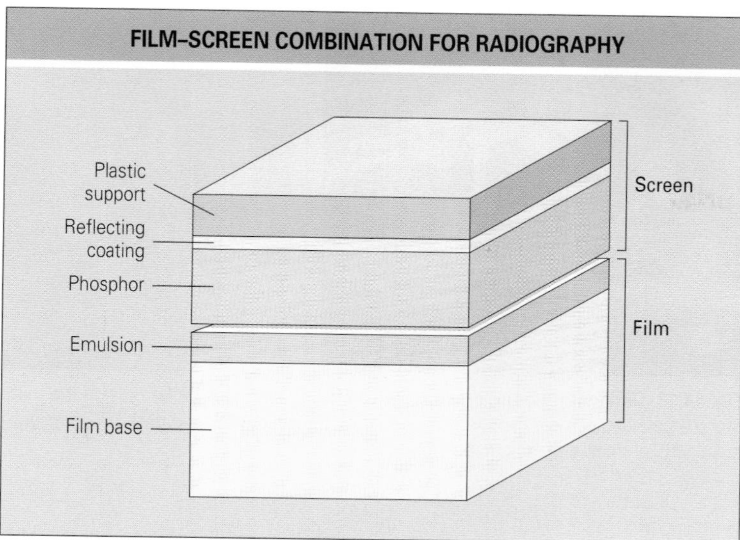

Fig. 14.9 **Film–screen combination for radiography.**

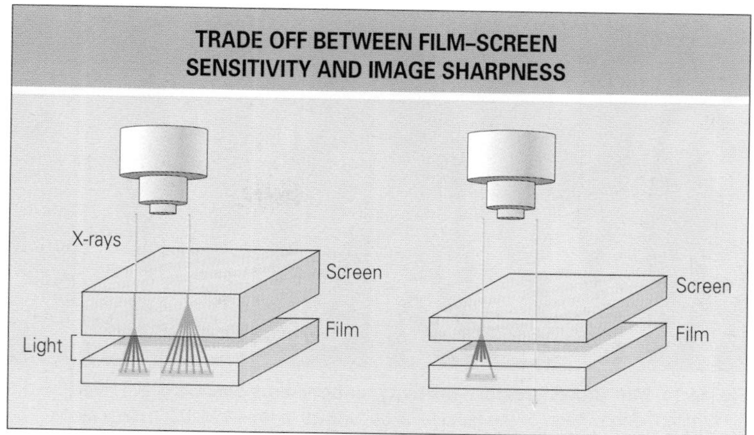

Fig. 14.10 Trade off between film–screen sensitivity and image sharpness. The thick screen on the left absorbs more X-rays than the thin screen on the right, and is therefore more sensitive (fast). However, many of the X-rays (yellow) are converted into light (purple) farther from the film, which allows greater lateral spread of the divergent light rays and consequent blurring of the radiographic image.

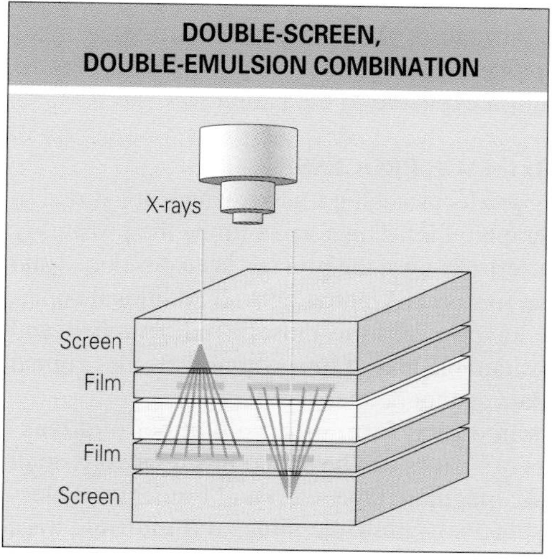

Fig. 14.11 Double-screen, double-emulsion combination. Double-emulsion film is more sensitive (fast) but allows more divergence of the light between emulsions and therefore produces images with more blurring.

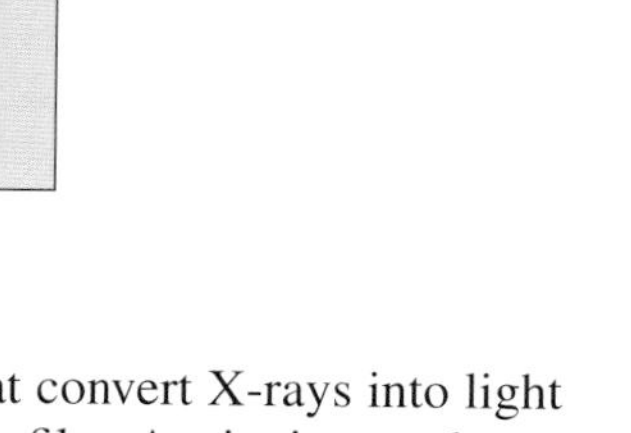

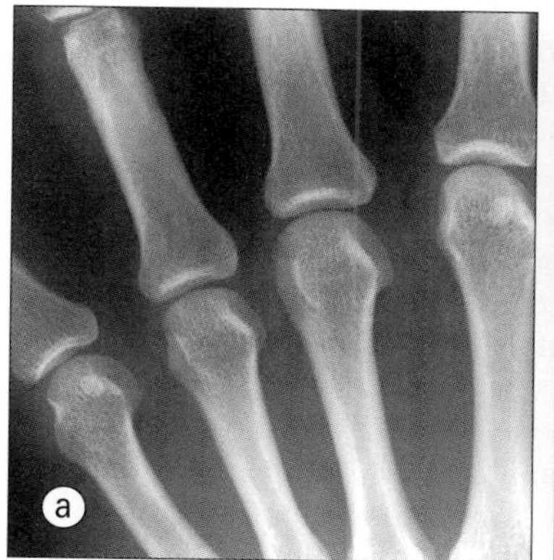

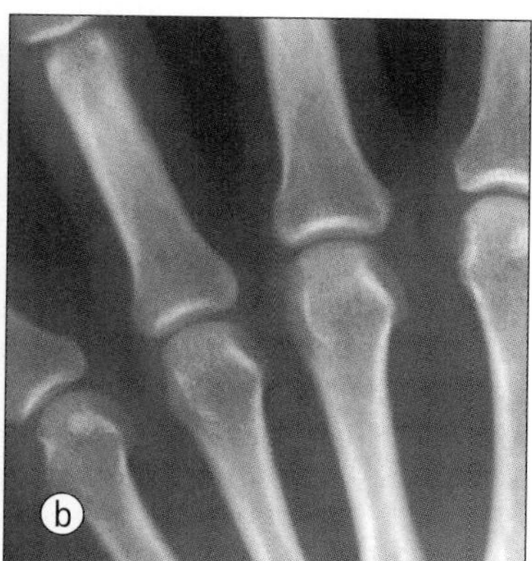

Fig. 14.12 High-quality single-emulsion, single-screen radiography. Radiograph of the hand shows less blurring with single-emulsion, single-screen film (a) than with double-screen, double-emulsion film (b), although 30-fold greater exposure is necessary in the former case.

Intensifying screens contain phosphors that convert X-rays into light that more efficiently exposes the underlying film. Again, image sharpness is maximized by using thin single-screen systems. The phosphor should thus be as efficient as possible (Fig. 14.10). Rare-earth phosphors (e.g. lanthanum, gadolinium) are optimal in this respect.

Accordingly, high-efficiency, single-screen, single-emulsion film–screen combinations or single-emulsion film without any screen are preferred when high-quality radiography is essential, as in the setting of a therapeutic trial of a potential antiarthritic agent (Figs 14.11 & 14.12). For routine clinical radiography, however, double-screen, double-emulsion film–screen systems are often used because of their greater overall sensitivity, despite the increased noise and geometric unsharpness associated with their use.

RADIOGRAPHY: RELATIVE STRENGTHS AND LIMITATIONS

Strengths	Limitations
High contrast and resolution for cortical and trabecular bone Widely available Inexpensive	Superimposition of overlying structures Poor soft-tissue contrast Radiation exposure

Fig. 14.13 Radiography: relative strengths and limitations.

STRENGTHS AND LIMITATIONS

Radiography is the oldest imaging modality and there is considerable experience with its use. It is also the least expensive and most widely available imaging technique (Fig. 14.13), and offers higher spatial resolution than any other modality, providing extremely high contrast for cortical and trabecular bone. One important limitation of radiography is its projectional viewing perspective. Projection of three-dimensional anatomy onto a two-dimensional film results in morphologic distortion and superimposition of overlapping structures, which can conceal even large abnormalities. Nondisplaced fracture lines are easily obscured in a haystack of linear densities on a radiographic image, and erosions viewed en face can be extremely challenging to delineate for even the most experienced eyes (see Figs 14.14 & 14.15). This can be improved somewhat by obtaining additional views of the anatomy, although this does not always solve the problem entirely. Despite a lower inherent spatial resolution, CT and MRI have been shown to be approximately twice as sensitive as radiography for detecting osseous erosions in rheumatoid arthritis (RA) or osteophytes in osteoarthritis (OA).

Another approach to dealing with the problem of superimposition is stereoradiography. In this technique, two images of the structure of interest are obtained at slightly different angles to simulate binocular vision. The two stereo images are then viewed side by side either with a specially designed pair of goggles containing compensatory mirrors, or the eyes crossed to fuse the two images.

A more serious limitation of conventional radiography is its relatively poor sensitivity for trabecular bone loss. As much as 30–50% of

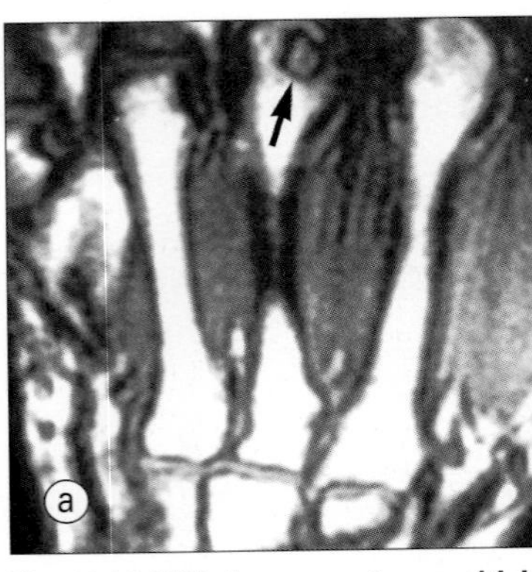
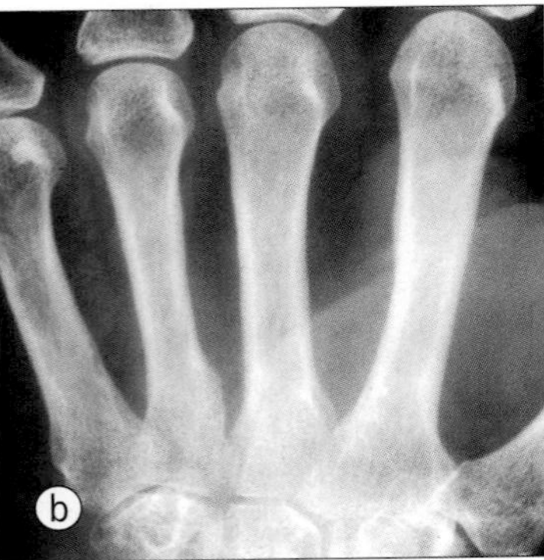

Fig. 14.14 MRI shows greater sensitivity for bone erosions. Coronal T1-weighted 3D gradient-echo image of the hand (a) acquired with a low-field (0.2T) dedicated-extremity MRI system (Artoscan) shows a large erosion (arrow) in the metacarpal head that is not visible on a radiograph of the same region (b).

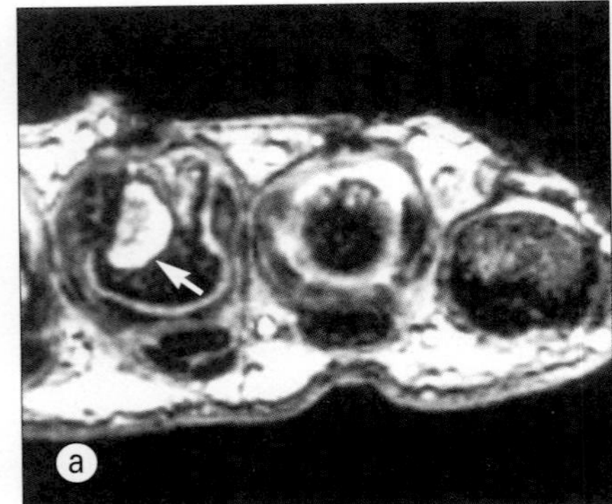
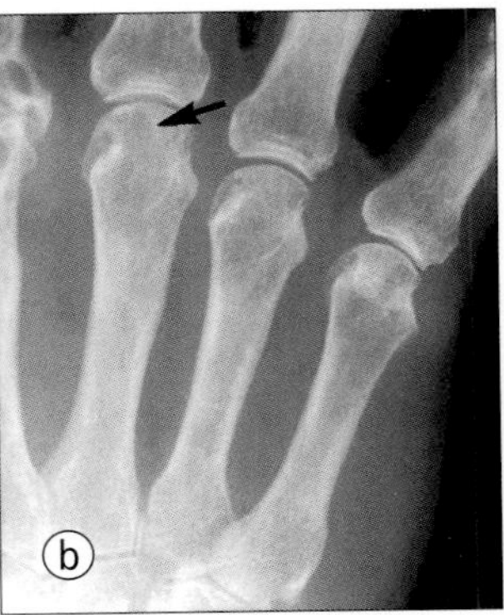

Fig. 14.15 Delineating bone erosions with MRI. A large erosion (arrows) in the third metacarpal head is more clearly delineated with transverse T2*-weighted 3D gradient-echo MRI (a) than with radiography (b).

trabecular bone must be removed before the change becomes perceptible on conventional radiographs. High-detail radiography using a small focal spot, geometric magnification and a single-emulsion film without any screen offers at least a partial solution to the problem, but it is not as widely available and often still leaves some uncertainties.

However, the most important limitation of conventional radiography is its relatively poor contrast for soft tissues that are not calcified or fatty. This lowers the sensitivity of radiography for detecting changes in the marrow cavity of the bones (e.g. stress fracture or nondisplaced insufficiency, osteonecrosis, osteomyelitis and infiltrating neoplasm), as well as for evaluating injuries to the soft tissues themselves. Radiography thus provides only a keyhole view of the complex disease process affecting the arthritic joint as a whole organ. Radiography cannot directly visualize the articular cartilage, inflamed synovial tissue, joint effusion, bone marrow edema, intra-articular menisci, labra, ligaments or periarticular tendons and muscles. Indirect evaluation of these structures through the displacement of intra-articular fat pads (Fig. 14.16) or by narrowing of the distance between two opposing subcortical cortexes viewed in tangent can be helpful, but is relatively unreliable unless special techniques are used.

One technique that can improve the evaluation of intra-articular structures, such as the articular cartilage and menisci of the knee, is arthrography. In this technique, radiopaque contrast material is injected into the joint, occasionally in combination with air (double-contrast arthrography), to delineate the surfaces of these structures. This can be helpful, but is subject to all of the problems typically associated with projectional imaging. Arthrography of the knee, for example, necessitates numerous different views and uncomfortable manipulation of a sometimes already painful joint in order to ensure complete coverage of all important structures. Moreover, intra-articular injection is a mildly invasive procedure, and fluoroscopy increases significantly the degree of radiation exposure to the patient.

DIGITAL IMAGING AND IMAGE PROCESSING

Conventional radiography produces analog images which are stored in hard-copy form on radiographic film. This format limits the possibility of modifying image characteristics once the film has been developed and requires considerable space to store the radiographs. If additional copies of the images are wanted, the original films must be radiographed, and this is associated with considerable loss of image quality. If the original films are lost, the image data cannot be recovered.

Storage of image data in digital form offers a number of advantages. First, large numbers of images can be stored in a relatively small space (e.g. on optical disk, magnetic tape, etc.) and transmitted electronically over great distances to multiple sites, and multiple hard copies can be generated as needed. Digital image data can also be processed by computer to alter the characteristics of the image (e.g. noise reduction, contrast modification, edge enhancement and image subtraction; Fig. 14.17), as well as to obtain quantitative information, such as the distance between morphologic structures (e.g. the joint space between apposing articular cortexes), or the mean pixel value within a specified ROI. More sophisticated morphometric analyses, such as determination of the volume or 3D geometry of an anatomic structure are also possible.

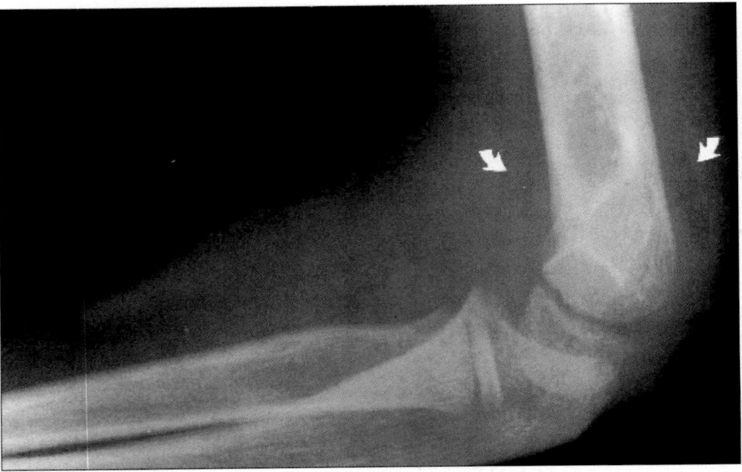

Fig. 14.16 Displacement of fat pads in the elbow by joint effusion. Lucencies (arrows) flanking the distal humerus on the lateral projection of the elbow represent intra-articular but extrasynovial fat pads displaced by joint effusion. This is the only abnormality visible on this radiograph of a nondisplaced supracondylar fracture of the humerus.

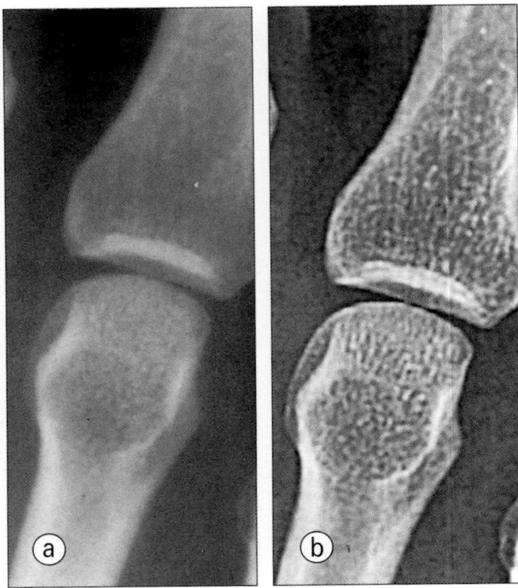

Fig. 14.17 Digital radiography: edge enhancement. Edge-enhanced digital image (a) of the second metacarpophalangeal joint shows considerably greater detail than the original digital image (b) (pixel size was 100μm).

Digital images consist of a matrix of pixels (picture elements), each with a numerical value. The matrix is in multiples of two because of the binary nature of digital systems: 64 × 64, 128 × 128, 256 × 256, etc. Analog image data, on radiographs, for example, can be converted into digital form with an electronic device called an analog-to-digital converter (ADC). This device converts each line of video image into a row of pixels, measures the brightness or signal level of each pixel and converts it into a digital number stored in computer memory. These data can then be processed and archived in a variety of ways, but for viewing the images must first be converted (or in the case of digitized radiographs, reconverted) to analog form using a digital-to-video converter (DVE). This image is then adjusted by windowing (see below). Computed image processing is the basis not only for digital radiography, but also for such powerful tools as CT, real-time ultrasonography and MRI.

COMPUTED TOMOGRAPHY

BASIC PRINCIPLES

Unlike the single-step process of projectional imaging, image formation in CT is a multi-step process in which multiple planar projections are mathematically combined to produce cross-sectional images (tomogram). This is fundamentally the same approach that is used in real-time ultrasound and MRI. As in radiography, X-rays are the energy source in CT although a pencil or fan-shaped beam is used to restrict the exposure to a single slice. Multiple exposures of this slice are acquired from different angles, and the fractional transmission is measured using electronic X-ray detectors (ionization chambers or scintillation detectors). Signals from the X-ray detectors are then digitized by the ADCs and transferred to the computer for image reconstruction. The technique used to reconstruct the CT image is called filtered back projection (Fig. 14.18).

Like MRI and real-time ultrasonography, CT images are structured in an array of individual picture elements or 'pixels' (Fig. 14.19). The size of each pixel is determined by the field of view and the matrix size. For example, an image with a 20cm field of view divided into a matrix of 512 × 256 has pixels measuring 391μm × 781μm. This determines the in-plane resolution of the image. The slice thickness, or through-plane resolution, is determined by the beam width, and typically ranges from 1.0mm to 10mm. The pixel size multiplied by the slice thickness gives the voxel size, which is the fundamental element of the CT image. Each voxel in a CT image is assigned a CT number corresponding to the average linear attenuation coefficient of all structures within the voxel. This value is normalized to the attenuation coefficient of water and expressed in Hounsfield units ranging from –1000 to +1000. Typical values are air, –1000; fat, –100; water and other non-hemorrhagic fluid collections (urine, bile, lymph and cerebrospinal fluid), 0; soft tissues, +10; fresh blood, +50; dense bone, +1000.

There are 2000 different levels in this scheme. However, since the human eye can perceive only 16–20 gray levels, it is necessary to combine or 'bin' these CT image data. Exactly how many CT numbers are combined in each gray level is determined by window settings selected by the user to optimize the visibility of those structures which are of greatest diagnostic importance. These settings can be adjusted freely while viewing the images on a monitor, but must be specified before filming hard copies of the images. The window width defines the range of CT values (e.g. 500) converted into the full gray scale, or brightness range. The window level determines the position of the center of the window along the CT value scale. Pixels above the upper window limit are depicted as white while those below the lower limit are black; those in between span the full scale of gray. Decreasing the window width increases the contrast between structures that are relatively close in CT number. However, this also eliminates contrast between more tissues with CT numbers beyond the upper or lower limits of the window (Fig. 14.20).

Converting an image into an array of pixels is inherently blurring since all structures within a pixel (or voxel) are reduced to a single gray scale value, i.e. there is no detail within a pixel. This effect is known as partial-volume averaging, and is fundamental to all digital images. The larger the voxel, the greater the number of structures averaged and, accordingly, the lower the image detail. Reducing voxel size increases spatial resolution, but also increases the relative image noise. Image noise is defined as the standard deviation of pixel numbers in the background or a water standard. Clarity of image detail ultimately depends

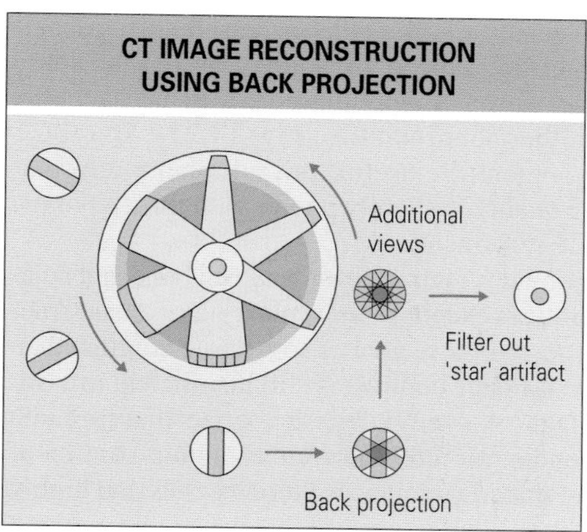

Fig. 14.18 CT image reconstruction using back projection. Back projection combines CT density profiles from several different projections to generate a cross-sectional image of the anatomy.

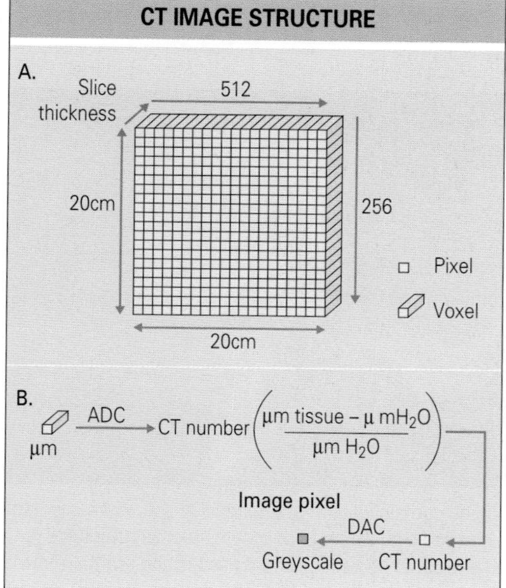

Fig. 14.19 CT image structure. The CT image is an array of voxels (a). Voxel dimensions are defined by the field of view, the matrix size, and slice thickness. Attenuation in a voxel is converted to a CT number normalized to the attenuation of water using an ADC and stored in computer memory (b). The CT numbers must be converted to greyscale values with a digital–to–analogue converter (DAC) for the image to be viewed on a monitor or filmed.

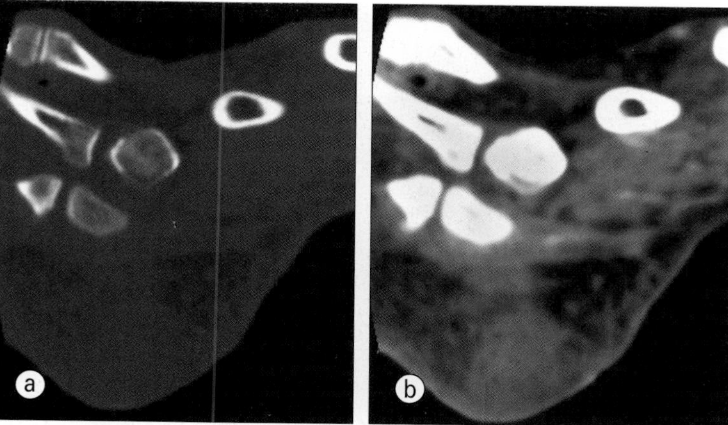

Fig. 14.20 Windowing the CT image. CT image of the foot filmed using 'bone windowing' optimally delineates bone morphology but shows poor contrast between the soft tissues in the same region (a). Decreasing the upper gray scale threshold for CT attenuation increases soft-tissue contrast (b). However, in doing this, bone attenuation values above the threshold are assigned the same maximal gray scale value and thus show no contrast.

CT: RELATIVE STRENGTHS AND LIMITATIONS	
Strengths	Limitations
Cross-sectional imaging	Limited planes of section (axial)
High bone contrast	Relatively poor soft-tissue contrast
Improved soft-tissue contrast	Radiation exposure
	Expensive

Fig. 14.21 CT: relative strengths and limitations.

on the balance between voxel size and noise. Image noise is particularly problematic in visualizing low-contrast tissue differences. Noise on a CT image can be reduced by increasing the exposure settings although this increases patient exposure to radiation as well. Digital filtration can also be used to reduce noise although this adds some blur. Finally, noise can be reduced by widening the window width.

STRENGTHS AND LIMITATIONS

The greatest advantage of CT over conventional radiography is its tomographic nature (Fig. 14.21). This eliminates the spatial distortions and magnification associated with projectional radiography, but more importantly obviates the problem of overlapping structures obscuring important findings. Nevertheless, CT is relatively restricted in terms of the planes that it can support. The CT sections must be transverse to the bore of the gantry (i.e. axial). This limits tomography of the chest, abdomen and pelvis to the transverse anatomic plane. In some instances, however, the structure of interest (e.g. the wrist or ankle) is small enough to be positioned in the opening of the gantry in such a way as to allow sagittal, coronal or oblique planes of section. This is true of the head and the distal upper and lower extremities, but not the spine, shoulder, hip or knee.

Contiguous axial images can be reformated into different planes (Fig. 14.22), but reformatted images are generally of inferior quality for a number of reasons. Firstly, spatial resolution is generally highest in the original plane of section (i.e. axial), as the through-plane resolution is limited by the slice thickness. The minimum slice thickness used clinically is 1mm, although thicknesses of 3–5mm are most common. Thick slices produce a so called 'pixely' appearance to reformated images. It is important therefore to acquire very thin contiguous slices if a need for multiplanar reformating is anticipated. Thin slices, of course, create their own problems. The use of very thin slices may pose a problem in terms of anatomic coverage. To cover a 5cm region of the cervical spine at 1mm requires a total of 50 slices. Although this is at the upper limit of reasonable, to cover the thoracic or lumbar spine in this manner is not feasible. Moreover, thin slices

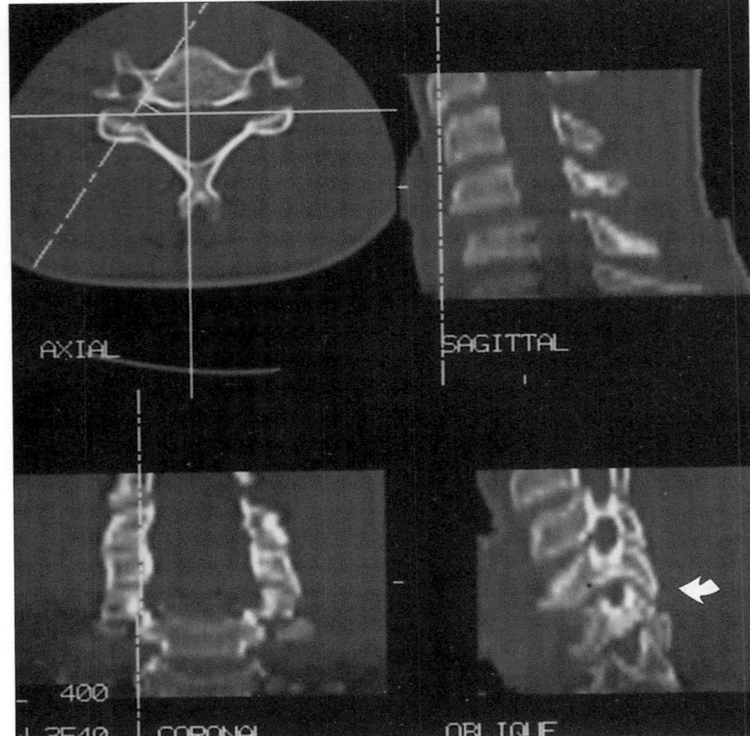

Fig. 14.22 Multiplanar reformation of CT images. Oblique sagittal reformation from contiguous transverse CT images of the cervical spine shows narrowing of the C5–C6 neural foramen (arrow). Sagittal and coronal reformations are also shown.

require greater patient exposure to offset the increased noise associated with their use. Also, movement by the patient during the study can produce a shift in the position of individual slices in the stack that can mimic a fracture or other abnormalities (Fig. 14.23). Spiral CT offers greater speed and is therefore useful for multiplanar reformations. However, the image quality is slightly poorer with this technique than with conventional CT reformations.

Like radiography, CT provides high contrast between bone and adjacent tissues and, accordingly, is excellent for evaluating osseous structures. Additionally, CT offers slightly greater soft-tissue contrast than does radiography. However, image contrast is still insufficient to visualize the articular cartilage or synovial tissue, or to discriminate between tendonitis and tendon rupture. Intravenous administration of iodine-containing contrast material enhances blood vessels and highly vascularized soft tissues on CT, but in general this has not been found to be as useful in musculoskeletal applications as it has been for evaluating the brain, chest, abdomen and pelvis. Direct injection of

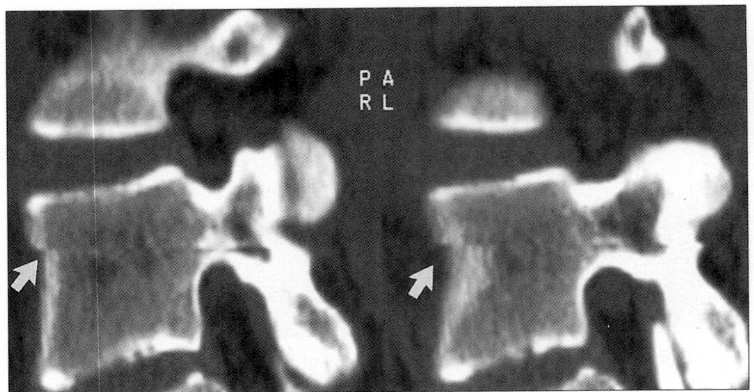

Fig. 14.23 Misregistration in reformated CT images. High-resolution sagittal reformation of the lumbar spine shows a misregistration artifact through the vertebral body (arrows). Such artifacts are caused when the patient moves slightly between slices during the examination, and can be misinterpreted as a fracture.

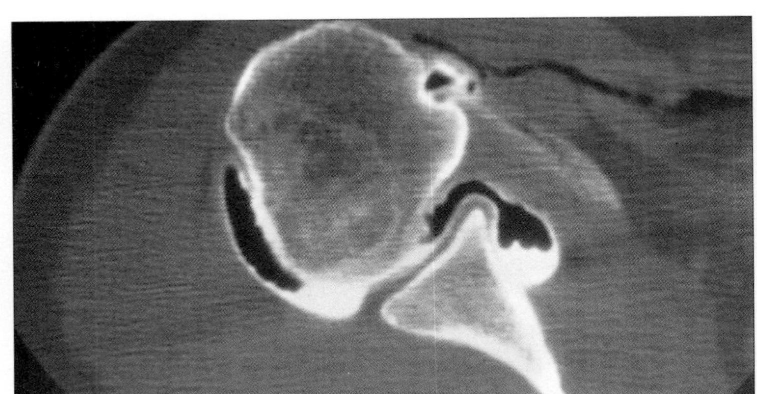
Fig. 14.24 CT arthrography. Iodine-containing contrast material and air were injected into the shoulder joint under fluoroscopic guidance to delineate articular structures, such as the glenoid labrum, that are isodense with adjacent tissues and are therefore otherwise difficult to discriminate.

iodinated contrast and/or air into a joint (CT arthrography), on the other hand, can separate otherwise isodense intra-articular structures and delineate their surfaces (Fig. 14.24). In the shoulder CT arthrography has been found to be useful for evaluating labrocapsular structures in patients with joint instability, but has not been used with any great frequency in other joints. Axial CT arthrography of the knee can delineate the articular cartilage over the patella, but offers poor visualization of the femorotibial structures, including the cartilage, menisci and cruciate ligaments, on axial images. Sagittal and coronal reformations are better for viewing these components of the joint, but are limited by poor spatial resolution. Finally, this approach reveals only the surfaces of these structures; it does not disclose intrasubstance changes that may precede gross morphologic disruption. As is discussed below, MRI is the optimal technique for imaging hyaline cartilage, synovium, menisci, ligaments and tendons.

RADIONUCLIDE SCINTIGRAPHY (EMISSION IMAGING)

BASIC PRINCIPLES

Scintigraphy offers a unique approach to imaging. Unlike other modalities which provide primarily morphologic information about the body, scintigraphy has the capacity to probe the physiologic and biochemical attributes of tissues through differential uptake of certain radiopharmaceuticals. Also, changes in radiopharmaceutical uptake over time offer information about the dynamics of these processes in tissues, and the technique can be used not only for medical imaging but also for radiation therapy with radiopharmaceuticals that emit high-energy β particles.

Numerous radionuclides can be used for scintigraphic imaging (e.g. ^{67}Ga, ^{111}In, ^{123}I, ^{131}I, ^{133}Xe, ^{169}Yb, ^{201}Tl). However, ^{m99}Tc is particularly well suited for the purpose. Indeed, it is as though this radionuclide were specifically designed by nature to serve medicine. The γ-radiation emitted by ^{m99}Tc is of sufficiently high energy (140keV) to penetrate the body, but low enough to be absorbed by the scintillation crystal. The half-life of 6h is adequate for synthesis, delivery and imaging of the radiopharmaceutical, but short enough to keep patient radiation exposure relatively low (94% is gone within 24h). Moreover, ^{m99}Tc is easily chelated to various different compounds that affect its biodistribution. For example, diethylenetraminepenta-acetic acid (DTPA) directs ^{m99}Tc to the kidney where it is readily excreted, whereas ^{m99}Tc-pyrophosphate localizes in infarcted tissue and inflamed synovium, ^{m99}Tc-methylene or hydromethylene diphosphonate targets bone and ^{m99}Tc-sulfur colloid accumulates in reticuloendothelial cell-containing tissues such as liver, spleen and bone marrow. Monoclonal antibodies are a particularly intriguing class of chelates for more selective tissue targeting.

To generate a scintigraphic image, primary γ-rays emitted from the body must be detected and spatially defined. The receptor for scintigraphy is a crystal most commonly composed of thallium-activated sodium iodide (NaI[Tl]) and coupled to numerous photomultiplier tubes; γ-rays are absorbed by the scintillation crystal and converted into visible light photons, which are in turn converted into electrons by the photomultiplier tubes. The magnitude of the amplified voltage pulse produced is proportional to the light intensity, which is in turn proportional to the energy of the absorbed γ-rays. Scattered γ-rays and background radiation tend to be of lower energy than primary γ-rays, and can therefore be filtered out, or rejected, from the image to increase the signal-to-noise ratio. Scatter radiation is more of a problem in imaging photopenic, or 'cold', lesions than 'hot' lesions. If two different radionuclides are used simultaneously, image contrast depends on the extent to which their energy spectra differ.

Scintigraphy tends to produce images with less detail and more noise than other modalities. This is primarily because relatively fewer photons are used to generate scintigraphic images. Quantum mottle (random distribution of photons across the image) is thus the major cause of noise in scintigraphy. As with other modalities, quantum mottle is reduced by increasing the number of photons, or counts, in the image. This, however, increases the imaging time and the opportunity for patient motion blurring. Thicker crystals capture more photons and are, therefore, more sensitive. However, receptor blurring due to diffusion of light in the scintillation crystal is also proportional to the crystal thickness. This compromise between receptor sensitivity and image blur is analogous to that described above for intensifying screens in conventional radiography.

Conventional scintigraphic images are projectional, and therefore show morphologic distortion and superimposition (Fig. 14.25). Using a technique analogous to that of CT, single photon emission

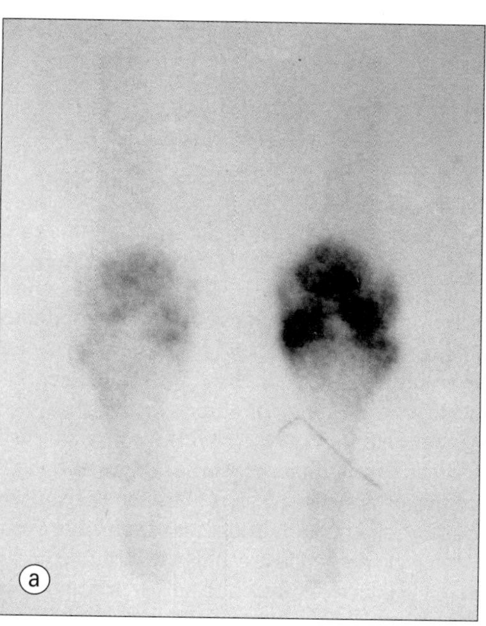

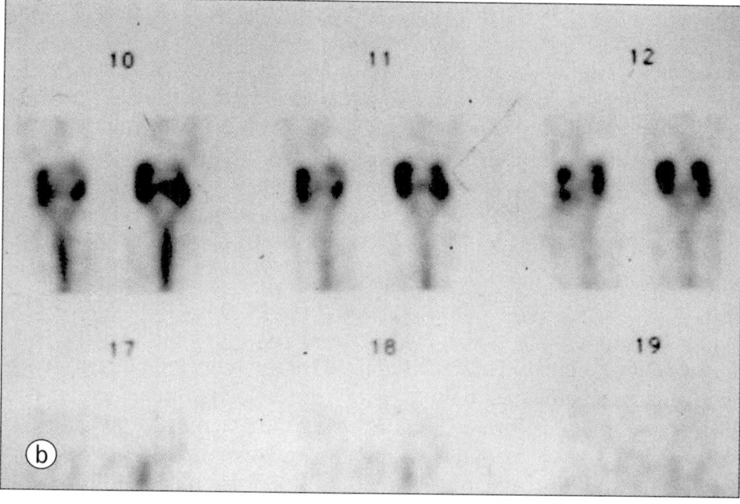

Fig. 14.25 Projectional and tomographic (SPECT) scintigraphy. Frontal projection bone scan of both knees of a patient with a previous partial left medial meniscectomy shows increased uptake in the medial and lateral femoral condyles of the left knee (a). SPECT is better for localizing these changes but requires several images to cover the same anatomy (b).

SCINTIGRAPHY: RELATIVE STRENGTHS AND LIMITATIONS	
Strengths	**Limitations**
Whole-body coverage	Very poor spatial resolution
Highly sensitive to bone pathology	Relatively nonspecific
Physiologic imaging	Time demanding for patient
Tissue /process targeted	Radiation exposure
	Expensive

Fig. 14.26 Scintigraphy: relative strengths and limitations.

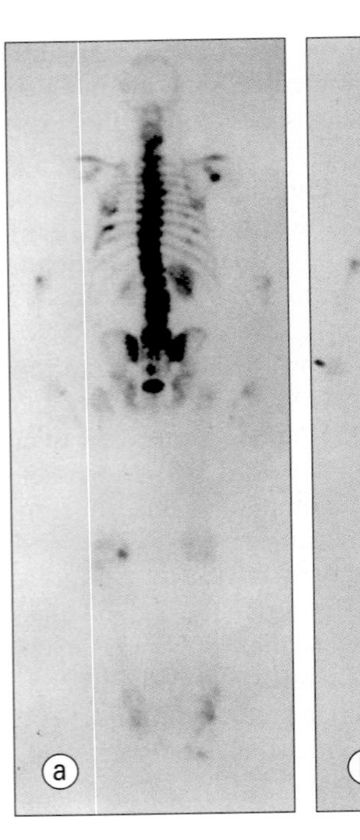

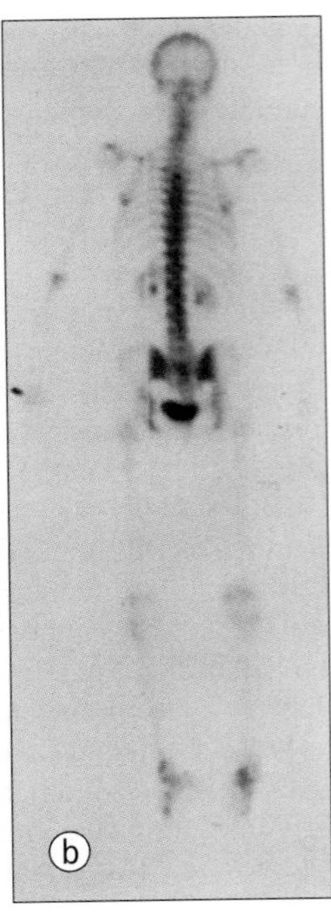

Fig. 14.27 Whole body scintigraphy. Posterior projection whole body bone scan of a patient with metastatic prostate cancer shows multiple foci of increased uptake in the spine and several ribs (a). Abnormal uptake in the right shoulder and left knee may be related to degenerative changes rather than metastatic disease, and must therefore be correlated with radiography or MRI. A normal bone scan is shown for comparison (b).

COMPARATIVE COSTS OF JOINT IMAGING	
Radiography	**Area**
Knee	
(3 views + weight-bearing or patellofemoral)	1
with arthrography	4
C-spine (4 views + flexion / extension)	2
L-spine (4 views + flexion / extension)	2
CT	
Knee	7
with sagittal / coronal reformations	11
Scintigraphy*	
Single joint	4
Multiple joints	8
Whole body	6
with tomography (SPECT)	8
Triple phase	7
MRI†	
Conventional whole body	14

* Values are for imaging a single joint and include radiopharmaceutical administration.
† Values are for conventional whole-body MRI. Dedicated extremity MRI is less expensive but, at present, Medicare reimbursements do not distinguish between the different types of MRI.

Fig. 14.28 Comparative costs of joint imaging. Values are normalized to the cost of a three-view radiographic series of the knee, and estimated from the 1995 Medicare reimbursement rates (technical and professional components) for California (area 5) in US dollars.

tomography (SPECT) can be performed with a rotating scintillation camera. The resulting cross-sectional images obviate the problems of morphologic distortion and overlapping structures (Fig. 14.25).

STRENGTHS AND LIMITATIONS

The principal advantage of scintigraphy over other imaging modalities is its ability to identify tissues or organs with abnormal physiologic or biochemical properties (Fig. 14.26). The most common scintigraphic technique for evaluating musculoskeletal disease is the bone scan, which uses ^{99m}Tc chelated to methylene diphosphonate (MDP) to target bone. Exactly how this radiopharmaceutical is incorporated into the bone is controversial, but recent studies suggest that ^{99m}Tc and MDP moieties are actually dissociated and incorporated into organic and inorganic phases respectively. Regardless, increased skeletal uptake can be seen at sites of elevated blood flow (increased delivery of tracer) or increased bone metabolism (increased retention of tracer). Both of these processes are affected in a large variety of bone disorders, including trauma, infection, ischemia, neoplasms and arthritis. Accordingly, whereas bone scintigraphy is highly sensitive for these conditions, it is also relatively nonspecific. Foci of increased uptake in the spine, for example, typically require close correlation with radiography or MRI to differentiate metastases from degenerative changes or insufficiency fractures. The high-energy radionuclides ^{99m}Tc-MDP, ^{67}Ga citrate and ^{111}In chloride are more specific markers for the inflammatory compartment of the joint. However, poor spatial resolution with these radionuclides compounded by low target-to-background activity ratios limits their utility, particularly in small joints.

Although projectional imaging has its disadvantages (e.g. obscured anatomic detail), it does enable large areas of anatomy to be depicted in a single image. Scintigraphy is thus a convenient way of surveying the entire skeleton for multifocal processes such as metastatic disease or polyarthritis (Fig. 14.27). Greater anatomic detail is achieved with SPECT, but at the cost of increased numbers of images.

Bone scintigraphy can be time-consuming for the patient, as a lag period of 2 or more hours after the injection of radiotracer may be necessary to achieve acceptable tissue-to-background ratio (i.e. contrast). Scintigraphy also exposes patients to ionizing radiation. The whole body exposure associated with bone scan is approximately equivalent to that of a lumbar spine radiographic series. Finally, bone scintigraphy is a relatively expensive test, costing almost the same as CT (Fig. 14.28).

ULTRASONOGRAPHY (REFLECTION IMAGING)

BASIC PRINCIPLES

Unlike other energy transfer phenomena used for imaging, sound requires a medium through which to propagate a signal. It cannot pass through a vacuum as can X-rays used in radiography or CT, γ-radiation used in scintigraphy or electromagnetic induction used in MRI. Sound waves are simply vibrations passing through matter, yet they can be focused and reflected like light. The human ear can detect sound frequencies between 0.02 and 20kHz. However, ultrasound operates at frequencies of 1–15MHz, and is therefore beyond the range of human hearing.

Sound vibrations used in ultrasonography are produced by a transducer containing a piezoelectric crystal that deforms in the presence of an electric charge. Electric pulses are thus converted by the transducer into ultrasound pulses of a specific frequency. These pulses are conveyed to the body through a gel, enter the body and are attenuated, reflected or scattered by internal structures. Reflected ultrasound pulses that return to the transducer deform the crystal and are reconverted into electrical pulses used to generate the image. The transducer is thus also the receiver.

Each transducer emits sound at only one frequency (the resonant frequency). Higher-frequency waves generate images with greater spatial detail but are attenuated to a greater degree and therefore penetrate tissues over relatively shorter distances (Fig. 14.29). Most clinical systems thus use several different transducers of differing frequencies (typically 3MHz, 5MHz, 7MHz and 10MHz).

When an ultrasound pulse propagating through the body encounters an interface between two substances of differing acoustic impedance, a portion of the pulse is reflected back to the transducer while the remainder continues on. The greater the acoustic impedance mismatch between the two adjacent substances, the greater the magnitude of the reflected pulse. The time required for the reflected pulse to reach the transducer indicates how far away the reflective interface is. The ultrasound image is formed by converting the magnitude of each echo into a gray-scale value, and translating the relative timing between successive echoes into spatial distances. With the aid of high-speed

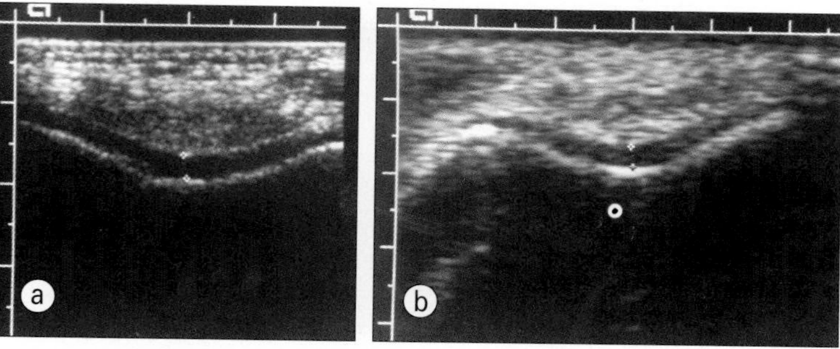

Fig. 14.29 Effect of transducer frequency on ultrasonography of the articular cartilage. Transverse ultrasonography of the knee in flexion shows the articular cartilage over the femoral trochlear groove as a hypoechoic band. The images acquired with a high-frequency (7MHz) transducer (a) show greater spatial resolution than those obtained with a low-frequency (3MHz) transducer (b), although the low-frequency transducers provide deeper tissue penetration.

computers, volleys of closely spaced ultrasound pulses can be used to provide a continuously updated image in so-called 'real time'.

One intriguing quality of ultrasonography is its sensitivity to blood flow. By determining the change in frequency produced by the flowing blood (Doppler effect), the direction and velocity of the flow can be deduced. On state-of-the-art scanners, these parameters can be color coded (e.g. flow towards transducer = blue, flow away from transducer = red) and superimposed on a real-time gray-scale image of the anatomy. The ability to evaluate blood flow raises the possibility of assessing the severity of synovitis in patients with arthritis using Doppler ultrasound[1]. However, only preliminary work has been conducted thus far in this area, and it remains controversial[2].

STRENGTHS AND LIMITATIONS

As with MRI, ultrasonography offers direct multiplanar tomography without any need for image reformating, as would otherwise be necessary with CT (Fig. 14.30). Ultrasonography can also provide images in real time, without any exposure to ionizing radiation. The modality is inexpensive and widely available. It offers relatively good soft-tissue contrast, and is particularly effective at identifying fluid collections such as bursitis and abscesses. However, ultrasound waves cannot penetrate bone. Accordingly, acoustic shadows cast by overlying bones can obscure important articular structures, such as the hyaline articular cartilage, menisci, synovial tissue and intra-articular ligaments (Fig. 14.31). Through the acoustic windows that are available, however, the ultrasonographer can peer into the joint and examine at least portions of these structures.

ULTRASONOGRAPHY: RELATIVE STRENGTHS AND LIMITATIONS

Strengths	Weaknesses
Multiplanar imaging	Bone shadows obscure anatomy
Good soft-tissue contrast	Limited soft-tissue contrast
Excellent for fluid collections	Operator dependent
Widely available and accessible	
No ionizing radiation	

Fig. 14.30 Ultrasonography: relative strengths and limitations.

MAGNETIC RESONANCE IMAGING

Although it has developed only within the past 15 years, MRI has emerged as the imaging modality of choice for a variety of musculoskeletal indications, including meniscal tear, cruciate ligament injury and other internal derangements of joints. The clarity and detail with which MRI depicts cross-sectional anatomy makes interpretation of the images appear deceptively simple. In reality, MRI is a highly sophisticated technology, and while a detailed understanding of quantum physics may not be necessary to view the images, some background knowledge is essential to understand the findings as well as critically to assess conclusions drawn from investigations that employ this technology. The following brief review of basic principles and terminology used in MRI is provided, therefore, to help individuals outside the discipline of radiology take better advantage of the growing number of studies in the literature that use MRI. For the interested reader, there are several excellent books and articles that delve deeper into the physics of MRI and its applications in medicine[3–8].

BASIC PRINCIPLES

Magnetic resonance imaging is based on the natural magnetic behavior of atomic nuclei as they spin about their axes. Although a number of different nuclei (e.g. sodium, phosphorus, hydrogen) could theoretically be used to generate images with MRI, only hydrogen is present in adequate quantities within tissues to be employed for clinical imaging. When the nuclei within a tissue are placed in the very high magnetic field in the bore of an MRI magnet, they show a net tendency to align their nuclear magnetic moments along this static magnetic field (longitudinal magnetization; Fig. 14.32). Exposure of these protons to a second field [radiofrequency (rf) pulse] that rotates and is perpendicular to the original static field of the magnet (90° rf pulse) realigns the protons transversely (transverse magnetization; see Fig.

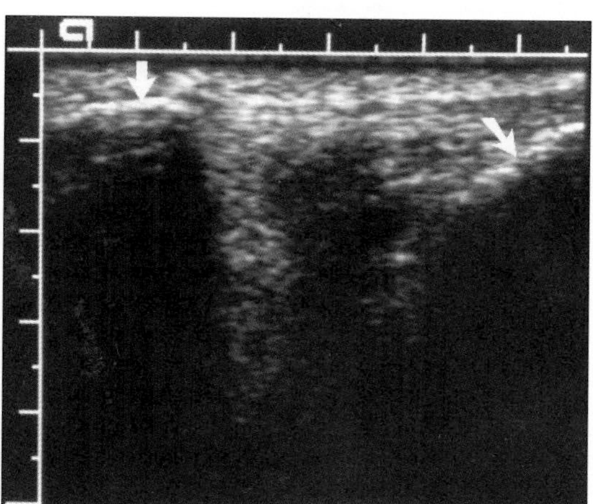

Fig. 14.31 Bone shadowing in ultrasonography of joints. Sagittal sonogram of the knee shows acoustic shadows from the patella (straight arrow) and tibia (oblique arrow) obscuring underlying anatomy.

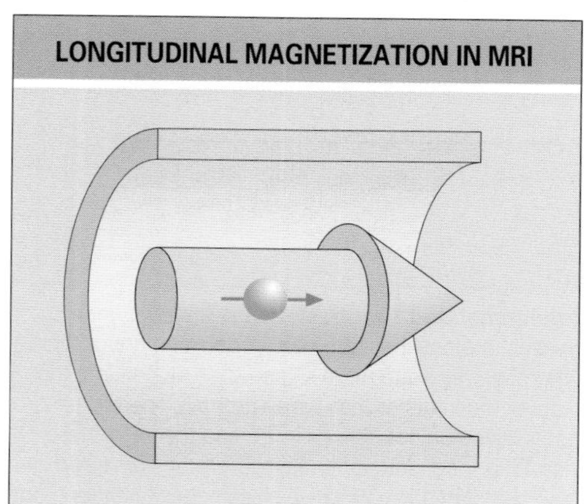

Fig. 14.32 Longitudinal magnetization in MRI. Hydrogen nuclei in tissues placed within the large magnetic field of the MRI magnet align their magnetic moments (small arrow) with the static field (large arrow). This process is called longitudinal magnetization.

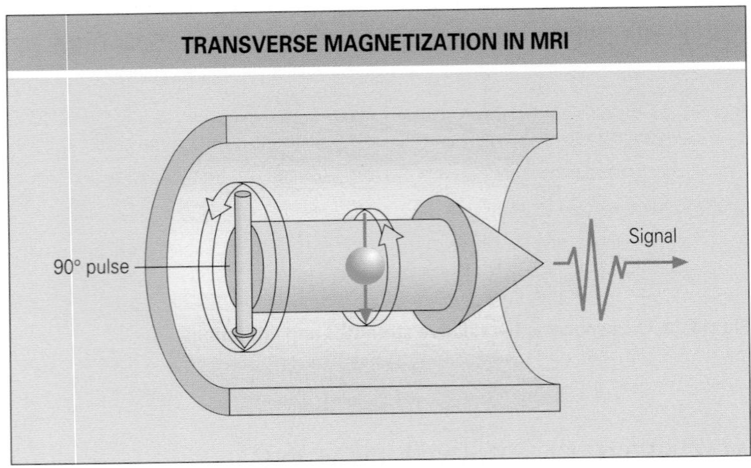

Fig. 14.33 Transverse magnetization in MRI. Exposing the longitudinally magnetized protons to a second oscillating magnetic field realigns the magnetic moments and induces an electrical current in wire coils placed near the patient.

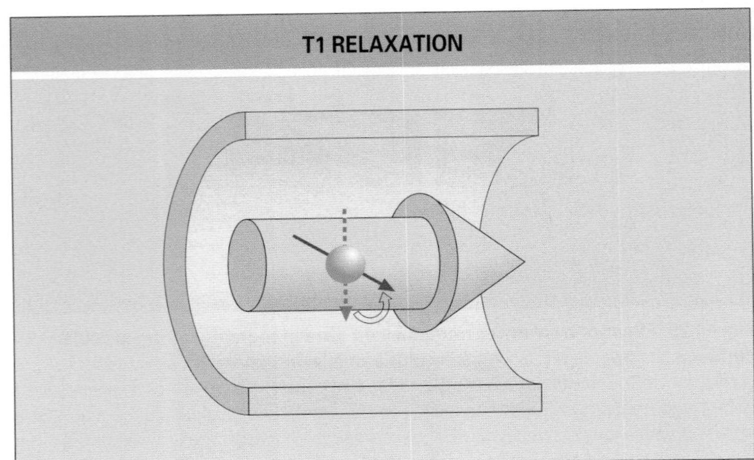

Fig. 14.34 T1 relaxation. Once the transverse field is turned off, protons relax to their original alignment with the static magnetic field. The rate of this T1 relaxation depends on the local microenvironment of the protons.

14.33). This rotation of one magnetic field against another induces an alternating electrical current in receiver coils near the patient in proportion to the magnitude of the net magnetic moment of these transversely aligned protons. This signal is then used to generate the images by computerized Fourier transformation.

Once the rf pulse is turned off, the protons relax to their original alignment with the static field of the magnet (see Fig. 14.34). This process of recovering longitudinal magnetization is called T1 relaxation. This varies from tissue to tissue depending on the microenvironments of the different proton populations. In general, fat shows rapid T1 relaxation, whereas water shows slow T1 relaxation (see Fig. 14.35). Under conditions of rapid rf pulsing (typically, a sequence of 192–512 rf pulses is used to generate an image), slow-T1 substances, such as water, are not given sufficient time to recover between the pulses and therefore exhibit low signal intensity, while fast-T1 substances, such as fat, show high signal intensity (see Fig. 14.5). Short-TR sequences therefore generate contrast among tissues on the basis of differences in T1 and are accordingly referred to as T1-weighted.

Subtle T1 contrast (e.g. between articular cartilage and synovial fluid) is usually overshadowed on T1-weighted images by the far greater difference in signal intensity that exists between fat and most other tissues. However, by selectively suppressing the signal intensity of fat, it is possible to expand the scale of image intensities across smaller differences in T1 and thus to augment residual T1 contrast (Fig. 14.36). Another application of fat suppression is to increase contrast between fat and other substances, such as methemoglobin and gadolinium (Gd)-enhanced tissue, which also show rapid T1 relaxation. The most widely used technique for fat suppression is based on the chemical-shift phenomenon: as the frequency of protons in fat differs from that of protons in water the magnetization of fat (or water) can be selectively suppressed by a specifically tuned rf pulse at the beginning of the sequence (Fig. 14.37).

A similar technique can also be used to suppress the signal of water indirectly through a mechanism called magnetization transfer.

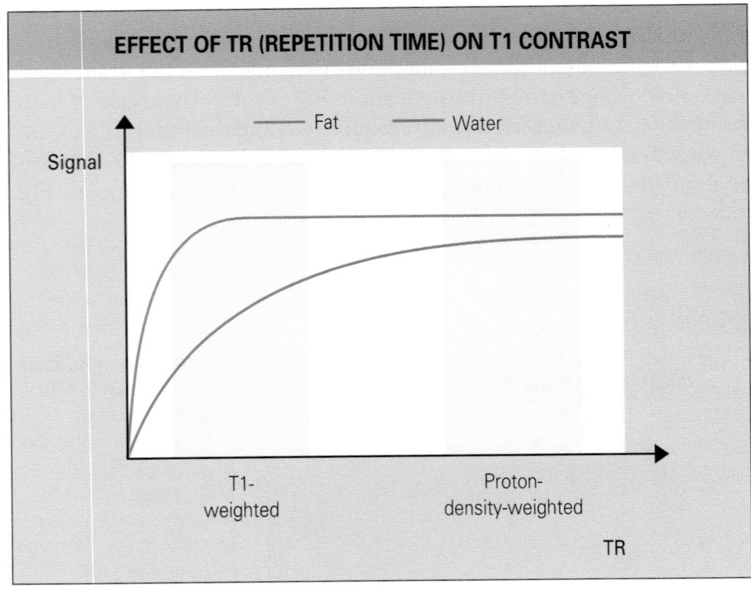

Fig. 14.35 Effect of TR (repetition time) on T1 contrast. As the time between successive excitations (TR) increases, protons in fat and water recover more of their longitudinal magnetization and therefore generate more signal when flipped into the transverse plane. Fat protons recover much faster than water protons. Therefore, when TR is short, tissue contrast is based on differences in T1, and the images are referred to as T1 weighted. When TR is long, both fat and water protons have had sufficient time to recover, and contrast depends on relative proton density rather than relative T1. Long TR images are accordingly called proton-density weighted.

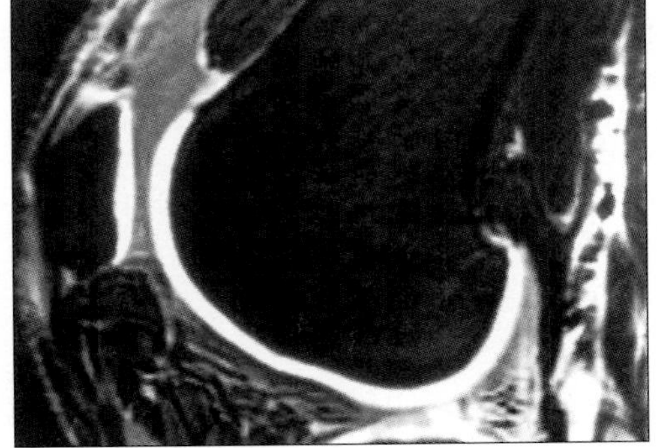

Fig. 14.36 Augmentation of T1 contrast with fat suppression. Sagittal fat-suppressed T1-weighted gradient echo image of the knee depicts cartilage as an isolated band of high signal-intensity tissue in sharp contrast with adjacent low signal-intensity synovial fluid and suppressed fat.

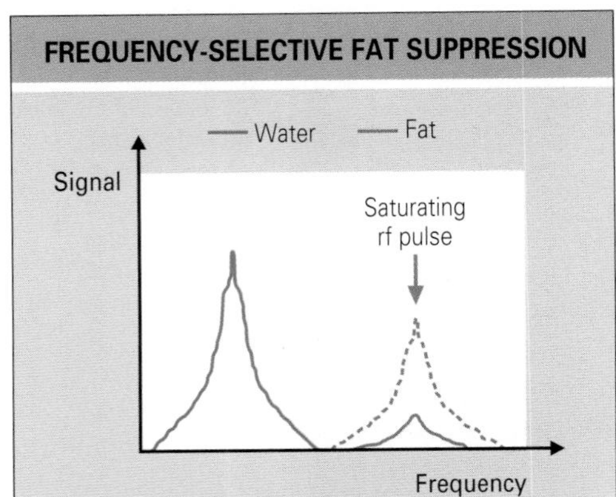

Fig. 14.37 Frequency-selective fat suppression. Hydrogen spectrum in MRI shows different frequencies for protons in fat and water (chemical shift phenomenon). Because of this spectral separation, it is possible selectively to excite or suppress one group of protons (e.g. fat).

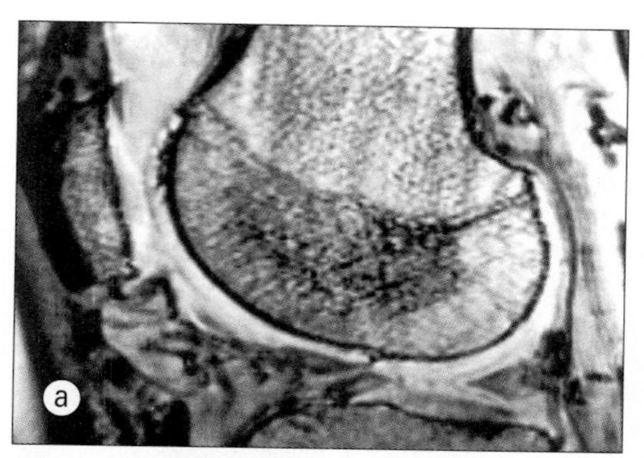

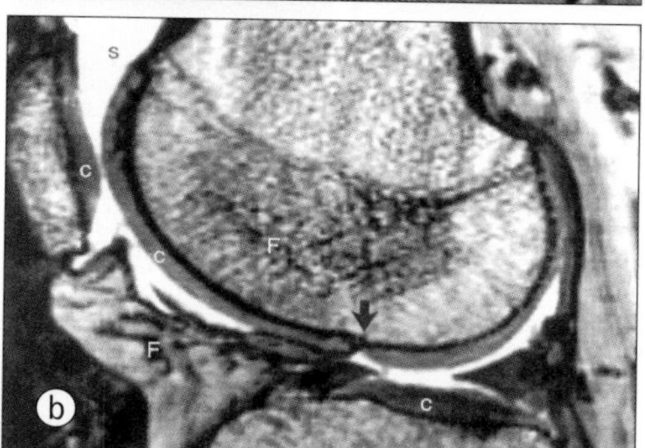

Fig. 14.38 Magnetization transfer effects in articular cartilage. Sagittal T2-weighted 3D gradient echo image of the knee shows poor contrast between cartilage and adjacent synovial fluid (a). The addition of a magnetization-transfer pulse evokes a loss of signal from structures containing both collagen and water, such as cartilage (C) but not synovial fluid (S) or fat (F). This creates contrast between cartilage and adjacent structures, and allows small morphologic defects in the cartilage (arrow) to be seen (b). Adapted from Peterfy C *et al.*[10].

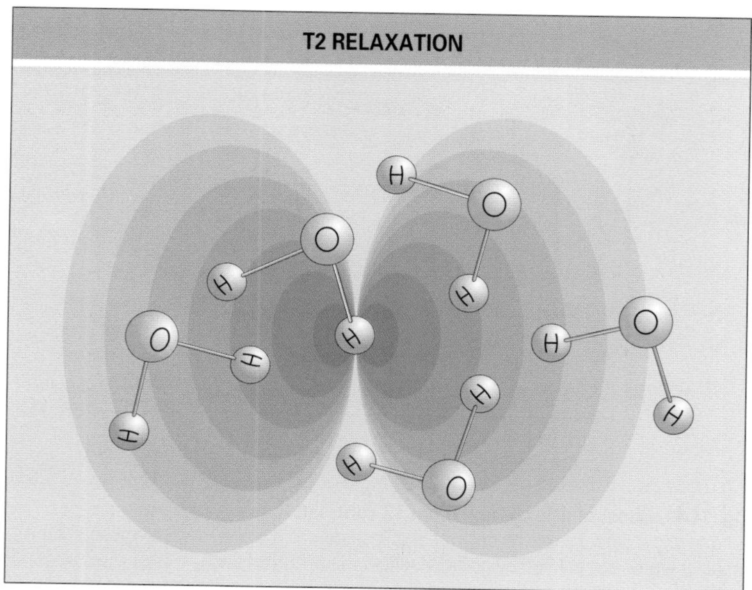

Fig. 14.39 T2 relaxation. Exposure of individual protons to the magnetic fields produced by neighboring protons alters individual spin frequencies and causes protons to fall progressively out of phase with each other. The resulting decay of signal from the proton pool is termed T2 relaxation.

In this case, direct suppression of tightly constrained protons in macromolecules like collagen, which are thermodynamically coupled to freely mobile protons in bulk water, evokes a transfer of magnetization from the water proton pool to the macromolecular pool to maintain equilibrium. This manifests as a loss of longitudinal magnetization, and therefore signal intensity, from water in proportion to the relative concentrations of the two proton pools in the tissue and the specific rate constant for the equilibrium reaction. Since collagen (unlike fat) is strongly coupled to water in this way, cartilage and muscle exhibit pronounced magnetization transfer effects[9–12]. Magnetization transfer techniques are therefore useful for imaging the articular cartilage, and could potentially be used to quantify the collagen content of this tissue (Fig. 14.38).

Image contrast is also influenced by T2 relaxation. This phenomenon manifests as a loss of transverse magnetization, and therefore signal, over time as neighboring protons fall out of phase with each other (Fig. 14.39). As with T1 relaxation, the rate of T2 relaxation, or 'dephasing', of a group of protons depends on their local microenvironment and therefore varies among different tissues. Freely mobile water protons (e.g. in synovial fluid) show slow T2 relaxation, and therefore retain signal over time, while constrained or 'bound' water protons (e.g. by collagen or proteoglycan) show rapid T2 relaxation and signal decay (Figs 14.40 & 14.41).

In addition to the effects of neighboring protons on each other (T2 relaxation), fixed magnetic field heterogeneities in a specimen also cause protons to dephase and lose transverse magnetization. The combined effects of these two causes of proton dephasing is called T2* relaxation. Signal lost to fixed magnetic heterogeneity, but not that lost to T2 relaxation, can be recovered by rephasing the protons with a 180° rf pulse (spin echo) or to a lesser extent by rapidly reversing the magnetic gradient (gradient echo). Long echo time (TE) sequences thus generate contrast among tissues on the basis of T2 (see Fig. 14.41), and when combined with a long TR to minimize the effects of T1 on contrast, are referred to as T2 weighted.

Local perturbations of the magnetic field typically arise at interfaces between substances that differ considerably in magnetic susceptibility (the degree to which a substance magnetizes in the presence of a magnetic field), such as between soft tissue and gas, metal or heavy calcification. Severe T2* at these sites is referred to as magnetic susceptibility artifact. Spin echo technique corrects for fixed magnetic heterogeneities and therefore can provide images with true T2 contrast. Gradient echo technique is faster than spin echo, but does not

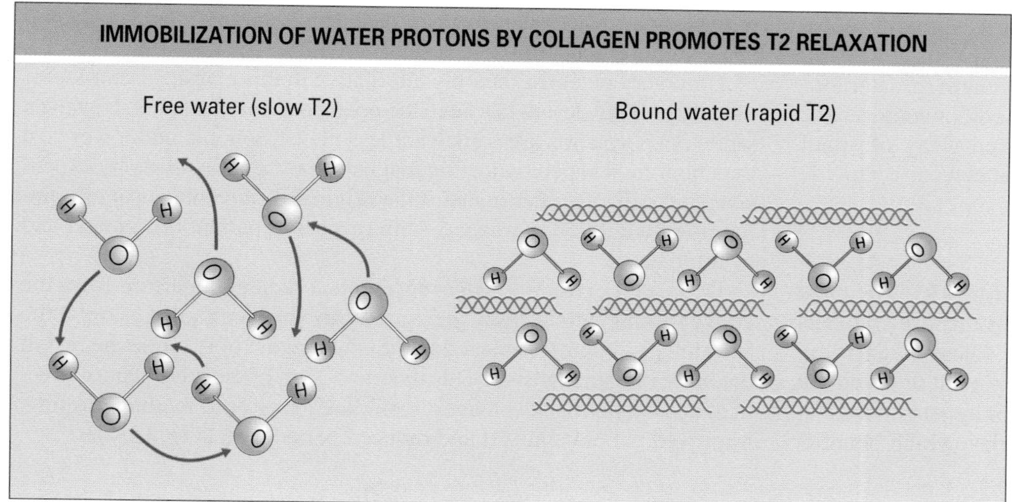

Fig. 14.40 Immobilization of water protons by collagen promotes T2 relaxation. Collagen fibrils tend to constrain water molecules and thus promote internuclear interactions and T2 relaxation. In some collagen-containing tissues (e.g. tendons and menisci) T2 relaxation is so rapid that even the shortest TE used in conventional clinical imaging is too late to detect any signal.

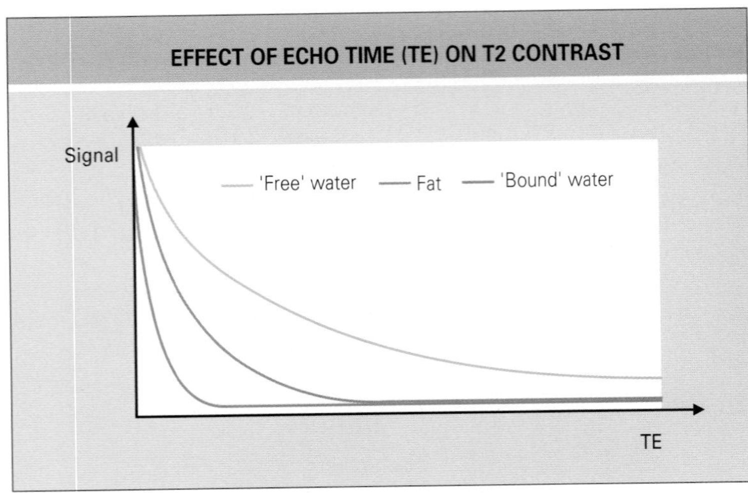

Fig. 14.41 Effect of echo time (TE) on T2 contrast. Freely mobile water protons tend to show slow T2 relaxation, whereas less mobile protons, such as those in fat or those in water constrained by collagen, show rapid T2 relaxation.

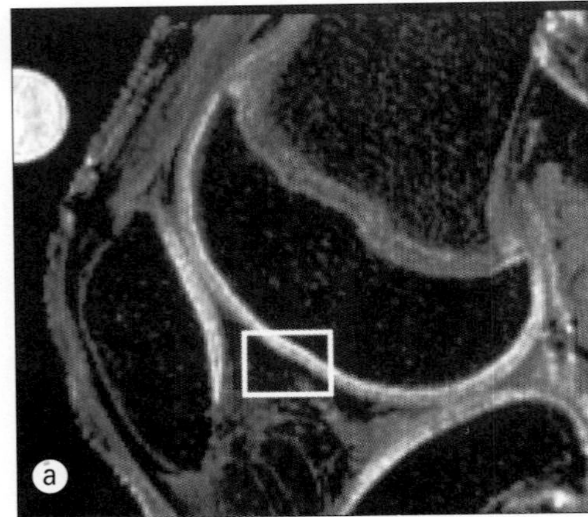

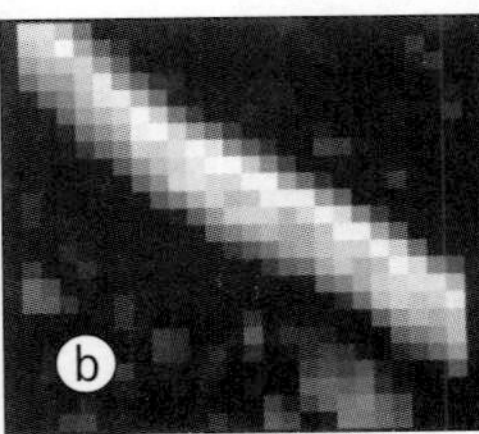

Fig. 14.42 Partial volume averaging. Sagittal fat-suppressed T1-weighted gradient echo image of the knee acquired with a resolution of 0.6mm × 0.6mm × 1mm delineates cartilage with relatively good clarity (a). Magnification of a portion of the image reveals how edge detection is limited by pixel size as well as the contrast between adjacent structures (b).

correct for these effects and therefore provides only T2*-weighted images, which are vulnerable to magnetic susceptibility effects, such as those caused by metallic prostheses. Magnetic susceptibility effects are more severe on high field-strength magnets (see below).

Finally, diffusion of protons (i.e. water) within a specimen during the acquisition of an image will result in loss of phase coherence among the protons and therefore a loss in signal. This effect is usually insignificant in conventional MRI but can be augmented with the use of strong magnetic field gradients such as those employed in MR microimaging. Water diffusivity is thus an additional tissue parameter measurable with MRI[13,14].

Both T1 weighting (short TR) and T2 weighting (long TE) involve discarding MRI signal. If these effects are eliminated, signal intensity reflects only the proton density. Accordingly, long-TR/short-TE images are often referred to as proton-density weighted. However, even the shortest finite TE attainable is too long to escape T2 relaxation completely, and extremely long TRs (>3500msec) are not practical for imaging in vivo. Therefore, even so called proton-density-weighted images contain some T1 and T2 contrast.

The spatial resolution of an MRI image is defined by the dimensions of the voxels which make it up. As with CT, all signal within a voxel is averaged. Therefore, if an interface with high signal intensity on one side and low signal intensity on the other side passes through the middle of a voxel, the interface is depicted as an intermediate signal intensity band the width of the voxel (Fig. 14.42). This effect is known as partial volume averaging. The smaller the voxel, the greater the spatial resolution. However, as voxel size decreases, so does signal-to-noise ratio. Accordingly, high-resolution imaging requires sufficient signal-to-noise ratio to support it. Signal-to-noise ratio can be increased by shortening TE (less T2 decay), increasing TR (more T1 recovery), imaging at higher field strength (greater longitudinal magnetization) or utilizing specialized coils which reduce noise (small surface coil, quadrature coil, phased array of small coils)[15]. Specialized sequences such as 3D gradient echo also provide greater signal-to-noise ratio.

DIFFERENT MAGNET TYPES

A variety of different magnet types are available for MRI. The most widely used are superconducting high-field systems that use cryogens and supercooling to improve magnet performance. These magnets are cylindrical and have a central bore into which the patient or specimen is placed. Scanners constructed with permanent magnets operate at room temperature and can be made with open sides, which benefits patient tolerance in some cases. These systems are less expensive than superconducting magnets but provide lower field strength, which necessitates longer imaging times to achieve comparable signal-to-noise ratio and spatial resolution (Fig. 14.43). MRI at low field strength also exhibits less chemical-shift phenomenon, which limits the ability to perform frequency-selective fat suppression. An alternative method of fat suppression [i.e. short-tau inversion recovery (STIR)] must, therefore, be used at low field strength. Metallic artifacts are less severe at low field strength. Accordingly, patients with internal fixation hardware, shrapnel or other metallic objects may produce better images on MRI at low field strength.

The most common configuration for both high- and low-field MRI has been the whole-body scanner (Figs 14.43 & 14.44). In order to image a knee, ankle, elbow or wrist with such a system, the entire body must be placed within the bore of the magnet. This has a number of important implications. First, it provokes feelings of claustrophobia in some patients. Although a only minority (<10%) of patients cannot complete the examination due to claustrophobia, a larger percentage find the experience unpleasant and may have to be sedated in order to cope. This is particularly true of children who often require heavy sedation or anesthesia, which may necessitate the involvement of an anesthesiologist, thus increasing the variable costs of MRI. Exposing the entire body to the magnetic field within the bore of even relatively low field strength magnets also poses a potential health risk to patients with pacemakers, vascular clips, cochlear implants or various other metallic implants. Relatively high stray fields associated with most MRI magnets extend this risk to include metallic objects, such as oxygen tanks, wheelchairs or i.v. poles inadvertently brought into the examination room. Moreover, the purchase price, maintenance costs and space requirements of these systems are high.

Until very recently, the only alternative to this classic circumferential whole-body design has been the open permanent magnet. However, while open systems are somewhat less claustrophobic and lower cost than high-field superconducting magnets, they remain relatively expensive, and still engender many of the original disadvantages of circumferential, whole-body imagers with respect to patient discomfort and health risk.

Dedicated extremity MRI represents a radical departure from the conventional whole-body design. With this technology, only the extremity of interest is placed within the magnet bore while the rest of the body remains outside. This unique design offers a number of practical and economic advantages, including lower cost, facilitated siting, improved patient comfort and reduced patient risk (Fig. 14.44).

IMAGING TRADE OFFS RELATED TO MRI FIELD STRENGTH		
	High-field	Low-field
Signal-to-noise ratio*	++	+
Contrast-to-noise ratio	?	?
Spatial resolution*	++	+
Imaging time	+	++†
Contrast		
T1 relaxation	+	+++
T2 relaxation	+++	++
Magnetic susceptibility	++	+
Fat suppression		
–chemical shift	yes	no
–STIR	yes	yes
Cost	++	+

Fig. 14.43 Imaging trade offs related to MRI field strength.
(* Improved by increasing imaging time or use of superconducting coils;
† Depends on trade off between faster T1, allowing shorter TR, and weaker longitudinal magnetization necessitating greater signal averaging to maintain signal-to-noise ratio and spatial resolution;
STIR = Short tau inversion recovery.)

IMAGING ARTICULAR TISSUES WITH MRI

Diarthrodial joints are particularly suitable for MRI. Not only does the modality provide direct multiplanar tomography with relatively high spatial resolution, but it is unparalleled in its ability to depict soft-tissue detail (Fig. 14.45). Thus, MRI is the only modality that can examine all components of the joint simultaneously and therefore the joint as a whole organ. Moreover, in addition to morphologic parameters, MRI is capable of measuring a variety of compositional and functional tissue parameters relevant to the arthritic process. Because MRI is noninvasive and generally well tolerated by patients, frequent serial examinations can be performed even on asymptomatic patients.

High cost and limited availability have been the principal impediments to acceptance of MRI for evaluating patients with arthritis. However, with approximately 9000 MRI systems currently available worldwide, lack of availability is a less serious limitation than in the past. Moreover, as with any maturing technology, the cost of MRI is decreasing. This is because of both market forces and technical developments such as dedicated extremity scanners, which can provide imaging at only a fraction of the cost required for conventional whole-body MRI. As discussed above, low-field dedicated extremity MRI also eliminates the risk of claustrophobia and the potential hazards of metal in the room or in the patient.

Bone

Because of the absence of hydrogen protons in cortical and trabecular bone, these structures are depicted as linear signal voids silhouetted on either side by signal-containing marrow and periosseous tissues. Osseous contours are thus well delineated on MRI. This inherent contrast combined with multiplanar tomographic capability makes MRI more sensitive than radiography for detecting bone erosions (see Figs 14.14 & 14.15) and osteophytes (Fig. 14.46). It is also highly sensitive to conditions that alter the composition of marrow, such as trauma, infection, ischemia and neoplasms. Accordingly, MRI is the most sensitive modality for detecting insufficiency fractures and stress fractures (Fig. 14.47), osteomyelitis, osteonecrosis and metastatic and primary bone tumors. Independent loss of cortical or trabecular bone, as can be seen in involutional osteoporosis, hyperthyroidism or hyperparathyroidism, on the other hand, is relatively inconspicuous on conventional MRI. Modalities based on X-rays, particularly dual X-ray absorptiometry (DXA), are potentially more sensitive in such cases.

Hyaline articular cartilage

Normal hyaline articular cartilage has a relatively high proton density, and because of the presence of collagen exhibits intermediate T1 relaxation and rapid T2 relaxation. Adjacent synovial fluid also has a high proton density, but shows slow T1 and T2 relaxation. Accordingly, contrast between cartilage and synovial fluid is poor on proton-density-weighted images but high on T2-weighted images, in which the cartilage is depicted as a low signal intensity structure adjacent to high signal intensity synovial fluid and intermediate signal intensity marrow fat. Early matrix damage can also be seen on T2-weighted MRI, as collagen loss and increased water content within the diseased cartilage result in increased signal intensity (Fig. 14.48)[16]. A complete set of heavily T2-weighted fast spin echo images of the knee can be acquired in as little as 3–4 minutes using routine clinical MRI scanners.

On T1-weighted images, low to intermediate signal intensity cartilage shows poor contrast with adjacent low signal-intensity synovial fluid but excellent contrast with high signal-intensity bone marrow fat and adipose tissue. Addition of fat suppression augments T1-contrast on these images and makes the articular cartilage appear as a band of high signal-intensity against low signal-intensity synovial fluid and adjacent fat (Fig. 14.36)[17]. Combining this technique with thin-section 3D gradient-echo imaging provides high-resolution, high-contrast images of the articular cartilage, which correlate well with arthroscopy[10,12,18–20].

Synovial tissue and synovial fluid

Synovial fluid in joint cavities and bursae are most saliently depicted on fat-suppressed T2-weighted images or STIR images. Synovial tissue lining these structures is generally too thin to be depicted with conventional MRI. As synovial tissue thickens and becomes fibrotic, it

COMPARISON OF MAGNET CONFIGURATIONS			
	Whole body – closed	Whole body – open	Dedicated extremity
Field strength	High/low	Low	Low*
Coverage	Full	Full	Limited
Cost	++++	+++	+
Space	++++	+++	+
Claustrophobia	++	+	-
Safety	+	+	++

* High-field potentially available in closed, circumferential configuration, but not currently used for dedicated extremity MRI.

Fig. 14.44 Comparison of different magnet configurations.

MRI: GENERAL STRENGTHS AND LIMITATIONS	
Strengths	Limitations
Multiplanar and 3D imaging	May induce claustrophobia
Unparalleled soft-tissue contrast	Metal implants in body may be hazardous
Morphologic, compositional and functional measures	Technical sophistication required
Widely available	Can be expensive*
No radiation	

* Recently introduced dedicated extremity MRI is relatively inexpensive.

Fig. 14.45 MRI: General strengths and limitations.

may develop a short T2 and thus lose signal more rapidly than the adjacent joint fluid on T2-weighted images. This increases the contrast with adjacent joint fluid but not the articular cartilage, which also shows low signal intensity on T2-weighted images. Nonfibrotic synovial tissue, on the other hand, may not be distinguishable from joint fluid without intravenous administration of Gd-DTPA, which increases the signal intensity of this highly vascular tissue on T1-weighted images. Moreover, the rate of enhancement of synovial tissue following bolus intravenous injection of Gd-DTPA correlates with the histologic severity of the synovitis[21]. This offers a useful way of identifying patients with arthritis before radiographic changes become apparent (Fig. 14.49). In a study of 27 patients with joint pain but negative radiographs[22], Gd-enhanced MRI showed a sensitivity and specificity of 100% and 73%, respectively, for diagnosing RA, whereas the revised American Radiology Association (ARA) criteria offered only 69% sensitivity and 64% specificity, respectively, in this group. Gadolinium-enhanced MRI also offers a potential way of monitoring treatment in patients with RA, although longitudinal data are limited.

Other intra-articular and periarticular structures

Intra-articular and periarticular ligaments (e.g. cruciates, collaterals) normally exhibit low signal intensity on T2-weighted images because of the abundance of collagen within them (Fig. 14.50). Disrupted ligaments appear discontinuous and/or contain high signal-intensity edema and hemorrhage. The menisci of the knee and labra of the shoulder also appear low in signal intensity on MRI because of the presence of collagen. As with ligaments, the emergence of linear high signal within these structures is indicative of tear (Fig. 14.50), although it must be emphasized that nondisplaced tears are most sensitively detected on short TE images (i.e. T1-weighted or proton-density-weighted spin echo, all gradient echo). Adding Gd-containing contrast material into the joint (MR arthrography; Fig. 14.51) increases the sensitivity of MRI for meniscal tears and especially labrocapsular abnormalities.

Tendons and muscles

Because of their highly collagenous nature, normal tendons have a very short T2 (<1msec) and, therefore, generate little signal on MRI. This provides an inherent contrast between most tendons and the surrounding tissues, and makes tendon imaging with MRI relatively straightforward. Magnetic resonance imaging is highly sensitive to the full spectrum of tendon abnormalities that affect patients with arthritis. Fluid within a tendon sheath is easy to visualize on T2-weighted images, and increased signal intensity within the tendon itself is indicative of tendonitis or tear, as can arise from either direct tenosynovial invasion or attrition from rubbing across the jagged margins of osseous erosions. The utility of MRI for evaluating tendons in the shoulder and ankle is well established; however, MRI is also highly sensitive for detecting tendon abnormalities within the hands and wrists of patients with RA[23]. Significant tendon abnormalities can go clinically undetected in such patients for some time. Dedicated extremity MRI now offers a relatively inexpensive means of assessing these patients.

Skeletal muscle also contains collagen and therefore appears dark on T2-weighted images. Muscular strain, contusion and rupture all show high signal intensity on T2-weighted images. Strain appears as a feathery high signal intensity at or along the musculotendinous junction and pericapsular region of the muscle, while contusion from direct trauma produces local edema and interstitial hemorrhage at the site of impact. Muscular rupture can produce a localized hematoma, which may contain high-signal intensity methemoglobin for several weeks on T1-weighted images. Denervation atrophy from compartment syndrome or

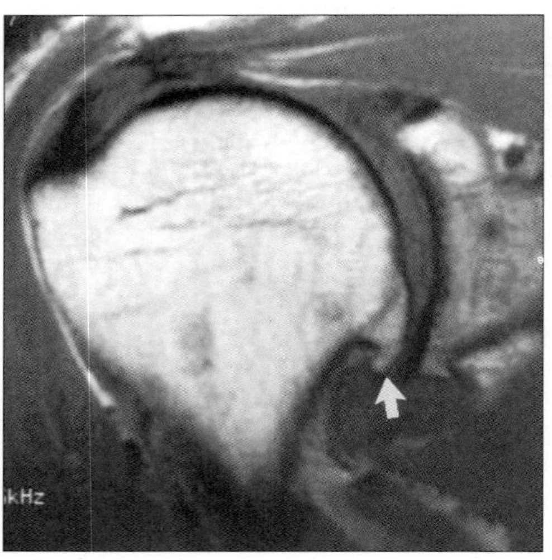

Fig. 14.46 Imaging osteophytes with MRI. Oblique coronal T1-weighted MRI of the shoulder shows a large osteophyte (arrow) of the inferior margin of the humeral head.

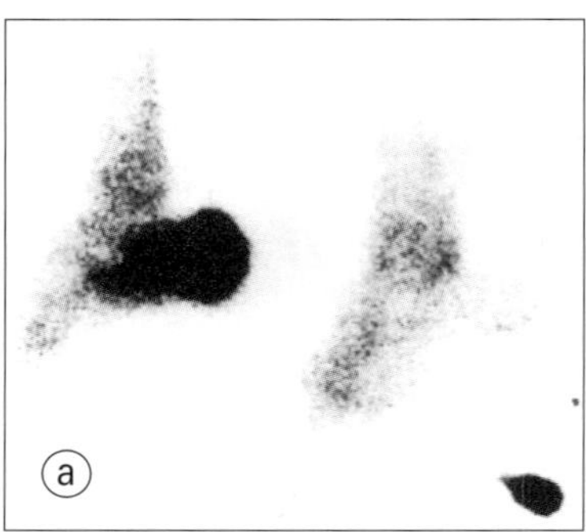

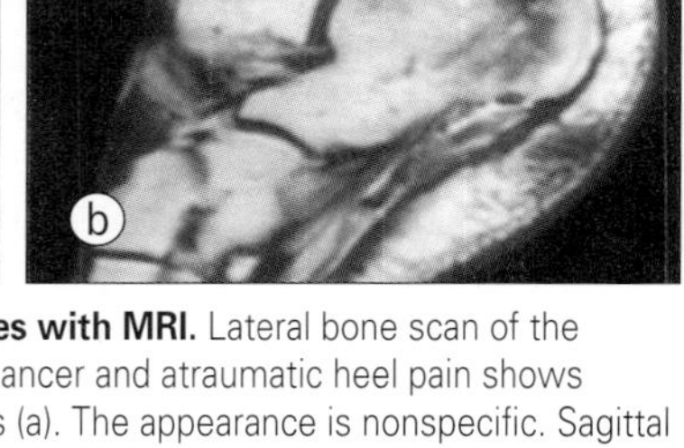

Fig. 14.47 Imaging insufficiency fractures with MRI. Lateral bone scan of the calcaneus of an elderly woman with lung cancer and atraumatic heel pain shows diffusely increased uptake in the calcaneus (a). The appearance is nonspecific. Sagittal T1-weighted spin echo MRI of the calcaneus shows a vertical band of low signal replacing the normal marrow fat, a pattern pathognomonic for fracture, and very different from that seen with metastasis, osteonecrosis or osteomyelitis (b).

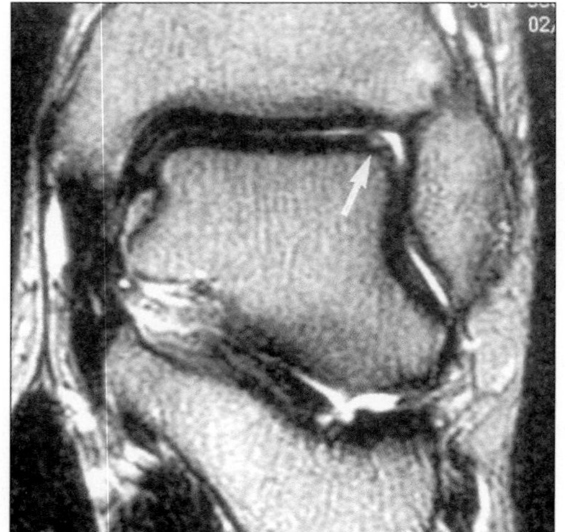

Fig. 14.48 Imaging cartilage matrix damage with MRI. Coronal T2-weighted fast spin echo MRI of the ankle shows a focus of increased signal (arrow) within the cartilage over the lateral talar dome, indicative of matrix damage.

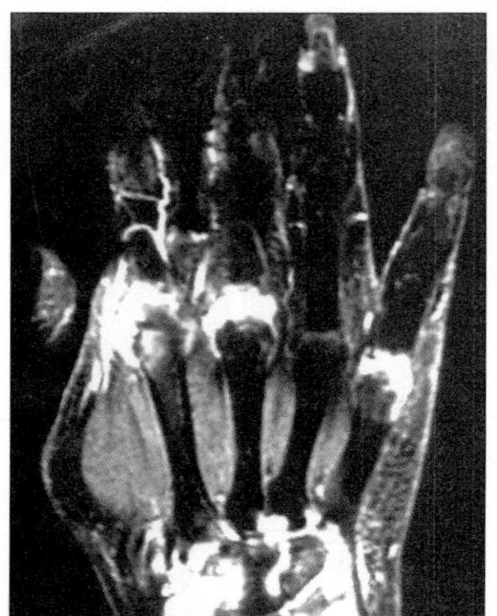

Fig. 14.49 Identifying early synovitis with Gd-enhanced MRI. Coronal Gd-enhanced, fat-suppressed, T1-weighted MRI of a patient with RA without radiographic findings shows marked synovitis of the wrist and the second, third and fifth, but not the fourth, metacarpophalangeal joints. From Sugimoto *et al.*[22].

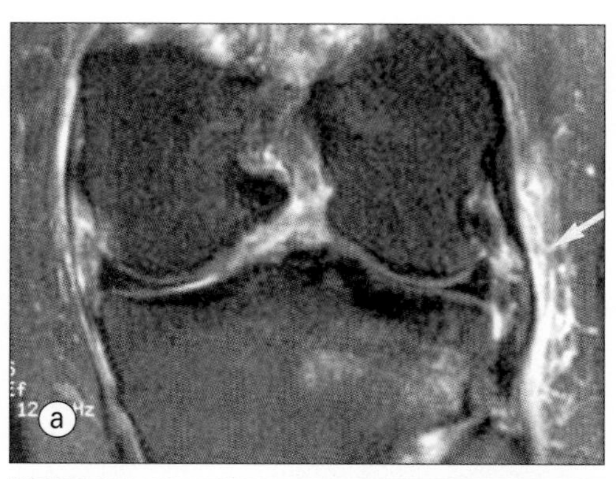

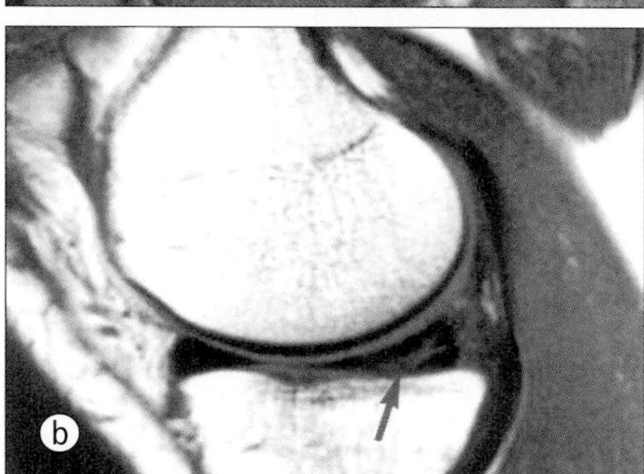

Fig. 14.50 Imaging ligaments and menisci with MRI. Coronal fat-suppressed T2-weighted image of the knee shows an intact fibular collateral ligament (white arrow) (a). Surrounding high signal intensity fluid is indicative of sprain. Meniscal tear appears as a linear band of increased signal (black arrow) within the otherwise low signal-intensity meniscus on sagittal T1-weighted MRI (b).

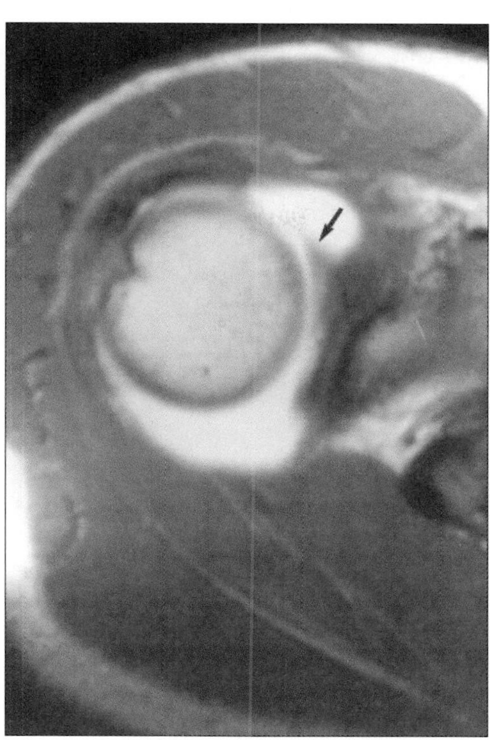

Fig. 14.51 MRI arthrography of the shoulder. Transverse T1-weighted MRI of the shoulder following intra-articular injection of 20ml dilute Gd-containing contrast material delineates the anterosuperior labrum (arrow), which would otherwise be indistinguishable from the isointense anterior capsule and adjacent muscle.

other causes results in diffuse muscle edema and fatty atrophy. Both T1-weighted and T2-weighted images are, therefore, useful in this setting.

CONCLUSIONS

The myriad of imaging tools available today offers unprecedented opportunities to rheumatologists to explore and combat arthritis. However, with this growing armamentarium comes a greater need for technical sophistication on the part of the clinician. This is compounded by growing pressures to contain costs and for clinicians to play a more central role in directing diagnostic testing. These demands necessitate a deeper understanding of the trade-offs associated with choosing one modality over another, and a clear sense of the immediate and downstream costs associated with each approach. There is a particular need for rheumatologists to become familiar with the newer imaging modalities, such as MRI, not only better to understand the growing number of studies that utilize them, but also to assist in directing their development to serve the needs of rheumatologists and their patients.

REFERENCES

1. Newman JS, Laing TJ, McCarthy CJ, Adler RS. Power Doppler sonography of synovitis: assessment of therapeutic response – preliminary observations. Radiology. 1996;198:582–4.
2. Cardinal E, Lafortune M, Burns P. Power Doppler US in synovitis: reality or artifact? Radiology. 1996;200:868–9.
3. Abragam A. The principles of nuclear magnetism. London: Oxford University Press; 1983.
4. Budinger T, Lauterbur P. Nuclear magnetic resonance technology for medical studies. Science. 1984;226:288–98.
5. Haacke E, Tkach J. Fast MR imaging: techniques and clinical applications. AJR 1990;155:951–64.
6. Pykett I. NMR imaging in medicine. Sci Am. 1982;246:78–88.
7. Young S. Magnetic resonance imaging: basic principles. New York: Raven Press; 1988.
8. König S, Brown R. Determinants of proton relaxation in tissue. Magn Reson Imag. 1984;1:437–49.

9. Woolf SD, Chesnick S, Frank JA, Lim KO, Balaban RS. Magnetization transfer contrast: MR imaging of the knee. Radiology. 1991;179:623–8.
10. Peterfy CG, Majumdar S, Lang P, *et al.* MR imaging of the arthritic knee: improved discrimination of cartilage, synovium and effusion with pulsed saturation transfer and fat-suppressed T1-weighted sequences. Radiology. 1994;191:413–19.
11. Hall LD, Tyler JA. Can quantitative magnetic resonance imaging detect and monitor the progression of early osteoarthritis? In: Kuetner KE, Goldberg VM, eds. Osteoarthritic disorders. Rosemont: American Accadamy of Orthopaedic Surgeons; 1995:67–84.
12. Peterfy CG, van Dijke CF, Janzen DL, *et al.* Quantification of articular cartilage in the knee by pulsed saturation transfer and fat-suppressed MRI: optimization and validation. Radiology. 1994;192:485–91.
13. Xia Y, Farquhar T, Burton-Wuster N, Ray E, Jelinski LW. Diffusion and relaxation mapping of cartilage–bone plugs and excised disks using microscopic magnetic resonance imaging. Magn Reson Med. 1994;31:273–82.
14. Burstein D, Gray ML, Hartman AL, Gipe R, Foy BD. Diffusion of small solutes in cartilage as measured by nuclear magnetic resonance (NMR) spectroscopy and imaging. J Orthop Res. 1993;11:465–78.
15. Kneeland JB, Hyde JS. High-resolution MR imaging with local coils. Radiology. 1989;171:1–7.
16. Peterfy CG, Genant HK. Emerging applications of magnetic resonance imaging for evaluating the articular cartilage. Radiol Clin North Am. 1996;34:195–213.
17. Chandnani VP, Ho C, Chu P, Trudell P, Resnick D. Knee hyaline cartilage evaluated with MR imaging: a cadaveric study involving multiple imaging sequences and intraarticular injection of gadolinium and saline solution. Radiology. 1991;178:557–61.
18. Recht MP, Pirraino DW, Paletta GA, Schils JP, Belhobek GH. Accuracy of fat-suppressed three-dimensionl spoiled gradient-echo FLASH MR imaging in the detection of patellofemoral articular cartilage abnormalities. Radiology. 1996;198:209–12.
19. Disler DG, McCauley TR, Kelman CG, *et al.* Fat-suppressed three-dimensional spoiled gradient-echo MR imaging of hyaline cartilage defects in the knee: comparison with standard MR imaging and arthroscopy. AJR. 1996;167:127–32.
20. Peterfy CG, van Dijke CF, Lu Y, *et al.* Quantification of articular cartilage in the metacarpophalangeal joints of the hand: accuracy and precision of 3D MR imaging. AJR. 1995;165:371–5.
21. Tamai K, Yamato M, Yamaguchi T, Ohno W. Dynamic magnetic resonance imaging for the evaluation of synovitis in patients with rheumatoid arthritis. Arthritis Rheum. 1994;37:1151–7.
22. Sugimoto H, Takeda A, Masuyama J, Furuse M. Early-stage rheumatoid arthritis: diagnostic accuracy of MR imaging. Radiology. 1996;198:185–92.
23. Rubens DJ, Blebea JS, Totterman SMS, Hooper MM. Rheumatoid arthritis: evaluation of wrist extensor tendons with clinical examination versus MR imaging – a preliminary report. Radiology. 1993;187:831–8.

3

PRINCIPLES OF MANAGEMENT

Peter M Brooks

PRINCIPLES OF MANAGEMENT OF PATIENTS WITH RHEUMATIC DISEASE

Peter M Brooks & Joseph A Buckwalter

Management of chronic rheumatic disease

- Diagnosis should include the assessment of activity, prognosis and goal setting.
- Treatment is adjusted in the light of evaluation of the response.
- Coordination of a multidisciplinary approach and re-evaluation of disease are essential.

Therapeutic issues

- Which drugs should be used and when?
- What surgical procedures and when?
- Which physical therapies are appropriate?
- Continuing re-evaluations of the patient's disease status, disability and expectations and requirements are essential.

Management of patients with rheumatic disease remains a significant challenge and one that requires careful consideration, judgment and an adherence to the principles of evidence-based medicine[1]. Some rheumatic diseases are acute and settle completely with early and appropriate treatment. These include infectious arthritis and gout – diseases for which we are well aware of the pathogenesis and treatment. Even in these conditions, however, damage may occur to the joint during that acute phase which can lead on to progressive degenerative arthritis later in life. The process is complex because of:

- the chronicity of these diseases and the need for ongoing monitoring of disease activity,
- functional status and patient response to the disease and treatment (see Chapter 3.14),
- the need to coordinate a multidisciplinary therapeutic approach, including a variety of medical specialties as well as allied health care providers.

The doctor providing rheumatologic management must coordinate specialist input in a variety of areas and must be knowledgeable about management options, their applications and their risks and benefits. Orchestrating these various approaches and monitoring their efficacy requires knowledge of what each offers, but, as importantly, requires the doctor to think in terms of the influence of life stages on disease and treatment and how they may relate to disease expression and modulation (for example, the effect of aging on drug metabolism and toxicity). Of great importance here is the establishment of realistic goals for the various treatments. Although doctors can give patients information on the likely outcomes of treatment, the final decision on a particular therapy should be made in consultation with the patient (see Chapter 3.03). It is generally recognized that the goals of the patient and the physician are often different and this must be acknowledged by the treating 'team'. The ability to communicate with patients is extremely important when caring for any patient with a chronic disease, particularly a rheumatic condition, and emphasizes the importance of attainment of these skills in undergraduate and postgraduate education[2,3].

The problem of involving the patient in therapeutic decisions is the very different experiences of the doctor and the patient. The doctor can appreciate the long-term disability that is likely to result if the disease is not treated immediately, whereas the patient has little understanding of what is likely to occur in 10 or 20 years. The patient is much more likely to be influenced by the potential for immediate adverse consequences of a therapy (an adverse drug reaction, risks of surgery or anesthetic) than by a 'potential' reduction of disability (decreased pain or joint erosion) 10 years later. Optimal management of patients will increasingly involve them in making decisions regarding risk factors such as weight and a range of lifestyle modifications.

Pharmacologic interventions, rehabilitation, orthoses and other devices, nonpharmacologic modalities and surgery should be considered to influence both disease and the patient, and these are mutually interdependent. They cannot be seen as isolated intervention points in a disease process because they may significantly alter the course of the disease – and the patient – sometimes permanently. Other life issues which are very important and have to be considered in treatment include the changes with age and development, be they childhood, adolescence or the influence of occupations such as school, work and home tasks. Rheumatic diseases are invariably chronic and are characterized by unpredictable remissions and relapses. The course of these diseases can be influenced by many factors, including biological processes, family and societal interactions, education and treatment. Good management requires acknowledgment of all and attention to most. A critical thing to remember is that expectations for what a therapy will or will not do may differ substantially between the treating health care professional and the patient[4,5]. Great care must be taken to inform patients of the benefits and risks of various therapies and to respect their ultimate treatment choices.

The major therapeutic strategies in rheumatic diseases are shown in Figure 1.1. It is very rare in chronic rheumatic diseases that these interventions are used singly and a critical issue in good management comes with the timing of each of the interventions. This is particularly

THERAPEUTIC STRATEGIES IN RHEUMATIC DISEASES	
Pharmacotherapy	**Nonpharmacologic**
Analgesics NSAIDS Antirheumatic drugs Corticosteroids Immunosuppressive agents Biological modifiers Specific antigout preparations Radiotherapy • Direct • Radiopharmaceutical	**Rehabilitation** **Education** Knowledge • General • Specific Behavioral modification • Relaxation techniques • Stress management **Physical therapy** Exercise • General preventive • Specific therapeutic Rest
Surgery	Light • Ultraviolet • Laser Heat/cold Hydrotherapy Electricity • Transcutaneous • Nerve stimulation Ultrasound Mobilization/manipulation Devices • Splints • Orthoses • Household modifications • Home/work/walking devices
Reconstruction • Tendon • Ligament Arthroplasty Arthrodesis Synovectomy Osteotomy Joint debridement Decompression • Spinal cord • Peripheral nerve	

Fig. 1.1 Therapeutic strategies in rheumatic diseases.

so with drug therapy and with surgery where a decision to use one modality may preclude others. Surgical management may also be complicated by multiple joint involvement and the need to consider surgery on some joints before others (see Chapter 3.12).

ASSESSMENT OF DISEASE AND MANAGEMENT

A range of outcome measures[6,7] has been proposed for the assessment of rheumatic diseases and is summarized in Figure 1.2. The outcome measures will vary with the disease under review. Although primarily designed for use in clinical trials, they do have applications in everyday clinical practice. These outcomes should be measured in a reliable and valid way, but just how many should be included in any particular study will depend on a variety of factors including the study objectives, the interests of the investigator, registration requirements and budget. With the increasing number of scales to measure outcome, it is important that those selected are reliable, valid and able to detect a clinically important change (see Chapter 3.14).

Professional groups such as the American College of Rheumatology (ACR) and the International League of Associations for Rheumatology, the OMERACT group and the Osteoarthritis Research Society have recently addressed some of the problems of lack of consistency in trials and are currently developing core sets of end points for rheumatic diseases such as osteoarthritis (OA) and osteoporosis. These groups have already considered the development of end points for testing new interventions for rheumatoid arthritis (RA)[6] and have recommended a core set of outcomes which include clinician and patient global assessment, a disability measure, an acute phase reactant, joint counts both tender and swollen, a visual analog pain scale and radiographs for long-term studies. The American Academy of Orthopedic Surgeons and the Council of Musculoskeletal Specialty Societies have developed instruments to assess outcomes of treatment based on region-specific musculoskeletal function, including instruments for the upper extremities, the spine and the lower extremities[8–10]. These groups have also developed a specific outcome instrument for children with musculoskeletal injuries and disorders. Currently these instruments are being used to collect data in the US on outcomes of a variety of musculoskeletal diseases and injuries.

Some of these outcomes will also be useful in clinical practice for routinely monitoring patients. Because clinical disagreement and observer variability are common throughout medicine, clinicians need to recognize the necessity for explicit, objective criteria for clinical outcomes of interest. Training can help reduce the level of clinical disagreement but in clinical trials the criteria should be applied by observers who are unaware of whether the patient is being treated with an active compound or not.

OUTCOME MEASURES IN RHEUMATIC DISEASES

Attribute	Example
Death	Mortality rate
Disease	Imaging CT, radiograph Biochemical Serologic C-reactive protein rheumatoid factor DNA binding
Distress	Pain assessment Joint count Range of motion
Disability	Health Assessment Questionnaire Western Ontario MacMaster Arthritis Impact Measurement Scale
Dysfunction	Psychosocial questionnaires
Disposition	Risk factor assessment
Debt	Cost of disease/therapy Resource consumption
Drug effect/toxicity	Side effects/toxicity index
Disharmony	Family function scales

Fig. 1.2 Outcome measures in rheumatic diseases.

PRINCIPLES OF MANAGEMENT STRATEGIES

The timing and type of intervention used in rheumatic diseases will depend on the disease and the therapy.

NONPHARMACOLOGIC TREATMENT

Nonpharmacologic treatments can be relatively harmless but are costly in terms of time and resources. Their efficacy needs to be assessed like any other treatment. If outcome is not improved, the therapy should be discontinued or not used (see Chapter 3.11). Nonpharmacologic treatments will vary in their sophistication, from massage of a painful area in soft tissue rheumatism to careful mobilization of a lumbar apophyseal joint by a well-trained manipulative physical therapist. Educational activities can be generic or specific and may involve the imparting of new knowledge or a specific behavioral modification program[11]. Exercises, again, may be specific for particular muscles or muscle groups or they may be generalized. The importance of low-impact general exercise programs is seen throughout life; even the elderly can benefit in terms of musculoskeletal symptoms from a general aerobic exercise program[12]. A variety of devices for patients afflicted by musculoskeletal disease assist in performing activities of daily living, ranging from turning on faucets, getting on and off a toilet and opening jars to remaining mobile.

PHARMACOTHERAPY

Pharmacotherapy is disease specific. In metabolic diseases such as hyperuricemia, drugs to lower the serum uric acid (allopurinol or a uricosuric agent) can be combined with a specific anti-inflammatory drug [e.g. colchicine or a nonsteroidal anti-inflammatory drug (NSAID)] to suppress pain and inflammation. In OA, purely analgesic agents such as acetaminophen are often more appropriately used initially since NSAIDs are associated with significant morbidity. In several recent studies, acetaminophen has been shown to be of benefit in up to 30% of patients with OA of the knee previously treated with NSAIDs[13–15]. These agents may be beneficial if inflammatory episodes arise in OA, but therapy should be reviewed frequently and the dose reduced or discontinued as appropriate. In OA, advice on changes in lifestyle, such as weight reduction and exercise, may be extremely beneficial when combined with simple analgesics.

'Aggressive' pharmacotherapies

Rheumatoid arthritis and the other major inflammatory connective tissue diseases require aggressive therapies. Patients need to be carefully monitored with both clinical and disease-specific laboratory parameters, including imaging, biochemical and serologic markers. These diseases may progress slowly, but there is increasing evidence that, in conditions such as RA, damage to cartilage occurs at an early stage, which is when the disease should be aggressively treated[16]. Indeed, there is a good argument now for treating RA from the outset (at least at diagnosis) with specific antirheumatic drugs since some of the less potent agents such as antimalarials and sulfasalazine have a relatively low incidence of severe side effects. In RA it is important continually to re-assess the patient and determine whether disease activity is really being suppressed, to prevent development of significant deformity.

Combinations of pharmacologic agents tend to be the norm now in the management of many inflammatory rheumatic diseases, but a frequent review of therapy is required to ensure that the drugs being used actually suppress disease activity. Of interest is a recent study from tenWolde *et al.* which assesses whether patients with RA who have a good response to long-term treatment with antirheumatic drugs would benefit from continuation of therapy[17]. In this 12-month study the cumulative incidence of a flare was 38% for patients continuing on placebo and 22% for those continuing on their specific antirheumatic drug. A number of other studies in the literature have also suggested that patients with RA on long-term treatment are not able to continue on a single agent for long periods of time either because they develop side effects or because the disease becomes active again[18] (Fig. 1.3). In practice, very few patients achieve remission on antirheumatic drugs and the disease (RA) continues its inexorable progression to long-term disability.

The 'pyramid' and 'stepdown' or 'sawtooth' approaches

As important as the individual or combined action of drugs used is the way in which they are used in the clinical setting (see Chapters 3.06 – 3.10). In RA, for example, the conventional 'pyramid' approach (Fig. 1.4) has been largely superseded by the 'stepdown' (Fig. 1.5) or 'sawtooth' models (Fig. 1.6). Although both have considerable merit[19,20], these novel approaches need to be assessed in formal clinical trials. In a recent study of the 'sawtooth' strategy in patients with early RA, Möttönen *et al.*[21] demonstrated that, over a 6-year period, 32% of 142 patients attained ACR remission criteria[22]. Although this study was not randomized, results do suggest a better outcome for RA with this approach than with less formalized strategies.

SURGERY

In the chronic rheumatic diseases, physicians should work closely with surgeons in attempting optimally to time surgical intervention (see Chapter 3.12). Modified interventions such as arthroscopic debridement, tendon synovectomy and synovectomy need to be reviewed carefully to see if they could reduce the need for arthroplasty in the future. Timing of surgery needs to be assessed carefully and, in particular, the sequence of surgery performed on various joints, particularly in the chronic rheumatoid, needs to be carefully evaluated. These topics are discussed in depth in Chapter 3.12.

ALTERNATIVE MEDICINE

Alternative and traditional medications are used by an extraordinarily large number of patients with musculoskeletal conditions (see Chapter 3.15). A recent study from Australia has estimated the cost to the Australian population for alternative medicine in 1993 to be in excess of Aus$621 million and that of alternative therapists to be in excess of Aus$300 million[23]. This combined amount is nearly three times the

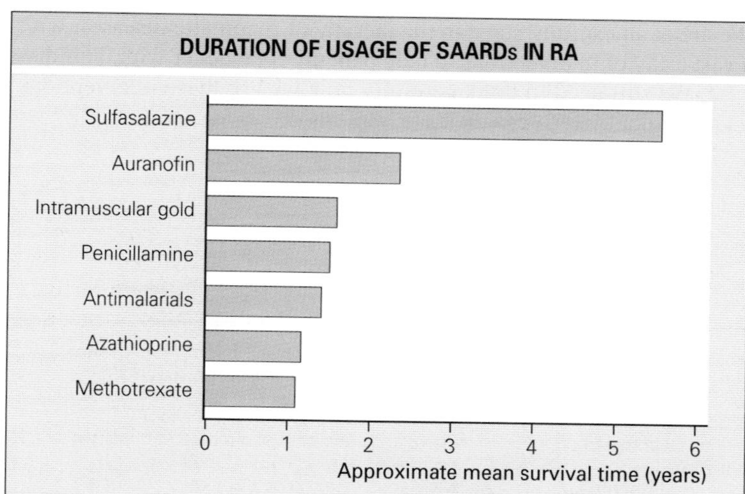

Fig. 1.3 Approximate median survival time for seven disease-modifying antirheumatic drugs (SAARDs). From Wolfe[18].

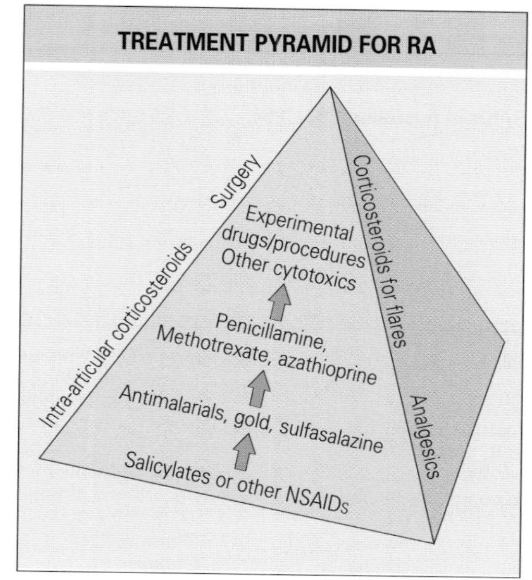

Fig. 1.4 Treatment pyramid for RA.

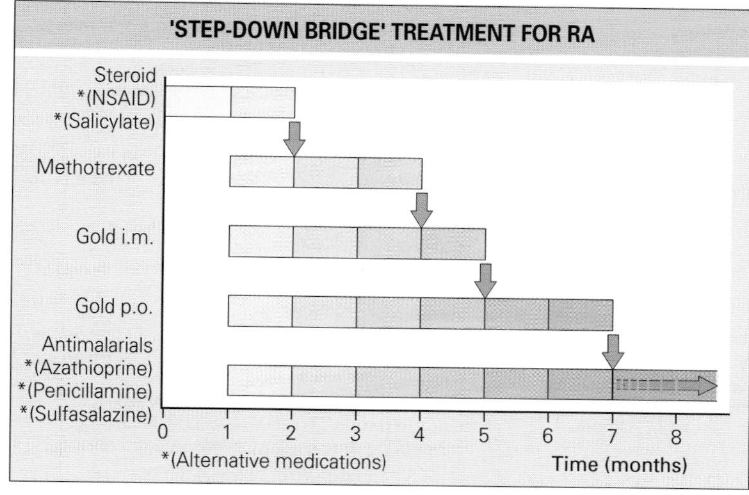

Fig. 1.5 'Step-down bridge' treatment for RA. From Wilske and Healey[19].

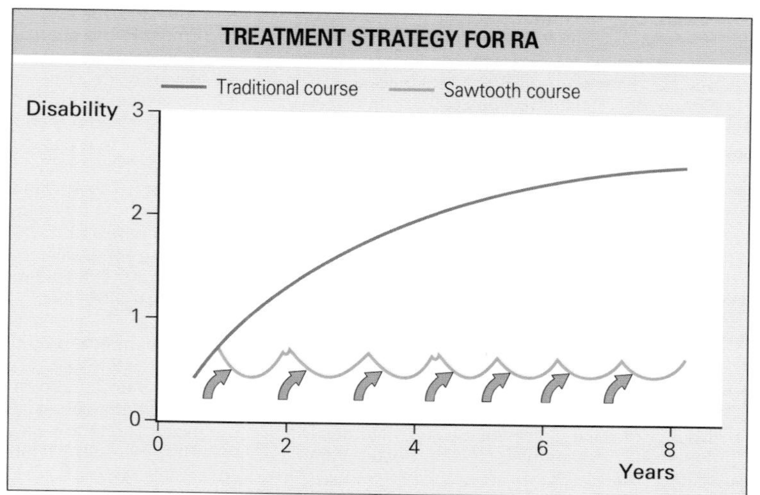

Fig. 1.6 'Sawtooth' treatment strategy for RA. Arrows indicate the administration of slow-acting antirheumatic drugs singly or in combination. Modified from Fries[20].

total amount of patient contributions for all classes of pharmaceutical drugs purchased in Australia for 1992–1993. These data should be viewed in the light of the absence of properly evaluated safety or efficacy data for the vast majority of these therapies.

CHANGING THERAPEUTIC PRACTICES

Management of rheumatic diseases has changed dramatically over the past 10 years. There has been much less emphasis on the use of NSAIDs, particularly in OA and soft tissue disorders. This is reflected by recent data[24] from Australia showing a significant decrease in community use of these drugs over the years 1990–1994 (Fig. 1.7). These data are reflected on the international scene. The reduction in NSAID use is due to a number of factors, including recognition of the toxicities of NSAIDs[25], earlier and more aggressive use of slow-acting antirheumatic drugs in the treatment of RA and data suggesting that, for OA, acetaminophen should be used initially before commencing a NSAID. It has also been appreciated over the past few years that different NSAIDs vary in their potential for gastrointestinal toxicity: ibuprofen is least likely to be associated with this adverse event[26].

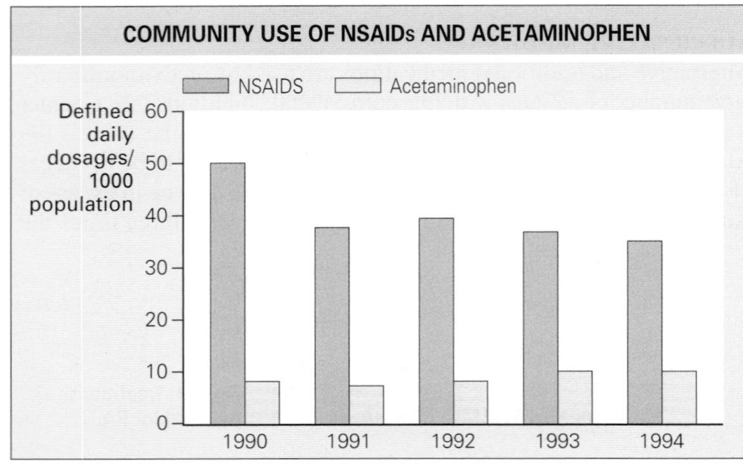

Fig. 1.7 Community use of NSAIDs in Australia 1990–1994. From McManus *et al.*[24].

A new generation of specific cyclo-oxygenase (COX)-2 inhibitors now being developed is certainly likely to change the use of NSAIDs in the future[27]. More aggressive approaches to the early treatment of inflammatory arthritis and the development of specific biological agents will also impact significantly on management strategies. Evolving surgical approaches – with arthroscopic surgery, early intervention and new prostheses with different fixations – will also change practices. Changes in health care systems, including a much greater emphasis on the evaluation of interventions and on cost effectiveness, are also beginning to influence the way we treat patients and have led to the development of a series of guidelines for the management of OA[28,29] and RA[30] and the monitoring of antirheumatic therapy[31]. These guidelines will need to be reviewed continually and updated as therapeutic advances are made.

CONCLUSIONS

We are at an exciting stage in the therapy of rheumatic diseases, with a vast array of interventions to help patients cope better with their disease. We still need to think carefully how we use these interventions and continually reassess their efficacy.

REFERENCES

1. Cochrane's legacy (editorial). Lancet. 1992;340:1131–2.
2. Brooks PM. Undergraduate education in rheumatology. Br J Rheumatol. 1996;35:203–4.
3. Branch WT, Arky RH, Woo B, S *et al.* Teaching medicine as a human experience: a doctor–patient relationship course for faculty and first year medical students. Ann Intern Med. 1991;114:482–9.
4. Lorig K, Cox T, Cuevas Y, Kraines RG, Britton M. Converging and diverging beliefs about arthritis: Caucasian patients, Spanish speaking patients and physicians. J Rheumatol. 1984;11:76–9.
5. Donovan J. Patient education and the consultation: the importance of lay beliefs. Ann Rheum Dis. 1991;50:418–21.
6. Boers M, Tugwell P, Felson D, *et al.* WHO–ILAR core endpoints for symptom modifying antirheumatic drugs in RA clinical trials. J Rheumatol. 1994;41(suppl):86–9.
7. LeQuesne M, Brandt K, Bellamy N, *et al.* Guidelines for testing slow acting drugs in OA. J Rheumatol. 1994;41(suppl):65–74.
8. American Academy of Orthopaedic Surgeons/ Council of Musculoskeletal Speciality Societies. Disabilities of the Arm, Shoulder and Hand Outcomes Data Collection Package (Version 1.3). Rosemont: Illinois, 1996:1–7.
9. American Academy of Orthopaedic Surgeons/ Council of Musculoskeletal Speciality Societies. Lower Limb Outcomes Data Collection Package (Version 1.3). Rosemont: Illinois, 1996:1-40.
10. American Academy of Orthopaedic Surgeons/ Council of Musculoskeletal Speciality Societies/ Council of Spine Societies. Spine Outcomes Data Collection Package (Version 1.3). Rosemont: Illinois, 1996:1–25.
11. Hawley DJ. Psycho-educational interventions in the treatment of arthritis. Baillière's Clin Rheumatol. 1995;9:803–23.
12. Fiatrone M, Marks BC, Ryan ND, *et al.* High intensity strength training on nonagenarians. JAMA. 1990;263:3029–34.
13. Dieppe P, Cushnagan J, Jasani MK, McCrae F, Watt I. A two-year placebo-controlled trial of non-steroidal anti-inflammatory therapy in osteoarthritis of the knee joint. Br J Rheumatol. 1993;32:595–600.
14. Williams HJ, Ward JR, Egger MJ, *et al.* Comparison of naproxen and acetaminophen in a two year study of treatment of osteoarthritis of the knee. Arthritis Rheum. 1993;36:1196–206.
15. March LM, Irwig LM, Schwarz J , *et al*, . *N*-of-1 trials comparing a non-steroidal anti-inflammatory drug with paracetamol in osteoarthritis. Br Med J. 1994;309:1041–6.
16. Emery P. The optimal management of early rheumatoid arthritis: the key to preventing disability. Br J Rheumatol. 1994;33:765–8.
17. tenWolde S, Breedveld FC, Hermans J, *et al.* Randomised placebo-controlled study of stopping second-line drugs in rheumatoid arthritis. Lancet.1996;347:347–52.
18. Wolfe F. The epidemiology of drug treatment failure in rheumatoid arthritis. Baillière's Clin Rheumatol. 1995;9:619–32.
19. Wilske KR, Healey LA. Remodelling the pyramid – a concept whose time has come. J Rheumatol. 1989;16:565–7.
20. Fries JF. Re-evaluating the therapeutic approach to rheumatoid arthritis: the 'saw tooth' strategy. J Rheumatol. 1990;17:12–15.
21. Möttönen T, Paimela L, Ahonen J, *et al.* Outcome in patients with early rheumatoid arthritis according to the 'saw tooth' strategy. Arthritis Rheum. 1996;39:996–1005.
22. Pinals RS, Masi AT, Larsen RA. The Subcommittee for Criteria of Remission in Rheumatoid Arthritis of the American Rheumatism Association Diagnostic and Therapeutic Criteria Committee. Preliminary criteria for clinical remission in rheumatoid arthritis. Arthritis Rheum. 1981;24:1308–15.
23. MacLennan AH, Wilson PH, Taylor AW. Prevalence and cost of alternative medicine in Australia. Lancet.1996;347:569–73.
24. McManus P, Primrose JG, Henry DA, *et al.* Pattern of non-steroidal anti-inflammatory drug use in Australia 1990–1994. Med J Aust. 1996;164:589–92.
25. Somervaile K, Faulkner G, Langman M. Non-steroidal anti-inflammatory drugs and bleeding peptic ulcer. Lancet.1986;i:462–4.
26. Henry D, Kim L-Y, Garcia-Rodriquez LA, *et al.* Variability in risk of gastrointestinal complications with individual non-steroidal anti-inflammatory drugs: results of a collaborative meta-analysis. Br Med J. 1996;312:1563–6.
27. Richardson CE, Emery P. New cyclo-oxygenase and cytokine inhibitors. Baillière's Clin Rheumatol. 1995;9:731–58.
28. Hochberg MC, Altman RD, Brandt KD, *et al.* Guidelines for the medical management of osteoarthritis. Part I – Osteoarthritis of the hip. Arthritis Rheum. 1995;38:1535–40.
29. Hochberg MC, Altman RD, Brandt KD, *et al.* Guidelines for medical management of osteoarthritis. Part II – Osteoarthritis of the knee. Arthritis Rheum. 1995;38:1541–6.
30. American College of Rheumatology Ad Hoc Committee on Clinical Guidelines. Guidelines for management of rheumatoid arthritis. Arthritis Rheum. 1996;39:713–22.
31. American College of Rheumatology Ad Hoc Committee on Clinical Guidelines. Guidelines for monitoring drug therapy in rheumatoid arthritis. Arthritis Rheum. 1996;39:723–31.

2

THE PROVISION OF RHEUMATOLOGIC SERVICES

Elizabeth M Badley

- Musculoskeletal disorders are the major cause of long-term disability, with a prevalence of 4–10%. A quarter to a third of the adult population suffer from problems with the joints, neck or back.
- The prevalence of these disorders increases with age, with implications for their future impact in an aging population.
- Comprehensive care needs to have a range of components: public and patient education, community services, good primary care, specialist care, particularly orthopedics and rheumatology.
- There is not one ideal system of rheumatology care: it can range from a sole office-based practitioner to a full rheumatic disease unit, comprising comprehensive in- and outpatient services supported by a team of health professionals.
- Rheumatology is increasingly becoming an ambulatory care specialty, and in many countries there are strong moves to increased care in the community.

INTRODUCTION

The provision of rheumatologic services has to be set in the context of the need for services for people with rheumatic disorders as a whole. This has several aspects which includes the nature of rheumatic disorders, how many people are affected and might need such services, and what kind of services should be provided.

Rheumatic and musculoskeletal disorders include the arthropathies, connective tissue disorders, back disorders, soft tissue rheumatism, bone disorders and sprains and strains. Rheumatic disorders range in severity from minor aches and pains affecting the joints and related structures, to serious and potentially life-threatening conditions, such as complicated rheumatoid arthritis (RA) and connective tissue disorders. The conditions can be relatively short-lived and self-limiting, episodic, or ongoing, progressive and disabling. Medical care may or may not be sought, and who is consulted will depend not only on the nature of the condition but also on local aspects of the health care delivery system.

Rheumatologic services may refer to the services provided by the rheumatologist or the services that are required to meet the needs of those with rheumatic disorders. The mandate of the former is more circumscribed and puts the rheumatologist in the central role. With the latter emphasis, rheumatologic input is but one of a possible range of responses, and the focus is on the needs of a particular population or community. This chapter addresses both aspects.

THE NEED FOR RHEUMATOLOGIC SERVICES

Much of what we know of the burden of rheumatic disorders in the community comes from general surveys of the population. These have the advantage of providing comprehensive coverage of those with rheumatic disorders, independently from their contacts with formal services. From the point of view of the clinical rheumatologist, one of the major drawbacks is that data are based on self-report. However, the American HANES I survey showed good agreement between reported symptoms and those confirmed by clinical examination[1]. The identification of specific disorders, for example, differentiation between RA and osteoarthritis (OA), is more of a problem. Where information is available, approximately 1 in 20 of those reporting chronic arthritis with symptoms have RA[1]; the ratio for those reporting activity limitation is about 1 in 8[2]. The majority within the category are designated as having OA or another arthropathy.

MORBIDITY AND DISABILITY DUE TO RHEUMATIC DISORDERS

Although the overall mortality from musculoskeletal disorders (MSD) is low[3,4], it can be significant in some of the more serious inflammatory disorders, such as RA in which it has been estimated to reduce lifespan by 5–7 years. The major impact in the population is in terms of morbidity and disability. It has been estimated that a quarter to a third of the adult population suffer from problems with the joints, neck or back[1,5–7]. The prevalence of symptoms and number of sites affected increases markedly with age. The major sites are the back and knee (see Fig. 2.1)[1,5]. Women are affected more frequently than men. The female preponderance is greater for 'arthritis' and less so for back and soft tissue disorders.

In the 1990 Ontario Health Survey (OHS), which referred to the household population, 29% of people aged 16 years and older reported MSD and 22% reported long-term health problems due to musculoskeletal disorders [7]. A similar figure was found for the USA, and indicated that some 13% of the population reported arthritis as a chronic condition, with a further 8% reporting back disorders[2]. Of those with musculoskeletal disorders in the 1990 OHS, about 60% reported arthritis and rheumatism, and slightly more than a third reported back disorders, with the remainder reporting other associated conditions[7]. The prevalence of chronic musculoskeletal disorders increases almost linearly with age from 7.5% in the 16–24 age group to 47.6% in those aged 75 years and older. This age-related increase is seen in other population surveys. Generally, the prevalence of arthritis affecting the limb joints increases with age, whereas back disorders show an increase in prevalence to middle age with a leveling-off or slight decline in old age (see Fig. 2.1). Notwithstanding their high population frequency, musculoskeletal disorders cannot be dismissed as aches and pains. In the 1990 OHS, the median duration of all musculoskeletal disorders was 5 years, and 80% had a duration of 1 year or longer. Overall, 82% of respondents reported pain, and 50% reported pain that limited activities[7]. Musculoskeletal disorders are the number one type of chronic condition reported in the population, followed closely by allergies (prevalence 19.7%) and by circulatory disorders (13.5%)[8].

Musculoskeletal disorders are the major cause of long-term disability in the population[2,8–10]. Data from the 1990 OHS show that musculoskeletal disorders represent over 54% of all long-term disability[8]. The next most frequent causes of long-term disability, circulatory and respiratory disorders only have population prevalences of 1.4 and 0.6%, respectively[8], whereas the prevalence of disablement in association with MSD is of the order of 4–10%[5,9,11–13]. The prevalence of disability increases markedly with age, with over 20% of the population aged 65 years and older reporting MSD as a cause of disability (see Fig. 2.2)[12,13]. The way the prevalence of MSD-associated disability changes with age is similar to that for morbidity from these conditions.

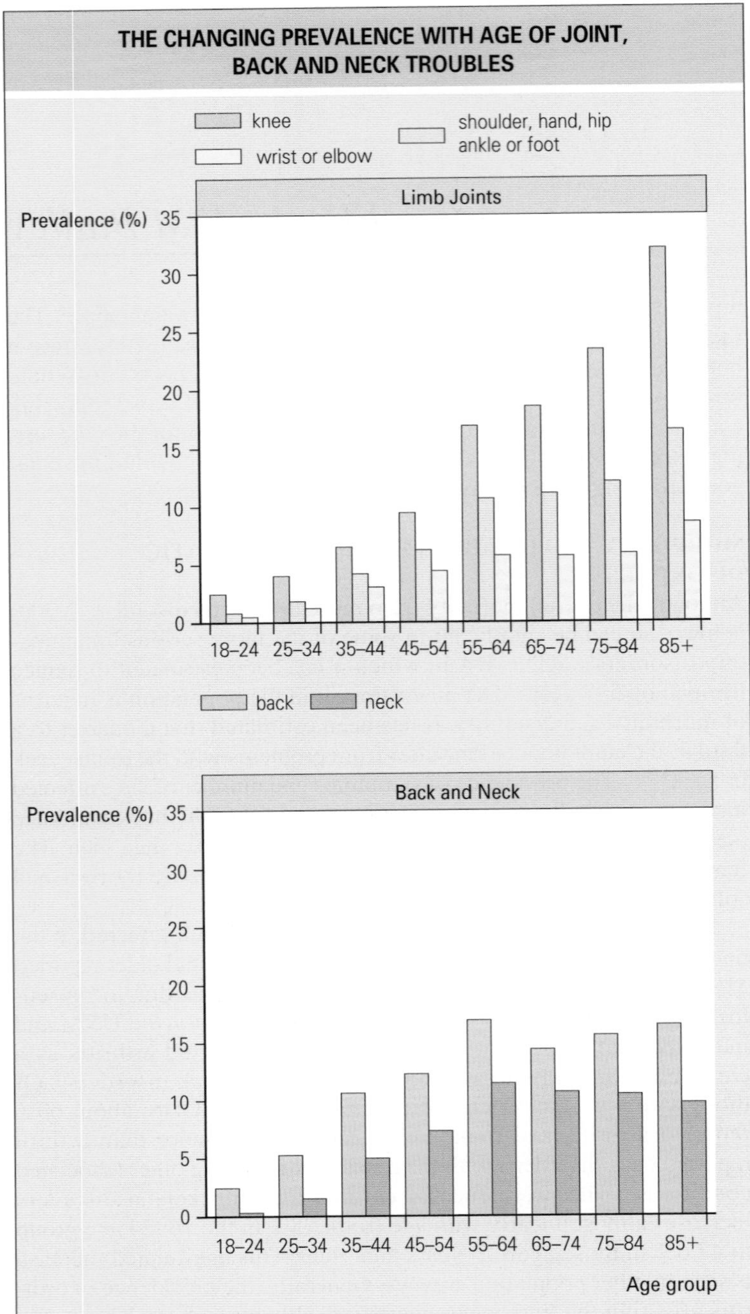

Fig. 2.1 The changing prevalence with age of joint, back and neck troubles. Data on self-reported pain, swelling or stiffness in the joints, neck or back from the postal screening questionnaire of the Calderdale Rheumatic Disablement Survey[5].

ASSESSMENT OF CURRENT HEALTH CARE UTILIZATION

Musculoskeletal disorders are an important reason for health care utilization. Figure 2.3 uses data from the 1990 OHS to summarize the prevalence of morbidity and health care use associated with musculoskeletal disorders. A health professional had been consulted within the previous 2 years for 79% of the musculoskeletal disorders reported in the OHS, which represents a 2-year consultation rate of 23% of the adult population. The corresponding consultation rate for a 1-year period was 21% of the adult population. The proportion of those with MSD consulting in the previous year varied slightly depending on the duration of the condition. It was 86% for those with MSD of duration 1 year or less, and declined with duration to 60% for those with duration of 10 years or longer. So over half of those individuals with MSD of long duration had consulted a health professional within the previous year. Only 8% of respondents reported never having consulted a health professional for these conditions.

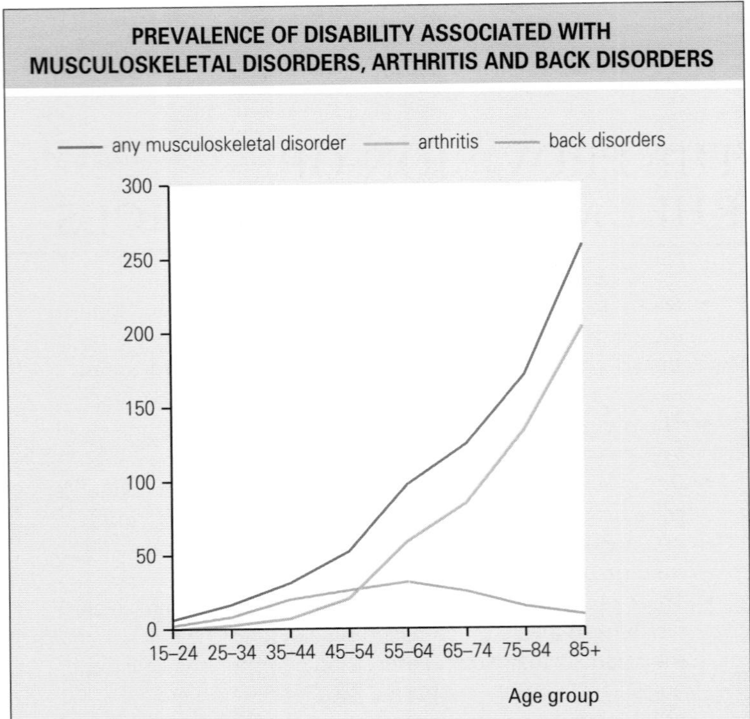

Fig. 2.2 Prevalence of disability in association with musculoskeletal disorders, arthritis and back disorders. By 10-year age-groups in the 1986 Canadian population[12].

In terms of more immediate impact, about 40% of those with MSD reported some type of health care utilization or illness from their condition in the previous 2 weeks. This represents a prevalence of 12% of the household population. The two most frequently reported types of 2-week impact were the use of prescription medication for MSD and health professional consultation (Fig. 2.3). Unfortunately, data are not available about the type of MSD medication. Compared with conditions of other major body systems, MSDs were the number one reason for consulting health professionals within the previous 2 weeks, and the second most frequently reported reason for prescription and non-prescription drug use, and for restricted activity days8.

From the point of view of the health care system, the US National Health Survey found that in each year about 15% of the population have episodes of musculoskeletal disorders of sufficient severity to warrant medical care or restriction of activity[9]. This is second in magnitude only to respiratory conditions. Data from the UK show that a similar proportion of the population (15%) consult their general practitioner with a musculoskeletal complaint each year[14,15]. Musculoskeletal disorders account for 9% of all physician visits, 5% of all hospital discharges and 10% of all hospital procedures in the US[10], which is similar to data from the UK and Canada[4,15,16,17]. Although these proportions may appear substantial in absolute terms, the rate of hospital admission for rheumatologic disorders is low, especially compared with the population prevalence. The rate of hospital admissions is thought to be decreasing as a result of cuts in hospital services and the impact of changes in health care systems. Thus rheumatology has increasingly becoming an ambulatory care specialty. Data from the UK suggests that on average about 15% of patients presenting in primary care with a rheumatologic condition are referred to a specialist[14]. Unfortunately, there is a large gap in available information on ambulatory services, as data on outpatient or office visits to rheumatologists are lacking.

IMPACT OF RHEUMATIC DISORDERS

A summary of the importance of musculoskeletal disorders in the adult population is given in Fig. 2.4[13]. This summary is restricted to the developed countries of the world.The age-related increase in prevalence of MSD has implications for the future impact of these disorders

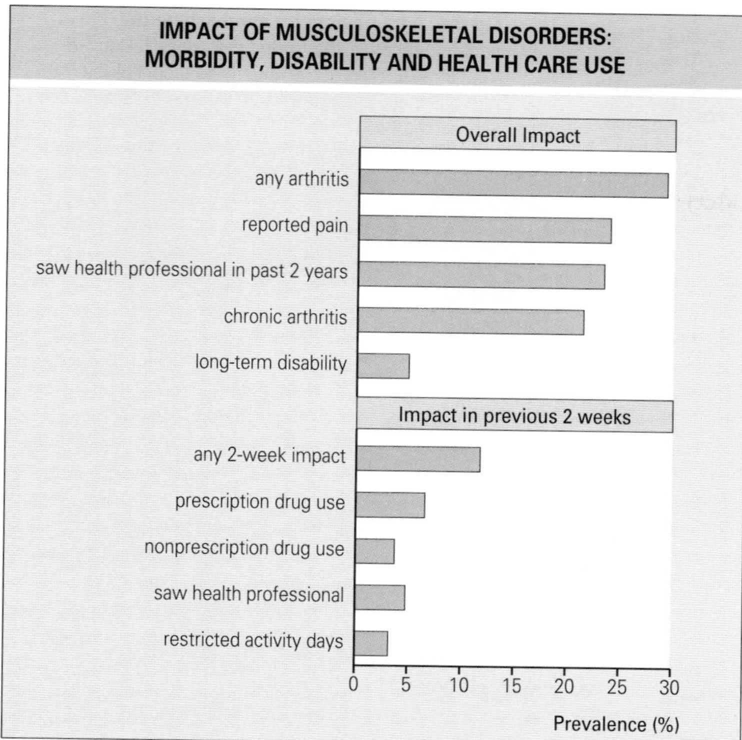

Fig. 2.3 The population impact of musculoskeletal disorders: morbidity, disability and health care use. Percentage prevalence in the Ontario population[7].

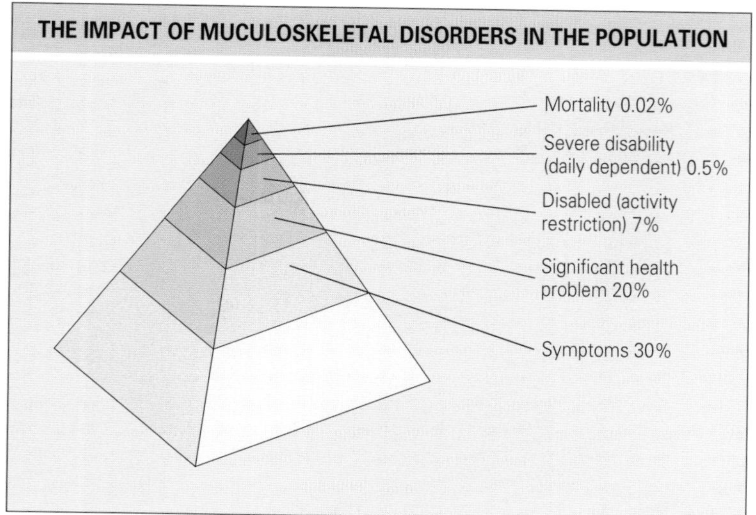

Fig. 2.4 A summary of the impact of musculoskeletal disorders in the population.

with the aging of the population[18,19]. Age has an effect particularly on the increasing prevalence of joint disorders, especially OA and osteoporosis, as revealed by increasing incidences of hip and other fractures[9]. An international comparison of the projected prevalence of disabilities associated with MSD in western countries shows an increase in both prevalence and numbers due to the aging of the population[19]. This projected increase is greatest in countries of the New World, for example, the USA, Canada and Australia, particularly the latter two countries. The situation in the developing countries is even less well documented. The burden of rheumatic disorders is likely to be very different. Partly this relates to the spectrum of morbidity, with a higher burden of communicable diseases, nutritional disorders and trauma, which in turn may give rise to associated musculoskeletal disorders. A further factor is the younger demographic structure of the population. The developing countries are 'aging' at a greater rate than the developed countries, and it is to be expected that the frequency of musculoskeletal disorders in these countries will increase dramatically, and the overall spectrum will move towards that found in the more developed countries. The response to these problems are part of a much larger picture and are not dealt with here.

SERVICES TO COVER THE SPECTRUM, SEVERITY AND CHRONICITY OF RHEUMATIC DISORDERS

The chronicity and uncertain outcome of many of the rheumatic disorders means that there is a need to respond to the disabling consequences experienced by individuals, and their families. The question is how does one organize services to meet the needs of this very diverse client group? A key issue must be that of triage, making sure that the appropriate level of care is available for different types and severity of MSD-associated problems.

RESPONDING TO THE BURDEN OF CHRONIC, DISABLING DISORDERS

Consideration of services for chronic and disabling rheumatic disorders requires a framework which extends the traditional medical model. Such a framework is offered by the WHO International Classification of Impairments, Disabilities and Handicaps[20] (see Fig. 2.5.)

The disease or the disorder, in this case arthritis, may result in impairment. This represents the consequences of arthritis for the performance of the body or parts of the body, such as restricted joint movement, deformity or loss of strength or endurance. Impairment may then result in disability, i.e.the restriction in the performance of activities. For example, disability may result in an individual having difficulty or inability in activities of daily living, such as walking, dressing or any of the other activities that make up the daily life of the person. Impairment or disability may result in handicap which is the disadvantageous consequence for the individual. Handicap can be experienced in a number of different dimensions. For people with arthritis, there may be loss of physical independence, with the need to rely on the help of other people. There may be an impact on mobility, the ability to move around effectively in the environment, and also on occupation, including work, leisure and obligations in the home. Social integration and relationships with other people may be affected. Finally, there may be reduced economic self-sufficiency, not only through reduced earning power, but also because of the extra expenses incurred because of the disease.

Figure 2.5 also indicates that handicap is not an inevitable and direct consequence of impairment and disability. More social consequences of arthritis arise from an interaction of the impairment and disability with other external factors[21]. The physical environment, such as steps or stairs, architectural barriers and housing, is one such factor. For example, the impact of disabilities in climbing stairs will be less for someone who lives in a single-story house with no external or internal steps or stairs. Other interacting factors include the availability of resources, such as assistive devices, personal help, education, personal attributes, money and possessions. What might be termed the social setting also has a part to play. This would include the attitudes of others (both within the family and more generally), cultural background and values, and expectations.

LESSENING THE IMPACT OF DISEASE

It may be reasonable to wonder what all this has to do with rheumatologic services. If the needs of those with rheumatic disorders are to be addressed then all these factors are of relevance. It is clear that the rheumatologists cannot do everything. Medical care is mainly concerned with controlling the underlying disease or disorder. This is perhaps the most important role for the clinical specialist. The assumption is that if the underlying disorder can be controlled then the adverse consequences of impairment, disability and handicap will be avoided.

There have been calls for the objectives of health care to be on the quality of life rather than on its duration, to minimize loss of fitness and to prevent unnecessary loss of physical disability[22]. With this in

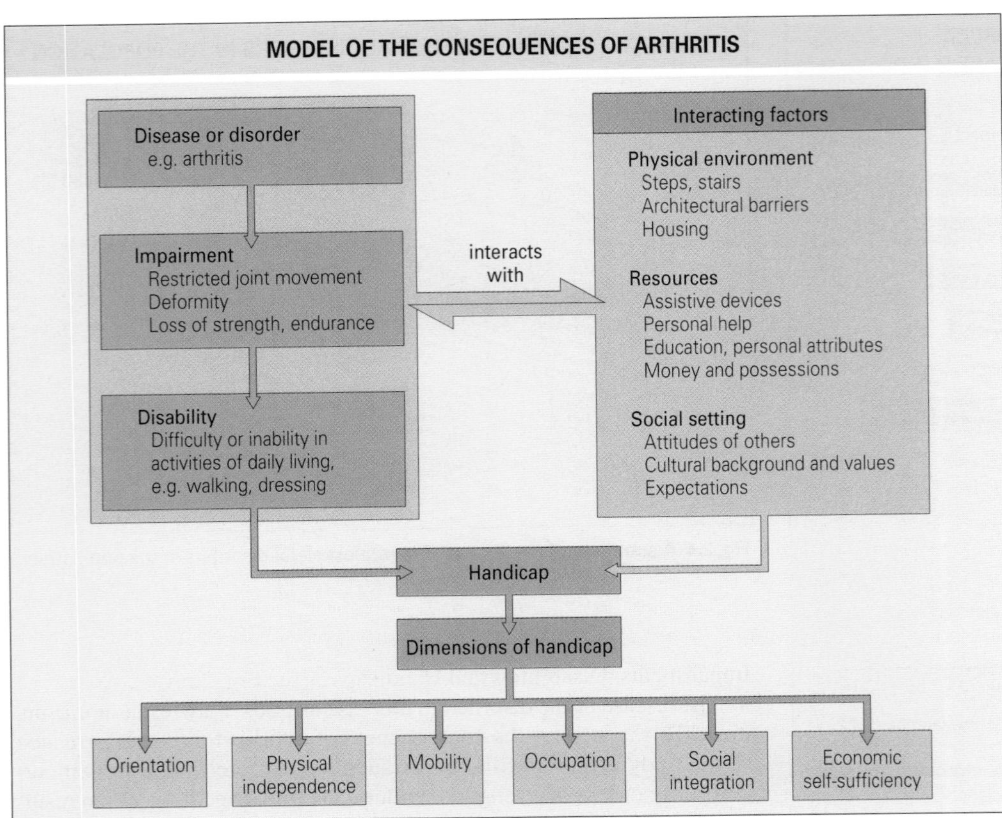

Fig. 2.5 A framework for approaching the consequences of rheumatic disorders[21]. Derived from an extension of the underlying model of the International Classification of Impairments, Disabilities and Handicaps[20].

mind, an important aspect of care becomes the postponement of the disabling aspects of morbidity. Arguably, the most important outcome is to prevent handicap and its adverse impact on the life of the individual and family. A range of modalities may need to be used to achieve these objectives, many of which are more the province of rehabilitation and community services, but all are services to which referral might need to be made. Some of the other factors that might influence outcome are indicated on the right-hand side of Figure 2.5. The range of potential interventions is wider than those normally thought of as mainstream medical services. Depending on how services are organized, the rheumatologist may have an important role to play in the coordination of these interventions for the benefit of the patient. For example, consideration may have to be made of the needs of older people so that they can remain in their own homes, and to prevent the breakdown of informal support offered by relatives and friends. Similarly, the rheumatologist may have to interact with employers to advocate for modifications to the working environment.

A COMPREHENSIVE STRATEGY FOR SERVICE FOR RHEUMATIC DISORDERS

A comprehensive strategy for rheumatic disorders would need to have a number of different components to address different aspects of care (Fig. 2.6). It would need to relate to all people in the population (the large box in Fig. 2.6) and provide information about what can be done, about the importance of these disorders as health problems and about the need for services.

A most important focus of any strategy for rheumatic disorders is people with these disorders and their families. Many of rheumatic disorders will be minor and self-limiting and not require medical intervention. The frequency of musculoskeletal symptoms as a cause of ill-health is in the same league as colds, coughs and stomach upsets[8,9]. Information about self-medication and the criteria for consultation are readily available for these latter conditions. In contrast, information about musculoskeletal symptoms, for example, adequate dosage of aspirin and pain-relievers, simple physical remedies and when it is important to seek medical care, is not so much part of 'common knowledge'. It is clear that the magnitude of the morbidity is such that the system would be overwhelmed if all who are affected sought consultations, yet there is a need to ensure that those who need help receive it. Use of so-called alternative therapies by people with musculoskeletal disease is also enormous, although largely unevaluated, and this needs to be taken into account when considering strategies for care at the community level.

For those with established or serious MSD there is a need for education about 'self-management' strategies. Self-management education includes techniques for controlling pain and other symptoms, use of exercise, use of assistive devices and adaptations, as well as medication and appropriate consultation with health professionals. Musculoskeletal disorders in general, and arthritis in particular, can be facilitated by 'self-management' strategies. For example, evaluation of a formal program, the Arthritis Self-Management Program (ASMP), first developed in the USA, has shown significant decreases in pain and medical consultation as well as increases in self-efficacy among participants [23]. Exercise has been shown to be beneficial in reducing pain and stiffness and in maintaining function[24,25].

Ideally a range of community support and rehabilitation services need to be in place both for formal treatment and to facilitate so-called 'self-management'. Both physical and occupational therapy have important and complementary roles in the maintenance of function and the control of disability for people with rheumatic disorders. People with arthritis may also need orthotics and perhaps special shoes. Services to facilitate 'self-management' could range from structured community-based programs, such as the ASMP, to support groups. An important community-level provision is the availability of appropriate classes or other facilities that offer exercise programs appropriate for people with rheumatic disorders, including exercise in water.

Sooner or later most people with rheumatic disorders consult primary care physicians or health professionals, including nurse practitioners. It is important that these professionals have the training and experience to carry out appropriate investigations to make a correct diagnosis and to prescribe appropriate treatment. The latter might include advice about self-management techniques. In many ways the primary care practitioner can be viewed as a gatekeeper. The practitioner may manage the problem or a referral may be made. It is reasonable to expect that, for example, nonarticular rheumatism, low back pain, most OA, and some uncomplicated and established RA could be managed at the primary care level. There are also roles for the general

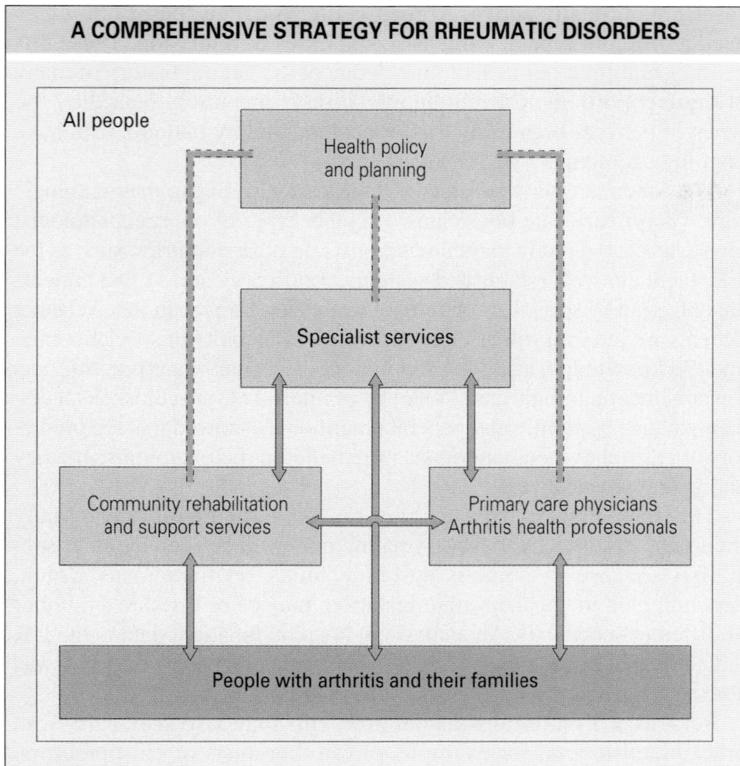

Fig. 2.6 A comprehensive strategy for rheumatic disorders.

practitioner in the long-term management and monitoring of the more chronic rheumatic disorders with specialists. Unfortunately, the literature suggests that primary care training in musculoskeletal conditions is deficient, and this is supported by evidence that the primary care diagnosis, treatment and referral of patients with musculoskeletal conditions has been found to be suboptimal in some cases[26–30]. Educational responses are discussed in Chapter 3.3.

Patients with severe, unusual or refractory conditions may be referred to specialist care. Rheumatology services are discussed below. However, rheumatologists are only one part of the care delivery system for the person with rheumatic disorders. The complementary surgical specialty is orthopedics. In terms of our model outlining the consequences of disease (Fig. 2.5), the orthopedic surgeon makes an important contribution in the treatment of impairment and the restoration of function. The most notable success in the musculoskeletal field is, of course, joint replacement. Good liaison with the rheumatologist can help to ensure planned and timely surgery. However, orthopedics may also be the primary referral for the management of many disorders.

All these services, including those provided at the local level or to the population as a whole, need to be viewed within the framework of health policy and planning. This means that there is a need for information to support the development, provision and funding of appropriate services. In this context, health professionals in the field of rheumatic disorders have important roles as advocates about issues of the provision of services at the local and also at the national levels.

RHEUMATOLOGIST CARE

Figure 2.6 shows the specialist as central to a strategy for rheumatic disorders. Specialist care ideally would be located at the 'local' hospital, and serve as a consultant to primary care practitioners and be readily accessible to the population. A medical consultant[31] ideally provides a diagnosis and specialist advice and deals with chronic, complex diseases necessitating long-term specialist follow-up. It has been suggested that the areas where the rheumatology consultant might contribute are as follows[31]:

- Reversible conditions – to initiate treatment with nil or short-term follow-up for self-limiting conditions, i.e. soft tissue problems, acute back problems, etc.
- Irreversible disease – where a musculoskeletal condition gives rise to chronic symptoms but the majority of which do not require long-term follow-up, only re-referral for acute episodes, i.e. spondylosis, OA, etc.
- Fluctuating disease – this would include any chronic inflammatory disease of the musculoskeletal system characterized by episodes of disease exacerbation which may have significant sequelae unless correctly managed, i.e. RA, seronegative arthropathies, connective tissue diseases, etc. These diseases necessitate monitoring of both disease and therapies. This may be totally hospital-based but the development of shared care with primary health care is the more worthwhile objective. Before this can be implemented, standard guidelines on how to monitor diseases and drugs would be useful. The long-term management of these patients is an area where primary care physicians may have problems because of a lack of training.

Specialist care may also be provided at the tertiary care level. This type of care would most often be found in the larger centers and in teaching hospitals. A problem with individual rheumatologists working in small units at the secondary care level is that, although they provide a service, the rheumatologist has little exposure to rare conditions[32]. The danger is that patients with special needs may not receive optimum care unless special facilities are set up, both to treat these patients and to offer their physicians the advice and support of clinicians with specialist experience. One of the challenges facing those planning rheumatology services is the need to ensure that these special facilities are available, at least at a regional level. Such centers may develop on an ad hoc basis, for example, a teaching center may evolve into a tertiary or quaternary referral center when physicians have a special interest in rare or complicated disorders. Referrals will often be from other practicing rheumatologists, particularly those who have trained in that center. Other areas for which special regional services may need to be planned include arthritis in children. This is the case in the UK, but in other countries it happens on an ad hoc basis. Tertiary care services may also function at the secondary care level. They may need to do this in order to train the next generation of trainees and to give exposure to the spectrum of patients seen in 'ordinary' practice.

CURRENT PATTERNS OF RHEUMATOLOGIC CARE

Existing patterns of care are not well documented. There is no single ideal system. As well as structural differences between health care systems organization and methods of payment, there are also variations in patterns of rheumatologic care both between countries and cultures and in different communities. This applies to what are considered to be the treatments of choice, and how and in which order treatment modalities are applied. Any rheumatologist who has worked in more than one center, and especially those who have gone to other countries, can attest to this. Examples of major differences include the use of spa therapy in Germany, use of manipulation for low back pain, and the primary choice of second-line drugs for the treatment of RA.

It is uncertain to what degree variations in the funding and delivery of care account for the differences in the national rates of provision of rheumatology services. There are also different practices with regard to accreditation and certification as specialists[33]. The number of rheumatologists per 1000 population varies between and within most western countries. For example, within the European Community per capita rheumatologic provision is estimated to vary 10-fold from 0.3/100,000 (in Eire) to 3.5/100,000 in Denmark[33], with big variations within countries[33–37]. A 1990 estimate for the US is 1.2/100,000 with a projection that there will be 1.5/100,000 by the year 2000[38]. The per capita rheumatology provision may actually overestimate the amount of rheumatologic care available. In many cases, teaching, research and administrative commitments, particularly in University centers, may reduce the real availability of clinical care from what is apparent from a mere counting of heads[36].

RHEUMATOLOGY SERVICES NEEDED TO MEET HEALTH CARE NEEDS

This section looks in more detail at assessing the magnitude of need for specialist rheumatologic provision[39].

CONDITIONS CARED FOR BY RHEUMATOLOGISTS

The need for rheumatologists will depend on the range of conditions normally treated, and this varies between countries. For example, in France osteoporosis is part of the normal spectrum of rheumatologic practice, whereas this is not universally the case in English-speaking countries. There are other differences in the degree to which rheumatologists manage soft tissue and localized joint complaints and low back pain. For example, the main thrust in Sweden is on inflammatory diseases and soft tissue problems whereas low back disorders and OA are handled by other specialists or in primary care[32].

The content of the practice also depends on the nature and location of the rheumatologic practice. A survey in the UK[40] highlighted the very different natures of rheumatologic practice in teaching hospitals and district general hospitals. In teaching hospitals, there was a greater emphasis on inflammatory arthropathies, whereas patients with localized joint problems and back disorders were more likely to be seen by rheumatologists in general hospitals. There are also differences in the scope of the tasks undertaken by the rheumatologist, the most notable being whether physical medicine and rehabilitation is included or not. There are also changes over time, for instance, the increasing recognition of fibromyalgia as part of the rheumatologic caseload[39].

NATIONAL PREVALENCE OF THESE CONDITIONS

In planning services for a particular locality, an approximate indication of the number of people with rheumatic disorders can, in principle, be derived by applying age- and sex-specific prevalence rates to the population of interest. In practice it is very difficult to ascertain the prevalence of conditions needing treatment owing to the lack of suitable published statistics. Figure 2.7 lists the conditions included in the 1990 ACR study, together with their estimates of prevalence. The ACR Manpower Study drew heavily on the work of a US task force which considered both epidemiologic and US national health survey data. Other data from developed countries indicate a similar picture, at least in terms of morbidity and disability. It is when one needs data for specific conditions that there are considerable uncertainties. As indicated above, factors which will affect the prevalence of rheumatic disorders include the age and sex composition of the population. This will to some degree determine workload; arthropathy increases in prevalence with age, whereas low back pain plateaus in late middle-age. As the proportion of old people in the community rises, so will the total burden of rheumatic disease and the need for specialist services[18,19].

REFERRAL TO A RHEUMATOLOGIST

Estimating the proportion of people with each of these conditions who should see a physician and the percentage of those who should see a rheumatologist calls for judgment and it is likely that this judgment will vary between countries. There are few data on what proportion of referrals are practitioner or patient driven. Patient driven referrals might be expected to increase with greater community knowledge. A major influence on referral is the organization of health care. In many countries general practitioners are the first port of call for patients with rheumatic disorders, and many patients will be managed at this level. The 1990 ACR Manpower Study assumed that 100% of RA cases need ongoing medical care, 87% of it from rheumatologists (Fig. 2.7). Quite apart from whether this is a reasonable estimate, it supposes that all cases are clinically active. Arguably, the so-called 'burnt out' cases need a different type of care, as would cases in remission. These difficulties highlight our lack of knowledge of the natural history of many of these conditions. Current appreciation is inevitably biased by the types of patients seen in the major centers, and by patients who have ongoing problems.

The American study considered three tracks leading to rheumatologic care: via primary care physicians, via other types of nonrheumatologist physicians and directly to rheumatologists. In other countries, such as the UK, there are well-established systems of primary care, so that patients are only seen by specialists on referral by the general practitioner. Whether patients are referred will also depend on the availability of specialist care, and the knowledge, attitudes and beliefs of primary care practitioners towards rheumatologic care. A survey of referral of musculoskeletal disease patients by family and general practitioners showed that the predictors of referral to rheumatologists were belief in rheumatologist efficacy and young physician age[41].

The specialist referred to may not be a rheumatologist. Many rheumatic diseases by their very nature may well be seen by other specialists. A case in point is systemic lupus erythematosus which, depending on the primary manifestation, may be referred to a number of different specialists. An analysis of hospital inpatient data in the UK indicated that of the range of major rheumatic diagnoses, only RA was admitted to rheumatology beds more than 50% of the time.

Persons with musculoskeletal problems may also seek care from other practitioners, for example, physiotherapists or chiropractors. There is relatively little documentation of the rate of usage of these practitioners, although one important factor is likely to be related to payment systems. For example, the Workers' Compensation Board of Ontario, Canada, has a system whereby musculoskeletal injuries such as sprains and strains are treated primarily by physiotherapists, rather than by physicians.

NUMBER OF VISITS PER YEAR

Judgment is also required in estimating the annual number of visits to a rheumatologist for each condition. A lot depends on whether the rheumatologist assumes full responsibility for care or whether the role is more as a consultant. In some instances, this will be determined by the nature of the disease and the availability of other services. For example, the monitoring of second-line drugs could be carried out by other health professionals. The organization of services will also be important. To use the example of the UK once again, a well-established system of primary care, in theory at least, offers the possibility of complete management of straightforward rheumatic disorders at this level. A further important influence in determining the frequency with which patients consult is what is reimbursed or allowed by the health insurance system.

ORGANIZATION OF RHEUMATOLOGY SERVICES

Geographical factors need to be taken into account when considering the organization of rheumatology services. It has been suggested that the requirement for rheumatologists is higher in less densely populated countries on account of the geographic dispersion of the population[34]. This raises the problem of devising a service for populations remote from specialist care. In this situation other physicians need to take over the day-to-day management, ideally with a specialist as a resource. The specialist input can be managed in a number of ways. One alternative is referral of patients to major centers which would need to have adequate inpatient facilities to accommodate patients who may have to travel long distances. A variant on admission to hospital beds is the provision of associated hotel or hostel facilities. A further alternative is to have the rheumatologists travel, and make regular visits to community clinics or hospitals in the remote areas. The comparative effectiveness, efficiency and impact on care of the patient of these different models of care have not been systematically evaluated.

Arrangements for rheumatologic care can range from a single-handed practitioner with an office-based practice, using external radiologic and

PATIENT CARE REQUIREMENTS MODEL					
Rheumatic condition*	Prevalence per 100,000 population †	Requiring medical care (%)	Requiring rheumatologic care (%)	Average annual rheumatology visits‡	Estimated annual rheumatology visits per 100,000 population
Arthropathy					
Rheumatoid arthritis	500	100	87	8	3468
Residual arthritides	800	80	50	3.5	1389
Osteoarthritis	3500	60	17	2	1213
Crystalline arthritis	1090	50	20	3	646
Connective tissue disease	100	100	94	6	562
Ankylosing spondylitis	200	85	70	4	560
Psoriatic arthropathy	62	100	71	6	262
Acute nonpyogenic arthritis	100	100	47	4	186
Pyogenic arthritis	28	100	50	8	112
Gonococcal infection of joint	7	100	55	4	15
Dorsopathy					
Neck and back pain	10,000	20	2	2	364
Disc displacement	1300	90	13	2	331
Soft tissue rheumatism					
Fibromyalgia	2000	60	16	6	1951
Bursitis/tendinitis	5500	50	9	2	979
Internal joint derangement	100	80	7	2	4
Bone disorders					
Osteoporosis	7000	80	6	2	889
Paget's disease	2000	10	3	4	248
Osteomyelitis	136	100	25	1	34
Other musculoskeletal disorders	1351	45	< 1.0	1.5	7

* Residual arthritides include Lyme arthritis, polymyalgia rheumatica and arthritis unspecified.
† Rate per 100,000 population aged 17 years and older.
‡ Number of medically necessary rheumatology visits per year for the average patient with the given rheumatic condition.

Fig. 2.7 Patient care requirements model. Adapted from Marder *et al.*[39].

laboratory services, to a full rheumatic diseases unit. This would comprise a comprehensive inpatient and outpatient service, supported by a team of health professionals including doctors, physiotherapists, occupational therapists, social workers and so on.

There have been significant advances in the investigation and treatment of these diseases, together with a growing understanding of the prevention of disability. It is thus possible for the rheumatologist to treat a greater proportion of patients with rheumatic diseases than ever before. Rheumatology has always been in demand. It has been suggested that considerable expansion is required to provide an optimal service even before allowances are made for the aging population and technological advances[42].

IMPLICATIONS

Rheumatologic services have to cover a wide range of conditions, with a range of outcomes. There are many different systems of care already in operation, both between and within countries. It is clear that what is understood as the mandate of rheumatology varies and is evolving. This evolution is being driven on the one hand by technologic developments and increases in knowledge, and on the other by the impact of financial constraints on the health care system. Rheumatology is becoming increasingly an ambulatory care specialty. There are also strong moves in many countries to increased care in the community. This implies new roles for the rheumatologists as a specialist resource in a consultative service, and increased partnership and shared care with family physicians and other health professionals. Care in the community also means new roles for other health professionals, and one of the associated developments is the increasing autonomy of other professionals, such as nurses and rehabilitation therapists.

There is a lack of comparative studies looking at outcome of care in relation to specialty of treatment, the type of treatment package or the organization of care. There is enormous potential for studies to investigate whether different patterns of care have an impact on outcome, with scope for direct comparison of different modalities and different methods of care delivery. Outcomes could include not only benefit in terms of the management of the disease, but also aspects such as patient satisfaction and preference, and cost effectiveness.

There is little hard evidence on which to plan services rationally. Arguably, the introduction of new or improved services needs to build on, or at least take note of existing services. Even if formal rheumatology services have not been available there will still have been people in the catchment area who will have been receiving at least some form of assistance for their rheumatic disorders. The planned introduction of new or reorganized services also creates opportunities for evaluation.

A vital issue for the future and for the maintenance of services is what is variously called quality assurance or audit. Does the service do any good? One of the problems in many countries is that, while there may be data on inpatient services available for diagnostic groups as a by-product of hospital statistics, there are few, if any, routine sources of data on outpatients. Therefore, it is difficult even to document the workload and contribution of rheumatology, let alone the benefit. In times of increasing financial constraint there is a need to be able to describe, or better still, quantify the contribution of rheumatology services in relation to resources consumed.

This chapter has briefly touched on a number of issues in relation to the provision of rheumatology services. There are two ways of approaching this; by considering the burden of rheumatic disorders in the population and how the needs of those affected might be met, and from the narrower perspective of rheumatology. It is clear that the rheumatologist is only one part of the bigger picture, and that there are many variations on the overall theme. There is still much to be done in understanding the different ways in which this picture might be painted, and much to be learnt from study of the ways in which care is currently delivered, both within and between different countries and health care systems.

REFERENCES

1. Cunningham LS, Kelsey JL. Epidemiology of musculoskeletal impairments and associated disability. Am J Public Health. 1984;74:574–9.
2. LaPlante M. Data on disability from the National Health Interview Survey, 1983–85. An InfoUse report. Washington, DC: US National Institute on Disability and Rehabilitation Research; 1988.
3. Reynolds MD. Prevalence of rheumatic diseases as causes of disability and complaints by ambulatory patients. Arthritis Rheum. 1978;21:377–82.
4. Wood PHN, Badley EM. Rheumatic disorders. In: Miller DL, Farmer RDT, eds. Epidemiology of diseases. Oxford: Blackwell Scientific Publications; 1982:333–46.
5. Badley EM, Tennant A. Changing profile of joint disorders with age: findings from a postal survey of the population of Calderdale, West Yorkshire, United Kingdom. Ann Rheum Dis. 1992;51:366–71.
6. Lee P, Helewa A, Smythe HA, Bombardier C, Goldsmith CH. Epidemiology of musculoskeletal disorders (complaints) and related disability in Canada. J Rheumatol. 1985;12:1169–73.
7. Badley EM, Webster GK, Rasooly I. The impact of musculoskeletal disorders in the population: are they just aches and pains? Findings from the 1990 Ontario Health Survey. J Rheumatol. 1995;22:733-9.
8. Badley EM, Rasooly I, Webster GK. Relative importance of musculoskeletal disorders as a cause of chronic health problems, disability, and health care utilization: Findings from the 1990 Ontario Health Survey. J Rheumatol. 1994;21:505–14.
9. Kelsey JL. Epidemiology of musculoskeletal disorders. New York: Oxford University Press; 1982.
10. Felts W, Yelin E. The economic impact of the rheumatic diseases in the United States. J Rheumatol. 1989;16:867–84.
11. Martin J, Meltzer H, Elliot D. The prevalence of disability among adults. OPCS surveys of disability in Great Britain, Report 1. OPCS Social Survey Division. London: HMSO; 1988.
12. Reynolds DL, Chambers LW, Badley EM, *et al.* Physical disability among Canadians reporting musculoskeletal diseases. J Rheumatol. 1992;19:1020–30.
13. Badley EM. The impact of musculoskeletal disorders in the Canadian population (Editorial). J Rheumatol. 1992;19:337–40.
14. Office of Population Censuses and Surveys. Morbidity statistics from general practice. Second National Survey 1970–71. The Royal College of General Practitioners, Office of Population Censuses and Surveys, Department of Health and Social Security, Studies on Medical and Population Subjects No.26. London: HMSO; 1974.
15. Wood PHN, Badley EM. Epidemiology of locomotor disorders in general practice. In: Jayson MIV, Million R, eds. Locomotor disability in general practice. Oxford: Oxford University Press; 1983:3–29.
16. Wood PHN. The basis of rheumatological practice, including nomenclature and classification. In: Scott JT, ed. Copeman's Textbook of Rheumatic Diseases, 6E. London: Churchill Livingstone; 1986:19–58.
17. Hospital statistics 1987/88, Ministry of Health, Ontario; 1988.
18. Badley EM. Population projections and the effect on rheumatology. Ann Rheum Dis. 1991;50:3–6.
19. Badley EM, Crotty M. An international comparison of the estimated effect of the aging of the population on the major cause of disablement, musculoskeletal disorders. J Rheumatol. 1995;22:1934–40.
20. World Health Organization (WHO). International Classification of Impairments, Disabilities, and Handicaps. Geneva: WHO; 1980.
21. Badley EM. The genesis of handicap: definition, models of disablement, and role of external factors. Disability and Rehab. 1995;17:53–62.
22. Fries JF. Aging, natural death, and the compression of morbidity. N Engl J Med. 1980;303:130–5.
23. Lorig K, Holman H. Arthritis self-management studies: A twelve-year review. Health Educ Q. (1993);20:17–28.
24. Kovar PA , Allegrante JP, MacKenzie CR, Peterson MGE, Gutin B, Charlson ME. Supervised fitness walking in patients with osteoarthritis of the knee. A randomised controlled trial. Ann Intern Med. 1992;116:529–34.
25. Minor MA, Hewett JE, Webel RR, Anderson SK, Kay DR. Efficacy of physical conditioning exercise in patients with rheumatoid arthritis and osteoarthritis. Arthritis Rheum. 1989;32:1396–1405.
26. Goldenberg DL, Meenan RF, Allaire S, Cohen AS. The educational impact of a rheumatology elective. Arthritis Rheum. 1983;26:658–63.
27. Renner BR, DeVellis BM, Ennett ST, *et al.* Clinical rheumatology training of primary care physicians: the resident perspective. J Rheumatol. 1990;17:666–72.
28. Strosberg MA, Strasberg JM. Do family practice residents in the United States learn clinical rheumatology? An important question. J Rheumatol. 1980;7:923–6.
29. Stross JK, Bole GG. The impact of a new rheumatologist on the management of rheumatic disease patients in community hospitals. Arthritis Rheum. 1983;26:1033–6.
30. Glazier RH, Dalby DM, Badley EM, Hawker GA, Bell MJ, Buchbinder R. Determinants of physician confidence in the primary care managment of musculoskeletal disorders. J Rheumatol. 1996;23:351–6.
31. Bird H. Workshop 4: Follow up and monitoring of patients. In: Scott DL, Baillie K, eds. Measuring performance in clinical rheumatology. Proceedings of the joint meeting between The British Society for Rheumatology and CASPE Research. London: Arthritis and Rheumatism Council Research Conference. Proceeding No. 7;1990:148–51.
32. Wollheim F. Commentary. Br J Rheumatol 1991;30:122. Comment on: Rheumatology manpower in the 1990s. Br J Rheumatol. 1991;30:119–22.
33. Symmons DPM, Jones S, Silman AJ. Manpower. Brit J Rheum 1993;32(suppl 4):18–21.
34. Davis P. Rheumatology manpower in the 1990s in Canada. Br J Rheumatol. 1991;30:234–8.
35. Brooks P, Edmonds J. Rheumatology manpower in Australia (letter). Br J Rheumatol. 1991;30:316–7.
36 Hawker GA, Badley EM. The provision of specialist rheumatology care: implications from a survey of rheumatologists in Ontario, Canada. J Rheumatol. 1995;22:959–66.
37. Symmons DPM, Bankhead CR, Griffiths I, Shipley M. Changing patterns of rheumatology manpower and practice in the UK in the 1990s. Br J Rheumatol. 1996;35:483–8.
38. Meenan RF. Rheumatology manpower – The US perspective. (Editorial). Br J Rheumatol. 1991;30:81.
39. Marder WD, Meenan RF, Felson DT, *et al.* The present and future adequacy of rheumatology manpower. A study of health care needs and physician supply. (Editorial). Arthritis Rheum. 1991;34:1209–17.
40. Bamji AN, Dieppe PA, Haslock DI, *et al.* What do rheumatologists do? A pilot audit study. Br J Rheumatol. 1990;29:295–8.
41. Felson DT, Meenan RF, Dayno SJ, Gertman P. Referral of musculoskeletal disease patients by family and general practitioners. Arthritis Rheum. 1985;28:1156–62.
42. Symmons DPM, Jones S, Hothersall TE. Rheumatology manpower in the 1990s. Br J Rheumatol. 1991;30:119–22.

3

HEALTH PROMOTION AND PATIENT EDUCATION FOR PEOPLE WITH ARTHRITIS

Adrian Bauman, Ylva Lindroth & Lawren H Daltroy

- Arthritis patient education is an important adjunct to traditional clinical management.
- The context and meaning of the illness for each patient are important, as well as the expectations of those who care for and support the patient with arthritis.
- Patient education goals for physicians include improved physician–patient communication, to increase patient understanding of the condition and the reasons for adherence to therapeutic advice.
- Even brief attention to patient education at every clinic visit or consultation may have an important impact.
- Additional patient education activities may be carried out by doctors, or by a multidisciplinary team of health professionals in the clinical or community setting.
- The main outcomes of patient education include information and awareness, improved behavioral skills and enhanced psychologic outcomes.
- Population strategies are needed to ensure access to education programs for all patients with arthritis, including the socially disadvantaged and those with less common and multisystem forms of arthritis.

INTRODUCTION

Early definitions of patient education focused on information transfer, usually from physician to patient, and upon teaching patients about the body, how it works and how to care for it. During the 1970s, radical social movements advocated the concept of patient self-care, defined as 'a process whereby lay people could function effectively on their own behalf in health promotion and disease prevention ... at the level of the primary health resource in the health care system'[1]. The concept of patient education grew during the 1980s and extended information transfer, but moved beyond 'self-care'. Consensus-derived definitions described patient education as 'a planned learning experience using a combination of methods such as teaching, counseling, and behavior modification techniques which influence patients' knowledge and health behavior . . . (and) involves an interactive process which assists patients to participate actively in their health care, and provides them with information about available health services and their use'[2]. This definition has lasted over a decade, as it develops the principles of patient responsibility but not self-care, the notion of behavioral learning rather than information alone and the concept of shared responsibility and collaborative decision-making with health care providers.

The term 'patient education' is generally restricted to people with chronic disorders, which distinguishes it from primary prevention programs (cervical cancer screening), and health education and health promotion programs (smoking cessation, physical activity programs). There is a role for primary prevention of some forms of arthritis, with a reduction in obesity [osteoarthritis (OA)], and an increase in calcium intake and in physical activity (osteoporosis) is of clear benefit[3], but requiring whole community, as well as patient education strategies.

The principles of patient education are relevant to diseases which vary markedly over time and among individuals in their clinical symptoms and effects on the patient's life. As well as for arthritis, patient education has been shown to be effective for patients with other chronic diseases, including asthma and diabetes[4–6].

RATIONALE FOR ARTHRITIS PATIENT EDUCATION

The aims are to develop and deliver patient education as a low-cost adjunct to clinical arthritis management, with few or no adverse effects. It is part of the development of multidisciplinary and integrated health care, extending clinical and medical management[7]. Given the increasing prevalence of arthritis with an aging population in developed countries, innovative methods of improving management in an era of constrained costs are required. Arthritis patient education is likely to be useful not only where health care costs and physician time are being constrained or rationed (as in the US or Europe), but also where health systems have limited resources and expertise (as in many developing countries).

Patient education is concerned with involving the patient in management decisions to more efficiently meet patients' needs. It is also concerned with improving the communication between health care providers and patients. In addition, patient education focuses upon better patient adherence with recommended advice, and with improving functional status, patient and family coping and improved quality of life among those with arthritis.

SETTINGS FOR PATIENT EDUCATION

Arthritis patient education may be delivered in several ways in different contexts[8]. These include clinical and community settings as well as distance learning, the use of new technologies, including telephone counseling, structure mailed materials and even possibly the internet. The range of settings for arthritis education is shown in Figure 3.1. All the modalities listed may emphasize collaborative management, shared responsibility and the psychosocial context for chronic disease, but the depth of education provided is the greatest in the most intensive structured education modes, which provide substantial opportunities for practice, feedback and behavioral reinforcement.

WORKING WITH PATIENTS' BELIEFS ABOUT ARTHRITIS

PATIENTS' BELIEFS

Patients develop a concept of their arthritis which is quite different from a clinical perspective[9]. Patients see illness in terms of the restrictions imposed upon them, and their beliefs about their condition. Beliefs about arthritis causation, unproved treatments and folk remedies persist in the community[10,11]. Informal social networks, as well as the lay press and mass media, interest patients in other approaches to their illness, including alternative treatments and (fictitious) 'cures'.

According to attribution theory, individuals construct modes of illness to explain their symptoms[3]. In this way, patients with arthritis describe and conceptualize their disease and their symptoms in terms of their lifestyle. Patients assess disease severity in terms of specific things they can and cannot do, rather than in terms of pathologic processes. Pain is perceived in terms of the way it limits their activity, not in terms of biochemical measures or measured length along a visual analog pain scale. This may mean that clinicians need to deal with patients' experience of pain, as well as with objectively measured parameters. Finally, patients' beliefs may influence what they recall from consultations, as well as what they do with clinical advice.

When patients attend for medical care, they are already influenced by a broad range of opinions about arthritis and how it should be managed. Physicians may have a different set of beliefs about what patients should know. Clinical encounters should begin with the process of identifying and understanding these patient-held beliefs about arthritis.

NEEDS ASSESSMENT

Needs assessment is the process of defining the problems, barriers to adherence and environmental factors which influence individual patients with a disease in their social context. Although important, an appraisal of patient needs is infrequently reported in arthritis education research[8]. This concept of defining the perceptions, beliefs and needs of patients is an important first step in arthritis patient education[12]. Needs may differ across cultures and health systems, and by socioeconomic characteristics.

Patients often perceive their needs differently from clinicians[9,13–15]. Needs assessment will define the parameters for individualized patient education. Some will need detailed information; others will already know about arthritis, but will need the skills to manage daily domestic tasks. Patients with arthritis often are concerned about their therapy, its adequacy and the possible usefulness of alternative treatments. Some patients, especially those with systemic disease, are fearful about the consequences of their condition. Although patients usually regard physicians as the primary source of advice, they are often concerned about the quality of doctor–patient communication and of the explanations they receive. Other patient concerns include fatigue, psychologic effects, depression, emotional and family difficulties rather than concerns about medication side effects[13]. Addressing these patient-held concerns and beliefs about their arthritis forms the main focus of the initial stages of arthritis education[11,16].

THEORETIC FOUNDATIONS AND STRUCTURE OF ARTHRITIS PATIENT EDUCATION PROGRAMS

THEORETIC FOUNDATIONS OF ARTHRITIS EDUCATION

Arthritis patient education is well grounded in behavior change theory, derived from a range of disciplines including psychology and the principles of adult learning. Other psychologic theories, including attribution and decisional balance theories, help explain patients' beliefs about their disease. The attributions that patients make (*post hoc* reasons and explanations for symptoms and illness manifestations) may influence their behavior (see below).

A unified model for arthritis education comes from social learning theory (SLT). This posits that health-enhancing behaviors result from the interplay between physiology (underlying disease severity), social and physical environments, and an individual's cognitions about his or her disease[17]. This approach integrates program components erroneously thought to be separate, such as cognitive behavior change strategies and a self-management framework[18]. One of the dimensions of the cognitive part of the model is self-efficacy, an individual's situation-specific confidence in carrying out a task. Efficacy is an important antecedent of many behaviors. Perceptions of the possible consequences of carrying out the behavior are also thought important in the process of adopting health behaviors (outcome expectancies). Increases in self-efficacy are considered important objectives of arthritis education, as they usually lead to increases in appropriate health behaviors and health outcomes[19–22], although these associations are not always apparent[23].

Figure 3.2 shows some of the general dimensions of social learning theory. A range of factors across environments may contribute to the adoption of self-management behaviors. These in turn may lead to

SETTINGS FOR ARTHRITIS PATIENT EDUCATION

Setting	Type of patient education
Medical care	Patient education delivered by physicians as part of the medical consultation
Inpatient surgical education	Pre- or perioperative education for patients with arthritis undergoing joint surgery (may be individual or small group)
Ancillary to medical care	Patient education delivered by a team approach, involving allied health professionals, often including physical therapists, occupational therapists and nurses; this occurs in practice settings, outpatient clinics and hospital settings
Structured small group education	Patient education delivered by trained patient educators as well as other clinicians and health professionals, usually through multisession, multidisciplinary education; this can occur in the outpatient or community setting
Other forms of individual education	Other methods of individual contact, including telephone counseling and advice programs
Public and community education	Broader program reaching a wider target audience, comprising other forms of arthritis education, such as books, pamphlets and other resources, written self-instructional material, audiovisual material, computer assisted learning, internet resources
Community resources	Dissemination, public education and mass media campaigns and activities, and support group development; activities carried out by national arthritis foundations and societies

Fig. 3.1 Settings for arthritis patient education.

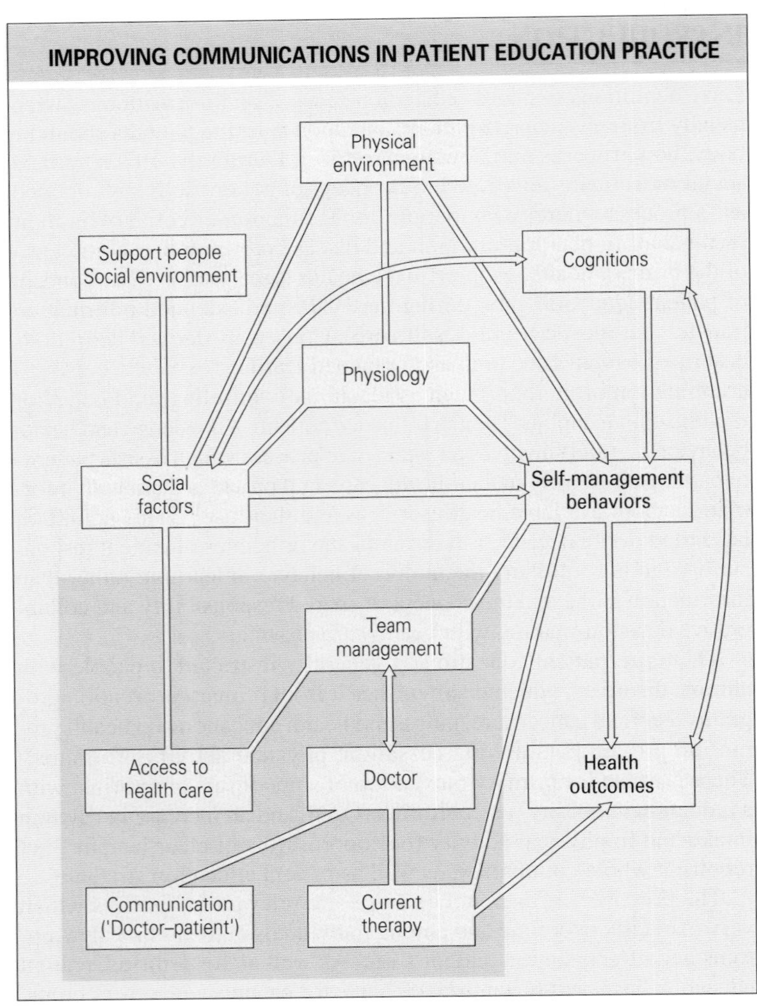

Fig. 3.2 Arthritis patient education: a social learning framework.

improved health outcomes, although the model is schematic rather than evidenced by causal research. Arrows tend to point in a single direction, but may in reality be bidirectional. Improved health outcomes, such as reduced pain, may reinforce and increase the behaviors contributing to it, such as medication adherence or joint protection behaviors. Similarly, some of the psychosocial concomitants of arthritis are consequent upon physical disease severity, especially pain and disability[8].

The lower half of Figure 3.2 (shaded) depicts the health system and health provider factors which contribute to patient education, and to the adoption of health behaviors and to health outcomes. Health service provision varies across countries, depending on health system financing, reimbursement mechanisms for physicians, the availability of ancillary staff and a 'team' approach to case management, and the availability and cost of medications and devices to assist daily task performance.

DEVELOPING APPROACHES TO ARTHRITIS EDUCATION

The development and conduct of arthritis patient education programs require achievable educational and behavioral goals and objectives. Patients should understand program goals and perceive them as relevant.

Adult learning approaches are used throughout patient education programs. Lifestyle and coping skills are taught not via didactic means but by experience and through interactions with other patients and their problems (vicarious learning). Small group programs usually have 6–10 members to allow enough time for individual needs as well as group processes. This approach focuses on problem solving; solutions tailored to the needs of the individual may have relevance for the whole group. Groups comprised of patients of similar ages with the same diagnosis allow discussion and cross-fertilization of ideas and skills to occur.

As indicated above, theoretical approaches, including cognitive behavioral and self-management programs, hold the most promise for successful arthritis education[18]. Other approaches are often tried, but the results of programs using biofeedback, psychotherapeutic interventions or hypnosis are not consistent[24].

The length of the program should be determined, as well as the need for reinforcement sessions at patient follow-up. The short-term benefits of arthritis education programs (AEPs) should be realistic, as only knowledge transfer could be expected immediately following a brief or minimal intervention. The costs of patient education, measured in terms of direct program and instructor costs, should be assessed per patient who attends.

CONTENT OF ARTHRITIS EDUCATION PROGRAMS

Knowledge change

Structured arthritis patient education is based around three areas: increasing knowledge, increasing skills and improving psychologic outcomes (Fig. 3.3). The first task is to inform patients about their rheumatic condition, although knowledge transfer alone is insufficient for cognitive or behavioral changes. Patients need to develop the same general view of the disease process as the physician, and to be able to judge deterioration or improvement and the need to monitor their own condition. Patients need a clear understanding of complex clinical concepts (such as 'joint erosion', 'synovectomy' or 'vasculitis'). The elements of anatomy, inflammation, muscle function and nutrition are important prerequisites for an understanding of the role of anti-inflammatory therapy, daily muscle exercise, joint protection and weight reduction programs. Patients' understanding of medical advice and clinical states is enhanced if simple, nonthreatening language is used, and clear written instructions are provided for later review. For example, the concept of a 'vertebral disk rupture' may have frightening connotations for some patients. Time spent providing a detailed explanantion may help patients with subsequent coping and pain management.

An important goal of patient education is to promote a healthy skepticism among patients, so that they understand the prognosis of their condition and can critically appraise new information, particularly that which promises a cure or describes unproved therapies. A related component is to allow patients access to community-based information and resources. These include access to government support, including financial and material assistance, as well as to lay helpers and non-governmental arthritis foundations and societies.

Behavior change

Most programs emphasize the development of self-management skills. These include specific behaviors, such as daily exercise regimens and joint protection skills, which are learned through observation, participation (trialing of the behaviors themselves) and subsequent practice. Behaviors are also learned by patients' observing their consequences, for example being able to carry out more domestic tasks if medication regimens are adhered to and joint conservation practiced.

Medication use is a good example of patient self-management. The complexity of the medication adherence issue is illustrated by patients who need to self-regulate analgesic use while adhering to less flexible regimens of arthritis-suppressing medication. Self-management is illustrated by patients' needs to adjust their activity levels, to learn when to rest or wear splints and when to seek additional support, such as physical therapy or transcutaneous electrical nerve stimulation (TENS).

Psychosocial support and coping

There are emotional dimensions to all facets of patient education and skills development. Many programs aim to help patients cope with their arthritis, to feel more confident about being able to manage it and to function in the conduct of daily tasks. The role of carers and social supports is also included in many programs, but does not consistently improve outcomes[24]. Nonetheless, family members and partners may have a role in emotional support, and in allowing more of the program material to be understood, remembered and subsequently practiced at home.

CONTENT AREAS OF STRUCTURED ARTHRITIS PATIENT EDUCATION

Content area	Examples of specific content
Knowledge	Anatomy, disease process, inflammation Symptoms and signs for improvement or deterioration in disease; understanding of disease monitoring Pharmacologic therapy: use, effects, side effects; alternative therapy Understanding of benefits of surgical intervention Use of heat and cold, joint protection, podiatry Understanding of nutrition, diet and hazardous diets, weight control Understanding of where to find community resources, helping agencies, potential assistance from government agencies
Skills and behaviors	Role of exercise; rest; joint protection skills, TENS, acupuncture Specific goal setting, daily routines established Making domestic tasks easier; domestic environmental modifications Self-monitoring or adherence; when to take additional medication Pain management: use of hot/cold, relaxation, other pain management behaviors Work and occupational simplification (where possible) Problem-solving (linked to self-management skills)
Psychosocial and communication dimensions	Communicating with health care providers; learning assertiveness and when to ask questions Reducing anxiety, increasing confidence (efficacy) for specific tasks, reducing feelings of helplessness and fear Learning to cope with chronic illness and depression Eliciting support from spouse/family members; learning to cope with disease management in the domestic context

Fig. 3.3 Content areas of structured arthritis patient education.

OUTCOMES OF ARTHRITIS EDUCATION PROGRAMS

The expectation that patient education can reduce mortality or morbidity is difficult to prove. This leads to some negativity regarding the putative effects expected of patient education programs in the short and long term. In this context, outcomes need to be achievable and specific and to use established measures. Most chronic disease education has substantial proximal effects, particularly upon knowledge and psychologic outcomes, with less well-defined effects upon behaviors and health care utilization. Effects are generally smaller, but still significant, for the better designed, randomized controlled studies[4].

A range of knowledge measures is used to assess arthritis education, testing knowledge about the content of the interventions, including the disease process and its therapy. The next level of outcomes includes cognitive and other psychologic measures, such as self-efficacy, helplessness and sense of control, anxiety, depression and coping styles. Behavioral measures include adherence measures, physical activity, pain management strategies and joint protection behaviors. Scales measuring disability, functional status and the ability to carry out tasks are common [using the Health Assessment Questionnaire (HAQ) or Arthritis Impact Measurement Scales (AIMS)][25]. Pain can be measured using a visual analog scale (VAS). Reliability and validity information is available for these categories of outcome measurements[25]. Measures of family support, patient concerns and objective health care utilization measures (such as physician visits) are also used. Generic measures of quality of life (SF-36, Nottingham Health Profile, Sickness Impact Profile) are becoming more commonplace, to allow cross-disease comparisons in outcomes[26].

TEAM AND SYSTEM APPROACHES

Shared care involves patients, physicians and other health professionals[27]. In some countries, specialist rheumatologists provide most arthritis care, whereas in others it is shared with primary medical health care providers (general practitioners) who are pivotal in coordinating community and ongoing care for most patients. Shared care involves a team approach which may include nurses, physical therapists, occupational therapists, social workers or counselors and sometimes dietitians, podiatrists and pharmacists[27,28].

Team members should reinforce each other. For example, complex therapeutic regimens may need regular reinforcement, with medication interactions and side effects reviewed and administration devices demonstrated to reduce patient confusion. Community-based follow-up for older patients may facilitate adherence. A team approach, with multiple professional visits, may be required to deal with patient denial of the condition or its severity[11]. Examples of education tasks are shown in Figure 3.4, to illustrate the varying skills and roles of different professionals.

In some countries, integrated rheumatology centers may have access to a full range of health professionals. Here, primary care comprises family practitioners working with other health professionals. In some centers, the role of rheumatology specialist nurse or nurse practitioner has been developed to provide community-based care. In other settings, family practitioners work only with community nurses and/or practice visitors.

The team approach is increasingly seen as part of the 'managed care' phenomenon in health care delivery. In theory, it can maximize the potential for patients to integrate their illness into their lifestyles, allowing different professionals to motivate and reinforce the patients' learning. In practice, few professionals have direct experience or training in patient education, and this approach risks becoming 'an orphan treatment – espoused by most health professionals, but the responsibility of none'[29].

Team functioning is important, whether by way of routine care systems or by structured patient education. Teams need to demarcate their professional responsibilities, to prevent overlap and omission[16]. Weekly team meetings are one way of overcoming this problem. More difficult is the sensitive issue of interprofessional rivalry and conflict, and the perceived or real hierarchical relationships among team members. Good communication among team members, as well as with patients, can overcome this problem and allow patient education to be integrated across a range of patient care settings.

DOCTOR–PATIENT INTERACTIONS

OVERVIEW

Individual patient education activity is an important part of the doctor–patient interaction during the clinical consultation. This section describes the potential of this setting for effective patient education. Good communications between patient and provider can significantly affect patient outcomes[30–34]. Most physicians believe that patient education is an important part of what they do, but many feel unprepared for, and/or uncomfortable providing, patient counseling[35].

Randomized trials show that both patients and physicians can improve their communication skills with brief training, resulting in improved patient adherence and health outcome[30,32,36–38].

COMMUNICATION IN THE CONSULTATION

The physician has three major communication goals to be achieved with the cooperation of the patient:

- to listen to the patient so as to arrive at a diagnosis;
- to negotiate the optimal treatment regimen which is acceptable to the patient; and
- to counsel the patient regarding management of the disease and treatment regimen, so these may be carried out effectively.

Despite considerable attention given to the medical interview, physicians frequently fail to uncover important patient concerns. Time may be short and the patient reluctant to 'bother' the doctor. From 20% to 50% of

INDERDISCIPLINARY ROLES: TEAM APPROACHES TO ARTHRITIS EDUCATION

Professional	Role in patient education (examples)
Nurse/pharmacist	Primary care role in explaining and demonstrating medication use, actions, interactions, side effects; medication administration devices
Rheumatologist and/or family physician	Explain the disease, its physiology, natural history and range of therapies available; the need for disease monitoring; the place of intra-articular injection, surgery, etc. In some countries, this is the role of community general practitioners, especially for uncomplicated and prevalent conditions (most OA, osteoporosis), and providing adjunctive care for complicated or multisystem disease
Physical therapists	Static and dynamic exercises, mobility, prevention of contractures or weakness, acupuncture, TENS; modification of physical activity during active phases of disease; pain management strategies
Nutritionist	Role of diet; 'alternative' diets and their potential risks; weight control strategies
Occupational therapist	Training in relearning routine activities of daily living, recreation and leisure pursuits; use of technical devices; joint support, when to rest and partially to immobilize joints
Social workers	'Patients rights' for treatment, arranging time off work, support from carers in the family and community, and government; sometimes, provision of individual or family counseling
Counselor or psychologist	Anxiety and/or depression counseling, dealing with denial or with disease crises; coping with sexuality

Fig. 3.4 Interdisciplinary roles: team approaches to arthritis education.

arthritis patients at a typical clinic visit experience psychosocial or work problems which are attributable to their disease but are infrequently detected by their physicians. Failure to recognize and treat, reassure or refer for these problems may limit patients' satisfaction and their ability to take advantage of other treatments the physician has to offer.

A primary task of the clinician is to select a treatment regimen and recommend it to the patient. Numerous treatment options are available for many rheumatic patients. Discussion of patient goals and consideration of patient preferences may help the doctor and patient set priorities for treatment approaches, simplify the regimen and encourage adherence to treatment. However, patients often feel left out of the decision-making process[39]. Although many may not wish actively to be involved in the actual decision-making process about treatments[40,41], even patients who would rather be passive are more satisfied with their physician when they participate more fully in negotiations about treatments[42]. Research into the decision-making process indicates that low adherence to treatment plans may result when problems arise. For example, patients require a detailed plan which specifies increases in anti-inflammatory medication when a flare in systemic illness occurs[43].

The risks of recommended treatments are often underdisclosed[32]. Despite the apprehension of some physicians, disclosure of potential side effects has not been found to make patients anxious, more likely to report side effects or be noncompliant[44,45].

PATIENT ADHERENCE TO THERAPEUTIC REGIMENS

Patient adherence to therapeutic regimens is essential to achieve therapeutic goals. However, arthritis patients adhere to only 50–75% of prescribed treatments[46,47]. Problems with adherence are so common that physicians should anticipate them as a matter of course. Various techniques improve adherence to therapeutic regimens[34,48]. Once a treatment has been agreed upon, the doctor should be sure that the patient understands its purpose, knows how to carry it out correctly, will remember it, has the necessary confidence, skills and resources, and is prepared for problems.

Patients frequently misunderstand the purpose of treatment. Daltroy *et al.*[49] found that 15% of patients failed to understand the purpose of their prescriptions. At 4 months, patients were compliant with 29% of misunderstood prescriptions, but were compliant with 58% of prescriptions whose purpose they had understood. Arluke[50] found that arthritis patients' therapeutic expectations may differ from those of their physician (for example, function improvement compared with pain relief), and different concepts of what constitutes adequate duration of therapy.

Patients typically forget half of medical instruction in a very short time[32]. The use of repetition, written instructions and reinforcing materials such as brochures and self-help materials may increase patients' understanding of and adherence to therapeutic regimens.

As half of all regimens are not followed adequately, it is sensible to anticipate problems so they can be dealt with before they interfere with the effectiveness of therapy, or with the doctor's ability accurately to assess the efficacy of a given treatment in a patient. Patients who anticipate problems are more likely to adhere to their plans, because:

- they are more realistic,
- they are better able to make contingency plans to deal with potential negative outcomes and
- they are better prepared psychologically to deal with negative outcomes that they cannot avert[43].

Reinforcement of patient confidence may increase adherence to treatment[51].

IMPLICATIONS FOR COMMUNICATION IN PRACTICE

A summary of the major issues in physician–patient communication research is presented in Figure 3.5. The doctor–patient interaction has a strong emphasis upon adherence with recommended therapy. The table summarizes current recommendations for improving education in clinical practice and for integrating it with other settings for patient education.

EFFECTIVENESS OF ARTHRITIS PATIENT EDUCATION

CRITERIA FOR PROGRAM EFFECTIVENESS

Before recommending arthritis education, it is important for clinicians and administrators to be confident of the program's effectiveness. Given the differences in education programs, different target groups and diverse conditions subsumed under the title of 'arthritis', it is difficult to determine whether arthritis patient education is unequivocally effective. The evidence for effectiveness emanates from the diversity and extent of programs evaluated, as well as the development and use of reliable and validated outcome measures. Although some of these measures are of subjective phenomena, such as pain, sense of control or quality of life, they have generally been been subjected to both psychometric and external validation[25,52], providing clinicians with more confidence in these measures.

Evaluation standards suggest that randomized designs and comparable interprogram outcome measures are necessary to develop a clear understanding of program effects. Effective programs need to have been developed to meet patients' needs, have a strong theoretic grounding in applied behavior change and be developed and delivered in a replicable manner. An educational appraisal of the components of the curricula of structured education programs is required to determine if a program has achievable objectives which are likely to be met[8].

The duration of program effects is important, as many educational programs produce short-term changes which are not maintained. Other considerations include the potential for sampling bias in the recruitment of patients who attend arthritis education. Are they better educated, younger or earlier in the natural history of their condition? These factors influence program generalizability, and it is important to consider whether similar results would be obtained with a general community sample of arthritis patients.

EVIDENCE FOR EFFECTIVENESS OF ARTHRITIS EDUCATION

Several reviews of patient education have been conducted, with overall study effects showing trends favoring those exposed to arthritis education. One formal meta-analysis pooled these data[53], and noted that arthritis patient education resulted in a significant 16% improvement in interventions subjects' joint pain [effect size (ES) 0.21, 95% confidence interval (CI) 0.08–0.31], a 22% improvement in mood disturbance (ES 0.28, 95% CI 0.15–0.42), but a nonsignificant effect upon disability (ES 0.09). The ES of arthritis patient education upon pain scores was significant, and 25% as large as that attributed to treatment with nonsteroidal anti-inflammatory drugs (NSAIDs)[53]. These effects

IMPROVING COMMUNICATIONS IN PATIENT EDUCATION PRACTICE	
Key strategy	**Principles for clinical practice**
Address patient concerns	Listening to patient; doctor to write down concerns with patient
Set patient goals	Set realistic priorities and goals for the patient (based on above), and develop management plan for each
Inform patient of treatment options	Explain all therapies, their risks, benefits and costs; identify and discuss patient preferences
Adherence enhancing strategies	Identify individual barriers to adherence, including time, cost, convenience, memory; develop simple strategies (written instructions, medication dosettes, etc.) for each patient to overcome potential problems with adherence
Integrate clinical practice with multidisciplinary patient education	Identify allied health personnel, specific professionals who may help the patient, local structured group patient education programs, community resources and agencies

Fig. 3.5 Improving communications in patient education practice.

were supplemental to clinical therapy. One limitation of these findings is that most program evaluations are conducted for patients with rheumatoid arthritis (RA) or OA, with less research evidence available for other conditions[14].

A recent review of arthritis patient education described 32 intervention studies, just over half of which used a randomized experimental design[15]. Of these studies, 25 were reviewed in detail. Most studies which measured knowledge reported favorable effects of intervention, a finding similar to those for other chronic diseases[4–6]. In spite of improvements in knowledge, several studies still report that many patients could not name their rheumatologic diagnosis[3]. Another review conducted a more formal meta-analysis of program effects, analyzing data from 34 arthritis education interventions[18].

In the review by Hirano *et al.*[15], a total of 34 measures of behavior were reported in 25 studies, with 29 showing effects favoring the intervention groups. Of 11 studies with exercise or physical activity measures, 10 reported favorable effects and six reported outcomes which significantly improved. Of six studies assessing adherence, one showed significant effects and five out of 13 showed significant effects upon other behavioral outcomes, including relaxation, pain relief techniques and joint protection. Among psychologic outcomes, five of eight showed significant effects upon depression and none showed adverse effects. Other psychologic outcomes included improvements in cognitions (self-efficacy) and decreased perceived helplessness. Many studies assessed health status measures, with seven out of 14 showing significant effects upon measures of pain and three of 10 showing significant differences in disability. Only two studies reported by Hirano had assessed general measures of quality of life, and neither reported intervention effects. An encouraging trend was seen in the increase in behaviorally based intervention since 1980, as these have been shown to be more effective than instructional programs alone[4].

The review by Hawley[18] showed similar findings, with the largest effect sizes for measures of improved knowledge, and clearly significant effects for increases in exercise behaviors, coping and self-efficacy. Results for pain, functional status and depression were generally, but not always, positive, and stronger for OA than RA patients. Only one study assessed reductions in health care utilization, and suggested the potential for cost-effective arthritis education[19]. Some studies are now reporting longer-term outcomes at 4–5 years following arthritis programs[20,54].

Potential limitations in interpretation need to be considered in any appraisal of the effectiveness of AEPs. Evaluations are often based on small sample sizes, limited to OA or RA patients, usually volunteers who are often more educated than their source populations[18]. Other limitations include the possibility of inclusion of some subjects with other diagnoses, the range of reliable and validated but self-reported outcomes (seldom assessing physiologic measures of disease severity), and the general observation that effects weaken at 12 months[18]. These concerns are very similar to those reported in meta-analyses of other behavioral interventions for chronic disease. They warrant further investigation in subsequent evaluation designs, but do not negate the role and importance of arthritis education.

PUBLIC HEALTH APPROACHES

The increasing proportion of elderly in the population, and increasing longevity, are contributing to increased prevalence of, and health costs associated with, arthritis[7,55]. A population-wide approach generally observes that only a small fraction of affected individuals actually attend or receive any substantial patient education[56]. This approach assumes that all affected individuals are likely to need some degree of patient education, and that strategies should be developed to reach them. Such strategies include health professional and physician training, community education programs and the use of mass media and public service announcements to provide low-intensity but widely disseminated messages about arthritis. It may include changes to the physical environment or to regulations so that it is easier for patients to access facilities, functional aids or other devices, or domestic modifications to allow them to lead normal lives.

Public health has an equity dimension, with the objective of reaching all population segments, including socially disadvantaged groups, those who speak minority languages and those who cannot access specialist medical care. These groups may be disadvantaged through poor understanding of their illness, less defined social supports and poorer psychosocial health. In addition, public health implies that patients with all types of arthritis may require education and support, so programs and materials should be developed for the less common but serious varieties of rheumatic disease. Community agencies, such as arthritis foundations and societies, have an important role in community support, as well as in the development and dissemination of educational materials and resources[57]. Arthritis foundations have central roles in community networking, fostering support groups and communicating through newsletters and other media with patients and their carers.

Several innovative attempts to provide community-based arthritis education have been reported. One example in Java (Indonesia) was developed by the International League Against Rheumatism (ILAR)[58]. It used a culturally relevant ‘puppet shadow play’ to inform nonliterate communities about arthritis and ways of performing activities of daily living. Another example was a distance education approach to arthritis education developed for indigenous populations in northern Canada[59]. Other approaches are used to achieve greater population reach, including professional education. A recent initiative trained public health nurses about arthritis, in order to add dissemination of arthritis education to their community-based activities[60].

These approaches involve physicians in program development and in the delivery and dissemination of program content. Political commitment and advocacy are required on the part of rheumatologists for such programs to be developed, and to reach the majority of those with arthritis in the population in a cost-efficient and cost-effective manner.

THE FUTURE OF ARTHRITIS PATIENT EDUCATION

The next generation of patient education programs will be subject to increasing health system accountability. A substantial increase is expected in cost-effectiveness comparisons among different approaches[55]. Programs of different lengths, using different educational modes, will be compared. For example, the effects of telephone counseling versus better physician advice or community support groups versus multisession structured education will be compared and costed using standard outcome measures. Some results of the newer methods are being reported, including a controlled trial of telephone counseling for RA and OA, which show promising results[61]. This further research will define the health-cost savings attributable to different types of arthritis patient education, and enable specific formats to be recommended.

Future programs will be linked more effectively to behavior change and adherence theory, and directed to meet patients needs and concerns. Patient education will extend to hospital-based and perioperative settings for rheumatologic patients. Education will be integrated and funded as part of inpatient and outpatient clinical care, through trained physicians, or via team approaches or ‘managed care’[7]. Health professionals, including medical students, may receive training in interdisciplinary health care and patient education as part of under- and postgraduate curricula.

The evolution of patient education continues. Educational materials are being developed which are more appropriate to the general reading age of the population[62]. New approaches to educational material development and dissemination are required to reach minority and disadvantaged populations, and those with rarer forms of arthritis. Innovative programs being developed in the US have extended the concept of partly trained lay-led programs, and have developed 'Patient Partners in Arthritis™', a system of highly trained patients acting as medical and peer educators[63].

Finally, evaluation research will provide ongoing evidence for program effectiveness. New studies, using representative samples of the target population, will provide findings which are more generalizable, and a standardized evaluation method. A recommended minimal data set of outcomes may be developed. For example, programs could agree by consensus to use standard measures of disability and pain (HAQ, VAS pain measure) so that comparisons can be made across programs.

The net sum of activity over the next decade should result in improved technologies for arthritis patient education, and provide evidence for effectiveness and cost efficiency for health service decision-makers. Regional and international dissemination strategies may be needed for effective, low-cost arthritis patient education programs, which span the spectrum of rheumatologic disorders.

REFERENCES

1. Levin L. The lay resource in health and health-care. Health Promotion. 1986;1,(3):285–91.
2. Bartlett EE. Forum: patient education. Eight principles from patient education research. Prevent Med. 1985;14:667–9.
3. Daltroy L, Liang M. Arthritis education: opportunities and state of the art. Health Educ Q. 1993;20:3–16.
4. Mazzuca SA. Does patient education in chronic disease have therapeutic value?. J Chron Dis. 1982;35:521–9.
5. Brown SA. Studies of educational interventions and outcomes in diabetes adults: a meta-analysis revisited. Patient Educ Counsel. 1990;16:189–215.
6. Bauman A. Effects of asthma patient education upon psychological and behavioral outcomes. In: Maes S, Leventhal H, Johnston M, eds. International review health psychology. Chichester: Wiley; 1993:199–212.
7. Winfield J. Arthritis patient education – efficacy, implementation and financing. Arthritis Rheum. 1989;32:1330–3.
8. Tucker M, Kirwan J. Does patient education in rheumatoid arthritis have therapeutic potential? Ann Rheum Dis. 1991;50:422–8.
9. Silvers I, Hovell M, Weisman M, Mueller M. Assessing physician/patient perceptions in rheumatoid arthritis. Arthritis Rheum. 1985;28:300–7.
10. Donovan JL, Blake DR, Fleming WG. The patient is not a blank sheet; lay beliefs, and their tolerance in patient education. Br J Rheumatol. 1989;28:58–61.
11. Donovan J. Patient education and the consultation: the importance of lay beliefs. Ann Rheum Dis. 1991;50:418–21.
12. Price J, Hillman K, Toral M, Newea S. The public's perceptions and misperceptions about arthritis. Arthritis Rheum. 1983;26:1023–8.
13. Bauman A, Barnes C, Schrieber L, Brooks P, Dunsmore J. The unmet needs of patients with systemic lupus erythematosus: planning for patient education. Patient Educ Counsel. 1989;14:235–42.
14. Lorig K, Konkol L, Gonzalez V. Arthritis patient education: a review of the literature. Patient Educ Counsel. 1987;10:210–52.
15. Hirano P, Laurent D, Lorig K. Arthritis patient education studies. 1987–1991: a review of the literature. Patient Educ Counsel. 1994;24:9–54.
16. Hill J, Bird H, Hopkins P, Lawton C, Wright V. The development and use of a patient knowledge questionnaire in rheumatoid arthritis. Br J Rheumatol. 1991;30:45–9.
17. Bandura A. Social diffusion and innovation. In: Social foundations of thought and action: a social cognitive theory. Englewood Cliffs, NJ: Prentice-Hall; 1986:142–81.
18. Hawley, D. Psycho-education interventions in the treatment of arthritis. Ballière's Clin Rheumatol. 1995;9:803–23.
19. Lorig K, Manzonson P, Holman H. Evidence suggesting that health education for self management in patients with chronic arthritis has sustained health benefits while reducing health care costs. Arthritis Rheum. 1993;36:439–46.
20. Lorig K, Holman H. Arthritis self management: a twelve year review. Health Educ Q. 1993;20:17–28.
21. Davis P, Busch A, Lowe J. Evaluation of a rheumatoid arthritis patient education program: impact on knowledge and self-efficacy. Patient Educ Counsel. 1994;24:55–61.
22. Taal E, Rasker JJ, Seydel ER, Wiegman O. Health status, adherence with health recommendations, self-efficacy and social support in patients with rheumatoid arthritis. Patient Educ Counsel. 1993;20:63–76.
23. Simeoni E, Bauman A, Stenmark J, O'Brien J. An evaluation of a community arthritis education program in Australia: the dissemination of a developed program. Arthritis Care Res. 1995;8:102–6.
24. DeVellis RF, Blalock SJ. Psychological and educational interventions to reduce arthritis disability. Ballière's Clin Rheumatol. 1993;7:397–416.
25. Bowling A. Measuring disease. Buckingham: Open University Press; 1995:209–32.
26. Scott D, Long A, Silman A. Disease outcomes in rheumatology. B J Rheumatol. 1995;34:704–6.
27. Maycock J. Role of health professionals in patient education. Ann Rheum Dis. 1991;50:429–34.
28. Ahlmen M, Sullivan M, Bjelle A. Team versus non team outpatient care in rheumatoid arthritis. Arthritis Rheum. 1988;31:471–9.
29. Lorig K. Patient education: treatment or nice extra (editorial). Br J Rheumatol. 1995;34:703–4.
30. Roter D, Hall J. Doctors talking with patients,

patients talking with doctors: improving communication in medical visits. Westport, CN: Auburn House; 1992.
31. Stewart M, Roter D. Communicating with medical patients. Newbury Park: Sage; 1989.
32. Daltroy LH. Doctor–patient communication in rheumatological disorders. Ballière's Clin Rheumatol. 1993;7:221–39.
33. Haynes RB, Taylor DW, Sackett DL (1979). Compliance in health care Baltimore, Johns Hopkins Press.
34. Joos SK, Hickam DH. How health professionals influence health behavior: patient–provider interaction and health care outcomes. In: Glanz K, Lewis FM, Rimer BK, eds. Health behavior and health education: theory, research, and practice. San Francisco: Jossey-Bass; 1990:216–41.
35. Merkel WT, Margolis RB, Smith RC. Teaching humanistic and psychosocial aspects of care: Current practices and attitudes. J Gen Intern Med. 1990;5:34–41.
36. Kaplan SH, Greenfield S, Ware JE Jr. Impact of the doctor–patient relationship on the outcomes of chronic disease. In: Stewart M, Roter D, eds. Communicating with medical patients. Newbury Park: Sage; 1989:228–45.
37. Thompson SC, Nanni C, Schwankovsky L. Patient-oriented interventions to improve communication in a medical office visit. Health Psychol. 1990;9:390–404.
38. Anderson LA, Sharpe PA. Improving patient and provider communication: a synthesis and review of communication interventions. Patient Educ Counsel. 1991;17:99–134.
39. Katz JN, Daltroy LH, Brennan TA, Liang MH. Informed consent and the prescription of nonsteroidal antiinflammatory drugs. Arthritis Rheum. 1992;35:1257–63.
40. Strull WM, Lo B, Charles G. Do patients want to participate in medical decision making? JAMA. 1984;252:2990–4.
41. Beisecker AE, Beisecker TD. Patient information-seeking behaviors when communicating with physicians. Med Care. 1990;28:19–28.
42. Brody DS. The patient's role in clinical decision-making. Ann Inter Med. 1980;93:718–22.
43. Janis I. The patient as decision-maker. In: Gentry WD, ed. Handbook of behavioral medicine. New York: Guilford Press; 1983:326–68.
44. Quaid KA, Faden RR, Vining EP, Freeman JM. Informed consent for a prescription drug: impact of disclosed information on patient understanding and medical outcomes. Patient Educ Counsel. 1990;15:249–59.
45. Morris LA, Kanouse DE. Informing patients about drug side effects. J Behav Med. 1982;5:363–73.
46. Deyo RA. Compliance with therapeutic regimens in arthritis: issues, current status, and a future agenda. Semin Arthritis Rheum. 1982;12:233–44.
47. Bradley LA. Adherence with treatment regimens among adult rheumatoid arthritis patients: Current status and future directions. Arthritis Care Res. 1989;2(Suppl3):33–9.
48. Sackett DL. A compliance practicum for the busy practitioner. In: Haynes RB, Taylor DW, Sackett DL, eds. Compliance in health care. Baltimore: Johns Hopkins University Press; 1979:286–96.
49. Daltroy LH, Katz JN, Liang MH. Doctor–patient communication and adherence to arthritis treatments. Arthritis Care Res. 1992;5(Suppl3):S19.
50. Arluke A. Judging drugs: patients' conceptions of therapeutic efficacy in the treatment of arthritis. Hum Org. 1983;39:84–7.
51. Holman H, Lorig K. Perceived self-efficacy in self-management of chronic disease. In: Schwarzer R, ed. Self-efficacy: thought control of action. Washington: Hemisphere; 1992:305–24.
52. Fries J, Spitz P, Kraines R, Holman H. Measurement of patient outcome in arthritis. Arthritis Rheum. 1980;23:137–45.
53. Mullen P, Laville E, Biddle A, Lorig K. Efficacy of psychoeducational interventions on pain, depression and disability in people with arthritis: a meta analysis. J Rheumatol. 1987;14:33–9.
54. Lindroth Y, Bauman A, Brooks PM, Priestley D. A 5 year follow up of a controlled trial of an arthritis education programme. Br J Rheumatol. 1995;34:647–52.
55. Mazzuca S. Economic evaluation of arthritis patient education. Bull Rheum Dis. 1994;43:6–8.
56. Bauman A. An asthma education perspective – is hospital-based education sufficient? Patient Educ Counsel. 1991;17:159–60.
57. MacFarlane A, Gaffin J, Jones R, Seifert M. General public education. Ann Rheum Dis. 1991;50:435–8.
58. Darmawan J, Muirden K, Wigley R, Valkenburg H. Arthritis community education by leather puppet shadow play in rural Indonesia. Rheumatol Int. 1992;12:97–101.
59. McGowan P, Green L. Arthritis self management in native populations in British Columbia: an application of health promotion and participatory research in chronic disease control. Can J Aging. 1995;14:201–12.
60. Mazzuca S, Brandt K, Katz B, Weinberger M. A behaviorally effective model for training of general health professionals by a rheumatology team. J Rheumatol. 1991;18:53–8.
61. Maisiak R, Austin J, Heck L. Health outcomes of two telephone interventions for patients with rheumatiod arthritis or osteoarthritis. Arthritis Rheum. 1996;39:1391–9.
62. Larsen I, Schumacher H. Comparison of literacy level of patients in a VA arthritis center with the reading level required by educational materials. Arthritis Care Res. 1992;5:13–16.
63. Nieman T, Branch V, Wood H, Lipsky P. Impact of an intervention by arthritis educators on arthritis patients health status (abstract). Presented at the American College of Rheumatology, 1994.

4

PRINCIPLES OF PAIN AND PAIN MANAGEMENT *Milton L Cohen*

- Pain is best appreciated in a biopsychosocial framework, which identifies nociceptive, neuropathic, cognitive–perceptual and socioenvironmental determinants.
- Pain is the major contributor to the morbidity, disability and socioeconomic costs of musculoskeletal disorders.
- The fundamental clinical feature in the assessment of pain is hyperalgesia (tenderness) which allows inference of the anatomic origin and mechanism of production of pain.
- Management of pain includes influencing nociception where possible, treating the pain itself as a symptom, and addressing the consequences of pain on mood, beliefs and behavior.
- Treatment modalities include opioid, nonopioid and adjuvant analgesic drugs, physical programs and a variety of cognitive and behavioral approaches, tailored to the individual.

INTRODUCTION

MUSCULOSKELETAL PAIN IN A BIOPSYCHOSOCIAL FRAMEWORK

The cardinal clinical feature of musculoskeletal problems is pain.The International Association for the Study of Pain[1] defines pain as an unpleasant sensory and emotional experience associated with actual or potential tissue damage or described in such terms. This links pain not only to nociception (the detection of tissue damage) but also to the threat or apprehension of nociception, thus involving factors governed by perception or belief. Despite the tradition of clinical method as a quest for an underlying disease process of which the pain is merely a symptom, some clinical problems characterized by arthralgia and myalgia, such as various forms of 'soft-tissue rheumatism' or 'nonspecific spinal pain', do not resolve into clear pathologic entities. This is also reflected in the well-documented but poorly recognized discordance between radiologic signs of altered musculoskeletal anatomy and the clinical picture. This is a challenge to the biomedical model of illness which, if not addressed, can lead to inappropriate assessment, labeling and therapy. Furthermore, as has been discussed in Chapters 1.2 and 1.5, the morbidity, disability and socioeconomic costs of rheumatologic disorders are attributable largely to the pain which characterizes them.

Pain may be driven by nociception initially, but may persist in situations where nociception is no longer readily detectable. Pain then becomes not only a problem in its own right as a form of distress but also a source of disability or loss of function. These concerns underline the importance of a biopsychosocial framework for analyzing

BIOPSYCHOSOCIAL MODEL FOR PAIN		
Biopsychosocial hierarchy	Clinical determinants	Example
Society	Socioenvironmental	Unemployment
Interperson	Cognitive–perceptual	Depression
Person	Cognitive–perceptual	Inability to write or type
Nervous system	Neuropathic	Pain
Tissue	Nociceptive	Arthritis of hands

Fig. 4.1 Biopsychosocial model for pain.

rheumatologic disorders. This embraces both the somatic reductionist direction (considering the person as a collection of organs, tissues, cells and molecules) and the broader psychosocial direction (reflecting the interaction of the person with family, friends, workplace, local community, national community and the biosphere itself)[2].

A simplified approach (Fig. 4.1) identifies, in ascending biopsychosocial hierarchical order:

- tissue damage (nociceptive level),
- processing of nociceptive information by the nervous system (neuropathic level),
- the whole person in terms of affect, cognition and behavior (cognitive–perceptual level) and
- society at large (sociologic and environmental levels).

This chapter presents a framework for appreciating rheumatologic disorders as problems of pain, from the somatic basis for nociception through understanding the clinical phenomenon of tenderness (allodynia) to appreciating the role of disrupted psychosocial function arising out of the attendant distress.

NOCICEPTION IN MUSCULOSKELETAL TISSUES

BASIC OUTLINE OF NOCICEPTION

Nociceptors[3] are primary afferent neurons which respond to noxious (tissue-damaging) stimuli. Cutaneous nociceptors have been the best described and in humans include those subserved by lightly myelinated (Aδ) and nonmyelinated (C) fibers. Aδ afferents, also classified as mechanoheat receptors, are considered to transduce pain of sharp, pricking quality as experienced initially following insult, while the more slowly conducting C afferents – polymodal nociceptors – are responsible for the dull, deep quality of prolonged pain following injury. As nociceptive afferents enter the spinal cord, those of smaller diameter segregate laterally and terminate in the more superficial layers of the dorsal horn (laminae I and II); the larger non-nociceptive afferents segregate medially and terminate in deeper laminae (see Fig. 4.2). Of the many neuropeptides which are candidates for transmitter function in primary nociceptive afferents, substance P (SP) and excitatory amino acids such as glutamate and aspartate have received most attention.

In the dorsal horn, primary afferent neurons interact with interneurons and descending supraspinal pathways to modulate incoming nociceptive information. The interneurons comprise both nociceptive-specific and wide dynamic-range cells, the latter in particular receiving convergent input from cutaneous and deep structures, providing a substrate for the phenomenon of referred pain. The pharmacology of this interaction is complex, serotonin, norepinephrine (noradrenaline) and enkephalin in particular being described in descending inhibitory pathways.

The myelinated axons from the majority of second-order nociceptive neurons terminate in the contralateral thalamus via the anterolateral quadrant of the spinal cord. A minor spinothalamic projection ascends ipsilaterally. Spinothalamic axons terminate in several distinct thalamic nuclei: the lateral (ventrobasal) nuclei project to the somatosensory cortex, while the medial nuclei, which also receive input from the reticular formation, project to wide areas of the ipsilateral cortex. This division is held to underlie respectively the sensory–discriminative and motivational–affective aspects of pain.

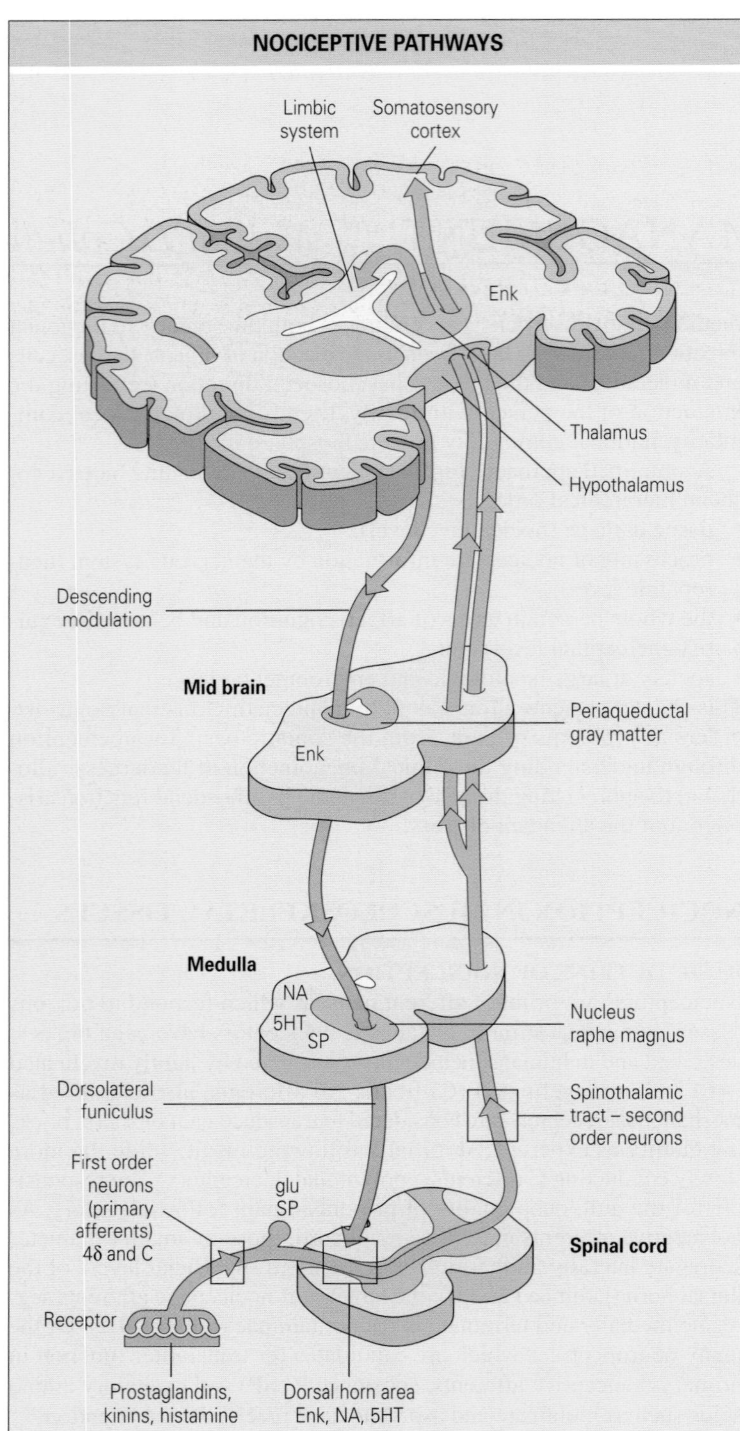

Fig. 4.2 Nociceptive pathways. (Enk, enkephalins and other opioids; NE, norepinephrine (noradrenaline); 5HT, 5-hydroxytryptamine; SP, substance P and other tachykinins; glu, glutamate and other excitatory amino acids.)

RECEPTORS AND PRIMARY AFFERENTS IN JOINT, BONE AND MUSCLE

Animal studies have been the predominant source of information concerning nociception in musculoskeletal tissues[4,5]. Mammalian joints have a rich array of receptors potentially able to signal nociception. Nociceptors homologous with polymodal cutaneous nociceptors subserved by unmyelinated C afferent fibers are found in a diffuse lattice throughout the joint capsule, while free nerve endings found in internal and external joint ligaments correspond to high-threshold Aδ cutaneous nociceptors. These receptors may also respond to non-noxious mechanical and chemical stimuli. Joint cartilage does not contain such receptors. The human synovium itself is now known to contain postganglionic sympathetic efferent fibers and unmyelinated C nociceptive afferents[6]. These fibers may be relevant in the process of neurogenic inflammation, if not also in signaling nociception.

Little is known about bone nociception. Structurally, the periosteum and bone marrow have been shown to be richly innervated in normal (but not arthritic) rats by fibers containing neuropeptides, suggesting that they may be nociceptive.

Pain in muscle may be difficult to localize and is often referred to other deep somatic structures. Specific nociceptors are probably present in skeletal muscle, of which the majority may be free nerve endings, again subserved by Aδ and C afferents. The degree of specificity of muscle nociceptors has been difficult to assess, as there appears to be heterogeneity not unlike cutaneous nociceptors. A relatively high proportion of slowly conducting muscle afferents is non-nociceptive, responding to low-threshold mechanical stimuli including muscle contractions. Similar endings are present in tendons. These receptors may signal pressure, force or movement.

Mechanically insensitive afferents (MIAs), which do not normally respond even to noxious mechanical stimulation, have been described in feline joints. In the presence of an experimental arthritis, these MIAs acquire new response properties, characterized by spontaneous activity and discharge during non-noxious movement. No such receptors have been found in skeletal muscle.

SPINAL AND SUPRASPINAL CONNECTIONS

At the spinal cord level, nociceptive-specific and wide dynamic-range neurons in the dorsal horn receive nociceptive inputs from articular tissues and may also respond to non-noxious mechanical stimulation of limb joints. These dorsal horn neurons receive convergent inputs from cutaneous, muscle and visceral afferents. Dorsal horn neurons responding exclusively to activation of muscle nociceptors are very rare.

Noxious joint and muscle inputs can reach thalamic and cortical levels. In models of experimental arthritis, the populations of neurons and ascending pathways activated by inflamed joints appear to be different from those signaling noxious cutaneous inputs. Tonic descending inhibitory influences have been described on dorsal horn neurons which receive convergent input from deep tissues. Such inhibition affects both the excitability of dorsal horn neurons in response to external stimuli and the degree of convergence from different sources.

BIOCHEMISTRY OF MUSCULOSKELETAL NOCICEPTION

The major role of activation and sensitization of joint afferents appears to be played by prostaglandins, in a manner similar to that of inflammation itself. Prostaglandin E (PGE) reverses the depressing effect of cyclooxygenase inhibitors on the spontaneous and movement-evoked activity of nociceptive afferents from inflamed joints. Leukotrienes sensitize nociceptors in animals and humans. Bradykinin, serotonin and histamine also activate these afferents, although the effects are of short duration. These inflammatory mediators may act synergistically: bradykinin, PGE_2 and serotonin enhance responsiveness of joint afferents to mechanical stimuli. Substance P may stimulate the release of prostaglandins from synovial cells[3,5].

Muscle nociceptors are activated particularly by mechanical stimulation and by bradykinin. They can be sensitized by increase in temperature, increase in acidity and exposure to substances such as bradykinin, serotonin and PGE_2. Once irritated by a noxious mechanical stimulus, muscle nociceptors develop sensitivity to epinephrine (adrenaline).

CLINICAL CORRELATES

In microneurographic studies in humans, Aδ and C afferents subserving muscle nociceptors have been found, which respond to local pressure and to algesic substances similarly to receptors in animals. Repetitive electrical stimulation of these muscle afferent units has been associated with cramp-like sensations; however, it remains difficult to assess whether different qualities of muscle pain are mediated by different types of muscle nociceptors. Intrafascicular microstimulation of single joint afferents has been associated with innocuous deep sensations in humans.

The degree of convergence of deep afferents at the spinal level provides an anatomic basis for the poor localization and discrimination which may attend joint and muscle pain, and the referral of pain and hyperalgesia that may accompany pathology.

PATHOPHYSIOLOGY OF MUSCULOSKELETAL PAIN AND HYPERALGESIA

HYPERALGESIA, ALLODYNIA AND SENSITIZATION

The cardinal clinical phenomenon attending musculoskeletal pain is tenderness, which encompasses two clinicopathologic phenomena, hyperalgesia and allodynia. Consistent with the definition of pain above, hyperalgesia is defined as increased pain in response to a noxious stimulus[1], allodynia as pain in response to an innocuous stimulus[1]. In clinical examination, both hyperalgesia and allodynia can be elicited, depending on the nature and intensity of the stimulus used: for example, palpation (pressure) is potentially noxious; light touch or brush is not.

The clinical characteristics of hyperalgesia and allodynia are:

- decreased threshold to noxious stimuli (which may include responding to innocuous stimuli),
- increased pain from suprathreshold stimuli and
- spontaneous pain.

The neurophysiologic correlates of these phenomena at the receptor or afferent fiber level, called sensitization, are:

- decreased response threshold,
- increased response to suprathreshold stimuli and
- spontaneous activity.

In the context of cutaneous injury, the most extensively studied model, two types of hyperalgesia have been described. Primary hyperalgesia occurs in an area of injury whilst secondary hyperalgesia may be found in the undamaged tissue surrounding the injury. The psychophysical characteristics and mechanisms of these two types are distinct[7] (Fig. 4.3).

PRIMARY HYPERALGESIA – PERIPHERAL SENSITIZATION

The main mechanism of primary cutaneous hyperalgesia to thermal stimuli is sensitization of Aδ and C fiber afferents. Primary mechanical hyperalgesia may be attributable to sensitization of some nociceptors to mechanical stimuli or to enlargement of the mechanical receptive field of the primary afferent nociceptor, although sensitization of central nociceptive pathways may also be relevant (see below).

Sensitization of joint nociceptors has been shown in both cat and rat models of joint inflammation: MIAs and afferents previously responding only to intense joint movement develop increased resting activity and begin to respond to non-noxious movements[5]. - Experimental myositis in these animals is associated with an increase in resting discharge in both presumed nociceptors and receptors responding to weak mechanical stimuli, with an increased proportion of the latter[4].

DISTINCTION BETWEEN PRIMARY AND SECONDARY HYPERALGESIA IN SKIN		
	Primary	Secondary
Clinical	Tissue inflamed or damaged	Absence of obvious tissue inflammation or damage
	Allodynia in region of inflammation or damage	Provokable hyperesthesias (including allodynia) in region of pain
Psychophysical	Reduced threshold to stimulation	Normal threshold to stimulation
	Reduced tolerance to thermal and mechanical stimulation	Reduced tolerance to mechanical stimulation only
Mechanism	Sensitization of nociceptors (thermal; possibly mechanical)	'Axon reflex'
	Enlarged receptive fields (mechanical)	Sensitization of central nociceptive pathways

Fig. 4.3 Distinction between primary and secondary hyperalgesia in skin.

NEUROGENIC INFLAMMATION

The involvement of the nervous system in inflammation[8,9] has been recognized since the demonstration of the 'axon reflex', localized vasodilatation and exudation which can be induced by antidromic stimulation of primary C nociceptive afferent fibers, which release neuropeptides at their peripheral terminals. These peptides are synthesized proximally in cell bodies in the dorsal root ganglia and are transported distally as well as centrally. They include SP, calcitonin gene-related peptide (CGRP), somatostatin, vasoactive intestinal peptide (VIP), neurokinin A and neurokinin B. As a group, they exert a variety of influences on inflammation, including changes in vascular tone and permeability, activation of neutrophils, proliferation and function of T- and B-lymphocytes, release of cytokines, production of oxygen-free radicals and release of prostaglandins.

Neurogenic inflammation contributes to acute and chronic arthritis. Intra-articular injection of SP in rats induces local inflammation, while capsaicin, which selectively depletes SP from primary afferent fibers, attenuates the development of experimental arthritis in the rat. In animal models of chronic arthritis, injection of SP increases the local severity of inflammation, and the severity of arthritis and the density of SP-containing nociceptive afferents are directly related.

In humans, immunohistochemical techniques reveal at least SP and CGRP in synovium, found in patterns suggesting local release in inflammatory arthritis compared with osteoarthrosis. Clinically, afferent or sympathetic interruption influences inflammatory joint disease. These observations together establish the relevance of the efferent influence of primary nociceptive afferents on joint inflammation.

SECONDARY HYPERALGESIA – CENTRAL SENSITIZATION

Allodynia occurring outside an area of tissue damage or inflammation ('secondary hyperalgesia') is usually defined by the response to mechanical stimuli. There are three potential mechanisms:

- peripheral sensitization (nociceptor),
- central sensitization (spinal) and
- reduced descending inhibition (supraspinal).

Microneurographic studies in humans have provided some evidence for the first of these.

The major mechanism invoked to explain secondary hyperalgesia is the phenomenon of neural plasticity at the spinal cord level. This refers to the changes in connectivity resulting from persistent nociceptive input (injury, noxious stimulation or C-fiber afferent electrical stimulation), characterized by increased activity, enhanced responsiveness to peripheral stimuli and enlarged receptive field size of dorsal horn cells[10]. The clinical correlates of this are spontaneous pain, allodynia, hyperalgesia and an increase in the size of the region from which pain can be elicited.

In rats, changes in dorsal horns following peripheral nerve injury, including trans-synaptic degeneration and reorganization with the formation of new synaptic connections, provide an anatomic basis for the phenomenon of sensitization[11]. Its proposed biochemical basis is the release of neuropeptides and excitatory amino acids (EAAs) into the dorsal horn, leading to slow depolarization, then persistent changes in excitability and ultimately excessive depolarization with EAA-induced cytotoxicity. This cell dysfunction, with possible loss of inhibitory mechanisms, could lead to persistence of changes in the absence of further noxious input.

CENTRAL CHANGES IN EXPERIMENTAL ARTHRITIS AND MYOSITIS

Acute or chronic arthritis or myositis can induce changes in central nociceptive pathways (dorsal horn, thalamus and primary somatosensory cortex), manifest as increased background discharge and enhanced responsiveness to afferent activity both from the site of inflammation and from other convergent inputs[4,5]. Reduction in tonic descending inhibition of spinal cord neurons which receive articular afferent input has been shown in association with acute feline arthritis.

INITIATION AND MAINTENANCE OF CENTRAL SENSITIZATION

An extensive literature, both in animals and clinically and experimentally in humans, supports the concept that sustained C-afferent nociceptive input from peripheral inflammation or nerve damage is associated with central hyperexcitability[12]. In humans, duration and extent of secondary hyperalgesia in skin are dependent on the intensity of the initiating nociceptive stimulus. It has been suggested that central excitability may be a physiologic accompaniment of ongoing nociception. Whether central sensitization needs ongoing afferent 'drive' or may become autonomous has yet to be determined.

ASSESSMENT OF PAIN AT THE SOMATIC LEVEL

At the clinical level the presenting feature is pain. A rational approach is to determine:

- what is the anatomic origin of pain
- what are the mechanisms of pain production and
- is there an associated disease process?

The first two can be addressed through dissection of the accompanying allodynia and hyperalgesia: whether primary (implying peripheral sensitization) or secondary (implying central changes) (Fig. 4.4).

PRIMARY HYPERALGESIA: NOCICEPTIVE PAIN – INFLAMMATORY AND MECHANICAL MODELS

Conceptually, inflammation may be seen as the combination of:

- pain, attributable to activation of nociceptors,
- primary hyperalgesia, due to sensitization of nociceptors, and
- swelling, which reflects the vascular effects of neuropeptide release.

This conceptualization accounts for inflammation occurring in response to both immunologic and neurogenic processes[8], as well as being influenced by ischemia[13]. This inflammatory model accounts for most (but not all) of the pain and hyperalgesia of active (but not inactive) inflammatory disease. As inflammation is known to sensitize nociceptors and MIAs, a scenario for subsequent persistent sensitivity to movement of damaged joints and muscles may well be created.

Nociceptors and mechanoreceptors in musculoskeletal tissues may also be activated by increased intra-articular pressure or abnormal posture of joints. Although not usually considered to transduce nociception, mechanoreceptors may become involved in the generation and maintenance of spinal cord plasticity such that mechanoreceptive information is processed as noxious.

The relevant clinical observation is that joints which do not move properly (usually hypomobile or, less commonly, hypermobile) may be painful whether or not they are anatomically abnormal. This model implies that changes in joint biomechanics *per se* may be responsible for pain and primary hyperalgesia without invoking inflammatory processes. It follows that mechanical nociception may be particularly relevant in joints which have been damaged by a pathologic process (e.g. osteoarthritis), especially if nociceptors have been sensitized by prior influences (see also Chapter 1.11).

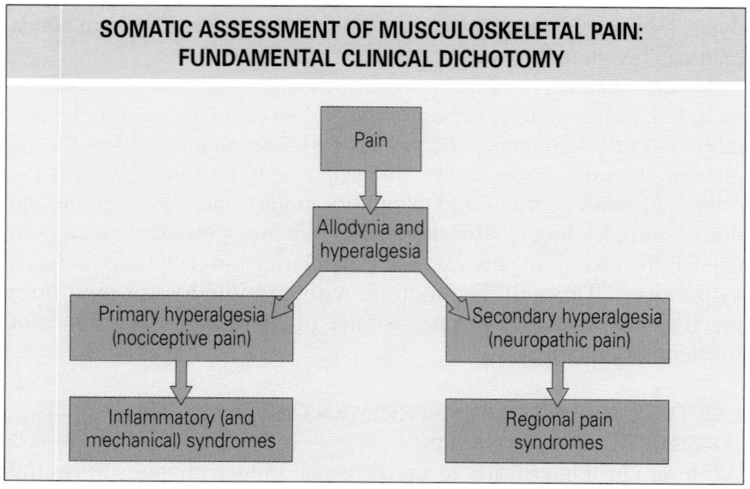

SECONDARY HYPERALGESIA: NEUROPATHIC MODEL

The well-recognized phenomenon of referred pain is considered to depend on neuroanatomic convergence at a spinal level and on perceptual divergence at thalamic and cortical levels[14]. The finding of (mechanical) allodynia in regions of referred pain argues in favor of altered central function as well: the psychophysical characteristics of referred pain are those of secondary hyperalgesia[7,10].

Referred pain is recognized in chronic arthropathy. For example, pain from an osteoarthritic hip is commonly referred to the knee. Considering the chronicity of many rheumatologic diseases and the attendant potential for sustained nociception over time, the role of altered function of central nociceptive pathways in the pathogenesis of musculoskeletal pain should be considered. Clinically this would be expressed as regions of secondary hyperalgesia.

The constructs of fibromyalgia and related syndromes (Chapter 4.15) are built on the assumption that peripheral musculoskeletal pathology accounts for the pain. In the absence of convincing evidence for such pathology, the concept of secondary hyperalgesia and central sensitization must be invoked for physiologic plausibility of this construct and to avoid circular arguments.

In humans, however, the question remains of how the perception of these presumed central changes may in turn influence them. The occurrence of clinical allodynia in the absence of 'hard' signs has led to considerable controversy. On one side of the debate are the proponents of specific clinical entities such as 'fibromyalgia syndrome' and 'myofascial pain syndrome' (Chapter 4.15); the critics on the other side describe these as examples of 'pseudoneuropathies' of implied psychogenic origin[15]. Given that primary psychogenic hypotheses are as untestable as the human central nociceptive system is at present inaccessible, the role of perception by conscious, sentient humans confronted with a nociceptive event which fails to settle must be taken into account. In these situations of joint and muscle pain where the pathology is not readily attributable to (peripheral) nociception, clinical assessment may depend even more on understanding the biopsychosocial hierarchical levels of the 'nervous system' and above (see Fig. 4.1).

SOMATIC ASSESSMENT OF MUSCULOSKELETAL PAIN: FUNDAMENTAL CLINICAL DICHOTOMY

Pain → Allodynia and hyperalgesia → Primary hyperalgesia (nociceptive pain) → Inflammatory (and mechanical) syndromes

Allodynia and hyperalgesia → Secondary hyperalgesia (neuropathic pain) → Regional pain syndromes

Fig. 4.4 Somatic assessment of musculoskeletal pain: fundamental clinical dichotomy.

ASSESSMENT OF PAIN AT THE COGNITIVE–PERCEPTUAL AND SOCIOLOGIC LEVELS

Pain disrupts the life of the individual in terms of relationships with others, self-esteem, ability to complete tasks of daily living and to work and function as a member of the community. Identification of the somatic processes leading to musculoskeletal pain forms only part of the clinical picture. The consequences for function and for mood are of at least equal importance, especially with respect to the patient's ability to perform activities of daily living. In chronic musculoskeletal illnesses where the pathology is known and rational therapy available, such as the inflammatory joint diseases, the three major determinants of overall health are psychologic status, physical functioning and pain itself[16]. Anxiety and depression are common in cohorts of patients with rheumatoid arthritis, chronic low back pain and chronic neck pain, their development being related more to socioeconomic than to clinical indices. Disability is strongly correlated with attitude to illness: these considerations underlie the importance of assessing patients' beliefs regarding the nature and prognosis of their pain[17–19].

FACTORS IN THE COGNITIVE–PERCEPTUAL AND SOCIOLOGIC ASSESSMENT OF PAIN
Affective
Anxiety Anger Depression
Behavioral
Posture and usage patterns Reinforcement of inactivity Role changes Interference with sleep Interpersonal relationships Treatment seeking: doctor shopping; drug usage
Cognitive
Beliefs and expectations regarding causation, pathology and prognosis Influence of industrial, financial and legal issues Intercurrent stressors

Fig. 4.5 Assessment of musculoskeletal pain at cognitive–perceptual and sociologic levels.

PRINCIPLES OF PAIN MANAGEMENT
Aims
Minimize distress Maximize function
Modalities
Pharmacologic (see Fig. 4.7) Analgesics Anti-inflammatories Adjuvant analgesics Physical Ergonomic analysis of posture and function Exercise regimens Avoidance of passive treatments 'Psychological' (cognitive–behavioral) Validation Goal-setting Pacing of activity Self-regulatory skills (relaxation, distraction) Stress management skills Problem-solving skills

Fig. 4.6 Principles of pain management.

Assessment of pain at this cognitive–perceptual level includes effects on mood, activity and rest patterns, consequences of pain on ability to work and to function socially, on self-esteem and on beliefs (Fig. 4.5). Of many instruments which have been developed for the assessment of these aspects of pain[20], the Westhaven Yale Multidimensional Pain Inventory (WHYMPI) has been most utilized. Cognitive factors, such as pain coping strategies, modulate health status in both inflammatory and noninflammatory musculoskeletal disease. A number of these instruments both correlate with changes in pain intensity and physical functioning and respond to cognitive–behavioral therapy[21].

These outcome measures can be used in assessing the efficacy of a variety of interventions, including pharmacologic, and may also be used in determining prognosis, especially in musculoskeletal diseases, where impairment may not always be reflected in disability for which, in turn, there is no simple single measure.

MANAGEMENT OF PAIN

A management plan based on an understanding of physical and psychosocial pathology is optimal for the patient with musculoskeletal pain. In both inflammatory and noninflammatory conditions, it has been shown that prognosis may be affected as much by cognitive, behavioral and socioeconomic factors as by specific treatments. With respect to chronic musculoskeletal pain, however, both nociception (peripheral or central) and the pain itself (as a problem in its own right) need to be addressed. A rational approach to pain management includes treatments directed at the mechanisms of nociception, at the affective and evaluable components of the pain, aspects of the underlying disease and at the consequences in terms of personal and sociologic function (Fig. 4.6).

TREATMENT OF MECHANISMS OF NOCICEPTION

The traditional approach to the management of inflammatory disease has included the use of a range of drugs often prescribed in a rather hierarchical fashion. Nonsteroidal anti-inflammatory drugs (NSAIDs) tend to be used initially, followed after some period of time by the use of second-line agents (see Chapters 3.5–3.10). Specific antagonists to non-prostaglandin mediators have yet to be developed for the clinical setting.

The role of altered central nociception in the production of pain and (secondary) allodynia and/or hyperalgesia in chronic musculoskeletal disorders awaits further elucidation. This phenomenon does suggest the usefulness of agents that may interfere with excitatory EAAs and monoamines in these conditions, where sensitization of dorsal horn neurons is highly likely to have occurred. Currently available agents include anticonvulsant and tricyclic antidepressant drugs.

Two interacting groups of neurochemical mediators, colocalized to the terminals of fine primary afferent fibers in the dorsal horn, are held responsible for the mechanism of plasticity induced by noxious stimulation. These include C-fiber neuropeptides and EAAs [L-glutamate, L-aspartate, *N*-methyl-D-aspartate (NMDA)][10]. Antagonists to these mediators have been shown in experimental animals to suppress or prevent sensitization of dorsal horn neurons in response to nociceptive input. In humans, experience is limited to postoperative and experimental pain.

TREATMENT OF PAIN ITSELF

The use of opioid and nonopioid analgesics is rational in these disorders, to reduce the distress of pain itself, over and above the physical consequences of disease (Fig. 4.7). Acetaminophen (paracetamol) is an undervalued effective analgesic agent. Its mechanism of action remains poorly understood, although there is evidence for direct effects on the central nervous system[22]. A major advantage is its lack of upper gastrointestinal toxicity, especially ulceration and bleeding. The well-

RATIONAL PHARMACOTHERAPY FOR PAIN		
Target	**Drug**	**Proposed action**
Inflammation; peripheral sensitization	NSAID	Antiprostaglandin
	Corticosteroids (systemic or local)	Vascular and cellular effects
Neuropathic pain; central sensitization	Tricyclic antidepressants	Effects on monoamine [serotonin and norepinephrine (noradrenaline)]-mediated central pathways
	Anticonvulsants	Suppression of paroxysmal discharges
	Local anesthetics (oral)	Nondepolarizing neural blockade
	Neuropeptide antagonists*	Opposition to SP, CGRP, etc.
	NMDA receptor antagonists*	Opposition to EAAs
Pain itself	Acetaminophen (paracetamol)	Central
	Opioid agonists	Activation of μ-receptors (brain), δ- and κ-receptors (spinal cord); possible peripheral action

Fig. 4.7 Rational pharmacotherapy for pain. (* Under development)

known hazard of hepatotoxicity, seen virtually only with drug overdose, is increased with liver disease and alcoholism, and the daily dose should be carefully monitored in these situations. The risk for nephrotoxicity with chronic dosing remains uncertain but is probably very small.

The role of opioids in the management of chronic, moderate to severe musculoskeletal pain is controversial. Although certain patients may indeed benefit, without toxicity and without developing addiction (which remains the main concern in both medical and administrative circles), the question of true efficacy has not yet been answered[23]. Although they are considered to work mainly through opiate receptors in the central nervous system, either by inhibition of transmission of nociceptive messages to higher centers or through activation of descending antinociceptive pathways[24], increasing evidence points to peripheral analgesic actions of opioids, especially in conditions characterized by inflammatory (primary) hyperalgesia[25]. It is important that analgesics are taken regularly rather than in pain-contingent regimens and that the reduction in distress associated with their use be linked with increased activity.

Antidepressant drugs may enhance the analgesia induced by other drugs. The presumed site of action is at the spinal cord level (as for their putative effect on central sensitization), although their beneficial effect on sleep and on mood, where appropriate, suggests action elsewhere in the neuraxis. Debate continues over possible modes of action and whether or not these drugs induce analgesia in the absence of depression in chronic pain generally[26].

PHYSICAL THERAPY

The goals of physical therapy include increasing and maintaining muscle strength and endurance, increasing joint motion, reducing joint instability and improving capacity to perform activities of daily living. As with pharmacologic agents, physical prescriptions should be individualized, ideally based on a biopsychosocial evaluation, to take into account comorbidity, issues of pain control and compliance (see Chapter 3.11).

COGNITIVE–BEHAVIORAL THERAPY AND PAIN CLINICS

Chronic pain management programs emphasize therapies which seek to change behavior and belief systems. The recognition that the clinical problem of chronic pain should be processed in a biopsychosocial framework (see Fig. 4.1) has led to the development of multidisciplinary management programs which incorporate both physically and psychologically based components. The latter include operant de-conditioning, cognitive restructuring, problem solving, coping skills training, relaxation and biofeedback.

Many publications proclaim the effectiveness of such programs which are commonly delivered through interdisciplinary pain clinics. A meta-analysis of 65 such studies concluded that the benefits can extend to variables such as return to work or usage of the health care system[27]. 'Neglected' issues in the treatment and outcome studies of chronic pain patients, discussed in a landmark trilogy[28], included:

- the bases on which treatment modalities are offered,
- the failure of patients to attend or to complete programs,
- the problem of treatment termination and relapse and
- a lack of agreement on the criteria for success.

Pain control is not yet a unified field, with diversity among centers, including diagnostic and etiologic frames of reference, professional background of staff, selection criteria used and treatment modalities offered[29]. The processes of improvement in the context of multidisciplinary programs have yet to be clarified: efficacy may be related to changes in belief and cognitive coping strategies rather than to the use of specific techniques such as exercise, suggesting that improvements may be more closely associated with what patients think about their pain than with what they do about it[30].

SUMMARY

An understanding of the sociobiology of pain is integral to the practice of musculoskeletal medicine. Recognition of the interaction of the somatic components (nociception and its central transmission) with the cognitive and perceptual components (belief, mood and behavior) provides a framework for comprehensive assessment and management. At the somatic level, this includes insight into the mechanisms of the fundamental clinical phenomena of allodynia and hyperalgesia, while at the cognitive–perceptual level, it may be appreciated that not all the observed distress need be nociceptive. A combination of pharmacologic and cognitive–behavioral therapies, appropriate to the individual patient, is recommended.

REFERENCES

1. Merskey H, Bogduk N, eds. Classification of chronic pain, 2E. Seattle: IASP; 1994.
2. Steig RL, Williams RC. Chronic pain as a biosociocultural phenomenon: implications for treatment. Semin Neurol. 1983;3:370–6.
3. Portenoy RK. Basic mechanisms. In: Portenoy RK, Kanner RM, eds. Pain management: theory and practice. Philadelphia: FA Davis Company; 1996:19–39.
4. Mense S. Nociception from skeletal muscle in relation to clinical muscle pain. Pain. 1993;54:241–90.
5. Schaible H-G, Grubb BD. Afferent and spinal mechanisms of joint pain. Pain 1993;55:5–54.
6. Mapp P. Innervation of the synovium. Ann Rheum Dis. 1995;54:398–403.
7. Treede R-D, Meyer RA, Raja SN, Campbell JN. Peripheral and central mechanisms of cutaneous hyperalgesia. Prog Neurobiol. 1992;38:397–421.
8. Matucci-Cerini M, Partsch G. The contribution of the peripheral nervous system and the neuropeptide network to the development of synovial inflammation. Clin Exp Rheumatol. 1992;10:211–15.
9. Levine JD, Goetzl EJ, Basbaum AI. Contribution of the nervous system to the pathophysiology of rheumatoid arthritis and other polyarthritides. Rheum Dis Clin N Am. 1987;13:369–83.
10. Coderre TJ, Katz J, Vaccarino AL, Melzack R. Contribution of central neuroplasticity to pathologic pain: review of clinical and experimental evidence. Pain. 1993;52:259–85.
11. Woolf CJ, Shortland P, Coggeshall RE. Peripheral nerve injury triggers central sprouting of myelinated afferents. Nature. 1992;355:75–7.
12. Dubner R. Neuronal plasticity and pain following peripheral tissue inflammation or nerve injury. In: Bond MR, Charlton JE, Woolf CJ, eds. Proceedings of the VIth World Congress on Pain. Amsterdam: Elsevier; 1991:263–76.
13. Blake DR, Merry P, Unsworth J. Hypoxic reperfusion injury in the inflamed human joint. Lancet. 1989;i:289–93.
14. Ruch TC. Pathophysiology of pain. In: Ruch TC, Patton HD, eds. Physiology and biophysics. Philadelphia: Saunders; 1965:345–63.
15. Ochoa JL. Essence, investigation and management of 'neuropathic' pains: hopes from acknowledgement of chaos. Muscle Nerve. 1993;16:997–1008.
16. Kazis LE, Meenan RF, Anderson JJ. Pain in the rheumatic diseases: investigations of a key health status component. Arthritis Rheum. 1983;26:1017–22.
17. McFarlane AC, Brooks PM. An analysis of the relationship between psychological morbidity and disease activity in rheumatoid arthritis. J Rheumatol. 1988;15:926–31.
18. Weiser S, Cedrashi C. Psychosocial issues in the prevention of chronic low back pain – a literature review. Balliere's Clin Rheum. 1992;6:657–84.
19. Radanov BP, Sturzenegger M, Di Stefano G. Long-term outcome after whiplash injury. A 2-year follow-up considering features of injury mechanism and somatic, radiologic and psychosocial findings. Medicine (Baltimore). 1995;74:281–97.
20. Turk DC, Melzack R, eds. Handbook of pain assessment. New York: Guildford; 1992.
21. Parker JC, Bradley LA, DeVellis RM, *et al.* Biopsychosocial contributions to the management of arthritis disability. Arthritis Rheum. 1993;36:885–9.
22. Piletta P, Porchet HC, Dayer P. Distinct central nervous system involvement of paracetamol and salicylate. In: Bond MR, Charlton JE, Woolf CJ, eds. Proceedings of the VIth World Congress on Pain. Amsterdam: Elsevier; 1991:181–4.
23. Jamison RN. Comprehensive pretreatment and outcome assessment for chronic opioid therapy in nonmalignant pain. J Pain Symptom Manage. 1996;11:231–41.
24. Ferrante FM. Opioids. In: Ferrante FM, Vade-Boncoeur TR, eds. Postoperative pain management. New York: Churchill-Livingstone; 1993:145–209.
25. Stein C. Peripheral analgesic effects of opioids. J Pain Symptom Manage. 1991;6:119–24.
26. Watson CPN. Antidepressant drugs as adjuvant analgesics. J Pain Symptom Manage. 1994;9:392–405.
27. Flor H, Fydrich T, Turk DC. Efficacy of multidisciplinary pain treatment centers: a meta-analytic review. Pain. 1992;49:221–30.
28. Turk DC, Rudy TE, Sorkin BA. Neglected factors in chronic pain treatment outcome studies – determination of success. Pain. 1993;53:3–16.
29. Csordas TJ, Clark JA. Ends of the line: diversity among chronic pain centers. Soc Sci Med. 1992;34:383–93.
30. Jensen MP, Turner JA, Romano JM. Correlates of improvement in multidisciplinary treatment of chronic pain. J Cons Clin Psychol. 1994;62:172–9.

5

NSAIDs

Peter M Brooks

Summary

- NSAIDs continue to provide 'background' anti-inflammatory therapy for rheumatic diseases.
- Newer NSAIDs with selective inhibition of COX 2 (inducible) enzyme are associated with a lower incidence of gastrointestinal and renal adverse events.
- Variability in response to NSAIDs is seen both in terms of anti-inflammatory activity and adverse events.

INTRODUCTION

Nonsteroidal anti-inflammatory drugs (NSAIDs) remain the principal pharmacologic agents for symptom relief in patients with the rheumatic diseases. They constitute the largest single group of drugs used worldwide and annually have total sales in excess of $US 2 billion. The NSAIDs are prescribed in the full range of rheumatic diseases and in many countries can now be purchased over the counter for symptomatic relief of headaches, dysmenorrhea and sports injuries. Over the past few years there has been a broadening in the traditional use of NSAIDs to their prescription for such things as renal colic, biliary colic, headache and other painful disorders.

The number of NSAIDs available continues to proliferate, and although subtle differences exist in pharmacokinetics, adverse reaction profiles and mechanisms of action, none of these parameters alone explains the marked variability in response noted with these agents in clinical practice. The question as to how many NSAIDs are required is a vexed one but is continually asked by rheumatologists, pharmaceutical manufacturers and drug regulators. Quite marked differences exist internationally in the availability of NSAIDs, with six to seven NSAIDs being available in many Scandinavian countries and up to forty in Italy. Despite the fact that the slow-acting antirheumatic drugs (SAARDs) are being used earlier in the management of inflammatory rheumatic diseases, NSAIDs will continue to provide symptomatic relief in the foreseeable future.

In this chapter we explore new insights into the mechanism of action of NSAIDs, cover the range of drugs available, discuss their major pharmacokinetic and pharmacodynamic differences, and raise some of the issues relevant to variability in response to these drugs. Adverse drug reactions produced by NSAIDs still pose a major problem, and strategies for reducing these to a minimum, together with practical prescribing points, are discussed.

MECHANISM OF ACTION

Inflammation in the rheumatic disease is extremely complex, involving a multiplicity of interactions between cells, mediators and other factors. Over the past few years it has been realized that the traditional principal mechanism of action of NSAIDs, i.e. inhibition of cyclooxygenase (COX), only partly explains their success in suppressing inflammatory responses. A simple schema of the inflammatory process in rheumatoid arthritis (RA) is shown in Figure 5.1, along with the sites of possible action of NSAIDs [1]. It is now clear that prostaglandins have a significant influence on many of the cells and other mediators involved in the immune response. Interfering with prostaglandin synthesis will, therefore, have far-reaching effects on these activities, and NSAIDs can be said to have some mild immunomodulatory activity. In this respect the differentiation between NSAIDs, SAARDs and immunosuppressive drugs is becoming less clear.

The major actions of NSAIDs are summarized in Figure 5.2. The effect of NSAIDs on prostaglandin production is well known, but it is

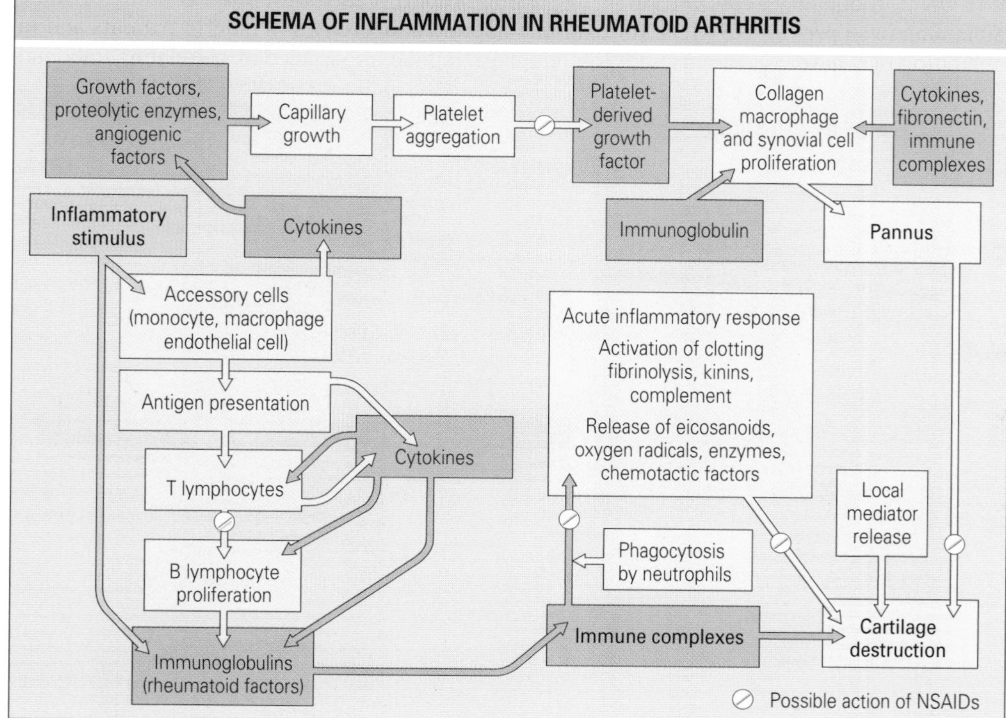

Fig. 5.1 Schema of inflammation in RA, and the possible sites of action of NSAIDs.

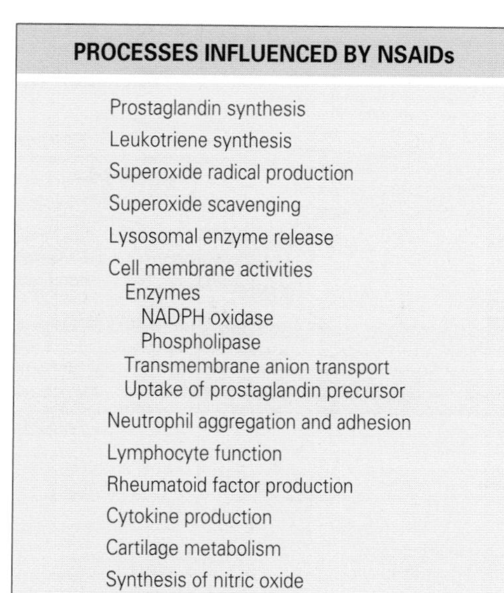

Fig. 5.2 Processes influenced by NSAIDs.

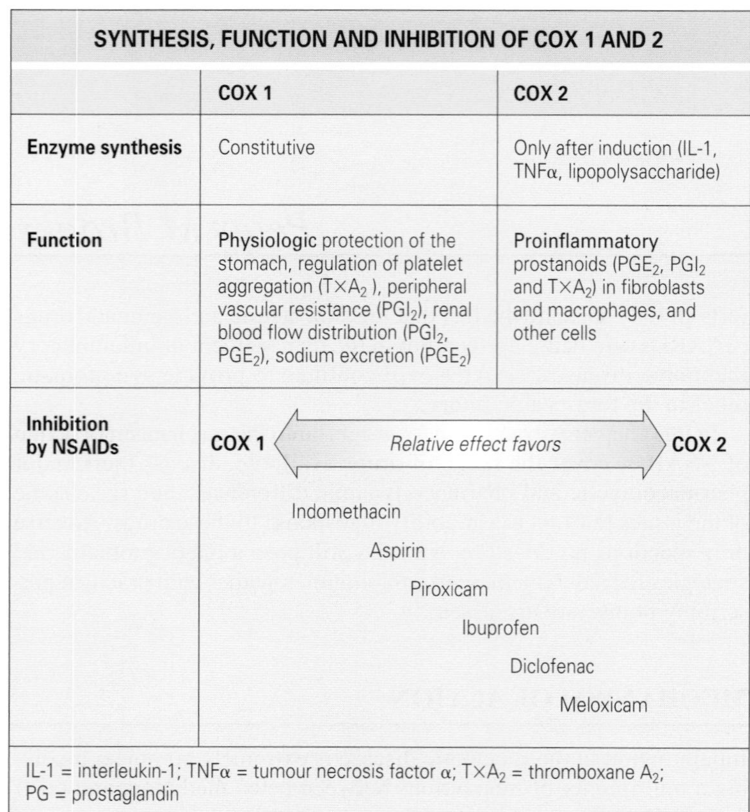

SYNTHESIS, FUNCTION AND INHIBITION OF COX 1 AND 2

	COX 1	COX 2
Enzyme synthesis	Constitutive	Only after induction (IL-1, TNFα, lipopolysaccharide)
Function	**Physiologic** protection of the stomach, regulation of platelet aggregation ($T{\times}A_2$), peripheral vascular resistance (PGI_2), renal blood flow distribution (PGI_2, PGE_2), sodium excretion (PGE_2)	**Proinflammatory** prostanoids (PGE_2, PGI_2 and $T{\times}A_2$) in fibroblasts and macrophages, and other cells
Inhibition by NSAIDs	COX 1 ⟵ *Relative effect favors* ⟶ COX 2 Indomethacin Aspirin Piroxicam Ibuprofen Diclofenac Meloxicam	

IL-1 = interleukin-1; TNFα = tumour necrosis factor α; $T{\times}A_2$ = thromboxane A_2; PG = prostaglandin

Fig. 5.3 Synthesis, function and inhibition of cyclooxygenases (COX)1 and 2. Adapted from Frölich [4].

interesting to note that salicylate, which has little effect on this parameter, is as effective in patients with RA as aspirin (a potent prostaglandin synthesis inhibitor) [2]. NSAIDs differ in their affects on neutrophils, lymphocytes and chondrocytes [3]. Care must be taken, however, in the interpretation of the data relating to NSAID action on chondrocyte function, since many of the studies were carried out *in vitro* and at nonphysiologic concentrations. Carefully conducted long-term studies in man are required to assess the influence of NSAIDs on cartilage function.

Recently it has been shown that COX has two distinct isoenzymes – a constitutive form (COX 1) and an inducible form (COX 2) found at sites of inflammation [4]: COX 1 is responsible for maintaining renal perfusion and normal gastric mucosa. Selective COX 2 inhibition may have the advantage of reducing renal and gastric adverse events, as suggested with some of the newer NSAIDs such as meloxicam [5] (Fig. 5.3).

The available NSAIDs come from a variety of chemical classes (Fig. 5.4). Differences in their physicochemical parameters may influence the pharmacokinetics and give rise to differences in their beneficial and adverse effects. For example, the more lipid-soluble NSAIDs, such as ketoprofen, naproxen and ibuprofen, penetrate the central nervous system (CNS) more easily and are associated with mild changes in mood and cognitive function. The majority of NSAIDs are weakly acidic and will preferentially concentrate in inflamed tissues.

PHARMACOKINETICS

The pharmacokinetic parameters of a drug are dependent on its absorption and bioavailability, its distribution throughout the body and its half-life. An understanding of the pharmacokinetics of a drug is only relevant to patient care if the therapeutic response and adverse reactions are related to the plasma concentrations achieved with that drug [6]. Dose–and/or plasma concentration–response relationships have been demonstrated in RA for a number of NSAIDs, including naproxen, carprofen and ibuprofen [3,6]. As can be seen from Figure 5.5, the percentage of patients responding to naproxen increases with the plasma concentration. Linear relationships between plasma concentration of NSAIDs and toxicity have also been demonstrated.

Most NSAIDs are completely absorbed from the gastrointestinal tract, but this can be slowed by food. NSAIDs are now generally presented as enteric-coated tablets or as a sustained-release preparation. These have been developed together with the longer half-life NSAIDs in an attempt to provide more stable plasma concentrations throughout a 24-hour period. It should be appreciated, however, that NSAIDs diffuse more slowly into synovial fluid and that the synovial fluid concentrations are more much stable and show fewer fluctuations than plasma concentrations, even for short half-life drugs (Fig. 5.6). This fluctuation in synovial fluid concentrations may in part be responsible for the dosing interval of short half-life drugs being longer than their plasma half-lives [7].

NSAIDs are highly bound to plasma proteins, and the amount of free drug (the active component) is relatively small. The binding of NSAIDs to plasma proteins can be reduced in various diseases, or in subjects with hypoalbuminemia. For most NSAIDs the unbound fraction does not change in relation to the plasma concentration, but naproxen, phenylbutazone and salicylate do have dose-dependent protein binding, unbound concentrations increasing proportionally with dose. Binding of some NSAIDs, for example naproxen, decreases in elderly patients and in patients with RA, emphasizing the importance of correlating unbound

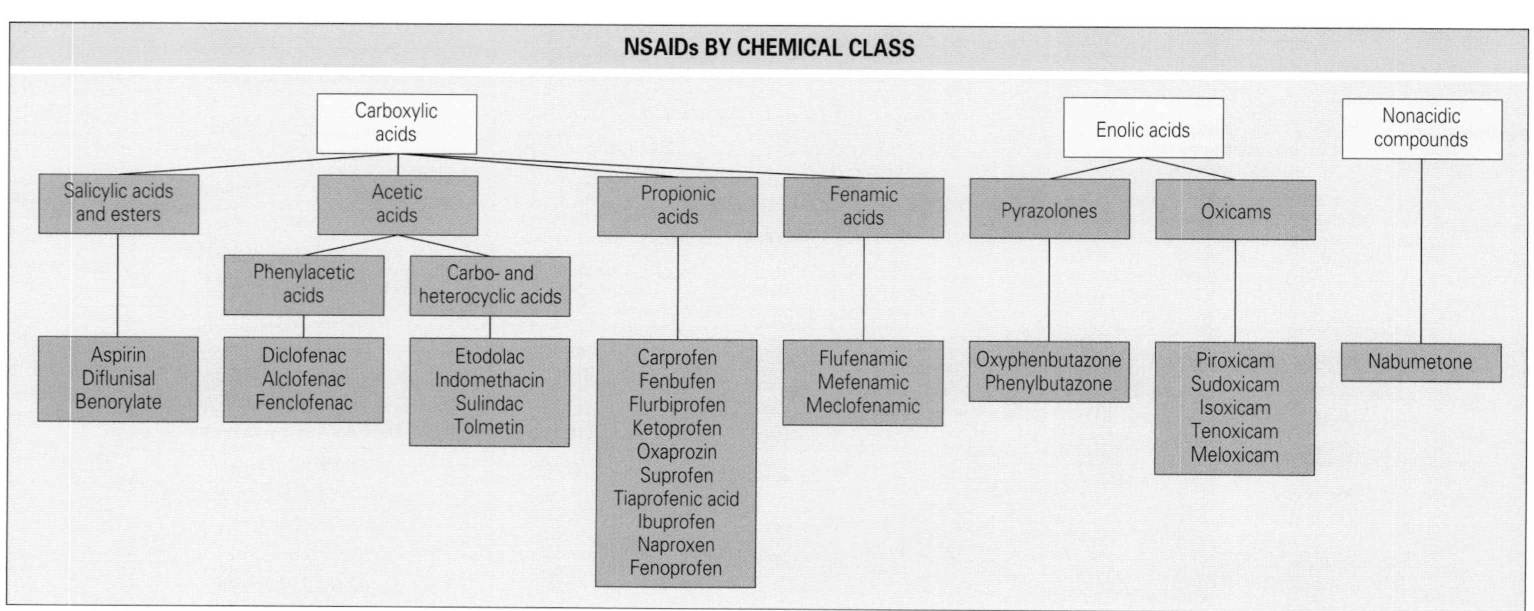

Fig. 5.4 The classification of NSAIDs by chemical class.

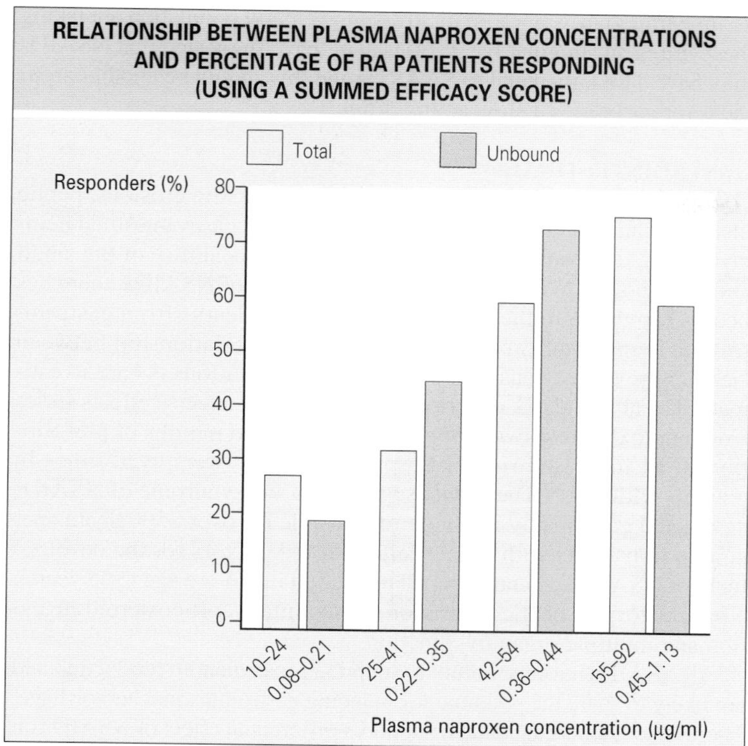

Fig. 5.5 Relationship between plasma naproxen concentrations and response of RA patients (summed efficacy score). Adapted from Tonkin and Wing[24].

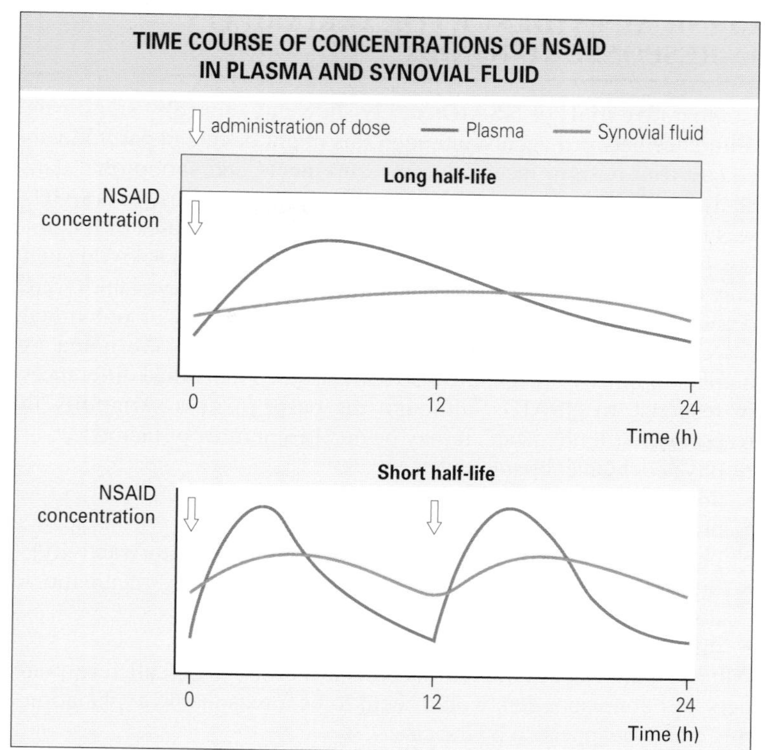

Fig. 5.6 Time course of plasma and synovial fluid NSAID concentrations.

concentrations with effect rather than total plasma concentrations. The NSAIDs can be divided into two groups on the basis of their plasma elimination half-life (Fig. 5.7). Those drugs with a long half-life, such as piroxicam and tenoxicam, take a long time to reach steady state in the body and, therefore, a longer period of treatment is required before a maximum clinical response can be expected.

The clearance of NSAIDs is predominantly by hepatic metabolism, with production of inactive metabolites. These inactive metabolites are then excreted in the urine. The clearance of some NSAIDs, including diflunisal, ketoprofen, fenoprofen, naproxen and indomethacin, is decreased in renal failure and inhibited by probenecid. The main reason for this decrease is the fact that the acylglucuronide metabolites of these drugs are retained and are then hydrolyzed back to the parent compound.

Some NSAIDs, such as aspirin, nabumetone, fenbufen and sulindac, are converted into active metabolites, which produce the major anti-inflammatory pharmacologic effect. Sulindac is particularly interesting since the active metabolite (the sulfide) is produced in the large intestine and the process seems to be reversible. Conversion of the active sulfide metabolite into the inactive sulindac occurs in the kidney and has been proposed as the explanation for the reported renal sparing effects of this drug. Enterohepatic recycling of certain NSAIDs, particularly indomethacin and sulindac, can occur.

Some of the NSAIDs of the propionic acid class, including ibuprofen, ketoprofen, fenoprofen, naproxen, tiaprofenic acid and flurbiprofen, exist as two optical isomers, or enantiomers. Interestingly, it is only the *S* enantiomer which inhibits cyclooxygenase, while the *R* enantiomer is inactive. Unidirectional conversion of the *R* into the *S* form of the NSAID can occur to a variable degree *in vivo*, depending on the drug and the individual subject. Naproxen is marketed as the *S* enantiomer only, but the other arylpropionic acids, such as ibuprofen, ketoprofen and flurbiprofen, exist as equal mixtures of the inactive *R* and active *S*.

The pharmacokinetics of some NSAIDs can be affected by liver disease, renal disease or old age[8]. Because of the complex nature of the metabolism of NSAIDs, these factors may potentially affect the disposition of these agents but, unfortunately, no generalizations can be made and the effect of disease states must be considered for each individual agent. The principal effects are shown in Figure 5.8.

HALF-LIVES OF NSAIDs

Short (< 6 hours)		Long (> 12 hours)	
NSAID	Half-life (h)	NSAID	Half-life (h)
Aspirin	0.25	Azapropazone	15.0
Diclofenac	1.1	Carprofen	12.0
Etodolac	6.0	Diflunisal	13.0
Fenoprofen	2.5	Fenbufen	11.0
Flufenamic acid	1.4	Meloxicam	20.0
Flurbiprofen	3.8	Nabumetone	26.0
Ibuprofen	2.1	Naproxen	14.0
Indomethacin	4.6	Oxaprozin	58.0
Ketoprofen	1.8	Phenylbutazone	68.0
Mefenamic acid	2.0	Piroxicam	57.0
Pirprofen	3.8	Salicylate	2.0–15.0
Suprofen	2.5	Sulindac	14.0
Tolmetin	1.0	Tenoxicam	60.0
Tiaprofenic acid	3.0		

Fig. 5.7 The half-lives of NSAIDs.

THE EFFECTS OF DISEASE STATES AND AGING ON THE ELIMINATION OF NSAIDs

	Renal failure	Hepatic failure	Old age
Azapropazone	↓	↓	↓
Indomethacin	–	↓	↔
Sulindac	–	↓	↓
Naproxen	↓	↓	↓
Ketoprofen	↓	–	↓
Tiaprofenic acid	↓	–	↓↔
Piroxicam	↔	–	↓↔
Salicylate	–	–	↓

Fig. 5.8 The effects of disease states and aging on the elimination of NSAIDs.

CLINICAL EVIDENCE FOR VARIABILITY IN RESPONSE TO NSAIDs

Comparative trials of NSAIDs rarely show any clinically significant difference between agents, although this might be due in part to inadequate trial design, insensitive measurements and suboptimal data analysis. The first demonstration of variability in response to NSAIDs was made by Huskisson *et al.*[9], who compared fixed doses of ibuprofen, fenoprofen, ketoprofen and naproxen in patients with RA. Although only minor differences in mean values of disease activity variables were demonstrated between the drugs, marked variations in individual response, with preferences for particular NSAIDs, were noted. A number of other workers have also demonstrated individual differences in response to NSAIDs, although the basis for this variability in response is still not clear[3]. It may be due to a number of factors:

- physicochemical parameters;
- dosage selection and timing of dose;
- pharmacokinetic variation;
- pharmacodynamics (i.e. variability in anti-inflammatory activity);
- intersubject variability in pathophysiology of various rheumatic diseases;
- different adverse reactions.

Although differences in pharmacokinetics between so-called responders and nonresponders would seem to be a reasonable explanation, this does not appear to be the case[3].

ADVERSE DRUG REACTIONS

Adverse drug reactions to NSAIDs are frequently reported to drug evaluation authorities[10] and cover a broad spectrum of reactions, from the common gastrointestinal problems to rare side effects such as aseptic meningitis[11,12] (Fig. 5.9). Gastrointestinal adverse events are usually mild but are seen most often (in approximately 10% of patients on NSAIDs), followed by renal events, skin rashes and CNS reactions. Serious adverse reactions to NSAIDs are relatively rare, but they do assume importance since up to 30% of the elderly population are taking these drugs on a regular basis. Fries *et al.* have suggested that NSAIDs may have a toxicity equal to SAARDs and this should be another argument for early use of slow acting drugs[13].

ADVERSE REACTIONS TO NSAIDs	
Gastrointestinal	Indigestion Gastroesophageal reflux Erosions Peptic ulcer Gastrointestinal hemorrhage and perforation Small and large bowel ulceration
Hepatic	Transaminitis Hepatocellular Cholestasis
Renal	Transient rise in serum creatinine Hyponatremia Acute renal failure Interstitial nephritis Hyperkalemia Analgesic nephropathy
Hematologic	Thrombocytopenia Neutropenia Red cell aplasia Hemolytic anemia
Cutaneous	Photosensitivity Erythema multiforme Urticaria Toxic epidermal necrolysis
Respiratory	Bronchospasm Pneumonitis
Central nervous system	Headache Dizziness Personality change Aseptic meningitis

Fig. 5.9 Adverse reactions to NSAIDs.

GASTROINTESTINAL

Gastrointestinal reactions to NSAIDs include gastric erosions, peptic ulcer formation and perforation, upper and lower gastrointestinal hemorrhage, and inflammation and changes in permeability of the small and large bowel. With the increased prescribing of NSAIDs, there has been a rapid rise in the incidence of reported deaths from gastrointestinal hemorrhage and perforation. The true relationship between NSAID use and serious gastrointestinal complications is hard to estimate. The absolute risk of serious gastrointestinal adverse effects varies from approximately two cases per 10,000 person months of prescription to an increased risk of hospitalization of over seven times in patients with RA[14]. These data suggest that the syndrome of NSAID-associated gastropathy might be responsible for over 2500 deaths per annum in patients with RA[15]. Particular risk factors for the development of NSAID-associated peptic ulceration in RA are age (>65 years), a past history of peptic ulceration, concomitant corticosteroid ingestion and multiple organ dysfunction.

All NSAIDs have the ability to suppress prostaglandin production and are likely to share the potential for inducing gastrointestinal hemorrhage. There is now emerging data to support a differential effect of NSAIDs on gastric mucosa. Studies have shown a clear relationship between bleeding peptic ulcer and dose of NSAID, but also a suggestion that NSAIDs such as ibuprofen and diclofenac may be less likely to cause peptic ulceration than others[17]. One of the problems with assessing the incidence of side effects is the fact that, in patients with RA, up to 50% of peptic ulcers are asymptomatic.

NSAID-induced ulcers should be treated like any other gastric lesion. If possible, the NSAID should be ceased, but if that cannot be done, continued use is only likely to slow healing of the ulcers. The ulcers may be treated with H_2-receptor antagonists, proton pump inhibitors such as omeprazole or prostaglandin analogues such as misoprostol[18,19]. Risk factors for NSAID-associated peptic ulcer complications include age over 65, prior ulcer disease, high dose and multiple NSAIDs, concurrent steroid therapy and duration of therapy. Smoking, alcohol and infection with *Helicobactor pylori* may also play a role. Prophylaxis with histamine receptor antagonists, prostaglandin analogs and proton pump inhibitors reduces ulcer formation and other gastrointestinal complications as well[19]. If a patient with peptic ulceration is known to be infected with *H. pylori*, this should be treated although there is no data to support widespread elimination of *H. pylori* at this time. In summary, peptic ulceration should be treated and NSAIDs withdrawn if possible. Prophylaxis with a proton pump inhibitor or misoprostol should be offered to those at-risk patients who genuinely require long term NSAIDs.

RENAL

Since prostaglandins modulate many of the physiologic activities of the kidney, including renal blood flow and glomerular filtration, renin release, tubular ion transport and water exchange, it is not surprising that NSAIDs commonly produce renal toxicity[20]. These prostaglandin-driven renal functions are of particular importance in patients with underlying renal disease, and great care must be taken in prescribing NSAIDs to people with even mild renal dysfunction. NSAIDs can cause reversible impairment of glomerular function, edema, interstitial nephritis and papillary necrosis, acute renal failure and hyperkalemia.

Although there is a strong link between analgesic intake and renal disease, this involves compound analgesic agents rather than NSAIDs. It is quite common to see a transient rise in the serum creatinine level within two weeks of commencing an NSAID, but this returns to normal, despite continuation of the drug. The particular risk factors for NSAID-induced renal disease are a past history of renal disease, volume depletion in association with diuretic therapy or hypoalbuminemia, and hepatic disease.

It has been suggested that sulindac might have a lesser effect on renal function, but it is clear that no NSAID can be prescribed with absolute safety with respect to renal adverse effects. Sodium retention, edema and hypertension are often precipitated by NSAIDs, and NSAIDs might also interfere with the action of a number of antihypertensive and diuretic medications. NSAIDs interfere with blood pressure control on an individual basis, and patients commenced on these drugs should have their blood pressure monitored at regular intervals [21,22].

HEPATIC

A transient rise in liver enzyme levels is commonly seen with NSAIDs, but this usually settles despite continuing therapy. Occasionally, significant hepatitis may occur, and this is seen particularly with aspirin in association with acute viral illnesses (Reye's syndrome). Cholestasis is associated with sulindac and diclofenac therapy but is usually mild [23].

HEMATOLOGIC

A broad spectrum of hematologic adverse reactions to NSAIDs has been described, including anemia, thrombocytopenia, neutropenia and aplastic anemia. Aplastic anemia has a high mortality but is rarely associated with NSAIDs, except with phenylbutazone or oxyphenbutazone. Thrombocytopenia has been associated with most NSAIDs, while all NSAIDs will interfere with platelet aggregation. With aspirin this effect on platelet function is irreversible and seen throughout the life of the platelet, but with other NSAIDs the effect is most often seen while the drug is present in the bloodstream in significant quantities. From a practical point of view, this means platelet function will return to normal approximately three half-lives after an NSAID is ceased, and approximately four days after aspirin is ceased.

DERMATOLOGIC

Most dermatologic side effects are relatively mild and settle quickly once the drug is ceased, but fatal reactions, including erythema multiforme, have been described with most NSAIDs. Dermatologic side effects seem to be most commonly associated with those NSAIDs which have long half-lives.

RESPIRATORY

Asthma is most common with salicylate, but may be precipitated or exacerbated by NSAIDs. Symptoms may be mild or severe, and fatal attacks of bronchospasm have been precipitated by a single dose of NSAID. If aspirin-sensitive asthmatic patients require an NSAID, then a low dose should be administered in a controlled environment equipped with facilities to reverse bronchospasm. Pulmonary alveolitis has also recently been reported with NSAID therapy and, although rare, should be considered when an illness suggestive of pulmonary infecton, but failing to respond to antibiotic therapy, develops in a patient on an NSAID.

ADVERSE REACTIONS IN THE CENTRAL NERVOUS SYSTEM

Side effects in the CNS are probably more common with NSAID therapy than is normally appreciated. Headaches might occur with indomethacin, and an aseptic, meningitis-like picture has been described with ibuprofen in systemic lupus erythematosus. Many patients report drowsiness and alteration in mood. Aspirin has effects on the electroencephalogram and it might be that some of the nonulcer dyspepsia (nausea) commonly seen in association with NSAIDs has its basis in the CNS rather than the gastrointestinal tract. Tinnitus is commonly seen in patients on salicylate therapy and can be used as a method of monitoring treatment. This particular side effect has recently been shown to be dose-related.

DRUG INTERACTIONS

Since NSAIDs are commonly taken by the elderly, who generally have many diseases, the potential for drug interaction is enormous. The common interactions of NSAIDs are shown in Figures 5.10 and 5.11.

NSAIDs AFFECTING OTHER DRUGS

Drug affected NSAID implicated	**Effect**	**Approach to management**
Oral anticoagulants Phenylbutazone, Oxyphenbutazone, Azapropazone	Inhibition of metabolism of S-warfarin, increasing anticoagulant effect.	Avoid NSAIDs if possible. Careful monitoring where unavoidable.
Lithium Probably all NSAIDs	Inhibition of renal excretion of lithium, increasing lithium serum concentrations and increasing risk of toxicity.	Use sulindac or aspirin if NSAID unavoidable. Careful monitoring of lithium concentration and appropriate dose reduction.
Oral hypoglycemic agents Phenylbutazone, Oxyphenbutazone, Azapropazone	Inhibition of metabolism of sulfonylurea drugs, prolonging half-life and increasing risk of hypoglycemia.	Avoid this group of NSAIDs if possible; if not, monitor blood sugar closely.
Phenytoin Phenylbutazone, Oxyphenbutazone	Inhibition of metabolism of phenytoin,increasing plasma concentration and risk of toxicity.	Avoid this group of NSAIDs if possible; if not, intensify therapeutic drug monitoring.
Other NSAIDs	Displacement of phenytoin from plasma protein, reducing total concentrations for the same unbound (active) concentration.	Careful interpretation of phenytoin total concentration; measurement of unbound concentration may be helpful.
Methotrexate Probably all NSAIDs	Reduced clearance of methotrexate (mechanism unclear) increasing plasma concentration and risk of severe toxicity.	This is only relevant to high dose methotrexate used in cancer chemotherapy.
Sodium valproate Aspirin	Inhibition of valproate metabolism increasing plasma concentration.	Avoid aspirin; close monitoring of plasma concentration if other NSAID used.
Digoxin All NSAIDs	Potential reduction in renal function (particularly in very young and very old) reducing digoxin clearance and increasing plasma concentration and risk of toxicity (no interaction if renal function normal).	Avoid NSAIDs if possible; if not, frequent checks of digoxin plasma concentration and plasma creatinine.
Aminoglycosides All NSAIDs	Reduction in renal function in susceptible individuals, reducing aminoglycoside clearance and increasing plasma concentration.	Close plasma concentration monitoring and dose adjustment.
Antihypertensive agents β-blockers, diuretics, ACE inhibitors, vasodilators Indomethacin, Other NSAIDs	Reduction in hypotensive effect, probably related to inhibition of renal prostaglandin synthesis (producing salt and water retention) and vascular prostaglandin synthesis (producing increased vasoconstriction).	Avoid all NSAIDs in treated hypertensive patients if possible; if not monitor carefully. May need additional antihypertensive therapy.
Diuretics Indomethacin, other NSAIDs	Reduction in natriuretic and diuretic effects; may exacerbate congestive cardiac failure.	Avoid NSAIDs in patients with cardiac failure; monitor clinical signs of fluid retention.
Anticoagulants All NSAIDs	Gastrointestinal tract mucosal damage, together with inhibition of platelet aggregation, increasing risk of GI bleeding in patients on anticoagulants.	Avoid all NSAIDs if possible.
Hypoglycemic agents Salicylate (high dose)	Potentiation of hypoglycemic effects (mechanism unknown).	Monitor blood sugar level.

Fig. 5.10 Interactions between NSAIDs and other drugs: NSAIDs affecting other drugs.

DRUGS AFFECTING NSAIDS		
Drug implicated NSAID affected	**Effect**	**Approach to management**
Antacids Indomethacin ? other NSAIDs	Variable effects of different preparations: aluminum-containing antacids reduce rate and extent of absorption of indomethacin sodium bicarbonate increases rate and extent of absorption of indomethacin.	No action required unless marked reduction in absorption results in poor response to NSAID; dose may need to be increased in this case. Not as important with those NSAIDs that have enteric coating or slow release profiles.
Probenecid Probably all NSAIDs	Reduction in metabolism and renal clearance of NSAIDs and acyl glucuronide metabolites which are hydrolyzed back to parent drug.	May be used therapeutically to increase the response to a given dose of NSAID.
Cholestyramine Naproxen and probably other NSAIDs	Anion exchange resin binds NSAIDs in gut reducing rate (? and extent) of absorption.	Separate dosing times by 4h; may need bigger than expected dose of NSAID.
Metoclopramide NSAIDs Aspirin	Increased rate and extent of absorption of aspirin in patients with migraine.	May be used therapeutically.

Fig. 5.11 Interactions between NSAIDs and other drugs: drugs affecting NSAIDs.

Interactions can be pharmacokinetic or pharmacodynamic, as described by Tonkin and Wing [24]. The most important potential interactions occur between NSAIDs and diuretic and hypotensive agents, anticonvulsants, lithium and anticoagulants. The potential interaction with methotrexate and NSAIDs is not seen with the low doses of methotrexate prescribed for RA or seronegative arthropathies. With care, most significant interactions can be avoided.

PRACTICAL PRESCRIBING

Patients with rheumatic disease continue to show variability in their response to NSAIDs. The therapeutic challenge in each case is to find the right NSAID in terms of providing pain relief without significant adverse reactons. The vast majority of patients will respond to an NSAID within 7–10 days of commencing therapy, and if this does not occur the NSAID should be ceased and another one commenced. To date there is no evidence that combinations of NSAIDs are more efficacious than adequate doses of single agents. Because NSAIDs are primarily anti-inflammatory, they should be reserved for those patients who do have evidence of inflammation and not used long-term in those with non-inflammatory degenerative disease. The dose of NSAID should be kept to a minimum, possibly with supplementation of analgesics such as paracetamol (acetaminophen). Patients on NSAIDs should be continually assessed for the development of adverse drug reactions and to establish whether or not they are continuing to respond to the NSAIDs. When NSAIDs are ceased, this should be done over a period of a few days to prevent any rebound in pain and inflammation.

REFERENCES

1. Forrest M, Brooks PM. Mechanism of action of nonsteroidal anti-inflammatory drugs. Baillière's Clin Rheumatol. 1985;2:275–94.
2. Preston SJ, Arnold MH, Beller EM, Brooks PM, Buchanan WW. Comparative analgesic and anti-inflammatory properties of sodium salicylate and acetyl salicylic acid (aspirin) in rheumatoid arthritis. Br J Clin Pharmacol. 1989;27:607–11.
3. Brooks PM, Day RO. Non-steroidal anti-inflammatory drugs differences and similarities. N Engl J Med. 1991;324:1716–25.
4. Frölich JC. Prostaglandin endoperoxide synthetase isoenzymes: The clinical relevance of selective inhibition. Ann Rheum Dis. 1995;54:942–3.
5. Richardson C, Emery P. New cyclooxygenase and cytokine inhibitors. Baillière's Clin Rheumatol. 1995;9:731–58.
6. Day RO, Graham GG, Williams KM. Pharmacokinetics of non-steroidal anti-inflammatory drugs. Baillière's Clin Rheumatol. 1988;2:363–93.
7. Graham GG. Pharmacokinetics and metabolism of non-steroidal anti-inflammatory drugs. Med J Aust. 1987;147:597–602.
8 Verbeek RK. Pathophysiologic factors affecting the pharmacokinetics of non-steroidal anti-inflammatory drugs. J Rheumatol. 1988;15:44–57.
9. Huskisson EC, Woolf PC, Baume HW, Scott J, Franklyn S. Four new anti-inflammatory drugs – responses and variations. Br Med J. 1974;1:1084–9.
10. Committee on Safety of Medicines Update. Non-steroidal and anti-inflammatory drugs and serious gastrointestinal adverse reactions. Br Med J. 1986;292:614.
11. Brooks PM. Side effects of non-steroidal anti-inflammatory drugs. Med J Aust. 1988;148:248–81.
12. O'Brien WM, Bagby GF. Rare adverse reactions to non-steroidal anti-inflammatory drugs. J Rheumatol. 1985;12:13–20, 347–83, 562–7, 785–90.
13. Fries JF, Williams CA, Ramey DR, Bloch DA. The relative toxicity of alternative therapies for rheumatoid arthritis: Implications for the therapeutic progression. Semin Arthritis Rheum. 1993;23(Suppl 1):68–73.
14. Langman MJS. Epidemiological evidence on the association between peptic ulceration and anti-inflammatory drugs use. Gastroenterology. 1989;96:640–6.
15. Fries JF, Miller SR, Spitz PW. Towards an epidemiology of gastropathy associated with non-steroidal anti-inflammatory drug use. Gastroenterology. 1989;96:647–55.
16. Langman MJS, Weil J, *et al.* Risks of bleeding peptic ulcer associated with individual non-steroidal anti-inflammatory drugs. Lancet 1994;343:1075–8.
17. Rodriguez LAG, Jick H. Risk of upper gastrointestinal bleeding and perforation associated with individual non-steroidal anti-inflammatory drugs. Lancet. 1994;343:769–72.
18. Lichtenstein DR, Syngal S, Wolfe MM. Non-steroidal anti-inflammatory drugs and the gastrointestinal tract. Arthritis Rheum. 1995;1:5–18.
19. Silverstein FE, Geis GS, Struthers BJ and the Mucosa Study Group. NSAIDs and gastrointestinal injury: Clinical outcome. The Mucosa Trial. Gastroenterol. 1994;106:A180.
20. Schlondorff D. Renal complications of non-steroidal anti-inflammatory drugs. Kidney Int. 1993;44:643–53.
21. Pope JE, Anderson JJ, Felson DT. A meta analysis of the effects of non-steroidal anti-inflammatory drugs on blood pressure. Arch Intern Med. 1993;153:477–84.
22. Simon LS. Actions and toxicity of non-steroidal anti-inflammatory drugs. Curr Opin Rheum. 1995;7:159–66.
23. Carson JL, Strom BL, Duff A, Gupta A, Das K. Safety of non-steroidal anti-inflammatory drugs with respect to acute liver disease. Arch Intern Med. 1993;153:1331–6.
24. Tonkin AL, Wing LMH. Interactions of non-steroidal anti-inflammatory drugs. Baillière's Clin Rheumatol. 1988;2:455–83.

6

SYSTEMIC CORTICOSTEROIDS IN RHEUMATOLOGY

John R Kirwan

Definition

- Corticosteroids act through specific cytoplasmic receptors and control of gene transcription.
- Corticosteroid treatment increases lipocortin production and induces changes in lymphocyte function, Fc receptor suppression and downregulation of many proinflammatory enzymes produced by macrophages.
- Low dose oral corticosteroids only transiently reduce symptoms of inflammation in rheumatoid arthritis but inhibit bony erosion in the longer term.
- In polymyalgia rheumatica the main pitfalls are the use of too high an initial dose of corticosteroid and too rapid a reduction in treatment thereafter.
- The potential adverse effects of corticosteroids require careful consideration before initiating high dose or long-term therapy.

MECHANISM OF ACTION

STRUCTURE

The principal corticosteroid hormone of the human adrenal cortex is cortisol (hydrocortisone), derived from hydroxylation of cortisone (Fig. 6.1). The 11β and 17α hydroxyl groups are important for corticosteroid activity and prednisone, a synthetic analog of cortisone, is also hydroxylated before becoming biologically active. The additional double bond in ring A of the resultant prednisolone enhances corticosteroid activity without increasing mineralocorticoid activity, an effect which is increased by 6α methylation (to produce methylprednisolone) or 9α fluorination (triamcinolone) or both (dexamethasone)[1].

PLASMA LEVELS

Plasma cortisol is normally maintained at a concentration of 5–25μg/ml by the hypothalamic–pituitary–adrenal feedback control mechanism. Most (80%) is bound to the α-globulin transcortin and some (10%) to albumin[2]. The remaining 10% provides biological activity. As the synthetic analogs do not compete for transcortin binding sites, and are less extensively bound to plasma albumin, they are able to diffuse into tissues more completely. The duration of anti-inflammatory action of cortisol and its analogs given orally is similar to the duration of suppression of the hypothalamic–pituitary–adrenal axis, suggesting that the molecular binding sites used by the hypothalamic sensory mechanism are the same as those needed for attachment to receptors in peripheral tissues.

CORTICOSTEROID RECEPTORS

Free cortisol diffuses into individual cells where specific receptor proteins are found in the cytoplasm of corticosteroid-responsive tissues (Fig. 6.2). The human corticosteroid receptor is a 95kDa phosphorylated protein with corticosteroid-binding, deoxyribonucleic acid (DNA)-binding

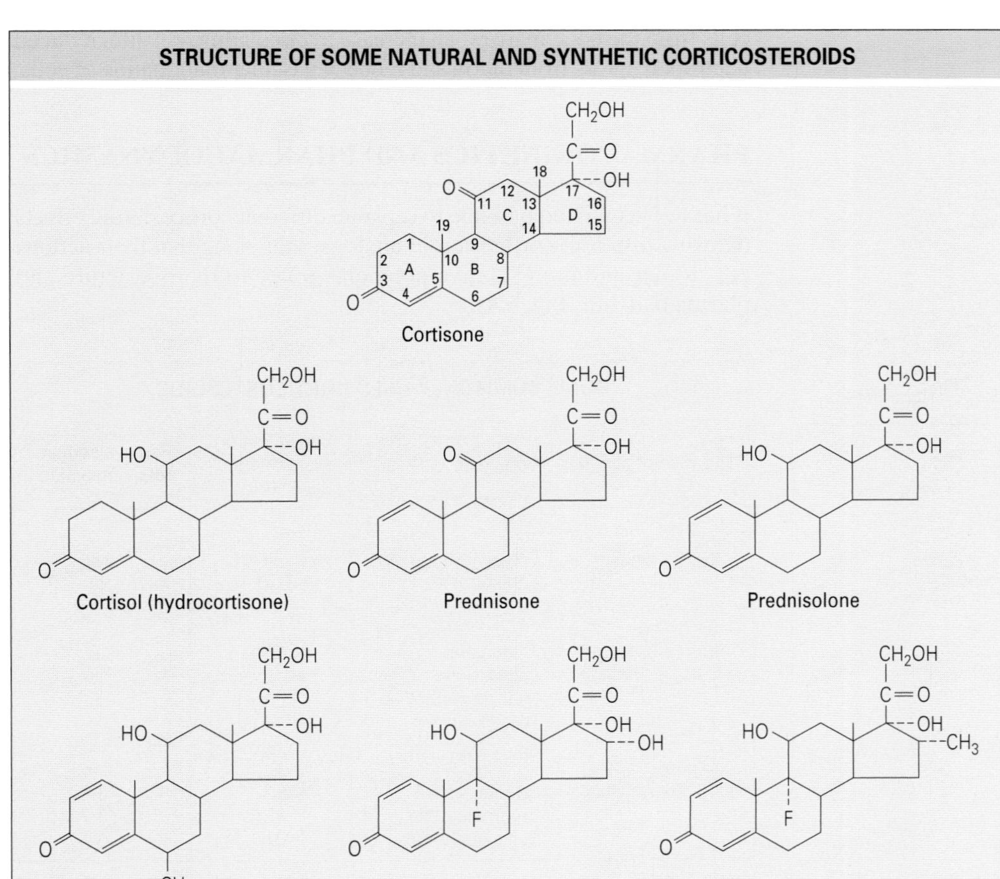

Fig. 6.1 Structure of some natural and synthetic corticosteroids.

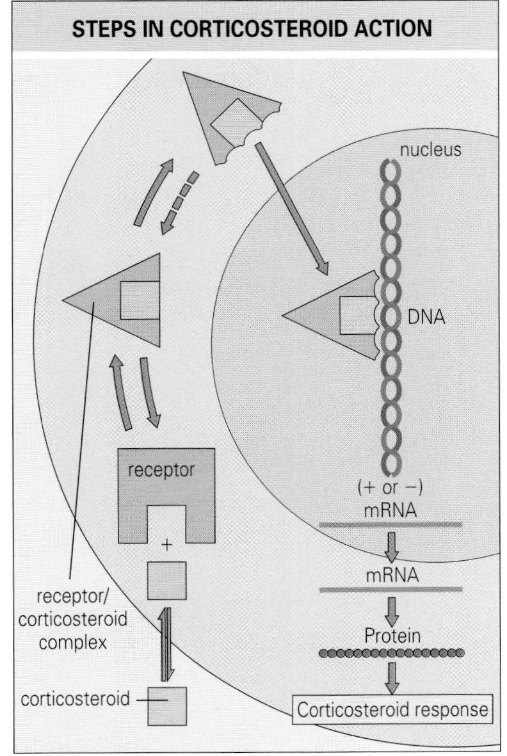

Fig. 6.2 Steps in corticosteroid action. Unbound corticosteroid diffuses across the cell membrane and binds to a specific cytoplasmic receptor. The corticosteroid–receptor complex undergoes a conformational change and moves into the nucleus attaching to chromosomal DNA, thereby increasing (or reducing) the synthesis of corresponding messenger RNA.

and strongly antigenic regions, each of roughly equal size. The receptor gene has now been cloned and sequenced, confirming and extending the general description of this protein. The corticosteroid receptor belongs to a superfamily of regulatory proteins that include receptors for thyroid hormones and the vitamin A-related metabolite, retinoic acid[3].

The corticosteroid and receptor form a complex that undergoes a conformational change, leaves the cytoplasm and moves to the nucleus, where it binds reversibly to specific sites on chromatin. This results in the production of messenger ribonucleic acid (mRNA), which codes for enzymes or other proteins that produce the hormonal effects. Most cellular responses can be detected within 2 hours of corticosteroid exposure and some within 10 minutes[2]. In general, corticosteroid response is not observed if RNA synthesis is inhibited. In addition, the concentration of a specific corticosteroid required for optimal response is lower when it has a higher affinity for the corticosteroid receptor.

ACTION THROUGH PROTEIN SYNTHESIS

Although reduced protein synthesis has been recognized in some tissues (e.g. lymphoid cells, muscle, bone and skin), the main corticosteroid effect is through increased rates of synthesis of certain proteins, especially of lipocortin. The anti-inflammatory effect of lipocortin is mediated through its inhibition of the enzyme phospholipase A_2 which converts membrane-bound phospholipids into arachidonic acid, with the subsequent intracellular production of prostaglandins, leukotrienes and oxygen radicals (Fig. 6.3)[4]. These products leave the cell and are themselves able to stimulate the release of phospholipase A_2 from adjacent cells. By stimulating lipocortin production, corticosteroids inhibit proinflammatory cytokine production, including that of interleukin-1 (IL-1), IL-2, the IL-2 receptor, interferon-α (IFN-α) [5], tumor necrosis factor (TNF)[6] and, perhaps, various colony stimulating factors (CSFs) such as IL-3 [5].

In addition, corticosteroids even in very low concentrations inhibit the synthesis of a variety of proinflammatory enzymes, including the macrophage products collagenase, elastase and plasminogen activator[7]. Corticosteroids also stimulate the production of a protein that controls the cyclooxygenase-2-gene (activated in inflammatory cells).

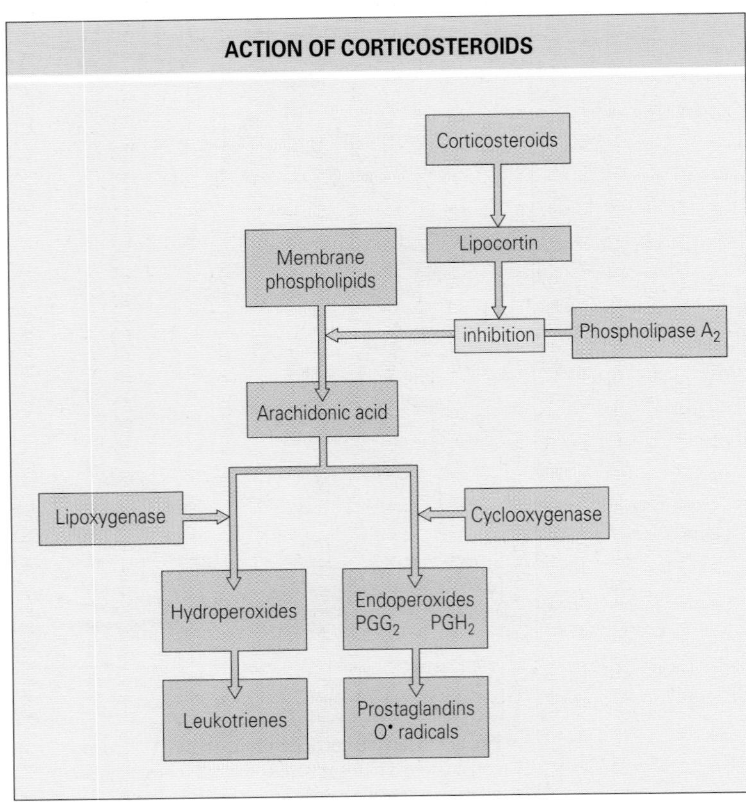

Fig. 6.3 Corticosteroids induce the synthesis of lipocorti), which inhibits the enzyme phospholipase A_2. Arachidonic acid release from membrane phospholipids is blocked and the production of proinflammatory substances via cyclooxygenase and lipoxygenase is reduced.

LYMPHOCYTE FUNCTION

Although corticosteroids inhibit the expression of murine MHC class II antigens and may inhibit antigen presentation by human monocytes, there seems to be no relation in man between the reduction in class II expression and suppression of antigen presentation[8]. Lymphocyte proliferation *in vitro*, and delayed-type hypersensitivity *in vivo*, are inhibited by corticosteroids although information about the differential effects of corticosteroids on particular T-cell subsets is scarce.

Information about corticosteroid effects on B lymphocytes and antibody production in man is contradictory. A 5-day course of methylprednisolone (96mg/day) lowered serum immunoglobulin levels by 20%[9] but in more chronic experiments specific antibody production was not reduced in corticosteroid-treated patients[10]. Also, *in vitro* immunoglobulin production by cells taken from patients on high-dose corticosteroids is decreased although B cells from normal subjects given a bolus of corticosteroids actually produce more immunoglobulins[11].

Fc RECEPTOR SUPPRESSION

Many cells, including red blood cells (RBC), carry a surface receptor for the Fc portion of immunoglobulin – the Fc receptor (FcR). Corticosteroids inhibit FcR expression[12] which may explain the prompt improvement seen when patients with autoimmune hemolytic anemia or autoimmune thrombocytopenia are given corticosteroids. By inhibiting FcR (and C3 receptors) in the mononuclear–phagocyte system (MPS) (reticuloendothelial system), the clearance of antibody-coated RBCs and platelets is reduced.

CHANGES IN WHITE CELL TRAFFIC

Large intravenous (i.v.) doses of corticosteroids given to normal human volunteers increase the numbers of circulating neutrophils but decrease peripheral lymphocytes, eosinophils and monocytes[13]. These changes reach their maximum in 4–6 hours and generally return to normal by 24 hours. Most of these effects reflect changes in patterns of cell traffic rather than changes in bone marrow function. Neutrophilia, for example, results from a combination of increased release of immature cells from the bone marrow, an increase in circulating half-life, reduced neutrophil egress from blood and reduced vascular margination of cells.

PHARMACOKINETICS AND PHARMACODYNAMICS

It has not yet proved possible to separate different corticosteroid effects by using different corticosteroid analogs, indicating that their actions are similar and their relative potencies relate to their structure and plasma half-life (Fig. 6.4).

SOME COMMONLY USED CORTICOSTEROIDS

Duration of action	Corticosteroid	Equivalent oral or intravenous doses (mg)	Relative sodium-retaining action
Short ($t_{1/2}$ 8–12 hours)	Cortisone	25	0.8
	Cortisol	20	1
Intermediate ($t_{1/2}$ 12–36 hours)	Prednisone	5	0.8
	Prednisolone	5	0.8
	Methylprednisolone	4	0.5
	Triamcinolone	4	0
Long ($t_{1/2}$ 36–72 hours)	Paramethasone	2	0
	Dexamethasone	0.75	0
	Betamethasone	0.60	0

Fig. 6.4 Some commonly used corticosteroids.

Prednisolone is rapidly absorbed from the gastrointestinal tract and is reversibly bound to plasma proteins. At low or normal plasma concentrations, binding is largely to globulins, but at higher concentrations there is an increase in albumin-bound and free corticosteroid. In hypoalbuminemic patients, high dosage leads to high levels of free corticosteroid and increased side effects. Prednisolone is rapidly metabolized in the liver, conjugated and excreted in the urine. It disappears from the blood within 1.5–3 hours, having a half-life of about 1 hour[14]. However, its action at the tissue level lasts considerably longer.

Drug interactions with corticosteroids may occur. Enhancement of the rate of metabolism of some corticosteroids has been noted with concurrent administration of phenobarbital, phenytoin and rifampicin, probably by inducing hepatic microsomal drug-metabolizing enzymes[15]. Giving aspirin and corticosteroids concurrently decreases salicylate levels owing to an increased rate of salicylate metabolism. A reduction in corticosteroid dosage in such patients may result in increased plasma salicylate levels with symptoms of salicylate overdosage[16]. Corticosteroids may make control of diabetes mellitus with insulin or oral hypoglycemic drugs more difficult and potassium loss may be increased by giving corticosteroids and thiazides or related diuretics concurrently.

EFFICACY

CORTICOSTEROIDS IN RHEUMATOID ARTHRITIS

Corticosteroids are the only drugs which reliably, effectively and rapidly suppress synovitis in rheumatoid arthritis (RA). This effect was demonstrated long before their mechanism of action was investigated and cannot be fully explained by the factors described earlier. In a recent review of the main clinical trials of corticosteroids in RA it was concluded[17] that in both short- and long-term studies corticosteroids are effective anti-inflammatory agents, significantly better than placebo in the relief of pain and stiffness, and superior to nonsteroidal anti-inflammatory drugs (NSAIDs). However, benefits are not sustained unless increasingly high doses are employed, so that side effects and adrenal suppression preclude their long-term use in RA except in specific circumstances.

In early studies there was a suggestion that corticosteroids may be able to reduce the rate of radiologic progression[18]. Uncontrolled long term follow-up of some of these patients appeared to show the inhibition of continued erosion development over a 4 year treatment period[19]. A randomized, placebo-controlled trial of the addition of a fixed daily dose of 7.5mg prednisolone to existing standard treatment has now been conducted in 128 patients with active disease of less than 2 years duration[20]. Radiologic progression was assessed by changes in the Larsen score, which were halved in those patients taking prednisolone.

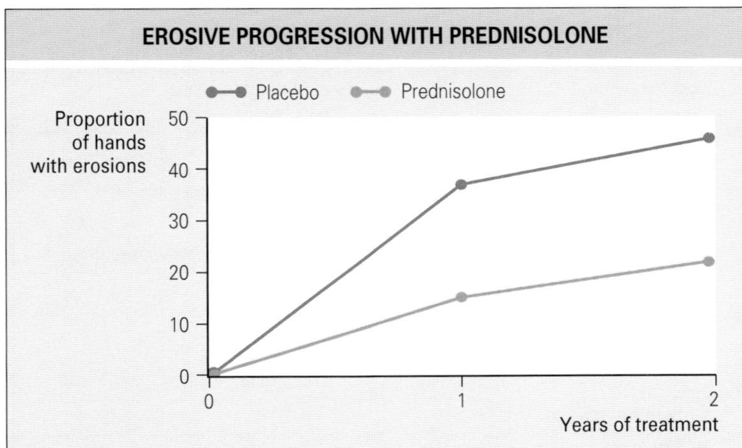

Fig. 6.5 Development of erosions in hands which had no erosions at the start of a trial of 7.5mg prednisolone daily, compared to placebo, in patients with rheumatoid arthritis for less than 2 years.

Of hands in both groups, 69% did not have erosions at the start of the study. Of these 46% of placebo treated hands had developed erosions by 2 years, while only 22% of prednisolone treated had done so (Fig. 6.5). Most patients received NSAIDs and specific antirheumatoid drugs in addition to their study medication, and clinical symptoms improved in both groups. Symptoms improved more rapidly in the prednisolone group, but this added benefit of corticosteroid treatment lasted only 6–9 months. There was no difference between the groups in changes in the acute phase response (although measurements were not made during the first 3 months of treatment). No significant short-term corticosteroid-related adverse effects were reported. In view of these findings, treatment can be advocated for two years in patients early in the disease and probably for patients who have had arthritis for up to 4 years (Fig. 6.6). Nonerosive patients who have had the diagnosis for more than 2 years are unlikely to ever develop erosions and therefore do not require prednisolone therapy. Patients will experience a 'bonus' of short-term symptomatic control, but should be warned that this will eventually subside even though the corticosteroids will continue to protect against joint destruction at least for the 2-year period. Longer periods of treatment would raise the specter of adverse events such as osteoporosis and atherosclerosis (see later).

PULSED CORTICOSTEROIDS

Pulse therapy involves the i.v. infusion of a large dose of corticosteroid (usually 1g of methylprednisolone) over a short time – perhaps 30 minutes. A variety of regimens are used currently, but most entail a course of three pulses on alternate days, followed by a resting phase of around 6 weeks. This form of treatment was initiated in renal transplant recipients, but gradually spread to the treatment of other renal disorders, most notably lupus nephritis. The observation was made in such patients that synovial inflammation responded rapidly, and for prolonged periods, with i.v. therapy. Following anecdotal reports of benefit in RA, controlled studies were performed through the 1980s which suggested beneficial effects lasting 6–12 weeks from this regimen with relatively few side effects[21]. These trials are small, however, and therefore limited in statistical power.

Methylprednisolone has been used in a number of studies to produce an early initial response in RA patients commencing second-line agents, thus effectively bridging the gap between initiation and response with these agents. A recent review[22] of the use of pulsed methylprednisolone stresses the impressive favorable risk:benefit ratio of this therapy with few or minor adverse effects. Most of the serious adverse effects – cardiovascular collapse, myocardial infarction, severe infection—have occurred in patients with compromised cardiovascular or immune systems as a result of their disease, or due to concomitant drug treatment. The minimal effective dose of methylprednisolone is uncertain at present. It has been reported that doses as low as 320mg may be as effective as 1g[23] although others[24] have concluded that using only 500mg results in substantial loss of efficacy. If equivalent oral doses are as effective as i.v. treatment[25], this will allow pulsed treatment to become an outpatient procedure with reduced costs and less patient discomfort, although Choy *et al.*[26] found that intramuscular methylprednisolone was superior to equivalent oral doses in their study of corticosteroids and gold therapy.

TREATMENT STRATEGIES FOR LOW-DOSE PREDNISOLONE

Disease duration	Patients with erosions	Patients without erosions
Less than 2 years	Treatment effective	Treatment effective
2–5 years	Treatment likely to be effective	Treatment unnecessary
Over 5 years	Treatment not tested	Treatment unnecessary

Fig 6.6 Efficiacy of low-dose prednisolone therapy for the prevention or reduction of progressive joint destruction in rheumatoid arthritis.

CORTICOSTEROIDS IN VASCULITIS

In experimental models of vasculitis, such as serum sickness, circulating immune complexes activate platelets, deposit in blood vessel walls fixing complement and induce chemotaxis and phagocytosis by polymorphonuclear leukocytes with the release of enzymes that cause tissue damage. Aggregates of activated platelets form a nidus for blood coagulation and release thromboxane, which itself propagates further platelet activation, vasoconstriction and thrombus formation. In some vasculitides, such as Kawasaki's syndrome and Takayasu's disease, there is evidence of such a coagulopathy with hyperfibrinogenemia and hypofibrinolytic activity, which may result in luminal occlusion[27]. Corticosteroids are widely used to treat systemic vasculitis in RA, systemic lupus erythematosus (SLE) and other autoimmune diseases and are clearly powerful inhibitors of the inflammatory processes. However, corticosteroids may not inhibit subsequent organization of the platelet and fibrin thrombus and induction of endothelial cell and smooth muscle cell proliferation. Thus, in spite of clinical and laboratory improvement after corticosteroid treatment, patients may go on to develop evidence of progressive ischemia, such as blue digits. Conn *et al.*[27] suggest that where there is no clinical evidence of active inflammation indicated by fever, myalgia, arthralgias or active skin lesions, and no laboratory evidence of inflammation such as elevation of the erythrocyte sedimentation rate (ESR), a more plausible management strategy would be the use of vasodilators and inhibitors of platelet activation. They postulate that corticosteroids fail to control the generation of platelet-derived thromboxane (possibly because platelets do not possess a nucleus and cannot form lipocortin), but it may be that this deficiency is often offset by the concomitant, widespread use of (platelet suppressing) NSAIDs.

CORTICOSTEROIDS IN POLYMALGIA RHEUMATICA AND TEMPORAL ARTERITIS

The signs and symptoms of polymyalgia rheumatica (PMR) and temporal arteritis (TA) overlap and can often be confused, but both are treated with corticosteroids. No controlled trials have been conducted which allow an adequate definition of the best treatment regimen, but three cohorts of patients and their use of corticosteroids have been reported in the literature[28–30]. Although there are some differences, the overall pattern suggests the need to treat PMR initially with about 15mg prednisolone daily, reducing slowly over 18–24 months. About twice that dose of corticosteroids will be required to treat coexisting or separate TA and for perhaps 6 months longer. All series reported a few complications, including some patients with PMR who become more definite cases of TA while on treatment. The main pitfalls seem to be the use of too high a dose of corticosteroids initially, with a too rapid reduction in treatment thereafter[31].

VARIABILITY OF RESPONSE

BIOAVAILABILITY

Enteric coated (EC) prednisolone is often prescribed on the assumption that it reduces gastrointestinal adverse reactions, although there is no clear documentation of this in the literature There are, however, concerns that bioavailability may be variable and that dissolution of the plant extract coating may be affected by factors such as food intake and gastrointestinal motility. Moreover, absorption of enteric coated preparations may be unreliable[32].

ANTILIPOCORTIN ANTIBODIES

Hirata[33] observed that a high proportion of patients with chronic rheumatic diseases had autoantibodies to lipocortin whereas disease-free people did not. Levels were particularly high in patients with SLE and RA. This has led to the concept that the presence of these autoantibodies may contribute to the etiology of these diseases by removing 'protective' proteins that regulate eicosanoid generation.

Using recombinant human lipocortin-1 as a target, Podgorski *et al.*[34] devised an assay for measuring antilipocortin autoantibodies. They confirmed the presence of both IgG and IgM antilipocortin autoantibodies in patients with SLE and RA. They observed that in patients with SLE the antibodies were present whether or not the patient had already received any corticosteroid therapy, but in the group with RA, significantly raised titers were only seen in patients who had received oral corticosteroid therapy. In both groups, high titers of autoantibodies correlated strongly with the clinical phenomenon of corticosteroid 'resistance'. This was not seen with other inflammatory diseases for both those who were receiving corticosteroids or those who were 'corticosteroid resistant'.

The idea that administration of corticosteroids may stimulate the formation of autoantibodies to lipocortin in certain susceptible groups, and possibly corticosteroid resistance, may have important implications for corticosteroid therapy.

ADVERSE DRUG REACTIONS

GENERAL

The clinical complications which may occur during the use of corticosteroid therapy are protean (Fig. 6.7) and have been further elaborated in recent observational studies[35]. Corticosteroids induce alterations of fat distribution that account for the classic Cushingoid appearance. These include truncal obesity, 'buffalo hump' and moon faces, which occur in 13% of patients who receive corticosteroids for 2 months and almost half of patients treated for 5 years or more. Other localized fat deposits may be found in the mediastinum and temporal fat pads. Obesity and Cushingoid features often resolve rapidly when patients are switched to alternate-day therapy.

Exogenous corticosteroids also influence glucose, protein and electrolyte metabolism, and hepatic enzyme function resulting in a tendency towards hyperglycemia and insulin resistance, protein catabolism in muscle and bone, sodium retention and potassium loss.

INFECTIONS

Corticosteroid therapy predisposes to a wide range of infections. Among bacterial agents, staphylococcal, Gram-negative, tuberculous and *Listeria* infections appear most frequently associated. Certain viral, fungal and bacterial infections also occur often.

ADVERSE EFFECTS OF SYSTEMIC CORTICOSTEROID THERAPY	
Metabolic	obesity glucose/protein metabolism electrolyte imbalance enzyme induction
Predisposition to infection	
Musculoskeletal	myopathy osteoporosis osteonecrosis tendon rupture corticosteroid withdrawal syndrome
Gastrointestinal	peptic ulcer disease pancreatitis
Ophthalmic	cataract glaucoma
Central nervous system	psychosis depression benign intracranial hypertension
Dermatologic	acne striae alopecia bruising skin atrophy
Growth retardation	
Hypothalamic–pituitary–adrenal axis suppression	

Fig. 6.7 Adverse effects of systemic corticosteroid therapy.

Clinical data to support a large increase in the risk of infection during corticosteroid therapy are harder to obtain. In many published clinical trials, patients also have diseases that predispose to infection and are exposed to atypical organisms in a hospital environment[36]. The putative association between corticosteroid therapy and reactivation of tuberculosis provides a good example. In large studies of patients receiving corticosteroids in low doses over long periods of time for chest conditions, no increased risk of developing active tuberculosis has been observed. Likewise, cohorts of patients with positive tuberculin skin tests have been followed up for prolonged periods without development of active disease. Those studies reporting an increased risk of tuberculosis in patients treated with corticosteroids have often included patients treated with several immunosuppressive agents or with diseases predisposing to infection. These findings have led many authors to conclude that the risk of developing active tuberculosis during corticosteroid therapy is much lower than initially suspected[37].

PEPTIC ULCERATION

Peptic ulceration is not a common occurrence in endogenous Cushing's disease yet it is widely held that corticosteroid therapy is frequently complicated by the appearance or reactivation of peptic ulcers. The basis for this view resides in a number of anecdotal reports of the development of peptic ulcers in patients receiving corticosteroids and several series of corticosteroid-treated patients with a high incidence of ulcers. Close scrutiny of the evidence from controlled studies of corticosteroid therapy suggests that the increased risk of peptic ulceration – if it exists at all – is considerably lower than is widely believed[21], but corticosteroids may exacerbate the ulcerogenic properties of NSAIDs[38].

OSTEOPOROSIS

The bone loss associated with corticosteroid therapy principally affects trabecular bone. Studies using photon absorptiometric measurement of bone mineral density have shown that bone loss is greater in the lumbar spine, less in the proximal femur and least in the forearm. Vertebral wedge and crush fractures are a frequent complication of corticosteroid-treated RA, with prevalence rates from 11–20% reported[21].

The increased risk of fractures at other skeletal sites in such patients, however, remains unclear. In a case-control study of hip fracture in the UK[39], current use of corticosteroids was associated with a doubled hip fracture risk. Studies of bone loss in patients treated with corticosteroids do not clearly suggest a threshold dose below which osteoporosis can be avoided. Bone loss has been reported with prednisolone doses of 10mg daily, reducing to zero over 20 weeks [40], other studies suggest maintenance of bone stock on doses up to 7.5mg daily[41]. There appears to be a consistent relationship between doses above 7.5mg daily and rate of bone loss.

ATHEROSCLEROSIS

Information is beginning to accumulate that prolonged corticosteroid therapy may accelerate the development of atherosclerosis[21]. Lower limb atherosclerosis may occur in as many as 60% of corticosteroid-treated patients with RA.

Several studies of mortality in RA and other connective tissue diseases have detected an increased cardiovascular mortality among sufferers, suggesting an approximate doubling in the death rate from ischemic heart disease. Although data on corticosteroid use in these studies are often incomplete, one study reported an excess of coronary artery deaths in a corticosteroid-treated group when compared with a noncorticosteroid-treated control group[19]. The evidence linking corticosteroid therapy with atherosclerosis falls far short of proof, but if true, even a small effect would have considerable clinical significance.

PULSED INTRAVENOUS THERAPY

Reports of complications following pulse corticosteroid therapy[21] have usually arisen in renal transplant patients (Fig. 6.8). Most important among these is sudden death, most probably arising as a result of ventricular dysrhythmia and consequent myocardial infarction. In three such cases, the i.v. bolus was administered rapidly (in one case over only 20 seconds) and all were taking furosemide (frusemide), which may have induced hypokalemia. It has been suggested that increasing the infusion time to at least 30 minutes might prevent such events. Nevertheless, the incidence of such sudden death appears to be extremely low, given that well over 10,000 renal transplant patients are likely to have been treated with pulse corticosteroids. Other reported complications include transient arthralgias and synovitis, hyperglycemia, pancreatitis, gastrointestinal bleeding, visual disturbance and acute psychosis.

ADVERSE EFFECTS OF PULSE METHYLPREDNISOLONE THERAPY
Sudden death/ventricular dysrhythmia
Severe infection
Transient arthralgia/synovitis
Hyperglycemia
Pancreatitis
Gastrointestinal bleeding
Acute psychosis

Fig. 6.8 Adverse effects of pulse methylprednisolone therapy.

Severe fatal infections have also been reported. However, these are rare, and have occurred in transplant patients on daily doses of azathioprine, often following continued, long-term use of 1g pulses. *In vitro* studies indicate, however, that methylprednisolone pulses fail to reduce bacterial phagocytosis or killing by human neutrophils.

PRACTICAL PRESCRIBING TIPS

GENERAL APPROACH

It may be helpful to consider the prescription of corticosteroids in three broad dose ranges. Low daily doses, in the region of 15mg prednisolone or less, are used to treat polymyalgia, symptomatic arthritis and relatively quiescent SLE. High doses (20–60mg daily) are helpful in vasculitis (particularly involving larger arteries as in temporal arteritis or polyarteritis nodosa) or active, systemic SLE. Very high doses, particularly of pulsed methylprednisolone, are used to treat severe acute crises such as widespread vasculitis or nephritis.

CORTICOSTEROIDS IN CHILDREN

Growth retardation may occur in children receiving corticosteroids as these agents inhibit linear bone growth and delay epiphyseal closure (see Chapter 5.24). Regular daily administration of 7.5mg prednisolone or above is associated with inhibition of linear growth. The mechanism of action is unknown although suppression of growth hormone secretion and other metabolic effects may contribute. Alternate day administration of the same total dose may reduce this effect[42] and is now preferred.

REDUCING THE DOSE

High doses of corticosteroids are often used for only short periods and can be reduced rapidly with little adverse effect provided the underlying disease remains controlled. The precise pattern of reduction will depend upon the particular clinical circumstances under consideration, but control of short, severe exacerbations of, for example, vasculitis can be achieved with high doses over several days to a week or two, followed by rapid reduction to moderate levels (15–20mg daily). Patients treated in the longer term with moderate or low doses of corticosteroid may develop a 'corticosteroid withdrawal syndrome' if their treatment is then reduced. The constellation of complaints includes myalgia, fatigue, malaise, anorexia, nausea and weight loss[43] and has been reported in as many as 70% of patients treated with 30mg prednisone daily for longer than 3 months. There appears to be no correlation between symptoms and adrenal function. In certain clinical settings, however, such as polymyalgia rheumatica and polymyositis, it may be difficult to differentiate from poor control of the primary disease.

One approach to avoiding this is to reduce the corticosteroid treatment only slowly – perhaps by as little as 2.5mg daily every 6–10 weeks down to 7.5 mg daily, then by about 1mg daily over the same time interval, and in some patients by 1mg on alternate days to gradually stop the final few milligrams.

CORTICOSTEROID-SPARING AGENTS

This term is used to describe drugs which are prescribed in order to make it easier to reduce the corticosteroid dose, while at the same time controlling the underlying disease. Azathioprine, cyclophosphamide and methotrexate are each used for this purpose, commonly in doses lower than when used as single agents (for example, azathioprine maybe prescribed at 50mg daily rather than the 2.5mg/kg/day target dose used to treat RA). This use of 'combination' therapy to reduce adverse reactions is well recognized in other fields of medicine.

FUTURE DIRECTIONS

Corticosteroids, acting through their receptor molecule, clearly play a central role in the control of the inflammatory process. Other cytoplasmic receptor molecules with similar properties and effects on immune function regulation are now being identified, particularly in relation to therapeutic immunomodulators[44]. Furthermore, the primary and tertiary structures of human phospholipase A_2 have now been determined[45], raising the prospect of designing specific inhibitors for the active site which may be more powerful than lipocortin. Evidence is now emerging that some rheumatic diseases may in themselves blunt the normal anti-inflammatory response of the hypothalamic–pituitary–adrenal axis, resulting in inappropriately low corticosteroid levels[46]. Attempts are also being made to develop tissue-specific effects which may reduce potential adverse reactions[47]. Rapid developments can be expected in this field.

REFERENCES

1. Jenkins D. Pharmacology of prednisone, prednisolone, 6-CH_3 prednisone and prednisolone and triamcinolone. In: Mills LC, Mayer JE, eds. Inflammation and disease of connective tissue. A Hakremann Symposium. Philadelphia: WB Saunders; 1961:328–35.
2. Baxter HD, Forssham PH. Tissue effects of glucocorticoids. Am J Med. 1972;53:573–89.
3. Gehring U. Genetics of glucocorticoid receptors. Mol Cell Endocrinol. 1986;48:89–96.
4. Rothbut B, Russo-Marie F. Novel concepts in the mode of action of anti-inflammatory steroids. Agents Actions. 1984;14(Suppl):171–80.
5. Grabstein K, Dower S, Gillis S, *et al.* Expression of interleukin-2, interferon-gamma and the IL-2 receptor by human peripheral blood lymphocytes. J Immunol. 1986;15,136(12):4503–8.
6. Beutler B, Krochen N, Milsark IW, *et al.* Control of cachetin (TNF) synthesis mechanism of endotoxin resistance. Science. 1986;232:977–80.
7. Werb Z. Biochemical actions of glucocorticoids on macrophages in culture-specific inhibition of elastase, collagenase and plasminogen activator secretion and effects on other metabolic functions. J Exp Med. 1978;147(6):1695–1712.
8. Gerrard TL, Volkman DJ, Jurgensen CH, *et al.* Activated human T cells can present antigens but cannot present soluble antigens. Cell Immunol. 1985;95(1):65–74
9. Butler WT, Rossen RD. Effects of corticosteroids on immunity in man. 1. Decreased serum IgG concentrations caused by 3 or 5 days of high doses of methylprednisolone. J Clin Invest. 1973;52:2629–40.
10. Tuchinda M, Newcomb RW, Devald BL. Effect of prednisone treatment on the human immune response to keyhole limpet haemocyanin. Int Arch Allergy Appl Immunol. 1972;42:533–44.
11. Cupps TR, Edgar LL, Thomas CA, *et al.* Multiple mechanisms of B cell immunoregulation in man after administration of *in-vivo* corticosteroids. J Immunol. 1984;132(1)170–5.
12. Crabtree GR, Munck A, Smith KA. Glucocorticoids inhibit expression of Fc receptors on the human granulocytic cell line. HL-60. Nature. 1979;279:338–9.
13. Parillo JE, Fauci AS. Mechanisms of glucocorticoid action on immune processes. Annu Rev Pharmacol Toxicol. 1979;19:179–201.
14. Oluhy RG, Newmark SR, Lauler DR, *et al.* Pharmacology and chemistry of adrenal glucocosteroids in steroid therapy. In: Azarnoff DL, ed. Philadelphia: WB Saunders; 1975:8.
15. Brooks SM, Werk EE, Ackerman SJ, *et al.* Adverse effects of phenobarbital on corticosteroid metabolism in asthmatics. N Engl J Med. 1972;286:1125.
16. Klinenberg JR, Mullen R. Effect of corticosteroids on blood salicylate concentrations. JAMA. 1965;194:601.
17. George E, Kirwan JR. Corticosteroid therapy in rheumatoid arthritis. Bailliere's Clin Rheumatol. 1990;4:621–47.
18. Bryon MA, Kirwan JR. Corticosteroids in rheumatoid arthritis: is a trial of their disease modifying potential feasible? Ann Rheum Dis. 1986;46:171–3.
19. West HF. Rheumatoid arthritis. The relevance of clinical knowledge to research activities. Abstr World Med. 1967;41:401–17.
20. Kirwan JR and the Arthritis and Rheumatism Council Low-Dose Glucocorticoid Study Group. The effect of glucocorticoids on joint destruction in rheumatoid arthritis. New Engl J Med. 1995;333:142–6.
21. Cooper C, Kirwan JR. The risk of local and systemic corticosteroid administration. Baillière's Clin Rheumatol. 1990;4:305–32.
22. Weusten BLAM, Jacobs JWG, Bijlsma JWJ. Corticosteroid pulse therapy in active rheumatoid arthritis. Semin Arthritis Rheum. 1993;23:183–92.
23. Radia M, Furst DE. Comparison of three pulse methylprednisolone regimens in the treatment of rheumatoid arthritis. J Rheumatol. 1988;15:242–56.
24. Shipley ME, Bacon PA, Berry H, *et al.* Pulsed methylprednisolone in active early rheumatoid disease: A dose ranging study. Br J Rheumatol. 1988;15:242–6.
25. Needs CJ, Smith M, Boutagy J, *et al.* Comparison of methylprednisolone (I gram IV) with prednisolone (I gram orally) in rheumatoid arthritis: a pharmokinetic and clinical study. J Rheumatol. 1988;15:224–8.
26. Choy EHS, Kingsley G, Corkhill MM, Panayi GS. Intramuscular methylprednisolone is superior to pulse oral methylprednisolone during the inducton phase of chrysotherapy. Br J Rheumatol. 1993;32:734–9.
27. Conn D, Tomkins RB, Nichols WL. Glucocorticoids in the management of vasculitis–a double edged sword? J Rheumatol. 1988;15(5):1181–3.
28. Salvarini C, Macchioni PL, Tartoni PL, *et al.* Polymyalgia rheumatica and giant cell arteritis: a 5-year epidemiologic and clinical study in Reggio Emilia, Italy. Clin Exp Rheumatol. 1987;5:205–15.
29. Delecoeuillerie G, Joly P, de Lara AC, Paolaggi JB. Polymyalgia rheumatica and temporal arteritis: a retrospective analysis of prognostic features and different corticosteroid regimens (11 year survey of 210 patients). Ann Rheum Dis. 1988;47:733–9.
30. Lundberg I, Hedfors E. Restricted dose and duration of corticosteroid treatment in patients with polymyalgia rheumatica and temporal arteritis. J Rheumatol. 1990;17(10):1340–5.
31. Kirwan JR. Treatment of polymyalgia rheumatica. Br J Rheumatol. 1990;29:316.
32. Henderson RG, Wheatlev T, English J, *et al.* Variation in plasma prednisolone concentrations in renal transplant recipients given enteric-coated prednisolone. Br Med J. 1971;1:1534–6.
33. Hirata F. The regulation ot lipomodulin, a phospholipase inhibitory protein in rabbit neutrophils bv phosphorylation. J Biol Chem. 1981;256:7730–3.
34. Podgorski MR, Goulding NJ. Hall ND, *et al.* Autoantibodies to recombinant lipocortin in RA and SLE. Br J Rheumatol. 1987;26(suppl. 2):54–5.
35. Weisman MH. Corticosteroids in the treatment of rheumatologic diseases. Curr Opin Rheumatol. 1995;7:183–90.
36. Grieco MH. The role of corticosteroid therapy in infection. Hosp Pract. 1984;18:131–43.
37. Haanaes OC, Bergman A. Tuberculosis in patients treated with corticosteroids. Eur J Respir Dis. 1983;64:294–7.
38. Piper JM, Ray WA, Daughery JR, Griffen MR. Corticosteroid use and peptic ulcer – role of non-steroidal anti-inflammatory drug. Annals if Internal Medicine 1991;114:735–40.
39. Cooper C, Barker DJP, Wickham C. Physical activity, muscle strength and calcium intake in fracture of the proximal femur in Britain. Br Med J. 1988;297:1443–6.
40. Laan RFJM, Van Reil PLCM, van de Putte LBA, van Erning LJTO, van't Hof MA, Lemmens JAM. Low dose prednisolone induces rapid reversible axial bone loss in patients with rheumatoid arthritis: a randomized controlled study. Ann Intern Med, 1993;119:963–8.
41. Sambrook PN, Eisman JA, Yeates MG, Pocock NA, Eberl S, Champion GD. Osteoporosis in rheumatoid arthritis: Safety of low dose corticosteroids. Ann Rheum Dis. 1986;45:950–3.
42. Reimer LG, Morris HG, Ellis EF. Growth of asthmatic children during treatment with alternate-day steroids. J Allergy Clin Immunol 1975;55:224–31.
43. Dixon R, Christy N. On the various forms of corticosteroid withdrawal syndrome. Am J Med. 1980;68:224–30.
44. Moore JM, Peattie DA, Fitzgibbon MJ, *et al.* Solution structure of the major binding protein for the immunosuppressant FK506. Nature. 1991;351:248–50.
45. Wery JP, Schevitz RW, Clawson DK, *et al.* Structure of recombinant human rheumatoid arthritis phospholipase A_2 at 2.2Å resolution. Nature. 1991;352:79–82.
46. Chikanza IC, Petrou P, Kingsley G *et al.* Defective regulation of the hypothalamic–pituitary–adrenal axis in rheumatoid arthritis is not a consequence of chronic inflammation per se. Br J Rheumatol. 1992;31 (Suppl. 2):28.
47. Messina OD, Barreira JC, Zanchetta JR, *et al.* Effect of low dose deplazacourt rheumatoid vs prednisolone on bone mineral content in premenopausal rheumatoid arthritis. J Rheumatol. 1992;19:1520–6.

7

INTRA-ARTICULAR AND INTRALESIONAL THERAPY

Howard A Bird

- Corticosteroids available for intra-articular injection vary in chemical structure and solubility. Fluorinated compounds have greatest potency. The least soluble have a longer period of action.
- Triamcinolone hexacetonide is the most effective corticosteroid for relieving inflammatory arthritis localized to a small number of joints. Evidence for the efficacy of corticosteroids in osteoarthritis remains controversial.
- Intra-articular corticosteroids have largely superseded radionuclide synovectomy.
- The evidence for the efficacy of facet joint and epidural injections to relieve back pain remains controversial.
- Intra-articular 'chondroprotective' therapies are under investigation, and intra-articular injections of hyaluronic acid derivatives can cause prolonged symptomatic relief in osteoarthritis.

INTRODUCTION

For patients with monoarthritis, oligoarthritis or isolated soft tissue lesions, intra-articular or intralesional injection therapy may avoid the necessity of systemic drug therapy. With localized disease, consideration should always be given to whether local rest, perhaps enforced by a splint, might obviate the need for injection. Sometimes local injection therapy may be required to supplement systemic drug therapy which is failing to control a particularly troublesome joint.

Injection therapy is probably safer than is sometimes alleged but is certainly not localized in pharmacokinetic terms. Most compounds injected into an inflamed joint leave it rapidly. There is undoubtedly a placebo effect associated with a needle, and patients may develop an emotional attachment to it. This is analogous to the beneficial effect obtained when a nonsteroidal anti-inflammatory drug (NSAID) is applied as a topical application to the skin over a painful joint, a route for which pharmacokinetic studies also imply relative lack of localization of response. In addition, the skill and cost of the physician's time must be added to the price of the injected drug in the final cost–benefit equation. A detailed description of injection techniques appropriate to the various joints and soft tissue sites commonly requiring injection is provided elsewhere (see Chapter 2.12). Available intra-articular therapies are shown in Figure 7.1.

AVAILABLE INTRA-ARTICULAR THERAPIES	
Corticosteroids:	**Radioisotopes:**
Hydrocortisone Prednisolone and its salts Methylated prednisolone (methylprednisolone) Chlorinated prednisolone (triamcinolone, with its salts)	Colloidal gold Yttrium Rhenium Erbium
	Dysprosium
Liposomes	**Chondroprotective agents:**
Osmium	Dona-200S Glycosaminoglycan polysulfate Glycosaminoglycan peptide complex

Fig. 7.1 Available intra-articular therapies.

INJECTABLE CORTICOSTEROID THERAPY

PHARMACOLOGY OF AVAILABLE PREPARATIONS

Hydrocortisone is the most physiological of available corticosteroids and can be synthesized. Prednisolone is less soluble and is available as a variety of salts. The addition of a methyl group to provide methylprednisolone only slightly reduces solubility but may prolong duration of action. The introduction of a fluorine atom to produce triamcinolone enhances pharmacologic potency, and the complexing of this as an acetonide salt further reduces solubility, which in turn prolongs action. Figure 7.2 shows a list of commonly used corticosteroids together with the ratio of doses needed to produce comparable benefit and the average duration of pain relief after standard therapeutic dosing [1]. The relative solubility, when quoted by manufacturers, is also listed. In general, the more recently manufactured

DURATION OF ACTION AND SOLUBILITY OF COMMONLY USED INTRA-ARTICULAR CORTICOSTEROID PREPARATIONS			
Preparation	**Relative doses required to provide equivalent pharmacological effect**	**Average duration of pain relief (days)**	**Solubility***
Hydrocortisone acetate	× 6.25	6.0	0.0018
Hydrocortisone *tert*-butyl acetate	× 6.25	12.1	–
Prednisolone acetate	× 5	7.8	–
Prednisolone *tert*-butyl acetate	× 5	14.5	<0.0010
6-methylprednisolone acetate	× 5	8.2	0.0014
Dexamethasone acetate	1	7.6	–
Dexamethasone *tert*-butyl acetate	1	14.9	–
Triamcinolone diacetonide	× 5	7.7	0.0056
Triamcinolone acetonide	× 5	14.2	0.0040
Triamcinolone hexacetonide	× 5	21.2	0.0004

* Percentage w/v in H_2O at 25°C.

Fig.7.2 Duration of action and solubility of commonly used intra-articular corticosteroid preparations.

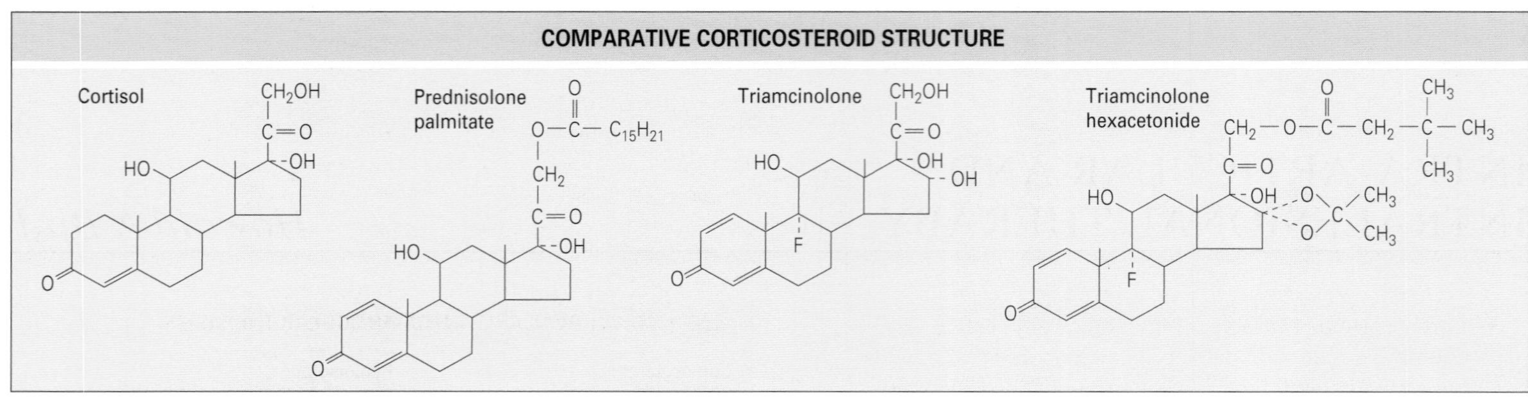

Fig. 7.3 Comparative corticosteroid structure.

the molecule, the greater the cost. The enhanced efficacy of triamcinolone is also matched by an increased tendency to cause side effects, particularly local tissue necrosis if injected into the wrong place by unskilled hands.

The comparative corticosteroid structure of these molecules is shown in Figure 7.3. The normal initial step in the metabolism of these corticosteroid salts is hydrolysis of the ester. This and the relative solubility of the compound both contribute to the duration of local effect.

PHARMACOKINETICS OF INTRA-ARTICULAR INJECTION

The synovium is extremely vascular in inflammatory arthritis. Small molecules such as methotrexate injected into one knee joint leave it quickly. The molecule can normally be found in the opposite noninjected knee joint within 10–15 minutes [2]. Corticosteroids fare a little better because of their larger size and lesser solubility, but it is a myth that significant systemic absorption does not occur from the intra-articular route. Studies using radiolabeled exogenous corticosteroids are not available, but the endogenous cortisol depression caused by intra-articular injection therapy (Fig. 7.4) gives an idea of the speed with which the corticosteroid leaves the joint [3]. Studies in which serum methylprednisolone levels have been followed after intra-articular injection of methylprednisolone acetate show that the maximum serum concentration of methylprednisolone is more closely related to the number of joints injected than to the total dose used. By implication, the total area of synovium across which corticosteroids can be transported is important.

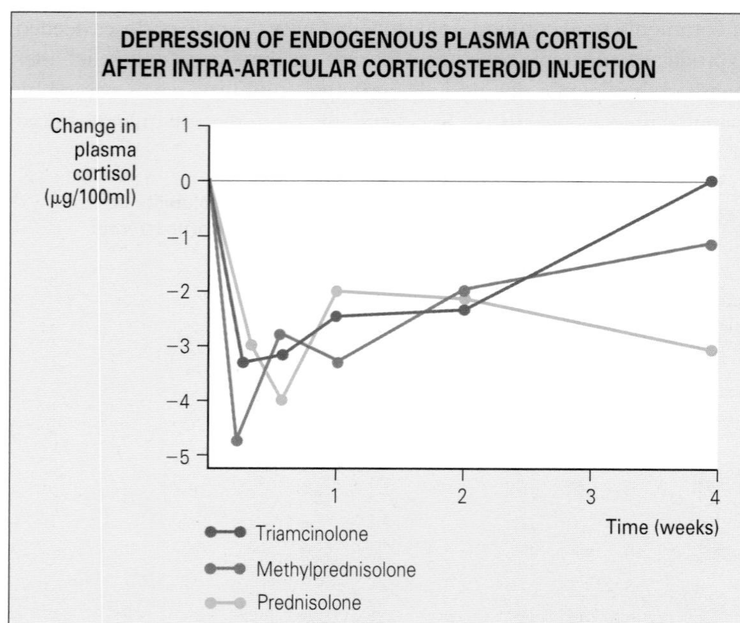

Fig. 7.4 Depression of endogenous plasma cortisol after intra-articular corticosteroid injection.

CHOICE OF CORTICOSTEROID PREPARATION

A variety of early studies, each using different clinical assessments suggests that whatever the indication, the ranking order for potency starts with hydrocortisone. Then follow prednisolone salts, with prednisolone *tert*-butyl acetate being the most efficacious and methylprednisolone only slightly superior. Triamcinolone is the most effective corticosteroid preparation, with its duration of action determined by the size of the esterified side chain [3,4]. Triamcinolone hexacetonide therefore provides maximum benefit, but this has to be set against the greater tendency of this compound to cause local tissue necrosis if it is not injected into a cavity or if it is accidentally infiltrated into the skin. My own practice is to recommend hydrocortisone for intralesional use, even in unskilled hands. Failure to respond to hydrocortisone would then be an indication to use prednisolone, possibly as prednisolone *tert*-butyl acetate, and these compounds alone should be used for the infiltration of tendon sheaths, however skilled the clinician. Inflammatory arthritis is more likely to respond to triamcinolone hexacetonide, the injection of choice in the hands of an experienced clinician.

INDICATIONS AND DOSES OF CORTICOSTEROIDS

For soft tissue rheumatism (fibrositis) an injection of hydrocortisone mixed with 1% or 2% lidocaine (there being no drug interaction between these compounds) can be successfully infiltrated into tender sites and trigger points with relative safety. A dose of 10–25mg hydrocortisone would be typical. For epicondylitis, particularly at the elbow, a smaller volume of steroid, probably prednisolone *tert*-butyl acetate, should be injected directly onto the most tender site. A typical dose of prednisolone would be 10–25mg, and a little lidocaine could be added. The volume of fluid that can successfully be injected into a tendon sheath is limited, normally restricting the dose of prednisolone salt to about 10mg. The volume of corticosteroids that can be injected into interphalangeal joints and metacarpophalangeal joints with inflammatory arthritis is also limited, effectively restricting the dose of triamcinolone to 5–10mg. For larger joints, such as the knee or ankle, 20mg of triamcinolone would be a reasonable starting dose, increasing to 30mg or occasionally 40mg if the first injection remains ineffective after 1–2 weeks. The joint size allows the simultaneous injection of 1% or 2% lidocaine, though the benefit derived from this is unlikely to last more than a few hours. The presence of an inflammatory effusion tends to cushion the joints, and although, in general, fluid that can be removed easily and without discomfort to the patient should be aspirated prior to corticosteroid injection, aspiration to dryness may unmask substantial crepitus that was previously unnoticed by the patient.

COMPLICATIONS

Suppression of the hypothalamic–pituitary–adrenal axis undoubtedly occurs (Fig. 7.4) and increases with the number of joints injected [5,6]. The risk of tissue necrosis with triamcinolone has already been mentioned; in addition a postinjection 'flare' occurs in a small number of patients receiving this drug by the intra-articular route [7].

The risk of joint disorganization after steroid injection to the hip and knee may be exaggerated [8]. Experimental joint damage described in rabbits is probably irrelevant, and in a large survey of patients receiving multiple intra-articular steroid injections for osteoarthritis (OA) and rheumatoid arthritis (RA), only two out of 65 patients demonstrated radiologic deterioration, and even this might have been consistent with the natural progression of the disease. It has been argued [8,9] that, providing the interval between injections is not less than 4 weeks for a weight-bearing joint in man, the benefit is likely to outweigh the damage that might accrue by leaving the inflammatory arthritis untreated. A thermographic comparison of the different long-acting corticosteroid preparations has suggested that benefit from triamcinolone hexacetonide in the knee with rheumatoid synovitis would normally last 6 weeks [3]. Although it has been argued that a period of 48 hours bed rest after corticosteroid injection in weight-bearing joints might reduce side effects, a controlled study[10] suggests that this is not the case. Opinions vary on whether benefit is [11] or is not [10] enhanced by resting the joint after injection.

Infection may occasionally occur but this is exceptional if a strict aseptic technique is observed. It needs to be distinguished from the occasional postinjection flare.

CLINICAL EFFICACY

Inflammatory joint disease responds best to the anti-inflammatory effect of corticosteroids. In a comparison of methylprednisolone, triamcinolone acetonide and triamcinolone hexacetonide in rheumatoid arthritis, at 12 weeks the proportion of patients still gaining pain relief was 59% for the hexacetonide salt and 44% for the acetonide salt, hydrocortisone being hardly effective [12]. In early juvenile chronic arthritis presenting at the knee, intra-articular injections (sometimes repeated) of triamcinolone hexacetonide have induced remission of 2 years or more in 40% of children.

The evidence for efficacy in osteoarthritis is less clear, the advantages of corticosteroid injection often being short-lived [13]. Most investigators agree that the more marked the joint destruction, the less the benefit.

A variety of soft tissue lesions respond to corticosteroid injections to tendon sheaths, particular trigger finger and thumb. Corticosteroids are also advocated for painful shoulder syndromes though not all are convinced of their superiority over alternative treatments such as physiotherapy and mobilization [14]. Corticosteroids are superior to the use of lidocaine alone in the treatment of lateral epicondylitis [15].

FUTURE TRENDS

Improved localization would provide substantial clinical benefit. Liposomes have been suggested as a new approach [11,16]. The corticosteroid is incorporated into a bilayer of phospholipids which is absorbed by phagocytes in the synovium. Arguably, the drug remains physiologically encapsulated at the site it is most needed. There is some evidence that cholesterol-rich liposomes are specifically taken up by inflammatory tissue of rats with adjuvant arthritis [16] but the liposome technique has not yet found widespread application in routine clinical practice. The next decade will bring the advent of monoclonal antibodies and these may provide an alternative and more specific way of targeting drugs at the cartilage, the synovium, and particularly the site of pannus formation, where they are most needed.

OTHER INJECTABLE DRUGS

Intra-articular NSAIDs have been evaluated [17] but their use lacks relevance. Compounds leave the joints just as quickly as they are likely to be absorbed into the joint from the systemic circulation after oral administration, and the injectable route is more expensive and carries a slight risk of infection. Moreover, intra-articular injection demands the presence and cost of a physician. Osmium tetroxide is a chemical agent that can induce a chemical synovectomy. It is a toxic compound and has been superseded by the use of the more efficient corticosteroid preparations. Benefit has been claimed for some disease-modifying drugs injected into joints. Superoxide dismutase is said to be as efficacious as intra-articular methylprednisolone in OA [18] and in RA [19], though the rationale for its use has been questioned and the placebo effect of such repeated injections must be strong. Rifampicin has also been given by intra-articular injection with claims of benefit. Although intra-articular methotrexate appeals for a patient with monoarthritis who cannot tolerate the oral route of delivery, the drug leaves the joint cavity quickly [2], this route differing little pharmacokinetically from an intramuscular injection which can be given by a nurse.

RADIONUCLIDE SYNOVECTOMY

Several isotopes are available. Colloidal gold-198 (^{198}Au) has been replaced in most centers by the powerful beta-emitter yttrium-90 (^{90}Y). The greater beta emission of ^{90}Y provides greater irradiation for a very thick synovium, particularly at the knee, and the absence of gamma emissions makes it safer for the patient and administrator. For medium sized joints rhenium-186 (^{186}Re) is used in Europe. Erbium-169 (^{169}Er) is probably the isotope of choice for the small joints of the hands [20]. Recently a short half-life beta-emitter (dysprosium) has also been shown to be efficacious [21].

There are stringent regulations governing the use of radiocolloids in most countries, and often a special licence must be held by the physician injecting the compound. Disposal of waste should be meticulous. There is a risk to the patient of extra-articular spread of the radioisotope, and immobilization for a period after injection (typically a plaster cast for 1 week) has been advocated, though this may err on the side of caution. There is also a theoretic risk to the patient of chromosomal damage.

Controlled trials have suggested that intra-articular radiocolloids are more beneficial than surgical synovectomy [22] though a comparison of erbium and intra-articular corticosteroid injections to the fingers [23] showed no difference between the two treatments. Triamcinolone has even been shown to be superior to erbium [24]. For these reasons, the risks of radiocolloid use are increasingly felt to outweigh the advantages.

FACET JOINT AND EPIDURAL INJECTIONS

Injections of steroid and lidocaine are sometimes given for low back pain alongside other treatments (varying from physiotherapy and traction to transcutaneous electrical nerve stimulation and even lengthy bed rest). The term low back pain covers a variety of diagnoses ranging from coccydynia to lumbar disc protrusion. Chymopapain enjoyed an explosive growth for this last indication in the 1980s though is now used much less [25].

Apart from the nonspecific infiltration of hydrocortisone and anesthetic for nonspecific lumbar myalgia, which probably has a placebo effect though may help to break up fibrosis in soft tissue, two particular syndromes are said to benefit specifically from local corticosteroid injection. If pain on palpation can be localized to the posterior facet joints of the lumbar spine, which are the only synovial joints that occur in the spine at this level and which are copiously innervated, local injection of corticosteroid may theoretically relieve inflammation. Even if fluoroscopic control is provided, the results are controversial and a recent carefully controlled study suggested no significant benefit when the injection of methylprednisolone acetate was compared to placebo at this site [26].

Epidural injections may also relieve low back pain. They are rationally restricted to unilateral back pain of nerve route distribution and the standard anesthetic technique of giving an epidural injection is used. A little hydrocortisone is mixed with 1% or 2% lidocaine. With practice, accurate localization can be achieved, but sometimes fluoroscopic control is required. Opinions differ on the efficacy. A controlled trial showed no statistically significant improvement at 20 months when patients with radiographically confirmed lumbar nerve route compression were treated with methylprednisolone acetate and procaine [27]. However 80mg of methylprednisolone in 10ml of physiological saline produces significant improvement in pain relief at 2 weeks compared to saline placebo when given to patients with sciatica [28]. The benefit was sustained at 6 months in only two thirds of these patients. Recently intrathecal midazolam has been claimed to be as effective as epidural corticosteroid for chronic mechanical low back pain in a pilot sudy [29].

CHONDROPROTECTIVE AGENTS

So-called ‘chondroprotective’ agents, designed to slow or prevent cartilage damage, have caused much controversy. A variety of oral, intramuscular or intra-articular agents have been widely prescribed in some European countries for the treatment of OA, without there being good, definitive data to establish their efficacy, and in spite of a variety of side effects. The agents that have been most popular for intra-articular use have been glycosaminoglycan derivatives such as Dona-200S and glycosaminoglycan polysulphate [30]. More recently, other intra-articular therapeutic approaches have been investigated as possible ways of preventing joint damage, or stimulating the repair of joints. These include the injection of matrix precursor cells into cartilage defects and the use of intra-articular growth factors[31, 32]. As yet these interventions remain experimental.

Intra-articular injections of hyaluronic acid derivatives have also been widely used in the treatment of OA [33]. Most preparations are derived from cockscomb (*Celosia cristata*) and have minimal allergenicity after purification. The molecular weight of different products varies from 50×10^4 to 700×10^4. Several different agents have now been licensed for use in many parts of the world, including Canada, Japan, and some European countries, and are variously classified as drugs or devices. Most are given as a course of two to five intra-articular injections at weekly intervals, with possible repeat courses at about 6-month intervals. Side effects appear minor, although flares of synovitis occur in some cases [34]. These agents have been investigated for two possible activities – a long-acting symptomatic benefit, and a ‘chondroprotective effect’. In spite of difficulties with trial design when repeated intra-injections are used as an intervention, producing a large placebo effect, there is a lot of data to support the contention that hyaluronate inections are efficacious, and it may be that the higher molecular weight products are the most effective[35,36]. However, their relative benefits in comparison to other interventions for OA remain unclear, and there is, as yet, no evidence to support any effect on disease progression.

REFERENCES

1. Hollander JL. Symposium on intra-synovial corticosteroid therapy of rheumatic diseases. Held at XVII Nordic Congress of Rheumatology. Elsinore: Denmark;1978.
2. Bird HA, Ring EFJ, Daniel R, *et al.* Comparison of intra-articular methotrexate with intra-articular triamcinolone hexacetonide. Curr Med Res Opin. 1977;5:141–6.
3. Bird HA, Ring EFJ, Bacon PA. A thermographic and clinical comparison of three intra-articular steroid preparations in rheumatoid arthritis. Ann Rheum Dis. 1979;38:36–9.
4. Esselinckx W, Bacon PA, Ring EFJ, *et al.* A thermographic assessment of three intra-articular prednisolone analogues given in rheumatoid synovitis. Br J Clin Pharmacol. 1978;5:447–51.
5. Esselinckx W, Kolanowski J, Nagant de Deuxchaisnes CH. Adrenocortical function and responsivenesss to tetracosactrin infusions after intra-articular treatment with triamcinolone acetonide and hydrocortisone acetate. Clin Rheumatol. 1982;1:176–84.
6. Reid DM, Eastmond C, Rennie JAN. Hypothalamic–pituitary–adrenal axis suppression after repeated intra-articular steroid injection. Ann Rheum Dis. 1986;45:87.
7. Berger RG, Yount WJ. Immediate ‘steroid flare’ from intra-articular triamcinolone hexacetonide injection: case report and review of the literature. Arthritis Rheum. 1990;33:1284–6.
8. Intra-articular steroids (leading article). Br Med J. 1987;1:600–1.
9. Balch HW, Gibson JNC, El-Ghobarey AF, Bain LS, Lynch MP. Repeated corticosteroid injections into lame joints. Rheumatol Rehab. 1977;16:137–40.
10. Chatham W, Williams G, Moreland L, *et al.* Intra-articular corticosteroid injections: should we rest the joints? Arthritis Care Res. 1989;2:70–4.
11. de Silva M, Hazleman BL, Page Thomas DP, Wraight P. Liposomes in arthritis: a new approach. Lancet. 1979;i:1320–2.
12. Blyth T, Hunter JA, Stirling A. Pain relief in the rheumatoid knee after steroid injection. A single-blind comparison of hydrocortisone succinate and triamcinolone acetonide or hexacetonide. Br J Rheumatol. 1994;30:35–8.
13. Dieppe PA, Sathapatayavongs B, Jones HE, Bacon PA, Ring EFJ. Intra-articular steroids in osteoarthritis. Rheumatol Rehab, 1980;19:212–7.
14. Bulgen DY, Binder AI, Hazleman BL, Dutton J, Roberts S. Frozen shoulder: prospective clinical study with an evaluation of three treatment regimens. Ann Rheum Dis. 1984;42:353–60.
15. Price R, Sinclair H, Heinrich I, Gibson T. Local injection treatment of tennis elbow – hydrocortisone, triamcinolone and lignocaine compared. Br J Rheumatol. 1991;30:39–44.
16. Love GW, Amos N, Kellaway IW, Williams BD. Specific accumulation of cholesterol-rich liposomes in the inflammatory tissue of rats with adjuvant arthritis. Ann Rheum Dis. 1990;49:611–4.
17. Rylance HJ, Chalmbers TM, Elton RA. Clinical trials of intra-articular aspirin in rheumatoid arthritis. Lancet. 1980;ii:1099–122.
18. Gammer W, Broback LG. Clinical comparison of orgotein and methylprednisolone acetate in the treatment of osteoarthrosis of the knee joint. Scand J Rheumatol. 1984;13:108–12.
19. Goebel KM, Storck U, Neurath F. Intra-synovial orgotein therapy in rheumatoid arthritis. Lancet. 1981;i:1015–17.
20. Gumpel JM. Radiosynoviorthesis. In: Huskisson EC, ed. Anti-rheumatic drugs (Clinical Pharmacology and Therapeutics Services, Vol 3). New York: Praeger, Eastbourne; 1983:647–63.
21. Edmonds J, Smart R, Laurent R, Butler P, Brooks P, *et al.* A comparative study of the safety and efficacy of dysprosium-165 hydroxide macro-aggregate and yttrium-90 silicate colloid in radiation synovectomy – A multicentre double blind clinical trial. Brit J Rheum. 1994;33:947–53.
22. Gumpel JM, Roles NC. A controlled trial of intra-articular radiocolloids versus surgical synovectomy in persistent synovitis. Lancet. 1975;i:488–9.
23. Gumpel J, Matthews SA, Fisher M. Synoviorthesis with erbium-169: a double-blind controlled comparison of erbium-169 with corticosteroid. Ann Rheum Dis. 1979;38:341–3.
24. Menkes CJ, Aignan M, Calmiche B, Le Go A. Le traitement des rhumatismes par les synoviorthèses. Choix des malades, choix des articulations, modalités practiques, resultats, indications, contre-indications. Rhumatologie. 1972;2(Suppl 1):61.
25. Deyo RA. Fads in the treatment of low back pain. N Eng J Med, 1991;325 (14):1039–40.
26 Carette S, Margoux S, Ruchon R, Grondin C, Gagnon J, Allard Y, Latulippe M. A controlled trial of corticosteroid injections into facet joints for chronic low back pain. N Eng J Med. 1991;325 (14):1002–7.
27. Cuckler J, Bernini PA, Wiesel SW, Booth RE, Rothman RH, Pickenns GT. The use of epidural steroids in the treatment of lumbar radicular pain. J Bone Joint Surg, 1985;67A (1):63–6.
28. Ridley MG, Kinsley RH, Gibsonn T, Grahame R. Outpatient lumbar epidural corticosteroid injection in the managemennt of sciatica. Br J Rheumatol,1988;27:295-9.
29. Serrao JM, Marks RL, Morley SJ, Goodchild CS. Intrathecal midazolam for the treatment of chronic mechanical low back pain: a controlled comparison with epidural steroid in a pilot sudy. Pain. 1992;38:5–12.
30. Brandt KD. Towards pharmacologic modification of joint damage in osteoarthritis. Ann Intern Med. 1995;122:874–5.
31. Brittberg M, Lindahl A, Nilsson A, Ohlsson C, Isaksson O, Peterson L. Treatment of deep cartilage defects in the knee with autologous chondrocyte transplantation. New Eng J Med. 1994;331:889–95.
32. Howel DS, Altman RD. Cartilage repair and conservation in osteoarthritis: state of the art review. J Rheumatol. 1993;19:713–24.
33. Peyron JG. Intra-articular hyaluronan injections in the treatment of osteoarthritis: state of the art review. J Rheumatol. 1993;20(suppl 39):10–15.
34. Puttick M, Wade P, Chalmers A, Connell D, Rango K. Acute local reactions after intraarticular hylan for osteoarthritis of the knee. J Rheumatol. 1995;22:1311–4.
35. Adams ME, Atkinson MH, Lussier AJ *et al*. The role of viscosupplementation with hylan G-F 20 in the treatment of osteoarthritis of the knee. Osteoarthritis and Cartilage. 1995;3:213–226
36. Lohmander LS. A controlled randomised, double-blind multicentre trial ofintra-articular hyaluronan treatment in osteoarthritis of the knee. Acta Orthop Scand. 1995;66(suppl 265):25-36.

8

SAARDs

Richard O Day

Summary

- Definitive, early drug therapy with appropriate slow-acting antirheumatic drugs (SAARDS) including methotrexate within 3 months of diagnosis may improve the outcome of rheumatoid arthritis (RA) by reducing joint damage.
- Gold and D-penicillamine are used less with the advent of methotrexate; insight into their modes of action on transcription factor AP-1 binding to DNA provides important clues to effective drug therapy in RA.
- Sulfasalazine and hydroxychloroquine have an important role in the treatment of early disease and as part of combination regimens some of which are now showing considerable promise.
- Authoritative consensus guidelines for the safe use of SAARDs now set the standard for surveillance of patients treated with these drugs.

INTRODUCTION

There is no universally accepted classification scheme for the many drugs used in the management of chronic, inflammatory rheumatic conditions. The drugs have been classified based on presumed mechanisms of action (antimetabolites, cytotoxics or immunosuppressives), alleged benefit (disease-modifying or remission-inducing) or their observed onset of clinical effects. Typically several or more weeks elapse after initiation of these drugs before clinical improvements are noted. Thus, the term slow-acting antirheumatic drugs (SAARDs) represents a convenient way to describe these compounds.

Studies of the efficacy of SAARDs in RA are difficult because of the variability of the disease, the wide range of responses to SAARDs, the generally slow onset of effect and considerable toxicity of some SAARDs. These factors are a formidable test of the quality of design of clinical trials of SAARDs and unfortunately, relatively few good studies exist. Common faults include insufficient numbers of patients and inappropriate analysis of data, particularly the treatment of data from subjects who fail to complete the study[1]. It has become apparent that studies of efficacy restricted to 6–12 months do not provide answers to the more important questions concerning the effect of SAARDs on the patient's long-term outcome, particularly quality of life and ability to continue working[2]. Indeed, some authors have suggested that we have been deluded as to the value of SAARDs in patients with RA because closer study reveals evidence of few sustained remissions, high levels of cessation of SAARD therapy over 2–4 years, increased mortality and inexorable progression to disability and deformity in the majority of patients[2,3].

A more optimistic assessment of the merits of SAARDs has emerged which suggests considerable contribution to the quality of life of patients although the end result is often disability and deformity (Fig. 8.1). However, it is agreed that there is much room for improvement. It has been emphasized that substantial damage to joints occurs in the first 2 years of RA and that the degree of suppression of inflammation during this early period of disease is postulated to be the best correlate of eventual joint damage. Newer regimens of antirheumatic therapy which stress earlier commencement of SAARDs, prediction of outcome for individual patients based on clinical, bone density and laboratory (rheumatoid factor, genetic markers) features and use of various combinations and cycles of SAARDs are under investigation and promise improved long-term outcomes[5]. The benefits of prompt commencement of SAARDs in early RA are now becoming apparent with fewer erosions appearing in the early treatment groups[6]. It is now recommended that SAARD therapy should not be delayed beyond 3 months for any patient with an established diagnosis of RA[7].

The mechanisms of action of SAARDs are poorly understood and any proposed mechanism needs to account for some of the common features of this group of drugs (see Fig. 8.2). The proposed mechanism should be demonstrable selectively in those patients that respond, and ought to be detectable before clinical improvement is apparent, proving that the mechanism is causal with respect to suppression of RA[8].

GOLD

The place of gold therapy in the treatment of RA has been re-evaluated. There is clear evidence for the short-term efficacy of injectable gold but less certainty about the long-term benefits. Auranofin (oral gold) appears to be less effective than other SAARDs[9]. The majority view is that gold therapy remains a useful option in RA[10,11], probably able to retard the radiologic progression and decline in quality of life due to this disease. However, gold along with the other SAARDs is decreasingly used in favor of methotrexate.

MECHANISM OF ACTION

Gold in antirheumatic drugs is maintained in oxidation state I and is usually bound to sulfhydryl groups which can exchange with other sulfhydryl ligands (see Fig. 8.3), reactions that are critical to the localization and therefore action of these drugs. Injectable gold compounds, such as sodium aurothiomalate, are polymeric, water soluble and not absorbed orally whereas auranofin is monomeric, lipid soluble and at least partially absorbed following oral administration.

The entry of gold into cells occurs via a sequence of ligand exchange reactions involving sulfhydryl groups on the cell surface[12].

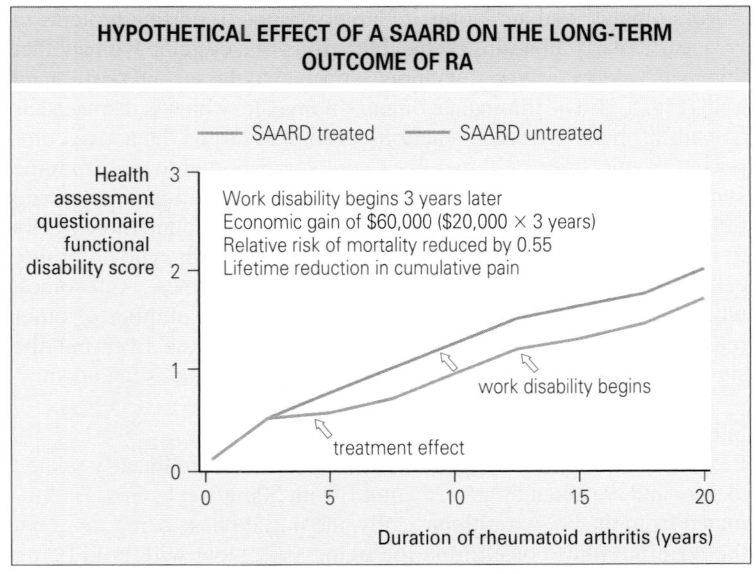

Fig. 8.1 The hypothetical effect of a SAARD on the long-term outcome of RA including quality of life, ability to work and longevity. Adapted from Wolfe[4].

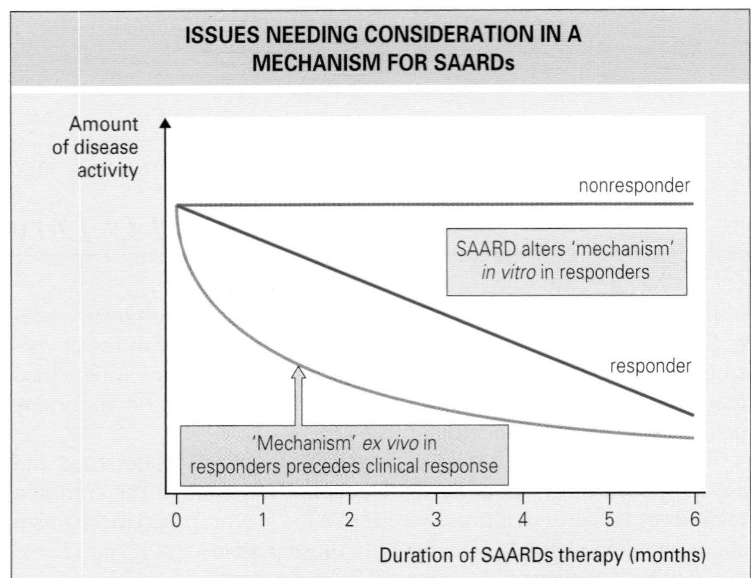

Fig. 8.2 Some issues to be considered when proposing a mechanism for the antirheumatic properties of SAARDs. Proposed mechanisms of action of SAARDs should be present in responders and absent in nonresponders and precede clinical improvement. The slow onset and offset of action of SAARDs and the variable efficacy between individuals ranging from no effect to remission should also be explained. Adapted from Day *et al.*[8].

The cellular actions of polymeric injectable gold may relate to the formation of monomeric aurocyanide from cyanide released during polymorph phagocytosis[11]. Aurocyanide is particularly able to enter cells compared to polymeric gold complexes. If aurocyanide is the active form of polymeric gold complexes, it would be formed preferentially in the vicinity of activated polymorphs and macrophages.

An important new finding is that aurothiomalate may regulate gene expression by inhibiting the binding of specific transcription factors to their response elements in DNA. Binding of the transcription factor AP-1, a dimer of the proto-oncogenes *jun* and *fos*, is specifically inhibited by very low concentrations of gold at about 1–5μmol/l [13]. The expected consequences of reduced AP-1 transcriptional activity is a reduction in the expression of a number of cytokines, metalloproteinases and cell adhesion molecules.

Other potential mechanisms of action commonly require unrealistic concentrations of gold *in vitro* or are likely to be artefactual and a consequence of gold-induced disease suppression *in vivo* (Fig. 8.4).

PHARMACOKINETICS AND PHARMACODYNAMICS

Aurothiomalate and auranofin are largely bound to plasma proteins *in vivo*, particularly albumin, via the thiol group of a cysteine with another thiol, such as cysteine or glutathione, attached to the second position on gold (Fig. 8.3). The thiomalate of aurothiomalate, which is displaced as a result of these exchange reactions, is unlikely to be the active component of injectable gold therapy. Gold is transported to and from the synovial fluid as a complex with albumin, concentrations in synovial fluid being about 50% of those in plasma[11]. Gold is bound more avidly to inflamed synovial tissue, most gold being found in synovial lining cells and more deeply placed macrophages in 'aurosomes'. Aurosomes, which are derived from lysosomes, are found in a number of other macrophage-type cells such as Küpffer cells of the liver but the significance of aurosomes for efficacy or toxicity remains unknown.

Injectable gold complexes

Peak concentrations are achieved in about 2 hours, are linearly related to dose and are about 5mg/l (25μmol/l) with 50mg/week. Gold is eliminated from the body multiphasically, the initial phase being rapid but the terminal phase of elimination being very slow with gold being detected in tissues up to 23 years post-therapy.

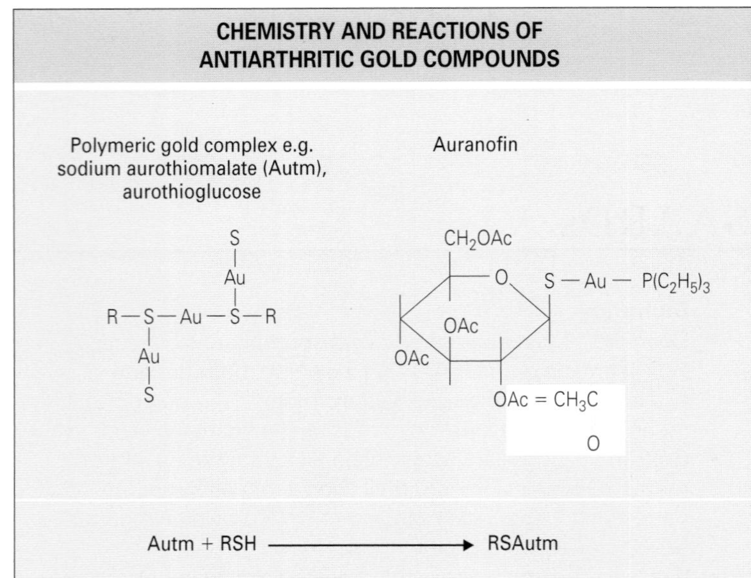

Fig. 8.3 Chemistry and reactions of antiarthritic gold compounds. The reaction of a subunit of polymeric sodium aurothiomalate and endogenous thiols. (AC is acetyl.)

Auranofin

Absorption of gold from auranofin following a single dose is about 20–25%. Most gold is eliminated in the feces with 15% excreted in urine over 3 months. The plasma half-life of gold following auranofin is 11–31 days but there is less retention of gold in tissues than following injectable gold[17].

POSSIBLE MECHANISMS OF ACTION OF GOLD COMPOUNDS IN RA

Target	Effect
Transport to tissues/cells	Polymeric gold metabolized to aurocyanide (AuCN) Auranofin (AF) already monomeric[11]
Gene transcription	Regulation of gene expression/protein synthesis[13]
Polymorphonuclear cells	Aggregation, phagocytosis, chemiluminescence and reactive oxygen species (ROS) release Aurothiomalate (Autm) weakly inhibits AF and AuCN strongly inhibit
Synovial cells in culture	Inhibition of growth and collagen synthesis
Monocytes	Cytokine production, e.g. IL-1 Autm no effect AF inhibits Chemotaxis, phagocytosis, chemiluminescence, ROS production Autm little or no effect AF inhibits Inhibit accessory cell function for lymphocyte proliferation [14] HLA class II expression Autm enhances (low dose) and inhibits (high dose) expression[15]
Lymphocytes	*In vivo* studies: Generally few effects of gold compounds; no changes in T-cell subset ratios; no effects on antibody-dependent cytotoxicity or killer T-cell function; increases in mitogen responses *ex vivo* and delayed hypersensitivity *In vitro* studies: High concentrations inhibit lymphocyte proliferation to a range of mitogens secondary to monocyte effects; Autm and AF inhibit IL-1 induced proliferation[16]
Immunoglobulins	*In vivo* studies: Levels of immunoglobulin, RF and immune complexes fall

Fig. 8.4 Possible mechanisms of action of gold compounds in RA. Targets in bold may be most significant. *In vitro* unless stated. Adapted from Champion *et al.*[11].

SUMMARY OF PERFORMANCE OF GOLD COMPOUNDS IN RA

Injectable gold compounds

1. Intramuscular gold 10–50mg/week for 1–2 years is effective but no dose–response relationship is evident.
2. Response cannot be predicted.
3. Excellent responses occur in 20–35% of patients after 6–12 months treatment.
4. Excellent responses are sustained beyond 1 year in only 50%.
5. Sustained remission occurs in very few patients.
6. Gold slightly retards radiologic progression of RA.
7. Only about 20% of patients are still taking gold after 4 years therapy.
8. Gold has similar efficacy to D-penicillamine, sulfasalazine, azathioprine and methotrexate and may be slightly more efficacious than antimalarials.

Auranofin

1. Auranofin 6mg/day is superior to placebo and improves RA over 6–9 months, is slightly less effective than aurothiomalate and D-penicillamine (750mg/day) but causes fewer serious adverse effects than these SAARDs.
2. Remissions are less common than with aurothiomalate and improvements are usually not sustained.
3. Diarrhea is dose-limiting.

Fig. 8.5 Summary of performance of gold compounds in RA. Adapted from Champion *et al.*[11].

EFFICACY

Gold therapy is of value in the treatment of RA (Fig. 8.5) and of possible value in psoriatic arthritis, particularly the nonspondylitic form. Gold also has efficacy in juvenile arthritis with positive rheumatoid factor but not the systemic form[11]. Gold therapy not only improves the symptoms and signs of RA but decreases erythrocyte sedimentation rate (ESR) and rheumatoid factor (RF) levels while increasing hemoglobin concentrations. Unfortunately, the benefits of gold therapy are usually not sustained long-term, the drug only being able to slow progression in most instances.

TOXICITY

Toxicity with injectable gold is common, occurring in about 30–40% of patients (Figs 8.6 & 8.7). However, with careful surveillance most serious toxicity can be avoided. Doses greater than 50mg/week are associated with more toxicity. Aurothioglucose appears to be less likely to cause skin reactions. Auranofin is safer and less toxic than injectable gold, diarrhea being the commonest problem, followed by mucocutaneous reactions, conjunctivitis, proteinuria and thrombocytopenia[19]. Diarrhea declines with continued use and responds to dosage reduction.

PRACTICAL PRESCRIBING TIPS

Considerable effort is needed to educate patients concerning efficacy, toxicity and requirements for follow-up visits when injectable gold is to be used. Although aurothioglucose is less likely to cause postinjection reactions than aurothiomalate, a wider bore needle is required to inject the former. If injection pain is a problem, lidocaine (lignocaine) can be added. A test dose (1mg) is followed by 5, 10 then 10–50mg/week, to a total dose of about 1g – or about 6 months therapy, when a decision about continued therapy can be made. Maintenance therapy is continued at 10–50mg every 2–4 weeks and can be given indefinitely while there is perceived benefit. Concomitant nonsteroidal anti-inflammatory drugs (NSAIDs) are usual and, increasingly, so are combinations with other SAARDs.

Monthly assessments of disease activity with some clinical and laboratory measurements such as joint tenderness, morning stiffness, pain, global assessment of symptoms, ESR [or C-reactive protein (CRP)] and hemoglobin will indicate if improvement is occurring. Inquiry concerning skin itching or mouth ulcers should precede each injection. A complete blood count weekly for the first month and then every 2–4 weeks for the next 5 months is the commonest regimen with careful attention to downward trends in platelets or neutrophils which require increased surveillance and possible dosage reduction or cessation. Precipitous drops in white cells or platelets demand immediate cessation of gold. Eosinophilia warns that an adverse reaction (allergic type) is likely, e.g. a skin reaction, and it is sensible to reduce the dose of gold or even stop temporarily if counts are high. Urine testing for protein should be performed before each injection. Blood count frequency may drop somewhat (e.g. every 4–6 weeks) after 6 months according to dose and regimen selected and previous responses of the patient.

Skin itch or minor rashes or mouth ulcers will usually recede quickly although sometimes topical, but rarely oral, corticosteroids are

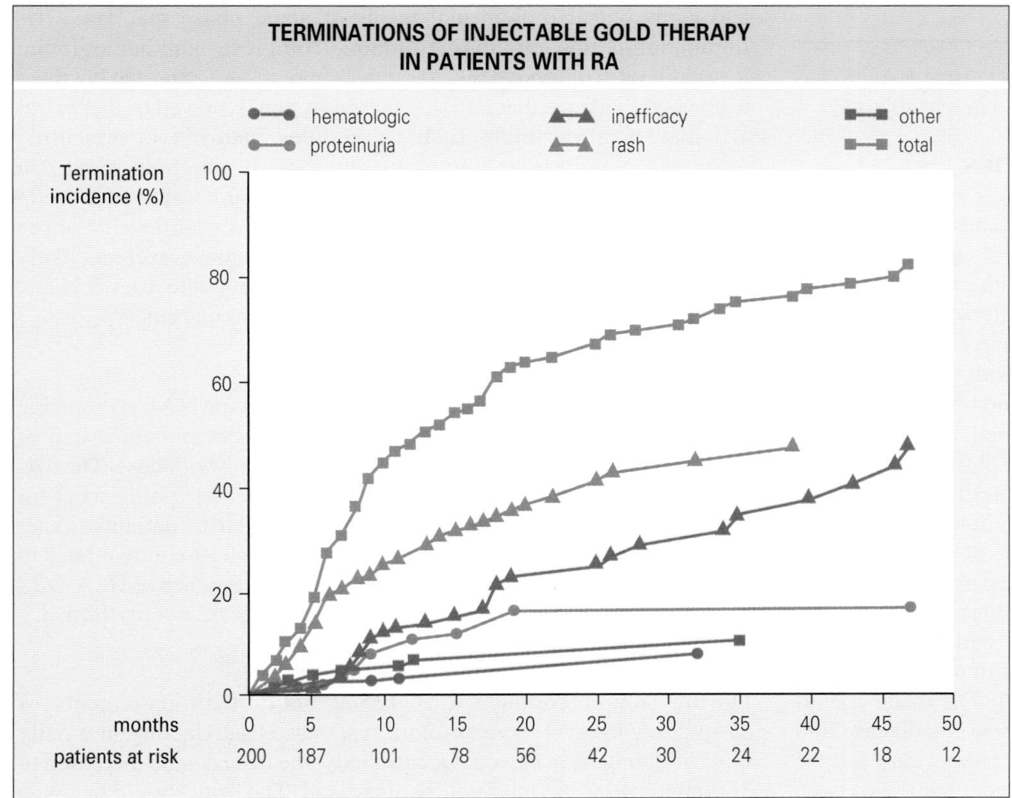

Fig. 8.6 Terminations from injectable gold therapy in patients with RA. A life-table analysis. Adapted from Sambrook *et al.*[18].

TOXIC EFFECTS OF GOLD COMPOUNDS	
Organ	Notes
Mucocutaneous (60–80% of toxicity)	Dermatitis and mouth ulcers; pruritus commonest; rashes usually erythematous and macular but rarely can exfoliate.
Vasomotor	Within minutes usually of aurothiomalate injection and include sweating, flushing, nausea, faintness, hypotension and weakness; malaise, fatigue and myalgia can follow injections.
Kidney	Transient and minor proteinuria commonly; occasional membranous glomerulonephropathy; rarely nephrotic syndrome which usually recovers in months to years; weak association with HLA-DR3/HLA-B8.
Blood	Eosinophilia occurs often prior to a toxic reaction. Neutropenia due to gold, as opposed to RA itself, is suggested by rapid or progressive fall in neutrophils. Thrombocytopenia (occurs in 1–3%); usually minor but can be precipitate and serious. Aplastic anemia rare but has a high fatality rate. Recombinant DNA-derived human hemopoietic growth factors have improved outcome somewhat.
Lung	Hypersensitivity pneumonitis reversible on cessation of gold. Case reports of bronchiolitis obliterans.
Liver	Case reports of cholestasis, fatty and inflammatory cell infiltrates.
Bowel	Case reports of enterocolitis with some deaths.
Nervous system	Case reports of peripheral and cranial neuropathies, Guillain–Barré syndrome, encephalopathy, myokymia

Fig. 8.7 Toxic effects of gold compounds.

needed. Gold can be reintroduced once the reaction has been absent for some weeks, using extremely small doses of aurothiomalate or, preferably, aurothioglucose.

D-PENICILLAMINE

D-Penicillamine (DPA) has been used for 25 years to treat RA and has been shown to have some benefit in progressive systemic sclerosis.

MECHANISM OF ACTION, PHARMACOKINETICS AND PHARMACODYNAMICS

The D enantiomer of penicillamine is employed because of the greater toxicity of the L enantiomer. Plasma concentrations of DPA reach a peak between 1.5 and 4 hours following oral dosage with bioavailability of between 50–70% which can be reduced substantially with enteric coating of the DPA, concurrent food, antacids and oral iron preparations[20]. The drug has a volume of distribution of 57–93 l, with little uptake into cells, in keeping with its low lipid solubility, and avid binding to plasma albumin from which it dissociates slowly[21]. D-Penicillamine is cleared largely through oxidation to form disulfides with plasma albumin, L-cysteine, homocysteine and itself resulting in penicillamine disulfide (Fig. 8.8). D-Penicillamine albumin disulfide accumulates in the first weeks of therapy to concentrations five times those of DPA in plasma, making it a 'sink' for DPA for a considerable time period[21]. *S*-methyl-DPA and *N*-acetyl-DPA are minor urinary metabolites of DPA.

D-Penicillamine readily forms thiazolidines with aldehydes or ketones and this could be important in its actions in progressive systemic sclerosis and the cutaneous toxicity of DPA. The metal chelating property of DPA underlies its efficacy in Wilson's disease and heavy metal poisoning. Transition metals such as copper catalyze the oxidation of DPA to disulfides and in the process reactive oxygen

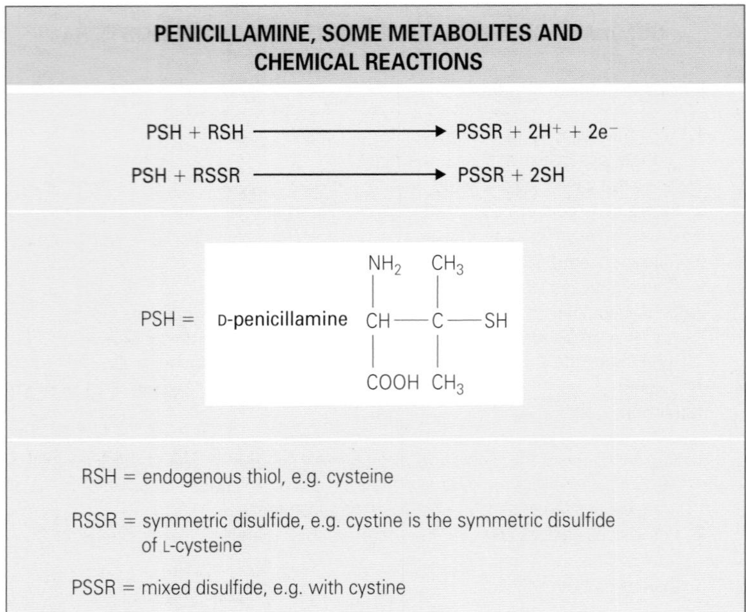

Fig. 8.8 D-Penicillamine and its chemical reactions.

species such as hydrogen peroxide are formed which may be responsible for some of the biological actions of DPA.

Although the mode of action of DPA is uncertain it seems likely that the drug could modulate the immune system via sulfhydryl exchange reactions on or in various cells. Thus, the activities of T-lymphocytes, natural killer (NK) cells, monocytes and macrophages may be modulated by whether cell surface receptor sulfhydryl groups are oxidized or reduced, these reactions being influenced by DPA therapy. Recent data reveal DPA-induced inhibition of the binding of the transcription factor AP-1 to DNA, analogous to the effect of gold, sustaining the long-held belief that the two drugs may have a common mode of action related to shared sulfhydryl reactivities[22].

EFFICACY

D-Penicillamine is efficacious in RA, improving not only symptoms and signs but also abnormal levels of acute phase reactants, RF, immunoglobulins, circulating immune complexes and hemoglobin. Response rates of around 60–70% after 6 months are expected but there is no good evidence that radiologic progression is slowed or that extra-articular manifestations such as nodules, neuritis or vasculitis respond[20]. Similarly to gold treatment, there is a high drop-out rate over time due to lack or loss of efficacy and also because of toxicity (Fig. 8.9). D-Penicillamine seems as effective as azathioprine, more effective than chloroquine and auranofin, and patients were as likely to be taking DPA as sulfasalazine and aurothiomalate after 5 years; however overall the differences demonstrated are marginal[20].

TOXICITY

Toxicity is common with about 50% of patients with RA experiencing an adverse effect in the first 6 months of treatment and about half of these having to cease DPA, the incidence increasing with dose. The toxicity profile is similar to that observed with injectable gold except for the autoimmune phenomena (Fig. 8.10). Similar to patients taking injectable gold therapy, there is an increased risk for toxicity related to a low metabolic capacity for sulfoxidation or the presence of HLA-DR3 or -B8. However, practically, these investigations are not performed.

PRACTICAL PRESCRIBING TIPS

Dosing should commence at 125mg daily with increments of 125mg/day every 4–8 weeks until response is satisfactory or a daily dose of 750mg is achieved. Occasionally, the dose can be increased to 1500mg/day but toxicity will be increased. The drug should be taken

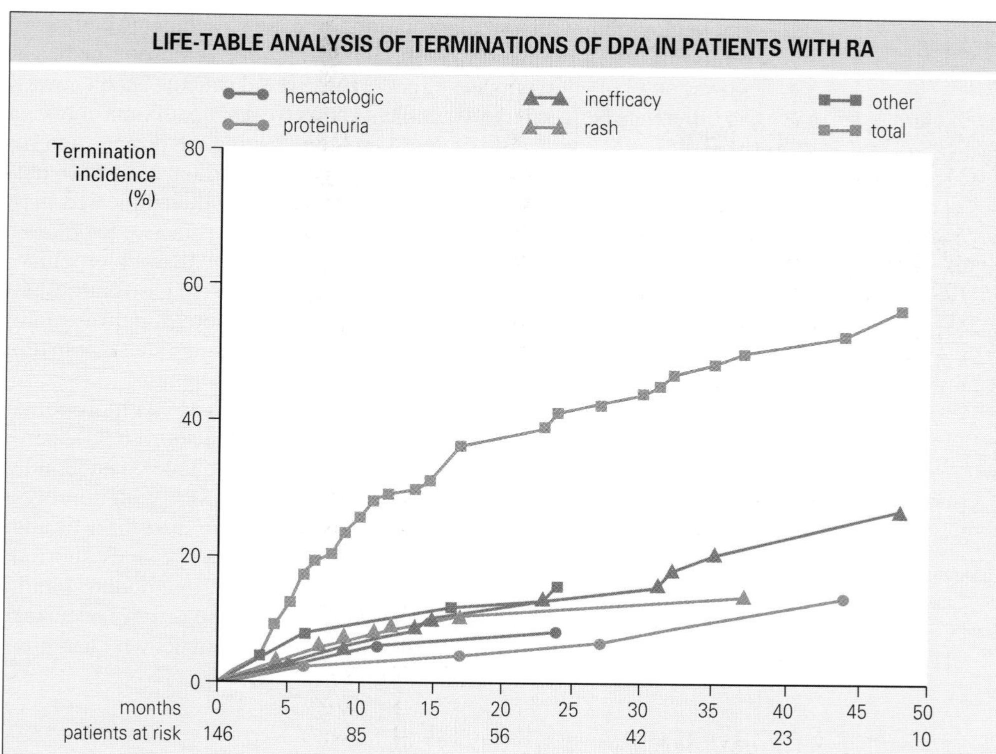

Fig. 8.9 Life-table analysis of terminations of D-penicillamine in patients with RA. Adapted from Champion *et al.*[23].

preferably in a nonenteric form and away from meals (e.g. 1–2 hours before), antacids and iron preparations. Dosage should be continued for 4–6 months before deciding if the drug has efficacy.

Mild skin rashes and pruritus can resolve with continued therapy but severe urticaria or pemphigus require immediate cessation of DPA.

A complete blood count and urinalysis should be performed regularly after 1 then 2 weeks and then at intervals of 2–4 weeks. Platelet counts of less than 150×10^9/l require dose reduction and weekly complete blood counts to determine appropriate action. Counts less than 100×10^9/l demand immediate cessation with careful reinstitution of therapy once the platelet count recovers to greater than 150×10^9/l. Significant leukopenia also demands permanent cessation of DPA and if there is a clear decline in leukocyte count, even within the normal range, the drug should be stopped and only very carefully reintroduced with increased frequency of surveillance. Patients need to be aware of symptoms that could indicate serious blood dyscrasias (e.g. fever, significant mouth ulceration, bleeding and abnormal bruising), so they can stop DPA and seek urgent medical attention.

Urine protein should be measured if the dipstick test is greater than a trace, but therapy can continue if 24 hour urine output is less than 1.0g. Dosage reduction or cessation and careful observation are required for greater amounts of proteinuria but very gradual reintroduction is possible in less severe cases. Heavy proteinuria and nephrotic syndrome may require investigation such as renal biopsy to rule out other causes and should respond to cessation of drug. Microscopic hematuria needs investigation because of the possibility of glomerulonephritis.

If patients have responded well to a carefully established dosage regimen with DPA, it is best to maintain that dose rate. If control of rheumatoid disease activity is lost, consider compliance or reduced bioavailability before gradually increasing the dose up to 750mg/day.

TOXICITY OF D-PENICILLAMINE

Organ	Notes
Mucocutaneous	Pruritic and urticarial rash commonest; oral ulcers and stomatitis; possible increased risk in penicillin allergy. Pemphigus.
Gastrointestinal	Nausea. Dysgeusia or metallic taste especially early in therapy which usually resolves slowly.
Kidney	Proteinuria common; occasional hematuria may indicate rapidly progressive glomerulonephritis, e.g. Goodpasture's syndrome or SLE, and is life-threatening requiring corticosteroids and immunosuppressives; membranous or proliferative glomerulonephritis; rarely nephrotic syndrome which usually recovers in months to years; weak association with HLA-DR3/HLA-B8.
Blood	Gradual or rapid effects at any time. Thrombocytopenia which can be precipitate and serious. Neutropenia due to D-penicillamine, as opposed to RA itself, is suggested by rapid or progressive fall in neutrophils. Aplastic anemia has a high fatality rate.
Lung	Case reports of bronchiolitis obliterans.
Autoimmune	Myasthenia gravis. Polymyositis/dermatomyositis. Goodpasture's syndrome (antiglomerular basement membrane antibody may be present). Drug-induced SLE. Pemphigus (oral involvement common); dangerous and requires cessation of drug, glucocorticosteroids and, perhaps, plasmapheresis.
Pregnancy	Teratogenesis.

Fig. 8.10 Toxicity of D-penicillamine in RA.

ANTIMALARIALS

Chloroquine and hydroxychloroquine (see Fig. 8.11) have been used to treat RA and systemic lupus erythematosus (SLE) since the 1950s and responses in RA are similar but somewhat less than observed with most other SAARDs except for auranofin. The antimalarials have a major advantage in their lack of life-threatening toxicity compared to other SAARDs. Thus, antimalarials are increasingly being used early in the course of RA and in combination regimens with other SAARDs.

MECHANISM OF ACTION

The massive accumulation of chloroquine and hydroxychloroquine in the important intracellular, acid vesicular lysosomal system of lymphocytes, macrophages, fibroblasts and polymorphs may be instrumental in the antirheumatic activity of these drugs in RA and SLE. The various functions of this system, such as glycosylation of proteins,

ANTIMALARIALS USED IN RHEUMATIC DISEASES

(Structure: 7-chloroquinoline with 4-position $HN-CH(CH_3)-CH_2-CH_2-CH_2-N(R_1)(R_2)$)

	R_1	R_2
Chloroquine	CH_2CH_3	CH_2CH_3
Hydroxychloroquine	CH_2CH_3	CH_2CH_2OH
Desethylchloroquine	CH_2CH_3	H
Desethylhydroxychloroquine	H	CH_2CH_2OH
Bisdesethylchloroquine	H	H

Fig. 8.11 Antimalarials used in the treatment of the rheumatic diseases. Chloroquine is formulated as a phosphate salt and hydroxychloroquine is formulated as either sulfate or phosphate salts. Hydroxychloroquine tablets contain 200mg of the sulfate and 155mg of the base while chloroquine tablets contain 250mg of the phosphate or 200mg of the sulfate and 150mg of the base.

digestion of membrane lipids, turnover of cell surface receptors, etc., may be changed as a result of alkalinization of the lysosome and/or by effects on acid protease function and release[24]. Antimalarials may inhibit the antigen-processing ability of monocytes and macrophages thereby inhibiting responses of lymphocytes to antigens *ex vivo*. Additionally, interleukin-1 (IL-1) release from monocytes and macrophages is inhibited at realistic concentrations and this may have important effects[25].

PHARMACOKINETICS AND PHARMACODYNAMICS

Chloroquine and hydroxychloroquine should be administered with food as, although the rate of absorption is slowed, bioavailability is not substantially affected and gastrointestinal adverse effects are reduced[24,26]. The bioavailability of hydroxychloroquine in patients with RA is about 80% but varies three-fold and therefore may contribute to variability in patient response[27].

The antimalarials have exceptionally long half-lives of the order of 40 days which indicates that there will be a 3–4 month delay before steady-state concentrations are achieved. The antimalarials accumulate in tissues and white and red blood cells extensively[28]. Tissue accumulation is explained in large part by the avid uptake of antimalarials by lysosomes due to the relative acidity of these cellular structures (pH 4.8) versus plasma and the basic nature of the drugs. This explains the high tissue concentrations in liver, which is lysosome rich, and the low concentrations in muscle, which is lysosome poor.

Chloroquine and hydroxychloroquine are metabolized primarily by dealkylation. About 40% and 25% of doses of chloroquine and hydroxychloroquine respectively are excreted unchanged in urine indicating the need for adjustment of dosages downward in substantially renally impaired patients. Higher blood concentrations of hydroxychloroquine were associated with less disease activity in a retrospective, cross-sectional study of patients with RA[29]. Recent data indicate that there is substantial intersubject variability in steady-state blood concentrations of hydroxychloroquine and chloroquine suggesting potential value in blood concentration monitoring.

EFFICACY

Well-controlled, double-blind studies of hydroxychloroquine and chloroquine against placebo in patients with RA demonstrate efficacy in 60–80% of patients apparent over 4–6 months treatment in standard parameters of disease activity including functional class, joint count, pain, grip strength, morning stiffness, patient and observer's assessments, ESR and hemoglobin with a small proportion of patients achieving complete remission[30,31]. Compared to sulfasalazine, hydroxychloroquine has a slower onset of antirheumatic effect in rheumatoid patients but there was no difference between these treatments at 48 weeks[32]. Sulfasalazine was more effective than hydroxychloroquine in slowing the progression of bony erosions around joints in a recent study[33]. Antimalarials have not been proven to retard erosion formation. Older studies indicated that hydroxychloroquine 200–600mg/day was similarly effective to chloroquine 250–500mg/ day in patients with RA, with hydroxychloroquine having a slight advantage with respect to fewer adverse gastrointestinal effects. However, a meta-analysis revealed that chloroquine was more effective than hydroxychloroquine at the usual dosing rates employed for both drugs[9], a surprising finding requiring confirmation.

Children with juvenile RA were treated with hydroxychloroquine 6mg/kg/day for 12 months in a double-blind trial but showed little benefit compared to placebo[34]. A number of studies indicate considerable efficacy of hydroxychloroquine and chloroquine in SLE with improvement in malaise and tiredness, disease flare-ups, skin rash, arthritis and pleuritic pain. However, a recent double-blind, 48-week-study showed a significant effect on joint pain only[35]. Moreover, in a double-blind, placebo-controlled study significant flares in disease activity occurred when hydroxychloroquine was withdrawn from patients who had previously been stabilized on the drug[36].

TOXICITY

In contrast to other SAARDs, the majority of adverse effects of antimalarials are transient and not serious and generally cessation of drug is unnecessary (Fig. 8.12). Hydroxychloroquine in the usual doses employed is less likely to be associated with adverse effects than chloroquine.

Irreversible retinopathy, characterized by progressive decrease in visual fields and irreversible blindness, in combination with characteristic fundal changes have been reported in a number of patients taking chloroquine at higher doses than is now recommended. Relatively very few reports incriminate hydroxychloroquine, but in part this may reflect the relative use of chloroquine and hydroxychloroquine. Consensus opinion is that retinal toxicity correlates with daily dose of drug and that upper dosage limits for adults should be 4mg base/kg/day for chloroquine and 6mg base/kg/day for hydroxychloroquine.

PRACTICAL PRESCRIBING TIPS

Response to antimalarials is slow and, although initial effects may be seen around a month, full effects may not be apparent until around 6 months of therapy has elapsed. Dosage limits of around 6mg

TOXICITY OF ANTIMALARIALS IN RA AND SLE

Organ	Notes
Mucocutaneous	Pruritic and urticarial rash; stomatitis.
Gastrointestinal	Anorexia; nausea; vomiting; abdominal pain, diarrhea.
CNS	Dizziness; tinnitus; headache.
Eyes	Blurred vision and accommodation difficulty, especially early in therapy which resolves with continued therapy. Photophobia. Retinal damage (bull's eye retinopathy).
Pregnancy	Crosses placenta; theoretically hazardous therefore avoid if possible; some cases of fetal abnormalities reported but little data.
Overdose	Chloroquine more dangerous; cardiorespiratory failure occurs rapidly; emphasize importance of keeping medication away from children.

Fig. 8.12 Toxicity of antimalarial therapy in the treament of RA and SLE. (CNS, central nervous system.)

base/kg/day for hydroxychloroquine or 4mg base/kg/day of chloroquine in practice mean 400mg/day of hydroxychloroquine sulfate (2 tablets) and 250mg of chloroquine phosphate (1 tablet). If body weight is substantially outside the 60–70kg range then alterations in dosing either up or down should be instituted. If clearly beneficial, then antimalarial therapy should be continued. In the most common situation encountered of partial response, the addition of a second SAARD is increasingly being considered despite lack of evidence from trials[37].

Careful ophthalmologic screening at baseline and every 6–12 months is recommended to identify retinal damage which is extremely uncommon but reversible if identified early. This includes funduscopy and visual field charting by an ophthalmologist. Patients should be advised to report any visual symptoms especially decreased night vision, loss of central or peripheral vision and intolerance of glare. A complete blood count and urinalysis can be performed at intervals coinciding with ophthalmological review.

SULFASALAZINE

In the late 1930s, Professor Nanna Svartz of Stockholm, in collaboration with the Pharmacia company, synthesized sulfasalazine which consists of salicylic acid joined to sulfapyridine by an azo bond (Fig. 8.13). After a long period of indifference to the value of sulfasalazine as an antirheumatic drug, studies by McConkey, Amos and others in the late 1970s rekindled interest in its rheumatologic potential. Sulfasalazine is an effective and relatively safe antirheumatic drug in RA and uniquely has efficacy in ankylosing spondylitis and HLA-B27 related arthropathies. Also, the drug appears to have efficacy in juvenile arthritis and psoriatic arthritis.

MECHANISM OF ACTION

The mode of antirheumatic action of sulfasalazine is unknown but sulfasalazine and/or sulfapyridine may suppress immunologic processes in the gut of relevance to the pathogenesis of RA and spondyloarthropathies. Potentially important mechanisms include the ability of sulfasalazine to scavenge proinflammatory reactive oxygen species released from activated phagocytes. Effects on prostanoid levels may be important, synthesis of leukotriene B_4 in polymorphs and thromboxane A_2 in platelets being inhibited[38].

The numbers of activated lymphocytes circulating are reduced after 12 weeks sulfasalazine therapy. This is accompanied by significant falls in IgM and RF titers, but there are no changes in lymphocyte subsets and lymphocyte responses to concanavalin-A *ex vivo* are restored to normal. These effects could be a consequence of decreased rheumatoid disease activity via other mechanisms.

PHARMACOKINETICS AND PHARMACODYNAMICS

There is little absorption of intact sulfasalazine (10–20%) as the drug is quite insoluble. Sulfapyridine and 5-aminosalicylic acid are liberated in the colon following bacterial reduction of the azo bond (Fig. 8.13) and virtually no sulfasalazine is found in stools. Concomitant cholestyramine is likely to reduce the availability of sulfapyridine as it binds sulfasalazine rendering it unavailable for bacterial digestion. Sulfasalazine is highly protein bound (>95%), peak plasma concentrations occurring 3–5 hours postdose with an apparent plasma elimination half-life of 6–17 hours, probably reflecting the absorption half-life (Fig. 8.14).

About 50% of 5-aminosalicylic acid is recovered in feces while 30% is excreted in urine as its *N*-acetylation product. Sulfapyridine, which appears in plasma 4–6 hours postdosing, is subject to extensive metabolism to N^4-acetylation and ring hydroxylation products and subsequent glucuronidation of these metabolites. Genetically determined variation in 'acetylation' and 'oxidative' capacities, respectively, leads to substantial contrasts in rates of metabolism of sulfapyridine and steady-state plasma concentrations.

Sulfapyridine may be the antirheumatic principle of sulfasalazine while 5-aminosalicylic acid is the anti-inflammatory species in inflammatory bowel disease. However, sulfasalazine could have important antirheumatic actions either in the gut or systemically in its own right. To date, no plasma concentration response relationships for sulfapyridine have been discerned[38,40].

EFFICACY

Sulfasalazine exhibits specific antirheumatic actions and is about as effective as gold and DPA. It is slightly more effective than antimalarials but works more rapidly, benefits becoming apparent at 4 weeks. Sulfasalazine has less serious adverse effects but discontinuation rates are similar to other SAARDs[8,39]. Radiologic progression of RA was significantly less for sulfasalazine than hydroxychloroquine at 24 and 48 weeks, this advantage being still sustained at 3 years[34,41], supporting other studies suggesting sulfasalazine retards radiologic progression in RA.

Uncontrolled studies of sulfasalazine combined with DPA and gold respectively suggest increased efficacy but increased discontinuations due to toxicity.

Sulfasalazine is considered an effective SAARD in juvenile arthritis despite the lack of controlled studies[42]. Controlled, double-blind studies in ankylosing spondylitis, up to 52 weeks duration, indicate efficacy of sulfasalazine with a slightly slower onset of action than in

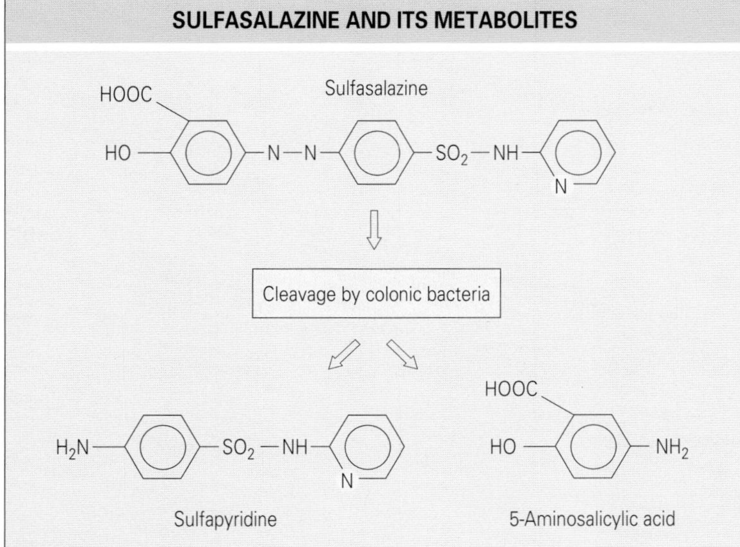

Fig. 8.13 Sulfasalazine and its metabolites. The role of the colon in liberation of sulfapyridine is illustrated.

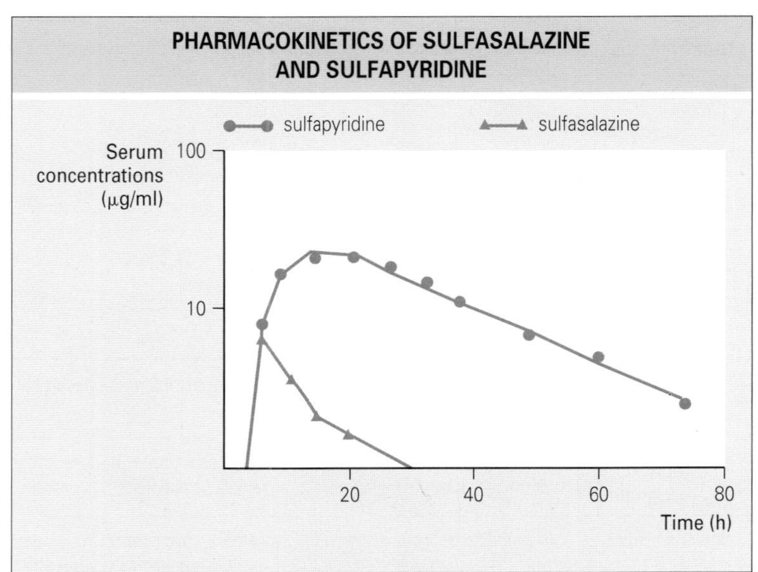

Fig. 8.14 Pharmacokinetics of sulfasalazine and sulfapyridine. Sulfasalazine and sulfapyridine concentrations following a single 2g oral dose of sulfasalazine. Adapted from Taggart *et al.*[39].

RA[43]. Sulfasalazine appeared highly effective in patients with HLA-B27 associated asymmetric, pauciarticular arthritis in an open, uncontrolled study[44]. Sulfasalazine shows efficacy in patients with psoriatic arthritis without exacerbation of skin disease[45].

TOXICITY

Sulfasalazine ranks with antimalarials and auranofin as the best tolerated of the SAARDs. Thus, in a study of 774 RA patients followed for 1–11 years there were no deaths or long-term adverse effects[46]. Adverse effects are commonest in the first 2–3 months of therapy. The commonest side effects involve the gastrointestinal tract, hematologic, skin and central nervous system (Fig. 8.15). Dose reduction is often effective in reducing these adverse effects. Nausea and upper abdominal discomfort, often in association with headache and dizziness, are the commonest adverse effects in the first months of therapy and are less likely if dosage is increased gradually. An enteric-coated formulation of sulfasalazine is better tolerated than uncoated formulations. Despite sulfasalazine being ranked as relatively well tolerated, reports of continuation rates on the drug vary from 40–70% after 2 years, attrition due to adverse effects and inefficacy. After 5 years around 20% of patients were still taking sulfasalazine, similar to rates for gold and DPA.

Leukopenia is most likely in the first 6 months of treatment but can occur at any time indicating the need for continued review, particularly because early recognition and dosage cessation or reduction leads to reversal in most cases.

Although no teratogenetic or perinatal morbidity or mortality has been observed in the progeny of male or female patients taking sulfasalazine at conception or during pregnancy, this drug should be avoided in these circumstances if possible. Little sulfasalazine enters milk and sulfapyridine levels are 40% of plasma levels. Sulfasalazine is considered safe for breast-feeding infants. Rapidly reversible male infertility occurs in association with sulfasalazine due to reduction in sperm count, sperm motility and also morphologic abnormalities of the sperm. This effect has not been considered a contraindication to the use of sulfasalazine in males but the drug should be withdrawn in males wishing to father children.

PRACTICAL PRESCRIBING TIPS

Adult dosage for rheumatic diseases is around 2g (range 1.5–3g/day) of the enteric-coated formulation, usually 1g twice a day with meals. Tolerance is improved if starting doses of 500mg to 1g/day are selected incrementing by 500mg/day at minimum intervals of a week. Increases above 2g/day are rarely helpful. Neutropenia is likely to occur suddenly and monitoring policies designed to avoid this are difficult. Many rheumatologists perform blood counts every 2–4 weeks during the first 3 months of therapy and then reduce the frequency. It is important that patients understand that there is a possibility of serious hematologic effects and that they learn to recognize the important signs such as sore throat, fever and significant malaise.

COMBINATIONS

Many rheumatologists are using combinations of SAARDs including methotrexate[47] despite lack of objective evidence of efficacy from the few studies performed[48]. Recent data from a 2-year study indicate that a combination of methotrexate, sulfasalazine 1g/day and hydroxychloroquine 400mg/day with methotrexate dosing from 7.5mg to 17.5mg/week in order to induce remission is substantially more effective than methotrexate alone or sulfasalazine plus hydroxychloroquine[49]. Undoubtedly, such results will stimulate further analysis of the potential of combinations of SAARDs.

CONCLUSION

There is uniform support for the early introduction of SAARD therapy once RA has been diagnosed, the conception being that effective suppression of disease activity in the first few years will prevent the long-term deleterious effects of RA[7]. A major meta-analysis revealed that there was little difference between methotrexate, injectable gold, DPA and sulfasalazine with regard to efficacy, members of this group being slightly more effective than antimalarials, and clearly more effective than auranofin, while antimalarials and auranofin were best tolerated (Fig. 8.16). Safe use of SAARDs requires careful monitoring. Authoritative guidelines have recently become available[50]. Increasingly, rheumatologists are commencing therapy with methotrexate[7]. Also, combinations of SAARDs including methotrexate are being employed in RA that is persistently active although there is as yet little trial evidence to underpin the practice[7]. Early assessment with decisive selection of therapy based on an individual patient's risk for poor outcome combined with an aggressive approach to non-response to therapy are essential components of the contemporary approach to the management of RA.

TOXICITY OF SULFASALAZINE	
Common adverse effects	
Gastrointestinal	Nausea, vomiting, malaise, anorexia, abdominal pain, dyspepsia, indigestion.
CNS	Headache, pyrexia, light headedness, dizziness.
Less common and some serious adverse effects	
General	Hypersensitivity reactions.
Skin	Rash (pruritic, macular papular) 1–5%, alopecia, Stevens–Johnson syndrome and related serious skin disorders. Rarely serum sickness.
Hepatic	Hepatic enzyme elevations; acute hepatic reactions; more serious damage has been described.
Lung	Fibrosing alveolitis; rarely reversible pulmonary infiltrates accompanied by eosinophilia, fever and weight loss have been described.
Hematologic	Leukopenia (1–3%); thrombocytopenia (less frequent than leukopenia); hemolysis, MCV increased; methemoglobinemia; aplastic anemia; agranulocytosis.
Nervous system	Irreversible neuromuscular and CNS effects rarely reported.
Kidney	Serious kidney damage has occurred rarely.

Fig. 8.15 Toxicity of sulfasalazine.

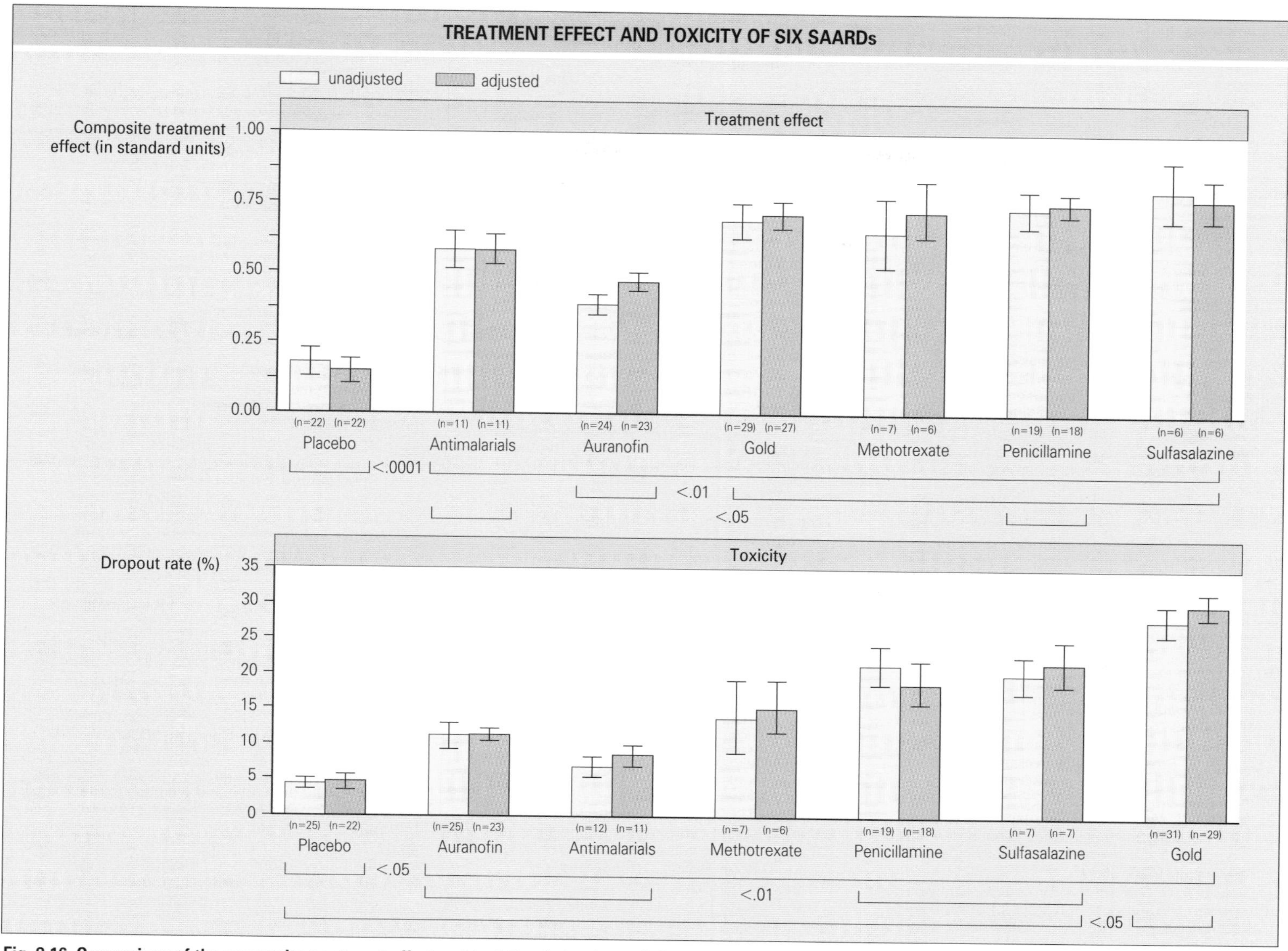

Fig. 8.16 Comparison of the composite treatment effect and toxicity of placebo and six second-line antirheumatic drugs. n = the number of treatment groups included. Adapted from Felson *et al.*[9].

REFERENCES

1. Paulus H, Egger M, Ward J, Williams HJ and the Cooperative Systematic Studies of Rheumatic Diseases Group. Analysis of improvement in individual rheumatoid arthritis patients treated with disease-modifying antirheumatic drugs, based on the findings in patients treated with placebo. Arthritis Rheum. 1990;33:477–88.
2. Pincus T. Rheumatoid arthritis: disappointing long-term outcomes despite successful short-term clinical trials. J Clin Epidemiol. 1988;41:1037–41.
3. Wolfe F, Hawley D, Cathey M. Termination of slow acting antirheumatic therapy in rheumatoid arthritis: a 14-year prospective evaluation of 1017 consecutive starts. J Rheumatol. 1990;17:994–1002.
4. Emery P. The optimal management of early rheumatoid disease: the key to preventing disability. Br J Rheumatol. 1994;33:765–8
5. Wolfe F. 50 years of antirheumatic therapy: The prognosis of rheumatoid arthritis. J Rheumatol. 1990;17(Suppl 22):24–32.
6. Van der Heide A, Jacobs JWG, Bijlsma JWJ, *et al.* The effectiveness of early treatment with second-line antirheumatic drugs: a randomized, controlled trial. Ann Intern Med. 1996;124:699–707.
7. American College of Rheumatology Ad Hoc Committee on Clinical Guidelines. Guidelines for the management of rheumatoid arthritis. Arth Rheum. 1996;39:713–22
8. Day R, Breit S, Cairns D, Champion G. Aspects of the clinical trials of slow acting anti-rheumatic drugs. In: Brooks P, Day R, Williams K, Graham G, eds. Basis for variability of response to anti-rheumatic drugs. Agents Actions. 1988;:121–35.
9. Felson D, Anderson J, Meenan R. The comparative efficacy and toxicity of second-line drugs in rheumatoid arthritis. Arthritis Rheum. 1990;33:1449–61.
10. Felson D, Anderson J, Meenan R. The use of short-term efficacy/toxicity tradeoffs to select second-line drugs in rheumatoid arthritis: a metaanalysis of published clinical trials. Arthritis Rheum. 1992;35:1117–25.
11. Champion G, Graham G, Zeigler J. The gold

complexes. In: Brooks P, ed. Slow-acting antirheumatic drugs and immunosuppressives. Ballière's Clin Rheumatol. 1990;4:491–534.
12. Snyder RM, Mirabelli C, Crooke S. Cellular association, intracellular distribution, and efflux of auranofin via sequential ligand exchange reactions. Biochem Pharmacol. 1986;35:923–32.
13. Handel ML, Watts CKW, Day RO, Sutherland RL. Inhibition of AP-1 binding and transcription by gold and selenium involving conserved cysteine residues in *Jun* and *Fos*. Proc Natl Acad Sci. 1995;92:4497–501.
14. Lipsky P, Ziff M. Inhibition of antigen- and mitogen-induced human lymphocyte proliferation by gold compounds. J Clin Invest. 1977;59:455–66.
15. Sanders K, Carlson P, Littman B. Effects of gold sodium thiomalate on interferon stimulation of C2 synthesis and HLA-DR expression by human moncocytes. Arthritis Rheum. 1987;30:1032–9.
16. Haynes D, Garrett I, Whitehouse M, Vernon-Roberts B. Do gold drugs inhibit interleukin-1? Evidence from an *in vitro* lymphocyte activating factor assay. J Rheumatol. 1988;15:775–8.
17. Blocka K, Furst D, Landaw E, Dromgoole S, Blomberg A, Paulus H. Single dose pharmacokinetics of auranofin in rheumatoid arthritis. J Rheumatol. 1982;9(Suppl 8):110–19.
18. Sambrook P, Browne C, Champion G, *et al.* Terminations of treatment with gold sodium thiomalate in rheumatoid arthritis. J Rheumatol. 1982;9:932–4.
19. Heuer M, Pietrusko R, Morris R, Scheffler B. An analysis of worldwide safety experience with auranofin. J Rheumatol. 1985;12:695–9.
20. Joyce D. D-Penicillamine. In: Brooks P, ed. Slow-acting antirheumatic drugs and immunosuppressives. Ballière's Clin Rheumatol. 1990;4:553–74.
21. Joyce D. D-Penicillamine pharmacokinetics and action. In: Brooks P, Day R, Williams K, Graham G, eds. Basis for variability of response to anti-rheumatic drugs. Agents Actions. 1988:197–206.
22. Handel ML, Watts CKW, Sivertsen S, Day RO, Sutherland RL. D-penicillamine causes free radical dependent inactivation of AP-1 DNA binding. Mol Pharmacol. 1996; 50:1–5.
23. Champion G, Sambrook P, Browne C, Day R, Vallance J, Warwick N. Influence of previous gold on d-penicillamine toxicity. In: Dawkins R, *et al.* Immunogenetics in rheumatology. Amsterdam: Excerpta Medica; 1982:311–16.
24. Tett S, Cutler D, Day R. Antimalarials in rheumatic diseases. In: Brooks P, ed. Slow-acting antirheumatic drugs and immunosuppressives. Ballière's Clin Rheumatol. 1990;4:467–89.
25. Salmeron G, Lipsky P. Immunosuppressive potential of antimalarials. Am J Med. 1983;75(Suppl IA):19–24.
26. McLachlan AJ, Tett SE, Cutler DJ, Day RO. Absorption and *in vivo* dissolution of hydroxychloroquine in fed subjects assessed using deconvolution techniques. Br J Clin Pharmacol. 1993;36:405–11.
27. McLachlan AJ, Tett SE, Cutler DJ, Day RO. Bioavailability of hydroxychloroquine tablets in patients with rheumatoid arthritis. Br J Rheumatol. 1994;33:235–9.
28. Tett S, Cutler D, Day R, Brown K. Dose-ranging study of the pharmacokinetics of hydroxychloroquine following intravenous administration to healthy volunteers. Br J Clin Pharmacol. 1988;26:303–13.
29. Tett SE, Day RO, Cutler DJ. Concentration–effect relationship of hydroxychloroquine in rheumatoid arthritis – a cross sectional study. J Rheumatol. 1993;20:1874–9.
30. Clark P, Casa E, Tugwell P, *et al.* Hydroxychloroquine compared with placebo in rheumatoid arthritis. A randomised controlled trial. Ann Intern Med. 1993;119:1067–71.
31. HERA Study Group. A randomised trial of hydroxychloroquine in early rheumatoid arthritis: The HERA Study. Am J Med. 1995:98:156–68.
32. Nuver-Zwart I, Van Riel P, Van De Putte L, Gribnau F. A double blind comparative study of sulphasalazine and hydroxychloroquine in rheumatoid arthritis: evidence of an earlier effect of sulphasalazine. Ann Rheum Dis. 1989;48:389–95.
33. Van Der Heijde D, Van Riel P, Nuver-Zwart I, Gribnau F, Van De Putte L. Effects of hydroxychloroquine and sulphasalazine on progression of joint damage in rheumatoid arthritis. Lancet. 1989;i:1036–8.
34. Brewer E, Giannini E, Kuzmina N, Alekseev L. Penicillamine and hydroxychloroquine in the treatment of severe juvenile rheumatoid arthritis. N Engl J Med. 1986;314:1269–76.
35. Williams HJ, Egger MJ, Singer JZ, *et al.* Comparison of hydroxychloroquine and placebo in the treatment of the arthropathy of mild systemic lupus erythematosus. J Rheumatol. 1994;21:1457–62.
36. The Canadian Hydroxychloroquine Study Group. A randomized study of the effect of withdrawing hydroxychloroquine sulfate in systemic lupus erythematosus. N Engl J Med. 1991;324:150–4.
37. Paulus H. Antimalarial agents compared with or in combination with other disease-modifying antirheumatic drugs. Am J Med. 1988;85:45–52.
38. Porter D, Capell H. The use of sulphasalazine as a disease modifying antirheumatic drug. In: Brooks P, ed. Slow-acting antirheumatic drugs and immunosuppressives. Ballière's Clin Rheumatol. 1990;4:535–51.
39. Taggart A, McDermott B, Delargy M, *et al.* The pharmacokinetics of sulphasalazine in young and elderly patients with rheumatoid arthritis. Scand J Rheumatol. 1987;64:29–36.
40. Chalmers I, Sitar D, Hunter T. A one-year, open, prospective study of sulfasalazine in the treatment of rheumatoid arthritis: Adverse reactions and clinical response in relation to laboratory variables, drug and metabolite serum levels and acetylator status. J Rheumatol. 1990;17:764–70.
41. Van der Heijde D, van Riel P, Nuver-Zwart E, *et al.* Sulphasalazine versus hydroxychloroquine in rheumatoid arthritis: 3-year follow-up. Lancet. 1990;335:539.
42. Grondin C, Malleson P, Petty R. Slow-acting antirheumatic drugs in chronic arthritis of childhood. Semin Arthritis Rheum. 1988;18:38–47.
43. Ferraz M, Tugwell P, Goldsmith C, *et al.* Meta-analysis of sulfasalazine in ankylosing spondylitis. J Rheumatol. 1990;17:1482–6.
44. Mielants H, Veys E, Joos R. Sulphasalazine (salazopyrin) in the treatment of enterogenic reactive arthritis and ankylosing spondylitis with peripheral arthritis. Clin Rheumatol. 1986;5:80–3.
45. Farr M, Kitas G, Waterhouse L, *et al.* Sulphasalazine in psoriatic arthritis: a double-blind placebo controlled study. Br J Rheumatol. 1990;29:46–9.
46. Amos R, Pullar T, Capell H, *et al.* Sulphasalazine for rheumatoid arthritis: toxicity in 774 patients monitored for one to 11 years. Br Med J. 1986;293:420–3.
47. Cash JM, Klippel JH. Second-line drug therapy for rheumatoid arthritis. New Eng J Med. 1994;330:1368–75.
48. Felson DT, Anderson JJ, Meenan RF. The efficacy and toxicity of combination therapy in rheumatoid arthritis: a meta-analysis. Arthritis Rheum. 1994;37:1487–91.
49. O'Dell JR, Haire CE, Erikson N, *et al.* Treatment of rheumatoid arthritis with methotrexate alone, sulfasalazine and hydroxychloroquine, or a combination of all three medications. New Eng J Med. 1996;334:1287–91.
50. American College of Rheumatology ad hoc Committee on Clinical Guidelines. Guidelines for monitoring drug therapy in rheumatoid arthritis. Arthritis Rheum. 1996;39:723–31.

IMMUNOSUPPRESSIVES

Daniel E Furst & Philip J Clements

- Of the immunosuppressive SAARDS, methotrexate is the most frequently used.
- There is some evidence that methotrexate, cyclophosphamide and cyclosporin inhibit bony damage resulting from RA.
- Cyclophosphamide and cyclosporin are associated with the most serious toxicity of these SAARDS.
- Combination SAARD therapy may be effective in aggressive RA.

INTRODUCTION

This chapter reviews the use of slow-acting antirheumatic drugs (SAARDs) not covered in Chapter 3.8, namely: antibiotics, azathioprine, chlorambucil, cyclophosphamide, cyclosporin, methotrexate and combination therapy.

Since the mechanisms of action of these drugs demonstrate some similarities (as well as differences), their mechanisms of action are addressed together (Fig. 9.1). Likewise, the pertinent pharmacokinetics of these medications are discussed in a single section. Thereafter, the evidence that these drugs are effective, their toxicity and tips on their use are separately addressed. The suggestions regarding therapeutic use represent a generally accepted approach that is typically not often fully tested.

MECHANISMS OF ACTION

SAARD	Active agent(s)	Mechanism	Reference
Azathioprine	6-Thioinosinic acid 6-Thioguanylic acid	Interferes with adenine and guanine ribonucleosides	5–10
Chlorambucil	Phenylacetic acid mustard (metabolite)	Cross-links DNA	7–10
Cyclophosphamide	Phosphoramide mustard (metabolite)	Cross-links DNA	5–12
Cyclosporin	Parent compound and up to 15 metabolites	Suppresses IL-2 synthesis and release Suppresses T-cell response and interaction	10–13
Methotrexate	Parent compound and metabolites, including 7-OH-methotrexate and methotrexate polyglutamates	Inhibition of dihydrofolate reductase, thymidylate synthetase and phosphoribosyl-aminoimidazole-carboxamide-transformylase activity IL-1 and IL-2 suppression	14–16
Tetracyclines	Parent compound	Metalloproteinase inhibition: possible effects on PMN and lymphocyte function	2–4

Fig. 9.1 Mechanisms of action.

MECHANISMS OF ACTION

ANTIBIOTICS

A persistent hypthosis exists that rheumatoid arthritis (RA) is caused by an infectious agent. Some antibiotics have been used to treat this disease. Despite lack of clear evidence supporting an 'infective hypothesis' for RA, these antibiotics might be effective because they have mechanisms of action independent of their antimicrobial effects. This section addresses the nonantimicrobial mechanisms that might account for activity in RA[1].

Dapsone is a drug used to treat leprosy, and may inhibit polymorphonuclear activity. *In vitro* studies indicate that dapsone, at concentrations achievable *in vivo*, reversibly inactivates myeloperoxidase, inhibits the release of prostaglandin E_2 by polymorphonuclear cells, inhibits polymorphonuclear neutrophil leukocyte (PMN) chemiluminescence and oxygen radical release *in vitro*, and prevents the activity of leukotriene B_4[2]. In animal adjuvant arthritis models, dapsone is antipyretic, analgesic and inhibits β-glucuronidase release[3].

Rifampin (rifampicin), in contrast, has a greater effect on lymphocytes. In early studies rifampin suppressed T-cell rosettes in humans and, at high doses, decreased lymphoid organ structure and suppressed T-cells in mice and guinea pigs[4].

Tetracycline has multiple immunomodulating and anti-inflammatory effects which include: decreased PMN phagocytosis, chemotaxis and migration and decreased phagocytosis in human monocytes; inhibited lymphocyte proliferative responses; inhibition of interferon-gamma ((IFN-γ) production and possibly calcium sensitive antibody production[1,2]. Tetracyclines clearly inhibit matrix metalloproteins from neutrophils, macrophages, osteoblasts, chondrocytes, epithelial cells and rheumatoid synoviocytes[1]. Minocycline and doxycycline are more effective in this latter regard than tetracycline, and their metalloproteinase-inhibiting activities may mediate a reduction in bone resorption[1].

AZATHIOPRINE

Azathioprine (AZA) interferes with adenine and guanine ribonucleotides via suppression of inosinic acid synthesis[5]. Its main active metabolite is 6-thioinosinic acid. This, in turn, is a metabolite of azathioprine's principal metabolic product, 6-mercaptopurine (6-MP)[6]. In RA, azathioprine reduces the numbers of circulating B and T-lymphocytes (particularly suppressor, or CD8, cells)[6], mixed lymphocyte reactivity[5], IgM and IgG synthesis[6,7] and interleukin (IL)-2 secretion[8].

CHLORAMBUCIL

Chlorambucil's mechanism of action is probably similar to that of cyclophosphamide: it cross-links deoxyribonucleic acid (DNA) and proteins, and thereby prevents cell replication[9]. Chlorambucil itself is not cytotoxic but is rapidly and almost completely metabolized to phenylacetic acid mustard, its principal and most active metabolite[10].

CYCLOPHOSPHAMIDE

Active metabolites (principally phosphoramide mustard) cross-link DNA so that it cannot replicate. Cyclophosphamide (CTX) is cytotoxic to both resting and dividing lymphocytes[9–11]. In RA patients cyclophosphamide suppresses helper cell functions, decreases the number of activated T-cells by 30–40% (which correlates with clinical improvement) and dramatically decreases B cells for months[12]. Low doses (20mg/kg) in mice affect mainly suppressor T-cells.

Cyclophosphamide readily suppresses primary cellular and humoral immune responses, especially if administered immediately after the antigen challenge, but can also inhibit an established humoral or immune response. It effectively suppresses many cell-mediated immune responses, such as delayed hypersensitivity skin test, graft-versus-host reactivity of lymphoid cells, cell-mediated cytotoxicity, mitogen- and antigen-induced blastogenesis and production of soluble mediators. It also has anti-inflammatory properties[9,10].

CYCLOSPORIN

Cyclosporin (CSA) complexes with cyclophilin (a cytoplasmic protein) which then binds calcineurin, an intracellular phosphatase. This, in turn, regulates gene transcription coding for IL-2 and other cytokines[10,12,13].

The major mechanisms of action of cyclosporin are related to:

- inhibition of IL-2 and IL-1 receptor production,
- inhibits macrophage–T-cell interactions and T-cell responsiveness.

Cyclosporin blocks the amplification of cellular immune responses and the generation of T-cell effectors and other functions dependent on IL-2. It inhibits the B cell production of antibody to T-cell-dependent antigens, the production of IFN-γ and natural killer (NK) cell activity. Growth of bone marrow-derived myeloid, erythroid or B lymphocyte cell lines is not inhibited, and B lymphocyte responses to T-cell-independent antigens are not affected. Although cyclosporin is a strong inhibitor of delayed hypersensitivity, it does not impair macrophage responses to lymphokines[10].

METHOTREXATE

Methotrexate (MTX) inhibits dihydrofolate reductase (DHFR), thus interrupting purine biosynthesis, as well as the synthesis of thymidylic and inosinic acids[14,15]. However, methotrexate is metabolized intercellularly to methotrexate polyglutamates and these long-lived metabolites inhibit DHFR plus other folate-dependent enzymes, such as thymidylate synthetase and 5-aminoimidazole-carboxamide-ribonucleotide-transformylase (AICAR)[14,16]. Kremer recently found normalization of low IL-2 through an effect on polyamine synthesis[16]. Other anti-inflammatory effects of methotrexate include reduced IgM-rheumatoid factor production, decreased IL-1 production, secretion or binding, and decreased IL-6 activity[15].

PHARMACOKINETICS

The most pertinent pharmacokinetics of the SAARDs are summarized in Figure 9.2. Additional comments regarding the pharmacokinetics of each drug are outlined below.

AZATHIOPRINE

Azathioprine is chemically cleaved to 6-MP, which is metabolized inside cells to thioinosinic and thioguanylic acid through the action of hypoxanthine phosphoribosyltransferase (HGPRT). The inosinic and thioguanylic acids, in turn, affect ribonucleotide synthesis. Thus, secondary intracellular metabolites are the source of azathioprine's activity, making blood or plasma levels of azathioprine unlikely to be very useful[17]. There are two populations of azathioprine metabolizers – with rapid metabolizers having four times the azathioprine clearance of slow metabolizers (mean total clearance: approximately 2 *vs* 8 l/kg/h)[17]. Very large intraindividual variability [variability of area under the concentration curve (AUC), day 1 *vs* day 2, as large as 257%] makes it hard to use kinetics productively[18].

A major pathway of 6-MP metabolism is via thiopurine methyltransferase (TM). This enzyme exhibits genetic polymorphism, and is found in very low concentrations in one out of 300 individuals, resulting in elevated thioguanylic acid when azathioprine is used. Escousse *et al.* support the contention that patients with low TM are at increased risk of myelosuppression[19].

CHLORAMBUCIL

Oral bioavailability of chlorambucil is adequate (0.70). It is rapidly and almost completely metabolized, at unknown sites, to phenylacetic acid mustard and several other poorly characterized metabolites[20,21]. Phenylacetic acid mustard is further metabolized, also at unknown sites. Each dose of chlorambucil is almost completely metabolized and renally excreted within 24 hours[20,21].

CYCLOPHOSPHAMIDE

Cyclophosphamide itself is not cytotoxic but is enzymatically converted by hepatic microsomal enzymes into multiple metabolites of which phosphoramide mustard is thought to be the most active cytotoxic agent[11,22,23]. Cyclophosphamide and its metabolites are excreted largely by the kidney[22]. The drug is extensively metabolized before excretion, with less than 25% of the administered dose appearing unchanged in the urine[22]. Of the urinary metabolites, about 50% consist of carboxyphosphamide and about 15% of 4-ketophosphamide[11,22,23]. Acrolein, a metabolite excreted in the urine, is thought to be responsible for urologic toxicity and the use of 2-mercaptoethanesulfonate (mesna) may detoxify acrolein, reducing bladder toxicity[24]. Only small amounts of radioactive label appear in stool, expired air, spinal fluid, sweat, breast milk, saliva and synovial fluid[11,25].

Dialysis removes 72% of cyclophosphamide so the drug should be administered after dialysis[23].

Allopurinol and cimetidine (but not ranitidine) inhibit hepatic

PHARMACOKINETICS OF SAARDs							
SAARD	Bioavailability	Clearance (ml/min/kg)	Serum elimination half-life (hours)	Unbound fraction	Routes of elimination	Site of metabolism	Reference
Azathioprine	0.8 (6-MP)	21–200 (AZA) 114 (6-MP)	1.7 (AZA) 1.2–1.5 (6-MP)	0.30 0.80 (6-MP)	Renal (20–45%)	Liver>renal	17–19
Chlorambucil	0.7	20	1.3–1.7 1.9–2.6 (mustard)	0.01	Renal (20–70%)	?	10, 20, 21
Cyclophosphamide	0.97	1.2	2–8 8.7 (mustard)	0.87 0.45 (mustard)	Renal (cyclophosphamide 50%, metabolites 8–35%)	Liver	10, 22, 23, 25
Cyclosporin	0.2–0.5	2-32	10–30	0.10	Renal (6%) Bile (94%)	Liver	26–35
Methotrexate	0.25-1.0	1.2	6–55 (MTX) 116 (7-OH-MTX)	0.35–0.60	Renal (30–80%) Bile (3–23%)	Liver	14, 36–43

Fig. 9.2 Pharmacokinetics of SAARDs.

microsomal enzymes, resulting in increased cyclophoshamide-alkylating metabolites[23].

CYCLOSPORIN

Absorption of the usual cyclosporin formulation is erratic and incomplete, although a new cyclosporin microemulsion is both more consistently and better absorbed (by 30–143%)[26–29]. Grapefruit juice, too, increases absorption (by 62% in one study) [30]. The drug is largely distributed outside the blood volume (body fat, liver, pancreas, lungs, kidneys, adrenal glands, spleen and lymph nodes have higher concentrations than serum). It is highly bound to plasma proteins, erythrocytes and lipoproteins[26,27]. About 11% of a cyclosporin dose is found in infant cord blood[31]. It is metabolized in the liver by cytochrome P-450 mixed-function oxidase to at least 15 known metabolites, some of which have immunosuppressive properties[26,27]. CYP3A (an hepatic metabolizing enzyme) activity correlates with cyclosporin dosing requirements after renal transplant ($r = 0.55$) [32]. At steady state colonic tissue cyclosporin concentrations are 50–250 times those of blood levels, indicating significant tissue concentration of cyclosporin. Elimination of cyclosporin is primarily via the biliary system, with only small amounts appearing in the urine[26,27].

Inducers of hepatic enzyme metabolism (e.g. rifampin, phenobarbital and phenytoin) lower cyclosporin concentrations, while drugs that inhibit hepatic metabolism (e.g. ketoconazole, fluconazole[33]) raise cyclosporin blood concentrations[26,27]. In five renal transplant patients, azathioprine halved cyclosporin AUCs[28]. Neither famotidine nor meprazole changed cyclosporin kinetics. Diltiazem regularly increases cyclosporin levels by inhibiting cyclosporin metabolism while neither verapamil nor nifedipine affected cyclosporin kinetics[34,35]. Administration of cyclosporin with other nephrotoxic agents, such as aminoglycosides and nonsteroidal anti-inflammatory agents (NSAIDs), may increase cyclosporin's nephrotoxic potential[26,27].

METHOTREXATE

Methotrexate bioavailability is the same whether the drug is given as a solution, tablet or as a subcutaneous or intramuscular injection[36,37]. Bioavailability is adequate although large interindividual variability exists (bioavailability: 0.2–1.0) and food does not affect bioavailability[14,16,38]. After long-term treatment synovial membrane and bone concentrations are about 10 times plasma concentrations although plasma kinetics are not affected[39,40]. Methotrexate AUC increases by a factor of about three as age increases from 7 to 15 years[41]. This explains why some children require larger doses than adults. In children both renal and metabolic methotrexate clearance are decreased (by 50% and 14% respectively) at night compared to daytime[42]. Renal excretion of the drug and its metabolites is the main pathway of disposition, although biliary excretion may be significant (10–31%)[14]. This drug's activity is dependent on the parent compound, its principal hydroxy-metabolite and its intracellular glutamates, which means the relationship between blood concentration and effect or toxicity is complex and, probably, indirect.

It is probable that all NSAIDs, including aspirin, decrease methotrexate clearance, although clinical effects are uncommon, particularly when using low dose methotrexate[43,44].

EFFICACY, TOXICITY AND THERAPEUTIC USE

ANTIBIOTICS

Efficacy

Dapsone

Dapsone has been used in several studies of RA[1,45]. Swinson and Ziosnich compared 22 dapsone-treated and 19 placebo-treated patients in a 14-week, double-blind trial and dapsone appeared moderately effective and showed improvement in erythrocyte sedimentation rate (ESR), C-reactive protein (CRP) and five of seven clinical measures[46]. In contrast, an 80-patient, randomized study comparing hydroxychloroquine, dapsone and their combination was unable to show clinical improvement in any of the three groups[47]. Hemolytic anemia, unfortunately, was not uncommon and is a limiting toxicity[47]. Dapsone's potential beneficial effects may be outweighed by its toxicity (particularly hemolytic anemia).

Rifampin

Intra-articular rifampin seemed effective in some patients with joint effusions[1]. However when given orally in controlled studies, rifampin appeared ineffective[1,36]. In a small, open, randomized study comparing hydroxychloroquine and rifampin, the hydroxychloroquine group improved while the rifampin group did not[36].

Tetracycline

After some initial encouraging open studies of minocycline and other tetracyclines, two double-blind studies were undertaken[48,49]. A European study examined 80 RA patients given minocycline 200mg daily or placebo for 26 weeks. Fifteen patients in the minocycline group improved by at least 25% compared to only seven in the placebo group. Laboratory tests also improved[48]. A 219 patient trial in the US compared minocycline 200mg daily and placebo during 48 weeks[49]. A 50% improvement in joint swelling was detected in 54% of the minocycline group compared to 39% in the placebo group ($P = 0.02$). Both trials showed drug effect despite the fact that the European study utilized patients with more severe disease. Minocycline 200mg daily appears effective in some patients with RA, although comparisons with other SAARDs, delineation of the 'responder' population and testing with other tetracycline derivatives has not yet been done.

Toxicity

Dapsone and rifampin

Dapsone is associated with hemolytic anemia and with numerous skin rashes, peripheral neuropathies, gastrointestinal (GI) symptoms, central nervous system (CNS) symptoms and an SLE-like syndrome. Rifampin is associated with liver dysfunction, GI effects, thrombocytopenia, CNS effects, renal insufficiency and some rashes. Numerous drug interactions are also possible (Physicians' Desk Reference (PDR)).

Tetracyclines

In comparisons during the double-blind studies, nausea, dizziness, light-headedness and photosensitive skin rashes were the principle side effects of concern[48,49]. Rare hepatotoxicity is always possible with tetracyclines. Of more concern is the possible effect of long-term antibiotics on microbial resistance, although there have been no reports of such an effect thus far.

Therapeutic use

Dapsone

Dapsone dosing regimens of 50–150mg/day are recommended. Close follow-up is required for toxicity, especially hemolytic anemia. Many patients cannot tolerate more than 75–100mg/day without decreases in hemoglobin.

Rifampin

Rifampin, 600mg daily, is the usual dose that has been used in published studies. Numerous side effects can occur including hepatic, hematologic, CNS and renal toxicity. Patients need regular observation for these potential side effects.

Minocyline

Minocycline, 100mg taken twice daily on an empty stomach, is usually recommended. Ingestion of food or iron within 2 hours after medication is not advised. Some practitioners caution patients about sun exposure. Liver function tests and complete blood counts (CBCs) should be drawn every 4–12 weeks[48,49].

AZATHIOPRINE

Efficacy

Azathioprine, 1.25–3.0mg/kg/day, is clearly more effective than

EFFICACY OF SAARDs IN RHEUMATOID ARTHRITIS (CONTROLLED TRIALS ONLY)						
SAARD	Placebo (P)	AZA	CTX	DPA	Gold	HCQ/CQ*
Azathioprine (AZA)	AZA>P	–	AZA=CTX	AZA=DPA	AZA=Gold	AZA=CQ
Chlorambucil (CHL)	CHL>P	–	–	–	–	–
Cyclophosphamide (CTX)	CTX>P	CTX=AZA	–	–	CTX≥Gold	–
Cyclosporin (CSA)	CSA>P	–	–	CSA=DPA	–	–
Methotrexate (MTX)	MTX>P	MTX>AZA	–	–	MTX=Gold	–
* hydroxychloroquine (HCQ) or chloroquine (CQ)						

Fig. 9.3 Efficacy of SAARDs in rheumatoid arthritis.

placebo in RA[6,10]. There appears to be a dose–response relationship for this drug in RA, comparing placebo, azathioprine 1.25mg/kg/day and 2.5mg/kg/day (although the data are not completely consistent)[6].

There have been at least 11 double-blind controlled trials comparing azathioprine to other SAARDs[6,50,51]. The largest of these trials compared azathioprine 1.25–1.50mg/kg/day and D-penicillamine (DPA) 10–12mg/kg/day over 24 weeks in 206 RA patients[52]. The analysis concentrated on the 70 azathioprine and 64 DPA patients who completed the trial (only 65% of the patients). Both drugs were associated with improvement in 'nearly all efficacy variables ... in both groups.' Only the rise in hemoglobin and decrease in ESR were statistically better for DPA patients. There have been three trials published comparing methotrexate and azathioprine[6,50,51]: two demonstrated a trend favoring methotrexate, and one demonstrated statistical differences favoring methotrexate. Cyclosporin 4.2mg/kg/d equalled azathioprine in a 6 month, double-blind trial, although blood pressure and creatinine rose more after cyclosporin than azathioprine[51]. Thus, it appears that there are no major differences between the clinical efficacies in RA of azathioprine, cyclosporin, (1.0–3.0mg/kg/day), cyclophosphamide, organic gold, D-penicillamine and chloroquine (Fig. 9.3).

Placebo-controlled trials of azathioprine have also been completed in psoriatic arthritis, Reiter's syndrome, Behçet's syndrome, polymyositis and SLE[6,53,54]. Small placebo-controlled trials of psoriasis (six patients in a cross-over trial) and Reiter's syndrome (eight patients in a cross-over trial) showed positive results over 4–6 months[6,54]. A placebo-controlled, 2-year study of 73 patients with Behçet's syndrome (37 of whom received azathioprine) concluded that 'azathioprine was effective in controlling the progression of Behçet's syndrome, especially in its most serious manifestation, eye disease'[54]. Conflicting results are available from five small placebo-controlled trials of azathioprine plus prednisone versus prednisone alone in SLE nephritis. Although each trial contained too few subjects to be convincing by itself, a meta-analysis by Felson and Anderson suggested a marginal benefit for azathioprine over placebo, especially in lessening renal deterioration[55].

Toxicity

The principle toxicities of azathioprine include bone marrow suppression and gastrointestinal disturbances (Fig. 9.4). A few observers indicate an increased incidence of viral infections in RA patients using azathioprine[56], although not all authors agree with this conclusion[10]. A 50-fold increase in relative risk of malignant disease has been documented in azathioprine-treated renal transplant patients (particularly non-Hodgkin's lymphoma)[1]. In RA, the azathioprine-related risk of lymphoma (and non-Hodgkin's lymphoma) is confounded by an increased relative risk secondary to RA *per se*[6]. Overall, there is probably a small added risk of developing some malignancy when using azathioprine in RA (relative risk of 1.3)[10]. This relative risk is between 2.2 and 8.7 for developing a lymphoproliferative disorder[6,10]. Reversible lymphoma has been documented after azathioprine[57]. Bone marrow toxicity has been associated with low levels of purine methyltransferase (which occurs in 0.3% of the population) both in renal transplant and RA patients[19].

Interactions with allopurinol, cyclophosphamide and neuromuscular blockers (e.g. succinylcholine) have been known to require decreasing

THE TOXICITY OF SAARDs (RANGES IN %)					
	Shared				
	AZA	CHL	CTX	CSA	MTX
Dose-related marrow suppression					
Leukopenia	4–27	14–50	6–32	2–6	1–4
Thrombocytopenia	0–5	8–37	0–4	≤2	1–2
Susceptibility to infection					
Overall	0–9	18–27	0–22	0–6	–
Herpes zoster	0–6	4–27	5–30	0–3	–
GI intolerance					
Nausea, vomiting	9–23	4	19–45	4–40	10–18
Diarrhea	≤1	–	3–18	2–18	5–12
Rash	1–6	0–18	0–2	0–2	1–2
	Not shared				
	AZA	CHL	CTX	CSA	MTX
Hair					
Alopecia	–	2	7–80	–	≤6
Hypertrichosis	–	–	–	7–49	–
Stomatitis	0–5	–	–	–	6–10
Gum hyperplasia	–	–	–	4–12	–
Hepatic					
Abnormal liver function	0–5	–	–	0–8	8–38
Fibrosis/cirrhosis	–	–	–	–	4–20
Azoospermia/oligospermia	–	≤100	60–100	–	±
Amenorrhea	–	2–8	0–53	–	–
Cystitis	–	–	4–45	–	–
Teratogenesis	±	↑	↑	±	30–83
Neoplasia	↑	↑	↑	↑	–
Decreased GFR	–	–	–	50–87	–
Hypertension	–	–	–	33	–
Neurotoxicity	–	–	–	10–40	–
Pneumonitis	–	–	–	–	0–5

Fig. 9.4 The toxicity of SAARDs.

the dose of azathioprine significantly (50–75% decrease when using allopurinol)[6]. One study suggested that azathioprine-associated hepatitis increases the risk of cyclophosphamide-induced hepatitis, although these data have not been replicated[7].

Therapeutic use

Before using azathioprine, discussion of risks, treatment goals and laboratory testing are appropriate. To test for possible acute azathioprine sensitivity, 25–50mg doses are suggested for the first week. Thereafter doses are increased by 0.5mg/kg/day, with the goal of reaching 2–3mg/kg/day. The dose may then be adjusted to the minimum effective dose.

Monitoring should include hemoglobin, white blood cell (WBC) and platelet counts every 2 weeks while dosing regimens are being changed, and every 4–6 weeks during stable regimens. Liver function tests can be performed every 6–8 weeks.

CHLORAMBUCIL

Efficacy

One double-blind, placebo-controlled study of chlorambucil has been reported in RA (25 patients received chlorambucil, and 23 received placebo over 3 months)[10,58]. Multiple clinical and serologic parameters improved significantly in the chlorambucil-treated group compared with the placebo-treated group. Most of the reported experience comes from France, Australia and Russia[10,59]. In uncontrolled series, the overall response rate in RA has been about 70%[55,10].

A controlled trial of chlorambucil was reported in 40 patients with Behçet's syndrome[60]. In an 'evaluator-blinded' trial versus cyclosporin, chlorambucil was more effective for extraocular disease (skin, arthritis) while cyclosporin was more effective for ocular Behçet's syndrome.

Although chlorambucil has been used in SLE, polyarteritis nodosa, Wegener's granulomatosis, multiple sclerosis, sarcoidosis, dermatomyositis and amyloidosis, no controlled study has substantiated its effectiveness in these disorders[58,60].

Toxicity

The most common toxicities with chlorambucil use are dose-related bone marrow suppression and infertility. Even though chlorambucil suppresses lymphocytes, its usual dose-limiting bone marrow toxicities are granulocytopenia and/or isolated thrombocytopenia[4,23]. Cumulative bone marrow toxicity occurs regularly with chlorambucil and often requires drug discontinuation. In Cannon *et al.*'s study, only one of the 28 subjects was able to continue the drug for longer than 21 months[59].

The risk of infertility, azoospermia and amenorrhea increases with increasing duration of therapy, as well as with increasing doses, although spermatogenesis has returned 15 to 17 years after discontinuing chlorambucil[10,24]. In Chapman's review, irreversible azoospermia was regularly produced in adult males who received >400mg of the drug although hormonal function was maintained[61]. In postpubertal females, both gametogenesis and hormonal function are altered adversely and menopause occurs[10]. While the frequency of infertility in males is quite high, it is lower in females.

The risk of neoplasia is clearly increased in subjects receiving chlorambucil, particularly of the skin and hematologic systems[10,24,62]. An acute leukemia incidence of 0.93% (relative risk of developing acute leukemia is 10 times that of the normal population (RR-10)) was reported by Kahn *et al.* in a group of 1711 RA patients treated with chlorambucil for 1–13 years[61].

Therapeutic use

Discussion of risks, treatment goals and laboratory testing are appropriate. Regular monitoring should include hemoglobin, WBC and platelet counts every 1–2 weeks while dosing regimens are being changed, and every 2–4 weeks during stable regimens.

Chlorambucil can be instituted orally in doses of between 0.1 and 0.2mg/kg/day[23,24]. Once response or toxicity has occurred (one or the other often occurs within 3–4 months of instituting therapy), it is suggested that the drug be continued at a lower dose that controls the disease and maintains the WBC between 3000 and 4000/mm^3 (usually a dose between 3 and 4mg daily)[23,24]. Since oral contraceptives and inhibitors of gonadotropin-releasing hormone protect ovarian function from cytotoxic damage in animal models, consideration might be given to the use of one or the other agent in female subjects interested in preserving fertility[61,63,64,65]. Their use in humans is purely exploratory.

CYCLOPHOSPHAMIDE

Efficacy

Oral cyclophosphamide has consistently been better than placebo, both clinically and in terms of ESR and rheumatoid factor, in five placebo-controlled trials when used in doses >1.5mg/kg/day[24]. It has not been consistently effective in doses <1.0mg/kg/day. Cyclophosphamide reaches its peak of effectiveness after approximately 16 weeks[24]. Two small studies have shown that cyclophosphamide can retard bone destruction (one study of cyclophosphamide at 1.5mg/kg/day for 18 months and a second of cyclophosphamide at 2.0mg/kg/day for 8 months)[24].

When compared with other SAARDs, cyclophosphamide is clinically equal to azathioprine, clinically equal to, or superior to, intramuscular gold[24] and equal to azathioprine but superior to intramuscular gold in retarding bone destruction[24]. Uncontrolled studies generally support the efficacy of cyclophosphamide in the treatment of RA[24]. These studies suggest several additional characteristics:

- once peak effectiveness is reached, after 16 weeks of drug therapy, that level of efficacy remains constant for at least 25 months;
- although remission may be maintained for several years after withdrawal of cyclophosphamide, most patients will have a recurrence of RA symptoms;
- nonarticular complications of RA, such as interstitial lung disease, cutaneous ulcers and peripheral neuropathy, may respond to oral cyclophosphamide.

Systemic lupus erythematosus is the only other rheumatic disease in which placebo-controlled trials of cyclophosphamide have been performed. Two placebo-controlled studies in the 1970s suggested that oral cyclophosphamide plus prednisone was marginally superior to placebo plus prednisone in treating SLE[66,67]. Austin *et al* have shown that the development of renal failure in subjects with diffuse proliferative glomerulonephritis is delayed by i.v. cyclophosphamide given in doses of 0.75g/m^2 every 3 months coupled with high-dose prednisone[68].

Even though no placebo-controlled studies have been performed in the necrotizing systemic vasculitides, cyclophosphamide is considered by most authorities to be the drug of choice for the management of polyarteritis nodosa and Wegener's granulomatosis[24,68]. Intravenous cyclophosphamide (up to 900mg/m^2) has real but limited usefulness in Wegener's granulomatosis because, despite response, 52% of patients relapse[68]. The most favorable outcomes were patients who received oral cyclophosphamide on a daily basis. Recent open studies of cyclophosphamide in scleroderma with pulmonary involvement demonstrated encouraging effects[7,69]. Intravenous cyclophosphamide has been used in anectodal series combining cyclophosphamide with prednisone and/or plasmapheresis in SLE and CNS angiitis, with good response[58].

Toxicity

Cyclophosphamide's significant toxicity is the major factor limiting its clinical use in the rheumatic diseases. Major toxicities include its carcinogenicity, propensity to cause infertility, frequent cumulative bone marrow toxicity and association with hemorrhagic cystitis[24]. Kinlen's experience with 643 RA patients suggests a relative risk of 12.8 for all cancers combined, a risk of 10.9 for non-Hodgkin's lymphoma and a 10-fold increase in bladder cancer[70].

The risk of infertility, azoospermia and amenorrhea with cyclophosphamide rises with increasing duration of therapy, increasing drug doses and with increasing age in women. Irreversible azoospermia was regularly produced in adult males receiving a total dose of cyclophosphamide >18g. In men, plasma testosterone levels tend to remain normal, as does the histologic appearance of Leydig and Sertoli cells, suggesting sparing of hormonal function[65]. In postpubertal females, however, both gametogenesis and hormonal function are altered adversely, and menopause occurs. In one study of 92 women with SLE who were treated with cyclophosphamide, 36% developed amenorrhea and 27% had sustained amenorrhea (>12 months). A further 19% had oligomenorrhea[71]. In the Damewood experience, the total mean dose of cyclophosphamide needed to produce amenorrhea was 5.2g in women over 40 years of age, 9.3g in women aged 30–39 years, and 20.4g in women aged 20–29 years[72]. Reappearance of fertility following drug discontinuation has been documented, but azoospermia and amenorrhea are usually permanent once they have appeared[72].

The urologic adverse effects of cyclophosphamide are thought to be related to its urinary metabolite, acrolein. Hemorrhagic cystitis has been reported in about one third of subjects receiving oral cyclophosphamide daily, and there is a significant but lesser incidence of bladder fibrosis and bladder carcinoma[8,10]. In a cohort study of 119 RA patients, nine developed bladder cancer during an average 13.1 years of follow-up although three of the nine occurred after a delay of 14, 16 and 17 years[73]. The incidence of cystitis and bladder carcinoma is markedly reduced when cyclophosphamide is used on an intermittent, i.v. basis. Bladder toxicity can also be reduced by the concomitant administration of mesna[74].

Other problems include GI side effects and infections. Omdal *et al.* documented nausea in 68% of 25 patients and severe infections in 24%[75].

Therapeutic use

Laboratory evaluation for toxicity is very important with cyclophosphamide. Complete blood count, platelet count or estimate and urinalysis with microscopic examination should be obtained every 7–14 days initially and can be reduced to every 2–4 weeks once the disease and the dose have been stabilized for 2–3 months[71]. Because of cyclophosphamide's significant toxicity, its use in RA should be limited to patients having cutaneous ulcerations, neuropathy and/or vascular complications suggestive of polyarteritis-like disease, and those subjects who have failed all other SAARDs but who still have active, severe RA. In these instances, oral cyclophosphamide at a dose of 2mg/kg/day might be considered[24]. An i.v. regimen of cyclophosphamide has been suggested for management of rheumatoid vasculitis. In this regimen 500–1000mg of cyclophosphamide and 500–1000mg of methylprednisolone are given intravenously on days 1, 8, 29 and 58[24]. Patients are then continued on oral SAARDs. In either case, once the disease has come under control, switching to less toxic SAARDs over a longer period should be considered.

Intravenous cyclophosphamide is the preferred cytotoxic in the management of diffuse proliferative glomerulonephritis and SLE[68]. It is usually started at 0.75g/m^2 when glomerular filtration rate (GFR) is greater than one third of predicted normal. When renal function is less than one third of normal, the starting dose is 0.5g/m^2. Cyclophosphamide can be administered in 150ml of a 5% glucose solution over 30–60 minutes. Diuresis should be ensured by increased i.v. and oral fluids, and possibly diuretics. Nausea and vomiting are common and may require antiemetic therapy. Intravenous pulse methylprednisolone may also be given at about the same time in 1g doses daily for 3 consecutive days. This helps decrease nausea and is also part of the treatment for glomerulonephritis. Oral daily prednisone is usually instituted at the same time. Intravenous pulse cyclophosphamide (with or without i.v. methylprednisone) is usually given once every 1–3 months thereafter for up to 2–5 years' total therapy[68].

Cyclophosphamide given orally is usually the preferred method for the management of polyarteritis and Wegener's granulomatosis[48]. It should be instituted in doses of 2mg/kg/day (75–125mg/day) and the dose altered to maintain the WBC between 3000 and 3500/mm^3.

Monitoring for lymphoproliferative disease and other malignant disease is appropriate but undefined. Avoidance of pregnancy is strongly recommended. Again, consideration might be given to the use of oral contraceptives or gonadotropin-releasing hormone inhibitors in subjects interested in preserving fertility, although their use in humans is purely exploratory[62,65,66].

CYCLOSPORIN

Efficacy

Three placebo-controlled trials, and one trial comparing medium dose with very low dose cyclosporin, have been performed and show that cyclosporin is an efficacious drug in RA[76]. In these studies, 146 subjects with definite or classic RA received cyclosporin in initial doses of 1–10mg/kg/day. These studies continued for 4–6 months, at which time the final cyclosporin dose ranged from 3.8–7.4mg/kg/day. Analysis demonstrated that cyclosporin improved clinical symptoms and signs; however, no significant improvement was noted in many laboratory parameters such as ESR or rheumatoid factor titers. Nephrotoxicity has been the major limiting factor preventing the use of higher doses. Based on these studies, patients treated with 2.5–4.0mg/kg/day of cyclosporin should show substantial response within 3–4 months; in some instances the response occurs within the first month. Double-blind, controlled trials show cyclosporin (up to 5mg/kg) to be effective as D-penicillamine, chloroquine or azathioprine in RA[13,77].

Two blinded trials found cyclosporin superior to 'conventional therapy' in the management of Behçet's syndrome, particularly its ocular complications[26,59]. Two placebo-controlled trials have shown cyclosporin to be effective in clearing the cutaneous lesions of psoriasis[13,78], but no study has been reported on its efficacy in psoriatic arthritis. An open trial of cyclosporin in systemic sclerosis appeared to show improvement in skin involvement[79] but acute renal failure has also occurred in 3 of 8 systemic sclerosis patients receiving cyclosporin[80].

Toxicity

When cyclosporin is used to treat rheumatic disease, side effects are generally mild and reversible at low doses[13,26,76,77]. Dose-related decreases in GFR with corresponding increases in serum creatinine (the principal adverse effect) are common during cyclosporin immunosuppression. In patients using greater than 5mg/kg/day, cyclosporin renal biopsies sometimes showed focal interstitial fibrosis, tubular atrophy and/or arteriolar lesions. However these did not occur if the dose of cyclosporin remained at 5mg/kg/day or less and if serum creatinine did not rise more than 50% above baseline[8,13,26]. In male rats there was a close correlation between tissue cyclosporin concentrations and decreased creatinine clearance ($r = -0.9967$)[81]. In Tugwell *et al.*'s study (average dose: 3.8mg/kg/day) serum creatinine rose over the first 4 months but then stabilized; after discontinuation of cyclosporin, serum creatinine returned to within 15% of baseline in all except two patients[76].

Elevation of blood pressure is another common side effect of cyclosporin therapy, and new onset hypertension has been reported in about one third of rheumatoid and psoriatic patients[82]. Although antihypertensive therapy may be required, potassium-sparing diuretics should be avoided because cyclosporin may cause hyperkalemia[21]. Calcium channel blockers may increase cyclosporin levels by decreasing its metabolism, and changes in cyclosporin dosage may be required[34,35].

Significant hepatotoxicity manifests as elevated hepatic enzymes and bilirubin may be seen, but usually only with higher cyclosporin doses[26,25]. In 154 RA patients treated for up to 12 months, creatinine increased at some point >30% in 48%, hypertrichosis occurred in 35%, paresthesias were seen in 29%, gum hyperplasia was demonstrated in 14% and GI complaints (mostly nausea) occurred in 47%[83]. Thus far, there is no indication that cyclosporin predisposes to malignancies.

Therapeutic use

Cyclosporin therapy may be instituted after a thorough discussion of the risks (particularly nephrotoxicity). Cyclosporin use should be avoided in patients with pre-existing renal disease. It may be instituted at doses of 2.5mg/kg/day given in two divided doses every 12 hours. The dose may be cautiously increased 25–50% every 2–4 weeks until a maximum dose of 5mg/kg/day is reached, unless this is prevented by a rise in creatinine of 30% or greater. Dosage reductions of 25–50% are warranted if serum creatinine increases above baseline by 30% or if uncontrollable hypertension appears. Hypertension can usually be managed with beta-blockers and angiotensin-converting enzyme (ACE)-inhibitors. Introduction of drugs known to interact with cyclosporin (diltiazem, ketoconazole, rifampin, phenytoin) may require adjustment of cyclosporin dose. Weekly or every other week serum creatinine determinations are warranted as long as the cyclosporin dose is being adjusted. Once the cyclosporin dose is stable, a serum creatinine measurement every 2–4 weeks may be adequate. Chemistry screens, CBCs and urinalysis should be done at the time of serum creatinine determinations. Periodic monitoring for lymphoproliferative disease and other malignancy is appropriate but undefined, as is monitoring for pregnancy.

Testing for cyclosporin levels is possible, but the levels obtained often do not clearly reflect cyclosporin toxicity or efficacy. The clearest recommendation is that toxicity is best monitored by frequent serial serum creatinine levels (every 7–14 days). If cyclosporin levels are monitored, trough values >300ng/ml (using a radioimmunoassay method employing a monoclonal antibody specific for cyclosporin in plasma) should be avoided[26].

METHOTREXATE

Efficacy

The anti-inflammatory efficacy of methotrexate in RA has been repeatedly demonstrated, including a study showing that the effect is dose-related[14]. The meta-analysis of Tugwell *et al.* demonstrated a 27% lowering of the ESR, a 27% decrease in joint swelling count and an improvement of 26–39% in joint tenderness count and pain visual analog scale[84].

There is a trend for patients to remain on methotrexate longer than on comparative SAARDs (e.g. 45–62% on methotrexate after 3 years, versus 18–62% on intramuscular gold, 35% on hydroxychloroquine, and 11–39% on sulfasalazine). The evidence that methotrexate retards bony damage in RA is building, with four studies supporting such effects and two studies unable to do so[85]. A meta-analysis was relatively persuasive showing that methotrexate slowed the appearance of new erosions as well as intramuscular gold therapy and better than azathioprine treatment[86].

Controlled trials in asthma and psoriatic arthropathy also show some evidence of efficacy[8,87]. A meta-analysis of three controlled trials of methotrexate in juvenile rheumatoid arthritis showed that 10mg methotrexate was more effective than placebo[88].

While methotrexate is being used in other diseases as well, including SLE, polymyositis, inflammatory bowel disease, biliary cirrhosis, sarcoidosis, ankylosing spondylitis, childhood dermatomyositis, giant cell arteritis, Wegener's granulomatosis and systemic sclerosis, well-controlled trials in these indications have not yet been published.

Toxicity

The most common toxicities when using methotrexate are gastrointestinal, with stomatitis and dyspepsia being the most frequent (see Fig. 9.4). Folic acid minimizes stomatitis[14]. Open studies indicate that infections may occur more commonly in patients using methotrexate, although controlled studies have been unable to corroborate this[89].

While leukopenia can occur with methotrexate, as with most other SAARDs, the principal areas of concern when using this drug are its pulmonary and hepatic toxicity. Pulmonary hypersensitivity, with severe hypoxia, seems to occur in 2–6% of patients on low-dose methotrexate therapy for RA, and this can be life threatening. Luckily, it is usually reversible. Transaminitis is common, occurring in up to 67% in one study[14]. While some fibrosis, and even progressive fibrosis, has been reported in liver biopsies[14], progression to cirrhosis in RA is quite rare. The consensus appears to be that pretreatment liver biopsies are not usually necessary (see below) [14]. An American College of Rheumatology (ACR) *ad hoc* committee recommended liver function testing every 4–8 weeks and liver biopsies only after 5 years or if liver function tests were frequently elevated[90].

Teratogenicity is an accepted side effect of methotrexate, while oncogenicity does not seem to be a problem[86,88]. Recently reports of pseudo-lymphomas, associated with methotrexate (sometimes also coincident with EBV infection) have been published[91]. Drug interactions promoting toxicity such as renal failure, bone marrow aplasia and severe GI toxicity have been documented, although rarely, for sulfamethaxisole-trimethoprine and NSAID (not only aspirin)[92].

Therapeutic use

Appropriate discussion of the eventual need for liver biopsy and the need to prevent pregnancy are mandatory before starting methotrexate[90]. The use of alcohol should be minimized and should remain less than two ounces a week[14].

Baseline liver biopsies are not usually needed before beginning methotrexate unless there is a history of alcohol abuse, elevated liver function texts or chronic hepatatis B or C[14]. Liver biopsies need not be done until after about 5 years of therapy[90].

Follow-up consists of CBCs and liver function tests, done every 2–4 weeks initially and then every 4 to 8 weeks. Serum creatinine (or creatinine clearance) every 4–12 weeks is also useful[90].

COMBINATION SAARD THERAPY

Twelve of 14 open studies seemed to show that combination SAARD therapy was more effective than single therapy[83]. However, well-controlled, double-blind studies have been much less encouraging (Fig. 9.5).

Most studies, when comparing each drug alone to the combination in a standard, randomized, double-blind, controlled study, were unable to demonstrate the superiority of a combination when compared to the more effective of the single drugs (Fig. 9.5) [83,93–95].

The three positive trials, interestingly, used differing and unconventional designs or doses[83,93–95]. Of 101 patients entering a trial of HCQ plus gold versus placebo plus gold, Scott *et al.* compared only patients who completed the trial (27 on sodium aurothiomalate plus HCQ, versus 32 on sodium aurothiomalate plus placebo). Two of 13 measures favored the combination; the other 11 measures showed no difference[93]. Tugwell *et al.* added cyclosporin (mean dose: 2.79mg/kg/day) or placebo to patients who 'failed' methotrexate[95]. He found that 32% more patients improved by a stringent combined index (the ACR improvement criteria) on the combination than on methotrexate alone. This study, clearly, applies to a subset of RA patients albeit an important one. Ferraz *et al.* compared a low dose of methotrexate (7.5mg/week) plus 250mg chloroquine to 7.5mg weekly methotrexate plus placebo in 82 RA patients[94]. This study favored the combination

DOUBLE-BLIND TRIALS OF SAARD COMBINATIONS

Combination	Outcome	Comparator	*N*
HCQ + SSZ	=	HCQ or SSZ	91
HCQ + SSZ	<	Dpen	56
MTX + AF	=	MTX or AF	335
MTX + AZA	=	MTX	209
HCQ + Dapsone	=	HCQ or Dapsone	80
HCQ + MTX	=	MTX	141
HCQ + Gold	±>	Gold or placebo	101
MTX + CSA	≥	MTX	148
CQ + MTX	≥	MTX	82
HCQ + SSZ + MTX	>	MTX or HCQ + SSZ	100

Fig. 9.5 Double-blind trials of SAARD combinations[93–98]. (HCQ, hydroxylchloroquine; SSZ, sulfasalazine; Dpen, D-penicillamine; MTX, methotrexate; AF, auronofin; CSA, cyclosporine; AZA, azathioprine.

IMMUNOSUPPRESSIVE AGENTS				
Drug	Toxicity risks requiring monitoring	Baseline evaluation	Clinical monitoring	Laboratory monitoring
Azathioprine	Bone marrow suppression, hepatoxicity, lymphoproliferative disorders	Blood count, creatinine, liver enzymes	Symptoms of myelosuppression	Blood count every 1–3 months, and within 1–2 weeks if any dose change
Chlorambucil	Bone marrow suppression, malignancies, including lymphoproliferative disorder	Blood count, urinalyses, creatinine liver enzymes	Symptoms of myelosuppression	Blood count every 1–3 months, and within 1–2 weeks if any dose change
Cyclophosphamide	Hemorrhagic cystitis, bone marrow suppression, malignancy and lymphoproliferative disorders	Blood count, urinalyses, creatinine, liver enzymes	Symptoms of myelosuppression, and hemorrhagic cystitis	Blood counts every 1–3 months, urinalysis and urine cytology every 6–12 months (and after cessation)
Cyclosporin	Renal insufficiency, anaemia and hypertension	Blood pressure, blood count, creatinine and uric acid	Edema	Blood pressure and creatinine monthly
Methotrexate	Hepatic fibrons, pulmonary infiltrates bone marrow suppression	Blood count, chest radiograph, liver function tests, renal function	Dyspnoea, oral ulceration, nausea, vomiting, myelosuppression	Blood count , liver and renal function tests every 4–8 weeks

Fig. 9.6 Guidelines for monitoring some immunosuppressive agents (after the ACR ad hoc committee)

but used unusually low methotrexate doses. All the positive studies seem to have been designed to test subpopulations of patients, such as 'completers', methotrexate 'failures' and low dose methotrexate users, somewhat limiting the generalizability of the results.

Excellent results in an open study of 31 RA patients using HCQ, azathioprine and cyclophosphamide were mitigated by significant toxicity[96]. Four malignancies (three in predisposed patients), 14 significant infections and five cases of subclinical macular degeneration were found. The results of a double-blind, 2 year study comparing methotrexate (7.5–17.5mg/week), HCQ (400mg/day) plus sulfasalazine (1g/day) versus HCQ and sulfasalazine versus variable dose methotrexate was recently published[97]. The triple combination was effective (>50% improvement in tenderness and swelling for at least 3 months) in 78% of patients, and only 28% or 31% of the other two groups improved by the same definition, respectively. Toxicity requiring discontinuation occurred half as frequently in the combination as the methotrexate group. These very encouraging results require corroboration.

While the data regarding combination SAARD therapy are conflicting, its use is increasingly based on studies such as the above. It is hoped that the use of combination SAARD therapy represents a step forwards in treating more aggressive RA.

RECOMMENDED MONITORING STRATEGIES

The American College of Rheumatology ad hoc committee on clinical guidelines has recently produced some recommendations for monitoring therapy with these agents[98], as shown in Figure 9.6. These recommendations may need some modification according to local circumstances and the clinical states of individual patients.

REFERENCES

1. Kloppenberg M, Dijkmons BA, Breedveld FC, *et al.* Antimicrobial therapy for rheumatoid arthritis In: Innovative treatment approaches for rhuematoid arthritis. Brooks PM and Furst DE), eds. Clin Rheum. 1995;9:759–69.
2. Wozel G, Barth J. Current aspects of modes of action of dapsone. Int J Derm. 1988:27:547–52.
3. Lewis AJ, Gemmell DK, Stimson WH. The anti-inflammatory profile of dapsone in animal models of inflammation. Agents Act. 1978;8578–86.
4. Gupta S, Grieco MH, Siegel I. Suppression of T-lymphocyte rosettes by rifampin. Studies in normals and patients with tuberculosis. Ann Int Med. 1975;182:844–8.
5. Elion GB, Hitchings GH. Azathioprine. Handbook Exp Pharmacol. 1975;38:404–25.
6. McKendry RJR. Purine analogs. In: Dixon J, Furst DE, eds. Second line agents in the treatment of rheumatic diseases. New York: Marcell Dekker; 1991.
7. Cannon GW, Ward JR. Cytotoxic drugs and sulfasalazine. In: McCarty DJ, ed. Arthritis and allied conditions, 11E. Philadelphia: Lea and Febiger; 1989:563–91.
8. Bacon PA, Salmon M. Modes of action of second line agents. Scand J Rheum. 1987;64(Suppl):17–24.
9. Klinenberg JR, Reichman R, Clements PJ. Investigational therapy for rheumatoid arthritis. In: Cohen AS, ed. Progress in clinical immunology, Vol 1. Orlando: Grune & Stratton; 1984:111–44.
10. Tsokos GC. Immunomodulatory treatments in patients with rheumatic diseases: mechanism of action. Semin Arthritis Rheum. 1987;17:24–38.
11. Clements PJ. Cytotoxic immunosuppressive drugs. In: Paulus HE, Furst DE, Dromgoole SH, eds. Drugs for rheumatic disease. New York: Marcel Dekker; 135–56.
12. Lacki, JK, Schochat T, Sobieska M. Immunological studies in patients with rheumatoid arthritis treated with methotrexate or cyclosphosphamide. Z Rheumatol. 1994;53:76–82.
13. Furst DE. Cyclosporin, leflunomide and nitrogen mustard. In: Innovative treatment approaches for rheumatoid arthritis. Clin Rheum. 1995;9:711–729.
14. Songsiride N, Furst DE. Methotrexate – the rapidly acting drug. Clin Rheum. 1990;4:575–94.
15. Segal R, Yaron M, Tartakovsky B. Methotrexate: mechanism of action in rheumatoid arthritis. Semin Arthritis Rheum. 1990;20:190–99.
16. Kremer JM. The mechanism of action of methotrexate in rheumatoid arthritis: The search continues. J Rheum. 1994;21:1–5.
17. El-Yazigi A, Wahab FA. Pharmacokinetics of azathioprine after repeated oral and single intravenous administration. J Clin Pharmacol. 1993;33:522–6.
18. Ohlman S, Albertioni F, Peterson C. Day-to-day variability in azathioprine pharmacokinetics in renal transplant recipients. Clin Trans. 1994;8(Suppl 3):217–23.

19. Escousse A, Mousson C, Santona L, *et al.* Azathioprine-induced pancytopenia in homozygous thiopurine methyltransferase-deficient renal transplant recipients: a family study. Transplant Proc. 1995;27:1739–42.
20. McLean A, Woods RL, Catovsky D, Farmer P. Pharmacokinetics and metabolism of chlorambucil in patients with malignant disease. Cancer Treat Rev. 1979;6(Suppl):33–42.
21. Loos U, Musch E, Malek M, Riedel E. Comparative pharmacokinetics of chlorambucil and prednimustine after oral administration. Oncology. 1991;48:334–42.
22. Grochow LB, Colvin M. Clinical pharmacokinetics of cyclophosphamide. Clin Pharmacol. 1979;4:380–94.
23. Moore JM. Clinical pharmacokinetics of Cyclophosphamide. Clin Pharmacokin. 1991;20(3):194–208.
24. Clements PJ. Alkylating agents. In: Dixon J, Furst DE, eds. Second line agents in the treatment of rheumatic diseases. New York: Marcel Dekker; 1991.
25. Duncan IH, Colvin OM, Fenselau C. Mass spectrometric study of the distribution of cyclophosphamide in humans. Toxicol Appl Pharmacol. 1973;24:317–23.
26. Kowal A, Carstens Jr JH, Schnitzer TJ. Cyclosporin in rheumatoid arthritis. In: Furst DE, Weinblatt ME, eds. Immunomodulators in the rheumatic diseases. New York: Marcel Dekker; 1990:61–98.
27. Ptodronski RJ, Veukataramaman R, Burckart GJ. Clinical pharmacokinetics of cyclosporin. Clin Pharmacokin. 1986;11:107–32.
28. Grekas D, Nikolaidis P, Karamonzis M, Alivanis P, Tourkantonis A. Effects of azathioprine on cyclosporin metabolism. Nephron. 1992;60:489 (letter).
29. Bokenkamp A, Offner G, Hoyer PF. Improved absorption of cyclosporin A from a new microemulsion formulation: implications for dosage and monitoring. Ped Nephrol. 1995;9:196–8.
30. Ducharme MP, Warbasse LH, Edwards DJ. Disposition of intravenous and oral cyclosporin after administration with grapefruit juice. Clin Pharm Ther. 1995;57:485–91.
31. Claris O, Picaud JC, Brazier JL, *et al.* Pharmacokinetics of cyclosporin A in 16 newborn infants of renal or cardiac transplant mothers. Devel Pharm Ther. 1993;20:180–5.
32. Turgeon DK, Leichtman AB, Lown KS. P450 3A activity and cyclosporin dosing in kidney and heart transplant recipients. Clin Pharm Ther. 1994;56:253–60.
33. Lopez-Gill JA. Fluconazole–cyclosporin interactions: a close dependent effect. Ann Pharmacother. 1993;27:427–30.
34. Wagner K, Philipp TH, Heinemeyer G, *et al.* Interactions of cyclosporin and calcium antagonists. Transplant Proc. 1989;21:1453–6.
35. Sketris IS, Methot ME, Nicol D. Effect of calcium-channel blockers on cyclosporin clearance and use in renal transplant patients. Ann Pharmacother. 1994;28:1227–31.
36. Borg AA, Davis MJ, Fowler PD. Rifampicin in early rheumatoid arthritis. Scand J Rheum. 1993;22:39–42.
37. Jundt JW, Browne BA, Fiocco GP, *et al.* A comparison of low dose methotrexate bioavailability: oral solution, oral tablet, subcutaneous and intramuscular dosing. J Rheum. 1993;20:1845–9.
38. Hamilton RA, Kremer JM. The effects of food on methotrexate absorption. J Rheum. 1995;22:630–4.
39. Bologna C, Edno L, Anaya JM, *et al.* Methotrexate concentrations in synovial membrane and travecular and cortical bone in rheumatoid arthritis patients. Arthritis Rheum. 1994;37:1770–3.
40. Kremer JM, Petrillo GF, Hamilton RA. Examination of pharmacokinetic variables in a cohort of patients with rheumatoid arthritis beginning therapy with methotrexate compared with a cohort receiving the drug for a mean of 81 months. J Rheum. 1995;22:41–4.
41. Albertioni F, Flato B, Seideman P, *et al.* Methotrexate in juvenile rheumatoid arthritis. Eur J Clin Pharmacol. 1995;47:507–11.
42. Koren G, Ferrazzini G, Sohl H, *et al.* Chronopharmacology of methotrexate pharmacokinetics in childhood leukemia. Chrono Int 1992;9:434–8.
43. Tracy, TS, Worster T, Bradley JD, *et al.* Methotrexate disposition following concomitant administration of ketoprofen, piroxicam and flurbiprofen in patients with rheumatoid arthritis. Br J Clin Pharm. 1994;37:453–456.
44. Combe B, Edno L, Lafforgue P, *et al.* Total and free methotrexate pharmacokinetics with and without piroxicam in rheumatoid arthritis patients. Br J Rheum. 1995;34:421–8.
45. McConkey B, Davies P, Crockson RA, *et al.* Effects of gold, dapsone, and prednisone on serum C-reactive protein and haptoglobin and the erythrocyte sedimentation rate in rheumatoid arthritis. Ann Rheum Dis. 1979;38:141–4.
46. Swinson D, Ziosnich JLJ. Double-blind trial of dapsone against placebo in the treatment of rheumatoid arthritis. Ann Rheum Dis. 1981;40:235–9.
47. Haar D, Solvkjaer M, Unger B, *et al.* A double-blind comparative study of hydroxychloroquine and dapsone alone and in combination in rheumatoid arthritis. Scand J Rheum. 1993;22:113–18.
48. Kloppenburg M, Breedveld FC, Terwiel JP, *et al.* Minocycline in active rheumatoid arthritis. Arthritis Rheum. 1994;37:629–36.
49. Tilley BC, Alarcon GS, Heyse SP, *et al.* Minocycline in rheumatoid arthritis, a 48 week, double-blind, placebo-controlled trial. Ann Int Med. 1995;122:81–9.
50. Jeurissen MEC, Boerbooms AMTh, Van de Putte LBA, Doesburg WH, Lemmens Am. Influence of methotrexate and azathioprine on radiologic progression in rheumatoid arthritis. A randomized double-blind study. Ann Intern Med. 1991;114:999–1004.
51. Kruger K, Schattenkirchner M. Comparison of cyclosporin A and azathioprine in the treatment of rheumatoid arthritis – results of a double-blind multicentre study. Clin Rheum. 1994;13:248–55.
52. Paulus HE, Williams HJ, Ward JR, *et al.* Azathioprine versus D-penicillamine in rheumatoid arthritis patients who have been treated unsuccessfully with gold. Arthritis Rheum. 1984;27:721–7.
53. Calin A. A placebo controlled cross-over study of azathioprine in Reiter's syndrome. Ann Rheum Dis. 1986;45:653–5.
54. Yazici H, Pazarli H, Barnes C, *et al.* A controlled trial of azathioprine in Behçet's disease. N Engl J Med. 1990;322:281–5.
55. Felson DT, Anderson J. Evidence of the superiority of immunosuppressive drugs and prednisone alone in lupus nephritis: results of a pooled analysis. N Engl J Med. 1984;311:1528–33.
56. Whisnant JK, Pelkey J. Rheumatoid arthritis: treatment with azathioprine ?. Clinical side effects and laboratory abnormalities. Ann Rheum Dis. 1982;41(Suppl 1):44–7.
57. Larval L, Soule J-C, LeTourneau A. Reversible lymphoma in the setting of azathioprine therapy for Crohn's disease. N Engl J Med. 1994;331:883–4.
58. Clements PJ, Davis J. Cytotoxic drugs: their application to the rheumatic diseases. Semin Arthritis Rheum. 1986;4:231–54.
59. Cannon GW, Jackson CG, Samuelson CO Jr, *et al.* Chlorambucil therapy in rheumatoid arthritis: clinical experience in 28 patients and literature review. Semin Arthritis Rheum. 1985;15:106–18.
60. Sinoway PA, Callen JP. Chlorambucil: An effective corticosteroid-sparing agent for patients with recalcitrant dermatomyositis. Arthritis Rheum. 1993;36:319–24.
61. Chapman RM, Sutcliffe SB. Protection of ovarian function by oral contraceptives in women receiving chemotherapy for Hodgkin's disease. Blood. 1981;58:849–51.
62. Kahn MF, Arlet J, Bloch-Michel H, *et al.* Leucemies aigues apres traitement par agents cytotoxiques en rheumatologies: 19 observations chex 2006 patients. Nouv Presse Med. 1979;8:1393–7.
63. Glode LM, Robinson J, Gould SF. Protection from cyclophosphamide-induced testicular damage with an analogue of gonadotropin-releasing hormone. Lancet. 1981;i:1132–4.
64. Nseyo UO, Huben RP, Klioze SS, Pontes JE. Protection of germinal epithelium with luteinizing hormone-releasing hormone analogue. J Urol. 1985;34:187–90.
65. Schilsky RL, Lewis BJ, Sherins RJ, Young RC. Gonadal dysfunction in patients receiving chemotherapy for cancer. Ann Intern Med. 1980;93:109–14.
66. Austin HA, Klippel JH, Balow JE, *et al.* Therapy of lupus nephritis: controlled trial of prednisone and cytotoxic drugs. N Engl J Med. 1986;314:614–19.
67. Klippel JH, Austin HA, Barlow JE, *et al.* Studies of immunosuppressive drugs in the treatment of lupus nephritis. Rheum Dis Clinics North Amer. 1987;13:47–56.
68. Reinhold-Keller E, Kekow J, Schnabel A, *et al.* Influence of disease manifestation and antineutrophil cytoplasmic antibody titer on the response to pulse cyclophosphamide therapy in patients with Wegener's granulomatosis. Arthritis Rheum. 1994;37:919–24.
69. Silver RM, Warick JH, Kinsella MB, Standt LS, Baumann MH, Strange C. Cyclophosphamide and low-dose prednisone therapy in patients with systemic sclerosis (scleroderma) with interstitial lung disease. J Rheum. 1993;20:838–44.
70. Kinlen LJ. Incidence of cancer in rheumatoid arthritis and other disorders with immunosuppressive treatment. Am J Med. 1985;78(Suppl 1A):44–9.
71. Wang CL, Wang F, Bosco JJ. Ovarian failure in oral cyclophosphamide treatment for systemic lupus erythematosus. Lupus. 1995;4:11–14.
72. Damewood MD, Grochow LB. Prospects for fertility after chemotherapy or radiation for neoplastic disease. Fertil Steril. 1986;45:443–58.
73. Radis CD, Kahl LE, Baker GL, *et al.* Effects of cyclophosphamide on the development of malignancy and on long-term survival of patients with rheumatoid arthritis. Arthritis Rheum. 1995;38:1120–7.
74. Ehrlich RM, Freedman A, Goldsobel AB, Stiehme ER. The use of sodium-2-metcaptoethane sulfonate to prevent cyclophosphamide cystitis. J Urol. 1984;131:960–2.
75. Omdal R, Husby G, Koldingsnes W. Intravenous and oral cyclophosphamide pulse therapy in rheumatic diseases: side effects and complications. Clin Exper Rheum. 1993;11:283–8.
76. Tugwell P, Bombardier C, Gent M, *et al.* Low-dose cyclosporin versus placebo in patients with rheumatoid arthritis. Lancet 1990;335:1051–55.
77. International Kidney Biopsy Registry of Cyclosporin in Autoimmune Diseases. Renal morphology after cyclosporin A therapy in rheumatoid arthritis patients. Br J Rheum. 1993;32:65–71.
78. VanJoost TL, Box JD, Heule F, Meinard, MMHM. Low-dose cyclosporin A in severe psoriasis. A double-blind study. Br J Dermatol. 1988;118:183–90.
79. Clements PJ, Lachenbruch PA, Sterz M, *et al.* Cyclosporin in systemic sclerosis. Results of a forty-eight week open safety study in ten patients. Arthritis Rheum. 1993;36:75–83.
80. Denton CP, Sweny P, Abdulla A, *et al.* Acute renal failure occurring in scleroderma treated with cyclosporin A: a report of three cases. Br J Rheum. 1994;33:90–2.
81. Mead JC, Brown PAJ, Whiting PH. The relationship between total kidney cyclosporin A concentrations, trough drug levels and renal function in the rat following withdrawal of treatment. Human Exp Tox. 1994;13:506–11.
82. Krupp P, Monka C. Side-effect profile of cyclosporin A in patients treated for psoriasis. Br J Dermatol. 1990;122(Suppl):47–56.
83. Borgini MJ, Paulus HE. Combination therapy. In: Brook PM , Furst DE, ed. Innovative treatment approaches for rheumatoid arthritis. Bailliere's Clin Rheum. 1995;9:689–710.
84. Tugwell P, Bennerr K, Gent M. Methotrexate in rheumatoid arthritis. Annals Int Med. 1987;107:358–66.

85. Alarcon GS, Lopez-Mendez A, Walter J, *et al.* Radiographic evidence of disease progression in methotrexate treated and non-methotrexate disease modifying antirheumatoid drug treated rheumatoid arthritis. J Rheum. 1992;19:1868–73.
86. IARC Working Group. Methotrexate. IARC Monogr. 1982;26:282–5.
87. Mullarkey MF, Blumenstein BA, Andrade P, *et al.* Methotrexate in the treatment of cortico-dependent asthma. N Engl J Med. 1988;318:603–7.
88. Nyfors A, Jensen H. Frequency of malignant neoplasms in 248 long-term methotrexate-treated psoriatics. Dermatologica. 1983;167:260–1.
89. Escalante A, Beardmore TD. Risk factors for early wound complications after orthopedic surgery for rheumatoid arthritis. J Rheum. 1995;22:1844–51.
90. Kremer JM, Alancon GS, Lightfoot RW, *et al.* Methotrexate for rheumatoid arthritis. Suggested guideleines for monitoring liver toxicity. American College of Rheumatology. Arthritis Rheum. 1994;37:316–28.
91. Davies JMS, Eastman A, Furst DE, *et al.* Lymphoma in two patients on low dose methotrexate therapy with identification of Epstein–Barr virus. Arthritis Rheum (in press), 1996.
92. Furst DE. Practical clinical pharmacology and drug interactions of low-dose methotrexate therapy in rheumatoid arthritis. Br J Rheum. 1995;34(Suppl 2):20–5.
93. Scott DL, Dawes PT, Tunn E, *et al.* Combination therapy with gold and hydroxychloroquine in rheumatoid arthritis: a prospective, randomized, placebo-controlled study. Br J Rheumatol. 1989;28:128–33.
94. Ferraz MB, Pinheiro GR, Helfenstein M, *et al.* Combination therapy with methotrexate and chloroquine in rheumatoid arthritis. A multicenter randomized placebo-controlled trial. Scand J Rheum. 1994;23:231–6.
95. Tugwell P, Pincus T, Yocum D, *et al.* Combination therapy with cyclosporin and methotrexate in severe rheumatoid arthritis. N Engl J Med. 1995;333:183–4.
96. Csuka M, Carrera GF, McCarty DJ. Treatment of intractable rheumatoid arthritis with combined cyclophosphamide, azathioprine, and hydroxychloroquine. A follow-up study. JAMA. 1986;255:2315–19.
97. O'Dell JR, Haire CE, Erickson N, *et al.* Treatment of rheumatoid arthritis with methotrexate alone, sulfasalazine and hydroxychloroquine, or a combination of all three medications. N Engl J Med. 1996;334:1287–91.
98. ACR ad hoc committee on Clinical Guidelines. Guidelines for Monitoring Drug Therapy. Arthritis Rheum. 1996;39:723–31.

10

IMMUNOTHERAPIES

Ernest HS Choy, Gabrielle H Kingsley & Gabrielle S Panayi

- Immunotherapy usually involves the use of biologic agents such as monoclonal antibodies, soluble receptors or peptides, though immunoactive drugs are increasingly being developed.
- Cytokines, particularly TNF and IL-1, and T-cells have been the major therapeutic targets in arthritis.
- Anticytokine therapy has excellent anti-inflammatory properties but its effects are generally short-lived so long-term or repeated treatment is needed.
- Anti-T-cell therapy shows a much more limited short-term effect but may have the potential to effect a more fundamental alteration in the disease process.
- There have been no long-term immunotherapy studies so the effects of these agents on disease outcome is unknown.

INTRODUCTION

Immunotherapies are reviewed below under three main headings, anticytokine treatments, agents targeting adhesion processes and anti-T-cell agents. However, other therapies, such as oral tolerance and bone marrow transplantation, which do not fit easily into these groups are also discussed. One temptation is to focus exclusively on intellectual aspects, that is to say, what individual agents reveal about pathogenesis. Although this role as an immunologic probe is vital, immunotherapeutic agents must ultimately be judged by the same standards as any other treatment for a chronic disease. The ideal treatment needs to be highly effective yet cheap, easy to use and nontoxic. It should induce long-term disease remission after a single or short course of treatment and it should be appropriate for a substantial proportion of those with the disease. Application of the criteria shown in Figure 10.1 will enable the reader to judge whether a new agent is really a breakthrough.

DIFFERENT TYPES OF BIOLOGIC AGENTS

These are a number of possible biologic approaches to immunotherapy (Fig. 10.2). The commonest biologic treatments used so far have been monoclonal antibodies (MABs). A MAB is a single immunoglobulin clone produced using hybridoma technology. Hybridomas are generated by the fusion of a single B cell to a myeloma cell. The B cell determines antibody specificity; the myeloma cell confers immortality and the antibody isotype. Therefore, MABs target a single antigen with high affinity and specificity, which makes them attractive therapeutic tools. Furthermore, by selecting specific antibody isotypes, MABs can mediate desired functions such as complement-mediated cytotoxicity or Fc receptor binding. Most MABs are murine in origin so their use has been hampered by the development of human anti-mouse antibodies with the risk of anaphylaxis and reduced efficacy on retreatment (see Fig. 10.3). Genetic engineering has reduced this problem by developing chimeric and humanized MAB. Chimeric antibodies are murine immunoglobulins the Fc of which has been substituted by human sequences. When the framework region of the Fab is also replaced by human sequences, leaving only the antigen-binding site as a murine sequence, the antibody is known as a humanized antibody. These 'man-made' MABs are less antigenic and have therefore largely superseded murine MABs in the therapy of human diseases.

THERAPIES AGAINST CYTOKINES

ANTI-TNF-α MONOCLONAL ANTIBODIES

The potent proinflammatory cytokine tumor necrosis factor (TNF)-α is found in the joints and blood of RA patients. It induces mesenchymal cells to produce IL-1, IL-6, granulocyte macrophage colony–stimulating factor (GM-CSF) and matrix metalloproteinases which degrade cartilage and bone. Some researchers have argued that TNF-α is the major pathogenic cytokine in RA[2]. In placebo-controlled trials, both chimeric and humanized anti-TNF-α MABs produced immediate improvement in disease activity[3,4]. Disease activity measures such as erythrocyte sedimentation rate (ESR), C-reactive protein (CRP) and the number of tender and swollen joints dropped rapidly after treatment. The therapeutic effect of anti-TNF-α MAB relates closely to the serum concentration. However, high dose anti-TNF-α MAB treatment (10mg/kg) produced only a transient clinical improvement lasting 4–8 weeks. Repeated treatments have been shown to be feasible but the duration of clinical response shortens[5] and there is an increased incidence of infection and the development of anti-double stranded DNA (dsDNA) antibodies. There have also been case reports of lymphoproliferative diseases associated with anti-TNF-α therapy which may be a major stumbling block for this treatment strategy.

The anti-TNF-α MAB trials are good examples of how biologic

JUDGING NEW TREATMENTS FOR CHRONIC DISEASES
Significance of the results
How clinically significant are the stated benefits?
Are any adverse effects appropriate to the level of efficacy?
Does the agent induce remission or merely suppress disease?
Is there any effect on long-term disease outcome?
Is this treatment practicable in a normal clinical setting?
Is the treatment cost-effective?
Can the agent be combined effectively with other treatments?
Aspects of trial design
Was the trial design relevant to normal clinical practice?
Do the patients studied reflect an average patient population?
Is the result relevant only to a subgroup of patients?
What was the level of the placebo response?
Other factors
Are there fundamental lessons for disease pathogenesis?
Ethical aspects related to the study and future use of the agent

Fig. 10.1 Judging new treatments for chronic diseases.

DIFFERENT TYPES OF BIOLOGICAL TREATMENTS

Treatment type	Examples
Monoclonal antibodies	
Murine antibodies	Anti-ICAM-1 monoclonal antibody, BIRR
Chimeric antibodies	Anti-TNF-α monoclonal antibody, cA2
Humanized antibodies	Anti-TNF-α monoclonal antibody, CDP571
Soluble receptors (conjugated to human immunoglobulin)	Soluble IL-1 receptor TNF receptor fusion protein
Immunotoxins	
Antibodies conjugated to toxin	Anti-CD5 conjugated to ricin
Cytokine conjugated to toxin	IL-2 DAB
Immunosuppressive/ regulatory cytokines	IL-10 IL-4
Natural cytokine antagonists	IL-1 receptor antagonist
Small molecule inhibitors inhibiting cytokine release	Metalloproteinase inhibitors
Peptides	Vβ17 peptide vaccination
Immunomodulation	T-cell vaccination Oral tolerance

Fig. 10.2 Different types of biologic treatments.

treatments may provide useful information on disease pathogenesis. After treatment with anti-TNF-α MAB, IL-6 decreased in parallel with ESR and CRP, suggesting that TNF-α via IL-6 has an important role in the acute phase response. Anti-TNF-α treatment also transiently increased circulating lymphocyte numbers, probably due to reduced expression of synovial vascular adhesion molecules which are known to be upregulated by TNF-α[6]. One other important observation is a difference in the biologic effect between the two antibodies, cA2 and CDP571. Whereas cA2 led to a reduction in monocyte number, CDP571 did not. The reason for this is that chimeric antibody, cA2 (Centocor), is conjugated to a human IgG_1 which is complement fixing and therefore kills TNF-α-bearing cells (including monocyte–macrophages) while the humanized antibody, CDP571 (Celltech Therapeutic Ltd), is conjugated to a human IgG_4 and is therefore noncomplement fixing. This illustrates the importance of specific IgG classes in mediating different functions.

These data confirm the *in vitro* actions of TNF-α and indicate that it is a major mediator of inflammation in RA. Interestingly, although inflammatory markers improved after treatment, there was no change in serum levels of the lymphocyte activation workers, soluble CD4 and soluble IL-2 receptor. Further studies are needed to assess the effect on long-term disease modification and joint destruction.

SOLUBLE TNF RECEPTORS

'Man-made' antibodies, though less immunogenic, still provoke an immune response; other biologic agents which may be less antigenic have therefore been developed (see Fig. 10.2). Soluble cytokine receptors are receptor molecules which have been cleaved off their normal site on the cell surface. They compete with cell-bound receptors for cytokines and therefore act as competitive inhibitors. Unfortunately, soluble cytokine receptors have very short half-lives although these can be prolonged by grafting them to human immunoglobulin Fc.

There are two types of cellular receptor for TNF-α, p55 and p75. Both types also have soluble forms. These have been conjugated to human immunoglobulin Fc and are being tested in RA[7]. A placebo-controlled trial of such a fusion protein administered by subcutaneous injection showed significant benefit over placebo at a dose of $16mg/m^2$. Such fusion proteins may be less antigenic than 'man-made' antibodies and may improve retreatment efficacy. However, the problems of nonspecific immunosuppression and oncogenesis remain.

MURINE, CHIMERIC AND HUMANIZED MONOCLONAL ANTIBODIES

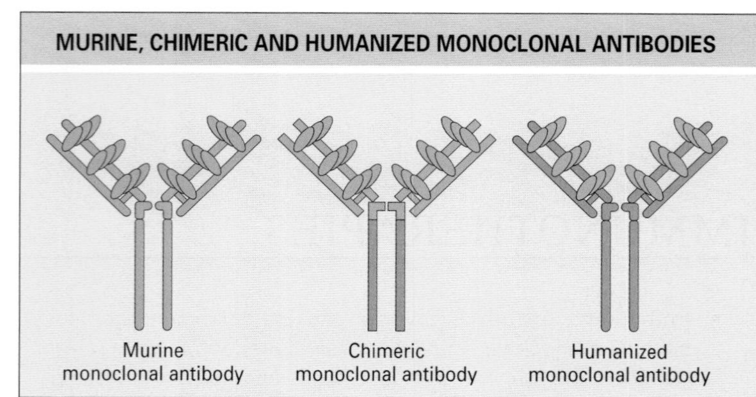

Fig. 10.3 Murine, chimeric and humanized monoclonal antibodies. Blue indicates murine sequences; green indicates human sequences.

Anti-interleukin-1 reagents

Interleukin-1 is a pro-inflammatory cytokine thought to be particularly important in mediating joint damage in RA. It binds to two types of receptors: IL-1 receptor type I (IL-1RI) and IL-1 receptor type II (IL-1RII). However, only IL-1RI transmits signals intracellularly, leading to cell activation, whereas IL1-RII is a decoy receptor; both can exist as soluble forms. These soluble receptors and cell surface IL1-RII compete with cell-bound IL-1RI for IL-1, thus inhibiting IL-1-mediated cell activation (Fig. 10.4). There is also a naturally occurring antagonist: IL-1 receptor antagonist (IL-1ra), which binds to IL-1RI almost irreversibly. Since it does not deliver an active signal, it inhibits IL-1 by competing for IL-1RI.

When recombinant human soluble IL-1RI was administered to patients with RA, it failed to produce significant clinical improvement although there was reduction in monocyte surface IL-1[8]; in many cases, the disease worsened. This may be due to recombinant soluble IL-1RI binding to IL-1ra. If this binding occurs, less IL-1ra will bind to cell surface IL-1RI. These free IL-1RI molecules will therefore engage with IL-1 itself, augmenting IL-1-induced cell activation and inflammation. As soluble IL-1RII does not bind to IL-1ra, it may be a better therapeutic choice. Recombinant human IL1-ra (Amgen), administered as subcutaneous injections, has been tested in a double-blind placebo-controlled multicenter trial[9]. A dose of 150mg/day administered subcutaneously produced significant clinical improvement and slowed the progression of erosions. The commonest side effect was a reaction at the injection site.

The results with IL-1ra confirm that blocking IL-1 is also an effective treatment strategy for RA. However, both IL1-ra and soluble IL-1 receptors have short half-lives so frequent dosing is necessary. One way currently being examined to circumvent this problem is to use gene therapy techniques[10]. In animal models, synoviocytes transfected with the human IL1-ra gene and re-injected into the joint produce IL1-ra continuously in the synovium with consequent clinical improvement. A human study is in progress.

OTHER CYTOKINE-BASED TREATMENTS

Immunosuppressive cytokines such as IL-4 or IL-10 may be used to suppress inflammation. Collagen-induced arthritis is inhibited by IL-10 and a multicenter, placebo-controlled trial of IL-10 in RA is in progress. Interferon (INF)-γ produced only minimal therapeutic benefit in RA; its use has been abandoned. Anti-IL-6 MAB, used by Wendling *et al.* in a open study[12], showed promising results but no placebo-controlled trials have been performed to assess its true efficacy.

There are many alternative strategies[13] to inhibit cytokines, including drugs such as tenidap and intravenous γ-globulin. The efficacy of the latter is doubtful; at least at low doses, placebo-controlled studies show no benefit[14]. Many cytokines are expressed on the cell surface and released through enzymatic cleavage by specific metalloproteinases. Thus another way of inhibiting cytokine action is to use small

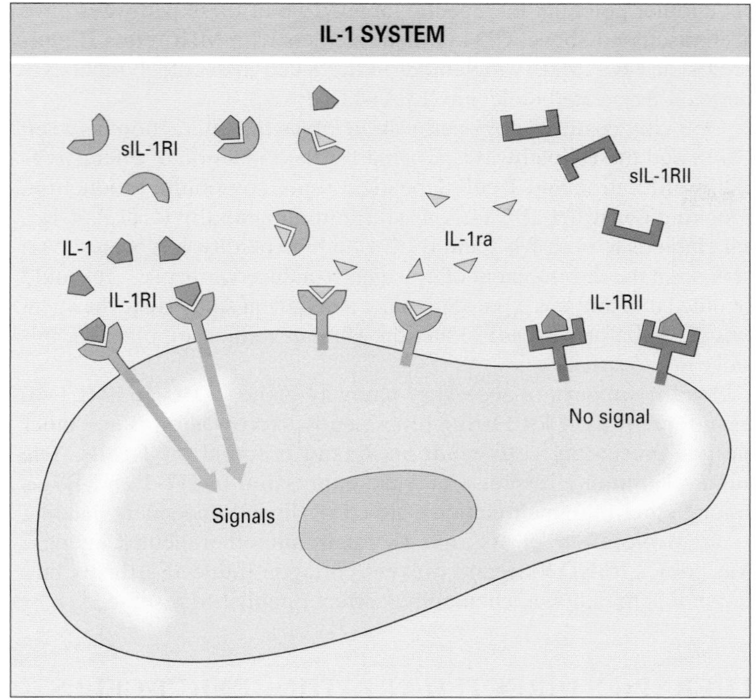

Fig. 10.4 IL-1 system.

molecule metalloproteinase inhibitors. In addition, yet another possibility would be to use antisense oligonucleotides which, by binding to the cytokine complementary DNA and/or RNA, inhibits transcription and translation.

SUMMARY

Anticytokine therapies have been intensively investigated as treatment for RA. The advantages and disadvantages of this approach are summarized in Figure 10.5.

THERAPIES AGAINST ADHESION MOLECULES

Leukocyte migration plays a central role in the generation of synovitis, implying that its inhibition might be an effective therapeutic strategy in RA. Some antirheumatic drugs, including corticosteroids and methotrexate, inhibit leukocyte adhesion to endothelium. Furthermore, as already discussed, anti-TNF MABs may, in part, exert their effect by inhibiting adhesion molecule expression in the joint[6].

Leukocytes migrate into tissues using a multistep process, initially binding to endothelium, then migrating between the endothelial cells and finally entering and being retained within the tissue. Each step is regulated by multiple specific adhesion molecules (homing receptors) on leukocytes which interact with their counterparts (addressins) on the endothelial or target organ cells (see Chapter 5.12). All these homing receptor–addressin pairs are potential immunotherapeutic targets. One important consideration is how much of the migration process is general for all inflamed peripheral tissues and how much is organ specific. The inhibition of synovium-specific adhesion processes would obviously be the ideal way to achieve efficacy and selectivity in arthritis.

To date, only one antiadhesion agent has been studied *in vivo* in RA, a murine MAB directed against the important but widely utilized adhesion molecule intercellular adhesion molecule (ICAM)-1 (CD54); this molecule also has an accessory function in T-cell activation. Two open studies have been carried out by a single group, one in 32 patients with active disease refractory to treatment[15] and the other in 10 patients with active but 'early or indolent' disease, defined as previous treatment with no more than one disease-modifying drug[16]. The treatment was well tolerated and appeared to be effective, especially in early RA,

ADVANTAGES AND DISADVANTAGES OF ANTICYTOKINE THERAPY

Advantage	Disadvantage
Excellent anti-inflammatory targets	Transient effect, therefore long-term treatment necessary
Many targets to choose from	Nonspecific and therefore risk of immunosuppression
Rapidly effective	Many treatments have short half-lives

Fig. 10.5 Advantages and disadvantages of anticytokine therapy.

although a placebo-controlled study is required. The mechanism of action has not been fully defined, but both an alteration in T-cell recirculation and a transient T-cell hyporesponsiveness may contribute.

ANTI-T-CELL MONOCLONAL ANTIBODIES

In rheumatoid arthritis, T-lymphocytes, in particular $CD4^+$ T-lymphocytes, are thought to be an ideal target for therapy[14,17].

EARLY T-CELL IMMUNOTHERAPY

Therapies such as thoracic duct drainage, total lymphoid irradiation and lymphocytopheresis have been abandoned because of side effects and impracticability, although some studies suggested efficacy. More recently, cyclosporin, a T-cell inhibitor, has been shown to be effective.

Based on these successes, anti-T-cell treatments aimed at depleting different T-cell subsets have been tested in RA (see Fig. 10.6). The first anti-T-cell MAB used was anti-CD7. It was ineffective[18], probably because it targeted a subset of T-cells now thought to be unimportant in RA. A second anti-T-cell MAB, CD5-plus, is an immunoconjugate of murine anti-CD5 MAB and the cellular toxin, ricin. It deletes $CD5^+$ T- and B cells. Despite promising open studies the placebo-controlled trial result was negative[19], possibly because of both an unexpectedly high placebo response rate and the use of a lower dose than was used in the open study (to avoid profound lymphopenia). Another immunotoxin is IL2-DAB in which IL-2 is joined to a diphtheria toxin A chain. As IL-2 receptors are only found on activated T-cells, IL2-DAB was potentially a more specific treatment. Placebo-controlled trials[20] showed that it was superior to placebo but only 18% of patients responded, compared with no responders in the placebo group. Furthermore, in the treatment group, the withdrawal rate was high (12 out of 45 patients) and half the patients showed an abnormal rise in liver transaminases after treatment. As a result, anti-CD7, CD5-plus and IL2-DAB have been abandoned as treatments for RA.

CAMPATH-1H (ANTI-CDW52)

Campath-1H is an IgG1 humanized MAB[21]. It targets a panlymphocyte antigen CDw52 (of unknown function), fixes complement and is extremely lytic. Clinical improvement was observed after intravenous Campath-1H[22] but there were significant side effects. Campath-1H induced a cytokine release syndrome in all patients which was characterized by high fever, rigors, chills, diarrhea and hypotension. Intravenous treatment led to profound and persistent peripheral blood lymphopenia which did not correlate with disease improvement; indeed, disease often relapsed long before the lymphocyte count returned to normal. Biopsy studies show that a large number of lymphocytes persist in the joint[23] after treatment, suggesting that either synovial lymphocytes are resistant to lysis or Campath-1H did not penetrate the joint. Worryingly the prolonged lymphopenia was associated with increased incidence of opportunistic infections. The severity of the cytokine release syndrome can be reduced by administering Campath-1H subcutaneously[24] although

ANTI-T-CELL TREATMENTS AND THEIR TARGET T-CELL SUBSETS		
Anti-T-cell treatment	Cells surface target	Targeted T-cell subset
Murine and chimeric anti-CD7 MABs	CD7	CD7⁺-activated T-cells
CD5-plus (murine anti-CD5 MABs conjugated to ricin)	CD5	CD5⁺ T- and B cells
IL2-DAB (recombinant human IL-2 conjugated to the A chain of diphtheria toxin)	IL-2	IL-2 receptor positive activated T-cells
Campath-1H (humanized anti-CDw52 MAB)	CDw52	All T- and B cells
Murine anti-CD4 MABs	CD4	CD4⁺ T-cells
Chimeric depleting anti-CD4 MABs	CD4	CD4⁺ T-cells
Nondepleting humanized anti-CD4 MABs	CD4	CD4⁺ T-cells

Fig. 10.6 Anti-T-cell treatments and their target T-cell subsets.

this also reduces efficacy. Campath-1H has been withdrawn from development for RA.

ANTI-CD4 MONOCLONAL ANTIBODIES

Open studies of murine anti-CD4 MAB showed promising results in RA[17]. As a result, the chimeric anti-CD4 MAB, cM-T412 (Centocor), was tested in several clinical trials. Neither a single nor repeated weekly treatments produced any clinical improvement although there was a dose-related peripheral blood CD4 lymphopenia. When cM-T412 was administered in an open study daily for 5 days, 10 out of 12 patients appeared to improve; in 3 this was prolonged[25]. The degree of lymphocyte depletion and the percentage of lymphocytes coated with cM-T412 were less in the joint than in peripheral blood but, interestingly, the degree of synovial T-cell coating correlated with clinical response[25]. One explanation for the prolonged clinical response seen in some patients may be the induction of apoptosis in etiologic antigen-specific cells[26]. Despite these interesting preliminary studies, a placebo-controlled trial of cM-T412 in early RA did not show any significant benefit[27]. However, the dose of cM-T412 used in this study was less than the previous study because treatment was not given when the CD4 lymphocyte number was less than 250×10^6/l. Although no clinical benefit was seen, when the synovia of these patients were examined, there were reductions in the degree of inflammation[28]. Clearly, higher doses and more prolonged therapy may achieve a more significant clinical benefit. However, this would also lead to an unacceptably profound CD4 lymphopenia with the risk of severe immunosuppression. Hence, the strategy of depleting $CD4^+$ lymphocytes as a treatment for RA has been abandoned.

Another MAB-related therapeutic strategy is to induce immunologic tolerance using nondepleting anti-CD4 MABs. This has been shown to be effective in animal models of RA such as streptococcal cell wall and collagen-induced arthritis. A number of nondepleting anti-CD4 MABs are currently being tested in RA patients and early results suggest they are effective[29,30].

THERAPY DIRECTED AGAINST OTHER T-CELL ACCESSORY MOLECULES

The primary interactions in antigen processing by the immune system involves the formation of a complex of T-cell receptor, antigenic peptide and MHC molecule. However, a number of other accessory or costimulatory pathways are also required for optimal effect; these provide yet another potential therapeutic target. Two of these pathways have been discussed above: CD4 (which interacts with MHC class II molecules) and ICAM-1 [which binds to the T-cell molecule, lymphocyte function-associated molecule (LFA)-1].

One vital costimulatory pathway involves the interaction between CD28 and the B7 pathway[14], crucial for the induction of effective T-cell proliferation and T-cell dependent immunoglobulin production. Blocking construct of CTLA-4 with immunoglobulin (CTLA-4-Ig), which binds to both B7-1 and B7-2 with high avidity, has been shown to prevent the development of collagen II-induced arthritis[31]. It should be noted that this was a prevention not a treatment study since the agent was given before disease induction. Human studies are planned, initially in psoriasis.

Another important accessory pathway is the CD40-gp39 (CD40 ligand) pathway, CD40 being prominently expressed on B and other antigen-presenting cells while its ligand is found on T-cells. The humoral immune response and the expression of B7-1 and B7-2, among other immune functions, are CD40 ligand-dependent, leading to an exploration of its role as an immunotherapeutic agent[32]. Antibodies to CD40 ligand prevent collagen-induced arthritis but, again, it is not known whether they affect established disease.

THERAPIES DIRECTED AT PATHOGENIC T-CELLS

The holy grail for those seeking to use T-cells as therapeutic targets in RA is to develop a treatment which affects, primarily or exclusively, the arthritogenic T-cells. If such were possible, it might only be effective in early disease, before the immune–inflammatory cascade of synovitis has been initiated. Alternatively, without the initiating T-cells, even late-stage synovitis might ultimately settle.

In animal models, it is fairly easy to identify the arthritogenic clones which induce disease since they can be transferred from one animal to another. This led to the development of the technique of T-cell vaccination[17], analogous to bacterial vaccination, in which animals are immunized with pathogenic T-cells attenuated by chemicals or radiation such that they no longer induce disease. The animals develop an antivaccine immune response which also inhibits the nonattenuated but otherwise immunologically identical pathogenic T-cells responsible for the disease. T-cell vaccination in animal models is able both to prevent and to treat established disease. Attempts have been made to apply this technique to humans using synovial T-cells which are postulated to contain a higher proportion of pathogenic T-cells than those in the blood; studies have been small and no firm conclusions can be drawn. No further studies are currently planned in RA though more success has been reported in multiple sclerosis where a good candidate exists for the disease-causing antigen, myelin basic protein, enabling identification of possible disease-inducing T-cells.

An alternative approach to the identification of pathogenic T-cells examined whether T-cells with particular T-cell receptor Vβ chains were expanded in lesional sites, such as the synovium, compared with blood. It was proposed that such expanded T-cells would be pathogenetically relevant. It was further suggested, by analogy with experiments in animals, that vaccination with peptides from T-cell receptors on pathogenic T-cells would inhibit disease[17]. Many different Vβ populations were reported as expanded by various groups of investigators. However, one group looked at Vβ usage by recently activated T-cells, defined as T-cells expressing the IL-2 receptor, on the basis that these recently activated cells were more relevant to disease pathogenesis. As the results showed an increase of $V\beta17^+$ usage by IL-2 receptor-positive (IL-$2R^+$) T-cells in the synovium, the investigators embarked on a clinical trial of a Vβ17-derived peptide in RA[33]. This was an uncontrolled open dose-finding study, so evidence of clinical and biologic efficacy must be treated cautiously although the investigators note that patient joint scores decreased at all follow up visits as did $V\beta17^+$ IL-$2R^+$ T-cells in the blood. Approximately 40% of patients developed a

T-cell response to the vaccinated peptide. No toxicity was observed, but further studies are clearly needed.

Other ways of interfering with the activation of the trimolecular complex of T-cell receptor, peptide and MHC molecule, have been examined either *in vitro* or in animal models *in vivo*. Monoclonal antibodies against MHC molecules have been used to block antigen presentation. Soluble MHC peptide–autoantigenic peptide complexes have been developed with the aim of inducing T-cell anergy by binding to the T-cell receptor in the absence of costimulatory signals. Synthetic T-cell receptor binding peptides have also been identified which aim to anergize the T cell or deflect its secreted cytokines from a proinflammatory to an immunosuppressive pattern; these have so far only been tested *in vitro*.

ORAL TOLERANCE

The phenomenon of oral tolerance was first demonstrated in the early years of this century but analysis of the underlying immunologic mechanisms and therapeutic application are much more recent, the first studies in humans being performed only in the past 5 years. Oral tolerance was initially defined as the capacity to decrease immunologic reactivity to an antigen by administering that same antigen via the gut. However, more detailed study has shown that, in certain systems, oral antigens may induce tolerance, not only to themselves but also to other antigens from the same tissue. This phenomenon, known as 'bystander suppression', is critical to therapy for human diseases since the causative antigen is usually unknown. Also crucially for treating humans, tolerance can be induced where an immune reaction is ongoing. One interesting recent development is that highly effective tolerance can also be induced by inhalation of antigen.

The mechanisms underlying oral tolerance are still unclear[34]. Immunologic tolerance potentially involves three main processes: deletion of specific T-cell clones, clonal anergy and active suppression. Both the two latter mechanisms have been shown to operate in different oral tolerance systems. A currently popular model suggests that exposure to low-dose oral antigen, for example type II collagen, induces antigen-specific regulatory (TH2) T-cells in the gut lymphoid tissue to produce suppressive cytokines such as transforming growth factor (TGF)-β, IL-4 and IL-10. These cells then migrate from the gut to the target organ; in the case of T-cells specific for type II collagen this would be the joint. There they would encounter their cognate antigen, again leading to the local release of TGF-β, IL-4 and IL-10. This local release of suppressor cytokines would suppress any immune process in the target tissue whether triggered by the original cognate antigen or by any other antigen present in the diseased tissue, hence bystander tolerance. In contrast, higher doses of oral antigen, perhaps because they are partially absorbed systemically, directly induce unresponsiveness (anergy) of pathogenic (TH1, INF-γ-producing) T-cells. Such clonal anergy is antigen-specific and thus of less use in treating human disease due to unknown pathogens. It is currently unclear whether the mechanisms underlying tolerance to inhaled antigen are the same as those in oral tolerance.

In animal models of arthritis, oral administration of type II collagen before or after disease onset has been shown to be effective in preventing or ameliorating collagen-induced arthritis (type II collagen). Bystander suppression has also been demonstrated since adjuvant arthritis, induced by mycobacterial proteins, can be suppressed by feeding with type II collagen.

In RA, a placebo-controlled, randomized study showed a clinical improvement in patients treated with chicken-derived type II collagen compared to placebo[35]. There was also an increase in the number of patients who went into remission in the active group. No side effects were seen. Disappointingly, a study from a different group, using bovine type II collagen, failed to demonstrate any significant difference between active and placebo groups, although a minority of patients were said to respond, and, again, there was no toxicity[36]. The cause of this variation is not clear although both studies were significantly underpowered. Larger studies, in progress, may resolve the issue.

BONE MARROW TRANSPLANTATION AND STEM CELL THERAPY

Despite the intensive research described above, most of the new immunotherapies are still a long way from practical use. The pressure remains on clinicians to do something for patients who have severe and unremitting connective tissue diseases and who do not respond to standard therapy. Case reports have shown that allogeneic bone marrow transplantation for leukemia or aplastic anemia often induces remission of coincident autoimmune disease. These observations led to consideration of autologous bone marrow transplantation (with or without selection for stem cells) as a therapy for critically ill connective tissue patients[37]. It is unclear whether this therapy produces permanent remission. If the primary defect is in the stem cell, recurrence is likely; if the disease is due to an abnormal response to antigen, the possibility exists of tolerance developing (particularly if memory T-cells are ablated). Only time will tell if the major dangers associated with this type of treatment are outweighed by the benefit.

OTHER NEW THERAPEUTIC APPROACHES

This chapter has primarily concentrated on interventions directed against the fundamental immune processes involved in RA. Many other novel therapeutic approaches are being examined which may be complementary to those mentioned above or suitable for patients at different stages of the disease. One such approach is the use of drugs able to inhibit metalloproteinases, the enzymes now thought to be largely responsible for bone erosion. Another is the use of agents which inhibit angiogenesis (new blood vessel formation), which is critical in the proliferation of the synovium and the formation of pannus. A third approach is the use of recombinant cytokines or growth factors to treat particular manifestations, for example erythropoietin for anemia or granulocyte colony-stimulating factor (G-CSF)/GM-CSF to treat the neutropenia of Felty's syndrome.

REFERENCES

1. Kingsley GH, Lanchbury J, Panayi G. Immunotherapy in rheumatic disease: an idea whose time has come – or gone? Immunol Today. 1996;17:9–12.
2. Feldmann M, Brennan FM, Maini RM. Role of cytokines in rheumatoid arthritis. Annu Rev Immunol. 1996;14:397–440.
3. Elliott MJ, Maini RN, Feldmann M, *et al.* Randomised double-blind comparison of chimeric monoclonal antibody to tumour necrosis factor α (cA2) versus placebo in rheumatoid arthritis. Lancet. 1994;344:1105–10.
4. Rankin EC, Choy EH, Kassimos D, *et al.* The therapeutic effects of an engineered human anti-tumour necrosis factor alpha antibody (CDP571) in rheumatoid arthritis. Br J Rheumatol. 1995;34:334–42.
5. Elliott MJ, Maini RN, Feldmann M, *et al.* Repeated therapy with monoclonal antibody to tumour necrosis factor α (cA2) in patients with rheumatoid arthritis. Lancet. 1994;344:1125–7.
6. Tak PP, Taylor PC, Breedveld FC, *et al.* Decrease in cellularity and expression of adhesion molecules by anti-tumour necrosis factor α antibody treatment in patients with rheumatoid arthritis. Arthritis Rheum. 1996;39:1077–81.
7. Baumgartner S, Moreland LW, Schiff MH, *et al.* Double-blind placebo-controlled trial of tumour necrosis factor receptor (p80) fusion (TNFR:Fc) in active rheumatoid arthritis. Arthritis Rheum.

1996;39(Suppl):74A.
8. Drevlow BE, Loris R, Haag MA, *et al.* Recombinant human interleukin-1 receptor type I in the treatment of patients with active rheumatoid arthritis. Arthritis Rheum. 1996;39:257–65.
9. Bresnihan B on behalf of the collaborating investigators, Lookabaugh J, Witt K, Musikic P. Treatment with recombinant human interleukin-1 receptor antagonist (rhIL-1ra) in rheumatoid arthritis: results of a randomised double-blind placebo-controlled multicenter trial. Arthritis Rheum. 1996; 39(Suppl):73A.
10. Evans CH, Robbins PD. Pathways to gene therapy in rheumatoid arthritis. Curr Opin Rheumatol. 1996;8:230–4.
11. Walmsley M, Katsikis PD, Abney E, *et al.* Interleukin-10 inhibition of the progression of collagen-induced arthritis. Arthritis Rheum. 1996;39:495–503.
12. Wendling D, Racadot E, Wijdenes J. Treatment of severe rheumatoid arthritis by anti-interleukin 6 monoclonal antibody. J Rheumatol. 1993;20:259–62.
13. Henderson B. Therapeutic modulation of cytokines. Ann Rheum Dis. 1995;54:519–23.
14. Kalden JR, Manger B. Biologic agents in the treatment of inflammatory rheumatic diseases. Curr Opin Rheumatol. 1996;8:195–200.
15. Kavanaugh AF, Davis LS, Nichols LA, *et al.* Treatment of refractory rheumatoid arthritis with a monoclonal antibody to intercellular adhesion molecule 1. Arthritis Rheum. 1994;37:992–9.
16. Kavanaugh AF, Davis LS, Jain RI, Nichols LA, Lipsky PE. Phase I/II open-label study of the safety and efficacy of an anti-ICAM-1 (intercellular adhesion molecule-1; CD54) monoclonal antibody in early rheumatoid arthritis. J Rheumatol. 1996;23:1338–44.
17. Choy EHS, Kingsley GH, Panayi GS. T-cell regulation. In: PM Brooks, DE Furst, eds. Innovative treatment approaches for rheumatoid arthritis. London: Baillière Tindall; 1995:653–71.
18. Kirkham BW, Pitzalis C, Kingsley GH, *et al.* Monoclonal antibody treatment in rheumatoid arthritis: Clinical and immunological effects of a CD7 monoclonal antibody. Br J Rheumatol. 1991;30:459–63.
19. Olsen NJ, Brooks RH, Cush JJ, *et al.* A double-blind, placebo-controlled study of anti-CD5 immunoconjugate in patients with rheumatoid arthritis. Arthritis Rheum. 1996;39:1102–8.
20. Moreland LW, Sewell KL, Trentham DE, *et al.* Interleukin-2 diphtheria fusion protein (DAB486IL-2) in refractory rheumatoid arthritis. A double-blind, placebo-controlled trial with open-label extension. Arthritis Rheum. 1995;38:1177–86.
21. Isaacs JD, Watts RA, Hazelman BL, *et al.* Humanised monoclonal antibody therapy for rheumatoid arthritis. Lancet. 1992;340:748–52.
22. Isaacs JD, Manna VK, Rapson N, *et al.* Campath-1H in rheumatoid arthritis – an intravenous dose-ranging study. Br J Rheumatol. 1996;35:231–40.
23. Ruderman EM, Weinblatt ME, Thurmond LM, Pinkus GS, Gravallese EM. Synovial tissue response to treatment with Campath-1H. Arthritis Rheum. 1995;38:254–8.
24. Matteson EL, Yocum DE, St Clair EW, *et al.* Treatment of active refractory rheumatoid arthritis with humanized monoclonal antibody CAMPATH-1H administered by daily subcutaneous injection. Arthritis Rheum. 1995;38:1187–93.
25. Choy EH, Pitzalis C, Cauli A, *et al.* Percentage of anti-CD4 monoclonal antibody-coated lymphocytes in the rheumatoid joint is associated with clinical improvement. Implications for the development of immunotherapeutic dosing regimens. Arthritis Rheum. 1996;39:52–6.
26. Choy EH, Adjaye J, Forrest L, Kingsley GH, Panayi GS. Chimaeric anti-CD4 monoclonal antibody cross-linked by monocyte Fc gamma receptor mediates apoptosis of human CD4 lymphocytes. Eur J Immunol. 1993;23:2676–81.
27. van der Lubbe PA, Dijkmans BA, Markusse HM, Nassander U, Breedveld FC. A randomized, double-blind, placebo-controlled study of CD4 monoclonal antibody therapy in early rheumatoid arthritis. Arthritis Rheum. 1995;38:1097–106.
28. Tak PP, van der Lubbe PA, Cauli A, *et al.* Reduction of synovial inflammation after anti-CD4 monoclonal antibody treatment in early rheumatoid arthritis. Arthritis Rheum. 1995;38:1457–65.
29. Levy R, Weisman M, Weisenhutter C, *et al.* Results of a placebo-controlled multicentre trial using a primatised non-depleting anti-CD4 monoclonal antibody in the treatment of rheumatoid arthritis. Arthritis Rheum. 1996; 39(Suppl):122A.
30. Panayi GS, Choy EHS, Connolly DJA, *et al.* T cell hypothesis in rheumatoid arthritis (RA) tested by humanised non-depleting anti-CD4 monoclonal antibody (mAb) treatment. I: Suppression of disease activity and acute phase response. Arthritis Rheum. 1996;39(Suppl):244A.
31. Knoerzer BD, Karr RW, Schwartz BD, Mengle-Gaw LJ. Collagen-induced arthritis in the BB rat: prevention of disease by treatment with CTLA-4-Ig. J Clin Invest. 1995;96:987–93.
32. Buhlmann JE, Noelle RJ. Therapeutic potential for blockade of the CD40 ligand, gp39. J Clin Immunol. 1996;16:83–96.
33. Moreland LW, Heck Jr LW, Koopman WJ, *et al.* Vβ17 T cell receptor peptide vaccination in rheumatoid arthritis: results of phase I dose escalation study. J Rheumatol. 1996;23:1353–62.
34. Weiner HL, Friedman A, Miller A, *et al.* Oral tolerance: immunologic mechanisms and treatment of animal and human organ-specific autoimmune disease by oral administration of autoantigens. Annu Rev Immunol. 1994;12:809–37.
35. Trentham DE, Dynesius-Trentham RA, Orav EJ, *et al.* Effects of oral administration of type II collagen on rheumatoid arthritis. Science. 1993;261:1727–30.
36. Sieper J, Kary S, Sorensen H, *et al.* Oral type II collagen treatment in early rheumatoid arthritis. A double-blind, placebo-controlled, randomized trial. Arthritis Rheum. 1996;39:41–51.
37. Tyndall A, Gratwohl A. Haemopoietic stem and progenitor cells in the treatment of severe autoimmune disease. Ann Rheum Dis. 1996;55:149–51.

11

PRINCIPLES OF REHABILITATION

Gerold Stucki and Oliver Sangha

- Rehabilitation is the management of disease consequences.
- These include impairments (e.g. pain, muscle imbalance, limited range of motion), functional limitations (e.g. reach, grip) and disability (e.g. household activities).

A structured approach to rehabilitation management involves the following:
- Identify problems and needs most relevant to the patient.
- Relate the problem to modifiable impairments, personal and environmental factors.
- Select appropriate measures to follow the result of the intervention.
- Plan, implement and coordinate interventions.
- Treat impairment by restoring organ structures and function; compensate for functional limitations; address psychosocial factors; prevent further impairment and disability.

DEFINITION AND GOALS OF REHABILITATION

Medical interventions focus on causation and disease processes, while rehabilitation is concerned with the consequences of disease. Rehabilitation is defined as the management of disease consequences. Its goals are to reduce symptoms, improve function and minimize disability. The key to successful disability management is the identification of individualized problems and needs and of potentially modifiable and limiting components in the disabling process. Rehabilitation options are to:
- treat impairments by restoring organ structures and function (a treatment strategy),
- overcome functional limitations (a rehabilitative strategy) and
- prevent further impairment and disability (a preventive strategy).

Attention is given to potentially disabling behaviors and environmental factors that increase disablement. Although the condition may not be cured or prevented, rehabilitation can improve function and minimize disability and health care costs, making it successful for both the individual and society[1].

MODELS OF DISABILITY

Models of the disabling process differ in their perspective and taxonomy. The WHO International Classification of Impairments, Disabilities and Handicaps (ICIDH)[2] provides a framework for the consequences of disease. A similar, though distinct, model of the disabling process was first proposed by Nagi[3].

The comprehensive framework of disability laid out by the US Committee on a National Agenda for the Prevention of Disabilities emphasizes the interaction between the disabling process, quality of life and individual risk factors[1] (Fig. 11.1).

Pathology refers to the interruption or interference with normal bodily processes at the level of cells and tissues. Impairment is defined as a discrete loss of or abnormality of anatomic structures (e.g. deformity) and/or function [e.g. reduced range of motion (ROM), muscle weakness] and resulting symptoms (e.g. pain, fatigue). The level of reference is the organ (e.g. joint unit) or organ system (e.g. musculoskeletal system).

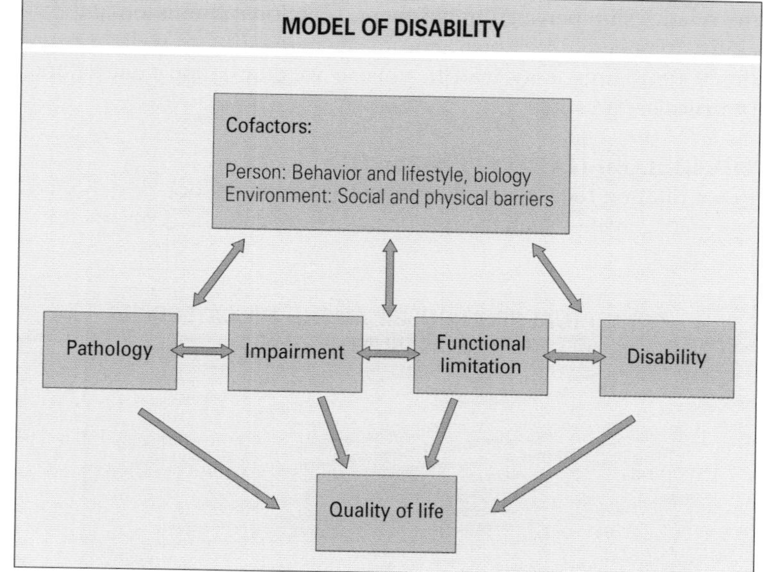

Fig 11.1 Model of disability[1,2]. Adapted from Pope and Tarlov[1].

Functional limitation refers to the restriction on, or lack of, ability to perform an action or activity (e.g. reaching, gripping, walking, carrying) within the range considered normal that results from single or multiple impairments. Disability is the inability to perform or limitation in performing socially defined activities (e.g. activities of daily living, leisure, sport and play) and roles (e.g. mother, employee) within a social and physical environment. It is the gap between the capabilities of an individual and the demands of the environment. In contrast to impairment and functional limitation, the concept of disability is relational (between the person and the environment) and not attributional (the person).

Quality of life refers to total well-being, encompassing both physical and psychosocial determinants. Quality of life closely approximates the WHO's definition of health as a state of complete physical, mental and social well-being, and not merely the absence of disease or infirmity. Quality of life is affected by each stage of the disabling process (e.g. in patients with scleroderma the quality of life may be decreased due to esthetics of the skin disease, pain, restricted grip function and consequent inability to shop). Within the disabling process, each stage affects an individual's quality of life; it is not a finite endpoint but an integral part of the disabling process.

Risk or cofactors include biological (e.g. HLA), environmental (e.g. architectural barriers, living and work conditions), lifestyle and behavioral characteristics (e.g. diet) which are associated with musculoskeletal conditions. Risk factors are not only associated with the onset of impairment, but interact with the disabling process at each stage. Bidirectional arrows in Figure 11.1 indicate the possibility of 'feedback'. Risk factors also affect the progression of disability and may include, depending on the stage, treatment, rehabilitation, age of onset, financial resources, expectations and environmental barriers.

The relationship of the various components of the disabling process are shown in Figure 11.2. There is no universal threshold of impairment or functional limitation at which someone becomes disabled and at which people experience a diminution of their quality of life.

Whether people with defined functional limitations are disabled depends on their expectations, personal resources and the demands of their physical environment such as their living conditions. Patients tend to have diminished expectations with increasing age, severity or chronicity of the problem. A young, healthy physician may thus ascribe a greater degree of disability than is perceived by the patient himself[4]. Furthermore, patients do not attach the same value to pain, fatigue, functional limitations and disabilities. This might explain why younger, educated patients view reduced physical function due to osteoarthritis (OA) as less important than do elderly, less educated patients[5]. Also, the relationship between impairment, functional limitation and disability may be bidirectional. For instance, inability to walk (a functional limitation) may lead to muscle weakness and contractures (impairments)[6].

THE REHABILITATION PERSPECTIVE

Rehabilitation focuses on disease consequences as opposed to medical management which focuses on pathology with the goals of curing or interfering with the disease processes. In rehabilitation, the goal is to address the individual problem and the rehabilitation options are to treat impairments, functional limitations and psychosocial factors, and to modify the physical and social environment (Fig. 11.3).

In rheumatology the rehabilitation perspective is central to patients with back pain, soft tissue and age-related musculoskeletal problems. However, it is also an important perspective in inflammatory diseases.

In inflammatory diseases anatomic and functional rehabilitation management includes joint protection and the maintenance of physical fitness and is important to prevent impairments. With the destruction of individual joints the diagnosis of anatomic and functional deficits (ROM, strength, stability) guides rehabilitative or surgical management.

In patients with back pain, soft-tissue and age-related musculoskeletal conditions, the diagnosis of anatomic and functional impairments is keyClinically these patients present with typical clusters or patterns of anatomic and functional impairments which may be summarized as syndromes or conditions[7].

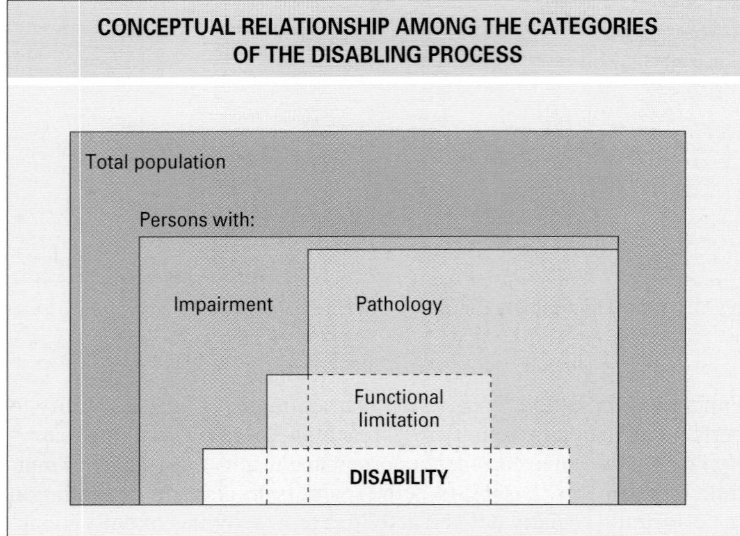

Fig. 11.2 Conceptual relationship among the categories of the disabling process. According to Nagi[3], all impairment is associated with pathology, but not all impairments lead to functional limitations. Similarly, all functional limitation and disability is associated with impairment, but not all functional limitations lead to disability. Disability can exist in the absence of functional limitation (e.g. disfigurement in a patient with scleroderma)[1,2]. With permission from Pope and Tarlov[1].

A STRUCTURED APPROACH TO REHABILITATION MANAGEMENT

Rehabilitation is a continuous process and involves the identification of problems and needs, the relation of problems to impairments and factors of the person and the environment, the planning and coordination of treatments, and the assessment of effects (Fig. 11.4).

IDENTIFY PATIENT PROBLEMS AND NEEDS

The goal of rehabilitation management is to address the patient's problems and needs as fully as possible. Accordingly, the end points of rehabilitation management are successful problem solving or individual goals achieved. Patients with musculoskeletal conditions typically suffer from an array of problems, including pain, fatigue, functional limitations and physical, mental and social disability. It is necessary to set priorities and goals and a realistic time frame for achieving them.

While individual goals achieved are the primary end points of any rehabilitation intervention, it is useful to review disease consequences systematically. A profile provides information about change and difficulty level in activities that might have been unrecognized. It is important to recognize and address a loss in physical function or the development of depression at an early stage when an intervention may be more successful.

REHABILITATION MANAGEMENT OF DISEASE CONSEQUENCES VS TREATMENT OF DISEASES

	Rehabilitation perspective	Medical perspective
Level of reference	Disease consequences Impairment Functional limitation Disability	Disease process
Treatment approach	Empiric, individualized	Evidence–based
Type of intervention	Multidisciplinary, nonpharmacologic techniques	Physician–directed, pharmacological and surgical medications
Involvement of the patient	Active (cooperation)	Passive (compliance)

Fig. 11.3 Rehabilitation management of disease consequences versus treatment of diseases.

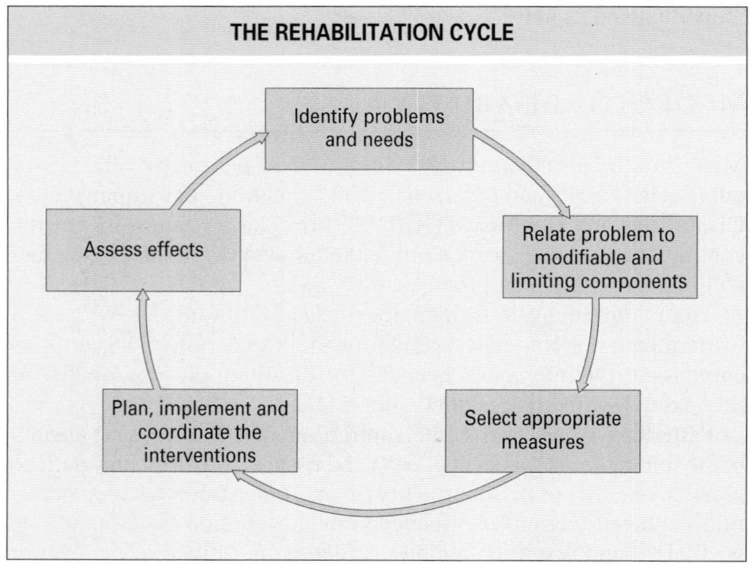

Fig. 11.4 The rehabilitation cycle. A structured approach to rehabilitation management.

RELATE THE PROBLEM TO MODIFIABLE AND LIMITING COMPONENTS

The key to successful rehabilitation management is understanding the relationship between the target problem and the impairments, functional limitations and psychosocial and environmental factors which exacerbate it[8]. The goal is to address the individual's problem and the rehabilitation program seeks to:

- treat impairments and compensate for functional limitations,
- address psychosocial factors and
- modify the physical and social environment.

Improvement in these parameters are fine, but the ultimate goal is to improve the person's health status and their quality of life.

Not all impairments, functional limitations and psychosocial factors relevant to the problem are modifiable or of equal importance. When planning the rehabilitation intervention, it is necessary to identify and address the factors with the greatest potential for improvement. The contribution of psychosocial and environmental factors to problems is discussed in detail in the sections on 'How to overcome functional limitations' and 'How to recognize and address psychosocial factors'. The following focuses on the diagnosis of impairments. The rehabilitation intervention is guided by the most relevant impairments and the stage of tissue injury and repair rather than the underlying disease (Fig. 11.5).

Which impairments contribute to the problem?

Impairments of the musculoskeletal organ include ROM, muscle strength, flexibility and endurance, tenderness of tendons and ligaments and synovitis.

Impairments in the musculoskeletal system are rarely restricted to one anatomic structure for long. An example is acute weakness of the extensor hallucis longus caused by lumbar disc herniation and sciatic nerve compression. However, coexisting back pain will often cause involvement of segmental structures of the spine (muscles, tendons, ligaments, etc.). Muscle imbalance, reduced joint mobility and irritation of ligaments, tendons and subcutaneous tissues may persist and interact in a vicious circle even after the triggering event has disappeared.

In most situations the clinical evaluation will reveal a cluster of impairments and it is impossible to identify which came first. Because musculoskeletal structures react in a finite number of ways similar patterns of impairments are found with a variety of underlying pathologies or triggering factors. For example, a radial epicondylitis may be from overuse and repetitive microtrauma but may also result from a painful cervical spine syndrome with chain involvement of muscles and tendons of the upper extremity.

Common patterns of impairments are seen around peripheral joints and the spine. Clusters of impairments around the joints are referred to as periarthropathies. Periarthropathies commonly occur around the knee, the hip, the shoulder and the elbow.

The pattern of periathropathy of the knee is found, for example, in patients with OA or crystal arthropathies. Anatomic and functional changes may include inflammation of tendons inserting at the pes anserinus and of the medial collateral ligament, anserine bursitis, atrophy of the medial, lateral and deep part of the quadriceps and reduced flexibility of the hamstrings and rectus femoris.

Clusters of anatomic and functional impairments of the spine are often referred to as 'low back pain' or 'vertebral syndrome'. Most vertebral syndromes share patterns of impairment, including muscle imbalance, joint dysfunction, reduced spinal mobility and irritation of tendons and ligaments. For example, weak and atrophied abdominal muscles and shortening of the lumbar erector trunci may be found in patients with static problems of the spine (e.g. scoliosis, hyperlordosis), segmental joint hypomobility, degeneration of the intervertebral joints or chronic improper positioning with a repetitive task.

The pattern of impairments with periarthropathies and vertebral syndromes is influenced by personal characteristics, coexisting illness and a variety of other cofactors. For instance, the impairment found in a periarthropathy of the knee varies with joint alignment (varus or valgus

PROBLEM-ORIENTED TREATMENT OF IMPAIRMENTS

Impairment	Examples of underlying pathologies	Treatment options
Acute inflammation of the joint and/or periarticular structures	Crystal arthropathy, inflammatory OA, reactive arthritis, RA, overuse, trauma	Relieve intra-articular pressure Aspiration of joints Relieve pain; reduce inflammation Immobilization Local cooling Iontophoresis (topical NSAID) NSAID, corticosteroids Maintain joint function Active or active-assisted ROM exercise Static (isometric) muscle strengthening
Chronic inflammation of the joint and/or periarticular structures	RA, psoriatic arthritis and other spondyloarthropathies, crystal deposition disease	Maintain joint function Active ROM exercise Dynamic (low load) muscle strengthening Cautious stretching Joint protection Education Functional immobilization: splints Aids and devices Modify physical environment Correct deformities Splints and orthotics Muscle relaxation Heat (moist packs) Hydrotherapy Cardiovascular fitness Controlled physical activity Aerobic exercise Adapted recreational and sports activities
Joint hypermobility	Constitutional tendon and ligament laxity, pregnancy, Marfan's syndrome, Ehler–Danlos syndrome, ligament injury	Stabilization Dynamic, concentric and eccentric exercise Corrective splinting Functional immobilization Selective: preventive taping Nonselective: brace, abdominal binder or corset, collar
Joint hypomobility	Intra-articular problems: meniscus lesion, effusion, hemarthrosis, chondromatosis, loose body; reduced ROM due to muscle shortening, capsule retraction, osteophytes	Eliminate intra-articular obstruction Aspirate effusion, hemarthrosis Arthroscopic removal of meniscus, loose body Restore transversal gliding of surfaces Transversal mobilization Consider impulse mobilization
Muscle dysfunction (strength, endurance, flexibility)	Unbalanced exercise, deconditioning, repetitive movements at work or with sports activities, joint pathologies	Restore muscle balance (include antagonists) Stretching Strength and endurance exercises Muscle relaxation Heat Hydrotherapy
Acute sensorimotor loss	Radicular or nerve compression, e.g. acute disc herniation	Relieve pain; reduce inflammation Analgesics, NSAIDs Cold or galvanization therapy along irradiation (e.g. leg) Rest (limit to few days) Functional immobilization (e.g. hip flexion to reduce ischiadic tension) Muscle relaxation Muscle relaxants Hydrotherapy Local cooling or heat Mobilization Start without gravity (pool exercise)
Chronic sensorimotor loss	Carpal or tarsal entrapment, disc herniation, spinal stenosis	Address inflammatory component to reduce edema Local corticosteroid injection or oral corticosteroid therapy NSAIDs Immobilization (e.g. wrist splint, abdominal binder) Restore muscle balance Coordinated strengthening and stretching exercises General fitness Musculoskeletal and aerobic exercise

Fig. 11.5 Problem-oriented treatment of impairments. (NSAIDs, nonsteroidal anti-inflammatory drugs.)

deformity), coexisting varicosities or panniculitis. While tendinitis and bursitis of the pes anserinus are common to most patients with a knee periarthropathy, tendinitis and muscle imbalance of either the tractus iliotibialis or the adductors are more prominent in individuals with varus or valgus deformity.

Which impairments are limiting?

Someone is either capable of performing a task, or can do it with some difficulty, with a lot of difficulty or not at all but impairments, e.g. muscle strength and ROM, are on a continuum.The clinician must be knowledgeable about what impairment is the most limiting for particular functional activities. Trial and error may be necessary. A small loss in strength or ROM[9] may be the straw that breaks the camel's back. For instance, a small loss of knee flexion from 90° to 80° can limit sit-to-stand transfers[10]. A patient with degenerative spinal stenosis may not be able to climb stairs because of weakened quadriceps muscles. A strengthening program (e.g. on a stationary bicycle) to increase strength from 50 to 80 Newton may enable the patient to climb stairs and stay in their own apartment.

Assessing stage of tissue injury and healing

The stage of tissue injury and repair sets up or establishes what the treatment objectives are. A useful concept from sports medicine describes four phases[11]:

- treatment of inflammation;
- mobilization;
- strengthening; and
- functional restoration.

Inflammation, is a local response to cellular injury with capillary dilatation and leukocyte infiltration. It manifests clinically with redness, heat and pain. The goal is to control swelling and pain. Typical modalities include rest of the involved joint and application of cold. As inflammation comes under control, restoring function is important to avoid secondary impairments. Prolonged rest should be avoided because it causes loss of muscle strength and, in the long run, loss of connective tissue strength, length and flexibility (e.g. joint capsule contractions and tendon strength). Range of motion exercises and isometric exercise therapy are introduced.

The goal during the strengthening phase is to increase performance without exacerbating inflammation. Isometric training should be supplemented with dynamic, low-weight, high-repetition exercises. Response to strengthening exercise is highly dependent on physical characteristics, training status and, most importantly, phase of recovery. Thus, the program needs to be individualized and reassessed and adjusted frequently, progressing to higher weight, low-repetition exercises as tolerated. The final treatment step focuses on restoration of complex functions and tasks. Defined complex functions may be demonstrated with occupational therapy techniques, sport and play.

This approach is an important guide in acute musculoskeletal injury and in formulating an approach to rheumatic diseases. With persistent inflammation, particularly in inflammatory rheumatic disorders, pharmacologic and nonpharmacologic approaches to reduce inflammation need to be prescribed for longer periods of time and therapeutic progression towards higher performance exercise and complex function training may be limited. It is critical to prevent loss of organ function. Systematic mobilization of all joints along the physiologic ROM (active or active-assisted ROM exercise) several times a day is essential for joint nutrition and to avoid capsule or, tendon contractures, and muscle atrophy and shortening. At the same time, controlled static exercises of all muscle groups maintain muscle strength.

In some situations, direct treatment of the impaired structures is not tolerated. An example is the patient with reflex sympathetic dystrophy. The involved area is hypersensitive and would react to heat with more pain and swelling. Modalities such as baths with increasing temperature are initially applied to the contralateral extremity (consensual treatment) to stimulate regulation processes.

PLAN, IMPLEMENT AND COORDINATE THE INTERVENTION

Spectrum of techniques

While the medical treatment of diseases involves pharmacologic agents primarily, rehabilitation management uses a wide array of nonpharmacologic techniques including physical and occupational therapy, physical modalities, psychosocial interventions and modifications of the environment. Cultural background, personal preferences and beliefs of both the health care professional and the patient are important to treatment success[12]. For instance, self-consciousness may limit a patient's willingness to comply with wrist splints or to exercise in a public pool.

Coordinated, longitudinal, multidisciplinary team care

Many rheumatic diseases are chronic and affect many aspects of a person's life. Access to and coordination of rehabilitation services seem more important to health status and quality of life than which individual treatments are used. Not all patients need all services and the intensity and frequency of individual services will vary over the lifetime of a patient. Therefore, it is critical to ensure access to a full array of comprehensive and coordinated services. Continuity of care provides security in the face of an uncertain future.

Coordinated longitudinal care involves a number of disciplines, including physical medicine, rheumatology, orthopedics, physical therapy, occupational therapy, social work, podiatry, vocational counseling and clinical psychology. There is evidence that multidisciplinary team care benefits patients with RA and ankylosing spondylitis. In RA, comprehensive team care seems to improve function and minimize functional loss, impaired function and amount of synovitis. Controlled studies that compared the benefits of inpatient and outpatient therapy for rheumatic diseases[13–16] have generally found only modest or no differences with respect to disease activity, whereas pain, quality of life and mental well-being appeared better with inpatient treatment. In a recent study involving patients with active RA, a short period of inpatient multidisciplinary treatment as compared with routine outpatient care had a direct beneficial effect on disease activity and emotional status; the favorable effect on disease activity was still present after 52 weeks[17]. In ankylosing spondylitis a program of physical therapy and patient education led to improved function and mobility[18]. Bakker *et al.* demonstrated a significantly higher level of mobility, fitness and health status in ankylosing spondylitis patients who underwent supervised group therapy in addition to a home exercise program[19].

Involvement of the patient and family

Rehabilitation interventions usually require the active involvement and understanding as well as motivation of the patient. It is important to involve and to empower the patient and, if appropriate, the family in the decision making process.

Ideally, a rehabilitative effort should commence with a 'contract' between patient and therapist to define the goals, expectations, strategy and commitment of both parties. Successful rehabilitation will heavily depend on the relationship between the health care professional and patient. Patient–health care professional communication is critical.

ASSESS EFFECTS

To adjust treatment, interventions need to be related to results during the rehabilitation process. Results should be monitored periodically[30]. This seems particularly important in preventive interventions, where effects usually cannot be assessed immediately. Among patients in coordinated longitudinal team care, systematic follow up may detect slowly developing problems. The more comprehensive the assessment, the more information that can be obtained with regard to physical, mental and social health.

Feedback to improve the process and results of care

Measurement of goals attained or simple repeated measurement of pain on a visual analog or numerical rating scale can be done easily in clinical practice. Analyses of self-administered health status profiles may require computer scoring. Ideally, the results should be available and used during the patient visit.

Assessments of processes and results (measurement–improvement systems) may also be used to monitor and improve rehabilitation interventions for groups of patients. Feedback of information on structure, process and outcomes for individual patients and providers can be used for the development and maintenance of quality in rehabilitation services[20–22].

Structures refer to characteristics of the health care setting. Processes refer to the intervention itself, from the details and steps taken in the planning, implementation and execution of rehabilitation interventions. Outcomes refer to effects. In rehabilitation, they typically include problems solved and disease consequences. Impairments and functional limitations and behaviors are, but common intermediate end points of rehabilitation interventions.

TECHNIQUES TO TREAT IMPAIRMENT

Central to musculoskeletal function are joint and muscle biomechanics and neuromuscular functioning. This section illustrates joint mobilization and immobilization techniques, together with methods to increase muscle strength, endurance and neuromuscular functioning. Modalities help improve musculoskeletal functioning by reducing pain and inflammation, stimulating reparative processes and improving muscle tone. Figure 11.5 summarizes techniques useful in the rehabilitative management of specific anatomic and functional impairments.

ANGULAR JOINT MOBILIZATION

Active range of motion exercise

The most elementary joint mobilization technique is angular movement of a joint along the physiologic axes (ROM exercise) by the patient themselves[23]. ROM exercise is thought to be important for the nutrition of joints and for maintaining the range of motion within physiologic limits. It is crucial for patients who are confined to bed or who have a single joint or group of joints immobilized. Thus, it is an integral part of a daily exercise program for patients with RA and other systemic rheumatic disorders with reduced physical ability and activity.

Assisted range of motion exercise

If the patient is too weak or if active exercise causes too much pain, assisted ROM exercise may be carried out by a therapist. Assisted ROM exercise should be limited to the active range within physiologic limits. Going beyond physiologic limits may injure an already inflamed joint. A special technique of assisted ROM exercise, passive continuous motion for the knee using automated machines, can reduce length of hospital stay after joint arthroplasty[24].

Passive range of motion exercise

Passive ROM exercise by a therapist can go beyond physiologic limits towards the anatomic limits defined by muscles, tendons, ligaments, the joint capsule and articular bones. Accordingly, restriction of the anatomic ROM may be due to muscle and tendon shortening, reduced capsule flexibility or bone proliferation (e.g. osteophytes in OA). The typical joint where physiologic and anatomic structures coincide is the elbow joint. A hard end feel can be appreciated with maximum extension, when the olecranon touches the fossa olecrani. For most other joints, the anatomic limits have soft end feel due to the periarticular structures. With passive ROM exercise, the periarticular structures can be stretched and pathogenic limits extended towards the physiologic limits. Figure 11.6 shows the limitation of ROM with shortening of tendons (soft end feel) or osteophytes (hard end feel).

The patient may be instructed to conduct a daily passive ROM program to increase and/or maintain ROM most relevant to function. In patients with chronic arthropathies, daily passive ROM is critical to prevent a slow deterioration in joint mobility. For example, in patients with hip OA the joint capsule tends to contract, resulting in a decreased hip extension. A few degrees' loss in hip extension may interfere with walking and cause low back pain. While it is not possible to overcome the restriction of joint mobility by osteophytes, daily ROM exercises prevent further restriction due to capsule contraction.

JOINT PLAY TECHNIQUES

Mobilization (gliding of joint surfaces)

While active and passive angular mobilization has been the main technique for many decades it has constraints for improving ROM. Gliding of joint surfaces against each other (joint play or accessory movements[25,26]) must also be improved.

These accessory movements are not under voluntary control. They are necessary for full painless function of the joint and full ROM. Often, it is advantageous to improve joint gliding rather than force angular mobility, which may cause pain and considerable pressure to the joint surfaces.

Reduced joint play movement has been called 'joint dysfunction'. It can be improved with traction or transversal movements in the direction of the restriction (Figs 11.7 & 11.8). To avoid pain and allow for better execution of the maneuver it is preferable to perform transversal stress only after traction. Indeed, traction itself may be sufficient to enlarge the joint capsule and periarticular structures. Moreover, for some joints (e.g. the hip joint), traction may be applied more easily than transversal movements.

Because of joint biomechanics, restriction and direction of mobilization generally differ for convex or concave joints. In the case of convex joints such as the metacarpophalangeal or knee joint, mobilization is in the same direction as the restricted angular movement. This is because angular movement, for example volar flexion, is associated with volar gliding of the phalanx with respect to the metacarpus. In concave joints such as the wrist, mobilization is in the opposite direction to the restricted angular movement. Angular movement, such as volar flexion, is also associated with dorsal gliding of the carpal bones in the wrist with respect to radius and ulna.

While these rules are generally applicable, angular movement and joint play movements need to be tested in all directions and mobilization planned according to the dysfunctions found.

To test and improve joint play movements, the examiner places the joint in a resting position (loose packed position), which is the position of a joint in its range of motion where it is under the least amount of stress. It is also the position in which the the joint capsule has its greatest capacity. The resting position of the metacarpophalangeal joint is slight flexion; for the knee it is at about 25 degrees of flexion[25].

To test and improve joint play movements a close packed position should be avoided. For the knee joint this is in full extension and for the metacarpophalangeal joint it is full flexion. In this situation the two joint surfaces fit together precisely; that is, they are fully congruent and the joint surfaces are tightly compressed, the ligaments and capsule are maximally tight and the joint surfaces cannot be separated by distractive forces.

Impulse mobilization

Based on the concept of joint play, schools of manipulative therapy believe that a reversible restriction of joint movement due to pain, functional joint incongruence or muscle dysfunction may be resolved by an impulse mobilization following the rules for convex and concave joints.

If the distal joint surface is convex, the impulse mobilization is directed towards the opposite of the restricted angular movement, whereas in the case of a concave distal joint, the impulse should point towards the side of the restricted angular movement. Under defined conditions (fixation of the proximal part of the peripheral joint and traction of the distal part in functional position), a high-velocity, low-amplitude thrust force is applied to the joint. While the amplitude of the movement exceeds the restriction and restores physiologic limits,

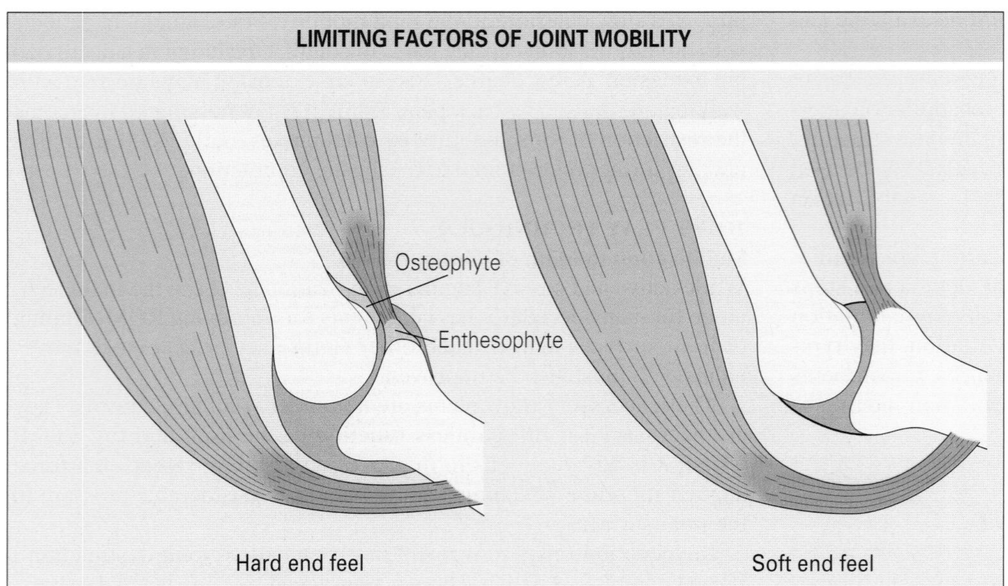

Fig. 11.6 Limiting factors of joint mobility. Left: hard end feel – ROM limited by structural obstruction. Right: soft end feel – ROM limited by capsular contraction or shortening of musculotendinous unit. (Adapted from Dvorac *et al.*[35])

impulse mobilization should never exceed the anatomic joint range; this could cause irreversible structural damage to the capsule and/or periarticular tissues. Consequently, the amplitude is usually very small. Although manipulation therapy is one of the best studied, its mechanism and benefits are still a matter of debate[27]. Manipulative therapy, which has been used not only for peripheral joints but also successfully for the treatment of vertebral syndromes, requires extensive training, experience and caution.

TRACTION

Traction improves angular movement by stretching articular and periarticular structures[23] and is applied manually or by traction equipment. Manual traction is used for peripheral joints and the cervical spine. For larger joints, including the hip, the patient's own body weight may be utilized with slings. Mechanical appliances facilitate traction for the cervical spine but should be used only under close supervision and adjustment of defined weights. Mechanical traction has been used for treating low back pain with or without radicular symptoms but is not of value in most patients[23].

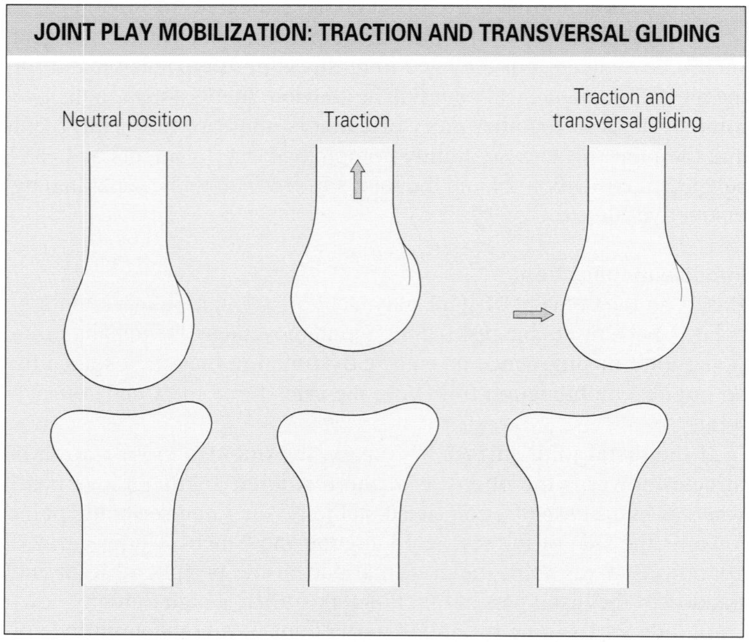

JOINT PLAY MOBILIZATION: TRACTION AND TRANSVERSAL GLIDING

Neutral position

Traction

Traction and transversal gliding

Fig. 11.7 Joint play mobilization: traction and transversal gliding.

JOINT IMMOBILIZATION

Rest

Bed rest or immobilization of joints with splints is used to treat joint inflammation from injury or inflammatory, crystalline, degenerative or metabolic arthropathies. The dilemma with rest is that, if prolonged, it causes adverse systemic and local effects, including osteoporosis, muscle weakness and reduced strength of tendons, ligaments and other periarticular tissues. Therefore, immobilization should be used as little as possible.

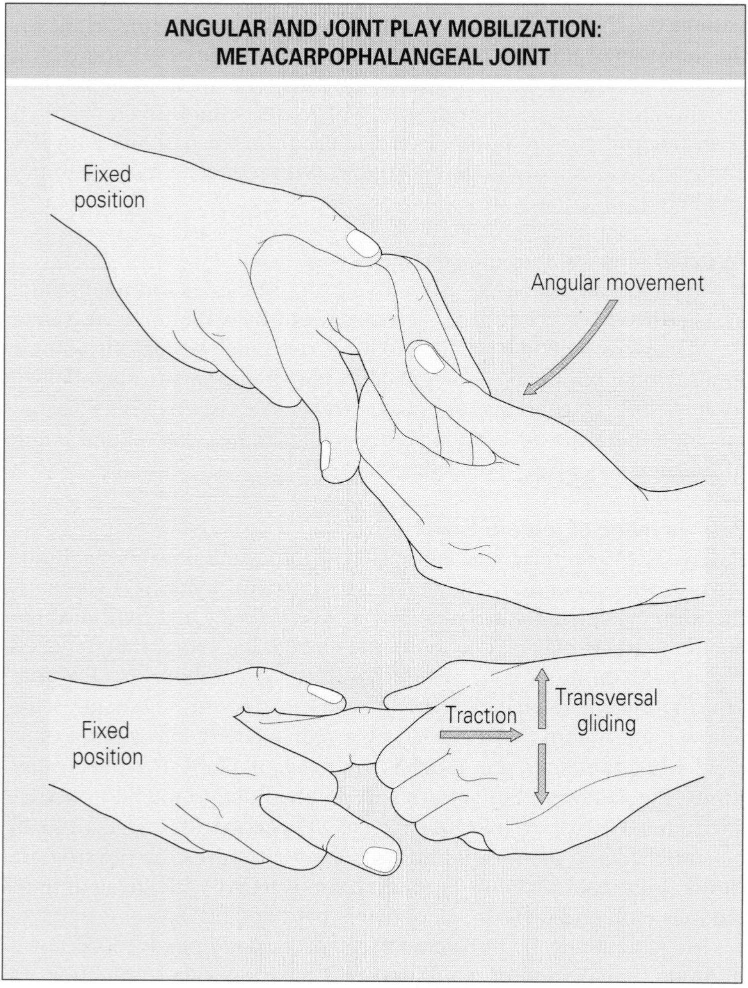

Fig. 11.8 Angular and joint play mobilization of a metacarpophalangeal joint.

Rest may involve the whole body (bed rest), a joint (by means of a cast or splint) or functional immobilization along joint axes (e.g. restriction of supination and pronation of the ankle with tape). While bed rest may be used as an adjunct for short periods to reduce systemic inflammation, complete bed rest should be avoided. Selective functional immobilization of defined joints is appropriate to most other situations.

Selective functional immobilization

Functional immobilization is commonly used in rehabilitation after orthopedic surgery. For example, after cruciate ligament repair, knee flexion is restricted using orthotics to unload healing ligaments. With increasing ligament strength, flexion is gradually increased. Despite selective immobilization, joint nutrition and flexibility of periarticular structures can be maintained, allowing for a much faster recovery. In inflammatory rheumatic diseases, selective immobilization using splints is particularly helpful along with muscle strengthening in treating joint instability. Wrist splints reduce joint swelling and pain in patients with synovitis of the wrists.

Nonselective functional immobilization

A common application of nonselective functional immobilization is the abdominal binder or corset, which increases intra-abdominal pressure, reduces back symptoms and helps stabilize the lumbar vertebral spine. With an abdominal binder no particular joint or joint axis is restricted but there is general restriction of the physiologic ROM. In the elderly with rectus diastasis where strengthening of abdominal muscles is difficult, an abdominal binder is a helpful adjunct to therapy. An abdominal binder may also reduce pain in patients with segmental instability – for instance, due to spondylolisthesis. In spinal stenosis, an abdominal binder or an orthopedic three-point corset restricts spine extension which reduces the spinal canal space and induces spinal claudication.

A cervical collar restricts the movement of the cervical spine to various degrees depending on the material used (soft or hard). Muscle spasm is an important contributor to symptoms in nonspecific cervical pain syndromes. A collar can promote muscle relaxation and may be effective in pain relief. However, after whiplash injury cervical mobilization does not seem to be effective and may delay recovery[28].

Except for cost, there are no substantial drawbacks to the short-term use of immobilizing corsets and collars. However, long-term use requires caution. Muscles which are not used lose strength, endurance and flexibility. This may result in muscular imbalance or instability. It is generally advisable to strengthen specifically the immobilized muscles and/or use these devices intermittently for a few hours at a time.

Change of vector of forces

Parts of muscles may be immobilized with devices applied to change the vector of forces. By placing pressure on the brachioradialis muscle it is possible to redistribute the forces to the musculotendinous unit. For instance, forearm band is a helpful adjunct therapy in patients with a chronically irritated and inflamed epicondylus humeri lateralis (tennis elbow).

Taping is a simple, safe and cheap way to change the vector of forces. For example, medial taping of the patella (Fig. 11.9) may improve malalignment causing abnormal force distribution on the lateral facet and reduce pain in patients with OA patellofemoral OA of the lateral facet[29].

MUSCLE TECHNIQUES

Muscle function is a critical component of the functioning of the musculoskeletal organ. Muscle balance results from opposing forces generated across joints by muscle groups and is a reflection of muscle strength, length, tension, endurance and coordination. In muscle diseases such as polymyositis general muscle weakness is the main concern; in conditions such as periarthropathies and vertebral syndromes diagnosis and treatment of muscle imbalance is most useful.

Restoring muscle balance

Muscle imbalance is regularly found in periarthropathies and vertebral syndromes[30]. In periathropathies, muscle imbalance is often associated with tendinitis, bursitis and altered joint biomechanics. In knee and hip OA, the hamstrings, adductors and the rector femoris tend to have reduced flexibility, while the lateral, medial and deep quadriceps tend to be weakened. Weakening of the latter muscle groups can result in diminished control of patellofemoral tracking during movement. This promotes joint irritation and contributes to the degenerative process. Accordingly, quadriceps strengthening and stretching of the hamstrings, adductors and rectus femoris often reduce pain and improve function in patients with hip and knee OA[31].

Inadequate exercise focusing unilaterally on strengthening is an important cause of muscle imbalance. Sedentary lifestyle leads to reduced flexibility, poor endurance and spasm, shortening of spinal muscles and weakened abdominal muscles. Both inadequate exercise and sedentary lifestyle contribute to back pain. Reduced flexibility of postural muscles leads to the typical protraction of the shoulder and hyperlordosis. An exercise program should address the postural muscles of the spine, together with the abdominal muscles and the muscles of the shoulder girdle.

Strengthening exercises

Reduced muscle strength is a major problem in primary muscle disorders, in corticosteroid myopathy and in painful conditions leading to disuse atrophy. Techniques for building muscle strength employ high-resistance loads against which a muscle must work[11]. Resistance to motion can be applied manually by a therapist, by using weights or through various types of equipment. Strengthening exercises take one of three forms: isometric, isotonic or isokinetic. They can be varied in velocity of movement or contraction type: eccentric versus concentric. Isometric exercise is static by definition and both isokinetic and isotonic exercises may be used in a concentric (shortening contraction) or eccentric (lengthening contraction) mode with varying levels of load and velocity.

Complex modern exercise programs, also known as medical training therapy[7], systematically train muscle groups according to their postural or action-oriented work, but these are costly. Simple home exercise or supervised programs[32] seem effective for localized problems including knee and hip OA[33].

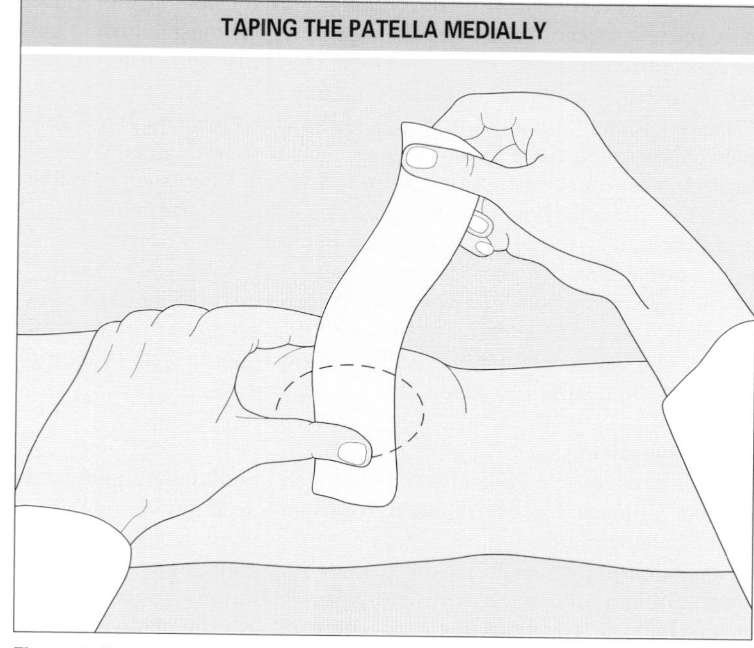

Fig. 11.9 Taping the patella medially. The tape pulls the patella to the medial side of the knee joint[38].

Static exercise

An isometric contraction is a muscle contraction that does not produce movement of the joint[11]. Peak isometric strength is the maximum force that can be exerted against an immovable object. Isometric contractions can generate a large amount of force, and daily isometric exercise at 50% of maximal strength may retard disuse atrophy. It may help build strength, especially in those who are far removed from their peak strength potential[34].

One drawback to isometric exercise is that gains in strength are made primarily at the joint angle at which the muscle is exercised. It is unclear how far the gains in strength can be further improved and there may be little transference of strength to other activities. On the other hand, isometrics have the advantage of being relatively easy to perform and they require little or no equipment. Because of the lack of joint motion, they are useful in maintaining strength and muscle mass in the immobilized limb and when joint motion is painful or otherwise contraindicated (e.g. the acute inflammatory phase of RA). With control of inflammation and healing of tissues, dynamic exercise can be introduced.

Dynamic exercise

Fast, shortening (concentric) contractions develop the lowest muscle tensions. Fast, lengthening (eccentric) contractions develop the highest muscle tensions. Isometric contractions develop tension in between. At its extremes, high velocity, low load may exclusively increase muscle endurance. High-load, low-frequency techniques on the other hand will almost exclusively increase muscle strength. Thus, dynamic exercise can improve both endurance and strength although the extent may vary depending on velocity and load[7].

Isotonic exercises involve moving a constant load through a full ROM with or without changing the velocity of movement. Lighter weights can be lifted through more repetitions than heavier ones.

One problem with isotonic exercise is that maximal muscle torque varies with the length of the muscle. The muscle can contract at its maximum capacity at only one point in the full ROM, at a point slightly longer than resting length. However, to lift a weight through a full ROM requires that the muscle must be able to lift it even at its weakest point. Thus true isotonic exercise is inefficient because it does not cause muscle overload throughout the whole contraction. The use of cams and pulleys attempts to circumvent this problem by varying the resistance of the load to match the average torque curve for specific muscle groups.

Most isotonic exercises involve concentric and eccentric exercises. Eccentric contractions, while developing more tension, also produce more muscle soreness and more damage to type II muscle fibers than do concentric contractions[35]. The advantages of isotonic training are its effectiveness and its universal availability.

Isokinetic exercises employ special machines which have lever arms that rotate around fixed axes. The user pushes or pulls the lever arm through a set range of motion at a preset speed. The speed remains constant, no matter how hard the subject pushes. By maintaining the speed (velocity), the user can generate maximal force (torque) at all angles of the range.

The biggest drawback to isokinetic exercise is the reliance on special equipment. These machines may be unavailable to the general public. The newer isokinetic machines allow training with eccentric as well as concentric resistance.

Flexibility training

Flexibility of muscle depends on ambient and body temperature and whether a muscle has been trained. A program to improve flexibility can be beneficial in a number of ways. It may lessen the likelihood of injury, minimize postexercise soreness, reduce contractures, decrease joint pain and alleviate myofascial pain. Techniques for stretching include ballistic stretching, static stretching, passive stretching and proprioceptive neuromuscular facilitation[7,11,30]. There are many different stretching techniques for individual joints.

Ballistic stretching involves repeated, rapid, forceful stretching maneuvers such as bouncing or twisting. This technique is no longer recommended for routine stretching due to the high risk of injury caused by the rapid generation of force.

In static stretching, the body part is positioned to provide a gradual stretch over a duration of at least 15 seconds. Alternatively, a muscle may be stretched by contracting its antagonist. The stretch is usually repeated several times. It is the easiest stretch to perform and is widely used for pre-exercise stretching (after a warm up). It also helps reduce muscular soreness following exercise. The best results are obtained when stretching is combined with an increase in tissue temperature into the therapeutic range (42–45°C). This may be accomplished by using heating modalities or warm up exercises.

Passive stretching is performed by a partner applying stretch to the patient's relaxed muscle or extremity. The most effective methods for stretching are contract–relax or hold–relax techniques (proprioceptive neuromuscular facilitation)[36]. For example, the gastrocnemius–soleus complex may be stretched by isometric contraction of the muscle for 5 seconds followed by slow duration passive or static stretching[37]. The initial contraction may decrease muscle activity by affecting the neural elements or it may help stretch the fascia and tendons. Partners are often utilized for this technique.

At the beginning of a training session, stretching should be performed in a slow, progressive manner to avoid injuries[30]. In the therapeutic situation the application of superficial heat prior to stretching techniques may be helpful. In the training situation, more intense stretching should be performed after the training.

FUNCTIONAL REHABILITATION

Functional rehabilitation extends traditional physical therapy to restore highly complex movement patterns[38]. In addition to improving strength and flexibility, a functional rehabilitation program incorporates agility and proprioceptive and/or kinesthetic training. It is a challenging task to analyze and permanently alter neuromuscular functioning which occurs subconsciously.

A functional rehabilitation program gradually takes the patient from simple to highly complex activities requiring refined proprioceptive acuity. Functional or neuromuscular rehabilitation is most often applied to patients after stroke or brain injury but modified techniques are often helpful in the rehabilitation of patients with musculoskeletal conditions. For instance, if intensive treatment of periarticular structures, joint play and muscle balance in a painful tennis elbow does not help, addressing neuromuscular regulation may be a superior alternative.

Neuromuscular techniques share the following common characteristics:

- consciousness of posture, tension of muscles and soft tissue structures and movements;
- training of movement sequences relevant to complex functions; and
- interplay between conscious and unconscious movement sequences.

While physiologic knowledge and evidence about treatment efficacy of different joint and muscle techniques are expanding, there is limited data about neuromuscular coordination. An important exception is gait, where much progress has been made through gait analyses. Many neuromuscular techniques remain purely empiric.

Recreational activities

Recreational activities are useful to improve neuromuscular functioning. They may contribute to body perception, expand skills, aid general conditioning and recruit social supports. Also, they are more enjoyable than repetitive therapeutic exercises. For instance, the traditional Chinese technique tai chi chuan[39] is an enjoyable alternative to improving strength in patients with knee OA. Training of hand and finger muscles or strengthening of shoulder or hip muscles can be facilitated with loom weaving. Some sports activities are particularly suited to musculoskeletal rehabilitation. Examples include volleyball and swimming (particularly the crawl stroke) for patients with spondyloarthropathies. Activities like walking, golf, low impact aerobics and cross country skiing can be done by many patients with musculoskeletal conditions. Jogging places a high impact upon the joints in the lower extremities and should be avoided in patients with arthropathies of weight-bearing joints, but walking can be done safely in mild to moderate disease. Contact sports such as football or soccer should be avoided.

Some general precautions should be given with respect to sports. The difficulty level is defined in the way that movement of individual joints and execution of complex functions are controlled. For instance, in sports like skiing unexpected, demanding terrain may force uncontrolled movements which could damage joints. Certain sports need to be modified to accommodate functional limitations in patients with certain conditions (e.g. avoiding serving overhead in volleyball for patients with spondyloarthropathies).

Biofeedback

Biofeedback techniques are used in patients who have difficulty perceiving and controlling muscle and joint function. For instance, biofeedback in quadriceps strengthening allows the patient to sense a muscle contraction and to improve control of defined muscle groups. Biofeedback is also useful in Raynaud's phenomenon.

PHYSICAL FITNESS

Patients with musculoskeletal conditions manage to live with their disabilities, but a significant portion of their physical capacity may be spent fulfilling daily routines. For example, numerous studies document that RA patients have reduced muscular strength[40] and decreased aerobic capacity[41].

All patients with chronic musculoskeletal conditions should have a comprehensive training program to maintain and improve general and musculoskeletal fitness. These components should include flexibility (ROM exercises), muscle balance (static and/or dynamic strengthening exercises and stretching exercises), musculoskeletal endurance and training of coordination (e.g. play and modified sports activities), as well as cardiovascular training to maintain or improve aerobic capacity and prevent deconditioning.

For patients with normal aerobic capacity exercise will maintain fitness. For patients with low aerobic capacity training may improve it. Physical training in patients with systemic rheumatic disorders requires supervision since patients may have coexisting conditions, such as lung disease, which will require modification of the program. Studies have shown that rheumatic patients can perform aerobic exercises without negative effects.

Supervised aerobic training may improve symptoms, function and work capacity and reduce fatigue in a host of rheumatic conditions, including fibromyalgia[42], OA of the knee[32], SLE[41] and RA[40,43]. Regular aerobic exercise is also an important adjunct to the treatment of myofascial pain and chronic pain states. Aside from improving cardiovascular fitness aerobic training aids in weight control and improves the person's sense of well-being.

For cardiovascular fitness, the American College of Sports Medicine recommends aerobic exercise using large muscle groups which causes an elevation of training heart rate to 60–90% of the maximum heart rate or reaching 50–85% of VO_{2max} for 20–60 minutes three to five times per week[44]. Training heart rate is calculated by taking 60–90% of predicted maximum heart rate, which is approximately 220 minus age (in years). An endurance training program should start with low-intensity sessions to allow the exercise novice to maintain an appropriate training heart rate for the minimal length of time required for cardiovascular adaptation.

JOINT PROTECTION AND ENERGY CONSERVATION

Joint protection and energy conservation are educational interventions to help patients to use their joints in the most comfortable way, thus reducing pain and conserving energy[45]. Energy conservation also involves splints and other aids. Central to the question of whether behavioral change results in improved symptoms is the question of which educational method is most effective in changing and maintaining optimum behavioral change[46]. A large controlled study documented a significant improvement in many aspects of joint protection and function in a 6-week trial[47]. Principles of joint protection with a focus on the wrist and hand are listed in Figure 11.10.

MODALITIES

Modalities to apply heat or cold to musculoskeletal areas have been used in the management of patients with musculoskeletal conditions throughout history. Today's techniques are based on the application of energy through heat, light, cold or electric therapy, the stimulation of slow fibers and gate control effects through transcutaneous electrical nerve stimulation (TENS).

Whether a therapy is hot or cold is related to normal body temperature. If the local application is 34–35°C (body temperature), the body does not absorb or lose energy. If the therapy is cooler or warmer than body temperature, compensating mechanisms produce heat through muscle contraction or increased motor activity or give up energy through vasodilatation and sweating.

While modalities are simple and rather inexpensive some caution is required. Dermal injury from hot or cold application may occur in patients with reduced sensibility (e.g. diabetic neuropathy) or peripheral vascular disease.

Studies of the effects of hot or cold in patients with inflammatory arthritis show benefits in terms of pain, joint stiffness, strength and function. Controlled studies in small numbers of patients do not indicate superiority of either superficial heat or cold in OA or RA[48].

Heat

Heat is prescribed for muscle relaxation, to reduce stiffness and improve local circulation[49]. These mechanisms may contribute to pain relief. Muscle relaxation is achieved through reflexive relaxation and a direct effect. Heat can be delivered by radiation (light), conduction (hot pack, paraffin, water) or conversion (diathermy, ultrasound). Radiant and conductive heat sources are forms of local or superficial heat; short wave and microwave diathermy and ultrasound are classified as deep heat.

There are few experimental studies of the effects of superficial heat in arthritis. Dellhag *et al.*[50] performed a randomized controlled trial of active hand exercise and paraffin treatments. The groups receiving paraffin were the only ones to report less pain immediately after treatment; however, paraffin without exercise produced no therapeutic benefit. Exercise, with or without paraffin, produced significant improvements in pain, stiffness and function; the group that received paraffin and exercise showed the most improvement in grip strength. Other studies of paraffin have also reported positive results from combined paraffin and exercise programs. Short-term pain reduction, but

PRINCIPLES OF JOINT PROTECTION IN PATIENTS WITH ARTHRITIS
To do
Use the strongest and largest joints available for a specific task Carry objects close to the body Spread the weight of objects over many joints Slide objects using both hands Plan work areas so that the most frequently used equipment is reached easily Use appropriate aids and devices
To avoid
Prolonged static positions Force in the direction of flexion and ulnar deviation of hands and fingers Lateral deviating pressures on the hand and the wrist Pressure against the volar surface of the fingers Activities involving tight grasp Force and constant pressure against the pad of the thumb

Fig. 11.10 Principles of joint protection in patients with arthritis.

without functional gains, was shown when paraffin was used alone[48].

Deep heat is used to treat chronic irritated structures with a low metabolic activity such as tendons. Ultrasound is used in managing adhesive capsulitis but its effectiveness could not be confirmed for either pain relief or increased motion[51]. In controlled trials ultrasound was no better than placebo in an exercise program for knee OA[52].

Microwave electrotherapy is the only modality which delivers energy to the bone and joints and may theoretically be useful in the treatment of joint diseases. However, a study of short wave diathermy for knee OA demonstrated that this mode of electrotherapy did not improve function, strength, endurance or pain from exercise alone[33]. Microwave diathermy did not produce significant pain relief or improve function in controlled trials with arthritis patients[53].

It is controversial whether heat can and should be applied to inflamed joints. There is agreement that heat is contraindicated in acute arthritis (e.g. gout) because it produces increased and sustained inflammation and pain. However, heat might enhance pain reduction and muscle relaxation in patients with moderate joint inflammation. Many patients with RA find mild heat with moisture helpful. For degenerative joint diseases and soft tissue syndromes without prominent inflammation, more intense heat modalities are usually well tolerated. Similarly, patients with spondyloarthropathies seem to prefer intense heat over applications with mild heat.

The selection of a modality needs to include the personal preferences of the patient. While some patients feel comfortable and perceive an effect only with hot mud packs others react to this regimen with anxiety and discomfort, preferring mild heat from moisture packs or infrared lamps. When prescribing or applying heat, a pragmatic approach based on trial and error is preferable to strict adherence to standard 'cookbook' recipes.

Hydrotherapy

Whole body heat can be accomplished with a tub or heated pool. Hydrotherapy has a long history. The Romans cultivated bathing in thermal stations; Hapsburg princes regularly visited thermal spas; and other celebrities from Goethe to Kafka used thermal stations to improve or maintain their health. Nowadays, whole body heat is frequently integrated in sports (e.g. saunas in health clubs).

While there is no scientific evidence as to the effects of hydrotherapy (and it is difficult to imagine a controlled blinded evaluation), conventional wisdom has it that bathing in warm waters relaxes body and mind and patients find it very useful. Hydrotherapy is best tolerated with temperatures close to body indifference temperature of 34–35°C. Patients fatigue relatively fast in water above the indifference temperature. Below the indifference temperature, patients will perceive water as cold because they have to produce heat with muscle contractions to maintain body temperature. To avoid fatigue and skin problems, hydrotherapy should be limited to about 20 minutes.

Hydrotherapy can be an adjunct to many treatment programs. In elderly patients with degenerative joints or spine diseases, thermal hydrotherapy is an efficient way to reduce tense muscles. Combined with a program to improve muscle balance, the effect may be maintained.

Hydrotherapy may be used in RA patients where systemic disease activity is under control to decrease muscle tension and reduce pain. To avoid exacerbation of inflammatory activity, hydrotherapy in RA needs to be introduced carefully and should not exceed 10–15 minutes to avoid fatigue.

Hydrotherapy may be harmful to patients with cardiovascular and vascular problems. Because of vasodilation, blood may pool and induce hypotension when patients exit the warm bath, placing them at risk of fainting. Thus, patients need to be advised to leave the water slowly, ask for assistance and sit down for a while after leaving the pool.

Local cooling

The major physiologic effects of local cooling are vasoconstriction in both superficial and intra-articular tissues, reduction of local metabolic rate and slowed nerve conduction and nerve firing rates. Cooling has a local analgesic effect and reduces inflammatory responses to tissue trauma. Cold is applied by cold packs, ice massage, immersion or vapocoolant sprays. There are no data that any one type of cold application consistently produces superior results.

Cold therapy needs to be applied with caution. Cold packs out of the freezer with temperatures below 0°C may cause serious burns if applied directly to the skin. It is advisable to cover the pack with a towel.

Cooling with ice massage or ice packs empirically is a highly effective analgesic therapy (e.g. in acute shoulder periarthritis). Cold appears to be effective and well tolerated by persons with all sorts of arthritis, especially with acute inflammation. It reduces edema and pain. Cold packs applied three times a day for one month to one knee of patients with RA decreased pain and increased motion in the treated knee compared with the contralateral knee[54]. Patients also reported improved sleep and decreased use of analgesics[54]. However, in chronic mild inflammation (for instance, in patients with RA), mild moist heat which reduces pain through muscle relaxation is often preferred. In knee OA, cold provided significant pain relief more quickly than heat[55].

Increasing temperature and contrast baths

Increasing temperature and alternating hot and cold baths (contrast baths) may help decrease edema in treating reflex sympathetic dystrophy[11]. Baths with increasing temperature are often started at 28°C. Addition of warm water gradually increases the temperature (about 1°C per minute). Initially, only treatment (of the contralateral extremity) may be tolerated and the highest temperature may be limited to not more than 30°C. With less severe symptoms, direct treatment of the symptomatic side, higher temperature differences and contrast baths can be applied.

Massage

Massage is a common technique to relieve muscle spasm, pain and stiffness. Massage can boost blood flow in muscles, increase lymph flow, relax muscles and decrease blood pressure[11]. In many situations massage is used after application of heat and cold to augment the effect on muscle relaxation and to decrease pain before stretching or strengthening exercises. There are a variety of massage techniques[33] but little rigorous data since controlled clinical trials would be difficult if not impossible to conduct.

Electrotherapy

There are two basic rationales for electrotherapy in pain control. Galvanic electrotherapy is used to exhaust pain conducting, slow, unmyelinated nerve fibers. Low to middle frequency electrotherapy (e.g. TENS) is based upon the 'gate' theory of pain. Stimulation of slow nerve fibers through stimulation of larger, myelinated nerve fibers inhibits pain impulses carried more slowly by unmyelinated nerve fibers at the level of the dorsal column of the spinal cord. The faster impulses arrive at the dorsal column first and 'close the gate', forestalling propagation of the slower pain impulses

Galvanic electrotherapy should be used with particular caution because they may cause serious burns. This is of particular concern in patients with impaired pain sensation (e.g. diabetics). Galvanic current is mainly indicated for the treatment of acute radicular pain and inflammation of periarticular structures such as tendons and ligaments. Because galvanic electrotherapy enhances transport of substances with dipolar characteristics through the skin, it is used to promote resorption of topical nonsteroidal anti-inflammatory drugs (NSAIDs) or corticosteroids (iontophoresis).

The most common form of therapeutic electrical stimulation used for pain control is TENS of cutaneous and peripheral nerves via surface skin electrodes. Despite widespread use, controlled evaluations in low back pain[56] and OA of the knee[57,58] do not show superiority to placebo treatment[59]. A small battery-powered current is used to apply TENS; after appropriate instruction this can be controlled by the patient.

There are few contraindications to TENS. To avoid vagal stimulation, it should not be placed over the anterolateral aspect of the neck.

Theoretically, it may cause malfunction of cardiac pacemakers. Hypersensitivity to the electrodes (skin irritation) occasionally necessitates discontinuation but can be minimized if different electrodes are used.

STRATEGIES TO COMPENSATE FOR FUNCTIONAL LIMITATIONS

Despite optimal treatment of impairments it might not be feasible to restore organ function to the extent necessary to perform functional tasks and roles. Using multiple strategies it is possible to accommodate or compensate for functional deficits or help the patient to accept more realistic expectations.

BRACES

Braces are external devices that aid simple or complex body functions. Splints and orthotics support or stabilize a body part, while prosthetics replace a body part. Splints and orthotics are used:

- to immobilize a joint that is inflamed to reduce swelling (for instance, wrist splints in RA);
- to correct a malalignment which may be inducing symptoms (for instance, a foot orthotic to correct valgus stress on the medial collateral ligament of the knee);
- as an interim measure to assess whether surgical fusion would be useful; and
- rarely, to facilitate natural fusion of an inflamed joint.

Progressive splinting is sometimes used as an alternative to surgery to reduce a severe joint contracture. Splints and orthotics can be fixed or dynamic to accept some movement in the joint. Splints and orthotic devices need to be tested empirically on the individual and there is no method to predict which patients will benefit. Callinan *et al.*[60] compared soft and hard wrist–hand resting splints. The soft splint reduced pain more effectively and was worn more often than the hard splint.

Few braces and indications have been evaluated critically but their use is considered best practice. Most studies have been conducted in RA patients, examining the effect of wrist and hand splinting on reducing inflammation. Splints reduce inflammation[61], increase motion[61] and hand function[62], improve grip and pinch strength, decrease both day and night pain, and increase the person's ability to carry out daily activities[63].

AIDS AND DEVICES

While braces, splints and orthotics target the person, aids and devices aim to improve interaction with the environment. Such devices probably do not influence the natural history of a joint condition but they are among the most effective aids for people with disabilities.

The key to the successful prescription and use of aids and devices is to identify the functional limitations or complex functions most relevant to the problem and to work with the patient on adjusting the appliance or aids. Many aids and appliances are also useful as preventive measures. Devices can be as simple and cheap as a long handle for a comb or as expensive as specially designed equipment[23,64,65]. Occupational therapists should be consulted to develop a specific prescription. Useful aids and devices for walking, climbing or gripping are given in Figure 11.11.

MODIFYING THE ENVIRONMENT OR THE NATURE OF A TASK

The limiting factors to an activity are often external, including financial limitations, social circumstances, architectural barriers and the attitudes of other people. Some of these are amenable to change and may require the coordinated efforts of a number of health care professionals[66]. Although dramatic societal changes have taken place in this century, we remain a long way from having a disabled user-friendly environment. Health care professionals should be advocates for this.

For many patients, it might be advisable to adjust the environment or to change the nature of a task. For instance, an individual with difficulty in transferring to the upright position from a standard high toilet at work may be treated by increasing knee and hip flexion range (the intrinsic limiting factor). If this is impractical or impossible, the addition of an elevated toilet seat or armrests may allow independence to be achieved. Architectural barriers are found not only in bathrooms but also in kitchens, on stairways and on public transportation.

For a patient with severe RA domiciliary services may be essential.

RECOGNIZING AND ADDRESSING BIOPSYCHOSOCIAL FACTORS

DEPRESSION

The humane and effective care of patients with chronic musculoskeletal conditions requires health care professionals to recognize and address psychosocial needs and be personally engaged and empathetic[8,67]. Like patients with other chronic diseases, people with rheumatic diseases experience psychological morbidity[68]. The impact of depression and depressive symptoms not diagnosable as frank depression on worsening function and pain should not be underestimated[68,69]. Depression bears a significant relationship to pain (see Chapter 3.4). In RA patients, however, the causal direction is still unknown[69]. Depression may be the most important cofactor in the disabling process and its effect on functional disability is additive[68]. It increases utilization of health services, and contributes to the amplification of somatic symptoms. Reduced quality of life may be as strongly influenced by psychologic disturbances associated with impairments as by the impairment itself. Depression interferes with optimal treatment and requires motivation, cooperation and active behavior. Early recognition and treatment of depressive symptoms is crucial to minimize disability associated with musculoskeletal problems.

PERSONALITY CHARACTERISTICS AND PATIENT BEHAVIOR

Global functioning, pain and fatigue, sleep and even disease activity seem to be influenced by personality characteristics and behavior. For instance, patients who are active participants in the management of their disease show better outcomes[70].

Psychoeducational interventions (individual or group) provide patient education and support, and teach coping skills and pain management. These are a critical component of patient care in any disease but are particularly important in chronic disease where the patient and health care providers have a lifelong relationship and share decision making. In arthritis, medications offer a 20–50% improvement in arthritis symptoms and a variety of psychoeducational interventions provides a further 15–30%[70] improvement in function and quality of life. For example, Holman *et al.* randomized 280 patients with RA, OA and other forms of arthritis into six 2-hour arthritis self-management courses. After 4 years, OA and RA patients reported 18% less pain and less depression, with 34% fewer medical visits and substantial cost savings[71].

RECOGNIZING RISK FACTORS FOR WORK DISABILITY

In RA high rates of work disability appear to be a function of physical impairments, the interactions between impairments and the physical requirements of work, and the flexibility with which work can be accomplished[72]. For work-related back pain early recognition of some other regional musculoskeletal disorders and risk factors and addressing potential problems is more rewarding than the reintegration of patients who have lost their job and hope[72].

The following are some predictors of work incapacity and work loss in lower back pain[73,74]:

- incoherent presentation of pain localization, and stable symptoms over time;
- inability to influence pain and function by movement or change of position, physical modalities, posture, behavior or exercise;
- relapse of a pre-existing condition and lack of response in previous episodes;
- dissatisfaction with work;
- problems of articulating, communicating or contracting realistic and problem-oriented treatment goals (setting of goals);

STRATEGIES TO COMPENSATE FOR FUNCTIONAL LIMITATIONS			
Functional limitation	Potential disability	Underlying impairments	Adaptive aids and devices
Tipping head	Drinking	Pain and limited cervical ROM	Use straw or glass with cutout for the nose
Turning head	Driving	Reduced ROM with ankylosis of vertebral joints or hyperostosis, C1–2 arthritis	Larger rear view mirror
Reaching	Eating, cooking, hygiene, washing hair	Shoulder or elbow pain, limited ROM, weakness (Milwaukee shoulder; RA)	Use long-handled or angled utensils (combs and brushes, spoon) and back-scrubbing aids
Grip	Eating, cooking, personal hygiene, dressing, shopping	Arthritis of wrist and finger joints, atrophy of musculi interossei, stiffness, limited ROM, weakness and decreased sensorium	Replace small knobs with big handles Replace buttons, shoelaces, belts, bra hooks with Velcro fasteners Select clothes that are easy to put on: slip-on shoes, clip on ties, zippers with big ring pulls Use large and sharp chef's knife or knife with vertical grip; wall-mounted electric opener for cans; and lid lifter to break the suction on vacuum lids
Carrying	Shopping, household activities	Pain, weakness and reduced endurance upper extremity	Use wheeled carriers or carts for carrying small loads
Balance and stability with standing and moving	Going out, shopping traveling	Weakness, numbness and balance disturbance, joint dysfunction	Use a cane Use attachments to canes and crutches to improve stability and grip Prevent slipping with suction-cup mat or nonskid tape on the bottom of the tub Use single lever faucets and shower caddys Use terry-cloth robe to dry after bathing Shower seat
Rising from sitting	Bathing, sitting	Hip or knee pain and quadriceps weakness	Raised toilet seat and stool; safety rails or bars on the wall; toilet armrest
Walking	Moving around apartment, shopping, traveling	Hip and/or knee pain and muscle weakness	Canes, crutches and walkers Wheelchair for longer distances
Climbing stairs	Moving around the house, shopping, traveling	Hip or knee pain, weakness (RA, OA, degenerative spinal stenosis, spondyloarthropathies)	Consider home elevator and ramps Install rails and split-risers to raise half of each step
Bend or lift (while standing)	Household activities	Pain, reduced ROM of spine or hip	Long-handled reaching aids, dust pans, dusters and mops
Bend knee (while sitting)	Dressing	Pain, muscle weakness, limited ROM of knee or hip	Use long-handled shoehorn, garter snaps or spring clothespins on a piece of tape for helping to put on socks

Fig. 11.11 Strategies to compensate for functional limitations.

- poor self-perceived prognoses, particularly when associated with an unrealistically high perception of impairment;

VOCATIONAL COUNSELING

Vocational counseling is extremely important in patients with chronic arthritis and covers a multitude of specific skills, including job modification, retraining and adaptation of the work environment. However, arthritis patients as a group are not referred to these services. For example, less than 0.5% of the estimated 100,000 plus work-disabled persons in Massachusetts with rheumatic conditions are served by the State's Vocational Rehabilitation Services (VRS)[75]. Studies albeit uncontrolled suggest that VRS is effective in rheumatic conditions. For example, 52 patients with RA followed for one year after VRS showed increased employment from 35% to 75%, but at one year only 57% maintained their job[76]. Another study showed a 41% return to work rate after VRS[77].

Successful management of work disability usually requires both mobilization of patient resources and modification of the workplace. It is critical to find the right balance between the requirements of the job and the limitations imposed by the condition[72] and to develop realistic goals within a defined and reasonable time frame. Most workplace interventions require a cooperative effort between patients, health care professionals and employers. Ideally, a detailed, quantitative job description is worked out. Following this a workplace evaluation can identify modifiable factors including work ergonomics, the modification of tasks, and the use of aids and devices. Comprehensive rehabilitation efforts can then focus on training of specific requirements of the job (work hardening) and improvement of global fitness.

SUMMARY

Rehabilitation is the area of medicine which deals with the practical consequences of disease on the patient's ability to be independent, productive, grow and enjoy life. To make a difference, the physician must understand what is limiting and the patient's priorities, what are realistic goals, what is likely to be modifiable; and to assess, try something and reassess. It is important to engage the patient in both active and passive processes to achieve a reduction in symptoms, improvement in function and the best possible quality of life.

REFERENCES

1. Pope AM, Tarlov AR. Disability in America: toward a national agenda for prevention. Washington: National Academy Press; 1991.
2. World Health Organization (WHO). The international classification of impairments, disabilities, and handicaps. A manual relating to the consequences of disease. Geneva: WHO; 1980.
3. Nagi SZ. A study in the evaluation of disability and rehabilitation potential: concepts, methods, and procedures. Am J Public Health. 1964;54:1568–79.
4. Ouslander JG, Beck JC. Defining the health problems of the elderly. Ann Rev Public Health. 1982;3:55–83.
5. Katz JN, Phillips CB, Fossel AH, Liang MH. Stability and responsiveness of utility measures. Med Care. 1994;32:183–8.
6. Kirby RL. The nature of disability and handicap. In: Basmajian JV, Kirby RL, eds. Medical rehabilitation. Baltimore: Williams & Wilkins; 1984:13–8.
7. Guccione AA. Geriatric physical therapy. Boston: Mosby–Year Book; 1993.
8. Lorish CK, Abraham N, Austin J, Bradley LA, Alarcon GS. Disease and psychosocial factors related to physical functioning in rheumatoid arthritis. J Rheumatol. 1991;18:1150–7.
9. Ferraz MB, Oliveira LM, Araujo PM, Atra E, Walter SD. EPM-ROM scale: an evaluative instrument to be used in rheumatoid arthritis trials. Clin Exp Rheumatol. 1990;8:491–4.
10. Fleckenstein SJ, Kirby RL, MacLeod DA. Effect of limited knee-flexion range on peak hip joint moments of force in humans transferring from sitting to standing. J Biomech. 1988;21:915–8.
11. Buschbacher RM. Musculoskeletal disorders. A practical guide for diagnosis and rehabilitation. Boston: Andover Medical Publishers; 1994.
12. Battie MC, Cherkin DC, Dunn R, Ciol MA, Wheeler KJ. Managing low back pain: attitudes and treatment preferences of physical therapists. Phys Ther. 1994;74:219–26.
13. Spiegel JS, Spiegel TM, Ward NB, *et al.* Rehabilitation for rheumatoid arthritis patients. A controlled trial. Arthritis Rheum. 1986;29:628–37.
14. Anderson RB, Needleman RD, Gatter RA, Andrews RP, Scarola JA. Patient outcome following inpatient vs. outpatient treatment of rheumatoid arthritis. J Rheumatol. 1988;15:556–60.
15. Ahlmen M, Sullivan M, Bjelle A. Team versus non-team outpatient care in rheumatoid arthritis. A comprehensive outcome evaluation including an overall health measure. Arthritis Rheum. 1988;31:471–9.
16. Helewa A, Bombardier C, Goldsmith CH, Menchions B, Smythe HA. Cost-effectiveness of inpatient and intensive outpatient treatment of rheumatoid arthritis. A randomized controlled trial. Arthritis Rheum. 1989;32:1505–14.
17. Vliet Vlieland TPM, Zwinderman AH, Vandenbroucke JP, Breedveld FC, Hazes JMW. A randomized clinical trial of in-patient multidisciplinary treatment versus routine out-patient care in active rheumatoid arthritis. Br J Rheumatol. 1996;35:475–82.
18. Kraag G, Stokes B, Groh J, Helewa A, Goldsmith CH. The effects of comprehensive home physiotherapy and supervision on patients with ankylosing spondylitis: an 8 month followup. J Rheumatol. 1994;21:261–3.
19. Bakker C, Hidding A, van der Linden S, van Doorselaer E. Cost-effectiveness of group physical therapy compared to individualized therapy for ankylosing spondylitis. A randomized controlled trial. J Rheumatol. 1994;21:264–8.
20. Granger CV. A conceptual model for functional assessment. In: Granger CV, Gresham GE, eds. Functional assessment in rehabilitation. Baltimore: Williams & Wilkins; 1984:14–25.
21. Nelson EC. Using outcome measures to improve care delivered by physicians and hospitals. In: Heithoff KA, Lohr KN, eds. Effectiveness and outcomes in healthcare. Washington DC: Institute of Medicine, National Academy Press; 1990.
22. Stucki G, Sangha O. Clinical quality management: putting the pieces together. Arthritis Care Res. 1996;9:405–12.
23. Hicks JE, Nicholas JJ, Swezey RL. Handbook of rehabilitative rheumatology. Atlanta: American Rheumatism Association; 1988.
24. McInnes J, Larson MG, Daltroy LH, *et al.* A controlled evaluation of continuous passive motion in patients undergoing total knee arthroplasty. JAMA. 1992;268:1423–8.
25. Magee DJ. Orthopedic physical assessment, 2E. Philadelphia: WB Saunders; 1992.
26. Dvorac J, Tritschler T, Schneider W. Manual medicine therapy. New York: Thieme Medical Publishers; 1988.
27. Assendelft WJ, Koes BW, Knipschild PG, Bouter LM. The relationship between methodological quality and conclusions in reviews of spinal manipulation. JAMA. 1995;274:1942–8.
28. Cassidy JD, Duranceau J, Liang MH, *et al.* Quebec Task Force on whiplash-associated disorders. Redefining 'whiplash' and its management (abridged). Spine 1995;20(suppl.):s1–s73.
29. Cushnaghan J, McCarthy C, Dieppe P. Taping the patella medially: a new treatment for osteoarthritis of the knee joint? Br Med J. 1994;308:753–5.
30. Spring H, Illi U, Kunz HR, Rothlin K, Schneider W. Stretching and strengthening exercises. New York: Thieme Medical Publishers; 1991.
31. Adler S. Self-care in the management of the degenerative knee joint. Physiotherapy. 1985;71:58–60.
32. Kovar PA, Allegrante JP, MacKenzie CR, *et al.* Supervised fitness walking in patients with osteoarthritis of the knee. Ann Intern Med. 1992;116:529–34.
33. Chamberlain MA, Care G, Harfield B. Physiotherapy in osteoarthritis of the knees. A controlled trial of hospital vs. home exercises. InteRehabil Med. 1982;4:101–6.
34. Muller EA. Influence of training and of inactivity on muscle strength. Arch Phys Med Rehabil. 1970;51:449–62.
35. Stanish WD, Rubinovich RM, Curwin S. Eccentric exercise in chronic tendinitis. Clin Orthop Rel Res. 1986;208:65–8.
36. Knott M, Voss DE. Proprioceptive neuromuscular facilitation. New York: Harper & Row; 1968.
37. Moore MA, Hutton RS. Electromyographic investigation of muscle stretching techniques. Med Sci Sports Exerc. 1980;12:322–9.
38. Lephart SM, Henry TJ. Functional rehabilitation for the upper and lower extremity. Orthop Clin N Am. 1995;26:579–92.
39. Kirsteins AE, Dietz F, Hwang SM. Evaluating the safety and potential use of a weight-bearing exercise, tai-chi chuan, for rheumatoid arthritis patients. Am J Phys Med Rehabil. 1991;70:136–41.
40. Ekblom B, Lovgren O, Alderin M, Fridstrom M, Satterstrom G. Effect of short-term physical training on patients with rheumatoid arthritis: a six-month followup study. Scand J Rheumatol. 1987;4:87–91.
41. Robb-Nicholson LC, Daltroy L, Eaton H, *et al.* Effects of aerobic conditioning in lupus fatigue: a pilot study. Br J Rheumatol. 1989;28:500–5.
42. McGain GA. Role of physical fitness training in the fibrositis/fibromyalgia syndrome. Am J Med. 1986;81:73–7.
43. Harkcom TM, Lampman RM, Banwell BF, Castor CW. Therapeutic value of graded aerobic exercise training in rheumatoid arthritis. Arthritis Rheum. 1985;28:32–9.
44. American College of Sports Medicine: Guidelines for exercise testing and prescription, 4E. Philadelphia: Lea & Febiger; 1991.
45. Liang MH, Logigian MK. Rehabilitation of early rheumatoid arthritis. Boston: Little Brown, 1992.
46. Gerber LH, Furst G, Shulman B, *et al.* Patient education program to teach energy conservation behaviors to patients with rheumatoid arthritis. A pilot study. Arch Phys Med Rehabil. 1987;68:442–5.
47. Kraag G, Stokes B, Groh J, Helewa A, Goldsmith CH. The effects of comprehensive home physiotherapy and supervision on patients with ankylosing spondylitis – a randomized controlled trial. J Rheumatol. 1990;17:228–33.
48. Michlovitz SL. The use of heat and cold in the management of rheumatic diseases. In: Michlovitz S, ed. Thermal agents in rehabilitation, 2E. Philadelphia: Davis; 1990:158–74.
49. Backlund L, Tiselius P. Objective measurement of joint stiffness in rheumatoid arthritis. Acta Rheum Scand. 1967;13:275–88.
50. Dellhag B, Wollersjo I, Bjelle A. Effect of active hand exercise and wax bath treatment in rheumatoid arthritis patients. Arthritis Care Res. 1992;5:87–92.
51. Falconer J, Hayes KW, Chang RW. Therapeutic ultrasound in the treatment of musculoskeletal conditions. Arthritis Care Res. 1990;3:85–91.
52. Falconer J, Hayes KW, Chang RW. Effect of ultrasound on mobility in osteoarthritis of the knee. A randomized clinical trial. Arthritis Care Res. 1992;5:29–35.
53. Spiegel TM, Hirschberg J, Taylor J, Paulus HE, Furst DE. Heating rheumatoid knees to an intra-articular temperature of 42°C. Ann Rheum Dis. 1987;46:716–9.
54. Kangilaski J. Baggie therapy: simple pain relief for arthritic knees. JAMA. 1981;246:317–8.
55. Clarke GR, Willis LA, Stenners L, Nichols PJ. Evaluation of physiotherapy in the treatment of osteoarthritis of the knee. Rheumatol Rehabil. 1974;13:190–7.
56. Deyo RA, Walsh NE, Martin DC, Schoenfeld LS, Ramamurthy S. A controlled trial of transcutaneous electrical nerve stimulation (TENS) and exercise for chronic low back pain. N Engl J Med. 1990;322(23):1627–34.
57. Lewis D, Lewis B, Sturrock RD. Transcutaneous electrical nerve stimulation in osteoarthrosis: a therapeutic alternative? Ann Rheum Dis. 1984;43:47–9.
58. Griffin MR, Brand KD, Liang MH, Pincus T, Ray WA. Practical management of osteoarthritis. Arch Fam Med. 1995;4:1049–55.
59. Puett DW, Griffin MR. Published trials of nonmedicinal and noninvasive therapies for hip and knee osteoarthritis. Ann Intern Med. 1994;121:133–40.
60. Callinan N, Mathiowetz V, Fransen J. Soft versus hard resting splints in rheumatoid arthritis. Arthritis Care Res. 1993;6(suppl 5):A281.
61. Gault SJ, Spyker JM. Beneficial effect of immobilization of joints in rheumatoid arthritis and related arthritidies. Arthritis Rheum. 1969;12:33–44.
62. Kjeken I, Moller G, Kvien TK. Use of commercially produced elastic wrist orthosis in chronic arthritis: a controlled study. Arthritis Care Res. 1995;35:108–13.
63. Biddulph SL. The effect of the futuro wrist brace in painful conditions of the wrist. S Afr Med J. 1981;60:389–91.
64. Cochrane GM, Wilson AK, eds. Arthritis – an equipment guide. London: Arthritis and Rheumatism Council; 1991.
65. Fries JF. Arthritis. A take care of yourself health guide for understanding your arthritis, 4E. Addison-Wesley; 1995.
66. Zola IK. Toward the necessary universalizing of a disability policy. Milbank Q. 1989;67:401–28.
67. Bradley LA. Psychosocial factors and disease outcomes in rheumatoid arthritis: old problems, new solutions, and a future agenda. Arthritis Rheum. 1989;32:1611–4.
68. De Vellis B. The psychological impact of arthritis: prevalence of depression. Arthritis Care Res. 1995;8:284–9.
69. Parker JC, Wright GE. The implications of depression for pain and disability in rheumatoid arthritis. Arthritis Care Res. 1995;8:279–83.
70. Hirano PC, Laurent DD, Lorig K. Arthritis patient education studies. 1987–1991: a review of the literature. Patient Education and Counseling 1994;24:9–54.
71. Holman H, Mazonson P, Lorig K. Health education for self-management has significant and early and sustained benefits in chronic arthritis. Trans Assoc Am Physicians. 1989;102:204–8.

72. Yelin E. Musculoskeletal conditions and employment. Arthritis Care Res. 1995;8:311–7.
73. Bongers PM, De Winter CR, Kompier MAJ, Hildebrandt VH. Psychosocial factors at work and musculoskeletal disease. Scand J Work Environ Health. 1993;19:297–312.
74. Abenhaim L, Rossignol M, Gobeille D, *et al.* The prognostic consequences in the making of the initial medical diagnosis of work-related back injuries. Spine. 1995;20:791–5.
75. Allaire SH, Partridge AJ, Andrews HF, Liang MH. Management of work disability. Resources for vocational rehabilitation. Arthritis Rheum. 1993;36:1663–70.
76. Booth G, Goldklang G, Roth H. Rehabilitation of indigent arthritis patients in the District of Columbia. Med Ann District of Columbia. 1971;40:304–8.
77. Cochran GM. Rheumatoid arthritis: vocational rehabilitation. Int Rehabil Med. 1982;4:148–53.

12

PRINCIPLES OF ARTHRITIS SURGERY

Joseph A Buckwalter, W Timothy Ballard & Peter Brooks

- Appropriately selected and performed surgical treatments can relieve pain and improve function for patients with arthritis.
- Provides benefits for hundred of thousands of patients each year.
- Replacement of arthritic hips, knees and shoulders.
- Procedures including synovectomies, joint fusions, and debridements can also be useful.
- The success of surgical treatment of patients with arthritis depends on coordination of care among different specialists and health care providers.
- All patients being considered for surgical treatment require thorough preoperative evaluation and preparation and careful postoperative treatment and evaluation.

INTRODUCTION

All physicians providing care for patients with arthritis need to understand the role of surgical procedures in optimal care. For selected patients, current operative treatments, including joint debridement, synovectomy, osteotomy, soft tissue arthroplasty, resection arthroplasty, fusion and joint replacement effectively relieve pain and improve function (Fig. 12.1). In addition, patients with rheumatoid arthritis (RA) may benefit from tenosynovectomy and transfer, repair or reconstruction of ruptured tendons (Fig. 12.1). Experimental surgical procedures, performed with the intent of restoring lost or damaged articular cartilage, include osteochondral allografts, implantation of synthetic matrices that may incorporate growth factors, transplantation of chondrocytes or mesenchymal stem cells and joint distraction (Fig. 12.2). The appropriate roles of these procedures have not yet been clearly defined[1,2].

Pain that is not relieved by other treatments is the most common indication for operative treatment of arthritis. Loss of joint function is a less common indication because restoration of function by operative treatment is usually less predictable than pain relief. Surgeons also perform certain procedures with the intent of delaying or preventing future joint degeneration (e.g. acetabular redirectional osteotomy for congenital hip dysplasia in children, osteotomies of long bones to correct joint and limb malalignment and reconstruction of ligaments to improve joint stability). These procedures, and surgical treatment of septic arthritis, are not discussed in this chapter.

Although operative treatments of arthritis can produce excellent results, they also expose patients to serious risks. Potential operative and perioperative complications include extensive blood loss, cardiac arrhythmia and arrest, nerve and blood vessel injury, infection, venous thrombosis and pulmonary embolism. Late postoperative complications include delayed infection and loosening and wear of implants. Furthermore, even in the absence of complications, the results obtained with surgical procedures, including joint debridements and synovectomies, tenosynovectomies and osteotomies, may deteriorate with time. For these reasons, the potential risks and expected short- and long-term outcomes of operative treatment must be carefully considered for each patient. Nonetheless, individuals who fail to gain satisfactory results

CURRENT SURGICAL PROCEDURES FOR THE TREATMENT OF PATIENTS WITH ARTHRITIS

Surgical procedure	Common indications	Expected outcome
Joint debridement[3]	Loose bodies and other causes of mechanical joint dysfunction (knee, shoulder, hip, ankle)	Improved mechanical function and decreased pain
Joint debridement and penetration of subchondral bone[3]	Joint pain associated with loss or degeneration of articular cartilage (knee)	Variable
Joint synovectomy	RA, PVNS, synovial chondromatosis, hemophilia (knee, elbow, wrist, shoulder, ankle)	Temporary and, in some cases, long-term decrease in synovitis and possibly reduced rate of articular cartilage destruction
Tenosynovectomy[4,5]	RA and rarely other causes of tenosynovitis, including PVNS (wrist and hand)	Reduced pain and swelling, improved muscle tendon unit function
Tendon, ligament and joint capsule reconstruction[6–8]	Joint subluxation due to RA (MCP joints)	Improved joint stability and alignment
	Tendon ruptures due to RA (wrist and hand)	Improved muscle tendon unit function
Osteotomy[9–11]	OA (hip and knee)	Reduced pain and, in some cases, formation of a new articular surface and regression of osteophytes
Joint replacement[12–15]	Advanced joint degeneration due to OA, trauma, inflammatory diseases, bone necrosis (shoulder, elbow, hip, knee)	Pain relief, improved function
Joint fusion (including spinal fusion)[16,17]	Advanced joint degeneration or instability due to OA, trauma, inflammatory diseases, bone necrosis (hand, wrist, shoulder, hip)	Pain relief, restoration of alignment and stability (loss of motion and possible increased risk of degeneration of other joints)
Peripheral nerve decompression or transposition[18]	Localized nerve compression (ulnar and median nerves)	Reduced pain, improved function
Spinal cord and nerve decompression[19,20]	Existing or impending spinal cord and nerve root compression (cervical spine)	Decreased pain, improved function

Fig. 12.1 Current surgical procedures for the treatment of patients with arthritis. PNVS = Pigmented villonodular synovitis.

EXPERIMENTAL SURGICAL TREATMENTS FOR PATIENTS WITH LOSS OR DEGENERATION OF ARTICULAR CARTILAGE		
Surgical procedure	Common indications	Expected outcome
Osteochondral grafts[21–23]	Focal articular surface defects usually due to trauma (hip, knee)	Restoration of articular surface in selected patients with focal posttraumatic cartilage defects
Articular cartilage regeneration (periosteal and perichondrial grafts, chondrocyte transplants, artificial matrices)[3]	Focal articular surface defects usually due to trauma (knee and hand joints)	Results in small series of patients indicate that these approaches can restore an articular surface in localized defects
Joint distraction[30,61]	Ankle, hip OA	Limited evidence indicates that joint distraction can reduce joint pain

Fig. 12.2 Experimental surgical treatments for patients with loss or degeneration of articular cartilage.

from nonsurgical therapy or who have progressive disease should be evaluated by a surgeon before they develop deformity, joint instability, contractures or advanced muscle atrophy. Delaying surgery until these problems develop can compromise the results and increase the risk of complications.

PREOPERATIVE EVALUATION

With the exception of patients in whom arthritic disorders have caused or may cause spinal instability and neurologic damage, operative treatment of patients with arthritis is elective. Patients should undergo preoperative evaluation and should understand the full range of therapeutic options. Consideration of surgical intervention requires a thorough understanding of the degree of pain and functional limitation which the patient perceives and the possible surgical and nonsurgical treatments, as well as an understanding of the patient's social and occupational needs and expectations. Before planning surgery, patients should understand the potential benefits and risks of operative treatment. In general, the patients most likely to notice significant lasting benefit from operative treatment are those with joint pain not relieved by nonsurgical treatment. Patient age, overall health status and ability to comply with postoperative rehabilitation and precautions also help determine the outcome of operative treatment.

It is important to discuss with patients reasonable expectations for activity following surgery. For example, individuals who have joint fusions should understand how the fusion may limit their ability to perform certain types of tasks. Individuals being considered for joint replacement should appreciate that, in most instances, although they may expect significant pain relief, they still will not be able to perform certain types of high-demand activities without increased risk of implant failure. A reasonable expectation for many patients with osteoarthritis (OA) who undergo joint replacement is the potential for participating in low-impact activities such as swimming or golf. They should be advised against participating in high-impact and loading activities such as recreational or competitive sports that require running and jumping. Reviewing these expectations for postoperative level of function can be extremely helpful in enabling patients to make decisions concerning surgical intervention and in their acceptance of any appropriate activity limitations following surgery.

Even in patients with obvious joint disease and complaints of pain and loss of function, failure to carefully evaluate the cause of the symptoms can lead to disappointing results despite technically excellent operative treatment. Common diagnostic dilemmas include differentiating hip joint pain from lumbar radicular pain and shoulder joint pain from cervical radicular pain. Rheumatoid arthritis and other types of inflammatory arthritis may cause such severe joint deformity that detection of neurologic involvement becomes difficult. Patients with these disorders may develop joint sepsis that is not readily apparent because of the inflammatory nature of their underlying disease and the use of medications that suppress the inflammatory response to infection. Patients with joint disease and other causes of limb pain, such as Paget's disease, diabetic neuropathy or insufficiency fractures, also present difficult diagnostic problems. A careful history, physical examination and plain radiographs are sufficient to define the cause of symptoms for most of these patients, but in some cases joint aspiration, electrodiagnostic studies and additional imaging studies are needed to clarify the cause of pain and loss of function.

The importance of a thorough preoperative history and physical examination, as well as careful perioperative medical management, cannot be overemphasized. Many patients who could benefit from surgical treatment of arthritis, especially patients with OA, are elderly and may have decreased cardiac, pulmonary, renal or peripheral vascular function. These conditions require evaluation and in some cases treatment before planning surgery. Carious teeth, pharyngitis, cystitis, skin infections, including infected nodules in RA, and other potential sources of infection should be treated prior to surgery. Men with symptoms of prostatic hypertrophy need a urologic evaluation before surgery and women should be evaluated for asymptomatic urinary tract infections. Preoperative laboratory evaluation should include a measure of hemoglobin and hematocrit, urinalysis and other diagnostic tests as indicated by the individual's medical history. In addition, preoperative albumin levels provide information regarding the patient's overall nutritional status.

PREPARATION FOR OPERATIVE TREATMENT

The success of operative treatment in part depends on careful preoperative preparation. All patients should be well-informed about the planned procedure, the risks and common complications, the type and extent of postoperative rehabilitation and expectations for postoperative pain relief and function. To reduce the risks of operative and postoperative complications, including excessive bleeding and compromised healing, nonsteroidal anti-inflammatory drugs (NSAIDs) should be withdrawn, at least 3 half-lives prior to surgery, and in the case of aspirin, one week prior to surgery. For long half-life NSAIDs such as piroxicam this means stopping the drug approximately 5 days prior to surgery or, in the case of short half-life NSAIDs such as diclofenac or ibuprofen, 2 days preoperatively. Pain relief during the immediate preoperative interval can be provided with acetaminophen. This is important as a postoperative flare in inflammatory arthritis may compromise the results of surgery. Preoperative evaluation and instruction by physical and occupational therapists facilitates rehabilitation for some patients. Preoperative physical therapy is important for many patients, both as a method of increasing strength and range of motion, and for the educational benefits that help them prepare for postoperative rehabilitation.

In selected patients, delaying surgery will make it possible to achieve optimal management of cardiovascular or other systemic disorders, allow an improvement in their nutritional status and muscle strength, or a reduction in weight. Physicians may be reluctant to recommend weight reduction for obese patients, but this can produce relief of symptoms and increase the probability of a successful outcome. There is some evidence of an increased incidence of infection in obese patients following total joint arthroplasty[24], as well as increased intraoperative blood loss[25]. Obesity does not appear to increase the risk of implant loosening, but this may be because heavier patients are less active. For some overweight patients the pain and loss of mobility caused by arthritis make it more difficult to reduce their weight or avoid gaining weight. In these individuals, surgeons may recommend proceeding with operative treatment despite the increased risks associated with obesity.

POSTOPERATIVE COMPLICATIONS

In the immediate postoperative period patients must be monitored carefully for potential complications, including neurologic and vascular damage, excessive bleeding, infection, venous thrombosis and pulmonary embolism, cardiac, pulmonary and renal disorders and, in patients with joint replacements, joint dislocation and periprosthetic fracture. Although the majority of serious postoperative complications, including infection, nerve and blood vessel injury, pulmonary embolus and joint dislocation, occur within the first postoperative weeks, complications may occur at any time after surgery. In some patients heterotopic bone which restricts motion may form following surgery (Fig. 12.3). Patients with ankylosing spondylitis and some patients with OA have an increased risk of developing postoperative heterotopic bone[26,27]. Prophylactic postoperative irradiation treatment can decrease the risk of heterotopic bone formation[28]. Arthroplasty patients must be monitored indefinitely for subtle radiographic evidence of periprosthetic osteolysis, which, when treated early, may halt progression to massive bone loss and catastrophic failure (Fig. 12.4). The vast majority of failures among lower extremity total joint prostheses occur after the first decade postoperatively[29], and most patients remain asymptomatic until substantial bone loss, subsidence and even fracture have occurred. It is therefore imperative that routine follow up, including careful standardized clinical and comparative radiographic evaluation, continue on a regular basis throughout the patient's life. In addition, patients must be carefully monitored for early signs of infection. Early detection of infection in a prosthetic joint may make it possible to save the implant. However, treatment of chronic joint infections without removal of the implants rarely succeeds. Patients with multiple joint arthroplasties who develop sepsis in one prosthetic joint should be treated aggressively and observed closely because they have a substantial risk of developing a metachronous infection in another artificial joint.

POSTOPERATIVE REHABILITATION

For many patients the rehabilitation program has a major influence on the outcome of their surgical treatment. Physicians have a critical role in the education of patients concerning the importance of rehabilitation and close monitoring of the rehabilitation program. Rehabilitation should begin as soon as possible postoperatively and patients should not be discharged until their rehabilitation program has been established. In some instances patients will need regular rehabilitation therapy following discharge or even a period of time in a rehabilitation facility.

DISEASE-RELATED FACTORS THAT INFLUENCE OPERATIVE TREATMENT

Operative treatment options, indications for surgical treatment, preoperative evaluation and preparation, complications and outcomes vary considerably among arthritic diseases. Thus, the physician must consider the unique features of each disease in making decisions or advising patients concerning operative treatment.

OSTEOARTHRITIS

Although most patients with OA are elderly, young adults can present with posttraumatic OA or localized articular surface defects. A number of current surgical procedures are intended to reduce symptoms for both groups of patients by preserving or restoring a cartilaginous articular surface (see Fig. 12.1). These include arthroscopic joint debridement, resection or perforation of subchondral bone to stimulate formation of cartilaginous tissue, and use of grafts to replace degenerated articular cartilage (Fig. 12.2)[3]. By removing loose fragments of cartilage, bone and meniscus, and in some instances osteophytes, joint debridement may improve joint mechanical function and may reduce pain in some patients. Penetration of subchondral bone in regions of advanced cartilage degeneration stimulates formation of cartilaginous

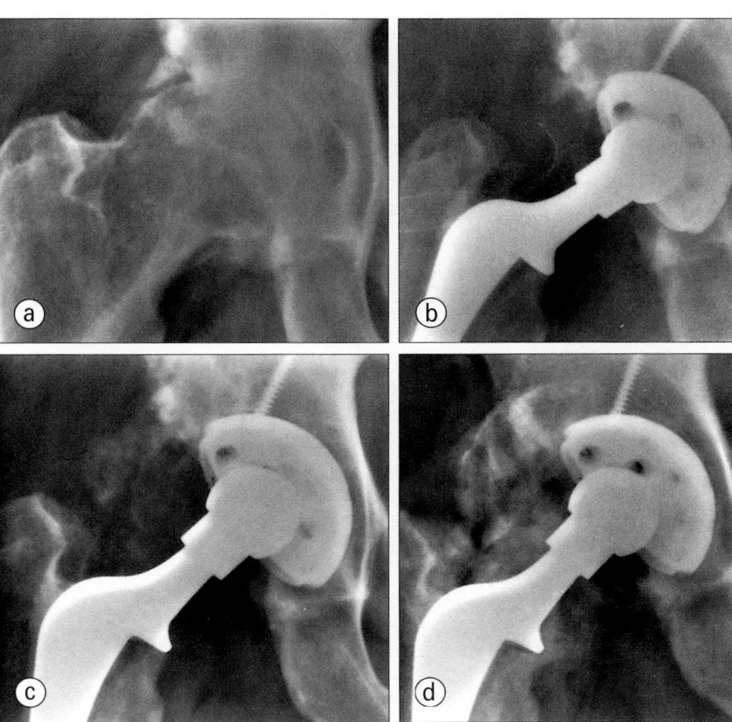

Fig. 12.3 Radiographs showing formation of heterotopic bone following hip replacement. (a) The right hip of a 59-year-old man with advanced OA. Notice the prominent osteophytes. (b) Immediately after surgery the majority of the osteophytes have been removed. (c) Six months later heterotopic bone has formed in the periarticular soft tissues. (d) Twelve months later extensive heterotopic bone limits hip motion. Patients with hypertrophic OA (i.e. extensive osteophyte formation) and anklyosing spondylitis have increased risk of heterotopic bone formation following joint replacement.

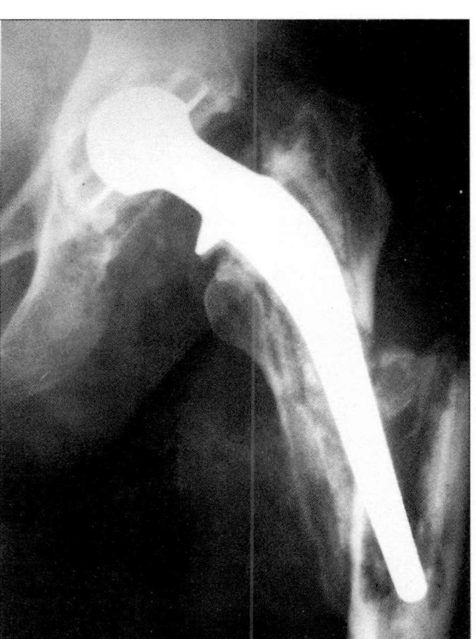

Fig. 12.4 Radiograph showing a left hip replacement with bone resorption around the femoral bone cement, loosening of the prosthesis and a fracture through the proximal femur. This 67-year-old man had a hip replacement 14 years ago. He had not been evaluated during the last seven years. Despite the development of severe periprosthetic osteolysis he did not notice any problems with his hip until he tripped on an electrical cord and sustained the fracture. Earlier detection of the asymptomatic osteolysis followed by surgical revision would have prevented the fracture and extensive loss of bone.

repair tissue, but because it lacks the properties of normal articular cartilage, this tissue frequently degenerates. Replacement of localized regions of degenerated cartilage with osteochondral, perichondrial, periosteal and chondrocyte grafts has produced promising short-term results in small series of patients. Overall, current procedures performed with the intent of preserving or restoring a cartilaginous articular surface and reducing symptoms are not likely to be beneficial in patients with advanced joint degeneration, although they may be helpful in selected patients with less severe disease[3].

Osteotomies realign joints and thereby redistribute joint loads. Surgeons plan these procedures to correct malalignment and shift loads from severely degenerated regions of the articular surface to regions where there is remaining articular cartilage. In selected patients with OA, osteotomies of the hip and knee relieve pain[9,10,11], but in general the results are less predictable than joint replacement and the reasons for the reduction in pain remain poorly understood[9]. For these reasons surgeons most commonly recommend osteotomies for young active people who have a stable joint with a functional range of motion, good muscle function and some remaining articular cartilage.

Joint fusion, i.e. arthrodesis, can relieve pain and restore skeletal stability and alignment in patients with advanced OA[16,17]. Because this procedure eliminates joint motion it has limited application. Furthermore, fusion of one joint increases the loading and motion of other joints and thereby may accelerate degeneration of these joints[13,15]. For example, fusion of the hip increases the probability of developing degenerative disease in the lumbar spine and ipsilateral knee joints[13] and fusion of one segment of the spine may increase the risk of degenerative changes in other segments[31]. Currently, surgeons most commonly perform fusions for treatment of degeneration of cervical and lumbar spine, hand interphalangeal, first metatarsophalangeal (TP), wrist and ankle joints.

For selected joints, resection of degenerated articular surfaces and replacement with implants fabricated from polyethylene, metal or other synthetic materials can relieve pain and allow the patient to maintain joint mobility (Fig. 12.5). Over recent decades, replacement of the hip and knee have proven to be effective methods of relieving pain and maintaining or improving function[12–14,32–34]. Further advances have led to better methods and implants for replacement of the hip, knee, shoulder and elbow. Unfortunately, joint replacements have limitations, primarily because they do not restore an articular surface with the mechanical properties and durability of articular cartilage and because the prostheses must be fixed to the patient's bone. None of the currently available synthetic materials duplicates the ability of articular cartilage to provide a durable low-friction gliding surface and to distribute loads across the synovial joint, nor can current implants achieve the stability and durability of the bond between articular cartilage and bone. Thus, wear of implants limits their lifespan, and loosening can lead to failure. For these reasons, current joint replacements cannot be expected to provide a lifetime of normal function for young, active patients.

RHEUMATOID ARTHRITIS

Compared to most patients with OA and the general population, patients with RA have increased risk of surgical complications. Increased mortality among patients undergoing cervical spine surgery has been associated with severe extra-articular manifestations of the disease, especially interstitial lung disease. It is important to consider the increased probability of local and systemic surgical complications associated with RA in counseling patients about the risks of surgery and to make certain that they receive appropriate preparation and planning for operative treatment. In particular, patients with RA require careful evaluation to prevent operative and perioperative neurologic injury, establish the sequence and timing of joints to be treated surgically (Fig. 12.6), and reduce the risks of infection and other complications.

Soft tissue inflammation and destruction causes a variety of problems for many patients with RA, including joint subluxations and dislocations due to involvement of joint ligaments and capsules and tendon ruptures due to involvement of the tenosynovium[4–6]. Joint synovectomies and tenosynovectomies may help relieve symptoms in selected patients. Soft-tissue reconstructions and synovectomies can realign and stabilize some affected joints, but fusion or replacement arthroplasty is necessary to restore alignment and stability in others.

Patients with RA commonly have cervical spine involvement that can lead to spinal instability and increased risk of neurologic deficits (Fig. 12.6b). The reported prevalence of radiographic changes in the cervical spine of patients with RA varies from less than 20% to more than 80%. Atlantoaxial subluxation is the most common type of cervical instability in patients with classic rheumatoid disease, occurring in more than 20% of patients. Typically, rheumatoid involvement of the cervical spine progresses slowly. Neurologic changes may be difficult to recognize due to limited joint motion and associated disuse muscle atrophy. To evaluate the risk of neurologic injury, patients with RA should have had active flexion and extension lateral cervical radiographs within the year prior to surgery. In a retrospective review of 113 patients with RA who underwent total hip or knee arthroplasty,

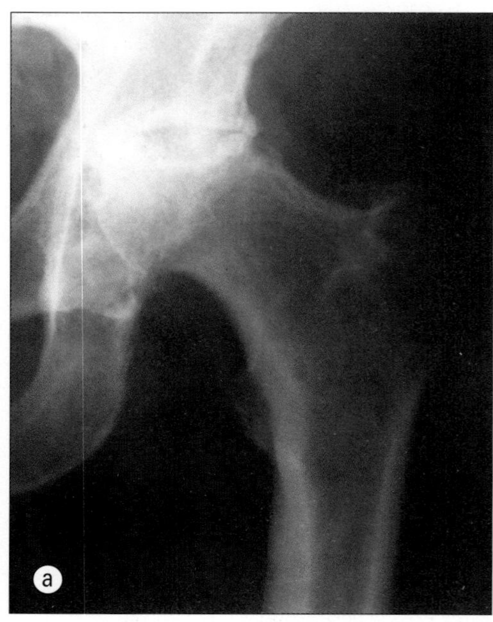

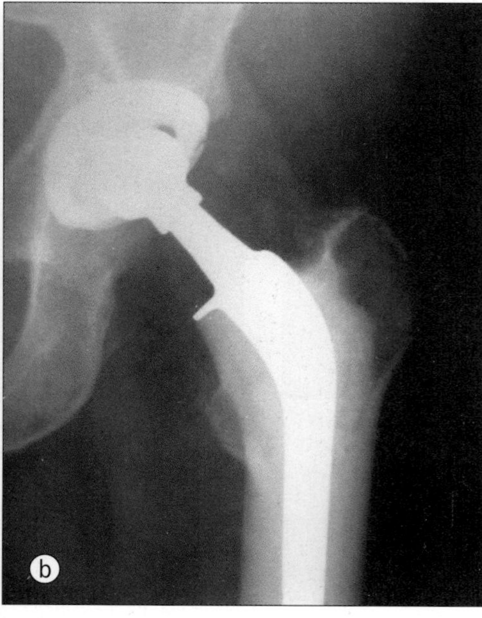

Fig. 12.5 Radiographs showing a hip replacement. The left hip of a 52-year-old man with osteonecrosis and advanced OA. Loss of articular cartilage has reduced the radiographic joint space to a thin line. The patient has severe hip pain and minimal hip motion. Notice the flattening of the femoral head as a result of collapse of bone in the necrotic region (a). The joint has been resected and replaced with a metal femoral component fixed with methylmethacrylate (cement) and an uncemented metal acetabular component containing a polyethylene liner. The patient no longer has hip pain and lacks only a few degrees of normal hip motion (b).

Collins *et al.*[35] reported significant atlantoaxial subluxation, atlantoaxial impaction and/or subaxial subluxation in 69 patients (61%). Of these 69 patients, 35 (50%) had no clinical signs or symptoms of instability at the time of admission for joint replacement arthroplasty. Instability of greater than 7–10mm at the atlantoaxial joint or greater than 4mm at subaxial levels on flexion and extension lateral radiographs generally requires stabilization prior to other elective surgery. Patients with lesser degrees of atlantoaxial and subaxial involvement should be evaluated preoperatively by the anesthesiologist and consideration given to an awake intubation.

Patients with multiple joint involvement require careful planning and timing of surgical procedures in order to allow optimal rehabilitation (Fig. 12.6). Patients indicated for lower extremity surgery may require surgical stabilization of the upper extremity first in enable crutch ambulation and use of the upper extremities to assist in transferring, rising from a chair and stair climbing. For example, the rheumatoid patient with severe wrist involvement as well as hip involvement may benefit from wrist arthrodesis prior to total hip arthroplasty. The patient with multiple lower extremity joint involvement may benefit from sequential or simultaneous treatment, depending on the joints involved and the severity of the disease. The patient with severe disease and contractures of both knees may benefit from having bilateral joint replacment. If only one knee is replaced, a flexion contracture in the untreated knee will cause the patient to keep the operatively treated knee flexed when standing and thereby compromise rehabilitation following surgery. Foot and ankle disease are generally addressed prior to hip and knee arthroplasty in order to give the patient a stable lower extremity on which to stand and rehabilitate the hip and knee.

Long-term use of corticosteroids increases the complexity of surgical treatment of patients with RA. In general, the common clinical practice has been to give these patients 'stress dose' corticosteroids perioperatively with the intention of preventing adrenocortical insufficiency. However, a recent study suggests that supplemental exogenous 'stress' glucocorticoids may not be needed for many of these patients[36]. Long-term corticosteroid use combined with the effects of disease can cause connective tissue changes which make the skin and superficial blood vessels friable. Extreme caution must be used in physically handling such patients. For example, in severely affected patients mild pressure can cause a hematoma or skin ulceration and adhesive tape can tear the skin. In addition, chronic corticosteroid use in patients with RA has been correlated with an increased incidence of fracture, infection and gastrointestinal hemorrhage or ulcer. Series of patients treated with total joint arthroplasties have demonstrated a higher incidence of infection in patients with RA than in patients with OA[24]. Whether these infections are due to corticosteroids or immunologic complications of RA itself is unclear. Patients with RA frequently have more than one joint arthroplasty, and infection of one arthroplasty is associated with an increased incidence of subsequent infection of another total joint[37].

Many patients with RA are treated with NSAIDs and/or methotrexate preoperatively. According to a review of 165 patients undergoing total hip arthroplasty[38], patients who are taking NSAIDs at the time of hospital admission were more likely to have postoperative

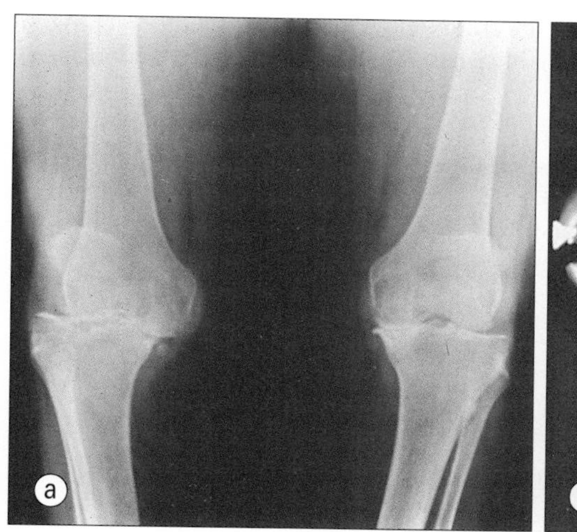

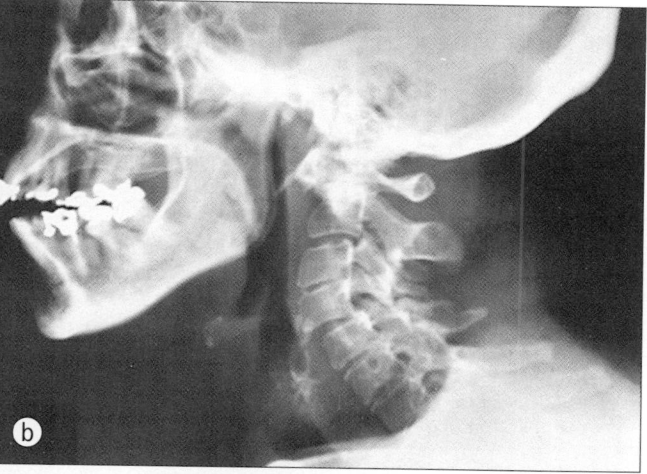

Fig. 12.6 Radiographs illustrating the sequence of surgical procedures in the treatment of a patient with multiple diseased joints including the neck, knees and feet. This woman presented with progressive deterioration in her ability to walk. Evaluation demonstrated that she had severe involvement of both knees (a), C1–C2 instability causing myelopathy (b) and foot deformity (c). Her spine was stabilized with posterior fusion of C1–C2 (d). This procedure was followed by a triple arthrodesis to stabilize her foot (e), and then by knee replacements (f & g). This sequence of procedures restored her ability to walk.

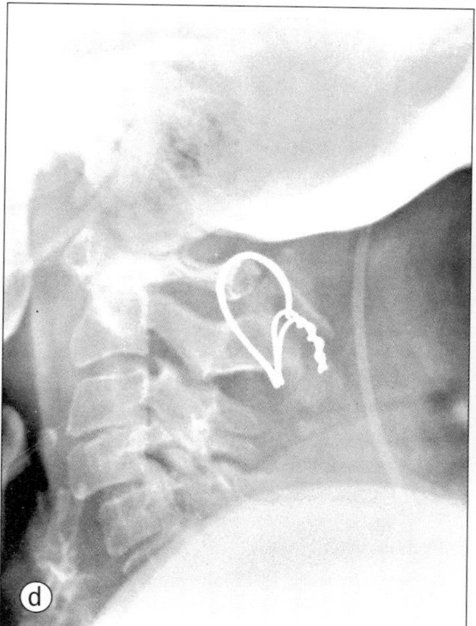

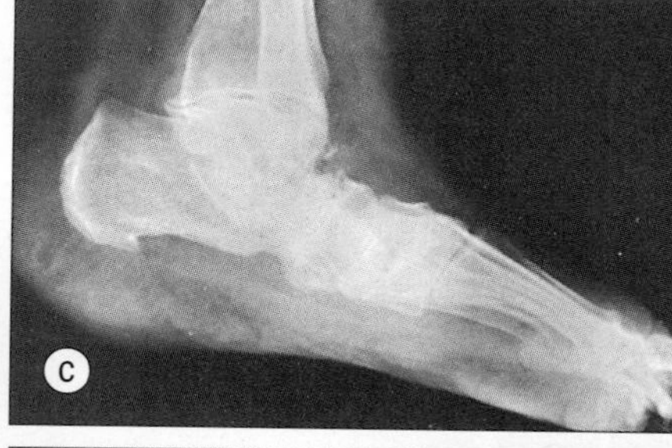

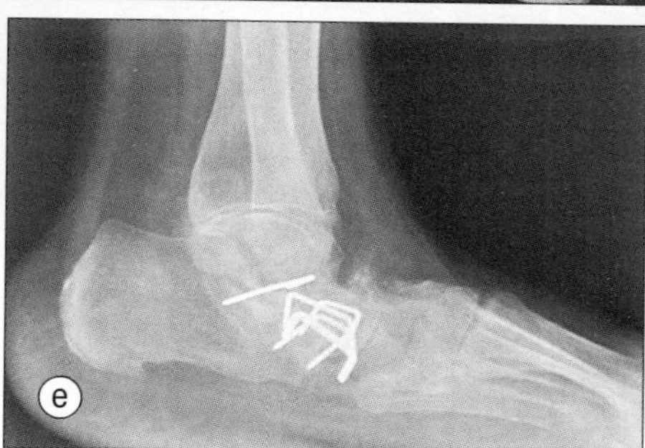

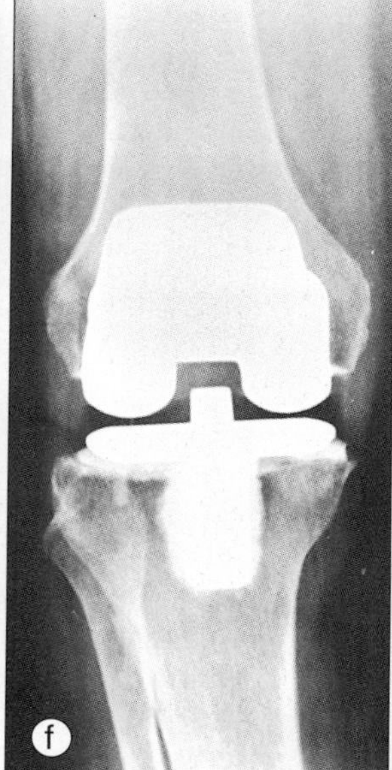

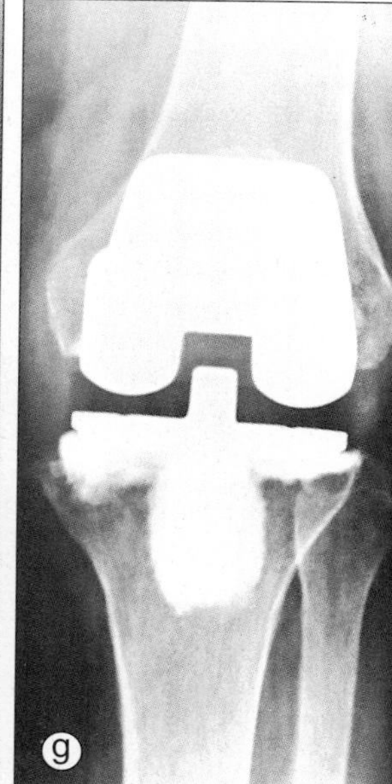

gastrointestinal bleeding and/or hypotension, particularly with agents which have a half-life of longer than 6 hours. Whereas many physicians have withheld methotrexate therapy prior to and immediately following surgery, recent data indicate no increase in wound or other postoperative complications in patients who continue methotrexate therapy perioperatively. Perhala *et al.*[39] compared 60 patients with RA who underwent a total of 92 joint arthroplasties without interruption of methotrexate therapy with a group of 61 patients not receiving methotrexate who underwent a total of 110 joint arthroplasties. Eight patients on methotrexate had a total of eight wound complications (8.7%) versus five patients with a total of six wound complications in the nonmethotrexate group (5.5%). In a prospective, randomized, nonblinded study of 64 patients with RA on methotrexate therapy, Sany *et al.*[40] reported no infections and no difference in wound healing between patients whose therapy was discontinued seven days before an orthopedic procedure and those whose therapy was continued perioperatively.

JUVENILE CHRONIC ARTHRITIS

Unlike patients with OA and RA, many patients with juvenile chronic arthritis (JCA) are skeletally immature and therefore can develop growth disturbances as a consequence of their disease (see Chapter 5.18). Limb length discrepancy is not uncommon, particularly in younger patients who have growth acceleration around an involved joint. Functional limb length may be compromised by joint contractures. Fortunately, the great majority of limb length discrepancies stabilize by adulthood and do not require equalizing procedures. As in other patients with arthritis, joint replacement arthroplasty is reserved for patients who are debilitated by pain and/or reduced function (Fig. 12.7), and is generally delayed until patients are skeletally mature. Joint replacement is also delayed because the life expectancy of young patients is greater than that of current prostheses. Moreover, each subsequent revision procedure necessarily involves greater periprosthetic bone loss and less predictable long-term results. Patients with JCA are often recommended for tendon lengthening to correct contractures, and prophylactic procedures, such as synovectomy, to alleviate symptoms and possibly delay articular cartilage destruction.

Patients with JCA present significant anesthetic risks. Although cervical spine involvement and accompanying neurologic deficits are not as common as in adults with RA, these problems do occur in association with JCA. Therefore, patients with JCA require preoperative screening radiographs as described for patients with RA. Unilateral collapse of the lateral mass of the atlas with or without axis involvement may result in a fixed rotational head tilt deformity that makes it difficult to establish an airway for general anesthesia. Micrognathia associated with temporomandibular joint involvement can also make endotracheal intubation difficult. Restricted motion of the axial and appendicular skeleton can make regional anesthesia difficult as well.

OSTEONECROSIS

Osteonecrosis (ON) is the leading cause of joint degeneration in young adults, particularly in the hip (see Fig. 12.5a). Although most cases of osteonecrosis are idiopathic, known risk factors for ON include corticosteroid use, alcoholism, hemoglobinopathies, collagen-vascular diseases, trauma and dysbaric or Caisson's disease in persons such as deep-sea divers who breathe compressed air (see Chapter 8.47). The most frequently involved site appears to be the femoral head, although involvement of the medial femoral condyle, humeral head, talus and second metatarsal head are not uncommon.

Treatment of ON in the absence of joint degeneration remains controversial, partly because the natural history of the disorder remains poorly understood. Nonsteroidal anti-inflammatory agents and decreased joint loading are commonly employed for temporary symptomatic relief, though neither has been shown to affect the long-term

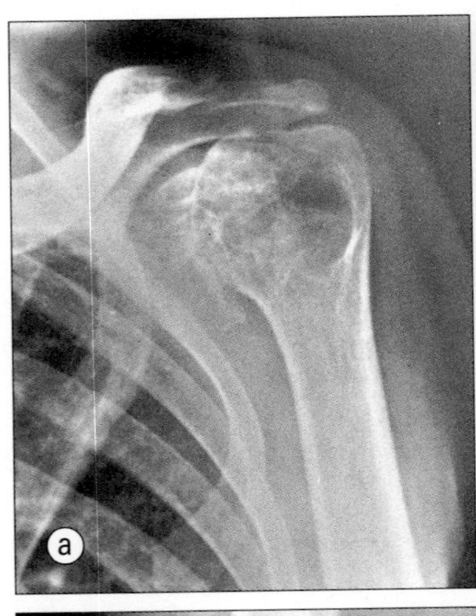

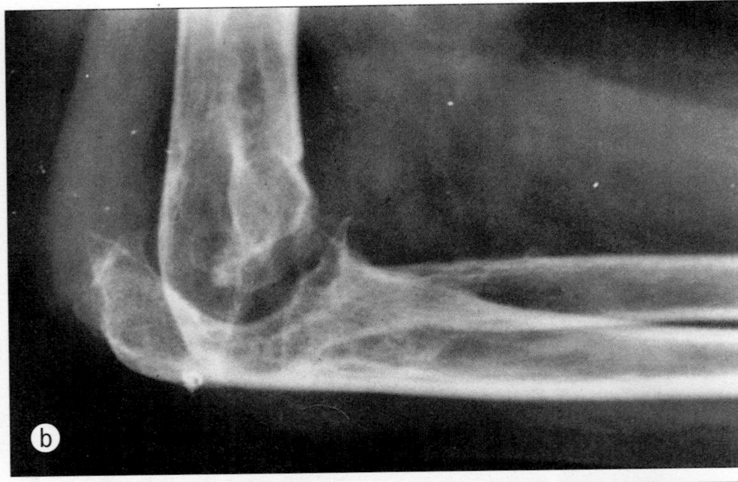

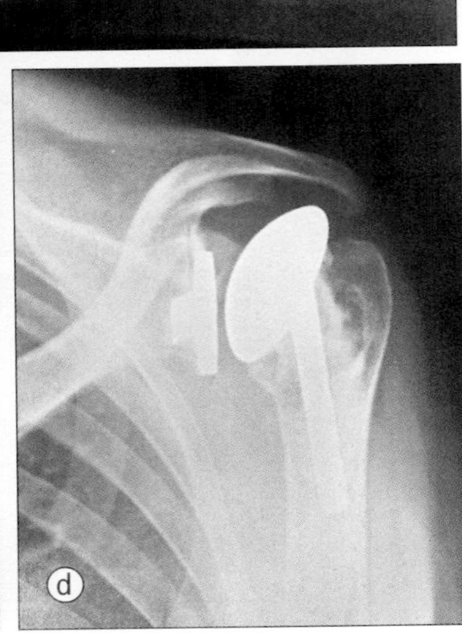

Fig. 12.7 Radiographs illustrating the surgical treatment of a 23-year-old woman with JCA. Destruction of the shoulder and elbow joints made it impossible for her to perform her activities of daily living (a & b). Replacement of her elbow and shoulder joints, followed by a rehabilitation program, restored her upper limb function (c & d).

results. Electromagnetic stimulation has also been employed on an experimental basis. Most surgical treatments of ON have been developed for treatment of the hip. Core decompression, i.e. drilling a channel from the lateral surface of the femur into the necrotic region of the femoral head, with or without bone grafting, has been advocated for patients who have femoral osteonecrosis without collapse or acetabular changes. In most series these procedures have reduced pain in a high percentage of patients. This treatment is generally considered ineffective in patients in whom the femoral head shows signs of collapse or who have evidence of joint degeneration. Other surgical procedures may be helpful, however. Less commonly employed treatments include femoral osteotomies, designed to place an intact segment of the femoral head in a weight-bearing position, and hip arthrodesis. Femoral head and total hip replacement arthroplasty have met with excellent results in this population (see Fig. 12.5), but durability of the prosthesis is a concern, particularly in young patients.

ANKYLOSING SPONDYLITIS

Joint replacements decrease pain and improve function for patients with advanced joint disease due to ankylosing spondylitis (AS) (see Chapter 6.16). In addition, some of these patients can benefit from osteotomies that correct spinal deformities. As with patients with adult RA and JCA, patients with AS carry a substantial risk of operative and perioperative complications. Spinal involvement can lead to extensive ligamentous calcification and heterotopic ossification which make regional anesthesia difficult, if not impossible. Patients with prolonged disease also can develop severe kyphotic deformities of the cervical, thoracic and lumbar spine which impede endotracheal intubation. Restricted chest excursion may further complicate intraoperative and postoperative care.

Patients with AS, and patients with diffuse idiopathic skeletal hyperostosis (see Chapter 8.10), and posttraumatic OA, are at increased risk for postoperative heterotopic ossification[27,41] (Fig. 12.3). Whereas excellent pain relief is obtained in AS patients after total hip arthroplasty, gains in total range of motion are often limited due to periarticular heterotopic ossification, as well as long-standing soft tissue contractures and muscle atrophy. Various regimens have been tried to prevent postoperative soft tissue ossification, but radiation therapy is the only treatment delivered locally instead of systemically, and appears to be the most effective means of preventing heterotopic bone formation after surgery[28]. Prospective evaluations have proved the efficacy of fractionated and single low-dose radiation therapy to the hip and abductor musculature when begun early in the postoperative period.

PSORIATIC ARTHRITIS

The perioperative concerns with NSAIDs and methotrexate discussed for RA apply to patients with psoriatic arthritis as well. A unique perioperative risk in patients with psoriatic arthritis is the development of a flare of psoriasis at the operative site due to the physiologic and/or psychological stress of surgery. Also known as isomorphic or Koebner's phenomenon, this process may predispose the patient to a generalized flare of psoriasis (see Chapter 6.21). Patients with psoriatic arthritis may have an increased incidence of postoperative infection. Menon and Wroblewski[42] reported superficial wound infection in 9.1% and deep wound infections in 5.5% of their 38 patients with psoriasis treated with total hip arthroplasty. The incidence of infection was significantly higher than for historical controls with OA and RA.

HEMOPHILIC ARTHROPATHY

Despite the risk of excessive bleeding, operative treatment can benefit patients with hemophilic arthropathy. Synovectomy is commonly performed in the knee and elbow, and improves range of motion and reduces pain for the majority of patients. Total knee and total hip replacements can improve function and relieve pain in hemophilic patients with advanced joint degeneration[43,44].

Patients with hemophilic arthropathy may be particularly difficult to manage perioperatively. Factor replacement has important risks and must be carefully monitored. A thrombotic event may be precipitated by repeated factor infusions, and resultant disseminated intravascular coagulation after elective surgery has been reported. Major elective surgery is generally contraindicated for the subgroup of patients with high levels of factor antibody (see Chapter 8.24).

Whether or not well-controlled hemophilic patients without AIDS are at increased risk for nontransfusion-related infection is unclear. Septic arthritis has been reported as a rare complication of hemophilia, but one which must be promptly diagnosed and definitively treated. Hemophilic patients infected by HIV-1 who have not progressed to AIDS do not appear to have an increased incidence of infection after surgery when compared with patients who are seronegative for HIV-1.

ENTEROPATHIC ARTHROPATHY

Although the relationships between inflammatory bowel disease and arthritis remain poorly understood, sacroiliitis develops in about 15% and a spondylitis indistinguishable from AS in about 5% of patients with inflammatory bowel disease (see Chapter 6.24). The majority of reports indicate that 6–8% of patients develop peripheral joint disease. Patients with inflammatory bowel disease are at increased risk of perioperative and late infections, particularly when orthopedic implants are utilized. This may occur by hematogenous seeding or direct contamination via a fistula or colostomy.

PIGMENTED VILLONODULAR SYNOVITIS

Pigmented villonodular synovitis (PVNS) most commonly involves the knee and has been reported in patients ranging in age from the second to the ninth decades (see Chapter 5.29). It also occurs in the ankle and shoulder as well as other joints, where it may be more difficult to detect. Arthroscopy may allow early diagnosis; and synovectomy, by arthrotomy or arthroscopy, usually provides symptomatic relief, and may be curative in patients with the localized form of the disease[45]. The diffuse form of the disease responds less favorably to synovectomy, with recurrences in about 30% of patients[46].

SYNOVIAL CHONDROMATOSIS

Synovial chondromatosis, a rare condition that results in the formation of cartilaginous nodules or fragments that may lie in synovial joint cavities, the synovium or in some instances in the periarticular soft tissues, causes joint pain, joint catching and locking and loss of motion, and can lead to degeneration of the articular surfaces (see Fig. 12.8). Removal of intra-articular loose bodies and, in some cases, synovectomy can relieve symptoms and improve motion in patients who have not developed advanced degenerative joint disease[47]. However, in many joints the cartilage fragments re-accumulate. In patients with advanced degenerative joint disease, joint replacement combined with synovectomy is curative.

SITES OF SURGICAL INTERVENTION

The operative treatments that provide the best results vary not only among arthritic diseases and patients, but also among anatomic sites. Thus, making decisions concerning surgical treatment must include consideration of the unique characteristics of the joint involved as well as the type of arthritis, patient age and social and medical factors.

HIP

The most commonly employed operative treatments for arthritis of the hip are cemented (i.e. inserted with polymethylmethacrylate cement) and uncemented total hip arthroplasty. More than 120,000 hip prostheses are implanted in the United States each year (Fig. 12.5)[32]. Osteotomies and fusions are performed less often than hip replacements, but can produce good results in selected patients.

Nearly 30 years of clinical studies now document the success of total hip replacement (see Fig. 12.5) for the treatment of disabling pain and impairment due to chronic hip diseases including, but not limited to, OA, RA, osteonecrosis, traumatic arthritis, AS, arthritis associated with Paget's disease and JCA. Recent long-term follow up studies show that total hip replacements will provide excellent function for more than 20 years in appropriately selected patients[8]. Initially, surgeons tended to limit hip replacement to patients between 60 and 75 years of age, but studies in the last decade have shown that both younger and more elderly patients also can benefit from this procedure[17,18]. Although most patients who have a hip replacement increase their level of physical function, patients with limited expectation for improved function can also benefit from the procedure.

The risks of postoperative venous thrombosis and infection in patients treated with hip replacements have significantly decreased in the last two decades. Early series of hip replacements reported a high rate of failure due to infection, but modern aseptic techniques and prophylactic antibiotic cover have reduced the incidence of infection to less than 1% of patients in recent series[48]. Loosening remains the predominant cause of long-term failure of hip replacements, but recent research has shed light on the causes of this problem. Particulate debris, most of which appears to be generated from wear of polyethylene surfaces, stimulates osteoclastic bone lysis at the bone–cement interface in prostheses fixed with methylmethacrylate and at the prosthesis–bone interface in uncemented implants. The osteolysis can lead to loosening of the prostheses, bone loss and bone fractures (see Fig. 12.4).

Improvements in cement techniques have decreased the incidence of aseptic femoral loosening from as high as 40% to less than 5% 10 years after the procedure for many groups of patients[15]. Even in a group of patients who were less than 50 years old at the time of cemented hip arthroplasty, only 8% had evidence of femoral component loosening 16–20 years after the procedure[49]. In contrast, cemented acetabular components continue to have a high rate of loosening despite improved cement techniques[15]. Preliminary reviews of the results with uncemented acetabular components (see Fig. 12.5b) suggest that they may produce better results. Although uncemented femoral components have been associated with postoperative thigh pain, some surgeons use them in young patients in an effort to increase prosthetic durability. Uncemented femoral components may also have a potential advantage in revision surgery where there is hope of regaining lost bone stock with bone growth into and around the prosthesis.

Despite its great success, total hip arthroplasty has important limitations, particularly for young patients who are likely to outlive the prosthesis. Alternatives to arthroplasty include osteotomy, arthrodesis and resection arthroplasty. Femoral and pelvic osteotomy have been shown to be effective in relieving pain in young patients with acetabular dysplasia and minimal or no radiographic degenerative change. Whether or not they alter the natural history of hip dysplasia is unclear. Results are less favorable in adults over 40 years of age and in patients with significant degenerative change. Arthrodesis of the hip offers young patients with hip arthritis a dependable, durable, pain-free hip. Once fusion is obtained, the patient may return to vigorous activity without the limitations imposed on arthroplasty patients. However, some patients find the prospect of a stiff hip unacceptable. At long-term follow up, patients complain of some difficulty sitting in a chair and using public transportation, but otherwise perform activities of daily living well with excellent pain relief. Patients who develop associated lumbosacral or knee pain later in life may be considered for conversion of the arthrodesis to a total hip arthroplasty.

Resection arthroplasty, originally described for treatment of tuberculous arthritis of the hip and osteomyelitis, is seldom employed today as a primary procedure. It remains an option for patients with recalcitrant infection involving a total hip arthroplasty and for low-demand patients who are not candidates for more extensive reconstruction. After resection arthroplasty, the proximal femur is allowed to articulate with the acetabulum or the ilium. The majority of otherwise healthy patients are ambulatory, but generally they require one or two crutches and a substantial heel lift in order to walk. Today, surgeons usually reserve resection arthroplasty for salvage of a failed or infected hip arthroplasty which is not amenable to revision.

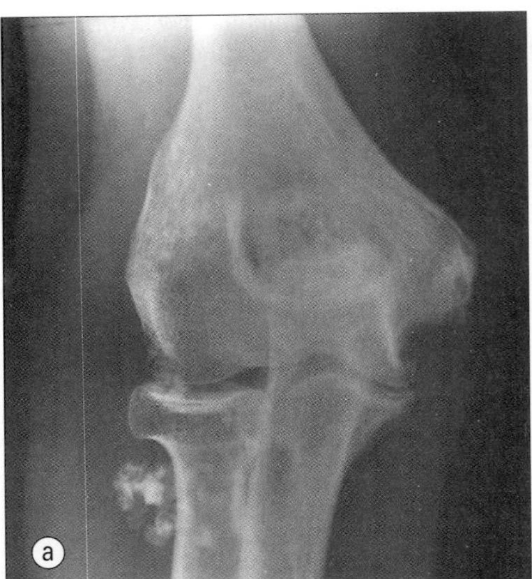

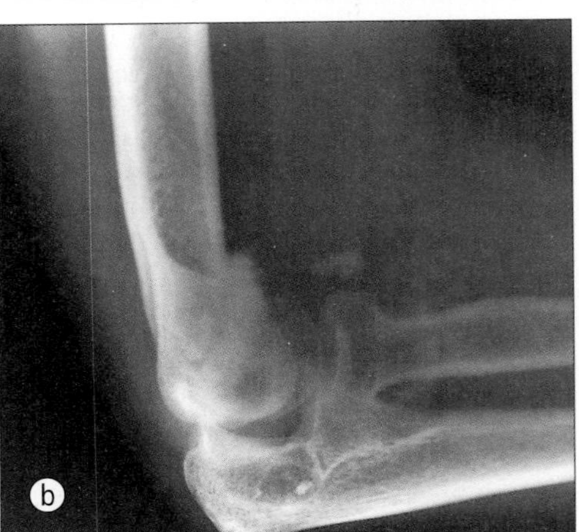

Fig. 12.8 Radiographs of the elbow of a 26-year-old woman with joint swelling, catching and restriction of motion. Anteroposterior radiograph showing multiple calcified chondral fragments surrounding the radial neck. Notice the osteophytes on the ulnar margin of the ulnar-humoral trochlea joint (a). Lateral radiograph showing calcified chondral fragments in the elbow joint. Removal of loose bodies and synovectomy can improve symptoms, but recurrence is likely (b).

KNEE

A variety of operative procedures have been described for treatment of the arthritic knee, including arthroscopy, osteotomy and replacement arthroplasty (see Fig. 12.1). The indications for these procedures differ significantly.

Arthroscopy has advanced the diagnosis and treatment of many forms of knee arthritis. It is particularly useful for patients whose symptoms may be attributed to a specific mechanical etiology, such as a meniscus tear or loose body. Arthroscopic synovectomy can reduce pain and swelling in patients with hemophilia, PVNS, synovial chondromatosis and early RA without significant cartilage erosion. Whether or not it alters the long-term course of these diseases is unclear. Arthroscopic debridement or chondroplasty for degenerative knee arthritis, except in the case of a degenerative meniscal tear or intra-articular loose bodies, does not appear to affect the natural history of the disease, although in some patients it may provide short-term relief of symptoms[3].

Osteotomy about the knee is intended to redirect the weight-bearing axis away from a degenerative portion of the tibiofemoral joint, and may also stimulate development of fibrocartilage in the unloaded degenerative compartment[3]. The majority of knee osteotomies are valgus osteotomies of the proximal tibia, performed to redirect weight bearing forces from a degenerative medial tibiofemoral articulation through a better preserved lateral compartment. Femoral osteotomies are preferred for valgus and excessive varus deformities of the knee. Osteotomies are generally chosen over total knee arthroplasties for young, heavy, active patients and, as a rule, should be reserved for patients with noninflammatory disease. Appropriate candidates have less than 5° of flexion contracture, greater than 90° of flexion and isolated medial or lateral tibiofemoral arthritis without significant patellofemoral involvement. Good results have been reported in 80–90% of patients for 6–9 years postosteotomy, with 60–70% good results at 10–15-year follow up[11]. It is difficult to compare these results with those of total knee arthroplasty, where the patients are generally older and less active.

As with total hip arthroplasty, total knee arthroplasty may be performed with cement or bone ingrowth as the means of fixation. Several large series reveal that tibial and femoral results are excellent regardless of the type of fixation, with 97% survival of prostheses at ten and 12-year analysis[50]. Despite excellent results with cement fixation, some surgeons reserve cemented tibial and femoral components for patients older than 50 or 60 years, or patients with poor bone stock, based on the assumption that uncemented components will last longer in young patients and preserve their bone stock. Patellar problems are the leading cause of failure after total knee arthroplasty. Unlike tibial and femoral results, results of uncemented patellar components, which require a metal backing for bone ingrowth, are substantially inferior to results of cemented all–polyethylene patellar components, and have thus fallen out of favor in recent years.

Knee arthrodesis is an option for patients with recalcitrant infection or failed total knee arthroplasty that cannot be effectively revised. Despite loss of knee motion, a functional lower extremity which permits painless weight bearing can be expected using current techniques. Resection arthroplasty has also been used for patients with failed total knee arthroplasty, but instability is a significant problem for many patients.

FOOT AND ANKLE

Arthritic involvement of the foot and ankle is not uncommon in RA and JCA as well as following traumatic injuries. Surgical options include cheilectomy (resection of an osteophyte or osteophytes), arthroscopic debridement, osteotomy, arthrodesis, replacement arthroplasty and, in advanced RA, resection of metatarsal heads.

Osteophytes may develop at the periphery of a joint and cause symptoms related to impingement during normal walking. These are not uncommon on the dorsum of the first MTP joint and the anterior aspect of the tibiotalar joint. While not curing the underlying disease, cheilectomy often provides relief of mechanical symptoms and associated pain[51]. Loose bodies may also be a source of mechanical symptoms and are amenable to arthroscopic removal.

Supramalleolar tibial osteotomy allows realignment of the weight-bearing axis through the tibiotalar joint. This can help preserve the joint in various congenital and posttraumatic degenerative conditions of the ankle. Low tibial osteotomy has been shown effectively to relieve symptoms in long-term relief with intermediate-stage primary OA[52]. Osteotomy is generally reserved for non-inflammatory arthritides, but it may also provide relief of pain and decreased frequency of intra-articular bleeding in patients with hemophilic arthropathy[53].

Arthrodeses of foot and ankle joints offer pain relief and stability to patients with severe arthritis (Fig. 12.6c & d). Fusions of these joints are well tolerated, even by children, despite some restriction of stressful activities such as hill climbing and running. While the vast majority of patients with ankle and/or peritalar arthrodeses obtain excellent pain relief and increased function, initial nonunion of the arthrodesis occurs in 5–30 per cent of cases[54–58]. Infection and delayed wound healing have been reported in 25–40% of patients with RA who undergo tibiotalar arthrodesis, yet the majority have an excellent long-term result[56,58].

Unlike replacement arthroplasty of the hip and knee, ankle replacement arthroplasties have not produced predictable results. Some 60–90% of these prostheses have reportedly failed by five to ten years after the procedure[59]. Most surgeons limit the use of this procedure to treatment of inflammatory arthritis in minimally active elderly patients who have multiple joint involvement[59].

A recent preliminary report describes encouraging results of joint distraction and motion as a treatment for patients with posttraumatic ankle OA. van Valburg and colleagues treated advanced posttraumatic OA of the ankle with joint distraction in 11 patients[60]. At an average of 20 months after treatment none of the patients had proceeded with an arthrodesis. All 11 patients had less pain, and five were pain-free; six had more motion; and the three of six that had radiographic studies had increased joint space. The authors concluded that distraction of an OA ankle joint delays arthrodesis, and that it may stimulate repair of OA cartilage.

HAND AND WRIST

Inflammatory arthritis and OA tend to have different patterns of joint involvement in the hand and wrist. Osteoarthritis most commonly affects the distal interphalangeal (DIP) joints and thumb carpometacarpal (CMC) joints, while RA most commonly involves the proximal interphalangeal (PIP), MTP, CMC, radiocarpal and distal radioulnar joints. In addition, the soft tissue damage caused by RA leads to joint subluxation and dislocation, tenosynovitis, tendon subluxation and tendon ruptures.

When evaluating the wrist and hand in patients with RA, it is imperative to obtain a history of the patient's functional abilities and carefully note any recent changes. Inability to actively flex or extend interphalangeal and/or MCP joints with preservation of passive motion usually signals a ruptured tendon. There is greater susceptibility to rupture in flexor and extensor tendons of patients with rheumatoid disease than in normal tendons. Underlying ultrastructural changes associated with the inflammatory process weaken the tendons and abnormal bony prominences, particularly at the distal radioulnar joint, abrade the weakened tendons making them prone to rupture. Tenosynovectomy not only reduces pain and increases range of motion and grip strength, but it may also help protect the tendons from rupture, particularly when combined with resection of abnormal bony prominences. Acute tendon ruptures should be evaluated early by a surgeon for consideration of reconstruction prior to the development of fibrosis and contractures. In the rheumatoid hand, the MCP joints of the fingers are generally reconstructed with silicone implants that function as flexible spacers. Ulnar drift of the digits with resultant ulnar subluxation of the extensor tendons may be at least partially corrected by surgical centralization of the extensor tendons and transfer of the intrinsic hand muscle insertions from one digit to the adjacent digit on the ulnar side[6].

Surgeons commonly treat advanced degeneration of the interphalangeal joints, carpus and wrist due to OA or inflammatory arthritis by arthrodesis. Interphalangeal joints should be fused in a partially flexed position. Arthrodesis may also be performed at the radiocarpal joint or selectively at diseased intercarpal joints. While some reduction in wrist motion and grip strength are commonly noted with limited intercarpal arthrodeses, long-term pain relief and stability are excellent.

Surgeons rarely recommend arthrodesis of arthritic thumb CMC joints, because motion of these joints is particularly important for overall hand function. The degenerative thumb CMC joint is amenable to interposition arthroplasty (resection of the joint surfaces and interposition of soft tissue, usually a portion of the abductor pollicis longus or flexor carpi radialis tendons), which yields excellent pain relief and increased grip strength.

Surgeons do not usually recommend wrist arthroplasty, partially because wrist arthrodesis has produced more predictable results. A review of the results of silicone spacer wrist implants showed a greater than 50% incidence of implant fracture, a revision rate of nearly one third, radiographic evidence of prosthesis settling and bony resorption in more than 75% of patients, and overall fair or poor clinical results in about half the patients[61]. Wrist arthroplasty designs have improved clinical outcome, but component failure remains a problem and has been reported in 22% of wrists 8.6 years postoperatively[50]. In selected patients with degenerative disease of the wrist, resection of the proximal row of carpal bones, i.e. proximal row carpectomy, can reduce pain while retaining functional wrist motion[62].

ELBOW

Routine activities of daily living require a wide range of elbow flexion and extension as well as pronation and supination. While elbow fusion can be reliably obtained with internal fixation, this results in substantial impairment since shoulder and wrist motion cannot adequately compensate for loss of elbow motion. Fortunately, radial head excision, synovectomy, arthroscopy and arthroplasty are alternatives which have yielded good results.

Arthritis involving primarily the radiohumeral articulation is not uncommon with RA and posttraumatic OA. Radial head resection offers increased range of motion and decreased pain in appropriately selected patients. Resultant proximal migration of the radius is minimal after this procedure, and elbow instability is seldom a concern if the medial collateral ligament complex is intact. Patients generally have good intermediate-term pain relief with increased range of motion. In one series, 84% of patients with RA reported good pain relief 6 months after the procedure[63]. Synovectomy may be performed alone or in conjunction with other procedures, such as radial head resection. Patients with hemophilia likewise have decreased pain and swelling following synovectomy, as well as a decreased incidence of hemarthrosis. Arthroscopy has been used effectively to perform synovectomies as well as removing loose bodies and osteophytes from arthritic elbows.

Elbow joint replacement arthroplasty, while a more recent development than hip and knee arthroplasty, has evolved rapidly. The rate of loosening in young active patients with posttraumatic arthropathy approaches 50% at 5–8-year follow up; but intermediate-term results in low-demand patients with inflammatory disease are promising, with survival of the components and good or excellent results reported in greater than 90% of rheumatoid patients at 3–8-year follow up[64].

SHOULDER

The high degree of compensatory movement in the scapulothoracic articulation as well as elsewhere throughout the upper extremity may be responsible for the relatively low incidence of patients with debilitating arthritis of the glenohumeral joints. Nonetheless, some patients with advanced shoulder arthritis can benefit from surgical treatment.

Shoulder arthrodesis relieves pain and provides a stable upper extremity with long-term durability for patients with severe glenohumeral arthritis[65]. Fusion is reliably obtained in the majority of patients with relatively few complications. Despite rigid fusion of the glenohumeral joint, abduction of 50° and flexion of 40° in the shoulder girdle is possible via scapulothoracic motion.

The majority of shoulder arthroplasties are performed for inflammatory arthritis of the glenohumeral joint (Figs 12.7c & 12.5d). Pain relief and improved general activities of daily living are reported in more than 90% of patients using contemporary techniques[66]. The most common long-term complication reported is glenoid component loosening[67]. To this end, recent studies have explored the use of hemiarthroplasty, which is a replacement of the humeral head without resurfacing the glenoid. This method has proved effective in selected patients, including those with rotator cuff tear arthropathy – chronic, massive rotator cuff tears with secondary superior migration of the humeral head and resultant erosive changes of the glenohumeral joint and inferior surface of the acromion.

SPINE

The clinical problems caused by arthritic disorders of the cervical spine, primarily RA and OA, are pain, compromised neurologic function and mechanical instability that causes or has the potential to cause pain and neurologic deficits. Spinal fusions can reduce pain, restore stability and in some instances prevent development of neurologic deficits. Surgical decompression of the spinal cord and nerve roots can relieve pain and improve neurologic function in selected patients.

Although patients with advanced RA of the cervical spine usually have pain, neurologic signs are reported in only 30% or less. However, signs of central nervous system (CNS) compromise may be mistakenly attributed to more overt effects of the disease, including joint deformity, pain, decreased range of motion and secondary muscular atrophy. The natural history of cervical involvement is unclear, but radiographic progression appears to be more common than neurologic progression (see Chapter 5.16).

Generally accepted indications for surgical intervention in RA patients with cervical spine involvement are pain refractory to nonoperative modalities, neurologic deterioration and radiographic evidence of impending spinal cord compression[68]. Whereas the anterior atlantodental interval has been conventionally used to determine the degree of atlantoaxial instability, recently the posterior atlantodental interval has been shown to be an important predictor of the potential for postoperative neurologic improvement[69]. The available evidence also suggests that patients who undergo cervical arthrodesis earlier in the course of their disease have more satisfactory results than those in whom arthrodesis is delayed[68]. Some authors have recommended that patients with atlantoaxial subluxation and a posterior atlanto-odontoid interval of 14mm or less, patients who have atlantoaxial subluxation and at least 5mm of basilar invagination and patients who have subaxial subluxation and a sagittal spinal canal diameter of 14mm or less, even in the absence of neurologic findings, undergo posterior surgical fusion at the involved levels. Pain is relieved in the majority of patients, but neurologic improvement is variable and closely related to preoperative radiographic instability and neurologic status[69].

In contrast to patients with RA involving the cervical spine, patients with OA of the cervical spine rarely have instability. However, they may develop pain and neurologic signs as a result of degenerative stenosis. Posterior decompression may be accomplished via laminectomy or laminaplasty. Laminectomy, or removal of part or all of one or more cervical laminae, allows excellent visualization and decompression at the expense of potentially destabilizing the spine with resultant kyphosis. Laminaplasty may be performed by one of many techniques, but in general involves cutting through the laminae completely on one side at the involved levels of the spine and cutting about 80% of the way through the contralateral laminae at the same levels. The cervical spinal canal may then be opened on the hinge of the partially cut laminae. This allows excellent multilevel decompression at the expense of decreased cervical motion. The choice between these two procedures remains controversial[19].

Osteoarthritis of the lumbar spine may also produce pain and neurologic symptoms and signs associated with spinal stenosis. In addition, some patients with degenerative disease of the lumbar spine develop spondylolisthesis. The majority of patients with OA of the lumbar spine should be treated by methods other than surgery, but decompression of the spinal cord and nerve roots and spinal fusion can improve symptoms for carefully selected patients.

EXPERIMENTAL SURGICAL TREATMENTS

Replacements of the hip and knee predictably relieve pain and provide stability and motion for large numbers of patients. Unfortunately, wear and loosening can cause these implants to fail. Other current operative treatments also relieve or reduce pain for many patients with arthritis. However, they are generally less successful in restoring joint function. Joint fusions and even joint replacements place important limits on function and other current treatments do not reliably arrest or reverse joint degeneration. Thus, there is a clear need for new therapeutic approaches. Advances in surgical techniques, implant materials and methods of fixing implants to bone may reduce the frequency and severity of long-term wear and loosening of joint replacements, making it possible to provide more patients with joint replacements that last a lifetime. Improved results of wrist and ankle joint replacement may be possible with new implant designs. Although they have not yet been shown to be effective in arthritic joints, operative approaches intended to preserve or restore cartilaginous articular surfaces that include surgical debridement of degenerated tissue and correction of mechanical abnormalities combined with implantation of artificial matrices, growth factors and transplanted chondrocytes or mesenchymal stem cells, have the potential to restore a joint surface[3]. In small groups of patients with advanced OA, joint distraction using external fixation devices has reduced pain and may have allowed partial reformation of an articular surface[30,60].

CONCLUSIONS

Surgical treatment can dramatically improve the quality of life for selected patients with arthritis by relieving pain and improving function. Replacement of the hip, knee or shoulder benefits hundreds of thousands of patients each year, but other procedures, including synovectomies, joint fusions and debridements, also have important roles in the treatment of patients with arthritis. The success of surgical treatment of patients with complex rheumatologic disorders depends on coordination of care among different specialists and other healthcare providers including nurses and physical therapists. All patients require careful preoperative evaluation and preparation, including education and postoperative rehabilitation. In recent decades the results of joint replacements have improved considerably and the rate of complications decreased. Better understanding of the wear of prosthetic joint surfaces and the relationships between wear and loosening of the prosthesis–bone interfaces should lead to implants and surgical techniques that improve the durability and long-term function of joint replacements. New approaches to the restoration of biologic articular surfaces have the potential to improve the treatment of disorders that lead to loss or degeneration of articular cartilage.

REFERENCES

1. Buckwalter JA. Joint distraction for osteoarthritis. Lancet. 1996; 347:279–80.
2. Mankin HJ, Buckwalter JA. Restoring the osteoarthritic joint. J Bone Joint Surg. 1996;78A:1–2.
3. Buckwalter JA, Lohmander S. Operative treatment of osteoarthrosis: current practice and future development. J Bone Joint Surg. 1994;76A:1405–18.
4. Brown FE, Brown ML. Long-term results after tenosynovectomy to treat the rheumatoid hand. J Hand Surg.1988;13:704–8.
5. Brumfield R, Kuschner SH, Gellman H, Liles DN, Winckle GV. Results of dorsal wrist synovectomies in the rheumatoid hand. J Hand Surg. 1990;15:733–5.
6. el-Gammal TA, Blair WG. Motion after metacarpalphalangeal joint reconstruction in rheumatoid disease. J Hand Surg. 1993;18:504–11.
7. Brown FE. Wrist deformity in rheumatoid arthritis. Extensor carpi ulnaris tendon transfer. Ann Plast Surg. 1984;13:121–5.
8. Ertel AN, Millender LH, Nalebuff E, McKay D, Leslie B. Flexor tendon ruptures in patients with rheumatoid arthritis. J Hand Surg. 1988;13:860–6.
9. Coventry MB, Ilstrup DM, Wallrichs SL. Proximal tibial osteotomy. A critical long-term study of eighty-seven cases. J Bone Joint Surg. 1993;75A:196–201.
10. Weisl H. Intertrochanteric osteotomy for osteoarthritis. A long-term follow-up. J Bone Joint Surg. 1980;62B:37–42.
11. Insall JN, Joseph DM, Msika C. High tibial osteotomy for varus gonarthrosis. A long-term follow-up study. J Bone Joint Surg. 1984;66A:1040–8.
12. Ballard WT, Callaghan JJ, Johnston RC. Revision of total hip arthroplasty in octogenarians. J Bone Joint Surg. 1995;77A:585–9.
13. Ballard WT, Callaghan JJ, Sullivan PM, Johnston RC. The results of improved cementing techniques for total hip arthroplasty in patients less than fifty years old. A ten year follow-up study. J Bone Joint Surg. 1994;76A:959–64.
14. Rand JA, Ilstrup DM. Survivorship analysis of total knee arthroplasty. Cumulative rates of survival of 9200 total knee arthroplasties. J Bone Joint Surg. 1991;73A:397–409.
15. Mulroy RD, Harris WH. The effect of improved cementing techniques on component loosening in total hip replacement. J Bone Joint Surg. 1990;72B:757–60.
16. Callaghan JJ, Brand RA, Pederson DR. Hip arthrodesis. A long-term follow-up. J Bone Joint Surg. 1985;67A:1328–35.
17. Hagan HJ, Hastings H. Fusion of the thumb metacarpalphalangeal joint to treat posttraumatic arthritis. J Hand Surg. 1988;13:750–3.
18. Stevens JC, Beard CM, O'Fallon WM, Kurland LT. Conditions associated with carpal tunnel syndrome. Mayo Clin Proc. 1992;67:541–8.
19. Herkowitz HN. The surgical management of cervical spondylotic radiculopathy and myelopathy. Clin Orthop. 1989;239:94–108.
20. Yoshida M, Otani K, Shibasaki K. Expansive laminoplasty with reattachment of spinous process and extensor musculature for cervical myelopathy. Spine. 1992;17:491–7.
21. Gross AE, Beaver RJ, Mohammed MN. Fresh small fragment osteochondral allografts used for posttraumatic defects in the knee joint. In Finerman GAM, Noyes FR, eds. Biology and biomechanics of the traumatized synovial joint: the knee as a model. Rosemont, IL: American Academy of Orthopaedic Surgeons; 1992:123–41.
22. Garrett JC. Fresh osteochondral allografts for treatment of articular defects in osteochondritis dissecans of the lateral femoral condyle in adults. Clin Orthop. 1994;303:33–7.
23. Meyers MH. Resurfacing of the femoral head with fresh osteochondral allografts: long-term results. Clin Orthop. 1985;197:111–4.
24. Wymenga AB, Horn JR, Theeuwes A, Muytjens HL, Slooff TJ. Perioperative factors associated with septic arthritis after arthroplasty. Prospective multicenter study of 362 knee and 2651 hip operations. Acta Orthop Scand. 1992;63:665–71.
25. Lehman DE, Capello WN, Feinberg JR. Total hip arthroplasty without cement in obese patients. J Bone Joint Surg. 1994;76A:854–62.
26. Goel A, Sharp DJ. Heterotopic bone formation after hip replacement. The influence of the type of osteoarthritis. J Bone Joint Surg. 1991;73B:255–7.
27. Kilgus DJ, Namba RS, Gorek JE, Cracchiolo A, Amstutz HC. Total hip replacement for patients who have anklyosing spondylitis. The importance of heterotopic bone and the durability of fixation of cemented components. J Bone Joint Surg. 1990;72A:834–9.
28. Healy WL, Lo TC, DeSimone AA, Rask B, Pfeifer BA. Single-dose irradiation for the prevention of heterotopic ossification after hip arthroplasty. A comparison of five hundred and fifty and seven hundred centigray. J Bone Joint Surg. 1995;77A:590–5.
29. Schulte KR, Callaghan JJ, Kelley SS, Johnston RC. The outcome of Charnley total hip arthroplasty with cement after a minimum twenty-year follow-up. The results of one surgeon. J Bone Joint Surg. 1993;75A:959–75.28.
30. Aldegheri R, Trivella G, Saleh M. Articulated distraction of the hip. Clin Orthop. 1994;301:94–101.
31. Lee CK. Accelerated degeneration of the segment adjacent to a lumbar fusion. Spine. 1988;13:375–7.
32. National Institutes of Health. Total hip Replacement. NIH Consensus Statement. 1994;12:1–31.

33. Callaghan JJ. Results of primary total hip arthroplasty in young patients. In Schafer M, ed. Instructional course lectures. Rosemont IL: American Academy of Orthopaedic Surgeons; 1994:315–21.
34. Mulroy WF, Estok DM, Harris WH. Total hip arthroplasty with use of so-called second-generation cementing techniques. J Bone Joint Surg. 1994;77A:1845–52.
35. Collins DN, Barnes CL, FitzRandolph RL. Cervical spine instability in rheumatoid patients having total hip or knee arthroplasty. Clin Orthop. 1991;272:127–35.
36. Friedman RJ, Schiff CF, Bromberg JS. Use of supplemental steroids in patients having orthopaedic operations. J Bone Joint Surg. 1995;77A:1801–16.
37. Murray RP, Bourne MH, Fitzgerald RH. Metachronous infections in patients who have had more than one total joint arthroplasty. J Bone Joint Surg. 1991;73A:1469–74.
38. Connelly CS, Panush RS. Should nonsteroidal anti-inflammatory drugs be stopped before elective surgery? Arch Intern Med. 1991;151:1963–6.
39. Perhala RS, Wilke WS, Clough JD, Segal AM. Local infectious complications following large joint replacement in rheumatoid arthritis patients treated with methotrexate versus those not treated with methotrexate. Arthritis Rheum. 1991;34:146–52.
40. Sany J, Anaya JM, Canovas F, *et al.* Influence of methotrexate on the frequency of postoperative infectious complications in patients with rheumatoid arthritis. J Rheumatol. 1993;20:1129–32.
41. Sundaram NA, Murphy JC. Heterotopic bone formation following total hip arthroplasty in anklyosing spondylitis. Clin Orthop. 1986;207:223–6.
42. Menon TJ, Wroblewski BM. Charnley low-friction arthroplasty in patients with psoriasis. Clin Orthop. 1983;300:127–8.
43. Kelly SS, Lachiewicz PF, Gilbert MS, Bolander ME, Jankiewicz JJ. Hip arthroplasty in hemophilic arthropathy. J Bone Joint Surg. 1995;67A:828–34.
44. Lachiewicz PR, Inglis AE, Insall JN, *et al.* Total knee arthroplasty in hemophilia. J Bone Joint Surg. 1985;76A:1361–6.
45. Flandry FC, Hughston JC, Jacobson KE, *et al.* Surgical treatment of diffuse pigmented villonodular synovitis of the knee. Clin Orthop. 1994;300:183–92.
46. Schwartz HS, Uni KK, Pritchard DJ. Pigmented villonodular synovitis. A retrospective review of affected large joints. Clin Orthop. 1989;247:243–55.
47. Ogilvie-Harris DJ, Saleh K. Generalized synovial chondromatosis of the knee: a comparison of removal of the loose bodies alone with arthroscopic synovectomy. Arthroscopy. 1994;10:166–70.
48. Fitzgerald RH. Total hip arthroplasty sepsis. Prevention and diagnosis. Orthop Clin North Am. 1992;23:259–64.
49. Sullivan PM, MacKenzie JR, Callaghan JJ, Johnston RC. Total hip arthroplasty with cement in patients who are less than fifty years old. J Bone Joint Surg. 1994;76A:863–9.
50. Bosco JA, Bynum DK, Bowers WH. Long-term outcome of Volz total wrist arthroplasties. J Arthroplasty. 1994;9:25–31.
51. Vogler HW, Stienstra JJ, Montgomery F, Kipp L. Anterior ankle impingement arthropathy. The role of anterolateral arthrotomy and arthroscopy. Clin Podiatr Med Surg. 1994;11:425–47.
52. Takura Y, Tanaka Y, Kumai T, Tamai S. Low tibial osteotomy for osteoarthritis of the ankle. Results of a new operation in 18 patients. J Bone Joint Surg. 1995;77B:50–4.
53. Pearce MS, Smith MA, Savidge GF. Supramalleolar tibial osteotomy for haemophilc arthropathy of the ankle. J Bone Joint Surg. 1994;76B:947–50.
54. Abdo RV, Wasilewski SA. Ankle arthrodesis: a long-term study,. Foot Ankle. 1992;13:307–12.
55. Cracchiolo A, Cimino WR, Lian G. Arthrodesis of the ankle in patients who have rheumatoid arthritis. J Bone Joint Surg. 1992;74A:903–9.
56. Moran CG, Pinder IM, Smith SR. Ankle arthrodesis in rheumatoid arthritis. 30 cases followed for 5 years. Acta Orthop Scand. 1991;62:538–43.
57. Gruen GS, Mears DC. Arthrodesis of the ankle and subtalar joints. Clin Orthop. 1991;268:15–20.
58. Kitaoka HB, Romness DW. Arthrodesis for failed ankle arthroplasty. J Arthroplasty. 1992;7:277–84.
59. Lachiewicz PF. Total ankle arthroplasty. Indications, techniques, and results. Orthop Rev. 1994;23:315–20.
60. Valburg AA, Roermund PM, Lammens J, *et al.* Can Ilizarov joint distraction delay the need for an arthrodesis of the ankle? A preliminary report. J Bone Joint Surg. 1995;77A:720–5.
61. Jolly SL, Ferlic DC, Clayton ML, Dennis DA, Stringer EA. Swanson silicone arthroplasty of the wrist in rheumatoid arthritis: a long-term follow-up. J Hand Surg. 1992;17:142–9.
62. Tomaino MM, Delsignore J, Burton RI. Long-term results following proximal row carpectomy. J Hand Surg. 1994;19:694–703.
63. Ewald FC, Simmons ED, Sullivan JA, *et al.* Capitellocondylar total elbow replacement in RA. The Journal of Bone Joint Surgery. 1993;75:498–507.
64. Rowe CR. Arthrodesis of the shoulder used in treating painful conditions. Clin Orthop. 1983;173:92–6.
65. Summers GD, Talor AR, Webley M. Elbow synovectomy and excision of the radial head in rheumatoid arthritis: a short term palliative procedure. J Rheumatol.1988;15:566–9.
66. Brostrom LA, Wallensten R, Olsson E, Anderson D. The Kessel prosthesis in total shoulder arthroplasty. A five-year experience. Clin Ortho. 1992;277:155–60.
67. Kraay MJ, Figgie MP, Inglis AE, Wolfe SW, Ranawat CS. Primary semiconstrained total elbow arthroplasty. Survival analysis of 113 consecutive cases. J Bone Joint Surg. 1994;76B:636–40.
68. Ranawat CS, O'Leary P, Pellici P, *et al.* Cervical spine fusion in rheumatoid arthritis. J Bone Joint Surg. 1979;61A:1003–10.
69. Boden SD, Dodge LD, Bohlman HH, Rechtine GR. Rheumatoid arthritis of the cervical spine. J Bone Joint Surg. 1993;75A:1282–97.

13

UNPROVEN REMEDIES, ALTERNATIVE AND COMPLEMENTARY MEDICINE

G David Champion

Summary

- Scientifically influenced orthodox medicine has made only a relatively recent and partial intrusion into the healing and health practices of the world's population. It is unrealistic to consider that evidence-based medicine can satisfy the needs and desires of the population with arthritis and rheumatism.
- Enquiry about alternative treatments being applied, and non-judgemental discussion of the evidence about efficacy and risks, are important in the conduct of medical care in rheumatology.
- Controlled trials of many alternative treatments are difficult in concept and implementation, and are relatively low in priority, but the pursuit of truth is fundamental in medicine.

ALTERNATIVE, UNORTHODOX, COMPLEMENTARY AND HOLISTIC MEDICINE

Alternative and complementary medicine is the aggregate of diagnostic and therapeutic practices and systems that are separate from, and in contrast to, conventional scientific medicine. Scientific or orthodox medicine may be simply described as the prevention and management of illness using methods that have been subjected to the same kind of rigorous experimental, statistical and observational scrutiny that are applied in other branches of science[1]. McCormick[2] considers that medicine is not (primarily) a science, but rather has a social function. Science contributes to this primarily social function by providing a body of relatively secure knowledge, contributing to the development of technologies and offering a way of thinking. 'Alternative' appears to describe the nonspecific beliefs and practices in a neutral, nonjudgmental way. However the term is seen by some as vaguely perjorative, rather like talking about 'foreigners', a heterogeneous category defined by what it is not, rather than by what it is. Although these alternative or unorthodox practitioners of medicine can be differentiated according to training, skill, and type of practice, they do not constitute a distinct community. They represent a heterogeneous population promoting disparate beliefs and practices that vary considerably from one movement or tradition to another, and form no consistent or complementary body of knowledge. However within each movement or tradition, a great deal of consensus may be observed[3].

'Alternative' is often considered to imply conflict with orthodox medicine, while 'complementary' indicates that some potential cooperation with orthodox practitioners may occur. Some of the psychologic, physical, dietary and pharmacologic practices are part of the conventional medical repertoire and are only 'alternative' when they are applied by nonmedical personnel or when claims for their value are greatly extended. There is an increasing acceptance in the UK and Europe of the term 'complementary' and of its practices[4]. The users of alternative medical practices seek to expand the medical model by adding selected therapies and treatments to its methodology. The boundaries between scientific medicine and alternative medicine are not fixed, but are socially and historically determined and depend to a large extent on the relative power of competing medical professionals. The division between orthodox and alternative systems had its origin in political, social and historic as well as scientific factors. Holistic medical practice is the combined use of conventional medicine, complementary medicine, psychotherapy and health education by medical and other practitioners, often within a general practice setting. Alternative practitioners have a variety of concepts of holism, but emphasize the individual and the interplay of mind, body and spirit in diagnosis and management. Alternative practitioners point out that *heal* comes from the same root as *whole* and *holiness*.

The extent of current alternative (unconventional) medical use in modern industrialized societies, as exemplified by a recent study in the USA, is impressive[5]. A representative population survey of 3,004 persons by interview in (multicultural) Australia showed that expenditure on alternative medicine was considerably greater than the patient contributions for pharmaceutical drugs, and that 20.3% had at some time visited at least one alternative practitioner[6]. Widespread alternative medicine use appears more likely in chronic rheumatic conditions for which orthodox treatments are relatively inadequate such as fibromyalgia syndrome[7]. Consumer surveys consistently show positive public attitudes to complementary medicine[4]. In countries for which statistics are available, alternative or complementary therapies are used by 20–50% of the population. There are some intriguing national idiosyncrasies, e.g. reflexology is popular in Denmark; anthroposophical medicine is popular in German-speaking countries; the Dutch are keen on spiritual healers; and massage is very popular in Finland[4]. It has been estimated that 75–80% of the world's population has limited access to orthodox scientific medicine and is reliant on traditional medicine, and the World Health Organization (WHO) has estimated that some five hundred million people utilize homeopathy.

PUBLICATIONS ON ALTERNATIVE AND COMPLEMENTARY MEDICINE

The British Library database is said to contain 55,000 articles on research into alternative and complementary medicine, to which 150–300 are added each month. Conventional literature searches do not adequately identify relevant studies. The public has an insatiable appetite for publications on alternative medicine and health. Articles on these topics boost the sales of magazines. There are reasonably comprehensive books[8,9] of which *Alternative Medicine: The Definitive Guide* is a major text[9], and vast numbers of specialized publications. Reader's Digest has recently published an appealing and well illustrated family guide, *Alternative Medicine*, an encyclopedic compilation of disorders and treatments[10]. Regrettably, the comments under the headings 'an orthodox view' are naive and inadequate. Pietroni has also written a family guide to alternative health care[11]. The current trend to holistic general medical practices has been described by Pietroni[12], and journals such as *Holistic Medicine*, *Complementary Therapies in Medicine (UK)*, *The Journal of Alternative and Complementary Medicine (USA)* and *Alternative Therapies in Health and Medicine (USA)* are supported by holistic medical practitioners. *The Journal of Ethnopharmacology* is a useful resource. There is, however, no satisfactory comprehensive textbook review written from a scientific perspective. Two recent publications have been firmly disparaging of alternative health and holistic medicine but generally there is not much scholarly criticism to be found in book form[13,14]. The colloquia conducted under the auspices of The Royal Society of Medicine was a major contribution to conciliation, or at least understanding, between conventional and complementary medicine[15]. The British

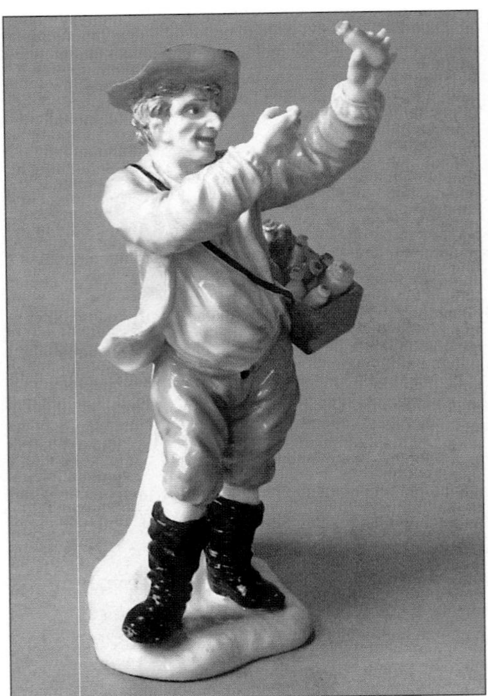

Fig. 13.1 The theriac vendor or 'quack medicine man'. Modeled by Simon Feilner, 1952. Conceived by Mithridates VI Eupator, King of Pontus (132–63 BC) and his physician, developed by Galen and others, theriac became the panacea for curing all diseases. Opium was one of the multiple ingredients and this may have accounted for its popularity which continued until the late 18th century. Reproduced with permission from Lydia Mez-Mangold. A history of drugs. Basel: Editiones Roche; 1971.

Medical Association's publication *Complementary Medicine: New Approaches to Good Practice*[16] has also been influential. The book by Fernandez-Madrid is useful to recommend to patients[17].

ALTERNATIVE MEDICINE ORIGINS, HISTORY, ILLNESS MODELS AND BELIEFS

Current alternative therapies and systems can be traced to traditional medicinal, psychotherapeutic and religio-magical practices[18], symbolic magic[19], metaphysical notions and to logical and empirical procedures. The theriac vendor (Fig. 13.1) is symbolic of 'quackery', a term historically used by the dominant Western practitioners since the 17th century to describe most, if not all, of their challengers. The mainstream of traditional and community healing practices has continued to evolve from antiquity to the present day, while conventional and scientific medicine did not gain much momentum until the 18th century. Paracelsus (Fig. 13.2), the subject of a number of recent biographic reappraisals, is a notable figure in the early emergence of science from magical, traditional and authoritarian medicine. The herbal magical principle, The *Doctrine of Signatures*, (Fig. 13.3), is of special interest to rheumatologists because it was invoked in the discovery of salicylates and hence the development of nonsteroidal anti-inflammatory drugs (NSAIDs).

Orthodox medical practitioners are often perplexed by the firmness of belief of alternative practitioners and the patients who attend them. Often these beliefs appear to lack logic and rationality. It is naive for physicians to expect our patients to make judgments consistently in favor of orthodox (scientific) medicine. After all, people believe in the paranormal, follow astrology, gamble for money against the odds, have false perceptions of risk, are overly influenced by single-case examples in the face of contrary statistics, resist changing beliefs despite empirical challenges that seem logically devastating and generally use judgmental heuristics that are simplistic and subject to bias and errors[22]. Belief is, at least in part, determined by the believer's environment. The social, including linguistic, context helps fix the content of belief. While beliefs are ideally logically based on evidence, the powerful impact of tradition, authority, revelation and hope are often overriding influences (even in those trained in science). These influences are at the heart of belief in unproven remedies, alternative and unconventional therapies. The remarkable influence of media personalities and other prominent figures is an example of authority, sometimes revelation. The acceptance by alternative therapists that the ideas, conjectures and theories are actual fact requires a substantial act of faith. The maintenance of faith would explain the apparent firm convictions and the evangelistic fervor of the healers that impresses many patients.

Orthodox medical practitioners often refer to alternative beliefs and practices as (scientifically) irrational, but care should be taken in considerations of rationality. Rationality is a normative concept that philosophers have generally tried to characterize in such a way that, for any action, belief or desire, if it is rational we ought to choose it. No such positive characterization has achieved anything close to universal acceptance. Often several competing actions or beliefs count as rational. An irrational belief is one that obviously conflicts with a fact that one knows. But a belief which obviously conflicts with what is known by one person need not obviously conflict with what is known by another. Acting rationally simply means acting in a way that is maximally efficient in achieving one's goals. If a patient's goal is to accept the illness to some extent and to minimize additional (imposed) problems, the choosing of an unproven but highly safe remedy might be rational. An important anthropological perspective on medicine and rationality has been presented by Byron Good[23].

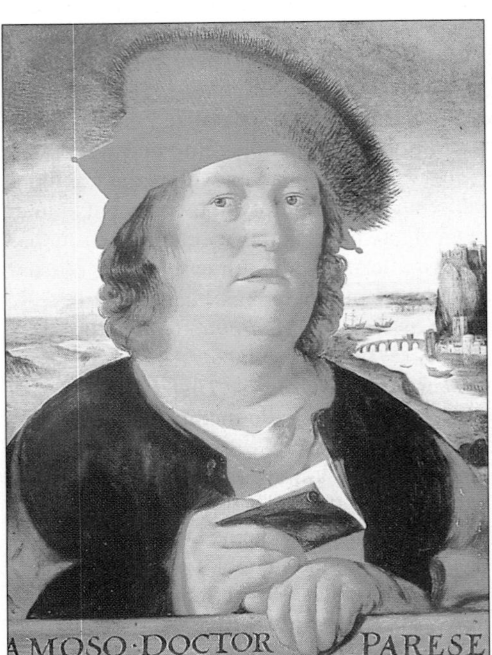

Fig. 13.2 Paracelsus, painted by Jan van Scorel (The Louvre, Paris). Paracelsus contributed to pharmacology, taught reliance on one's own observations, formalized the *Doctrine of Signatures* and subscribed to astrology and the occult sciences. While often regarded as the 'father of pharmacology', he could equally be regarded as a father figure for alternative medicine. Reproduced with permission from Reunion des Musées Nationaux, Paris[20].

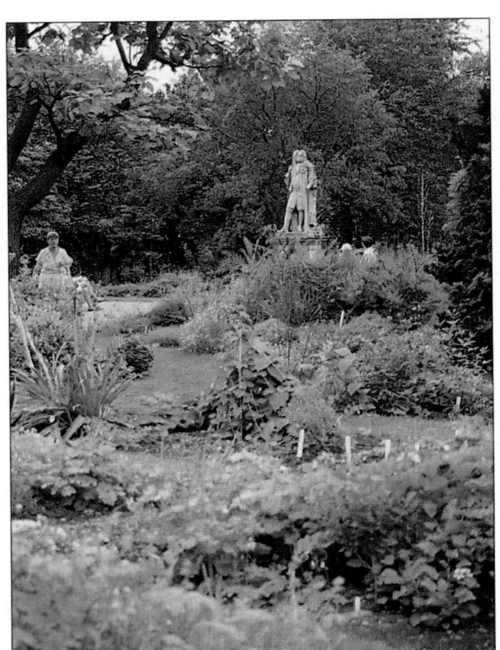

Fig. 13.3 Chelsea physic garden. Established in 1673 by the Society of Apothecaries, containing medicinal plants including a section commemorating the *Doctrine of Signatures*[21] (like cures like and each medicinal product from nature indicates by an obvious and well marked character the disease for which it is a remedy or the object for which it can be employed). Reproduced with permission from the curator.

NONSPECIFIC THERAPEUTIC RESPONSE AND THE PLACEBO EFFECT

Placebo is derived from the Latin ('I shall please or be acceptable'). The first antiphon at Vespers of the office of the Dead began with the words, *Placebo Domino in regione vivorum* ('I will walk before the Lord in the land of the living'). As sycophants and those who hoped to get something out of the relatives of the departed used to make a point of attending this service and singing the *Placebo,* the phrase *'To Sing Placebo'* came to mean to play the flatterer or sycophant[24].

Placebo principles and effects have been of major continuing interest in medicine[25–29]. The view commonly expressed by physicians is that the perception of therapeutic response to unproven remedies by the patient is attributable to a placebo effect. 'Placebo' is simply an inert substance or treatment. More comprehensively, a placebo is any therapy or component of therapy that is deliberately used for its nonspecific psychologic or psychophysiologic effect (intentional placebo), or is used for its presumed specific effect but is without specific activity for the condition being treated (inadvertent placebo). The term is also employed to describe a substance or procedure without specific activity for the condition being evaluated which is used as a control in experimental studies. 'Placebo effect' is an outcome occurring within the sociocultural context of the healing process. The main three possible theoretical mechanisms for the placebo effect, conditioning, learned expectancy and endogenous opiates, have been reviewed by Peck and Coleman[30]. They referred also to the symbolic meaning which anthropologists regard as important in therapeutic effect. A rigorous philosophical articulation of the placebo notion by Grünbaum is important basic reading for those contemplating a critical review of the placebo effect in alternative medicine[31]. People who are predisposed to trust others, to accept socially defined symbols of healing, those who are dependent and/or exhibit generalized chronic anxiety, are the most responsive to placebo, while the authority and enthusiasm of the healer and the nature of the therapy contribute importantly to the response.

The application of the placebo effect consciously and honestly by doctors presents a dilemma. On the one hand, scientific integrity is a compelling, indeed essential, attribute. To offer a therapy under false pretences is to violate patients' rights of informed consent. On the other hand, to quote Richard Asher, 'If you admit to yourself that the treatment you are giving is frankly inactive, you will inspire little confidence in your patients ... but if you can believe fervently in your treatment ... then your results are much better, your patients are much better and your income is much better, too'. Alternative practitioners have no such dilemma. The treatments are regarded as effective, or at least as having utility in the healing process, whatever the mechanism. The physician, in consideration of the use of a deliberate placebo, must determine where autonomy, health and truthfulness stand in relation to each other in the patient's scheme of basic values[32].

Joyce has comprehensively reviewed the complex issue of nonspecific aspects of treatment, considering the treatment and the patient–doctor (or healer) interaction[33,34]. Reasons for perception of benefit from an inert treatment include the *post hoc ergo propter hoc* fallacy of logic (after this therefore because of this), regression towards the mean[35], the wish bias and generalizations from small experiences. Not all nonspecific effects are advantageous. Many medical treatments are falsely perceived as unreasonably risky and this may result in a nocebo effect. The term 'nocebo' has been invoked to describe a 'negative placebo response', a self-contradictory term. The nacebo effect in the context of inert (even efficacious) treatments evidently results from complex responses to previous adverse therapeutic experiences. Useful treatment can be neglected because of inappropriate fears of adverse reactions. This has been whimsically referred to as 'the tomato effect'. Tomatoes were regarded by the Americans as poisonous for about 100 years after popularity had been achieved in Europe. Everyone in North America knew they were poisonous; it was obvious, tomatoes belonged to the nightshade family. Alternative practitioners often amplify potential nocebo and 'tomato' effects from orthodox treatments.

THE RESPONSE OF MEDICAL PRACTITIONERS AND REGULATORY AUTHORITIES

Surveys of physicians show that although views are highly varied, there is an overall belief that complementary (alternative) medicine is moderately effective[36]. The surveys do not answer the question whether physicians consider complementary medicine as a nonspecific powerful placebo or as specifically effective. Acceptance of complementary medicine is greater among younger physicians and does not appear to be increasing over time.

There are a number of problems which may arise from a *laissez-faire* attitude by doctors and the community to alternative medicine. The lack of diagnostic expertise may delay recognition of potentially treatable diseases. Inappropriately negative thoughts may be reinforced. Some people become passive body work 'junkies'. Orthodox practices and treatments are denigrated. Patients with disease seem often to have a conviction of relative invulnerability while anticipating that any drug side effects will occur to them. These views are enhanced by alternative practitioners. There is, however, apparent under-recognition of the adverse effects of alternative therapies and of the dangers of deceptive practices. The fundamental issues of objective evidence-based truth, integrity and scientific rationality are important in a civilized society. There is a community ambivalence towards science which we must recognise and analyze.

The therapies generally most acceptable to physicians are acupuncture, manipulation and homeopathy. Considering the therapies and ideas of alternative and complementary medicine, interested physicians could well further explore and test the value of manipulative treatments, traditional medicinal and herbal products, and acupuncture and its variants. Rheumatologists generally could justifiably focus more effectively on nutritional principles and on integrated posture and musculoskeletal function. The initiative to conduct trials should come from orthodox medicine. The investigation of single alternative therapies or of systems is difficult, but scientifically acceptable methods are available. The differences in the concepts and standards of evidence, knowledge, truth and ethics are considerable. Thus, for physicians maintaining rigid scientific integrity, only very limited rapprochement is conceivable. Physicians interested in and respectful of other philosophies and cultures and who are aware of the limits of science will establish more rapprochement. It is reasonably sensitive to accept that there will be occasions when our patients' needs will be better met by alternative practitioners. This view does not apply to overt charlatanism or quackery. However, are we able to draw a clear distinction between sincere belief by a 'healer' in an unproven remedy and deliberate deception, and is the former ethically acceptable when it may require considerable self-deception? This is a major philosophical difficulty.

There are limits to the progress which can be made by alternative practitioners. By emphasizing the uniqueness of the individual, they fail to identify or they accept clinical anomalies and thus exclude a major mechanism of biomedical discovery. Many alternative diagnostic and causal concepts and procedures are not credible in any critical scientific sense. Any treatments which appear promising are subjected by orthodox investigators to controlled trials which may lead to incorporation into orthodox medicine. Without research there can be no real progress. Without research-based knowledge of prognosis there can be no credible guidance, a point of particular importance in serious disease. There is no structural community support base such as foundations. There are no mechanisms for effective peer review. There is no transferable and valid medical record. The treatments are usually inapplicable or unwise in the more serious disorders, although studies for example of traditional Chinese medicine are occurring in cancer and acquired immunodeficiency syndrome (AIDS). Also alternative and complementary practices serve a support function when all else has failed. Patients and the community see alternative practitioners as having little authoritative responsibility in matters of public health care.

Notwithstanding these cautionary statements about the acceptance of alternative and complementary medicine, we should be mindful of the limits of biomedicine which were highlighted by Helmann[37]. Every day we are reminded in our practice that our ability to relieve arthritis and rheumatism is modest. The perceived failure of orthodox medicine or of its practitioners is the main reason for consulting alternative practitioners, according to surveys in industrialized countries.

One of the growing issues in medical practice is the influence of evidenced-based principles in which much of the evidence is based on outcomes research and randomized trials which lead to consensus statements and therapeutic guidelines. In turn, these guidelines are picked up by authorities concerned with the implementation of managed care. While the evidenced-based movement has considerable merit, there is concern in regard to judgment of appropriate treatment and implementation of that treatment for individual patients. There is an allied concern about the lack of attention to patient's preferences and attitudes. We shall need to be careful not to lose sight of individual attention, judgment and caring. The evolution towards patient-centered medicine is progressing[38]. Shortcomings of orthodox practitioners with regard to comprehensive individual attention is one of the criticisms of the alternative movement, for which there is some justification. Evidenced-based approaches can be effectively utilized in individualized treatment[39]. While science mainly deals with generalities, the tradition of medicine is that it has to do with individuals.

There has been increasing acceptance by governments of inclusion of alternative medical practice in the US. This has led for example to the NIH Office of Alternative Medicine. This in turn has led to critical consideration of the testing of alternative medicine. This topic was reviewed by Stalker[40] who presented a well argued and highly sceptical appraisal of the testing of alternative hypotheses by clinical trials, concluding that the majority of hypotheses had low probability ranking compared with orthodox hypotheses. With so much to be done on a limited number of patients by a limited number of investigators, Stalker concluded that few alternative therapies should be tested. Others have argued that there are cogent theoretical reasons for disproving popular, but ineffective or ill-advised therapies, and potentially finding additional useful methods, but the reality is that orthodox medicine's capability of testing many therapies is limited. A major criticism by alternative practitioners of therapeutic testing by controlled trials is that the alternative methods have frequently not been tested in their proper therapeutic setting. Isolated modalities are frequently tested in controlled trials whereas the treatment in reality is individualized and multimodal. For example acupuncture is not practised in isolation by traditional Chinese practitioners. There is some justification in this criticism. It is possible in a randomized trial to test alternative treatments which are individualized and in their proper therapeutic setting, although this cannot be done on a double-blind basis (observer blinding is feasible). The strength of belief should be assessed and may need to be considered in stratification or in analysis.

Ernst has cautioned that we should be sensitive to common misconceptions in arguments used against complementary medicine as well as arguments for complementary medicine[41]. Alpert in a recent editorial advised a five-point approach to alternative medical practices[42], as summarized in Figure 13.4. One might reasonably add that, in multicultural societies, it is increasingly imperative that we be conscious of the belief systems of our patients[43].

APPROACH TO ALTERNATIVE MEDICAL PRACTICES

1. Maintain open-minded attitude about potentially therapeutic interventions, including alternatives.
2. Encourage controlled trials.
3. Do not ignore or ridicule the potential of the placebo effect.
4. Do not accept all new therapies as efficacious on first acquaintance.
5. Avoid hubristic and arrogant attitudes towards alternative medical practices.

Fig. 13.4 Approach to alternative medical practices. Adapted from Alpert[42].

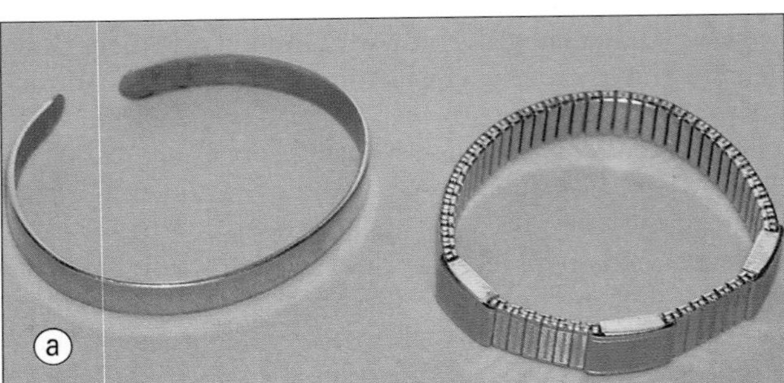

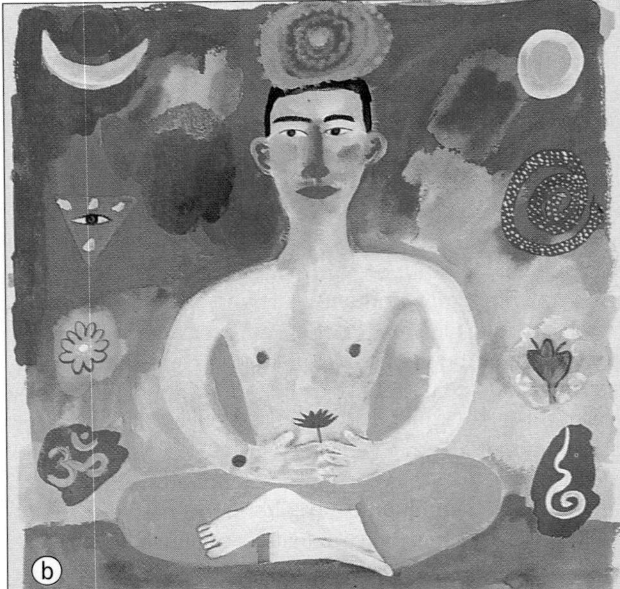

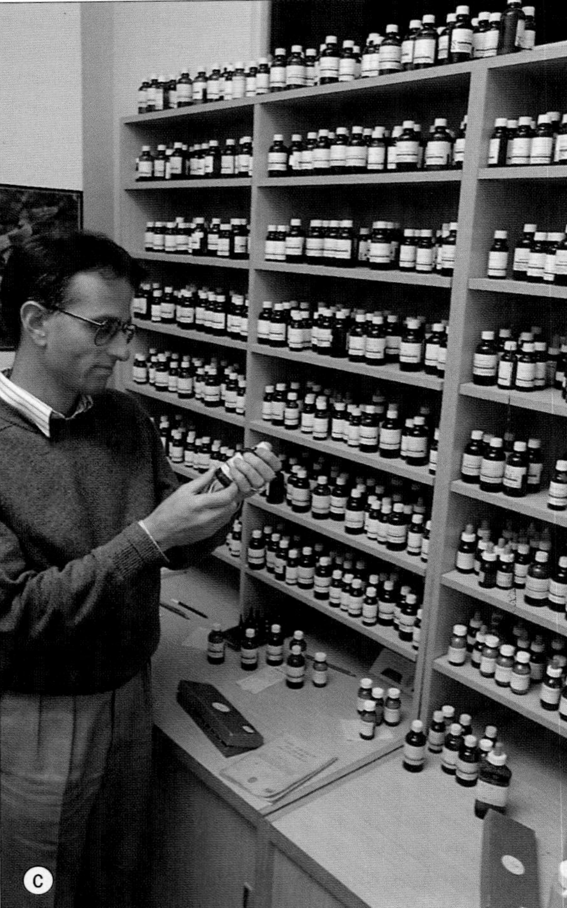

Fig. 13.5 Images of popular folk and alternative medicine. Copper bracelet, plain and with magnets (a). Illustration by Chris Corr, reproduced with permission from *Is Meditation Good for You* by S Blackmore[81] (b). Homeopathic medicines at the Wholistic Medical Centre, Sydney.

There is much that can be learnt from alternative practitioners. They are often socially and culturally in tune with their patients and with popular social movements. The treatments often satisfy needs and are sensitive to the patients' goals. Anecdotal evidence is powerful and, in addition to presenting statistics, it is often useful to illustrate a point by anecdote. In endeavoring to be objective, one should not lose sight of the value of compassion and empathy. Optimism is important, but has to be realistically constrained by scientific integrity. It has been suggested that some safe forms of alternative medicine, for example homeopathy, could be increasingly practised alongside orthodox medicine in a manner similar to the side-by-side relationship between chaplains and doctors. The contrary view however is that chaplains understand and accept the limitations of their participation, while alternative practitioners frequently do not.

A particular difficulty which presents to rheumatologists is the management of patients with medically unexplained somatic symptoms[44]. One perspective is that doctors overinvestigate and apply inappropriate symptomatic treatment. Another view is that doctors apply terms such as somatization which may be interpreted as perjorative, do not achieve a mutually agreed understanding with the patients and thereby deflect them towards alternative or complementary medicine. A reasonable guideline may be to maintain personal interest, to undertake more enlightened observation and to incorporate such patients into clinical research protocols.

In medical practice, particularly in rheumatology, it is usually desirable to discuss alternative therapies. One way of encouraging patients to acknowledge their alternative treatments is to have on the desk or in the consulting room an item, for example from traditional Chinese medicine, that can be a discussion point. In making therapeutic recommendations it may increasingly be regarded as appropriate to present the level of evidence for orthodox therapies and for the most popular of the alternative therapies.

The regulation of alternative practitioners varies widely. In some countries only registered health professionals may practice, while in others there is very little regulation of alternative health care and products. Legal reforms are proceeding in many countries[4]. Concern about the safety of herbal products has been one of the major determinants of increasing attention to regulation[45]. There appear to be double standards in litigation against orthodox medical practitioners and the alternative practitioners. In most countries it appears that malpractice by an alternative practitioner is more difficult to define and less likely to result in a successful suit. This no doubt results from the learned profession status of orthodox medicine in contrast to alternative practice.

ALTERNATIVE, COMPLEMENTARY AND UNPROVEN MEDICAL SYSTEMS, PRACTICES AND THERAPIES

A classification with summary of the origins and the concepts of the practitioners and of the systems and therapies is presented in the boxes on pages 3.13.6–3.13.12. The classification is based on the belief systems of the proponents rather than on biomedical science. Thus acupuncture, which appears as a component of the Chinese traditional medical system, is also classified with vital force (energy) therapies despite our recognition of neurophysiologic effects. Additionally, in the boxes the potential application to arthritis and rheumatism is briefly reviewed, along with any biomedical evidence. Figure 13.5 is a reminder of the magical origins of some alternative treatments, and Figure 13.6 emphasizes the powerful influence of tradition, in particular Chinese tradition, in popular alternative and complementary medicine throughout the world today. Other treatments which are periodically applied to patients with arthritis and rheumatism include cell therapy, chelation therapy, neural therapy and reconstructive therapy[11]. Some psychologic techniques such as guided imagery and humour and laughter have sufficient evidence for benefit in pain management to be increasingly used in hospitals. A more detailed, referenced review is available from the author.

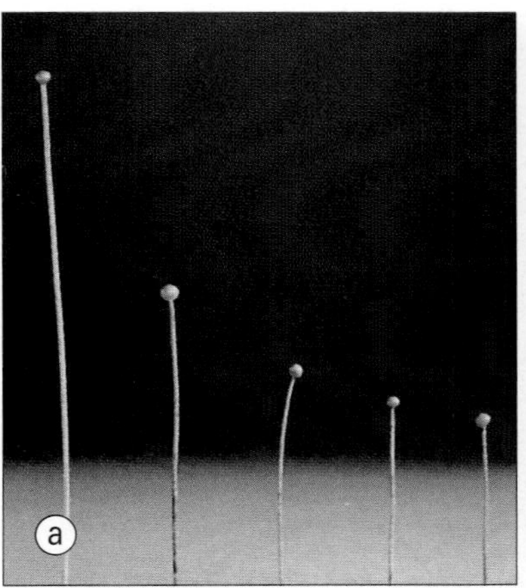

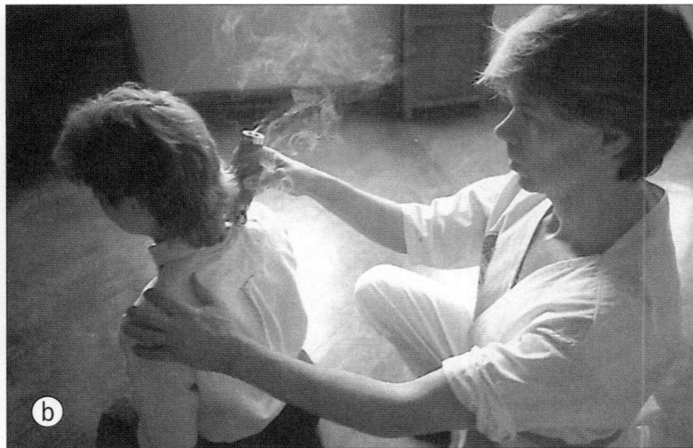

Fig. 13.6 Traditional Chinese medical practices popular today. Chinese 19th century acupuncture needles. Reproduced with permission from *Devils, Drugs and Doctors, A Wellcome History of Medicine* (a). Moxibustion. Reproduced from Nature and Health (Australia) with permission from the publishers and author (Penny Hemphill) (b). Patient with SLE attending traditional Chinese herbalist to supplement her medical treatment (c). Herbs imported from China and ceramic pot for infusion (d).

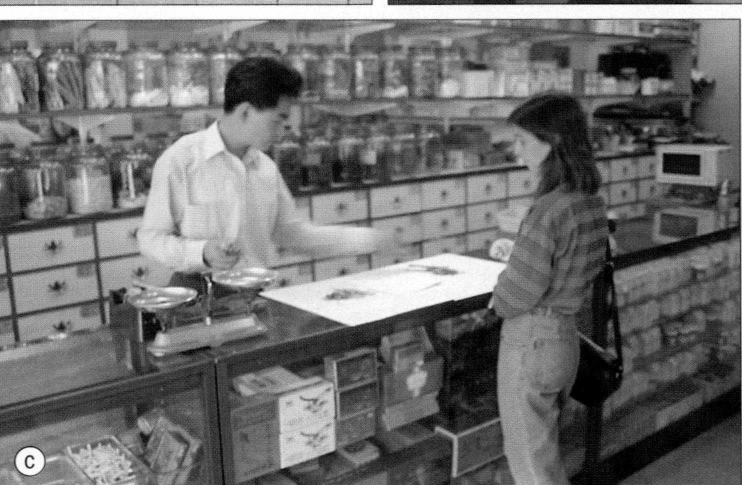

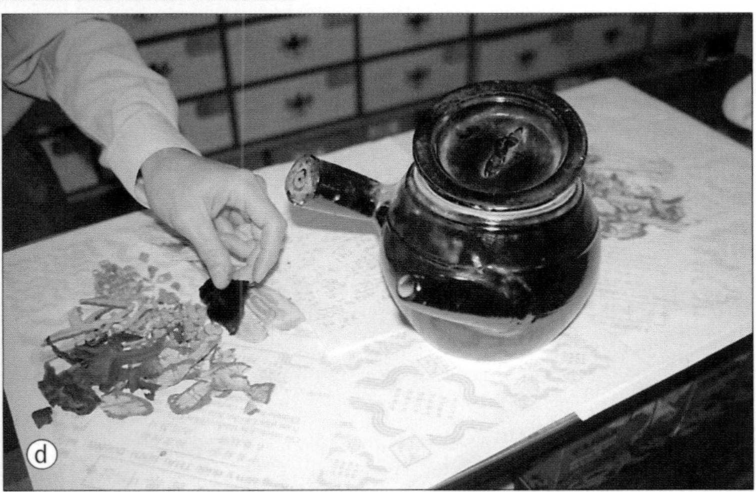

TRADITIONAL MULTIDIMENSIONAL MEDICAL AND HEALTH SYSTEMS

Origin, concepts and practices	Application and evidence in musculoskeletal medicine
Chinese traditional and derivative oriental	
The original primary health care providers were shamans. Physicians and shamans, though not identical, were linked (BC). The Yellow Emperor's Inner Classic (c.> 200 BC–100 AD) is the source of medical theory and was influenced by traditional Chinese naturalistic and Taoist thought. The Divine Husbandman's Classic of the Materia Medica (c. 100 AD) was the primary source of materia medica with a focus on individual herbs and freedom from supernatural references. The Chinese tradition was a major influence on other Oriental–Asian medical and health systems. The universe is composed of various forces: the complementary opposites of *yin* and *yang* and the five phases (elements). The human microcosm is a miniature of these forces. In the five-phase theory, each organ either nourishes or inhibits the function of another organ, just as the basic elements (fire, earth, metal, water, wood) also act adversely or beneficially on each other. *Yin* organs are solid (e.g. liver) while *yang* organs (e.g. stomach) are hollow and functional. Life is activated by *chi* (*qi*), vital life force or energy, which in health flows freely along meridians at the surface of the body and through organs. Illness is a disharmony of the whole body. Rheumatism is a wind and moisture disease, a numb disorder characterized by increased pain due to cold and damp. Mind–body–spirit are indivisible. The concept of cause (specific) is unimportant. Diagnosis is by history, inspection, hearing, smell and palpation of pulse, abdomen, and meridians. *T'ai Chi* exercises encourage free flow of *chi*. Acupuncture uses the meridian system and its corresponding surface points to correct and rebalance *chi*. 'Hot' medicines are used to treat 'cold' diseases such as arthritis[46–50].	Traditional Chinese Medicine (TCM) addresses the full range of illness and is best known for treating chronic disorders including rheumatic and psychosomatic conditions. The methods of treatment include herbal medicine (also animal, earth and mineral products), diet, acupuncture and its derivatives (see meridian-based energy therapies), physical therapies (*T'ai chi*, *Qigong* and other exercises, manipulation, massage), and meditative relaxation (Fig. 13.6). The Chinese Government has recently encouraged Western doctors to learn TCM and there has been a proliferation of medical and nonmedical practitioners in many countries, particularly in multicultural societies with many Asian people. Concerns about increased usage, products from endangered animal species, adulteration with potent drugs and other aspects of quality control have stimulated calls for regulation in some countries[50]. The Chinese materia medica[49] is a rich source for ethnopharmacologists, but antirheumatic research has lagged. TCM practitioners point out the fundamental inadequacies of controlled trial evaluation of a single therapeutic modality from a complex diagnostic and therapeutic system. In traditional Chinese practice, acupuncture is not used in isolation. The rebalance of vital energy (*chi*) has little credibility among Western scientists and is losing its grip on Asian researchers (see Acupuncture section). Extensive Chinese, Asian and Western research has supported the application of acupuncture, particularly for pain relief. *T'ai chi* is an applicable exercise regimen in arthritic patients, and in one study did not aggravate rheumatoid arthritis (RA). Research is published in the *Journal of Traditional Chinese Medicine*, the *American Journal of Chinese Medicine* and the *International Journal of Oriental Medicine.*
Indian traditional Ayurveda, Unani (Ayurveda + ancient Arabic), Siddha (Ayurveda + south Indian indigenous)	
Ayurveda, which comes from two Sanskrit roots and means 'The science of life', is a section in the last of the *vedas* (knowledge or science) written in c. 2000 BC. The main Ayurvedic texts, the *Susruta samhita* and *Charaka samhita* were written in the 5th and 2nd century BC. The science of medicine was presented as an amalgam of religious mysticism and magic together with an empirico-rational system of drugs. The texts contained remarkable insights into surgery, microbiological ideas, herbal and medicinal treatments and ethics[51]. A modern revival is Maharishi Ayurveda[52]. Biological individuality and the harmony of mind and body are fundamental. Imbalance from disruption of homeostatis or immunity are primary factors in the etiology of disease. Three physiologic principles called *doshas* (*vata, pitta, kapha*) regulate the function of the mind and body, e.g. chronic	pain results from *vata* imbalance. Combinatons of *doshas* and *subdoshas* are felt as patterns in the radial artery (pulse diagnoses). Treatment aims to restore the balance in the *doshas* by mental techniques, diet, exercise, sensory modalities, herbs, medicines and purification procedures. Traditional Indian practice has influenced meditation, relaxation and other psychic healing techniques, some of which help with rheumatic disease, especially control of pain. Ayurvedic medicine is said to be effective in arthritis, is practised in ethnic medicine and is being increasingly explored in complementary and holistic practice. There is an extensive body of research literature published in India in *The Journal of Research into Indian Medicine.*
Indigenous traditional Asian, African, American Indian, Australian, other	
Of the world's population, 80% relies on traditional medicine. The WHO definition of traditional medicine is the sum total of all the knowledge and practices, whether explicable or not, used in diagnosis, prevention and elimination of physical, mental or social imbalance and relying exclusively on practical experience and observation passed down from generation to generation, whether verbally or in writing. The difference depends on the cultures.	Religion, magic and medical treatments were inseparable. Primitive belief focused on sorcery and witchcraft, taboos, intrusion of disease objects, the action of disease spirits and loss of soul. There was a gradual emergence of empirico-rational surgical and medicinal practices and effective psychologic interventions. Religious beliefs and healing practices (including bone setters, herbalists) play an important role in current ethnic medicine.

DIETARY AND GASTROINTESTINAL CLEANING THERAPIES

Origins, concepts and practices	Application and evidence in musculoskeletal medicine
Fasting	
Fasting is a very old traditional therapy. It has symbolic religio-magic connotations. Links between eating, bowel function and diseases are deeply entrenched in folk lore. Fasting is considered by its proponents to provide physiologic rest, enabling the body to divert its energy to the process of removing metabolic waste, toxins and restoring homeostasis.	Naturopaths and some chiropractors are the main proponents of fasting, often as part of a detoxification program, in treating arthritis. Fasting has been used in research and treatment prior to challenge with potential dietary allergens. Fasting has been shown to lead to brief improvement in RA. Mechanisms which have been investigated include elimination of dietary allergens, rise in plasma cortisol, altered polymorph and immune function and modification of arachidonic acid function.
Purgation, intestinal antisepsis, colonic irrigation	
The idea that the bowel is an important source of toxins, microbial and chemical, is fundamental in folk medicine. Aqueous enemas were described in Ebers Papyrus, c. 1500 BC. Hippocrates mentioned enemas for fever and Galen referred to enemas. Medicinal purging, used since antiquity in traditional medicine, has a potent symbolic magic background. The intestine is believed to be an important source of stagnated fecal material resulting in toxins and gases. These occur because of insufficient water, stress, bad elimination habits, and illness. Hence bowel cleansing by laxatives, purging, antisepsis (as with herbs, acidophilus milk) or washouts should heal toxin-induced disorders including arthritis.	These treatments are occasionally applied in arthritis and rheumatism but the need, opportunity and sufficient gullibility infrequently come together. There is no scientific research available but there have been suggestions that replacement of bowel flora in patients with RA may not be as strange as it sounds.
Dietary modification	
Beliefs about dietary influence on arthritis by traditional healers and by the community was based on symbolism and empirical observation. Thus, celery and garlic acquired the status of remedies. Dietary therapy was more emphasized in early Western medicines, e.g. Hippocrates, than in Chinese medicine. Thomas Eddison spoke for the alternative nutritionists of today 'If doctors of today will not become nutritionists of tomorrow, the nutritionists of today will become the doctors of tomorrow'. Sound nutrition and 'virtuous' (raw, unprocessed) foods encourage the natural preventative and healing mechanicms. Current sociology of the health food industry was critically reviewed by Coward[13]. As food is responsible for just about everything, personal responsibility and group allegiances are emphasized. A thorough, rational, individual trial of diet to eliminate allergens or items promoting hypersensitivity is arduous and can be risky. Such an undertaking may be justifable occasionally in cases of inflammatory arthritis with clinical clues to food intolerance such as mouth ulcers, urticaria or irritable bowel. Reduction of obesity is sound in arthritic and in hyperuricemic patients. Adequate nutrition is particularly important in juvenile arthritis.	The extensive research into dietary treatments of RA has been reviewed by Buchanan *et al.*[71]. Kjeldsen-Kragh *et al.*[72] presented evidence that a vegetarian diet following fasting may help maintain the initial benefit from fasting, but other studies have not shown benefit from vegetarian diets. Well documented case reports of aggravated disease as a result of antigen–antibody reactions involving milk products and cereal have been reported. Exclusion diets appear to help only a very small percentage of patients but evaluation has been difficult. Diets rich in fish oil containing n-3 fatty acids, along with reduction of n-6 fatty acid intake have, on average, been associated with minor improvement in the symptoms of RA. Dietary fish oils may prove to be more effective when used in combination with specific anti-inflammatory agents. No important guidelines have come from research into dietary trace elements. Apart from the advantages of weight reduction, no dietary regimens have been shown to be significantly helpful in OA. Weight reduction, and reduction of high purine foods and alcohol, lower plasma urate in patients with gout.

MULTIDIMENSIONAL OR EXTENSIVELY TEXTUAL MEDICAL AND HEALTH SYSTEMS

Origins, concepts and practices	Application and evidence in musculoskeletal medicine
Anthropsophical medicine	
Rudolph Steiner published the philosophical basis in *The Philosophy of Freedom* (1894). Medical applications came later. Etymology: *anthropos* (man), *sophia* (wisdom). The phenomena of life, feeling, consciousness and spirit are not explained by scientific reductionism. Disciplined thought can extend perceptions and reveal other levels of reality. Four aspects of humans are proposed: physical body, 'etheric' body (life), 'astral' body (soul), and 'I' (human intelligent self). Degenerative conditions result from excessive activity of 'I'.	Anthroposophical physicians (based mainly in Europe) emphasize the comprehensive body–mind approach and the quality of healing which can be directed at any medical problem. The system is considered applicable especially to psychosomatic disorders. The treatments include medicine from natural sources, homeopathy, oil dispersion baths, rhythmical massage, artistic therapies, and 'eurythmy' ('visible' speech and 'visible' music). Steiner's works comprise 20 books and 60,000 published lectures. Fulder lists the more recent research but little of apparent applicability in rheumatology[7].
Chiropractic	
Chiropractic was derived from charismatic and observant lay bone-setters. The oldest references to manipulation are in the Bible, on a statue in a Buddhist temple >2000 years ago, the writings of Hippocrates and Avicenna. DD Palmer, grocer and healer, 'cured' a deaf patient by cervical manipulation in 1895. Greek origin: *keir* (hand), *praktikos* (practice). Palmer's view: subluxed vertebrae interfere with the proper flow of nervous impulses, prevent the 'innate intelligence' (vital force?) from passing through the body. Thus, the affected tissue or organ undergoes dysfunction, disease. Currently subluxations are believed to be structural or functional and are caused by physical or psychic stress, chemical factors. They lead to disease susceptibility, e.g. infection. 'The nervous system holds the key to the body's potential to heal itself'. The diagnostic technique involves history, static palpation of muscles and vertebrae, motion palpation of individual vertebral segments, measurements especially limb length, posture analysis, skin temperature analysis and spinal radiography. Treatment includes massage, vertebral and soft tissue mobilization, vertebral thrusting, stretching, and applied kinesiology. Reference 53.	There are some statistical data from the US suggesting that chiropractic is perceived as satisfactory by consumers, is relatively low in cost, and facilitates early return to work after back injury[54]. The social function and appeal of chiropractic was well reviewed by Firman and Goldstein[55]. Meade *et al.* conducted a randomized comparison of chiropractic and hospital outpatient treatment (including vertebral mobilization) of low back pain of mechanical origin[56]. The long-term outcome slightly favored the chiropractic therapy but it had been continued longer. Further comparative studies are indicated. The chiropractic and manipulative management of low back pain was reviewed by Haldemann[57]. There is no scientifically convincing research to support the subluxation–organ dysfunction theory, nor a recent proposal of neurohormonal (endorphin) action. There remain concerns about forceful treatment by isolated chiropractors with limited diagnostic capacity, and about patients becoming dependent on passive therapies.
Energy (vital force) medicine	
The idea of energy or vital force in one guise or another pervades alternative medicine, having its origins in ancient traditional medicine, notably Chinese (*chi*) and Indian (*gunas*). Energy principles have been applied in herbal medicine, homeopathy, acupuncture, chiropractic, reflexology, radionics, naturopathy, medical ecology, spiritual healing and in new age healing practices such as color therapy. The energy, vital force concept could reasonably be regarded as a theme rather than a health care system. However, with the coming together of new age ideas as pseudoscience, especially physics, it is likely that these practices will be more systemically developed[8]. The ancient and new age (crystals, other energies from nature, psychic influences) ideas have been developed to an amazing level of science fiction by Gerber[58] and this text leads the way into the next decade. The essence is to use subtle energy healing to restore balance and harmony of body, mind and spirit. Metaphysics rules.	The vital force therapies are to be found in one way or another in most alternative and holistic practices. The new age ideas such as crystal energy and new forms of psychic healing are more readily located in the US. The techniques are applied to all forms of arthritis and rheumatism. Watch for the development of comprehensive practices or the increasing application of these ideas in holistic practices. Most research has been directed to acupuncture meridians (see Acupuncture section). The pseudoscientific and esoteric conjectures are, in the main, presented in a manner that is virtually untestable. The book by Gerber is of interest as a highly referenced and plausible pseudoscientific text with notable sections on an Einsteinian paradigm of healing[58].
Environmental medicine	
The complex relationship between individuals and the environment was explored and popularized by T G Randolph whose book *Human Ecology and the Susceptibility to the Chemical Environment* (1962) was the first textbookof environmental medicine. In addition to a general medical recognition, enviromental medicine has been a special interest of some physicians, naturopaths and other practitioners. Many illnesses are believed to be caused or aggravated by allergy or sensitivity to ingested, inhaled or applied chemicals, toxins and pollutants. These include chronic fatigue, RA, systemic lupus erythematosus (SLE) and many forms of arthritis and rheumatism. Suspectibility is increased by inheritance, poor nutrition, infection and stress, drugs. Testing is by elimination diet, skin testing, provocation, Radio Allergo Sorbent Test, electroacupuncture feedback, blood tests.	Many patients with major rheumatic diseases and those with idiopathic chronic disorders characterized by fatigue and aches and pains will report their experiences with environmental medicine practitioners. Pursuit of environmental causes is inherently appealing and seems to offer a pleasing solution. Regrettably such solutions are infrequent, often illusory. There have been many studies of food hypersensitivity (see Diet section), and environmental potential toxins in RA, SLE, scleroderma and other rheumatic disorders. Rheumatologists have been attentive to environmental issues, often under pressure from the patients. There is a recent textbook[59].
Folk, domestic and self-help remedies	
Common knowledge, family and folk beliefs are acquired from elders, word-of-mouth, magazines, lay books, pharmacies, doctors, arthritis organizations, self-help groups, advertisements. The origins of many beliefs and practices go back to antiquity and include a rich variety of symbolic magic, common sense, orthodox and discredited medical ideas and applications from alternative medicine. The over-riding concept is – if it worked on someone and is not too silly or risky, try it (the power of anecdote). The practices range from common sense and empiric to magic. Common treatments are: rest, heat, ice, supports, exercises, analgesics, liniments, patent medicines, herbs, minerals, vitamins, diets, copper bracelets, amulets, psychic practices including prayer and relaxation, hydrotherapy, potato or camphor in bed, magnets, vibration, purging. The Reader's Digest text is a useful general reference[10], also the book by Pietroni[11].	Virtually all patients and many nonpatients with arthritis and rheumatism apply self-help remedies. It is wise to enquire routinely, e.g. over-the-counter aspirin increases the risk of gastrointestinal disorders in patients taking NSAIDs. Some remedies, e.g. over-the-counter analgesics, are of established efficacy. Arthritis Foundations can assist by providing guidelines for self-help remedies. Research on diet and other individual remedies is covered separately. The efficacy of salicylate and NSAIDs containing topical applications requires further study. The distribution to the affected joint may be predominantly by the systemic circulation. With increasing access to medical information, including on the Internet, it is expected that many individuals will seek to have more control over the selection of therapies, i.e. extension of self-help further into the medical domain.
Herbal medicine	
The medicinal, aromatic and savory properties of plants (leaf, seed, stem, flowers, root, bark) have been valued by humans for aeons. In traditional and tribal medicine, herbs have had religio-magical uses, often with ceremony, and also empirically-based therapeutic roles. Healers passed on knowledge orally and by text. Many herbs were identified by the application of symbolic magic (e.g. willow bark), others by 'intuitive revelations'. The first 'physic gardens' of medicinal plants that are known were in Egypt in 1400 BC. Herbal medicine constitutes a large part of traditional medicine[60], is relied on by the majority of the world's population and is extensively used also in the industrialized nations[61]. While symbolic magic and placebo effects are important, herbalists believe in several therapeutic principles (applied to rheumatism) including detoxification: • restoration of balance of the 'vital force' • nourishment and stimulation • antirheumatic actions. The whole plant should be used in herbal remedies, not an isolated pure active drug extract, because the other active substances are necessary for efficacy and safety. In Chinese and other herbal practices each patient requires a different combination of herbs prepared or administered by different methods. Herbal preparations are available from naturopaths, traditional and other nonmedical practitioners, natural product stores and pharmacies. They may be taken or used as whole herbs, powders, teas (infusions, decoctions) capsules, tablets, extracts, tinctures, oils, salves and ointments, enemas and baths. Proprietary herbal mixtures are frequently combined with nutritional supplements, fish oils, minerals and vitamins. Some popular herbs for rheumatism include aloe vera, alfalfa, celery, comfrey, dandelion, devil's claw, evening primrose oil, feverfew, garlic, ginger, horseradish, kelp, parsley, Paraguay tea, willow bark, wintergreen and yucca.	Herbal derivatives are widely used in orthodox rheumatology, e.g. salicylates (willow bark), colchicine (autumn crocus), opiaties (opium poppy), quinine (cinchona bark). Retrieval of controlled trials of other herbal products tested in rheumatic disease is not very rewarding. There was a negative trial of tipi (*Petiveria alliacea*), a popular 'analgesic' tea in osteoarthritis (OA). Certain plant seed oils, notably evening primrose, borage and blackcurrent contain relatively large amounts of gammalinolenic E, an eicosanoid with known anti-inflammatory and immunoregulating properties. Evening primrose oil and blackcurrent seed oil have shown marginal benefits in trial in RA. The folk belief that nightshade vegetables aggravate arthritis does not appear well founded (see 'tomato effect' mentioned earlier). Most of the peer-reviewed journal literature on herbal medicine (phytomedicine) relevant to rheumatology has focused on toxicity including adulterating chemicals, prescription drugs, heavy metals and illegal substances, and on other quality-control issues such as substituted herbs. The *Journal of Ethnopharmocology* and the journal *HerbalGram*, published by the American Botanical Council and the Herb Research Foundation, are potentially useful resources for investigative rheumatologists. WHO has published guidelines for the assessment of herbal medicines[62]. The teaching and prescribing of phytomedicine is rapidly increasing, having been particularly prominent in Europe. At least 13 multinational drug companies have started to buy or collaborate with European phytomedicine firms[45]. The regulatory issues are complex and important and are discussed elsewhere. It is of concern that, although there is no practical difference in concept between chemicals in plants and synthetics, consumers think otherwise. *(continued)*

MULTIDIMENSIONAL OR EXTENSIVELY TEXTUAL MEDICAL AND HEALTH SYSTEMS (continued)	
Origins, concepts and practices	**Application and evidence in musculoskeletal medicine**
Holistic medicine	
Holistic medicine is an alternative movement which has also been evolving within the medical profession in response to perceived shortcomings in scientific ('reductionist') medicine and in response to the popular appeal of respecting and treating the whole person[63]. In fact, orthodox medicine is inherently holistic, although individual practices and pracitioners fall short of the ideal. New ideas have been derived from traditional medicine, complementary practitioners, revival of Hippocratic principles and social movements (greening, Gaia, general systems theory, new age). Holistic medicine is a system of health care which emphasizes personal responsibility and fosters a cooperative relationship among all those involved, leading towards optimal attunement of body, mind, emotions and spirit. The focus is on prevention, life style, psychotherapeutics, social context of illness causation, diet, exercises, meditation, family involvement, clinical ecology, assisting nature and the promotion of good health. The concept of holism differs between alternative practitioners (who apply it to diagnosis and management of individuals) and medical complementary services and practices, which is the main focus of this section.	Holistic practices provide a comprehensive, if scientifically uncritical, service which is applicable to chronic arthritis and rheumatism and potentially appealing to many patients. The holistic movement claims superior attention to and care in relation to body, mind and spirit but has no construct to demonstrate efficacy, cost-effectiveness or validity. Orthodox medicine has been slow and ineffective in responding to those aspects of the holistic propaganda which may be viewed as inappropriate. The individual practitioners vary in training and in associates, but homeopathy, acupuncture, naturopathy, chiropractic and new age (energy) ideas are prominent. There is often focus on mind–body medicine[64] and psychoneuroimmunology. Scientific research is notably absent and indeed is frequently regarded as irrelevant or inappropriate. There are some descriptive research publications[12] and journals such as Holistic Medicine.
Homeopathy	
Homeopathy is a system of treatment developed from the natural 'law' (magic) of *similia similibus curantur* (like is cured by like). That is, a substance which can cause symptoms in the healthy can cure similar symptoms occurring in the sick. The principle was recognized by Hippocrates and by Paracelsus, but was developed as a system of healing by S. Hahnemann (*Materia Medica Pura*, 1811). He observed that cinchona bark, used to treat intermittent fever (malaria) produced similar symptoms when he took some himself. Greek roots: *homoios* (similar), *pathos* (suffering). Hahnemann went on to discover that potency could be retained in high dilution ('potentization'). Hering formulated the law of cure: during cure, the symptoms move from vital to less vital organs, also disappear downwards. Homeopaths believe that cure requires stimulation of the natural healing processes and that the organism becomes sensitive to that which will stimulate the cure. They emphasize the 'vital force' conjecture (doctrine). Symptoms are interpreted as curative efforts being made by the body. The art lies in matching the symptom spectrum ('picture') with the appropriate remedy spectrum ('picture'), matching 'vibrational frequencies'. A single remedy, the similimum, the most similar, is sought. The experiments in healthy volunteers were called 'provings'. Remedies may be toxin releasing, toxin eliminating, liver-stimulating or constitutional. Practitioners consult compendiums called repertories and *materia medicas* to determine the remedy which best matches the total picture of the symptoms. Healing begins by eliminating the immediate symptoms then progressing to the older underlying symptoms. Remedies are prepared from plant and other sources in alcohol, then filtered to give a 'mother tincture' from which dilutions are made. The shaking of each dilution is thought to be important. About 500 remedies are in regular use. Classic homeopaths use a similimum and not a potentization of an apparent causal agent, while modern homeopaths use combinations of several or many substances and may include low dilutions of herbal products.[65]	Hahnemann allegedly initially had more success with acute disorders, but homeopathic treatments have become widely used in chronic arthritis and rheumatism. Some homeopathic remedies for rheumatic symptoms include *actea spicata, ammonium carbonicum, antimonium tartaricum, arnica montana, arsenicumalbum, bryonia alba, calcarea, caulophyllum, causticum, colchicum, gelsemium, nux vomica, pulsatilla, rhus toxicodendron, ruta graveolens, sulphur*. The safety and symbolism are appealing to many. The extreme dilution of dose has aroused much scientific controversy. The theory that homeopathic remedies do not transmit chemicals but information is difficult to test. The idea is that a dissolved substance leaves an imprint on the water which is then replicated in the body. It has been suggested that the remedy may contain a specific qualitative capacity (analogous to pheremones) to trigger the autoregulation of healing and control mechanisms. Hill and Doyon reviewed 40 randomized trials of homeopathic remedies and found no acceptable evidence of efficacy[66]. The study by Kleijnen *et al.*[67], a survey of trials, was important in showing the difficulty of literature retrieval in discussing publication bias, in highlighting difficulties in trials where treatment should be individualized and in evaluating outcomes. Trials in RA, OA, fibrositis, and musculoskeletal pain and trauma generally scored low by criteria for design. There was a trend for poorer trials to be positive. The main general conclusion, applicable to the studies in rheumatology, is that there were sufficient positive studies to encourage further research. The scientific jury is still out on homeopathy. There appear to be no replicated positive controlled trials. However the practitioners are often 'walking placebos' with good communication skills and safe treatment, therefore the utility of homeopathic (medical) practice has quite wide support. In the wider world the population who receive homeopathy has been estimated to be 500 million.
Hydrotherapy, balneotherapy, spas	
Hydrotherapy is one of the most ancient of all treatments for rheumatism[68]. Aztecs used steam baths and masseurs. Public baths were popularized by the Romans who had been influenced by the Greeks. Hippocrates in 400 BC described watering places in 'Airs, Waters and Places'. Pliny in 77 AD wrote about the mineral springs in Europe. The term 'spa' was derived from the Walloon word '*espa*' meaning fountain. Spa, in the Belgain Ardennes, was a famous mineral spring. Priessnitz (1798–1858) extended the treatments, administering water in every possible way. Mineral springs supply natural water containing salts and gases derived from the rocks and soils through which they flow. Hydrotherapy, as an all-purpose therapy, was based on the ancient concept of the humors – the necessity for expelling excesses. Empirical and symbolic benefits come from water which may be hot, vaporized, with salts, with bubbles, with mud, with radioactivity or holy; water which is applied, sprayed, used from immersion, drunk and injected into various orifices. The alternative practices include whirlpools, sitz baths, steam, hot and cold compresses and rubs, hyperthermia and colonic irrigation. Additives for rheumatism: salt, Epsom salts, ginger, oat straw and various oils.	Hydrotherapy is employed by physiotherapists as an appealing and effective method of exercise therapy. The buoyancy is useful and the heat and the diuretic effects may add to the benefit. The spas, where multiple additional therapies (physical, dietary, homeopathic, electrical, psychic) are applied, retain some popularity but the cost-effectiveness of long-term outcomes is uncertain. A very appealing book about spas has been published[68]. There is no scientific evidence that the chemical content of the water is therapeutically relevant in arthritis and rheumatism. Immersion for prolonged periods has a diuretic effect and this may be a factor in the facilitation of movement of arthritic joints. The case for immersion in baths and the application of mud packs was covered by Sukenik *et al.* and subsequent correspondence. Elkayam et al. showed that mud packs and mineral baths could be partially beneficial in RA and OA. Konrad *et al.* found balneotherapy, underwater traction and underwater massage very little better than no treatment for low back pain. Psoriasis and psoriatic arthritis improved as a probable result of bathing in Dead Sea water and exposure to sun, especially with the addition of mud packs, and sulphur baths. Significant and lasting improvement in low back pain as a result of spa therapy in Saint-Nectaire, France, was shown in a randomized controlled trial.
Naturopathy	
Naturopathy is a system of treatment of ailments which utliises the 'vital curative force' and employs nature's agencies, forces, processes and products. Nature-based treatments date back to the dawn of healing. The philosophical roots can be traced back to the Hippocratic school of medicine. The revival of vitalism in the 19th century was combined with empirical natural methods. The term was coined by John Scheel, 1895. Progress followed the Kneipp Committee in 1900 and B. Lus in 1902, also H. Lindlahr (philosophy of natural therapeutics). 'Taking the cure' at natural springs and spas was a major influence. After a suppressed period earlier this century, naturopathy has recently flourished. Naturopathy is a mixture of traditional folk wisdom, empiricism and selections of biomedical science. The basic principles are: • the healing power of nature is fundamental, • treat the cause rather than the effect (disease), • ill health results from lowering of resistance due to diet, spinal displacement, stress, etc.; accumulation of toxins; deficiencies of vitamins, minerals and other essentials, • promotion of harmony of body, mind and emotion (treat the whole person), • new principles of living (various old and new therapies) with focus on prevention. Diagnosis is by history, observation, iris examination, assessment of 'vital reserve', nutritional assessment, hair analysis. Naturopaths frequently treat rheumatic symptoms by employing a selection of counseling with modification of life style, diet and nutritional advice, herbal medicine, homeopathy Bach flower remedies, supplements (vitamins, minerals, biochemical remedies), exercises, massage and manipulation, hydrotherapy, and numerous other therapies, including acupuncture.	The apparent success relates to the ideas and idioms of the population and the concepts seem to make sense. Furthermore, there are plausible themes, e.g. pain control using hot pepper (capsaicin), clove oil (eugenol), wintergreen oil (methyl salicylate). While components of treatment used by naturopaths have been subjected to research, there has been no formal scientific evaluation of the system. Baer has recently published an historical and descriptive review from an American perspective[69]. Naturopaths argue that scientific method is inapplicable to this form of therapy which is individualized. It is however possible to perform a scientifically acceptable randomized study comparing a comprehensive individualized naturopathic regimen with standard medical treatment, but not on a double-blind basis. In the treatment of RA, the following have at least undergone some scientific evaluation: fish oils (EPA), evening primrose oil, selenium, vitamin E, zinc, vitamin C, copper, flavonoids, phenylalanine and feverfew. Naturopathy is, in some respects, an alternative system which is a cause for concern because of the plausible presentation of potentially misleading pseudoscience. Information with low-level evidence is presented confidently along with factual nutritional guidance. Evaluation is slow, and is difficult for the patient who may be impressed by the process and confused about the outcome.

(*continued*)

MULTIDIMENSIONAL OR EXTENSIVELY TEXTUAL MEDICAL AND HEALTH SYSTEMS (continued)	
Origins, concepts and practices	**Application and evidence in musculoskeletal medicine**
Osteopathy	
Anrdew T. Still lost three sons in an epidemic of meningitis and felt induced to seek another healing system. He reasoned that humans became ill because the structure was out of adjustment (the ideas of a skilled mechanic), 1874. In 1892 he founded the first school of osteopathy in Missouri. J. M. Littlejohn expressed osteopathy in holistic terms and set up the British School of Osteopathy in 1917. Osteopathic practice covers the spectrum from strong links with orthodox medicine, albeit with a 'holistic' emphasis (especially DOs from the US and medically qualified oestopaths in the UK), to lay therapists and practitioners who combine osteopathy with naturopathy. The basic principle is that abnormal musculoskeletal function ('somatic dysfunction') causes symptoms independently of structural pathology. Inappropriate muscle tension and restriction joint motion are important. The 'pain-spasm' cycle is emphasized. A wide range of psychologic, nutritional and physical causes are identified. Structural pathology often interacts with mechanical dysfunctions. Some osteopaths offer a 'complete' diagnostic and assessment service either medical or naturopathic–holistic[70].	Almost all patients attending osteopaths have pain and about 85% is spinal. Specific patterns of segmental spinal dysfunction are said to correlate with visceral disorders, but such claims may in part be explained by mechanisms of somatic referred pain. The manual techniques include: soft tissue massage, stretching, kneading, 'neuromuscular techniques'; passive movements and high velocity thrusts of joints or spinal segments; and a variety of other soft tissue and skeletal procedures, both active and passive. Osteopaths claim the most comprehensive range of manipulative techniques characterized by minimum force and greatest specificity. Osteopathy is evidently the first alternative health care system to achieve legal statutary recognition in Europe (UK). There is surprisingly little evalution of osteopathy in biomedical journals. Descriptive research indicates that there is an apparently acceptable level of safety. Most research has been on neuromuscular physiology. Controlled trials have not been easy to perform. A trial by Gibson *et al.* showed no difference in outcome of back pain between treatment by an osteopath, shortwave diathermy and placebo but this is insufficient evidence to refute the efficacy of osteopathy. See also Skeletal Manipulation.

MEDICINAL TREATMENTS INCLUDING NUTRITIONAL SUPPLEMENTS	
Origins, concepts and practices	**Application and evidence in musculoskeletal medicine**
Herbal remedies* Homeopathic remedies* Home remedies* (*See tables of Textual Medical and Health Systems)	
Liniments, rubefacients, topical analgesics	
Liniment is derived from the Latin *linere* (to smear). The use of liniments and ointments (salves) for pain relief has been recorded from the Babylonians and Assyrians in 3000–5000 BC. One explanation of 'quack' is derived from quacksalver, a seller of salves advertised vocally (by quacking). The alleged benefits come from the human touch (if applied by another), the symbolic effects of disappearance of the application and of the skin reaction and from penetration of the 'active' ingredient to the painful tissue (no doubt also placebo effects).	Common ingredients used for rheumatic disorders are: menthol, oil of wintergreen, methyl salicylate, herbs such as aloe vera, copper and more recently NSAIDs, as well as a variety of oils. The studies have until recently generally been of low standard. Recent research on unbound concentration of an NSAID from both knees when the application was applied to one knee suggests that bioavailable drug at deep sites comes mainly via the general circulation. The pharmaceutical companies marketing NSAIDs have been developing topical preparations enthusiastically.
Minerals, inorganic biochemicals	
The majority of these remedies have been quasi-scientific interpretations by naturopaths of biomedical data. Many products were devised by M. Blackmore, combing Schuessler's early 20th century German homeopathic idea of small doses of essential minerals and trace elements with Hahnemann's homeopathic principles (Blackmore's Celloid Minerals). Silica is a 'vital element to our human scaffolding'. Sodium phosphatase is a 'metabolic acid remover'. Potassium sulfate is a 'cell oxygenator'. Potassium chloride 'removes congestion'. Zinc, copper, and manganese 'enable the production of the protective antioxidant superoxide dismutase'. Selenium also 'plays a valuable role as an antioxidant'. These examples do not begin to do justice to the imaginative pseudoscience of biochemical remedies. Calcium is regarded as a key mineral in arthritis.	Many of our patients are taking minerals and salts for their arthritis, fortunately usually in small doses. The average patient will not see much conceptual distinction between the orthodox rationale for iron and calcium supplements and the proposed rationales for minerals and salts by a naturopath. Most research has been directed to possible anti-inflammatory and/or antirheumatic effects of zinc and copper. While some rationale exists, the clinical studies have not shown convincing evidence of efficacy.
Organic remedies other than herbs	
Organic 'cures' taken orally have been derived from traditional and folk medicine, ethnic medicine, orthodox and unorthodox biomedical science, and homeopathy and have been developed especially by naturopaths. It is in this field that quacks with secret ingredients are frequently to be found. Amino acids (D-phenylalanine and tryptophan) 'increase endorphine activity and so relieve pain'. Fish oil, cod liver oil, rich in omega-3 series long-chain polyunsaturated fatty acids, have potentially anti-inflammatory actions. Proteolytic enzymes (pancreatic bromelain) are believed to be anti-inflammatory. Glycosaminoglycans 'stimulate cartilage', but are not bioavailable orally. Marine products are thought to be anti-inflammatory, while royal jelly is treated as if magic and honey with apple cider vinegar is an old favorite.	Patients with major inflammatory forms of arthritis appear to be especially likely to try these treatments. Orthodox physicians and naturopaths commonly suggest fish oil supplements, along with reduction of saturated (animal) fat intake. Most of the treatments are in the domain of alternative and complementary practitioners. Vegetable sources of minerals are frequently advised, e.g. kelp for calcium, sodium chloride, iron and magnesium; lettuce, brown rice, spinach, cucumber and barley for silica. There are proponents of vaccines, hormones and cellular therapy. Fish oil supplements are of established, though modest, efficacy in RA and thus are used in orthodox medicine. Interestingly, the composition of snake oil, perjoratively symbolic of quackery, is very similar to fish oil. Trials have shown that the greenlipped mussel extract (Seatone) does not work but its sales continue.
Patent, proprietary medicines	
The two principal sources of proprietary formulations are pharmacies stocking pharmaceutical lines and health stores purveying naturopathic products. The pharmaceutical products include established analgesics, also minerals and salts, vitamins, topical applications and a variety of old favorite patent medicines with actions along homeopathic and naturopathic lines. The naturopathic products are essentially those referred to in this box.	This is a large industry, usually regulated, well supported by the vast population of sufferers from arthritis and rheumatism. By definition, the treatments of proven efficacy [salicylates, paracetamol (acetaminophen), ibuprofen, codeine] are not 'alternative'.
Vitamins including megadose therapy	
Vitamins are a group of unrelated organic compounds that, in trace amounts, are essential for normal metabolic functioning, but must be obtained from the environment. F. G. Hopkins developed the concept of accessory food factors in 1906. The use of doses above minimal requirements is an 'alternative' concept, although the anti-oxidant action of vitamins C and E is lately being explored in orthodox medicine . The theoretical basis for megavitamin therapy stems from L. Pauling's work on vitamin C. The naturopathic beliefs about the role of vitamins in musculoskeletal disorders may be summarized: A: inhibits collagenase and thus is important for the structure of cartilage, tendon, ligament and bone, B5 (pantothenic acid): considered important in cartilage growth, B6 (pyridoxin): required for collagen, hence cartilage synthesis, C: low in osteoarthritis, important in cartilage, connective tissue repair and as an antioxidant, E: antioxidant, anti-inflammatory, membrane stabilizer, anabolic for cartilage. Orthomolecular medicine practitioners believe in the primacy of nutrition, biochemical individuality, that blood tests do not necessarily reflect tissue concentratons of nutrients and in the prescription of megavitamin therapy.	Vitamins are frequently prescribed by holistic and naturopathic practitioners for the treatment of arthritis and rheumatism. Vitamin D in cod liver oil is also popular. Either supplementary tablets or dietary guidance is given as components of the nutritional regimen. Megavitamin therapy has been applied to arthritis but the following is small. There is no sound evidence that the pharmacologic doses of the vitamins used to treat arthritis have definite therapeutic efficacy. However, there are early indications that high dose vitamin C (perhaps also E) as an oxidant could slow the progression of osteoarthritis. As adjunctive therapy, vitamin E may have anti-inflammatory action but more research is needed.

MUSCULOSKELETAL THERAPIES UTILIZING MANUAL AND/OR BODY AWARENESS TECHNIQUES ('BODY WORKS')	
Origins, concepts and practices	**Application and evidence in musculoskeletal medicine**
Body awareness and movement methods	
Alexander technique[73] The techique was created by an Australian actor FM Alexander (1869–1955). Concerned about habitual loss of voice, he observed that even the thought of speaking was sufficient to pull his head back and down and tighten his throat. Other actors were observed to respond to instruction in posture and movement in voice and health. Suboptimal muscle awareness (kinesthesia, proprioception) leads to defects in posture, function, and to fatigue, tension, depression. The aim is to restore kinesthetic awareness, neuromuscular control, lengthen the spine and improve efficiency.	Alexander technique This is a potentially useful technique to prevent and treat musculoskeletal disorders, especially those with spinal pain and pain in the supporting muscles. The techniques utilize many common sense principles in tune with scientific physiology. Postural defects are shown; then, with instruction and touch, an improved pattern of posture, movement and balance is achieved. Much practice is required. The published research is descriptive and related to physiologic principles. There are evidently no sound controlled trials of Alexander techniques in the treatment of musculoskeletal disorders.
*Feldenkrais technique[74] M. Feldenkrais was a Russian-born Israeli physicist and engineer who was motivated by a painful disorder of his knee. In learning to walk without pain, he studied biomedical science and was influenced by judo, yoga, Gurdjieff's spiritual philosphy and Freud's psychology. Awareness of the skeleton and its muscles and of its orientation and movement in space is learnt through experience which invoIes curiosity and pleasure. Restricted movements imprint distorted images in the mind but aware, efficient and free movements will transmit new patterns and ways of moving. While Alexander focused on posture, Feldenkrais emphasized natural, pleasurable and instinctive motion.	Feldenkrais technique Like the Alexander technique, Feldenkrais methods are widely applicable to musculoskeletal disorders, particularly those involving the spine. Through sessions of awareness through movement (active) and on functional integration (passive manipulation), patients are said to conserve energy and avoid strain. Those who persevere frequently report good results (otherwise they would not persevere). The literature is plausible and appealing to many but does not have much scientific content. It would be difficult to perform and assess a controlled trial because the Feldenkrais group is likely to experience positive bias in reporting outcome.
Meridian-based therapies (acupressure, shiatzu, reflexology)	
* Acupressure * *Shiatzu* * Reflexology Acupressure seems to have arisen from the human instinct to hold or massage parts of the body that hurt. Chinese Taoist monks began to formalize this reaction over 5000 years ago into a system called Tao-Yinn. This has come down to the present as *Do In*, the art of rejuvenation through self massage. *Shiatzu* is a an ancient Japanese adaptation, also incorporating massage. Reflexology is an ancient Chinese treatment using pressure on points in the feet. It was known also to other old cultures and was rediscovered by American ear, nose and throat consultant W. Fitzgerald. In acupressure and *shiatzu*, the aim is to unblock the energy paths by manipulating acupuncture (meridian) points and thus restore balance and recuperation. The techniques are milder than acupuncture and were incorporated into family and folk medicine. In acupressure, the stages of therapy are general energy balancing, specific attention to blocked meridians and closing techniques. In *shiatzu*, the massage is added to promote the flow of energy in the required directions. The reflexology concept is that there are reflexes in the feet for all parts of the body and thus one can influence blood flow and nervous tension in the affected region.	These techniques are claimed to be useful as health maintenance systems to reduce stress, increase circulation and tune up energy and balance. They are applied in a variety of musculoskeletal disorders, usually minor complaints. Acupressure and *shiatzu* are applied in folk medicine as first aid in pain relief. Scientific research is not readily identifiable. It is difficult to conceive how a reflexology theory such as segments of the feet correspond to pre-birth stages and that 'metamorphic' therapy will aid problems acquired during gestation might be tested. However, at a simpler level it is quite feasible to test, for example, reflexology treatment of sciatica.
Skeletal manipulation	
* Chiropractic * Osteopathy Because of the extensive training required, textual documentation and claims to be comprehensive systems of healing, these therapies are covered in the accompanying box on medical and health systems. They are included here as they are frequently applied specifically as manual treatments for musculoskeletal disorders, especially with spinal pain.	There has been research into the outcome of various forms of manipulation, especially for low back pain. Koes *et al.*[75] reviewed randomized controlled trials of spinal manipulation and mobilization for back and neck pain and concluded that, although there was some evidence of efficacy, methodological limitations reduced the strength of the conclusions. The same group recently conducted a randomized controlled trial which showed that manipulative therapy was better than general practitioner and placebo treatment, and slightly better than conservative physiotherapy after 12 months[76]. Manipulation is of short-term benefit in some patients, particularly those with uncomplicated acute low back pain. The efficacy for chronic low back pain remains uncertain. A clinical trial of manipulative therapy for chronic low back pain by Triano *et al.*[77] provided useful guidelines for researching this type of therapy and references to studies of manipulation.
Other body work therapies	
Therapeutic massage is an ancient and very widely used therapy with extensive variations. Claims are made that massage promotes relaxation, overcomes fatigue, lessens fibrosis and adhesions, relieves pain, reduces swelling, improves circulation, breaks up metabolic wastes in muscles. Rolfing (structural integration) is based on the idea that human function is improved when the segments of the body are properly aligned. 'A person's emotional state may be seen as the projection of his or her structural imbalances' (Ida Rolf). The treatment involves manipulating and stretching the fascial tissues.	While the apparent benefit and utility of these forms of treatment are widely accepted by the public as treatments for rheumatic and other disorders, evaluation from a critical medical perspective is very limited. The scientific basis for the ancient art of massage was reviewed by Goats[78].
*See boxes of Textual and Health Symptoms.	

REFERENCES

1. Weatherall DJ. Scientific method and the art of healing. In: Weatherall DJ, Ledingham JGG, Warrell DA, eds. Oxford Textbook of Medicine. 3E. Oxford: Oxford University Press; 1996:7–10.
2. McCormick J. The contribution of science to medicine. Persp Biol Med. 1993;36:315–22.
3. Gevitz N. Alternative medicine and orthodox canon. Mt Sinai J Med. 1995;62:127–31.
4. Fisher P, Ward A. Complementary medicine in Europe. Br Med J. 1994;309:107–11.
5. Eisenberg DM, Kessler RC, Foster C, Norlock FE, Calkins DR, Delbanco TL. Unconventional medicine in the United States. Prevalence, costs, and patterns of use. N Engl J Med. 1993;328:246–52.
6. MacLennan AH, Wilson, DH, Taylor AW. Prevalence and cost of alternative medicine in Australia. Lancet. 1996:347:569–73.
7. Piori-Boisset M, Esdaile M, Fitzcharles M-A. Alternative medicine use in fibromyalgia syndrome. Arthritis Care Res. 1996;9:13–17.
8. Fulder S. The handbook of complementary medicine, 2E. Oxford: Oxford University Press; 1988.
9. Strohecker J, ed. The Burton Goldberg Group. Alternative medicine: the definitive guide. Puyallup, Washington: Future Medicine Publishing, Inc.; 1994.
10. Henderson JM, ed. The Reader's Digest family guide to alternative medicine. Sydney: Reader's Digest (Australia) Pty. Ltd.; 1992.
11. Pietroni P. The family guide to alternative health care: how to treat everyday ailments with complementary remedies. London: Simons and Schuster: 1995.
12. Pietroni P. The greening of medicine. London: Victor Gollancz Ltd.; 1990.
13. Coward R. The whole truth. The myth of alternative health. London: Faber and Faber; 1989.
14. Stalker D, Glymour C, eds. Examining holistic medicine. New York: Prometheus Books; 1989.
15. Watt J, Wood C, eds. Talking health. Conventional and complementary approaches. London: Royal Society of Medicine Services; 1988.
16. British Medical Association. Complementary medicine: new approaches to good practice. Oxford: Oxford University Press; 1993.
17. Fernandez-Madrid F. Treating arthritis: medicine,

PSYCHIC, PSYCHOSOMATIC AND VITAL FORCE (ENERGY) THERAPIES

Origins, concepts and practices	Application and evidence in musculoskeletal medicine
Acupuncture and its variants	
Acupuncture is derived from Latin words *acus* (needle) and *punctura* (a pricking). The Chinese refer to 'needle effect', 'needle skill' or 'needle therapy'. Acupuncture dates back more than 5000 years. The Inner Classic Yellow Emperor (Nei Jing), 200–100 BC, is the source of medical theory. Acupressure is a formalized version of instinctive holding or massaging hurting places developed by Taoist monks over 5000 years ago, influenced by the meridian energy flow concept. Moxibustion is a related ancient Chinese technique. Acupuncture [46-48,50,79] is believed to change the vital energy (*Ch'i* or *Qi*) which flows in the 'meridians', a network of 'channels' which connect the internal organs with the superficial parts of the body. The acupuncture points are accessible regions where the channels (meridians) can be needled and stimulated mechanically or electrically so that the smooth flow of *Ch'i* (*Qi*) and blood regulate *Yin* and *Yang*, moisten the tendons and bones and benefit the joints (*Nei Jing*). Acupuncture is a *Yang* treatment because it moves from the exterior to the interior. It is a compilation of three different philosophical concepts. The traditional Chinese view is that acupuncture is but one component of a complex and comprehensive healing art, while in the West its application is selective and is mainly for the relief of musculoskeletal pain. Mechanical or electrical stimulation of the needle at acupuncture points produces characteristic sensations including 'numbness'[80]. Variations and modern adaptations include acupressure, laser acupuncture, auricular acupuncture, moxibustion (the heating of moxa, i.e. mugwort or *Artermisia vulgaris*, at acupuncture points), cupping (suction by cups containing heated air) and 'touch for health'. Acupuncture is currently widely used for painful musculoskeletal disorders by orthodox, complementary and alternative practitioners.	Contemporary acupuncture as practised in the West is a mixture of Eastern and Western concepts, neither truly classic TCM nor fully scientific. This duality is reflected in recent useful publications[81,82]. The scientific evaluation of acupuncture is beset with conceptual and practical difficulties. The clinical trials have, in the main, studied the single modality 'Western' acupuncture. Among many deficiences in trial design, an important and inadequately resolved issue is the choice of placebo control[83]. The treatment and control are usually not demonstrably equivalent in psychologic impact. There is no sound evidence that acupuncture influences the underlying rheumatic process and the US National Council Against Health Fraud, in an assertive and somewhat controversial paper, concluded that the better the design of the study, the less the evidence that acupuncture is more than a placebo. On the other hand, many authorities and medical bodies accept evidence for analgesic effects. WHO provisionally lists intercostal neuralgia, cervicobrachial syndrome, frozen shoulder, tennis elbow, sciatica, low back pain and osteoarthritis as conditions that may be amenable to acupuncture. There are numerous studies of acupuncture in the pain of RA and OA. While there are positive results compared with controls, it is difficult to conclude that acupuncture has clinically significant efficacy when psychologic benefits are demonstrably nullified or controlled. There is a view that if acupuncture is mainly a placebo it is a powerful one. Research into the mechanisms of analgesia in acupuncture from the Shanghai College of TCM[80] in major Asian and Western centers has not supported the traditional *chi* and meridian concepts but has moved to peripheral and central neurophysiology. Acupuncture points have no specific morphologic features. The points generally correspond to tender and trigger points. A nociceptive stimulus is required, and the analgesic effects can be blocked by local anesthetic. Needles activate polymodal receptors (thinly myelinated and unmyelinated fibers). Central effects, presumably acting on the descending pain modulation system, are blocked by systemic naloscone. The International Association for the Study of Pain classifies acupuncture as a peripherally applied neuroaugmentative and counter-irritation technique.
Healing by faith, spiritualism, energy, magnetism, psychic, metaphysical and magic means	
Healing is really the oldest profession.The primitive roots of healing are shamanism and magic. The laying on of hands to heal was recorded in the Ebers Papyrus (c. 1500 BC). The Greeks used therapeutic touch therapy in their Asklepian temples for centuries BC. The Bible has many references, especially concerning Jesus. A major function of early religions was to heal disease. As the power of the church declined, royal touch became prominent. Magnetic energy theories were promulgated by Paracelsus, Fludd, and Mesmer. The characteristics of folk healers were well described by Hand[18]. In faith healing of religious type, the power of God is invoked. Apart from the concept of divine intervention, placebo, suggestion and psychoneuroimmunologic effects have been invoked. Other healers believe in the transmission of some form of energy (magnetic, cosmic, etheric, paranormal). Spiritual healing has been described as the re-creation of the flow of life energy between body, soul and consciousness so that the whole person may return to balance and harmony. Thus, self-healing is often emphasized, the healer acting as a channel. It is an important prerequisite for healing that there is a strong desire by the healer to do so. Spiritual and energy-invoking healers state that it does not matter if the recipient is sceptical.	Controlled clinical trials are difficult to conduct and Fulder states that there have never been any significant trials[8]. It is, however, surprising that Benor was able to cite 122 controlled experiments on healing, of which 68 were claimed to demonstrate significant effects[84]. The results have been published mainly in parapsychology journals and would, no doubt, make interesting reading for a scientifically trained sceptic. Generally, believers in parapsychologic phenomena produce positive results, while disbelievers produce negative ones (the 'sheep or goat' effect). A psychotherapeutic and anthropologic viewpoint of religio-magical healing was published by Frank and Frank[85]. A randomized trial recently resulted in data supporting some efficacy for healing by laying-on-of-hands, compared with psychotherapy and no treatment, for chronic back pain. A trial of spiritual healing in chronic idiopathic pain showed minor benefits compared to randomly assigned controls on no treatment. Strategies for research into spiritual healing were outlined by Hodges and Schofield[86].
Mind–body therapies	
Yoga positions have been observed engraved on seals from about 3000 BC in India. *T'ai chi ch'uan* mythology states that a Taoist monk Chang Sanfeng invented the movements after dreaming about a strange fight–dance between a snake and a bird. Primitive healers used the receptivity to suggestions which occurred in a trance. Mesmer is the founder of modern hypnotism. Several of the body-orientated psychotherapies were offshoots of Freudian ideas developed as turn-of-the-century European society turned from repression to openness. W. Reich is considered a forerunner of much modern 'body work' (bioenergetics, Rolfing, Feldenkrais). Relaxation therapy, meditation and biofeedback have moved from ancient origins to modern science. These mind–body therapies require more active participation by the subjects than is so in spiritual healing. The therapies include: autogenic training, bioenergetics, biofeedback, breathing, chanting, hypnotherapy, meditation, relaxation, *T'ai chi ch'uan* and yoga.	Each of these therapies have been claimed to have application to arthritis and rheumatism. Relaxation therapy, biofeedback, meditation and hypnotherapy in particular are used in psychologic, medical and paramedical practices, especially for the control of chronic pain. Alternative proponents of the therapies claim control over the underlying disorders. *T'ai chi ch'uan* for example is proposed to improve blood and lymph circulation, increase energy flow, massage organs, calm body and mind, deepen breathing and enhance oxygenation, 'open' joints and thereby alleviate arthritis. It may, in reality, provide useful low stress exercise. Many patients appear to benefit from yoga meditation but these practices require much time in a busy world. A modest controlled trial suggested benefit in painful OA of hands. While warning the reader not to be unduly sceptical about the benefits of meditation because of extravagant claims, Blackmore reviewed the scientifically revealed limitations[87]. Controlled studies have confirmed that pain, including rheumatic pain, can be reduced by relaxation therapy, biofeedback, meditation practices and hypnotherapy. Several studies have shown hypnotherapy to be more effective than acupuncture. Biofeedback has been shown to reduce Raynaud's phenomenon.
Parapsychologic (energy) therapies	
Many of these therapies are new age developments or derivaties of ancient healing arts. Some are used in energy medicine, naturopathy and other alternative practices. A selective list includes: aromatherapy, Bach flower remedies, color therapy, crystals and pyramids, ion generators, magnetic field therapy, radionic and psionic medicine, sound therapy.	Desperate and intrigued patients will often optimistically pursue these therapies, feeling that there is little to lose. Magnetic healing and the health effects of electromagnetic fields were reviewed by Macklis[88].

myth and magic. Detroit: Plenum Press; 1991.
18. Hand WD. Magical medicine. The folkloric component of medicine in the folk belief, custom and ritual of the peoples of Europe and America. Berkeley: University of California Press; 1980.
19. Camp J. Magic, myth and medicine. London: Priory Press Ltd.; 1973.
20. Lyons AS, Petrucelli RJ. Medicine. An illustrated history. New York: Harry N Abrams, Inc.; 1978.
21. Court WE. The doctrine of signatures or similitudes. Trends Pharmacol Sci. 1985;6:225–7.
22. Kahneman D, Slovic P, Tversky A, eds. Judgement under uncertainty: heuristics and biases. Cambridge: Cambridge University Press; 1982.
23. Good BJ. Medicine, rationality and experience. An anthropological perspective. Cambridge: Cambridge University Press; 1994.
24. Brewers Dictionary of Phase and Fable. London: Cassell; 1970.
25. Chaput de Saintonge DM, Herxheimer A. Harnessing placebo effects in health care. Lancet. 1994;344:995–8.
26. Gotzsche PC. Is there logic in the placebo? Lancet. 1994;344:925–6.
27. Oh VMS. The placebo effect. Can we use it better? Br Med J. 1994;309:69–70.
28. Richardson PH. Placebo effects in pain management. Pain Rev. 1994;1:15–32.
29. Turner JA, Deyo RA, Loeser JD, Von Korff M, Fordyce WE. The importance of placebo effects in pain treatment and research. JAMA. 1994;271:1609–14.
30. Peck C, Coleman G. Implications of placebo theory for clinical research and practice in pain management. Theor Med. 1991;12:247–70.
31. Grünbaum A. The placebo concept in medicine and psychiatry. In: Shepherd M, Sartorius N, eds. Non-specific aspects of treatment. Toronto: Hans Huber; 1989:7–38.
32. Kluge E-H. Placebos: some ethical considerations. Can Med Assoc J. 1990;142:293–5.
33. Joyce CRB. Non-specific aspects of treatment from the point of view of a clinical pharmacologist. In: Shepherd M, Sartorius N, eds. Non-specific aspects

of treatment. Toronto: Hans Huber; 1989:57–94.
34. Joyce CRB. Placebo and complementary medicine. Lancet. 1994;344;1279–81.
35. Bland JM, Altman DG. Some examples of regression towards the mean. Br Med J. 1994;309:780.
36. Ernst E, Resch K-L, White AR. Complementary medicine: what physicians think of it: a meta-analysis. Arch Intern Med. 1995;155:2405–8.
37. Helman CG. Limits of biomedical explanation. Lancet. 1991;337:1080–3.
38. Laine C, Davidoff F. Patient-centered medicine. A professional evolution. JAMA. 1996;275:152–6.
39. Glasziou PP, Irwig LM. An evidenced based approach to individualising treatment. Br Med J. 1995;311:1356–8.
40. Stalker DF. Evidence and alternative medicine. Mt Sinai J Med. 1995;62:132–43.
41. Ernst E. Complementary medicine: common misconceptions. J Roy Soc Med. 1995;88:244–7.
42. Alpert JS. The relativity of alternative medicine. Arch Intern Med. 1995;155:2385.
43. Bowman KW, Lee RNF. Cultural issues in critical care: a Chinese case study. Annals RCPSC. 1995;28:228–40.
44. Mayou R. Medically unexplained physical symptoms. Do not overinvestigate. Br Med J. 1991;303:534–5.
45. Sears C. The easy way to sell drugs. New Scientist. 1995;4 Nov:36–40.
46. Kaptchuk TJ. Chinese medicine. The web that has no weaver. London: Rider; 1983.
47. Van Alphen J, Aris A, eds. An illustrated guide to the Asian arts of healing. London: Serina Publications: 1995.
48. Beinfield H, Korngold E. Between heaven and earth: a guide to Chinese Medicine. New York: Ballentine; 1992.
49. Bensky D, Gamble A, Kaptchuk T, complilers and translators. Chinese herbal medicine. Materia medica. Seattle: Eastland Press; Revised edition 1993.
50. Patrick H. Traditional Chinese medicine and public health: the Yin and the Yang. J Roy Soc Med. 1995;88:485–6.
51. Deavin A. Subtle secrets of a 5,000-year tradition. J Alternative Complementary Med. 1989;7:15–18.
52. Sharma HM, Triguna BD, Chopra D. Maharishi Ayur-Veda: modern insights into ancient medicine. JAMA. 1991;265:2633–7.
53. Haldemann S. Principles and practice of chiropractic. Norwalk: Appleton & Lange; 1992.
54. Jarvis KB, Phillips RB, Morris EK. Cost per case comparison of back injury claims of chiropractic versus medical management for conditions with identical diagnostic codes. J Occup Med. 1991;33:847–52.
55. Firman GJ, Goldstein MS. The future of chiropractic: a psychosocial view. New Engl J Med. 1975;293:639–42.
56. Meade TW, Dyer S, Browne W, Townsend J, Franks AO. Low back pain of mechanical origin: randomised comparison of chiropractic and hospital outpatient treatment. Br Med J. 1990;300:1431–7.
57. Haldemann S. Manipulation and massage for the relief of back pain. In: Wall PD, Melzack R, eds. Textbook of pain. Edinburgh: Churchill-Livingstone; 1994:1251–62.
58. Gerber R. Vibrational medicine. New choices for healing ourselves. Santa Fe, New Mexico: Bear and Company; 1988.
59. Brooks SM, Gochfeld M, Herzstein J, Schenker MB, Jackson RJ. Environmental medicine. St Louis: Mosby: 1995.
60. Farnsworth NR, Akerele O, Bingel AS, Soejarto DD, Guo Z. Medicinal plants in therapy. Bulletin of the World Health Organization. 1985;63/6:965–81.
61. Bellamy D, Pfister A. World medicine. Plants, patients and people. Oxford: Blackwell; 1992.
62. Ekerele O. Summary of WHO guidelines for the assessment of herbal medicines. HerbalGram 1992;28:13–20. Available as Classical Botanical Reprint 234.
63. McKee J. Holistic health and the critique of western medicine. Soc Sci Med. 1988;26:775–84.
64. Goleman D, Gurin J, eds. Mind body medicine. How to use your mind for better health. Sydney: Choice Books; 1995.
65. Lockie A, Geddes N. The complete guide to homeopathy. The principles and practice of treatment. New York: Readers Digest Press;1995.
66. Hill C, Doyon F. Review of randomized trials of homoeopathy. Rev Epidemiol Sante Publique. 1990;38:139–47.
67. Kleijnen J, Knipschild P, ter Riet G. Clinical trials of homoeopathy. Br Med J. 1991;302:316–23.
68. Croutier AL. Taking the waters. Spirit, art, sensuality. New York: Abbeville Press; 1992.
69. Baer HA. The potential rejuvenation of American naturopathy as a consequence of the holistic health movement. Med Anthropol. 1992;13:369–83.
70. Chaitow L. Osteopathy: a complete health care system. London: Thorsons; 1982.
71. Buchnanan HM, Preston SJ, Brooks PM, Buchanan WW. Is diet important in rheumatoid arthritis? Br J Rheumatol. 1991;30:125–34.
72. Kjeldsen-Kragh J, Haugen M, Borchgrevink CF et al. Controlled trial of fasting and one-year vegetarian diet in rheumatoid arthritis. Lancet 1991;338:899–902.
73. Alexander FM. The use of the self. London: Gollancz; 1985.
74. Feldenkrais M. Awareness through movement. Health exercises for personal growth. London: Penguin Books; 1977.
75. Koes BW, Assendelft WJ, van der Heijden GJ, Bouter LM, Knipschild PG. Spinal manipulation and mobilisation for back and neck pain: a blinded review. Br Med J 1991;303:1298–303.
76. Koes BW, Bouter LM, van Mameren H et al. Randomised clinical trial of manipulative therapy and physiotherapy for persistent back and neck complaints: results of one year follow-up. Br Med J 1992;304:601–5.
77. Triano JJ, McGregor M, Hondras MA, Brennan PC. Manipulative therapy versus education programs in chonic low back pain. Spine
78. Goats GC. Massage – the scientific basis of an ancient art. Br J Sports Med. 1994;28:149–52,153–6.
79. Shanghai College of Traditional Medicine. Translated and edited by O'Connor J, Bensky D. Acupuncture. A comprehensive text. Seattle: Eastland Press; 1989.
80. Wu D-Z. Acupuncture and neurophysiology. Clin Neurol Neurosurg. 1990;92:13–25.
81. Liao SJ, Lee MHM, Ng LKY. Prinicples and practice of contemporary acupuncture. New York: Marcel Dekker, Inc.; 1994.
82. Stux G, Pomeranz B. Basics of acupuncture. Berlin: Springer; 1995.
83. Vincent C, Lewith G. Placebo controls for acupuncture studies. J Roy Soc Med. 1995;88:199–202.
84. Benor DJ. Spiritual healing research. Holistic Med. 1990;5:87–94.
85. Frank JD, Frank JB. Religiomagical healing. In: Persuasion and healing. A comparative study of psychotherapy. Baltimore: The John Hopkins University Press, 1991: 87–112.
86. Hodges RD, Scholfield AM. Is spiritual healing a valid and effective therapy? J Roy Soc Med. 1995;88:203–7.
87. Blackmore S. Is meditation good for you? New Scientist. 1991;131:24–7.
88. Macklis RM. Magnetic healing, quackery, and the debate about the health effects of electromagnetic fields. Ann Intern Med. 1993;118:376–83.

14

PRINCIPLES OF OUTCOME ASSESSMENT

Nicholas Bellamy

- The assessment of health status in individuals provides information on disease severity and can guide therapy.
- Health status measures can also be of value to disability insurers, litigators and health care agencies concerning the impact of diseases and effect of interventions in individuals and in disease groups.
- Good outcome measures must be ethical, valid, reliable and responsive.
- Measurements of pain, impairment, disability, handicap, patient and physician global assessments, multidimensional health status instruments and adverse treatment reactions are all commonly used in rheumatology.
- Core sets of outcome measures have been recommended for use in trials in specific rheumatic diseases.
- The choice of outcome measures will depend on several factors, including whether they are being used for research purposes, or in general practice.

INTRODUCTION

Outcome assessment is the measurement process whereby the consequences of a decision are evaluated. It is an essential component of health care at all levels, regardless of specialty, from policy making to the treatment of individual patients. While the focus of this chapter is on individual patients, formal assessment of the impact of health care decisions on health care costs, quality of care, quality of life, morbidity and mortality in the population is equally important. Such assessments are an integral part of health care delivery systems.

OUTCOME ASSESSMENT: A CONCEPTUAL FRAMEWORK

The basic sequence of most chronic diseases is that an etiologic event triggers a pathologic response, which results thereafter in a number of clinical manifestations and outcomes. Two types of measures may be used to assess events in that sequence: process measures and outcome measures. Process measures include histologic and biochemical analyses, the measurement of biological markers in various body fluids, imaging procedures [either direct, such as arthroscopy, or indirect, such as magnetic resonance imaging (MRI)] and function tests (e.g. pulmonary function, nerve conduction). In contrast, outcome measures examine the clinical consequences of a disease. Several years ago Fries popularized a paradigm in which outcome was categorized according to five dimensions: the 5Ds – Death, Disability, Discomfort, Drug (or other iatrogenic) reactions and Dollar (or economic) costs[1] (Fig. 14.1). These outcomes are all relevant to patients, are discernible consequences of disease and represent the ultimate outcomes of the disease process and its clinical manifestations. However, the components of health are many and diverse, and it is now possible to measure many different aspects of a patient's condition[2]. A conceptual framework for structuring outcome assessment is shown in Figure 14.2. Although elements such as function and coping have been depicted as separate and distinct entities there is often overlap and interaction between component measures. Furthermore, measurement requirements will differ in different situations, such as epidemiologic research, clinical trials and routine clinical practice.

It is important to appreciate that in the discipline of clinical measurement, or clinical metrology, there is variable and sometimes inap-

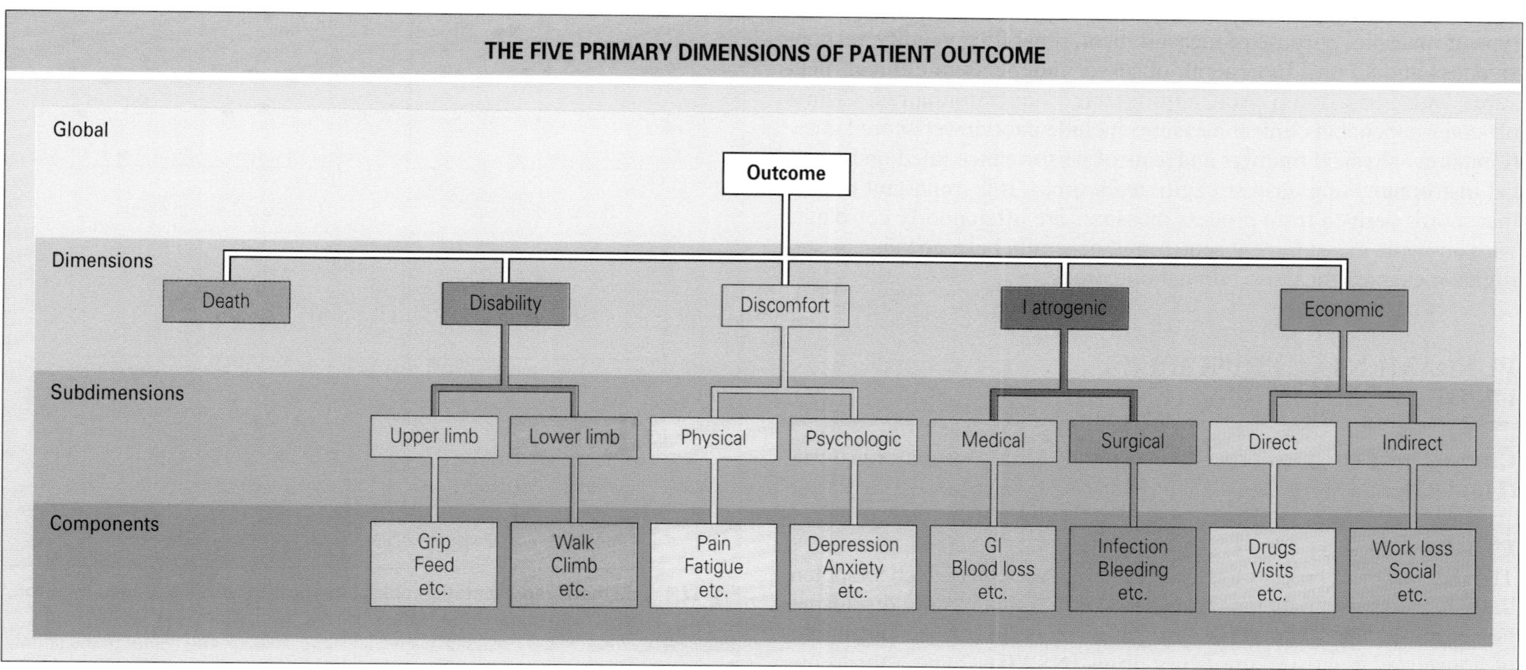

Fig. 14.1 The five dimensions of musculoskeletal outcome. Adapted with permission from Fries and Bird[1].

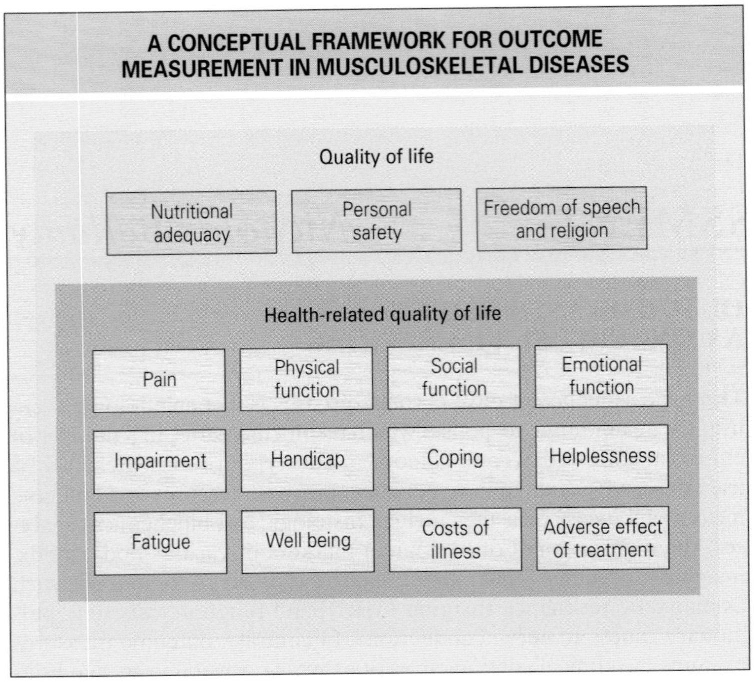

A CONCEPTUAL FRAMEWORK FOR OUTCOME MEASUREMENT IN MUSCULOSKELETAL DISEASES

Quality of life

Nutritional adequacy | Personal safety | Freedom of speech and religion

Health-related quality of life

Pain | Physical function | Social function | Emotional function

Impairment | Handicap | Coping | Helplessness

Fatigue | Well being | Costs of illness | Adverse effect of treatment

Fig. 14.2 A conceptual framework for outcome measurement in musculoskeletal diseases.

propriate use of common terminology. Outcome measures may be divided into two broad categories: observer dependent (or assessor rated) and observer independent (or self-rated). Although the terms 'subjective' (soft) and 'objective' (hard) are frequently used to categorize outcome measures, they should be avoided, since the term 'subjective' may imply that the measurement properties of a technique are inferior, while the term objective may imply erroneously that the technique has greater validity[3]. In fact, some so-called 'subjective' measures have better reliability, validity and responsiveness than other so-called 'objective' measures. Furthermore, certain techniques, such as face-to-face interview, walk time, grip strength and articular index, involve an interaction between the assessor and the patient, so that these techniques are not easily classified as either purely subjective or purely objective. It is more appropriate, therefore, to refer to a measurement technique according to its measurement characteristics (i.e. type of measure, purpose of measurement, reliability, validity, responsiveness and so on). In general, observer-independent clinical measures are based on self-administered questionnaires, while observer-dependent clinical measures include interviewer-scored questionnaires, physical findings and tests of performance rated on technical instruments (e.g. grip strength, walk time). It is important to note that scores derived from process measures are often poorly correlated with outcome measurement scores, and generally have no value as surrogate measures for those clinical outcomes.

FUNDAMENTAL PRINCIPLES OF OUTCOME ASSESSMENT

Outcome measurement procedures should fulfill four major criteria[2] (Fig. 14.3).

ETHICS

The measurement process must be ethical [2]. Processes which are potentially hazardous to patients raise ethical issues that require disclosure. For example, the inherent risks of gastroscopy [in endoscopic studies of nonsteroidal anti-inflammatory drugs (NSAIDs)] and arthroscopy (in chondroscopy studies) must be explained to, and accepted by, study participants. Where possible, less invasive procedures should be

MAJOR CRITERIA FOR OUTCOME ASSESSMENT TECHNIQUES FOR MUSCULOSKELETAL DISEASES

- The measurement process must be ethical.
- Validity should be adequate for achieving measurement objectives.
- Reliability should be adequate for achieving measurement objectives.
- Responsiveness must be adequate, i.e. the technique must be able to detect a clinically important improvement or deterioration.

Fig. 14.3 Major criteria for outcome assessment techniques for musculoskeletal diseases. Adapted with kind permission of Bellamy[2] and Kluwer Academic Publishers.

employed. Finally, the importance and necessity of acquiring new information should be weighed against any attendant risks.

VALIDITY

Validity is a measure of the extent to which an instrument specifically measures the phenomenon of interest[2]. In contrast, reliability defines the extent to which the measurement procedure yields the same result on repeated determinations. Validity and reliability are separate clinimetric issues, and it does not follow that because a measure is reliable it is also valid or *vice versa* (Fig. 14.4). More specifically, validity is concerned with sources of nonrandom error (i.e. systematic error or bias) whereas reliability is concerned with sources of random error, also known as noise. Systematic error or bias may prevent an instrument from truly measuring what is intended, which results in inaccuracy. A number of different strategies may be employed to determine

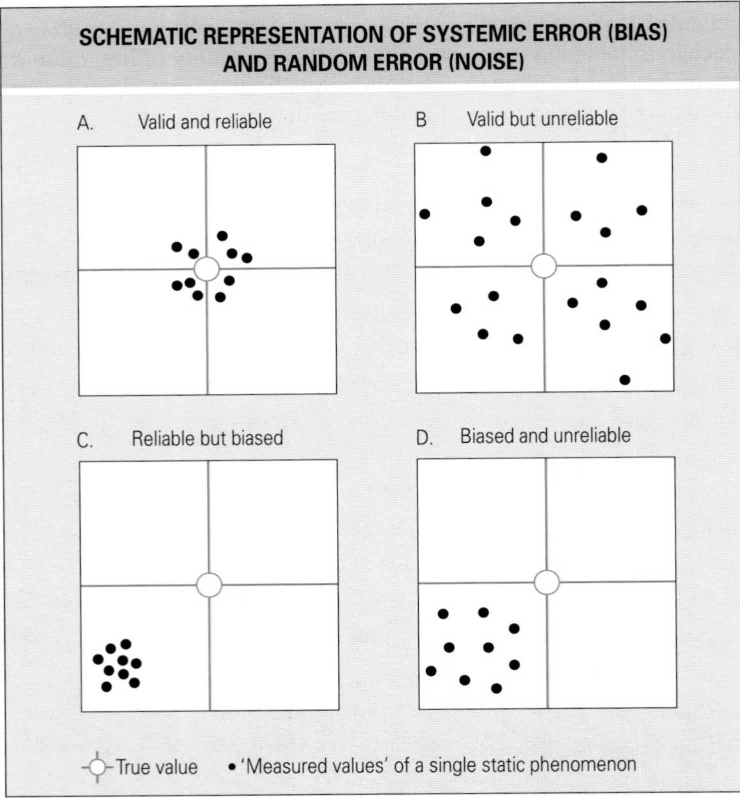

Fig. 14.4 Schematic representation of systematic error (bias) and random error (noise). A comparison of measurements which are: valid and reliable (a); valid but unreliable (b); reliable but biased(c); biased and unreliable (d). The center of the target (0) represents the true value and the black circles(•) represent the 'measured values' of a single static phenomenon. Adapted with kind permission of Bellamy[2] and Kluwer Academic Publishers.

validity, each conceptually different and relying on different methods of assessment. There are four types of validity: face, content, construct and criterion.

Face validity

A measure has face validity if experts judge that it measures at least part of the defined phenomenon[2]. In many instances this is self-evident, whereas in others, particularly in measures of functional status, it may not be entirely obvious whether the measurement reflects physical, social or emotional function.

Content validity

An instrument can have face validity but fail to capture in its entirety the dimension of interest[2]. Content validity, therefore, is a measure of comprehensiveness – the extent to which the measure encompasses all relevant aspects of the defined attribute. Content validity is generally determined by group consensus (e.g. nominal or Delphi techniques). The decision regarding which items should be included in an instrument and which excluded is critical, because it defines the nature of the instrument and its future applicability. Any subsequent addition or deletion results in an instrument that requires further validation.

Given the variability in symptom expression by patients, one of two approaches can be employed to achieve comprehensiveness. The first is to include a standard battery of measures that probes frequently occurring symptoms which are clinically important to the majority of patients. In the second approach, the measurement process is tailored to the individual by measuring only those items which are important to each person. The issue of importance can be decided by patients, who rate the importance of their symptoms, or by clinical assessors, whose decision is based on their perception of the patient's symptoms.

Construct validity

Construct validity is of two types: convergent and discriminant[2]. Both are tested by demonstrating relationships between measurement scores and a theoretical manifestation (i.e. construct or consequence of an attribute) of the disease. Convergent construct validity testing is assessed by the statistical correlation between scores on a single health component, as measured by two different instruments. If the correlation coefficient is positive and appreciably above zero, the new measure is said to have convergent construct validity[2]. In contrast, discriminant construct validity testing compares correlation coefficients between scores on the same health component, as measured by two different instruments (e.g. separate measures of physical function), and between scores on that health component and each of several other health components (e.g. measures of social and emotional function). A measure has discriminant construct validity if the proposed measure correlates better with a second measure, accepted as more closely related to the construct, than it does with a third, more distantly related measure[2].

Criterion validity

Criterion validity is assessed by statistically testing a new measurement technique against an independent criterion or standard (concurrent validity) or against a future standard (predictive validity)[2]. Criterion validity is an estimate of the extent to which a measure agrees with a 'gold standard' (i.e. an external criterion of the phenomenon being measured). The major problem in criterion validity testing is the general lack of gold standards. Indeed, some purported gold standards may not provide completely accurate estimates of the true value of a phenomenon.

RELIABILITY

Consistency, reproducibility, repeatability and agreement are synonyms for reliability[2]. Reliability is the extent to which a measurement procedure yields the same result on repeated determinations (Fig. 14.4). This determination may either be the result of different measurements performed at the same time, or the same measurements performed at different times. Repeated measurements are rarely exactly the same, since there is always some random error, noise or degree of inconsistency. There are various methods of calculating reliability, each method reflecting a different aspect of instrument performance such that different coefficients are derived using different methods. Defined sources of measurement error include the subject, the assessor and the measuring instrument. Patient variability often arises from normal variation in symptoms or from fatigue or inattention. Observer variability may be the result of inadequate standardization, the necessity for complex judgments, perceptual elements or fatigue. Technical instruments may also vary, such as the cuff configuration of the modified sphygmometer or mechanical resistance in a dynamometer or dolorimeter.

RESPONSIVENESS (SENSITIVITY TO CHANGE)

The primary goal of outcome assessment is to detect clinically important changes in some aspect of a condition[2]. In order to detect change, a measurement technique needs to be targeted on aspects of the disease amenable to change, using scaling methods that allow detection of change, and be applied at a point in time when change might have occurred. Validity and reliability are important aspects of measurement techniques, but the capacity to detect change is the quintessential requirement of a successful outcome measure. It is important to note that an assessment technique may fail to record any clinical improvement for a number of reasons (e.g. patient lacks response potential, lacks compliance with the treatment program, has inefficacious treatment, insensitive outcome measure or a Type II error occurs due to inadequate sample size).

The precise definition of a minimum clinically important change in health status is elusive. The magnitude of the difference depends on a number of factors including:

- the assessment technique being used (mainly due to differences in scale lengths);
- the nature of the intervention (drugs, physical therapy, surgery);
- the comparison being made (active or placebo comparisons);
- the adverse effect profile of the intervention; and
- the cost and convenience of the treatment program.

Preliminary estimates of minimum clinically important differences for some outcome measures have been published[2].

OUTCOME ASSESSMENT TECHNIQUES

There are literally hundreds of techniques for assessing the beneficial and adverse outcomes of treatment. A number of health status instruments have been developed to assess particular conditions (see Fig. 14.5) (see also Appendix: selected measures for outcome assessment of rheumatic diseases). Readers interested in specific measurement issues should consult one or more standard measurement texts[2,4,5]. This section will briefly review the measurement of pain, impairment, disability, handicap, patient and physician global assessments, multidimensional health status instruments (quality of life, utility), process measures and adverse drug reactions.

PAIN

Pain is an entirely subjective phenomenon, the perception of which is modulated by a variety of influences, and results in pain behaviors which may be observed[2]. The severity of perceived pain can only be rated by the sufferer. In contrast, pain behavior can be rated by a trained assessor. Individuals who deliberately either augment or minimize their reported pain are probably in the minority. Pain can be assessed using a variety of techniques, including the Likert (LK) or adjectival scale, visual analog (VA) scale, ladder scale, numerical rating scale, chromatic continuous analog scale, pain faces scale, McGill Pain Questionnaire[6] or behavioral observation techniques[7] (see Fig. 14.6). Of these, the LK and VA scales are most frequently employed – several valid, reliable and responsive pain scales having been developed.

When applying pain scales, it is important to specify the aspect of

CATEGORIZATION OF SELECTED HEALTH STATUS MEASURES FOR OUTCOME ASSESSMENT IN MUSCULOSKELETAL DISEASES
General arthritis measures
Health Assessment Questionnaire (HAQ): Arthritis Rheum. 1980;23:127–45. Arthritis Impact Measurement Scales (AIMS): Arthritis Rheum. 1980;23:146–52. Arthritis Impact Measurement Scales (AIMS2): Arthritis Rheum. 1992;35:1–10. Clinical Health Assessment Questionnaire (CLINHAQ): Arthritis Rheum. 1989;32:S99.
Rheumatoid arthritis related
Rapid Assessment of Disease Activity in Rheumatology (RADAR): Arthritis Rheum. 1992;35:156–62. McMaster Toronto Arthritis Patient Preference Disability Questionnaire (MACTAR): J Rheumatol. 1987;14:446–51.
Osteoarthritis related
Australian/Canadian Hand Index (AUSCAN): Scand J Rheumatol .1996;Suppl.106:5. Dreiser Algofunctional Index: Rev Rhum [Engl. Ed.] 1995;62(Suppl 1):43S–53S. Indices of Clinical Severity (Lequesne): Semin Arthritis Rheum 1991;20 (Suppl 2, June):48–54. Western Ontario and McMaster Universities (WOMAC) Osteoarthritis Index. J Rheumatol 1988;15:1833–40.
Ankylosing spondylitis related
Bath Ankylosing Spondylitis Indices: J Rheumatol. 1995;22:740–44. Dougados Functional Index: J Rheumatol. 1988;15:302–7. Dutch AS Index: Br J Rheumatol. 1994;33:842–6. HAQ-S: J Rheumatol. 1990;17:946–50.
Fibromyalgia related
Fibromyalgia Impact Questionnaire (FIQ): J Rheumatol. 1991;18:728–33.
Low back pain related
Low Back Pain Scale: Pain. 1978;4:273–81. Roland & Morris Scale: Spine. 1983;8:45–50;141–44. Oswestry Low Back Pain Disability Questionnaire: Physiotherapy. 1980;66:271–3. Million Instrument: Spine. 1982;7:204–12.
Systemic lupus erythematosus related
British Isles Lupus Assessment Group's Index (BILAG): Q J Med. 1988;69:927–37. Systemic Lupus Activity Measure (SLAM): Arthritis Rheum. 1989;32:1107–18. Systemic Lupus Erythematosus Disease Activity Index (SLEDAI): Arthritis Rheum. 1992;35:630–40.
Handicap
Disease Repercussion Profile (DRP): Br J Rheumatol. 1996;35:921–32.
Fatigue
Multidimensional Assessment of Fatigue: Nurs Res. 1993;42:93–9. Piper Fatigue Scale: Oncol Nurs Forum. 1990;17:661–2.
Coping
Coping with Rheumatic Stressors (CORS): Br J Rheumatol. 1994;33:1067–73. Coping Strategies Questionnaire: Pain. 1983;17:33–44. London Coping with RA Questionnaire: Psychol Health. 1990;4:187–200. Self Efficacy Scale: Arthritis Rheum. 1989;32:37–44.
Helplessness
Arthritis Helplessness Index: J Rheumatol. 1988;15:427–32. Rheumatology Attitudes Index: J Rheumatol. 1988;15:418–26.
Quality of life
SF-36: Med Care. 1992;30:473–81. NHP: Soc Sci Med. 1981;15A:221–9. EuroQol: Br J Rheumatol. 1994;33:655–62. Quality of Well-Being Scale: Health Services Res. 1976;11:478–507. Sickness Impact Profile: Med Care. 1981;19:787–805. HUI: J Clin Oncol. 1992;10:923–8. Standard Gamble: Socioecon Planning Sci. 1976;10:129–36. Time Trade-Off: J Health Econ. 1986;5:1–30.

Fig. 14.5 Categorization of selected health status measures for outcome assessment in musculoskeletal diseases.

pain which is being assessed (e.g. stair climbing, walking, rest, night, overall) and the time interval over which pain is being evaluated (e.g. 48 hours, 1 week, etc). Several segregated multidimensional health status instruments, including the Health Assessment Questionnaire (HAQ)[8], Arthritis Impact Measurement Scales (AIMS and AIMS2)[9,10] and Western Ontario and McMaster Universities Osteoarthritis Index (WOMAC)[11], contain distinct pain subscales (see Appendix: selected measures for outcome assessment of rheumatic diseases).

IMPAIRMENT, DISABILITY AND HANDICAP

The terms impairment, disability and handicap are often confused. Fortunately the World Health Organization (WHO) has characterized these three different entities[12]. Impairment is defined as any loss or abnormality of psychologic, physiologic or anatomic structure or function. It signifies that a pathologic state has reached a stage of detectability. In contrast, disability includes any restriction or lack of ability to perform an activity in the manner considered normal. Such disabilities include alteration in behavior, interactive processes such as communication, as well as strictly physical functions. A handicap is manifest as a disadvantage experienced by an individual as a result of an impairment or disability, such that it limits or prevents the fulfilment of a role considered normal for that individual. In essence, therefore, impairment occurs at an organ level (intellectual, sensory, visceral, musculoskeletal), disability at a personal level (behavior, self-care, locomotion, dexterity) and handicap at a social level (independence, geographic mobility, employability, social integration)[12].

Impairment

Examination-based measures are often directed at the assessment of abnormalities in structure (e.g. swelling, tenderness). As such they are categorized as measures of impairment. The most important examination-based measurement procedure is the separate enumeration of swollen and tender joints in patients with inflammatory polyarthritis[2]. There has been debate regarding the use of binary (present or absent) versus graded evaluations dependent on the degree of abnormality, total versus reduced joint counts, and area-weighted versus non weighted articular indices. By consensus, however, the preferred method is to

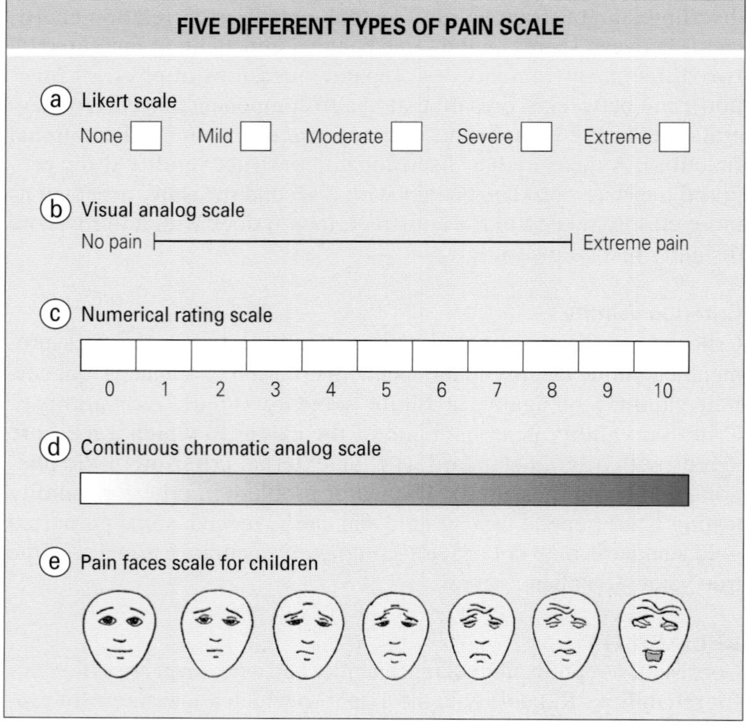

Fig. 14.6 Five different types of pain scales. Likert scale (a), visual analog scale (b), numerical rating scale (c), chromatic continuous analog scale (d), pain faces scale (e; Bieri[49]).

use separate counts of the number of swollen and tender joints, such as the American College of Rheumatology (ACR) 68 joint count, or the European League Against Rheumatism (EULAR) 28 joint count. It is convenient to chart individual joint involvement on a humunculus or mannequin (Fig. 14.7). Other methods have been developed for scoring joint involvement in osteoarthritis (OA), enthesopathy in ankylosing spondylitis (AS) and tender points in fibromyalgia[2]. Methods for assessing other clinical signs, such as heat, erythema and crepitus, have been less rigorously studied[13].

Disability

Functional measures can be subdivided into those based on observed tests of performance and questionnaires that assess functional capacity.

Performance-based measures

Performance-based measures might at first seem the most direct way to assess the patient's function[2]. However, such measures often involve an interaction between the assessor and subject which may augment or diminish the true performance. Furthermore, observer reliability may be a problem and a change in performance on the test may not correspond to a change in the performance of the related activities of daily living. Nevertheless, some measures, such as the modified Schober test in ankylosing spondylitis, grip strength in rheumatoid arthritis (RA), and range of movement in knee OA, remain in common usage. There are a large number of performance-based assessment techniques, some based on microprocessor technology. Several of the latter techniques have specific research applications but are not currently relevant to the clinical practice of rheumatology (e.g. dynamic measures of grip strength or joint movement)[2].

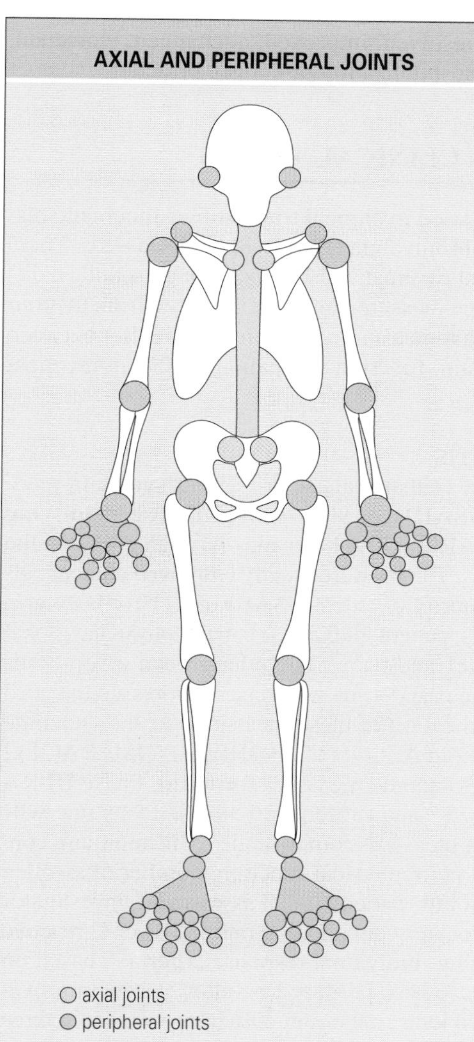

Fig. 14.7 A humunculus (or mannequin) for recording joint involvement due to arthritis in routine clinical care.

Capacity-based measurement

Musculoskeletal patients may suffer three types of functional disability: physical, emotional and social. All three forms are amenable to outcome assessment using valid, reliable and responsive questionnaires. Physical disability, in particular, has received considerable attention, some techniques being designed for a specific purpose while others have multipurpose applications (Fig. 14.5)[2]. Physical disablement is one of the two most important and immediate consequences of most musculoskeletal conditions. The capacity to measure this aspect of the disease, both in clinical trials and clinical practice, is paramount. Several fully validated health status instruments include separate measures of pain and function and are to be preferred over *ad hoc* scales. Disease-specific measures of function include the WOMAC Index (OA), the Bath Ankylosing Spondylitis Functional Index (BASFI)[14], the Dougados Index (AS)[15] and the Fibromyalgia Impact Questionnaire (FIQ)[16]. In contrast, measures such as the HAQ, AIMS and AIMS2 have multipurpose applications. It should be noted that the ACR Functional Classification Criteria were developed for the classification of global function not as outcome criteria[17]. As a result measures such as the HAQ, AIMS, AIMS2 and WOMAC are preferred as outcome measures in RA and OA studies, since their scaling properties are capable of detecting small, but nevertheless clinically important, changes in functional capacity.

The measurement of emotional disability in musculoskeletal disease is important, as considerable psychologic morbidity has been noted in patients with musculoskeletal disorders. Furthermore, it is not surprising, given the degree of pain, disability, anxiety, depression and diminished sense of well being, that many musculoskeletal disorders have social consequences.

Handicap

Measures of handicap reflect the social consequence of disease. Whether an individual is handicapped can be defined either by society or by an individual. Carr has recently illustrated this point as follows: '...a keen amateur musician with relatively mild RA may find that he is unable to play his instrument, but is able to continue work as a personnel manager. From society's perspective, he would not be considered handicapped, but at a personal level, the loss of what is to him a very important activity would represent considerable disadvantage'[18].

Until recently the measurement of handicap in the rheumatic diseases has attracted relatively little attention. The recent publication of the Disease Repercussion Profile, a valid and reliable measure of patient-perceived handicap, represents a significant advance in this previously underdeveloped area of musculoskeletal clinical measurement[18].

GLOBAL ASSESSMENTS

Global assessments by patient and physician of the patient's overall condition are commonly used in clinical trials and in clinical practice[2]. It is extremely important to specify in the wording of the global question which aspects of the patient's condition are being considered (e.g. overall health status, symptom severity, disease activity, etc.). The patient global assessment is particularly important as it can be phrased to assess current status or change in status and be focused on a particular anatomic area, the condition in general or the patient as a whole. Alternatively, it can be used to assess drug tolerability and/or efficacy or other aspects of the treatment program (palatability, compliance, affordability, convenience). The time frame over which the patient should consider his or her status should be defined (e.g. 48 hours, one week). It is debatable whether the physician global assessment adds anything to the measurement process over and above the patient global assessment. However, the physician (or other assessor) can consider in addition aspects of the condition which are not assessable by the patient (e.g. radiographic change, biochemical, hematologic, immunologic abnormalities) and may have insight into whether the patient tends to amplify or minimize reported symptoms. Again, the physician requires clear specification as to which aspects of the condition should be considered when making his or her assessment. The time frame for the physician global assessment usually should be specified as 'today' since the assessor generally has no knowledge of the patient's prior status, other than that described by the patient and captured by the patient global assessment.

MULTIDIMENSIONAL HEALTH STATUS INSTRUMENTS

In addition to unidimensional measurement techniques, a large number of disease-specific and generic multidimensional health status instruments (HSI) have been developed[2]. Many are very sophisticated instruments which have undergone extensive validation procedures and have high performance with superior levels of validity, reliability and responsiveness. They are either self-administered or interviewer administered. It is important for users to contact the originator prior to initial application for instructions regarding usage (e.g. presentation, scoring, analysis), permission for use and guidance regarding copyright and royalty issues. The latest version of the instrument should be obtained as well as a copy of the user's guide.

Some HSIs have been developed in the form of segregated multidimensional indices (SMIs) which contain separate, distinct subscales that explore different aspects of the condition, such as HAQ, AIMS, AIMS2 and WOMAC. They provide subscale scores on each of several separate dimensions. Others are in the form of aggregated multidimensional indices (AMIs), where scores from several different dimensions are weighted and aggregated into a single score, such as the Lequesne Clinical Severity Indices[19], Pooled Index[20], Disease Activity Score[21] and Stoke Index[22]. Health-related quality of life can be assessed either using a multi-item questionnaire, such as SF-36 and its derivative SF-12[23], Nottingham Health Profile (NHP)[24], EuroQol[25] (see also the Appendix: selected measures for outcome assessment of rheumatic diseases) or using a utility-based methodology, for example the Health Utilities Index (HUI)[26], Standard Gamble, Time Trade Off or Category Scaling. A utility is a holistic measure of the quality of life which rates an individual along a continuum from death (0.0) to full health (1.0).

Still other multidimensional HSIs assess not only musculoskeletal symptoms but also multisystem involvement by connective tissue diseases, such as the Systemic Lupus Erythematosus Disease Activity Index (SLEDAI)[27] (see Chapter 7.7), or use several scales to assess different aspects of a condition, for example the Bath Ankylosing Spondylitis Indices[14]. Many of the aforementioned instruments represent the current state of the art in musculoskeletal clinical metrology.

PROCESS MEASUREMENT TECHNIQUES

Plain radiographs are the most frequently employed process measure used in musculoskeletal outcome assessment. The method of scoring films must be standardized for comparative purposes. In RA, hand films are scored by either the Sharp or Larsen methods[28]. In OA, standard methods have been developed for taking radiographs (e.g. anteroposterior standing semiflexed views of the knees). The original scoring system for OA, developed by Kellgren and Lawrence[29], has been superseded by two recent atlases by Altman *et al.*[30] and Burnett *et al.*[31]. To assess joint space narrowing in the medial compartment of the knee, the microfocal method, scored by computer, currently represents the most refined technique[32]. Imaging methods, based on computer tomography (CT), ultrasonography, scintiscanning and thermography, have found application. Volumetric MRI may find future application in outcome assessment but is subject to ongoing validation. Dual energy X-ray absorptiometry (DEXA) is widely applied in bone mineral density (BMD) determination in patients with osteoporosis.

The most useful ancillary tests for repeated outcome assessments are those that are not invasive. Although a scoring system for chondropathy in OA (requiring direct arthroscopic visualization of the cartilage) is available for research purposes, it currently has limited applicability in routine clinical practice. Pulmonary function testing in patients with scleroderma and urinary sediment microscopy in patients with lupus are obvious applications of two harmless noninvasive procedures for monitoring visceral involvement. Other noninvasive markers of the disease process have potentially important future applications in diagnostic, prognostic and evaluative research.

ADVERSE REACTIONS

Adverse reactions caused by treatment can result in symptoms, clinical signs, laboratory abnormalities or death. Problems often arise in detecting, categorizing, attributing and grading adverse events. Adverse event rates differ significantly depending on whether the assessment is based on open-ended questioning or structured questionnaires, or is determined by a standard protocol. Two systems of categorizing adverse events in clinical trials are the Coding Symbols for Thesaurus of Adverse Reaction Terms (COSTART)[33], and the WHO Adverse Reaction Dictionary (WHOARD)[34]. Both systems categorize side effects according to defined structures. In addition, a subindex of COSTART provides a COSTART to WHOARD translation. The routine use of these coding systems to categorize adverse reactions is an important step in the international standardization of measurement procedures.

Attribution is the process of ascribing adverse reactions to interventions or other causes. The etiologic relationship is often graded as none, possible, probable or definite. A number of factors determine the assigned level of the relationship including prior knowledge of the patient, the pharmacodynamic profile of the intervention and the duration of treatment. The most difficult attribution decisions are in assigning the grades of 'none versus possible' and 'probable versus definite', and in grading the intensity of an adverse reaction. Often severity is rated as being mild, moderate or severe. A mild adverse reaction is one which is easily tolerated by the patient, causes minimal discomfort and does not interfere with every day activities. A moderate side effect is an adverse experience which causes sufficient discomfort to interfere with normal everyday activities, while a severe reaction is an adverse experience which is incapacitating and prevents normal everyday activities. Finally, it is important to categorize the outcome of an adverse reaction, for example as resolved, improved, unchanged, worsened, hospitalization required, hospitalization prolonged or death.

MEASUREMENT IN CLINICAL TRIALS

Measurement procedures used in clinical trials in four rheumatic diseases [RA, OA, AS and fibromyalgia (FM)] will be discussed[2]. There are more than 100 different rheumatic disorders, each presenting a different challenge in outcome measurement. It can be seen from the four disorders reviewed here that measurement preferences differ between different disorders, but pain, function and patient global assessment are often emphasized.

RHEUMATOID ARTHRITIS

In general, RA clinical trials either evaluate fast-acting, symptom-modifying drugs, such as NSAIDs or slow-acting disease modifying antirheumatic drugs (SAARDs). The latter may have an effect on the underlying disease process. The most frequently employed clinical outcome measures in the majority of recent NSAID trials have been grip strength, morning stiffness, patient global assessment, physician global assessment, articular index and pain[2]. There have been several outcome conferences over the past decade which have addressed the need for international standardization of these measures. At the Outcome Measurement in Rheumatoid Arthritis Clinical Trials (OMERACT) I conference, a core set of outcome measures for future Phase III RA clinical trials was proposed[35] and subsequently ratified[36] by the ACR (Fig. 14.8). The following measures comprise the ACR minimum core set for RA clinical trials: pain, physical function, number of swollen joints, number of tender joints, patient global assessment, investigator global assessment, erythrocyte sedimentation rate (ESR) or C-reactive protein (CRP), and imaging. Individual response criteria[37], based on these clinical variables, have been proposed as follows: 20% improvement in tender and swollen joint counts and 20% improvement in three of the five remaining ACR core set measures; patient and physician

CORE SETS OF OUTCOME MEASURES FOR RHEUMATOID ARTHRITIS AND OSTEOARTHRITIS CLINICAL TRIALS
Rheumatoid arthritis:
pain function number of tender joints number of swollen joints patient global assessment physician global assessment CRP or ESR radiographs (for disease-modifying studies)
Osteoarthritis:
pain function patient global assessment imaging (for studies of ≥1 year)

Fig. 14.8 Core sets of outcome measures for rheumatoid arthritis and osteoarthritis clinical trials.

global assessments; pain; disability; and an acute-phase reactant. The aforementioned variables should be assessed with validated methods using standardized techniques.

OSTEOARTHRITIS

Clinical trials in OA can be subdivided into those that assess symptom-modifying OA drug effects (SyMOAD) and those that assess structure-modifying OA drug effects (StMOAD). To date, no drugs prevent, arrest or repair structural damage in OA. A recent review of OA clinical trials demonstrated that the majority of studies have used clinical outcome measures of pain, physician global assessment and patient global assessment[2]. A core set for OA was proposed recently by participants at the OMERACT III conference[38], and has been endorsed at an Osteoarthritis Research Society (OARS) Task Force Workshop[39] (Fig. 14.8). The core set for future Phase III studies in hip, knee and hand OA is pain, function, patient global assessment and, for studies of 1 year or longer, joint imaging using validated methods and standardized techniques. No response criteria have yet been established for OA.

ANKYLOSING SPONDYLITIS

There has been no international consensus on a core set of outcome measures for Phase III studies in AS. However, the most frequently used measures in recent AS studies (≥50% of trials) have been pain, morning stiffness, chest expansion, the Schober test and finger to floor distance[2].

FIBROMYALGIA

There has been no international agreement on a core set of measures for future Phase III trials in FM. However, the most frequently used measures in recent FM studies (≥50% of trials) have been tender points, patient global assessment, fatigue, quality of sleep, pain and stiffness[2].

MEASUREMENT IN CLINICAL PRACTICE

Measurement procedures in clinical practice either support the research interests of investigator clinicians or underpin individual management decisions in routine clinical care. Unlike the randomized controlled clinical trial, data collection is not necessarily confined to a single disorder, a fixed number of patients, or a finite number of assessment points. As a result, the quantity of data may progressively increase. In the majority of rheumatology practices data collection has to be performed either by the rheumatologist or by a trained assistant, which produces significant constraints. For this reason, careful consideration needs to be given to the following four questions:

- Why is data collection necessary (i.e. what important questions will be answered)?
- How will data be collected?
- How will data be analyzed?
- How will the logistic requirements of an expanding data base be met?

OUTCOME MEASUREMENT FOR INVESTIGATOR CLINICIANS

Clinic-based studies may provide valid information regarding natural history, prognosis and the results of treatment programs[40]. Such studies are complex because clinic patients are less highly selected (comparable with randomized controlled trials), although in some health care systems they have already passed through a referral filter in order to access specialist care. Furthermore, such patients may be affected by comorbidities, take concomitant therapies, be exposed to multiple changes in antirheumatic therapy, or sometimes to combinations of drugs, and be followed over long periods of time. The success of clinic-based studies is often dependent on data acquired using Patient Self-Report Questionnaires (PSQs), since they can be completed by the patient while sitting in the waiting room and place less burden on clinic staff. Pincus has identified nine properties of PSQ data that make them particularly useful in routine rheumatology care[40]:

- Data are highly reliable, coefficients being among the highest seen in clinical medicine.
- Data are significantly correlated with joint counts, radiographs, laboratory tests and measures of functional status.
- Data at baseline effectively predict values several years later.
- Data are as, or more, effective than other data in predicting long-term functional declines, work disability and mortality in RA patients.
- Data indicate that mortality in RA is associated with greater disease severity.
- Data are as good or better than many other clinical, radiographic or laboratory measures in detecting change in status in clinical trials.
- Data are needed for accurate assessment of long-term outcomes since they may be overlooked by alternate measurement methods.
- Measurable insight is provided into important psychologic problems of patients.
- The tests are sensitive, simple, inexpensive and can be used in any rheumatologist's office to document and monitor clinical status.

It is essential for long-term success that the procedures and processes used are fast and simple, otherwise there is a high risk of frustration and fatigue on the part of the patient, the clinic staff or both. Wolfe and

CHARACTERISTICS OF HEALTH STATUS QUESTIONNAIRES FOR ROUTINE USE IN THE CLINIC

- Health status questionnaires (HSQs) must be short, not use more than minimal staff time and not disturb the routine of the clinic. They must fit into the routine of the clinic.
- HSQs must help the physician and staff with record keeping, not impede it. They must assist in documentation of clinical care.
- Cost must be minimal.
- The results must be available at the time the patient is seen.
- Comparison with previous data and with other patients must be contemporaneous.
- The results must be intuitive and interpretable.
- The information must be more than just additional data. It must be clinically useful.

Fig. 14.9 Characteristics of health status questionnaires for routine use in the clinic. (Reproduced with permission of Wolfe and Pincus[41].)

EXAMPLES OF QUANTITATIVE MEASUREMENT BATTERIES FOR ROUTINE ASSESSMENT IN AS, FM, OA AND RA PATIENTS IN ROUTINE CLINICAL CARE

Condition	Pain	Function	Patient global	Physician global	Articular index[a]	Quality of life[b]
Ankylosing spondylitis	BASI	BASI	Likert	Likert		SF-36/SF-12
Fibromyalgia	FIQ	FIQ	Likert	Likert		SF-36/SF-12
Osteoarthritis (hip or knee)	WOMAC	WOMAC	Likert	Likert		SF-36/SF-12
Osteoarthriits (hand)	AUSCAN	AUSCAN	Likert	Likert		SF-36/SF-12
Osteoarthritis (generalized)	HAQ	HAQ	Likert	Likert		SF-36/SF-12
Rheumatoid arthritis	HAQ	HAQ	Likert	Likert	ACR/EULAR*	SF-36/SF-12

Fig. 14.10 Examples of quantitative measurement batteries for outcome assessment in RA, OA, AS and FM patients in routine clinical care . It may be necessary to supplement the efficacy battery with specific procedures for monitoring drug toxicity or other adverse outcomes. [a] Useful in measuring response to disease-modifying antirheumatic drugs. [b] Optional at the time of writing.
BASI, Bath ankylosing spondylitis. These indices contain measures for function (BASFI), disease activity (BASDAI), global status (BASG), radiology (BASRI), psychology (BASPSYCH) and metrology (BASMI)[14].

Pincus have identified seven characteristics of PSQs for use in the clinic[41] (Fig. 14.9). The Modified Health Assessment Questionnaire (MHAQ) and Clinical Health Assessment Questionnaire (CLINHAQ) are two of several useful general purpose instruments. For certain types of patients, however, disease-specific questionnaires, such as the WOMAC, FIQ, BASI, or Dougados Functional Index may be required, as well as, or instead, of these more general measures. For the investigator clinician, data management will be more of a problem than outcome measurement. Interested readers are referred to the experience of Wolfe (CLINHAQ–ARION system) and Pincus (MHAQ–Vanderbilt system)[41] and to recent reviews regarding database issues for tracking patients with RA[42], systemic lupus erythematosus and other connective tissue disorders[43], FM[44] and back pain[45].

OUTCOME MEASUREMENT IN ROUTINE CLINICAL PRACTICE

The needs of the private practice rheumatologist, working alone or in a small group, may not easily be met by complex data management systems, particularly if the necessary logistic support and computer skills are not readily available, or if there is no investigational goal. For many practitioners the goal will be to efficiently track the progress of individual patients. In clinical practice, a decision must be made whether to formally assess all patients, or only patients with a certain disorder or only selected patients. The most obvious patients to assess are those with chronic disorders in whom long-term follow-up is anticipated, (e.g. RA, OA, seronegative spondyloarthropathies, FM and connective tissue disorders), rather than those in whom a cure, or complete recovery is anticipated in the short-term (e.g. gout or rotator cuff tendinitis). In recent surveys conducted in Canada[46] and Australia[47] rheumatologists were more likely longitudinally to follow patients with RA and AS than those with OA or FM.

Practitioners commonly evaluate patient outcomes on the basis of a combination of the interview and physical examination, radiographic and/or other ancillary data, and patient and physician global assessments. There is considerable variation in the clinical measurement techniques preferred by different rheumatologists in routine outpatient care when following patients with RA, OA, AS and FM[46,47]. The essential characteristics of a measure for outpatient care in Canada and Australia are simplicity, rapid completion, easy scoring, reliability, validity and sensitivity to change[46,47].

Despite excellent measurement properties many of the multidimensional health status instruments previously described are used infrequently in routine clinical care. Indeed, the major emphasis in clinical metrology has been on the development of instruments for clinical research rather than for routine clinical purposes. The challenge now is to apply these techniques in clinical practice as well as to build on clinical research experience in order to construct short, simple patient-centered questionnaires that are easily scored and can be used in office practice.

Some examples of measurement batteries that can be used to measure clinically relevant outcomes in RA, OA, AS and FM in routine practice are illustrated in Figure 14.10. Although the wording of global assessment questions has not been standardized internationally, they may be very useful in grading the overall condition in many different disorders. In addition, the SF-36 (or SF-12) may give useful information about health-related quality of life.

Four final issues deserve special consideration:

- Although measures of discomfort (pain), disability (function) and patient and physician global assessment are common to all rheumatic diseases, conditions with extra-articular consequences may require additional organ-specific assessments (e.g. skin scores in scleroderma).
- Outcome measurement in children is problematic. It is important to select scales which are valid, reliable and responsive in this particular group of patients[48,49].
- In addition to defining *a priori* a schedule for assessing the beneficial effects of a treatment program, it is equally important to establish a monitoring schedule for adverse events, particularly for pharmacologic interventions[50]. Such a schedule should be capable of detecting both clinical and nonclinical (laboratory) forms of toxicity in a timely fashion.
- Flow charts are particularly useful in documenting longitudinal change in clinical status, as well as for charting the nonclinical (laboratory) tolerability of antirheumatic drugs. It is important in routine clinical care not only to chart impressions but also to implement standard procedures for monitoring clinical benefit and adverse events in a standardized fashion, using valid, reliable and responsive outcome assessment techniques.

While implementation of what might be termed 'quantitative rheumatology' may require the development of new instruments or modification of existing instruments to meet demands in routine clinical practice, there is no reason why some of the shorter, user-friendly, patient self-administered questionnaires currently available cannot be used immediately. The ability to quantitate the clinical condition provides patients, medical practitioners, allied health professionals, third party payers and litigators with much important and useful information.

REFERENCES

1. Fries JF, Bird HA. The assessment of disability: From first to future principles. Br J Rheumatol. 1983;22(Suppl):48–58.
2. Bellamy N. Musculoskeletal clinical metrology. Dordrecht: Kluwer Academic Publishers; 1993:1–367.
3. Fries JF, Bellamy N. Introduction. In: Bellamy N, ed. Prognosis in the rheumatic diseases. Dordrecht: Kluwer Academic Publishers; 1991:1–10.
4. Spilker B. Quality of life and pharmacoeconomics in clinical trials, 2E. New York: Lippincott-Raven Press; 1996.
5. Streiner DL, Norman GR. Health measurement scales – a practical guide to their development and use, 2E. New York: Oxford University Press; 1995.
6. Melzack R. The McGill Pain Questionnaire: Major properties and scoring methods. Pain. 1975;1:275–99.
7. Anderson KO, Bradley LA, McDaniel LK, *et al.* The assessment of pain in rheumatoid arthritis – validity of a behavioural observation method. Arthritis Rheum. 1987;30:36–43.
8. Fries JF, Spitz P, Kraines RG, Holman HR. Measurement of patient outcome in arthritis. Arthritis Rheum. 1980;23:137–45.
9. Meenan RF, Gertman PM, Mason JH. Measuring health status in arthritis: The Arthritis Impact Measurement Scales. Arthritis Rheum. 1980;23:146–52.
10. Meenan RF, Mason JH, Anderson JJ, Guccione AA, Kazis LE. AIMS2 – the content and properties of a revised and expanded Arthritis Impact Measurement Scales health status questionnaire. Arthritis Rheum. 1992;35:1–10.
11. Bellamy N, Buchanan WW, Goldsmith CH, Campbell J, Stitt LW. Validation study of WOMAC: A health status instrument for measuring clinically important patient relevant outcomes to antirheumatic drug therapy in patients with osteoarthritis of the hip or knee. J Rheumatol. 1988;15:1833–40.
12. World Health Organization.Classification of impairments, disabilities and handicaps. Geneva: WHO, 1980.
13. ARA Glossary Committee, American Rheumatism Association. Dictionary of the rheumatic diseases, Vol 1. Signs and symptoms. New York: Contact Associates International Ltd; 1982.
14. Calin A. The individual with ankylosing spondylitis: Defining disease status and the impact of illness. Br J Rheumatol. 1995;34:663–72.
15. Dougados M, Gueguen A, Nakache J-P, Nguyen M, Amor B. Evaluation of a functional index for patients with ankylosing spondylitis. J Rheumatol. 1990;17:1254–5.
16. Burckhardt CS, Clark SR, Bennett RM. The fibromyalgia impact questionnaire: Development and validation. J Rheumatol. 1991;18:728–33.
17. Hochberg MC, Chang RW, Dwosh I, Lindsey S, Pincus T, Wolfe F. The American College of Rheumatology 1991 revised criteria for the classification of global functional status in rheumatoid arthritis. Arthritis Rheum. 1992;35:498–502.
18. Carr AJ. A patient-centred approach to evaluation and treatment in rheumatoid arthritis: The development of a clinical tool to measure patient-perceived handicap. Br J Rheumatol. 1996;35:921–32.
19. Lequesne MG, Mery C, Samson M, Gerard P. Indexes of severity for osteoarthritis of the hip and knee: Validation- value in comparison with other assessment tests. Scand J Rheumatol. 1987;65(Suppl):85–9.
20. Smythe HA, Helewa A, Goldsmith GH. 'Independent assessor' and 'pooled index' as techniques for measuring treatment effects in rheumatoid arthritis. J Rheumatol. 1977;4:144–52.
21. van der Heijde DMFM, van't Hof MA, van Riel PLCM, van Leeuwen MA, van Rijswijk MH, van de Putte LBA. Validity of single variables and composite indices for measuring disease activity in rheumatoid arthritis. Ann Rheum Dis. 1992;51:177– 81.
22. Davis MJ, Dawes PT, Fowler PD, *et al.* Comparison and evaluation of a disease activity index for use in patients with rheumatoid arthritis.

Br J Rheumatol. 1990;29:111–15.
23. Ware JE Jr, Sherbourne CD. The MOS 36-item Short-Form Health Status survey (SF-36): 1. Conceptual framework and item selection. Med Care. 1992;30:473–83.
24. Hunt SM, McKeena SP, McEwen J, Williams J, Papp E. The Nottingham Health Profile: Subjective health status and medical consultations. Soc Sci Med. 1981;15a:221–9.
25. Economic and Health Outcomes Research Group: Hurst NP, Jobanputra P, Hunter M, Lambert M, Lochhead A, Brown H. Validity of Euroqol – a generic health status instrument – in patients with rheumatoid arthritis. Br J Rheumatol. 1994;33:655–62.
26. Feeny D, Furlong W, Barr RD, Torrance GW, Rosenbaum P, Weitzman S. A comprehensive multiattribute system for classifying the health status of survivors of childhood cancer. J Clin Oncol. 1992;10:923–8.
27. Bombardier C, Gladman DD, Urowitz MB, Caron D, Chang CH. Committee on Prognosis Studies in SLE. Derivation of the SLEDAI – a disease activity index for lupus patients. Arthritis Rheum. 1992;35:630–40.
28. Cuchacovich M, Couret M, Peray P, Gatica H, Sany J. Precision of the Larsen and the Sharp methods of assessing radiologic change in patients with rheumatoid arthritis. Arthritis Rheum. 1992;35:736–9.
29. Kellgren JH. The epidemiology of chronic rheumatism, Atlas of standard radiographs Vol. 2. Oxford: Blackwell Scientific; 1963.
30. Altman RD, Hochberg M, Murphy WA Jr, Wolfe F, Lequesne M. Atlas of individual radiographic features in osteoarthritis. Osteoarthritis Cart. 1995;3(Suppl A):3–70.
31. Burnett S, Hart DJ, Cooper C, Spector TD. A radiographic atlas of osteoarthritis. Dorchester: Springer-Verlag London Ltd; 1994.
32. Buckland-Wright JC, McFarlane DG, Jasani MK, Lynch JA. Quantitative microfocal radiographic assessment of osteoarthritis of the knee from weight bearing tunnel and semiflexed standing views. J Rheumatol. 1994;21:1734–41.
33. US Department of Commerce, National Technical Information Service. COSTART: Coding symbols for thesaurus of adverse reaction terms. 3E. Springfield: US Department of Commerce, National Technical Information Service; 1989.
34. WHO. The WHO adverse reaction dictionary. Uppsala: WHO Collaborating Centre for International Drug Monitoring; 1990.
35. Boers M, Tugwell P, Felson DT, *et al.* World Health Organisation and International League of Associations for Rheumatology core endpoints for symptom modifying antirheumatic drugs in rheumatoid arthritis clinical trials. J Rheumatol. 1994;21(Suppl 41):86–9.
36. Felson DT, Anderson JJ, Boers M, *et al.* The American College of Rheumatology preliminary core set of disease activity markers for rheumatoid arthritis clinical trials. Arthritis Rheum. 1993;36:729–40.
37. Felson DT, Anderson JJ, Boers M, *et al.* American College of Rheumatology preliminary definition of improvement in rheumatoid arthritis. Arthritis Rheum. 1995;38:727–35.
38. Bellamy N, Kirwan J, Boers M, *et al.* Recommendations for a core set of outcome measures for future phase III clinical trials in knee, hip and hand osteoarthritis – consensus development at OMERACT III. J Rheumatol. 1997 [In Press].
39. Osteoarthritis Research Society (OARS) Task Force Report. Design and conduct of clinical trials in patients with osteoarthritis: Recommendations from a task force of the Osteoarthritis Research Society. Osteoarthritis Cart. 1996;4:217–43.
40. Pincus T. Why should rheumatologists collect patient self-report questionnaires in routine rheumatologic care? In: Wolfe F, ed. Rheumatic Diseases Clinics of North America: Data collection and analysis. Philadelphia: WB Saunders Company; 1995;2:271–319.
41. Wolfe F, Pincus T. Data collection in the clinic. In: Wolfe F, ed. Rheumatic Disease Clinics of North America: Data collection and analysis. Philadelphia: WB Saunders Company; 1995;21:321–58.
42. Wolfe F. A database for rheumatoid arthritis. In: Wolfe F, ed. Rheumatic Disease Clinics of North America: Data collection and analysis. Philadelphia: WB Saunders Company; 1995;22:481–500.
43. Edworthy SM. A database for systemic lupus erythematosus and systemic connective tissue disorders. In: Wolfe F, ed. Rheumatic Disease Clinics of North America: Data collection and analysis. Philadelphia: WB Saunders Company; 1995;21:501–25.
44. Littlejohn GO. A database for fibromyalgia. In: Wolfe F, ed. Rheumatic Disease Clinics of North America: Data collection and analysis. Philadelphia: WB Saunders Company; 1995;21:527–57.
45. Raspe H. A database for back (axial skeletal) pain. In: Wolfe F, ed. Rheumatic Disease Clinics of North America: Data collection and analysis. Philadelphia: WB Saunders Company; 1995;21:559–79.
46. Bellamy N, Kaloni S, Pope J, Coulter K, Campbell J. A survey of outcome measurement procedures used in routine rheumatology outpatient practice by Canadian rheumatologists. J Rheumatol, 1997;24:(in press).
47. Bellamy N, Muirden KD, Brooks P, Barraclough D, Tellus MM, Campbell J. A survey of outcome measurement procedures used in routine rheumatology outpatient practice by Australian rheumatologists. Med J Australia. 1997 (in press).
48. McGrath PA. Pain in children – nature, assessment, and treatment. New York: The Guilford Press; 1990.
49. Bieri D, Reeve R, Champion GD, Addicoat L, Ziegler JB. The faces pain scale for the self-assessment of the severity of pain experienced by children: development, initial validation, preliminary investigation for ratio scale properties. Pain. 1990;41:139–50.
50. American College of Rheumatology Ad Hoc Committee On Clinical Guidelines. Guidelines for monitoring drug therapy in rheumatoid arthritis. Arthritis Rheum. 1996;39(5):723–31.

4

REGIONAL PAIN PROBLEMS

Juan J Canoso & Simon Carette

1

INTRODUCTION

Simon Carette & Juan Canoso

- Nonarticular rheumatic disorders are widespread in the general population accounting for over 60% of new patient rheumatologic consultations.
- Skin, joint structures, arterial walls and periosteum are richly endowed with pain receptors.
- Chemical stimuli derived from inflamed or otherwise damaged tissue are the main signal of primary pain apparents.
- The affective dimension of pain results from connections of the C-fiber paleospinothalamic tract with the reticular formation, brainstem and cerebral cortex (particularly the frontal and temporal lobes).
- Knowledge of functional anatomy is essential in the diagnosis of regional pain syndromes.

Rheumatology traditionally has been associated with the concept of articular diseases. However, a recent survey of Canadian rheumatologists indicates that nonarticular disorders such as fibromyalgia, neck and back pain and local soft tissue rheumatism together account for 65% of disorders among new patient consultations[1]. This, by itself, is hardly surprising especially given how commonly some of these conditions occur in the adult population. For instance, population surveys conducted in various countries indicate a prevalence of back pain of about 40% for occurence of actual back pain, 75% for back pain during the previous year and more than 80% for back pain experiencing back pain at some point during their lifetime to date[2]. In a recent survey conducted in Cambridge, UK, the point prevalence of shoulder problems in people aged 70 years and over was 21%[3]. The prevalence of fibromyalgia in the general population of Wichita, Kansas, was 3.4% for females, with values higher than 7% in women between the ages of 60 and 79 years[4]. These statistics underline the importance for rheumatologists to be familiar with the diagnosis and management of these common conditions.

Since pain is a common denominator to all of these conditions, it is appropriate at the beginning of this section briefly to review some of the recent advances in our understanding of pain mechanisms.

Pain has been defined by the International Association for the Study of Pain as 'an unpleasant sensory and emotional experience associated with actual or potential tissue damage, or described in terms of such damage'[5]. Pain can be classified as:

- inflammatory, when associated with tissue damage, inflammation or both;
- neuropathic, when due to lesions of the peripheral or central nervous systems (CNS).

Altered central processing has been offered as an explanation for the pain felt by patients with fibromyalgia in whom there is no evidence of peripheral pathology[6].

PERIPHERAL NOCICEPTORS

The skin, joint structures, arterial walls and periosteum are richly supplied with pain receptors while the muscles and deep tissues are less extensively supplied. These so-called nociceptors are free nerve endings that can be activated by a variety of mechanical (stretching), thermal

EVENTS LEADING TO ACTIVATION AND SENSITIZATION OF PERIPHERAL NOCICEPTORS

A. K BK PG

B. SP BK Mast cell H SP 5HT Platelet

C. Histamine Mast cell 5HT SP Platelet

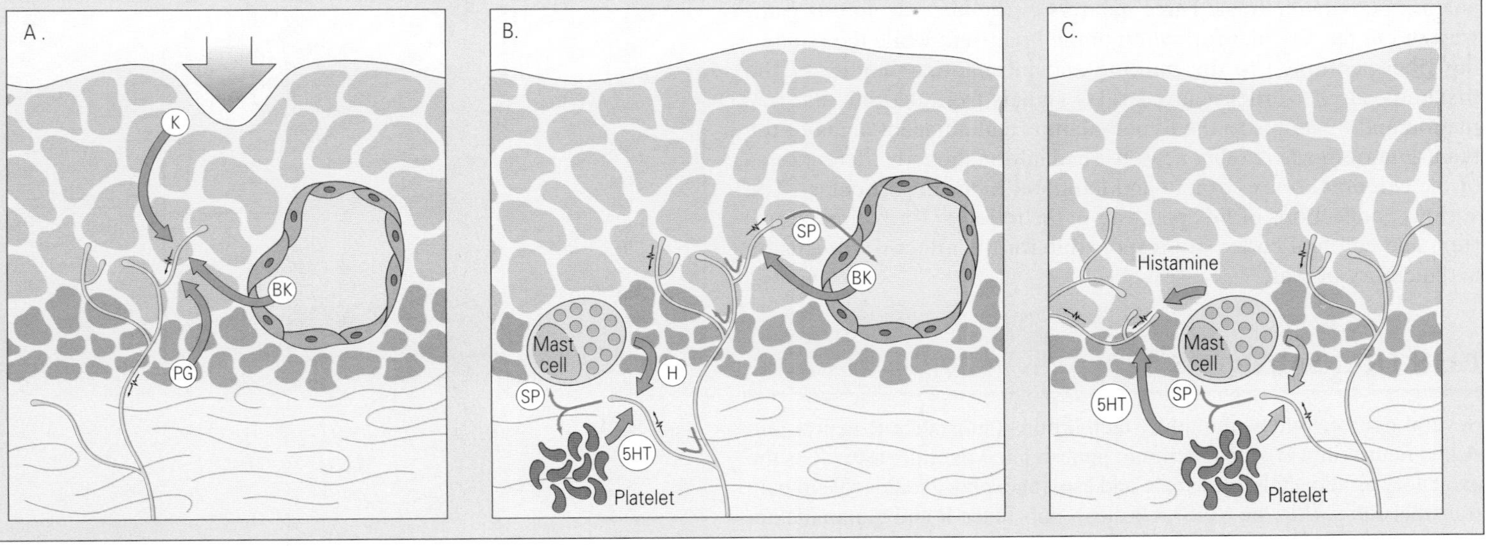

Fig. 1.1 Events leading to activation and sensitization of peripheral nociceptors. (a) A physical stimulus causes cell damage and release of potassium (K). Prostaglandins (PG) are synthesized and bradykinin (BK) is released from blood vessels. Prostaglandins increase the sensitivity of the nociceptors to bradykinin. (b) The nociceptor impulses propagate not only to the spinal cord but to other local nerve terminals where they stimulate the release of neuropeptides such as substance P (SP) in the damaged tissues. The latter stimulates the liberation of more bradykinin from blood vessels as well as histamine from mast cells and serotonin from platelets. (c) All these mediators activate more nociceptors leading to hyperalgesia. Reproduced from Fields H. (1987) Pain. With the kind permission of The McGraw-Hill Companies.

(heat and cold) and chemical stimuli. The latter constitute the most important source of signaling of primary afferents in inflammation and tissue damage and include a number of substances such as bradykinin, kallidin, oxygen free radicals, substance P, potassium, histamine, serotonin, prostaglandins, leukotrienes, cytokines and neuropeptides that are released by damaged cells or synthesized during the events that follow tissue injury (Fig. 1.1)[7].

PRIMARY AFFERENT FIBERS, DORSAL HORN AND ASCENDING TRACTS

The nociceptive information is transmitted to the CNS by two types of afferent fibers, classified on the basis of their conduction velocity: the thinly myelinated A-delta fibers, which conduct impulses at 5–15m/s and the smaller unmyelinated C fibers, which conduct impulses at 0.2–1.5m/s. The A-delta fibers are associated with the 'fast pain' which develops within a fraction of a second after a painful stimulus is applied. The pain is usually well localized and is described as sharp, pricking, tearing or electric. The C fibers are associated with 'slow pain'. This type of pain begins after 1 second or more and can increase in intensity over a period of seconds or even minutes as a consequence of the 'wind-up' phenomenon by which repeated constant stimulation of the C fibers causes an increased response of the dorsal horns. 'Slow' pain is usually poorly localized and is often described as dull, aching, burning or throbbing. Both A-delta and C fibers have their cell body in the dorsal root ganglion.

After entering the spinal cord, the A-delta fibers ascend or descend for one to three segments in the tract of Lissauer situated posteriorly to the dorsal horn before terminating in laminas I (substantia marginalis) and V of the dorsal horn. From there, they excite second-order neurons that cross to the contralateral side of the cord and ascend in the anterolateral neospinothalamic tract. While some of the fibers of this pathway terminate in the reticular formation of the brainstem, where they provide nociceptive information to the descending inhibitory pathways, most ascend to the thalamus (ventral posterolateral nucleus, medial part of the posterior complex, intralaminar nuclei and submedian nucleus), from where third-order neurons relay the nociceptive information to the somatosensory cortex.

After ascending or descending in the tract of Lissauser, the C fibers terminate in laminas I and II (substantia gelatinosa) of the dorsal horn where they synapse with short interneurons that end in lamina V from the same segment. From there, the majority of neurons cross to the contralateral side of the spinal cord where they ascend in the anterior paleospinothalamic tract. Three quarters of the fibers from this pathway end in the reticular formation of the brainstem while the remaining fibers continue to the midline and intralaminar nuclei of the thalamus. Higher-order neurons relay signals from the reticular formation and thalamus to the hypothalamus and adjacent areas of the brainstem from where other neurons send information to different areas of the cerebral cortex (frontal and temporal lobes in particular). The various connections of this pathway in the reticular formation, brainstem and cerebral cortex are responsible for the affective dimension and memory of pain.

PAIN TRANSMITTERS

Several neuropeptides, including tachykinins (substance P, neurokinin A and neurokinin B) and calcitonin gene-related peptide, as well as the excitatory amino acids, glutamate and aspartate, play a major role in pain transmission within the CNS[8]. Of these, substance P and glutamate are the two most important. Both are released from the peripheral and central terminals of C fibers following a noxious stimulus. The local application of capsaicin, the active ingredient of hot chili peppers, initially stimulates the release of these neurotransmitters and is therefore algesic. However, continued application blocks their release and leads to desensitization and analgesia[9]. Similarly, antagonists selective for the postsynaptic receptors for glutamate (NMDA) prevent the phenomenon of 'wind up' and show analgesic activity in several animal models[10].

Other neuropeptides such as somatostatin and galanin, as well as adenosine analogs, are also released by primary afferent neurons. They have mainly inhibitory actions in the dorsal horn and could therefore have potential analgesic properties[8].

PAIN INHIBITORY MECHANISMS

Pain transmission can be modulated by a number of endogenous mechanisms. The region in which these mechanisms have been best characterized is the dorsal horn of the spinal cord. Descending inhibitory pathways originating from the cerebral cortex, the thalamus and particularly the brainstem (the periaqueductal gray, raphe nuclei and locus ceruleus subceruleus complex) play an important role in this system. The main neurotransmitters involved in these pain inhibitory pathways are serotonin, norepinephrine and the endogenous opioids[11]. Intrinsic modulation of nociception can also occur at the peripheral terminals of afferent nerves through the interaction of the immune system with peripheral nociceptors[12]. Thus, in painful inflammatory conditions, stimulation with cytokine (interleukin-1) or corticotropin-releasing hormone will lead to the release of opioid peptides from macrophages and lymphocytes. These will activate opioid receptors on sensory nerves to inhibit the release of excitatory neuropeptides such as substance P and calcitonin-gene-related peptide.

The various pathways leading to the perception of pain are illustrated in Figure 1.2.

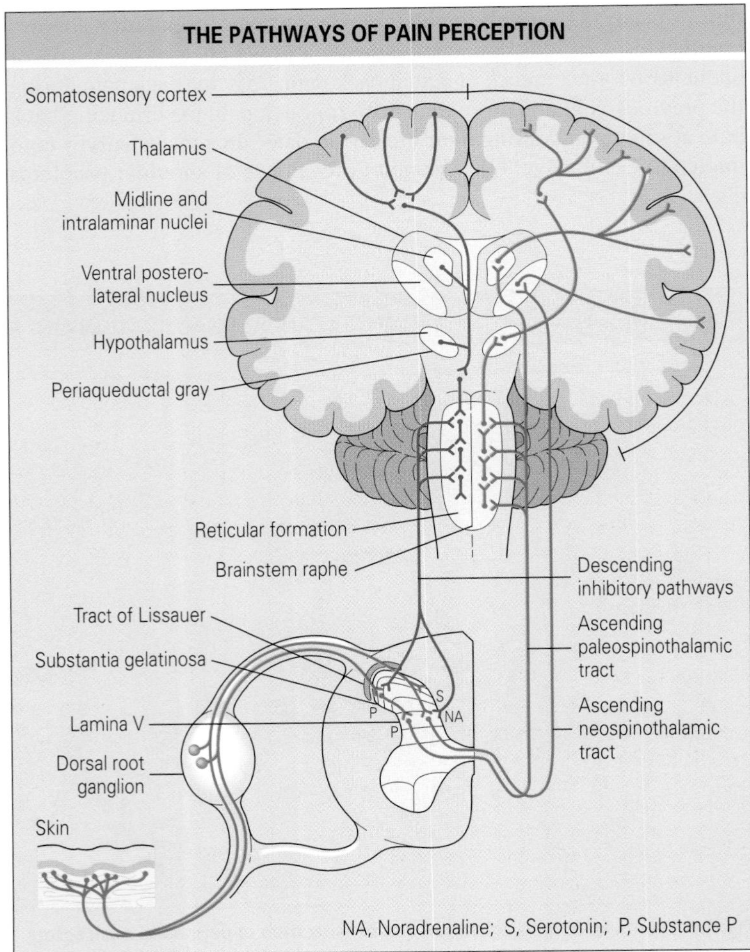

Fig. 1.2 The pathways of pain perception. NA, Noradrenaline; S, Serotonin; P, Substance P.

REGIONAL PAIN: DIFFERENTIAL DIAGNOSIS OF LOCAL CAUSES (FROM SUPERFICIAL TO DEEP)					
	Pain caused by	Site of tenderness	Swelling	Passive joint motion	Resisted motion
Cellulitis	Pressure; stretching	Erythematous patch	Diffuse	Normal unless involved area is stretched	Painless
Bursitis (superficial)	Pressure; opposite flexion in acute cases	Bursal sac	Bursal sac; peribursal swelling in acute cases	Normal extension may limit flexion	Painless flexion may have painful extension
Necrotizing fascitis*	Constant, excruciating	Involved site	Involved site; may be absent at first	Often splinted	? (probably painful)
Suppurative myositis	Pressure; stretching; contraction	Indurated muscle	Focal muscle induration	Limited opposite to muscle	? (probably painful)
Tendonitis/ tenosynovitis	Active motion	Tendon/sheath	Tendon/sheath	Normal except opposite to tendon	Painful
Enthesitis	Active motion	Tendon insertion	Tendon insertion	Normal except opposite to insertion	Painful
Bursitis (deep)	Motion; pressure	Bursal sac	Bursal sac	Varies with bursa	Varies with bursa
Nerve (various processes)	Pressure; stretching	Nerve (pain plus paresthesias)	Nerve	Normal extension; may limit flexion	Painless
Fibromyalgia	Pressure; stretching	Defined points	Subjective	Normal	Usually painless
Bone (various processes)	Constant; often nocturnal increase	Bone	May be present	Normal	Painless
Joint	With use	Around joint	Joint	Decreased/painful in all direction	Painless

Fig. 1.3 Regional pain. Differential diagnosis of local causes (from superficial to deep). (*Other superficial changes may be present at first. Systemic toxicity present. Patients are usually febrile. Physicians must be aware of this presentation.)

REGIONAL PAIN SYNDROMES

Regional pain may be caused by local lesions or may reflect pathology elsewhere, usually at a proximal site. Local sources include the soft tissues (skin, superficial bursae, fascia, muscle, tendon, enthesis, deep bursae), nerves, joints and bones (Fig. 1.3). Remote pain may reflect radiation from deep structures, ischemia, peripheral nerve or nerve root irritation, putative segmental neurovascular mechanisms (e.g. in sympathetic dystrophy and the thoracic outlet syndrome) and central mechanisms such as in the thalamic syndrome and fibromyalgia.

Needless to say, an adequate history followed by a thoughtful physical examination are essential to sort out this bewildering array of possibilities. More than in other areas of rheumatology knowledge of functional anatomy is essential, as shown by the two cases below.

KNEE PAIN WITH NORMAL KNEE EXAMINATION

In a patient complaining of knee pain, absence of localized tenderness (bone, joint capsule, ligaments, tendons, adjacent muscles), normal motion and/or and lack of pain upon stressing para-articular tendons/ligaments and joint compartments should direct the clinician's attention to the hip, a notorious source of referred pain to the knee. To test the hip in isolation (and further prove a non knee origin of pain) the joint is rotated, adducted, and abducted keeping the knee in extension. If these motions are also painless the examination is extended to the femoral nerve, lumbar plexus and upper lumbar spine. Pinprick sensation, patellar reflex, the reversed Lasègue sign and lumbar motion are appropriate maneuvers for these possible involvements.

RADIAL WRIST PAIN

In a patient complaining of radial wrist pain, attention is first focused on the distal radius (periosteal tenderness). The wrist is then flexed, extended and stressed at the radiocarpal component to detect arthritis of the radiocarpal joint, scaphoid osteonecrosis or scaphoid–lunate dissociation. The basal joint of the thumb is next stressed by applying axial pressure and torque motions to the metacarpal (pain usually indicates osteoarthritis involving this joint). The Finkelstein maneuver follows to assess extensor pollicis brevis/abductor pollicis longus tenosynovitis. The smooth surface of a dorsal ganglion should not be missed. Finally, the investigator searches for possible neuropathic causes: carpal tunnel syndrome, compressive neuropathy of the superficial branch of the radial nerve at the lateral forearm, compression neuropathy of the deep branch of the radial nerve at Froshe's arcade and a C6 radiculopathy.

REFERENCES

1. White KP, Speechley M, Harth M, Ostbye T. Fibromyalgia in rheumatology practice: a survey of Canadian rheumatologists. J Rheumatol. 1995;22:722–6.
2. Raspe HH. Back pain. In: Silman AJ, Hochberg M, eds. Epidemiology of the rheumatic diseases. Oxford: Oxford University Press; 1993:330–4.
3. Chard MD, Hazleman R, Hazleman BL, King RH, Reiss BB. Shoulder disorders in the elderly: a community survey. Arthritis Rheum. 1991;34:766–9.
4. Wolfe F, Ross K, Anderson J, Russell IJ, Hebert L. The prevalence and characteristics of fibromyalgia in the general population. Arthritis Rheum. 1995;38:19–28.
5. Merskey H. Pain terms: a list with definitions and notes on usage. Recommended by the IASP Subcommittee on Taxonomy. Pain. 1979;6:249–52.
6. Woolf CJ. Somatic pain-pathogenesis and prevention. Br J Anaesth. 1995;75:169–76.
7. Dray A. Inflammatory mediators of pain. Br J Anaesth. 1995;75:125–31.
8. Dickenson AH. Spinal cord pharmacology of pain. Br J Anaesth. 1995;75:193–200.
9. Winter J, Bevan S, Campbell. Capsaicin and pain mechanisms. Br J Anaesth. 1995;75:157–68.
10. Rang HP, Urban L. New molecules in analgesia. Br J Anaesth. 1995;75:145–56.
11. Stamford JA. Descending control of pain. Br J Anaesth. 1995;75:217–27.
12. Stein C. The control of pain in peripheral tissue by opioids. N Engl J Med. 1995;332:1685–90.

2

ANATOMY AND BIOMECHANICS OF THE SPINE

Nikolai Bogduk

Anatomy
- The design of vertebrae and their joints
- Muscles of the vertebral column
- Spinal nerves, dermatones, myotomes

Biomechanics
- Movements of the cervical and lumbar spine
- LIfting, fatigue failure
- Instability

ANATOMY

The term 'spine' has no formal status in anatomic nomenclature. However, in colloquial usage it refers to that part of the body that surrounds the vertebral column. Accordingly, the spine can be defined as the vertebral column, its contents and immediate adnexa, the latter being the muscles, nerves and blood vessels of the vertebral column.

THE VERTEBRAL COLUMN

The vertebral column is a series of individual bones – the vertebrae, which when articulated constitute the central, axial skeleton of the body. Its primary function is to endow the body with longitudinal rigidity – the hallmark of all vertebrates. Secondly, the vertebral column constitutes a firm base from which structures can be suspended, such as the ribs and abdominal muscles which allow the body to maintain cavities of relatively constant size and shape. Thirdly, the vertebral column in humans is able to sustain longitudinal compressive forces from the head, trunk or upper limbs to the lower limbs, and to allow movements between its parts, which are essential for assuming and maintaining the upright posture.

Textbooks of anatomy emphasize the role of the vertebral column in protecting the spinal cord, but this is not its primary role. The relationship between the spinal cord and vertebral column is only adventitious; the vertebral column constitutes a convenient route for the spinal cord to follow in order to gain access to distant parts of the trunk and to the limbs. The primary role of the vertebral column is musculoskeletal, as outlined above; it is designed primarily to subserve mechanical functions, and only fortuitously does the column protect the spinal cord.

REGIONS OF THE VERTEBRAL COLUMN

Along its length the vertebral column is divided into distinct regions each with different functions and demands (Fig. 2.1).

- The cervical region is the most cephalad region and constitutes the axial skeleton of the neck, responsible for supporting and moving the head.
- The thoracic region, from which the ribs are suspended, supports the thoracic cavity, i.e. the respiratory cavity.
- The lumbar region lies opposite the abdominal cavity, and allows for mobility between the thoracic portion of the trunk and the pelvis.
- The sacral region is strongly incorporated into the pelvis, and unites the vertebral column with the bones of the lower limb girdle.
- The coccyx is a rudimentary structure in humans, representing a vestigial tail, which nevertheless retains a function in supporting the pelvic floor.

Typically the cervical region is made up of seven vertebrae, the thoracic region of twelve vertebrae, the lumbar region of five, the sacral region of five fused vertebrae and the coccyx of four fused rudimentary segments. In each region the vertebrae are named by a number from above downwards, i.e. C1 to C7, T1 to T12, L1 to L5, S1 to S5.

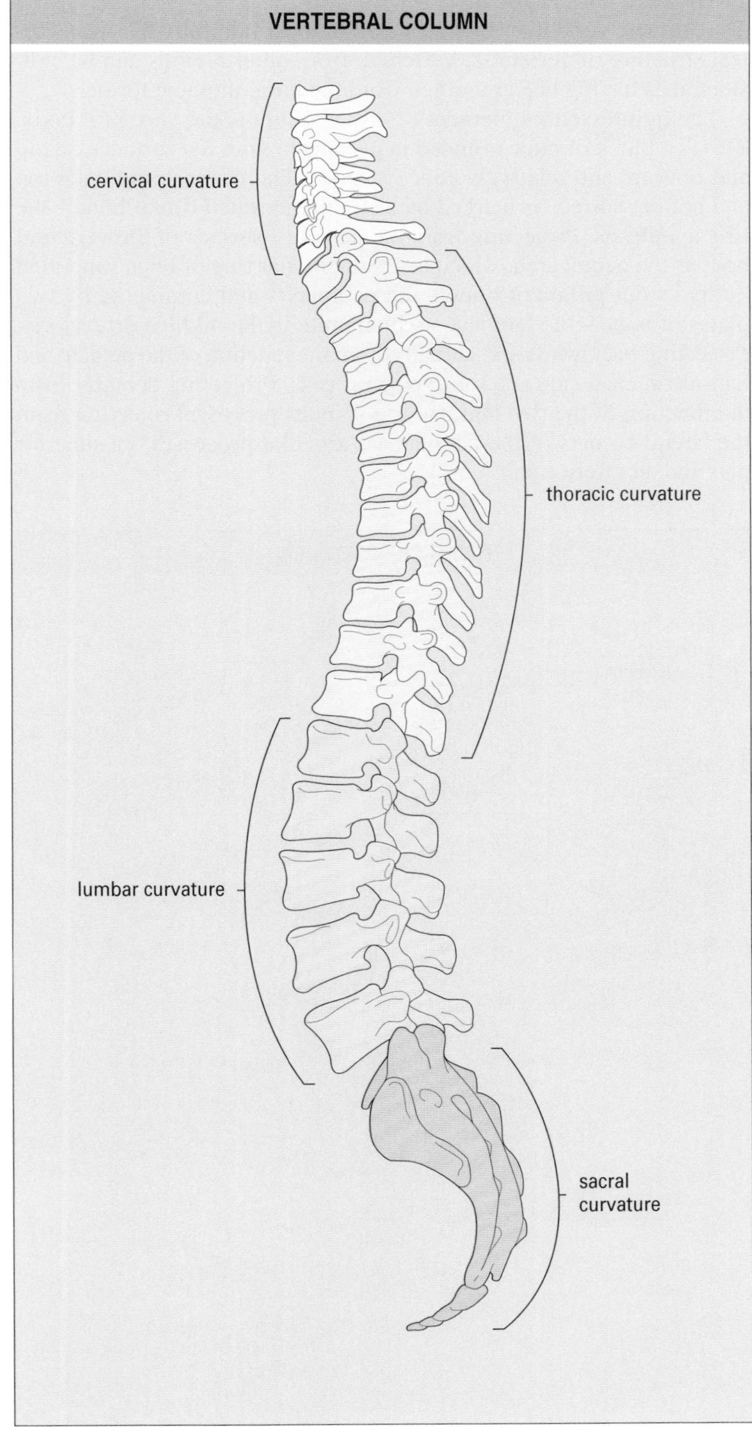

Fig. 2.1 The vertebral column.

When fully articulated, the vertebral column exhibits four curves; the cervical and lumbar regions are lordotic (convex forwards), and the thoracic and sacral regions are kyphotic (concave forwards). The two kyphotic curves are primary, being present at birth, and are dictated largely by the shape of the constituent vertebrae; they lie opposite the thoracic and pelvic visceral cavities respectively. The two lordotic curves are secondary, arising during infancy as weight bearing is assumed; they characterize the regions of the vertebral column with the greatest mobility. The lordotic curves enhance the compliance of the vertebral column in weight bearing. Compressive loads exerted through these regions tend to accentuate the curve, whereupon the compressive load can be resisted, in part, by tension developed in ligaments along the convex aspect of the curve; variations or oscillations in compressive loads can therefore be partly buffered by variations in ligamentous tension, instead of being wholly absorbed by the crystalline (bony) structure of the vertebrae.

THORACIC VERTEBRAE

The thoracic vertebrae (Fig. 2.2) exhibit most faithfully the archetypical structure of vertebrae. Vertebrae from other regions can be considered as having been modified from the basic thoracic form.

The quintessential element of any vertebra is the vertebral body. This is a block of bone rounded in perimeter, with flat surfaces on top and bottom, and relatively concave sides. The perimeter of each top and bottom surface is marked by a slightly elevated rim of bone – the ring apophysis. Projecting from the posterior surface of the vertebral body is the neural arch, which is a semicircular ring of bone supported by two stout pillars of bone – the pedicles – and completed by two plates of bone – the laminae – which unite in the midline posteriorly. Projecting backwards and laterally from the junction of the pedicle and lamina on each side is a transverse process. Projecting dorsally from the junction of the two laminae is a spinous process. Projecting from the lateral corners of the laminae are articular processes – a superior pair and an inferior pair.

The transverse and spinous processes constitute levers to which muscles are attached, while the articular processes form joints connecting consecutive vertebrae. The articular surface of each articular process is known as the articular facet and is covered by hyaline cartilage. The body and transverse processes of thoracic vertebrae are marked by facets that allow for the articulation of the ribs. Each rib articulates by its head to a vertebral body and by its tubercle to a transverse process.

The transverse and spinous processes and the articular processes sustain forces exerted by gravity and by muscles, and serve to stabilize the vertebral column. The neural arch primarily serves to transmit the stabilizing forces from the articular and muscular processes to the vertebral bodies. However, in forming an arch it produces an aperture through which the spinal cord is transmitted. In a single vertebra the aperture surrounded by the neural arch and the posterior surface of the vertebral body is known formally as the vertebral foramen (Fig. 2.2). When a series of vertebrae are connected, their neural foramina are aligned to form a longitudinal canal known as the vertebral canal (Fig. 2.3).

Spinal nerves leaving the spinal cord emerge from the vertebral column by passing between consecutive vertebrae. They do so through an aperture known as the intervertebral foramen which is bounded superiorly by the pedicle of the upper vertebra, inferiorly by the pedicle of the lower vertebra, anteriorly by the intervertebral disc and adjacent vertebral bodies, and posteriorly by the joint formed between the inferior and superior articular processes of the two vertebrae.

Externally, all the surfaces of a vertebra are formed by compact, cortical bone. Internally, the vertebra is formed by trabeculated, cancellous (or spongy) bone. In the vertebral body the trabeculae are positioned basically as vertical and transverse struts whose arrangement reinforces the surfaces and walls of the vertebral body to allow it to sustain large weights with a minimum expenditure of bone. From the vertebral body, trabeculae sweep into the posterior elements to form buttresses that reinforce the articular processes and transverse processes in a manner corresponding to the direction of forces that these processes habitually sustain.

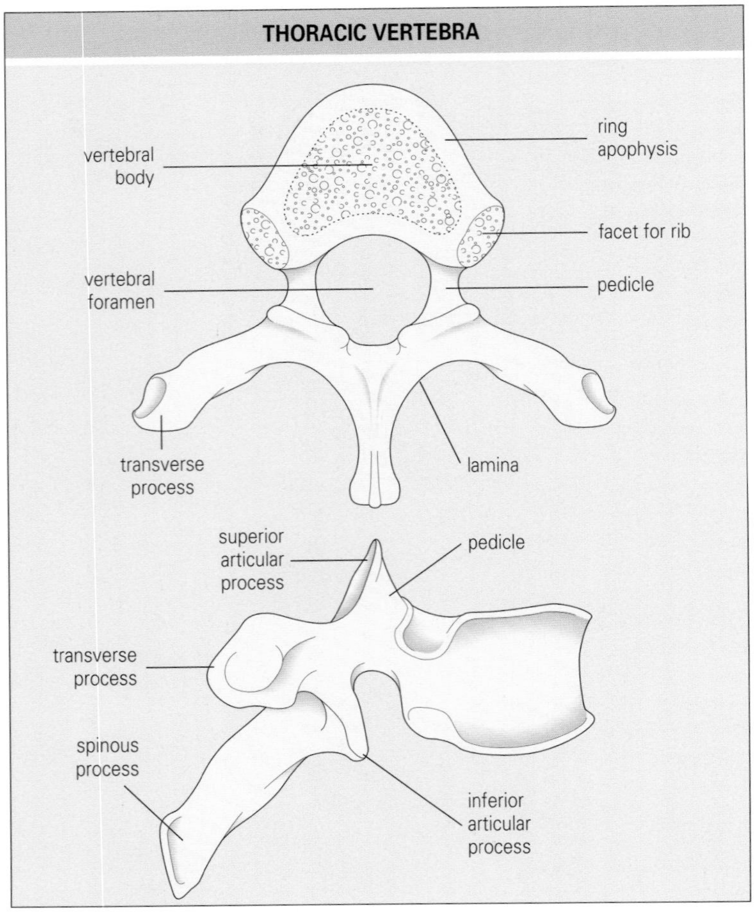

THORACIC VERTEBRA

vertebral body
ring apophysis
facet for rib
vertebral foramen
pedicle
transverse process
lamina
superior articular process
pedicle
transverse process
spinous process
inferior articular process

Fig. 2.2 Thoracic vertebra.

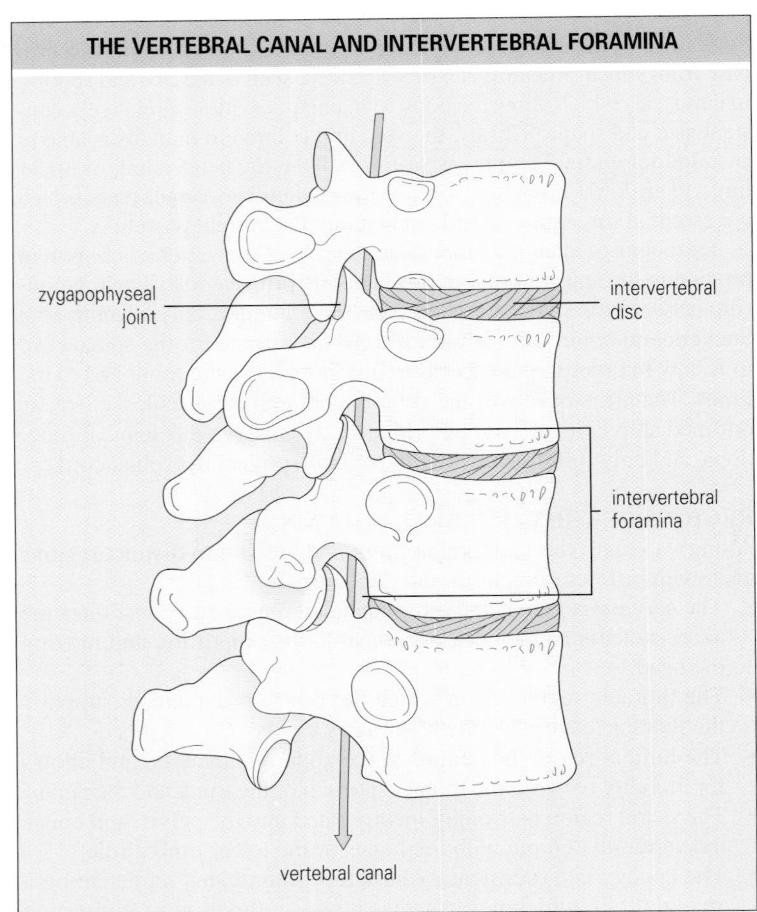

Fig. 2.3 Alignment of vertebrae. The vertebral canal and intervertebral foramina in relation to an articulated series of thoracic vertebrae.

The upper and lower surfaces of the vertebral bodies are flat because the vertebral bodies are the essential weight-bearing elements of the vertebra. The flat design presents a maximal surface area dedicated to withstanding longitudinal compression forces. However, the legacy of this design is that the vertebral bodies themselves provide no bony features to stabilize them against sliding and axial rotatory movements. This missing stability is provided by the posterior elements of the vertebrae. The inferior articular processes of each vertebra constitute hooks which engage the superior articular processes of the next lower vertebra. The resistance to forward sliding offered by the superior articular processes is transmitted through the inferior articular processes via the laminae and pedicles to the upper vertebral body, thereby preventing forward sliding between vertebral bodies.

THE TYPICAL CERVICAL VERTEBRAE

The typical cervical vertebrae (Fig. 2.4) differ from the archetypical thoracic vertebrae in several key respects. The vertebral bodies are shorter and bear uncinate processes on their superoposterior lateral edges. The articular processes are supported on a stout column of bone: the articular pillar. The transverse processes are U-shaped in cross section, forming a gutter which lodges the ventral ramus that emerges above the vertebra. Proximally the floor of the transverse process is pierced by the foramen transversarium, which at levels C1–C6 transmits the vertebral artery.

AXIS AND ATLAS

In order to serve their particular function, the first and second cervical vertebrae, known as the atlas and axis, respectively, are greatly modified from the typical form of a cervical vertebra (Fig. 2.5).

The atlas vertebra resembles no other vertebra. It lacks a vertebral body and is basically a ring with a thickened lateral mass on each side. Each lateral mass bears a concave, superior facet and a flat, inferior facet through which the weight of the head is transmitted to the axis. The two lateral masses are joined anteriorly and posteriorly by arches

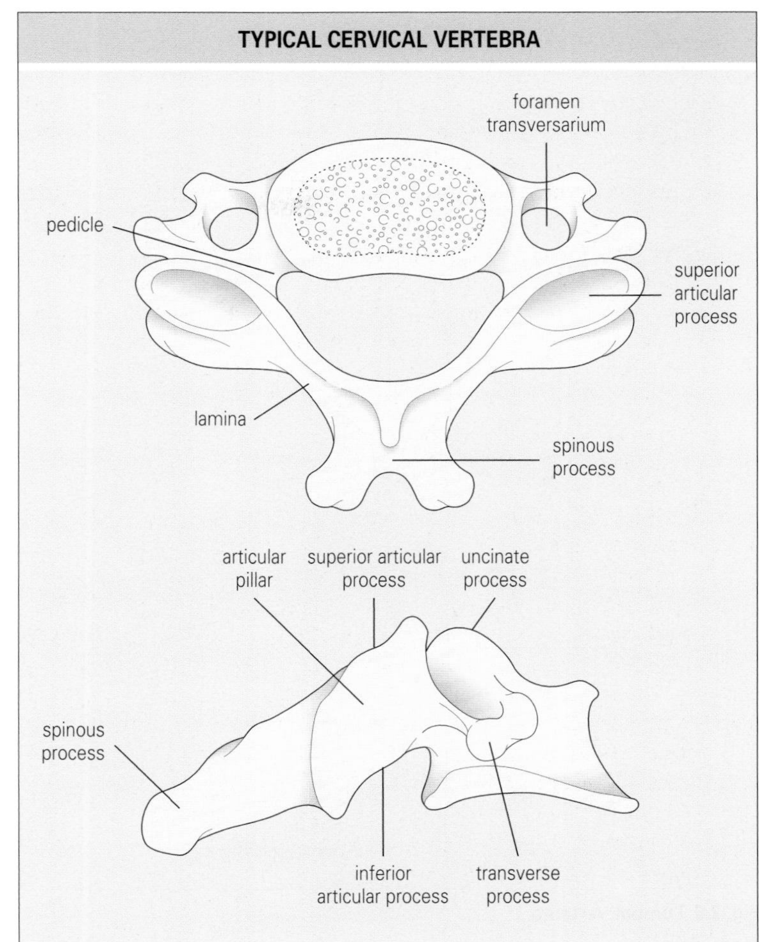

Fig. 2.4 Typical cervical vertebra.

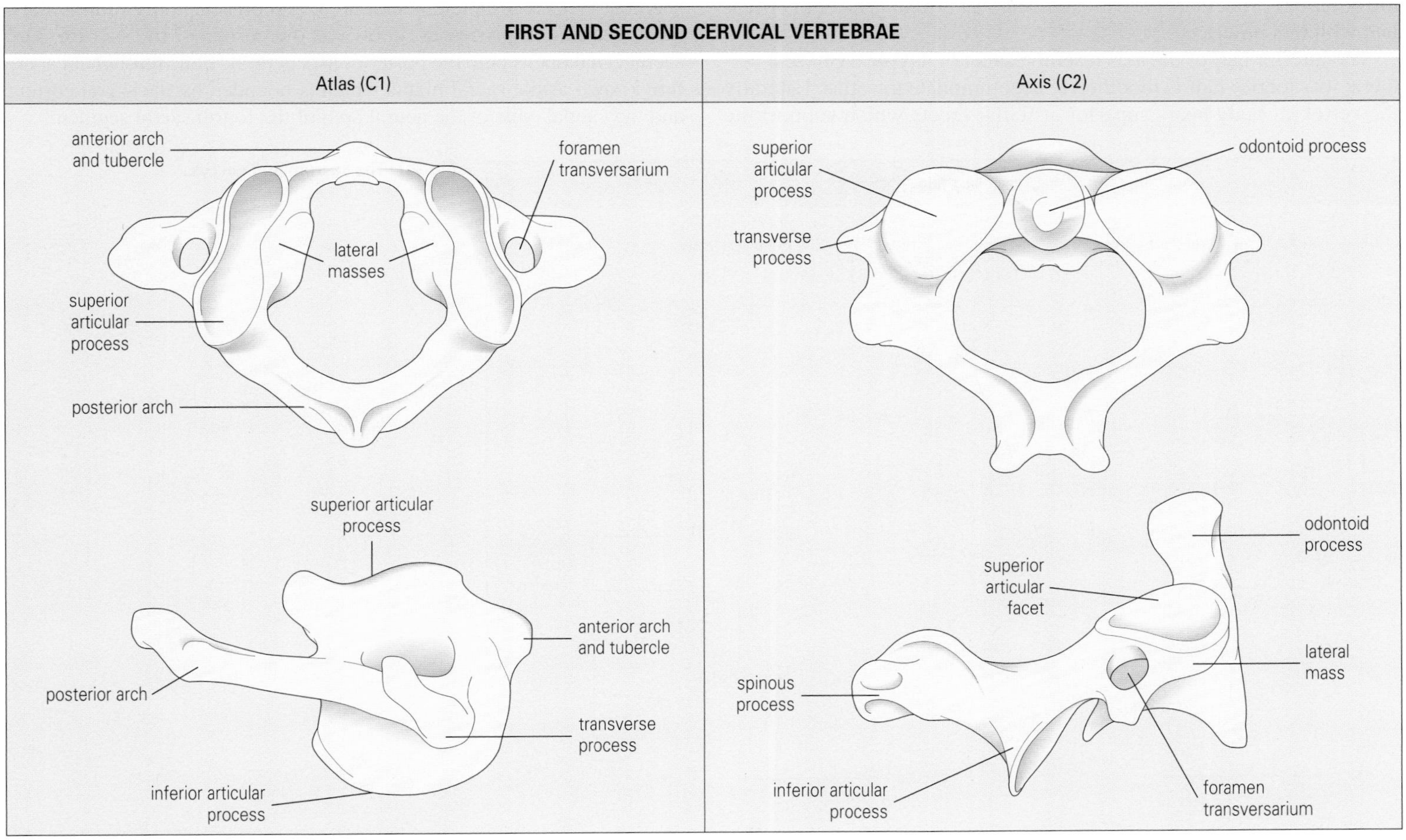

Fig. 2.5 The first and second cervical vertebrae.

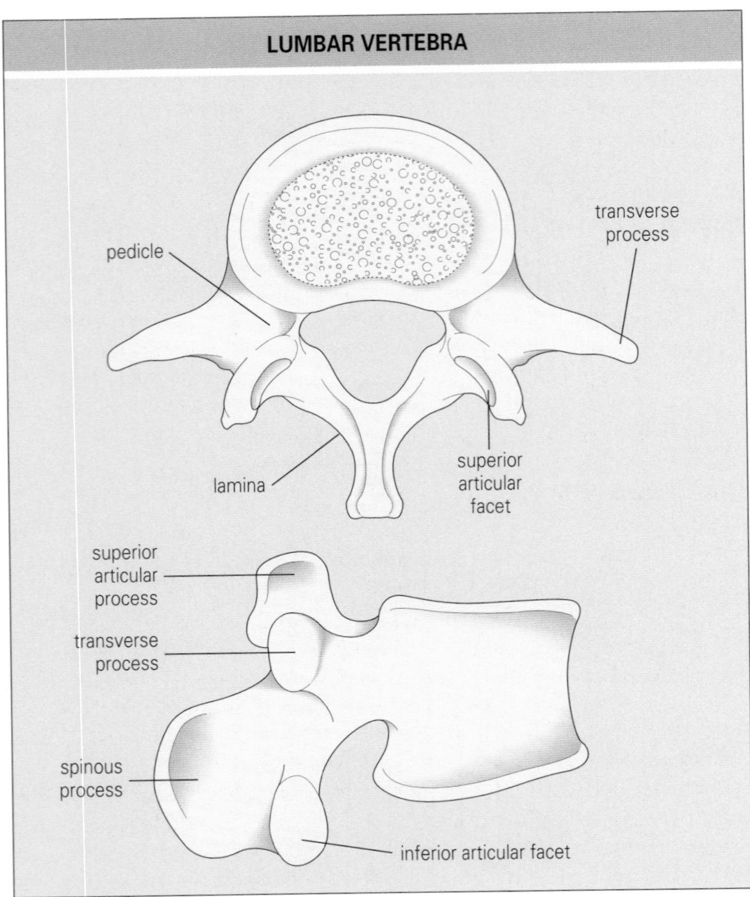

Fig. 2.6 Lumbar vertebra.

of bone. The posterior arch bears at its middle a tubercle that represents a rudimentary spinous process. The anterior arch lies in front of the odontoid process of the axis and bears an articular facet to articulate with this process.

The inferior half of the axis resembles that of a typical cervical vertebra; its superior half is modified to accommodate the atlas. Laterally the vertebral body bears superior articular facets which support the atlas. Anteriorly the vertebral body bears an odontoid process which constitutes a pivot around which the atlas can rotate.

LUMBAR VERTEBRAE

The lumbar vertebrae (Fig. 2.6) are robust bones designed to bear the weight of the trunk and to control its movements on the pelvis in the upright posture. Each consists of a large vertebral body endowed with stout posterior elements. Additional processes are present, which serve as special sites of muscle attachment. Each transverse process bears on its proximal, posterior surface an accessory process, and each superior articular process bears on its dorsal edge a rounded tubercle called the mamillary process.

The transverse processes of the lumbar vertebrae typically project from the junction of the pedicle and lamina, but the transverse process of L5 is distinct in that its base extends across the entire lateral surface of the pedicle on to the vertebral body. This feature allows the fifth lumbar vertebra to be recognized on CT scans without having to resort to scout films.

THE SACRUM

The sacrum is a mass of five fused vertebrae (Fig. 2.7). It is triangular in shape: slightly concave anteriorly, broad superiorly and tapering inferiorly. Each sacral segment presents what can be recognized as a vertebral body, a transverse projection forming a lateral mass on each side and a neural arch posteriorly that supports a rudimentary spinous process. The fused neural arches enclose the sacral portion of the vertebral canal. Anteriorly and posteriorly, consecutive segments are separated by the anterior and posterior sacral foramina which, respectively, transmit the ventral and dorsal rami of the sacral spinal nerves.

Opposite the first three sacral segments the lateral portion of the sacrum is thickened and bears an auricular (ear-shaped) surface on its lateral aspect, which constitutes the articular surface of the sacroiliac joint. Posterior to this, opposite the first sacral segment, lies a large pitted area for the attachment of the interosseous sacroiliac ligament.

Posteriorly the first sacral segment presents a pair of superior articular processes that articulate with the fifth lumbar vertebra. The fifth sacral segment lacks a complete neural arch, and presents only rudimentary inferior articular processes, known as the cornua of the sacrum. The sacral canal opens onto the posterior aspect of the bone through an aperture known as the sacral hiatus which is bounded by the sacral cornua and the caudal edge of the neural arch of the fourth sacral segment.

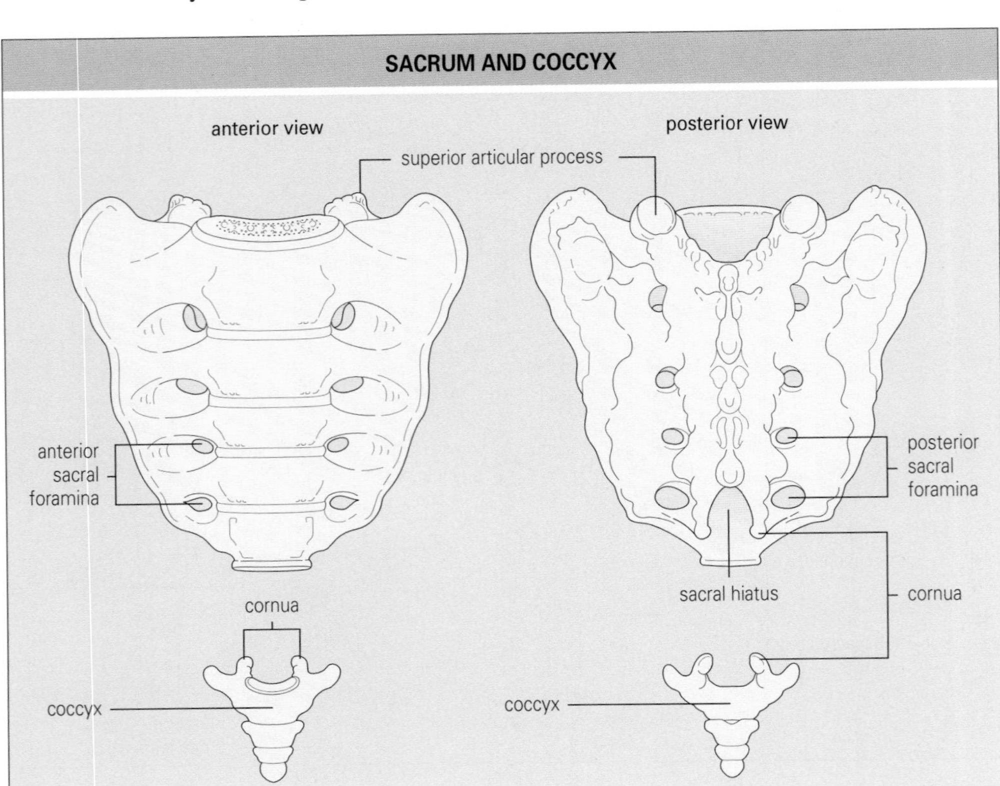

Fig. 2.7 The sacrum and coccyx.

COCCYX

The coccyx consists of the fused vertebral bodies of four or more small coccygeal vertebrae (Fig. 2.7). The first two segments carry rudimentary transverse processes and the first carries rudimentary superior articular processes known as the coccygeal cornua.

SPINAL JOINTS

Each vertebra is typically united to the next by three joints. The joint between the vertebral bodies is formed by an intervertebral disc; the joints between the articular processes are typical synovial joints known as the zygapophyseal joints.

THE INTERVERTEBRAL DISC

The intervertebral disc subserves several functions. Foremost, it separates the vertebral bodies allowing them to bend with respect to one another. For this function it must be pliable. Meanwhile, it must also sustain the compression loads exerted on the interbody joint by the weight of the body above the joint and by the back muscles when they act. For this function the intervertebral disc must also be strong.

An intervertebral disc typically consists of a nucleus pulposus surrounded by an anulus fibrosus, both sandwiched between superior and inferior vertebral end-plates (Fig. 2.8). Our knowledge of the detailed structure of the intervertebral disc is based on studies of lumbar discs[1]. The nucleus pulposus of a lumbar intervertebral disc consists of a central core of a well-hydrated proteoglycan matrix surrounded by fibrocartilage. The anulus fibrosus consists of 10–12 concentric lamellae of collagen fibers. In any given lamella the collagen fibers run in parallel at an angle of about 65° to the vertical, but the direction of this angle alternates in successive layers.

Within the anulus fibrosus, two portions can be identified. The outermost lamellae are attached to the ring apophyses of the two vertebrae and constitute the 'ligamentous' portion of the anulus fibrosus[1]. The inner lamellae of the anulus fibrosus do not attach to bone. Instead, they pass into the vertebral end-plates above and below the nucleus pulposus to form a complete spheroidal envelope around the nucleus[2]. Because of its bony attachments the ligamentous portion of the anulus fibrosus is designed primarily to limit movement between the vertebral bodies. By forming a capsule around the nucleus pulposus, the internal lamellae of the anulus fibrosus function to resist radial expansion of the nucleus pulposus under pressure.

The vertebral end-plates are layers of cartilage that bind the disc to the vertebral body. Towards its vertebral surface each end-plate consists of hyaline cartilage but towards its discal surface it consists of fibrocartilage because of the collagen fibres of the anulus fibrosus embedded in it.

Regional differences

Little is known of the detailed structure of thoracic intervertebral discs. The extent to which they conform or differ from the structure of lumbar discs is unknown. The study of the normal anatomy of cervical discs has only recently begun but has revealed conspicuous differences from lumbar discs. Foremost, the nucleus pulposus of a cervical disc constitutes a much smaller component of the disc than in lumbar discs[3]. Secondly, only in infants, children and adolescents is the nucleus pulposus of a cervical disc mucoid in nature, like that of lumbar discs. Beyond the age of 20 years, the nucleus pulposus of a cervical disc becomes quite fibrous[4]. Consequently, in young adults and into middle age a cervical disc is more like a fibrous, interosseous ligament than a buoyant, hydrodynamic structure such as a lumbar disc of the same age. Thirdly, there is emerging evidence that transverse fissures across the posterior half of a cervical disc occur increasingly frequently with age, and so regularly that they constitute a normal feature[5]. This feature is of significance in the context of the so-called uncovertebral joints and the movements of the cervical vertebrae.

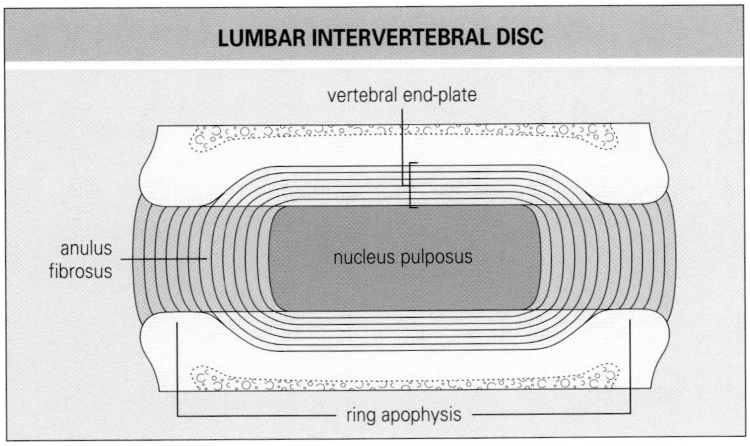

LUMBAR INTERVERTEBRAL DISC

vertebral end-plate
anulus fibrosus
nucleus pulposus
ring apophysis

Fig. 2.8 The lumbar intervertebral disc: schematic sagittal section.

THE LONGITUDINAL LIGAMENTS

The interbody joints are traditionally regarded as being reinforced by the anterior and posterior longitudinal ligaments, but the biomechanical significance of these ligaments has been overemphasized.

Throughout most of the vertebral column, the posterior longitudinal ligament constitutes little more than a thin carpet along the vertebral canal. In the craniocervical region, it expands to become the membrana tectoria, but this structure does not play any substantial ligamentous role; rather, it forms a protective, membranous barrier that separates the spinal cord from the odontoid process.

The anterior longitudinal ligament is prominent only in the thoracic region. In the neck it is attenuated to a thin, narrow strip lying between the prevertebral muscles on each side. In the lumbar region, most of what is regarded as the anterior longitudinal ligament comprises tendons of the crura of the diaphragm[1].

Anatomically, the longitudinal ligaments are relatively too thin to serve major mechanical roles. Such roles as have been attributed to them are more properly invested in the ligamentous portions of the anulus fibrosus of the intervertebral discs.

THE ZYGAPOPHYSEAL JOINTS

The zygapophyseal joints (Fig. 2.9) are formed by the inferior articular process of one vertebra and the ipsilateral superior articular process

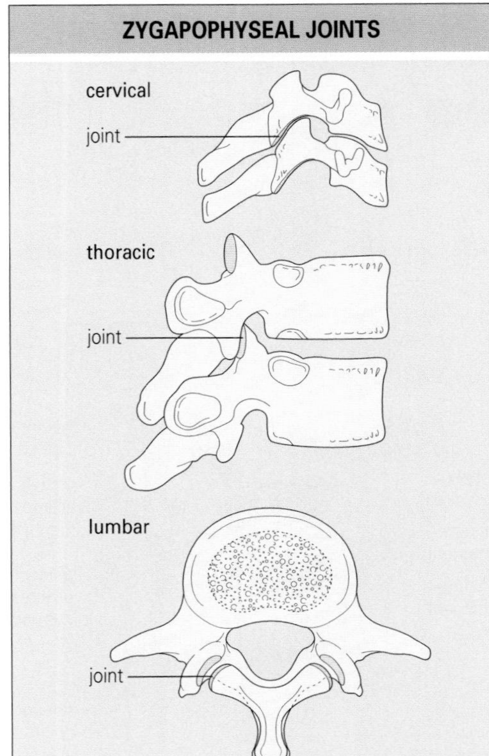

Fig. 2.9. The zygapophyseal joints. Regional differences in joint orientation are evident.

of the next. Each joint is enclosed by a fibrous capsule, and may contain a variety of intra-articular inclusions: intra-articular fat pads, fibro-adipose meniscoids and capsular rims[6,7].

Thoracic zygapophyseal joints are orientated basically in the coronal plane, and consequently serve to preclude forwards translation of the thoracic vertebrae. Cervical zygapophysial joints are oriented obliquely; the superior articular facets face upwards and backwards and thereby contribute to weight bearing as well as impeding forwards translation of the vertebra they support. Lumbar zygapophyseal joints are oriented longitudinally with their superior articular facets facing backwards and medially to prevent both forwards translation and axial rotation of the vertebra above[1].

THE POSTERIOR LIGAMENTS

Insofar as the zygapophyseal joints are the joints of the vertebral arches, they are said to be reinforced by the ligaments of the vertebral arches: the ligamentum flavum, the interspinous ligament and the supraspinous ligament. However, these ligaments offer insubstantial support for these joints and, indeed, paradoxically, the strongest of the posterior spinal ligaments prove to be the capsules of the zygapophyseal joints themselves[1].

The ligamentum flavum is represented from the C2–C3 level to the L5–S1 level and consists largely of elastic fibers that connect consecutive laminae. While offering some resistance to separation of the laminae in flexion of the vertebral column, the ligamentum flavum is too distensible because of its elastic nature to limit this movement. Its function is to provide a smooth posterior wall to the vertebral canal that accommodates, without buckling, large changes in interlaminar distance during flexion and extension of the vertebral column[1].

In the lumbar region, the interspinous ligament is formed by collagen fibers passing caudoventrally between adjacent spinous processes, but only the anterior two thirds of each ligament is truly ligamentous. The posterior third represents terminal tendons of the erector spinae muscle, finding attachment to a spinous process[1]. In the cervical region a definitive interspinous ligament is lacking. A cervical interspinous space is typically filled with fascial tissue derived from the so-called ligamentum nuchae.

The ligamentum nuchae has classically been portrayed as constituting a substantial supportive ligament of the neck. However, dissection reveals this structure to be only a midline fascial septum that separates the two semispinalis capitis muscles. It has no substantive mechanical function except dorsally where it forms a raphe for the origins of trapezius, splenius and rhomboid minor.

CRANIOCERVICAL JOINTS

The head is connected to the neck by a series of unique joints involving the atlas and axis vertebrae (Fig. 2.10). The atlas constitutes a platform which supports the skull. In turn, this platform is supported by the axis which is designed to permit axial rotation of the atlas and, thereby, the head.

The atlanto-occipital joints are paired synovial joints in which the concave facets of the superior articular processes of the atlas form stable sockets that accommodate the condyles of the occiput. The curvature of the sockets permits nodding movements of the head on the atlas, but largely precludes other movements. Consequently, during axial rotation of the head, the head and atlas move essentially as a single unit on the axis.

The atlas is supported on the axis by the lateral atlantoaxial joints. These are essentially planar, synovial joints which allow a large range of gliding movements for rotation of the head and atlas. During rotation, the anterior arch of the atlas slides around the anterior surface of the odontoid process, this movement being accommodated by the median atlantoaxial joint.

Backwards movement of the atlas is prevented by impaction of the anterior arch of the atlas against the odontoid process. The reverse movement is prevented by the transverse ligament of the atlas which constitutes a strong belt passing behind the odontoid process and connecting the left and right lateral masses of the atlas, and which forms a synovial joint between itself and an articular facet on the back of the odontoid process.

The transverse ligament of the atlas is the most important structure stabilizing the atlantoaxial joint[8]. The next most major ligaments in this region are the alar ligaments which pass laterally from the posterolateral surface of each side of the odontoid process to the lateral

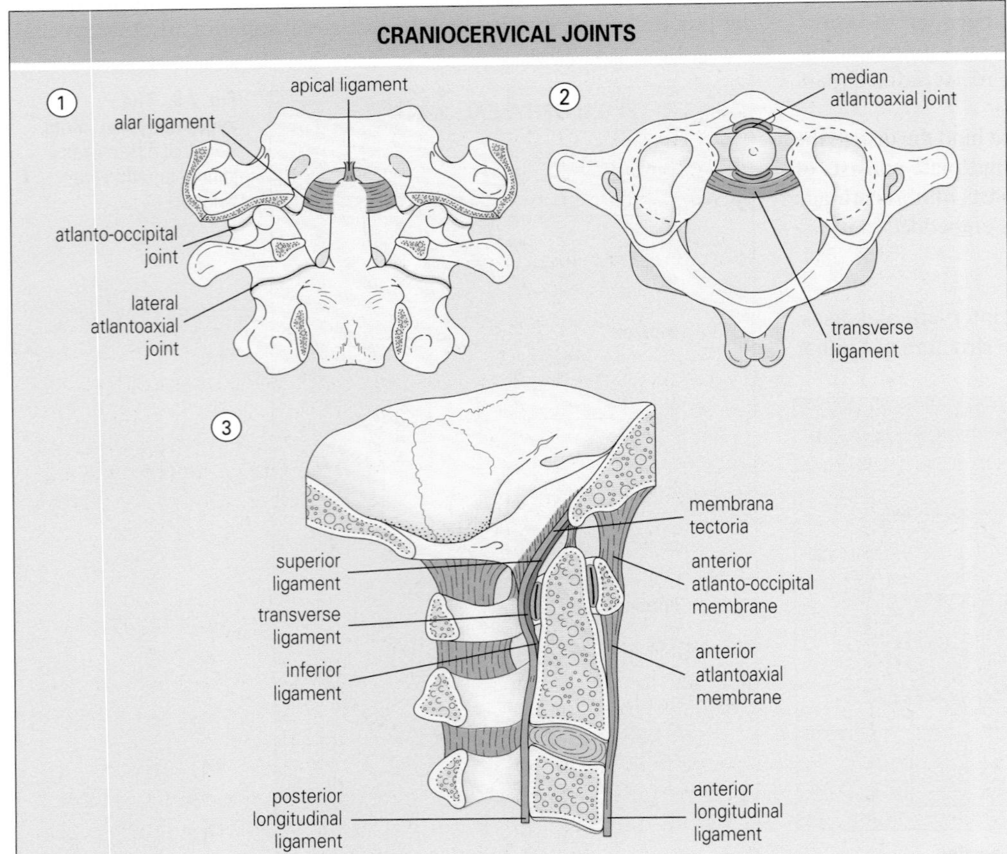

Fig. 2.10 The craniocervical joints. Posterior view of the atlanto-occipital joints and the lateral atlantoaxial joints with the posterior arch of the atlas and the laminae of the axis removed to reveal the alar ligaments (1). Top view of the atlas articulating with the axis to show the median atlantoaxial joint and transverse ligament (2). Sagittal section through the median atlantoaxial joint (3).

margin of the foramen magnum (Fig. 2.10). Because of their orientation the alar ligaments prevent distraction of the head from the axis, ipsilateral gliding of the head and atlas on the axis and excessive contralateral axial rotation of the head[9]. The alar ligaments are also sufficiently strong that, if the transverse ligament of the atlas is disabled, they can limit forward sliding of the skull with respect to the axis[8]. Complete forwards dislocation of the skull and atlas therefore requires destruction of both the transverse ligament and the alar ligaments.

Other ligaments in the craniocervical region, such as the apical ligament of the dens, the longitudinal band of the cruciate ligament and the accessory atlantoaxial ligaments, are not of any known mechanical significance. The anterior and posterior atlanto-occipital and atlantoaxial membranes constitute fascial septa separating the vertebral canal from the exterior regions of the vertebral column, rather than being structures of any dynamic mechanical importance.

UNCOVERTEBRAL JOINTS

The uncinate processes of the cervical vertebrae constitute a fascinating and hitherto mysterious feature of the vertebral column. They have been portrayed as forming a synovial joint with the vertebral body above – the so-called uncovertebral joints. But anatomic evidence refutes this interpretation. No such joints are present in embryos, infants or children. Rather, what develops in this region are adventitious clefts in the anulus fibrosus of the cervical intervertebral disc. What has been misrepresented as articular cartilage in these clefts in fact comprises layers of split collagen fibers of the anulus fibrosus that have undergone cartilaginous metaplasia[10].

SACROCOCCYGEAL JOINTS

The sacrum is united to the body of the coccyx by a rudimentary intervertebral disc in the form of a symphysis. Posteriorly, the superior articular processes of the coccyx are united to the cornua of the sacrum by fibrous joints reinforced by the posterior sacrococcygeal ligaments. The sacrococcygeal joint is mobile only in children, adolescents and young adults. With increasing age it undergoes ankylosis. In some individuals, particularly women, a mobile fibrous joint may persist between the first and second coccygeal segments.

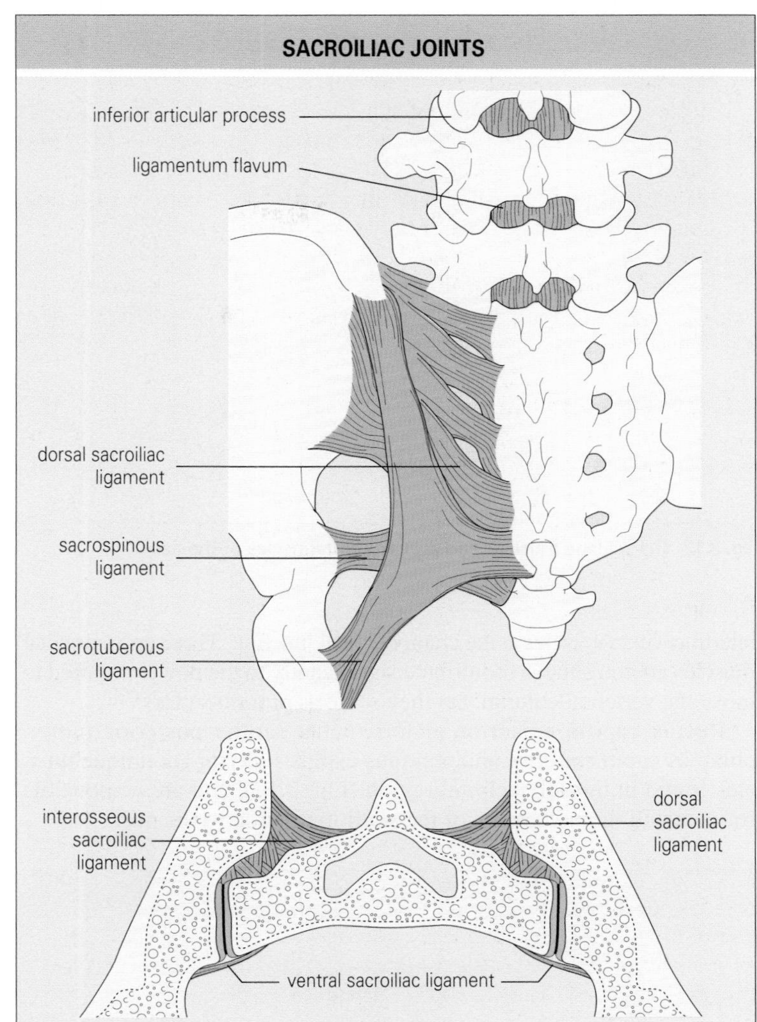

Fig. 2.11 The sacroiliac joints: poster view and coronal section.

SACROILIAC JOINT

The sacroiliac joint is a synovial joint between the sacrum and ilium on each side. The joint cavity is auricular and reaches the anterior margin of the sacrum. The joint is designed to connect the vertebral column firmly to the lower limb girdle but also to allow obligatory movements that occur during gait.

The stability of the sacroiliac joint lies in the nature of its articular surfaces and ligaments (Fig. 2.11). The ligaments are designed to clamp the sacrum between the two ilia. Cardinal in this role are the dense, interosseous ligaments lying dorsal to the joint, and the ventral sacroiliac ligament covering its anterior aspect. The clamping effect engages corrugations on the articular surfaces of the sacrum and ilia which locks the bones together, so preventing translations and rotations between them. Forwards rotation, or nutation, of the sacrum is further restricted by the sacrotuberous and sacrospinous ligaments, and symptoms may develop in these ligaments if the intrinsic sacroiliac ligaments are disabled.

The structure of the sacroiliac joint evolves with age. In children it is essentially a planar synovial joint; in young adults it develops its intra-articular corrugations; but in old age the joint undergoes fibrous and even osseous ankylosis[11].

MUSCLES OF THE VERTEBRAL COLUMN

A practical way to describe the muscles of the vertebral column is according to their topographic location in relation to the transverse processes of the vertebral bodies. While the entire vertebral column is endowed with muscles posteriorly, only the cervical and lumbar regions are covered by muscles anteriorly and laterally. The thoracic region lacks any lateral or prevertebral musculature.

ANTERIOR VERTEBRAL MUSCLES

The anterior vertebral muscles are those lying anterior to the plane of the transverse processes of the vertebral column.

Longus cervicis and longus capitis

The longus cervicis muscle covers the front of the bodies of the cervical and upper three thoracic vertebrae. The longus capitis muscle arises from the lower transverse cervical processes and inserts into the base of the skull (see Fig. 2.12). These muscles are not well developed and their lines of action lie close to the axes of sagittal rotation of the cervical vertebra. Consequently, they are not particularly strong flexors of the neck. At best they control small amplitude movements of the head and neck in the sagittal plane. Forced flexion of the neck is achieved by the sternocleidomastoid.

POSTERIOR VERTEBRAL MUSCLES

The posterior vertebral muscles are those lying behind the plane of the transverse processes of the vertebral column. They are best considered in groups: unisegmental muscles, multifidus, semispinalis, erector spinae and splenius.

Unisegmental muscles

The unisegmental muscles are the interspinales and intertransversarii, which are best developed in the cervical and lumbar regions (Fig. 2.13). Rectus capitis anterior and rectus capitis lateralis are homologues of the

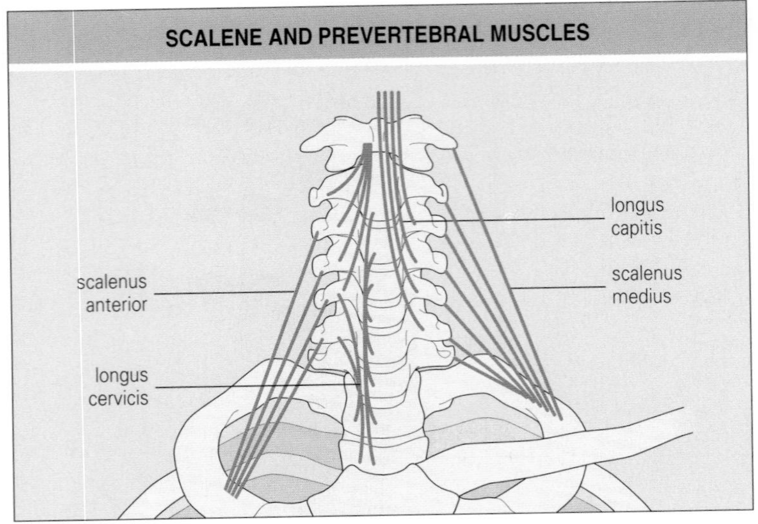

Fig. 2.12 The scalene muscles and prevertebral muscles of the neck.

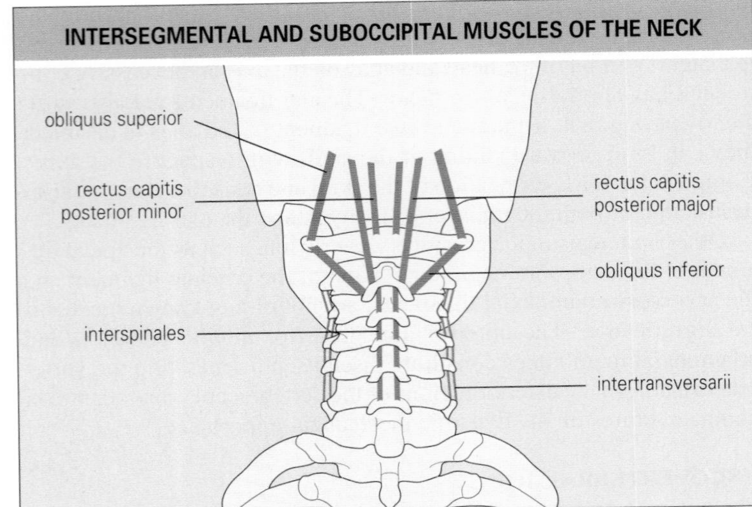

Fig. 2.13 The intersegmental and suboccipital muscles of the neck.

intertransverse muscles at the craniocervical junction. These unisegmental muscles are too small to contribute significantly to the power required to move the vertebral column, but they serve as proprioceptors[12,13].

Rectus capitis posterior major, rectus capitis posterior minor, obliquus capitis inferior and obliquus capitis superior are unique muscles found in the suboccipital region (Fig. 2.13), and are responsible for controlling movements of the skull in relation to the neck.

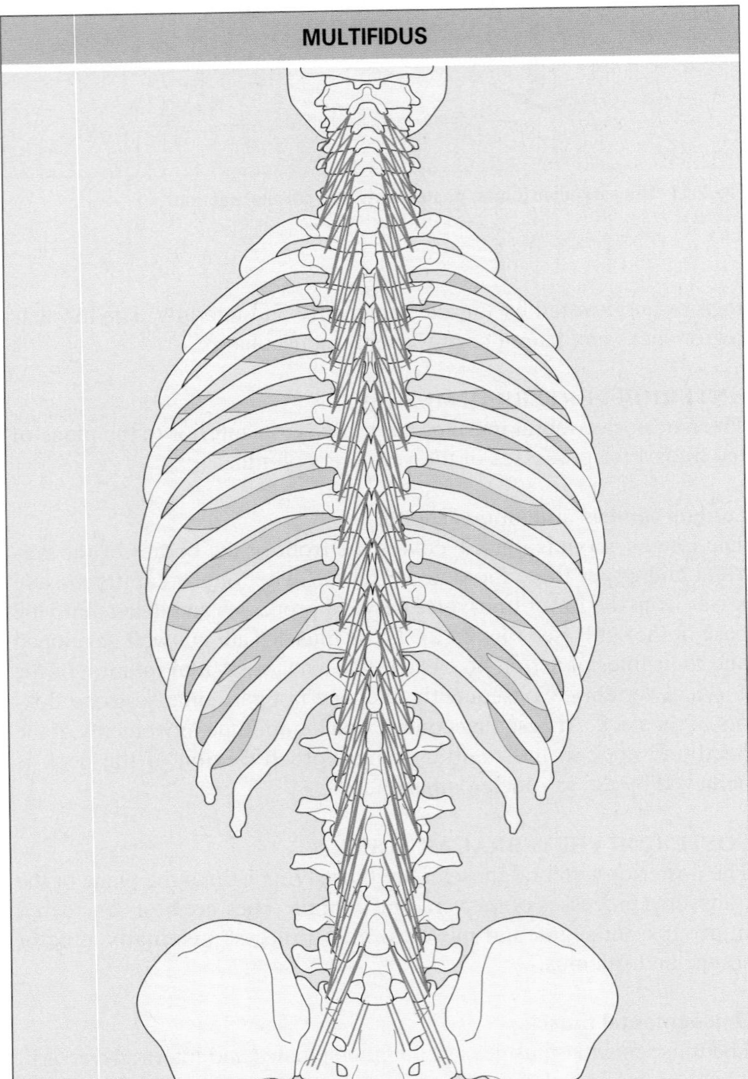

Fig. 2.14 Multifidus.

Multifidus

Multifidus is a series of multipennate muscles covering the laminae of the vertebral column, each stemming from a spinous process from level C2 to L5 (Fig. 2.14). Each spinous process is subtended by three or four fascicles that are anchored to articular processes in the cervical region, transverse processes in the thoracic region, mamillary processes in the lumbar region and to the back of the sacrum[1].

The fibers of multifidus execute posterior sagittal rotation of their vertebra of origin. The multifidus has been represented as a rotator of the vertebral column, but the orientation of its fibers means that any such rotation must occur simultaneously with extension, with extension being by far the dominant movement[1].

Semispinalis

The semispinalis system of muscles is characterized by fibers that arise from transverse processes and insert into spinous processes or their equivalent (Fig. 2.15). These fibers cover the multifidus muscle. Three

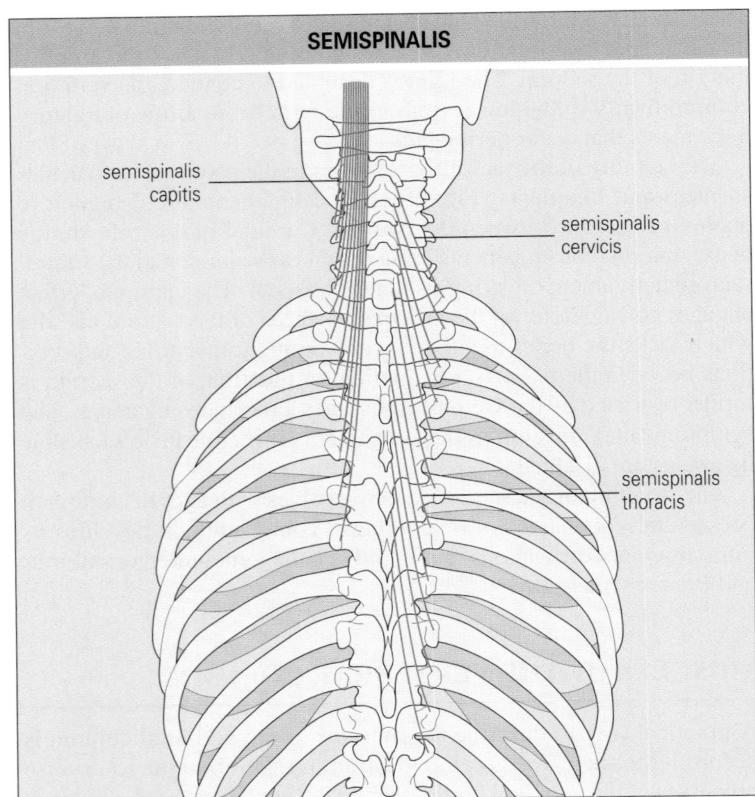

Fig. 2.15 The semispinalis muscles.

divisions of the semispinalis are recognized along the length of the vertebral column. Semispinalis thoracis inserts into the cervical (C7) and thoracic (T1 to T4) spinous processes; semispinalis cervicis into the spinous processes of C2 to C5; and semispinalis capitis into the occipital bone below the superior nuchal line. This last muscle constitutes the largest and strongest of the posterior neck muscles.

The semispinalis thoracis and semispinalis cervicis execute posterior sagittal rotation of those vertebrae to whose spinous processes they are attached, while the semispinalis capitis extends the head.

Erector spinae

The erector spinae consists of a minor portion, spinalis, and two major portions, longissimus and iliocostalis. The spinalis connects spinous processes while the longissimus and iliocostalis connect homologous portions of the costal and transverse elements of the lumbar, thoracic and cervical vertebrae and skull (Fig. 2.16). The spinalis is developed only in the thoracic region where its fibers connect the middle thoracic spinous processes to the lower thoracic and upper lumbar spinous processes.

The largest division of the longissimus is the longissimus thoracis, the fibers of which lie lateral to the semispinalis thoracis and the lumbar multifidus. It has lumbar fibers that anchor the lumbar vertebrae directly to the iliac crest, and thoracic fibers whose caudal tendons form the medial half of the erector spinae aponeurosis[1]. Two smaller divisions are the longissimus cervicis and longissimus capitis. The iliocostalis lies lateral to the longissimus and connects the costal elements of the vertebral column. It has three divisions: iliocostalis lumborum, iliocostalis thoracis and iliocostalis cervicis. The iliocostalis lumborum has lumbar fibers that anchor the lumbar transverse processes directly to the iliac crest, and thoracic fibers whose caudal tendons form the lateral half of the erector spinae aponeurosis[1].

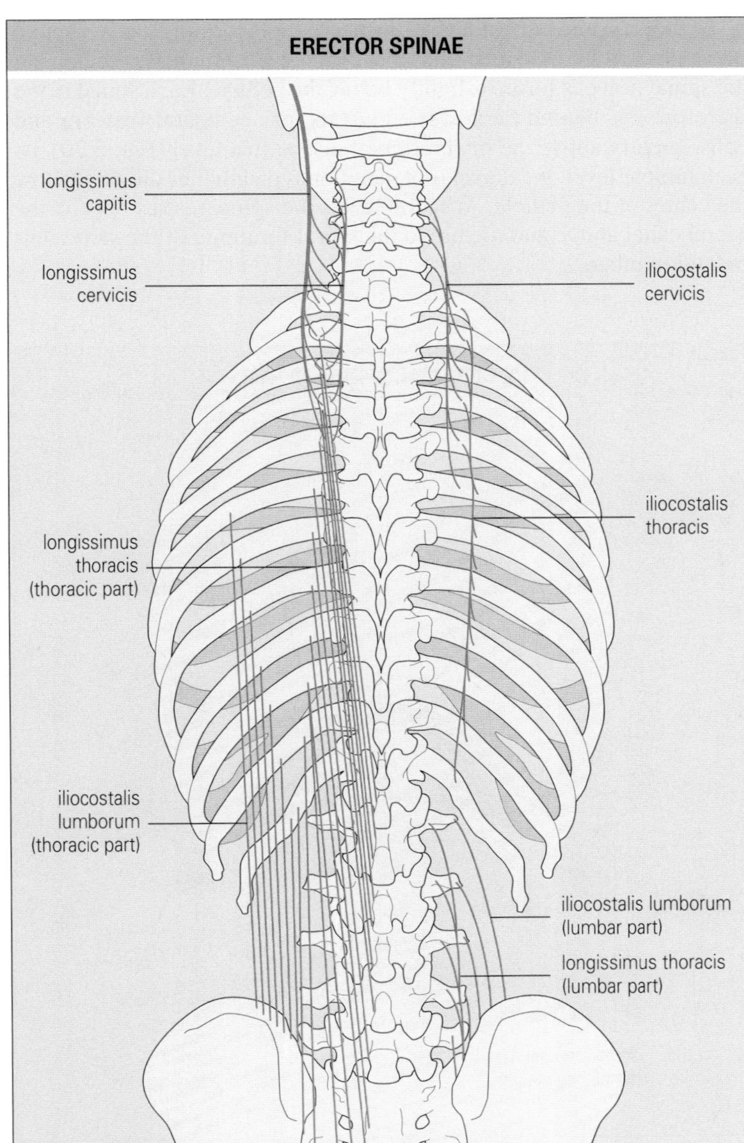

Fig. 2.16 Erector spinae.

Acting bilaterally, those fibers of the longissimus thoracis and iliocostalis lumborum that form the erector spinae aponeurosis are the most powerful extensors of the trunk, accounting for nearly 90% of the extensor moment at L1–L2 and nearly 50% of the moment at L5; at lower lumbar levels the multifidus and the lumbar fibers of erector spinae provide the remaining 50% of the extensor moment[14]. Acting unilaterally the longissimus thoracis and iliocostalis lumborum control lateral flexion of the lumbar spine.

The functions of iliocostalis thoracis, longissimus cervicis, iliocostalis cervicis and longissimus capitis have not been determined. They are all disposed to be extensors of their particular regions of the vertebral column but they are relatively very small in size compared to much stronger extensors such as semispinalis capitis.

Splenius

The splenius muscle wraps around the posterior and lateral aspects of the neck, covering all the other posterior neck muscles (Fig. 2.17). It consists of two parts: the splenius cervicis and splenius capitis. Both parts arise from the inferior half of the ligamentum nuchae and the spinous processes of C7 to T6. The splenius cervicis inserts into the transverse processes of the cervical vertebrae while the splenius capitis inserts into the mastoid process of the skull. Collectively, the splenius acts as an extensor of the neck and head. Unilaterally, the splenius acts synergistically with the opposite sternocleidomastoid to rotate the head and neck.

Thoracolumbar fascia

The thoracolumbar fascia consists of three layers. The anterior and middle layers surround the quadratus lumborum and psoas muscles. Critical to the function of the lumbar spine is the posterior layer. This layer covers the back of the lumbar erector spinae and multifidus, and is fused with the middle layer along the lateral border of the erector spinae.

The posterior layer is formed by the tendons of the aponeurosis of latissimus dorsi. These tendons cover the ipsilateral back muscles and reach the lumbar and sacral spinous processes in the midline where

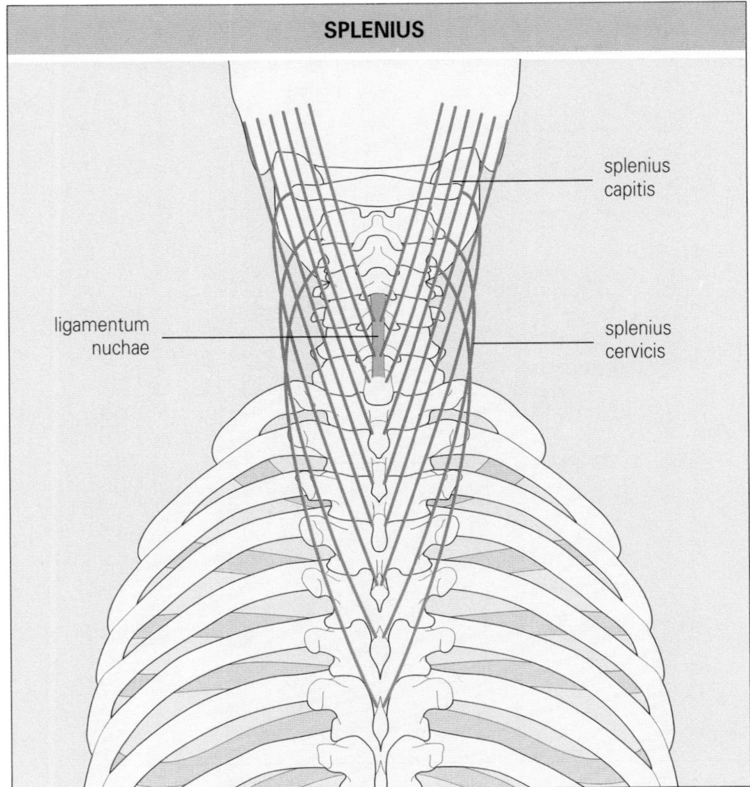

Fig. 2.17 The splenius muscles.

they interlace with fibers of the opposite side. Crossing the midline the tendons pass deep to the tendons of the opposite side producing a bilaminar structure to the posterior layer of thoracolumbar fascia[15,16].

The posterior layer of thoracolumbar fascia not only functions as a retinaculum for the back muscles but also, because of its attachments, acts passively as an extensive posterior ligament of the lumbar spine[1].

NERVES OF THE VERTEBRAL COLUMN

THE SPINAL CORD AND NERVE ROOTS

The spinal cord occupies the upper four fifths of the vertebral canal. It extends from the foramen magnum to the upper lumbar region. Its caudal end usually lies opposite the L1–L2 intervertebral disc but may lie one vertebral level above or below this. Its surface is intimately covered by the pia mater. The spinal cord is enclosed by the dural sac otherwise referred to as the theca, which extends from the foramen magnum as far as the S2 segment of the sacrum. The internal surface of the dural sac is lined by the arachnoid mater, and cerebrospinal fluid in the subarachnoid space bathes the spinal cord.

The spinal cord consists of 31 segments – eight cervical, twelve thoracic, five lumbar, five sacral and one coccygeal. Each gives rise to a pair of dorsal and a pair of ventral nerve roots. Each set of ventral and dorsal roots proceeds to converge and leave the dural sac as a spinal nerve. The cervical spinal nerves lie above their ipsisegmental vertebrae except for the C8 spinal nerve which lies below the seventh cervical vertebra. All other spinal nerves lie below their ipsisegmental vertebra (Fig. 2.18).

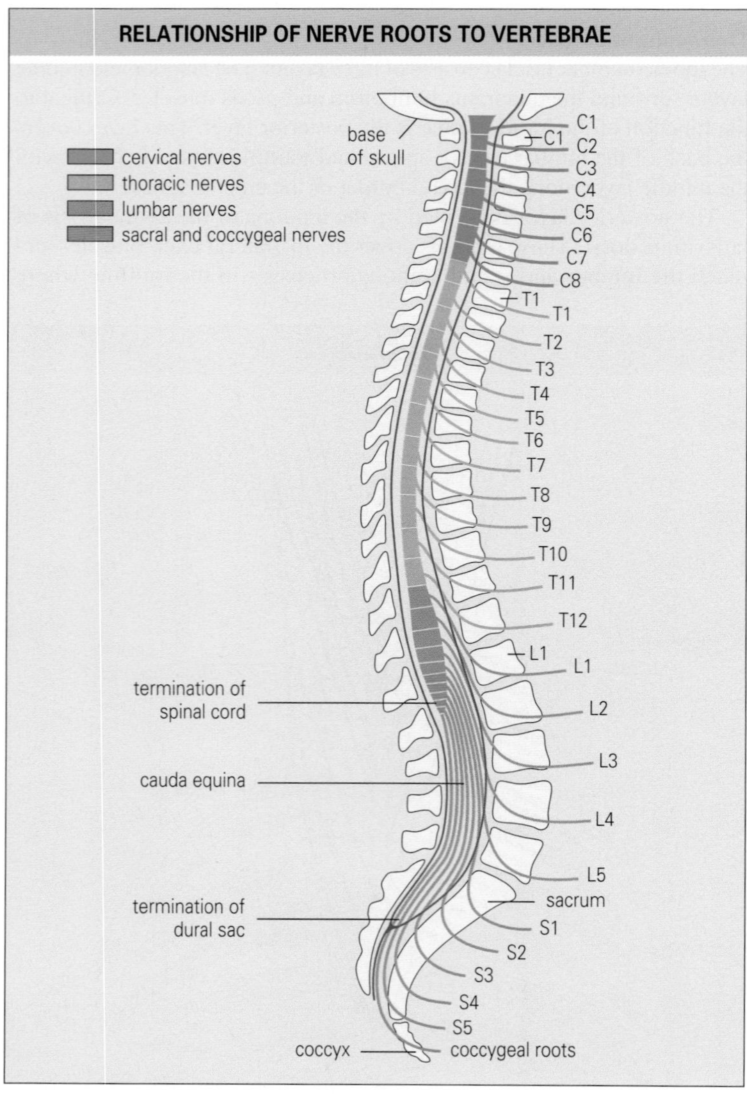

Fig. 2.18 The relationship of spinal nerves to vertebrae.

Within the dural sac, the upper cervical nerve roots tend to pass upwards towards their spinal nerve. Lower cervical nerve roots pass transversely or slightly downwards. Thoracic, lumbar and sacral nerve roots assume a progressively steeper, downwards course from the spinal cord to their respective spinal nerves. Below the caudal end of the spinal cord the lumbar, sacral and coccygeal nerve roots are aggregated in the dural sac as a leash of nerves known as the cauda equina. Within the cauda equina the nerve roots assume a constant topographic relationship. Those destined for more caudal locations lie medially and dorsally, while those about to leave the dural sac lie laterally and ventrally.

As each set of ventral and dorsal roots leaves the dural sac, it draws with it a sleeve of dura mater and arachnoid mater which distally blends with the epineurium of the spinal nerve. The dorsal root ganglia typically lie at the distal end of the dorsal root inside the apex of the dural sleeve.

SPINAL NERVES

Spinal nerves are mixed nerves consisting of motor fibers leaving the spinal cord in the ventral roots, and sensory fibers passing to the spinal cord along the dorsal roots. Some sensory fibers also enter the spinal cord along the ventral roots, and at segmental levels T1 to L2 the ventral roots convey preganglionic sympathetic efferent fibers, while the S2,S3 ventral roots convey preganglionic parasympathetic efferents.

At typical cervical levels the spinal nerves occupy the intervertebral foramen resting on top of the ipsisegmental pedicle. In this location they lie below the level of the intervertebral disc (Fig. 2.19). The C1 spinal nerve rests on the posterior arch of the atlas while the C2 spinal nerve lies behind or slightly below the lateral atlantoaxial joint.

At thoracic and lumbar levels, the nerve roots forming a given spinal nerve pass around the medial aspect of the ipsisegmental pedicle, and the spinal nerve is formed slightly below the pedicle. Each spinal nerve therefore lies behind the lower end of its ipsisegmental vertebra and consequently above the intervertebral disc at that level (Fig. 2.20). At each lumbar level, the dorsal root ganglion typically lies directly below the center of the pedicle. At sacral levels the spinal nerves occupy the sacral canal above and medial to the sacral foramina of the same segmental number.

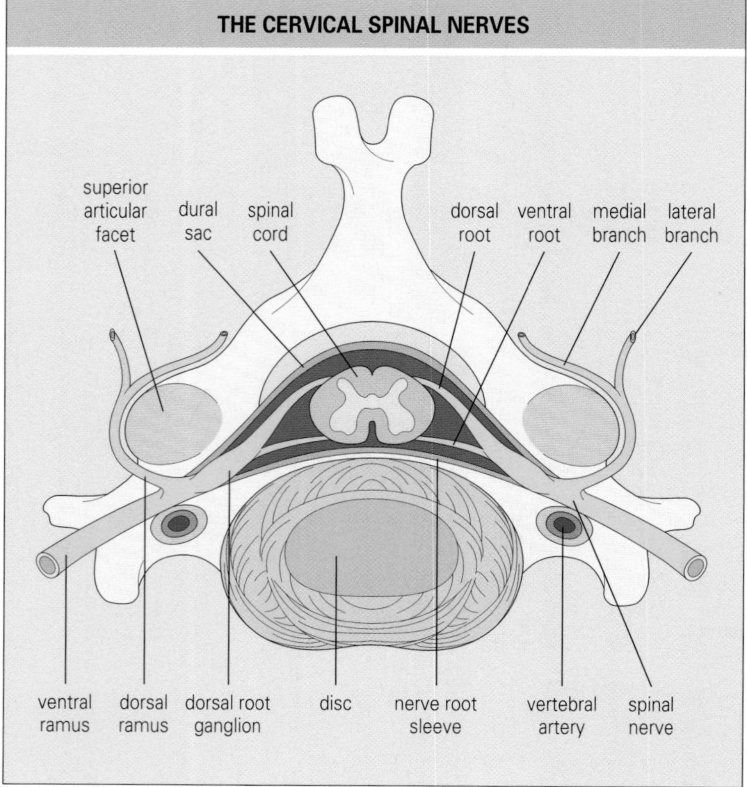

Fig. 2.19 The cervical spinal nerves. Schematic transverse section showing their ventral and dorsal roots and their rami.

Each spinal nerve is very short, being no longer than the intervertebral foramen is wide. At the lateral margin of the intervertebral foramen, the spinal nerve divides into a ventral ramus and a dorsal ramus. The C1 spinal nerve undergoes its branching on the posterior arch of the atlas; the sacral spinal nerves divide inside the sacral canal.

Dorsal rami

The dorsal rami of the spinal nerves are distributed to the posterior elements of the vertebral column and to the postvertebral muscles[17–19]. Upon leaving the intervertebral foramen, each dorsal ramus enters the posterior compartment of the spine by crossing the top edge of the transverse element of the subjacent vertebra, where it divides into medial and lateral branches (see Fig. 2.19) The C1 dorsal ramus is atypical. It leaves the posterior arch of the atlas to enter the suboccipital triangle, and innervates the suboccipital muscles. The lateral branches of the dorsal rami are distributed to the more lateral of the postvertebral muscle: splenius, longissimus and iliocostalis in the neck, and longissimus and iliocostalis in the thoracic and lumbar regions. The medial branches of the dorsal rami innervate the posterior joints of the vertebral column and the more medial of the back muscles: multifidus and semispinalis. Articular branches are distributed to each of the zygapophyseal joints above and below the course of the medial branch.

The medial branch of the C2 dorsal ramus is distinctive in that it forms the greater occipital nerve which winds around the inferior border of the obliquus inferior. This nerve enters and supplies semispinalis capitis before becoming cutaneous over the occiput[17]. The medial branch of the C3 dorsal ramus furnishes a similar branch, the third occipital nerve, which becomes cutaneous over the suboccipital region; it has the added distinction of innervating the C2–C3 zygapophyseal joint around whose capsule this nerve winds[17].

As a rule, at lower thoracic, lumbar and sacral levels, the lateral branches of the dorsal rami become cutaneous, the lateral branches of the S1, S2 and S3 dorsal rami forming the medial cluneal nerves. At cervical and upper thoracic levels the medial branches of the dorsal rami provide the cutaneous distribution, save that the dorsal rami of C5, C6 and C7 typically have no cutaneous branches.

Ventral rami

The thoracic ventral rami simply leave their intervertebral foramen and become intercostal nerves, each supplying the muscles of that intercostal space and the overlying skin. The lower six intercostal nerves are prolonged beyond the costal margin to supply the muscles and skin of the lateral and anterior abdominal wall in a segmental fashion.

The cervical, lumbar and sacral ventral rami form plexuses before being distributed peripherally (Fig. 2.21). The cervical plexus is formed by the C1–C4 ventral rami and supplies the sternocleidomastoid, trapezius, levator scapulae, the upper scalenes and prevertebral muscles of the neck, and cutaneous branches to the side of the face, auricle and neck.

The brachial plexus is formed by the C5–C8 and the T1 ventral rami, and supplies the lower scalenes, the muscles of the shoulder girdle and the muscles and skin of the upper limb. The lumbar plexus is formed by the L1–L4 ventral rami; it innervates the lower abdominal wall and

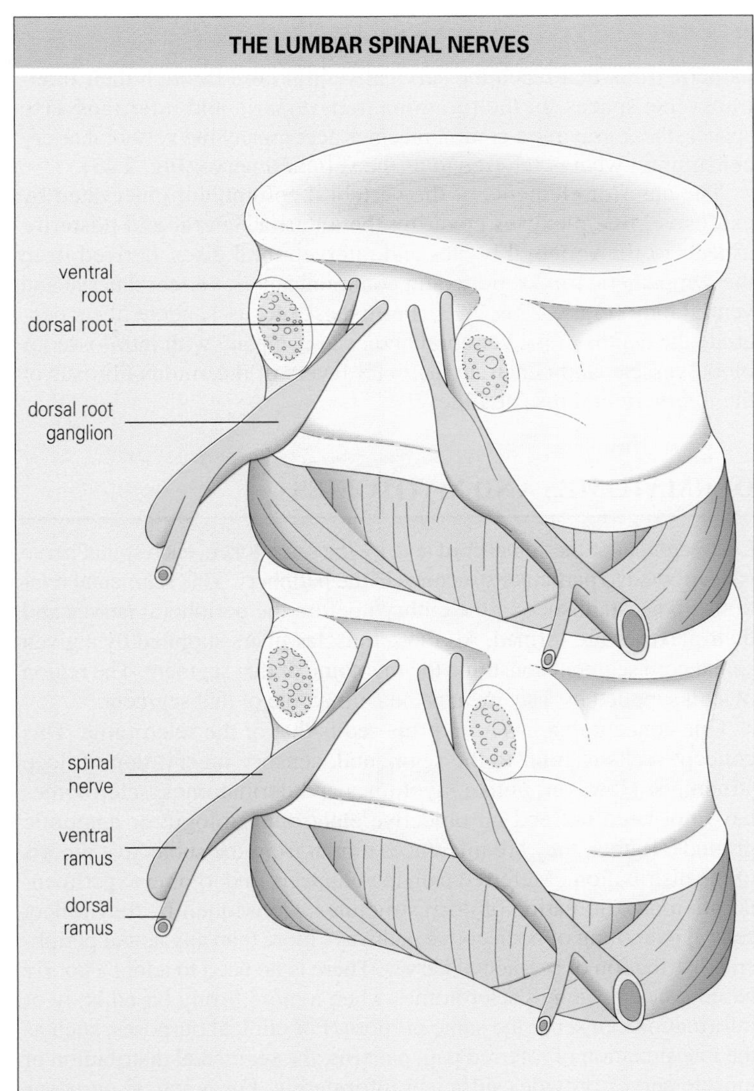

Fig. 2.20 The lumbar spinal nerves. The spinal nerve is formed by the junction of the dorsa and ventral roots immediately below the pedicle. The spinal nerve and roots lie behind the lower part of the vertebral body, not behind the disc.

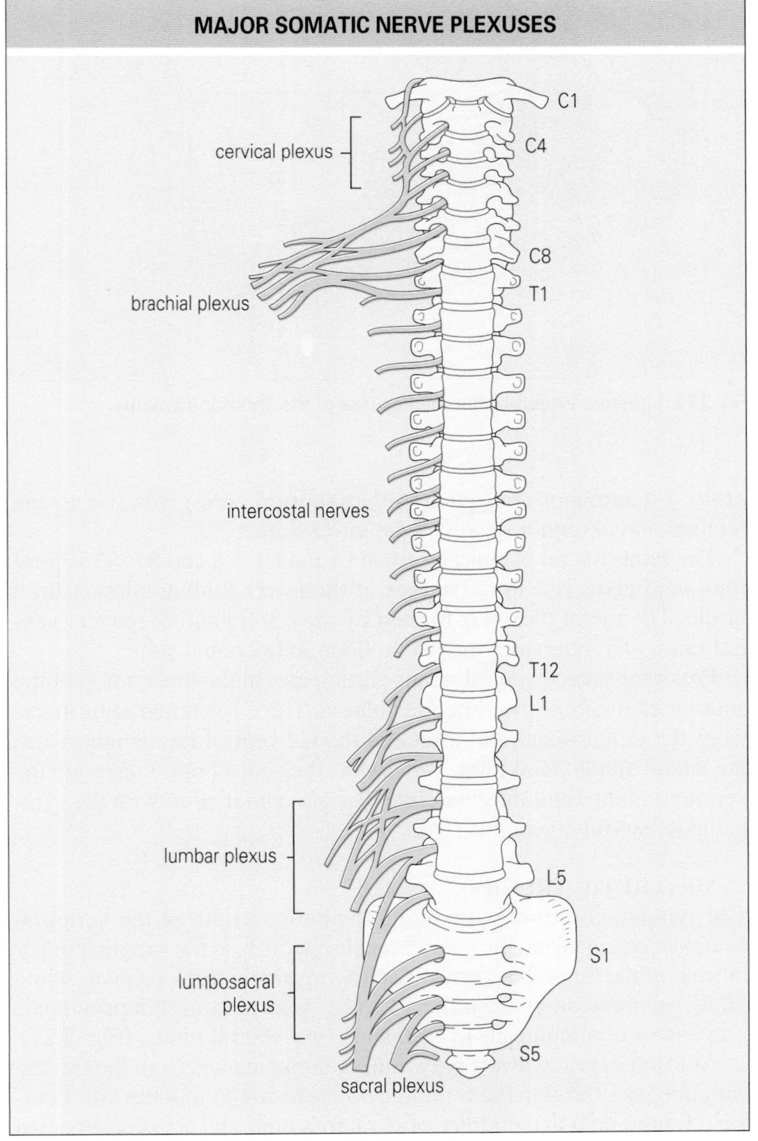

Fig. 2.21 Major somatic nerve plexuses.

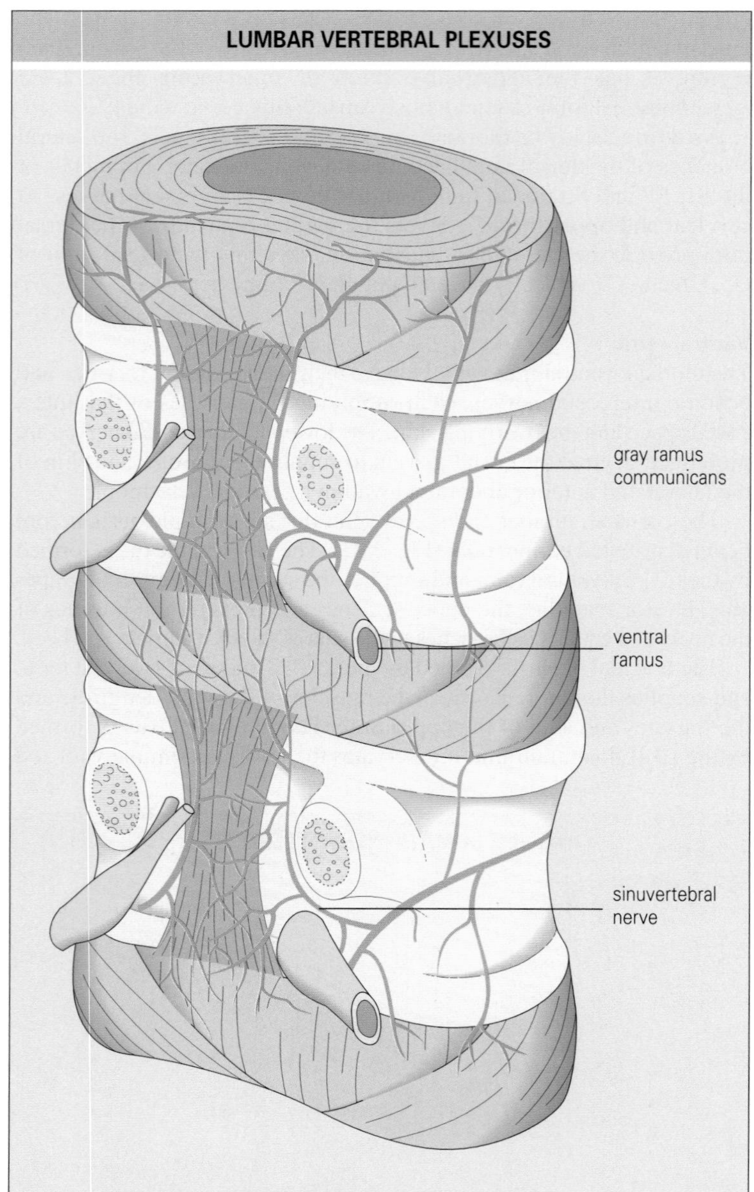

Fig. 2.22 Lumbar vertebral column: plexuses of the anterior elements.

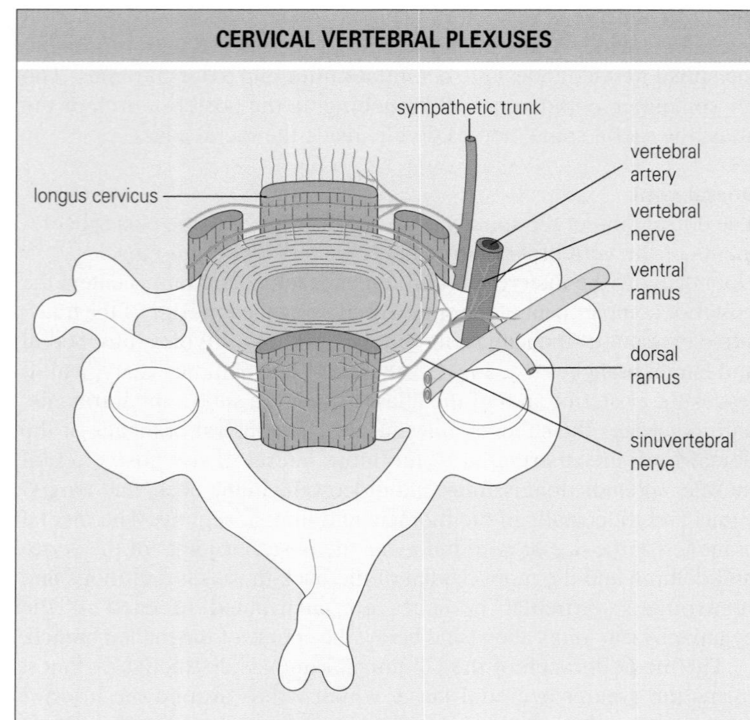

Fig. 2.23 Cervical vertebral column: plexuses of the anterior elements.

groin, psoas major and quadratus lumborum, and gives rise to the femoral and obturator nerves of the lower limb.

The lumbosacral plexus is formed by the L4, L5 and S1–S3 ventral rami, and gives rise to the nerves of the lower limb and lower limb girdle. The sacral plexus is formed by the S3–S5 and coccygeal ventral rami, and innervates the pelvic floor and perianal skin.

Proximally, each ventral ramus participates in the innervation of the anterior elements of the vertebral column. The C1 ventral ramus innervates the atlanto-occipital joint and the C2 ventral ramus innervates the lateral atlantoaxial joint. Otherwise, the ventral rami innervate the vertebral bodies and intervertebral discs in conjunction with the sympathetic nervous system.

SYMPATHETIC TRUNKS

The sympathetic trunks run along the entire length of the vertebral column spanning from the carotid canal superiorly to the ganglion impar in front of the tip of the coccyx. Each sympathetic trunk receives white rami communicantes from the T1 to L2 ventral rami, but provides a gray ramus communicans to each and every ventral ramus (Fig. 2.22).

At lower cervical levels gray rami communicantes from the stellate ganglion pass through the foramina transversaria to join the lower cervical ventral rami in their intervertebral foramina, and are supplemented by direct branches from the middle cervical ganglion and cervical sympathetic trunk that reach the cervical ventral rami through their intertransverse spaces. In the foramina transversaria and intertransverse spaces, these gray rami communicantes accompany the vertebral artery constituting what is referred to as the vertebral nerve (Fig. 2.23).

The anterior elements of the vertebral column are innervated by extensive, fine plexuses covering the anterior, lateral and posterior aspects of the vertebral bodies and intervertebral discs, derived from the sympathetic trunks, gray rami communicantes, vertebral nerve and ventral rami (Figs 2.22 & 2.23). From these plexuses, nerve fibers penetrate the depths of the vertebral bodies in company with intra-osseous blood vessels, and penetrate the outer layers of the anulus fibrosus of the intervertebral disc at all levels[20–23].

DERMATOMES AND MYOTOMES

Each segment of the spinal cord and, by the same token, each spinal nerve is distributed to particular structures in the periphery. This segmental relationship is established in the embryo before the peripheral nerves and their plexuses are formed. All those muscles fibers supplied by a given spinal cord segment constitute the myotome of that segment. The region of skin supplied by a segment is the dermatome of that segment.

One concept that has been proposed is that of the sclerotome. This concept seeks to refer to the segmental, sensory innervation of deep structures. However, unlike myotomes and dermatomes, sclerotomes have not been defined on objective electrophysiologic or anatomic grounds. Rather, they are inferences drawn from the subjective reports of the distribution of referred pain in volunteers undergoing experimental noxious stimulation of deep structures. Consequently, they reflect central patterning of nociceptive pathways more than any actual peripheral distribution of segmental nerves. There is no need to adopt a poorly based concept such as sclerotomes when a more firmly based body of information can serve the same purpose. For clinical purposes, such as the interpretation of referred pain patterns, the segmental distribution of muscle nerves provides sufficient information. For practical purposes one can assume that the segmental sensory distribution to muscles is the same as that of their motor distribution; and joints are supplied by the same segments as the principal muscles that act on them.

The basic pattern of dermatomes is depicted by the thoracic spinal nerves. Each nerve supplies the skin overlying the ipsisegmental intercostal space, with the addition that lower intercostal nerves project in the direction of their ribs onto the anterolateral abdominal wall. In the limbs, this basic parallel pattern of dermatomes is stretched and distorted by the longitudinal growth and rotation of the limb bud in the embryo. The systematic pattern is nonetheless evident in so far as consecutive segments are represented in order from proximal to distal along the cephalic border of the limb and then from distal to proximal along the caudal border of the limb (Fig. 2.24).

The myotomes of the body follow a similar systematic pattern (see Fig. 2.25). The muscles of the trunk are supplied by consecutive segments represented in the intercostal and first two lumbar nerves. In the limbs, two relationships apply. More proximal muscles are innervated by higher segments, and ventral muscles acting on a given joint are innervated by higher segments than the dorsal muscles acting on the same joint. The actual distribution of myotomes varies from individual to individual, but the modal pattern is summarized in Figure 2.25.

This pattern can be used as the basis for clinical testing of segmental motor deficits, but it serves equally well for the interpretation of deep and referred pain. Pain perceived in a region occupied by a particular muscle or joint does not necessarily imply an origin in that muscle or joint. Rather, it may indicate a source in any of the deep, somatic structures innervated by the same segments that innervate the muscle or joint in question.

For example, levator scapulae lies above the scapula and is innervated by C3 and C4. Pain overlying the levator scapulae may reflect an origin in levator scapulae but also may reflect a source in any structure innervated by C3 or C4. The posterior scapular muscles and the glenohumeral joint are both supplied by C5 and C6, but pain in the shoulder or over the scapula may reflect an origin in any of the structures innervated by C5 or C6, which includes not only shoulder muscles and shoulder joints but also C5 and C6 segments of the vertebral column.

The anterior chest wall provides a further illustrative example. Deeply, the upper chest wall is supplied by the T1–T4 segments but it is covered by the pectoralis major which is supplied by C5–C8. Consequently, chest wall pain may indicate an origin anywhere in the tissues supplied by C5 to T4. The T1–T4 component invites a consideration of the thoracic viscera, but the C5–C8 component invites a consideration of referred pain from the neck.

BIOMECHANICS

Biomechanics is the discipline that describes the operation of the musculoskeletal system. It embraces kinematics – which deals with the range and patterns of movements, and kinetics – which deals with the forces that cause and resist these movements. With respect to the vertebral column, much is known about its kinematics, but knowledge of its kinetics is limited because of the complexity of the system and difficulties in studying the moving vertebral column *in vivo*.

Of the various regions of the vertebral column, the cervical spine, lumbar spine and sacroiliac joints are the best understood. Little is known about how the thoracic spine operates, largely because this region and its movements are obscured by the rib cage which renders the thoracic vertebral column difficult to study radiologically.

SACROILIAC JOINT

Although firmly constrained by its ligaments, the sacroiliac joint exhibits movements that are small in magnitude and complex in nature. The amplitude of nutation of the sacrum is normally not more than 2°[24]. However, movements of greater amplitude occur, but in other planes. During flexion and extension of the hips, each hemipelvis rotates about an axis that passes from the pubic symphysis to the greater sciatic notch. During extension, each hemipelvis turns downwards about this axis, and during flexion it turns upwards[25]. The resulting movement of the sacroiliac joint involves an upwards gliding of the ilium on the sacrum during extension, coupled with an element of distraction between the two bones superiorly and anteriorly. A converse coupling occurs during flexion.

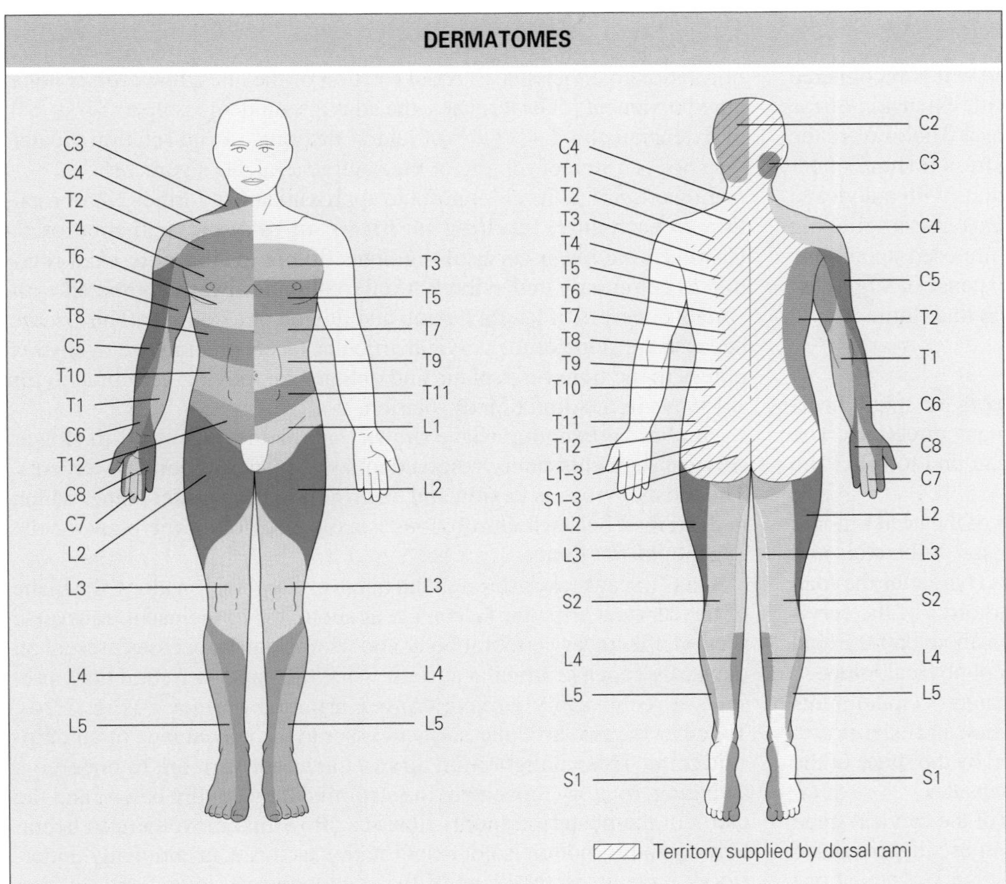

Fig. 2.24 The dermatomes.

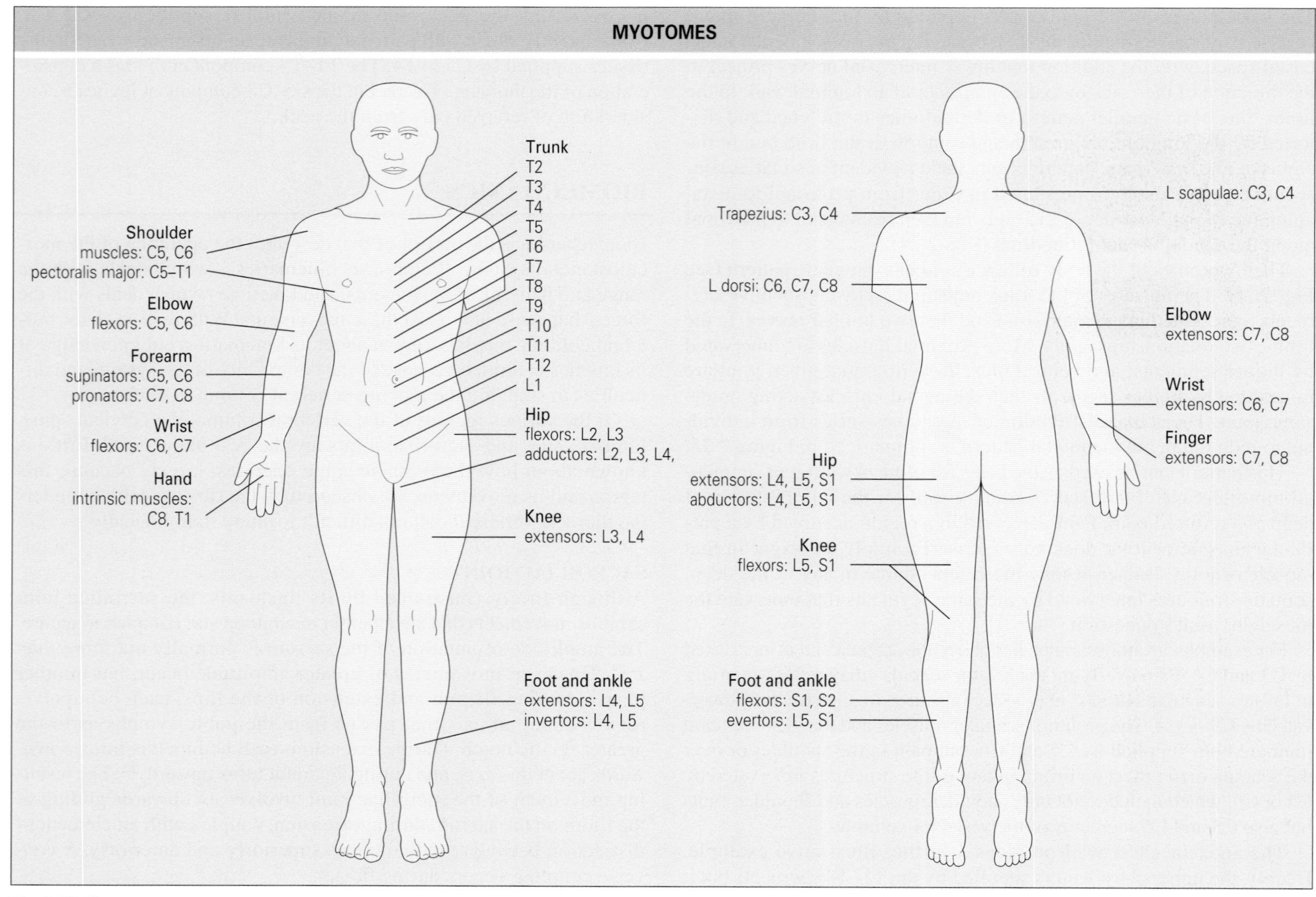

Fig. 2.25 The myotomes.

Perhaps these movements can be better appreciated if it is recognized that, during gait, the flexion of one hip coupled with extension of the other imposes severe twisting forces on the pelvis as a whole. Were the pelvis a solid, single ring of bone, it would suffer stress fracture under these conditions (as indeed it does in some individuals with ankylosed joints). The sacroiliac joint consequently serves as a stress-relieving joint, the tension that otherwise would have been imposed upon bone being absorbed by the sacroiliac ligaments, at the expense of slight distracting and sliding movements between the sacrum and ilium.

CERVICAL SPINE

The head is a sensory platform, carrying the receptors for smell, hearing and vision, which must be able to orientate in many directions. The function of the cervical spine is to support the head and to move the sensory platform in three-dimensional space.

In static loading in the upright posture, the weight of the head is borne through the atlanto-occipital joints, the lateral masses of the atlas and through the lateral atlantoaxial joints onto the axis. Thereafter the load is transmitted both through the vertebral bodies and discs of the cervical spine, and through the zygapophyseal joints, with about half the load passing through the discs and half through the zygapophyseal joints.

Nodding movements of the head occur at the atlanto-occipital joints which accommodate a total range of about 15° of flexion and extension[26]. Other movements at these joints are largely precluded by the shape of the atlantal sockets and tension developed in the joint capsules.

Essentially half of the total range of axial rotation of the cervical spine is accommodated by the atlantoaxial joints. Moving as single unit the head and atlas normally exhibit 43° ± 5.5° (mean ± standard deviation) of rotation to either side[27]. Axial rotation of the atlas, however, is not a pure movement for as it rotates, the atlas also undergoes up to 14° (± 6°) of extension and 2.4° (± 6°) of lateral flexion[28]. Axial rotation greater than 56° is a sign of rupture of the contralateral alar ligament[27].

Lower cervical levels contribute approximately a further 28° of rotation to each side, resulting in 70–80° of total cervical rotation[26]. However, the lower cervical segments do not exhibit pure axial rotation as commonly understood. Axial rotation is always combined with variable degrees of lateral flexion and flexion or extension. This occurs because the slope of the cervical articular facets precludes movements purely in the transverse plane and obliges the moving vertebrae to tilt sideways in the direction of rotation.

Studies by Penning[29] have shown that the movements of the lower cervical segments can be resolved into two planes of pure movements. The most obvious is flexion and extension in the sagittal plane, which is described below. Less obvious is axial rotation in the plane of the zygapophysial joints.

On CT scans taken through the uncovertebral region along the plane of the cervical articular facets, i.e. at about 45° to the usual transverse section, the lower vertebral body and its uncinate processes present an upwardly concave articular surface while the upper vertebral body presents a reciprocally curved, convex articular surface[29] (Fig. 2.26). Together the two articular surfaces assume the appearance of an ellipsoid joint. This configuration allows the upper vertebra to undergo a swinging, rotatory movement in relation to the vertebra below, and the clefts in the posterior anulus fibrosus allow this movement to occur. However, this motion is not axial rotation as it is conventionally understood; it occurs in the plane of the zygapophyseal joints, and rotation

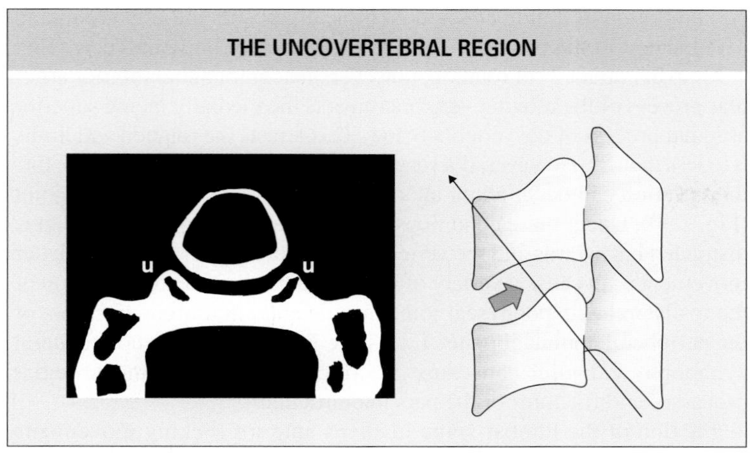

Fig. 2.26 The uncovertebral region as seen in a CT scan taken through the plane of the zygapophyseal joints. U = uncovertable joint.

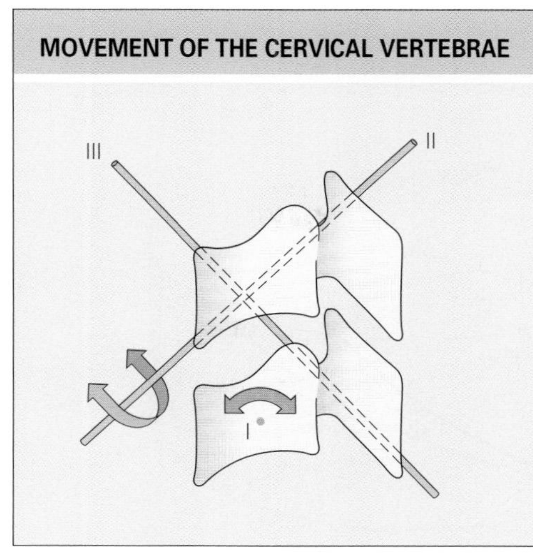

Fig. 2.27 Axes and planes of movement of the cervical vertebrae.

at right angles to this plane is precluded by impaction of the zygapophyseal joints. The structure of a cervical interbody joint is therefore that of a saddle joint allowing only two planes of movement: flexion and extension in the sagittal plane, and axial rotation in the plane of the zygapophyseal joints (Fig. 2.27). Under these conditions, lateral flexion of the cervical intervertebral joints does not occur. What appears to be lateral flexion is a composite of axial rotation of lower cervical vertebra coupled with contralateral rotation of the atlas.

Flexion of a typical cervical segment involves an anterior rocking movement of the moving vertebrae and an anterior translation. An opposite combination of movements occurs in extension. During flexion each vertebral body rocks and glides on the underlying disc while the inferior articular facets glide upwards and forwards over their opposed superior articular facets. As the facets move, the joints subluxate and the exposed articular surfaces are protected by the fibroadipose meniscoids of these joints. Failure of a meniscoid to re-enter the joint cavity after flexion or rotation of the joint can result in acute torticollis[6].

The total range of motion (mean ± sd) from full flexion to full extension for each segment is C2–C3, 10° ± 3°; C3–C4, 15° ± 3°; C4–C5, 19° ± 4°; C5–C6, 20° ± 4°; C6–C7, 19° ± 4°[30]. These ranges, however, are only indicative, for it has been shown that in normal individuals ranges of motion differ from day to day and according to whether flexion or extension is executed first; differences of 5–15° in a given segment can be recorded, along with differences of up to 30° in total range of neck motion[31]. These normal variations place serious limitations on the use of range of motion either as a diagnostic tool or as an index of success of therapy.

Notwithstanding differences in range of motion, flexion–extension occurs in normal individuals about axes whose location is tightly clustered. For each cervical segment the axis of rotation lies in a characteristic location with little variation between individuals[32] (Fig. 2.28). At C2–C3 the axis lies in the posteroinferior corner of the C3 vertebral body. At successively lower levels the axes progressively move towards the upper central region of the vertebral body. Neck pain is significantly associated with an abnormal location of one or more axes of rotation. Determining axes of rotation therefore provides an objective measure of disturbed cervical function secondary to pain[33].

LUMBAR SPINE

Pivotal to all movements of the lumbar spine are the intervertebral discs, which are designed to sustain static compression loads, yet to be sufficiently compliant to allow bending and twisting movements. Compression loads are exerted by the weight of the body above any given disc, plus any external load being carried. However, the greatest compression loads are those exerted on the disc by the back muscles.

In the first instance, compression loads are borne passively by the anulus fibrosus of the disc. Indeed, it has been shown experimentally that the ability of a disc to sustain brief compression loads is not reduced by removal of its nucleus pulposus[34]. However, without a nucleus, the tendency of a compressed anulus fibrosus is to buckle inwards. The role of the nucleus pulposus, therefore, is to brace the anulus fibrosus from within. Critical to this function is the water-binding capacity of the nucleus pulposus. If the nucleus pulposus is injured and loses its water-binding capacity, its bracing action is impaired, the anulus buckles and the disc narrows. In a normal disc, however, about half of any compression load is borne through the anulus and half directly through the nucleus.

In upright standing, most of the weight of the trunk is borne through the lumbar vertebral bodies and discs. However, the lordotic curve of the lumbar spine results in some of the load being borne by the zygapophyseal joints. The exact proportion varies from segment to segment and according to the tilt of the vertebra in the lordotic curve. The joints low in the curve (L3–L4, L4–L5 and L5–S1) bear about 19% of the load, while the upper joints take only 11% [35]. In sitting, the lordosis is flattened and the zygapophyseal joints take no load.

Bending in the sagittal plane, or in the coronal plane, involves deformation of the lumbar discs. On the side to which bending occurs the anulus fibrosus is compressed and tends to bulge outwards. On the opposite side the anulus fibrosus is stretched. Meanwhile, the nucleus pulposus is deformed and tends to displace away from the direction of maximum compression into the stretched zone of the anulus fibrosus. The disc is superbly designed to accommodate these movements; the criss-cross arrangement of the collagen fibers of the anulus ensures that all laminae of the anulus contribute to retaining the nucleus and

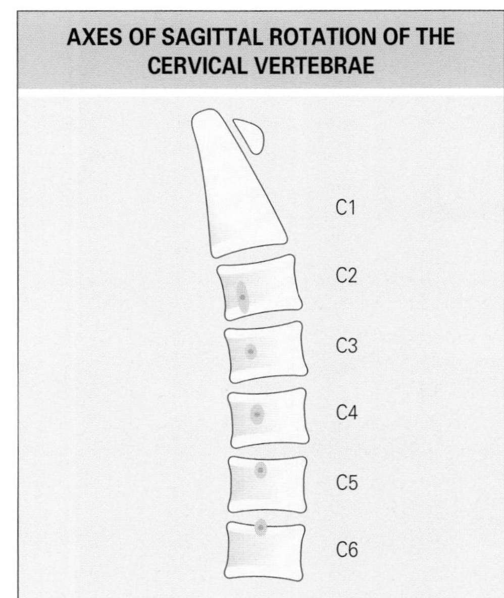

Fig. 2.28 Locations of the axes of sagittal rotation of the cervical vertebrae.

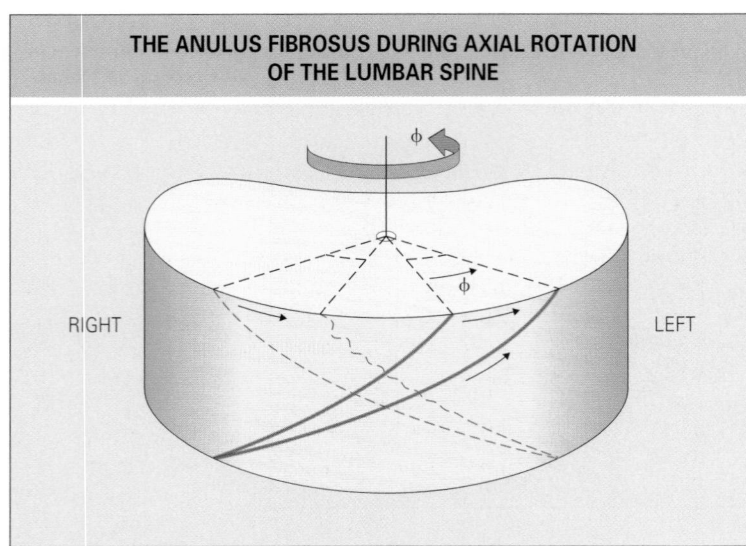

Fig. 2.29 The anulus fibrosus during axial rotation of the lumbar spine.

resisting separation of the vertebral bodies[36]. Indeed, so strong is a normal disc that it cannot be ruptured by compression loads; the vertebral end-plates fracture before the anulus fibrosus fails[37,38]. Even, if a channel is cut through the anulus a normal disc does not herniate under compression[34,39,40]. Disc herniation requires an antecedent degradation of the nucleus and weakening of the anulus fibrosus[1,41].

The lumbar disc is substantially weaker in axial rotation. As a vertebral body rotates, the underlying anulus fibrosus is twisted, but only half of the collagen fibers in the anulus resist this motion – those inclined in the direction of rotation; the other half are shortened and offer no resistance (Fig. 2.29). The collagen fibers that resist rotation are stretched, and it can be shown that only about 3° of rotation is required before these collagen fibers start to fail[36]. For this reason the lumbar disc must be protected against excessive rotation by the zygapophyseal joints.

Axial rotation of a lumbar segment typically occurs initially around an axis located in the posterior third of the vertebral body and disc (Fig. 2.30). After about 2° of rotation, however, the contralateral inferior articular process of the moving vertebra impacts the medially facing superior articular process of the vertebra below. This arrests the rotation and limits it to less than 3°. However, if a rotatory force continues to be applied, further rotation can occur about an axis now located in the impacted joint (Fig. 2.30). Under these conditions, the ipsilateral zygapophyseal joint is distracted backwards and the vertebral body shears laterally. These latter movements can cause a variety of injuries including fracture avulsion of the ipsilateral zygapophyseal joint capsule and circumferential tears of the peripheral anulus fibrosus. Excessive impaction of the contralateral zygapophyseal joint can cause fractures of its facets and articular processes and fractures of the pars interarticularis[1,42,43].

Flexion of the lumbar spine involves anterior rocking movements of the vertebral bodies combined with anterior translation. An opposite combination of movements occurs in extension. At each segment, as the vertebral body rocks and glides forwards on the underlying disc, the inferior articular processes are lifted out of the socket formed by the superior articular processes of the vertebra below. During this movement, the zygapophyseal joints subluxate and the exposed articular surfaces are covered by the fibroadipose meniscoids of these joints. Failure of the meniscoids to re-enter the joint space upon extension after flexion may result in a painful locked back as the meniscoid buckles under the joint capsule, acting like a loose body[1].

During flexion, excessive anterior translation is prevented by the tips of the inferior articular processes hooking onto the superior articular processes of the vertebra below. Tension in the anulus fibrosus is a secondary constraint. Anterior rotation is limited by tension in the posterior ligamentous system, which includes the capsules of the zygapophyseal joints, and is controlled by the posterior back muscles. Extension is limited either by impaction of consecutive spinous processes or by impaction of inferior articular processes on the lamina below[1]. Sudden severe extension can cause an inferior articular process to chisel into the lamina and cause a pars interarticularis fracture.

If one inferior articular process is longer than the other, impaction occurs on one side only. Continued extension is converted by this

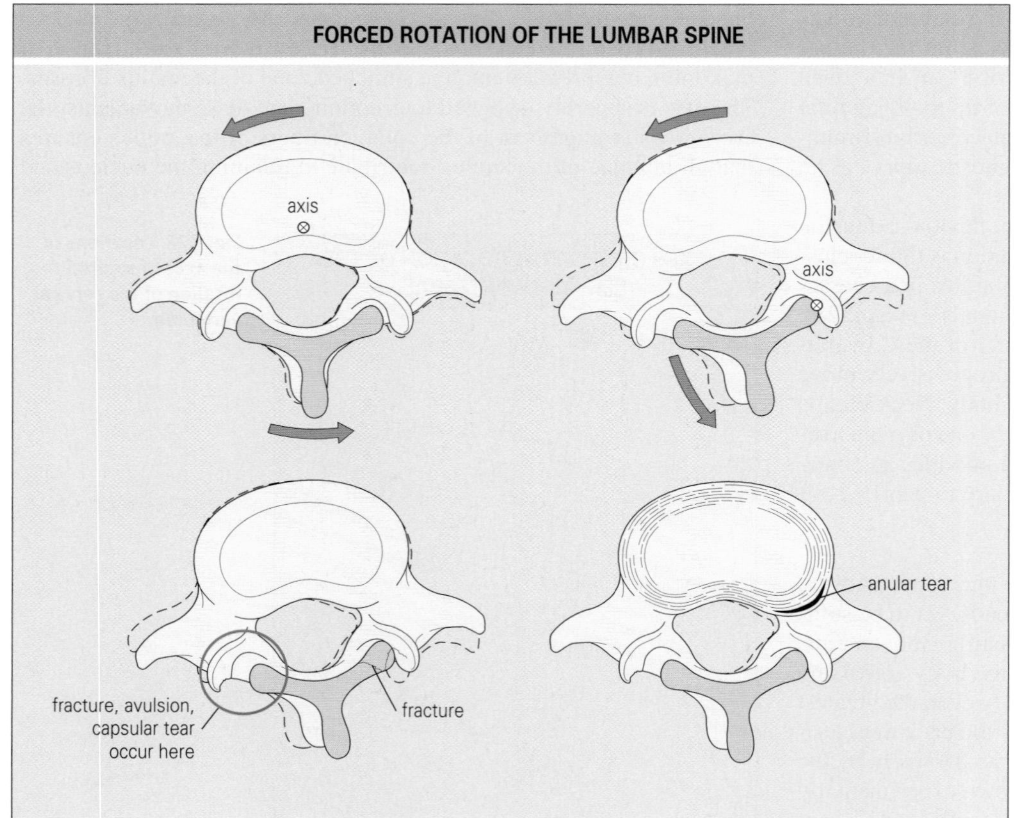

Fig. 2.30 Sequence of events during forced rotation of the lumbar spine.

impaction into a posterior rotation of the opposite side, which results in distraction and disruption of the zygapophyseal joint on that side[1]. In this way zygapophyseal joints can be injured by extension.

Flexion and extension of the lumbar vertebrae occur around axes that are typically located just below the intervertebral disc and slightly behind its midpoint[44] (Fig. 2.31). The location of these axes is governed by the balance of forces acting on the segment, which include the weight of the trunk, the force generated by muscles and the resistance to movement afforded by the zygapophyseal joints, disc and ligaments of the segment. Any change in these forces results in displacement of the axis from its normal location[45]. Injured and degenerated lumbar segments exhibit abnormal locations of these axes[46,47], and an abnormal axis is an objective sign of altered spinal function.

Lifting

Lifting is the major arduous task of the lumbar spine. In engineering terms it involves the balancing of flexion moments exerted by the trunk and the external load being lifted by extension moments generated within the body.

A moment is the work done by a force that tends to bend or rotate an object. Its magnitude is the product of the magnitude of the force (in newtons) and the perpendicular distance (in meters) from the center of rotation to the line of the force; the latter distance being known as the moment arm.

As a body stoops forwards several forces exert flexion moments. Gravity exerts a downwards force on the mass of the trunk, and the resulting moment is determined by the horizontal displacement of the center of the trunk from the lumbar spine (Fig. 2.32). The load to be lifted exerts an additional moment whose magnitude is determined by the displacement of the load from the lumbar spine. The sum of these moments must be overcome by mechanisms within the lumbar spine.

For example, the trunk of a 70kg individual weighs about 40kg. Under gravity it exerts a downwards force of 392N (40kg $\times$ 9.8 ms^{-1}). At about 90° of forward stoop the center of gravity of the trunk lies about 30cm from the lumbar spine, and exerts a moment of 118Nm. A mass of 30kg located 45cm in front of the lumbar spine exerts a moment of 132Nm (40 $\times$ 9.8 $\times$ 0.45). The total flexion moment that must be overcome for the lift is 250Nm.

In a stooped position, the lumbar vertebrae are fully flexed and the posterior ligaments of the lumbar spine are fully engaged; the back muscles are fully stretched. It is these structures that must generate an extension moment to overcome any flexion moment. However, their disadvantage is that they lie very close to the lumbar spine; their moment arms are only of the order of 0.05m (5cm). Therefore, they must exert very large forces in order to generate large moments.

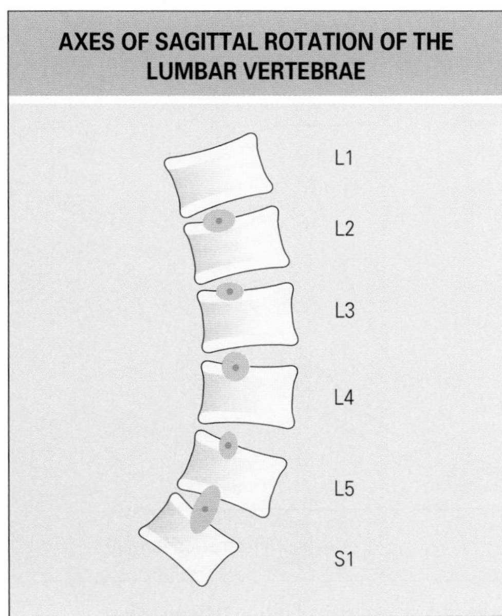

Fig. 2.31 Axes of sagittal rotation of the lumbar vertebrae.

The maximum strength of the back muscles is only about 4000N. Acting at 5cm behind the lumbar spine, the maximum moment that they can exert is only about 200Nm. Collectively the posterior ligaments (including the posterior layer of thoracolumbar fascia) can resist about 50Nm. Thus, the maximum total moment that the flexed lumbar spine can sustain is 250Nm; enough to raise a 30kg mass in a 90° stooped position. To lift greater loads, the load must be brought closer to the lumbar spine in order to shorten its moment arm.

In this regard, it should be noted that in a stoop lift the lumbar spine must act passively. If the back muscles were to shorten the posterior ligaments would be disengaged and their 50Nm contribution would be lost. The lumbar spine must stay fully flexed to benefit from the combined tension of the ligaments and the muscles. Under these conditions, the flexed lumbar spine, like the jib of a crane, is rotated upwards as a whole by the hip extensors acting on the pelvis. The back muscles shorten only when the moment arm of the external load is reduced to an extent that muscle contraction alone can balance the flexion moment.

In a squat lift, with the lumbar lordosis maintained, ligaments do not contribute to balancing the external load; the back muscles alone must oppose any flexion moment. This requires greater concentration than in a stoop lift in order to actively control the back muscles.

Whether a load is lifted with a stooped posture or a squat position (with the knees bent) is essentially immaterial. It is not the posture of the lumbar spine that counts. The critical element is the moment arm of the trunk and of the load to be lifted. Loads carried closer to the body exert smaller flexion moments; they are less likely to tear muscles or posterior ligaments, and require less muscular effort to balance them.

However, what should not be neglected is the compression load exerted by the back muscles, even for modest loads carried sensibly close to the body which may still require great effort by the back muscles. Lifting 30kg at 45cm, or 60kg at only 22.5cm still requires maximum tension in the back muscles – a force of 4000N. This force will be exerted longitudinally along the lumbar spine and is ten times greater than the body weight carried by the spine. An average vertebral body can sustain about 10,000N before its end-plates fracture, but the lower end of the normal range is around 4000N[37]. Thus, it is possible for an individual with strong back muscles but relatively weak

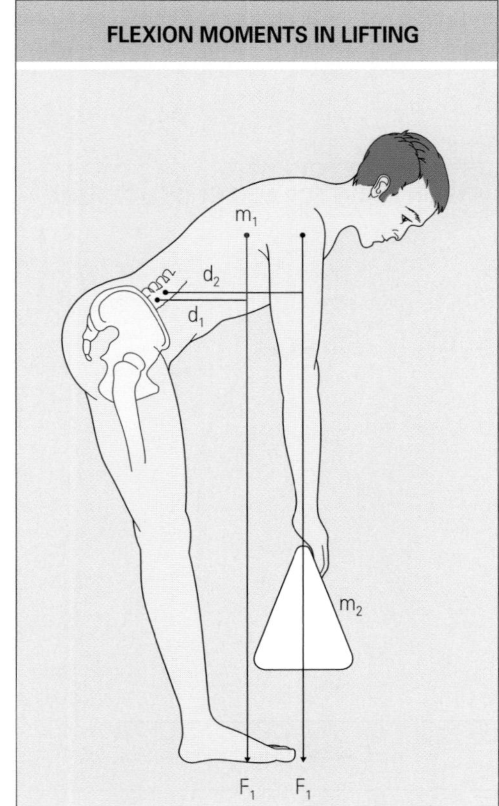

Fig. 2.32 Lifting. Flexion moments are generated by the trunk (m_1) acting at a distance d_1 from the lumbar spine, and by the external load (m_2) acting at a distance d_2.

vertebral bodies to sustain an end-plate fracture during a heavy lift involving maximum exertion of their back muscles. Such an injury can initiate a chain of events that leads to degradation of the nucleus pulposus and the development of internal disc disruption[41].

The risk of injury is greater when lifting is associated with rotatory movements of the trunk, as in swinging from left to right while in a stooped position. In this position the lumbar spine is prestressed by the flexion; in particular, the fibers of the posterior anulus fibrosus will have undergone near-maximum strain. Adding a twisting movement calls upon the anulus fibrosus to resist more force and undergo further strain. Beyond maximum strain lies injury. In particular, the posterolateral anulus is liable to tear under these conditions, resulting in a torsion injury to the disc[41].

The back muscles afford no protection against twisting; they lie essentially parallel to the axis of axial rotation and cannot control twisting movements[48]. Only the oblique abdominal muscles are able to control axial rotation. Failure to engage these muscles during a lift and twist renders the lumbar spine susceptible to injury by torsion.

Intra-abdominal pressure has long been touted as a means of resisting flexion moments and aiding the back muscles during a lift. The belief was that intra-abdominal pressure acts upwards on the diaphragm and thereby extends the trunk and relieves the back muscles of a proportion of the flexion load. Biomechanical studies and clinical studies, however, have dispelled this notion. The force required to produce any significant antiflexion moment exceeds the hoop tension of the abdominal muscles[1], and because the abdominal muscles lie in front of the lumbar spine, their contraction causes a flexion moment that negates any antiflexion moment produced by a rise in intra-abdominal pressure[1]. Nevertheless, although they do not oppose flexion, the abdominal muscles are critical for controlling the axial stability of the lumbar spine during a sagittal lift.

Fatigue failure

Of growing interest in lumbar spine biomechanics is the concept of fatigue failure. Whereas past studies focussed on the biomechanics of sudden injury and the strength at failure of various components of the lumbar spine, contemporary studies have been addressing the effects of repeated applications of forces whose magnitude is insufficient to damage tissues acutely.

When a structure is progressively stretched (or compressed) by applying to it progressively greater forces, it undergoes deformation (elongation or compression) referred to as strain, and measured as a fraction of the initial length of the structure. Plotting the relationship between the applied force (stress) and the resulting strain yields the characteristic stress–strain curve of the structure or tissue in question (Fig. 2.33). The initial region of this curve is referred to as the 'toe phase', and reflects any macroscopic slack in the tissue being taken up. The next region is the linear phase, and reflects the resistance to deformation exerted by the molecules that constitute the tissue. The slope of this segment, being the ratio between the change in force and the change in strain, measures the stiffness of the tissue. The final phase is failure, where the bonds between the molecules are totally disrupted and the tissue fails. The stress applied at the point of failure is known as the ultimate tensile stress.

A different behavior is manifest when moderate forces are repeatedly applied (Fig. 2.34). After many repetitions the tissue fails at a stress much less than that required to disrupt the tissue upon a single application. The implication is that each application of the moderate force disrupts a small proportion of the bonds within the tissue, but these are not repaired before the next application which disrupts a further proportion. Repeated applications of the force thus result in the accumulation of damage until sufficient bonds are disrupted and the tissue fails.

In the lumbar spine, the anulus fibrosus is resistant to failure when subjected to single stresses. However, when repeatedly stressed the anulus fails at stresses well below its ultimate tensile stress. When subjected to stress equal to about 60% of the ultimate tensile stress an anulus fails after fewer than 3000 repetitions, but in some cases, can fail after as few as 20 repetitions[49].

Vertebral bodies exhibit a similar behavior. When subjected to stresses equal to 50–80% of ultimate compressive strength, fractures of the vertebral end plate occur within 1000 repetitions, and in some cases after as few as 30–80 repetitions[50]. The forces involved are within the range of those encountered in activities of daily living, and these experimental studies warn that in the face of repetitive loading, elements of the lumbar spine can be injured by forces considerably less than those expected for an acute injury.

INSTABILITY

One of the most controversial and elusive concepts in spine medicine is that of instability. This rubric is often applied as a clinical diagnosis to patients whose back pain is brought on by certain movements. However, there is no universal consensus as to the diagnostic criteria[51]. The implication is that the patient has a lesion that somehow renders

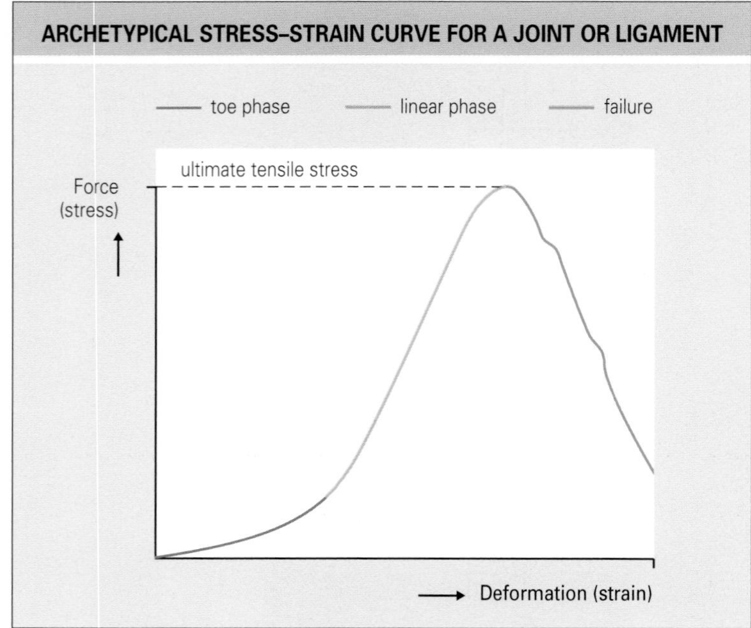

Fig. 2.33 Archetypical stress–strain curve for a joint or ligament.

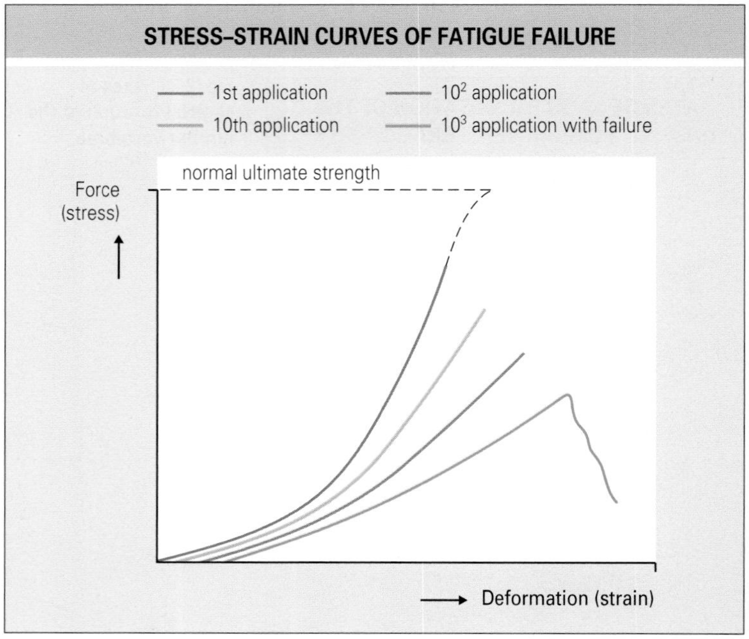

STRESS–STRAIN CURVES OF FATIGUE FAILURE

1st application
10th application
10^2 application
10^3 application with failure
normal ultimate strength
Force (stress)
Deformation (strain)

Fig. 2.34 The stress–strain curve of a structure exhibiting fatigue failure.

one of the motion segments 'looser' than normal. But no studies have shown any correlation between symptoms and objective evidence of a lesion or movement abnormality.

In the appendicular skeleton, instability is clinically apparent for the joint can be palpated and examined. An unstable joint is one that exhibits an excessive range of motion under physiologic conditions, such as clinical examination or during activities of daily living, particularly when the motion occurs in a plane or direction that is not normal for that joint. In the spine, such instability is less apparent for the vertebral joints are not visible or readily accessible to clinical examination. Consequently, spinal instability remains a theoretic concept or an abstract clinical impression. Nevertheless, biomechanists have ventured to define spinal instability.

One definition describes instability as decreased stiffness as manifested by the stress–strain curve for a spinal segment[52]. This definition, however, does not capture the implied essence of instability: that the joint feels as if it is about to fall apart. Another definition describes instability in terms of an increased neutral zone[53]. The neutral zone is virtually synonymous with the toe phase of a stress–strain curve. A joint with an increased neutral zone is one that exhibits an excessive range of movement when minimal forces are applied, although subsequently it exhibits normal stiffness. Essentially, the joint is looser than normal early in the range, but ultimately remains intact. Symptoms occur when the joint accelerates through the early phase and strikes resistance at a velocity greater than normal, later than expected. An analogy would be the sensation of walking down a series of 15cm steps only to encounter suddenly a step of 20cm; one might stumble but not fall, but the foot strikes the unexpected step harder than usual.

A more demanding definition has been based on the so-called instability factor, which is an integral of the ratio between the horizontal displacement of a moving vertebra and its angular displacement[54]. When a vertebra normally moves from extension to flexion the degree to which it rotates is matched with the extent to which it translates. Over the entire range of motion there is a harmonious relationship between rotation and translation, expressed by the ratio between linear displacement and angular displacement (Fig. 2.35a). An unstable segment is one in which the harmony between the two types of motion is disturbed, such as excessive rotation for a given translation, or excessive translation for a given amount of rotation (Fig. 2.35b).

The instability factor measures this harmony across the entire range of motion but requires multiple X-ray exposures and detailed and meticulous analysis of the films to calculate the ratios between linear displacement and angular displacement for each sequential increment of motion. Instability is deemed to be present when the instability factor exceeds 25[54]. Because the technique is demanding it has not gained popularity, but the concept of instability factor probably captures best the clinical impression that spinal instability is a disorder in which the quality of movement of a segment is disturbed but ultimately the segment is not at risk of frankly falling apart. What remains to be determined for this and other definitions of instability is the correlation between objectively documented instability, the source of pain and how best it should be treated.

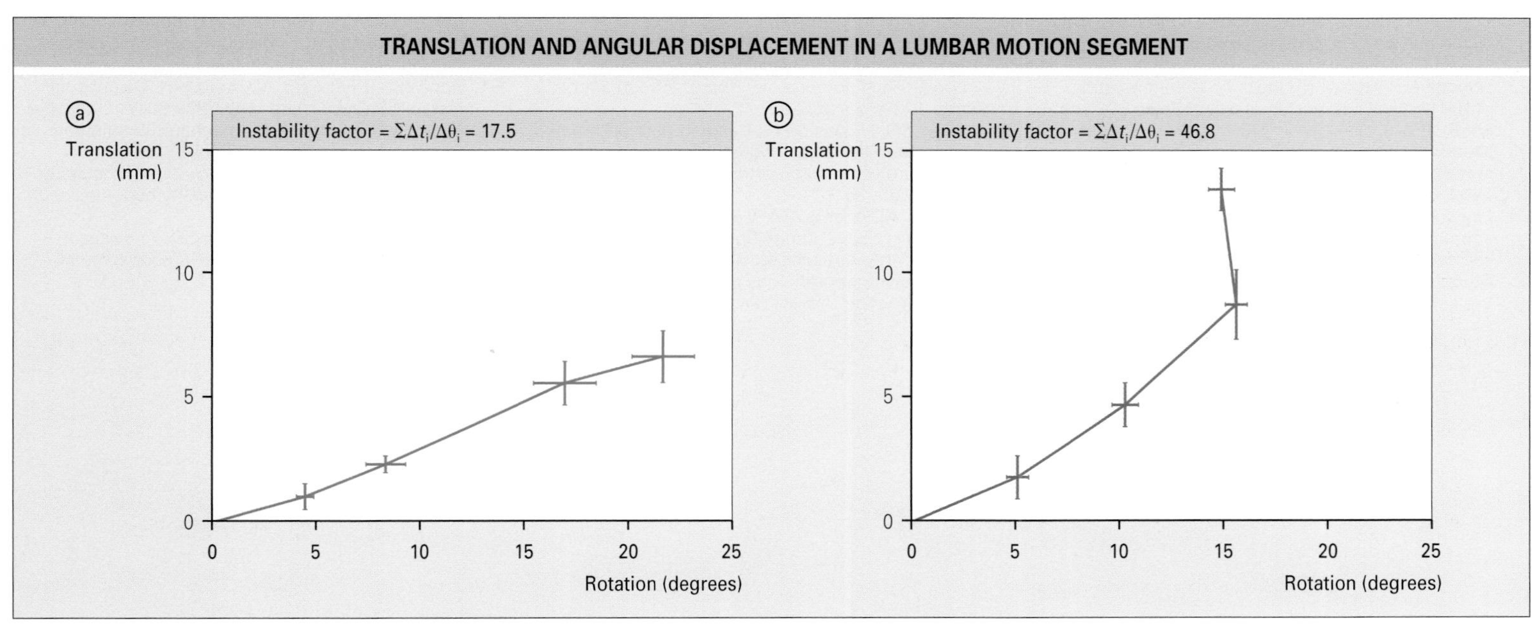

Fig. 2.35 The relationship between translation and angular displacement in a normal (a) and an ostensibly unstable (b) lumbar motion segment. (Based on Weiler *et al.*[54].)

REFERENCES

1. Bogduk N, Twomey LT. Clinical anatomy of the lumbar spine, 2E. Melbourne: Churchill Livingstone; 1991.
2. Inoue H. Three dimensional architecture of lumbar intervertebral discs. Spine. 1981;6:138–46.
3. Taylor JR. Growth and development of the human intervertebral disc. PhD Thesis, University of Edinburgh, 1973.
4. Oda J, Tanaka H, Tsuzuki N. Intervertebral disc changes with aging of human cervical vertebra. Spine. 1988;11:1205–11.
5. Taylor JR, Milne N. The cervical mobile segments. Proceedings of whiplash symposium. Adelaide: Orthopaedic Special Interest Group, Australian Physiotherapy Association, South Australian Branch; 1988:21–7.
6. Mercer S, Bogduk N. The menisci of the cervical zygapophysial joints. Brit J Rheumatol. 1993;32:705–10.
7. Bogduk N, Engel R. The lumbar zygapophysial menisci. A review of their anatomy and clinical significance. Spine. 1984;9:454–60.
8. Fielding JW, Cochran G van B, Lawsing JF, Hohl M. Tears of the transverse ligament of the atlas. J Bone Joint Surg. 1974;56A:1683–91.

9. Dvorak J, Panjabi MM. Functional anatomy of the alar ligaments. Spine. 1987;12:183–89.
10. Tondury G. The behaviour of the cervical discs during life. In: Hirsch C, Zotterman Y, eds. Cervical pain. Oxford: Pergamon Press; 1972:59–66.
11. Bowen V, Cassidy JD. Macroscopic and microscopic anatomy of the sacroiliac joint from embryonic life until the eighth decade. Spine. 1981;6:620–8.
12. Bastide G, Zadeh J, Lefebvre D. Are the 'little muscles' what we think they are? Surg Radiol Anat. 1989;11:255–6.
13. Nitz AJ, Peck D. Comparison of muscle spindle concentrations in large and small human epaxial muscles acting in parallel combinations. Am Surg. 1986;52:273–7.
14. Bogduk N, Macintosh JE, Pearcy MJ. A universal model of the lumbar back muscles in the upright position. Spine. 1992;17:897–913.
15. Bogduk N, Macintosh JE. The applied anatomy of the thoracolumbar fascia. Spine. 1984;9:164–71.
16. Vleeming A, Pool-Goudzwaard AL, Stoeckart R, van Wingerden JP, Snijders CJ. The posterior layer of the thoracolumbar fascia. Its function in load transfer from spine to legs. Spine. 1995;20:753–8.
17. Bogduk N. The clinical anatomy of the cervical dorsal rami. Spine. 1982;7:319–30.
18. Bogduk N, Wilson AS, Tynan W. The human lumbar dorsal rami. J Anat.1982;134:383–97.
19. Bogduk N, Valencia F. Innervation and pain patterns of the thoracic spine. In: Grant R, ed. Physical therapy of the cervical and thoracic spine, 2E. New York: Churchill Livingstone; 1994:77–87.
20. Groen GJ, Baljet B, Drukker J. Nerves and nerve plexuses of the human vertebral column. Am J Anat. 1990;188:282–96.
21. Bogduk N, Tynan W, Wilson AS. The nerve supply to the human lumbar intervertebral discs. J Anat. 1981;132:39–56.
22. Bogduk N, Windsor M, Inglis A. The innervation of the cervical intervertebral discs. Spine. 1988;13:2–8.
23. Mendel T, Wink CS, Zimny ML. Neural elements in human cervical intervertebra; discs. Spine. 1992;17:132–5.
24. Lavignolle B, Vital JM, Senegas J, et al. An approach to the functional anatomy of the sacroiliac joints in vivo. Anat Clin. 1983;5:169–76.
25. Sturesson B, Selvik, G, Uden A. Movements of the sacroiliac joints: a roentgen stereophotogrammetric analysis. Spine. 1989;14:162–5.
26. Bogduk N. Biomechanics of the cervical spine. In: Grant R, ed. Physical therapy of the cervical and thoracic spine, 2E. New York: Churchill Livingstone; 1994:27–45.
27. Dvorak J, Hayek J, Zehnder R. CT-functional diagnostics of the rotatory instability of the upper cervical spine. Part 2. An evaluation on healthy adults and patients with suspected instability. Spine. 1987;12:726–31.
28. Mimura M, Moriya H, Watanabe T, Takahashi K, Yamagata M, Tamaki T. Three-dimensional motion analysis of the cervical spine with special reference to the axial rotation. Spine. 1989;14:1135–9.
29. Penning L. Differences in anatomy, motion, development and aging of the upper and lower cervical disc segments. Clin Biomech. 1988;3:37–47
30. Dvorak J, Froehlich D, Penning L, Baumgartner H, Panjabi MM. Functional radiographic diagnosis of the cervical spine: flexion/extension. Spine. 1988;13:748–55.
31. Van Mameren H, Drukker J, Sanches H, Beursgens J. Cervical spine motion in the sagittal plane. (I). Range of motion of actually performed movements, an X-ray cinematographic study. Eur J Morph. 1990;28:47–68.
32. Amevo B, Worth D, Bogduk N. Instantaneous axes of rotation of the typical cervical motion segments: a study in normal volunteers. Clin Biomech. 1991;6:111–7.
33. Amevo B, Aprill C, Bogduk N. Abnormal instantaneous axes of rotation in patients with neck pain. Spine.1992;17:748–56.
34. Markolf KL, Morris JM. The structural components of the intervertebral disc. J Bone Joint Surg. 1974;56A:675–87.
35. Adams MA, Hutton WC. The effect of posture on the role of the apophyseal joints in resisting intervertebral compression force. J Bone Joint Surg. 1980;62B:358–62.
36. Hickey DS, Hukins DWL. Relation between the structure of the anulus fibrosus and the function and failure of the intervertebral disc. Spine. 1980;5:100–16.
37. Hutton WC, Adams MA. Can the lumbar spine be crushed in heavy lifting? Spine. 1982;7:586–90.
38. Jayson MIV, Herbert CM, Barks JS. Intervertebral discs: nuclear morphology and bursting pressures. Ann Rheum Dis. 1973;32:308–15.
39. Brinckmann P. Injury of the anulus fibrosus and disc protrusions: an in vitro investigation on human lumbar discs. Spine. 1986;11:149–53.
40. Virgin WJ. Experimental investigations into the physical properties of the intervertebral disc. J Bone Joint Surg. 1951;33B:607–11.
41. Bogduk N. The lumbar disc and low back pain. Neurosurg Clin North Am. 1991;2:791–806.
42. Farfan HF, Cossette JW, Robertson GH, Wells RV, Kraus H. The effects of torsion on the lumbar intervertebral joints: the role of torsion in the production of disc degeneration. J Bone Joint Surg. 1970;52A:468–497.
43. Sullivan JD, Farfan HF. The crumpled neural arch. Orthop Clin North Am. 1975;6:199–213.
44. Pearcy MJ, Bogduk N. Instantaneous axes of rotation of the lumbar intervertebral joints. Spine. 1988;13:1033–41.
45. Bogduk N, Amevo B, Pearcy M. A biological basis for instantaneous centers of rotation of the vertebral column. Proc Inst Mech Eng. 1995;209:177–83.
46. Gertzbein SD, Seligman J, Holtby R, et al. Centrode characteristics of the lumbar spine as a function of segmental instability. Clin Orthop. 1986;208:48–51.
47. Gertzbein SD, Seligman J Holtby R, Chan KH, Kapasouri A, Tile M, Cruickshank B. Centrode patterns and segmental instability in degenerative disc disease. Spine. 1985;10:257–61.
48. Macintosh JE, Pearcy MJ, Bogduk N. The axial torque of the lumbar back muscles: torsion strength of the back muscles. Aust NZ J Surg. 1993;63:205–12.
49. Green TP, Adams MA, Dolan P. Tensile properties of the anulus fibrosus II. Ultimate tensile strength and fatigue life. Eur Spine J.1993;2:209–14.
50. Hansson TH, Keller TS, Spengler DM. Mechanical behaviour of the human lumbar spine. II. Fatigue strength during dynamic compressive loading. J Orthop Res. 1987;5:479–87.
51. Pope MH, Frymoyer JW, Krag MH. Diagnosing instability. Clin Orthop. 1992;279:60–7.
52. Pope MH, Panjabi M. Biomechanical definitions of spinal instability. Spine. 1985;10:255–6.
53. Panjabi MM. The stabilizing system of the spine. Part II. Neutral zone and instability hypothesis. J Spinal Dis. 1992;5:390–7.
54. Weiler PJ, King GJ, Gertzbein SD. Analysis of sagittal plane instability of the lumbar spine in vivo. Spine. 1990;12:1300–6.

3

LOW BACK PAIN

David G Borenstein

Summary

- Low back pain represents one of the most common symptoms, being second only to the common cold.
- The anatomic source of 'mechanical back pain', which accounts for more than 90% of low back pain episodes, cannot be differentiated precisely.
- One of the most important roles of the physician is to recognize nonmechanical causes.
- Investigations should be limited to the few patients with persistent or progressive pain and those in whom a nonmechanical cause is suspected.

INTRODUCTION

Low back pain is a ubiquitous health problem. It represents the most frequent illness of mankind after the common cold[1,2]. Between 65% and 80% of the world's population develop back pain at some point during their lives. A review of three time periods studied by the National Ambulatory Care Survey in the United States revealed mechanical low back pain as the fifth most common reason (2.8%) for physician office visits. Of these visits, nonspecific low back pain was the most frequent diagnostic group at 56.8%[3]. Data from the US Health Interview Survey indicate that impairments of the back and spine are the chronic conditions that most frequently cause activity limitation among people aged 45 years or under and that they represent the third most common reason for impairment in people aged 45–64 years[4].

The surgical subspecialties of orthopedics and neurosurgery are most frequently associated with low back pain evaluation and treatment, despite the fact that the vast majority of patients do not require surgical intervention. Surgeons evaluate a large number of patients with nonsurgical lesions in order to identify the relative few who require back surgery. In regard to back pain, rheumatologists have concentrated their efforts on the spondyloarthropathies and have shied away from patients with mechanical low back pain. Since they are experts in the conservative management of musculoskeletal disorders, rheumatologists are in many ways the most appropriate physicians to complete the initial and subsequent evaluation of patients with low back pain of any etiology and to plan a treatment program. They constantly use patient education, physical modalities and drug therapy, which are the cornerstones for treatment of back patients.

EPIDEMIOLOGY

Most episodes of back pain are not incapacitating. Over 50% of all patients with back pain improve after 1 week, while more than 90% are better at 8 weeks[5]. The remaining 7–10% continue to experience symptoms for longer than 6 months. The high costs associated with low back pain are related to these individuals with chronic pain. For example, in the state of Tennessee in 1986, 10% of cases with chronic low back pain accounted for 57% of the total expenditures (US$31.8 million) on work-related sickness payments[6]. Frymoyer has estimated that the direct cost of back pain in the United States in 1990 was over US$24 billion[7]. This excludes the US$3.6 billion of indirect costs of work-related sickness payments, litigation and lost days from work.

Many risk factors described for back pain involve occupational or psychologic characteristics. Occupational factors include jobs that require lifting beyond the worker's physical capabilities, or in an awkward position. Workers involved in heavy duty labor who are aged over 45 years have a 2.5 times greater risk of absence from work secondary to back pain compared to workers aged 24 years or younger[8]. Those individuals with an initial episode of back pain lasting 3 months or more have a risk for recurrence of 26.7% in the year following an initial pain episode versus 19.9% for an initial episode of 1 day's duration[9].

A number of psychologic conditions are associated with back pain. Neurosis, hysteria and conversion reaction are more frequent than depression as primary causes of acute back pain[10]. Depression is a frequent complication of patients who develop chronic low back pain. Obesity and cigarette smoking are also associated with an increased risk of back pain[11].

As many as 90% of patients with back pain have a mechanical reason for their pain[12]. Mechanical low back pain may be defined as pain secondary to overuse of a normal anatomic structure or pain secondary to trauma or deformity of an anatomic structure. The remaining 10% of adults with back pain have the symptom as a manifestation of a systemic illness[13]. Over 70 nonmechanical illnesses may be associated with back pain[14]. Careful clinical evaluation helps separate patients with mechanical back pain from those with nonmechanical back pain.

CLINICAL EVALUATION

The evaluation of a patient with low back pain requires an organized and thoughtful approach that should be tailored to the specific complaints of the patient. In rare circumstances, a patient's symptoms and signs can be related to an identifiable pathologic process involving a specific anatomic structure. In these cases, specific therapy can be given. However, in most cases, the offending anatomic structure, be it bone, muscle, ligament, fascia or disc, cannot be identified as the specific source of back pain. Fortunately, the natural history of the symptom is resolution frequently over a short period of time, so all interventions seem to work whether it is limitation of activity, over-the-counter medications, temperature modalities or chiropractors. Although the diagnostic process is inexact for many patients, it nevertheless remains essential to identify a specific abnormality.

The physician plays an essential role in the evaluation and treatment of low back pain patients and their recovery. The very nature of the interaction of a person and a physician makes that individual view themselves as being sick. The physician may encourage this behavior by evaluating or treating an individual in too aggressive a manner. This may be a particular problem for individuals who have been injured at work. It is essential for the physician to downplay 'illness behavior' in these patients. Patients with low back pain need to be encouraged to resume normal activities as soon as possible and be constantly reminded that the vast majority of individuals improve over a 2–3 week period.

HISTORY

The clinical history is an essential step in evaluating patients with low back pain. The astute clinician allows the patients to tell their stories in their own words, but also steers them in directions that elicit the essential information needed for the diagnostic process. The age of a patient is helpful in determining the potential cause of his or her back pain.

Certain disorders occur more commonly in younger individuals while others are associated with older patients (Fig. 3.1). The sex of the patient may also help select potential causes of low back pain. Certain disorders occur more frequently in men while others are associated more commonly with women. Others occur equally in both sexes (Fig. 3.2).

The duration and location of pain help decide the subsequent kinds of questions that the evaluating physician will ask. Mechanical low back pain tends to have an onset associated with a physical task and is usually of short duration (days to weeks). Medical causes of low back pain tend to have a more gradual onset with no identifiable precipitating factor. These causes of low back pain are frequently present from weeks to months. Most back pain is limited to the lumbosacral area of the low back. Radiation of pain in the thighs or to the knees may be related to referred pain from elements of the spine (muscle, ligaments or apophyseal joints). Pain that radiates from the low back to below the knees is usually neurogenic in origin and suggests a pathologic process affecting spinal nerve roots.

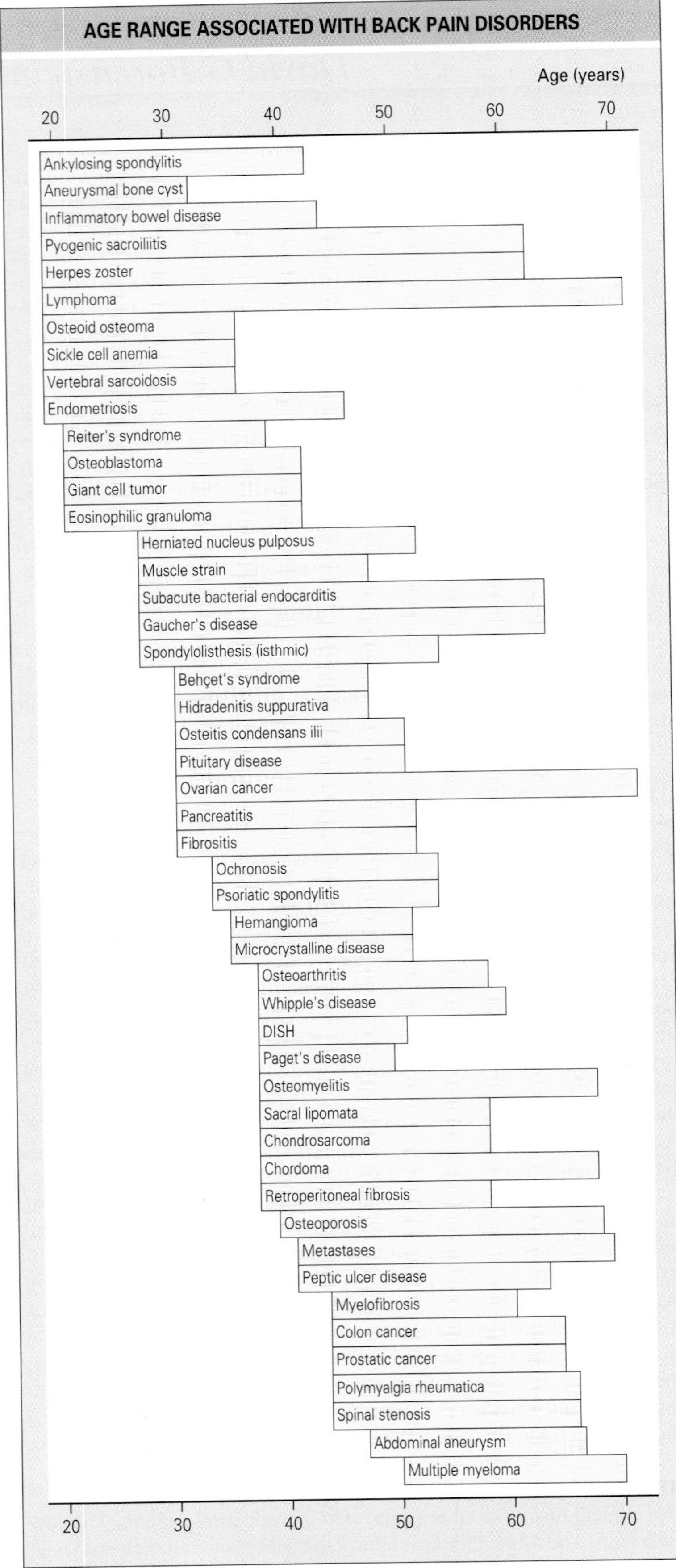

Fig. 3.1 Age range associated with back pain disorders. (Adapted with permission from Borenstein DG, Wiesel SW, Low back pain: medical diagnosis and comprehensive management, Philadelphia: WB Saunders; 1989.)

Present illness

Most of the time spent in obtaining the clinical history is used to elucidate the factors that affect the pain. The history is directed towards understanding the chronologic development of low back pain, its character and its response to therapy. The anatomic structures of the lumbosacral spine receive specific types of sensory innervation that are associated with distinct qualities of pain. The major categories of pain include superficial somatic, deep somatic (spondylogenic), radicular, neurogenic, visceral-referred and psychogenic (Fig. 3.3).

SEX PREVALENCE OF LOW BACK PAIN CONDITIONS
Male predominant
Spondyloarthropathies Vertebral osteomyelitis Benign and malignant neoplasms Paget's disease Retroperitoneal fibrosis Peptic ulcer disease Work-related mechanical disorders
Female predominant
Polymyalgia rheumatica Fibromyalgia Osteoporosis Parathyroid disease
Equal frequency
Inflammatory bowel disease Pituitary disease Subacute bacterial endocarditis

Fig. 3.2 Sex prevalence of low back pain conditions.

CATEGORIES OF LOW BACK PAIN

Category	Source/Pathologic Entity	Quality
Superficial somatic	Skin, subcutaneous tissues (cellulitis)	Sharp, burning
Deep somatic	Muscles, fascia, periosteum, ligaments, joints, vessels, dura (arthritis)	Sharp, dull ache, boring
Radicular	Spinal nerves (herniated disc, spinal stenosis)	Radiating, shooting, tingling
Neurogenic	Mixed motor sensory nerves (femoral neuropathy)	Burning
Visceral-referred	Abdominal viscera, pelvic viscera, aorta (autonomic sensory nerves)	Boring, colicky, tearing
Psychogenic	Cerebral cortex (conversion reaction, malingering)	Variable

Fig. 3.3 Categories of low back pain.

Superficial somatic pain

Superficial somatic pain is associated with disorders that affect the skin and subcutaneous tissues. These tissues are well innervated by cutaneous A fibers that cover very small fields. Pathogenic processes in these tissues cause sharp or burning pain. Areas of cellulitis are rapidly recognized because of their superficial location and are not diagnostically difficult. The exception may be in patients who present with the burning pain of herpes zoster prior to the appearance of vesicles. The acute onset and distribution in a dermatomal pattern should alert the clinician to this possibility.

Deep somatic pain

Deep somatic pain has its source in the vertebral column, the surrounding muscles, and the attaching tendons, ligaments and fascia. These structures are supplied by the sinuvertebral nerves and the unmyelinated pain fibers of the posterior primary rami of the spinal nerves. Deep somatic pain is characterized by a deep, dull ache that is maximal over the involved site and often radiates into the thighs but rarely below the knees. Acute injury to these tissues is associated with a sharp stab of pain at the moment of injury followed by a dull ache that may persist for weeks and may be associated with tenderness on palpation and reflex muscle spasm.

Radicular pain

Radicular pain is related to involvement of the proximal spinal nerves with inflammation, or any processes that decrease blood flow to the nerve. This type of pain is lancinating, shooting, burning, sharp and tender in quality and radiates from the low back to the lower extremity in the distribution of the compromised spinal nerve. In addition to the shooting pain, achiness and spasm may be experienced in the thigh and calf muscles. Herniated intervertebral discs are the most common cause of radicular pain. Other causes include overgrowth of bone from apophyseal joints intruding into the spinal canal, spinal stenosis, fracture-dislocation of the spine, infections and neoplasms.

Neurogenic pain

Neurogenic pain results from involvement of the sensory portion of a peripheral nerve. Diabetic neuropathy is a good example. This type of pain is described as burning, tingling, crushing, gnawing or skin crawling and tends to be sustained in most circumstances.

Visceral-referred pain

Visceral-referred pain arises from abnormalities in organs that share segmental innervation with the lumbosacral spine. The back pain may be gripping, cramping, aching, squeezing, crushing, tearing, stabbing or burning, depending on the affected organ. The wider distribution of viscerogenic pain differs from the more precise localization of somatic pain.

Psychogenic pain

Psychogenic pain is perceived at the level of the cerebral cortex. It does not follow any dermatomal pattern and may be of any quality. The patient may describe the pain in terms of suffering or punishment. Some terms used in this circumstance might include 'being hit', or 'being burned with a red hot poker'[15]. Duration may be extremely short or prolonged. In most circumstances psychogenic pain is resistant to all therapies. Patients who suffer from depression, hysteria or conversion reaction tend to exhibit psychogenic pain.

In addition to the quality of pain, elucidating factors that aggravate and alleviate pain are helpful in defining potential sources for the symptom. Typically, mechanical disorders worsen with activity, including prolonged sitting and standing, and improve with recumbency. The pain tends to occur on a recurring basis with the same degree of physical activity.

While some patients with medical disorders that affect the spine, such as compression, pathologic fractures or acute infection, may also find relief of their pain with recumbency and even complete immobility, most find no association with body position. Exceptions include patients with a spondyloarthropathy who classically report increased pain and stiffness when they remain in bed for a few hours; patients with tumors that involve the structures of the lumbar spine who are worse with recumbency; and patients with viscerogenic pain, in whom moving around trying to achieve a comfortable postion is characteristic.

Increases in cerebrospinal fluid pressure brought about by coughing or sneezing exacerbate radicular pain in patients with intervertebral disc herniation. Sudden motion may also cause reflex contraction of paraspinous muscles but no radiation of pain into the lower extremities.

The severity of pain may be measured by a number of means. The patient may describe how the pain has interfered with activities of daily living. The more severe the pain, the greater the intrusion on leisure time pursuits. Patients may fill in a diagram with the location, quality and severity of pain (Fig. 3.4). These pain diagrams are a helpful way of documenting the extent of pain involvement and subsequent response to therapy.

Family and social history

In addition to the present illness, other components of the history may help to identify any underlying abnormality which is a cause of back pain. Familial predisposition does occur in certain medical illnesses associated with back pain. Of particular importance is the group of illnesses that cause spondyloarthropathy. The ethnic background of the family may predispose individuals to specific illnesses. For example, Caucasian women of Northern European origins are at greater risk of developing osteoporosis. Mechanical disorders such as intervertebral disc herniation and spinal stenosis may have a familial predilection.

Occupational and social history are important for identifying those patients at risk of developing mechanical low back pain. The association

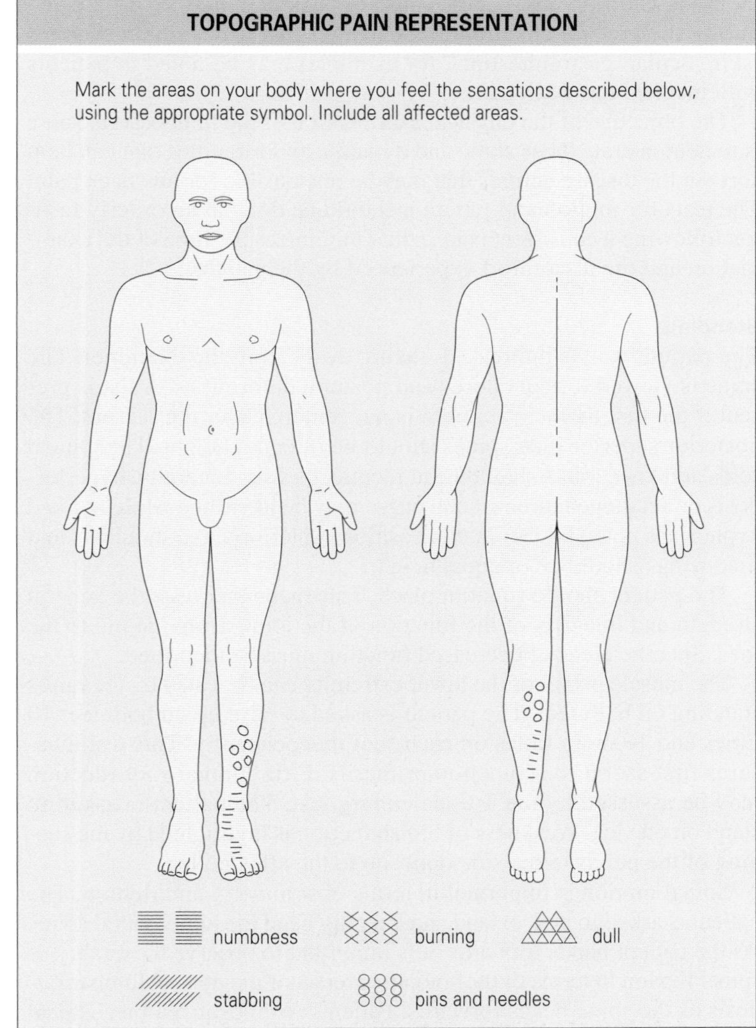

Fig. 3.4 Pain diagram. Pain distribution of a patient with radiculopathy secondary to a lumbar intervertebral disc herniation.

of work and the onset of pain is important in regard to compensation. The patient's opinion about the association of the pain and their work must be determined as well as their expectation of work-related sickness payments for injury and return to work. Some workers may be afraid to return to their job because of fear of reinjury. They may amplify their symptoms and may be slow to respond to therapy.

Social habits also need to be determined, particularly in regard to smoking, consumption of alcohol and the use of recreational drugs. Smoking is an independent risk factor for low back pain[11]. Increased use of alcohol is associated with osteoporosis, while illicit drug use causes immunosuppression and predisposition to infection.

Past medical history

Past medical history and a review of systems should be discussed briefly. In most circumstances, these components of the history add little additional information. However, for the patient with medical low back pain, these components of the medical history are particularly pertinent. Previous history of malignancy, arthritis or metabolic bone disease may be significant. The review of systems may identify the patient who has a systemic disorder causing back pain but does not realize the association between the two (skin rash and spondyloarthropathy).

PHYSICAL EXAMINATION

In patients with a history suggestive of mechanical low back pain, the physical examination should concentrate on the evaluation of musculoskeletal and neural tissues of the lumbosacral spine. However, a full examination should be completed at a subsequent visit if the patient does not improve in a short period of time.

When a medical cause of low back pain is suspected, a general medical physical examination should be completed before evaluation of the back. Clues to the specific cause of back pain may be discovered during the general examination. Changes in various organ systems (skin, ocular, gastrointestinal, for example) may be noted in patients with medical low back pain.

The objective of the physical examination of the lumbosacral spine is to demonstrate those static and dynamic abnormalities that can help sort out the disease entities that may be responsible for low back pain. The tests for motion and function should be done in an orderly fashion following a consistent pattern that minimizes the time of the examination and the discomfort experienced by the patient.

Standing

The patient stands undressed, facing away from the examiner. The spine is viewed for curvatures and postural deformities. A list is present if the first thoracic vertebra is not centered over the sacrum. The posterior superior iliac spines should be of equal height. The gluteal folds and knee joints should be at identical levels. Laterally, hyperlordosis or a flattened lumbosacral curve may be identified while marked kyphosis is noted best from this position. Anteriorly, the shoulders and iliac wings should be of equal height.

The patient should squat in place. This maneuver tests the general strength and integrity of the function of the joints from the hip to the toes. Specific areas of decreased function must be identified.

The muscle power of the lower extremity can be tested by toe raises standing on both feet. The patient is asked to raise up on both feet 10 times and 10 more times on each foot independently. This test measures first sacral root function primarily. Fifth lumbar root function may be assessed by the Trendelenburg test. The patient is asked to stand on one leg. Weakness of hip abduction is highlighted by the sagging of the pelvis to the side opposite to the affected leg.

Spinal motion is important in terms of symmetry and rhythm. The patient is asked to flex, extend and laterally bend the lumbosacral spine. As the patient bends forwards, it is important to observe the quality of spinal flexion in terms of the smooth reversal of the normal lumbar lordosis as the spine flexes forwards. Patients with localized mechanical disorders maintain the lordosis while bending from the hips when asked to flex forwards. Patients with injuries in musculoskeletal structures at the L4–L5 and L5–S1 interspaces will experience abnormal motion secondary to protective muscle contraction.

After full flexion, it is helpful to observe how the patient regains the erect posture. Patients with back lesions return to the erect position utilizing a fixed lordosis and rotating the pelvis with the help of knee and hip flexion. Pain that increases with forwards flexion suggests an abnormality in the anterior elements of the spine, including discogenic disease.

The patient should then be asked to extend the spine while limiting movement of the hip or knee. Pain that is increased by extension suggests disease in the posterior elements of the spinal column, including the apophyseal joints.

The exact source of pain with lateral bending is difficult to determine. Pain that is elicited on the same side as the bending motion suggests an apophyseal joint origin for the discomfort. Pain that is produced in a paraspinous location on the side opposite to the lateral bending motion may be of muscular, ligamentous or fascial origin. Spinal rotation is best examined when the patient is seated.

Bending forward over a table

Palpation of the spine and surrounding tissues with the back supported by the arms is possible with the patient bent forwards over a table. Palpation detects local tenderness, increased muscle tone or bony defects over the spinous processes. Sacroiliac tenderness may be elicited with direct percussion over these joints.

Kneeling

The ankle reflex is best determined in the kneeling position. It may also be elicited with the patient seated on the examining table.

Seated on a chair

Dorsiflexion power of the foot, a fifth lumbar nerve root function, is best tested by seating the patient on a chair and by pushing down on the patient's foot with the heel on the floor. The maneuver should be continued for a minute to allow for detection of weakness in the muscle. Patients who feign weakness may either resist pressure for a few seconds and then release the muscle suddently, or in a manner resulting in a 'cogwheel' effect. Function of the L5 nerve root may also be tested by asking the patient to dorsiflex the large toe of the foot.

Seated on the examining table

Reflexes may be elicited when the patient is seated on the examining table. The knee reflex reflects the integrity of the L4 nerve root. Asymmetry of the reflexes should only be accepted if the abnormality persists on repeated testing.

In the seated position, the plantar response may be tested by lifting the straight leg and stroking the lateral aspect of the foot. Patients with radicular abnormalities will experience pain down the leg below the knee to the ankle or foot. Patients will also lean backwards to minimize the traction on neural elements (tripod sign). Patients with hamstring tightness will experience thigh pain but no pain radiation below the knee. A Babinski reflex (extension of the large toe and spreading of the other toes) should be plantar, since the spinal cord conus is situated at L1–L2 level.

Hip flexor strength is tested by asking the patient to lift their thigh off the examining table. Downwards pressure by the examiner helps distinguish differences in strength from side to side.

Lying supine

The supine position is excellent for testing the status of the nerve roots, peripheral nerves and hip joints. Assessment of the neurologic status of the patient is very important in the overall back evaluation. A neurologic abnormality will give objectivity to a patient's subjective complaints. Any compression or traction on the dura surrounding a nerve will compress its contents and encroach upon the nerve and its blood supply. With inflammation of the nerve, pain is produced along the course of the peripheral nerve causing dysesthesias, motor weakness and decreased reflex function associated with the affected nerve root. Tests that increase nerve compression result in increased nerve pain or

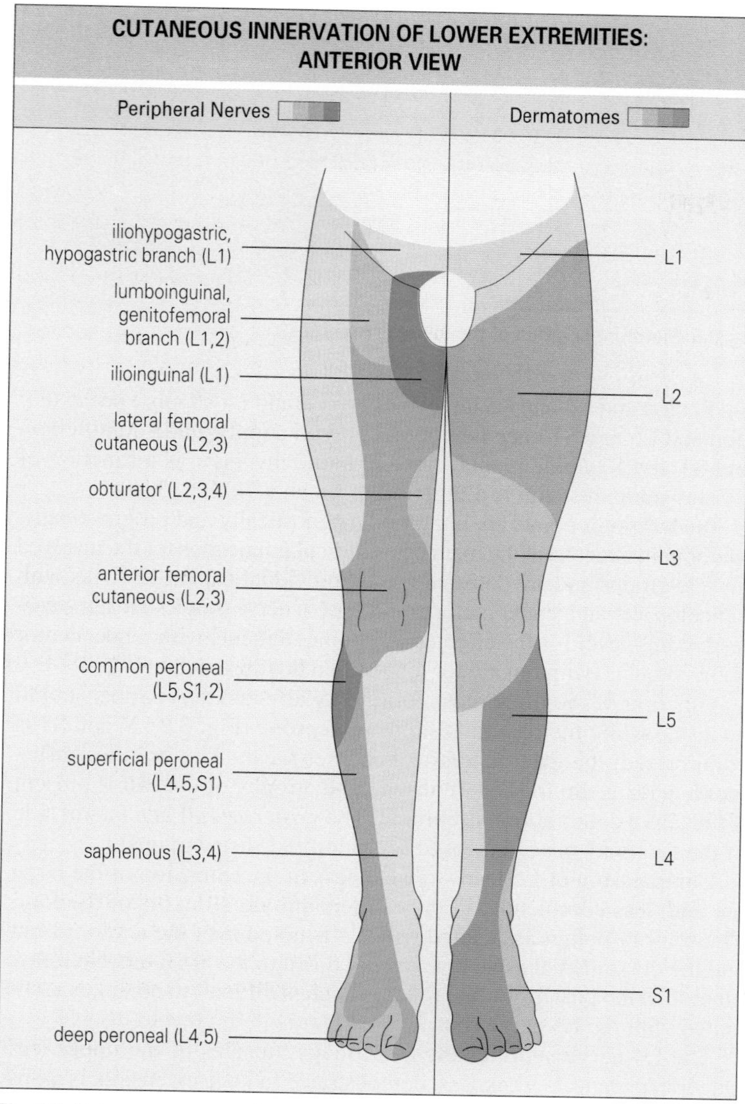

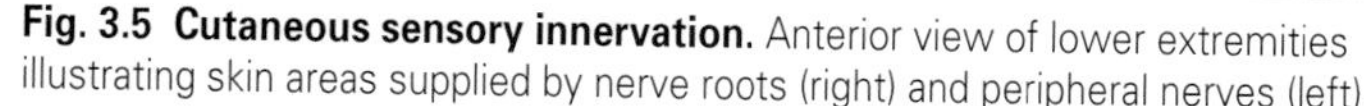
Fig. 3.5 Cutaneous sensory innervation. Anterior view of lower extremities illustrating skin areas supplied by nerve roots (right) and peripheral nerves (left).

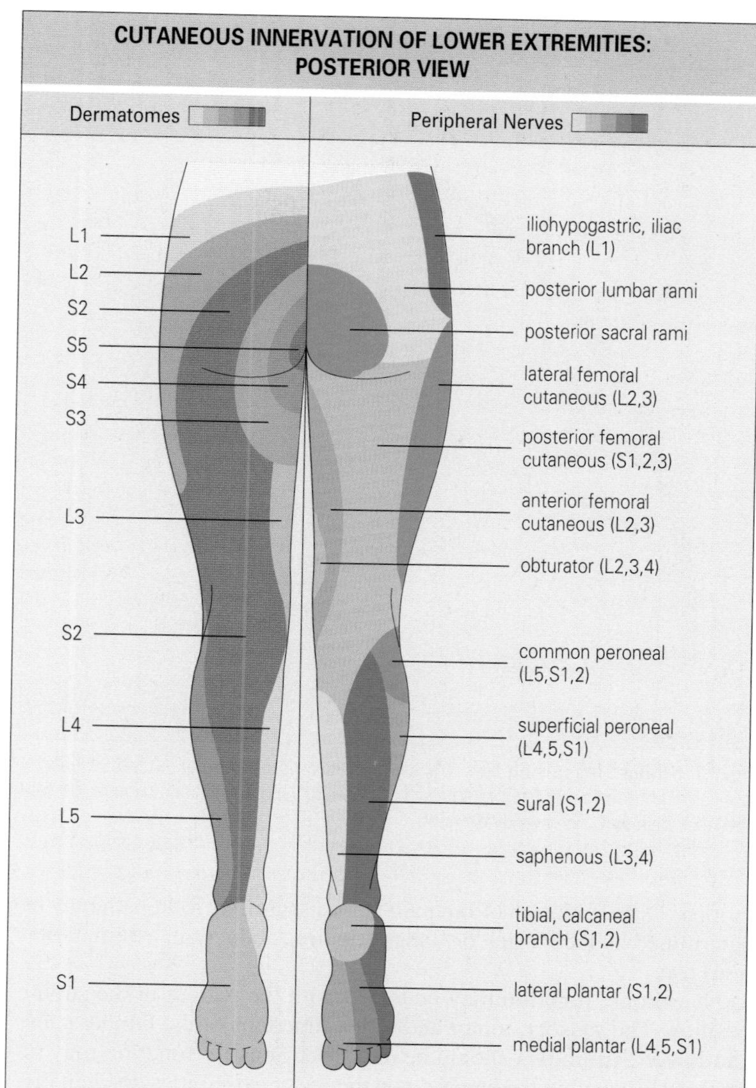

Fig. 3.6 Cutaneous sensory innervation. Posterior view of lower extremities illustrating skin areas supplied by nerve roots (left) and peripheral nerves (right).

dysfunction. Of the possible neurologic abnormalities, persistent muscle weakness is the most reliable indicator of persistent nerve compression with loss of nerve conduction[16]. Sensory findings are less reliable since they are affected by the state of fatigue and emotional state of the patient. Reflex changes are also not as reliable as motor function. Previous episodes of nerve compression may cause a loss of reflexes, which may not return even with recovery of motor and sensory function[17]. Older individuals may lose reflex function particularly in the ankles. The loss of reflexes is then symmetric. Patients who lose reflex function in both lower extremities acutely on the basis of compression have impingement of the cauda equina.

Upper motor neuron and peripheral nerve abnormalities may also cause neurologic dysfunction. Patients with upper motor neuron dysfunction develop muscle spasticity, hyperreflexia, and a Babinski reflex. Sensory and motor abnormalities associated with peripheral nerve injuries depend on the location of the damaged nerve. Peripheral nerves receive innervation from a number of nerve roots. An injury to a single nerve root may have little effect on motor or cutaneous function if the area is supplied by nerves from multiple levels. However, if a peripheral nerve is injured, a specific muscle may become paralyzed or specific skin areas become anesthetic (Figs 3.5 & 3.6) The distinction between upper motor, nerve root and peripheral nerve lesions is essential for the differential diagnosis of back pain. Different disease processes preferentially effect upper motor (multiple sclerosis), nerve root (disc herniation) or peripheral nerve (diabetes).

The straight leg raising test detects irritation of the sciatic nerve (L4, L5, S1). The passive raising of the leg by the foot with the knee extended stretches the sciatic nerve, its nerve roots and dural attachments (see Fig. 3.7). When the dura is inflamed and stretched, the patient will experience pain along its anatomic course to the lower leg, ankle and foot. Dural movement starts at 30° of elevation. Pain of dural origin should not be felt below that degree of elevation. Pain is maximum between 30° to 70° of elevation. Symptoms at greater degrees of elevation may be of nerve root origin, but may also be related to mechanical low back pain secondary to muscle strain or joint disease[18]. Dorsiflexion of the foot will exacerbate the radicular pain. Pain may also be experienced in the leg below the knee when the contralateral normal leg is raised. The presence of contralateral pain suggests a large central lesion in the spinal canal causing traction on the opposite nerve root when the normal leg is raised.

A bilateral straight leg raising test may also detect sciatic nerve irritation. The test is performed by lifting the legs by both ankles with the knees extended. This motion causes the pelvis to tilt upwards, diminishing the stretch on the neural elements. Pain that occurs in an arc of elevation of 70° is related to stress on the sacroiliac joints. Above 70°, pain is related to lesions in the lumbar spine. The bilateral straight leg raising test is useful to identify patients with psychogenic pain who frequently complain of pain at a lower elevation than noted during the unilateral straight leg raising test.

In the supine position, leg lengths should be measured to document discrepancies. The hip joints should be moved through their range of

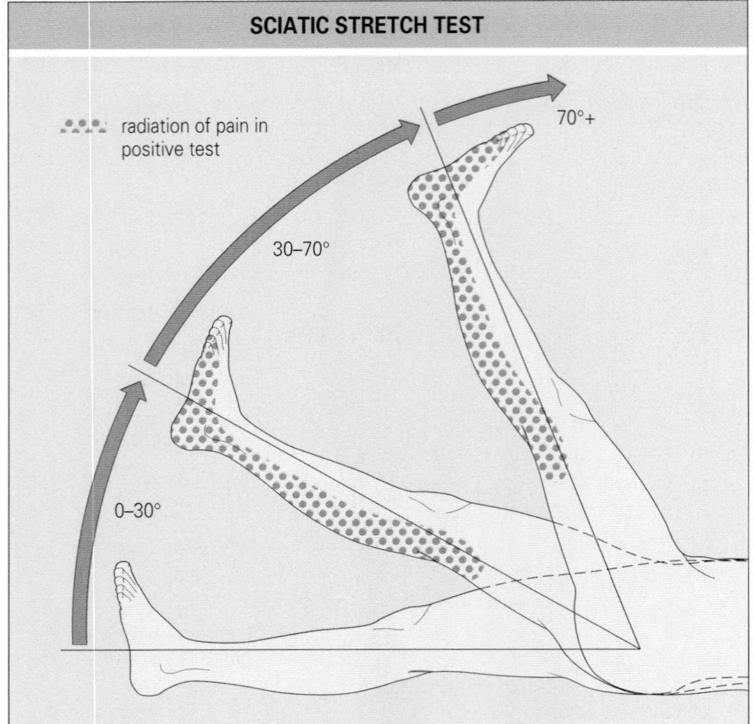

Fig. 3.7 Straight leg raising test. The leg is lifted with the knee extended. Sciatic roots are tightened over a herniated disc between 30° and 70°. Dorsiflexion of the foot increases pain with nerve impingement.

MOTOR INNERVATION OF LOWER EXTREMITIES

Region	Backward	Forward
Hip	L4,5 extension	Flexion L2,3
Knee	L5,S1 flexion	Extension L3,4
Ankle	S1,2 plantar flexion	Inversion L4 Dorsiflexion L4,5 Eversion L5,S1

Fig. 3.8 Motor innervation of the lower extremities.

motion. Differentiation of hip pain versus sacroiliac joint pain may be determined by the Patrick or 'faber' (flexion, abduction, external rotation) test.

Neurologic function may be tested with the patient in the supine position. The sensory, motor and reflex functions of the lumbar spine and lower extremities should be assessed. Sensory function may be assessed by running the hands down the lower extremities, to elicit differences in the legs. Any abnormality should result in a more detailed examination of pain, light touch and vibratory function.

Useful in screening is muscle testing of the legs, which measures strength on a five-point scale for: extension and flexion (knee); abduction and adduction (hip); and eversion and inversion and dorsiflexion and plantar flexion (foot).When testing muscle power, the intervening joints should be in a neutral position. Pressure is applied by the examiner to a nonarticular structure for a minimum of 5 seconds. When feasible, both sides should be tested simultaneously. The innervation of the muscles to the legs follows a sequential pattern. L2 and L3 supply hip flexion and L4 and L5 hip extension; L3 and L4 supply knee extension and L5 and S1 knee flexion; L4 and L5 supply ankle dorsiflexion and S1 and S2 ankle plantar flexion; ankle inversion is a function of L4 and ankle eversion is a function of L5 and S1 (Fig. 3.8).

Tender motor points are important diagnostically and prognostically. Motor points represent the main neuromuscular junctions for the involved muscle groups and are constant for an individual patient. Patients with radiculopathy and tender motor points have a nerve root lesion at the corresponding level for the affected myotome. Patients with tender motor points remain symptomatic for longer than do those without[19].

Function of the three most commonly affected nerve roots should be tested while the patient is supine and prone (Fig. 3.9). When S1 is compressed, the gastrocnemius becomes weak. The Achilles reflex (ankle jerk) is diminished or absent, and atrophy of the calf is present if the nerve compression is chronic. The posterior calf and lateral side of the foot may have decreased sensation (S1 distribution).

Compression of L5 leads to weakness in the extension of the large toe and, less completely, in the everters and dorsiflexors of the foot. The sensory deficit associated with L5 is noted over the anterior tibia and the dorsomedial aspect of the foot down to the great toe. No reflex other than the posterior tibial reflex, which is difficult to obtain, is associated with the L5 nerve root.

The L4 nerve supplies the quadriceps muscles of the upper leg. Quadriceps muscle weakness, demonstrated in knee extension, is associated with L4 nerve compression. The patient complaint associated with this lesion is frequently one of an unstable knee. Atrophy of the thigh musculature may be marked. Sensory loss affects the anteromedial aspect of the leg. The patellar tendon reflex is lost.

Prone position

The neurologic examination is completed by testing for higher lumbar and sacral nerve root function. Dural irritation of nerve roots from L2 to L4 are tested by the femoral stretch test (Fig. 3.10). With the knee bent, the thigh is elevated from the examining table. The test is positive if pain

LUMBAR ROOT LESIONS

Root	Muscle weakness/movement affected	Tendon reflex decreased
L2	Hip flexion/adduction	
L3	Hip adduction Knee extension	Knee jerk
L4	Knee extension Foot inversion/dorsiflexion	Knee jerk
L5	Hip extension/abduction Knee flexion Foot/toe dorsifexion	
S1	Knee flexion Foot/toe plantar flexion Foot eversion	Ankle jerk

Fig. 3.9 Lumbar root lesions. Cutaneous, motor, and reflex functions of the lower extremity.

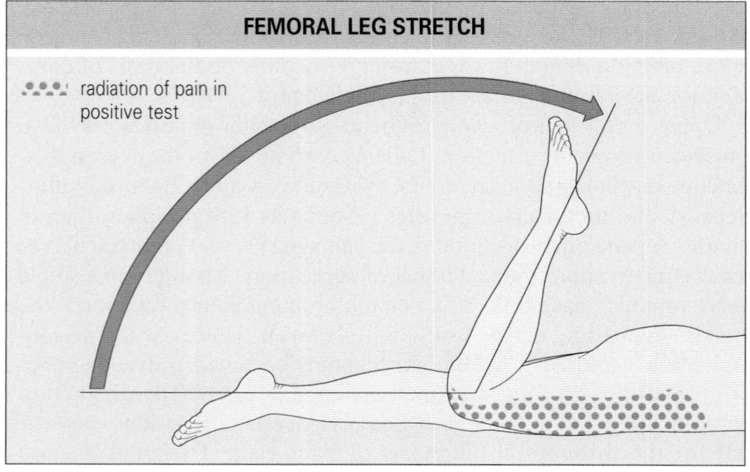

Fig. 3.10 Femoral stretch test. The knee is flexed and lifted superiorly. Sharp pain that is generated in the anterior thigh is considered a positive test.

is reproduced in the front of the thigh (L2 and L3) or the medial aspect of the leg (L4). Gluteus maximus strength is tested by having the patient contract the buttocks. Asymmetry of contraction or atrophy suggests an abnormality of S1.

Upper and lower sacral roots are tested by sensory examination of the skin over the lower legs, buttocks and perineum. If a patient has saddle anesthesia, a positive straight leg raising test in both legs, and abnormal sphincter tone, a cauda equina compression syndrome should be suspected.

The final part of the evaluation involves the genital and rectal examinations. This part of the examination is completed in patients who have symptoms and signs suggestive of medical low back pain. These examinations are helpful in detecting patients with prostatic abnormalities, rectal cancer or endometriosis.

A number of ancillary physical examination tests may be used to confirm abnormalities discovered during the routine examination. These tests are listed in Figure 3.11.

Non-organic physical signs

Patients who are involved with litigation or claims for work-related sickness payment occasionally exaggerate their symptoms. In these patients, the objective findings do not match the subjective complaints[20]. Close observation of the patients helps identify the inconsistencies. Waddell has described five tests that identify individuals with 'functional' or 'exaggerated' symptoms (Fig. 3.12)[21]. A finding of three or more of the five signs is clinically significant. Isolated positive signs are ignored. These tests can be incorporated unobtrusively into the physical examination. Using the tests on a consistent basis allows the examiner to become familiar with the spectrum of normal and abnormal findings. Once familiar with the tests, the physician will have less difficulty in identifying the patient who exaggerates symptoms for ulterior motives.

Value of results

Although the physical examination adds essential information for the evaluation of patients with low back pain, problems exist in the reproducibility and significance of abnormal findings. Part of the difficulty in the evaluation of low back pain is the lack of definition for physical signs. McCombe *et al.* evaluated the reproducibility between three observers of 54 physical signs used for back pain evaluation[22]. Reproducible signs included measurements of lordosis (by tape measure from the maximum kyphosis of the thoracic spine to that of the sacrum), and flexion range (Schober test); determination of pain location on flexion and lateral bend; straight leg raising test (pendulum goniometer measurement of the angle at which pain was first experienced and angle of maximum tolerance); determination of pain location in the thigh and legs, and sensory changes in the legs. Nerve root tension signs were reliable if the location of pain was described. Reproducibility of bone tenderness over the sacroiliac joints, spinous processes and iliac crests was greater than that associated with soft tissue structures. Although the better description of test results will allow greater agreement between physicians in regard to the presence or absence of physical signs, these descriptions do not have diagnostic validity.

The question of diagnostic validity was tested prospectively by Jensen in 52 patients with lumbar disc herniations confirmed at surgery for correlation of disturbed sensory and motor function and anatomic abnormalities[23]. The positive predictive value of disturbed sensation in the L5 dermatome and weakness of foot dorsiflexion was 76% for herniation from the fourth lumbar disc. The positive predictive value of altered sensation in the S1 dermatome was only 50%. Therefore, although the history and physical examination are important and may identify levels of nerve impingement, significant overlap exists between nerve root distribution in individuals, making a correct diagnosis of location of lesion based on physical signs alone difficult in some circumstances[24].

With information obtained from the history and physical examination the physician should be able to formulate a working diagnosis for the low back pain patient. The vast majority of patients (>90%) have low back pain on a mechanical basis. Since it is impossible in most of these patients to identify the precise anatomic source of the pain, the Quebec Task Force on Spinal Disorders has suggested to abandon the use of nonvalidated diagnostic terms such as lumbar sprain, lumbar strain, discopathy, facet syndrome, ligamentitis, etc. Instead, they have proposed a simple classification of activity-related spinal disorders in 11 categories, based on history, clinical and paraclinical examinations, and response to treatment[25] (Fig. 3.13).

Most patients with mechanical low back pain may be treated without any specific investigation during the initial visit. On the other hand, patients in whom the history and physical examination suggest a medical cause for their pain will require further diagnostic tests[26].

ANCILLARY TESTS FOR EVALUATION OF LOW BACK PAIN	
Schober test	Lumbosacral motion
Contralateral straight leg raising test	Nerve root compression
Bow string sign	Nerve root compression
Hoover test	Patient effort

Fig. 3.11 Ancillary tests for evaluation of low back pain.

WADDELL TESTS FOR FUNCTIONAL LOW BACK PAIN
Tenderness to superficial touch
Simulation tests Axial loading Spinal rotation in one plane
Distraction tests Inconsistent results on confirmatory testing
Regional disturbances Abnormalities not following neuroanatomic structures
Overreaction Disproportionate verbalization

Fig. 3.12 Waddell tests for functional low back pain.

CLASSIFICATION OF ACTIVITY-RELATED SPINAL DISORDERS		
Classification	Symptoms	Working status at time of evaluation
1	Pain without radiation	W (working)
2	Pain + radiation to extremity, proximally	I (idle)
3	Pain + radiation to extremity, distally*	
4	Pain + radiation to lower limb neurologic signs	
5	Presumptive compression of a spinal nerve root on a simple radiograph (i.e. spinal instability or fracture)	
6	Compression of a spinal nerve root confirmed by: specific imaging techniques (CT, myelography or MRI) Other diagnostic techniques (e.g. electromyography, venography)	
7	Spinal stenosis	
8	Postsurgical status, 1–6 months after intervention	
9	Postsurgical status, >6 months after intervention 9.1 Asymptomatic; 9.2 Symptomatic	
10	Chronic pain syndrome	W (working)
11	Other diagnosis	I (idle)

* Not applicable to the thoracic segment.

Fig. 3.13 Classification of activity-related spinal disorders. Modified with permission from Spitzer et al. [25]

INVESTIGATIONS

PLAIN RADIOGRAPHS

A plain radiograph of the lumbar spine is not a necessary part of the initial evaluation of patients with back pain unless they have a history of major trauma, or acute constitutional symptoms. The Quebec Task Force on Spinal Disorders suggested that, without neurologic dysfunction, plain radiographs should not be done during the first week of an acute episode of back pain[25]. Plain radiographs are associated with a number of drawbacks. Patients with back pain of a mechanical origin frequently have radiographs that are normal. In adults under the age of 50, the yield of unexpected findings can be as low as 1 in 2500 [12]. In addition, many individuals with radiographic abnormalities may be entirely asymptomatic[27]. Congenital abnormalities, including spina bifida, transitional vertebrae, Schmorl nodes, and mild scoliosis, are unlikely causes of back pain[28]. By age 50, 67% of normal individuals have evidence of intervertebral disc degeneration. Two thirds of patients with radiographic proof of lumbar disc degeneration are asymptomatic. Osteoarthritis of apophyseal joints noted on radiographs is not closely correlated with symptoms[29]. Conversely, abnormalities confirmed at operation are not identified by plain radiographs. In one study, plain radiographs predicted disc protrusion in only 34% of patients who underwent operations[30]. When abnormalities are found, radiologists may disagree over the clinical significance of the findings[31]. Plain radiographs deliver a significant amount of radiation to the skin and lumbar spine and add a significant cost to the initial evaluation of patients[32].

When lumbar radiographs are obtained, a single lateral film may be adequate (Fig. 3.14). Padley *et al.* reviewed lumbosacral spine radiographs of 200 patients with back pain and no neurologic signs[33]. The single lateral film was as satisfactory diagnostically as a three-film series. The single projection had the added benefit of reduced cost and exposure of the patient to radiation. Others have suggested that anteroposterior and lateral views are adequate for evaluation[34,35]. The coned lateral view of the lumbosacral junction and oblique views do not identify therapeutically important lesions that cannot be seen on the other views[36].

Plain radiographs may be recommended for patients who have a systemic medical illness such as an inflammatory arthropathy, infection, tumors or significant fractures. The clinical practice guidelines issued for the Agency for Health Care Policy and Research (AHCPR) for acute low back pain have recommended that criteria for obtaining plain films include older age, recent significant trauma, history of prolonged steroid use, prior cancer, recent infection, fever, drug abuse, unexplained weight loss or pain with recumbency[37].

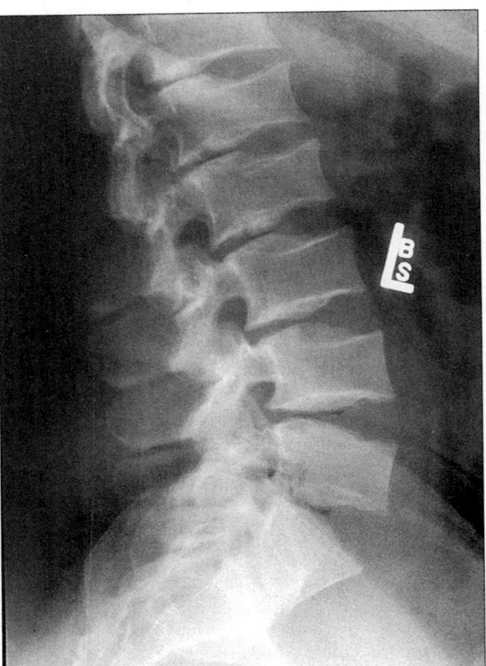

Fig. 3.14 Spondyloepiphyseal dysplasia. Plain radiograph, lateral view demonstrating elongation of vertebral bodies at multiple levels of the spine.

RADIONUCLIDE BONE SCINTIGRAPHY

Bone scintigraphy is of limited utility in low back pain patients. Bone scintigraphy detects increased bone turnover of any etiology. Mechanical and nonmechanical lesions associated with increased bone metabolism will result in a positive scan. Therefore, bone scintigraphy should be used selectively.

Technetium 99m diphosphonate scans are useful in detecting infection, tumors, inflammatory arthritis and fractures[38,39]. The sensitivity of bone scan is generally equal to magnetic resonance imaging (90% versus 96%), but for example is less specific in detecting vertebral osteomyelitis (78% versus 92%)[40]. Gallium and indium scans increase the specificity when used with a technetium scan, but are less sensitive when used alone[41]. Bone scintigraphy is better than magnetic resonance imaging (MRI) when evaluation of the whole skeleton is required[39]. Patients with metastatic disease may be unaware of bone lesions in other parts of the skeleton (Fig. 3.15). Increased activity in appendicular joints as well as in axial joints is suggestive of polyarthritis, usually associated with a spondyloarthropathy. Bone scan is best reserved for the patient with one of the following:

- Constitutional symptoms of fever and/or weight loss,
- Pain with recumbency,
- Failure to respond to conservative therapy, or
- Abnormal laboratory tests including elevated sedimentation rate or anemia.

COMPUTERIZED TOMOGRAPHY

Computerized tomography (CT) is useful for evaluating abnormalities of the lumbosacral spine, where the spatial anatomy is complex[42]. CT creates cross-sectional images of the internal structure of the spine at various levels and, with reformatting, can formulate sagittal and coronal images. The CT scan is the best technique for assessing the bony architecture of the spinal column, including the sacroiliac joints, before changes are noted on plain radiographs[43]. In addition, the structural relationships of soft tissues (ligaments, nerve roots, fat, intervertebral discs) can be evaluated as they relate to their bony environment. CT is an excellent technique for identifying mechanical disorders, including spinal stenosis, spondylosis, spondylolisthesis, trauma and congenital anomalies (Fig. 3.16)[44–47]. CT can visualize cortical bone destruction, calcified tumor matrix, soft tissue extension of tumors affecting the spine and is superior to MRI in this regard (Fig. 3.17)[48]. CT can also be used in an outpatient setting for percutaneous needle biopsy guidance of bony lesions[49].

Although CT is a very useful radiographic technique, it has its limitations. CT will not visualize intradural lesions unless radiographic contrast media is present intrathecally. CT is limited to only one slice of the skeleton at a time. Lesions located outside the imaged plane will not be viewed. CT slices are taken every 0.5cm. The radiologist must be informed about the area of the skeleton to be examined so that the duration of the test and exposure of the patient to radiation is limited. CT is associated with significant X-ray exposure (3–5rads).

The clinical significance of CT abnormalities must be evaluated in the setting of the patient's clinical findings. In a study of 53 asymptomatic and six symptomatic back pain patients with lumbar CT scans,

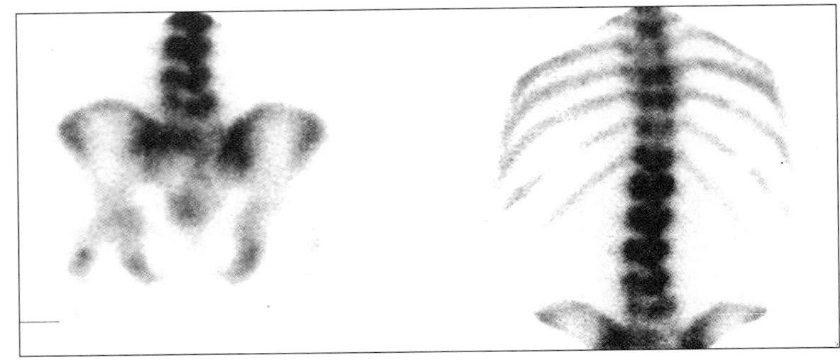

Fig. 3.15 Technetium bone scan. Increased tracer activity throughout the axial skeleton secondary to metastatic prostate cancer.

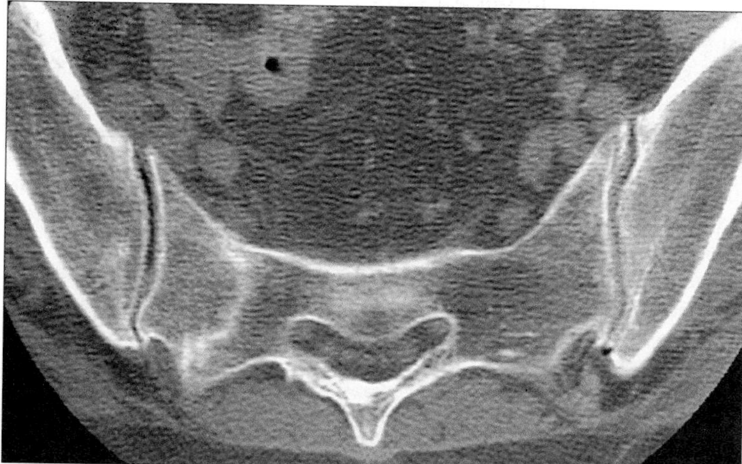

Fig. 3.16 Fracture. CT study of sacral spine demonstrating sacral fracture not visualized with plain radiographs.

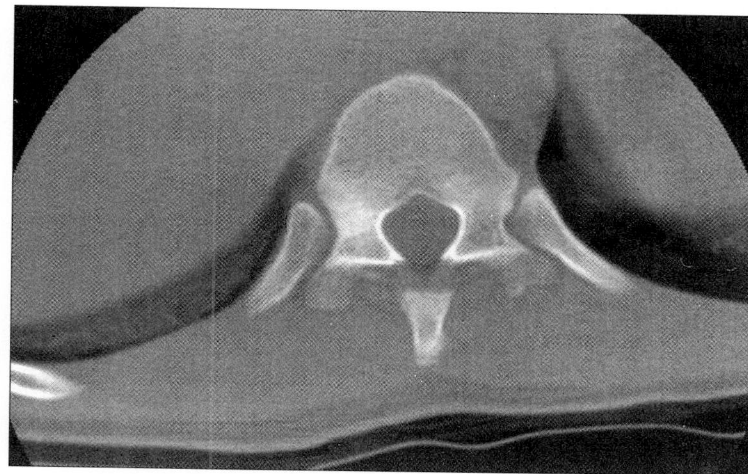

Fig. 3.17 Osteoid osteoma. CT study of thoracic spine demonstrating increased sclerosis associated with an osteoid osteoma.

abnormal findings were described in 34.5% of the asymptomatic individuals[50]. In patients aged under 40, 19.5% had a CT diagnosis of an intervertebral disc herniation. In patients aged over 40, 50% had abnormal findings, including disc herniation, spinal stenosis and apophyseal joint degeneration. In addition, there was agreement among the three neuroradiologists in only 11% of the cases. The implication of the study is that a patient with no historical or physical findings indicative of spinal pathology has a 1 in 3 chance of having an abnormal CT scan. Surgical intervention cannot be based upon anatomic abnormalities without clinical symptoms and physical signs that correlate with radiographic findings. CT should be used as a confirmatory, not diagnostic, test.

MYELOGRAPHY

Once the only means to identify spinal cord and nerve root compression, myelography has fallen out of favor as a radiographic technique, as it is associated with a number of drawbacks. Myelography is an invasive procedure requiring the injection of contrast media through a spinal needle. The procedure requires hospitalization for some patients. All the complications associated with a lumbar puncture may occur with a myelogram (headache, hematoma, infection, back pain and seizures)[51]. However, in combination with CT, myelography is helpful in detecting cord compression caused by fracture and soft tissue impingement associated with tumors. The use of a water soluble contrast agent, metrizamide, also provides information about the dynamic movement of cerebrospinal fluid. A complete block on myelography conclusively demonstrates pressure on neural elements. Cerebrospinal fluid may be removed for laboratory evaluation[52]. CT enhanced with contrast (CT myelogram) improves the accuracy of postoperative assessment of epidural fibrosis versus recurrent disc[53]. Arachnoiditis may also be evaluated by CT myelography. CT myelography is most helpful for these conditions when patients are unable to undergo magnetic resonance evaluation of these disorders[54].

Like the CT scan, the myelogram should be employed as a confirmatory study. An abnormal myelogram without associated clinical abnormalities is not significant. An abnormal iophendylate myelogram may be identified in 24% of individuals without back pain[55]. The myelogram should be reserved for the preoperative situation to confirm the presence of a damaged disc, a congenitally anomalous nerve root or an unsuspected tumor. Myelography is not as accurate as CT or MRI for the diagnosis of herniated nucleus pulposus that is corroborated at time of discectomy[56].

MAGNETIC RESONANCE IMAGING

Magnetic resonance imaging has revolutionized the radiographic evaluation of the lumbosacral spine. MRI has a number of advantages compared to other radiographic techniques. The procedure is noninvasive and uses magnetism and radio waves instead of ionizing radiation to generate its image. It is well tolerated by most patients except for claustrophobic individuals who may require sedation to remain in the limited confines of the machine. The entire length of the spinal cord and canal may be evaluated in multiple planes. MRI is able to define bony and soft tissue structures without intrathecal contrast. Patients who are not candidates for MRI evaluation include those on life support systems, and those who have a cardiac pacemaker, or ferromagnetic clips in the abdomen or on blood vessels. Pacemakers may revert to a fixed rate mode. Metal clips may migrate. Although nonferromagnetic appliances are not attracted to the magnets, the metal degrades the MRI image.

Many radiologists believe that MRI has become the primary imaging modality for the study of the spine[57]. MRI is an excellent technique to view the spinal cord. MRI identifies syringomyelia, atrophy, cord infarction, cord injury, multiple sclerosis and intramedullary tumors (Fig. 3.18)[58]. The development of contrast media (gadopentetate dimeglumine)

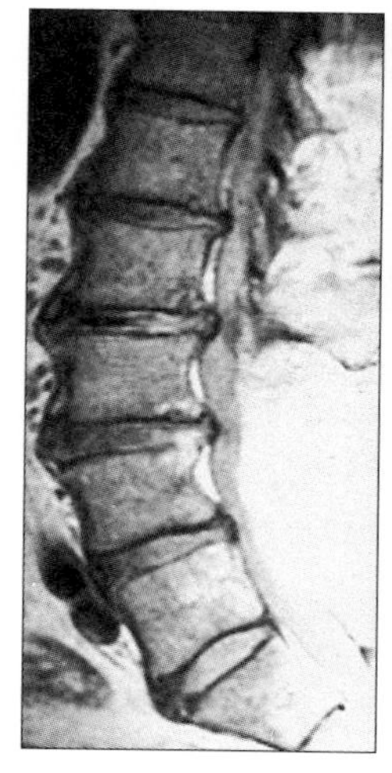

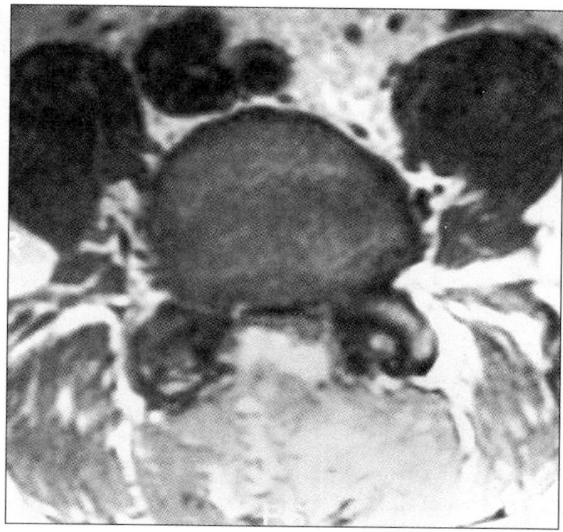

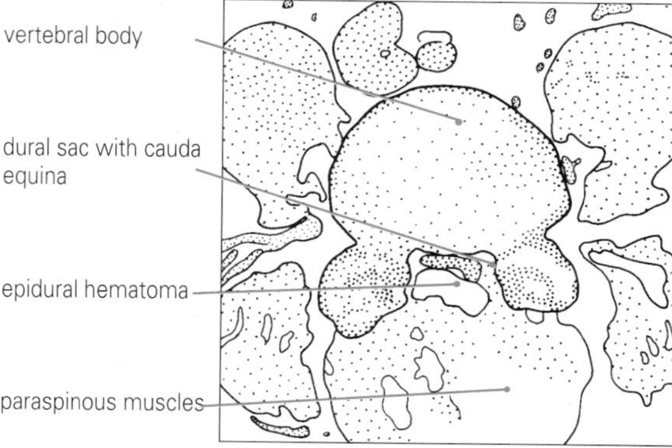

Fig. 3.18 Epidural hematoma. Postoperative sagittal and axial MRI studies showing an epidural hematoma compressing the cauda equina.

for MRI has improved the characterization of spinal cord tumors[59,60]. Contrast enhanced MRI is able to identify spinal cord pial metastases not visible by other radiographic techniques[61]. MRI delineates the extent of extradural tumor invasion of the spinal canal and compression or displacement of the spinal cord. MRI can identify the vertebral bodies in which bone marrow has been replaced with tumor (Fig. 3.19)[62,63].

MRI is an excellent technique for detecting infection of the spine, including discitis, osteomyelitis, epidural abscess, paraspinal abscess and myelitis[64]. MRI is more sensitive in the detection of vertebral osteomyelitis than are plain radiographs or CT [65]. Changes in the vertebral bodies and adjacent intervertebral disc spaces are visualized on T1-weighted images as areas of low signal intensity. On T2-weighted images, high signal intensity is seen crossing the involved bone and disc space.

MRI is also a useful technique for evaluating mechanical disorders of the lumbosacral spine. Disorders of the intervertebral disc are readily detected by MRI evaluation. Herniations can be identified in the sagittal plane and confirmed on the axial images[66]. Early degenerative changes are revealed by the loss of water indicated by the darkening of the disc on the T2-weighted image. MRI is also useful in the assessment of traumatic and nontraumatic fractures of vertebral bodies[67].

As with CT and myelography, MRI findings are only significant in patients with correlating clinical symptoms and signs. Boden *et al.* reported on a total of 104 MRI scans of 67 asymptomatic and 37 symptomatic individuals interpreted by three neuroradiologists for abnormalities[68]. The radiologists read 19 of 67 (28%) of the asymptomatic people as having substantial abnormalities. Herniated discs (24%) and spinal stenosis (4%) were the most common findings. Older persons (aged 60–80 years) had a majority of the abnormal findings. Therefore, the finding of an abnormal disc is more reliable in a symptomatic individual less than 60 years of age. Jensen *et al.* completed a MRI study on 98 asymptomatic individuals[69]. Only 36% of these individuals (mean age 42.3 years) had normal results. Fifty-two percent had a disk bulge at one level, 27% had a protrusion and 1% had an extrusion. An abnormality at two levels or more was noted in 38%[69].

Many questions remain over the optimal sequence of radiographic tests for the evaluation of the lumbosacral spine. A consensus is growing that MRI is the most useful technique for lumbar spine imaging. In the diagnosis of herniated discs and spinal stenosis, MRI has a sensitivity equal to or greater than those of CT or myelography[70]. In a study comparing MRI versus contrast CT for the diagnosis of herniated disc confirmed at surgery, 90.3% accuracy was associated with MRI while CT had an accuracy rate of only 77.4%[71]. MRI had greater sensitivity (88% accuracy) than myelography (75%) for the diagnosis of herniated discs[72]. MRI is also accurate in the diagnosis of spinal stenosis. A 96.6% agreement between MRI and contrast CT was identified for 41 patients evaluated for spinal stenosis in the central canal, lateral recess and foramens[73]. In addition, MRI was able to identify disc degeneration in 74 of 123 interspaces while CT identified only 27 of the 123 segments. Currently, MRI is the technique of choice for investigation of spinal stenosis and disc degeneration. The major limitation on MRI is the cost. The cost varies, and ranges from US$800 to US$1600 if contrast is required.

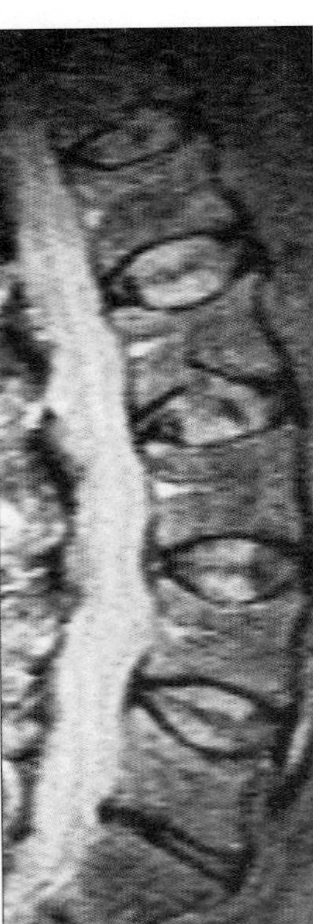

Fig. 3.19 MRI. Lumbar spine study of a multiple myeloma patient with abnormal bone marrow signal throughout the vertebral bodies, associated with remodeling of the vertebral bodies and pathologic fractures.

OTHER RADIOGRAPHIC TECHNIQUES

A number of other radiographic techniques are available for the evaluation of the lumbosacral spine. They are used infrequently compared to the techniques already discussed in this chapter. Spinal angiography permits the identification of the arterial origins and the venous drainage of vascular lesions of the spinal cord and column[74]. Arteriovenous malformations (AVM) are characterized by arteriovenous communication without an intervening capillary network. The extent of the lesion may encompass long distances even though the lesion originates from only one or few sites. Most of the abnormalities visualized by other radiographic techniques are produced by the enlargement of draining veins. A diagnostic spinal angiography may require evaluation of the entire spinal cord in order to identify the arterial supply to the lesion so that appropriate therapeutic decisions in regard to embolization or surgery can be made. Hemangioblastomas and hemangiomas may be more accurately visualized by angiographic techniques.

Lumbar discography is a procedure associated with the injection of contrast material through a percutaneous needle into the nucleus pulposus suspected of causing back pain. The reproduction of the patient's pain is considered a positive test. The test is used for patients with a degenerative disc who may be considered for spinal fusion because of persistent pain[75]. Its clinical significance remains controversial[76]. MRI is equally sensitive in detecting disc degeneration, but is unable to reproduce patient symptoms. The role of discography will be decided on its relevance to patient symptoms and the development of better, nonsurgical, therapies.

Thermography is a noninvasive procedure that records infrared radiation emitted from body surfaces. Thermographers believe that a close correlation exists between abnormal thermograms and surgically proven herniated discs[77]. However, meta-analysis of 28 studies evaluating the role of thermography in the evaluation of radiculopathy revealed significant methodologic flaws in 27. The one high quality study found no discriminant value for liquid–crystal thermography[78]. At present thermograms are not recommended for use in the routine decision-making for diagnosis of low back pain patients.

CLINICAL LABORATORY TESTS

The vast majority of individuals with low back pain do not require laboratory studies with their initial evaluation. However, patients who are elderly, who have constitutional symptoms or who have failed conservative therapy may benefit from a laboratory evaluation. The most useful test in helping to differentiate medical from mechanical low back pain is measurement of the erythrocyte sedimentation rate (ESR). An elevated ESR suggests the presence of inflammation in the body and, in the appropriate setting, should result in a more thorough evaluation of a patient for a systemic inflammatory disorder. In one study, an ESR of over 25mm/h had a false positive rate of only 6%[79].

Abnormalities in the complete blood count (hematocrit, leukocyte or platelet count) may be indicative of an inflammatory disorder including neoplasms. Alterations of calcium concentration and alkaline phosphatase activity suggest diffuse bone disease. Elevated acid phosphatase activity may mirror the extent of metastases from prostatic cancer. An urinalysis can identify the individual with renal abnormalities (nephrolithiasis). Detection of occult blood in the stool is a screening test for ulcers or gastrointestinal tumors.

ELECTRODIAGNOSTIC STUDIES

Electrodiagnostic studies are extensions of the neurologic examination and provide a means to identify nerve and muscle damage. These tests can confirm the clinical suspicion of nerve root compression, define the distribution and severity of involvement and document or exclude other illnesses of nerves or muscles that contribute to the patient's symptoms and signs. These tests include evaluation of electrical activity generated by muscle fibers at rest and during contraction (electromyography) and speed of conduction of impulses electrically generated in peripheral nerves (nerve conduction studies).

Electrodiagnostic tests are most helpful in documenting, objectively, neurophysiologic abnormalities in a patient where clinical examination (pain radiation, sensory changes, muscular weakness) does not necessarily indicate nerve root dysfunction[80]. Neurophysiologic tests can also document normal function where radiographic techniques have revealed anatomic abnormalities.

Electromyography (EMG) is the test most commonly ordered to document the presence of a radiculopathy[81]. Electromyography measures the action potentials of muscle fibers. As the nerve supplying a muscle becomes compressed, fibers to that muscle are lost and are eventually replaced with regenerated fibers. This process of denervation and reinnervation occurs over time (Fig. 3.20). Electromyography may not be able to document the hypersensitivity or the spontaneously generated electrical activity of the muscle until 3–4 weeks after the initial insult. Abnormalities associated with radiculopathy can include increased motor unit potentials, fibrillations and prolonged insertional activity. In a partially denervated muscle (the usual occurrence with herniated discs), the remaining axons from unaffected nerve roots grow to innervate more of the muscle fibers. The increase in the number of motor fibers per unit results in an asynchronous and prolonged muscle fiber depolarization. The result is a motor unit potential of longer duration and increased amplitude.

Fibrillations are action potentials that arise from small clusters of denervated, healthy muscle fibers awaiting reinnervation. Once present, fibrillations may persist for months. The amplitude of fibrillations diminishes over time. The finding of fibrillations is nonspecific since they are also associated with myopathic disorders.

Nerve fibers are damaged when entered by the EMG needle. This damage results in the production of electrical current, referred to as insertional activity. In normal fibers, insertional activity ceases once the needle electrode comes to rest. In radiculopathies, the insertional activity persists for seconds.

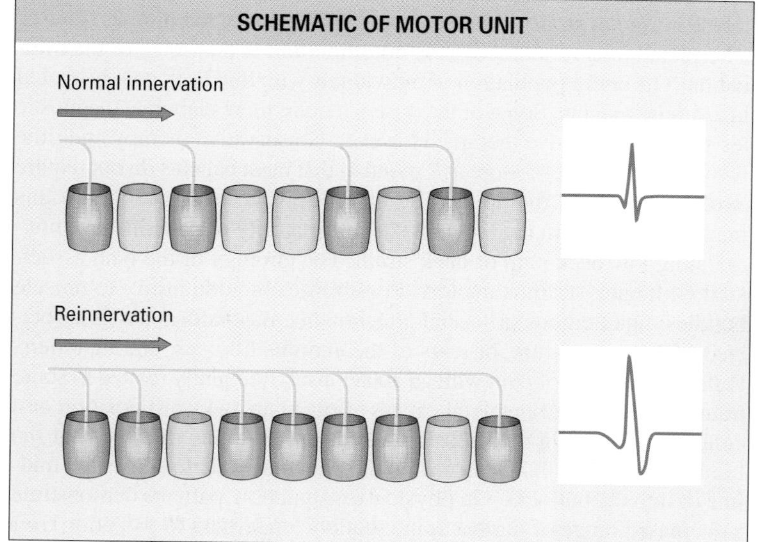

Fig. 3.20 Schematic of motor unit. A normal motor unit with four innervated muscle fibers and, below, reinnervation by terminal sprouting of an undamaged nerve fiber of fibers in a muscle partially denervated. Following reinnervation, corresponding action potentials (shown on the right) have greater duration and amplitude as a result of the increased number of innervated muscle fibers.

EMG findings are based upon the interpretation of the observer. The experience of the examiner is very important in obtaining the most accurate information from the EMG evaluation.

As opposed to EMG, nerve conduction tests become abnormal as soon as nerve damage occurs[82]. Nerve conduction tests include evaluation of H-reflex, F-response and somatosensory-evoked responses. The H-reflex is the electrical equivalent of a tendon reflex. It consists of a sensorimotor monosynaptic reflex arc that is measured over the gastrocnemius on stimulation of the posterior tibial nerve in the popliteal fossa. The H-reflex is commonly used for evaluation of S1 radiculopathy and is associated with a high degree of accuracy[83]. The time latency is standardized for age and the length of the limb. The time difference between the lower extremities should be 2ms or less.

An F-response exclusively measures motor nerve pathways between the point of stimulation and anterior horn cells in the spinal cord. It is not a reflex since no sensory nerves are involved. F-responses may be entirely normal in pure sensory radiculopathies. Unlike the H-reflex, the F-response is variable in latency and must be repeated to average the responses. In addition, many F-responses evaluate nerve roots of multiple levels. Single level radiculopathies may have normal F-responses[84]. F-response is reported as the minimal response or latency time; 2ms is the maximally allowed difference between the extremities.

Somatosensory-evoked responses measure the sensory pathways between the point of stimulation, the spinal cord and the scalp. The most commonly utilized means of eliciting the response for radiculopathies is by stimulation of specific nerves, such as the sural nerve (S1) or superficial peroneal nerve (L5). By standardizing the latency in normal individuals of the same height and leg length, disturbances in nerve conduction can be assessed. Dermatomal-evoked responses are another means to try and isolate one nerve root for evaluation. By stimulating specific areas of skin associated with dermatomes, it is possible to evaluate the integrity of sensory pathways. Abnormal dermatomal and small sensory nerve responses are correlated with the presence of a radiculopathy[85].

The limitations of electrodiagnostic studies must be considered when evaluating patients with low back pain. These studies do not determine a specific diagnosis. Localization of the lesion is not easy since most muscles in the lower extremity are innervated by two or more nerve roots. In a study of 20 patients with radicular symptoms secondary to disc herniation, 13 had EMG abnormalities that corroborated the affected disc level at surgery in five individuals only[86]. Despite these limitations, electrodiagnostic tests remain an important part of the investigation of low back pain patients. An abnormal EMG is corroborative evidence of organic disease and helps the physician determine who is a potential candidate for surgical intervention. Electromyography changes may recede with resolution of the nerve impingement. However, patients with a good operative decompression with relief of symptoms may have EMG abnormalities persist 1 year after surgery[86]. In patients without neurologic dysfunction, EMG and nerve conduction tests are normal.

DIFFERENTIAL DIAGNOSIS

Each patient with back pain presents to the physician a different set of complaints. These complaints may be associated with a broad range of disorders, from mechanical muscle strain, to spondyloarthropathy, to metastatic disease. The problem confronting the examining physician is to integrate the patient's symptoms and physical signs into a logical diagnosis and initial treatment plan and to identify those individuals with more serious ailments from the vast majority with mechanical disorders. With the myriad of symptoms, signs, laboratory tests, radiographic methods and possible diagnoses, the physician must be organized in his approach to the patient with low back pain. Most patients with low back pain will improve and will not require additional diagnostic testing. In times of increasing medical financial costs, diagnostic tests must be obtained in a thoughtful and time-efficient manner. A standardized approach to the diagnosis and treatment of low

MECHANICAL LOW BACK PAIN					
	Muscle strain	Spondylothesis	Herniated disc	Osteoarthritis	Spinal stenosis
Age (years)	20–40	20–30	30–50	over 50	over 60
Pain pattern					
Initial location	Back	Back	Back	Back	Leg
Onset	Acute	Insidious	Acute	Insidious	Insidious
Standing	+	+	–	+	+
Sitting	–	–	+	–	–
Flexion	+		+	–	–
Extension	–	+	–	+	+
Straight leg raising	–	–	+	–	+ (stress)
Plain radiograph	–	+	–	+	+

Fig. 3.21 Mechanical low back pain.

back pain is possible if basic rules are followed. This approach has been utilized in the evaluation of thousands of patients and has been useful in the vast majority of those individuals[87].

The primary objective for the physician is to return the patient with acute low back pain to regular activity as quickly as possible. Patients who continue with low back pain for six months or longer are unlikely to have resolution of pain and rarely return to their usual employment. The effort required to evaluate and treat patients effectively to prevent the evolution into a chronic pain syndrome is worthwhile. In achieving this goal, the physician must be concerned with making efficient and precise use of diagnostic studies, avoiding ineffectual surgery and making therapy available at a reasonable cost.

SYSTEMATIC APPROACH TO LOW BACK PAIN

Most patients with low back pain have a mechanical cause for their symptoms and do not require any diagnostic tests (Fig. 3.21). Individuals who must be evaluated more intensively are those with life-threatening disorders, such as cauda equina compression or expanding abdominal aneurysms (Fig. 3.22).

Patients with cauda equina compression have a symptom complex that may include low back pain, bilateral sciatica, saddle anesthesia,

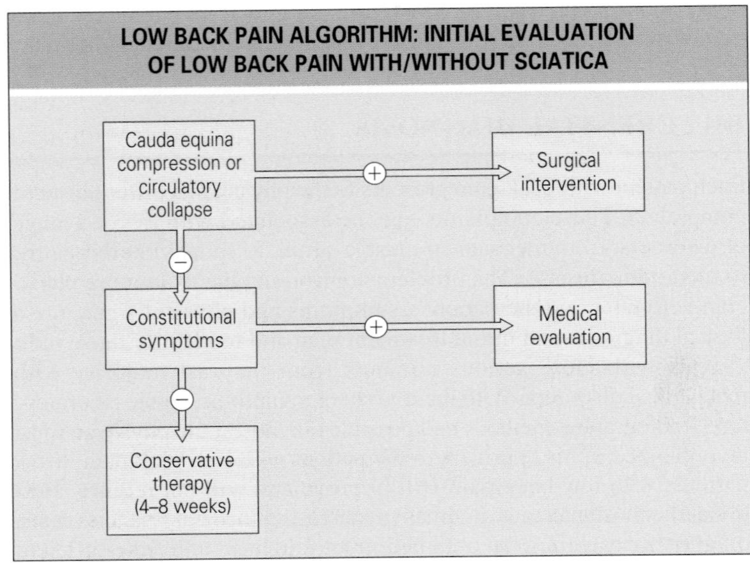

Fig. 3.22 Low back pain algorithm. Initial evaluation.

or bladder and bowel incontinence. The most common mechanical causes of cauda equina compression are central herniations of intervertebral discs, while epidural abscesses and tumor masses constitute the most frequent nonmechanical causes. Once the diagnosis is suspected, the patient should undergo a radiographic procedure to visualize the affected anatomic area of the lumbosacral spine. MRI is the most sensitive radiographic technique for detecting these lesions. Patients are treated appropriately for their underlying abnormalities.

A patient with tearing or throbbing back pain who has experienced acute dizziness may have an expanding abdominal aneurysm. Any change in the frequency, intensity or location of the pain suggests expansion in the size of the aneurysm. Patients with an abdominal aneurysm are usually older individuals who have had a history of lower extremity claudication. If patients complain of syncope or are hypotensive, they must be evaluated for an aneurysm on an emergency basis. Physical examination of the abdomen may reveal a pulsatile mass, abdominal bruits and decreased pulsations in the lower extremities. Patients with expanding aneurysms may be evaluated with CT or ultrasonography, depending on the patient's hemodynamic status. Patients with an expanding aneurysm require surgical correction of the aneurysmal defect.

Other patients with low back pain who need to be identified before therapy is initiated are those with medical low back pain. Most of these patients can be identified during the history portion of the evaluation since they usually present with one of the following:

- fever and/or weight loss;
- increased pain on recumbency (sleeping in a chair);
- morning stiffness lasting hours;
- acute, localized lumbosacral bone pain;
- visceral pain associated with alterations in gastrointestinal or genitourinary function.

Patients with any of these symptoms should be evaluated thoroughly.

Those without cauda equina syndrome or a medical illness may be started on conservative therapy without a laboratory or radiographic evaluation. One exception to this guideline is older individuals (aged over 50 years) with new onset back pain. These patients may benefit from a plain radiograph of the lumbar spine and ESR measurement to detect neoplastic or infectious disorders[37].

Conservative management for acute low back pain includes patient education, controlled physical activity, nonsteroidal anti-inflammatory drugs (NSAIDs), muscle relaxants or physical therapy. Any or all of these components of conservative management may be used in an individual patient.

The physician should decide on a course of therapy and continue it for a 4–6 week trial. The determination of a specific diagnosis, whether it be a muscular strain of the paraspinous muscles of the lumbar spine or a herniated intervertebral disc, is not important at this stage of the evaluation. The entire population of individuals with low back pain is treated in a similar manner. Some of these may require more elaborate diagnostic tests or more invasive therapy. However, conservative therapy and time is so effective (90% or more at 2 months) that most patients do not require expensive tests or therapies. The opportunity to treat patients in this manner results from the fact that the vast majority of patients have nonradiating low back pain or back strain. The etiology of the pain associated with back strain is unclear. Possibilities include injury to muscle bundles, ligamentous or fascial attachments, mechanical stress associated with poor posture, or tears of the annulus fibrosus, among others. Patients complain of pain with an acute onset, frequently related to some traumatic event that involved excess effort in an awkward position or a contusion. The pain is localized to areas lateral to the midline near the lumbosacral junction. On occasion the pain may radiate across the midline or into the buttocks. On physical examination, patients demonstrate a decreased range of lumbar spine motion, tenderness to palpation over the involved muscle and increased muscle contraction. Laboratory and radiographic evaluations of these patients are normal. Any variation from normal should result in an evaluation for alternative diagnoses.

After 4–6 weeks have passed, patients in whom the initial treatment regimen fails are sorted into four groups, based upon the location and

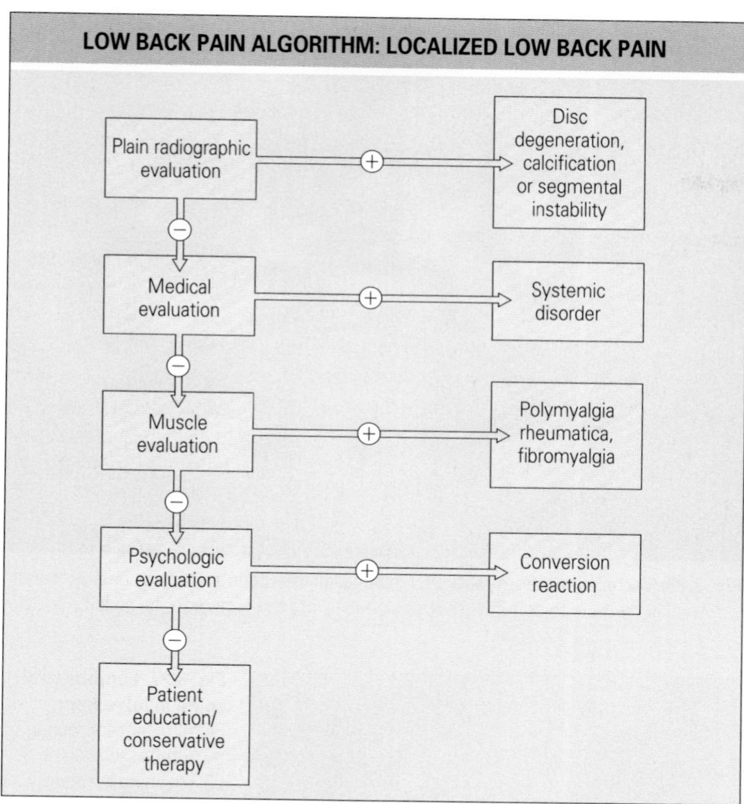

Fig. 3.23 Low back pain algorithm. Localized low back pain.

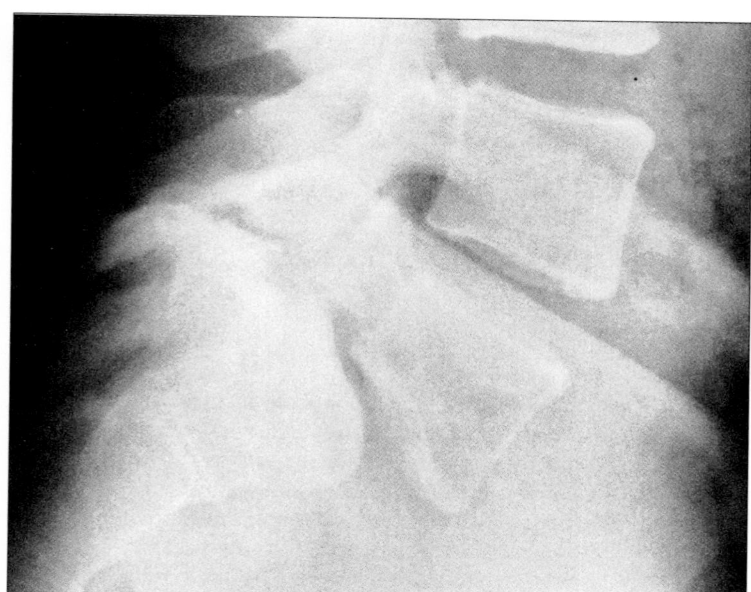

Fig. 3.24 Grade II developmental spondylolisthesis. At the L5–S1 level.

radiation of the residual pain. These groups include those with localized low back pain, leg pain below the knee (sciatica), anterior thigh pain and posterior thigh pain.

LOCALIZED LOW BACK PAIN

Patients with localized low back pain make up the largest group with residual pain (Fig. 3.23). Evaluation with plain radiographs of the lumbar spine is indicated, with flexion and extension views if spinal instability is suspected. Spondylolysis, with or without spondylolisthesis, is the most common structural abnormality to cause significant low back pain. Spondylolysis is a break in the pars interarticularis. If the defect permits displacement of one vertebra on another, it is termed a spondylolisthesis (Fig. 3.24). Individuals may have this abnormality without symptoms. Most patients with symptomatic spondylolisthesis complain of pain when their spine is placed in extension (increased displacement) as opposed to flexion (that tends to normalize vertebral body position). Most patients have a good response to nonoperative measures, including patient education, flexion exercises and a flexion back support. A small group will fail conservative management and require a fusion of the unstable segment.

Localized low back pain may also be associated with disorders of the intervertebral discs and related apophyseal joints. Abnormalities may be noted on plain radiographic evaluation of the lumbar spine. Decreased disc height and apophyseal joint sclerosis may not cause low back pain. However, articular degeneration with apophyseal joint sclerosis may be associated with decreased back motion and back pain[88]. Patients may have mild stiffness in the morning. During the day, these patients experience an improvement in their symptoms only to have a return of pain at the end of the day, after they have been physically active. Patients with osteoarthritis of the lumbar spine should be treated as other patients with this disorder affecting other joints in the skeleton. Therapy includes analgesics, NSAIDs and appropriate exercises. A point to remember is that older individuals who develop osteoarthritis are also more likely to develop more ominous causes of low back pain. These disorders (malignancy, infection, osteoporosis, for example) should be considered before the physician ascribes the patient's pain to osteoarthritis.

Another abnormality occasionally seen is disc calcification. This is associated with ochronosis, calcium pyrophosphate dihydrate disease, hemochromatosis, hyperparathyroidism and acromegaly. Patients with disc calcification should be evaluated for the associated endocrinologic or metabolic disorder.

Patients who fail to respond to conservative management and who have no specific radiographic abnormalities may improve with a local injection of a combination of an anesthetic and a semisoluble corticosteroid preparation into the area of maximal tenderness. Many patients with local muscle strain experience complete relief of symptoms with the injection. This therapy should be given to individuals who will be compliant with the instructions regarding limitation of activity. Patients who have undergone an anesthetic injection will not experience pain if they engage in physical activity that causes additional damage to musculoskeletal structures. These individuals should be cautioned to limit their activities for 24–48 hours to be sure that additional healing has occurred so that usual activities can be resumed.

Patients who persist with low back pain who do not have spondylolysis, disc calcification or osteoarthritis must be re-evaluated for the possibility of a systemic disorder causing their symptom. This re-evaluation should commence with a review of the patient's history and physical examination. The patient may have forgotten to mention an important symptom during the initial evaluation or may have developed a new one during the course of therapy. The histories of patients with medical low back pain may be divided into five groups according to symptoms. These groups include individuals with fever or weight loss, pain with recumbency, morning stiffness, acute localized lumbosacral bone pain or visceral pain.

Fever and/or weight loss

Patients with fever and/or weight loss frequently have an infection or tumor as a cause of their pain. Neoplastic lesions also cause pain with recumbency and will be discussed in the following section.

The clinical presentation of the patient with a spinal infection depends on the infecting organism (see Fig. 3.25). Bacterial infections cause acute, toxic symptoms, while tuberculous and fungal infections are indolent. The pain in bacterial infections is persistent, present at rest

INFECTIOUS DISORDERS AFFECTING THE LUMBOSACRAL SPINE
Vertebral osteomyelitis Bacterial Tuberculous Fungal Spirochetal Parasitic
Discitis
Pyogenic sacroiliitis

Fig. 3.25 Localized low back pain. Infectious disorders affecting the lumbosacral spine.

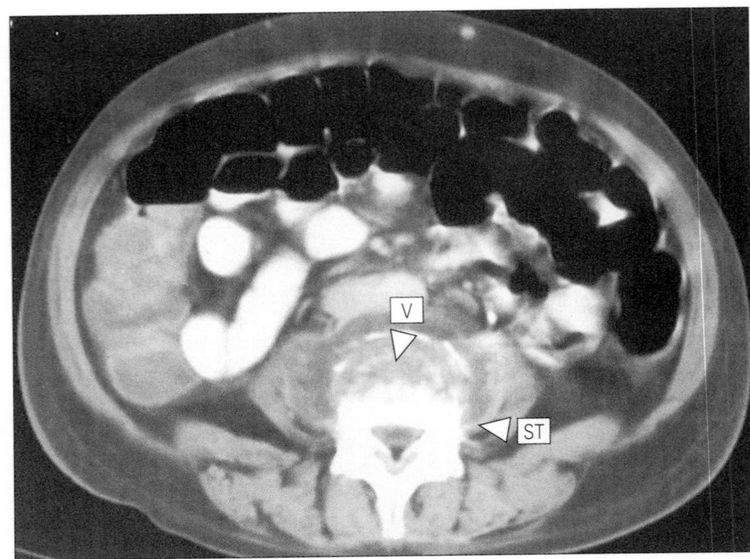

Fig. 3.26 Vertebral osteomyelitis. CT scan, axial view, demonstrating destruction of vertebral body (V) with soft tissue extension (ST) into the paravertebral space.

and is exacerbated by motion. Physical findings include decreased range of motion, muscle spasm and percussion tenderness over the involved bone. Plain radiographs may reveal localized areas of osteopenia. If radiographs are normal, technetium bone scintigraphy is indicated. MRI is a sensitive technique with which to investigate the entire lumbosacral spine for the presence of local infection. MRI also detects soft tissue extension of lesions beyond the bony confines of the vertebral column. CT should take place after MRI evaluation to delineate the bony architecture of lesions not visualized adequately by MRI (Fig. 3.26).

Vertebral osteomyelitis follows hematogenous spread from an extraosseous source and can be identified in 40% of patients[89]. Organisms may enter bone from nutrient arteries, or from the venous plexus of Batson, a valveless system of veins that supplies the spinal column. Organisms that cause osteomyelitis include bacteria, mycobacteria, fungi, spirochetes and parasites. The primary sources for spinal infections include the genitourinary tract, respiratory tract and skin. The most frequently encountered organism causing infection in 60% of cases is *Staphylococcus aureus*[90]. Gram-negative organisms are often grown from samples from the elderly and from parenteral drug abusers (*Escherichia coli* and *Pseudomonas aeruginosa*[91] respectively). In patients who have undergone surgery or trauma to the spine, nonpathogenic organisms (diphtheroids, *S. epidermidis)* may be associated with an indolent infection of the vertebral column[92]. Workers in the meat-processing industry may acquire a brucellosis infection[93]. Tuberculous and fungal infections of the vertebral column occur most often in the elderly and other immunocompromised individuals. Fifty to sixty percent of individuals with skeletal tuberculosis have axial skeletal disease. The clinical presentation of a patient with tuberculous spondylitis is pain over the involved vertebrae, low-grade fever and weight loss. The process is indolent and may be present for years before diagnosis (Fig. 3.27)[94].

The definitive diagnosis of infection is based on the recovery and identification of the causative organism from blood cultures, or from aspirated material or biopsy of the lesion. Antibiotic therapy is adequate to cure most spinal infections. Surgical intervention for drainage is needed if neurologic dysfunction has occurred secondary to the infection.

Other infections that affect the lumbosacral spine include discitis and pyogenic sacroiliitis. Infection of the intervertebral disc space in adults is most frequently associated with lumbar disc surgery. Approximately 3% of lumbar disc surgery patients develop disc space infections[95]. Diagnosis is confirmed by identifying the causative organism from blood cultures or aspirated disc material. Pyogenic sacroiliitis is an unusual form of septic arthritis[96]. The disease is associated with acute symptoms, severe sacroiliac joint pain and fever. Bone scinitigraphy with early perfusion views will identify the affected joint. Diagnosis of the causative organism may be obtained by blood cultures, fluoroscopic fine needle aspiration or open biopsy. Antibiotic therapy for 6 weeks is usually adequate to heal the infection without the need for surgical drainage.

Nocturnal pain/pain with recumbency

Tumors of the spinal column or spinal cord cause pain at night or with recumbency. Both benign and malignant neoplasms cause these symptoms. Nocturnal pain may be caused by swelling of neoplastic tissues associated with inactivity in the supine position or by stretching the neural tissues over the neoplastic mass.

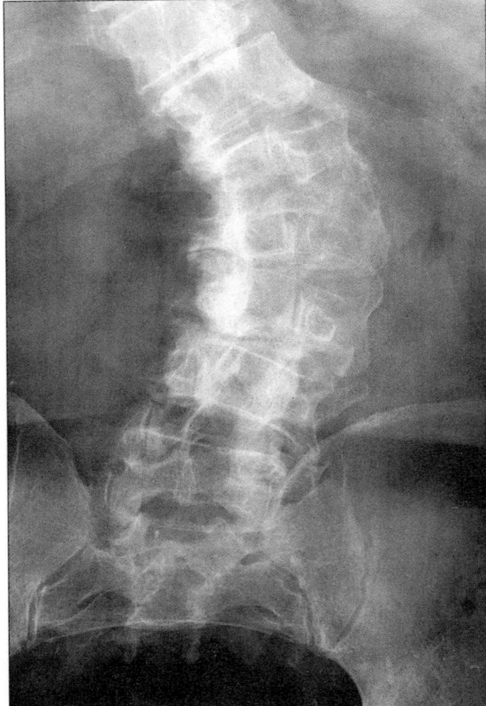

Fig. 3.27 Lumbosacral spine involvement. Pott's disease affecting the lumbosacral spine at L3, resulting in rotatory scoliosis and lateral calcification.

A number of benign and malignant tumors are associated with involvement of the lumbosacral spine (Fig. 3.28). Benign lesions tend to cause local pain and involve the posterior elements of vertebrae. Malignant lesions cause more diffuse pain, systemic symptoms and involve the anterior elements of vertebrae.

Patients with malignancies have pain that is gradual in onset but persistent in character and increasing in intensity. Physical examination shows localized tenderness over the lesion along with neurologic dysfunction if neural elements are compressed. Radiographic evaluation is very useful in detecting the location and characteristics of the neoplastic lesion.

An example of a benign tumor of bone that affects the lumbar spine is an osteoid osteoma. The tumor is most frequently found in young adults aged 20–30 years. Approximately 7% of osteoid osteomas occur in the spine, most frequently in the lumbar area[97]. The pain associated with this lesion is intermittent and vague initially, but with time becomes constant and aching, with a boring quality. The pain is not relieved with rest or application of heat. The pain is frequently exacerbated at night

NEOPLASTIC LESIONS OF THE LUMBOSACRAL SPINE		
Benign	**Malignant**	**Spinal cord tumors**
Osteoid osteoma Osteoblastoma Osteochondroma Giant cell tumor Aneurysmal bone cyst Hemangioma Eosinophilic granuloma Sacroiliac lipoma	Multiple myeloma Chondrosarcoma Chordoma Lymphoma Skeletal metastases	Extradural metastases Intradural–Extramedullary Neurofibroma Meningioma Intramedullary Ependymoma Astrocytoma

Fig. 3.28 Localized low back pain. Neoplastic disorders affecting the lumbosacral spine.

and disturbs sleep. In the spine, osteoid osteomas are associated with nonstructural scoliosis. The appearance of marked paravertebral muscle spasm and the sudden onset of scoliosis in a young adult requires an evaluation for the presence of this lesion. The lesion is on the concave side of the scoliosis. The symptoms of osteoid osteoma may be present for a considerable time before plain radiographic findings become evident. The pain is relieved with low doses of NSAIDs.

Physical examination reveals local tenderness. Scoliosis is reversible early in the course of the lesion. With prolonged spasm, muscle atrophy may occur. Vertebral deformity may occur in young individuals who are growing. Hyperemia of the tumor may cause swelling and erythema of the skin if the lesion is superficial in location.

The radiographic finding of a lucent nidus with a diameter of 1.5cm and a surrounding well-defined area of dense sclerotic bone is virtually pathognomonic of osteoid osteoma. The lesions are in the neural arch in 75% of vertebrae, articular facets in 18% and 7% in vertebral bodies (Fig. 3.29). Bone scans or CT scans should be utilized if an osteoma is suspected and not found on plain radiographs (Fig. 3.30)[98,99].

The treatment for an osteoid osteoma is simple excision of the nidus and surrounding sclerotic bone. If the nidus is not entirely removed, recurrence of the lesion is possible and symptoms may persist. On occasion, osteoid osteomas may undergo spontaneous healing.

Multiple myeloma is the most common primary malignancy of bone in adults (27% of biopsied bone tumors)[100]. Patients range in age from 50 to 70 years, with only a rare patient below the age of 40. Low back pain is the initial complaint in 35% of patients. The pain is aching and intermittent at onset, is aggravated by weight bearing and improved with bed rest. Some patients may have radicular symptoms that mimic those of sciatica and arthritis[101]. Significant neurologic dysfunction, including paraplegia, occurs more commonly with solitary plasmacytoma than with multiple myeloma[102].

Physical examination may demonstrate diffuse bone tenderness, fever, pallor and purpura in the later stages of the illness. Signs of spinal cord compression are present if vertebral body collapse has progressed to a significant degree.

Laboratory testing reflects the systemic nature of this malignancy. Included in the abnormal findings may be anemia, leukocytosis, thrombocytopenia, elevated ESR, hypercalcemia, hyperuricemia, elevated creatinine and a positive Coomb's test. An increase in serum proteins is secondary to the presence of abnormal immunoglobulins of any of the five classes. Urinalysis may detect Bence Jones protein formed by the production of excess immunoglobulin light chains. Bone marrow aspirate or biopsy reveals an excess number of plasma cells of varied histologic grades.

Plain radiographs demonstrate osteolysis without reactive sclerosis and sparing of the posterior elements of the spine (Fig. 3.31)[103]. Solitary plasmacytomas in the spine have variable radiographic appearances. They may be expansile, with or without reactive bone. They may invade an intervertebral disc space and mimic discitis. Bone scintigraphy does not detect myeloma since there is no reactive component of osteoblasts to the myeloma cells. MRI and CT are better techniques for identifying the presence and extent of myeloma lesions in the bone and soft tissues. MRI is able to detect spinal bone marrow involvement in asymptomatic myeloma patients[104].

The diagnosis of multiple myeloma is based upon clinical data, along with the detection of abnormal plasma cells on biopsy. Myeloma is treated with the use of chemotherapeutic agents to control the growth of the malignant plasma cells. In patients with cord compression, decompression laminectomy with or without local radiotherapy is indicated.

Skeletal metastases are 25 times more common than primary tumors as the cause of neoplastic lesions in the spine. Patients who are aged over 50 years are at greatest risk of developing metastatic disease. Autopsy results demonstrate that 70% of patients with primary tumors develop metastases to the thoracolumbar spine[105]. The common sources for skeletal metastases include tumors of the breast, prostate, lung, kidney, thyroid, colon, uterine cervix and bladder.

Lumbar pain is of gradual onset and increasing intensity. The symptoms are increased with motion, sneezing or coughing. The pain is local at the onset but may become radicular in character. Neurologic abnormalities may occur abruptly over a 4–6 month period.

Physical examination may demonstrate pain on palpation over the affected bone. Muscle spasm and limitation of motion are associated

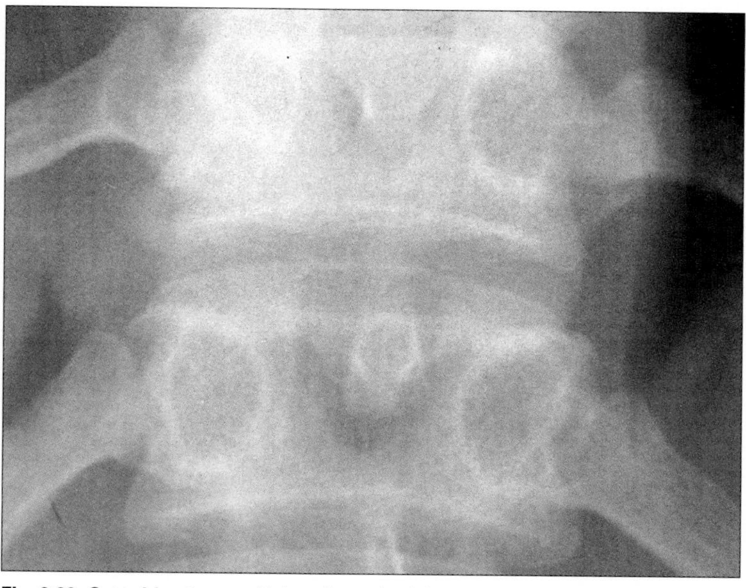

Fig. 3.29 Osteoid osteoma. Plain radiograph of thoracic spine demonstrating sclerosis affecting the right pedicle of T11.

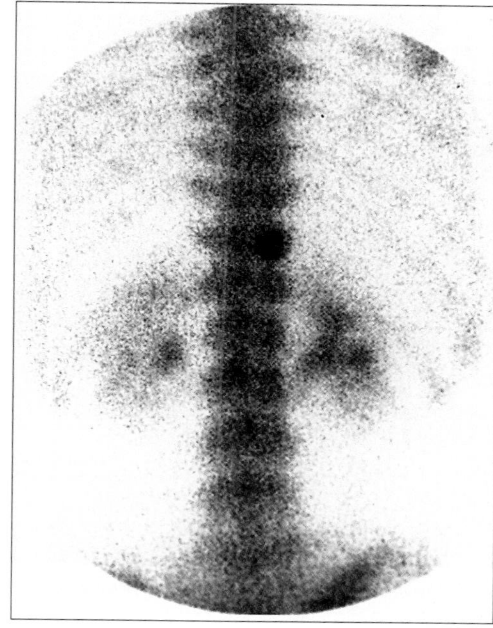

Fig. 3.30 Osteoid osteoma. Bone scintigraphy (posterior view) demonstrating increased uptake in T11. There is no other area of increased uptake in the skeleton.

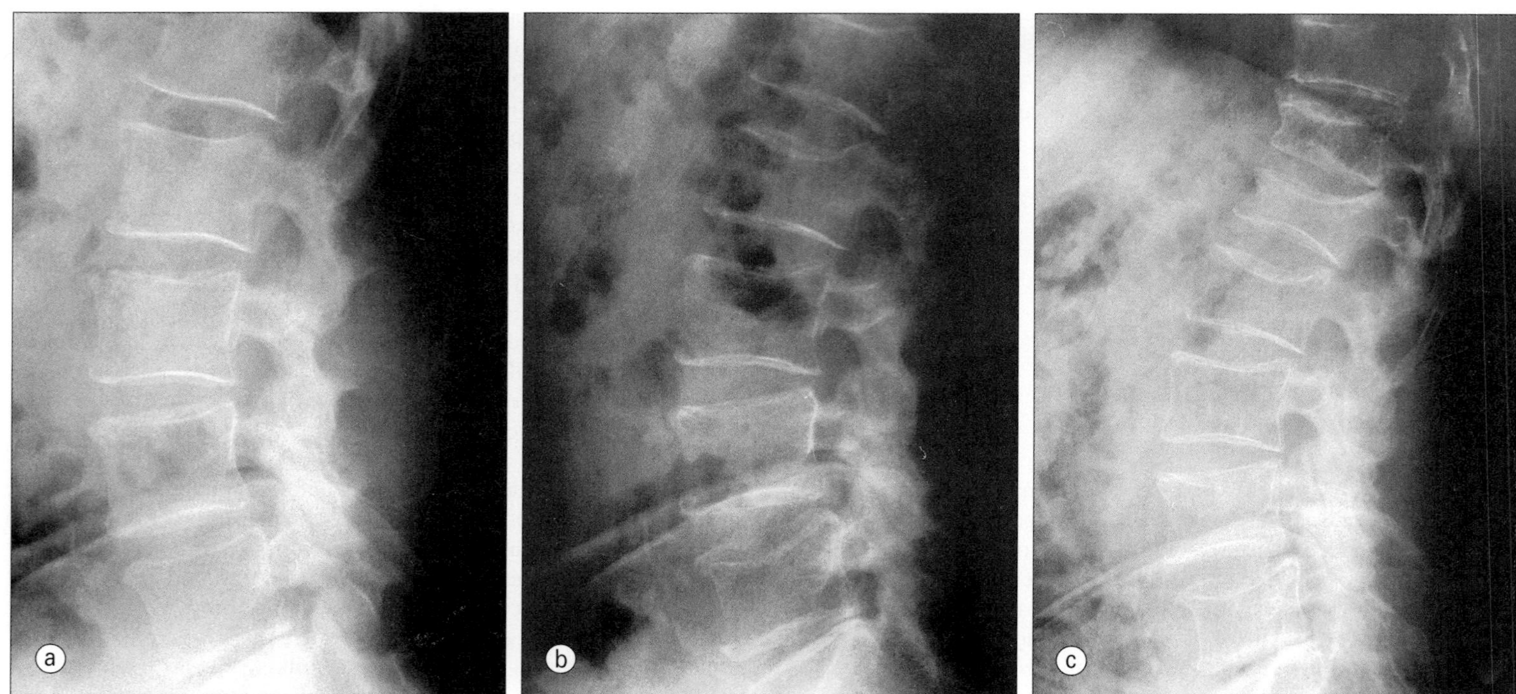

Fig. 3.31 Multiple myeloma. A series of plain radiographs taken over a 3-month period. Progressive osteopenia and pathologic compression fractures are noted. (a) Initial evaluation; (b) at 12 weeks; (c) at 14 weeks. Diagnosis was made at 12 weeks after initial presentation.

findings. Neurologic abnormalities are indicative of nerve root or spinal cord impingement.

Laboratory findings may include anemia, elevated ESR, abnormal urinalysis, increased alkaline phosphatase and, in metastatic prostate cancer, increased prostatic acid phosphatase. Histologic features of biopsy specimens may suggest the identity of the primary tumor, but some lesions are too undifferentiated for identification.

Radiographic abnormalities depend on the character of the underlying malignancy. Kidney and thyroid metastases are typically osteolytic while colon lesions are osteoblastic. Mixed lytic and blastic lesions are noted with breast, lung, prostate or bladder tumors (Fig. 3.32). Plain radiographs may not show any abnormalities until 30–50% of bone calcium is lost[106]. Bone scans are positive in over 85% of patients with metastases. MRI is able to show tumor in the spinal cord, extraosseous extension and bone marrow replacement, while CT is more helpful for detecting cortical bone involvement and bone mineralization[107].

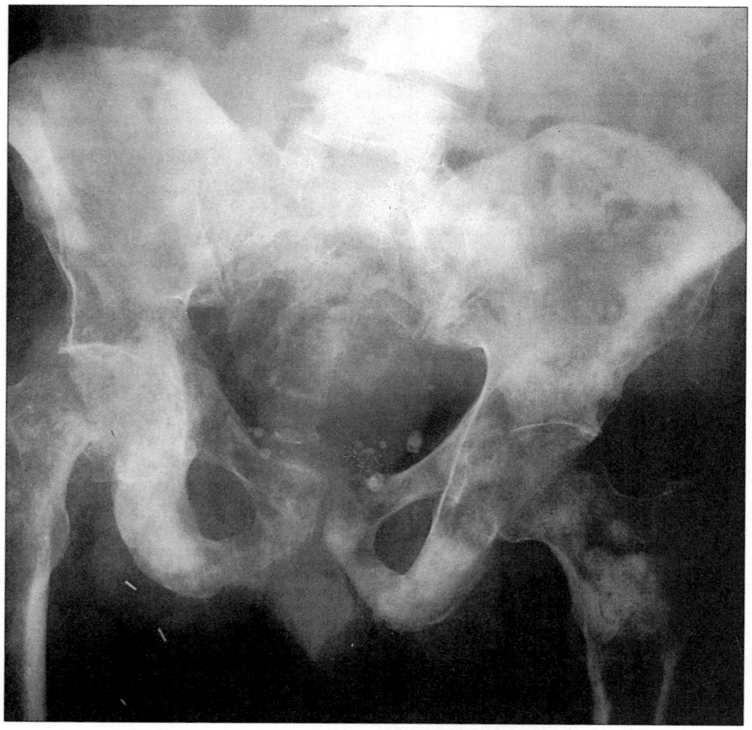

Fig. 3.32 Metastatic prostate cancer. Plain radiograph demonstrating osteoblastic lesions replacing lower lumbar vertebral bodies and most of the bony pelvis.

Neoplastic lesions may also occur inside the spinal canal. These intraspinal neoplasms may be extradural, between bone and the outermost covering of the spinal cord (the dura); intradural–extramedullary, between the dura and the spinal cord; and intramedullary, in the spinal cord proper. Extradural tumors are most commonly metastatic in origin. Intradural–extramedullary tumors are primarily meningiomas, neurofibromas or lipomas. Intramedullary tumors are ependymomas or gliomas. The neurologic abnormalities associated with these unusual neoplasms are dependent on their location in the spinal cord and cauda equina. MRI, by its ability to define the exact location, size and character of the lesions, has revolutionized the visualization of intraspinal lesions[59].

Treatment of metastatic disease of the spine is directed towards pain palliation. A cure is rarely possible since most metastatic lesions are rarely solitary. Radiotherapy is useful to control spinal pain. Decompressive laminectomy is recommended for patients who have recently developed neurologic dysfunction.

Morning stiffness

Morning stiffness of the lumbosacral spine is a frequent symptom in patients with inflammatory arthropathies that affect the axial skeleton (Fig. 3.33). While morning stiffness of mechanical origin may last an hour or less, stiffness associated with the spondyloarthropathies typically

RHEUMATOLOGIC DISORDERS AFFECTING THE LUMBOSACRAL SPINE

- Spondyloarthropathies
  - Ankylosing spondylitis
  - Reiter's syndrome
  - Psoriatic arthritis
  - Enteropathic arthritis

- Behçet's syndrome
- Familial Mediterranean fever
- Whipple's disease
- Diffuse idiopathic skeletal hyperostosis

Fig. 3.33 Rheumatic disease causing pain in the lumbosacral spine.

lasts for hours. The spondyloarthropathies include a group of arthritides that inflame the sacroiliac joints and the axial skeleton. Patients with a spondyloarthropathy may have unilateral or bilateral sacroiliac pain. Patients with ankylosing spondylitis or enteropathic spondylitis have sacroiliitis initially and subsequently develop spondylitis. On rare occasions, patients have pain that is primarily in the lumbar spine and spares the sacroiliac joints (Reiter's syndrome, psoriatic spondylitis). The spondyloarthropathy group of patients have great difficulty getting out of bed in the morning because of stiffness. They may also awaken during the night because of back pain.

Spondyloarthropathies are systemic illnesses that affect nonosseous organs. In these conditions, the extra-articular manifestations of the disease help characterize the specific form of arthritis causing the patient's low back pain. Iritis is associated with ankylosing spondylitis. Conjunctivitis, urethritis, keratoderma blennorrhagicum and circinate balanitis are seen in patients with Reiter's syndrome. Psoriatic skin and nail changes are noted in patients with psoriatic spondylitis. Patients with inflammatory bowel disease are also at risk of developing arthritis that affects the appendicular and axial skeleton joints.

Physical examination of the musculoskeletal system may demonstrate decreased mobility in the axial skeleton (i.e. Schober test, chest expansion). The general physical examination may discover physical findings unsuspected by the patient that help diagnose the specific spondyloarthropathy (oral ulcers, psoriatic skin lesions).

Laboratory tests may show a mild anemia and elevated ESR. Histocompatibility testing for the HLA-B27 haplotype is confirmatory but not diagnostic. Approximately, 8% of the Caucasian population is HLA-B27 positive but is unaffected by a spondyloarthropathy.

Plain radiographs of the sacroiliac joints represent the initial investigation of choice in patients suspected of having an inflammatory arthropathy of the axial skeleton (Fig. 3.34). Thoracolumbar radiographs are less helpful initially since squaring of the vertebral bodies and syndesmophytes rarely occur in the absence of sacroiliitis. Sacroiliac radiographs may show joint erosions in the lower third of the joints. Lumbar radiographs may show loss of lumbar lordosis and squaring of the vertebral bodies (Fig. 3.35). If plain radiographs are normal, tilting the radiography tube by 30° results in an image taken with the sacroiliac joint in one plane (Ferguson view). This view is helpful in detecting early changes of sacroiliitis. Bone scintigraphy can detect increased uptake in the sacroiliac joints but false positive results frequently occur. CT scan is the most sensitive test and may show early involvement of the sacroiliac joint when plain radiographs are normal or equivocal[108].

Patients with spondyloarthropathy are treated with a combination of NSAIDs and physical therapy. Additional therapies may be used to control the underlying illness that has caused the arthritis (topical preparations – psoriasis, corticosteroids – bowel disease).

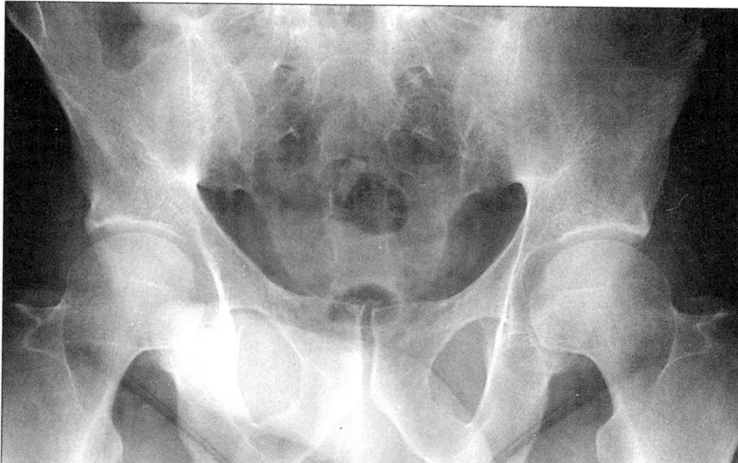

Fig. 3.34 Ankylosing spondylitis. Plain radiograph of the pelvis demonstrating bilateral sacroiliitis with fusion of the sacroiliac joints

Acute localized bone pain

Another group of patients with medical low back pain may present with acute onset of pain in the midline of the back. Pain localized to the midline is frequently associated with disorders that affect osseous structures of the lumbar spine. Acute localized bone pain is usually caused by a fracture or expansion of bone. Any systemic process that increases mineral loss from bone, causes bone necrosis or replaces bone cells with inflammatory or neoplastic cells will weaken vertebral bone to the point where fracture may occur spontaneously or with minimal trauma (Fig. 3.36). Patients with acute fractures experience sudden onset of pain localized to the affected bone. Bone pain may be the initial manifestation of disease or may occur in the setting of associated symptoms. A medical history, including the review of systems, may elicit responses that suggest the underlying cause of the patient's back pain (kidney stones – hyperparathyroidism, chronic cough – sarcoidosis).

Physical examination shows localized tenderness with palpation of the affected areas of the spine. Muscle spasm may surround the area of bony tenderness.

Laboratory evaluation of patients with acute localized bone pain may be quite extensive. Therefore, screening tests should suit the most likely causes of the patient's symptoms. Anemia or an increased ESR should raise the suspicion of an inflammatory process. Serum chemistries may detect abnormalities of calcium metabolism associated with vitamin D

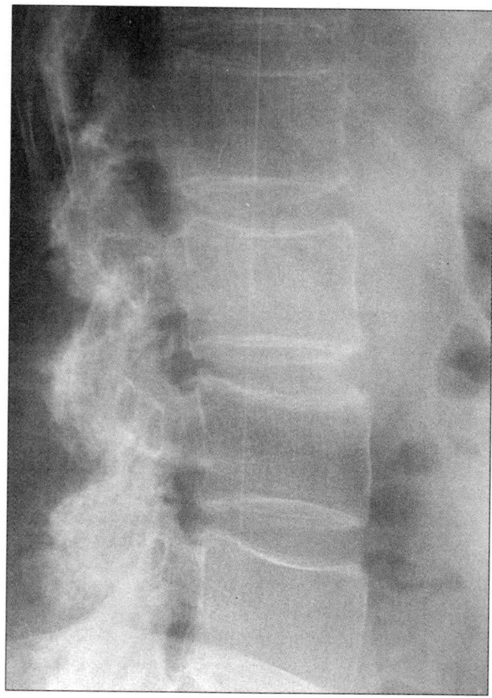

Fig. 3.35 Ankylosing spondylitis. Lateral view of lumbar spine demonstrates squaring of vertebral bodies, thin syndesmophytes, disc calcification and diffuse osteopenia.

ENDOCRINOLOGIC, HEMATOLOGIC AND MISCELLANEOUS DISORDERS AFFECTING THE LUMBOSACRAL SPINE

Endocrinologic/Metabolic
- Osteoporosis
- Osteomalacia
- Hyperparathyroidism

Hematologic
- Hemoglobinopathy
- Myelofibrosis
- Mastocytosis

Miscellaneous
- Paget's disease
- Subacute endocarditis
- Sarcoidosis
- Retroperitoneal fibrosis

Fig. 3.36 Endocrinologic, hematologic and neoplastic disorders that cause acute localized bone pain.

deficiency (osteomalacia) or elevated parathormone level (hyperparathyroidism). Elevations in alkaline phosphatase may suggest increased bone activity associated with neoplasms or Paget's disease.

Radiographic evaluation concentrates on the tender area noted with physical examination. Plain radiographs may show osteopenia if greater than 30–50% of the bone calcium has been lost (Fig. 3.37). Areas of sclerosis related to healed fractures or Paget's disease may be identified (Fig. 3.38). Microfractures cause significant pain and may not be detected with plain films. Bone scintigraphy is useful in this context for detection of increased bone activity associated with fractures. CT scans may identify the location of a fracture or an area of bone that has been replaced by inflammatory tissue.

Therapy for patients with acute localized bone pain must be tailored to the specific disease process causing their illness.

Visceral pain

Disorders of the vascular, genitourinary and gastrointestinal systems can cause stimulation of sensory nerves that results in the perception of pain both in the damaged area and in superficial tissues supplied by the same segments of the spinal cord (Fig. 3.39). Visceral sensory input travels to the brain in the same pathways as somatic sensory input. Sensory stimulation may result in pain felt only in somatic locations, or may stimulate anterior horn cells to produce muscular contractions. True visceral pain is felt at the site of primary stimulation and is dull, aching, diffuse and deep. Referred pain to the lumbosacral spine is sharp, well localized and may be associated with hyperalgesia.

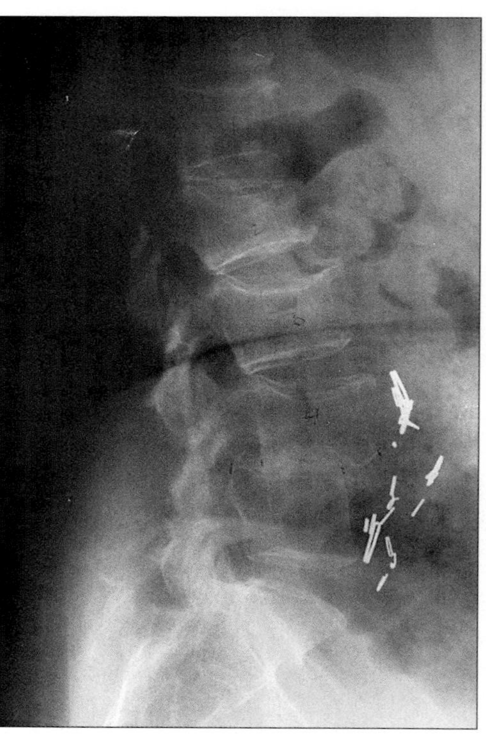

Fig. 3.37 Osteoporosis. Plain radiograph, lateral view, demonstrating diffuse osteopenia and multiple compression fractures.

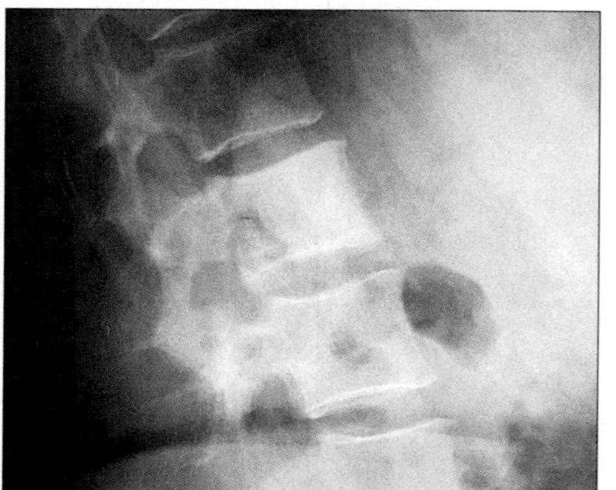

Fig. 3.38 Paget's disease. Plain radiograph demonstrating osteosclerotic alterations of bony trabeculae in L2 vertebral body. The body is slightly increased in size. This patient had elevation of serum alkaline phosphatase.

The duration and sequence of visceral pain follows the periodicity of the involved organ. Colicky pain occurs in peristaltic waves and is associated with a hollow viscus, such as the ureter, uterus, gall bladder, or colon. Throbbing pain is associated with vascular structures.

Back pain is rarely the only symptom of visceral disease. Changes in genitourinary or gastrointestinal function may be clues to the potential source of the patient's low back pain. Patients with viscerogenic pain get little relief from bed rest. Many patients prefer to move in order to find a comfortable position.

Vascular lesions cause dull, steady abdominal pain that is unrelated to activity. Back pain is usually associated with epigastric discomfort and may radiate to the hips or thighs if retroperitoneal structures are irritated. Rupture or acute expansion of the aneurysm is associated with tearing pain and circulatory collapse.

Back pain from genitourinary disorders may arise from the kidney, ureter, bladder or genital organs. Kidney pain is felt in the costovertebral angle. The pain is due to acute distension of the capsule of the kidney and is constant. Ureteral pain from nephrolithiasis may cause dull flank pain with chronic distention or colic if obstruction occurs at the ureteropelvic junction. Stones in the ureter or bladder may cause pain in the testicle or vulva. Patients with bladder infections may develop diffuse low back pain centered near the sacrum. Pain from genital organs may occur locally or in a referred pattern.

Back pain that recurs on a regular basis associated with eating or with alcohol intake is suggestive of a gastrointestinal source. Pain may be related to pancreatitis, peptic ulcer disease or colon or rectal disorders. Examination of the abdomen may be able to identify the maximum source of pain. Laboratory tests may be able to document the presence of pancreatic inflammation (elevated amylase). Endoscopic evaluation of the upper tract or colon may identify the presence of an ulcer or mass respectively.

Patients who do not have constitutional symptoms should be asked specifically about muscle pain and stiffness. Patients aged over 50 years may have proximal stiffness around the hips and shoulders. These patients may present with low back pain as well. Polymyalgia rheumatica must be considered in these older individuals. In younger individuals with more localized areas of pain, fibromyalgia may be the cause of low back pain[109]. Tender points are found in characteristic locations throughout the musculoskeletal system. Some patients may not even be aware of the tender points until they are pressed by the examiner.

The diagnosis of these disorders is a clinical one. Polymyalgia rheumatica is associated with an elevated ESR. Fibromyalgia has a normal ESR. The therapy for these illnesses is very different. Polymyalgia is treated with low-dose corticosteroids (prednisone, 10–15mg/day). Fibromyalgia is treated with mild aerobic exercise, and moderate doses of tricyclic antidepressants.

Some patients will remain undiagnosed. A surreptitious illness may be present but has not progressed to the point of detectability. These patients need to be watched carefully for the development of additional symptoms and signs while they continue to receive therapy for their low back pain. A repeat ESR is a cost-effective method to identify those patients who develop an inflammatory process.

VISCEROGENIC PAIN REFERRED TO THE LUMBOSACRAL SPINE
Vascular
Expanding aortic aneurysm
Genitourinary
Endometriosis
Tubal pregnancy
Kidney stone
Prostatitis
Gastrointestinal
Pancreatitis
Peptic ulcers
Colonic cancer

Fig. 3.39 Viscerogenic disorders that cause referred pain to low back.

If the medical evaluation remains unrevealing, the patient should be evaluated for any psychosocial difficulties. Drug habituation, depression, alcoholism and hysteria may be associated with low back pain. These patients will benefit from therapy directed at controlling their addiction or psychiatric difficulties.

Those patients who do not show any evidence of systemic medical illness or psychiatric difficulties should be educated about their back problem individually by the physician or in a back school. Back school reviews proper and efficient use of the body in work and recreation. Patients are given methods for dealing with the stresses of chronic pain. Many individuals are able to be more functional once they realize that their pain is not related to an acute illness. These individuals concentrate on maximizing their physical function in their daily activities as opposed to concentrating on the presence of pain.

LEG PAIN BELOW THE KNEE (SCIATICA)

Other patients who may continue to experience musculoskeletal pain despite a 4–6 week course of conservative management are those with sciatica. Further diagnostic tests are indicated to document the anatomic abnormalities associated with the patient's symptoms (Figs 3.40 & 3.41). Depending on the circumstances, the patient should undergo MRI or CT evaluation. Once the abnormality is identified (herniated disc, spinal stenosis) and medical disorders have been ruled out as possible causes of the patient's pain, additional therapy in the form of epidural corticosteroid injections may be given[110]. Long-acting corticosteroid is injected into the epidural space close to the location of nerve root compression. The procedure can be done in the outpatient setting. Although well-designed controlled studies are needed to prove the efficacy of this therapy, over 90% of patients with sciatica have described improvement in rest and walking pain over a 1-month period[111]. The maximum benefit is noted after 4 weeks. The injection may be given as a series of three over a 3 to 6 week period.

If epidural steroids are effective in alleviating the patient's leg pain, the patient should be encouraged to increase physical activity, although limiting activities that increase intradiscal pressure, such as heavy lifting or sitting for long periods of time. Patients with a disc herniation should be on restricted work for a 3-month period before resuming more typical physical activities.

If the epidural corticosteroid therapy has not been effective and the patient is considering surgical intervention, the individual must be re-evaluated for the persistence of a neurologic deficit and a positive tension sign. Electrodiagnostic tests may be obtained to confirm the presence of a radiculopathy and its level in the spinal cord. Some surgeons obtain a metrizamide myelogram before contemplating surgery, while others rely on the anatomic changes demonstrated by MRI (Figs 3.42 & 3.43).

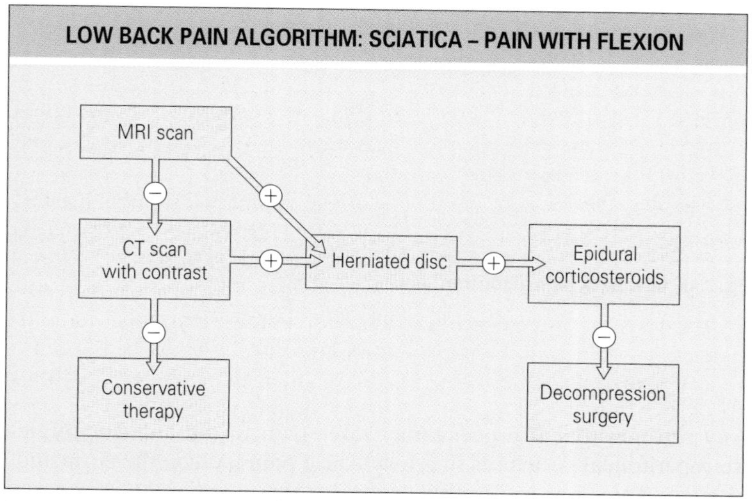

LOW BACK PAIN ALGORITHM: SCIATICA – PAIN WITH FLEXION

MRI scan
CT scan with contrast
Herniated disc
Epidural corticosteroids
Conservative therapy
Decompression surgery

Fig. 3.40 Low back pain algorithm. Sciatica – herniated disc.

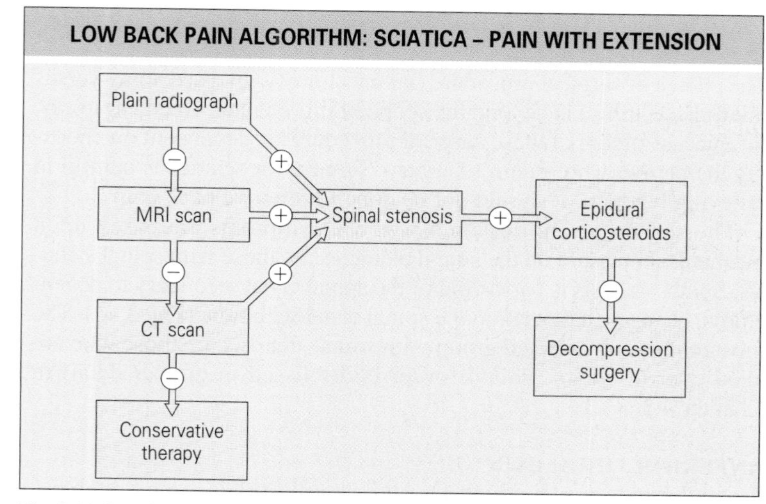

Fig. 3.41 Low back pain algorithm. Sciatica – spinal stenosis.

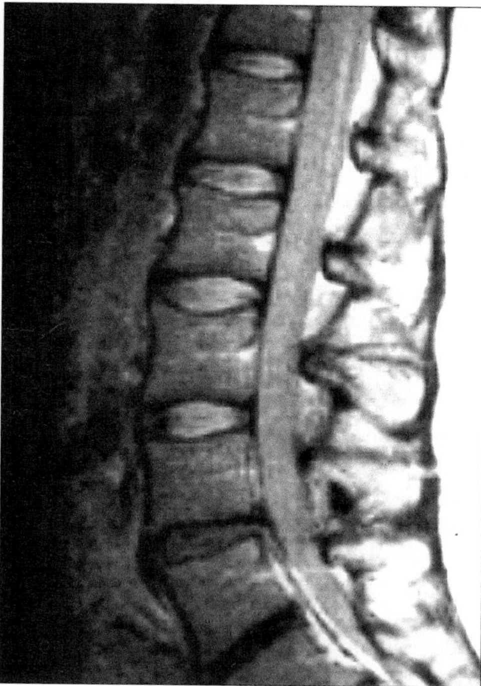

Fig. 3.42 Herniated intervertebral lumbar disc. Sagittal MRI demonstrates a herniated disc with caudal migration of the disc at the L4–L5 interspace.

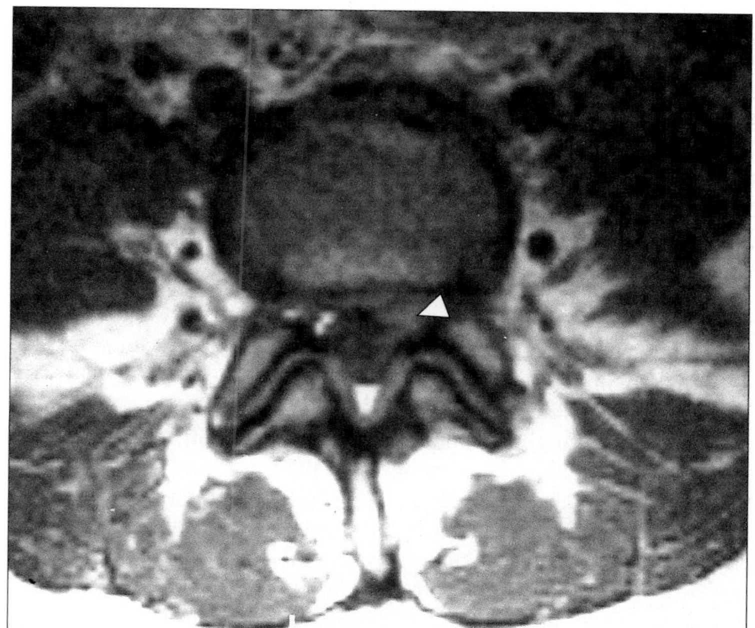

Fig. 3.43 Herniated intervertebral lumbar disc. Axial MRI demonstrates a herniated disc (arrow) blocking the left neural foramen.

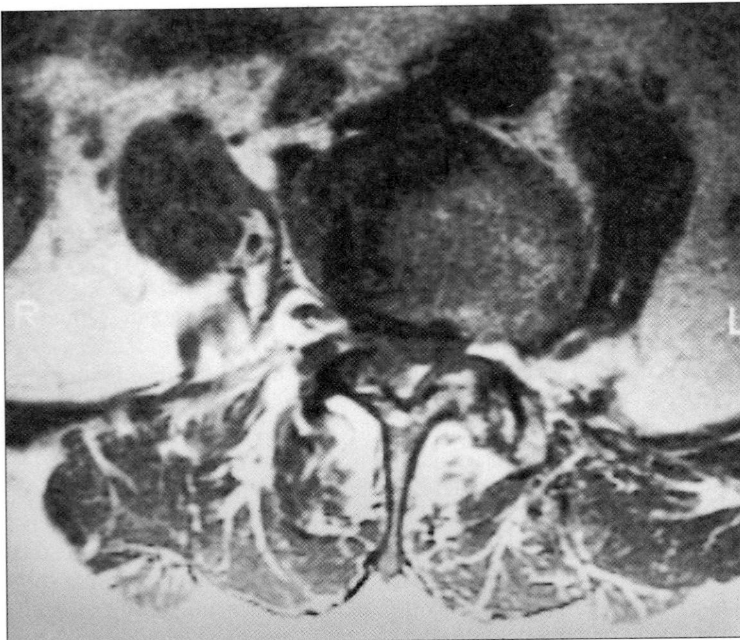

Fig. 3.44 Spinal stenosis. MRI, axial view, of the L3–L4 disc level demonstrating osteophytic overgrowth, disc degeneration and ligamentous hypertrophy. The cauda equina is compressed in the central area of the canal.

The choice of surgical procedure (laminectomy with discectomy versus microdiscectomy) is beyond the scope of this chapter. Needless to say, the success of any of these surgical procedures is dependent on choosing the patient who requires surgery. Surgery for sciatica is helpful in relieving leg pain. It should not be done to improve back pain.

The second group of patients whose symptoms are based upon mechanical pressure on the neural elements are those with spinal stenosis. Spinal stenosis is narrowing of the spinal canal secondary to degenerative changes that occur in the spinal canal with time (Fig. 3.44). The most commonly affected group with spinal stenosis are those who are aged over 60 years. This disorder is discussed in greater detail in Chapter 4.5.

ANTERIOR THIGH PAIN

A small group of individuals develop anterior thigh pain in conjunction with back pain. Such pain has a number of possible sources (Fig. 3.45). Pain in the anterior thigh is related either to hip disease, a hernia, kidney disorders, femoral neuropathy or retroperitoneal process (anterior). Hip arthritis causes pain that is primarily in the groin. However, the peripheral nerves that supply the hip joint also innervate muscles in the low back and anterior thigh. Hip disease may present as lateral low back and anterior thigh pain. A careful physical examination, including range of motion of the hips, will identify those individuals with decreased hip motion. The patient's pain should be recreated by putting tension on the hip joint. Plain films of the hips should document the presence of joint disease (Fig. 3.46).

An inguinal hernia can cause anterior thigh pain. Occasionally, the pain radiates into the lateral low back. Physical examination will identify patients with direct and indirect hernias.

Patients with kidney disease may present with anterior thigh pain. Nephrolithiasis will cause pain that radiates from the back into the genitalia or anterior thigh. A simple urinalysis may identify hematuria or pyuria suggesting a renal source for the pain. An intravenous pyelogram may be obtained to evaluate more fully the urinary system.

Disorders of the femoral nerve may be associated with anterior thigh pain. The anterior femoral cutaneous nerve (L2, L3) supplies the anterior thigh. Peripheral neuropathies may affect the femoral nerve. Diabetes is the most frequent cause of peripheral neuropathy. Evaluation for diabetes is appropriate for evaluating a patient with femoral neuropathy.

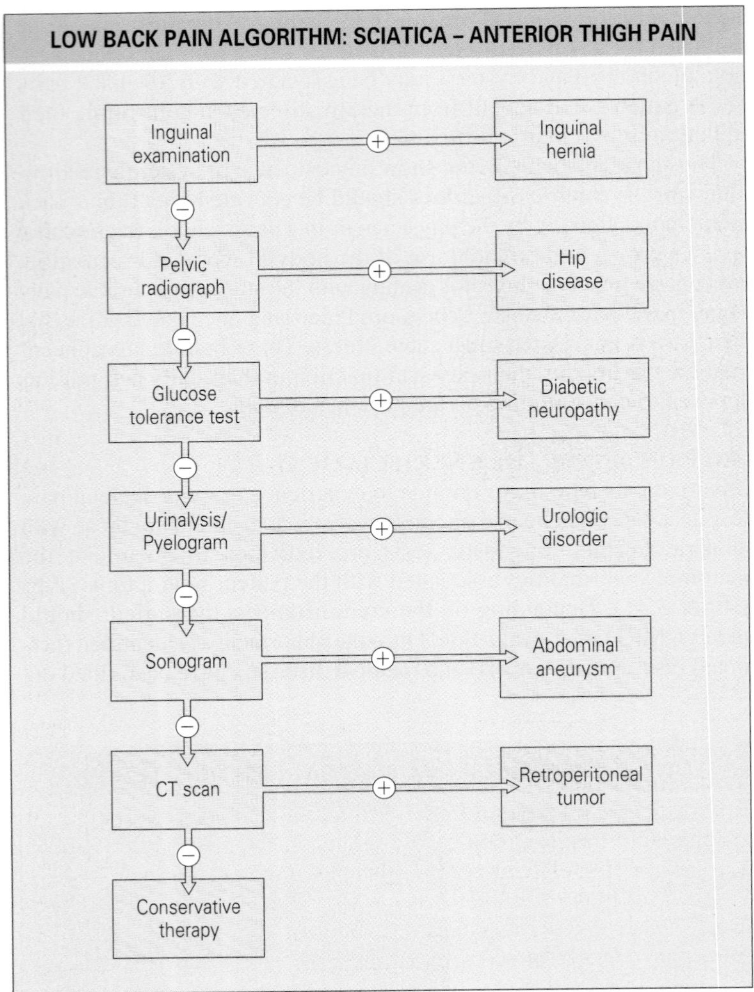

Fig. 3.45 Low back pain algorithm. Anterior thigh pain.

Any retroperitoneal process may refer pain to the anterior thigh. Retroperitoneal structures that may cause pain include the aorta and kidneys. Tumor or infiltrative processes that involve the retroperitoneum may also cause back and anterior thigh pain. If a retroperitoneal process is suspected, CT evaluation is appropriate to determine the status of the aorta, kidney and lymph nodes.

POSTERIOR THIGH PAIN

The fourth group of patients will complain of pain that radiates from the low back into the posterior thigh. These patients may have referred or radicular pain (Fig. 3.47). Patients with referred pain have it on the basis of injury to the bony, ligamentous and muscular components of the lumbar spine. The muscles of the posterior thigh and buttocks have the same embryologic origin as those of the lumbar spine. An injury to these structures in the lumbar spine may be referred to the posterior thigh. These patients may respond to a local injection of corticosteroid and anesthetic into the maximum point of tenderness in the lumbar spine. Patients with referred pain do not improve with surgical intervention.

Patients with lesions compressing the L2 and L3 nerve roots may experience pain on the medial and lateral portions of the posterior thigh. These areas are supplied with cutaneous nerves that have their origin at the L2 and L3 spinal cord levels. Occasionally, L4 lesions may also cause similar symptoms and signs. MRI evaluation can identify causes of nerve impingement at higher levels of the spinal cord. Electrophysiologic studies can corroborate the presence of a radiculopathy. Surgical intervention should only be contemplated when the clinical and laboratory data document a radiculopathy and conservative therapy has been ineffective.

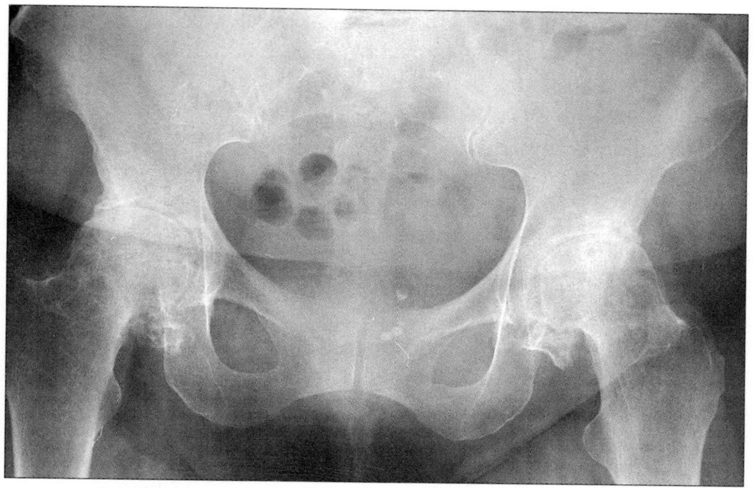

Fig. 3.46 Hip arthritis. Plain radiograph of pelvis demonstrating severe osteoarthritis of both hips. The patient had presented with back and knee pain. Hip examination revealed no motion of the joint. Back pain reduced with joint replacement.

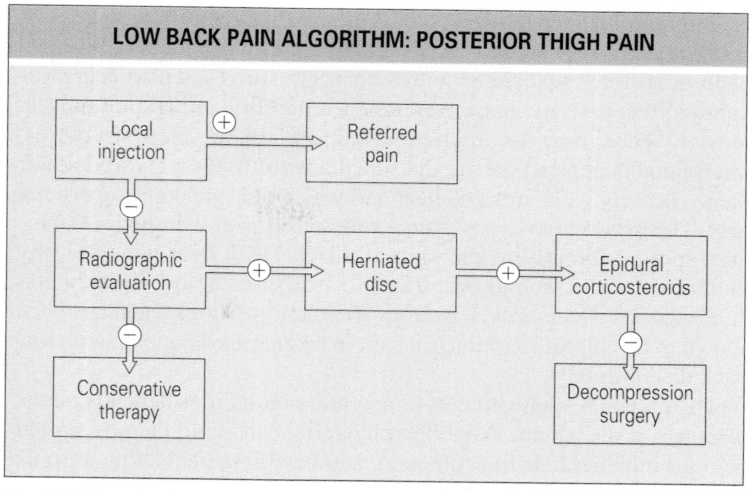

LOW BACK PAIN ALGORITHM: POSTERIOR THIGH PAIN

Local injection (+) → Referred pain

Local injection (−) → Radiographic evaluation

Radiographic evaluation (+) → Herniated disc (+) → Epidural corticosteroids (−) → Decompression surgery

Radiographic evaluation (−) → Conservative therapy

Fig. 3.47 Low back pain algorithm. Posterior thigh pain.

MANAGEMENT

No single form of therapy is effective for all forms of back pain. Patients with systemic causes for back pain must be treated with specific therapies effective for their underlying disease. Antibiotics are effective for osteomyelitis while chemotherapeutic agents are effective in slowing the growth of malignant plasma cells in multiple myeloma.

The vast majority of patients have low back pain on a mechanical basis. In most circumstances, the mechanical disorder causing the symptoms cannot be identified. Despite the inability to identify the specific source of the patient's pain, the physician is faced with treating the patient to decrease their symptoms. Ideally, therapy would decrease symptoms without any toxicities. This circumstance does not exist, and even conservative therapy has its potential risks. The risks associated with NSAIDs, muscle relaxants and injection therapy must be compared to the possibilities of infection, paralysis and death associated with surgical intervention. It is the role of the physician to maximize medical therapy so that surgical intervention is considered in the appropriate clinical setting. Only 1–2% of patients with low back pain will undergo lumbar spine surgery[37].

A panel of spine experts recently reviewed the medical literature concerning the efficacy of the components of therapy for low back pain[37]. In general, most components of back pain therapy were found to be without adequate studies demonstrating efficacy. The therapeutic recommendations of the panel include the following:

- Bed rest > 4 days is not helpful and may debilitate the patient. During the acute phase patients are encouraged to ambulate as tolerated.
- Relief of pain may be accomplished most safely with nonprescription analgesics or nonsteroidal medication. Spinal manipulation is helpful during the first 4 weeks in patients without radiculopathy.
- Low-stress aerobic acitivites can be safely started in the first 2 weeks of symptoms. Trunk muscle exercises should be delayed at least 2 weeks.
- Patients should be encouraged to return to usual activities, both vocational and recreational, as soon as possible.

The guidelines take into account the natural history of low back pain which is associated with symptom improvement in the vast majority of patients within 2 months of the onset of symptoms. Patients who have persistent or progressive pain or who have radicular pain may require additional interventions.

CONTROLLED PHYSICAL ACTIVITY

Components of a conservative management program for low back pain patients include patient education, 'controlled physical' activity, bed rest, exercise and drug therapy in the form of NSAIDs and muscle relaxants. Of all the therapies, controlled physical activity is utilized most frequently. Many patients spontaneously take to bed to assume a supine position when they develop mechanical back pain. The amount of scientific data to support this form of therapy is small[112,113]. Despite the lack of data, bed rest remains a mainstay of therapy.

The biomechanical rationale for bed rest is that intradiscal pressures are lower in the supine position. However, rolling over in bed may result in increased intradiscal pressure. In addition, the number of patients with herniated discs compared to muscle strain is small. The exact mechanism that causes improvement in pain associated with muscle and ligament injury is unknown.

Bed rest is not benign if it is continued for too long a duration. Muscles become deconditioned. Cardiovascular function diminishes. Individuals lose time from work and, with continuing bed rest, start to view themselves as ill[88].

Busy patients rarely stay in bed unless their back pain is severe. Most patients strictly limit their recreational activities and minimize the time lost at their job. A recent study reported the best outcome for low back pain is associated with those individuals who resume normal activity as opposed to extension exercises or bed rest. Resumption of normal activity is to be encouraged to improve the resolution of back pain[114].

PHYSICAL MODALITIES

Physical modalities may be used to diminish symptoms for short periods of time. These counterirritant forms of therapy include ice massage, hot packs, diathermy, ultrasound and transcutaneous electrical stimulation (TENS). These therapies may be applied by the patient themselves or by a therapist.

Patients with acute low back pain may experience analgesia with ice massage or cold packs. Cold temperatures decrease swelling, pain, and muscle spasm during the acute phase of an injury. Cold reduces metabolic activity locally, decreases muscle spindle activity, and slows nerve conduction. A cold pack may be placed in a towel and applied to the painful area of the back if the patient cannot tolerate the stroking of the skin with ice massage. Cold relieves pain and spasm for longer than superficial heat. Patients who experience increased alpha motor neuron discharges with cold application will experience increased muscle spasm and cannot tolerate this form of therapy. Patients may experience at least 33% reduction in pain following ice massage[115].

Heat is another form of counterirritant therapy that has utility in the treatment of low back pain patients. Heat should not be used in patients with back pain secondary to trauma. Heat causes vasodilatation and increased blood flow. This can cause increased damage to an area recently traumatized. However, heat increases the elastic properties of connective tissues and may be of particular utility in patients who complain of stiffness associated with their back pain. Heat also decreases gamma fiber activity, muscle spindle excitability and resting muscle tension. Heat may be applied to superficial or deep structures. Superficial heat penetrates to the subcutaneous tissues. Hydrocollator packs, heating pads, infrared heat and whirlpools generate superficial heat. The maximal safe exposure for these forms of therapy is 30 minutes applied directly to the skin at 45°C. Deep heat generated by diathermy or ultrasound penetrates to structures below the subcutaneous tissues. Deep heat is given in 20 minute sessions. Heat has been shown to be helpful for reducing pain in hospitalized patients with low back discomfort[116].

The practical application of temperature modalities depends on the response of the patient. Although physiologically cold therapy should be used in patients with acute pain, and heat in patients with chronic pain, these modalities may have the opposite effect. The recommendation should be cold for acute pain and heat for chronic pain initially. If the patient does not respond, or has an exacerbation of symptoms, the opposite temperature modality should be tried.

TENS therapy is based upon the gate control theory of pain that suggests that counterstimulation of the sensory system will modify pain perception in the cerebral cortex. TENS preferentially stimulates low-threshold alpha-A fibers. The stimulation of these fibers is thought to inhibit the nociceptive impulses of the small C unmyelinated and alpha-D fibers. The effect of TENS on pain is not mediated through opiate receptors. The electrical stimulation is produced by an electrical pulse generator which delivers current that can be varied in form, intensity and frequency to superficial electrodes. The optimal placement of the electrodes is proximal to the painful area. The average time for the onset of analgesia is approximately 20 minutes. Therapy should be given for at least 30 minutes. The pain relief from TENS may be present only during stimulation or may last for a considerable period of time. TENS is not indicated for patients with acute low back pain[37]. TENS has been shown to be superior to massage or equivalent to cold therapy[117]. However, a large, randomized, placebo-controlled study found no benefit of TENS for chronic low back pain[118]. The role of TENS in the therapy of low back pain is in question and should not be considered usual therapy for patients with low back pain.

DRUG THERAPY

A variety of drugs is widely used in the therapy of patients with acute and chronic low back pain. The types of medications that have been utilized have included analgesics, NSAIDs, muscle relaxants and antidepressants. Medications should be used for a limited period and monitored constantly. Additional analgesics or nonsteroidal medications should be tried if the initial drugs are ineffective. The potential toxicities of the agents must also be considered when choosing an agent for a patient.

Analgesics

Non-narcotic (acetaminophen) and narcotic (codeine, oxycodone, meperidine) analgesics have been utilized for low back pain. Patients who are intolerant of NSAIDs may benefit from acetaminophen, in doses of 500–650mg every 4 hours. A slow-release form of the drug may allow for a more prolonged analgesic effect in back pain patients. Acetaminophen is less effective than aspirin as an analgesic, but does not cause gastrointestinal bleeding, a frequently encountered toxicity of aspirin. The drug has a synergistic effect with the NSAIDs and may be used in combination to increase analgesia without increasing toxicity.

Narcotic analgesia should be reserved for patients with severe pain associated with a herniated disc. Codeine in doses of 30–60mg every 4–6 hours, in combination with an NSAID or acetaminophen, is an effective analgesic. This form of therapy may be used in an outpatient setting along with controlled physical activity and temperature modalities. However, codeine does have the potential to cause constipation that may exacerbate low back pain. Patients should be told to increase fiber in their diets and consume increased amounts of liquids to decrease the potential for this side effect. Stronger narcotic analgesia should be reserved for hospitalized patients. The continuation of narcotic analgesics in the outpatient setting should be discouraged. Addiction and tolerance frequently result from the continued use of narcotics. In addition, the efficacy of the narcotic analgesics diminishes over time. Narcotic analgesics have no role in chronic low back pain therapy.

NSAIDs

NSAIDs have analgesic properties in low doses and anti-inflammatory properties at higher doses. Different NSAIDs have greater potentials as analgesics or as anti-inflammatory agents. Some NSAIDs combine both characteristics. The onset of action of the agents is also an important characteristic. In acute back pain, a rapid onset of action is important to control symptoms quickly. In chronic pain, the onset of action is not as important as efficacy and safety over extended periods of time.

NSAIDs have been studied in patients with acute and chronic back pain. Naproxen, piroxicam and diflunisal have been reported to be more effective than placebo in relieving low back pain[119,120]. From a practical viewpoint, NSAIDs as a class of agents are effective in low back pain therapy. The problem that remains is that there is no specific selection criteria for the choice of a single agent for a specific patient with pain. The patient is given an NSAID with characteristics that fit the patient's symptoms and complicating medical problems (renal failure, gastric ulcer). The drug is given for a period of 2–4 weeks as a therapeutic trial, and is continued if efficacious and well tolerated. The drug is changed if the initial agent is ineffective or associated with serious toxicity. In that circumstance, an NSAID from a different chemical group is selected with the hope that it will be efficacious. The process is continued until an effective NSAID is identified.

The NSAID is continued while the patient increases physical activity and regains confidence. It is discontinued once the individual resumes their normal daily activities in work and recreation. Patients with chronic low back pain may require NSAIDs for extended periods of time. NSAIDs are not used so much to relieve pain as to support the patient's efforts to be physically active. Patients with chronic pain may not achieve a total resolution of pain, but should be encouraged to engage in as much physical activity as can be tolerated. NSAIDs help support the patient in this endeavor.

Muscle relaxants

Muscle relaxants are a group of drugs used to decrease muscle contraction present in patients with low back pain. The use of muscle relaxants in low back pain remains controversial[121]. The muscle relaxants used for low back pain patients work centrally to affect the activity of muscle stretch reflexes. Despite the skepticism concerning the pathophysiology of muscle spasm and the mechanism of action of these drugs, the muscle relaxants have been found to be effective for muscle contraction in the lumbar spine in scientific studies. Drugs, including cyclobenzaprine, carisoprodol, and chlorzoxazone, have been shown to be more effective than placebo in treating patients with muscle spasm[122]. Of interest is the lack of efficacy of diazepam, a benzodiazepine, as a muscle relaxant for low back pain. In appropriately selected patients with acute muscle spasm, the combination of an NSAID and a muscle relaxant is more effective than the same NSAID alone[123]. The major toxicity of muscle relaxants is drowsiness. Also noted are headache, dizziness and dry mouth. Muscle relaxants should be used only during the time the spasm is palpable. Once the spasm has subsided, the drug should be discontinued.

Antidepressants

Tricyclic antidepressants have been used for the treatment of chronic pain for patients with or without depression. A number of mechanisms have been suggested to explain the pain relief associated with the tricyclics. One theory suggests that tricyclic antidepressants increase serotonin levels in the pain inhibitory pathway in the central nervous system. Double blind studies have documented the role of tricyclics for relieving chronic pain. Low doses in the range of 10mg to 25mg may be needed to control symptoms[124]. Rare patients may require up to 150mg per day. The drug does not work immediately and may need to be continued for a number of weeks before decreased symptoms are noted. Newer antidepressants (sertraline, fluoxetine) are not as effective as tricyclics for chronic pain relief.

Injection therapy

Local or regional anesthesia given by injection is part of the therapeutic regimen for some patients with low back pain. By blocking peripheral pain input, the local area of pain can be eased as well as areas of referred pain and increased muscle tension. Patients who describe localized areas of muscle or ligamentous tenderness are candidates for local anesthetic therapy. The area injected may be an area of local trauma or a myofascial trigger point[125]. Trigger points are areas of the muscle that are painful at rest, prevent full lengthening of the muscle, weaken the muscle, refer pain in the muscle group on direct palpation and cause a local contraction when palpated. Trigger points may be found in the paraspinous muscles, the quadratus lumborum and the gluteal muscles. The point of maximum tenderness is injected with a combination of 1% lidocaine (lignocaine) and a depository form of corticosteroid[126]. A study by Garvey *et al.* suggests that needling the area with or without medication may have a beneficial effect[127]. Injections may be given on a weekly basis for 3–4 additional weeks. Controlled studies designed to evaluate the efficacy of this treatment modality have yet to be done.

Epidural corticosteroid injections are used for patients with nerve root compression who do not respond to conservative management. Corticosteroids are injected directly into the epidural space with the intention of increasing the anti-inflammtory effect in comparison to oral corticosteroids. The injections may be given on an outpatient basis. The course of therapy includes three injections given at variable intervals (days to weeks). The efficacy of these injections for the therapy of herniated discs and spinal stenosis with radiculopathy has been questioned. Epidural injections have been found to be effective in some patients[128]. Other studies have documented no improvement compared to a placebo group. Until larger studies are done, the utility of epidural corticosteroids is undetermined. In patients who have radiculopathy secondary to compression and are poor candidates for surgical intervention, epidural corticosteroids may be considered.

Patients who have apophyseal joint disease may develop pain on a referred basis that simulates radicular pain. In this circumstance, patients have received injections of anesthetic and corticosteroid to decrease pain[129]. The injections are done under fluoroscopic control to document the appropriate placement of the needle into the facet joint. Facets both at and above the level of the involved joint must be blocked in order to obtain adequate analgesia since each facet joint receives sensory innervation from two spinal levels. Injections are given every 2–4 weeks for three sessions. The efficacy of these injections has been questioned[130]. Even in studies reporting a good response, the mean pain relief is only 30%. No specific historical or physical factors identify those patients with zygapophyseal joint disease who may benefit from injection[131]. With the results of these studies, the use of facet joint blocks must be limited.

Exercise

Physical therapy, particularly in the form of therapeutic exercises, may be particularly helpful in controlling mechanical low back pain[132]. A number of different exercise programs are available for patients with low back pain. These include flexion exercises, extension exercises, stretching regimens and aerobic conditioning. As a generalization, patients with mechanical disorders of the discs prefer extension exercises, while those with posterior component disease prefer flexion exercises. In most circumstances patients eventually receive a combination of both forms of exercise.

A recent study suggests that with an exercise program, patients may feel worse before they feel better[133]. In this study, 2 months were required in patients with chronic low back pain before benefit was noted. The treating physician should find a physical therapist who is interested in taking care of back patients and communicate their concerns about patients to the therapist. The therapist can then try various exercise programs and modify them according to the response of the patient. The time spent in encouraging the patient to participate in exercises and becoming physically fit is well worth the effort.

Exercises may also play a significant role in preventing back pain in asymptomatic individuals. In a comparison with educational strategies, mechanical supports and risk modification, exercises that strengthen back and abdominal muscles were the only intervention associated with decreased frequency and duration of low back pain[134].

DOCTOR–PATIENT RELATIONSHIP

The importance of the interaction of the physician and patient education in the therapy of low back pain patients cannot be overlooked. Educational programs such as back school, where a number of individuals with back pain gather together to discuss ways of improving their situation, have been shown to be an effective way of controlling patients' symptoms. Some schools are directed at groups. Some are organized for individuals with acute or chronic back pain[135]. Back school has been shown to decrease pain and time missed from work compared to placebo interventions[136].

The significance of the doctor–patient relationship has been shown by the studies that have documented the benefit of chiropractic therapy for low back pain[137]. In this study of 215 patients who visited a physician and 242 who visited a chiropractor, overall satisfaction with care was three times greater with the chiropractors than with the physicians. Patients had greater satisfaction with the information imparted by the chiropractors, which included graphic descriptions of the causes of pain and instructions on physical measures to improve back pain. Physicians were perceived as being less concerned about the patient's condition and pain and were less confident about the underlying cause of the patient's discomfort. Chiropractic care is associated with the greatest number of visits per episode and the highest outpatient cost compared to other health care providers[138].

Many factors play a role in the therapy and outcome of patients with low back pain. A positive attitude about diagnosis and treatment play an important role in alleviation of pain. Physicians should not rely on machines alone to diagnose and treat patients with back pain. Communication between physican and patient that includes education about the patient's illness is an important part of back pain therapy.

REFERENCES

1. Kelsey JL, White AA III. Epidemiology and impact of low back pain. Spine. 1980;5:133–42.
2. Frymoyer JW, Pope MH, Costanza MC, Goggin JE, Wilder DG. Epidemiology studies of low back pain. Spine. 1980;5:419–23.
3. Hart LG, Deyo RA, Cherkin DC. Physician office visits for low back pain: Frequency, clinical evaluation, and treatment patterns from a U.S. national survey. Spine. 1995;20:11–19.
4. National Center for Health Statistics: Limitation of activity due to chronic conditions, United States 1969–1970. Vital and Health Statistics Series. 10, No. 80, 1973.
5. Dixon A StJ. Progress and problems in back pain research. Rheumatol Rehabil. 1973;12:165–75.
6. Federspiel CF, Guy D, Kane D, Spengler D. Expenditures for nonspecific back injuries in the workplace. J Occup Med. 1989;31:919–24.
7. Frymoyer JW, Cats-Baril WL. An overview of the incidences and costs of low back pain. Orthop Clin North Am. 1991;22:263–71.
8. Rossignol M, Suissa S, Abenhaim L. Working disability due to occupational back pain: three year follow-up of 2,300 compensated workers in Quebec. J Occup Med. 1988;30:502–5.
9. Rossignol M, Suissa S, Abenhaim L. The evolution of compensated occupational spinal injuries: A three-year follow-up study. Spine. 1992;17:1043–7.
10. Merskey H. The characteristics of persistent pain in psychological illness. J Psychosom Res. 1965;9:291–8.
11. Deyo RA, Bass JE. Lifestyle and low back pain: the influence of smoking and obesity. Spine. 1989;14:501–6.
12. Nachemson A. The lumbar spine: an orthopaedic challenge. Spine. 1976;1:59–71.
13. Hadler NM. Regional back pain. N Engl J Med. 1986;315:1090–2.
14. Borenstein DG, Wiesel SW, Boden SD: Low back pain: medical diagnosis and comprehensive management. 2E. Philadelphia: W.B. Saunders; 1995:181–589
15. Klein RF, Brown W. Pain descriptions in medical patients. J Psychosom Res. 1967;10:367–72.
16. Spengler DM, Freeman CW. Patient selection for lumbar discectomy. Spine. 1979;4:129–34.
17. Blower PW. Neurologic patterns in unilateral sciatica. A prospective study of 100 new cases. Spine. 1981;6:175–9.
18. Fahrni WH. Observation on straight leg raising with special reference to nerve root adhesions. Can J Surg. 1966;9:44–8.
19. Gunn CC, Chir B, Milbrandt WE. Tenderness at motor points: A diagnostic and prognostic aid to low back pain injury. J Bone Joint Surg. 1976;58A:815–25.
20. Vallfors B. Acute, subacute, and chronic low back pain: clinical symptoms, absenteeism, and working environment. Scand J Rehabil Med. 1985;11(suppl):1–98.
21. Waddell G, McCullogh JA, Kummel E, Venner RM. Non-organic physical signs in low back pain. Spine. 1980;5:117–25.
22. McCombe PF, Fairbank JCT, Cockersole BC, Pynsent PB. Reproducibility of physical signs in low back pain. Spine. 1989;14:908–18.
23. Jensen OH. The level-diagnosis of a lower lumbar disc herniation: The value of sensitivity and motor testing. Clin Rheumatol. 1987;6:564–9.
24. Nitta H, Tajima T, Sugiyama H, *et al.* Study on dermatomes by means of selective lumbar spinal nerve block. Spine. 1993;18:1782–6.
25. Spitzer Wo, LeBlanc FE, Dupier M. Scientific approach to the assessment and management of activity-related spinal disorders: a monograph for clinicians. Report of the Quebec Task Force on spinal disorders. Spine. 1987;12:S16–S21.
26. Deyo RA, Rainville J, Kent DL. What can the history and physical examination tell us about low back pain? JAMA. 1992;268:760–5.
27. Witt I, Vestergaard A, Rosenklint A. A comparative analysis of X-ray findings of the lumbar spine in patients with and without lumbar pain. Spine. 1984;9:298–300.
28. Deyo RA, Bigos SJ, Maravilla KR. Diagnostic imaging procedures for the lumbar spine. Ann Intern Med. 1989;111:865–7.
29. Lawrence JS, Bremmer JM, Bier F. Osteo-arthrosis. Prevalence in the population and relationship between symptoms and x-ray changes. Ann Rheum Dis. 1966;25:1–24.
30. Hakelius A, Hindmarsh J. The comparative reliability of preoperative diagnostic methods in lumbar disc surgery. Acta Orthop Scand. 1972;43:234–8.
31. Deyo RA, McNeish LM, Cone RO III. Observer variability in the interpretation of lumbar spine radiographs. Arthritis Rheum. 1985;28:1066–70.
32. Liang M, Komaroff AL. Roentgenograms in primary care patients with acute low back pain. A cost-effective analysis. Arch Intern Med. 1982;142:1108–12.
33. Padley S, Gleeson F, Chisholm R, Baldwin J. Assessment of a single spine radiograph in low back pain. Br J Radiol. 1990;63:535–6.
34. Eisenberg RL, Hedgcock MW, Williams EA, *et al.* Optimum radiographic examination for consideration of compensation awards. II.Cervical and lumbar spines. AJR. 1980;135:1071–4.
35. Gehweiler JA Jr, Daffner RH. Low back pain: the controversy of radiologic evaluation. AJR. 1983;140:109–12.
36. Scavone JG, Latshaw RF, Weidner WA. Anteroposterior and lateral radiographs: an adequate lumbar spine examination. AJR. 1981;136:715–7.
37. Bigos S, Bowyer O, Braen G *et al.* Acute Low Back Problems in Adults. Clinical Practice Guideline No. 14. AHCPR Publication No. 95_0642. Rockville, MD: Agency for Health Care Policy and Research, Public Health Service, US Department of Health and Human Services. December 1994.
38. Tumeh SS, Tohmeh AG. Nuclear medicine techniques in septic arthritis and osteomyelitis. Rheum Dis Clin North Am. 1991;17:559–84.
39. Pomeranz SJ, Pretorius HT, Ramsingh PS. Bone scintigraphy and multimodality imaging in bone neoplasia: strategies for imaging in the new health care climate. Semin Nucl Med. 1994;24:188–207.
40. Modic MT, Feiglin DH, Piraino DW. Vertebral osteomyelitis. Assesment using MR. Radiology. 1985;157:157–66.
41. Adatepe MH, Powell DM, Issacs GH, Nichols K, Cefola R. Hematogenous pyogenic vertebral osteomyelitis. Diagnostic value of radionuclide bone imaging. J Nucl Med. 1986;27:168–85.
42. Rosenthal DI, Mankin HJ, Bauman RA. Musculoskeletal application for computed tomography. Bull Rheum Dis. 1983;33(3):1–4.
43. Golimbu C, Firooznia H, Rafii M. CT of osteomyelitis of the spine. AJR. 1984;142:156–63.
44. Epstein BS, Epstein JA, Jones MD. Lumbar spinal stenosis. Radiol Clin North Am. 1977;15:227–39.
45. Faerber EN, Wolpert SM, Scott RM, Belkin SC, Carter BL. Computed tomography of spinal fractures. J Comput Assist Tomogr. 1979;3:657–61.
46. Wang A, Wesolowski DP, Farak J. Evaluation of posterior spinal structures by computed tomography. Spine: State Art Rev. 1988;2:439–65.
47. Carrera GF, Haughton VM, Syverstein A, Williams AL. Computed tomography of the lumbar facet joints. Radiology. 1980;134:145–8.
48. Beltran J, Noto AM, Chakeres DW, Christofordis AJ. Tumors of the osseous spine: staging with MR imaging versus CT. Radiology. 1987;162:565–9.
49. Herkowitz HN, Wesolowski DP. Percutaneous biopsy of the spine. Indications, techniques, results and complications. Update Spinal Disord. 1980;1:3–9.
50. Wiesel SW, Tsourmas N, Feffer HL, Citrin CM, Patronas N. A study of computer-assisted tomography. I. The incidence of positive CAT scans in an asymptomatic group of patients. Spine. 1984;9:549–51.
51. Baker RA, Hillman BJ, McLennan JE, Strand R, Kaufman S. Sequelae of metrizamide myelography in 200 examinations. AJR. 1978;130:499–502.
52. Weinstein JN. Differential diagnosis and surgical treatment of primary benign and malignant neoplasms. In: Frymoyer JW, ed. The adult spine: principles and practice. Raven Press: New York; 1991:832.
53. Braun IF, Hoffman JC, Davis PC, Landman JA, Tindall GT. Contrast enhancement in CT differentiation between recurrent disc herniation and post-operative scar. AJNR. 1985;6:607–12.
54. Byrd SE, Cohn ML, Biggers SL, Huntington CJ, Locke GE, Charles MF. The radiographic evaluation of symptomatic post-operative lumbar spine patient. Spine. 1985;10:652–61.
55. Hitselberger WE, Witten RM. Abnormal myelograms in asymptomatic patients. J Neurosurg. 1969;28:204–6.
56. Albeck MJ, Hilden J, Kjaer L, *et al.* A controlled comparison of myelography, computed tomography, and magnetic resonance imaging in clinically suspected lumbar disc herniation. Spine. 1995;20:443–8.
57. Erly WK, Carmody RF. MRI of the spine. Crit Rev Diagn Imaging. 1994;35:31377
58. Paushter DM, Modic MT, Masaryk TJ. Magnetic resonance imaging of the spine: applications and limitations. Radiol Clin North Am. 1985;23:551–62.
59. Sze G, Stimac GK, Bartlett C, *et al.* Multicenter study of gadopentetate dimeglumine as an MR contrast agent: evaluation in patients with spinal tumors. AJNR. 1990;11:967–74.
60. Parizel PM, Baleriaux D, Rodesch G, *et al.* Gd-DTPA-enhanced MR imaging of spinal tumors. AJNR. 1989;10:249–58.
61. Lim V, Sobel DF, Zyroff J. Spinal cord pial metastases: MR imaging with gadopentetate dimeglumine. AJNR. 1990;11:975–82.
62. Olson DO, Shields AF, Scheurich CJ, Porter BA, Moss AA. Magnetic resonance imaging of the bone marrow in patients with leukemia, aplastic anemia, and lymphoma. Invest Radiol. 1986;21:540–6.
63. Traill Z, Richards MA, Moore NR. Magnetic resonance imaging of metastatic bone disease. Clin Orthop. 1995;312:76–88.
64. Post MJD, Brown BC, Sze G. Magnetic resonance imaging of spinal infection. Rheum Dis Clin North Am. 1991;17:773–94.
65. Sharif HS, Morgan JL, al-Shahed MS, *et al.* Role of CT and MR in the management of tuberculous spondylitis. Radiol Clin North Am. 1995;33:787–804.
66. Jensen MC, Kelly AP, Brant-Zawadzki MN. MRI of degenerative disease of the lumbar spine. Magn Reson Q. 1994;10:173–90.
67. Kaplan PA, Orton DF, Russell JA. Osteoporosis with vertebral compression fracture, retropulsed fragments, and

neurologic compromise. Radiology. 1987;165:533–5.
68. Boden SD, Davis DO, Dina TS, Patronas NJ, Wiesel SW. Abnormal magnetic resonance scans of the lumbar spine in asymptomatic subjects: a prospective investigation. J Bone Joint Surg. 1990;72A:403–8.
69. Jensen MC, Brant-Zawadzki MN, Obuchowski N, *et al.* Magnetic resonance imaging of the lumbar spine in people without back pain. N Engl J Med. 1994;331:69–73.
70. Kent DL, Larson EB. Magnetic resonance imaging of the brain and spine. Is clinical efficacy established after the first decade? Ann Intern Med. 1988;108:402–24.
71. Fornistall RM, Marsh HO, Pay NT. Magnetic resonance imaging and contrast CT of the lumbar spine: Comparison of diagnostic methods and correlations with surgical findings. Spine. 1988;13:1049–54.
72. Szypryt EP, Twining P, Wilde GP, Mulholland RC, Worthington BS. Diagnosis of lumbar disc protrusion: a comparison between magnetic resonance imaging and radiculopathy. J Bone Joint Surg. 1988;70B:717–22.
73. Schnebel B, Kingston S, Watkins R, Dillin W. Comparison of MRI to contrast CT in the diagnosis of spinal stenosis. Spine. 1989;14:332–7.
74. Le Bras F, Wallman J, Barth MO, Gaston A. Spinal angiography. Spine: State Art Rev. 1988;2:379–94.
75. Troisier G, Cypel D. Discography: an element of decision: Surgery versus chemonucleolysis. Clin Orthop. 1986;206:70–8.
76. Walsh TR, Weinstein JN, Spratt KF, *et al.* Lumbar discography in normal subjects. A controlled, prospective study. J Bone Joint Surg. 1990;72A:1081–8.
77. Edeiken J, Wallace JD, Curley RF, Lee S. Thermography and herniated lumbar disks. AJR. 1968;102:790–6.
78. Hoffman RM, Kent DL, Deyo RA. Diagnostic accuracy and clinical utility of thermography for lumbar radiculopathy: A meta-analysis. Spine. 1991;16:623–8.
79. Waddell G. An approach to backache. Br J Hosp Med. 1982;28(3):187,190–1,193–4.
80. Eisen A. Electrodiagnosis of radiculopathies. Neurologic Clin. 1985;3:495–510.
81. Haldeman S. The electrodiagnostic evaluation of nerve root function. Spine. 1984;9:42–8.
82. Tonzola RF, Ackil AA, Shakani BT, Young RR. Usefulness of electrophysiological studies in the diagnosis of lumbosacral root disease. Ann Neurol. 1981;9:305–8.
83. Baylan SP, Yu J, Grant AE. H-reflex latency in relation to ankle jerk electromyographic, myelographic, and surgical findings in back pain patients. Electromyogr Clin Neurophysiol. 1981;21:201–6.
84. Fisher MA, Shivde AJ, Teixera C, Grainer LS. The F-response – a clinically useful physiological parameter for the evaluation of radicular injury. Electromyogr Clin Neurophysiol. 1979;19:65–75.
85. Scarff TB, Ballmann DE, Toleikis JR. Dermatomal somatosensory evoked potential in the diagnosis of lumbar root entrapment. Surg Forum. 1981;32:489–91.
86. Tullberg T, Svanborg E, Issacsson J, *et al.* A preoperative and postoperative study of the accuracy and value of electrodiagnosis in patients with lumbosacral disc herniation. Spine. 1993;18:837–42.
87. Wiesel SW, Feffer HL, Rothman RH. Industrial low back pain: a prospective evaluation of a standardized diagnostic and treatment protocol. 1984;9:199–203.
88. Borenstein DG, Burton JR. Lumbar spine disease in the elderly. J Am Ger Soc. 1993;41:167–75.
89. Ross PM, Flemming JL. Vertebral body osteomyelitis: Spectrum and natural history: A retrospective analysis of 37 cases. Clin Orthop. 1976;118:190–8.
90. Digby JM, Kersley JB. Pyogenic non-tuberculous spinal infection: an analysis of thirty cases. J Bone Joint Surg.1979;61B:47–55.
91. Kido D, Bryan D, Halpern M. Hematogenous osteomyelitis in drug addicts. AJR. 1973;118:356–63.
92. Schofferman L, Schofferman J, Zuckerman J, *et al.* Occult infection causing persistent low back pain. Spine. 1989;14:417–9.
93. Young EJ. Human brucellosis. Rev Infect Dis. 1983;5:821–42.
94. Gorse GJ, Pais MJ, Kusske JA, Cesario TC. Tuberculous spondylitis: a report of six cases and a review of the literature. Medicine. 1983;62:178–93.
95. Pilgaard S. Discitis following removal of lumbar intervertebral disc. J Bone Joint Surg. 1969;51A:713–6.
96. Vyskocil JJ, McIlroy MA, Brennan TA, Wilson FM. Pyogenic infection of the sacroiliac joint: Case reports and review of the literature. Medicine. 1991;70:188–97.
97. Cohen MD, Hanington DM, Ginsburg WW. Osteoid osteoma: 95 cases and a review of the literature. Semin Arthritis Rheum. 1983;12:265–81.
98. Winter PF, Johnson PM, Hilal SK, Feldman F. Scintigraphic detection of osteoid osteoma. Radiology. 1977;122:177–8.
99. Wedge HJ, Tchang S, MacFadyen DJ. Computed tomography in localization of spinal osteoid osteomas. Spine. 1981;6:423–7.
100. Dahlin DC, Unni KK. Bone tumors: general aspects and data on 8,542 Cases, 4E. Springfield: Charles Thomas; 1986:193–207.
101. Bayrd ED, Heck FJ. Multiple myeloma: a review of 83 proved cases. JAMA. 1947;133:147–57.
102. Valderrama JAF, Bullough PG. Solitary myeloma of the spine. J Bone Joint Surg. 1968;50B:82–90.
103. Jacobson HG, Poppel MH, Shapiro JH, Grossberger S. The vertebral pedicle sign: a roentgenographic finding to differentiate metastatic carcinoma from multiple myeloma. AJR. 1958;80:817–21.
104. Moulopoulos LA, Dimopoulos MA, Smith TL, *et al.* Prognostic significance of magnetic resonance imaging in patients with asymptomatic multiple myeloma. J Clin Oncol. 1995;13:251–6.
105. Fornasier VL, Horne JG. Metastases to the vertebral column. Cancer. 1975;36:590–4.
106. Edelstyn GA, Gillespie PG, Grebbel FS. The radiological demonstration of skeletal metastases: Experimental observations. Clin Radiol. 1967;18:158–62.
107. Galasko CSB. Diagnosis of skeletal metastases and assessment of response to treatment. Clin Orthop. 1995;312:64–75.
108. Kozin F, Camera GF, Ryan LM, Foley D, Lawson T. Computed tomography in diagnosis of sacroiliitis. Arthritis Rheum. 1981;24:1479–85.
109. Borenstein D. Prevalence and treatment outcome of primary and secondary fibromyalgia in patients with spinal pain. Spine. 1995;20:1055–60.
110. Ridley MG, Kingsley GH, Gibson T, Grahame R. Outpatient lumbar epidural corticosteroid injection in the management of sciatica. Br J Rheumatol. 1988;27:295–99.
111. Bush K, Hillier S. A controlled study of caudal epidural injections of triamcinilone plus procaine for the management of intractable sciatica. Spine. 1991;16:572–5.
112. Deyo RA, Diehl AK, Rosenthal M. How many days of bed rest for acute low back pain? A randomized clinical trial. N Engl J Med. 1986;315:1064–70.
113. Gilbert JR, Taylor DW, Hildebrand A, Evans C. Clinical trial of common treatment for low back pain in family practice. Br Med J. 1985;291:791–4.
114. Malmivaara A, Hakkinen U, Aro T, *et al.* The treatment of acute low back pain – bed rest, exercises, or ordinary activity? N Engl J Med. 1995;332:351–5.
115. Melzack R, Jeans ME, Stratford JG, Monks RC. Ice massage and transcutaneous electrical stimulation: Comparison of treatment of low back pain. Pain. 1980;9:209–17.
116. Landon BR. Heat or cold for the relief of low back pain? Phys Ther. 1967;47:126–30.
117. Melzack R, Vetere P, Finch L. Transcutaneous electrical nerve stimulation for low back pain. A comparison of TENS and massage for pain and range of motion. Phys Ther. 1983;63:489–93.
118. Deyo RA, Walsh N, Martin D, Schoenfeld L, Ramamurthy S. A controlled trial of transcutaneous electrical nerve stimulation (TENS) and exercise for chronic low back pain. N Engl J Med. 1990;322:1627–34.
119. Berry H, Bloom B, Hamilton EBD, Swinson DR. Naproxen sodium, diflunisal, and placebo in the treatment of chronic back pain. Ann Rheum Dis. 1982;41:129–32.
120. Videman T, Osterman K. Double-blind parallel study of piroxicam versus indomethacin in the treatment of low back pain. Ann Clin Res. 1984;16:156–60.
121. Johnson EW. The myth of skeletal muscle spasm. Am J Phys Med Rehabil. 1989;68:1.
122. Elenbaas JK. Centrally acting oral skeletal muscle relaxants. Am J Hosp Pharm. 1980;37:1313–22.
123. Borenstein DG, Lacks S, Wiesel SW. Cyclobenzaprine and naproxen versus naproxen alone in the treatment of acute low back pain. Clin Ther. 1990;12:125–31.
124. Hameroff SR, Crago BR, Cork RC, Schein K, Leeman E. Doxepin effects on chronic pain, depression and serum opiods. Anesth Analg. 1982;61:187.
125. Travell JG, Simons DG. Myofascial pain and dysfunction: the trigger point manual. Baltimore: Williams & Wilkins; 1983.
126. Swezey RL, Clements PJ. Conservative treatment of back pain. In: Jayson MIV, ed. The lumbar spine and back pain, 3E. Edinburgh: Churchill Livingstone; 1987:299–314.
127. Garvey TA, Marks MR, Wiesel SW. A prospective, randomized, double-blind evaluation of trigger point injection. Spine. 1989;14:962–4.
128. Dilke TFW, Burry HC, Grahame R. Extradural corticosteroid injection managment of lumbar nerve root compression. Br Med J. 1973; 2:635–7.
129. Jackson RP, Jacobs RR, Montesano PX. Facet joint injection in low back pain: a prospective statistical study. Spine. 1988;13:966–71.
130. Carette S, Marcoux S, Truchon R, *et al.* A controlled trial of corticosteroid injections into facet joints for chronic low back pain. N Eng J Med. 1991;325:1002–7.
131. Schwarzer AC, Wang S, Bogduk N, *et al.* Prevalence and clinical features of lumbar zygapophyseal joint pain: a study in an Australian population with chronic low back pain. Ann Rheum Dis. 1995;54:100–6.
132. Jackson CP, Brown MD. Is there a role for exercise in the treatment of patients with low back pain? Clin Orthop. 1983;179:39–45.

133. Manniche C, Hesselsoe G, Bentzen L, Christensen I, Lundberg E. Clinical trial of intense muscle training for chronic low back pain. Lancet. 1988;ii:1473–6.
134. Lahad A, Malter AD, Berg AO, *et al.* The effectiveness of four interventions for the prevention of low back pain. JAMA. 1994;272:1286–91
135. White AH. Back school and other conservative approaches to low back pain. St Louis: Mosby; 1983.
136. Mooney V. Alternative approaches for the patient beyond the help of surgery. Orthop Clin North Am. 1975;6:331–4.
137. Cherkin DC, MacCornack FA. Patient evaluations of low back pain care from family physicians and chiropractors. West J Med. 1989;150:351–5.
138. Shekelle PG, Markovich M, Louie R. Comparing the costs between provider types of episodes of back pain care. Spine. 1995;20:221–7.

4

NECK PAIN

Les Barnsley

Definition

- A common regional pain syndrome usually arising from undefined mechanical or musculoskeletal disturbance.
- Occurs acutely with marked hypomobility.
- Chronic symptoms are poorly understood.

Clinical features

- May rarely be a feature of serious underlying malignant, infective or inflammatory disorder.
- Can occur in association with neurologic involvement – myelopathy and radiculopathy.
- No examination or imaging findings are known that reliably identify the source of pain.
- Should be investigated with techniques targeting the pain, e.g. cervical zygapophyseal joint blocks and discography.

INTRODUCTION

The neck provides a link of great flexibility between the sensory platform of the head and the trunk. Simultaneously it protects vital conduits for nervous and vascular tissue between the brain and the rest of the body. These conflicting priorities are achieved through the structure of the cervical spine which combines strength with an extraordinary range of movement. The strength is achieved through a bony tube made up of the individual vertebrae. The range of movement is achieved through a complex articular system involving ligamentous intervertebral discs and paired posterior zygapophyseal joints in the lower neck, and loosely constrained synovial joints at the upper levels. The discs fissure posteriorly as part of the normal aging process[1], permitting rotatory movements through an oblique axis[2]. The posterior, zygapophyseal joints have no bony constraint and facilitate a broad range of movement through having flat surfaces that glide in concert to permit flexion and extension and in opposite directions to produce rotation. This complex is the subject of almost constant activity with the neck being reported to move over 600 times per hour or once every six seconds[1].

Pain perceived in the region of the neck arises as a result of noxious stimulation of any of the structures innervated by the cervical spinal nerves. These encompass local sources of pain among the intrinsic structures of the cervical spine, and distant sources that refer pain to the neck by virtue of being supplied by nerves that arise in the neck but leave the cervical region and enter the head or thoracic region. The majority of neck pain is acute and self-limiting and can be attributed to mechanical problems but a small percentage of neck pain becomes chronic, and it is these patients that are the focus of this chapter. Upon investigation, most instances of chronic neck pain will prove to be musculoskeletal in origin and are usually recognizable as such, but it is incumbent upon the physician assessing neck pain to exclude other serious and potentially treatable pathology. Fortunately, this rarely presents a dilemma as the history and physical examination typically permit ready differentiation of musculoskeletal causes from other causes of neck pain. Once nonmechanical conditions have been excluded the second responsibility is to provide a diagnosis as to the structure and pathology producing the neck pain. Only with a sound anatomic diagnosis can therapy be targeted and rational.

Frequently discussed in association with neck pain, but really a separate problem, is the question of cervical nerve root or cervical cord compression. These problems warrant assessment on their own merits, independent of any associated neck pain.

EPIDEMIOLOGY

Although less common than low back pain, neck pain represents a common human experience: its universality and unpleasantness is reflected by the colloquial use of the term 'pain in the neck' to describe a particularly disagreeable circumstance or individual. Population-based Finnish studies attest to a lifetime prevalence of chronic neck pain (pain lasting for more than three months) of 71%, with 41% of those surveyed reporting episodes of neck pain in the most recent month. The point prevalence was 9.5% for males and 13.5% for females[3]. The incidence of acute, self-limiting neck pain and stiffness is not known, but the general clinical impression is that it represents a common problem. Prevalence data indicate a frequency of 18% in a randomly sampled population[4]. The determinants of chronic, mechanical neck pain are still incompletely studied. There is no doubt that trauma, particularly whiplash injury (see Chapter 4.6), is an important cause of chronic neck pain with approximately 25% of those with neck pain following whiplash injury suffering chronic pain[5]. A clear relationship has been demonstrated between the nature of occupation and neck pain, with manual workers having higher frequencies of neck pain than those with sedentary jobs[6]. Other positive associations with neck pain include self-reported heavy workload, level of education[7] (probably a confounding factor with heavy workload) and depression[8]. Although often touted as a cause of neck pain, 'poor posture' has not been proved to be causally related to neck pain, largely because of difficulty in establishing a universal definition of what constitutes poor posture. It has been shown, however, that prolonged extreme flexion of the neck will precipitate neck pain, most likely through strain of the posterior zygapophyseal joint capsules[9]. It is unclear to what extent this can be extrapolated to less extreme postures. Neck pain is also more common with increasing age[10], so that neck pain in a young adult without a history of trauma should prompt a search for nonmechanical causes. The relationship of neck pain to body habitus has not been studied. Where neck pain is part of a systemic disease, its epidemiology will follow that of the underlying problem.

CLINICAL FEATURES

Neck pain may be classified as being referred from distant (noncervical structures), arising through involvement of cervical structures by neoplastic, inflammatory or infectious disease, or as being mechanical or musculoskeletal in origin. Diseases that may refer pain to the neck are outlined in Fig. 4.1. Fortunately, these conditions are usually readily recognized through their other clinical characteristics such as exertion-induced pain in angina, but the need for a complete history, including features other than those symptoms referrable to the neck, is highlighted. A cross tabulation of those conditions that can affect the components of the cervical spine is shown in Fig. 4.2. This approach, considering each structure and then the processes that may affect it, is

NON-MUSCULOSKELETAL SOURCES OF NECK PAIN	
Structure	Condition
Pharynx	Pharyngitis
Larynx	Laryngitis Carcinoma
Trachea	Tracheitis
Thyroid	Thyroiditis
Lymph nodes	Lymphadenitis
Carotid arteries	Carotidynia Dissection Inflammation
Aorta	Aneurysm Dissection
Heart	Angina Infarction
Pericardium	Pericarditis
Diaphragm	Inflammation by blood, infection

Fig. 4.1 Structures and example conditions that may refer pain to the neck.

more readily recalled than an exhaustive list of all candidate problems. The clinical history should cover those characteristics of the pain outlined in Figure 4.3. Each category reveals features that enable serious and distinctive conditions to be identified or, at least, strongly suspected.

ONSET OF PAIN

The setting in which the complaint of pain starts is most helpful in raising the suspicion of a diagnosis of nonmechanical neck pain. The patient's age and a past history of malignancy, particularly of the lung, breast, prostrate, thyroid or kidney, should raise the possibility of metastatic bone disease. Previous surgery, immunosuppression and past infections increase the risk of hematogenous osteomyelitis or septic arthritis. Inflammatory conditions such as ankylosing spondylitis, rheumatoid arthritis and polymyalgia rheumatica are suggested by involvement of areas other than the cervical spine, a history of pain and stiffness on first rising and after immobility ('gelling') and systemic features such as weight loss or sweats. Polymyositis and dermatomyositis may affect the neck muscles but the myalgias are widespread, are always associated with weakness and hence do not present a diagnostic problem in terms of neck pain.

Musculoskeletal pain typically arises following trauma or unaccustomed activity[11]. Acceleration and/or deceleration (whiplash) injuries in motor vehicle accidents are probably the most common cause of traumatic neck pain, although sports injuries and industrial accidents lead to similar symptoms. Occasionally, musculoskeletal pain can occur in the absence of a history of trauma, indicating that intrinsic disease processes, such as osteoarthritis, may be responsible for the development of pain.

Details of any trauma should be carefully documented so that the direction and magnitude of the forces that were applied to the neck can be estimated. Flexion imparts compressive forces to the vertebral bodies and discs and distractive forces on posterior spinal elements such as the zygapophyseal joint capsules and posterior neck muscles. Conversely, extension injuries compress posterior cervical structures such as the articular pillars and zygapophyseal joints while distracting anterior components such as the anterior annulus fibrosus of the disc, the vertebral end plates and anterior longitudinal ligament[5]. It has been noted that extension injuries appear to carry a worse prognosis for the development of chronic pain than flexion or lateral flexion injuries[12].

SITE OF PAIN

Musculoskeletal pain is typically perceived over the posterior aspect of the neck and rarely radiates past the anterior border of the sternomastoid muscle. Pain in the anterior part of the neck usually indicates disease of one of the anterior structures (Fig. 4.1) The anatomic significances of different patterns of pain are considered below.

QUALITY OF PAIN

The pain of mechanical, musculoskeletal derangement is typically dull, deep and aching. Exacerbations are usually short-lived, sharp pains superimposed on the chronic symptoms. Pain that does not follow this pattern, for instance pain that is shooting or electrical, should raise suspicion that neural structures are involved. Deep, unremitting pain with no periods of relief is a sinister sign implying ongoing distention, deformation or invasion of pain-sensitive structures such as those which may occur in malignancy.

RADIATION

Intrinsic neck pain can radiate into the head and down onto the shoulders. Headache is particularly common in those patients with upper cervical pathology, particularly at C3 and above. Pain from structures at these levels is often perceived in the distribution of the first division of the trigeminal nerve or the back of the head and neck, and is most likely mediated through the trigeminocervical nucleus in the upper spinal cord[13]. Pain from lower cervical levels can be referred to the shoulder girdle, arm, interscapular region and chest wall[14]. It has been observed that the more severe the pain, the larger the area of referral.

FREQUENCY AND DURATION OF EPISODES OF PAIN

Mechanical or noninflammatory musculoskeletal pain is typically experienced in episodes that are related to movement and exertion. This is particularly true in post-traumatic neck pain[15]. The pain is made worse by particular postures or exercises and is characteristically improved by rest and immobility. Pain that does not follow this pattern, that is not altered by movement and that worsens spontaneously, suggests a more sinister underlying cause.

MUSCULOSKELETAL STRUCTURES AND PATHOLOGIC PROCESSES							
	Muscles	Joints	Discs	Bone	Dura	Ligament	Other
Infectious		Septic arthritis	Discitis	Osteomyelitis	Abscess Meningitis		Epidural Abcess
Neoplastic				Primary Secondary	Neurofibroma Meningioma		Spinal cord tumor
Inflammatory	PM/DM, PMR	RA	Discitis? AS				
Metabolic				Paget's disease Osteoporosis Osteomalacia			

Fig. 4.2 Musculoskeletal structures of the neck and potentially painful pathologic processes that may affect them. PM = polymyositis, DM = dermatomyositis, PMR = polymyalgia rheumatica, RA = rheumatoid arthritis, AS = ankylosing spondylitis.

FEATURES OF PAIN TO BE ELICITED FROM THE CLINICAL HISTORY

Mode and time of onset
Site of pain
Quality of pain
Radiation of pain
Frequency and duration of episodes of pain
Pattern of episodes
If periodic, mode of onset and time of onset
Aggravating factors
Relieving factors
Associated features

Fig. 4.3 Features of pain to be elicited from the clinical history.

ASSOCIATED FEATURES

Infections are typically accompanied by fevers and malaise as well as specific features reflecting the tissues involved. Pain arising from malignant disease may be accompanied by paraneoplastic conditions such as peripheral neuropathy, hypercalcemia or features of metastatic disease elsewhere. Symptoms that may accompany primary neck pain are dizziness and visual disturbances which may be unaccompanied by abnormalities on conventional, neurologic examination. The exact pathophysiologic basis for these symptoms has not been elucidated but a variety of hypotheses and increasing volumes of experimental data suggest an organic basis for them[5]. These symptoms should not be interpreted as indicating a neurotic basis for the neck pain.

NEUROLOGIC ABNORMALITIES

Neurologic symptoms such as paresthesia and subjective weakness may occur in neck pain patients. Their significance depends on whether they are accompanied by definite neurologic signs. Weakness in the absence of neurologic signs may seem to suggest a nonorganic basis for the complaints, but a variety of experimental studies have shown that pain has an inhibitory effect on motor-neuron pools, resulting in a greater demand for effort and a consequent, subjective sensation of weakness-[16]. Paresthesia suggestive of nerve root irritation may arise, however, as a result of thoracic outlet syndrome caused by spasm of the scalene muscle[17]. This spasm seems to compress the lower trunk of the brachial plexus, causing the patient to experience paresthesia in the absence of clinical and imaging evidence of nerve root compression.

Hard neurologic signs are an uncommon finding in patients whose primary complaint is of neck pain, but if neurologic impairment is detected the thrust of investigation should be to determine the site and nature of the lesion. Coexistent neck pain and neurologic deficit may be due to intrinsic disease of the cord, dura or nerve roots by neoplasia or infection (see Fig. 4.2), or by compression of neural tissue by bone or discs that are themselves intrinsic sources of pain. The clinical assessment should establish whether the spinal cord, nerve roots or both are affected. The unexplained onset of, or presence of, impaired sphincter function, lower limb weakness and a sensory level are indicative of cord compression and demand urgent assessment by myelography [with or without computed tomography (CT) scan] or magnetic resonance imaging (MRI). These imaging modalities should determine whether a reversible cause of cord compression is present and allow the planning of any decompressive procedures.

Signs suggestive of a nerve root disorder, such as loss of a reflex or reflexes, dermatomal sensory loss or myotomic motor weakness may require confirmation by nerve conduction studies. Subsequent imaging of the course and origin of the nerve root(s) by myelography, CT or MRI often demonstrates the site and nature of the lesion and helps to ascertain whether the problem is intrinsic disease of the nerve or external compression. However, no mechanism is known to exist that permits the nerve roots themselves to be a cause of isolated neck pain[14]. Consequently, in the absence of neurologic signs, where neck pain alone is the clinical problem, there is no justification to perform nerve conduction studies, CT scans or MRI scans. Nothing evident in these studies correlates with the presence of mechanical pain let alone its source or cause.

In considering musculoskeletal or mechanical neck pain, the key issue is to determine the site of origin of the pain. However, there are no means by which a single structure such as the dura, cervical zygapophyseal joints or intervertebral discs can be singled out as the source on the basis of clinical history and examination. Studies of normal individuals have demonstrated the patterns of pain referral stemming from the noxious stimulation of cervical structures. The intervertebral discs were studied by Cloward, who showed that probing the anterior part of the cervical discs produced pain in the posterior neck, several segments below the level stimulated (Fig. 4.4a)[18]. Classic studies by Feinstein *et al.* in the 1950s revealed that injections of hypertonic saline into deep cervical muscles produced distinct patterns of pain, again over the posterior neck (Fig. 4.4b)[19]. More recent

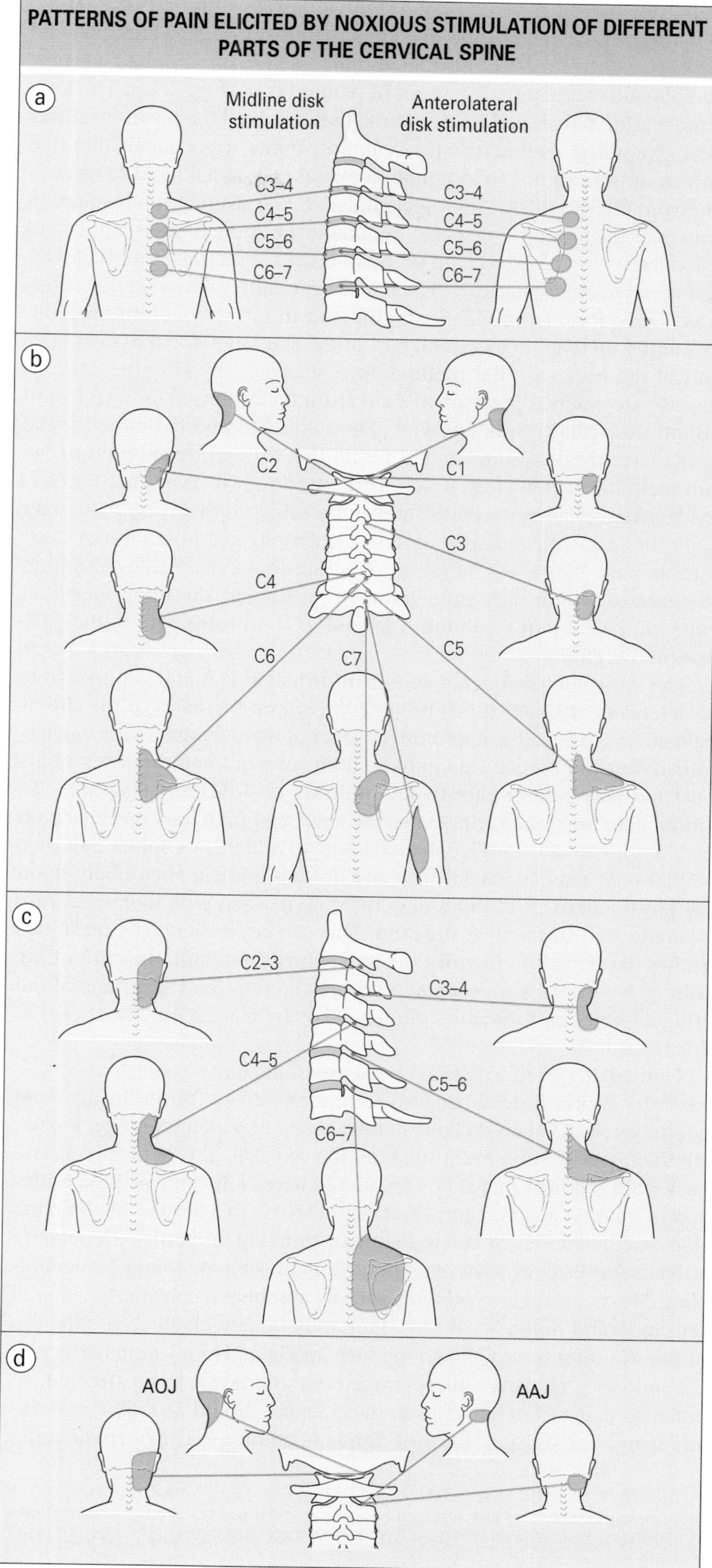

Fig. 4.4 Patterns of pain elicited by noxious stimulation of different parts of the cervical spine. (a) The back dot represents the site stimulated to produce the pain pattern. Intervertebral disks – probing of the disks in the midline anteriorly and lateral to the midline anteriorly (modified from Cloward[18]). (b) Deep musculoligamentous tissue – site of pain consistently produced by the injection of 6% saline into the interspinous region, just to the right of the midline, at cervical levels from C1 to C8 (modified from Feinstein *et al.*[19]). (c) Zygapophyseal joints – sites of pain consistently produced by distention of the cervical zygapophysial joints from C2/3 to C6/7 through intra-articular injections of contrast medium (modified from Dwyer *et al.*[20]). (d) Upper cervical synovial joints – sites of pain consistently produced by distension of the atlanto-occipital and atlantoaxial joints through intra-articular injections of contrast medium (modified from Dreyfus *et al.*[21]).

studies have concentrated on the synovial joints of the cervical spine. Dwyer *et al.* distended the capsules of the cervical zygapophyseal joints (C2–3 to C6–7) of normal volunteers[20]. Each joint had a reproducible and characteristic pattern of pain referral (Fig. 4.4c). The lowermost joint, C6–7, had a sclerotome that involved the posterior lower neck extending well across the scapula, so that it is conceivable that pain arising from this joint could be mistakenly considered to be arising from the shoulder. Moving cephalad, C5–6 stimulation resulted in pain over the crook of the neck, but above the spine of the scapula and C4–5 and C3–4 referred pain to the mid neck with biases to the lower and upper neck respectively. The uppermost joint assessed in this series was C2–3. Pain from C2–3 was located in the suboccipital region, extending up onto the occipital part of the skull and down to the upper half of the neck. Similar methodology was used by Dreyfus *et al.* to investigate referral patterns of pain from the atlantoaxial (AAJ) and atlanto-occipital joints (AOJ)[21]. They injected and distended these joints in normal volunteers and found that this produced pain in the suboccipital region (Fig. 4.4d). It is important to note that there is extensive overlap between different structures, so that 'disc pain' may occur in an identical distribution to zygapophyseal joint pain or deep muscle pain. Moreover, adjacent structures have extensive overlap in the area to which they refer pain. In particular, the upper cervical zygapophyseal joints and the AAJ and AOJ all refer pain to the suboccipital region.

The clinical consequence of this information is that it is impossible to determine the site of origin of neck pain on the basis of the site of pain alone. At best, the approximate level of involvement may be determined, but in practice this may be up to two or even three segments out, and may reflect pain from a number of different structures. To complicate the issue further, a single source of pain may produce pain over a wide area through enhanced receptive fields of spinal neurons, so that pain may appear diffuse and unfocused. It is incumbent upon the physician to carefully assess the core of such pain in considering where to start further investigation. This can be facilitated by questions asking the patient to identify the most consistent pain, the core of the pain or where the pain seems to start. Pain maps and diagrams of the affected body part that are completed by the patient may be useful in this regard.

Pain arising from irritation or disease of the nerve root typically follows the appropriate dermatome and is therefore felt in the arm and not the neck. As such it is outside the scope of a chapter on neck pain, but the historical and traditional linking of cervical root problems and neck pain requires that it be considered here. This pain will be radicular in quality, that is, pain which is perceived in a narrow band on the skin and that has electrical, radiating or shooting properties. Depending upon the severity of nerve root involvement, such pain may be accompanied by neurologic symptoms such as numbness, paresthesia, altered sensation and motor weakness. Pain may be perceived across the top of the shoulder from C4, and the face and head from lesions affecting C2 and C3[22]. However, these are uncommon levels to be affected, so much so that isolated lesions at these levels should prompt a systematic search for sinister, space-occupying pathology. The overwhelming majority of cervical root lesions occur at the lower levels, C6, C7 and C8, which all produce symptoms referrable to the forearm and hand and which have distinctive clinical features (Fig. 4.5). Because of the extensive overlap of dermatomes in the arm and the complex central representation of the upper limb, the pain referred to the arm through root irritation may be far more diffuse than the traditional diagrams of dermatomes would suggest. The usual etiology of cervical nerve root pain is from compromise of the exiting nerve root by so called 'spondylitic change'. This is a broad term the use of which should be discouraged. In general it is taken to mean degenerative changes that take place with increasing age in the cervical spine affecting the cervical vertebrae, the intervertebral discs, the uncinate processes and the zygapophyseal joints. Unlike the lumbar spine, disc prolapse itself is not the predominant cause of cervical nerve root irritation. This is because the nerve root in the lower cervical spine lies in the lower part of the foramen, at or below the level of the disc[23]. More typically, this part of the foramen is compromised by osteophytic involvement from the adjacent uncinate process or through hypertrophic changes in the adjacent zygapophyseal joint[1]. Where disc lesions do occur, the pathology is different to that affecting the lumbar spine. The discs fissure posteriorly as part of the normal aging process, so that there is no intact posterior annulus to 'bulge' in the manner described in the lumbar spine. Rather, disc contributions to neural encroachment are more likely to be discrete fragments of the disc that herniate into the foramen to cause neural compromise, either through direct pressure or through inciting a local inflammatory response. This has been demonstrated in a surgical study of radicular pain after whiplash injury which found that all patients with persistent neurologic features had disc fragments that had been misdiagnosed as prolapses on MRI[24].

COMMONLY AFFECTED NERVE ROOTS IN THE CERVICAL SPINE			
Root	Motor weakness	Reflex diminution	Sensory impairment
C6	Biceps Brachioradialis	Biceps, supinator (may be inverted) Triceps	Lateral forearm Thumb and index finger
C7	Triceps Forearm extensors	Triceps	Strip posteriorly along forearm, dorsum of middle and one other finger
C8	Thumb and finger extensor	None	Ulnar border of forearm, ring and little finger

Fig. 4.5 Commonly affected nerve roots in the cervical spine.

THE CLINICAL EXAMINATION

It is a time-honored belief that a careful clinical examination is an important and useful means of arriving at a diagnosis. For neck pain, this is only partly true. The principal role of the clinical examination is to exclude other conditions that may be present and contributing to the pain, such as infection, malignancy or inflammatory arthropathy, or to exclude neurologic involvement. Once these issues have been dealt with, and the diagnosis is that of isolated or mechanical neck pain, the diagnostic utility of a clinical examination of the neck is extremely limited.

GENERAL EXAMINATION

The general examination is performed to exclude nonmechanical causes of neck pain. This should be particularly focused on any system(s) where abnormalities have been suggested by history. In addition, examination of temperature, skin, joints, lymph nodes, abdomen and breasts should be performed. The yield from such assessment in the setting of neck pain is not known and is probably low, but the serious consequences of missing a potentially treatable systemic illness, malignancy or infection make the performance of such an examination mandatory.

NEUROLOGIC EXAMINATION

The aims of a neurologic examination in the presence of neck pain are to exclude cervical nerve root lesions or spinal cord lesions. The former requires a detailed examination of the arms. The muscles should be examined for wasting and fasciculation indicative of lower motor neuron lesions. Tone and power should then be assessed, before testing the biceps (C5–6), triceps (C6–7), supinator (C5–6) and finger (C8) jerks. Sensation to light touch and pain (pin prick) should then be checked, looking particularly for any dermatomal sensory loss. The lower limbs should be similarly examined, with the principal aim being the exclusion of any upper motor neuron signs indicative of cord compression due to the painful lesion in the neck. It is important to firstly examine the gait, and then the lower limbs for spasticity, clonus, up-going toes (Babinski sign), hyperreflexia and weakness. The trunk and lower limbs should be assessed for evidence of a sensory level.

LOCAL EXAMINATION

The neck examination again requires that nonmechanical causes such as local infection, bruising, lymphadenitis, etc. are excluded. This is readily accomplished with routine inspection and palpation. The other cervical structures, such as the larynx, thyroid, lymph nodes and carotid arteries, should be carefully palpated for evidence of swelling or tenderness. However, in the absence of suggestive history, the yield from such examination is likely to be small. The neck should be examined for tenderness. This is best achieved by exerting pressure first on a control area such as the occipital protuberance. This pressure should then be applied along the spinous processes and then the articular pillars as well as the trapezii. This at least provides some standardization of the stimulus and permits some grading of response, e.g. tender, very tender, exquisitely tender. Unfortunately, the localization of tenderness contributes little in the way of diagnostic information. There has been no demonstrated correlation between tenderness in a particular area and a specific anatomic diagnosis. At most, examination for tenderness permits the approximate level of any causative pathology to be estimated. Tenderness is also a subjective finding, so that it is subject to reporting biases from patients keen to either exaggerate or diminish their problems.

NECK MOVEMENT

Examination of the neck for mechanical problems traditionally incorporates the documentation of active and passive ranges of movement. The obsession with ranges of movement stems from a vain desire to provide a functional assessment of the patient and is no doubt fueled in part by most medicolegal assessments requiring detailed range of movement estimations to enable percentage impairments to be calculated. Indeed, the latest edition of the American Medical Association Guides to the Evaluation of Permanent Impairment advocates the use of motion pleniometers to determine the range of movement of the neck[25]. However, basic research casts grave doubts on the diagnostic utility and reliability of such assessments. Detailed cineradiographic techniques employed by Van Mameren *et al.* to assess flexion and extension have revealed that even normal individuals display marked variation in the pattern and amplitude of both segmental and total ranges of neck movement[26]. They concluded that, at least in the sagittal plane, range of movement was unsuitable as a parameter of cervical spine mobility. Such variability in controlled laboratory situations is likely to translate to a much larger error in clinical situations with the added variability of many observers and different measurement environments. Therefore, only gross abnormalities of range of motion, such as reproducible asymmetry of movement, are likely to be assessed reliably. Notwithstanding any concerns over the reliability of measurements of neck movement, their clinical utility is open to serious question. Biomechanical studies have shown that 50% of cervical rotation takes place at the atlantoaxial joints[27]. The remaining rotation occurs in approximately equal proportions below C2, so that each segment contributes less than 7° of movement. Therefore, even complete fusion of a segment below C1–2 may be clinically undetectable, and will most likely fall within measurement error. Even more fundamental is the diagnostic significance of any observed motion restriction. No correlations have been established between motion abnormalities and any specific anatomic diagnoses. Therefore, the measurement of ranges of motion in the neck provides no reliable or discriminatory diagnostic information. At best, restriction of movement in the neck indicates that there is one or more of: disturbance of the neuromuscular control of the neck, a painful lesion aggravated by movement or a mechanical restriction anywhere in the complex articular arrangements between two or more vertebrae. Similar concerns pertain to the observation of pain at extremes of range of movement.

INVESTIGATIONS

RADIOGRAPHS

Plain radiographs of the cervical spine are ordered almost universally for patients presenting with neck pain. This may be appropriate where there is a history suggestive of severe trauma likely to produce fracture or severe subluxation, or where major instability is suspected. The most useful views in these circumstances are lateral flexion and extension views, open mouth views and to a lesser extent the anteroposterior view. To assess for subluxation, lines linking the anterior vertebral bodies, posterior vertebral bodies and posterior border of the intervertebral canal in a lateral projection are constructed. These should describe a smooth arc (Fig. 4.6). The presence of a 'step' in this arc is a sign of subluxation, either through retrolisthesis or spondylolisthesis. Gross abnormalities of motion may be detected through comparing flexion and extension views, and instability demonstrated by comparing the construction lines described above on flexion and extension views. Of particular note is the issue of atlantoaxial instability. This occurs almost exclusively in RA but can occur in the presence of other destructive lesions affecting the odontoid peg or transverse or alar ligament complex. This is assessed by comparing the gap between the anterior part of the odontoid peg and the posterior margin of the anterior arch of the atlas as seen on lateral flexion and extension views. This should normally be less than 5mm (Chapter 5.5). Plain radiographs may also be useful in excluding primary bone disorders such as Paget's disease, significant sclerotic malignant infiltration of bone and destructive lesions such as osteomyelitis. However, standard views of the cervical spine are complex pictures with many structures being superimposed on all views, in contrast to a radiograph of a long bone. This means that radiographs tend to be insensitive in the detection of small abnormalities, such as purely lytic lesions without significant cortical bone destruction. Where such lesions are suspected but not detected on plain films, further imaging with CT, MRI or nuclear medicine techniques is desirable. Congenital lesions, such as hypoplastic vertebral bodies or fusion of segments (most typically between C2 and C3) are also detectable on plain films. It is not known what the true relationship of many of these abnormalities is to symptoms, but it would be tempting to argue that a fused segment places increased mechanical stress on the adjacent segment, which may in turn lead to pain. A more detailed description of these abnormalities can be found in Resnick's excellent monograph[28]. Rheumatic disorders affecting the spine, such as diffuse idiopathic skeletal hyperostosis (DISH) and ankylosing spondylitis, have characteristic radiographic appearances.The former causes large osteophytic linking between adjacent vertebrae but is more common in the lower thoracic spine. Ankylosing spondylitis is considered in detail in Chapter 6.17.

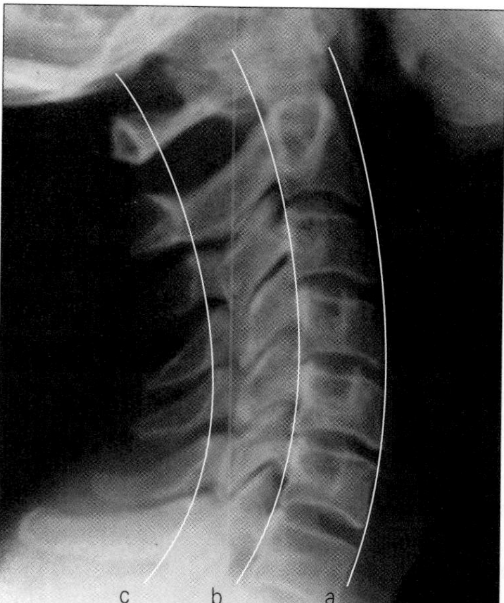

Fig. 4.6 Plain lateral radiograph of a normal cervical spine. Lines joining the anterior part of the vertebral body (a), the posterior aspect of the vertebral body (b), and the anterior border of the laminae (c), should describe a smooth arc.

For those patients with mechanical pain, the value of plain radiographs is much more limited. It is commonly stated that neck pain is due to cervical spondylosis, which is a radiologic diagnosis. However, it has been repeatedly demonstrated that the presence of degenerative or spondylitic changes in the spine does not correlate with symptoms of neck pain. In seminal work conducted over 30 years ago, Freidenburg and Miller studied 92 pairs of age- and sex-matched patients with and without neck pain[29]. Plain cervical films were obtained for all patients. The incidence of degenerative changes rose with age, was most common at the C5–6 level, both at the intervertebral disc and the zygapophysial joints, but bore no relationship to the presence of neck pain[29]. This finding was ratified by Heller *et al.* who failed to find any relationship between symptoms of neck pain and the presence of degenerative changes identified on lateral views of the cervical spine in patients undergoing barium swallows[30]. Therefore, the finding of degenerative or spondylitic changes on plain radiographs of the cervical spine has no discriminatory or diagnostic value: it is a sign of increasing age and provides no help for the physician seeking to explain a patient's neck pain.

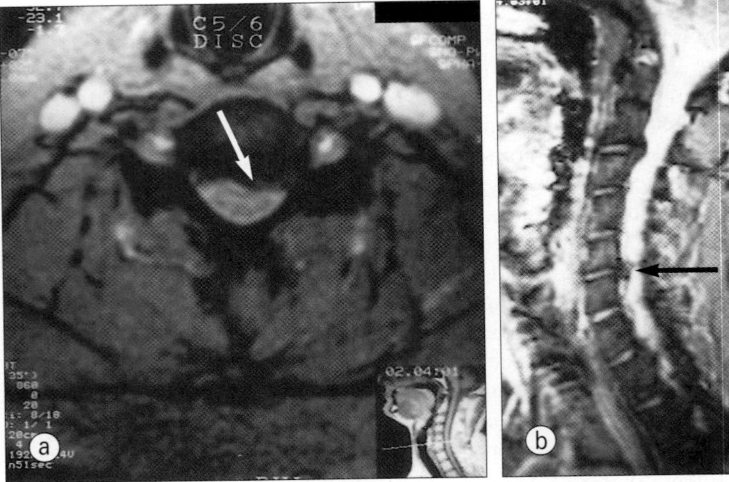

Fig. 4.7 Axial (a) and sagittal (b) MRI scans of a 47-year-old man with neck pain and decreased left biceps jerk with numbness over his thumb following a motor vehicle accident. The scans demonstrate a significant left posterolateral disk protrusion (arrow) at C5–6 which significantly compromises the exiting C6 nerve root.

COMPUTED TOMOGRAPHY

The principal value of CT in the assessment of cervical lesions is the visualization and measurement of the bony conduits through which the neural tissue must pass. This ability can be enhanced by the introduction of radiopaque contrast medium into the thecal sac (CT myelography), which permits direct visualisation of the nerve roots and sheaths and the spinal cord itself. Computed tomography is of less value in assessing soft tissues. The selection of these investigations would therefore be dictated by the clinical suspicion of a neurologic abnormality, either cervical myelopathy, cord compression or cervical nerve root compression. For neck pain alone, without neurologic symptoms or signs and without clinical or plain radiographic evidence of nonmechanical disorder, the role of CT remains to be determined. There are no extant studies relating CT abnormalities to symptoms in patients with neck pain. Therefore, in the presence of clinically benign neck pain, CT should only be obtained where there is a desire to clarify an abnormality detected on plain films or to assess neural compression or compromise.

An extension of static CT, functional CT, may yield more information in the future but studies of this technique in the neck have been limited to the atlantoaxial complex. The procedure requires that CT scans are obtained through the atlantoaxial joint during full left, then full right neck rotation. The intersegmental rotation between C1 and C2 is then measured and compared to normative data. Excessive ranges of motion imply disruption of the alar ligament complex, and have been documented in patients with chronic neck pain and headache following trauma[31,32]. However, the significance of these observations is not yet clear, and further progress awaits a gold standard test for pain stemming from the alar ligaments.

MAGNETIC RESONANCE IMAGING

Similar comments pertain to the use of MRI, which is highly specific and sensitive for disc herniations when compared to surgical findings and has results comparable to CT myelography (Fig. 4.7)[33]. Magnetic resonance imaging is particularly helpful in visualizing intra-cord pathology in the cervical region (such as demyelination, intra-axial tumors and spinal cord infarction) and enables accurate appraisal of developmental defects such as the Arnold Chiari malformation. It has high sensitivity (92%) and specificity (96%) for the detection of osteomyelitis, including that affecting the spine[34].

However, for the assessment of neck pain of mechanical origin, MRI, like CT, has not been validated. It has been shown that nearly one fifth of all asymptomatic patients had abnormalities on MRI scans, with 60% of older patients having abnormalities of their intervertebral discs[35]. Intra-discal lesions occurring in the anterior annulus have been found on MRI scans in patients with neck pain following whiplash injury[36], and would appear to match pathologic lesions reported in patients dying in motor vehicle accidents[37]. However, it has not yet been established that these 'rim lesions' seen on MRI are a source of pain. Surface coil MRI images of isolated cervical spines have revealed that, even with optimal imaging parameters, the soft tissue components of the zygapophyseal joints are seen poorly, if at all[38]. Therefore, it is unlikely that MRI will provide useful data in the assessment of subtle but painful injuries or other pathologic processes affecting these structures. This technique should be reserved for those patients in whom there is a clinical suspicion of intraspinal pathology, neural compromise or other neurologic disorder. It should not be a routine investigation in patients with a clinical history of uncomplicated, mechanical neck pain.

ISOTOPE SCANS

The most commonly used nuclear medicine technique in the assessment of neck pain is bone scanning using technetium labeled methylene-diphosphonate (^{99m}Tc MDP). This technique is highly sensitive for the detection of bony pathology with the notable exception of those lesions that have a purely lytic pathology, particularly multiple myeloma (Fig. 4.8). However, for the tumors that most commonly metastasize to bone – lung, breast, prostate, thyroid and kidney – the technique is the investigation of choice for the early detection of metastases. Bone scanning may also be useful in the detection of infection; it will often show avid uptake in the affected region. Using an early, angiographic assessment

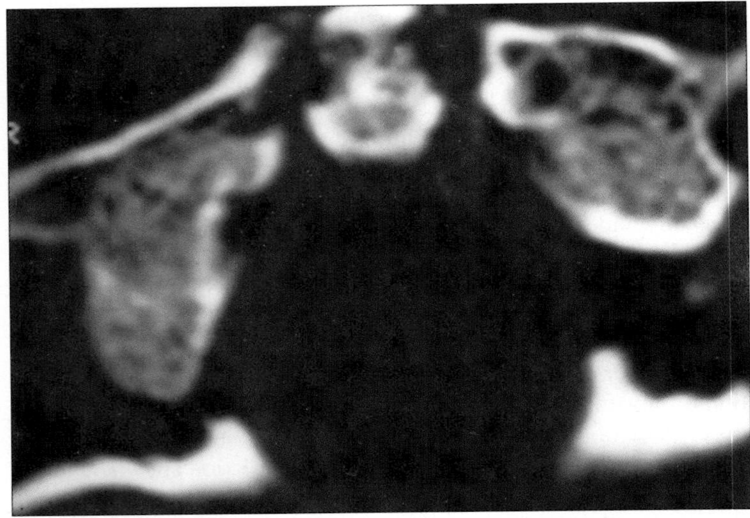

Fig. 4.8 CT scan of a 63-year-old man with known multiple myeloma who developed neck pain. Plain radiographs and bone scan failed to demonstrate the osteolytic lesions affecting the odontoid peg.

during the injection of the radiopharmaceutical and a blood pool image a short time later, increased vascularity can be assessed which can help differentiate infection or inflammation from degenerative change. Areas of increased radiopharmaceutical uptake in the cervical spine must be assessed with knowledge of the usual pattern of uptake. Notable in the cervical spine is the normal, physiologic increase in uptake over the C2 spinous process compared with lower cervical vertebrae. Only one study of the utility of bone scanning for a specific cause of neck pain has been undertaken[39]. This study assessed the sensitivity and specificity of single photon emission computed tomography (SPECT) and planar bone scans against a criterion standard of cervical zygapophyseal joint pain established by diagnostic blocks (see below). The study revealed bone scans to have negligible accuracy in the diagnosis of cervical zygapophysial joint pain after whiplash injury.

Bone scans have an important role in the assessment of patients where tumor or infection are suspected, but plain radiographs are normal or equivocal. In this setting their superior sensitivity to early disturbances in osteoblastic activity may reveal important pathology well before plain radiographic changes emerge. A difficult area is differentiating increased uptake from degenerative changes in the neck from other, more sinister, pathologies. This may require further imaging of the region of interest with CT or MRI where significant doubt exists. However, in the cervical spine, degenerative changes typically affect the intervertebral joints so that increased uptake in these regions should arouse less suspicion than uptake localized to, say, the vertebral body.

The role of other nuclear medicine techniques such as tumor thallium, indium-labeled white cell and gallium studies, is the pursuit of specific diagnoses suggested on history, examination, plain radiographs, other imaging modalities, or routine blood tests. They should not be used for screening patients with clinically benign neck pain.

BLOOD TESTS

Blood tests have no role in the assessment of pain that is mechanical on the basis of history and clinical examination. Where other problems such as tumor or infection are suspected they may provide supportive evidence. The most useful investigations would be complete blood count (CBC), erythrocyte sedimentation rate (ESR) and/or C reactive protein, and serum alkaline phosphatase. Infection and tumor are typically associated with an elevated ESR, infection with an elevated white cell count and Paget's disease with an increased alkaline phosphatase. It should be emphasized that these investigations have no role in the routine screening of patients where there are no historical or physical findings to suggest anything other than mechanical pain.

MYELOGRAPHY

Myelography is the introduction of radiographic contrast medium into the cerebrospinal fluid in the subarachnoid space with images then being collected as the contrast spreads, or is guided to the area of interest. The primary value of myelography is not the elucidation of a source of neck pain but the demonstration of the outline of the subarachnoid space, in particular the spinal cord and nerve root sheaths. This is of value in revealing intrusions upon the cervical spinal canal and intervertebral foramina, and compression of the cord or nerve roots by discs and disc fragments, infection or tumors. It may also reveal narrowing of the cervical spinal canal in patients with cervical myelopathy. Intraspinal lesions may be detected through the demonstration of expansion of the cord itself. However, all of these lesions would need to be suspected on the basis of neurologic symptoms and signs, and would rarely, if ever, present with neck pain alone.

INVESTIGATIONS TARGETING PAIN

In the absence of reliable morphologic correlates of mechanical neck pain on imaging, it is necessary to target the pain itself to identify the painful structure. This can be accomplished either by stimulating a potentially painful structure and determining whether pain is produced, or anesthetizing a structure and determining whether pain is relieved, thereby implicating that structure as a source of pain.

ZYGAPOPHYSEAL JOINT BLOCKS

The techniques for the diagnosis of cervical zygapophyseal joint pain rely on the simple principle that if a given joint is a source of pain, anesthetizing that joint will relieve the pain. There are two techniques by which the cervical zygapophyseal joints can be anesthetised. Local anesthetic can be injected into the joint or, alternatively, the nerves that convey pain from the joint can be anesthetized.

Intra-articular joint blocks

Intra-articular blocks of the cervical zygapophyseal joints are performed under fluoroscopic control. The procedure has been described using either a posterior or a lateral approach. In either case, a narrow gauge spinal needle is directed towards the center of the target joint. Once the needle is felt to have pierced the joint capsule, a minimal volume of contrast medium must be injected to confirm intra-articular placement (Fig. 4.9). Thereafter, 0.7–1.0ml of local anesthetic can be injected to anesthetize the joint.

The total injected volume should not exceed the joint capacity (generally accepted to be 1.0ml) since distention beyond this volume may cause capsular rupture. Nevertheless, even when smaller volumes have been employed, extra-articular leakage has been observed in up to 17% of cases[40]. The direction of spread, after extra-articular leakage, has not been reliably described. Epidural spread has been reported, but it is believed to be rare and has only been reported when more than 1.0ml of injectant was used.

Theoretically, extra-articular spread may compromise the specificity of an intra-articular block by anesthetizing structures other than the target joint. The risk of this is minimized by using minimal volumes to infiltrate the joint and by monitoring the spread of the contrast medium used to confirm intra-articular placement of the needle. Any significant spread to the epidural space or spinal nerve would result in numbness or other neurologic signs. A postprocedural, neurologic examination should be performed to detect any such inadvertent effects.

Medial branch blocks

Cervical medial branch blocks are a more expedient way to anesthetize a cervical zygapophyseal joint. They are easier to perform, are less painful to the patient and appear to provide the same diagnostic information[41]. They are performed under fluoroscopic control using either a posterior or a lateral approach. These blocks take advantage of the anatomy of the nerve supply to the cervical zygapophyseal joints.

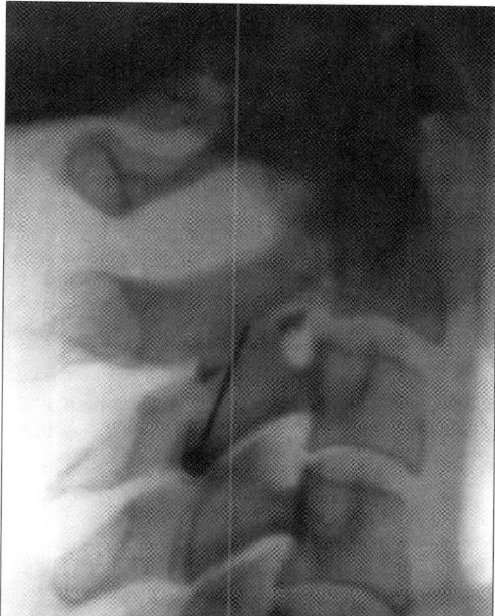

Fig. 4.9 Arthrogram of the C2–3 zygapophyseal joint. A needle has been placed into the center of the joint and injected contrast medium has filled the loose inferior and posterior recesses.

Innervation of the cervical zygapophyseal joints

The cervical zygapophyseal joints are innervated by articular branches derived from the medial branches of the cervical dorsal rami. The C4–C8 dorsal rami arise from their respective spinal nerves just outside the intervertebral foramina, and pass dorsally over the roots of the transverse processes. Lateral branches of the dorsal rami enter the lateral and superficial posterior neck muscles (splenius, iliocostalis and longissimus).

The medial branches of the typical cervical dorsal rami course posteriorly, hugging the waists of their ipsisegmental articular pillars. They are covered by the tendinous slips of origin of the semispinalis capitis (Fig. 4.10). Articular branches arise as the nerve approaches the posterior aspect of the articular pillar. An ascending branch innervates the zygapophyseal joint above, and a descending branch innervates the joint below (Fig. 4.10). Consequently, each typical cervical zygapophyseal joint receives a dual innervation, from the medial branch above and from the medial branch below its location. Beyond the zygapophyseal joints the medial branches of the cervical dorsal rami supply the semispinalis and multifidus muscles.

The medial branches of the C3 dorsal ramus comprise a deep medial branch which passes around the waist of the C3 articular pillar, as described above, and participates in the innervation of the C3–4 zygapophyseal joint. The superficial medial branch of C3 is larger and is known as the third occipital nerve. It winds around the lateral aspect and then the posterior aspect of the C2–3 zygapophyseal joint. As it does so, it furnishes from its deep aspect articular branches to the C2–3 zygapophyseal joint[42]. Articular branches may also arise from a communicating loop which crosses the back of the joint between the third occipital nerve and the C2 dorsal ramus. Beyond the C2–3 zygapophyseal joint, the third occipital nerve furnishes muscle branches to the semispinalis capitis and becomes cutaneous over the suboccipital region. In this respect the C3 dorsal ramus is the only cervical dorsal ramus below C2 that regularly has a cutaneous distribution. The dorsal rami of C4 and C5 may have cutaneous branches, whereas those from C6 to C8 rarely do.

The cervical medial branches below the third occipital nerve, i.e. those supplying C3–4 to C6–7, can be anesthetized by placing a small amount (0.5ml) of local anesthetic onto the nerve as it passes across the waist of the articular pillar. This is accomplished by placing a

CERVICAL ZYGAPOHYSEAL JOINT INNERVATION

Vertebral artery
Zygapophyseal joint
Ventral ramus
Semispinalis capitis
Articular branch of cervical dorsal rami
Medial branch of cervical dorsal rami

Fig. 4.10 A posterolateral view of the cervical spine illustrating the course of the medial branches of the cervical dorsal rami. All muscles except the origins of the semispinalis capitis at C4 and C5 have been removed. The medial branches of the cervical dorsal rami are seen to course across the waist of the articular pillars. At C4 and C5, they are shown covered by the tendinous origins of the semispinalis capitis. Articular branches arise from each medial branch, on the posterior aspect of the articular pillar, to innervate the zygapophyseal joints above and below. The medial branches are well away from the ventral rami of the spinal nerves and the vertebral artery.

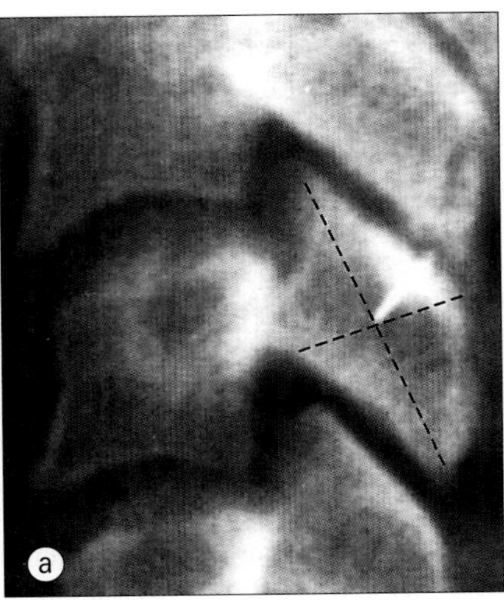

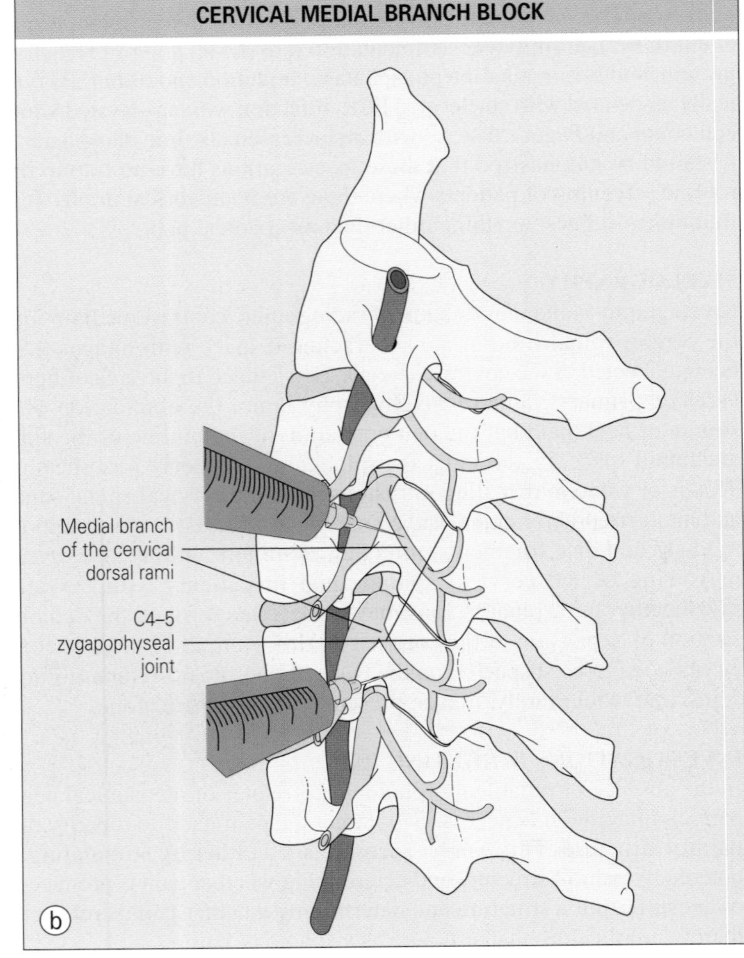

Fig. 4.11 Radiograph illustrating a needle correctly placed for an injection onto the medial branch of the C5 dorsal ramus. The target point is the centrode of the articular pillar as seen on a true lateral view (a). A schematic diagram of medial branch blocks of the C4 and C5 dorsal rami to anesthetize the C4–5 zygapophyseal joint. (b) Needles inserted from a lateral approach are positioned for infiltration of the medial branches of the cervical dorsal rami of C4 and C5. Note that the needle tips are proximal to the origins of the ascending and descending articular branches.

needle under image intensifier guidance onto the centrode of the articular pillar, usually from a lateral approach (Fig. 4.11). It has been shown that injections so placed do not spread laterally, posteriorly or inferiorly to affect any other diagnostically important structure; they remain constrained against the articular pillar, and hence the nerve, by the medial aspect of the semispinalis capitis tendon and muscle[43]. The third occipital nerve is anesthetized by placing local anesthetic onto the nerve as it passes across the C2–3 joint, which it ultimately innervates. Because of the more variable course of this nerve, lying on the convex aspect of the joint rather than the concavity at the waist of the lower articular pillars, three injections are placed to bracket its less consistent course (Fig. 4.12).

To fully anesthetize a given zygapophyseal joint at typical cervical levels, both medial branches that supply it must be blocked. Thus, in the case of a C5–6 zygapophyseal joint, the medial branches of C5 and C6 must be anesthetized. In the case of the C2–3 zygapophyseal joint, the third occipital nerve must be blocked. Adequate blockade of this nerve is indicated by the onset of numbness in its cutaneous territory.

Notwithstanding the correct technical execution of these blocks, their value as a diagnostic tool hangs on the correct interpretation of the patient's responses. This involves both the patient's reporting and the physician's interpretation of that report, which are necessarily subjective. Formal appraisal of the value of single blocks finds them wanting in accuracy, with a 27% false positive rate[44]. To circumvent this, two blocks should be used, administered on different occasions, using anesthetics with different durations of action, in random order under double-blind conditions. The veracity of the patient's response is then adjudicated through their report of the duration of pain relief afforded by the anesthetic given. Since the medial branches below the third occipital nerve do not have reliable cutaneous representation, the only way that a patient can tell which anaesthetic was used is through the duration of pain relief. It is therefore axiomatic that only a patient with pain can correctly identify the longer acting local anesthetic. This approach has been formally tested, and found to be a valid means of identifying cervical zygapophyseal joint pain[45].

A further refinement to this process is the addition of a third, placebo injection using normal saline as the injectant. Using a standard criterion of failure to respond to a double-blind administered placebo and any positive response to the local anesthetics reveals that simply using the two anesthetics results in high specificity but poor sensitivity[46]. Whichever approach is adopted depends on the aim of the investigation. Where aggressive neurolytic therapy is being considered, the extra accuracy afforded by triple, saline controlled blocks may be warranted.

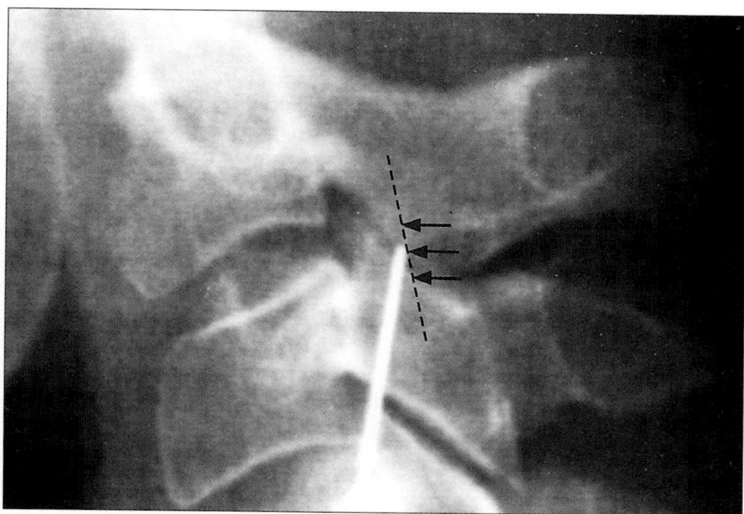

Fig. 4.12 Lateral radiograph of the cervical spine with arrows indicating the target points for injections to anesthetize the third occipital nerve, and therefore the C2–3 zygapophyseal joint. The points lie along a line that vertically bisects the articular pillar of C3 seen on a lateral projection. The middle point lies over the joint line, the upper point over the subchondral plate of the C2 inferior articular surface and the lower over the subchondral plate of the superior articular surface of C3.

Other situations, where less invasive therapy is being considered, may require only double blocks.

In summary, medial branch blocks are an exciting new tool for the diagnosis of cervical zygapophyseal joint pain. They are valid techniques that, when correctly and thoughtfully applied, provide a syndromic, anatomic diagnosis in many patients with otherwise undiagnosable neck pain. Studies using these techniques attest to a prevalence of cervical zygapophyseal joint pain of 54% in patients with chronic neck pain (whiplash) after motor vehicle accidents[47]. The prevalence in patients with spontaneous neck pain is not known, but clinical experience suggests that it is not a rare phenomenon.

OTHER ANESTHETIC BLOCKS

Anesthetic blocks of other structures, such as the greater occipital nerve and ventral rami of the spinal nerves, can occasionally be useful in confirming or eliminating structures in their territories as causes of pain, but in contrast to zygapophyseal joint blocks these procedures do not have documented reliability and specificity and do not currently have a place in the routine assessment of the neck pain patient.

PROVOCATION DISCOGRAPHY

The only regularly used provocative test in the neck is provocation cervical discography, in which a disc is punctured by a needle and distended by injecting contrast media. A positive discogram occurs when the procedure reproduces the patient's usual pain and implicates that disc as the source of pain[48]. The response can occasionally be confirmed by injecting local anesthetic in order to try to abolish the pain[49]. In practice the procedure itself can be quite painful and it is often difficult for the patient to judge whether it is their usual pain that is being reproduced.

The reliability of discography has been called into question by the observation that, in a significant proportion of patients, pain reproduced by discography can be completely eliminated by subsequent zygapophysial joint blocks at that level[50]. Since zygapophyseal joint blocks do not have any effect on pain perception from the disc, these observations must indicate that discograms are liable to false positive interpretations, wrongly incriminating the disc as a cause of pain when the true problem resides in the zygapophyseal joint. Furthermore, if zygapophyseal joint pain can be reproduced by stressing the disc at that segment, other structures with the same segmental nerve supply or mechanical relationships to the disc may be being falsely incriminated by seemingly positive discograms. On the basis of current evidence, discograms should only be considered as true positives if zygapophyseal joint blocks at that level are negative (i.e. no pain relief).

PATHOGENESIS OF NECK PAIN

The exact cause of most mechanical neck pain remains elusive. As it is not a life-threatening problem, there is a paucity of pertinent pathological data, and as the previous section suggests, currently available imaging modalities provide morphologic information that does not necessarily correlate with pain. In the case of acute neck pain, it has been suggested that the pain and hypomobility may stem from entrapment of the intra-articular menisci of the cervical zygapophyseal joint in the large capsular recesses of these joints, with inflammation, pain and stiffness ensuing before the meniscus is 'reduced'[51]. This may account for the rapid response of such acute hypomobility to mobilizing therapy. The source of more chronic neck pain remains arcane. The pathologic data concerning necks focuses on those problems that lead to neurologic compromise. Where pain alone is the clinical problem, there is little more than theory and deduction, a poor substitute for data. However, the use of the techniques such as zygapophyseal joint blocks and discography enables, at least, the anatomic source of pain to be identified in a number of cases. In the case of the disc, annular tears extending into the innervated outer third of the disc may well be the source of pain[52], but why the normal age-related changes, including extensive posterolateral fissuring, fail to cause pain is not understood. A variety of lesions resulting from trauma to the neck could affect the cervical zygapophyseal joints (see Chapter 4.6). Many of these could result in premature osteoarthritic change which can be expected to be painful. Alternatively, intra-articular adhesions and ongoing synovitis may be responsible for chronic zygapophyseal joint pain. For those patients without discogenic or zygapophyseal joint pain, the other candidate structure includes the dura. However, recent studies of rat dura suggest that below the tentorium, the dura are endowed with few nociceptive nerves[53]. A broader view of neck pain should also incorporate the possibility that some chronic neck pain is mediated within the spinal cord through 'wind up' of neuronal networks, principally in the posterior horn. The presence of these so called 'viscous circuits' has long been suspected but is still to be definitively demonstrated.

TREATMENT

The treatment of neck pain due to infection, tumor or inflammatory disease such as RA is necessarily the treatment of the underlying disorder, and is not further considered in this chapter. The treatment of mechanical neck pain can be divided into those treatments that are not targeted at any particular structure, and are therefore nonspecific, and those that are targeted at a particular, painful structure within the neck. The aim of treatment is to relieve pain and thereby improve function.

NONSPECIFIC TREATMENTS

Analgesics

The most commonly used nonspecific treatments for neck pain are simple analgesics such as acetominophen (paracetamol). These have an important role in acute neck pain and can also be used safely over long periods of time in more chronic problems where other treatment is ineffective. In patients with more severe pain, synthetic and nonsynthetic opioids, such as dextropropoxyphene or codeine, can be used but the potential for abuse and dependency needs to be considered before they are prescribed. These concerns should not prevent the physician from treating severe, refractory and incapacitating pain appropriately. Tricyclic antidepressants, in doses considerably less than those used in depression, can be used as co-analgesics. They are particularly useful where nocturnal sedation is desirable and where depression is present.

Exercises

In common with many treatments of neck pain, there are no extant studies dealing with exercise as a single treatment modality. Neck exercises have two principal aims. The first is to restore a normal range of motion. The second is to strengthen the neck musculature. Application of the latter approach may be useful in patients with recurrent episodes of acute pain with hypomobility. It has been suggested that these episodes are related to entrapment of the intra-articular menisci of the cervical zygapophyseal joints[51], and it seems reasonable to expect that stronger supportive musculature may help to prevent these episodes. Analogous to articular problems elsewhere in the body, there would be logic in preserving range of movement in the neck joints to prevent contracture and loss of range of motion. Whether the complexity of the cervical articular system permits individual joints to be actively mobilized by a patient is uncertain. However, the benign nature of the intervention and the potential benefits favor the inclusion of exercise in the treatment program for neck pain patients.

Physical therapy

Physical therapy incorporates a number of potentially therapeutic modalities such as heat, cold, interferential, ultrasound, traction, massage, passive and active range of motion exercises and muscle strengthening techniques. There are no controlled trials that have demonstrated unequivocal benefits for these techniques. Indeed, reviews of the physical therapy literature have concluded that there is little evidence for the efficacy of these modalities and call for further studies[54]. The undoubted fact that some patients report modest and temporary benefit from these approaches should encourage more formal appraisals, but whether any single modality or combination of modalities is definitely efficacious remains unknown. Current evidence suggests no benefit of nonmanipulative physical therapy over standard medical care[55].

Manual therapy/manipulation

A variety of 'hands on' techniques have been described in the treatment of neck pain. The best studied and most widely practiced are short lever high velocity 'adjustments', usually described as manipulations and used principally by chiropractors, the aim of which is to correct so-called vertebral subluxations. The other leading technique is known as mobilization and involves oscillatory movements both through the physiologic and accessory movements of spinal joints. The aim is to stretch tight joint capsules of symptomatic joints. The pathophysiologic basis for either of these approaches remains to be clearly demonstrated. Key issues of inter and intra-rater reliability for the diagnosis of vertebral subluxation or tight joints have yet to be resolved. Studies to date have therefore lumped together all patients with neck pain, and have also often included lumbar pain. At best, these studies show small benefit, of uncertain clinical significance, for manual techniques over conventional physical therapy modalities and best medical care[55]. A comprehensive meta-analysis of manual techniques for cervical pain and headache has concluded that mobilization was probably of benefit for acute neck pain, and that manipulation is slightly better than mobilization or physical therapy for chronic neck pain[56]. However, the most important message was that much more quality research is required before decisions on using manual techniques can be considered truly evidence-based. The same article attempted to quantify the risks of cervical manipulation and concluded on the basis of a number of assumptions that the risk of death or serious injury was in the order of less than one per 500,000–1,000,000 manipulations. However, the serious nature of the complications, such as cerebrovascular accident from carotid and vertebral artery dissection, requires that this treatment should not be considered benign. Although these serious complications are frequently cited as a reason why nonchiropractic trained practitioners shun cervical manipulation, it is sobering to note that the risk of life-threatening gastrointestinal hemorrhage from nonsteroidal anti-inflammatory drugs taken for one year is in the order of one per thousand.

Manipulation under anesthetic

The principle behind manipulation under anesthetic is that stiff and possibly painful joints are 'freed up' or intra-articular adhesions broken by passive manipulation of the neck unhindered by voluntary or involuntary muscle contraction. A single quality study has considered this treatment in which 21 patients were randomly assigned to receive manipulation and an amnesic dose of diazepam or the diazepam alone. The blinding was well maintained and no differences in postprocedural pain levels were observed between the control and treatment groups[57]. With the small but finite risks of anesthesia, this form of therapy cannot be recommended on the basis of available evidence.

Pillows and posture correction

There is a paucity of reliable data to show that either 'posture correction' or the use of variously profiled pillows helps patients with chronic neck pain. However, these are benign interventions and in the absence of proven efficacious treatment their use may be justified. Although again lacking empiric clinical trial evidence, the modification of workplace environments and practices to decrease extreme movements of the neck and decrease the amount of time that a fixed cervical posture is maintained are sensible adjuncts to other therapy, and have some basis in that extreme cervical postures have been shown to be associated with neck pain in normal individuals.

SPECIFIC TREATMENTS

Zygapophyseal joints

When a definitive diagnosis of cervical zygapophyseal joint pain has been made, therapy can be targeted at the specific joint. Injection of these joints with corticosteroids has been advocated on the basis of open studies, but a randomized controlled trial of corticosteroid injected into painful cervical zygapophyseal joints after whiplash injury has shown no benefit over injections of local anesthetic, with neither group obtaining useful relief[58]. It is not known whether patients whose pain arises spontaneously also fail to respond to intra-articular corticosteroids.

The other treatment modality proposed for cervical zygapophyseal joint pain is denervation of the joint, typically through percutaneous radiofrequency neurotomy of the medial branches of the cervical dorsal rami. Open studies have indicated that such techniques, when correctly performed, result in prolonged pain relief in around 70% of patients whose painful joint is below C2–3 and about 50% of patients with a painful C2–3 joint[59]. These results have been confirmed in a recent randomized controlled trial that demonstrated prolonged relief of zygapophyseal joint pain following percutaneous radiofrequency neurotomy. The active treatment group had a median duration of pain relief of 263 days, compared with 8 in the control group[60]. The long term effects of denervating a cervical zygapophysial joint are not known, but clinical experience on limited numbers of patients has indicated no lasting adverse effects, with the procedure being safely repeated at such time as the pain recurs over periods up to 3 years. Surgical intervention for proven cervical zygapophyseal joint pain has not yet been described.

Discs

The treatment options for proven disc pain are limited. By virtue of their diffuse innervation, they cannot be denervated to control pain in a manner analogous to that for the cervical zygapophyseal joints. Moreover, the exact site of pain production within a painful disc cannot yet be determined so that sclerosing or excising particular disc components is not currently a viable option. The current practice for the treatment of suspected or proven cervical disc pain is cervical disc excision, usually with fusion, carried out from an anterior approach. The rationale for this approach is simple – remove the part that hurts – but empirical efficacy studies on the effects of cervical spine surgery on neck pain are not available. The only studies available are open, nonrandomized and constitute retrospective reviews of individual practitioners' experiences[61,62]. Randomized, controlled studies of this operation on patients with proven disc pain are needed. For the time being, physicians contemplating such invasive intervention should ensure that the diagnosis of cervical disc pain is sound and that the patient is made aware of the potential risks of such operations, as well as the uncertainty of response.

CONCLUSION

Neck pain is a common and usually self-limiting disorder, but it is important to exclude serious underlying illness and neurological involvement. Future progress in the field of chronic and refractory pain will depend upon reliably identifying the source of pain, typically through invasive analgesic or provocation techniques. Many current treatments are not supported by properly constructed trials.

REFERENCES

1. Bland JH, Boushey DR. Anatomy and physiology of the cervical spine. Semin Arthritis Rheum. 1990;20:1–20.
2. Penning L. Normal movements of the cervical spine. AJR. 1978;130:317–26.
3. Mäkela M, Heliövara M, Sievers K, Impivaara O, Knekt P, Aromaa A. Prevalence, determinants, and consequences of chronic neck pain in Finland. Am J Epidemiol. 1991;134:1356–67.
4. Westerling D, Jonnson BG. Pain from the neck shoulder region and sick leave. Scand J Soc Med. 1980;8:131–6.
5. Barnsley L, Lord S, Bogduk N. Whiplash injuries. Pain. 1994;58:283–307.
6. Holt L. Frequency of symptoms for different age groups and professions. In: Hirsch C, Zotterman Y, eds. Cervical pain. New York: Pergamon Press, 1971:17–20.
7. Jacobsson L, Lindgarde F, Manthorpe R, Ohlsson K. Effect of education, occupation and some lifestyle factors on common rheumatic complaints in a Swedish group aged 50–70 years. Ann Rheum Dis. 1992;751:835–43.
8. Leino P, Magni G. Depressive and distress symptoms as predictors of low back pain, neck-shoulder pain, and other musculoskeletal morbidity: a 10-year follow-up of metal industry employees. Pain. 1993;53:89–94.
9. Harms Ringdahl K, Ekholm J. Intensity and character of pain and muscular activity levels elicited by maintained extreme flexion position of the lower-cervical-upper-thoracic spine. Scand J Rehabil Med. 1986;18:117–26.
10. Lawrence JS. Disc degeneration: its frequency and relationship to symptoms. Ann Rheum Dis. 1969;28:121–38.
11. Frykholm R. The clinical picture. In: Hirsch C, Zotterman Y, editors. Cervical Pain. Oxford: Pergamon Press, 1972:5–16.
12. Macnab I. Whiplash injuries of the neck. Manit Med Rev. 1966;46:172–4.
13. Bogduk N. Cervical causes of headache and dizziness. In: Grieve G, ed. Modern manual therapy of the vertebral column. Edinburgh: Churchill–Livingstone; 1986:289–302.
14. Bogduk N. Innervation and pain patterns in the cervical spine. Clin Phys Ther. 1988; 17:1–13.
15. Bring G, Westman G. Chronic post-traumatic syndrome after whiplash injury. A pilot study of 22 patients. Scand J Primary Health Care. 1991;9:135–41.
16. Stokes M, Young A. The contribution of reflex inhibition to arthrogenous muscle weakness. Clin Sci. 1984;67:7–14.
17. Capistrant TD. Thoracic outlet syndrome in whiplash injury. Ann Surg.1977;185:175–8.
18. Cloward RB. Cervical diskography: a contribution to the etiology and mechanism of neck, shoulder and arm pain. Ann Surg.1959;150:1052–64.
19. Feinstein B, Langton NJK, Jameson RM, Schiller F. Experiments on pain referred from deep somatic tissues. J Bone Jt Surg Am. 1954;36A:981–97.
20. Dwyer A, Aprill C, Bogduk N. Cervical zygapophyseal joint pain patterns. I: a study in normal volunteers. Spine. 1990;15:453–7.
21. Dreyfus P, Michaelsen M, Fletcher D. Atlanto-occipital and atlantoaxial joint pain patterns. Spine. 1994;19:1125–31.
22. Poletti CE. C2 and C3 radiculopathies: anatomy, patterns of cephalic pain and pathology. APSJ. 1992;1:272–5.
23. Pech P, Daniels DL, Williams AL, Haughton VM. The cervical neural foramina: correlation of microtomy and CT anatomy. Radiology. 1985;155:143–6.
24. Jonsson HJ, Cesarini K, Sahlstedt B, Rauschning W. Findings and outcome in whiplash-type neck distortions. Spine. 1994;19:2733–43.
25. American Medical Association. Guides to the assessment of permanent impairment, 4E. Chicago: American Medical Association, 1994.
26. Van Mameren H, Drukker J, Sanches H, Beursgens J. Cervical spine motion in the sagittal plane (I) range of motion of actually performed movements, an X-ray cinematographic study. Eur J Morphol. 1990;28:47–68.
27. Penning L, Wilmink JT. Rotation of the cervical spine. A CT study in normal subjects. Spine. 1987;12:732–8.
28. Resnick D. Additional congenital or heritable anomalies and syndromes. In: Resnick D, ed. Diagnosis of bone and joint disorders. 3E. Philadelphia: WB Saunders; 1995:4269–308.
29. Friedenberg ZB, Miller WT. Degenerative disc disease of the cervical spine: a comparative study of symptomatic and asymptomatic patients. J Bone Jt Surg (Am). 1963; 45A:1171–8.
30. Heller CA, Stanley P, Lewis-Jones B, Heller RF. Value of X-ray examinations of the cervical spine. Br Med J. 1983; 287:1276–8.
31. Dvorak J, Panjabi MM, Gerber M, Wichman W. CT-functional diagnostics of the rotatory instability of upper cervical spine. 1. An experimental study on cadavers. Spine. 1987;12:197–205.
32. Dvorak J, Hayek J, Zehnder R. CT-functional diagnostics of the rotatory instability of the upper cervical spine. Part 2. An evaluation on healthy adults and patients with suspected instability. Spine. 1987;12:726–31.
33. Mobic MT, Masyrak TJ, Mulopulos GP, Bundschuh C, Han JS, Bohlman H. Cervical radiculopathy: prospective evaluation with surface coil MR imaging, CT with metrizamide and metrizamide myelography. Radiology. 1986;161:753–9.
34. Unger E, Moldofsky P, Gatenby R, Hartz W, Broder G. Daignosis of ostemyelitis by MR imaging. AJR. 1988;150:605–10.
35. Boden SD, McCowin PR, Davis DO, Dina TS, Mark AS, Wiesel S. Abnormal magnetic-resonance scans of the cervical spine in asymptomatic subjects. J Bone Jt Surg (Am). 1990;72A:1178–84.
36. Davis SJ, Teresi LM, Bradley WGJ, Ziemba MA, Bloze AE. Cervical spine hyperextension injuries: MR findings. Radiology. 1991;180:245–51.
37. Taylor JR, Twomey LT. Acute injuries to cervical joints: An autopsy study of neck sprain. Spine. 1993;9:1115–22.
38. Fletcher G, Haughton VM, Khang-Cheng Ho, Shiwei Yu. Age-related changes in the cervical facet joints: studies with cryomicrotomy, MR, and CT. AJNR. 1990;11:27–30.

39. Barnsley L, Lord SM, Thomas P, Allen L, Southee A, Bogduk N. SPECT bone scans for the diagnosis of symptomatic cervical zygapophysial joints. Br J Rheumatol. 1993;32(Suppl. 2):52 Abst.
40. Dory MA. Arthrography of the cervical facet joints. Radiology. 1983;148:379–82.
41. Bogduk N, Marsland A. The cervical zygapophysial joints as a source of neck pain. Spine. 1988;13:610–17.
42. Bogduk N. The clinical anatomy of the cervical dorsal rami. Spine. 1982;7:319–30.
43. Barnsley L, Bogduk N. Medial branch blocks are specific for the diagnosis of cervical zygapophysial joint pain. Reg Anesth. 1993;18:343–50.
44. Barnsley L, Lord SM, Wallis BJ, Bogduk N. False-positive rates of cervical zygapophysial joint blocks. Clin J Pain. 1993;9:124–30.
45. Barnsley L, Lord SM, Bogduk N. Comparative local anaesthetic blocks in the diagnosis of cervical zygapophysial joint pain. Pain. 1993;55:99–106.
46. Lord SM, Barnsley L, Bogduk N. The utility of comparative local anaesthetic blocks versus placebo-controlled blocks for the diagnosis of cervical zygapophysial joint pain. Clin J Pain. 1995;11:208–13.
47. Barnsley L, Lord SM, Wallis BJ, Bogduk N. The prevalence of chronic cervical zygapophysial joint pain after whiplash. Spine. 1995;20:20–6.
48. Simmons EH, Segil CM. An evaluation of discography in the localization of symptomatic levels in discogenic disease of the spine. Clin Orthop. 1975;108:57–69.
49. Roth DA. Cervical analgesic discography: A new test for the definitive diagnosis of the painful-disk syndrome. JAMA. 1976;235:1713–14.
50. Bogduk N, Aprill C. On the nature of neck pain, discography, and cervical zygapophysial joint blocks. Pain. 1993;54:213–17.
51. Mercer S, Bogduk N. Intra-articular inclusions of the cervical synovial joints. Br J Rheumatol. 1993;32:705–10.
52. Bogduk N, Windsor M, Inglis A. The innervation of the cervical intervertebral discs. Spine. 1988;13:2–8.
53. Kumar R, Berger RJ, Dunsker SB, Keller JT. Innervation of the spinal dura. Myth or reality? Spine. 1996;21:18–26.
54. Tan JC, Nordin M. Role of physical therapy in the treatment of cervical disk disease. Orthop Clin North Am. 1992;23:435–49.
55. Koes BW, Bouter LM, Van Mameren H, *et al.* Randomised clinical trial of manipulative therapy and physiotherapy for persistent back and neck complaints: results of one year follow up. Br Med J. 1992;304:601–5.
56. Hurwitz EL, Aker PD, Adams AH, Meeker WC, Shekelle PG. Manipulation and mobilization of the cervical spine: a sytematic review of the literature. Spine. 1996;21:1746–60.
57. Sloop PR, Smith DS, Goldenberg E, Dore C. Manipulation for chronic neck pain: a double-blind controlled study. Spine. 1982;7:532–5.
58. Barnsley L, Lord SM, Wallis BJ, Bogduk N. Lack of effect of intra-articular corticosteroids for chronic cervical zygapophysial joint pain. N Engl J Med. 1994;330:1047–50.
59. Lord SM, Barnsley L, Bogduk N. Percutaneous radiofrequency neurotomy in the treatment of cervical zygapophysial joint pain: a caution. Neurosurgery. 1995;36:732–9.
60. Lord SM, Barnsley L, Wallis BJ, McDonald GJ, Bogduk N. Percutaneous readiofrequency neurotomy for chronic cervical zygapophyseal joint pain. NEJM. 1996;335:1721–6.
61. Whitecloud TS, Seago RA. Cervical discogenic syndrome. Results of operative intervention in patients with positive discography. Spine 1987;12:313–6.
62. Pawl RT. Headache, cervical spondylosis, and anterior cervical fusion. In: Nyhus LM, ed. Surgery Annual. 9E. New York: Appleton Century Crofts; 1977:391–408.

5

LUMBAR SPINAL STENOSIS

Stephen Hall & Peter J Lowthian

Definition

- A common condition of the elderly in which narrowing of the spinal canal results in compromise of the neural elements.

Clinical features

- Pseudoclaudication with activity related buttock, thigh or leg pain relieved by rest.
- Sciatica.
- Neurologic dysfunction of the cauda equina.

HISTORY

Although a pathologic picture of narrowing of the lumbar spinal canal was described by Morgagni in the 18th century, and a variety of clinical descriptions were offered for a similar condition in horses in the 19th century, it remained for Dejerinne and Sottas to provide an accurate clinical description of the lumbar spinal stenosis syndrome[1].

EPIDEMIOLOGY

The epidemiology of lumbar spinal stenosis is only partially characterized. It is clear that the prevalence of narrowing of the lumbar spinal canal rises with increasing age. However, there is no unanimity as to the precise dimensions at which narrowing in the midsagittal dimension is pathologic. Midsagittal narrowing to less than 12.0mm has been proposed as being probably pathologic and less than 10.0mm unequivocally pathologic[2]. Clinical recognition of the syndrome is very much age-related, with few cases diagnosed under the age of 50 years.

There is considerable variation in morphometry of lumbar vertebrae in various ethnic groups. Computed tomographic studies of adult human skeletons of black and white South Africans, Indians, and Italians have found a wide range of midsagittal diameters, with 5% of Italian and 10% of Indian skeletons having midsagittal diameters of less than 10.8mm[3,4].

Myelographic[5], computed tomographic[6] and magnetic resonance imaging (MRI) studies[7] of living patients have all shown that 20–25% of asymptomatic populations older than 40 years have marked narrowing of the lumbar spinal canal. These *in vivo* measurements support the conclusion drawn from postmortem morphometry studies that many cases of 'morphologic' lumbar spinal stenosis have no recognizable clinical expression. The natural history of this condition has not been studied longitudinally, and no data are available to assess the proportion of those people with narrowing of the lumbar spinal canal who will eventually develop symptoms of lumbar spinal stenosis syndrome.

Since clinical manifestations of this condition stem from nerve root compromise, it is not surprising that any disease process which can narrow the dimensions of the lumbar spinal canal may produce lumbar spinal stenosis syndrome. It has been recognized in association with Paget's disease[8], acromegaly[9], diffuse idiopathic skeletal hyperostosis[10], ossification of the posterior longitudinal ligament, ankylosing spondylitis[11], fluorosis, amyloidosis, following posterior element lumbar spinal fusion, as a late complication of osteoporotic and traumatic vertebral fractures, and as a result of a variety of benign spinal tumors and vascular spinal malformations[12,13].

CLINICAL FEATURES

The most characteristic symptom is pseudoclaudication, defined as any discomfort that occurs in the buttock, thigh or leg on standing or walking, which is relieved by rest and is not produced by peripheral vascular insufficiency. At times, similar symptoms can occur while lying down and are relieved only by walking around. Such discomfort is generally described as pain but occasionally is appreciated as numbness or weakness, with many patients experiencing various combinations of these symptoms[14].

Pseudoclaudication is generally relieved by lying down or sitting and adopting a posture of flexion at the waist. In daily life, such relief is achieved by, for example, leaning forwards on a shopping cart, leaning on a church pew or adopting a bent forwards position while walking (simian stance). Such pseudoclaudication typically affects multiple dermatomes and is difficult to ascribe to a single nerve root lesion. Forty percent of cases have bilateral symptoms[14].

Sciatica due to lumbar spinal stenosis is distinct from the sciatica which typically follows herniation of the nucleus pulposus. Objective neurologic signs are frequently absent. Restriction of straight leg raising (Lasègue's sign) is present in only 10% of cases of sciatica due to lumbar spinal stenosis. Ankle jerks are absent in 40%, knee jerks are absent in 10% and a small percentage have sensory loss or weakness[14,15]. A condition identical to meralgia paresthetica can be produced by stenosis at the upper lumbar levels[16].

Bowel and bladder sphincter disturbance can develop but are relatively uncommon. Their presence constitutes an absolute indication for surgery to stabilize the deficit and allow some potential for recovery of bladder function[17]. Rarely, intermittent priapism has been reported as a manifestation of lumbar spinal stenosis[18]. Men have been described who are unable to void in the standing position but are able to do so while sitting, a cauda equina equivalent of pseudoclaudication.

Restriction of lumbar spinal motion is common in this condition since most cases have significant and often severe spondylotic changes. It has been estimated that 65% of patients who undergo lumbar spinal surgery for lumbar spinal stenosis have significant mechanical lumbar pain[14]. This probably represents a substantial underestimate of the extent of lumbar pain in this context since the more mechanical lumbar pain a patient has the less likely they are to be offered lumbar spinal surgery.

INVESTIGATIONS

The purpose of investigation is to confirm the diagnosis in patients with a clinically defined lumbar stenosis syndrome, and, if necessary, to exclude other diseases. Imaging techniques and neurophysiologic investigations allow demonstration of the defined anatomy so that appropriate therapy can be planned. The imaging techniques are complementary and in most cases a combination of techniques is necessary.

Persistent back pain or atypical back pain with features such as night pain, fever or weight loss should be fully investigated to exclude causes other than degenerative changes. Tests such as blood chemistries, alkaline phosphatase and erythrocyte sedimentation rate are useful in excluding neoplastic and infectious conditions. Doppler studies of arterial pulses may be needed to exclude vascular causes of exertion-induced leg pains.

PLAIN FILM RADIOGRAPHS

Plain films usually show abnormalities in lumbar spinal stenosis, though they are not diagnostic of spinal canal narrowing. However, it is unusual to demonstrate absolutely normal lumbar plain films in this condition. Plain film changes which may be associated with stenosis include narrowing of disc spaces, apophyseal joint osteoarthritis and degenerative spondylolisthesis, particularly at L4/5[14]. These features are common in asymptomatic older individuals and their predictive value is limited. Measurement of interpedicular diameter and midsagittal measurements are of questionable clinical significance. Spondylolysis with spondylolisthesis frequently causes distortion of the nerve root exit foramen, which may lead to compromise of the exiting nerve but only rarely causes stenosis of the central lumbar canal.

COMPUTED TOMOGRAPHY

Computed tomograms (CTs) visualize structures localized to a single spinal level and can demonstrate articular facet hypertrophy, enlargement of laminae, hyperplasia and ossification of the ligamentum flavum, and disc prolapse (Fig. 5.1). The technique allows definition of the osseous margins and shape of the lumbar spinal canal. CT scanning provides better visualization of the lateral recesses and nerve root exit canals than does myelography and allows visualization of the spinal canal below the level of a myelographic block. Although abnormal dimensions are described, the clinical correlations with these are poor. A trefoil shape of the lumbar canal is typical of severe lumbar spinal stenosis. The presence of normal epidural fat makes significant mechanical nerve root compromise unlikely.

Most standard scanning protocols thoroughly cover the segments from L3 to the sacrum. Lumbar spinal stenosis is common at higher lumbar levels and up to 10% of cases will be inaccurately assessed with conventional CT scanning protocols alone[14]. Specific clinical information must be provided to the examining radiologist to maximize the usefulness of this technique.

MYELOGRAPHY

Contrast myelography remains valuable in defining the extent of lumbar spinal stenosis and the degree of nerve root entrapment, though it is better suited to definition of stenosis of the central lumbar canal than stenosis isolated to the lateral recesses. Demonstration of obstruction to dye flow can be dependent on posture, with compression of the dural sac by the ligamentum flavum and disk being more severe in extension (Fig. 5.2). Myelography can also be extended to allow demonstration of the conus medullaris and the lower thoracic levels.

The combination of contrast myelography and CT targetted at specific levels can demonstrate lateral recess and/or nerve root canal with greater definition than CT or myelography alone.

MAGNETIC RESONANCE IMAGING

Magnetic resonance imaging (MRI) is a valuable, noninvasive technique for imaging of the lumbar spine. However, studies using MRI have revealed changes of stenosis in 21% of asymptomatic subjects over the age of 60 years[7]. MRI and contrast CT are comparable in demonstrating spinal stenosis at any one segment (Fig. 5.3)[17].

There are few adequate studies comparing these various imaging modalities[19]. On balance MRI and CT myelography are comparable in establishing the radiologic (in contrast to clinical) diagnosis of lumbar spinal stenosis[20]. Which technique is to be employed will depend substantially on local experience, cost and availability of these technologies.

NEUROPHYSIOLOGIC INVESTIGATIONS

Electromyography is frequently abnormal if performed exhaustively. Thirty-four of 37 patients with surgically proven lumbar spinal stenosis had an abnormality on electromyogram with evidence of one or more radiculopathies[14]. These abnormalities can be difficult to interpret, with one study demonstrating that 11 of 36 patients with stenosis had electromyographic abnormalities at levels higher than those expected based on myelography[21]. The frequency of similar positive findings in an asymptomatic population is not known, and this complicates interpretation. Much of the usefulness of electromyography lies in excluding peripheral neuropathy and peripheral nerve entrapment syndromes[22]. Cortical somatosensory-evoked potentials provide a sensitive test of neurologic compromise and have been used in assessing the adequacy of neural decompression intraoperatively[23]. The specificity of this test is uncertain, and it is expensive and currently more of a research tool than a routine clinical procedure.

INVESTIGATIONAL APPROACHES

An algorithmic approach for investigation of lumbar spinal stenosis syndrome can be adopted (Fig. 5.4). The first step involves plain radiographs

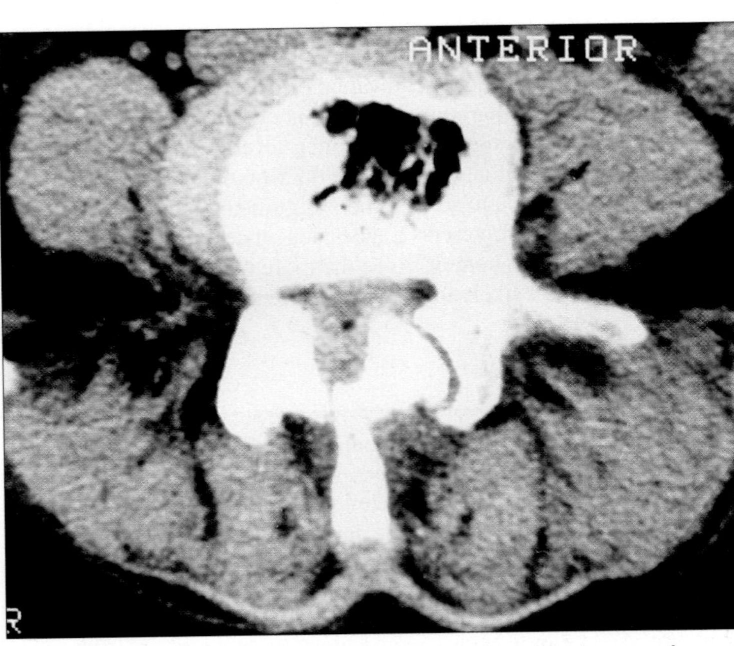

Fig. 5.1 CT showing thickened ligamentum flavum, facet joint hypertrophy and posterior disk bulging. Note absence of epidural fat with trefoil deformity of lumbar spinal canal.

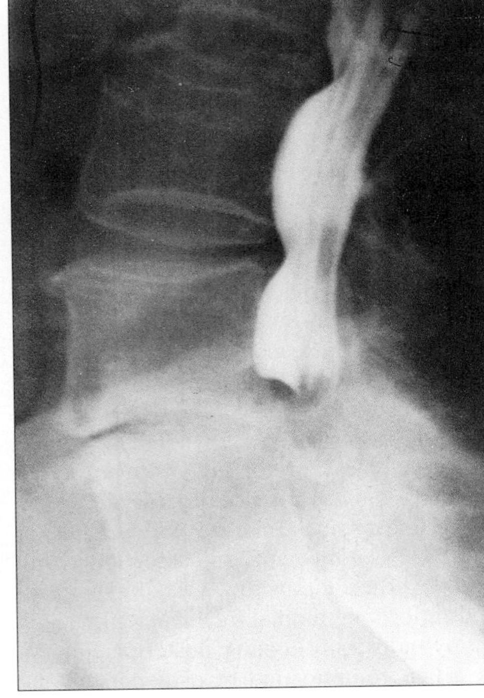

Fig. 5.2 Myelogram in extension. Note increased block with marked posterior indentation due to ligamentum flavum.

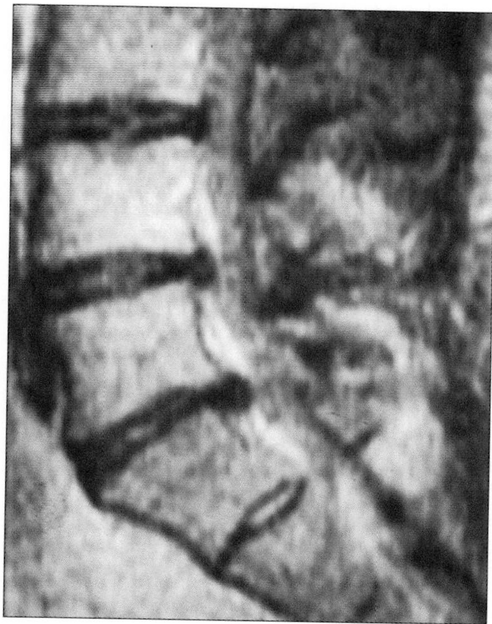

Fig. 5.3 MRI of lumbar stenosis with anterior impingement from disk bulging and posterior impingement from ligamentum flavum hypertrophy.

of the lumbosacral spine to assess the extent of lumbar spondylosis and consider alternative explanations for the patient's pain, particularly if back pain is a prominent feature. If the plain radiographs of the lumbar spine are absolutely normal the diagnosis is already considered doubtful. Many patients with mild symptoms require no further investigation.

The next step involves CT as a screening test. If plain radiographs show significant spondylotic change above L3 the CT will need to be extended to include investigation at the L1 and L2 levels. If CT demonstrates significant lumbar spinal stenosis consistent with the patient's symptoms, and surgery is contemplated, a more definitive imaging technique such as MRI or CT–myelography will be required.

If the CT does not demonstrate significant stenosis of the lumbar spinal canal, the diagnosis is doubtful and excluded in the majority of cases. But if clinical suspicion remains high, more extensive investigation with MRI or CT–myelography is warranted. If these are also normal, consideration should be given to electromyography to determine whether or not there is peripheral nerve entrapment or other neurologic problems.

DIFFERENTIAL DIAGNOSIS

There are a number of conditions which must be distinguished from lumbar spinal stenosis syndrome (Fig. 5.5).

PERIPHERAL VASCULAR DISEASE

Most patients with lumbar stenosis syndrome are in the seventh or eighth decade of life, the age group in which peripheral vascular disease is also common. At times there may be difficulty in distinguishing between exercise-related leg pain due to lumbar spinal stenosis and that resulting from occlusive vascular disease. However, a careful history and physical examination will usually allow a confident distinction, though at times vascular laboratory studies and vascular surgical consultation are required in complex cases[24]. Comorbidity is common in an elderly population, and a number of patients will require treatment directed at both their lumbar spine and their peripheral circulation to achieve successful restoration of functional status.

HERNIATED NUCLEUS PULPOSUS

Herniation of the nucleus pulposus typically produces unilateral sciatica. Such sciatica tends to occur in a younger population than that typically affected by lumbar spinal stenosis, and its clinical features are usually distinguishable from those due to narrowing of the lumbar spinal canal (see Fig. 5.6).

On occasion, a large central herniation of the nucleus pulposus will effectively narrow the contents of the lumbar spinal canal to produce a clinical picture absolutely indistinguishable from the lumbar spinal stenosis syndrome due to congenital narrowing or severe degenerative disease. This possibility would be suggested by an abrupt onset of neurologic symptoms.

REFERRED LUMBAR PAIN

Lumbar spondylosis may produce pain referred down one or both legs in addition to mechanical low back pain in the absence of nerve root compromise. This differential is of major importance in making decisions about decompression surgery.

TUMORS

Rarely, tumors of the spinal canal can totally mimic lumbar spinal stenosis by reducing the dimensions of the lumbar spinal canal with

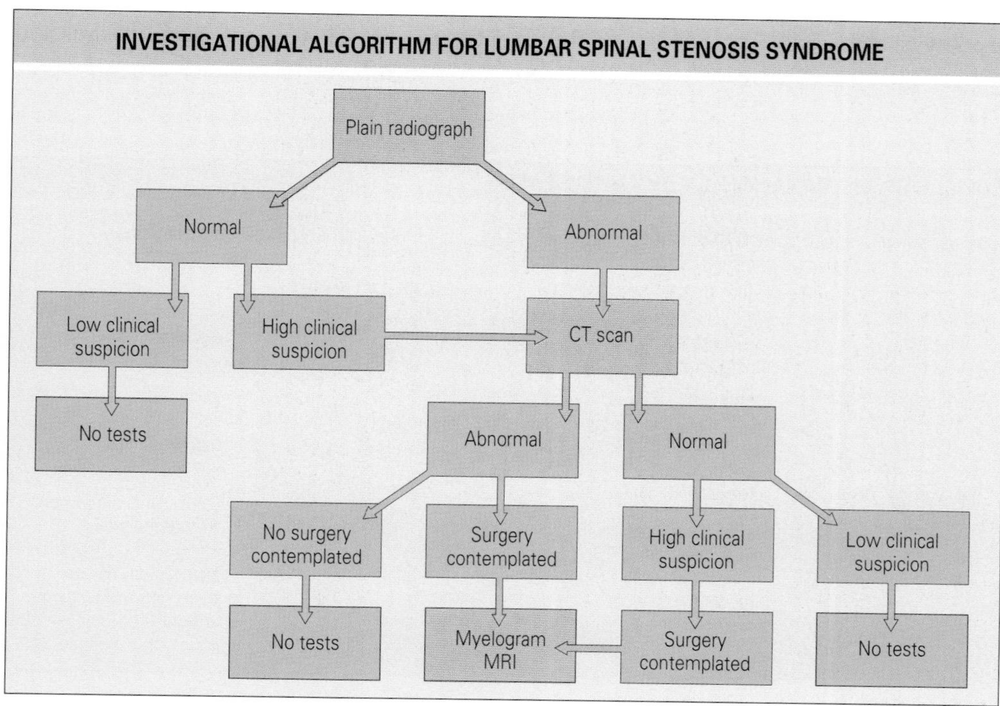

Fig. 5.4 Investigational algorithm for lumbar spinal stenosis syndrome.

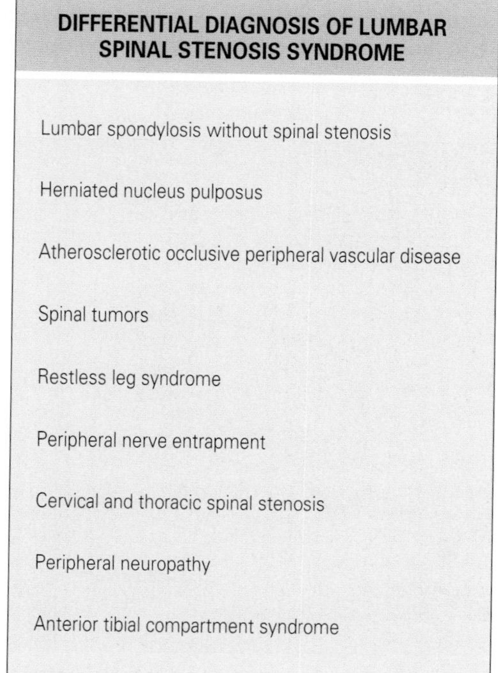

DIFFERENTIAL DIAGNOSIS OF LUMBAR SPINAL STENOSIS SYNDROME

- Lumbar spondylosis without spinal stenosis
- Herniated nucleus pulposus
- Atherosclerotic occlusive peripheral vascular disease
- Spinal tumors
- Restless leg syndrome
- Peripheral nerve entrapment
- Cervical and thoracic spinal stenosis
- Peripheral neuropathy
- Anterior tibial compartment syndrome

Fig. 5.5 Differential diagnosis of lumbar spinal stenosis syndrome.

COMPARATIVE CLINICAL FEATURES OF LUMBAR SPINAL STENOSIS SYNDROME			
Feature	Lumbar spinal stenosis	Herniated nucleus pulposus	Atherosclerotic occlusive peripheral vascular disease
Restricted straight leg raising	Occasional	Yes	No
Neurologic deficit	Occasional	Yes	No
Leg pain on walking	Yes	Occasional	Yes
Leg pain on sitting	No	Yes	No
Relief on standing still	No	No	Yes
Relief on sitting	Yes	No	Yes
Numbness/paresthesia	Yes	Yes	No

Fig. 5.6 Comparative clinical features of lumbar spinal stenosis syndrome.

resultant compromise of neurologic elements. In particular, epidural lipomatosis has frequently been reported to do this, both in the context of glucocorticoid excess – either iatrogenic or due to Cushing's disease – or rarely as an idiopathic phenomenon[25].

RESTLESS LEGS SYNDROME

This common condition produces a predominantly nocturnal discomfort which profoundly disturbs sleep and is relieved only by moving the legs either in bed or forcing the patient to arise and walk around to settle the discomfort. The etiology of this condition is unknown. Some cases have been attributed to lumbar spinal stenosis syndrome, though it is possible that these reports represent the coexistence of two common but unrelated problems.

PERIPHERAL NERVE ENTRAPMENT

While peripheral nerve entrapment syndromes are uncommon, they may produce radicular complaints indistinguishable from spinal disease. Electromyography with nerve conduction studies is usually required for their diagnosis[22].

CERVICAL AND THORACIC SPINAL STENOSIS

It is common for lumbar spinal stenosis to be associated with stenosis in the cervical and thoracic areas. This can produce diagnostic confusion, with some cases of thoracic spinal stenosis producing a pure pseudoclaudication syndrome[26]. Furthermore, myelopathy due to more rostral narrowing of the spinal canal will result in difficulty in walking and sphincter disturbance, symptoms which can easily be confused with those due to lumbar neurologic compromise[27].

ETIOLOGY AND PATHOGENESIS

The lumbar spinal canal is bounded anteriorly by lumbar discs, vertebral bodies and the posterior longitudinal ligament, laterally by the laminae and facet joints and posteriorly by the ligamentum flavum (Fig. 5.7). The nerve root canals through which spinal nerves exit the spinal canal are bounded anteriorly by the posterior surface of disks and vertebral body, posteriorly by facet joints and pars interarticularis and medially by the central vertebral canal[28]. Stenosis develops when there is a relative narrowing of the dimensions of the lumbar spinal canal due to either congenital or acquired factors. The midsagittal diameter of the spinal canal is narrowest at the bodies of the second, third and fourth lumbar vertebrae and widens at the level of the fifth lumbar vertebra.

Congenital spinal abnormalities tend to produce interpedicular narrowing such as that observed in achondroplasia, while acquired lumbar spinal stenosis is usually the result of spondylotic change and tends to cause midsagittal narrowing. Most cases of lumbar spinal stenosis syndrome are the result of both congenital and acquired narrowing of the lumbar spinal canal, thus limiting the utility of any rigid etiologic classification[29].

Pathologic studies of the lumbar nerve root canal show that lumbar spondylosis is associated with reduction in the vertical dimension due to disk space narrowing, posterior bulging of the intervertebral disks, retropulsion of annulus fibrosus remnants, and the formation of sclerotic ridges around the vertebral endplates (Fig. 5.7). Osteoarthritic facet joints project osteophytes anteriorly from the superior articular processes, and there are often synovial effusions, hemarthroses and

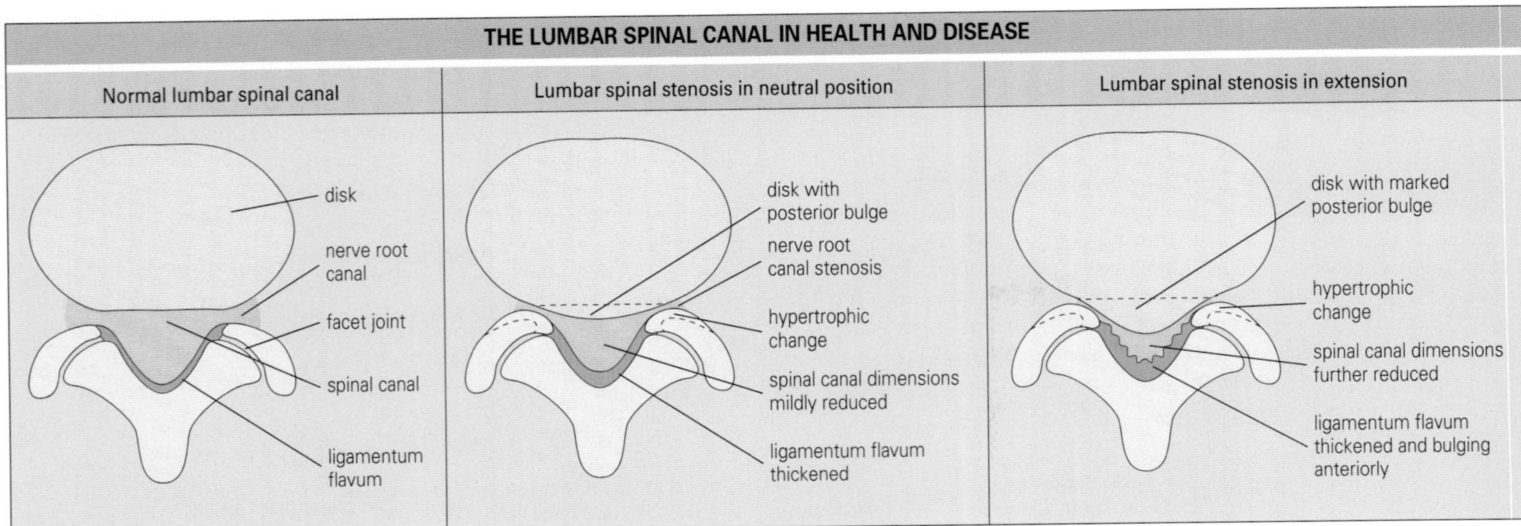

Fig. 5.7 Normal spinal canal, spinal canal in central spinal and nerve root canal stenosis in the neutral position, and the effect of lumbar extension on the spinal canal.

derangements of meniscal synovial folds. In extension and rotation there is significant encroachment on the nerve root complex (Fig. 5.7)[30]. Flexion-extension myelography has shown consistent anterior displacement of the entire lumbar dural sac on extension, caused by shortening and thickening of the ligamentum flavum[31]. Furthermore, the discs bulge posteriorly, particularly at the L3/4 and L4/5 levels, and with spinal extension there is also facet joint subluxation anteriorly, further compromising the dimensions of the lumbar spinal canal.

An experimental form of lumbar spinal stenosis in dogs suggests that 50% constriction of the cauda equina is required for any neurologic deficit[32]. With 75% constriction of the cauda equina the dogs progressively limped, reproducing lumbar spinal stenosis syndrome with pseudoclaudication.

The precise mechanisms which produce pseudoclaudication are poorly understood. The neuropathology of patients has shown chronic segmental compression of nerves at regular intervals corresponding to the site of myelographic obstruction, with confirmatory histologic features of nerve fiber damage[14]. Abnormalities of the pial vessels have been reported[33], and some patients have high cauda equina cerebrospinal fluid pressures[34]. Any or all of these factors may play a role in the genesis of pseudoclaudication.

MANAGEMENT

The key to effective management of this condition lies in drawing a clear distinction between the morphology of narrowing of the lumbar spinal canal due to either congenital or acquired disease (narrow spinal canal) and the symptoms which such neural compromise produces (lumbar spinal stenosis syndrome). Treatment of lumbar spinal stenosis involves assessment of the patient's back and radicular symptoms, and their general health.

Frequently the ability of the patients to cope with their symptoms can be helped by careful explanation of the cause of the symptoms. Not all patients with the clinical syndrome require surgical intervention. The key to conservative management lies in the patient's acceptance of mild disability, since most continue to be symptomatic in the longer term. Some patients improve spontaneously, presumably due to resolution of an acute disk prolapse in an already compromized canal. In one series of 32 untreated spinal stenosis patients followed for 4 years only 15% worsened with the remainder unchanged or improved[35].

Conservative management with drug therapy, physiotherapy, and bracing is indicated initially in patients presenting with back pain and radicular symptoms consistent with spinal stenosis[36]. Patients who continue to have disabling symptoms that severely restrict activity in spite of conservative therapy, and who are otherwise in good health, are offered surgery. Patients should be informed of the potential risks and benefits associated with surgery, and in particular that surgery may make their back pain worse.

DRUG THERAPY

Nonsteroidal anti-inflammatory drugs (NSAIDs) and analgesics are widely prescribed, and while they may be effective in the treatment of back pain their specific benefit in lumbar stenosis syndrome is unproven. Furthermore, considering that many of these patients are elderly and have substantial comorbidity, major risk factors for NSAID gastropathy, the potential for substantial toxicity is considerable. Narcotic analgesic use should be avoided if possible because of the risk of dependency.

Calcitonin is the initial treatment of choice in cases of lumbar spinal stenosis associated with Paget's disease[37]. Open studies have suggested that calcitonin may be effective in treating patients with neurogenic claudication without Paget's disease. A subsequent double blind study yielded less impressive results[38] and further studies indicate that such treatment is helpful but unlikely to be effective with severe neurogenic claudication with walking distances of less than 200 metres[39].

There are anecdotal reports of good results from epidural corticosteroid injections. However, the published trials in patients with radiculopathy provide conflicting results and have methodologic problems. The use of oral corticosteroids for up to 2 weeks for radicular symptoms has been suggested[40]. Nerve root block under radiographic control using local anesthetic may be a useful localizing investigation for patients with radicular pain prior to surgery[41]. There is minimal published data to support injection therapy despite its widespread use.

PHYSIOTHERAPY AND BRACING

Physiotherapy may be helpful in the treatment of back pain but there is no good evidence of its effectiveness for radicular symptoms. Specific exercises for abdominal bracing and stabilization programs can help back pain. The use of a lumbosacral orthosis may reduce low back pain, though in general these are poorly tolerated and the response of radicular pain to bracing is unpredictable and frequently unsatisfactory.

SURGICAL TREATMENT

The success of surgical approaches depends on adequate decompression of areas of absolute stenosis and good judgment with respect to adequacy of decompression of areas of relative stenosis. Preoperative assessment and planning using multiple imaging techniques is essential. Prior to surgery there must be demonstration of compression of spinal nerve structures which correspond to the patient's clinical symptoms and signs. Surgery should not be carried out for clinically asymptomatic stenosis.

Indications for surgery vary according to the patient characteristics but include sphincter and sexual dysfunction due to compression of conus medullaris or cauda equina, severe radicular symptoms, particularly if there are progressive neurologic motor deficits, and radicular symptoms failing to respond to conservative management[40]. There is debate among surgeons regarding the place of fusion procedures in addition to decompression, whether internal fixation devices should be used and how extensive the decompressions need to be[42].

Most patients require multiple level procedures, and in one study 72% of patients had three or more laminae removed. In the follow-up of those patients 4 years after surgery, 64% reported that surgery had yielded good to excellent results, but 36% still had more than half of their preoperative disability[14]. Similar results are reported for population-based series and from pooled series[43,44].

Factors associated with a poorer result include depression, significant comorbidity and single level lumbar decompression, the last suggesting the need for a decompression procedure able to correct all areas of stenosis[45,46]. The higher the degree of stenosis evident on preoperative myelography, the greater the chance of a good result after surgery[47]. An analysis of laminectomy failure of 45 patients found that only half had the clinical picture of neurogenic claudication and only 10 had radiologic evidence of severe lumbar canal stenosis. The most common technical problem was inadequate neural decompression[48]. This confirms earlier suggestions that the chance of a good postoperative result is higher in those patients who preoperatively described postural effects on symptoms[49]. In summary, the more the clinical picture is one of pseudoclaudication with convincing radiology of neural compromise and the less it is mechanical low back pain, the greater the chance of success with surgical intervention.

Bone regrowth is increasingly recognized in postoperative spines. The vast majority of patients will experience bone regrowth by 5–7 years with the more severe grades of bone regrowth being correlated with poorer functional outcome[50,51]. Repeat surgery for restenosis may be required.

Postoperative spondylolisthesis has been reported in up to 20% of patients who have surgery for acquired degenerative spinal stenosis. The factors that are associated with increased slipping remain uncertain, though it may be related to extent of the decompression involving trauma to the facet joints, size of the disk space preoperatively, presence of preoperative spondylolisthesis and the presence of scoliosis[52].

Some patients with lumbar spinal stenosis are left with persisting significant neurologic deficit, for example foot drop, despite maximal therapy, and such patients should have appropriate rehabilitation and orthoses to improve their functional status.

Unfortunately, in spite of adequate conservative and operative management, some patients are left with ongoing severe back pain and limitation. Multidisciplinary pain management and functional restoration techniques should be considered for these patients, and the management involves both physical and psychologic assessment and treatment[53].

REFERENCES

1. Verbiest H. Neurogenic intermittent claudication. In: Vinken PJ, Bruin GW. Handbook of clinical neurology. Vol 20. Amsterdam: North Holland; 1976.
2. Resnick D, Niwayama G. Degenerative disease of the spine. In: Resnick D, ed. Bone and joint imaging. Philadelphia: WB Saunders; 1989:413–39.
3. Eisenstein S. Lumbar vertebral canal morphometry for computerized tomography in spinal stenosis. Spine. 1983;8:187–91.
4. Postacchini F, Ripani M, Carpano S. Morphometry of the lumbar vertebrae. Clin Orthop. 1983;172:296–303.
5. Hitselberger WE,Witten RM. Abnormal myelograms in asymptomatic patients. J Neurosurg. 1968;28:204–6.
6. Weisel SW, Tsourmas N, Feffer HL, Citrin CM, Patronas N. A study of computer-assisted tomography I. The incidence of positive CAT scans in an asymptomatic group of patients. Spine. 1984;9:549–51.
7. Boden SD, Davis DO, Dina TS, Patronas NJ, Wiesel SW. Abnormal magnetic-resonance scans of the lumbar spine in asymptomatic subjects. J Bone Joint Surg. 1990;72–A:403–8.
8. Hadjipavlou A, Shaffer N, Lander P, Srolovitz H. Pagetic spinal stenosis with extradural pagetoid ossification. Spine. 1988;13:128–30.
9. Epstein N, Whelan M, Benjamin V. Acromegaly and spinal stenosis. J Neurosurg. 1982;56:145–7.
10. Kurihara A, Tanaka Y, Tsumura N, Iwasaki Y. Hyperostotic lumbar spinal stenosis. Spine. 1988;13:1308–16.
11. Weinstein PR, Karpman RR, Gall EP, Pitt M. Spinal cord injury, spinal fracture and spinal stenosis in ankylosing spondylitis. J Neurosurg. 1982;57:609–16.
12. McGuire RA, Brown MD, Green BA. Intradural spinal tumours and spinal stenosis. Spine. 1987;12:1062–6.
13. Madsen JR, Heros RC. Spinal arteriovenous malformations and neurogenic claudication. J Neurosurg. 1988;68:693–7.
14. Hall S, Bartleson JD, Onofrio BM, Baker HL, Okazak IH, O'Duffy JD. Lumbar spinal stenosis: Clinical features, diagnostic procedures and results of treatment in 68 patients. Ann Intern Med. 1985;103:271–5.
15. Jonsson B, Stromqvist B. Symptoms and signs in degeneration of the lumbar spine. A prospective consecutive study of 300 operated patients. J Bone Joint Surg [Br]. 1993;75–B:381–5.
16. Guo-Xiang J, Wei-Dong X, Ai-Haow. Spinal stenosis with meralgia paraesthetica. J Bone Joint Surg. 1988;70–B:272–3.
17. Deen HG, Zimmerman RS, Swanson SK, Larson TR. Assessment of bladder function after lumbar decompressive surgery for spinal stenosis: a prospective study. J Neurosurg. 1994;80:971–4.
18. Ram Z, Findler G, Spiegelman R, Shacked I, Tadmor R, Sahar A. Intermittent priapism in spinal canal stenosis. Spine. 1987;12:377–8.
19. Kent DL, Haynor DR, Larson EB, Deyo RA. Diagnosis of lumbar spinal stenosis in adults: A meta-analysis of the accuracy of CT, MR, and myelography. AJR. 1992;158:1135–44.
20. Bischoff RJ, Rodriguez RP, Gupta K, Righi A, Dalton JE, Whitecloud TS. A comparison of computed tomography–myelography, magnetic resonance imaging and myelography in the diagnosis of herniated nucleus pulposus and spinal stenosis. J Spinal Dis. 1993;6:289–95.
21. Seppalainen AM, Alaranta H, Soini J. Electromyography in the diagnosis of lumbar spinal stenosis. Electromyogr Clin Neurophysiol. 1981;21:55–66.
22. Saal JA, Dillingham MF, Gamburd RS, Fanton GS. The pseudoradicular syndrome. Lower extremity peripheral nerve entrapment masquerading as lumbar radiculopathy. Spine. 1988;13:926–30.
23. Herron LD, Trippi AC, Gonyeau M. Intraoperative use of dermatomal somatosensory-evoked potentials in lumbar stenosis surgery. Spine. 1987;12:379–83.
24. Dodge LD, Bohlman HH, Rhodes RS. Concurrent lumbar spinal stenosis and peripheral vascular disease. Clin Orthop. 1988;230:141–8.
25. Haddad SF, Hitchon PW, Godersky JC. Idiopathic and glucocorticoid-induced spinal epidural lipomatosis. J Neurosurg. 1991;74:38–42.
26. Yamamoto I, Matsumae M, Ikeda A, Shibuya N, Sato O, Nakamura K. Thoracic spinal stenosis: experience with 7 cases. J Neurosurg. 1988;68:37–40.
27. Dagi TF, Tarkington MA, Leech JJ. Tandem lumbar and cervical spinal stenosis. J Neurosurg. 1988;66:842–9.
28. Lee CY, Rauschning W, Glenn W. Lateral lumbar spinal canal stenosis: classification, pathologic anatomy and surgical decompression. Spine. 1988;13:313–20
29. Arnoldi CC, Brodsky AE, Cauchoix J, *et al.* Lumbar spinal stenosis and nerve root entrapment syndromes: definition and classification. Clin Orthop. 1976;115:4–5.
30. Rauschning W. Normal and pathologic anatomy of the lumbar root canals. Spine. 1987;12:1008–19.
31. Penning L, Wilmink JT. Biomechanics of lumbosacral dural sac: a study of flexion–extension myelography. Spine. 1981;6:398–408.
32. Delamarter RB, Bohlman HH, Dodge LD, Biro C. Experimental lumbar spinal stenosis. J Bone Joint Surg. 1990;72–A:110–20.
33. Watanabe R, Parke WW. Vascular and neural pathology of lumbosacral spinal stenosis. J Neurosurg. 1986;64:64–70.
34. Magnaes B. Clinical recording of pressure on the spinal cord and cauda equina. J Neurosurg. 1982;57:57–63.
35. Johnsson K-E, Rosen I, Uden A. The natural course of lumbar spinal stenosis. Clin Orthop. 1992; 279:82–6.
36. Nachemson A. Newest knowledge of low back pain. A critical look. Clin Orthop. 1992;279:8–16.
37. Herzberg L, Bayliss D. Spinal cord syndrome due to non-compressive Paget's disease of bone: a spinal artery steal phenomenon reversible with calcitonin. Lancet. 1980;ii:13–15.
38. Porter W, Miller CG. Neurogenic claudication and root claudication treated with calcitonin. A double-blind trial. Spine. 1988;13:1061–3.
39. Eskola A, Pohjolainen T, Alaranta H, Soini K, Slatis P. Calcitonin treatment in lumbar spinal stenosis: a randomized placebo-controlled, double-blind, cross-over study with one-year follow-up. Calcif Tissue Int. 1992;50:400–3.
40. Postacchino F. Lumbar spinal stenosis. In: Weinstein JN, Wiesel SW, eds. The lumbar spine. Philadelphia: WB Saunders; 1990:594–611.
41. Dooley JF, McBroom RJ, Takuchi T, MacNab I. Nerve root infiltration in the diagnosis of radicular pain. Spine. 1988;13:79–83.
42. Nasca RJ. Rationale for spinal fusion of lumbar spinal stenosis. Spine. 1989;14:451–4.
43. Tuite GF, Stern JD, Doran SE,Papadopoulos SM, McGillicuddy JE,Oyedijo DI *et al.* Outcome after laminectomy for lumbar spinal stenosis. J Neurosurg. 1994;81:699–706.
44. Turner JA, Ersek M, Herron L, Deyo R. Surgery for lumbar spinal stenosis. Attempted meta-analysis of the literature. Spine. 1992;17:1–8.
45. Herno A, Airaksinen O, Saari T. The long-term prognosis after operation for lumbar spinal stenosis. Scand J Rehab Med. 1993;25:167–171.
46. Katz JN, Lipson SJ, Larson MG, McInnes JM, Fossel AH, Liang MH. The outcome of decompressive laminectomy for degenerative lumbar stenosis. J Bone Joint Surg. 1991;73–A:809–16.
47. Herno A, Airaksinen O, Saari T, Miettinen H. The predictive value of preoperative myelography in lumbar spinal stenosis. Spine. 1994;19:1335–8.
48. Deen HG, Zimmerman RS, Lyons MK, Wharen RE, Reimer R. Analysis of early failures after lumbar decompressive laminectomy for spinal stenosis. Mayo Clin Proc. 1995;70:33–6.
49. Ganz JC. Lumbar spinal stenosis: post-operative results in terms of pre-operative posture-related pain. J Neurosurg. 1990;72:71–4.
50. Postacchini F, Cinotti G. Bone regrowth after surgical decompression for lumbar spinal stenosis. J Bone Joint Surg[Br]. 1992;74–B:862–9.
51. Chen Q, Baba H, Kamitani K, Furosawa N, Imura S. Postoperative bone re-growth in lumbar spinal stenosis. Spine.1994;19:214–9.
52. Johnsson K-E, Willner S, Johnsson K. Post-operative instability after decompression for lumbar spinal stenosis. Spine. 1986;11:107–10.
53. Mayer TG, Gatchel RJ, Kishino N, et al. Objective assessment of spine function following industrial injury. A prospective study with comparison group and one year follow-up. Spine. 1985;10:482–93.

6

PRACTICAL PROBLEMS

CERVICAL ROOT IRRITATION

Cyrus Cooper

DEFINITION OF THE PROBLEM

It is important to consider rare but potentially serious syndromes such as atlantoaxial subluxation and cervical myelopathy. Thereafter, the major distinction lies between soft tissue cervical spine disorders (which do not usually cause brachial neuralgia) and cervical spondylosis. Both of these are stable conditions, and management consists of an algorithm of sequentially applied conservative measures.

THE TYPICAL CASE

HD is an overweight 62-year-old woman with a 5-year history of progressively worsening neck pain. Symptoms begun after a fall while she was gardening and had a relapsing and remitting course with exacerbations lasting 4–5 weeks in every 3 months. She presented with a 2-week history of severe pain radiating from her neck to the radial aspect of her left forearm and hand. This pain initially woke her from sleep and had been continuous ever since. It was accompanied by numbness and tingling in the same area of the left arm and she had noticed weakness in lifting objects such as a full kettle. On examination, there was tenderness in the left paracervical region at the C5–C6 level, with a reduced left biceps tendon reflex. Neck movements were painful and restricted, especially right lateral flexion and rotation. Pain in the left arm was reproducible by vertical pressure on the head (Spurling's maneuver). The lateral cervical spine radiograph (Fig. 6.1) revealed disk-space narrowing at the C5–C6 level, with marginal osteophyte formation and subchondral sclerosis.

DIAGNOSIS

The cervical spine is one of the most complex articular systems in the body and numerous clinical syndromes have been associated with its dysfunction. The most frequent of these disorders is cervical spondylosis, a condition arising from a varying combination of cervical intervertebral disk degeneration and osteoarthritis (OA) affecting the apophyseal or intervertebral joints. The radiologic evidence of cervical spondylosis is almost universal above the age of 65 and there is no correlation between the presence of these changes on radiographs and the occurence of neck pain.

Radiculopathy results from disk or osteophyte encroachment on one or several cervical nerve roots, especially C6 (C5–C6 disk) and C7 (C6–C7 disk). It may result in pain or paresthesias affecting the upper limb dermatomes at the involved levels, with weakness and hyporeflexia (see Fig. 6.2).

Cervical myelopathy must be distinguished from brachial root compression as a cause of neurologic features in the arm. Cervical myelopathy may arise from disk prolapse as well as cervical spine instability. This latter cause is a potentially serious complication of inflammatory joint disorders such as rheumatoid arthritis (RA), requiring urgent evaluation [most usefully by magnetic resonance imaging (MRI)] and assessment for surgical stabilization. Cervical myelopathy usually manifests with a combination of upper and lower limb sensory and motor signs. In contrast, brachial root signs are confined to the upper limb.

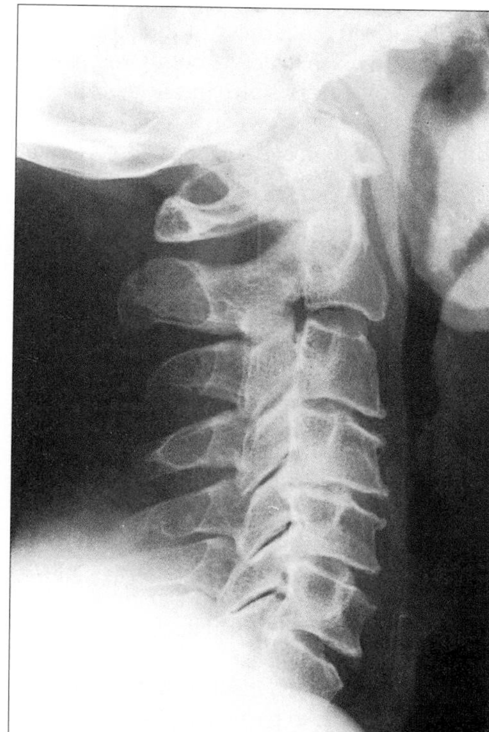

Fig. 6.1 Lateral cervical spine radiograph illustrating features of cervical spondylosis. There is loss of posterior disk height with irregularity of the disk margins at C4–C5 and C5–C6, with some subchondral sclerosis and osteophyte formation anteriorly and posteriorly at these levels.

CERVICAL ROOT LESIONS

Dermatome distribution
Anterior Posterior

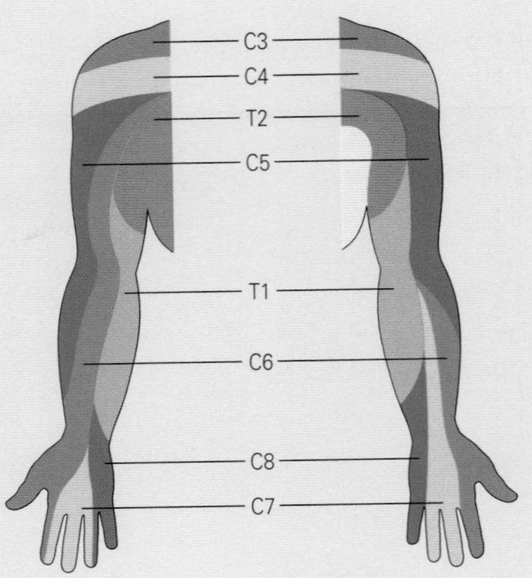

C3
C4
T2
C5
T1
C6
C8
C7

Root	Muscle weakness/ movement affected	Tendon reflex decreased
C5	Shoulder abduction Elbow flexion	Biceps jerk
C6	Wrist extension/ pronation	Supinator jerk
C7	Elbow/finger extension	Triceps jerk
C8	Wrist/finger extension	Finger jerk
T1	Finger abduction Thumb adduction/ opposition	

Fig. 6.2 Sensory and motor distribution of the cervical roots.

Inflammatory arthritides, such as RA, ankylosing spondylitis and juvenile chronic arthritis (JCA), commonly involve the cervical spine and enter the differential diagnosis of neck pain. It is extremely unusual for these disorders to result in brachial root irritation, so that neurologic symptoms and signs in the arm point towards a compressive lesion of the spinal cord or nerve roots.

Soft tissue disorders of the upper limb, such as frozen shoulder and tennis elbow, commonly result in referred pain and tenderness to more distant sites within the arm. The pattern of radiation may be difficult to distinguish from the dermatomal distribution in the arm, but it is not associated with neurologic signs in the upper limb.

A large proportion of cervical spine syndromes arises through disruption of the soft tissues supporting the neck. These include acceleration and deceleration (whiplash) injuries, musculoligamentous strains, tension myositis and acute neck strain. While these disorders frequently result in pain and localized tenderness of the paraspinal tissues, they do not usually irritate the brachial nerve roots. Osteophytic or diskal compression of roots, however, results in the neurologic picture outlined above.

A number of investigations may aid in localizing the cause of neurologic symptoms and signs in the upper limb. Cervical spine radiography and MRI provide important structural information as outlined above. Isotope scintigraphy may be useful in excluding rarer intrinsic bone abnormalities such as infection or tumor. Finally, nerve conduction studies may help differentiate between a peripheral polyneuropathy, focal radiculopathy and myopathy.

THERAPEUTIC OPTIONS

Disorders of the cervical spine are best treated with a program incorporating multiple approaches, each individualized for the specific patient (Fig. 6.3). These include patient education, physical therapeutic maneuvers to relieve pain and reduce nerve root compression, and drug therapy. While there is little controlled evidence by which to assess the success of these measures, clinical experience supports their efficacy in certain groups of patients and their widespread use is established. Surgery is only indicated in a few circumstances and the outcome of surgical intervention is moderate at best.

The more the patient understands about the mechanism of neck and arm symptoms, the more he or she is able to participate actively in the management program. Education must include postural training, the use of alternating rest (to diminish inflammation) and exercise (to maintain conditioning of muscles and ligaments), and advice about work and leisure activities.

The initial physical therapeutic interventions in a patient with cervical spondylosis and brachial root irritation comprise the use of a cervical collar, local pain-relieving measures and traction.

The desired degree of immobilization dictates the type of collar used. When structural displacement of the cervical spine is a concern, only a rigid collar succeeds in limiting neck movements by over 50%. In most cases of cervical spondylosis, however, a soft collar will suffice. Patients with root irritation often find relief during and after wearing a soft collar; those with disease at multiple levels do less well than those with single-level involvement.

The most usual pain-relieving maneuvers adopted are heat and cold applications, with the aim of relieving muscle spasm, and ultrasound

MANAGEMENT OF CERVICAL SPONDYLOSIS WITH BRACHIAL ROOT IRRITATION
Education
Reassurance Rest/exercise Occupational changes Psychotherapy
Physical therapy
Heat/cold Neck exercises Cervical collar Ultrasound/TENS/acupuncture Traction
Pharmacotherapy
Analgesics Muscle relaxants NSAIDs Local injection therapy

Fig. 6.3 Basic management program for cervical spondylosis with brachial root irritation.

and short-wave diathermy. If these modalities are ineffective, it is worth a trial of transcutaneous electronic nerve stimulation (TENS) or acupuncture. The gate theory of pain provides a rational basis for the use of TENS or acupuncture in intractable musculoskeletal pain, but neither measure has been shown predictably to provide relief.

Studies of traction have shown that at least 10kg is required to eliminate lordosis in the cervical spine. At this loading level, there is a 2–3mm increase in overall cervical length, which is preserved. Traction is reserved for situations where there are symptoms and signs of brachial root irritation.

In an otherwise healthy person, 10kg for 20min after local application of heat to relieve muscle spasm is usually effective. This treatment is usually repeated daily for a fortnight. Traction is contraindicated in patients with atlantoaxial subluxation or those with vertebrobasilar insufficiency.

Manipulation of the cervical spine is used by its devotees for those patients who have intractable symptoms, but disasters have been documented, especially when it is performed by the poorly trained or in situations of diagnostic uncertainty.

Analgesics, muscle relaxants and nonsteroidal anti-inflammatory drugs (NSAIDs) are useful in the management of cervical spine syndromes. Injection of local anesthetic and corticosteroid into areas of local tenderness about the lower neck, scapulae and shoulders may also be effective. As already stated, surgical intervention is rarely necessary. Indications include unremitting symptoms 4–6 months following documented disk prolapse, and clear progression of neurologic signs.

CONCLUSIONS

Brachial root irritation is a common rheumatologic problem that usually results from a combination of degenerative cervical disk disease and OA of the intervertebral joints. Once cervical myelopathy is excluded, pain and neurologic dysfunction in the arm are usually alleviated with conservative measures as part of a graduated program. Surgical intervention is rarely necessary.

REFERENCES

Bland JH. Disorders of the cervical spine. Diagnosis and medical management, 2E. Philadelphia: WB Saunders; 1994.

Holt L. Cervical, dorsal and lumbar spine syndromes. Acta Orthop Scand. 1954;(suppl 17):1–102.

Lawrence JS. Disc degeneration: its frequency and relationship to symptoms. Ann Rheum Dis. 1969;28:121–38.

Spurling RG, Seperberg LH. Intervertebral disc lesions in the lower cervical region. JAMA. 1953;151:354–9.

WHIPLASH INJURY

Les Barnsley

DEFINITION OF THE PROBLEM

Whiplash injury is common but lacks an accepted definition. The essential elements are that an injury occurs in a motor vehicle, the consequence of acceleration being applied to the head, which results in neck pain. Typically, neck pain following a whiplash injury is short-lived and settles with simple measures. However, a small proportion of patients have chronic, persistent, refractory and seemingly inexplicable symptoms, often without clear-cut physical findings or abnormalities on detailed imaging studies. These patients present major management and medicolegal problems.

THE TYPICAL CASE

BL is a 53-year-old steel worker. Three years ago, his car, while waiting at a stop light, was struck unexpectedly from behind by another vehicle. Over the next hour BL became aware of severe neck pain, centered at the base of his neck on the left. He was taken to the hospital where plain anteroposterior and functional lateral cervical spine radiographs were taken. These showed a loss of the normal lordosis but no bony injury. He had tenderness over the posterior neck, globally restricted neck movements but no neurologic abnormalities. He was prescribed a cervical collar and analgesics. However, he had no improvement and developed chronic neck pain centered to the left of the C6 spinous process. This was refractory to physical therapy, anti-inflammatory drugs and tricyclic antidepressants. He continued working but was unable to do any overtime and cut down on his usual leisure activities because of the pain. Several cervical computed tomography (CT) scans and repeat plain cervical radiographs were normal.

After 2 years, he was investigated with zygapophyseal joint blocks. Under double blind conditions, using contrasting local anesthetics, the medial branches of the left C5 and C6 dorsal rami were targetted to anesthetize the C5–C6 zygapophyseal joint. This relieved his neck pain for periods consistent with the anesthetics used. An intra-articular injection of betamethasone into the C5–C6 zygapophyseal joint provided incomplete relief for 2 weeks. He then had percutaneous radiofrequency neurotomy of the medial branches of the left C5 and C6 dorsal rami. This relieved his symptoms for 12 months, during which time his compensation case was settled in his favor. His pain has now returned and he is seeking a repeat procedure.

DIAGNOSTIC PROBLEMS

The investigation of whiplash injuries requires identification, in the first instance, of recognizable entities such as fracture, instability and spinal cord or nerve root compression. Fortunately these problems are usually apparent on routine clinical and radiologic assessment. However, some patients report chronic and disabling pain in the absence of obvious cause on physical examination or detailed imaging. It is now recognized that many serious bony, articular and ligamentous injuries can occur in whiplash (Fig. 6.4) and these may be undetectable on radiographs, CT

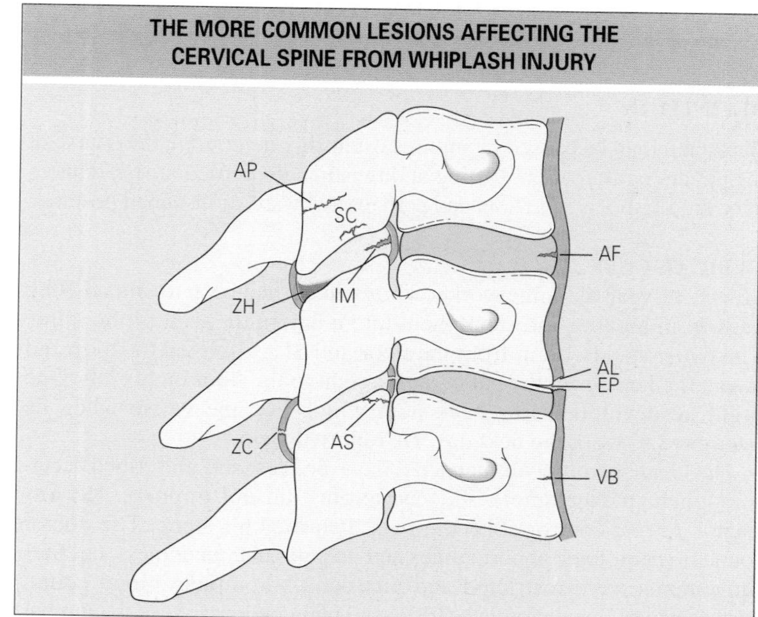

Fig. 6.4 A sketch of the more common lesions affecting the cervical spine from whiplash injury. AP: articular pillar fracture; SC: fracture of the subchondral plate; AF: tear of the annulus fibrosus of the intervertebral disk; ZH: hemarthrosis of the zygapophyseal joint; IM: contusion of the intra-articular meniscus of the zygapophyseal joint; AL: tear of the anterior longitudinal ligament; EP: end-plate avulsion and/or fracture; ZC: rupture of tear of the zygapophyseal joint capsule; AS: fracture involving the articular surface; VB: vertebral body fracture. Adapted with permission from Spine, State of the Art Reviews 1993;7.

or MRI. In particular, injuries to the cervical zygapophyseal joints and intervertebral disks have the potential to cause chronic symptoms with no obvious clinical or radiologic findings. These patients can be investigated with invasive techniques such as zygapophyseal joint blocks or diagnostic disk injection (diskography) that address the pain directly. Careful application of these techniques, with blinding and internal controls, permits the majority of patients with chronic pain following whiplash to be given a definitive, anatomic diagnosis, with over 50% of patients likely to have cervical zygapophyseal joint pain. Patients should always have this diagnosis explored first before embarking on diagnostic disk injection because of the latter technique's predilection to false-positive results.

It is inappropriate to investigate aggressively all patients with early whiplash, as approximately 75–80% will settle with conservative treatment, and should be reassured that this is the case. Where the cervical zygapophyseal joints are established as a source of pain, the patient can have their pain controlled with radiofrequency denervation (see Chapter 4.4). For discogenic pain, there are no validated, efficacious therapeutic options. However, establishing a legitimate anatomic diagnosis may provide reassurance and enable appropriate medicolegal settlement to be expedited.

There are some individuals who use a supposed whiplash injury as a lever for financial gain. However, fraudulent malingerers are in a small minority and may be identified by having inconsistencies between what is reported and what is observed, displaying exaggerated and inconsistent responses to examination, particularly palpation, and reporting responses to invasive investigations that are inexplicable on anatomic, physiologic or pharmacologic grounds. However, the overwhelming majority of patients with chronic neck pain after whiplash harbor genuine injuries that are not 'cured by a verdict'.

THERAPEUTIC OPTIONS

For those patients with cervical zygapophyseal joint pain, the use of intra-articular corticosteroid injections been shown to be ineffective in a controlled trial. Percutaneous radiofrequency neurotomy of the medial branches of the cervical dorsal rami has been shown to be effective in a randomised, placebo-controlled trial. No techniques have proven efficacy for the management of diskogenic pain, although diskectomy and fusion has been adopted by some. Patients being offered any of these treatments must have their diagnosis established beyond question, must be carefully counseled about the current status of these techniques and must be provided with realistic estimates of the likelihood of success and adverse effects.

For those patients without an anatomic diagnosis after the zygapophyseal joints and disks have been investigated, or who fail targeted treatment, there is no indication for further investigation. Their treatment should involve a multidisciplinary rehabilitation team, emphasizing improvement in fitness and function, encouraging return to work and providing strategies for pain management using psychologic, pharmacologic and physical techniques.

CONCLUSIONS

Patients with chronic neck pain after whiplash injury may have chronic painful injuries to the cervical zygapophyseal joints or intervertebral disks that can only be detected with invasive investigation. An anatomic diagnosis may assist in the just settlement of a compensation claim but the pathology underlying arthrogenic or diskogenic pain is not known. The diagnosis of cervical zygapophyseal joint pain should be sought as efficacious treatment is available. Otherwise treatment should be based on a rehabilitation model.

REFERENCES

Barnsley L, Lord S, Bogduk N. Whiplash injury. Pain. 1994;59:283–307.

Barnsley L, Lord S, Bogduk N. The prevalence of chronic cervical zygapophyseal joint pain after whiplash. Spine. 1995;20:20–5.

Jónsson H Jr, Bring G, Rauschning W, Sahlstedt B. Hidden cervical spine injuries in traffic accident victims with skull fractures. J Spinal Disord. 1991;4:251–63.

Spitzer WO, Skovron ML, Salmi LR, *et al.* Quebec Taskforce on Whiplash-associated Disorders. Redefining 'whiplash' and its management. Spine 1995;20(suppl.8):1–73.

WORK-RELATED LOW BACK PAIN

Nikolai Bogduk

DEFINITION

Back pain may be caused by injuries ostensibly incurred in the course of the patient's occupation. Lifting and twisting are particular risk maneuvers, but so, too, is vibration, and perhaps awkward or sustained postures.

TYPICAL CASE

SL is a 39-year-old mine worker whose duties had been to unload 10kg kegs from a pallet and stack them into a bay in the wall of the mine. The pallet stands 12cm from the floor and SL is obliged to stoop and swing the kegs from the pallet on his right to the floor on his left. One night he developed low back pain which became worse when he attempted to work the next day. He reported sick.

His local doctor recommended 2 days' bed rest and prescribed acetaminophen (paracetamol). SL's symptoms did not improve. He was unable to rest comfortably; the pain disturbed his sleep. The doctor found no neurologic abnormalities and no particular tenderness, but SL's movements were restricted and guarded. A complete blood count, erythrocyte sedimenation rate (ESR) and plain radiographs of the lumbar spine were all reported as normal. The doctor recommended physical therapy.

Hot packs and ultrasound were used to ease the pain, followed by ergonomic instruction and mobilizing exercises. A TENS machine afforded some relief but SL complained that the pain was still present 'deep inside'. Flexion and extension exercises were prescribed, but SL could not endure sit-ups because these aggravated his pain.

Seen by the company doctor, SL was instructed to attend a work-hardening program. Meanwhile, his local doctor ordered a CT scan, but this was negative. Although he enrolled in the work-hardening program, SL discharged himself after 3 days because he could not tolerate the aggravation of his pain. He turned to an acupuncturist who provided some relief during therapy but this wore off usually by the time SL arrived home. He received no greater pain relief from NSAIDs than from acetaminophen. When his pain was severe he had to call his local doctor to administer intramuscular meperidine (pethidine). Otherwise he became accustomed to taking 12 tablets a day of an acetaminophen–codeine mixture.

A board of insurance doctors found no abnormalities on physical examination and CT, and deemed SL fit for work. The company physician sought to find SL lighter duties, but all above-ground positions were fully occupied. SL was not able to tolerate his usual duties for more than an hour. He ceased work.

SL returned for more physical therapy. He tried chiropractic but felt worse after the treatment. Constipation became a problem. He was notified by his insurance company that they would no longer pay benefits. SL's lawyer advised him to persevere with physical therapy and arranged several consultations with specialists; CT scans were repeated but were reported as normal. One specialist recommended an intertransverse fusion; another advised against surgery. No working diagnosis was formulated, although all the specialists agreed that SL was suffering pain. However, the insurance doctors reaffirmed that there was nothing wrong with SL. A psychiatrist reported that SL was suffering abnormal illness behavior. The lawyer elected to proceed to trial in order to have SL's benefits reinstated.

DIAGNOSTIC PROBLEM

When back pain is the problem, and the patient has no history, signs or symptoms of a medical disorder, clinical examination cannot be diagnostic. Neither can radiographs or CT scans. Typically they show either no abnormalities or only false-positive findings. However, by the same token, neither can physical examination and investigations prove that a patient does not have an injury and does not suffer pain.

For occupational back pain the choice lies between relying on natural history or pursuing the diagnosis with advanced means. The chances are that in most cases back pain will resolve in a matter of days or weeks, regardless of investigation or treatment. However, persistence or increase of pain begs intensive investigation lest the patient become psychologically and socially disabled. In that case, the question is – what is the source of pain? Radiographs and CT do not answer this question; nor does electromyography.

THERAPEUTIC OPTIONS

The contemporary fashion is to treat idiopathic back pain empirically with a variety of techniques – physical therapy modalities, exercises of the flexion or extension variety, mobilization, manipulation or back school. Yet the evidence for the efficacy of any these techniques is either weak or missing. There is little evidence that the apparent success is due to anything more than the natural history or other factors. Interestingly, a supportive and welcoming personnel achieves much in reducing claims and achieving return to work. Functional restoration programs appear to have been successful in some centers of the United States, but there is no evidence that similar centers elsewhere offer the same quality of service, achieve the same apparent success or can do so at costs that other societies can afford.

Although many patients do respond to intervention, a proportion remain with pain and defy conservative programs. For these patients there is no established option, and most end up recycling through futile attempts at therapy; some undergo attempts at surgery without an anatomic diagnosis having been made.

For the pursuit of an anatomic diagnosis, a variety of invasive procedures are available. Putative sources of pain can be investigated using zygapophyseal joint blocks, sacroiliac joint blocks and disk stimulation. Collectively, these procedures can pinpoint the source of pain in over 60% of patients with chronic low back pain. However, although this may be satisfying intellectually or for medicolegal purposes, none of these diagnostic procedures at present leads to any proven therapy.

CONCLUSION

SL was eventually referred to a spine unit. Zygapophyseal joint blocks were performed but did not relieve his pain. An MRI, however, revealed a high-intensity zone in his L4–L5 intervertebral disk (Fig. 6.5). Provocation diskography and disko-CT confirmed the presence of painful internal disk disruption (IDD) (Fig. 6.6). SL was offered an anterior interbody fusion, but having been informed of the success rate he declined. He remains in pain, awaiting the outcome of his trial, hoping that the court will accept that his IDD was work-related.

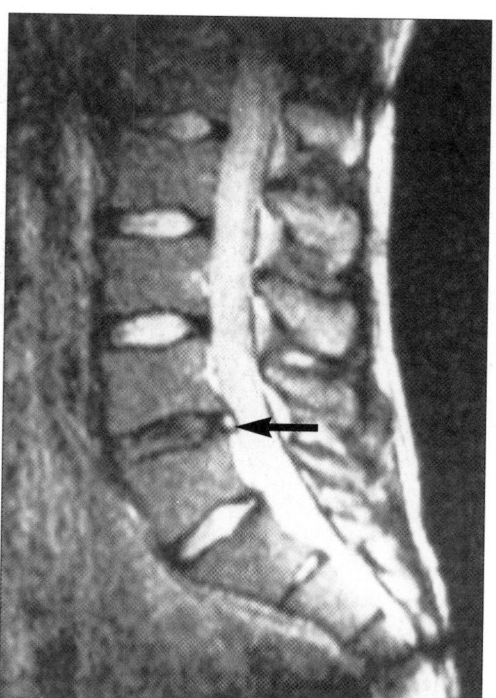

Fig. 6.5 MRI showing a high intensity zone lesion (arrow) in the L4–L5 intervertebral disc.

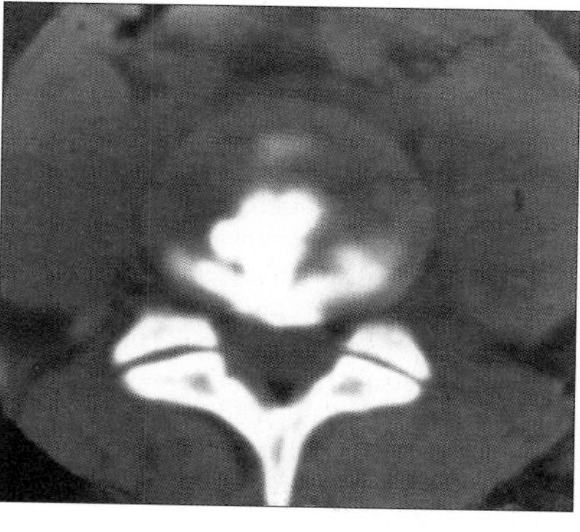

Fig. 6.6 Postdiscography CT scan of the disc in Fig. 6.5 showing a painful grade 4 disruption of the annulus.

REFERENCES

Aprill C, Bogduk N. High intensity zone: a pathognomonic sign of painful lumbar disc on MRI. Br J Radiol. 1992;65:361–9.

Bogduk N, Mercer S. Selection and application of treatment. In: Refshauge KM, Gass EM, eds. Musculoskeletal physiotherapy. Clinical science and practice. Oxford: Butterworth Heinemann; 1995:169–81.

Hazard RG. Spine update. Functional restoration. Spine. 1995;20:2345–8.

Schwarzer AC, Aprill CN, Bogduk N. The sacroiliac joint in chronic low back pain. Spine 1995;20:31–7.

Schwarzer AC, Aprill CN, Derby R, *et al.* Clinical features of patients with pain stemming from the lumbar zygapophyseal joints. Is the lumbar facet syndrome a clinical entity? Spine. 1994;19:1132–7.

Schwarzer AC, Aprill CN, Derby R, *et al.* The prevalence and clinical features of internal disc disruption in patients with chronic low back pain. Spine. 1995;20:1878–83.

Turner JA, Ersek M, Herron L, *et al.* Patient outcomes after lumbar spinal fusions. JAMA. 1992;268:907–11.

Wood DJ: Design and evaluation of a back injury prevention program within a geriatric hospital. Spine. 1987;12:77–82.

DEFINITION OF THE PROBLEM

Most patients who present with acute low back pain have a mechanical cause for their symptoms. Their pain is secondary to overuse of a normal anatomic structure (muscle strain), or to pathologic deformity of an anatomic structure (herniated nucleus pulposus). Diagnostic radiographic and laboratory tests are not required for the initial evaluation. However, the rapid evolution of progressive symptoms during follow up, or the occurrence of new physical findings suggesting increased neural compression or a systemic medical disorder, require prompt re-evaluation of the initial mechanical diagnosis.

THE TYPICAL CASE

AS, a 43-year-old man, presented with a 1-week history of acute low back pain. He was in his usual state of good health until he developed left-sided low back pain after a session of karate exercises. He noticed the pain onset after he had kicked with his left leg. The pain radiated into the thigh but not below the knee. The pain increased and he had difficulty getting out of bed. He was placed on ibuprofen and cyclobenzaprine without improvement. He denied any sensory or motor changes in the leg. He denied any constitutional symptoms.

His general physical examination was entirely within normal limits. Examination of the appendicular skeleton revealed a 1cm leg-length discrepancy that had been noted previously. Lumbosacral spine motion revealed flexion to 10° with marked bilateral paraspinous muscle contraction, extension of 5° without pain, lateral bending to 10° with paraspinous pain. Straight-leg raising tests in the seated and supine position were negative. The neurologic examination, including sensory, motor and reflex functions, was normal. The patient was given the diagnosis of acute musculoskeletal strain secondary to his exercises. His medical therapy was modified. He was told to contact his physician if there was an exacerbation of symptoms. He was to be re-evaluated in 2 weeks.

He returned 2 weeks later with increased pain in the low back and increasing pain in the right anterior thigh. He denied changes in constitutional symptoms or alterations in bowel or bladder habits. His physical examination revealed a markedly positive femoral stretch test, with pain radiating into the anterior thigh. He had a minimal decrease in the strength of the right thigh. An MRI scan was obtained within 24 hours.

The MRI demonstrated a mass lesion replacing the L4 vertebral body (Fig. 6.7). Soft tissue extension was present but the disk space was spared. The cauda equina was diffusely compressed centrally by the mass lesion (Fig. 6.8). The mass was biopsied by CT guidance. Malignant plasma cells were detected upon pathologic review of the biopsy. The diagnosis of a plasmacytoma was made. Concern about the stability of the spine and possible compression of the cauda equina necessitated the need for a surgical procedure to stabilize the spine with instrumentation (Fig. 6.9). The patient left the hospital 1 week after the stabilization without any back or leg pain.

DIAGNOSTIC PROBLEMS

The differential diagnosis for low back pain according to the patient's age is shown in Chapter 4.3 (Fig. 3.1). Mechanical abnormalities remain the most likely cause of back pain in a man in his fifth decade. Other possibilities include a late onset spondyloarthropathy, a benign bone tumor, an infection or referred pain (e.g. due to peptic ulcer disease). The patient originally presents with a history and physical examination suggestive of mechanical low back pain. However, within a short period of time he develops pain on the contralateral side. In addition, he develops neurologic signs of radiculopathy in a femoral nerve distribution. In a young individual, a herniated disk is the most likely cause of radiculopathy. The L3 and L4 nerve roots are less frequently affected than L5 and S1. Medical causes of low back pain must be considered in a patient with acute changes in neurologic function. Infections and neoplasms are the most likely medical disorders in a young patient. These disorders were thought to be unlikely in this instance because of the lack of constitutional symptoms.

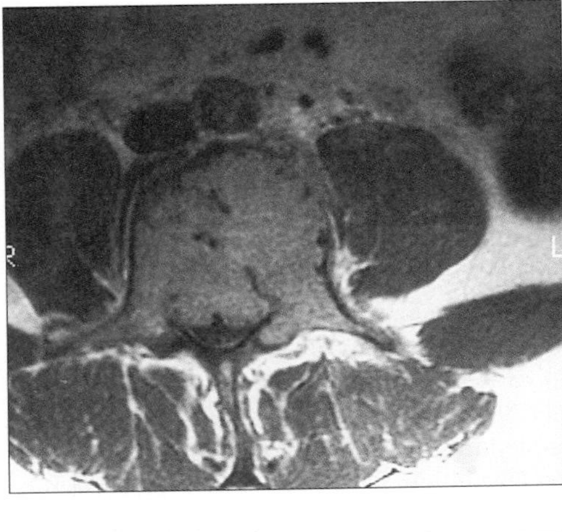

Fig. 6.8 Plasmacytoma. MRI scan, axial view, revealing replacement of the vertebral body and pedicles with a homogeneous mass. The mass has extended into the spinal canal, compressing the cauda equina.

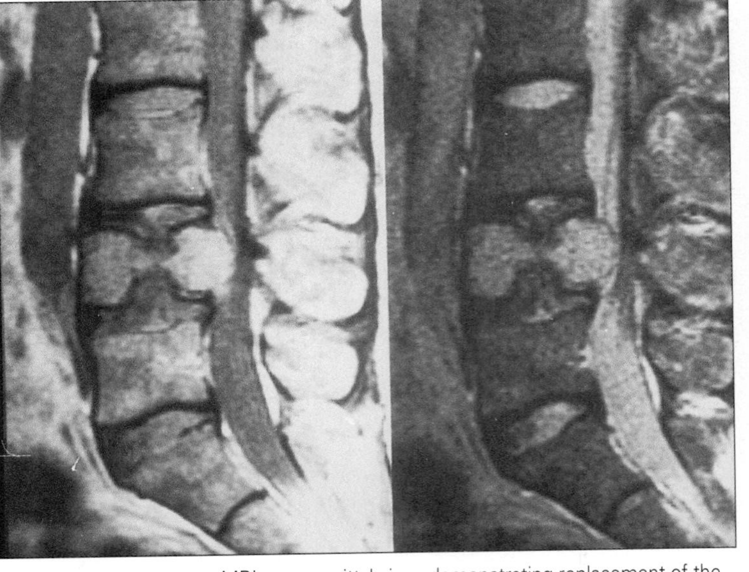

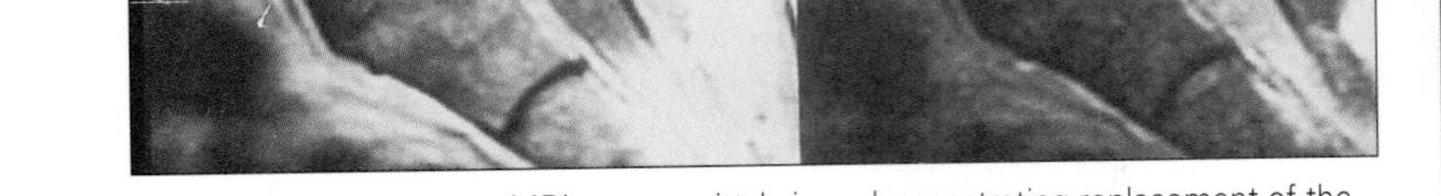

Fig. 6.7 Plasmacytoma. MRI scan, sagittal view, demonstrating replacement of the vertebral body with a mass lesion extending into the spinal canal.

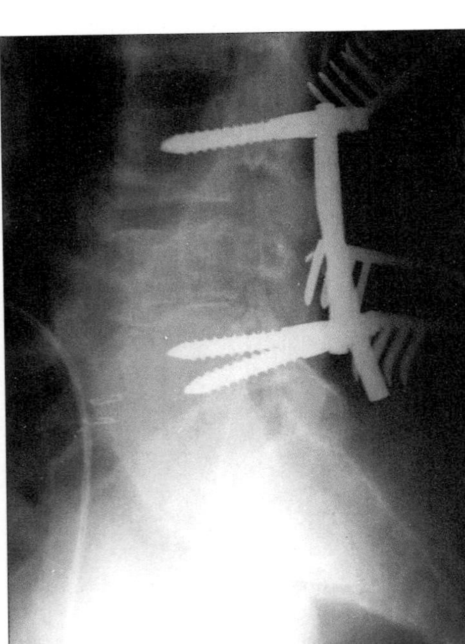

Fig. 6.9 Plasmacytoma. Postoperative plain radiograph, lateral view, demonstrating placement of rods to stabilize the spine and prevent neurologic damage.

Many imaging procedures are available for the diagnosis of low back pain. Plain radiographs are not helpful for most mechanical disorders but may provide a clue to the diagnosis of systemic disorders that affect older individuals. Plain radiographs in the present patient revealed diffuse osteopenia and disruption of the osseous borders of the L4 vertebral body. A MRI detects specific anatomic lesions in the lumbar spine with greater sensitivity than any other imaging modality. It is an excellent method for detecting both mechanical and medical disorders affecting the lumbar spine. An MRI scan images the cauda equina and vertebral column, documents the presence of herniated disk, and the extent of nerve root compression. However, the limitations to MRI include metal pins or clips in patients that may be dislodged because of the strong magnetic field created by the machine, claustrophobia and the cost of the procedure. In contrast to MRI, CT requires ionizing radiation and is sensitive only to the resolution of the radiographic cut. Computed tomography is more sensitive for defining the trabecular architecture of bone than for soft tissue structures surrounding the spinal column. Bone scan is a sensitive, but nonspecific, technique to detect increased bone metabolism caused by infection, tumor or inflammation. Bone scan is normal in most instances of myeloma of the spine secondary to the absence of osteoblastic activity.

THERAPEUTIC OPTIONS

The chief factor in the treatment of the patient with medical low back pain is the identification of the symptoms and signs as unrelated to a mechanical disorder. Establishing the diagnosis using laboratory and radiographic techniques is critical to the initiation of therapy. Choice of therapy will be dictated by the underlying medical condition giving rise to back pain.

CONCLUSIONS

A mechanical origin can be found for 90% of low back pain. A small but significant proportion of lumbosacral spine disorders are related to medical illnesses. The key to detecting the presence of a medical cause of low back pain is continuously re-examining the patient and being mindful of significant changes in history or physical examination. When these changes occur, expeditious evaluation of the patient using radiographic and laboratory techniques can result in a timely and appropriate diagnosis.

REFERENCES

Carlson K, Astrom G, Nyman R, *et al.* MR imaging of multiple myeloma in tumor mass measurement at diagnosis and during treatment. Acta Radiol. 1995;36:9–14.

Deyo RA, Bigos SJ, Maravilla KR. Diagnostic imaging procedures for the lumbar spine. Ann Intern Med. 1989;111:865–7.

Erly WK, Carmody RF. MRI of the spine. Crit Rev Diagn Imaging. 1994;35:313–77.

Schreiman JS, McLeod RA, Kyle RA, *et al.* Multiple myeloma: evaluation by CT. Radiology. 1985;154:483–6.

Steiner RM, Mitchell DG, Rao VS, *et al.* Magnetic resonance imaging of bone marrow. Diagnostic value in diffuse hematologic disorders. Magn Reson Q. 1990;6:17–34.

DISC SPACE INFECTION CAUSING LOW BACK PAIN

James Weinstein

DEFINITION OF THE PROBLEM

Spinal infections involving the vertebrae and the intervertebral discs, usually referred to as disc space infections because of the characteristic radiographic appearance, are rare causes of low back pain. However, they frequently mimic idiopathic low back pain. Because untreated spinal infection can result in systemic sepsis, neurologic deficit and spinal deformity, early diagnosis is critical.

THE TYPICAL CASE

DB, a 59-year-old farmer, presented with complaints of increasing lower back and vague abdominal pain, generalized weakness and malaise for 6 weeks. Eight weeks previously he had had dysuria and pyuria due to *Escherichia coli* which was treated successfully with antibiotics. Radiographs of the pelvis and lumbar spine at that time did not show any abnormalities. Four weeks ago he was evaluated by his physician and treated with analgesics and activity restriction for idiopathic low back. Despite this treatment his pain increased. He denied use of intravenous drugs and had no history of previous spine surgery or injections. He did report several episodes of chills followed by fever.

Examination showed a healthy man with a soft, nontender abdomen, normal rectal tone, no tenderness over his lumbar spine and no lumbar muscle spasm. Sensory examination did not show any abnormalities and motor examination revealed normal strength throughout his upper and lower extremities, with the exception of slightly decreased hip flexor strength bilaterally. Pulses and reflexes were symmetric, but he did have a bilateral positive straight leg raising test that caused back pain and abdominal discomfort. His temperature was 38.1°C, pulse 74 per min, respirations 20 per min and blood pressure 115/68mmHg. Hemoglobin was 11.3g/dL (113g/L), hematocrit 34%, white cell count 10,400mm^{-3} (10.4 × 10^{9}L^{-1}) with 79% neutrophils and ESR 121mm/h. Radiographs (Fig. 6.10) showed narrowing of the L5–S1 disc space with some irregularity of the end plates of L5 and S1 and anterior displacement of the bifurcation of the aorta, suggesting a disc space infection with a soft tissue abscess. A CT scan showed bilateral psoas abscesses (see Fig. 6.11).

Percutaneous aspiration of the left psoas abscess revealed purulent material. Cultures of the aspirate grew α-hemolytic streptococci, confirming the diagnosis of streptococcal L5–S1 disc space infection. The psoas abscesses were drained surgically and the patient treated with intravenous antibiotics. His symptoms resolved over the next 10 days with no residual disability at 6 months after surgical treatment.

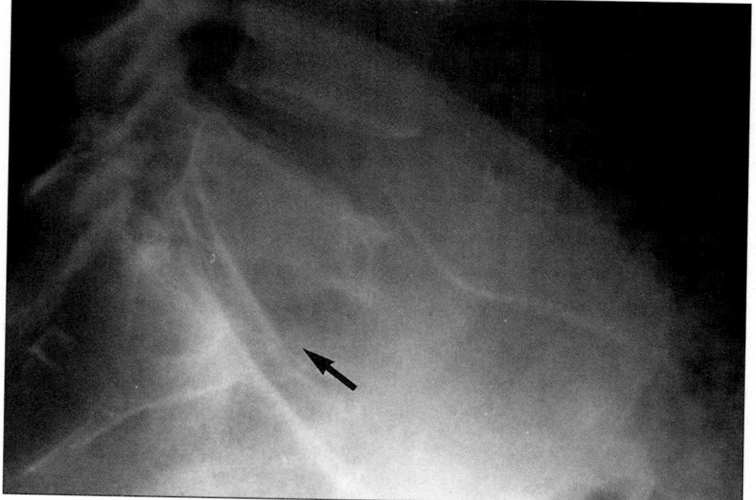

Fig. 6.10 Plain radiograph of the lumbar spine. Lateral radiograph showing narrowing of the L5–S1 disc space with new bone formation at the L5 end plate (arrow) and a soft tissue mass pushing the great vessels anteriorly. This finding of narrowing of the disc space and new bone formation with displacement of the great vessels strongly suggests the diagnosis of spinal infection with a soft tissue abscess.

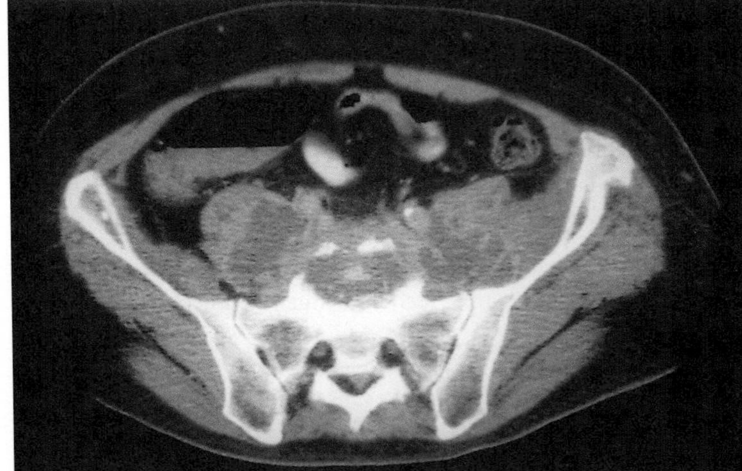

Fig. 6.11 CT of the lumbar spine. At the L5/S1 level lucent areas in both psoas muscles and destructive changes in the intervertebral disc space suggest the presence of spinal infection with bilateral abscesses.

DIAGNOSTIC PROBLEMS

Although a number of serious conditions, including benign and malignant tumors, Paget's disease, vascular disease, infections and fractures, cause discomfort in the lower back, most patients who present with low back pain do not have underlying medical disease and their symptoms will improve spontaneously. The history of a previous infection, and in particular a urinary tract infection with abdominal symptoms, suggests the possibility of disc space infection, although in this case the urinary tract infection was apparently not related to the spinal infection. Pyogenic infections of the lower spine usually present with persistent increasing pain. Pyrexia, local tenderness, muscle spasm, constitutional symptoms and neurologic deficits may or may not be present. Pain radiating to the abdomen or both legs and the presence of abdominal discomfort and symptoms may confuse the diagnosis. The prevalence of paraplegia or paraparesis varies from 3% to 15% in different series. In these patients radiculopathy may also be present.

In a recently reported series of 80 patients with spinal infection, *Mycobacterium tuberculosis* caused 31 (39%) of the infections, gram-negative bacilli 16 (20%), *Staphylococcus* species 15 (19%), *Streptococcus* species 15 (19%) and *Corynebacterium* species 1 (1%). The pathogens in the other 8 patients (10%) were not identified. The ESR is almost universally elevated in cases of established disc space infections, often exceeding 100mm/h. The white cell count may also be elevated and some patients may have positive blood cultures.

Early in the disorder radiographs may be normal. The radiographic evidence of established disc space infection includes:

- symmetric destruction of adjacent end plate surfaces of two vertebrae;
- loss of disc height;
- reactive new bone formation;
- sclerosis of bone end plates, with or without evidence of bone destruction or bone formation;
- soft tissue abscesses; and
- kyphosis or subluxation after there has been significant bone destruction.

On CT, changes in the disc space and vertebral end plates can be seen as can soft tissue abscesses. Needle biopsy of the disc space or a paraspinous abscess can make the diagnosis. However, the success rate for this procedure varies considerably among reported series. Needle biopsy may also be helped by CT imaging.

The early diagnosis of a disc space infection requires a high level of clinical suspicion. Any patient in whom this possibility is considered should have blood cultures, urine cultures, a complete blood count, ESR and AP and lateral radiographs of the spine. The radiographs may show evidence of soft tissue expansion around the disc before there is any evidence of bony change or loss of disc height. A bone scan may be helpful, showing a localized hot spot before radiographic change, and spinal MRI may show the abscess and disc space changes in the early stage of evolution. In addition, CT scans, as carried out in this case, may help delineate the anatomic changes.

THERAPEUTIC OPTIONS

Six weeks of parenteral antibiotics and possibly additional oral antibiotic therapy usually provides adequate treatment for patients with radiologic evidence of disc space infection and a positive culture. During the acute phase a short course of bed rest is also indicated and patients who have severe muscle spasm or pain may benefit from the use of a light corset. The ESR provides a method of assessing the efficacy of therapy in these patients.

Surgical intervention, including drainage and debridement of spinal infections, is indicated in patients who develop paraparesis or paraplegia. The following factors appear to increase the risk of neurologic deficits:

- older age,
- cervical or thoracic infection,
- staphylococcal infection as opposed to other organisms, and
- coexisting diabetes or RA.

Other possible indications for surgical debridement and possibly fusions in patients with spinal infections include severe back pain and muscle spasm that do not respond to appropriate antibiotic treatment, uncertainty as to the diagnosis, and extensive bone destruction with significant deformity, especially if bone destruction and deformity progress during antibiotic therapy. Use of bone grafts in an attempt to achieve bony fusion in spinal infections is controversial, although in one series of patients anterior debridement with or without bone grafting produced superior results as compared with nonsurgical management. The authors recommend resection of purulent material and necrotic bone followed by bone grafting.

CONCLUSIONS

Infection of the spine is an uncommon cause of low back pain. Pyogenic infections of the spine may present in otherwise healthy individuals with no history of previous spinal disorder or in patients with a history of other infections, spine or paraspinous injections or spinal surgery. They also present in individuals with a history of intravenous drug use. In individuals with a history of persistent low back pain, positive cultures and characteristic radiographic changes can establish the diagnosis of spinal infection. Prolonged antibiotic therapy and in some patients use of an orthosis are the essential elements of therapy. The principal controversy in the treatment of spinal infections concerns surgical versus nonsurgical treatment. When surgical treatment is selected there is also controversy about the use of bone grafts to achieve bony fusion.

REFERENCES

Bonfiglio M, Lange TA, Kim YM. Pyogenic vertebral osteomyelitis. Clin Orthop. 1973;96:234–47.

Eismont FJ, Bohlman HH, Soni PL, *et al.* Pyogenic and fungal vertebral osteomyelitis with paralysis. J Bone Jt Surg. 1983;65:19–29.

Krodel A, Sturz H, Siebert CH. Indications for and results of operative treatment of spondylitis and spondlyodiscitis. Arch Orthop Trauma Surg. 1991;110:78–82.

Perrone C, Saba J, Behloul Z, *et al.* Pyogenic and tuberculus spondylodiskitis (vertebral osteomyelitis) in 80 adult patients. Clin Infect Dis. 1994;19:746–50.

Ryan MD, Taylor TKF. The bacteriologic diagnosis and antibiotic treatment of hematogenous vertebral osteomyelitis in adults. Aust NZ J Surg. 1978;48:81–3.

DEFINITION OF THE PROBLEM

Coccydynia is a symptom not a diagnosis. It is defined as pain in and around the coccygeal region, particularly when sitting and rising from a sitting position. The female to male ratio is 5:1. The coccyx is more prominent in women and is more prone to injury or repetitive stresses. However, only 25% of patients give a history of direct trauma; 10% of cases present following childbirth.

THE TYPICAL CASE

CC is a 30-year-old woman who presented to her family physician with a 1-year history of increasing discomfort around the 'tailbone'. She was unable to sit on a chair for more than a few minutes and invariably perched on one buttock. The discomfort was such that she dreaded going to the theater or restaurants. There was no history of injury. Her physician prescribed NSAIDs and advised the use of a cushion. Her pain persisted and at subsequent consultations it was implied she was a very 'anxious' woman. She was told that nothing further could be done.

Finally, at her own insistence she was referred for a specialist opinion. On examination there was an exquisite tenderness on palpation of the coccyx. Movement of the coccyx at per rectum examination again caused pain but there was no other rectal abnormality. Lumbar spine movement was full, with no neurologic signs in the lower limbs. In view of the severity of the pain, radiographs of the sacrum and coccyx were taken. These were normal. A diagnosis was made of coccydynia due to localized musculoskeletal disorder. The option of outpatient cortisone and local anesthetic injection around the coccyx was discussed, but CC preferred to proceed with a manipulation and injection of the coccyx under general anesthesia. After infiltration around the coccyx with 10ml 0.5% bupivacaine and 2ml methylprednisone acetate, the coccyx was firmly extended and flexed for approximately 30 seconds using the index finger per rectum. Over the following 24 hours there was a moderate increase in discomfort but over the following 3 weeks there was progressive improvement. After 6 weeks CC was sitting normally and was particularly delighted that, after hearing so many negative comments from medical practitioners, she had finally been successfully treated. One year later she remained asymptomatic.

DIAGNOSTIC PROBLEMS

The key to successful treatment of coccydynia is to be precise about making the diagnosis. Pain radiating towards the buttocks from the lumbar spine is not coccydynia. The diagnosis of coccydynia should only be made if the pain is directly related to the coccyx. The overwhelming majority of cases are idiopathic in that no pathology can be demonstrated. There are rare causes such as chordoma and giant cell tumor, and unusual persistence of pain should alert the physician to these possibilities. Under such circumstances radiographs are indicated, but it has clearly been shown that the shape of the coccyx has no bearing on the incidence of idiopathic coccydynia. Particular care should be taken if there is pain around the coccyx with sensory changes and yet no tenderness to palpation. A cauda equina tumor is a possibility (Fig. 6.12). A high index of suspicion is needed when treating men with apparent coccydynia. Typical coccydynia is unusual in males and there is a high incidence of more sinister pathology, including prostatitis and rectal carcinoma.

Care also has to be taken in the interpretation of scans. It has been postulated that coccydynia is referred pain from the lumbosacral spine. Imaging of the lumbar spine will often reveal pathology but this will almost always be coincidental. The literature abounds with reports of asymptomatic disc prolapse and the demonstration of disc prolapse or degeneration in a patient with coccydynia is usually irrelevant. Pain around the coccyx and tenderness to palpation indicates a local problem. The overwhelming majority of women presenting with coccydynia fall into this category. Coccydynia has been likened to a 'tennis elbow of the "tailbone"'.

THERAPEUTIC OPTIONS

Coccydynia has an undeserved reputation as being difficult to treat. Patients have been labeled as neurotic, and yet it is really the symptoms that have not been understood. First, it must be established that the coccydynia is 'idiopathic' and not one of the cases where there is serious pathology. If the coccydynia is the result of recent trauma then analgesics or NSAIDs may suffice. Advice should be given to sit upright on a chair; slouching simply aggravates the coccygeal area. Physical therapy may be indicated in early cases, utilizing ultrasound or short-wave diathermy. Chronic coccygeal pain responds far less readily to physical therapy. Manipulative therapy as used by the physical therapist or chiropractor is often too painful to be tolerated. Some 60% of patients will respond to an injection of corticosteroid and local anesthetic, with infiltration generally around the coccyx. There is no need specifically to try to inject the sacrococcygeal joint. The most effective therapy is to perform a manipulation and injection under a short general anesthetic. Such treatment has an 85% success rate. Up to 20% of successfully treated patients will relapse within a year but the majority of such patients

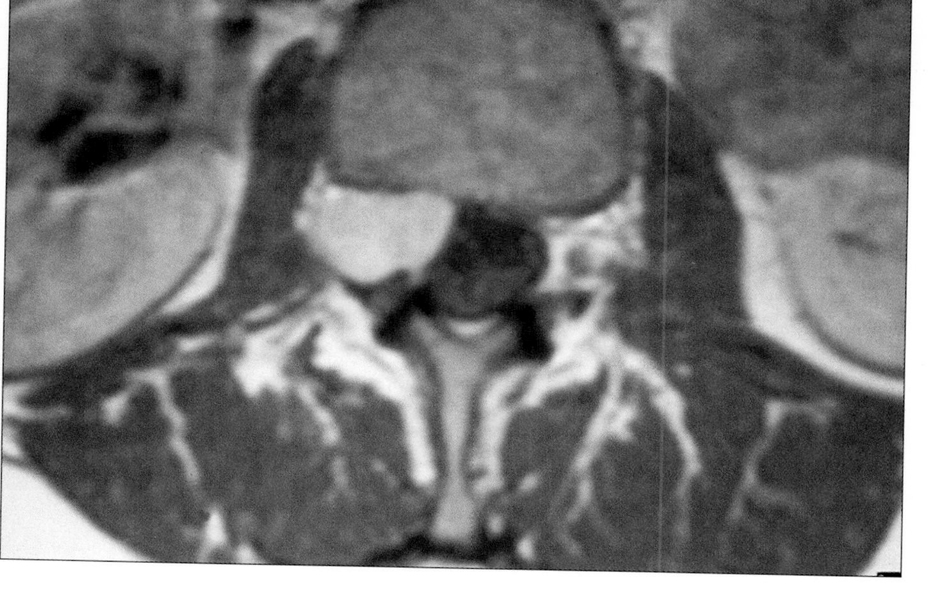

Fig. 6.12 MRI of caudal neurofibroma. Transverse T1-weighted MRI following intravenous gadolinium shows an enhancing mass occluding the right neural foramen of L2. Note how local bone erosion has widened the neural foramen.

respond well to further manipulation and injection.

If followed for prolonged periods, up to 20% of patients with chronic coccydynia continue with discomfort despite conservative therapy. If the pain is severe and typical (pain with sitting and tenderness to palpation), then coccygectomy is indicated. The mobile coccygeal segments are excised and any bony prominences smoothed down. It can take 3 months or longer for the tenderness following surgery to subside, but the overall success rate is over 90%. Patients with a particularly prominent coccyx can be considered for surgery without undue delay as there is a tendency for such patients to be resistant to conservative measures.

Persistent pain following coccygectomy is rare, but possibly relates to a neuralgic state. In such situations cryotherapy is an effective treatment, while neurosurgical ablation of the distal sacral nerves is the ultimate salvage procedure.

CONCLUSIONS

Coccydynia is a neglected problem for which there is treatment. A successful outcome depends upon a precise clinical diagnosis. Manipulation and injection offers the highest success rate. Beware of men with coccydynia.

REFERENCES

Bohm E, Franksson C. Coccygodynia and sacral rhizotomy. Acta Chir Scand. 1958;116:268–74.

Wray CC, Easom S, Hoskinson J. Coccydynia. Aetiology and treatment. J Bone Jt Surg. 1991;73B:335–8.

THE SHOULDER

Seamus E Dalton

- Shoulder motion involves four articulations: the glenohumeral, acromioclavicular, and scapulothoracic.
- The stability of the shoulder is provided by ligaments and the rotator cuff muscles.
- Common shoulder disorders include rotator cuff tendinitis, rotator cuff tears, capsulitis (frozen shoulder), glenohumeral arthritis, and acromioclavicular syndromes.
- Most shoulder conditions can be diagnosed clinically by a careful history and physical examination. In tendon conditions there is pain on active and resisted motion and passive range of motions tends to be normal. In early capsulitis and glenohumeral arthritis all active and passive motions are painful, there is no pain on resisted motion, and passive motion is decreased.

FUNCTIONAL ANATOMY

The clavicle, scapula and humerus make up the bony skeleton of the shoulder girdle, the relationship of which with the axial skeleton is maintained largely through muscular attachments and also the articulation of the clavicle with the thoracic cage at the sternoclavicular joint. Shoulder movement occurs through many planes and is achieved through motion at four articulations; the glenohumeral, acromioclavicular, sternoclavicular and scapulothoracic. Some constraint is also afforded to the head of the humerus through the subacromial joint by the overlying acromion and coracoacromial ligament. The glenohumeral joint is a multiaxial joint that allows the greatest freedom of movement of any joint of the body, although this is at the expense of stability. The bones of the shoulder girdle combine to provide a mobile framework upon which glenohumeral motion can take place.

Ligamentous support is important in maintaining the stability of the joints of the shoulder and allowing synchronous movements to take place. Muscles act as prime movers at the shoulder as well as providing some dynamic stability to the glenohumeral joint.

GLENOHUMERAL JOINT

The glenohumeral joint is not a true ball and socket joint and allows a certain amount of gliding movement, which is increased when there is laxity of the musculoligamentous support to the joint. Inherent bony stability is poor due to the shallow glenoid fossa and larger humeral head. The glenoid labrum is a rim of fibrocartilage at the periphery of the glenoid which effectively deepens the glenoid fossa and increases its diameter and contact with the humeral head, thereby affording some increased stability (Fig. 7.1). The joint capsule is lax, especially inferiorly, which allows rotation and elevation. In conditions where this capsule contracts there is restriction of glenohumeral motion. Restriction in this capsule posteriorly can aggravate or even give rise to secondary impingement.

The joint capsule is thickened anteriorly to form separate components known as the glenohumeral ligaments, which act to strengthen the anterior and inferior capsule. The superior glenohumeral ligament runs from the anterosuperior aspect of the glenoid to the proximal edge of the lesser tuberosity of the humerus, with the middle glenohumeral ligament running just below this.

The inferior glenohumeral ligament runs from the anteromedial aspect of the glenoid to the distal edge of the lesser tuberosity and proximal shaft of the humerus and has three components[1]. It is important in the provision of anteroinferior stability to the joint, particularly with the arm in abduction and external rotation, and has also been shown to provide some posterior stability[2]. Deficiencies in this ligament complex are important in the development of instability. However recent studies have described a number of anatomic variations in the glenohumeral ligaments which need to be differentiated from truly pathologic conditions[3,4]. The coracohumeral ligament runs from the coracoid process to the greater tuberosity and capsule and has a minor role to play in stabilizing the humeral head. The coracoacromial ligament extends from the undersurface of the medial acromion to the superolateral border of the coracoid process. Therefore, along with the acromion, it acts as a roof over the subacromial space under which the rotator cuff tendons slide, with the subacromial bursa lying between. This structure has been implicated in the pathology of impingement of the shoulder[5]. The transverse humeral ligament runs between the greater and lesser tuberosities, covering the long head of the biceps tendon (see Fig. 7.2).

The stabilizers of the shoulder can be divided into two groups; static and dynamic. The capsule, labrum, glenohumeral and, to a lesser

THE GLENOID FOSSA: ITS ATTACHMENTS AND RELATIONSHIP TO SCAPULAR STRUCTURES

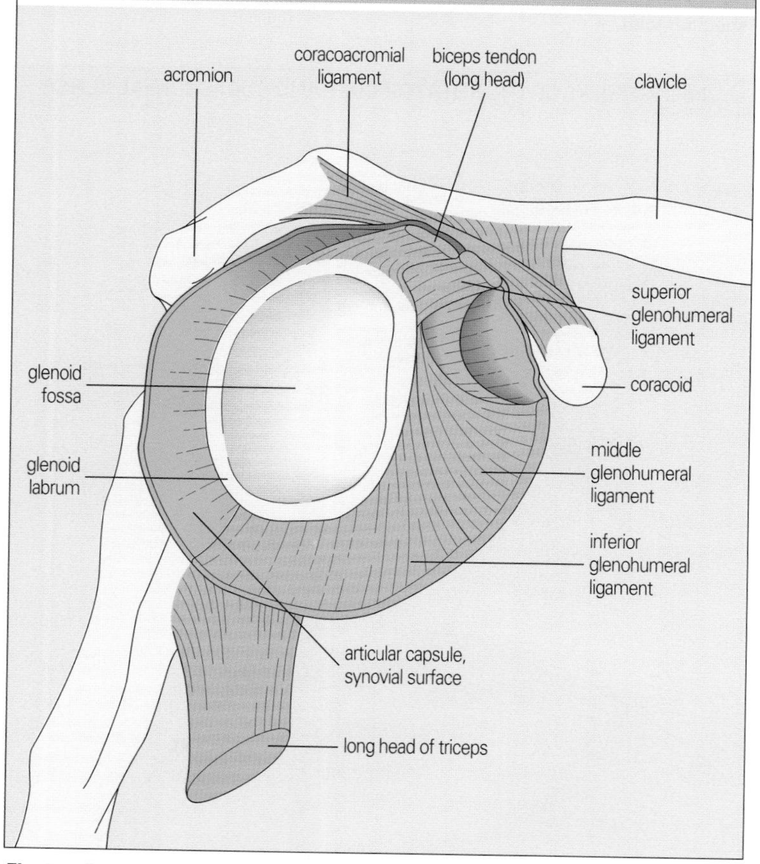

Fig. 7.1 The glenoid fossa. Its attachments and relationship to scapular structures.

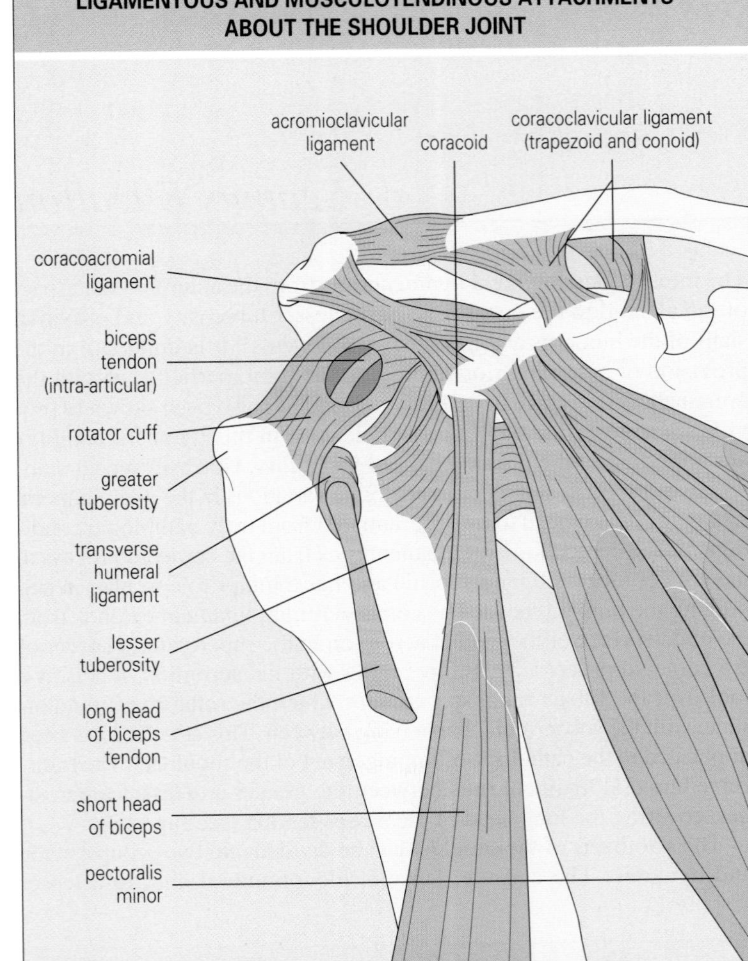

Fig. 7.2 Ligamentous and musculotendinous attachments about the shoulder joint.

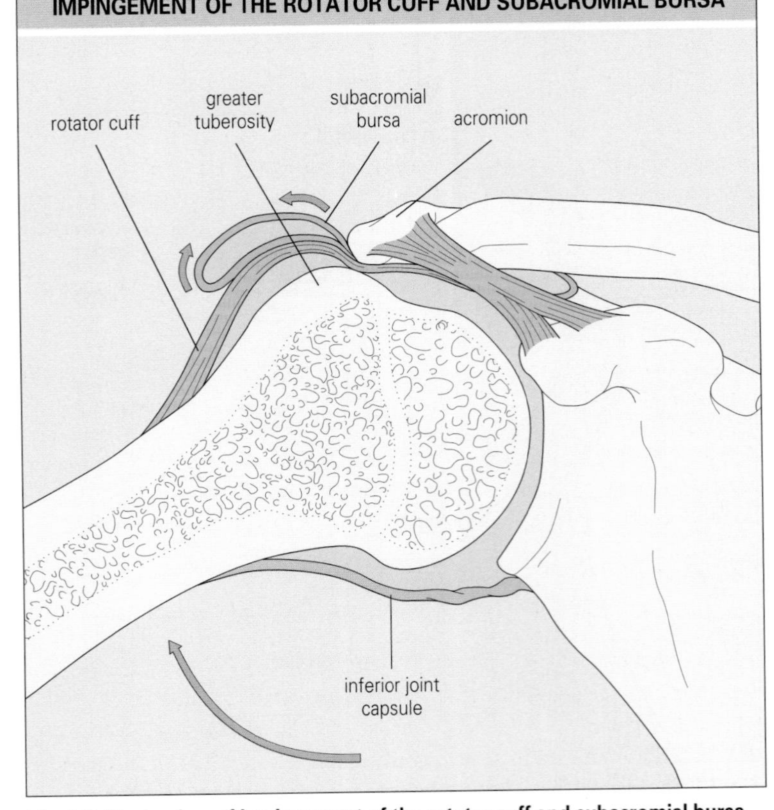

Fig. 7.3 Mechanism of impingement of the rotator cuff and subacromial bursa between the humeral head and overlying coracoacromial arch.

extent, coracohumeral ligaments can be thought of as static stabilizers of the glenohumeral joint. There are two sleeves of muscles about the shoulder; superficial and deep. The deep group comprises the rotator cuff muscles (supraspinatus, subscapularis, infraspinatus and teres minor) and the tendon of the long head of biceps. This layer acts dynamically to stabilize the humeral head in the glenoid fossa during shoulder movement, while simultaneously providing rotation (through subscapularis, teres minor and infraspinatus) and abduction (through supraspinatus). During the initiation of shoulder abduction or elevation, the larger more powerful deltoid muscle, if unopposed, would pull the humeral head superiorly towards the acromion. The rotator cuff muscles and the biceps tendon act as humeral head depressors to prevent this translational movement superiorly. This is known as the 'force-couple'. The subscapularis also acts to resist the tendency of the humeral head to sublux anteriorly in the upper ranges of abduction although its role is less important than previously thought[6]. Dysfunction of the rotator cuff muscles, either through weakness or a tear, results in diminished stabilization of the humeral head. This leads to weakness of the arm in elevation as well as superior migration of the humeral head, increasing the likelihood of subacromial compression or impingement (Fig. 7.3). Therefore, the four tendons of the rotator cuff grip the humeral head and act as guy-ropes to stabilize it during shoulder movement, resisting this sliding tendency within the joint. Also, there is a gap, or thinning of the cuff, between the supraspinatus and subscapularis tendons known as the rotator interval which is of variable size and may be implicated in some patients with anterior instability. The biceps tendon arises from the superior labrum or directly from the supraglenoid tubercle and acts as a humeral head depressor in full abduction. It has also been shown to contribute to anterior stability of the shoulder[7].

The outer sleeve of muscles comprises the deltoid, teres major, pectoralis major, latissimus dorsi and trapezius muscles. They act as prime movers of the humerus, although the trapezius acts through movement of the scapula and clavicle. The combination of these large muscles (which provide abduction, flexion, extension, adduction and a degree of rotation) with the deep layer of rotator cuff muscles (which provide more rotation of the humeral head) allows the expansive movement of the arm in actions such as reaching behind one's back or behind the head.

The deltoid muscle has three bellies; anterior, middle and posterior, producing respectively flexion, abduction and extension of the shoulder. All three muscles converge to an insertion on the deltoid tubercle on the lateral aspect of the humeral shaft. The rotator cuff muscles originate from the scapula and attach to the greater (supraspinatus, infraspinatus and teres minor) and lesser (subscapularis) tuberosities of the humerus.

Nerve supply to the glenohumeral joint is provided by those peripheral nerves supplying muscles acting upon the joint, namely the axillary, suprascapular, subscapular and musculocutaneous nerves. Innervation is via the fifth, sixth and seventh cervical roots, and the brachial plexus passes anterior and inferior to the glenohumeral joint.

ACROMIOCLAVICULAR JOINT

A fibrous disc separates the noncongruous surfaces of the distal end of the clavicle and the acromion and allows movement at this joint. During abduction and elevation the clavicle rotates through 30–40° and this largely occurs at the sternoclavicular joint[8]. There is a small amount of movement at the acromioclavicular joint and compressive force is applied to the joint in full elevation and horizontal adduction, which is the basis of stress tests applied to this joint. The joint is stabilized posteriorly by the posterior transverse ligament and inferiorly by the inferior ligament, and the deltoid and trapezius muscles act to provide some anterior and superior stability through their fascial layer. Of particular importance are the conoid and trapezoid, or coracoclavicular, ligaments which maintain the close relationship between the scapula and clavicle during shoulder movement.

SCAPULOTHORACIC JOINT

The scapula lies against the posterolateral aspect of the thoracic wall, rotating and sliding laterally in abduction, elevation and flexion. It provides the origin for the rotator cuff muscles as well as the deltoid muscle and the trapezius inserts along its superior aspect. The scapulothoracic joint represents that articulation between the scapula and thoracic cage, and motion here is important for normal functioning of the shoulder.

SCAPULOHUMERAL RHYTHM

Elevation and abduction of the arm involves synchronous motion at the glenohumeral and scapulothoracic joints. As elevation increases above 90° so does the proportion of scapulothoracic motion relative to glenohumeral motion. Scapulohumeral rhythm is representative of the ratio between movement at these two joints and is important in several shoulder disorders. Disturbance of the normal scapulohumeral rhythm affects the biomechanics of the shoulder joint and may result in secondary tendinitis of the shoulder. This is well demonstrated in elite swimmers, in whom muscle imbalances can give rise to tendinitis or impingement in this manner.

Several muscles (levator scapulae, serratus anterior, trapezius, rhomboids) act to stabilize and control movement of the scapula, and the balance between scapula elevators, rotators, depressors, retractors and protractors provides scapular control and determines scapulothoracic movement. Scapular control by these muscles is becoming better understood as an important factor in glenohumeral instability and rotator cuff dysfunction.

STERNOCLAVICULAR JOINT

Like the acromioclavicular joint the sternoclavicular joint contains an intra-articular fibrous disc which allows rotation of the clavicle during abduction and elevation. Strong ligaments stabilize this joint anteriorly and posteriorly.

BURSAE

Significant variation exists in regard to the number and extent of bursae around the shoulder. The subacromial bursa lies between the rotator cuff (mainly supraspinatus tendon) and overlying acromion. This bursa does not consist of a distinct sac and its synovial layers blend in with and are firmly attached to the acromion and rotator cuff. In subacromial impingement and rotator cuff tendinitis there is reactive inflammation of this bursa. The subscapularis bursa communicates with the synovial joint cavity between the superior and middle glenohumeral ligaments, and the synovial membrane of the joint invests the tendon of the long head of biceps. Other bursae include the subdeltoid, coracoid, infraserratus, and bursae at the insertion of the tendon of trapezius and at the tendon insertions on the humerus.

PHYSICAL EXAMINATION

HISTORY

Shoulder pain may be seen in association with several medical conditions and may be referred from cervical, thoracic or abdominal sources. Any history of diabetes, Raynaud's, cervical spondylosis, cerebrovascular or cardiac disease needs to be established. The mechanism of any injury will assist in making a diagnosis. A fall onto an outstretched arm can give rise to instability in the younger patient or a rotator cuff tear in the elderly. A fall onto the point of the shoulder may result in injury to the rotator cuff or acromioclavicular joint. Throwing injuries tend to stress the capsule and ligaments of the glenohumeral joint and can also give rise to rotator cuff or bicipital tendinitis. A good pain history is essential, since the location and type of pain varies between conditions. Pain referred from the cervical spine is often maximal over the suprascapular region with associated paresthesia or pain referred into the upper limb. Acromioclavicular and sternoclavicular pain is usually well localized to the involved joint. Pain from rotator cuff pathology is usually felt at the outer aspect of the upper arm or deltoid region. Adhesive capsulitis tends to give rise to an intense aching deep in the shoulder although features similar to rotator cuff pathology are common in the early stages. Radiating pain into the arm may indicate cervical pathology, thoracic outlet syndrome, compressive neuropathy, brachial neuritis or reflex sympathetic dystrophy. Night pain tends to be of two main types: either sharp pain associated with movement, indicative of a rotator cuff tendinitis or acromioclavicular pathology; or pain of a deep, constant aching nature more suggestive of capsulitis or a chronic tear of the rotator cuff.

INSPECTION

This should be carried out from anterior, posterior and lateral aspects and the patient's ability to undress may indicate functional limitations. Areas of erythema and bruising should be noted. Although uncommon, swelling of the shoulder joint will be seen anteriorly in the projection of the subscapularis bursa. Deformity of the shoulder girdle exists with acromioclavicular joint separation or fractures of the clavicle or humerus. It is important to look for positioning of the shoulder such as asymmetric elevation or overprotraction. Neck positioning should also be recorded. Rupture of the long head of biceps tendon is readily seen. Muscle wasting may be present in cases of cervical or brachial neuropathy (i.e. suprascapular nerve entrapment) but is also seen with chronic rotator cuff pathology in the supraspinatus and infraspinatus muscle bellies. Scapulohumeral and scapulothoracic rhythm during elevation should be assessed and any asymmetry noted. Winging of the scapula can be demonstrated by asking the patient to do a push-up against the wall. It is indicative of serratus anterior weakness (as in long thoracic nerve palsy) but can also occur with muscular dysfunction.

PALPATION

This should assess the presence of tenderness, swelling and instability of the acromioclavicular, sternoclavicular and glenohumeral joints. Tenderness over the tendon of the long head of biceps and the bicipital groove is common in bicipital tendinitis but comparison with the normal shoulder is necessary as this tendon is normally sensitive to touch. There may be tenderness over the rotator cuff insertions to the greater and lesser tuberosities but this is not always present in rotator cuff tendinitis. Acute calcific tendinitis is exquisitely tender over the involved tendon. The lateral margin of the subacromial joint can be palpated for swelling and tenderness and the glenohumeral joint itself may be tender in chronic or acute instability or capsulitis. An effusion of the glenohumeral joint should be differentiated from subacromial swelling, although communication between the two may exist in degenerative conditions where there is a full-thickness tear of the rotator cuff. Osteophytes can also be palpated at the margins of these joints, as can any crepitus present. Instability of the acromioclavicular and sternoclavicular joints is readily demonstrable but glenohumeral instability requires a more detailed examination combining assessment of laxity in anterior, posterior and inferior directions with stress and apprehension tests to determine the presence of symptomatic instability. This assessment needs to be carried out in the young adult presenting with shoulder pain since underlying instability is a frequent cause of tendinitis around the shoulder. Muscles of the shoulder girdle and neck region should be palpated for trigger points and tender points, typically present with myofascial syndromes and fibromyalgia respectively.

MOBILIZATION

Active and passive ranges of motion of both shoulders should be assessed in the planes of abduction, forward flexion and external rotation, both with the arm by the side and at 90° abduction. Internal rotation is frequently assessed as a combined maneuver with extension in bringing the arm up behind the back. This is limited in many periarticular conditions and a better assessment of true glenohumeral joint restriction is done by measuring true internal rotation with the arm by the side and the elbow extended, using the epicondyles as markers for comparison with the other shoulder. Any limitation of movement should be noted as well as any discrepancy between active and passive motion. Glenohumeral joint pathology is unlikely in the presence of a normal range of passive motion.

Further assessment should include passive adduction of the flexed and internally rotated shoulder to look for tightness of the posterior structures, namely the posterior capsule and external rotator cuff muscles, as this is often seen in chronic cuff pathology. Resisted shoulder movements are performed to assess involvement of muscles and tendons. The patient is asked to resist a specific movement in order to elicit an isolated, isometric contraction in the particular muscle group. The supraspinatus is tested with the arm abducted to 90°, flexed to 30° and internally rotated (i.e. thumb downwards). The examiner then resists abduction from this position. Resisted internal rotation tests the subscapularis and resisted external rotation tests infraspinatus and teres minor. Resisted abduction should also be carried out with the arm by the side. Biceps function can also be tested by resisting shoulder flexion with the elbow extended (Speed's test) or resisting supination with the elbow flexed to 90° (Yergason's test). Any assessment must include an examination of the cervical spine to assess range of motion and the presence of any referred upper limb pain (see Chapter 4.4).

SPECIAL MOVEMENTS

Specific examination techniques can be employed to further localize the source of pain in the shoulder region. Various tests for impingement have been described. In one of these the arm is flexed to 90°, adducted and then forcefully internally rotated and slightly elevated by the examiner, with the scapula stabilized by the examiner's other hand (Fig. 7.4a). In another variation the arm is placed in the adducted, flexed, internally rotated position and the patient is asked to externally rotate the arm against resistance (Fig. 7.4b). A further impingement test is carried out by passively forcing the arm into full forward flexion while the examiner stabilizes the top of the scapula with the other hand (Fig. 7.4c). In all situations a positive test is recorded if pain is felt as the subacromial bursa and the rotator cuff are forced against the undersurface of the acromion.

Apart from Speed's and Yergason's tests a further bicipital provocation test can be performed by asking the patient to abduct the arm to 90° with the palm upwards. The arm is then slowly adducted (with the elbow extended) across the midline and the chest against resistance[9]. In cases of bicipital tendon involvement a catching pain is felt in the region of the bicipital groove as the arm crosses in front of the shoulder joint (Fig. 7.5).

Pain at the acromioclavicular joint can be localized by performing various stress tests. In one the arm is held with the elbow and shoulder extended and then passively adducted across behind the back (Fig. 7.6). In another less specific maneuver the arm is abducted to 90° and then adducted across the patient's chest under the chin. In both tests pain is felt over an inflamed acromioclavicular joint at the limits of these movements. Assessment for a thoracic outlet syndrome is always difficult and several maneuvers are described which may provoke the symptoms of neurovascular compression (see Chapter 4.18).

The patient should be assessed for the presence of joint hypermobility. Laxity of the glenohumeral joint in anterior and posterior directions is determined by carrying out drawer tests in which the humeral head is gripped firmly and moved backwards and forwards in the glenoid fossa. This is best carried out with the patient lying supine and the abducted arm supported by the examiner's hand (Fig. 7.7). Inferior laxity is assessed by applying distal retraction to the arm while palpating the gap between the humeral head and acromion. Presence of a distinct gap can be felt and even seen, and is referred to as a positive sulcus sign. If present this is indicative of multidirectional laxity of the joint. Anterior apprehension and stress tests are carried out with the

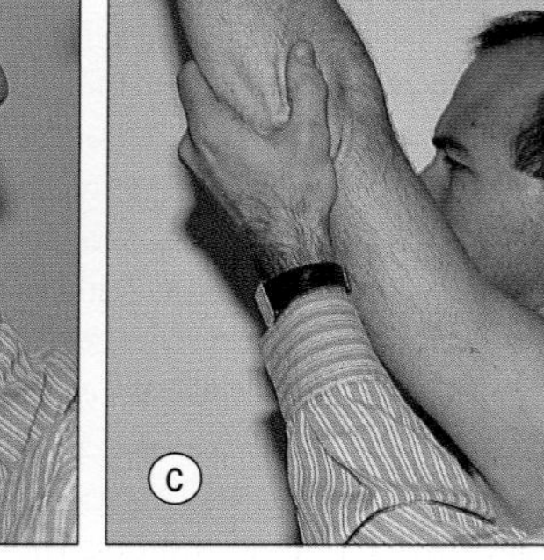
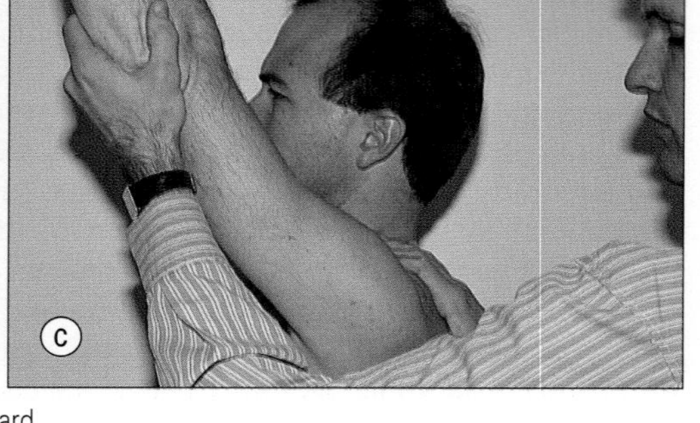

Fig. 7.4 Impingement tests: forced passive internal rotation (a); resisted external rotation (b); forced passive full forward flexion (c).

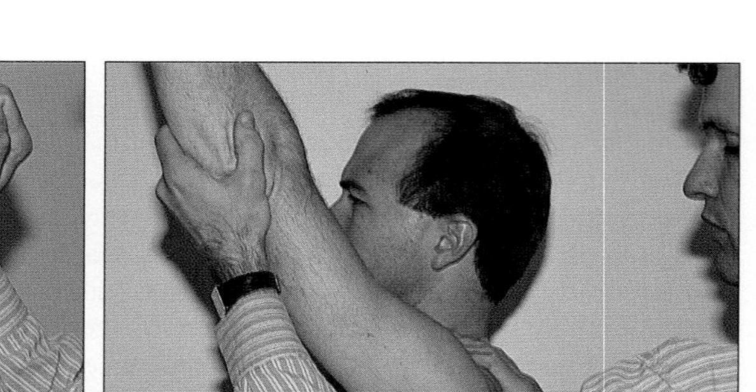

Fig. 7.5 Clinical tests for bicipital tendinitis: Speed's test (a); Yergason's test (b); bicipital provocation test (c).

Fig. 7.6 An adduction stress test of the acromioclavicular joint.

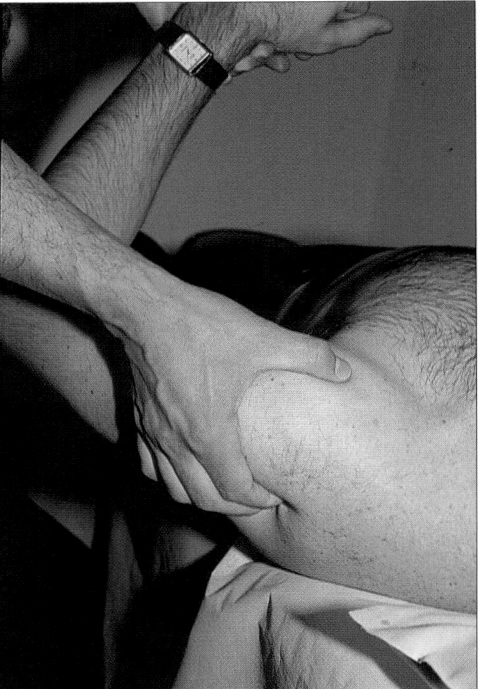
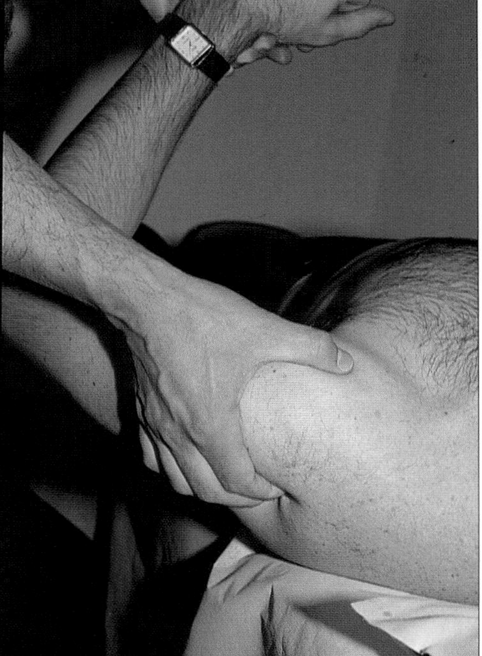

Fig. 7.7 The anterior drawer test.

examiner slowly extending and externally rotating the abducted arm with the patient supine. A positive test occurs when the patient experiences pain or apprehension during this maneuver and is confirmed when these symptoms disappear as the examiner's free hand applies a downward, i.e. stabilizing, force to the anterior aspect of the upper humerus. This often allows further external rotation of the arm (Fig. 7.8). Symptoms return as this stabilizing force is slowly withdrawn. The posterior stress test is carried out by applying gentle axial pressure to the humerus with the arm in the forward flexed, internally rotated and slightly adducted position, again in an attempt to reproduce pain and apprehension.

DIFFERENTIAL DIAGNOSIS OF SHOULDER PAIN

The glenohumeral joint may be affected as part of widespread joint disease, i.e., a polyarthropathy such as rheumatoid arthritis, crystal arthropathy, other inflammatory arthropathies or generalized osteoarthritis. Septic arthritis, neuropathic (Charcot's) arthritis, osteonecrosis and idiopathic destructive arthritis are all conditions which can affect the shoulder joint in isolation. In articular disorders of the shoulder there may be swelling or synovitis, and invariably there is an effect on passive and active motion of the glenohumeral joint with pain, restriction of motion and often crepitus.

Periarticular conditions affecting the shoulder can be loosely grouped into those with and those without capsulitis. If there is no capsular involvement then passive joint motion is largely unaffected, whereas active movement may be limited by pain and/or weakness (e.g. rotator cuff disorders). With capsulitis there is multidirectional restriction of passive motion, and differentiation from articular conditions of the shoulder is made on clinical and radiologic grounds.

Referred pain to the shoulder can occur with cervical disorders, Pancoast's tumor of the lung, subphrenic pathology, entrapment neuropathies and brachial neuritis. In these conditions passive and often active movements of the shoulder are largely unaffected and there is usually little or no pain when testing rotator cuff function. Again, differentiation from disorders of the shoulder is possible with an adequate history and examination (see Fig. 7.9).

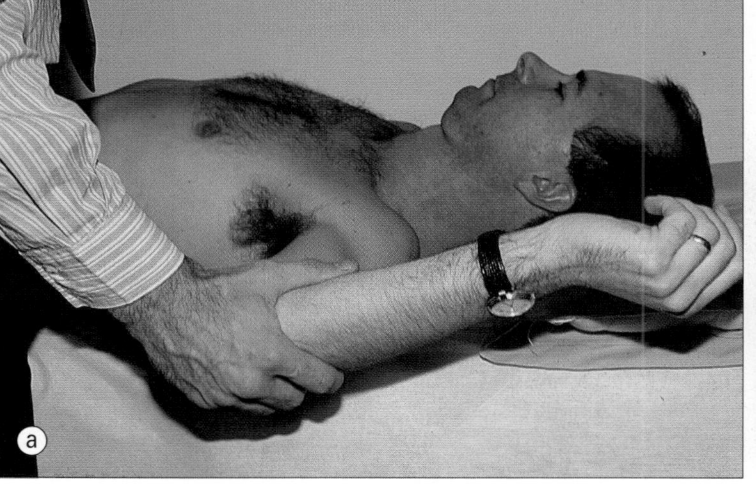
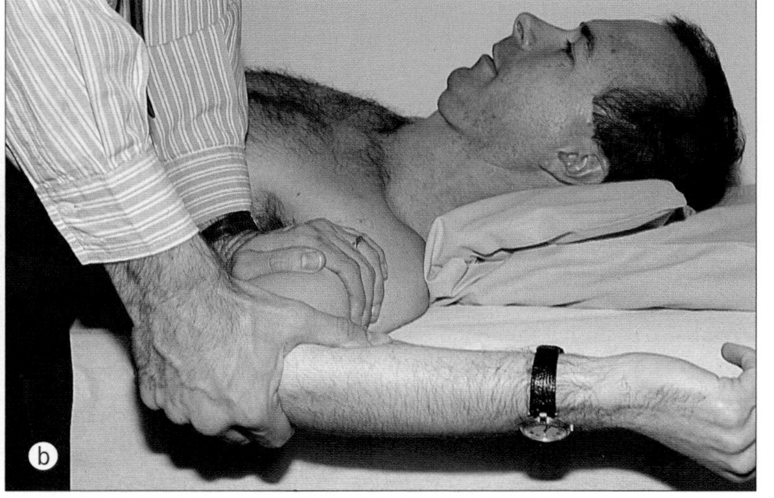

Fig. 7.8 A stress test for anterior glenohumeral instability (a). Containment sign: applying pressure anteriorly relieves the symptoms and allows further external rotation (b).

DIFFERENTIAL DIAGNOSIS OF SHOULDER PAIN

Diagnosis	Age	Type of onset	Location of pain	Night pain	Active range of motion	Passive range of motion	Impinge-ment signs	Radiation of pain	Paras-thesia	Weakness	Instability	Radio-graphic changes	Special features
Rotator cuff tendinitis	Any	Acute or chronic	Deltoid region	+	↓↓ guarding	Normal	+++	–	–	Only due to pain	Look for	In chronic cases	Painful arc of abduction
Rotator cuff tears (chronic)	Over 40 years	Often chronic	Deltoid region	++	↓↓↓	Normal (may ↓ later)	++	–	–	++	–	+	Wasting of cuff muscles
Bicipital tendinitis	Any	Overuse	Anterior	–	↓ guarding	Normal	+	Occasionally into biceps	–	Only due to pain	Look for	None	Special exam-ination tests
Calcific tendinitis	30–60 years	Acute	Point of shoulder	++	↓↓↓ guarding	Normal except for pain	+++	–	–	Only due to pain	–	++	Tenderness ++
Capsulitis 'frozen shoulder'	Over 40 years	Insidious	Deep in shoulder	++	↓↓	↓↓	+	–	–	–	–	–	Global range of motion ↓
Acromioclavicular joint	Any	Acute or chronic	Over joint	Lying on side	↓ full elevation	Normal	–	–	–	–	–	In chronic cases	Local tenderness
Osteoarthrosis of glenohumeral joint	Over 40 years	Insidious	Deep in shoulder	++	↓↓	↓↓	–	–	–	May have mild	–	+++	Crepitus
Glenohumeral instability	Usually <25 years	Episodic	Anterior or posterior	–	Only appre-hension	Only appre-hension	Possible	–	+ with acute episodes	+ with acute episodes	+++	Often	Stress tests
Cervical spondylosis	Over 40 years	Insidious	Supra-scapular	Often	Normal	Normal	–	++	+++	+	–	In cervical spine	Pain with neck movement
Thoracic outlet syndrome	Any	Usually with activity	Neck shoulder arm	–	Normal	Normal	–	++	++	++	–	–	Special exam-ination tests

Fig. 7.9 Differential diagnosis of shoulder pain: clinical and radiographic features of common causes of shoulder pain.

ROTATOR CUFF DISORDERS

The spectrum of disorders affecting the rotator cuff ranges from the mild transient tendinitis following an episode of glenohumeral instability in the young patient, to the complete tear in the degenerative rotator cuff of the older patient. The anatomic configuration of the shoulder joint is such that the cuff is subjected to stresses when the arm is in the elevated position. Impingement can occur as the supraspinatus tendon is compressed between the humeral head and the overlying anterior acromion, coracoacromial ligament and even the inferior border of the acromioclavicular joint[5,10]. Impingement may be structural due to the presence of an acromial spur or degenerative acromioclavicular joint, but it may also be functional, due to superior migration of the humeral head during abduction and elevation. Underlying glenohumeral instability is a frequent cause of rotator cuff tendinitis, particularly in the younger patient, as is eccentric overload in the throwing athlete, where the rotator cuff muscles act as decelerators of the throwing arm. As the rotator cuff becomes inflamed, thinned or torn, so its function as a humeral head depressor is compromised and superior migration of the humeral head can occur due to the unopposed action of the deltoid, giving rise to further impingement. In the degenerative cuff with a complete tear this can eventually result in a cuff arthropathy with degenerative changes taking place at the subacromial and glenohumeral joints. The subacromial bursa lies between the rotator cuff tendons and the overlying coraco-acromial arch and becomes inflamed with this impingement. This is a reactive process and is usually a secondary phenomenon, although primary subacromial bursitis can result from trauma.

ROTATOR CUFF TENDINITIS

Clinical presentation and features

Presentation depends to a degree on the age of the patient and the likely etiology. Tendinitis resulting from eccentric overload or glenohumeral instability in the young adult usually presents acutely following an activity such as throwing. In the middle-aged individual, onset may be more gradual, reflecting the underlying chronic changes seen in the involved tendon. The patient may present with aching and discomfort in the shoulder, pain on movement and a history of repetitive or strenuous upper limb activity. The elderly patient may present with no history of antecedent trauma or repetitive activity and there is usually a gradual history of increasing shoulder discomfort, night pain, pain with movement and weakness if a degenerative tear is present. Except in the young patient with a history of explosive arm activity or trauma, onset tends to be gradual and aggravated by movements into abduction and elevation or sustained overhead activity, which are commonly sports- or occupation-related. Patients frequently complain that they have difficulty reaching up behind their back when dressing. The pain at night usually occurs when rolling onto the affected side and is typically felt in the deltoid region rather than the point of the shoulder, although this can occur. Active movements may be restricted by pain and in the more severe or chronic cases a secondary capsulitis can develop, further restricting movement at the shoulder.

Findings on examination include a painful arc of abduction usually occurring between 70–120° abduction. When lowering from full abduction there is often a 'catch' of pain usually at midrange as impingement occurs. Passive motion tends to be full and pain-free if adequate muscle relaxation can be achieved. Point tenderness over the greater tuberosity can occur but is not always present and the diagnosis is confirmed by reproducing pain when resisting movement of the affected tendon and on impingement testing. In the older patient acromioclavicular joint involvement is often present and there may be early joint stiffness.

Pathology

Impingement has been shown to occur in forward flexion when the anterior margin of the acromion impinges on the supraspinatus tendon[5,11]. Vascular studies have demonstrated that there is a constant area of avascularity or 'critical zone' extending from a point approximately 1cm proximal to the point of insertion of the tendon into the greater tuberosity, and this compromise in microvascularity is seen with the arm in the adducted (neutral) position[12]. However, studies by Iannotti *et al.* have detected substantial blood flow in this critical zone using a laser Doppler[13]. It has long been supposed that this region of relative hypovascularity is compromised in elevation and abduction, thereby producing an inflammatory response and subsequent tendinitis. The pathology of this impingement syndrome has been classified by Neer into three stages:

- stage I, edema and hemorrhage of the tendon;
- stage II, fibrosis of the subacromial bursa and tendinitis of the rotator cuff;
- stage III, tendon degeneration, bony changes at the acromion and humeral head and eventual tendon rupture.

The bicipital tendon is frequently involved as part of this condition but is not usually the primary pathology. Generally, stage II occurs in patients aged 25–40 years, stage III in those aged over 40 years and stage I is the pathology found in those under 25 years of age.

There appears to be progressive tendon failure leading to cuff rupture with an incidence of up to 30% full-thickness and 20–30% partial thickness tears in the elderly population[14,15]. Possible etiological factors include trauma, attrition, ischemia and impingement. Recent work has looked at biochemical changes within the tendon matrix which may predispose to tendon rupture[16–18].

Investigations

Plain radiographs may show evidence of calcification in the rotator cuff tendons in chronic cases, and in longstanding cases there are changes suggestive of rotator cuff degeneration, i.e. cystic and sclerotic changes at the greater tuberosity insertion. Ultrasonography and magnetic resonance imaging (MRI) can be used to identify changes of rotator cuff tendinitis and partial tears but interpretation is fairly observer-dependent. Dynamic ultrasonography can also demonstrate thickening of the subacromial bursa and impingement[19].

Diagnostic pitfalls

Pain felt in the deltoid may suggest referred cervical pain, although this is more likely to present with upper trapezius or suprascapular pain referring down into the arm. Pain on active arm movement and impingement testing will assist in differentiation, and preservation of passive range of movement will differentiate a capsulitis from rotator cuff tendinitis. In cases of tendinitis due to underlying instability, and this must be suspected in patients under 25 years of age, examination should confirm symptomatic instability.

Management

The treatment of rotator cuff tendinitis is often difficult and usually made impossible by continued participation in aggravating activities. Rest and activity modification are necessary to prevent the problem becoming chronic. Initial treatment should be directed at reducing inflammation by means of physical modalities and a nonsteroidal anti-inflammatory drugs (NSAIDs) if required. When there is failure to settle symptoms by these means, a subacromial injection of corticosteroid can be used (see Chapter 2.12). As well as reducing pain, treatment should be directed at restoring range of motion and the normal biomechanics of shoulder movement, paying particular attention to scapular control and scapulohumeral rhythm. This is especially important in cases where such a disturbance in biomechanics has aggravated or even precipitated the problem. Once the pain has reduced and normal shoulder movement patterns have been restored, a strengthening program should be instituted concentrating on rotator cuff exercises in order to restore their function as humeral head stabilizers and depressors, thereby reducing the likelihood of further injury.

The younger patient with instability needs a full stabilization rehabilitation program and rarely requires injection to the shoulder. The older patient with a degenerative rotator cuff and associated acromioclavicular joint pathology may be resistant to conservative treatment.

Indications for surgery vary according to the age of the patient, stage of impingement or tendinitis, and the symptoms. The major indication for surgical intervention is pain, and in the presence of an intact rotator cuff, failure to respond to a conservative program within 1 year is a reasonable indication for surgery[20]. This involves subacromial decompression and encompasses an anterior acromioplasty and resection of the coracoacromial ligament, both of which can be carried out arthroscopically. Any impingement due to acromioclavicular joint pathology must also be addressed at operation.

Prevention

In the young patient or athlete attention to proper preparation for exercise and correct technique is important. Many athletes develop muscular imbalances about the shoulder, either through tightness or weakness, and if these are not corrected secondary impingement and tendinitis can result. In the older patient avoidance of sustained above-shoulder activities or explosive lifting will help prevent this condition from deteriorating or perhaps even developing.

ROTATOR CUFF TEARS

Clinical presentation and features

Rotator cuff tears may be acute or chronic, partial or full thickness. Partial tears may occur in any age group following trauma, but the full thickness (or complete) tear is rarely seen in the patient under 40 years of age. In the young adult a partial tear can result from a fall or explosive shoulder movement and presents very much as a rotator cuff tendinitis, although onset is acute. Also, full active range of motion may be preserved. The acute complete rupture after trauma should be readily diagnosed. The mechanism of injury is usually a fall onto the outstretched arm, a hyperabduction injury or a fall onto the side of the shoulder. Bruising is often delayed and occurs in the upper arm, and there is an immediate loss of active abduction with weakness of abduction and external rotation. There is a close association between dislocation of the shoulder in the patient over 40 years of age and partial or complete tears of the rotator cuff. In one review of 40 patients the incidence of full-thickness tears was 90%[21].

Chronic full thickness tears are found in 7–27%[22,23] of patients at autopsy, and many patients with a documented complete tear of the supraspinatus tendon have full active abduction, occasionally in the absence of pain. There may be no history of trauma and symptoms frequently become apparent with increased activity. The usual picture is one of pain on abduction and flexion with varying degrees of loss of active movement depending on the size of the tear. The patient may complain of weakness of abduction, flexion and internal or external rotation depending on the tendon involved.

Night pain is common and often severe. Examination reveals many of the features of rotator cuff tendinitis but there is often an inability to maintain the arm in abduction when lowering from the elevated position, i.e. a positive 'drop-off' sign. Subacromial crepitus and pain on impingement testing are present. A common clinical finding is wasting of the infraspinatus, and to a lesser extent supraspinatus, muscle bellies, together with weakness of abduction, but more often weakness of external rotation reflects the size of the tear. Rupture of the long head of the biceps tendon is frequently associated with chronic rotator cuff pathology.

Pathology

The incidence of degenerative cuff tears increases with age as does the size of tear[24]. Cuff arthropathy occurs when there is superior migration

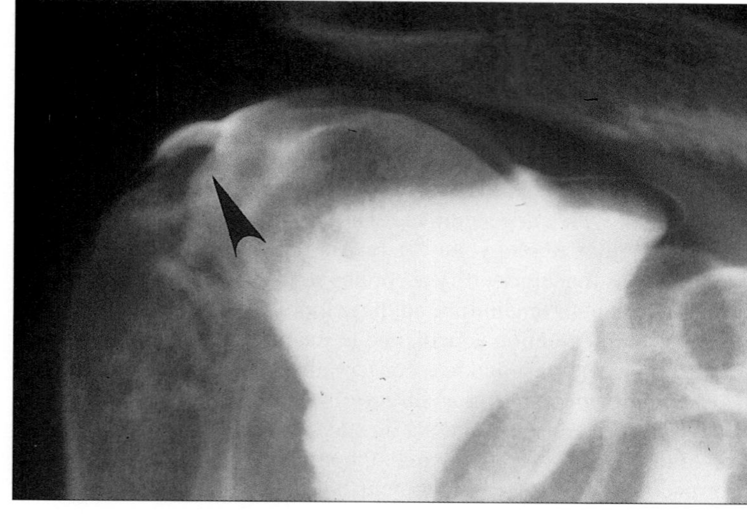

Fig. 7.10 Arthrogram of the shoulder showing leakage of dye into the supraspinatus tendon confirming a partial tear (arrow). This investigation is more accurate in the assessment of full thickness tears of the rotator cuff.

of the humeral head against the undersurface of the acromion. This occurs as the incompetent rotator cuff fails to stabilize and depress the humeral head and therefore counteract the pull of the deltoid. This leads to degenerative change both at the subacromial joint and secondarily at the glenohumeral joint. Management is difficult due to the combination of cuff deficiency and arthritic change. Neer estimates that 4% of cuff tears ultimately progress to a cuff arthropathy[25].

Investigation

Features of chronic rotator cuff degeneration can be seen on plain radiography with sclerosis and cystic changes at the greater tuberosity. Osteophyte formation may be present along the anterior inferior acromion, with possible acromioclavicular joint osteoarthrosis. With a complete tear there may be superior migration of the humeral head and narrowing of the subacromial space (less than 6mm indicates a tear). This finding is seen in cuff arthropathy where there is degenerative change in the subacromial compartment and glenohumeral joint.

Full thickness tears are readily demonstrated with single or double contrast arthrography, and although false negatives can occur, sensitivity approaches 90%. Partial tears can occasionally be seen (Fig. 7.10). Estimation of the size of the defect using this technique is unreliable. Ultrasonography can identify tears, both full and to a lesser extent partial thickness. Magnetic resonance imaging compares favorably with arthrography in the diagnosis of complete tears (Fig. 7.11) but is less consistent in the assessment of partial tears, and interpretation is difficult[26](Fig. 7.12). Arthroscopy is now readily available as a means of establishing the diagnosis in the patient with shoulder pain who requires further assessment. It is particularly useful in the assessment of instability while at the same time allowing visualization of the rotator cuff, subacromial bursa, intra-articular bicipital tendon and glenoid labrum. It also has a role in the estimation of the size of a cuff tear prior to more definitive surgery.

MANAGEMENT

Initially, partial rotator cuff tears should all be managed conservatively, as for rotator cuff tendinitis, although corticosteroid injection is probably not advisable within 4–6 weeks of an acute injury. The management of complete tears is somewhat controversial in terms of if and when to operate. Acute ruptures in the young or active patient should be managed surgically earlier rather than later. In the older or less active patient it is reasonable to have a trial of conservative management, but if there is no substantial improvement within 3 months then subacromial decompression and repair is advisable[27].

Chronic complete tears should all be treated with an adequate conservative program in the first instance. Failure to achieve pain relief is a major indication for surgical intervention. Any operative procedure should be directed primarily at relief of impingement, debridement of the cuff tear and usually, but not always, repair of the defect. Surgery should also be considered where there is an associated rupture of the biceps tendon as these cases appear more likely to develop a cuff arthropathy.

BICIPITAL TENDINITIS

CLINICAL PRESENTATION AND FEATURES

Although frequently diagnosed, bicipital tendinitis is not often seen in isolation and usually occurs in association with rotator cuff tendinitis or impingement, or with glenohumeral instability. Primary involvement of the tendon is seen as an overuse injury in sports such as weight-lifting where there is a repetitive stress placed upon the tendon, or after prolonged and repetitive carrying, e.g. of small children. The bicipital tendon acts as a secondary stabilizer of the humeral head and the translational movement seen with glenohumeral laxity can place

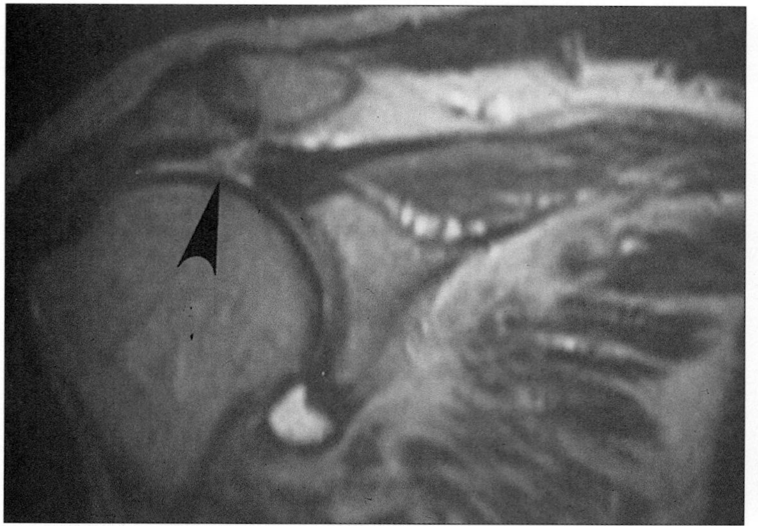

Fig. 7.11 MRI of complete rotator-cuff tear. T2-weighted MR image of the shoulder shows discontinuity of the supraspinatus tendon indicative of complete tear (arrow). The proximal tendon margin is frayed and retracted 1.5cm. Focal swelling and increased signal (arrowhead) in opposing articular cartilages of the glenhumeral joint are evidence of early degenerative disease.

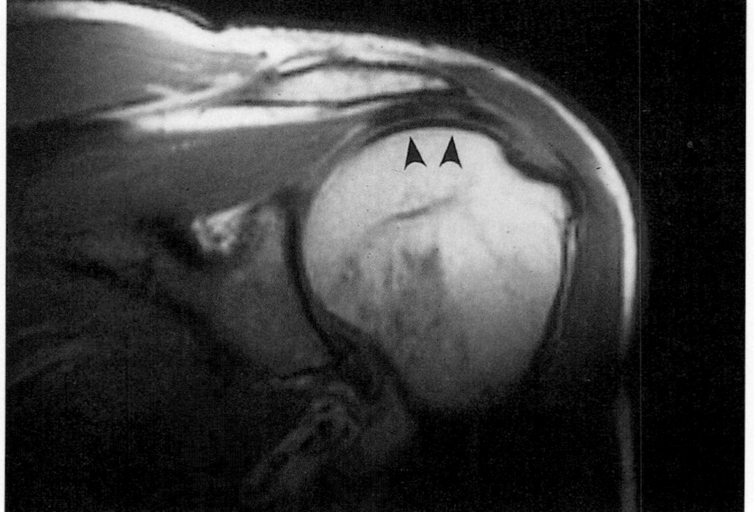

Fig. 7.12 MRI of partial rotator-cuff tear. T2-weighted MR image shows a focal defect in the undersurface of the supraspinatus tendon consistent with partial tear (arrow). Associated cartilage loss and subarticular cyst formation can be seen in the glenoid (arrowhead).

increased stress upon the tendon, leading to tendinitis. As with rotator cuff tendinitis the young patient with bicipital tendinitis should be assessed for instability. With chronic impingement or rotator cuff degeneration the biceps tendon may become fibrotic and attentuated and eventually rupture. Acute ruptures are also seen in young powerlifters and the diagnosis is made easy by the acute presentation.

Pain is usually felt over the anterior aspect of the shoulder, often radiating into the biceps muscle with well localized tenderness over the tendon as it runs in the bicipital groove. Pain is felt with overhead activities and often with shoulder extension and elbow flexion. Examination may reveal features of impingement, rotator cuff tendinitis and instability, all of which are important in determining the etiology of bicipital tendinitis. Pain may be reproduced with resisted elbow flexion, supination and shoulder flexion and various provocation tests are described, although none appears to be consistently positive. Passive shoulder extension stretches the biceps and may be painful. Rupture of the tendon is evident when there is the characteristic deformity of the upper arm with bunching up of the lateral muscle belly of the biceps best seen with resisted elbow flexion and supination.

Acute rupture of the transverse humeral ligament can result in subluxation or dislocation of the tendon. This can present with symptoms similar to bicipital tendinitis but often a more specific complaint is made of catching and a clicking sensation at the shoulder. Clinical examination may demonstrate subluxation of the tendon, which is felt as the arm is passively moved through internal and external rotation while in the 90° abducted position. Medial dislocation of the tendon is often found in association with tears of the subscapularis tendon.

PATHOLOGY

The tendon of the long head of biceps may be involved at several sites: its attachment to the superior glenoid labrum, which may be injured in a fall or throwing action (superior labrum anterior posterior (SLAP) lesion[28]); as it runs across the glenohumeral joint (intra-articular); or as it runs in the bicipital groove (extra-articular). The transverse humeral ligament stabilizes the tendon in the bicipital groove and if this mechanism is disrupted subluxation or dislocation of the tendon can result. This tends to occur as the arm is rotated in the abducted position. The tendon can become inflamed and thickened and fibrotic in chronic cases. In the older patient there may be attenuation and thinning of the tendon and eventual rupture. This latter presentation is almost always indicative of underlying rotator cuff degeneration as the bicipital tendon appears to become stressed in its attempt to act as a humeral head depressor in cases of rotator cuff incompetence. Also, the presence of a complete rotator cuff tear exposes the intra-articular portion of the bicipital tendon to the overlying acromion and further impingement.

INVESTIGATION

Special radiographic views demonstrate the bicipital groove, allowing assessment of its depth and the presence of any degenerative spurring. Filling of the synovial extension around the tendon is seen on arthrography and may be reduced in cases of chronic fibrosis. The tendon and any surrounding fluid can be seen well with ultrasonography, and this assists in the diagnosis of tears, both partial and complete, as well as tendinitis. It can also be used to demonstrate subluxation/dislocation of the tendon. MRI or arthroscopy allows visualization of the intra-articular portion of the tendon and its labral attachment.

MANAGEMENT

It is necessary to establish whether the tendinitis is primary or secondary, since a failure to address any underlying rotator cuff pathology or instability will lead to a recurrence of symptoms. The principles of management are rest, physical modalities, and NSAIDs as required. Low-power laser therapy has been reported to have a beneficial effect although this has been disputed[29,30].Corticosteroid injection is helpful in chronic cases but care should be taken not to inject the tendon itself (see Chapter 2.12). Since most cases of bicipital tendinitis are secondary, they usually settle as the primary condition is treated. The primary cases due to lifting or other activities respond to rest and simple anti-inflammatory measures. In chronic resistant cases surgery can be considered and this may involve subacromial decompression in cases of impingement, or tenodesis when there is chronic thickening of the tendon in the groove. Rupture of the tendon is normally treated conservatively except in the occasional young patient where upper arm strength is critical to their sport or profession. Usually, weakness following this injury is not significant. Subluxation of the tendon is usually treated conservatively, although occasionally surgery is necessary. Any conservative program must include range of motion exercises, stretches and, once symptoms have settled, a graduated eccentric and concentric biceps and rotator cuff strengthening program.

SUBACROMIAL BURSITIS

The close relationship between the subacromial bursa and the rotator cuff, specifically the supraspinatus tendon, is such that the term subacromial bursitis is frequently used when describing the pathology of impingement. In most cases inflammation of the bursa arises as part of the impingement process and coexists with an underlying rotator cuff tendinitis. This bursitis is therefore a reactive phenomenon. In chronic cases the bursa becomes thickened and fibrotic and surgical excision or debridement may be necessary. Treatment of rotator cuff tendinitis is directed at reducing the inflammation in the subacromial space or bursa as well as reducing the impingement.

Acute traumatic bursitis in the form of hemorrhage and edema can occur as a result of a fall or a direct blow to the point of the shoulder. Pain on abduction is present but differentiation from rotator cuff tendinitis is possible by the presence of increased tenderness and fluid at the subacromial space. A period of rest combined with simple measures, such as ice, usually allows resumption of normal activities, but occasionally persistent impingement develops, requiring further treatment.

CAPSULITIS

INTRODUCTION

Capsulitis of the shoulder remains a condition both difficult to define and universally awkward to manage. Many labels have been given to the situation where there is a painful restriction of shoulder movement apparently of soft tissue origin. These include frozen shoulder, periarthritis or pericapsulitis of the shoulder, adhesive capsulitis and adherent or obliterative bursitis. More recently there has been an attempt to classify patients with a painful stiff shoulder according to the presence or absence of capsular joint restriction as seen at arthrography[31]. Perhaps incorrectly, the term 'frozen shoulder' is applied to many conditions where restriction of movement is largely due to pain from an underlying condition, such as rotator cuff tendinitis, rather than to the classic global restriction of glenohumeral joint motion seen with a true adhesive capsulitis. Primary capsulitis of the shoulder can be defined as a condition of unknown etiology in which there is a painful global restriction of glenohumeral movement in all planes, both active and passive, in the absence of joint degeneration sufficient to explain this restriction. A condition known as secondary capsulitis exists in which is seen a similar clinical condition but in association with a clearly defined clinical disorder or precipitating event. Underlying diseases associated with this condition are diabetes mellitus, thyroid disease, pulmonary disorders such as tuberculosis or carcinoma, and cardiac disease or surgery. Myocardial infarct, cerebrovascular accident or shoulder trauma may precipitate the development of a shoulder capsulitis.

CLINICAL PRESENTATION AND FEATURES

Estimation of the prevalence of adhesive capsulitis is difficult due to variation in populations studied and diagnostic criteria used, but it appears to be in the order of 2–3% in nondiabetics[32–34]. Onset under the age of 40 years is rare, with the mean age of onset being in the sixth decade.

Women are slightly more affected than men. Involvement of the contralateral shoulder occurs in 6–17% of patients over the subsequent 5 years[35]. It is commonly stated that recurrence in the same shoulder does not occur. There is a frequent history of minor shoulder strain or injury prior to the onset of symptoms but whether this represents a true strain of the shoulder or simply the earliest awareness of pain is unclear. The natural history of this condition has been assessed by various authors and it appears that there are three phases in its development and progression. The shoulder moves from being simply painful, to being painful and stiff and eventually to being less painful but profoundly stiff. This last stage appears to be self-limiting and recovery is gradual and spontaneous. These stages have been termed painful, adhesive and resolution[36]. The duration of each stage in the overall condition varies considerably, but approximate durations are 3–8 months for the painful phase, 4–6 months for the adhesive phase and 1–3 years for the resolution phase. The extent of recovery is variable, with quoted figures of 33–61% of patients having a clinically detectable limitation of shoulder movement, and although many remain asymptomatic 7–15% of patients may have a persisting functional disability[37–40]. The extent to which the duration of the painful and adhesive phases determine the degree of residual disability remains controversial.

Painful phase

This is characterized by the insidious onset of symptoms, usually in the form of pain on shoulder movement and background ache in the shoulder region, often in the upper trapezius muscle. As the condition becomes established there is the development of increasing pain at rest and at night, the latter becoming quite disturbing and frequently waking the patient in the absence of a history of precipitative movement. Muscle spasm may develop, further limiting shoulder movement, which becomes restricted, with the increase in pain and stiffness at the shoulder. Towards the end of this phase stiffness becomes a major complaint.

Adhesive phase

Usually after several months the character of pain alters and becomes less severe. There is a reduction in pain at rest and at night but discomfort and a more severe pain at the limits of movement persist. Shoulder movement becomes more restricted during this phase.

Resolution phase

The pain is less evident and the dominant symptom is restriction of shoulder movement, which often appears less distressing for the patient now that the pain has eased. There is a slow and gradual improvement in range of motion, although this is frequently incomplete. The onset and rate of recovery are variable and unpredictable.

CLINICAL EXAMINATION

The physical signs alter to a degree as the condition progresses, with pain, often severe, present in the earlier stages. Differentiation from rotator cuff tendinitis is possible on the basis of there being a global restriction of passive movement rather than simply the loss of abduction and flexion which is often seen with chronic rotator cuff conditions. In the painful phase there is painful restriction of active and passive motion (often mild in the earlier stages). There may be pain on impingement testing and resisted movement, although this is less evident than in rotator cuff tendinitis. Associated findings are tenderness in the upper trapezius muscle and early scapula hitching in elevation. In the latter phases the important finding is significant restriction of glenohumeral movement with a compensatory increase in scapulothoracic motion during flexion and abduction. Pain may be present but there is less discrepancy between active and passive ranges. Disuse atrophy of the rotator cuff and deltoid muscles may exist. Joint line tenderness is not a universal finding but is common in the painful phase.

PATHOPHYSIOLOGY

The etiology of adhesive capsulitis is not known and the evidence for its association with the aforementioned conditions or trauma is unconvincing. Capsulitis is more prevalent in diabetics (prevalence 10–20%), usually occuring at a younger age and often associated with prolonged duration of the diabetes, insulin dependence, the development of limited joint mobility syndrome and widespread microvascular disease. Also bilateral involvement is more common in diabetes[32,33]. The links between diabetes and capsulitis may revolve around microvascular disease, abnormalities of collagen repair or predisposition to infection[36]. An association between capsulitis and thyroid disease and pulmonary conditions has been noted but provides little information regarding its pathogenesis[41–44]. Histologic studies have failed to demonstrate the presence of inflammatory cell infiltrates, granulomas or vasculitis in the joint capsule or synovium. Also, there is nothing to implicate infection, crystal arthropathy or trauma. Histologic studies of the joint capsule early in the disease are difficult to perform and the heterogenicity of patients loosely labeled as having capsulitis makes study of this condition difficult. However, Lundberg[32] noted an increase in fibrous tissue, fibroblast numbers and vascularity with no change in the synovial lining and no inflammatory cell infiltrate. To date there has been no association noted between capsulitis and histocompatibility antigen carriage in the population and no immunologic disturbance has been demonstrated. Several studies have looked at a variety of immunologic factors[45].

INVESTIGATION

Diagnosis is made largely on clinical grounds since there are few abnormalities found on investigation. Elevations of erythrocyte sedimentation rate (ESR), acute phase reactants and globulin levels are not usually seen, and calcium metabolism appears normal on testing. Plain radiographs are not helpful in making the diagnosis except to exclude widespread degenerative changes, calcific tendinitis or neoplasm. Classic features at arthrography are limitation of joint volume with a loss of the normal dependent axillary fold or pouch and irregularity of the capsular insertion to the anatomic neck of the humerus. Some authors insist that these changes need to be present in order to make a diagnosis of adhesive capsulitis. Ten to thirty percent of patients having arthrography have a demonstrable complete tear of the rotator cuff[31,39]. Other studies have suggested that a significant number of patients with a clinical diagnosis of adhesive capsulitis have normal findings at arthrography[39]. Arthroscopy allows further evaluation of these patients and different stages of synovitis and contracture have been described although variation in the patient population studied exists[31]. Bone scintigraphy may demonstrate increased isotope uptake in the affected shoulder region but this appears to have no predictive value in terms of outcome or response to treatment and is therefore of limited diagnostic value[46]. An average 50% reduction in bone mineral content in the affected humeral head has been demonstrated in bone densitometry studies, although again this is of little diagnostic or therapeutic value[32].

MANAGEMENT

Many therapies have been tried in an attempt to modify the natural history of capsulitis, and clinical studies of the efficacy of various treatment methods have been compromised by the difficulties with patient selection, diagnostic criteria and the variability in the natural resolution of the condition. The emphasis of treatment in the early stages should be on pain reduction and minimization of joint restriction. Analgesics and anti-inflammatory drugs provide limited relief of pain but do little to alter the course of the disorder. Physiotherapy utilizes physical modalities such as interferential to modify pain and reduce protective muscle spasm while attempting to encourage range of motion exercises early on in order to maintain joint mobility. Shoulder immobilization should be discouraged if at all possible, although in the painful phase the patient tends to minimize shoulder movement.

Intra-articular corticosteroid injections have been shown to improve pain and range of movement to a degree, although no long-term benefit has been demonstrated[47–50]. Oral corticosteroids have also been shown to improve pain but not affect the rate of recovery[51]. Few treatments have been shown to consistently affect rate of recovery or limit restriction of movement. Careful utilization of analgesic or anti-inflammatory drugs with physiotherapy may assist, although this may be due to a reduction in the protective spasm which is seen in the untreated patient. Judicious and occasional injection of corticosteroid to the affected joint may help but is of little benefit in the adhesive phase (see Chapter 2.12). Manipulation under anesthetic has been used to restore joint motion but may involve rupture of the inferior capsule and possibly the subscapularis tendon at its insertion. Care should be taken when carrying out this procedure, especially in the elderly patient, in order to avoid humeral fracture, shoulder dislocation or a significant rotator cuff rupture. Aggressive early rehabilitation in the immediate postmanipulation period is needed in order to maintain joint mobility, and patient cooperation with and tolerance of this treatment is essential. Manipulation during the painful phase is not recommended since painful recontraction of the capsule may occur and this treatment method is usually reserved for the adhesive phase once the pain has settled. Arthroscopy can be used as an adjunct to manipulation[52]. For many patients, however, once the painful phase of their condition has subsided the prospect of this painful procedure is not appealing. Improvement in range of movement following this procedure is variable and is perhaps dependent upon patient selection. Long-term recovery appears unchanged although resolution may be accelerated immediately following manipulation[31,38,40].

ACROMIOCLAVICULAR SYNDROMES

INTRODUCTION

Pain localized to the acromioclavicular joint is commonly seen either as an acute or a chronic condition. In the younger patient this joint is frequently subjected to trauma as a result of falls or contact sport. This may result in an acute injury and may also predispose the joint to further problems, such as instability or secondary osteoarthritis. Infection of this joint is rare but septic arthritis has been described[53].

TRAUMA

Disruption of the acromioclavicular joint may be seen in association with fractures of the outer end of the clavicle and often leads to the development of secondary osteoarthritis. More common are injuries to the joint itself, which are graded according to the degree of disruption of the joint capsule and supporting ligaments. Grade I injury involves minor sprain to the joint capsule without ligament disruption. Grade II injury involves subluxation of the joint with downward displacement of the acromion relative to the distal end of the clavicle. There is stretching of the inferior acromioclavicular ligaments, and stretching and possibly a partial tear, but not complete rupture, of the coracoclavicular ligaments. In a Grade III injury complete dislocation of the joint occurs due to rupture of the coracoclavicular ligaments. Grade III injuries can be further classified (often as Grades IV, V, and VI) according to the extent of disruption or perforation of the overlying deltotrapezius fascial or muscle layer by the displaced outer end of the clavicle.

Clinical presentation and features on physical examination

The mechanism of injury usually involves a fall directly onto the point of the shoulder. Pain is well localized to the top of the shoulder in the region of the involved joint, which is tender and often swollen to palpation. Abduction is often limited, both actively and passively, according to the degree of joint disruption. With a minor injury where there is good preservation of movement, acromioclavicular joint stress tests can be carried out to localize symptoms. In complete dislocation of the joint a visible step deformity is seen and examination will determine whether or not this dislocation can be reduced. This is important in the determination of the extent of any Grade III injury. The patient often describes a feeling of their shoulder having dropped due to the downward displacement of the acromion.

Management

For the Grade I or Grade II injury, treatment is largely symptomatic, with analgesics and provision of a sling for days to weeks depending on the symptoms. Shoulder movements should be encouraged as pain settles, and functional recovery is excellent. Controversy exists over the management of Grade III injuries. Provided perforation of the overlying muscle or fascial layer has not occurred, most patients settle with conservative treatment over a period of 6–10 weeks. Strapping of the joint has no effect on long-term stability and is not indicated in these patients[54]. Although effective, surgical stabilization by means of internal fixation is usually unnecessary, is associated with a significant complication and failure rate, and long-term results are not demonstrably better than for nonoperative treatment. Surgery should therefore be reserved for severe Grade III disruptions or where an individual's occupation may be compromised by persistent deformity or instability at that joint.

Late sequelae

Patients may present with persistent pain at the acromioclavicular joint. This represents low-grade joint inflammation and may be associated with an underlying instability, early development of secondary osteoarthritis, or osteolysis of the distal end of the clavicle. Persistent pain following joint injury may also result from damage to the intra-articular fibrocartilage sustained at the time of injury. Treatment is symptomatic, with anti-inflammatory medication or injection of intra-articular corticosteroid for resistant cases. Delayed surgical stabilization may be carried out in cases of gross instability and tears of the fibrocartilage can be debrided arthroscopically. Long-term treatment is as for osteoarthritis of the joint.

OSTEOLYSIS OF THE CLAVICLE

Osteolysis of the distal clavicle is a condition which may follow an acute injury or repetitive stress to the shoulder[55].

Symptoms are usually similar to those of acromioclavicular inflammation, with aching and pain at the limits of flexion and abduction. Radiographic changes typically show resorption of the distal clavicle, often with osteophyte formation, osteoporosis or tapering (Fig. 7.13). Response to activity modification and conservative treatment is usually satisfactory, but excision of the distal clavicle may be necessary. There may even be reconstitution of the distal clavicle with rest[56].

OSTEOARTHRITIS

Acromioclavicular joint morphology appears to be associated with the development of osteoarthritis[57]. A previous history of joint injury is common when osteoarthritis of this joint occurs in isolation, but the joint may also be involved as part of widespread osteoarthritic joint disease.

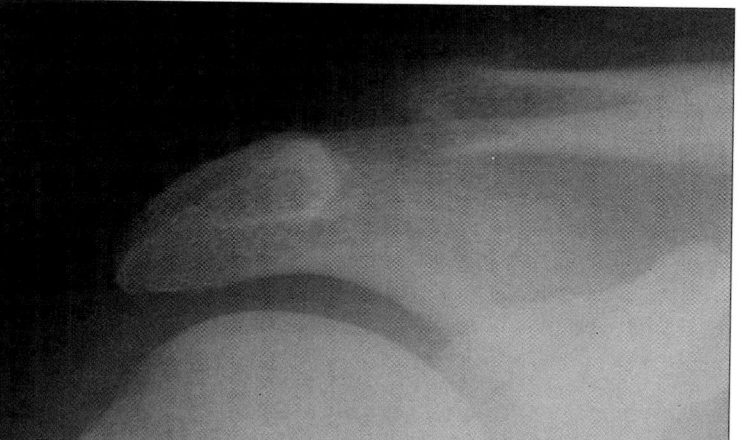

Fig. 7.13 Radiographic changes of osteolysis of the clavicle.

Clinical features

Pain and tenderness is well localized to the joint, which is often prominent due to osteophyte formation. Pain exists on full abduction or horizontal adduction and can also be reproduced with adduction of the extended arm. Crepitus is frequently localized to the joint. It is important to note that osteoarthritis of the joint is often seen in association with rotator cuff degeneration, and inferior osteophytes at the acromioclavicular joint may contribute to the development of a rotator cuff tear. Clinical features of both conditions frequently coexist, especially in the older patient.

Investigation

Degenerative change can be clearly seen on plain radiography and an arthrogram may reveal the presence of a complete tear of the rotator cuff. Traction or weight-bearing views can be taken in order to demonstrate joint instability.

Management

Initial management consists of local modalities and the use of analgesic or anti-inflammatory drugs. A suitable exercise program should be provided in order to restore normal scapulohumeral rhythm, glenohumeral range of motion and deltoid and rotator cuff strength once symptoms have settled. Cases resistant to conservative treatment may require surgery, which usually consists of excision arthroplasty of the joint while ensuring that instability is minimized. Careful assessment of rotator cuff function is important and in the presence of a significant tear rotator cuff repair or an acromioplasty may be indicated. Excision arthroplasty may also be indicated in the younger patient with chronic symptoms, whether due to degenerative change, osteolysis or instability.

CALCIFIC TENDINITIS

Radiologically detectable calcification in the rotator cuff tendons has a reported prevalence of 2.7–7.5%, occurring in symptomatic and asymptomatic shoulders[58,59]. It is common in the supraspinatus tendon and has been reported as being more common in women, housewives and sedentary individuals. Bosworth[60] estimated that 35–45% of individuals with calcification seen on radiography developed symptoms. Frequently bilateral, it usually occurs between the ages of 40 years and 60 years but can present as an acute condition in the younger patient. Patients may present with chronic symptoms of pain on movement with a catching sensation probably due to impingement. Acute calcific tendinitis has a quite different presentation with acute severe pain limiting passive or active shoulder movement almost completely, with exquisite point tenderness and occasionally erythema over the involved tendon. The onset of symptoms can be rapid with no history of injury or overuse and this occurs during the resorptive phase of calcification. Patients can therefore be divided into two groups. Firstly, those patients with an acute onset of severe pain and limitation of movement often in the absence of any previous shoulder symptoms. Secondly, patients who have a more chronic catching pain associated with movement presenting as an impingement problem.

PATHOPHYSIOLOGY

It has been argued by various authors that calcification occurs as part of a degenerative process involving the rotator cuff tendons, largely because it is rarely seen in people before the fourth decade[61]. Also, complete cuff tears have been found in 21% of patients with calcific tendinitis[62]. Histologic studies have confirmed that calcification follows on from tendon fibrosis and subsequent necrosis[62,63]. However Uhthoff and colleagues[64,65] have proposed a model for the pathogenesis of calcific tendinitis based on its clinical presentation as a self-healing condition in which the calcific process is actively mediated by cells in a viable environment. They classify the disease in three stages: precalcific, calcific and postcalcific. In the precalcific stage it is thought that there is fibrocartilaginous transformation in the avascular or 'critical' zone of the supraspinatus tendon. In the calcific stage calcium crystals are deposited in matrix vehicles to form large deposits (known as the formative phase). After a variable period of inactivity (resting period) there is spontaneous resorption of the calcium by means of peripheral vascularization and phagocytosis of the deposit (resorptive phase). Following removal of the calcium the space is filled with granulation tissue (postcalcific stage). Occasionally a deposit can rupture into the overlying subacromial bursa. There has been a reported association between this condition and HLA-Al[66].

INVESTIGATION

A plain radiograph will identify and localize the calcific deposit to a particular tendon, usually the supraspinatus. In the formative phase of calcification the deposit is well defined and homogenously dense. In the resorptive phase, usually presenting as the acute condition, the deposit is less well defined, irregular and has a fluffy, less dense appearance (Fig. 7.14). Degenerative rotator cuff disease and arthropathy may have radiologically detectable calcification but this is usually associated with other features of these conditions and the areas of calcification are usually small, stippled and close to the tendon insertion at the greater tuberosity.

Laboratory investigation usually does not reveal any abnormality of calcium or phosphate metabolism. There is no associated leukocytosis, raised ESR or change in serum alkaline phosphatase activity.

MANAGEMENT

Asymptomatic patients require no specific treatment. In patients with chronic symptoms conservative management should consist of mobility and strengthening exercises about the glenohumeral joint, physical modalities and NSAIDs for symptom relief if required. An injection of corticosteroid should only be given if there are clear-cut features of impingement and subacromial inflammation and should only be repeated with caution. In the acute stages treatment should include resting the arm in a sling, analgesics, anti-inflammatory medication and local application of ice. Injection of corticosteroid should be avoided as this may inhibit the resorption of calcium, but occasionally needling and aspiration of the deposit is possible with a subsequent reduction in pain. Injection of subacromial lidocaine should also be given for temporary relief of pain (see Chapter 2.12). Some authors advocate corticosteroid injection in the acute phase[65].

Surgical intervention is indicated when conservative management of the chronic condition has failed and there are persistent features of impingement. The deposit can be removed arthroscopically or at an open procedure and may be followed up by resection of the coracoacromial ligament and anterior acromioplasty although there is some evidence that these additional procedures are unnecessary .

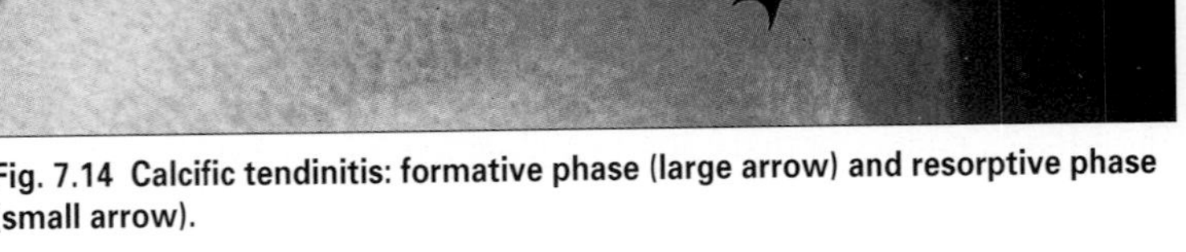

Fig. 7.14 Calcific tendinitis: formative phase (large arrow) and resorptive phase (small arrow).

SCAPULOTHORACIC BURSITIS

Scapulothoracic crepitus should by no means always be considered a pathologic symptom since it is found in 8–70% of the normal population[67]. Rarely, it may represent changes in the bony structure of the deep surface of the scapula or underlying ribs, such as an osteochondroma of the scapula or a rib exostosis. These lesions tend to give rise to a more pronounced snapping sound and may result in deviation of the scapula away from the chest wall. Soft tissue causes are more common, and frequently a diagnosis of scapulothoracic bursitis is made, although the exact pathology if present is difficult to define. Crepitus is frequently found in association with muscular complaints, such as fibrositis, and probably represents a frictional sound as the scapula glides across the underlying muscle layers. Treatment is probably best directed at relief of symptoms and postural exercises, although subscapular injections have been given with variable results and at considerable risk of pneumothorax. Arthroscopic debridement has been described.

GLENOHUMERAL INSTABILITY

Glenohumeral instability is becoming better understood as a major cause of symptoms and pathology of the shoulder joint. The more traditional orthopedic model of shoulder dislocation, whether acute or recurrent, has been expanded to encompass the more subtle but equally important subluxations and minor instabilities which can play an important role in the development of shoulder pain, especially in a young active population. Glenohumeral instability can be classified according to the etiology, direction, type and circumstance of the instability, although in reality this represents a spectrum of disorders ranging from the traumatic unidirectional dislocation with a Bankart lesion to the atraumatic multidirectional instability with bilateral glenohumeral laxity[68]. Symptomatic subluxation or instability often presents as a painful shoulder with all the signs and features of a rotator cuff or bicipital tendinitis, but a careful history and examination coupled with a high index of suspicion in the young adult should confirm the presence of instability.

Management of tendinitis in the young patient with instability should be directed at the resolution of symptoms, restoration of normal flexibility and scapular control, correction of faulty technique in athletes and then a suitable strengthening program for the dynamic stabilizers of the shoulder joint, notably the rotator cuff muscles. Also, correction of any muscle imbalance about the shoulder girdle is important. Arthroscopy allows closer evaluation of shoulder pathology and has an important role in the treatment of symptomatic instability, even to the extent of carrying out stabilization procedures.

REFERENCES

1. Turkel SJ, Panio MW, Marshall JL, Girgis FG. Stabilizing mechanisms preventing anterior dislocation of the glenohumeral joint. J Bone Joint Surg. 1981;63A(8):1208–17.
2. O'Brien SJ, Neves MC, Arnoczky SP, *et al.* The anatomy and histology of the inferior glenohumeral ligament complex of the shoulder. Am J Sports Med. 1990;18(5):449–56.
3. Gohlke F, Essigkrug B, Schmiz F. The pattern of the collagen fiber bundles of the capsule of the glenohumeral joint. J Shoulder Elbow Surg. 1994;3:111–28.
4. Williams MM, Snyder SJ, Buford D Jr. The Buford complex, the cord-like middle glenohumeral ligament and absent anterosuperior labrum complex: a normal anatomic capsulolabral variant. Arthroscopy. 1994;10:2417.
5. Neer CS. Anterior acromioplasty for the chronic impingement syndrome in the shoulder: a preliminary report. J Bone Joint Surg. 1972;54A:41–50.
6. Itoi E, Newman SR, Kuechle DK, Morrey BF, An K-N. Dynamic anterior stabilizers of the shoulder with the arm in abduction. J Bone Joint Surg Br. 1994;76:834–6.
7. Rodosky MW, Harner CD, Fu FH. The role of the long head of the biceps muscle and superior glenoid labrum in anterior stability of the shoulder. Am J Sports Med. 1994;22:121–30.
8. Inman VT, Saunders JB de CM, Abbott LC. Observations on the function of the shoulder joint. J Bone Joint Surg. 1944;26:1–30.
9. Dalton SE. Clinical examination of the painful shoulder. In: Hazleman BL, Dieppe PA, eds. The shoulder joint. Baillière's clinical rheumatology. London: Baillière Tindall; 1989:453–74.
10. Wuelker N, Plitz W, Roetman B. Biomechanical data concerning the shoulder impingement syndrome. Clin Orthop. 1994;303:242–9.
11. Sigholm G, Styf J, Korner L, Herberts P. Pressure recording in the subacromial bursa. J Orthop Res. 1988;6(1):123–8.
12. Rathbun JB, MacNab I. The microvascular pattern of the rotator cuff. J Bone Joint Surg. 1970;52B:540–53.
13. Iannotti JP, Swiontkowski M, Esterhafi J, Boulas HJ. Intraoperative assessment of rotator cuff vascularity using laser Doppler flowmetry. Abstract presented to AAOS Meeting, Las Vegas, 1989.
14. Fukuda H, Mikasa M, Yamanaka K. Incomplete thickness rotator cuff tears diagnosed by subacromial bursography. Clin Orthop.1987;223:51–8.
15. Yamanaka K, Fukuda H, Hamada K, Mikasa M. Incomplete thickness tears of the rotator cuff. Orthop Traumatol Surg (Tokyo).1983;26:713.
16. Riley GP, Harrall RL, Constant CR, Chard MD, Cawston TE, Hazleman BL. Tendon degeneration and chronic shoulder pain: changes in the collagen composition of the human rotator cuff tendons in rotator cuff tendinitis. Ann Rheum Dis. 1994;53:359–66.
17. Riley GP, Harrall RL, Constant CR, Chard MD, Cawston TE, Hazleman BL. Glycosaminoglycans of human rotator cuff tendons: changes with age and in chronic rotator cuff tendinitis. Ann Rheum Dis.1994;53:367–76.
18. Dalton S, Cawston TE, Riley GP, Bayley IJL, Hazleman BL. Human shoulder tendon biopsy samples in organ culture produce procollagenase and tissue inhibitor of metalloproteinases. Ann of Rheum Dis. 1995;54: 571–7.
19. Farin PU, Jaroma H, Harju A, Soimakallio S. Shoulder impingement syndrome: sonographic evaluation. Radiology. 1990;176:845–9.
20. Nielsen KD, Wester JU, Lorensten A. The shoulder impingement syndrome: the results of surgical decompression. J Shoulder Elbow Surg. 1994;3:12–16.
21. Hawkins RJ, Bell RH, Hawkins RH, Koppert GJ. Anterior dislocation of the shoulder in the older patient. Clin Orthop. 1986;206:192–8.
22. Grant JCB, Smith CG. Age incidence of rupture of the supraspinatus tendon. Anat Rec. 1948;100:666.
23. Hazlett JW. Tears of the rotator cuff. J Bone Joint Surg. 1971;53B:772.
24. Hijioka A, Suzuki K, Nakamura T, Hojo T. Degenerative change and rotator cuff tears: An anatomical study in 160 shoulders of 80 cadavers. Arch Orthop Trauma Surg. 1993;112:61–4.
25. Neer CS. Rotator cuff arthropathy. J Bone Joint Surg. 1983,65A:1232–44.
26. Stiles RG, Otte MT. Imaging of the shoulder. Radiology. 1993;188:603–13.
27. Hawkins RJ, Misamore GW, Hobeika PE. Surgery for full-thickness rotator cuff tears. J Bone Joint Surg. 1985;67A:1349–55.
28. Snyder SJ, Karzel RP, Del Pizzo W. SLAP lesions of the shoulder. Arthroscopy.1990;6:274–9.
29. England S, Farrell AJ, Coppock JS, Struthers G, Bacon PA. Low power laser therapy of shoulder tendonitis. Scand J Rheum. 1989;18:427–31.
30. Gam AN, Thorsen H, Lonnberg F. The effect of low-level laser therapy on musculoskeletal pain: a meta-analysis. Pain. 1993;52:63–6.
31. Neviaser RJ, Neviaser TJ. The frozen shoulder. Diagnosis and management. Clin Orthop. 1987;223:59–64.
32. Lundberg BJ. The frozen shoulder. Acta Orthop Scand. 1969;119(suppl.):1–59.
33. Bridgman JF. Periarthritis of the shoulder and diabetes mellitus. Ann Rheum Dis. 1972;31:69–71.
34. Satter MA, Luqman WA. Periarthritis: another duration-related complication of diabetes mellitus. Diabetes Care. 1985;8:507–10.
35. Rizk TE, Pinals RS. Frozen shoulder. Semin Arthritis Rheum. 1982;11(4):440–52.
36. Nash P, Hazleman BL. Frozen shoulder. In: Hazleman BL, Dieppe PA, eds. The shoulder joint. Baillière's clinical rheumatology. London: Baillière Tindall; 1989:551–66.

37. Lloyd-Roberts GC, French PR. Periarthritis of the shoulder. A study of the disease and its treatment. Br Med J. 1959;1:1569–71.
38. Reeves B. The natural history of the frozen shoulder syndrome. Scand J Rheumatol. 1976;4:193–6.
39. Binder A, Bulgen DY, Hazleman BL, Roberts S. Frozen shoulder: a long-term prospective study. Ann Rheum Dis. 1984;43:361–4.
40. Hazleman BL. The painful stiff shoulder. Rheumatol Rehabil. 1972;11:413–21.
41. Wohlgethan JR. Frozen shoulder in hyperthyroidism. Arthritis Rheum. 1987;30:936–9.
42. Bowman C, Jeffcoate W, Patrick M, Doherty M. Bilateral adhesive capsulitis, oligoarthritis and proximal myopathy as a presentation of hypothyroidism. Br J Rheum. 1988;27:62–4.
43. Johnson JTH. Frozen shoulder syndrome in patients with pulmonary tuberculosis. J Bone Joint Surg. 1959,41A:877–82.
44. Saha ND. Painful shoulder in patients with chronic bronchitis and emphysema. Am Rev Respir Dis. 1966;94:455–6.
45. Bulgen DY, Binder A, Hazleman BL, Park JP. Immunological studies in frozen shoulder. J Rheumatol. 1982;9(6):893–8.
46. Binder A, Bulgen DY, Hazleman BL. Frozen shoulder: an arthrographic and radionuclear scan assessment. Ann Rheum Dis. 1984;43:365–9.
47. Bulgen DY, Binder A, Hazleman BL. Frozen shoulder: prospective clinical study with an evaluation of three treatment regimens. Ann Rheum Dis. 1984;43:353–60.
48. Lee PN, Lee M, Haq AM, *et al.* Periarthritis of the shoulder: trial of treatments investigated by multivariate analysis. Ann Rheum Dis. 1974;33:116–9.
49. Richardson AT. The painful shoulder. Proc R Soc Med. 1975;8:731–6.
50. Rizk TE, Pinals RS, Talaiver AS. Corticosteroid injections in adhesive capsulitis: investigation of their value and site. Arch Phys Med Rehabil. 1991;72:20–2.
51. Binder A, Hazleman BL, Parr G, Roberts S. A controlled study of oral prednisolone in frozen shoulder. Br J Rheum. 1986,25:288–92.
52. Pollock RG, Duralde XA, Flatow EL, Bigliani LU. The use of arthroscopy in the treatment of resistant frozen shoulder. Clin Orthop. 1994;304:30–6.
53. Griffith PH III, Boyadjis TA. Acute pyoarthrosis of the acromioclavicular joint: a case report. Orthopedics. 1984;7(11):1727–8.
54. Rockwood CA, Young DC, Disorders of the acromioclavicular joint. In: Rockwood CA, Matsen FA, eds. The shoulder, Vol 2. Philadelphia: WB Saunders; 1990:413–76.
55. Cahill BR. Osteolysis of the distal part of the clavicle in male athletes. J Bone Joint Surg. 1982;64A(7):1053–8.
56. Levine AH, Pais MJ, Schwartz EE. Post traumatic osteolysis of the distal clavicle with emphasis on early radiologic changes. Am J Rheumatol. 1976;127:781–4.
57. De Palma AF. Surgery of the shoulder, 2E. Philadelphia: JB Lippincott; 1973.
58. Bosworth BM. Calcium deposits in the shoulder and subacromial bursitis: A survey of 12 122 shoulders. JAMA.1941;116:2477–82.
59. Welfling J, Kahn MF, Desroy M, Paolaggi JB, De Seze S. Les calcifications de l'epaule. II. La maladie des calcifications tendineuses multiples. Revue de Rhumatisme. 1965;32:325–34.
60. Bosworth BM. Examination of the shoulder for calcium deposits. J Bone Joint Surg. 1941;23:567–77.
61. McLaughlin HL. Lesions of the musculotendinous cuff of the shoulder. III: Observations on the pathology, course and treatment of calcific deposits. Ann Surg. 1946;124:354–62.
62. Hsu HC, Wu JJ, Jim YF, Chang CY, Lo WH, Yang DJ. Calcific tendinitis and rotator cuff tearing: a clinical and radiographic study. J Shoulder Elbow Surg. 1994;3:159–64.
63. MacNab I. Rotator cuff tendinitis. Ann R Coll Surg Engl. 1973;53:271–87.
64. Uhthoff HK. Calcifying tendinitis: An active cell-mediated calcification. Virchows Arch [A]. 1975;366:51–8.
65. Uhthoff HK, Sarkar K. Calcifying tendinitis. In: Hazleman BL, Dieppe PA, eds. The shoulder joint. Baillière's clinical rheumatology. London: Baillière Tindall; 1989:567–81.
66. Sengar DPS, McKendry RJ, Uthoff HK. Increased frequency of HLA-AI in calcifying tendinitis. Tissue Antigens.1987;29:173–4.
67. Milch H. Snapping scapula. Clin Orthop.1961; 20:139–50.
68. Dalton SE, Snyder SJ. Glenohumeral instability. In: Hazleman BL, Dieppe PA, eds. The shoulder joint. Baillière's Clinical Rheumatology. London: Baillière Tindall; 1989:511–34.

8

THE ELBOW

Michael D Chard

- The elbow is a complex hinge joint essential for the positioning and full use of the hand.
- Relevant anatomy includes the radiohumeral and ulnohumeral hinge, the connecting proximal radioulnar joint, the radial head, the medial and lateral epicondyles, the ulnar nerve groove, the muscles spanning the elbow and the olecranon bursa.
- Soft tissue lesions such as lateral epicondylitis and olecranon bursitis are far more frequent than joint disease.
- Diagnosis of elbow conditions is largely based on pain characteristics; location of swelling; presence of point tenderness; and the results of passive, active and resisted motion.

FUNCTIONAL ANATOMY

JOINT STRUCTURES

The elbow is considered to be a hinge joint but is more accurately classified as a trochleogi-glenoid joint since it is a hinged joint about a trochlea or pulley. This allows for motions of pronation and supination motion of the forearm. The combination of flexion and rotation at the elbow enables the hands to be brought into view and provides a steady but adjustable base for the hands to make best use of the highly mobile fingers and opposable thumb. It is a compound synovial joint since it is composed of articulation between the ulnar notch and trochlea of the humerus, and between the radial head and humeral capitellum (Fig. 8.1). In continuity with these is the proximal radioulnar joint [1].

At its distal end the humerus is expanded to form a modified condyle, widest transversely, and consists of articular and nonarticular parts. The capitellum on the lateral aspect is curved, forms less than half a sphere and contributes anterior and inferior surfaces. A shallow groove separates the capitellum from the medial trochlea, which has anterior, inferior and posterior surfaces. Its medial margin projects inferiorly and the edge is the main determinant of the angulation between the long axis of the radius and ulna in an extended supinated position. Medial and lateral bony projections of the lower humerus form the epicondyles which along with olecranon, coronoid and radial fossae make up the nonarticular part of the condyle. The fossae accept the relevant parts of the ulna and radius during extremes of extension and flexion movements. Above the larger medial and less prominent lateral epicondyle formed by the flexion of the distal humerus are the supracondylar ridges. The medial epicondyle provides a groove for the ulnar nerve as it crosses the elbow to enter the forearm.

At its proximal end the radius has a head, neck and tuberosity. The head is discoid with a proximal shallow cup for the humeral capitellum and an articular periphery which is deepest medially where it contacts the ulnar radial notch. Distal to this is the constriction of the neck which leads on medially to the bony prominence of the tuberosity. The large proximal ulna has large olecranon and coronoid processes, with a large trochlear and smaller radial notches to articulate with humerus and radius. The deep trochlear notch articulating with the humeral trochlea is a major contributor in making the elbow joint one of the most congruous and inherently stable. Together, the ulnohumeral and radiohumeral joints provide approximately 50% of the joint stability, the rest being due to soft tissue constraint.

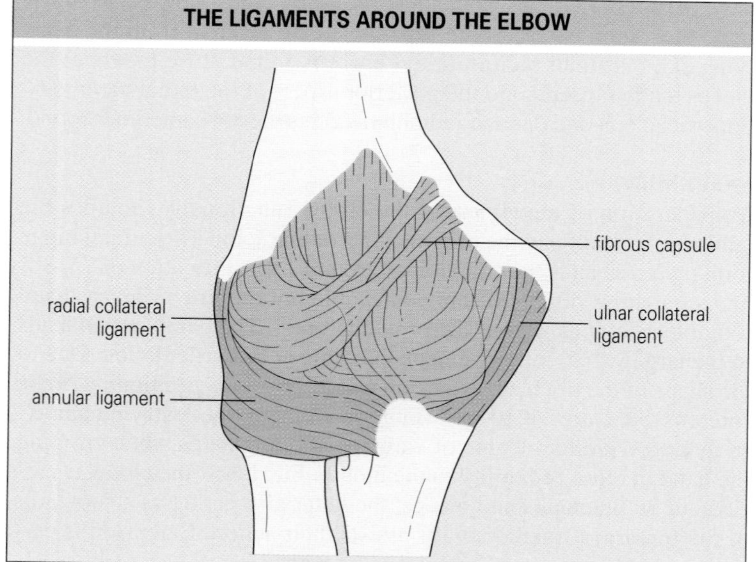

Fig. 8.1 Expanded view of the elbow joint showing the bony features.

LIGAMENTS, CAPSULE AND SYNOVIUM

Varus–valgus stability of the elbow is largely due to the collateral ligaments (Fig. 8.2) [2]. The medial (ulnar) collateral ligament has anterior, posterior and inferior (oblique) parts. It forms a triangular band with its apex attached around the medial epicondyle and extending in a fan-shaped fashion to insert into a proximal tubercle on the medial coronoid margin (anteriorly), and the medial margin of olecranon (posteriorly). The anterior portion is the most important elbow stabilizer. The lateral (radial)

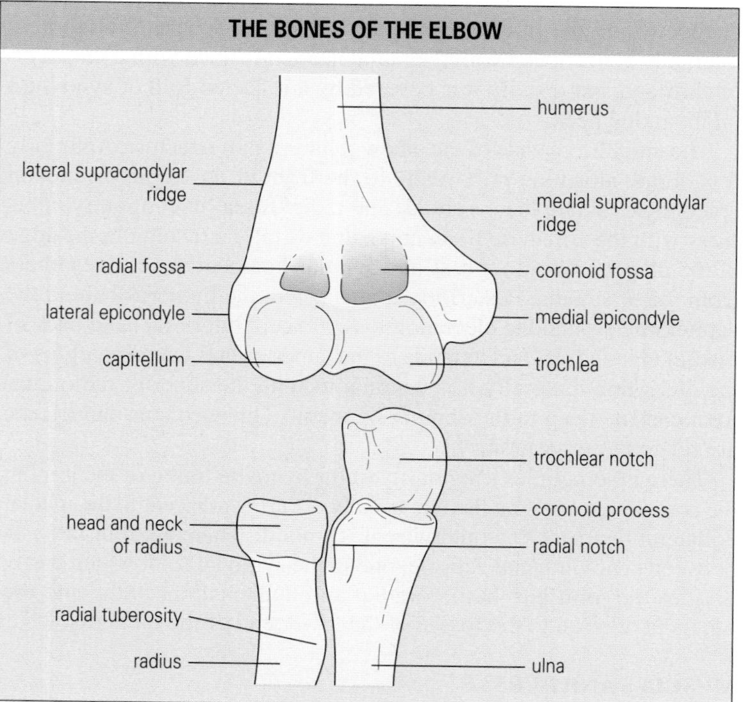

Fig. 8.2 Anterior view of the elbow joint showing the ligaments and capsule.

collateral ligament is attached low on the lateral epicondyle and extends to the annular ligament. Its superficial fibers are blended with those of the attachment of supinator and extensor carpi radialis brevis.

The annular ligament is a strong band that encircles the radial head, holding it against the radial notch of the ulna. It attaches to the edge of the notch anteriorly and on a ridge at or just behind the edge posteriorly. The proximal annular border is continuous with the cubital capsule except posteriorly where the capsule passes deep to it at the radial notch. The distal annular border attaches loosely to the radial neck after passing over a synovial reflection. Posterior to the ligament are the anconeus and the interosseus recurrent artery. Where the ligament internally is in contact with the radial head, it is lined with a thin layer of cartilage, but distally it is covered by a reflected fold of synovium on the radial neck.

The articular capsule of the elbow joint is a thin structure. Anteriorly it is broad, attaching proximally to the front of the humerus, medial epicondyle (above the coronoid) and radial fossa (in continuity on its sides with the collateral ligaments), and distally attaching to the edge of the ulna, coronoid process and annular ligament. It receives fibers from the brachialis. Posteriorly it attaches to the humerus behind the capitellum, around the olecranon fossa (except inferiorly) and back of medial epicondyle, and extends to the superior and lateral margins of the olecranon. Laterally it is continuous with the superior radioulnar joint capsule deep to the annular ligament. The anconeus and triceps are related to it posteriorly.

There is sometimes irregularity of the synovial lining of the joint in the coronoid process on flexion, usually occuring adjacent to the medial collateral ligament, but otherwise it is smooth. There are four fat pads between synovium and capsule; one in the synovial fold, which partly divides the joint into humeroradial and humeroulnar parts, and the others in relation to the fossae of the lower end of the humerus.

MUSCLES AND BURSAE

Muscles that are related to the elbow joint are the brachialis (in front) the triceps and anconeus (behind), the supinator and common extensor tendon (laterally) and the common flexor tendon and flexor carpi ulnaris (medially) (Fig. 8.3). Anterior to the brachialis, the biceps tendon passes on its way to insertion into the radial tuberosity. The common superficial flexor tendon is attached to the medial epicondyle and the common superficial extensor tendon to the lateral epicondyle, both exterior to the joint capsule. The anconeus attaches to the posterior aspect of the lateral epicondyle. Above the medial epicondyle on the supracondylar ridge is attached the humeral head of the pronator teres, while the lateral supracondylar ridge gives attachment to the extensor carpi radialis longus. The triceps passes posteriorly over the elbow joint to insert into the olecranon. Numerous bursal structures have been reported, but the main bursa around the elbow is the superficial olecranon bursa, which separates the olecranon from the overlying skin. A small bicipitoradial bursa is found close to where the biceps tendon inserts into the posterior aspect of the radial tuberosity. Superficial epicondylar and radiohumeral bursae are sometimes found.

MOVEMENT

Consideration of movement at the elbow functionally includes the cubital joint itself and the proximal radioulnar joint. The cubital hinge joint traverses an area of flexion of around 150°. Pronation of 75–80° and supination of 85–90° are achievable but require an intact distal radioulnar joint as well as the proximal one [3]. The combination leads to the large variety of movements possible at this articulation. Due to the shape of the trochlea, extension results in valgus positioning of the forearm to the arm of 10–15° (more in women), the 'carrying angle'. In flexion, a similar degree of varus positioning helps when bringing the hand in close proximity to the mouth. Flexion at the elbow is carried out by brachialis and biceps, the latter also acting as a supinator of the forearm. Brachioradialis assists their action. Extension is carried out by the triceps aided by the anconeus.

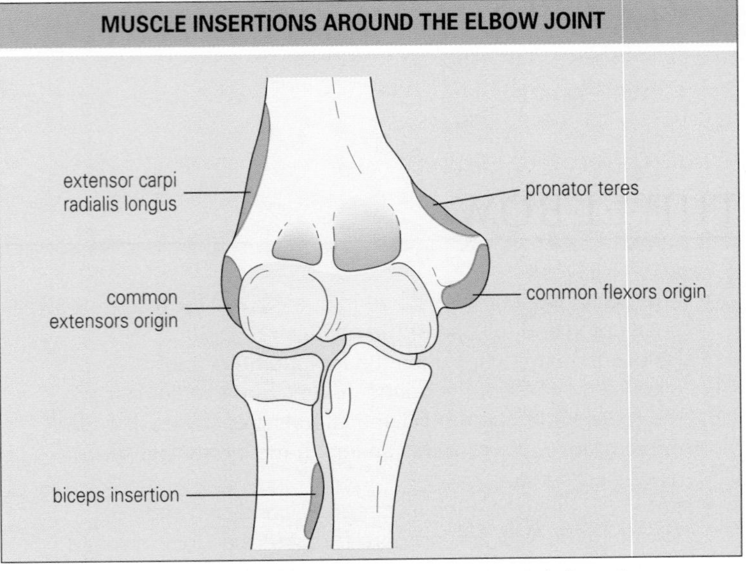

Fig. 8.3 Anterior view of the elbow joint showing the muscle insertions.

NEUROVASCULAR RELATIONSHIPS

The elbow joint receives articular arteries from numerous periarticular anastamoses that are supplied mainly by the brachial artery. Articular nerves are derived principally from the radial and musculocutaneous nerves, but the median, ulnar and sometimes the anterior interosseous nerves contribute as well. These nerves follow the supply of blood vessel and probably contain vasomotor fibers as well as pain and proprioception afferents. The neurovascular structures of the arm have an intimate relationship with the joint capsule. The brachial artery traverses the joint anteriorly, just medial to the biceps tendon in the antecubital space. The musculocutaneous nerve innervates the biceps and brachialis above the level of the elbow and terminates distally to form the lateral cutaneous nerve of the forearm. The course of the median nerve takes it anterior to the joint capsule and medial to the biceps tendon and brachial artery. The radial nerve passes anterior to the lateral epicondyle, descending beneath brachialis and brachioradialis muscles. The ulnar nerve traverses the elbow in the ulnar groove behind the medial epicondyle.

EXAMINATION

INTRODUCTION

The examination of the elbow must be preceded by a precise history to allow emphasis to be placed on particular areas. Complaints usually consist of pain, loss of movement, weakness, clicking or locking. There may be sharply localized pain, typical of extra-articular pathology, deep joint pain or the poorly localized pain of ulnar neuropathy with or without typical paresthesia extending to the hand. The functional interplay between elbow, shoulder and wrist means that examination of all these joints may be necessary. Referred pain in the elbow, especially from the neck or shoulder, is usually diffuse. Examination must include comparison of right and left arms (Fig. 8.4).

INSPECTION

Inspection is very important since much of the elbow joint is subcutaneous and so alterations in soft tissue or bony anatomy are easily seen. Anteriorly viewing the elbow in the extended, supinated position allows assessment of the carrying angle. It is increased in certain congenital conditions, such as Turner's syndrome, and may be altered by fractures around the elbow. Synovial proliferation and effusion are each detected as a fullness in the region of the lateral infracondylar recess. The swelling may be obliterated by pressure in the case of effusion. A hard bony swelling is detected where there is radial head

EXAMINATON OF THE ELBOW	
Inspection	Swelling joint bursa Deformity Carrying angle
Palpation	Synovial Joint line epicondyles/soft tissues Ulnar nerve
Movement	Active Passive Resisted
Other	Upper limb neurologic examination Neck and shoulder

Fig. 8.4 Examination of the elbow.

pathology, such as previous fracture. Posteriorly, swelling of the subcutaneous olecranon bursa may be detected, and in rheumatoid arthritis nodules often occur extending distally along the border of the ulna. Occasionally ulnar neuritis may result in enlargement of the ulnar nerve, which is seen medially.

PALPATION

Palpation is easily undertaken of the subcutaneous lateral and medial epicondyles and olecranon tip. Tenderness over the lateral epicondyle is typical of lateral epicondylitis. The radial head is palpated by gentle pressure over the radiocapitellar joint and assessed during pronation and supination movements. Loose bodies may be detected in the infracondylar recess. Medially the ulnar nerve may be palpated to detect thickening, and assessment with the elbow in flexion and extension detects ulnar nerve subluxation. The nerve may displace anteriorly during flexion, sometimes with an obvious snap, and be associated with ulnar nerve paresthesia. Posteriorly, the tip of the olecranon and the olecranon fossa above can be felt if the elbow is not in full extension. Flexion to around 15° also enables assessment of the collateral ligaments. These may be palpated. Varus stress with the humerus in full internal rotation, and valgus stress in full external rotation test for lateral and medial instability, respectively, but abnormality is often subtle and requires experience to detect [4].

MOVEMENT

Active and passive ranges of movement should be measured including flexion, extension and rotation. Most frequently, a reduced range of movement is due to pain. After injury, elbow joint extension is both the first movement to be lost and the last to recover. The normal range of flexion–extension, 0–150°, is in excess of that needed for everyday activity, which is of the order of 30–130°. Forcibly moving the joint beyond the pain-free range helps to identify the predominant cause of the restriction. In extension, posterior pain indicates a posterior impingement problem, whereas anterior pain indicates tightness of the anterior capsule. The reverse is true for loss of flexion. Early in arthritis flexion and extension are limited but rotational movements are often spared. Motion is best assessed with the elbow flexed to 90° and held to the side of the body, with supination often greater than 85° and a little less for pronation.

Pain should be sought on resisted active movements, particularly where there is no major intra-articular pathology. These are carried out with the elbow held at 90°. Flexion and supination strength is normally greater than extension and pronation. Passive, but not resisted, movements producing pain indicate intra-articular pathology, whereas pain on resisted movement alone indicates a musculotendinous pathology associated with that movement. To complete the assessment of muscles around the elbow, resisted flexion and extension of the wrist must be performed [5]. Neurologic examination must not be omitted, with particular attention paid to structures supplied by the C5, C6 and C7 nerve roots. Biceps jerk (C5), brachioradialis reflex (C6) and triceps jerk (C7) should be asssessed.

DIFFERENTIAL DIAGNOSIS OF ELBOW PAIN

Pain felt at the elbow may be due to either local pathology or referred pain (Fig. 8.5). As indicated above, shoulder and cervical problems frequently produce pain referred to the elbow. Although this pain is usually part of more generalized arm pain symptoms, which in the case of cervical spine lesions are often associated with frank neurologic symptoms, it may be localized. Examination of the neck and shoulder is therefore important in the assessment of elbow pain. Intrathoracic pathology can give rise to arm pain but is rarely localized to the elbow.

True elbow pain may be related to joint disease but is more commonly due to lesions of the soft periarticular tissues. These causes can usually be distinguished by history and appropriate examination. Primary osteoarthritis is not common, but elbow involvement frequently occurs in more generalized inflammatory arthritis. Traumatic effusions occur, and the joint may be involved by a fracture of the bones, minor fractures sometimes being missed and only presenting as an effusion. A traumatic/overuse form of osteochondritis of the radial head can occur in some throwing sports, especially in the teenage child. The joint may be affected by loose bodies and synovial osteochondromatosis. Traumatic partial subluxation of the radial head through the annular ligament occurs in children, especially if they have a hypermobile tendency. Plain anteroposterior and lateral radiographs are useful in assessing joint pathology. Further investigation of the joint is best carried out by arthroscopy rather than tomography or arthrography, although magnetic resonance imaging, where available, is a better noninvasive alternative.

SOFT TISSUE ELBOW LESIONS

INTRODUCTION

Apart from lateral epicondylitis ('tennis elbow'), medial epicondylitis ('golfer's elbow') and olecranon bursitis, soft tissue lesions at the elbow are relatively rare. Biceps tendinitis is characterized by local pain and tenderness in the region of the bicipital tuberosity of the radius, with pain on resisted flexion and supination. Pain on resisted flexion alone indicates the rarer brachialis muscle lesion with pain and tenderness which is less well localized and found behind the biceps tendon. Although uncommon, such a tear is particularly prone to develop myositis ossificans which in the early phases produces a warm, firm mass which can be mistaken for tumor [5]. Pain on resisted supination alone is said to indicate a supinator lesion, but this very rarely if

DIFFERENTIAL DIAGNOSIS OF ELBOW PAIN		
Local	Articular	Arthritis, osteochondritis, loose bodies, subluxation
	Periarticular	Lateral and medial epicondylitis, olecranon bursitis, ligamentous lesions, entrapment neuropathy
Referred		Cervical and shoulder disease

Fig. 8.5 Differential diagnosis of elbow pain.

ever occurs and pain would be felt further down the forearm. It is unusual to have a lesion at the site of triceps insertion into the olecranon (triceps tendinitis) but instead these occur higher in the arm at the musculotendinous junction. Ligamentous lesions do not usually occur in isolation, most often being associated with traumatic joint synovitis or effusion, if not frank joint derangement or fracture. Medially, a ligamentous lesion may form at least part of the elbow injury caused by some throwing sports, such as javelin.

OLECRANON BURSITIS

Bursal inflammation around the elbow can occur and principally affects the olecranon bursa (see Chapter 4.14). Both epicondylar and radiohumeral bursitis have been reported but are rare, producing vague symptoms around the elbow with swelling. They have in the past been suggested as causes of tennis elbow but rarely, if ever, have the same clinical features. Due to its superficial position over the olecranon, the olecranon bursa is prone to injury by friction or a blow. In addition, due to its position, swelling occurs easily and is readily visible. It may also be involved in crystal arthropathies (gout or rarely calcium pyrophosphate arthritis) or in generalized inflammatory arthritis, especially rheumatoid arthritis where swelling of the olecranon bursa may be seen in association with rheumatoid nodules on the ulnar border of the forearm (Fig. 8.6). There is often no obvious precipitating cause of olecranon bursitis. Infection of the bursa can occur.

In traumatic or idiopathic olecranon bursitis, pain is usually localized and typically does not occur on passive or resisted movement. It is usually provoked by leaning on the elbow or flexion with a constriction around the elbow such as a coat sleeve. Tenderness should be sought about the tip of the olecranon and will be present, sometimes with palpable thickening of the bursal wall, even in the absence of significant effusion; it is generally very sensitive to pressure. Septic olecranon bursitis occurs less frequently (around 25% of hospital cases) but it is important and should not be missed. Usually it occurs following an abrasion or it may be associated with an initial cellulitis of the skin. Septic olecranon bursitis usually causes pain with elbow flexion and sometimes with resisted extension, but it is different from acute arthritis as gentle passive extension is unimpaired [6]. Aspiration of the bursa both reduces symptoms and allows assessment of the fluid (see Chapter 2.12 for technical aspects). Along with gross visualization of blood staining, or turbidity of the fluid, white cell count and differential, and Gram stain with culture of the fluid should be undertaken to exclude infection. Polarizing light microscopy should be performed to reveal any crystals. If infection has been satisfactorily excluded by culture, local corticosteroid injection may be performed which is effective in speeding recovery [7]. A compressive elastic bandage will help to prevent recurrence of swelling. The finding of infection requires appropriate antibiotic therapy and reaspiration of pus as necessary.

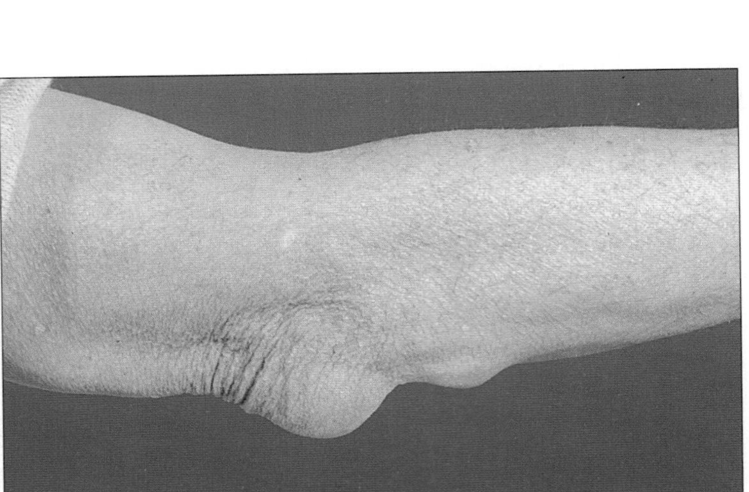

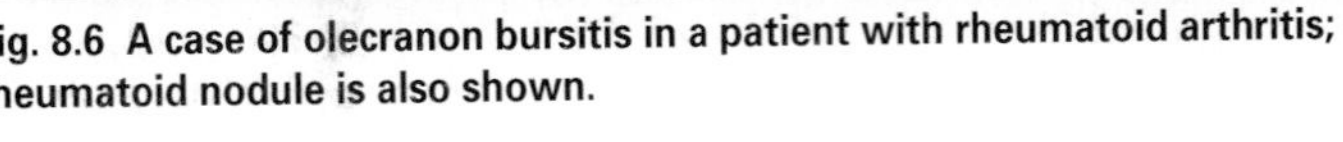

Fig. 8.6 A case of olecranon bursitis in a patient with rheumatoid arthritis; a rheumatoid nodule is also shown.

Staphylococcus aureus is the most frequently found organism although a streptococcus or *S. epidermidis* are less commonly found [6,8]. Other organisms are rarely implicated. If repeated non-infective bursitis occurs then surgical removal of the bursa should be considered.

LATERAL EPICONDYLITIS

Used synonymously with the term 'tennis elbow' this condition is one of the most common lesions of the arm. The first description is attributed to Runge in 1873 [9], but the name 'tennis elbow' is derived from Morris's description of 'lawn tennis arm' in the Lancet of 1882 [10]. Around 1–3% of the population are affected by it [11,12], mostly those aged between 40 years and 60 years, the dominant arm being affected most frequently. Some 40–50% of tennis players suffer with it, mainly older players [13,14], but in clinical practice less than 5% of cases are due to the game [15]. It is found most often in nonathletes and the majority are not manual workers. Many cannot describe any specific precipitating factors [16].

Etiopathology

There have been more than 25 suggested causes of the condition [17], and this reflects the use of the diagnosis nonspecifically for lateral elbow pain. Pathologic material for study is relatively rare as most cases do not come to surgery. Reported operative findings in relatively few chronic cases have included periostitis [9], infection [17], radiohumeral joint disease [18], radial nerve entrapment [19] and a lesion of the orbicular (annular) ligament [20]. It is believed, however, that the majority of cases are due to a musculotendinous lesion of the common extensor tendon at the attachment to the lateral epicondyle or nearby, especially that portion derived from extensor carpi radialis brevis [5,15].

Macroscopic tears in the common extensor tendon are sometimes found at operation [15], but repeated high dose local corticosteroid injections may have affected findings. Microfractures, cystic and fibrinoid degeneration and round cell infiltrations, immature fibrous tissue, hyaline degeneration and vascular plus fibroblastic proliferation ('angiofibroblastic tendinosis') sometimes with calcific debris and attempts at repair have been described [14,15,21,22,23]. Some cases show a chronic traction effect. Histologic evidence of inflammation has not been found. The relationship of such findings to the acute lesion is uncertain. Ischemic stress may be important because the tenoperiosteal junction (enthesis) and nearby tendon are relatively avascular, since the blood supply is a watershed of that derived from muscle and bone and working muscle takes up the blood supply at the expense of tendon.

Age is an important factor, since lateral epicondylitis rarely occurs before the age of 30 years. Adult maturity is associated with alterations in the enthesis, including changes in collagen content, reduction in cells and ground substance and increase in lipids, which then probably predispose it to injury [24]. Other possible changes that may be important, including those due to tendon elasticity, have yet to be elucidated. The onset of symptoms may be brought on by overuse and hence lateral epicondylitis is more often seen in the active middle aged than the less active elderly. In manual workers relative overuse of wrist and finger extensors may precipitate the condition, which most often affects the dominant arm. Sometimes there may be bilateral involvement either due to increased stress placed on the unaffected arm or resulting from a general tendency to soft tissue lesions which occurs in some individuals [14,16].

Clinical findings

Lateral epicondylitis usually arises slowly and apparently spontaneously; a blow or acute traumatic strains are relatively rarely remembered. Pain is localized to the lateral epicondyle but may spread up and down the upper limb. Grip is impaired due to pain, and this may result in restricted daily activities. Tenderness over the epicondyle is usual, although maximum tenderness is sometimes found at nearby sites [5,20]. The other cardinal sign is increase in pain on resisting wrist dorsiflexion with the elbow in extension (Fig. 8.7). Symptoms may also be precipitated by extending the elbow with the wrist flexed (Fig.

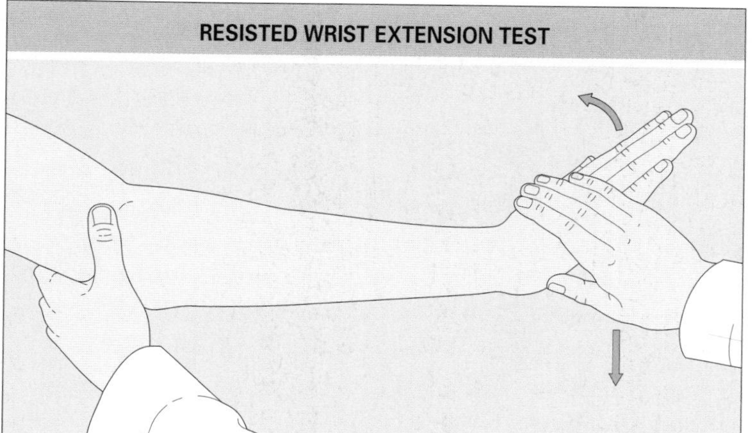

Fig. 8.7 Resisted wrist extension test.

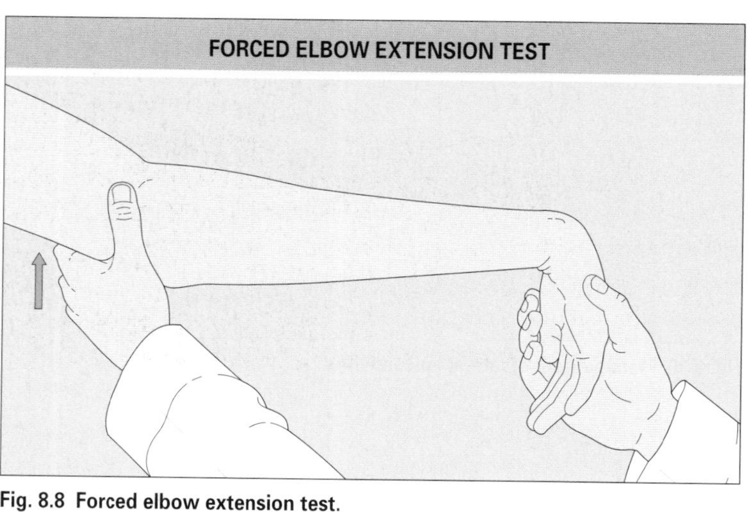

Fig. 8.8 Forced elbow extension test.

8.8) and by resisted middle finger extension. Resisted supination may also be painful. The range of movement of the elbow is usually normal but a few degrees of extension may be lost in some severe and chronic cases. It is important to exclude other conditions producing elbow pain, especially that referred from the cervical spine or shoulder, as well as arthritis of the elbow, although this is usually obvious.

A nerve entrapment around the elbow may produce diagnostic confusion. Radial tunnel syndrome or compression of the posterior interosseous nerve [19] can produce lateral elbow and upper forearm pain. It can be the cause of apparent lateral epicondylitis that is unresponsive to conservative treatment but is believed to be a rare cause of resistant cases [25]. These entrapments have been found to be due to compressive lesions caused by abnormal fibrous bands in front of the radial head, a sharp tendinous origin of extensor carpi radialis brevis, or a radial recurrent fan of vessels. More rarely, a lipoma or ganglion has been found to be the cause. Compression of the posterior interosseous nerve may occur where it passes through supinator muscle just below the elbow joint. A well defined arcade of Frohse is present in 30% of subjects [26] and makes a compression neuropathy more likely. Diffuse pain, symptoms distal to the lateral epicondyle and the presence of muscle weakness may be useful distinguishing features.

Investigations

Investigations are not usually required but radiographs of the elbow may be helpful in excluding joint disease and may occasionally show lateral soft tissue calcification. Electromyography may be helpful in excluding a nerve entrapment. Quantitative assessment of severity and response to treatment is difficult, but grading pain, tenderness and pain on resisted wrist extension can be helpful, and lifting graded weights and grip strength measurement aid objectivity [27]. A truly objective measurement is that of infrared thermography of the affected elbow which shows a discrete localized area of increased heat near the lateral epicondyle in 98% of affected elbows (Fig. 8.9). Analysis of the gradient across the abnormal area reveals a correlation with clinical severity [27]. Lack of general availability of this technique means it is mainly a research tool. Magnetic resonance imaging has been used to identify tissue abnormalities prior to surgery in chronic cases [28].

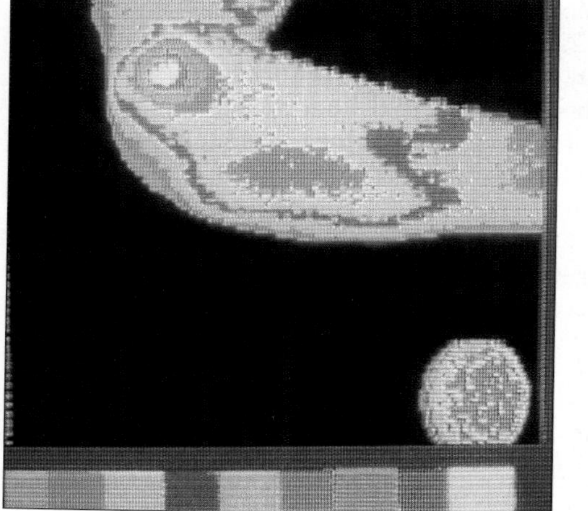

Fig. 8.9 An infrared thermographic pattern in lateral epicondylitis showing localized 'hot spot'.

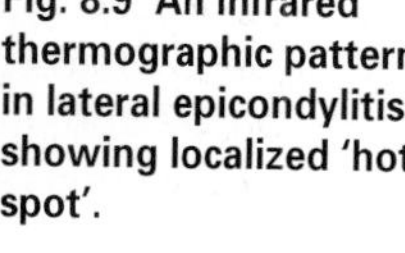

Management

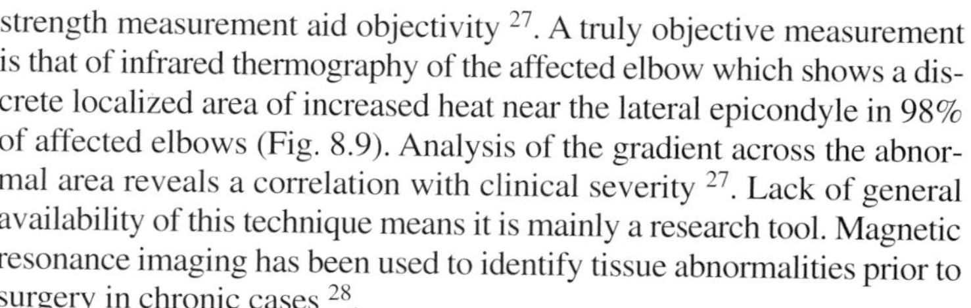

Over 40 treatment regimens for lateral epicondylitis have been described in the literature, ranging from the extremes of 'prolonged observation' to X-ray therapy. Reduced activity may result in resolution of symptoms in a few patients and may be effective in early cases especially with some form of splinting (see Fig. 8.10). A simple sling can be used but is unlikely to be effective as the forearm is usually held in position with the wrist flexed. A plaster cast or brace may be helpful, but since 4–6 weeks of immobility are required these risk a long term fixed flexion deformity. However, a hinged brace may be tried, which has a reduced risk of residual flexion deformity. A cock-up wrist splint reducing tension on forearm extensors is an alternative. Nonsteroidal anti-inflammatory drugs (NSAIDs) are often used, but evidence for their efficacy is tenuous. The new NSAID gels may be more useful and avoid the risk of systemic side effects. A trial of treatment in early or mild cases would be appropriate.

Numerous physical modalities of treatment have been used to treat lateral epicondylitis, but the efficacy of most of them remains unproven. Ultrasound, by its ability to cross myofascial planes and concentrate near bone, has theoretical advantages. A double blind controlled trial has confirmed an advantage for pulsed therapeutic ultrasound. Sixty-three percent of patients improved and the technique had the merit of being non-painful with a relapse rate lower than that after corticosteroid injection [29]. Medical laser light therapy has been used as treatment in recent years but published placebo controlled trials have not confirmed efficacy using varying techniques [30,31]. Acupuncture has also been used in treatment [32].

Local injections of corticosteroids have been widely used and have been shown to be superior to saline and local anesthetics [33]. Corticosteroids may not, however, produce a better outcome at six months after injection than lidocaine alone [34]. The newer preparations may produce a quicker response, but they may also lead to loss of subcutaneous fat, with dimpling and depigmentation, especially with repeated injection. Local corticosteroid injections (see Chapter 2.12) are both efficacious and cost effective, with around 90% of subjects responding. But the injection may cause increased pain for up to 72 hours afterwards and a significant number of patients relapse [16]. The injection may be repeated after 2–4 weeks, in the event of either failure to respond or relapse, but should not be repeated more than twice as it is unlikely then to be effective, increases risk of side effects and predisposes to chronic pain [35].

MANAGEMENT OF LATERAL EPICONDYLITIS	
Early/mild	Rest, splinting, NSAID
Established	Local corticosteroid injection Ultrasound
Resistant	Manipulation? Surgery – lateral release

Fig. 8.10 Management of lateral epicondylitis.

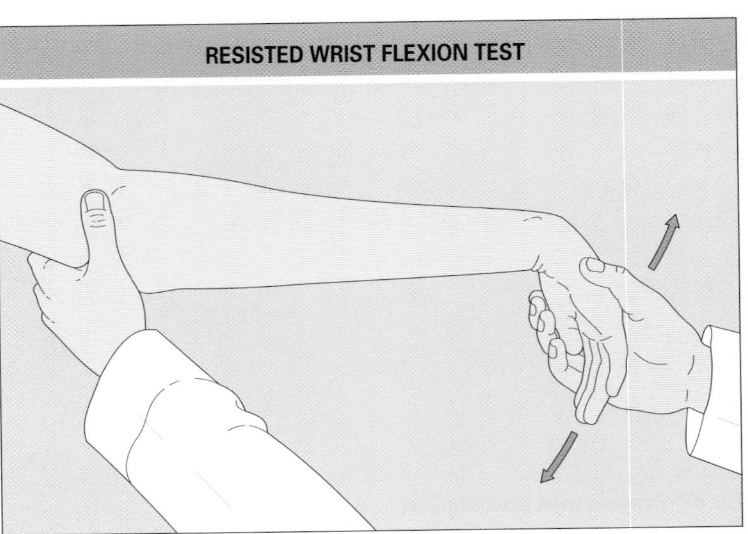

Fig. 8.11 Resisted wrist flexion test.

Prognosis

Lateral epicondylitis has been considered to be a self-limiting disorder with patients improving with or without treatment within 1 year [5]. This good prognosis contrasts with reported relapse rates of between 18% and 50% 6 months after conservative treatment [36,37]. In one study 40% of patients had prolonged minor discomfort, which in some persisted for 5 years. Manual workers, especially mechanics, builders and domestic workers, are most susceptible to recurrence on resumption of the activity which induced the initial pain [16]. Early treatment may improve prognosis. Firm strapping of the forearm muscles just distal to the elbow joint, or the use of one of the commercial elbow splints, may be helpful. Patients should be instructed to avoid straining the arm for at least 3 months. Although emphasis is on rest, graded exercises to strengthen forearm muscles may be prescribed, especially in the rehabilitation back to sport. In a few cases persistence of lateral elbow pain despite local treatment is due to a cervical lesion which was not originally clinically apparent, and re-examination may be necessary.

Resistant cases

Up to 10% of patients fail to respond to physical therapy and injections [38]. Surgical intervention is then considered. The value of manipulation as a means of avoiding surgery is controversial. It may be effective when performed under general anesthetic by an experienced practitioner, particularly using the method of Mills in conjunction with a local corticosteroid injection [38]. Approaches to surgical management have attempted to correct the presumed pathology. Excision of tissues around the epicondyle, removal of synovial fringe of the radiohumeral joint or partial removal of the annular ligament have all been advocated. Denervation of the lateral epicondyle has been used to relieve symptoms in a few cases. Most commonly either repair of tears [15], and removal of abnormal tendon is undertaken [22] or a procedure to lengthen the muscle tendon complex is carried out. Such lengthening has been achieved either by the less favored distal tenotomy [39] or by a 'lateral release' procedure involving division of the origin of the common extensor tendon [40,41]. Advocates of removal of abnormal tendon and repair claim a better response and are concerned about weakness caused by a 'lateral release'. Others believe the 'lateral release' gives as good long term results of around 90% using a simpler procedure which may even be carried out under local anesthetic. There is general agreement that extensive lateral release with resection of the proximal third of the annular ligament is best avoided due to risk of subsequent elbow instability [42].

MEDIAL EPICONDYLITIS

Otherwise known as 'golfer's elbow', this condition is around 15 times less commonly seen than lateral epicondylitis [15]. It is a lesion of the common flexor tendon at the medial epicondyle. As with 'tennis elbow', a sporting cause is relatively rare. The condition is usually milder and often pain and tenderness are less well localized to the medial epicondyle, being felt a little distal to the flexor origin. Pain on resisted wrist flexion with the elbow in extension is the most reliable sign (Fig. 8.11), although rarely flexion of the fingers rather than of the wrist best elicits symptoms. The pathology and management are essentially the same as those for lateral epicondylitis.

CONCLUSION

The elbow is a hinged joint to which is added the pronation and supination motion of the forearm, producing a steady adjustable base to make best use of the hands. Elbow pain is due either to joint disease or more commonly to a lesion of the soft periarticular tissues. Referred pain from the neck and shoulder can give rise to diagnostic confusion and must be excluded by appropriate examination. Nerve entrapment about the elbow can mimic the pain of a soft tissue lesion. Lateral epicondylitis is the most frequent periarticular lesion, affecting 1–3% of the population mainly in middle life, but despite its common name of tennis elbow it is rarely due to the sport. Medial epicondylitis and olecranon bursitis are the other common periarticular lesions. Diagnosis is clinical and straightforward, based on relevant history and examination. Olecranon bursitis and some elbow joint conditions may be effectively treated by aspiration and local corticosteroid injection but the possibility of an underlying infection must be considered and examination of synovial fluid is necessary before injection.

Epicondylitis can be successfully treated in 90% of cases by local corticosteroid injection into the tender tendon origin at the humeral epicondyle (see Chapter 2.12). The injection is not infrequently painful initially and relapse may occur requiring further injection. No more than two repeat injections should be given and the arm should not be strained for at least 3 months afterwards. Pulsed therapeutic ultrasound is an effective alternative which is nonpainful but is less frequently successful. For the 10% of resistant cases manipulation under general anesthetic may be tried but in general a surgical lateral release procedure should be considered.

REFERENCES

1. Williams PL, Warwick R, Dyson M, Bannister IH, eds. Gray's anatomy, 37E. Edinburgh: Churchill Livingstone;1989.
2. Morrey BF, An KN. Articular and ligamentous contributions to stability of the elbow joint. Am J Sports Med. 1983;11:315–9.
3. Boone DC, Azen SP. Normal range of motion in the joint in male subjects. J Bone Joint Surg. 1979;(AM)61:756–9.
4. Yocum LA. The diagnosis and non–operative treatment of elbow problems in the athlete. Clin Sports Med. 1989;8:439–51.
5. Cyriax J H. Diagnosis of soft tissue lesions. II Treatment by manipulation, massage and injection. In: Textbook of orthopaedic medicine. London: Balliere Tindall;1982.
6. Canoso JJ, Barza M. Soft tissue infections. Clin Rheum Dis. 1993;19:293–309.
7. Smith DL, McAfee JH, Lucas LM, Kumar KL, Romney DM. Treatment of nonseptic olecranon bursitis. A controlled blinded prospective trial. Arch Intern Med. 1989;149:2527–30.
8. Ho G, Su EY. Antibiotic therapy of septic bursitis: its implication in the treatment of septic arthritis. Arthritis Rheum. 1981;24:905–10.
9. Runge F. Zur Genese und Behandlung des Schreiberkrampfes. Berl Klin Woch. 1873;10:245–8.
10. Morris H. Riders sprain. Lancet. 1882;ii:557.
11. Allander E. Prevalence, incidence and remission rates of some common rheumatic diseases and syndromes. Scand J Rheumatol. 1974;3:145–53.
12. Kivi P. The aetiology and conservative treatment of humeral epicondylitis. Scand J Rehabil Med. 1982;15:37–41.
13. Gruchow HW, Pelletier BS. An epidemiologic study of tennis elbow. Am J Sports Med. 1979;7:234–8.
14. Nirschl RP, Pettrone FA. Tennis elbow. J Bone Joint Surg (Am). 1973;61:832–9.
15. Coonrad RW, Hooper WR. Tennis elbow: course, natural history, conservative and surgical management. J Bone Joint Surg. (Am). 1973;55:1177–87.
16. Binder AI, Hazleman BL. Lateral humeral epicondylitis – a study of natural history and the effect of conservative therapy. Br J Rheumatol. 1983;22:73–6.
17. Cyriax JH. The pathology and treatment of tennis elbow. J Bone Joint Surg. 1936;18:921–40.
18. Newman JH, Goodfellow JW. Fibrillation of the radial head as one cause for tennis elbow. Br Med J. 1975;2:328–30.
19 Roles NC, Maudsley RH. Radial tunnel syndrome: resistant tennis elbow as a nerve entrapment. J Bone Joint Surg (Br). 1972;54:499–508.
20. Bosworth DM. The role of the orbicular ligament in tennis elbow. J Bone Joint Surg (Am). 1955;37:527–33.
21. Sarkar K, Uhthoff HK. Ultrastructure of the common extensor tendon origin in tennis elbow. Vicrhows Arch A.1980;386:317–30.
22. Nirschl RP, Pettrone FA. Tennis elbow: the surgical treatment of lateral epicondylitis. J Bone Joint Surg (Am). 1979;61:832–9.
23. Regan W, Lester E, Coonrad R, Morrey BF. Microscopic histopathology of chronic refractory lateral epicondylitis. Am J Sports Med. 1992;20:746–9.
24. Neipal GA, Sitaj S. Enthesopathy. Clin Rheum Dis. 1979;5:857–62.
25. Van Rossum J, Buruma OJS, Kamphrisen HAC, Onvlee GJ. Tennis elbow – a radial tunnel syndrome? J Bone Joint Surg (Am). 1978;60:197–208.

26. Spinner H. The arcade of Frohse and its relationship to posterior interosseous nerve paralysis. J Bone Joint Surg (Am). 1968;50:809–12.
27. Binder A, Parr G, Page Thomas P, Hazleman B. A clinical and thermograhic study of lateral epicondylitis. Br J Rheumatol. 1983;22:77–81.
28. Potter HG, Hannefin JA, Morwessel RM, Di Carlo EF, O'Brien SJ, Altchek DW. Lateral epicondylitis: correlation of MR imaging, surgical and histopathological findings. Radiology. 1995;196:43–6.
29. Binder A, Hodge G, Greenwood AM, Hazlemanp BL, Page Thomas DP. Is therapeutic ultrasound effective in treating soft tissue lesions? Br Med J. 1985;292:512–4.
30. Lundberg T, Haker E, Thomas M. The effect of laser versus placebo in tennis elbow. Scand J Rehab Med. 1987:135–8.
31. Krasheninnkoff M, Ellitsgaard N, Rogvi–Hansen B, Zevthen A, Harder K, Larsen R, Gaardbo H. No effect of low power laser in lateral epicondylitis. Scand J Rheumatol. 1994;23:260–3.
32. Brattberg G. Acupuncture therapy for tennis elbow. Pain. 1983;16:285–8.
33. Day BH, Gordindasamy N, Patnaik R. Corticosteroid injection in the treatment of tennis elbow. Practitioner. 1978;220:459–62.
34. Price R, Sinclair H, Heinrich I, Gibson T. Local injection treatment of tennis elbow – hydrocortisone, triamcinolone and lignocaine compared. Brit J Rheum. 1991;30:39–44.
35. Coonrad RW. Tendinopathies of the elbow. Instructional course lectures of the American Academy of Orthopaedic Surgeons. 1991;40:25–32.
36. Clarke AK, Woodland J. Comparison of two steroid preparations used to treat tennis elbow, using the hypospray. Rheumatol Rehab. 1975;14:47–9.
37. Nevelos AB. The treatment of tennis elbow with triamcinolone acetonide. Curr Med Res Opin. 1980;6:507–9.
38. Wadsworth TG. Tennis elbow: conservative, surgical and manipulative treatment. Br Med J. 1987;294:621–4.
39. Garden RS. Tennis elbow. J Bone Joint Surgery (Br). 1961;43:100–6.
40. Calvert PT, Macpherson IS, Allum RL, Bentley G. Simple lateral release in treatment of tennis elbow. J Roy Soc Med. 1985;78:912–5.
41. Verhaar J, Walenkamp G, van Mameren H, van der Linden T. Lateral extensor release for tennis elbow. A prospective long term follow–up study. J Bone Joint Surg (Am). 1993;75:1034–43.
42. O'Neil J, Sarkar K, Uhthoff HK. A retrospective study of surgically treated cases of tennis elbow. Acta Orthop Belg. 1980;46:189–90.

9

THE WRIST AND HAND

Adel G Fam

- Pain in the wrist and hand may have its origin in the bones and joints, periarticular soft tissues (cutaneous and subcutaneous tissues, palmar fascia, tendon sheaths), nerve roots and peripheral nerves, and vascular structures or be referred from the cervical spine, thoracic outlet, shoulder or elbow.
- Precise diagnosis rests upon a meticulous history, a thorough examination and a few rationally selected diagnostic studies.

INTRODUCTION

The hand is the chief sensory organ of touch and is uniquely adapted for grasping. The radial side of the hand performs pinch grip between the fingers and thumb, while the ulnar side performs power grip between the fingers and palm.

FUNCTIONAL ANATOMY

The bones of the hand are divided into a central fixed unit for stability, and three mobile units for dexterity and power[1]. The fixed unit comprises the eight carpal bones tightly bound to the second and third metacarpals (Fig. 9.1). The three mobile units projecting from the fixed unit are:

- the thumb, the first carpometacarpal (CMC) joint which permits extension, flexion, abduction and adduction for powerful pinch and grasp, and fine manipulations;
- the index finger, endowed with independent extrinsic extensors and flexors and powerful intrinsic muscles for precise movements alone or with the thumb;
- the middle, ring and little fingers for power grip, a function enhanced by slight movements of the fourth and fifth metacarpals at their CMC articulations.

The axis of the wrist and hand is an extension of the longitudinal axis of the radius and the third metacarpal, with the wrist in the neutral position and the dorsal surface of the hand in the same plane as that of the distal radius[2].

WRIST (RADIOCARPAL) JOINT

This is an ellipsoid joint between the distal radius and articular disc proximally, and the scaphoid, lunate and triquetrum distally[1–3] (Fig. 9.1). The articular capsule is strengthened by the radiocarpal (dorsal and palmar), and collateral (radial and ulnar) ligaments. The articular disc, or triangular fibrocartilage of the wrist, joins the radius to the ulna. Its base is attached to the ulnar border of the distal radius and its apex to the root of the ulnar styloid process. The synovial cavity of the distal radioulnar joint is L-shaped and extends distally beneath the triangular fibrocartilage but is usually separated from the radiocarpal joint.

The radiocarpal, intercarpal, midcarpal (located between the proximal and distal rows of the carpal bones), CMC and intermetacarpal joints often intercommunicate through a common synovial cavity (Fig. 9.1).

The carpal bones form a volar concave arch or carpal tunnel, with the pisiform and hook of the hamate on the ulnar side and the scaphoid tubercle and crest of the trapezium on the radial side[1–3]. The four bony prominences are joined by the flexor retinaculum (transverse carpal ligament), which forms the roof of the carpal tunnel. The palmaris longus (absent in 10–15% of the population) partly inserts into the flexor retinaculum and partly fans out into the palm forming the palmar aponeurosis (fascia). The aponeurosis broadens distally and divides into four digital slips which attach to the finger flexor tendon sheath, metacarpophalangeal joint capsules and proximal phalanges. There is usually no digital slip to the thumb.

Tendons crossing the wrist are enclosed for part of their course in tenosynovial sheaths. The common flexor tendon sheath encloses the long flexor tendons of the fingers (flexor digitorum superficialis and flexor digitorum profundus) and extends from approximately 2.5cm proximal to the wrist crease to the mid-palm. It runs with the flexor pollicis longus tendon sheath and the median nerve through the carpal tunnel (see Fig. 9.2). The tendon sheath of the little finger is usually continuous with the common flexor sheath. The flexor pollicis longus tendon to the thumb runs through a separate tenosynovial sheath, but may join the common flexor sheath. The flexor carpi radialis is invested in a short tendon sheath as it crosses the volar aspect of the wrist between the split radial attachment of the flexor retinaculum. The flexor retinaculum straps down the flexor tendons as they cross at the wrist.

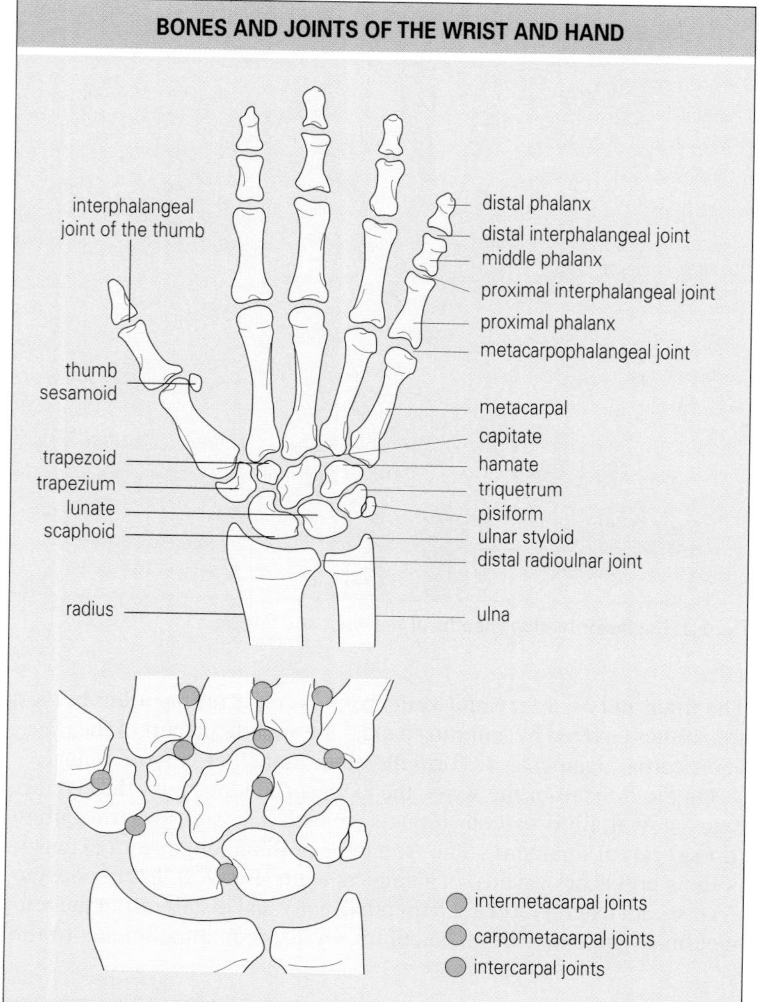

Fig. 9.1 The bones and joints of the wrist and hand.

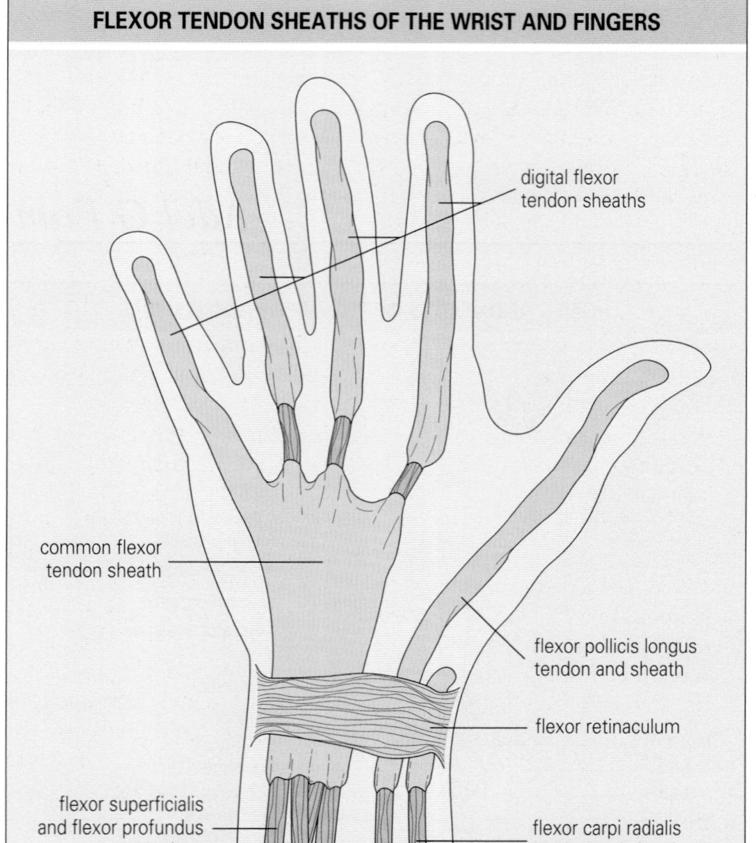

Fig. 9.2 The flexor tendon sheaths of the wrist and fingers.

The ulnar nerve, artery and vein cross over the retinaculum but are sometimes covered by a fibrous band – the superficial part of the transverse carpal ligament – to form the ulnar tunnel, or Guyon's canal.

On the dorsum of the wrist, the extensor tendons pass through six tenosynovial, fibro-osseous tunnels beneath the extensor retinaculum (dorsal carpal ligament). The Abductor pollicis longus and extensor pollicis brevis are usually in a single sheath (Fig 9.3). Each tenosynovial sheath extends about 2.5cm proximally and distally from the retinaculum. The extensor retinaculum, by its deep attachments to the distal radius and ulna, binds down and prevents bowstringing of the extensor tendons as they cross the wrist. The anatomic snuffbox corresponds to the depression between the extensor pollicis longus tendon and the tendons of the abductor pollicis longus and extensor pollicis brevis.

Movements of the wrist include palmar flexion, dorsiflexion (extension), ulnar deviation, radial deviation and circumduction. The intercarpal joints contribute to wrist movements, particularly palmar flexion. Prime wrist palmar flexors are the flexor carpi radialis, flexor carpi ulnaris and palmaris longus. The prime dorsiflexors are the extensor carpi radialis longus and brevis and the extensor carpi ulnaris.

Pronation (palm of the hand turned backward) to 90° and supination (palm turned forward) to 90° of the hand and forearm occur at the proximal and distal radioulnar joints.

THE CARPOMETACARPAL JOINTS

The first CMC joint is a saddle-shaped, very mobile joint between the trapezium and the base of the first metacarpal[1,3,4]. It allows 40–50° of thumb flexion–extension (parallel to the plane of the palm) and 40–70° of adduction–abduction (perpendicular to the plane of the palm). These movements are important in bringing the thumb in opposition with the fingers. The second and third CMC joints are relatively fixed, but the fourth and fifth are mobile, allowing the fourth and fifth metacarpals to flex forward (15–30°) toward the thumb during power grip.

THE METACARPOPHALANGEAL JOINTS

The metacarpophalangeal (MCP) joints are modified hinge joints which lie about 1cm distal to the knuckles (metacarpal heads)[1,4,5] (Fig. 9.1). Their capsule is strengthened by the radial and ulnar collateral ligaments on the sides and by the palmar (volar) plate on the volar surface. The collateral ligaments are loose in the neutral position, allowing radial and ulnar deviations, but become tight in the flexed position, preventing side-to-side motion (referred to as sagittal cam effect). The deep transverse metacarpal ligament joins the volar plates of the second to fifth MCP joints. The MCP joint of the thumb is large and has two sesamoid bones overlying its volar surface.

When the long extensor tendon of the digit reaches the metacarpal head, it is joined by the tendons of the interossei and lumbrical and expands over the dorsum of the MCP joint and digit forming the extensor hood or expansion (Fig. 9.4). The expansion divides over the dorsum of the proximal phalanx into an intermediate slip, which is inserted principally into the base of the middle phalanx, and two

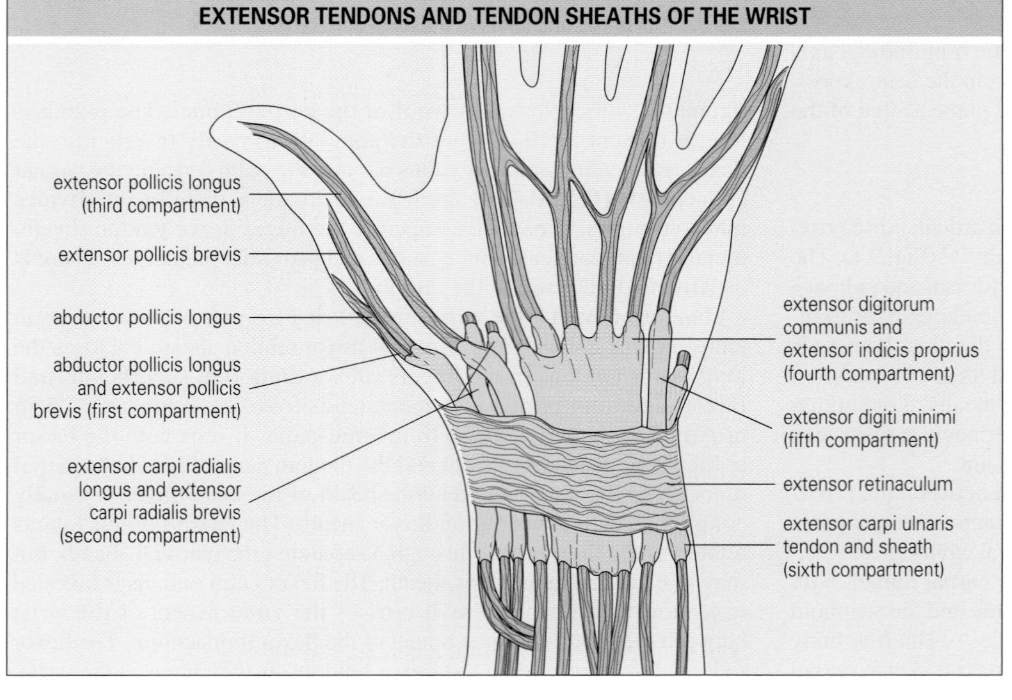

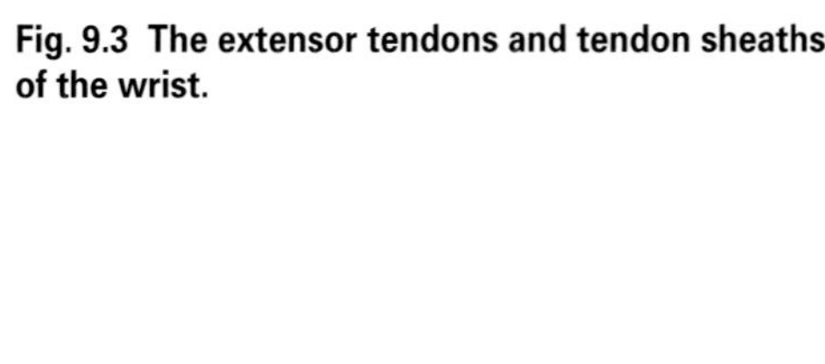

Fig. 9.3 The extensor tendons and tendon sheaths of the wrist.

collateral slips which are inserted into the base of the distal phalanx.

The first MCP joint permits 50–70° palmar flexion and 10–30° dorsiflexion. Radial and ulnar deviations are limited to <10–20°. The other MCP joints allow 90° palmar flexion, 30° dorsiflexion, and 35° of radial and ulnar movements. The extensor pollicis brevis, extensor indicis proprius, extensor digitorum communis and extensor digiti minimi dorsiflex the MCP joints. The palmar flexors are the flexor pollicis brevis, lumbricals, interossei and flexor digiti minimi brevis assisted by the long flexors. Radial and ulnar movements at the second to fifth MCP joints are a function of the intrinsic muscles.

THE INTERPHALANGEAL JOINTS

The proximal and distal interphalangeal (PIP and DIP) joints of the fingers and the IP joint of the thumb are hinge joints[1,4,5]. Their capsules are strengthened by the collateral ligaments on the sides and by the volar plates on the palmar surface, which serve to limit hyperextension, particularly at the PIP joints. Unlike the MCP joints, the radial and ulnar collateral ligaments remain taut in all positions, providing side-to-side stability throughout the range of movement.

The flexor tendon sheaths for the fingers enclose the tendons of flexor digitorum superficialis and profundus to their insertions on the middle and distal phalanges respectively. The sheaths extend from just proximal to the MCP joints to the bases of the distal phalanges (Fig. 9.2). The thumb flexor pollicis longus tendon sheath extends proximally to the carpal tunnel.

The flexor sheath of the little finger is often continuous with the wrist common flexor tendon sheath. Segmental condensations, or annular pulleys, in the digital flexor sheaths prevent bowstringing of the tendons and are mechanically critical for full digital flexion[1,4,6].

The PIP joints do not normally hyperextend. They allow 100–120° palmar flexion. The DIP joints permit 50–80° palmar flexion and 5–10° dorsiflexion. The IP joint of the thumb allows 80–90° palmar flexion and 20–35° dorsiflexion. The flexor digitorum superficialis flexes the PIP joints, and the flexor digitorum profundus flexes the DIP joints of the fingers. The prime dorsiflexors are the interossei and lumbrical muscles. The flexor pollicis longus flexes the IP joint of the thumb and the extensor pollicis longus dorsiflexes the joint.

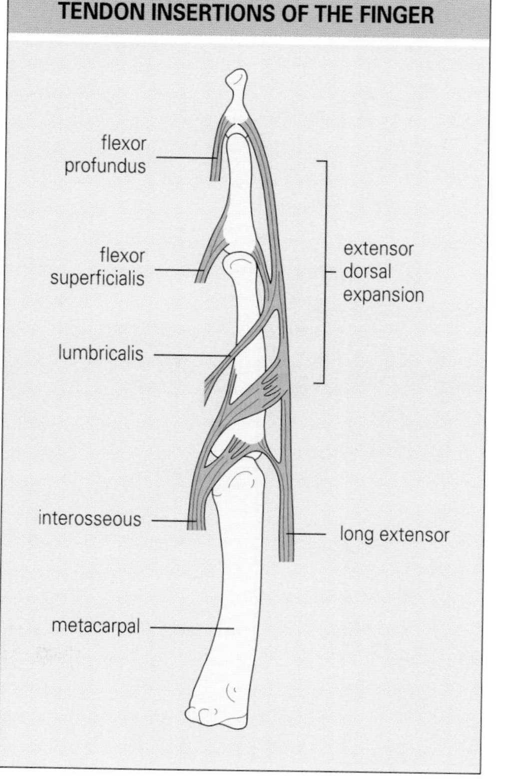

Fig. 9.4 Tendon insertions of the finger.

PHYSICAL EXAMINATION

INSPECTION

The wrist and hand are inspected for any swelling or deformity[2–5]. Arthritis of the radiocarpal joint produces a diffuse swelling distal to the radius and ulna. Extensor wrist tenosynovitis, by contrast, presents as a linear or oval-shaped dorsal swelling localized to the distribution of the tendon sheath. When the fingers are actively extended, the distal margin of the swelling moves proximally and folds in, like a sheet being tucked under a mattress (tuck sign)[2]. Tenosynovitis of the common flexor tendon sheath presents as a swelling over the volar aspect of the wrist just proximal to the carpal tunnel. The wrist is a common site for ganglia (Fig. 9.5). A ganglion is a cystic swelling arising from a joint capsule or from a tendon sheath. It is synovial lined and contains a clear, thick, jelly-like fluid.

Wrist deformities are common in rheumatoid arthritis (RA) and other chronic inflammatory arthritides. They include volar subluxation of the carpus with a visible step opposite the radiocarpal joint, carpal collapse (loss of carpal height to less than half the length of the third metacarpal, with inability to admit the tips of the patient's index and middle fingers), and radial posturing of the carpus (radial deviation of the carpus from the axis of the wrist and hand). Chronic arthritis of the distal radioulnar joint results in instability and dorsal subluxation of the ulnar head with a 'piano key' movement on downward pressure.

Entrapment of the median nerve in the carpal tunnel (carpal tunnel syndrome) can lead to atrophy of the thenar muscles (see Chapters 5.16 and 4.16). In RA, rupture at the wrist of an extensor tendon to the little or ring finger is associated with inability to actively dorsiflex the digit at the MCP joint.

Deformities of the fingers and thumb are common in RA. The fingers are inspected for swelling of the MCP, PIP or DIP joints, deformities, clubbing, subcutaneous RA nodules, gouty tophi, osteoarthritic Heberden's or Bouchard's nodes, sclerodactyly, telangiectasia, ischemic digital ulcers, pitted scars, nailfold infarcts, periungual erythema or psoriatic skin/nail lesions[5]. MCP synovitis produces a diffuse swelling of the joint that may obscure the valleys between the knuckles. Swelling of a PIP joint produces a fusiform or spindle-shaped finger. Digital flexor tenosynovitis produces a diffuse tender swelling over the volar aspect of the finger (sausage finger). MCP joint deformities include ulnar drift, volar subluxation (often visible as a step) and flexion deformities. Boutonnière deformity describes a finger with flexion of the PIP joint and hyperextension of the DIP joint (see Fig. 9.6). A swan-neck deformity describes the appearance of a finger in which there is hyperextension of the PIP joint and flexion of the DIP joint (Fig. 9.6). A Z-shaped deformity of the thumb is flexion of the MCP joint and hyperextension of the IP joint (Fig. 9.6). Telescoped shortening of the digits, produced by partial resorption of the phalanges secondary to psoriatic arthritis, RA or other destructive arthritis, is often associated

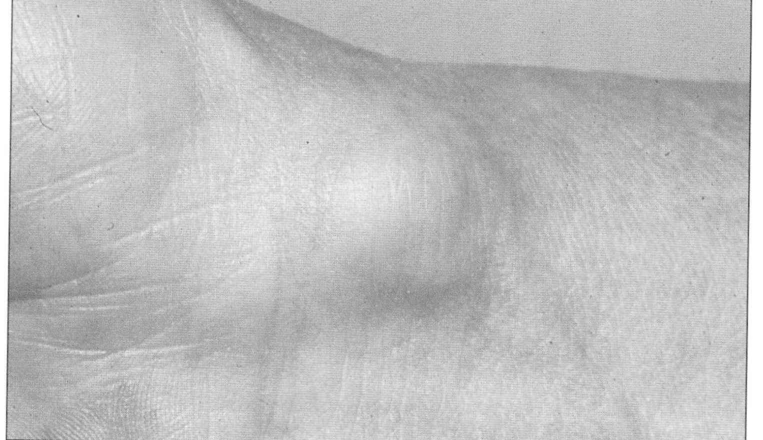

Fig. 9.5 A ganglion on the volar aspect of the wrist.

with concentric wrinkling of the skin (opera-glass hand).

Thickening and contracture of the palmar aponeurosis (Dupuytren's contracture) often produces flexion deformities of the ring and, less commonly, the little and middle fingers.

PALPATION

The wrist is palpated with the joint in slight palmar flexion[2,3]. The margins of a swollen synovium are detected most reliably by the thumbs firmly palpating the dorsal surface of the wrist while the fingers of both hands support the joint (Fig. 9.7). The joint is difficult to palpate from the volar surface because of the overlying flexor tendons. The presence of fluctuance indicates a large wrist effusion: pressure with one hand on one side of the joint produces a fluid wave transmitted to the second hand placed on the opposite side of the wrist.

Wrist tenosynovitis produces a superficial, linear, tender swelling extending beyond the joint margins. A crepitus may be palpable and movements of the involved tendon often produce pain.

The normal range of movement at the wrist comprises 80–90° palmar flexion, 70–80° dorsiflexion, 40–50° ulnar deviation and 15–20° radial deviation (Fig. 9.8).

The first CMC is palpated for tenderness, swelling or crepitus. Osteoarthritis is associated with crepitus and 'squaring' of the joint.

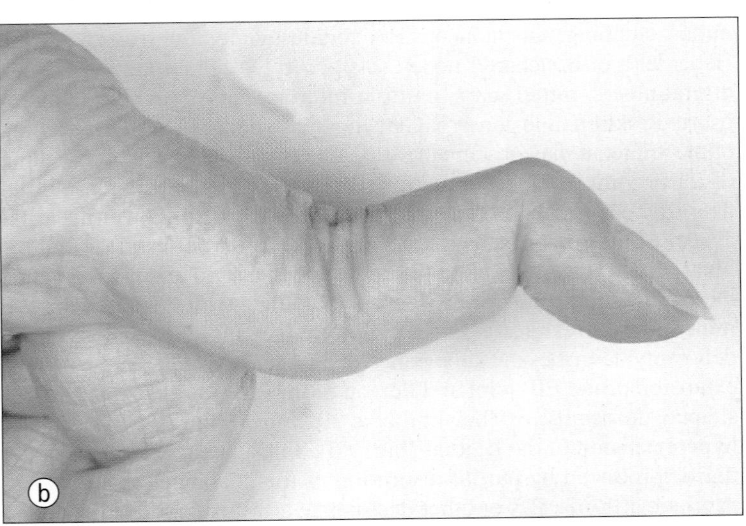

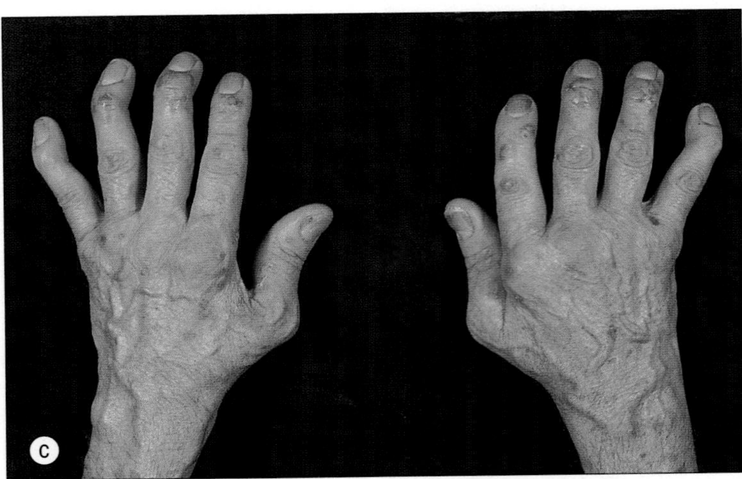

Fig. 9.6 Boutonnière (a) and swan-neck (b) deformities of the fingers, and 'Z'-shaped deformity of the thumb (c).

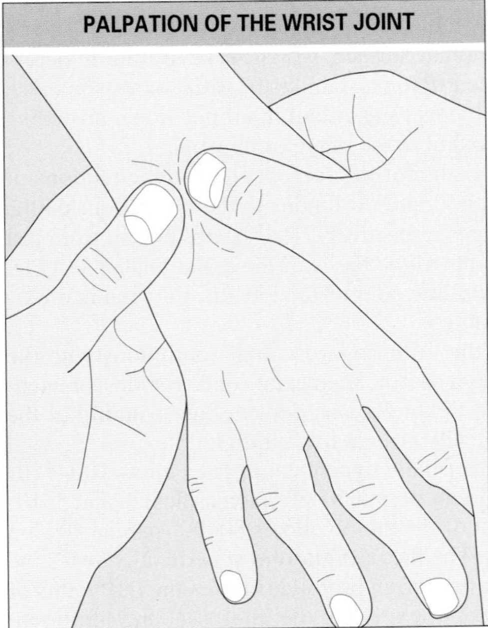

Fig. 9.7 Palpation of the wrist joint.

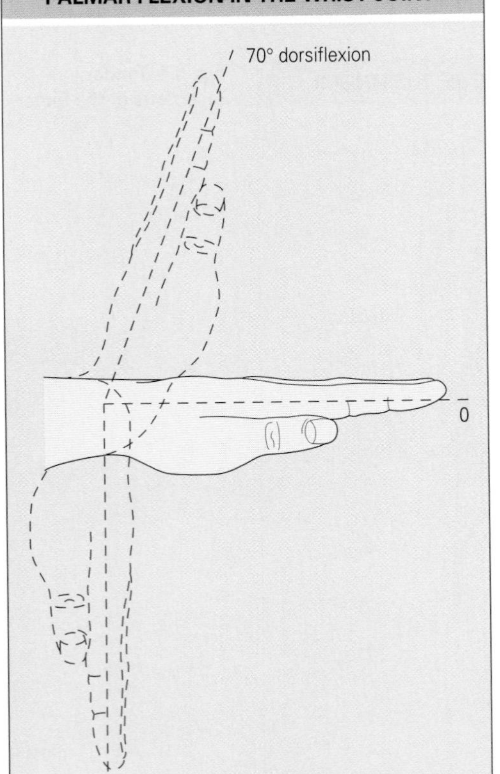

Fig. 9.8 Wrist joint: normal range of dorsiflexion and palmar flexion.

Synovitis of the MCP joint is detected most reliably by palpating firmly with the thumbs over the dorsal surface of the joint on each side of the extensor tendon, while the forefingers support the joint over the volar aspect (Fig. 9.9).

The joint is difficult to palpate from the volar aspect because of the thickened skin of the palm, overlaying fat pad and intervening flexor tendon sheath.

The PIP and DIP joints are palpated for tenderness, synovial thickening, or effusion using the thumbs and forefingers of both hands placed on opposite sides of the joint[3] (Fig. 9.10). To detect an effusion, compression of the joint by one hand produces ballooning or a hydraulic lift sensed by the other hand (balloon sign). Unlike PIP synovitis, dorsal knuckle pads produce a non-tender thickening of the skin localized to the dorsal surface of the PIP joints.

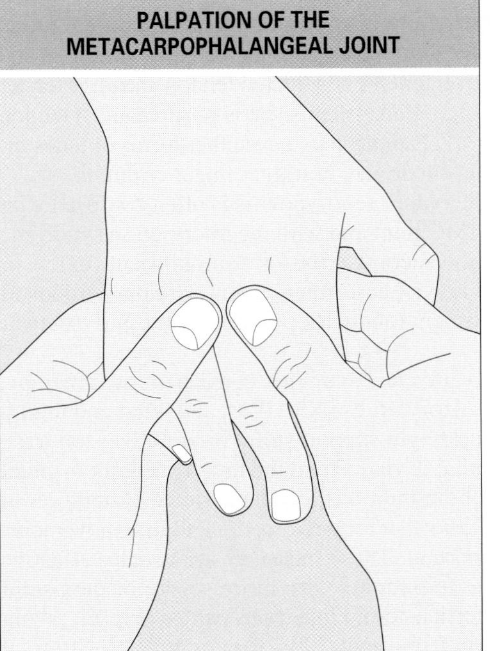

Fig. 9.9 Palpation of the MCP joint.

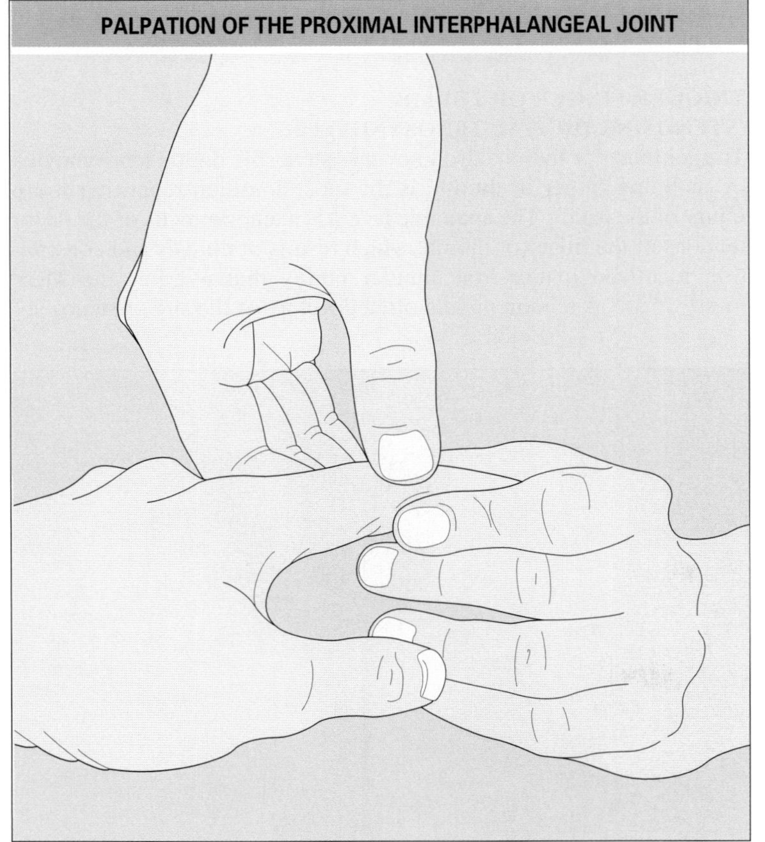

Fig. 9.10 Palpation of the proximal interphalangeal joint.

Finger tenosynovitis produces linear tenderness, volar swelling, thickening, nodules and/or crepitus of the flexor tendon sheath. Tendon nodules usually occur at the level of the metacarpal heads opposite the proximal annular pulley of the sheath. They can be palpated in the palm while the patient slowly flexes and extends the affected finger.

The range of movements at the MCP, PIP and DIP joints is assessed by asking the patient to extend the fingers, make a fist, then flex the fingers so that the fingertips touch the palm opposite the MCP joints. To test for stability of the MCP joint, the joint is palmar flexed to 90° to tighten the radial and ulnar collateral ligaments, and the corresponding metacarpal is then held in one hand while the other hand moves the finger from side-to-side to test the integrity of the collateral ligaments. The stability of the radial and ulnar collateral ligaments of the PIP and DIP joints can be assessed by applying side strain with the joint in the neutral position.

SPECIAL MANEUVERS

In carpal tunnel syndrome, percussion of the median nerve at the flexor retinaculum (just radial to the palmaris longus tendon at the distal wrist crease) produces paresthesia in the median nerve distribution: thumb, index and middle fingers and the radial half of the ring finger (Tinel's sign)[2,3]. Sustained palmar flexion of the wrist for 30–60 seconds may induce finger paresthesia (Phalen's wrist flexion sign). If the wrist cannot be flexed because of arthritis, pressure over the median nerve for 30 seconds often produces the same effect.

In de Quervain's stenosing tenosynovitis of the abductor pollicis longus and extensor pollicis brevis (vide infra), Finkelstein's test is a useful diagnostic maneuver. Passive ulnar deviation of the wrist with the fingers flexed over the thumb placed in the palm, stretches the tendons and reproduces the pain over the distal radius and the radial side of the wrist[2].

In vascular disorders of the hand, the patency of the radial and ulnar arteries can be assessed by Allen's test[1]. The patient elevates the hand and makes a fist while the examiner occludes both the radial and the ulnar arteries at the wrist. The patient then extends the fingers and repeats the maneuver until blanching of the hand is seen. Each artery is then released and the color of the hand returns to normal. If either artery is occluded, the hand remains blanched when this artery alone is released.

In swan-neck finger deformity, tightness and shortening of the intrinsic muscles (interossei and lumbricals) results in restriction of PIP flexion when the MCP joint is dorsiflexed. Thus, with the MCP joint dorsiflexed, the range of PIP flexion is less than that when the MCP joint is palmar flexed (positive Bunnell's test)[4].

DIFFERENTIAL DIAGNOSIS OF WRIST AND HAND PAIN

Pain in the wrist and hand is a relatively common symptom of diverse causes[7]. It may have its origin in the bones and joints of the wrist and hand, periarticular soft tissues (cutaneous and subcutaneous tissues, palmar fascia, tendon sheaths), nerve roots and peripheral nerves, or vascular structures, or be referred from the musculoskeletal structures of the cervical spine, thoracic outlet, shoulder or elbow. Figure 9.11 provides a classification of painful disorders of the wrist and hand based upon the site of origin of pain and its predominant location. Precise diagnosis rests upon a meticulous history, a thorough examination of the joints, periarticular structures, cervical spine, nerve and blood supplies to the hand, and a few rationally selected diagnostic studies. As with any other clinical problem, assessment begins with a complete history, which should take account of the onset, location, character, duration and modulating factors of pain. A history of unaccustomed, repetitive or excessive hand activity is particularly important in the diagnosis of wrist and/or finger tenosynovitis due to an overuse syndrome. Initial diagnostic studies include hematologic, biochemical and immunologic screening tests, and hand radiographs. Additional studies are sometimes required, including synovial fluid analysis, skeletal scintigraphy, nerve conduction studies, noninvasive vascular (Doppler) studies, arteriography, computed tomography, magnetic resonance imaging (MRI), arthrography and synovial biopsy.

DIFFERENTIAL DIAGNOSIS OF WRIST AND HAND PAIN
Articular
Arthritis of wrist, MCP, PIP and/or DIP due to Trauma, hypermobility, sprain RA (wrist, MCP, PIP joints) Osteoarthritis (first CMC, PIP and DIP joints) Other forms of arthritis: gout, psoriatic arthritis, infection Joint neoplasms
Periarticular
Subcutaneous RA nodules, gouty tophi, painful subcutaneous calcific nodules in scleroderma, glomus tumor of nail bed Palmar fascia Dupuytren's contracture Tendon sheath Wrist extensor tenosynovitis including de Quervain's tenosynovitis and extensor carpi radialis tenosynovitis Wrist volar flexor tenosynovitis (including carpal tunnel syndrome) Thumb flexor tenosynovitis (trigger or snapping thumb) Finger flexor tenosynovitis (trigger finger) Pigmented villonodular tenosynovitis (giant cell tumor of the tendon sheath) Acute calcific periarthritis: Wrist, MCP, and rarely PIP and DIP Ganglion
Osseous
Bone lesions Fractures, neoplasms, infection, osteonecrosis including Kienböck's disease (lunate) and Preiser's disease (scaphoid)
Neurologic
Nerve entrapment syndromes Median nerve Carpal tunnel syndrome (at wrist) Pronator teres syndrome (at pronator teres) Anterior interosseous nerve syndrome Ulnar nerve Cubital tunnel syndrome (at elbow) Guyon's canal (at wrist) Posterior interosseous nerve syndrome Radial nerve palsy (spiral groove syndrome) Lower brachial plexus Thoracic outlet syndrome, Pancoast's tumor Cervical nerve roots Herniated cervical disc, tumors Spinal cord lesion Spinal tumors, syringomyelia
Vascular
Vasospastic disorders with Raynaud's phenomenon Scleroderma, occupational vibration syndrome, etc. Small- or large-vessel vasculitis With digital ischemia, ischemic ulcers, e.g., SLE, RA, and Takayasu's arteritis
Referred pain
Cervical spine disorders Reflex sympathetic dystrophy syndrome (RSDS) e.g., shoulder–hand syndrome and causalgia Cardiac Angina pectoris

Fig. 9.11 Differential diagnosis of wrist and hand pain.

SPECIFIC DISORDERS OF THE WRIST AND HAND

DE QUERVAIN'S TENOSYNOVITIS

De Quervain's stenosing tenosynovitis of the abductor pollicis longus and extensor pollicis brevis typically represents an occupation- or avocation-related repetitive strain injury due to chronic overuse of the wrist and hand. It is most common in women between 30 and 50 years of age[8–10]. Repetitive activity, involving pinching with the thumb while moving the wrist in radial and ulnar directions, results in frictional inflammation with thickening and stenosis of the fibrous tendon sheath as it passes over the distal radius beneath the extensor retinaculum.

De Quervain's tenosynovitis may also occur in association with RA[11], psoriatic arthritis, other inflammatory synovitides, direct trauma, pregnancy and during the postpartum period[12].

Most patients report several weeks or months of pain on the radial aspect of the wrist and at the thumb base during pinch grip, grasping, and other thumb and wrist movements. The affected tendon sheath is tender and often swollen (Fig. 9.12). Finkelstein's test is positive and a tendon crepitus may be palpable[8–10]. Patients may have other forms of tenosynovitis such as carpal tunnel syndrome, or trigger finger or thumb.

The diagnosis of de Quervain's tenosynovitis is often confused with osteoarthritis of the first CMC joint and with the intersection syndrome due to tenosynovitis of the second extensor compartment (extensor carpi radialis longus and brevis) at its intersection with the tendons of the first extensor compartment (abductor pollicis longus and extensor pollicis brevis)[9].

Treatment of de Quervain's tenosynovitis consists of heat therapy, nonsteroidal anti-inflammatory drugs (NSAIDs), and wrist and thumb splinting[8–12]. A radial gutter light support splint immobilizes the wrist in slight extension and radial deviation and the first MCP joint in slight extension. The IP joint of the thumb is left unrestricted. Alteration of hand activities, avoiding tasks that require repetitive thumb movements or pinch grasping, is important. These measures are usually effective in alleviating symptoms. In patients with more severe or persistent pain, one or more local corticosteroid injections can be helpful, giving complete and lasting relief in about 70% of patients[11–15]. Surgical decompression of the first extensor compartment, with or without tenosynovectomy, is indicated in those with persistent or recurrent symptoms for more than 6 months[8–11,13–17].

TRIGGER FINGER OR THUMB (STENOSING DIGITAL TENOSYNOVITIS)

Trigger finger or thumb, also known as stenosing digital tenosynovitis or snapping finger or thumb, is the most common repetitive strain injury of the hand[9]. The anatomic lesion is a tenosynovitis of the flexor tendons of the finger or thumb, which results in fibrosis and constriction localized to the first annular pulley that overlies the MCP joint[9,13,17–21]. A tendon nodule often develops at the site of stenosis.

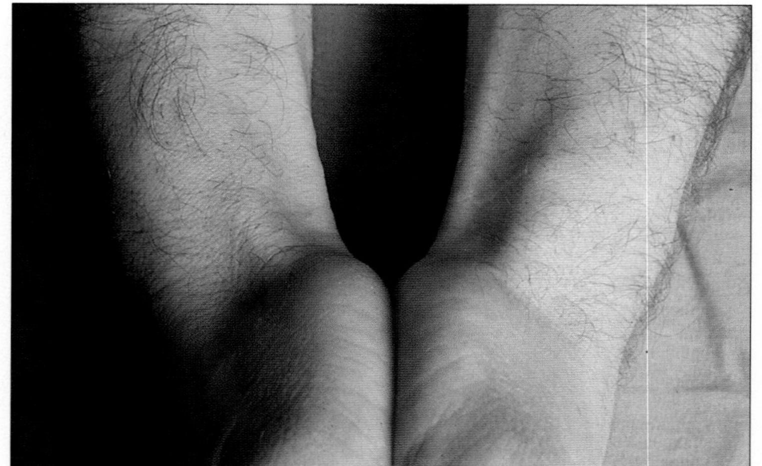

Fig. 9.12 De Quervain's tenosynovitis of the wrist.

The nodule and/or tendon sheath constriction interfere mechanically with normal tendon gliding, resulting in pain over the area of the pulley and 'snapping', 'triggering' or 'catching' movement of the finger or thumb. Pain along the course of the sheath with resisted flexion (performed isometrically), and pain on stretching the tendon passively in extension, are common. Intermittent locking of the digit in flexion may also develop, particularly upon arising in the morning. Passive extension of the PIP joint of the finger or IP joint of the thumb may produce a crepitus and a popping sensation as the digit is straightened. Examination reveals tenderness over the area of the proximal pulley often associated with linear tenderness and swelling of the flexor tendon sheath, and limitation of digital flexion and extension. A nodular tendon swelling can often be palpated in the palm just proximal to the MCP joint as it moves during finger or thumb flexion and extension.

The most common cause of trigger finger or thumb is overuse trauma of the hands from repetitive gripping activities with increased pull and friction on the flexor tendons[9,17–21]. One digit is often affected, usually the thumb, middle or ring fingers in this order. Other causes of flexor digital tenosynovitis include RA[11], psoriatic arthritis, diabetes mellitus[22], amyloidosis, hypothyroidism, sarcoidosis, pigmented villonodular tenosynovitis and infections, including tuberculosis and sporotrichosis A[18].

Management consists of modification of hand activities, local heat treatment, gentle exercises and NSAIDs as required[9,13,19–21]. Extension splinting of the affected digit at night prevents painful flexion during sleep. One or more corticosteroid injections of the affected flexor tendon sheath are effective and often curative in the majority of patients[13,18–21,23,24] (see Chapter 2.12). Surgical release with transection of the fibrous annular pulley of the finger or thumb flexor sheath is rarely required for those with chronic symptoms not responding to medical treatment[13,17,19–21,23,24].

DUPUYTREN'S CONTRACTURE

This is a relatively common condition characterized by nodular thickening and contraction of the palmar fascia drawing one or more fingers into flexion at the MCP joints[25–27]. In most patients, Dupuytren's contracture affects the ulnar side of both hands. The fourth finger is usually affected earliest, followed by the fifth, third, and second fingers in decreasing order of frequency. Fibrous nodules, resulting from contraction of proliferating fibroblasts and myofibroblasts in the superficial layers of the palmar fascia, are the earliest abnormality. The dermis is invaded by fibroblastic cells, resulting in puckering, dimpling and tethering of the overlying skin (Fig. 9.13). There is usually little pain, and if no further progression occurs the hand function is preserved and no treatment is required. However, after a variable period of months or years, the aponeurotic thickening may extend distally to involve the digits. The fingers become flexed at the MCP joints by taut fibrous bands radiating from the palmar fascia, and the hand cannot be placed flat on a table (positive table top test)[25]. Although there is no direct involvement of the joints or tendons, progressive flexion deformity of the fingers can lead to severe functional impairment.

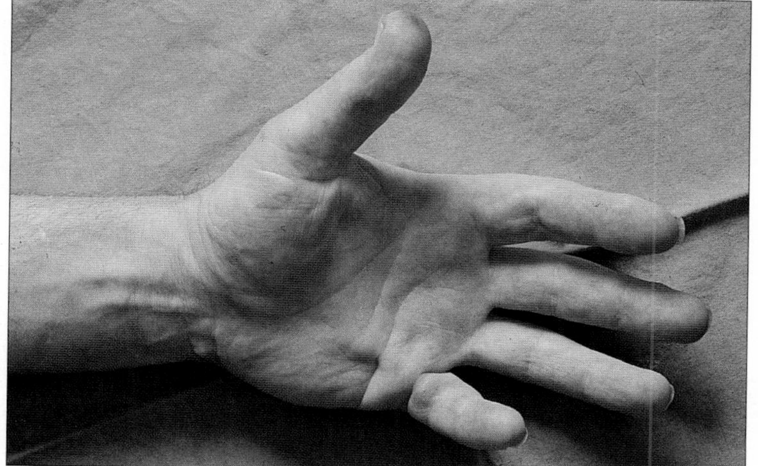

Fig. 9.13 Dupuytren's contracture of the palmar fascia.

The etiology of Dupuytren's contracture is poorly understood[25–27]. The disorder is rare in non-Caucasian individuals. Its incidence rises with increasing age, and the sex ratio is predominantly male (5:1). Familial predisposition is frequent, suggesting an autosomal dominant pattern with variable penetrance. Cytogenetic studies of Dupuytren's nodules have shown nonspecific chromosomal abnormalities, including numeric and structural clones and random aberrations, prophasing and premature centromere separation[28]. A pathogenetic role for local repetitive injury and occupational trauma remains unproven. A relationship to cigarette smoking, producing microvascular occlusion, has been suggested[29]. Dupuytren's contracture has been observed in association with idiopathic epilepsy, alcohol misuse, diabetes mellitus, chronic pulmonary disease and reflex sympathetic dystrophy syndrome[25–27]. The association of Dupuytren's disease with other localized fibroses, such as nodular plantar fibromatosis, nodular fasciitis of popliteal fascia, Peyronie's disease and knuckle pads, has led to the concept of a 'Dupuytren's diathesis'[27,30]. The cause of these fibrosing diseases is unknown but seems to be determined by a dominant gene with high penetrance in males, usually middle aged white men of Celtic ancestry[27].

Pathologically, Dupuytren's disease is initially characterized by marked fibroblastic proliferation and vascular hyperplasia. This is followed by dense, disorderly collagen deposition with thickening of the palmar fascia and nodule formation[25–27,31,32]. The abnormal fascia demonstrates elevated total amounts of collagen with increased content of reducible cross links and hydroxylysine[31]. About 25% of the collagen is type III which is not normally present in the palmar fascia[31]. Ultrastructurally, contractile, smooth-muscle-like fibroblasts or myofibroblasts, surrounded by bundles of disarrayed collagenous fibrils and completely or partially occluded capillaries are present in the fibrotic nodules and cords[31,32]. Although myofibroblasts are not specific to Dupuytren's contracture, they are believed to be responsible for contraction of the palmar fascia and finger deformities[31]. The finding of isolated foci of smooth muscles α-actin (an antibody marker for myofibroblasts) – positive fibroblasts dispersed in the dermis remote from the main Dupuytren's tissue – may explain the high recurrence rate of Dupuytren's disease after fasciectomy[33]. The vasoactive prostaglandins, PGE_2 and $PGF_2\alpha$, are present in increased concentrations in Dupuytren's nodules, and are thought to influence myofibroblast contractility and contribute to the etiopathogenesis of the disorder[34]. Increased expression of growth factors, such as platelet-derived growth factor-B, transforming growth factor-beta, and basic fibroblast growth factor in Dupuytren's fascial lesions, suggests that these polypeptides may play a role in fibroblastic proliferation[35–37]. Production of oxygen-derived free radicals may also be an important feature of the pathogenesis of Dupuytren's and other fibrotic conditions. Excessive formation of superoxide, hydrogen peroxide and hydroxyl radicals, resulting from microvascular occlusion and relative ischemia of the palmar fascia, can lead to tissue damage and enhanced fibroblastic proliferation[32,38]. Flow cytometry of inflammatory cells from Dupuytren's lesions has demonstrated predominance of CD3-positive T lymphocytes and increased expression of MHC class-II proteins[39]. An association between Dupuytren's contracture, HLA-DR3 and autoantibodies to type I–IV collagen has also been demonstrated[40]. Factor XIIIa-positive dermal dendrocytes of macrophage lineage, are present in and around Dupuytren's nodules[41]. These cells may be an important local source of fibrogenic cytokines[41]. These observations suggest that Dupuytren's disease may represent a T-cell mediated autoimmune disorder[39–41].

Dupuytren's contracture runs a variable course. Some patients show little change or incapacity over a period of many years, while in others fascial contraction progresses rapidly with severe deformity and impairment of hand function within a short period of time.

Treatment depends on the rate of progression and severity of the lesions. Recent observations suggest that MRI may be useful in assessing the extent and degree of cellularity, and hence 'activity' of the lesion[42]. In patients with mild disease, local heat, stretching exercises, and use of protective padded gloves during heavy manual grasping tasks, are often helpful[25–27]. Many patients learn the benign nature of the contracture, and adapt to the disorder. In more severe lesions with pain and inability to straighten the fingers, intralesional corticosteroid injections may be beneficial[25–27]. Preliminary observations suggest that intralesional infiltrations of interferon-γ, a lymphocyte-derived cytokine which inhibits fibroblastic proliferation and collagen formation, may be beneficial[43]. In those with advanced disease with progressive digital contracture of more than 30°, a positive table top test and functional impairment, limited or total palmar fasciectomy with or without skin graft replacement, is indicated[25–27,44,45]. The risk of recurrence is increased in young patients with active bilateral disease and cellular nodules, and in those with a strong family history and/or other ectopic fibrotic lesions[25,44,45].

REFERENCES

1. Markison RE, Kilgore ES. Hand. In: Davis JH, ed. Clinical Surgery. St. Louis: CV Mosby; 1987:2292–353.
2. McMurtry RY, Little AH. The wrist. In: Little AH, ed. The rheumatological physical examination. Orlando: Grune & Stratton; 1986:83–9.
3. Polley HF, Hunder GG. The wrist and carpal joints, metacarpophalangeal, proximal and distal interphalangeal joints, In: Polley HF, Hunder GG, eds. Physical examination of the joints, 2E. Philadelphia: WB Saunders; 1978;90–148.
4. McMurtry RY. The hand. In: Little AH. The rheumatological physical examination. Orlando: Grune & Stratton; 1986:91–100.
5. Williams PL, Warwick R, Dyson M, Bannister LH. Joints of the upper limb. In: Williams PL *et al.*, eds. Gray's Anatomy, 37e. Edinburgh, Churchill Livingstone; 1989:499–516.
6. Strauch B, de Moura W. Digital flexor tendon sheath: an anatomic study. J Hand Surg. 1985;10(A):785–810.
7. Bluestone R.A practical approach to hand pain. J Musculoskel Med. 1989:6(3):75–85.
8. Field JH. De Quervain's disease. Am Fam Physician. 1979; 20(1):103–4.
9. Thompson JS, Phelps TH. Repetitive strain injuries. How to deal with 'the epidemic of the l990s'. Postgrad Med. 1990;88(8):143–9.
10. Thorson E, Szabo RM. Common tendinitis problems in the hand and forearm. Orthop Clin N Am. 1992;23(1):65–74.
11. Gray RG, Gottlieb NL. Hand flexor tenosynovitis in rheumatoid arthritis. Prevalence, distribution, and associated rheumatic features. Arthritis Rheum. 1977;20(4):1003–8.
12. Nygaard IE, Saltzman CL, Whitehouse MB, Hankin FM. Hand problems in pregnancy. Am Fam Physician. 1989;39(6):123–6.
13. Lapidus PW, Guidotti FP. Stenosing tenovaginitis of the wrist and fingers. Clin Orthop. 1972;83:87–90.
14. Harvey FJ, Harvey PM, Horsley MW. De Quervain's disease: surgical or nonsurgical treatment. J Hand Surg. 1990;15(A):83–7.
15. Witt J, Pess G, Gelberman RH. Treatment of de Quervain's tenosynovitis: a prospective study of the results of injection of steroids and immobilization in a splint. J Bone Joint Surg. 1991;73(A):219–22.
16. Weiss A-PC, Akelman E, Tabatabai M. Treatment of De Quervain's disease. J Hand Surg. 1994;19A:595–8.
17. Sampson SP, Wisch D, Badalamente MA. Complications of conservative and surgical treatment of de Quervain's disease and trigger fingers. Hand Clinics. 1994;10(1):73–82.
18. Canoso JJ. Bursitis, tenosynovitis, ganglions, and painful lesions of the wrist, elbow and hand. Curr Opinion Rheumatol. 1990;2:276–81.
19. Freiberg A, Mulholland RS, Levine R. Nonoperative treatment of trigger fingers and thumbs. J Hand Surg. 1989;14(A):553–8.
20. Kraemer BA, Young VL, Arfken C. Stenosing flexor tenosynovitis. South Med J. 1990;83(7):806–11.
21. Rhoades CE, Gelberman RH, Manjarris JF. Stenosing tenosynovitis of the fingers and thumb. Results of a prospective trial of steroid injection and splinting. Clin Orthop. 1984;190:236–8.
22. Yosipovitch G, Yosipovitch Z, Karp M, Mukamel M. Trigger finger in young patients with insulin dependent diabetes. J Rheumatol. 1990;17:951–2.
23. Marks MR, Gunther SF. Efficacy of cortisone injection in treatment of trigger fingers and thumbs. J Hand Surg. 1989;14(A):722–7.
24. Anderson B, Kaye S. Treatment of flexor tenosynovitis of the hand 'trigger finger' with corticosteroids. A prospective study of the response to local injection. Arch Intern Med. 1991;151:153–6.
25. McFarlane RM. Dupuytren's disease. In: McCarthy JG, May JW Jr, Littler JW, eds. Plastic surgery, 2E. Philadelphia: WB Saunders; 1990: 5053–86.
26. Lynch M, Jayson MIV. Fasciitis and fibrosis. Clin Rheum Dis. 1979;5(3):833–55.
27. Wooldridge WE. Four related fibrosing diseases. When you find one, look for another. Postgrad Med. 1988;84(2):269–74.
28. Wurster-Hill DH, Brown F, Park JP, Gibson SH. Cytogenetic studies in Dupuytren's contracture. Am J Hum Genet. 1988;43:285–92.
29. An HS, Southworth SR, Jackson WT, Russ B. Cigarette smoking and Dupuytren's contracture of the hand. J Hand Surg. 1988;13(A):872–4.
30. Wheeler ES, Meals RA. Dupuytren's diathesis: a broad spectrum disease. Plast Reconstr Surg. 1981;68(5):781–3.
31. Gelberman RH, Amiel D, Rudolph RM, Vance RM. Dupuytren's contracture. An electron microscopic, biochemical and clinical correlative study. J Bone Joint Surg. 1980;62(A):425–32.
32. Murrell GAC, Francis MJO, Howlett CR. Dupuytren's contracture. Fine structure in relation to aetiology. J Bone Joint Surg. 1989;71(B):367–3.
33. McCann BG, Logan A, Belcher H, Warn A, Warn RM. The presence of myofibroblasts in the dermis of patients with Dupuytren's contracture. A possible source for recurrence. J Hand Surg. 1993;18B:656–61.
34. Badalamente MA, Hurst LC, Sampson SP. Prostaglandins influence myofibroblast contractility in Dupuytren's disease. J Hand Surg.1988;13(A):867–71.
35. Baird KS, Crossan JF, Ralston SH. Abnormal growth factor and cytokine expression in Dupuytren's contracutre. J Clin Path. 1993;46:425–8.
36. Terek RM, Jiranek WA, Goldberg MJ, Wolfe HJ, Alman BA. The expression of platelet-derived growth-factor gene in Dupuytren's contracture. J Bone Joint Surg. 1995;77-A:1–9.
37. Kloen P, Jennings CL, Gebhardt MC, Springfield DS, Mankin HJ. Transforming growth factor-beta: possible roles in Dupuytren's contracture. J Hand Surg. 1995;20A:101–8.
38. Duthie RB, Francis MJO. Free radicals and Dupuytren's contracure. J Bone Joint Surg. 1988;70(B):689–91.
39. Baird KS, Alwan WH, Crossan JF, Wojciak B. T-cell-mediated response in Dupuytren's disease. Lancet. 1993;341:1622–3.
40. Neumuller J, Menzel J, Millesi H. Prevalence of HLA-DR3 and auto-antibodies to connective tissue components in Dupuytren's contracture. Clin Immunology Immunopath. 1994;71(2):142–8.
41. Sugden P, Andrew JG, Andrew SM, Freemont AJ. Dermal dendrocytes in Dupuytren's disease: a link between the skin and pathogenesis? J Hand Surg 1993;18B:662–6.
42. Yacoe ME, Bergman AG, Ladd AL, Hellman BH. Dupuytren's contracture: MR imaging findings and correlation between MR signal intensity and cellularity of lesions. Am J Roentgenology. 1993;160:813–7.
43. Pittet B, Rubbia-Brandt L, Desmouliere A *et al.* Effect of gamma-interferon on the clinical and biologic evolution of hypertrophic scars and Dupuytren's disease: an open pilot study. Plast Reconstr Surg 1994;93:1224–35.
44. Ketchum LD, Hixson FP. Dermofasciectomy and full thickness grafts in the treatment of Dupuytren's contracture. J Hand Surg. 1987;12(A):659–63
45. Rombouts J-J, Noël H, Legrain Y, Munting E. Prediction of recurrence in the treatment of Dupuytren's disease: evaluation of a histologic classification. J Hand Surg. 1989;14(A):644–52.

THE HIP

Bernard Mazières & Simon Carette

- The hip joint is the best example in the human body of a ball-and-socket synovial joint. It is an exceptionally strong and stable articulation which also exhibits a wide range of multiaxial movements.
- These apparently contradictory properties of the hip joint allow a person to stand erect while also permitting complex activities such as walking, running, squatting and dancing.
- Degenerative and inflammatory diseases of the hip are common and can lead to severe functional disability.

FUNCTIONAL ANATOMY

The hip joint is formed by the rounded head of the femur which joins the cup-shaped cavity of the acetabulum (Figs 10.1 & 10.2). The femoral head forms about two thirds of a sphere and is entirely covered with hyaline cartilage, except for the fovea, to which the ligamentum teres is attached. The head is mounted on the 8–10cm neck which forms an angle of about 125–140° with the shaft of the femur. When the angle decreases below this range, either because of congenital or acquired disorders, this is referred to as coxa vara. When it is increased above this range, this is referred to as coxa valga (see Fig. 10.3). Two bony prominences project from the femoral neck: the greater trochanter, situated laterally, onto which are inserted several of the gluteal muscles; and the lesser trochanter, situated medially, onto which are inserted the hip flexors. Both trochanters are united anteriorly by a roughened ridge, called the intertrochanteric line, and posteriorly by a smoother crest, the intertrochanteric crest.

The acetabulum is formed by the union of the ilium, ischium and pubis. It faces laterally, downwards and slightly forwards to accommodate the femoral head. In contrast to the shallow glenoid fossa of the scapula, the acetabulum is deeper and therefore provides some intrinsic stability to the joint. In addition, its rim is reinforced by a strong lip of fibrocartilage, the acetabular labrum, which deepens the socket and forms a tight collar around the femoral head, adding significantly to the stability of the joint. The articular area of the acetabulum has the outline of a horseshoe (Fig. 10.2). The center of the cavity or acetabular fossa is occupied by a fat pad which is covered with synovial membrane. The lower margin of the acetabulum, or acetabular notch, allows passage to the ligamentum teres which contains a small branch from the obturator artery that supplies blood to the region of

MUSCULAR ATTACHMENTS OF THE LEFT PELVIS

1 – Obliquus abdominus externus
2 – Gluteus medius
3 – Gluteus maximus
4 – Piriformis
5 – Rectus femoris
6 – Semimembranosus
7 – Biceps femoris and semitendinosus
8 – Quadratus femoris
9 – Obturator externus
10 – Adductor magnus
11 – Gracilis
12 – Adductor brevis
13 – Adductor longus
14 – Pyramidalis
15 – Pectineus
16 – Rectus femoris
17 – Gluteus minimus
18 – Tensor fasciae latae

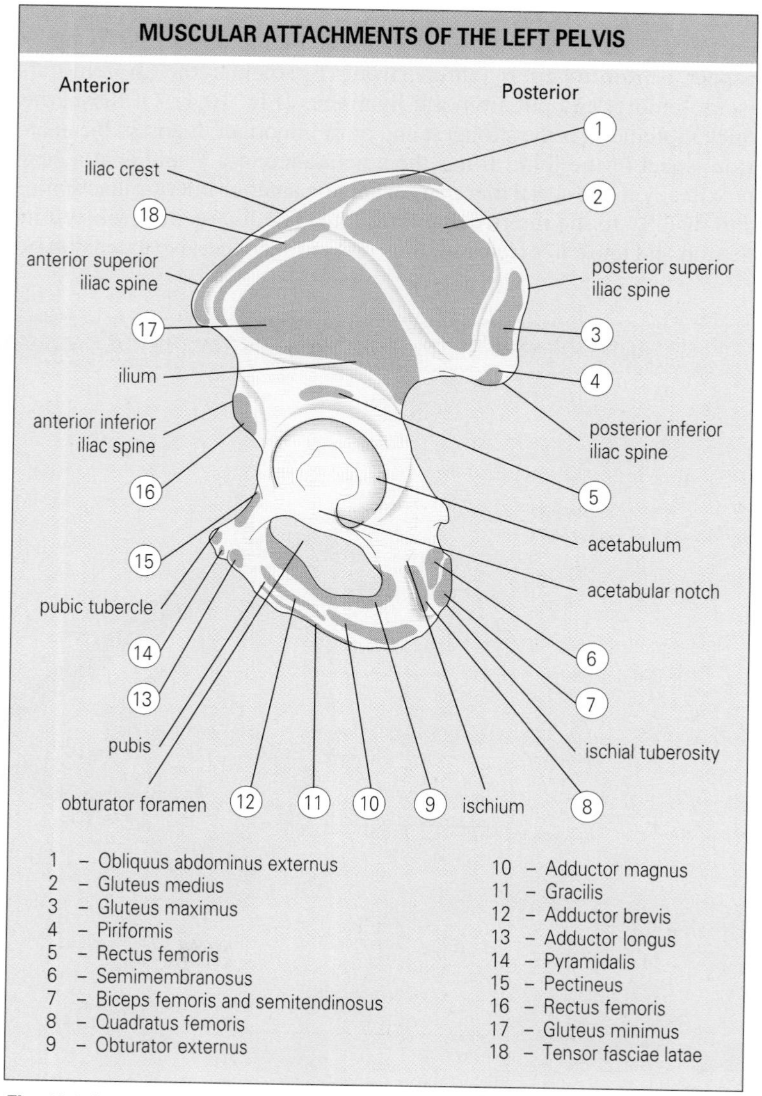

Fig. 10.2 Lateral aspect of the left pelvis. Muscle attachments are shown.

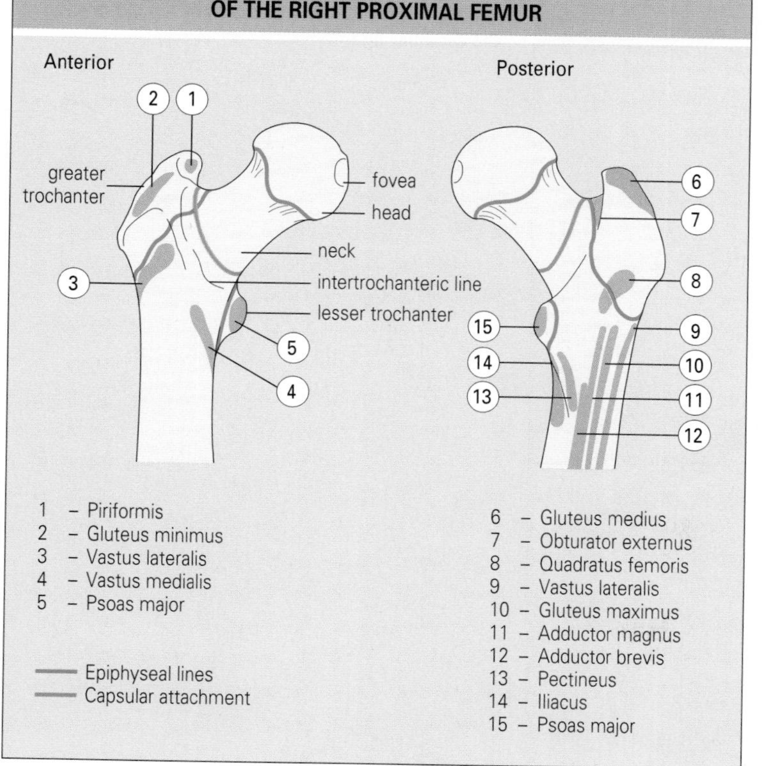

Fig. 10.1 Anterior and posterior aspects of the proximal right femur. The attachments of the muscles and hip capsule are shown.

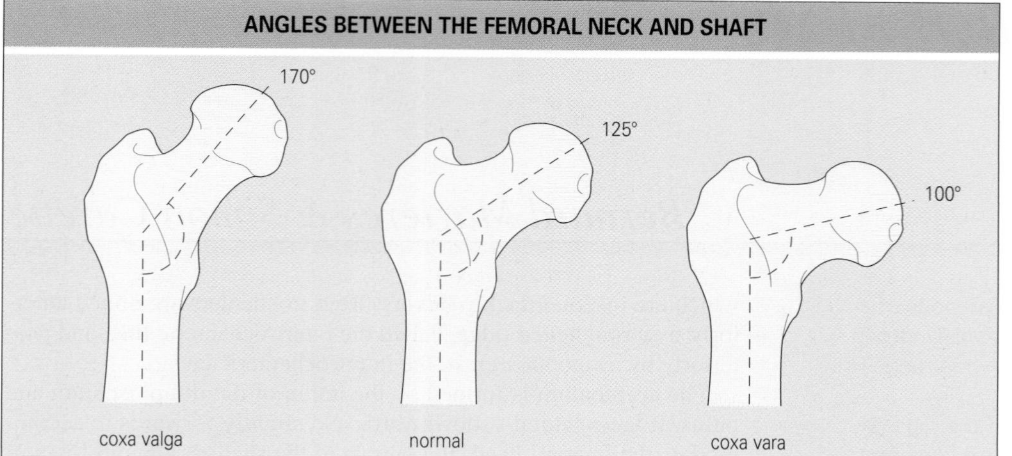

Fig. 10.3 Angles between the femoral neck and shaft in adults.

the fovea. The inferior margin of the acetabulum is closed in by the transverse acetabular ligament.

The thickness of the hyaline cartilage covering the femoral head varies significantly from one area to the other. It is thickest on the superior and posterior aspects of the head (3mm) and thins down to 0.5mm at the peripheral margin. Similarly, the acetabular cartilage ranges from 2–2.5mm in its posterosuperior segment to 1mm peripherally.

The fibrous articular capsule of the hip is attached proximally to the margin of the acetabulum and labrum and to the transverse acetabular ligament. Distally, it surrounds the head and neck of the femur and is attached anteriorly to the intertrochanteric line and posteriorly to the neck, slightly proximal to the intertrochanteric crest. The inner surface of the capsule is lined with the synovial membrane while its outer aspect is reinforced by three strong ligaments: the iliofemoral, ischiofemoral and pubofemoral ligaments (Fig. 10.4). Of these, the thick iliofemoral is the strongest and most important. It covers the anterior aspect of the joint. It has the appearance of a Y and is attached proximally to the acetabular margin and the anterior inferior iliac spine, and distally to the intertrochanteric line. The ligament is relaxed in flexion and tense in extension, thus preventing excessive extension of the hip and helping to maintain erect posture. The weaker ischiofemoral and pubofemoral ligaments strengthen the capsule posteriorly and inferiorly, respectively.

In the majority of individuals, the medial femoral circumflex artery, which is a branch of the common femoral artery, supplies most of the blood to the head and neck of the femur. Fracture of the femoral neck may therefore disrupt the blood supply to the femoral head and lead to osteonecrosis. In some patients, anastomoses with the small vessels of the ligamentum teres may prevent this from occuring [1].

The origin and insertion of the muscles of the hip region are shown in Figures 10.1 and 10.2. The main flexor of the thigh at the hip joint is the iliopsoas muscle. The chief extensors are the gluteus maximus and the hamstrings. The chief abductors are the gluteus medius and the gluteus minimus, while the chief adductors are the adductor longus, brevis and magnus. The main medial rotators are the tensor fasciae lata, gluteus medius and gluteus minimus and the main lateral rotators are the obturator muscles, gemelli and quadratus femoris.

Several bursae are found in the hip region. The three most important clinically include: the trochanteric bursa, which lies between the gluteus maximus muscle and the posterolateral aspect of the greater

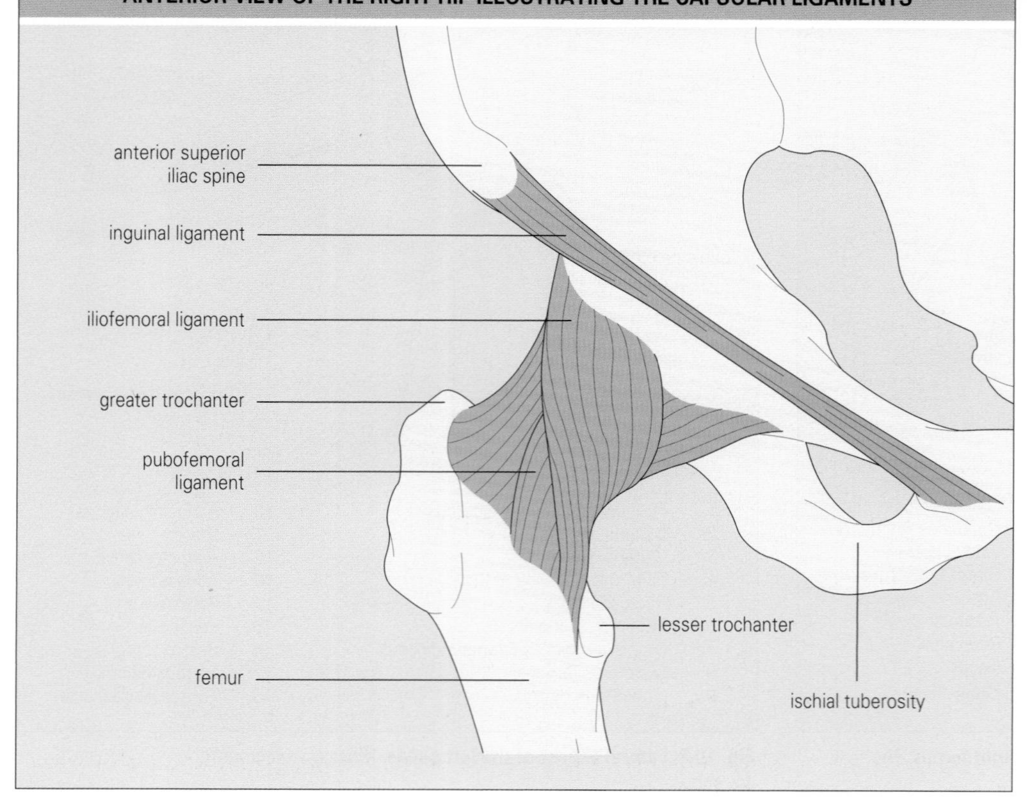

Fig. 10.4 Anterior view of the right hip illustrating the capsular ligaments.

trochanter; the iliopsoas bursa, which is located between the psoas tendon and the hip capsule, just lateral to the femoral vessels; and the ischiogluteal bursa, which lies between the gluteus maximus muscle and the ischial tuberosity.

PHYSICAL EXAMINATION

HISTORY

Hip pain is a common symptom with diverse etiologies. In the majority of instances, a diagnosis can be made with reasonable certainty by a careful history and physical examination.

Asking the patient to locate precisely the site of the pain is one of the most important aspects of the history, since it will narrow the diagnostic possibilities. Typically, hip disease manifests itself with pain in the groin which may radiate to the anterior, lateral or medial thigh, sometimes as far as the knee. However, not unusually, the pain may localize laterally to the greater trochanter, medially to the adductors, or posteriorly to the buttock. When these locations are associated with pain in the groin, it is usually easy to evoke hip pathology. The other etiologies of pain in the groin and anterior thigh area include iliopsoas bursitis, adductor tendinitis, hernias and pain from retroperitoneal structures.

Trochanteric bursitis is by far the most common cause of lateral trochanteric pain, although hip disease, as mentioned previously, and thoracolumbar pathology may also refer pain into this area. Buttock pain can be caused by referred back and sacroiliac pain, hip disease, ischiogluteal bursitis or vascular insufficiency.

Characterizing some of the alleviating and aggravating factors can help to differentiate certain disorders. For example, pain in the trochanteric area aggravated by lateral decubitus is highly suggestive of trochanteric bursitis, while pain in the ischiogluteal area aggravated by the sitting position should suggest an ischiogluteal bursitis. Groin pain aggravated by walking and relieved by rest is suggestive of a degenerative hip arthropathy, while pain in the same location, when associated with morning stiffness lasting more than 30 minutes and relieved by activity, is typical of an inflammatory arthropathy. Vascular insufficiency tends to present with buttock pain aggravated by walking and relieved within minutes by rest.

INSPECTION

The hip region should be inspected with the patient in both the standing and supine positions. In the standing position, the patient should be observed from the anterior, posterior and lateral aspects. Standing behind the patient, the presence of abnormal spinal curvatures should be noted. An exaggerated lumbar lordosis, especially if associated with a slight flexion of the knee, should alert the examiner to the possibility of a flexion deformity of the hip.

Pelvic tilting should also be noted. Tilting of the pelvis can be due to leg length discrepancy, scoliosis or hip disease. In the presence of leg length discrepancy, pelvic elevation will be present on the side of the longer leg when the patient stands with both legs parallel and the feet flat on the floor. The skin folds of the gluteal and popliteal regions will be higher on the longer leg. Hip disease may result in adduction or abduction deformities. An adduction deformity will be compensated by an upward tilt of the pelvis on the side of the adducted thigh, in order to allow the legs to be parallel during walking (Fig. 10.5). In contrast, an abduction deformity will be compensated by an elevation of the uninvolved side. In both cases, measurement of the actual length of the legs will be equal.

Rotational deformities of the hip are best evaluated with the patient facing the examiner. A vertical line drawn from the mid inguinal area should cross the middle of the patella and the middle of the ankle. Any deviation from this line defines a rotational deformity.

Particular attention should be paid to the patient's gait. There are two phases to the normal walking cycle: the stance phase, which begins with the heel strike and ends with the toe-off, and the swing phase, which begins with the toe-off and ends with the heel strike (see Chapter 1.12). During the stance phase, the hip joint loads three times the body weight. Pain in the hip may cause a patient to walk with an antalgic gait: in this case, the stance phase on the painful extremity is shorter than on the uninvolved side as the patient attempts to hurry off the painful limb as quickly as possible. Weakness of the gluteus medius will produce a Trendelenburg (abductor) gait: in this instance, the upper part of the body is thrown towards the weak limb during the stance phase in order to maintain balance because the abductors are unable to hold the pelvis level. Bilateral weakness of the gluteus medius will result in a waddling gait: the patient's upper body shifts laterally from side-to-side during the stance phase. Often, patients with a painful hip have components of both an antalgic and a Trendelenburg gait: the stance phase is shorter on the involved extremity and the upper part of the body is thrown towards the painful limb during the stance phase in order to avoid contraction of the gluteus medius, which might produce painful spasms.

With the patient lying supine, the examiner should observe the position of the lower extremities. Advanced hip diseases often cause the affected extremity to be held in flexion, abduction and external rotation, since this position relaxes the articular capsule and tends to lessen pain by reducing pressure in the joint.

Finally, the inguinal region should be inspected for any evidence of swelling. Enlargement of the iliopsoas bursa can cause inguinal swelling by one of two mechanisms: a localized bursitis, or extension of hip synovitis in the few individuals in whom the joint cavity communicates with the bursa. Such swelling has to be differentiated from adenopathies and hernias. In the absence of a communication with the iliopsoas bursa, synovitis of the hip will not usually cause any visible swelling or erythema, since the joint lies too deep to the skin surface. Similarly, trochanteric bursitis is only rarely associated with visible swelling in the greater trochanter region because of the thickness of the muscles and fat pad overlying the bursa.

ADDUCTION DEFORMITY OF THE RIGHT HIP CAUSING A FUNCTIONAL SHORTENING OF THE AFFECTED LEG

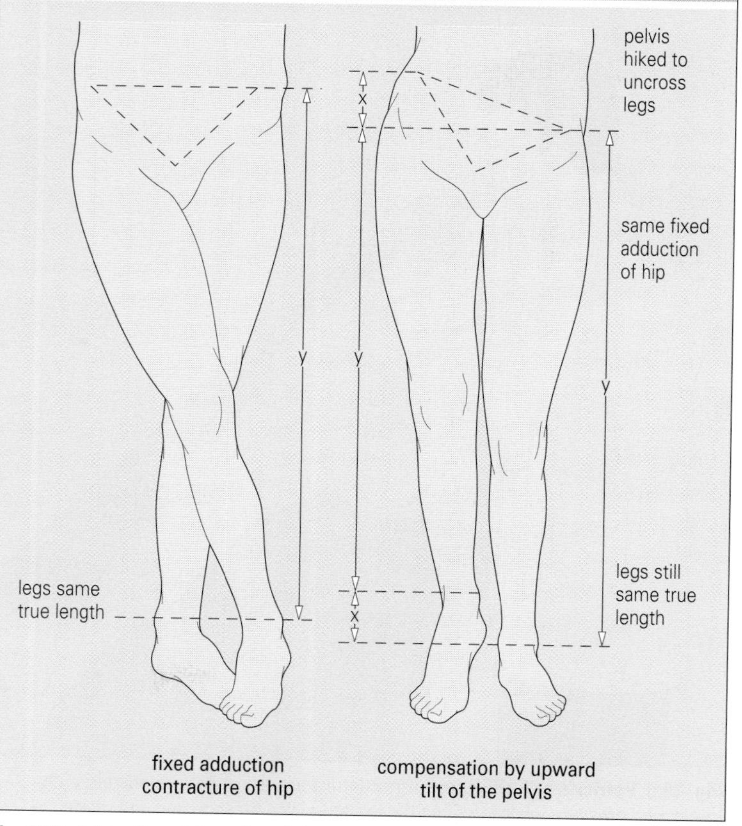

Fig. 10.5 Adduction deformity of the right hip causing a functional shortening of the affected leg.

PALPATION

Because of its deep location, the hip joint cannot be palpated directly. However, in the presence of hip disease, percussion of the heel or simultaneous firm compression of both trochanters may occasionally produce pain in the inguinal region. The bony landmarks and soft tissues of the hip area should be palpated systematically while noting any evidence of tenderness or swelling. With the patient in the supine position, these include:

- the anterior superior iliac spine;
- the contents of the inguinal area (from outside to inside: iliopsoas bursa, femoral nerve, artery and vein, lymph nodes, pubic tubercule and symphysis pubis);
- the muscles of the anterior thigh and the adductor muscles.

With the patient lying on one side, the greater trochanter and the iliotibial tract should be palpated. The ischial tuberosity is best examined in this position after passively flexing the hip and knee. Finally, with the patient in the prone position, the examiner will palpate the iliac crest, posterior superior iliac spine, sacroiliac joint, sciatic nerve and gluteus muscles.

MOBILIZATION

The hip joint is capable of movements in three planes: sagittal (flexion and extension), frontal (abduction and adduction) and horizontal (internal and external rotations). Similarly to the shoulder, the hip is capable of circumduction. With the exception of extension, all these movements are best assessed passively with the patient lying in the supine position on a firm table. Throughout the examination, the pelvis must be stabilized by the hand of the examiner in order to avoid including pelvic motion in the measurements. Inter-observer errors in the measurements are in the order of 5–10%, while intra-observer errors are somewhat less (1–5%). To measure the ranges of motion with an acceptable level of consistency and accuracy, certain procedural principles must be followed in a systematic fashion and the measurement of joints with multiple axes may require different positions for different motions [2].

With the knee flexed to 90°, the hip can be flexed to about 135°. However, when the knee is extended, hip flexion is limited to only 90°.

The hip can be abducted to 45–50°. By placing the hand on the opposite anterior superior iliac spine, the examiner can easily feel the pelvis beginning to move at the end point of hip abduction. The intermalleolar distance between full abduction of both hips is occasionally used as a quantitative measure of hip abduction, but it is a poorly reproducible measure.

Adduction of the hip is limited to 30–40° and is assessed similarly to abduction with the exception that the stabilizing hand of the examiner is placed on the ipsilateral anterior superior iliac crest.

External and internal rotation can be measured with the patient either in the prone or supine positions. In the latter, which is the most commonly used in practice, the knee and hip are flexed to 90°. The examiner holds the knee with one hand and the ankle with the other. The leg is then rotated inwards (external rotation) and outwards (internal rotation). Movements should be stopped as soon as the pelvis starts moving. External rotation is normally limited to 45° and internal rotation to 35°. In patients with very painful hip disorders (often in the context of trauma), it may be easier to evaluate movements of rotation with the legs extended by simply rolling one leg at a time internally (internal rotation) and externally (external rotation).

Hip extension is normally limited to 20–30°. It is the most difficult movement to measure. It can be done with the patient lying prone or sideways. Again, it is important to fix the pelvis to get an adequate measure.

Among all the movements of the hip, abduction and internal rotation are usually the first ones to be painful or limited in the presence of hip pathology.

SPECIAL TESTS

Patrick's test

Patrick's test is used as a screening test for hip joint pathology. The test is sometimes designated by the acronym FABER, based on the initial letters of the movements that it evaluates (flexion, abduction, external rotation).

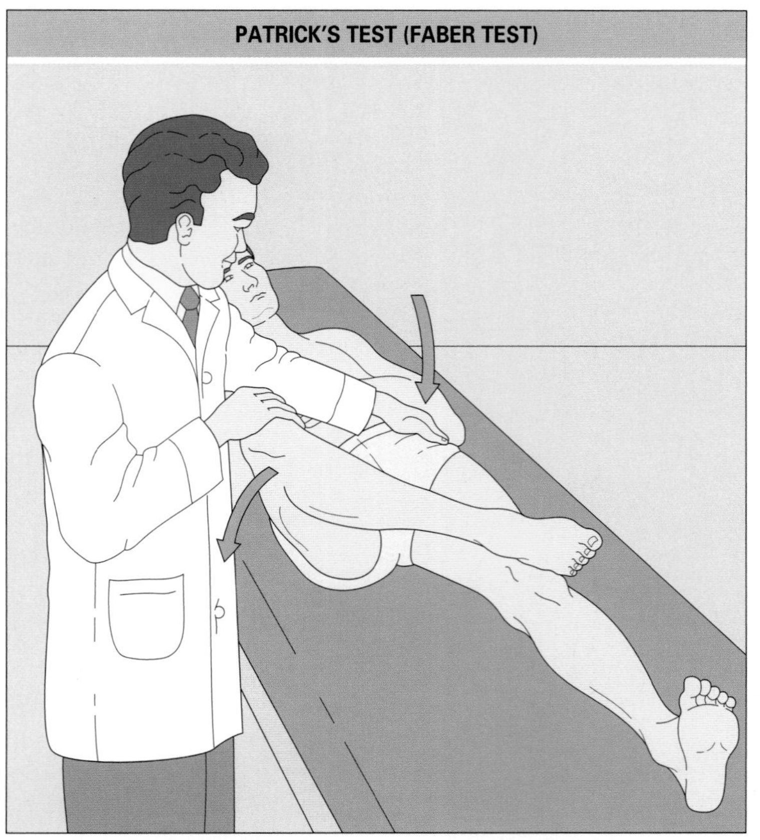

Fig. 10.6 Patrick's or FABER test. The contralateral iliac crest is stabilized with downward pressure while lowering the ipsilateral flexed, abducted and rotated leg. Rapid lowering tests the sacroiliac joint, while slow lowering tests the hip joint.

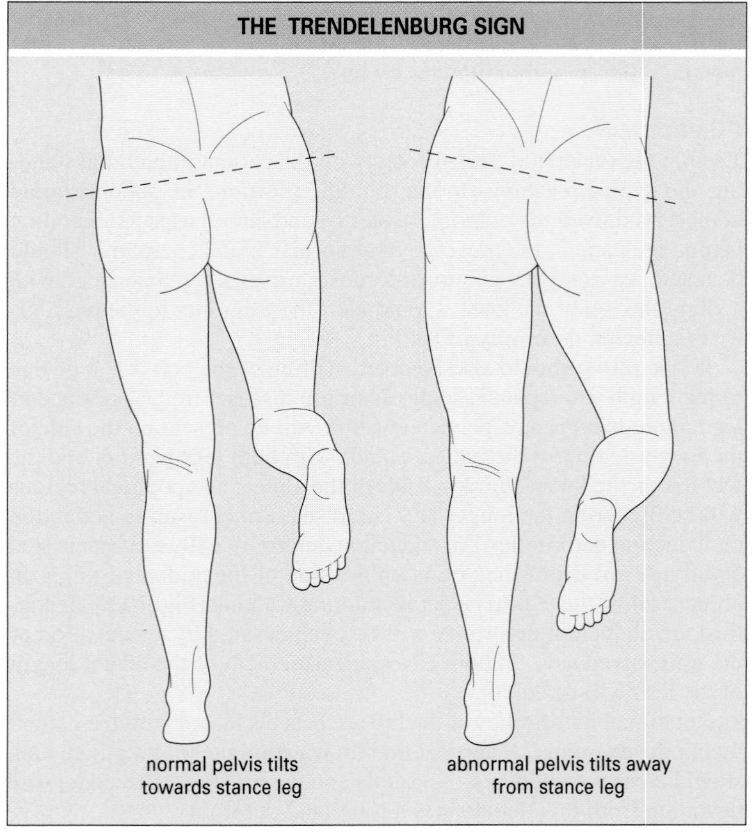

Fig. 10.7 The Trendelenburg sign. In a negative test, the pelvis tilts towards the stance leg because of adequate abductor contraction. In a positive test, the pelvis tilts away from the stance leg.

With the patient lying supine, the knee and hip are flexed to 90° and the foot of the examined extremity is placed on top of the opposite knee. The thigh is then slowly fully abducted and externally rotated towards the examining table (Fig. 10.6). The presence of groin pain, spasm or limitation of movement is suggestive of hip pathology. Patrick's test can also be used to stress the sacroiliac joints. To do so, one hand is placed on the abducted knee and the other on the opposite anterior superior iliac spine. Pain localized to the back when sudden pressure is applied simultaneously on each of these points, suggests sacroiliac pathology (see Chapter 6.16).

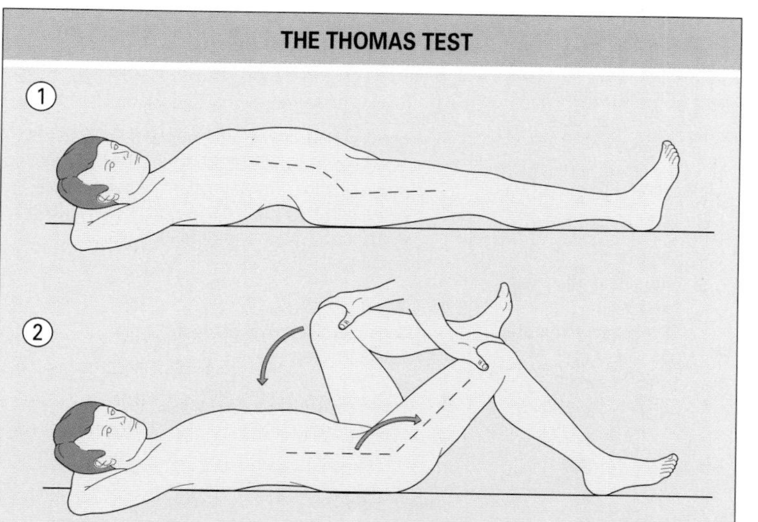

Fig. 10.8 The Thomas test. A flexion deformity of the hip is masked by an increased lumbar lordosis (1). Flexion of the contralateral hip flattens the lordosis and reveals the flexion deformity of the hip (2).

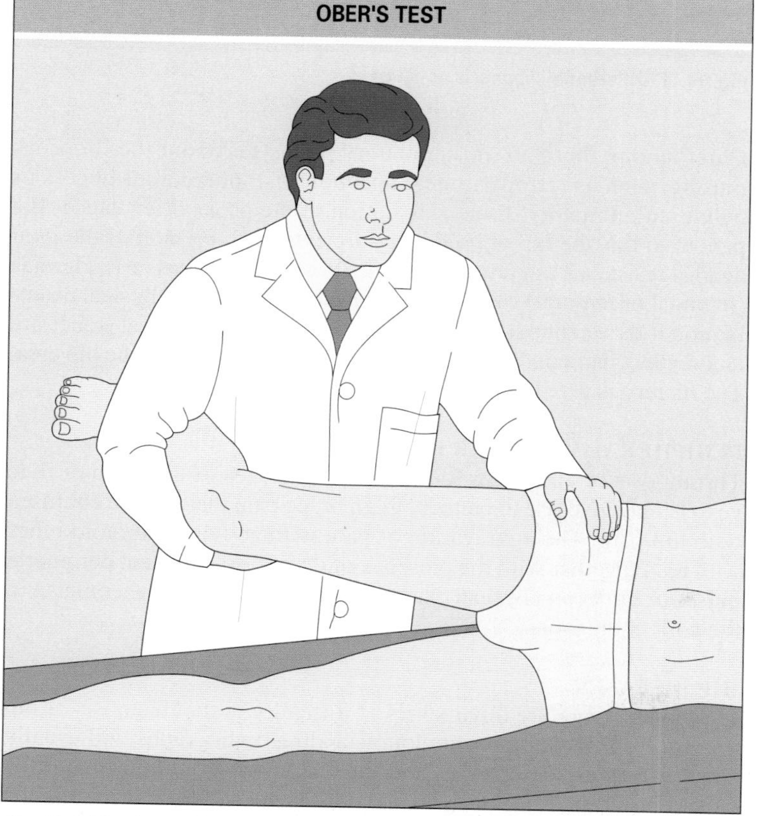

Fig. 10.9 Ober's test. In the presence of contraction of the iliotibial band, the uppermost hip remains abducted and does not drop back towards the table when the leg is released.

Trendelenburg's test

Trendelenburg's test is designed to evaluate the strength of the gluteus medius muscle. Normally, when a patient stands on one extremity, the abductor muscles on the weight-bearing side contract in order to maintain balance. This contraction causes the pelvis on the opposite side to rise slightly. In the presence of weak abductors or any condition which interferes with gluteus medius action (such as that caused by dislocation of the hip, coxa vara or arthritis), the pelvis on the contralateral side will not rise and may actually drop (Fig. 10.7). Patients with this sign will exhibit a Trendelenburg gait.

The Thomas test

The Thomas test is designed to evaluate the presence of a flexion contracture of the hip. With the patient lying supine, the thigh opposite the side to be tested is fully flexed on the abdomen in order to correct for any compensatory lumbar lordosis. Failure of the hip tested to lie flat on the examining table indicates the presence of a flexion contracture of that hip (Fig. 10.8).

Ober's test

Ober's test is designed to evaluate the presence of contracture of the iliotibial band. With the patient lying on one side, the lower knee and hip are flexed in order to eliminate lumbar lordosis, the upper leg is extended and abducted and then slowly lowered. Failure of the extremity to fall on the table when the supporting hand is withdrawn suggests the presence of contracture of the iliotibial band (Fig. 10.9).

Leg length measurement

Measurements of leg length are best performed with the patient lying supine with the legs fully extended and placed 15–20cm apart. Measurements are made from the anterior superior iliac spine to the middle of the lateral malleolus (Fig. 10.10). It is preferable to use the lateral malleolus as a landmark rather than the middle malleolus, in order to avoid measurement errors due to muscle wasting or obesity. A difference in length between the two legs of 1cm or less is not clinically significant.

Various radiologic techniques have been proposed to alleviate the lack of precision observed with clinical measurements of leg length. The simplest consists of obtaining a standing radiograph of the pelvis with the feet positioned 15–20cm apart [3]. In the absence of joint contractures, a difference in the height of the femoral heads indicates leg inequality. Scanography is a more complex method which requires taking radiographs of the hips, knees and upper ankles with the patient lying on a special calibrated frame [4]. Compared with the previous method, it has the advantage of identifying the bones which are shorter. An apparent (or functional) leg length discrepancy on inspection may result from a pelvic tilt due to a scoliosis or abduction or adduction contractures of the hip. In these situations, measurements from the

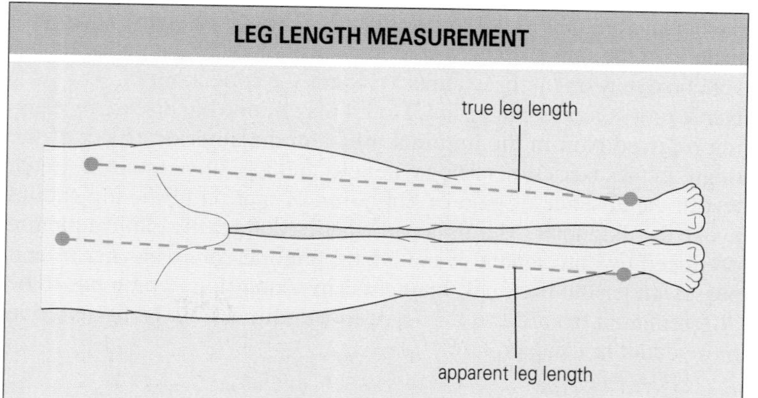

Fig. 10.10 Leg length measurement. The measurement is best made from the anterior superior iliac spine to the lateral malleolus.

umbilicus will show an apparent shortening of the leg on the side with the higher pelvis. However, when measured from the anterior superior iliac spine, the legs will have the same length.

True leg length discrepancy can be due to various congenital or acquired disorders, many of which occur during childhood. The most common of these include: congenital dislocation of the hip; acetabular dysplasia; Legg–Perthes disease; slipped capital femoral epiphysis; and congenital coxa vara. Leg length discrepancy is associated with an increased incidence of trochanteric bursitis on the longer side (see below). An increased incidence of osteoarthritis of the hip on the side of the longer leg has also been reported. The longer leg is typically held in adduction under a tilted pelvis. This results in decreased acetabular covering of the femoral head. The increased localized stress on the remaining weight-bearing area of the femoral head may contribute to the development of osteoarthritis [5].

DIFFERENTIAL DIAGNOSIS OF HIP PAIN

Pain in the hip region may arise from the hip joint itself, adjacent bones or periarticular soft tissues (cutaneous and subcutaneous tissues, muscles, tendons and bursae). In addition, thoracolumbar spine disorders, intra-abdominal pathologies and peripheral vascular diseases can present with referred pain in this region and should therefore be considered in the differential diagnosis. A classification of hip pain, based upon the tissues primarily involved, is outlined in Figure 10.11. Of these, osteoarthritis of the hip, trochanteric bursitis and spinal disorders account for the vast majority of conditions seen in clinical practice. A detailed history and careful physical examination of the joints (hip, pubis and sacroiliac), periarticular soft tissues, nerve and blood supply, abdomen and thoracolumbar spine are essential for a precise diagnosis.

LUMBAR SPINE DISORDERS

Pain in the posterior aspect of the hip is most often referred from the lumbar spine. The history and physical examination usually allow the examiner to separate hip disease from a low back disorder. Most patients with lumbar and/or buttock pain have a mechanical cause for their symptoms [6]. The value of imaging techniques is extremely limited in these patients [7], the great majority of whom fortunately improve with simple conservative measures [8].

Sacroiliac disorders can also cause buttock pain. When the patients present with an insidious onset of pain associated with severe morning stiffness that is relieved by activity, the diagnosis of sacroiliitis is usually considered. However, when these characteristics are lacking, the diagnosis may be missed, especially since the bedside techniques for sacroiliac joint examination are unreliable [9].

Mechanical disorders of the thoracolumbar junction (T12 and L1) may refer pain to the greater trochanter area and thus may mimic trochanteric bursitis. Such pain referral is due to the fact that the skin overlying the greater trochanter is innervated by a cutaneous branch originating from the dorsal rami of T12–L1 [10] (Fig. 10.12) . Pain on palpation and mobilization of the spinous processes of the lower thoracic and upper lumbar vertebrae may orient the examiner towards the correct origin.

Nerve root compression from L2 to L4 may mimic hip disease by causing referred pain in the inguinal area and the anterior aspect of the thigh. In these cases, neurologic deficits and a positive femoral stretch test in the absence of pain or limitation of motion of the hip should evoke the diagnosis. Meralgia paresthetica defines the clinical picture produced by entrapment of the lateral femoral cutaneous nerve as it passes under the inguinal ligament. This condition, which has to be differentiated from L2 to L4 nerve root compression, is discussed in more detail in Chapter 4.16.

INTRA-ABDOMINAL PATHOLOGIES

Various intra-abdominal and retroperitoneal conditions can refer pain to the hip region (the inguinal and anterior thigh areas especially).

DIFFERENTIAL DIAGNOSIS OF HIP PAIN	
Articular	**Periarticular**
Inflammatory joint diseases Rheumatoid arthritis Spondyloarthropathies Polymyalgia rheumatica	Bursitis Trochanteric Iliopsoas Ischiogluteal
Degenerative joint diseases Primary osteoarthritis Secondary osteoarthritis	Tendinitis Trochanteric Adductor
Metabolic joint diseases Gout Pseudogout Ochronosis Hemochromatosis Wilson's disease Acromegaly	Acute calcific periarthritis Heterotopic calcifications
	Osseous
Infections	Bone lesions Fractures, neoplasms, infection, osteonecrosis of the femoral head, metabolic bone disease (Paget's disease of bone, stress fractures, osteomalacia, hyperparathyroidism, renal osteodystrophy), reflex sympathetic dystrophy (transient migratory osteoporosis)
Tumors Benign Pigmented villonodular synovitis Osteochondromatosis Malignant Synovial sarcoma Synovial metastasis	In children Congenital dislocation of the hip (Usually not painful) Acetabular dysplasia (Usually not painful) Coxa vara (Usually not painful) Slipped capital femoral epiphysis (Usually not painful) Legg–Perthes disease Rickets
Hemarthrosis	
In children Transient 'toxic' synovitis Juvenile chronic arthritis	**Neurologic**
	Entrapment neuropathies Lateral femoral cutaneous nerve (meralgia paresthetica) Lumbar nerve root compression L2, L3 and L4
Referred pain	
Thoracolumbar spine Intra-abdominal structures Retroperitoneal structures	**Vascular**
	Atherosclerosis of aorta iliac vessels

Fig. 10.11 Differential diagnosis of hip pain.

Chief among these are inflammatory processes about the iliopsoas muscle, such as retroperitoneal appendicitis, tuberculous abcess or pelvic inflammatory disease. Irritation of the psoas often causes the patient to flex the hip or hold it rigidly extended. Flexion of the joint against resistance aggravates the pain (positive iliopsoas test). Hernias (inguinal or femoral) can usually be easily detected on physical examination if the examiner specifically looks for them. Ureteral stones are among the other conditions that can typically refer pain to the hip area. The history is usually characteristic.

PERIPHERAL VASCULAR DISEASES

Thrombosis or aneurysm formation of branches of the aorta or iliac vessels may give rise to buttock, thigh or leg pain that may be confused with hip pain. The aggravation of pain with activity and rapid relief with rest, together with the presence of decreased or absent peripheral pulses or bruits on physical examination, should orient the clinician to the correct diagnosis.

HIP DISEASES

In practice, there are three levels of difficulty in the diagnosis of hip disease. When symptoms are long-standing, radiographs will usually show characteristic changes and the diagnosis should pose no difficulty. For instance, it is easy to diagnose Paget's disease involving the femur and hip joint (see Chapter 8.45). Similarly, primary hip osteoarthritis is readily diagnosed in the presence of subchondral scle-

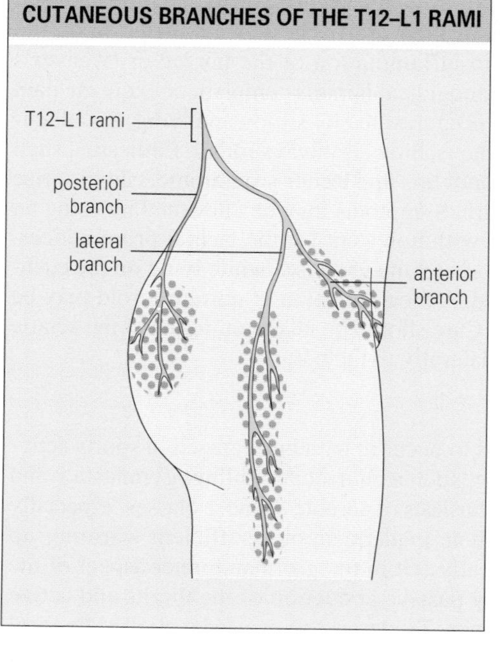

Fig. 10.12 Cutaneous branches originating from the T12–L1 rami innervate the skin overlying the iliac crest, the inguinal region and the greater trochanter area.

rosis, marginal osteophytes and superolateral joint space narrowing (see Chapter 8.3). The same applies to late stages of osteonecrosis when flattening of the femoral head has occurred (see Chapter 8.47) or to chondrocalcinosis when calcific deposits are visible in the hyaline cartilage and/or acetabular labrum.

In other more difficult cases, radiographs are abnormal but are not characteristic of a specific disorder. For example, localized or diffuse osteopenia or sclerosis of the femoral head, and/or neck and/or acetabulum may be observed, suggesting a bone pathology. Similarly, one may notice minimal joint space narrowing, sometimes with subchondral erosions and/or osteopenia, but without osteophytes or sclerosis. In these cases an inflammatory arthritis may be suspected. Radiographs are useful in confirming that the hip is affected but other investigations are usually needed to establish a definite diagnosis. In each circumstance, diagnostic modalities should be guided by the history and other physical findings. A clinical suspicion of early osteonecrosis may require bone scintigraphy, computed tomography or magnetic resonance imaging for confirmation. An arthrogram may be very helpful in documenting chondromatosis, synovial tumors, labrum tears or local thinning of the cartilage in the weight-bearing areas of an early osteoarthritic joint. The suspicion of a chronic septic or crystal-induced synovitis would require joint aspiration for synovial fluid analysis.

The most difficult diagnostic situation occurs when the patient presents with hip pain and a normal radiograph. All the conditions listed in Figure 10.11 must be considered. A careful history and physical examination become even more important in this situation. The presence of pain at the extremes of abduction and internal rotation suggest early hip disease caused by arthritis or osteonecrosis. Limitation of hip movements in all directions in a diabetic patient suggests an adhesive capsulitis of the hip joint which could be confirmed by an arthrogram. The presence of systemic symptoms, such as fatigue, fever, weight loss or worsening of pain at night, requires baseline laboratory tests and a radionuclide bone scan in search of a tumor or an indolent infectious process.

PERIARTICULAR SOFT TISSUES

Several problems of the hip are related to the soft tissue structures around the joint and its surrounding muscles. Although relatively common, many of these problems are poorly defined, misdiagnosed or both [10].

Bursitis and tendinitis

Numerous bursae are found in the hip region. Since they are lined with synovial tissue, they may be affected by all the inflammatory diseases affecting the hip joint, such as rheumatoid arthritis, and infectious or crystal-induced synovitis. Most commonly however, bursitis and tendinitis around the hip are induced by trauma or repetitive microtrauma.

Trochanteric bursitis

Trochanteric bursitis is the most common cause of pain about the hip region. The soft tissues that cross the bony posterior portion of the greater trochanter are protected from it by the three trochanteric bursae. The gluteus maximus bursa, which separates the fibers of gluteus maximus from the greater trochanter, is the most important of these bursae. It is not palpable unless it is distended or inflamed. Patients with trochanteric bursitis present with a deep, aching pain sometimes associated with a burning sensation on the lateral aspect of the hip and thigh. The pain increases with activities such as walking, squatting and climbing stairs, and is associated with a limp in 15% of patients [12]. Typically the pain decreases at rest, although it is frequently worse at night, especially when the patient is lying on the affected side. Tenderness can be elicited on palpation of the area around the greater trochanter which may feel boggy, at least in thin patients. Resisted abduction of the hip when the patient is lying on the opposite side may accentuate the discomfort. The movements of the hip are normal, but in severe cases discomfort can limit motion. Trochanteric bursitis is more common in women. It can occur as an isolated condition but is more frequently seen in association with damage to the ipsilateral hip joint, mechanical back strain and obesity [13]. The alteration in gait secondary to these conditions is often accompanied by a limitation of internal rotation of the hip and reflex tightening of the external rotators. These factors may increase the tension of gluteus maximus on the iliotibial band, and potentiate bursal inflammation [14]. Potential precipitating factors include local trauma, leg length inequalities, jogging and other athletic and stressful activities.

Slight irregularities of the greater trochanter or peritrochanteric calcifications of the bursa are sometimes seen on plain radiographs. Bone scintigraphy may show local increased uptake [13]. The differential diagnosis of increased radio-uptake in this region includes stress fractures, local infection and bone and soft tissue tumors. Clinically, however, hip disease and referred thoracolumbar pain are the two conditions that mimic trochanteric bursitis most commonly. The course of trochanteric bursitis is varied: an acute phase may last several days, followed by the gradual abatement of symptoms. However, in many patients, low-grade discomfort may persist for weeks or months.

Treatment includes continuous rest. Patients engaged in sports should be advised to reduce their level of activity, especially running and standing for prolonged periods on the affected limb. Nonsteroidal anti-inflammatory drugs can be used but results are often disappointing [12]. Ultrasound is useful only in a minority of patients. The efficacy of massages has not been studied. In uncontrolled series, infiltration of a local anesthetic and of a long-acting corticosteroid preparation in the trochanteric bursa has been shown to be helpful in confirming the diagnosis and bringing long-term relief [12–15]. It is considered by many to be the most effective treatment modality.

Failure of trochanteric bursitis to respond to conservative treatment may be due to tightness of the iliotibial band, as evidenced by a positive Ober's test. Referral to physiotherapy for exercises to stretch out the fascia lata femoris in these patients may be worthwhile. In patients with true leg length discrepancy, trochanteric bursitis tends to occur on the longer leg because of the increased stress imposed on the abductors. In these patients, a heel lift may be indicated. Various surgical procedures have been proposed for refractory cases of trochanteric bursitis but these are rarely, if ever, necessary [15,16].

Iliopsoas bursitis

Iliopsoas bursitis has been described in association with a variety of hip disorders, including osteoarthritis, rheumatoid arthritis, synovial chondromatosis, pigmented villonodular synovitis, osteonecrosis and septic arthritis [17]. While the bursa communicates with the hip cavity in only 15% of adults, a communication has been documented in most reported cases of bursitis. Several theories may explain this finding: hip

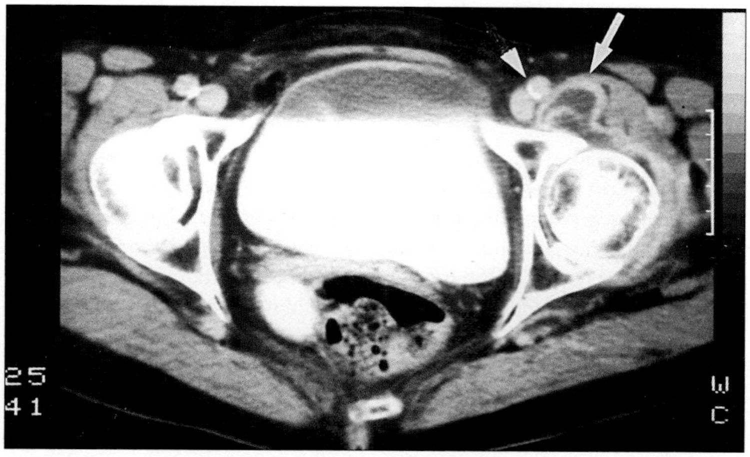

Fig. 10.13 **Computed tomographic scan of a patient with rheumatoid arthritis showing an enlarged fluid-filled iliopsoas bursa (arrow) communicating with the hip joint and displacing the neurovascular bundle (arrowhead).** Reproduced with permission from Letourneau *et al.*[21].

synovitis with excessive synovial fluid accumulation may cause enlargement of the iliopsoas bursa via a pre-existing communication; a weakened inflamed hip capsule may rupture into the adjacent bursa, creating a new communication; or the bursa itself may be enlarged by the inflammatory process[18].

The direction and degree of bursal enlargement are the most important factors in clinical presentation. The majority of patients are asymptomatic or present with a painful inguinal mass[18,19]. Others may present with leg swelling or varicosities secondary to femoral vein compression[20] or femoral nerve compression[21], thus making the diagnosis more difficult. Several cases of bladder and bowel compression have also been reported. Computed tomography has been proposed as the best diagnostic test to document iliopsoas bursitis (Fig. 10.13). Arthrography followed by the instillation of corticosteroids is also an effective diagnostic and therapeutic modality. Surgical excision of the bursa is occasionally necessary.

Ischiogluteal bursitis

Ischiogluteal bursitis is most commonly seen in patients engaged in jobs which favor repeated friction of the ischial bursae[22]. In the standing position, the gluteus maximus forms a thick pad over the ischial tuberosity. When the thigh is flexed, as in the sitting position, the distal border of the gluteus maximus moves superiorly, leaving the ischial tuberosity subcutaneous. Weavers repeatedly extend one limb and then the other in the practice of their craft. The repeated friction on the ischial bursa may lead to inflammation of the bursae or 'weaver's bottom'. Patients with ischiogluteal bursitis complain of exquisite pain over the ischions, which is aggravated by sitting and lying. Local tenderness on palpation of the ischions is always found. Enthesitis, such as seen in ankylosing spondylitis and Reiter's syndrome, can give rise to a similar clinical picture. Symptoms may be alleviated by using an 8–10cm rubber cushion with holes cut for the ischial prominences. Trunk and knee-to-chest stretching exercises while lying on the cushion should be encouraged. A local injection of corticosteroid may be used in refractory cases. Care should be taken not to inject the sciatic nerve which passes just laterally to the bursa.

Adductor tendinitis

Adductor tendinitis tends to occur in patients engaged in sports activities involving straddling, such as horseback riding, gymnastics and dancing, as well as in enthusiasts of aerobic exercise classes, especially in those individuals with an inadequate or insufficient warming-up period. The pain is typically felt in the groin and inner aspect of the thigh and is increased by passive abduction of the thighs and active adduction against resistance. Tenderness may also be elicited by local palpation of the adductor muscles, especially near their insertion on the front of the pubis. The differential diagnosis of adductor tendinitis include hernias, genitourinary afflictions (prostatitis, epidydimitis, urethritis, hydrocele, etc.), osteitis pubis and arthritis of the hip. Treatment consists of rest and ice during the acute phase. Nonsteroidal anti-inflammatory drugs, ultrasound and progressive stretching exercises are used in the subacute phase. Local corticosteroid injections are reserved for patients resistant to these conservative modalities.

Snapping hip syndrome

Some patients complain of pain in the hip region associated with an audible and palpable snapping sensation, usually felt in the lateral trochanteric area[23]. This is an uncommon entity reported most frequently in young individuals. Symptoms typically occur in activities such as climbing or walking upstairs during which a taut iliotibial band slips over the greater trochanter. On examination, the patient can usually reproduce the snapping sensation by flexing and internally rotating the thigh, and the examiner can sometimes feel the snapping sensation by applying a palm to the greater trochanter area. Treatment consists essentially of exercises to stretch the iliotibial band. Cases of snapping hip caused by slipping of the iliopsoas tendon over an osseous ridge on the lesser trochanter have been reported[23].

REFERENCES

1. Sevitt S. Avascular necrosis and revascularization of the femoral head after intracapsular fracture: a combined arteriographic and histological study. J Bone Joint Surg. 1964;46B:270–96.
2. Lea RD, Gerhardt JJ. Range-of-motion measurements. J Bone Joint Surg. 1995;77A:784–98.
3. Clarke GR. Unequal leg length: an accurate method of detection and some clinical results. Rheum Phys Med. 1982;11:385–90.
4. Morscher E, Figner G. Measurement of leg length. In: Hungerford DS, ed. Progress in orthopedic surgery, Volume 1, Leg length discrepancy: The injured knee. New York: Springer-Verlag; 1977:21–7.
5. Bjerkreim I. Secondary dysplasia and osteoarthritis of the hip joint in functional and in fixed obliquity of the pelvis. Acta Orthop Scan. 1974;45:873–82.
6. Spitzer WO, Leblanc FE, Dupier M. Scientific approach to the assessment and management of activity-related spinal disorders: a monograph for clinicians. Report of the Quebec Task Force on Spinal Disorders. Spine. 1987;12:S1-59
7. Witt I, Vestergaard A, Rosenklint A. A comparative analysis of x-ray findings of the lumbar spine in patients with and without lumbar pain. Spine. 1984;9:198–299
8. Berquist-Ullman M, Larsson U. Acute low back pain in industry. A controlled prospective study with reference to therapy and confounding factors. Acta Orthop Scand. 1977;170: S1–17.
9. Russell AS, Maksymowych W, LeClercq S. Clinical examination of the sacroiliac joints: a prospective study. Arthritis Rheum. 1981; 24:1575–7.
10. Maigne R. Low back pain of thoracolumbar origin. Arch Phys Med Rehabil. 1980;61:389–95.
10. Lotke PA. Soft tissue afflictions. In: Steinberg ME, ed. The hip and its disorders. Philadelphia: W.B. Saunders; 1991: 669–82.
12. Schapira D, Nahir M, Scharf Y. Trochanteric bursitis: A common clinical problem. Arch Phys Med Rehabil. 1986;67:815–7
13. Little H. Trochanteric bursitis: a common cause of pelvic girdle pain. Can Med Assoc J. 1979;120:456–8.
14. Swezey RL. Pseudo-radiculopathy in subacute trochanteric bursitis of subgluteus maximus bursa. Arch Phys Med Rehabil. 1976;57:387–90.
15. Gordon EJ. Trochanteric bursitis and tendinitis. Clin Orthop. 1961;20:193–202.
16. Zoltan DJ, Clancy WG, Keene JS. A new operative approach to snapping hip and refractory trochanteric bursitis in athletes. Am J Sports Med. 1986;14: 201–4.
17. Toohey AK, LaSalle TL, Martinez S, Polisson RP. Iliopsoas bursitis: clinical features, radiographic findings, and disease associations. Semin Arthritis Rheum. 1990;10:41–7.
18. Melamed A, Bauer CA, Howard Johnson J. Iliopsoas bursal extension of arthritic disease of the hip. Radiology. 1967;89:54–8.
19. Underwood PL, McLeod RA, Ginsburg WW. The varied clinical manifestations of iliopsoas bursitis. J Rheumatol. 1988;15:1683–5.
20. Helfgott SM. Unusual features of iliopsoas bursitis. Athritis Rheum. 1988;31:1331–3.
21. Letourneau L, Dessureault M, Carette S. Rheumatoid iliopsoas bursitis presenting as unilateral femoral nerve palsy. J Rheumatol. 1991;18:462–3.
22. Swartout R, Compere EL. Ischio-gluteal bursitis. JAMA. 1974; 227:551–2.
23. Schaberg JE, Harper MC, Allen WC. The snapping hip syndrome. Am J Sports Med. 1984;12:361–5.

11

THE KNEE

Geoffrey P Graham & John A Fairclough

- The knee, the largest of human joints, is comprised of two joints, the patellofemoral and the tibiofemoral.
- Knee stability is provided by capsular and accessory (cruciate, collateral) ligaments plus muscles that provide dynamic stability to the joint.
- The prepatellar and the pretendinous bursae are subcutaneous sacs independent from the joint. The gatrocnemius-semimembranosus bursa, which communicates with the joint in 50% of adults, when distended causes the Baker's cyst.
- Knee pain may arise from the joint itself, periarticular tissues such as tendons and bursae, or distant sites such as the hip or femur.
- An accurate diagnosis of knee conditions can usually be made based on the history and physical examination. Essential investigative techniques include synovial fluid analysis, X–ray analysis, MRI and arthroscopy.

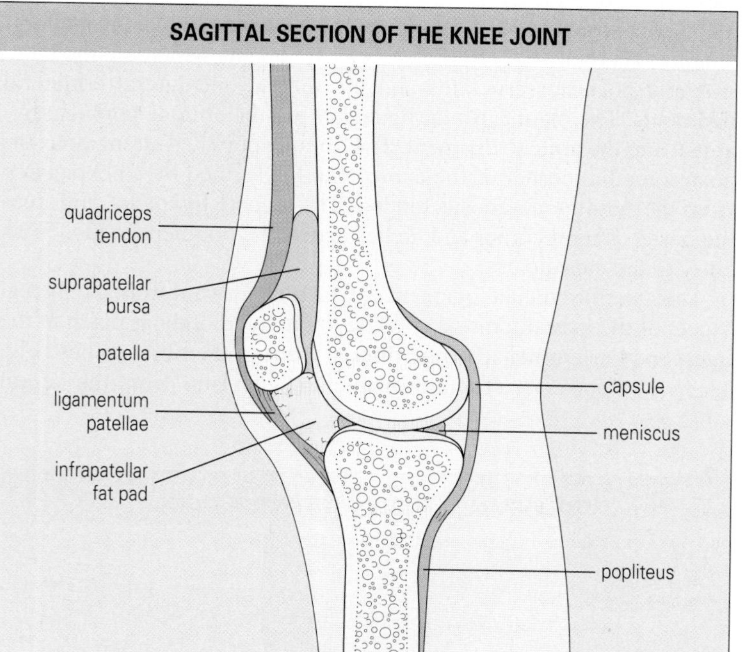

Fig. 11.1 Sagittal section showing the components of the knee joint.

FUNCTIONAL ANATOMY

The knee is the largest of the human joints in terms of the volume of its synovial cavity and the area of its articular cartilage. It actually consists of two joints, the tibiofemoral and the patellofemoral, which share a common synovial cavity. The synovial membrane of the joint is attached around the articular margins and the synovial cavity extends approximately one hand's breadth above the upper pole of the patella to form the suprapatellar pouch. Therefore, a collection of fluid in the joint or thickening of the synovium causes a characteristic swelling which extends above the patella.

The femoral and tibial condyles articulate with each other, with the fibrocartilaginous menisci interposed between them. The old name for the menisci was the semilunar cartilages, reflecting the fact that they are crescentic in shape. The lateral meniscus is nearly circular and the medial meniscus is semicircular. Their ends are attached to the intercondylar area of the tibia and their circumference to the meniscotibial and meniscofemoral ligaments, which are part of the capsule of the joint[1]. The lateral meniscus is attached to the femur posteriorly by the inconstant meniscofemoral ligaments of Wrisberg and Humphry. The popliteus tendon enters the joint through a deficiency in the capsule adjacent to the lateral meniscus and may be attached to it[2,3]. The menisci transmit approximately 60% of the force through the normal tibiofemoral joint and play a role in lubrication. They alter shape in order to maintain congruity of the joint as the knee flexes and extends. The peripheral 10–30% of the meniscus and the anterior and posterior horns receive a blood supply from the geniculate vessels and have the potential for repair[4]. The rest of the meniscus is avascular and is nourished from the synovial fluid, so there is little potential for healing in this area.

The knee is capable of flexion, extension and rotation. However, it is not a simple hinge joint with a single axis. The movements which occur are complex and involve both rolling and gliding of the femur on the tibia. The axis of rotation alters as the knee is flexed and extended. The normal motion of the knee is controlled by the shape of the articular surfaces and menisci and by the tension in the ligaments and capsule. Alteration in the configuration of any of these structures due to injury or disease can cause abnormal motion to occur. As the knee approaches full extension the shape of the joint surfaces and the tension in the ligaments cause the femur to internally rotate on the tibia, into the 'screwed home' position. Any further attempt to extend the knee simply increases the tension in the ligaments. On standing, the center of gravity passes in front of the axis of rotation of the knee, maintaining the ligaments in tension and so the muscles can relax. Standing requires very little energy expenditure due to this mechanism. No rotation is possible in the fully extended position; this can only occur in the flexed knee, when the ligaments are relaxed.

In health the center of the hip, the center of the knee and the center of the ankle lie in a straight line. Due to the medial inclination of the femur the long axes of the femur and tibia form a valgus angle of approximately 7°. Disease or an abnormality of growth may alter this angle – genu valgum represents an increase and genu varum a decrease.

The patella is a sesamoid bone lying in the quadriceps tendon (Fig. 11.1) and articulating with the trochlear groove of the femur. Its function is to increase the mechanical advantage of the quadriceps. It is triangular in section and has medial and lateral articular facets [5]. In full extension only the lower part of the patella is in contact with the articular cartilage of the femur. As the knee is flexed the patella enters the trochlea groove and sits centrally in it. A line drawn from the anterior superior iliac spine to the center of the patella represents the line of pull of the quadriceps which is lateral to the long axis of the femur. The angle formed by this line and a line drawn from the center of the patella to the tibial tubercle is called the Q angle (Fig. 11.2) [6]. The larger the Q angle, the larger is the force vector tending to pull the patella laterally. In a normal knee the Q angle measures approximately 15°, an angle exceeding 20° is abnormal. Genu valgum, persistent femoral anteversion and external tibial torsion increase this angle and therefore increase the tendency for the patella to dislocate. The factors acting against dislocation are the lower fibers of the vastus medialis, the shape of the patellofemoral joint and the fact that the lateral condyle is higher than the medial. The action of the lower fibers of the vastus medialis (the vastus medialis obliquus) is the most important factor. They originate from the medial intermuscular septum and run horizontally to the patella, controlling its lateral motion.

The knee gains little stability from the shape of the articular surfaces. The main stabilizers of the joint are the ligaments and the muscles, which provide dynamic stability. The capsule of the knee joint is a complex structure, parts of which are thickened to form named ligaments. There are also four accessory ligaments which are the anterior and posterior cruciates and the medial and lateral collateral ligaments. The main capsular ligaments are the oblique popliteal ligament and the arcuate ligament. The oblique popliteal strengthens the posteromedial corner of the capsule and is formed by an expansion from the semimembranosus tendon. The arcuate ligament reinforces the posterolateral corner and arches across the popliteus tendon at its entry to the capsule.

The anterior cruciate ligament (ACL) runs forward from the medial aspect of the lateral femoral condyle in the intercondylar notch to the intercondylar eminence of the tibia in front of the tibial spines (Fig. 11.3). The posterior cruciate ligament (PCL) runs from the lateral aspect of the medial femoral condyle in the intercondylar notch to insert at the back of the intercondylar area of the tibia and on its posterior aspect. The cruciate ligaments are complex structures composed of bundles of fibers of different lengths which twist around a main axis. This arrangement allows part of the ligament to be under tension in all positions of the joint. For convenience the ACL is described as being composed of two bands; an anteromedial which is taut when the knee is flexed, and a posterolateral, which is taut when the knee is extended [7]. From the orientation of the cruciate ligaments it can be seen that they are the main stabilizers of the knee in an anteroposterior direction: the anterior cruciate prevents anterior translation of the tibia on the femur and the posterior cruciate prevents posterior translation of the tibia on the femur. A further important function is to help provide rotatory stability and in particular to act as a check to internal rotation of the tibia. The medial collateral ligament runs forward and down from the medial femoral condyle to a broad insertion on the subcutaneous border of the tibia, deep to the pes anserinus. The ligament is a fan-shaped structure. Its anterior border is straight and easily identifiable, but its posterior border blends with the capsule of the knee joint[8,9]. The lateral collateral ligament is cord-like and is attached to the lateral femoral condyle. It runs down and slightly backwards to insert into the styloid process of the fibula where it blends with the insertion of the biceps femoris tendon. The collateral ligaments, in association with the capsule and the cruciate ligaments, provide varus and valgus stability. They also provide some rotational stability and in particular help to prevent external rotation of the tibia.

The quadriceps muscle consists of the rectus femoris and the three vasti: intermedius, medialis and lateralis. It is the main extensor of the knee and inserts into the patella via the quadriceps tendon (Fig. 11.4). Fibrous expansions from the vastus medialis and lateralis run obliquely to insert into the sides of the patella, the patella tendon and the tibia to form the medial and lateral patellar retinacula[9,10]. The iliotibial band is a thickening of the fascia lata on the lateral aspect of the thigh[11]. Proximally, the tensor fascia lata muscle inserts into it. Its distal insertion is into Gerdy's tubercle on the tibia and more proximally by oblique fibers which blend with the lateral patellar retinaculum. It helps to stabilize the lateral side of the joint and acts as an extensor when the knee is already near full extension. As the knee is flexed the iliotibial band moves backwards behind the center of rotation of the knee and acts as a flexor. The hamstrings are the main flexors of the knee, helped by the gastrocnemius, sartorius and gracilis. Medial rotation of the flexed knee is controlled by the medial hamstrings (semimembranosus and semitendinosus), popliteus, sartorius and gracilis. Lateral rotation is controlled by the biceps femoris alone.

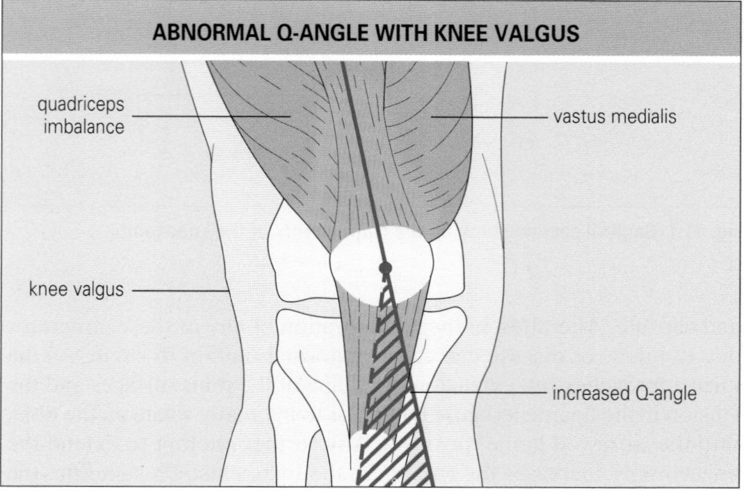

Fig. 11.2 The Q angle.

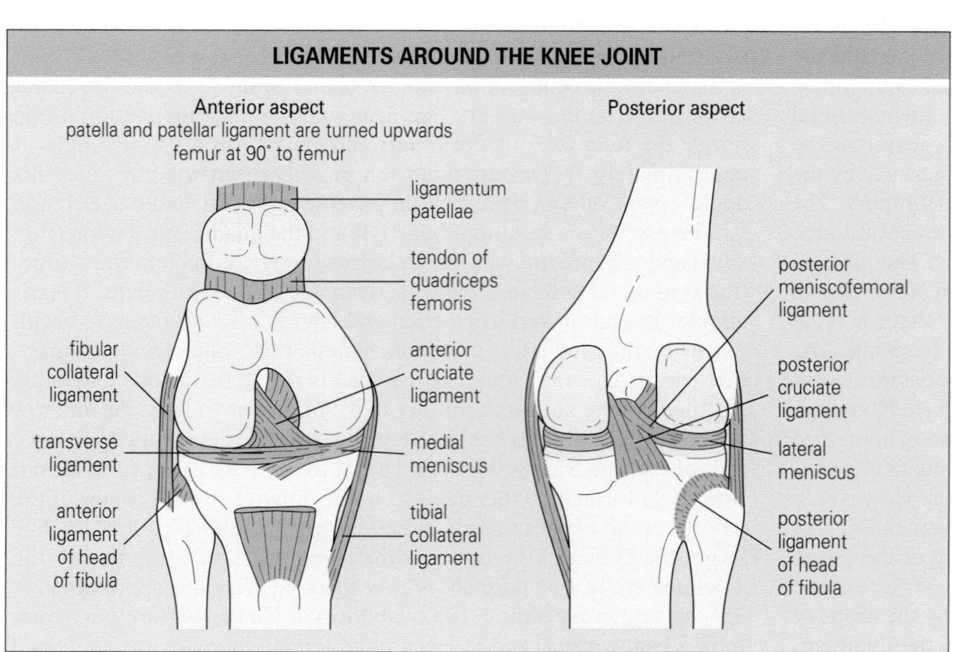

Fig. 11.3 Ligaments around the knee joint.

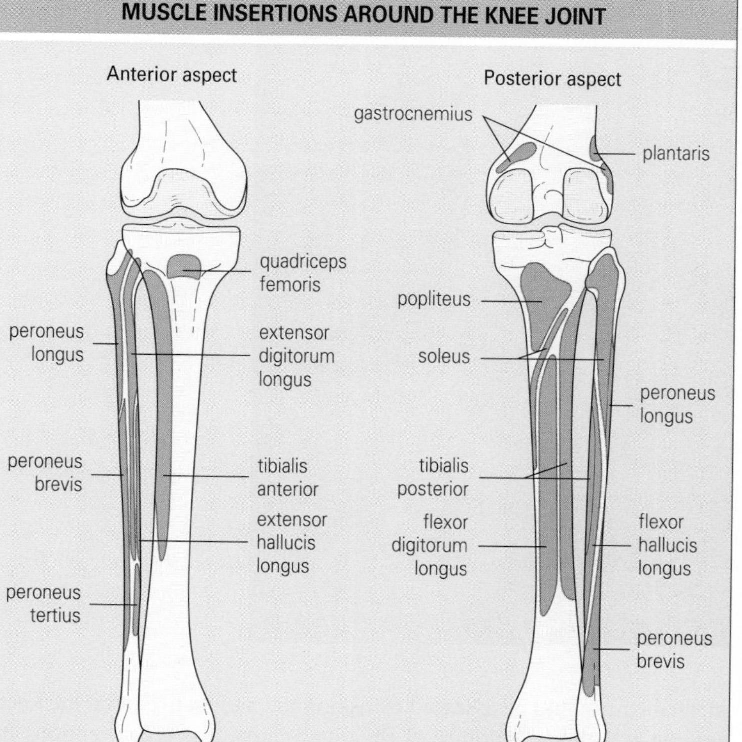

Fig. 11.4 Muscle insertions around the knee joint.

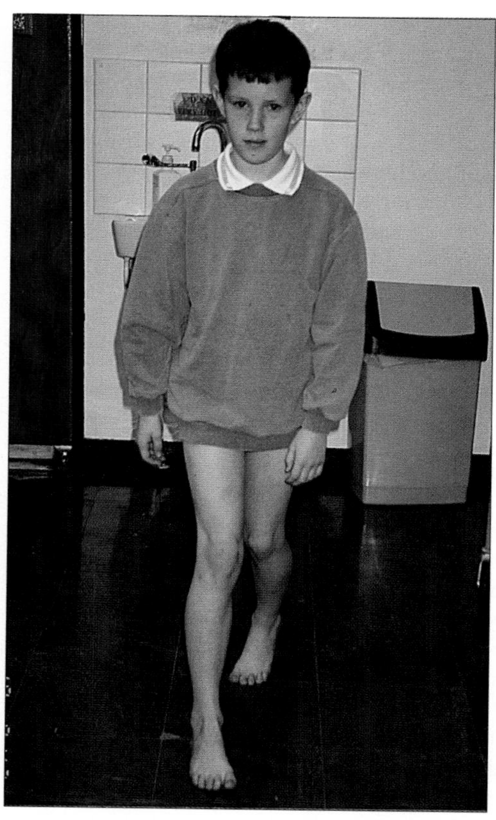

Fig. 11.5 Squinting of the patella caused by persistent femoral anteversion.

There are a number of bursae around the knee joint, all of which may become inflamed. The bursae in front of the knee are: the prepatellar bursa, which is subcutaneous and lies over the lower half of the patella; the infrapatellar bursa, which lies over the patella tendon and tibial tubercle; and the deep infrapatellar bursa, which separates the patella tendon from the upper tibia. On the medial side the anserine bursa is superficial to the medial collateral ligament and separates it from the tendons of sartorius, gracilis and semitendinosus. The common insertion of these three tendons lies superficial to the medial collateral ligament over the upper tibia and is called the pes anserinus. Other smaller bursae may be present deep to the medial collateral ligament[8,12]. Bursae lie deep to the semimembranosus and medial head of the gastrocnemius and may enlarge to form a swelling in the popliteal fossa[13]. On the lateral side, bursae may lie deep to the lateral head of gastrocnemius; between the lateral collateral ligament and the biceps femoris; and around the popliteus, separating it from the lateral femoral condyle and the lateral ligament.

EXAMINATION

The examination of the knee follows the standard pattern of inspection, palpation and movement[14]. Special tests for stability or meniscal pathology should be performed last. One of the most important aspects of examination of the knee which is often forgotten is to watch the patient standing and walking. It is important not to hurt the patient as this will increase muscle tone and make the rest of the examination more difficult. The examination should be modified in each individual case. Obviously the examination of a 75-year-old woman with rheumatoid arthritis differs from that of a 20-year-old who has a rugby injury.

INSPECTION

The patient should be asked to stand with the feet a few inches apart. The alignment of the knees and the presence of varus or valgus deformity on weight bearing should be noted. The degree of clinical varus is recorded by measuring the distance between the knees with the feet together and the degree of valgus is recorded by measuring the distance between the medial malleoli with the knees together. A recurvatum deformity is usually obvious on standing and persistent femoral anteversion causes 'squinting' of the patella (Fig. 11.5). The type of gait should be noted with and without aids.

Quadriceps wasting occurs very quickly with disuse, often within a few days. To assess this the patient should be asked to press the knees back into the examining table to contract the quadriceps and the tone and bulk should be judged and compared to the other side. The vastus medialis obliquus is often the first part of the muscle to waste. The circumference of the thigh 10cm above the upper pole of the patella should be measured and compared to the other side; this gives an objective measure of thigh wasting. The presence of swellings around the knee should be noted. Swelling within the synovial cavity is seen above the patella and on either side of the patella and patella tendon (Fig 11.6). A swelling which does not extend above the patella suggests

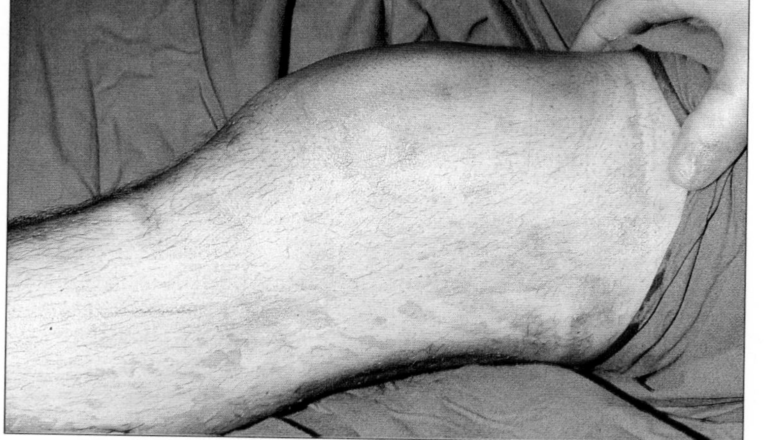

Fig. 11.6 Swelling within the synovial cavity.

local injury or an enlarged bursa. Inflammation of the pre- or infrapatellar bursae causes a characteristic swelling over the front of the knee. The presence of scars from previous surgery, injury or infection should be noted. Old scars fade and are easily missed, particularly arthroscopy scars which may be very small. They are usually situated on either side of the patella tendon, with another one superolateral to the patella. Bruising over the medial collateral ligament may indicate an injury to that structure and bruising in the calf may indicate rupture of the joint capsule. A swelling over the tibial tubercle in children indicates possible Osgood–Schlatter's disease. Tumors around the knee may present as a swelling particularly in children. Dilated veins over a swelling is an ominous sign, often indicating a neoplastic process.

PALPATION

The temperature of the joint should be compared to the other side; a localized increase in temperature suggests an inflammatory process but may also be caused by a recently removed bandage.

With the knee straight the presence of a large effusion or synovial thickening is usually obvious. A large, tense swelling indicates a hemarthrosis or a pyarthrosis. A lax swelling is usually due to an effusion associated with synovitis. Pain may be caused by capsular distension. A small amount of fluid in the knee may be detected by stroking one side of the knee and noting the appearance of a bulge caused by the displaced fluid in the sulcus on the opposite side of the patella. The test can be made more sensitive by pressing over the suprapatellar pouch with one hand to push fluid from there into the joint. On inspection synovial thickening may look like an effusion and often the two coexist. Synovial thickening can be distinguished from an effusion by its characteristic feel: fluid may be displaced and be ballotable from one side of the joint to the other, while thickened synovium cannot. Although it is possible to aspirate one or two milliliters of fluid from a normal knee, a clinically obvious effusion is always significant. A popliteal cyst may be palpated at the back of the knee and is usually more prominent on extension.

With the knee flexed the following should be palpated: the medial and lateral femoral condyles; the lower pole of the patella; the tibial tubercle; the medial and lateral joint lines; and the course and insertions of the collateral ligaments. Tenderness elicited at these sites suggests different problems depending on the history and age of the patient. In a young patient, tenderness over the medial femoral condyle may indicate osteochondritis dissecans. Tenderness at the lower pole of the patella indicates Sinding-Larsen–Johansson syndrome in a young patient or patellar tendinitis (jumper's knee) in an older patient. Tibial tuberosity tenderness in a young patient suggests Osgood–Schlatter's disease and a tender ossicle may be palpable. Swelling over the lateral joint line may indicate a meniscal cyst or a discoid meniscus. Osteophytes are often palpable along the joint line in osteoarthritis. A tender swelling just below the joint line on the medial side may indicate an inflamed bursa deep to the medial collateral ligament. Tenderness over the joint line after injury suggests a meniscal tear.

Tenderness over the insertions or course of the medial collateral ligament after injury is suggestive of a medial collateral ligament sprain, particularly if associated with localized bruising. The lateral collateral ligament may be palpated in the flexed knee when a varus stress is applied. Swelling and tenderness over its course is suggestive of a sprain.

MOVEMENT

With the patient supine the examiner should pick up both legs under the heels. A fixed flexion deformity or hyperextension of the knee will be obvious. A solid block to full extension is usually due to degenerative change and contracture, while a 'springy' block is usually due to a bucket handle tear of the meniscus. In a conscious patient with a medial collateral ligament sprain a block to full extension may be due to pain. The range of active and passive movement should be assessed. The normal range is from zero to approximately 140°, although a little hyperextension is not uncommon, particularly in young girls. The range of movement is best measured with a goniometer. The extensor

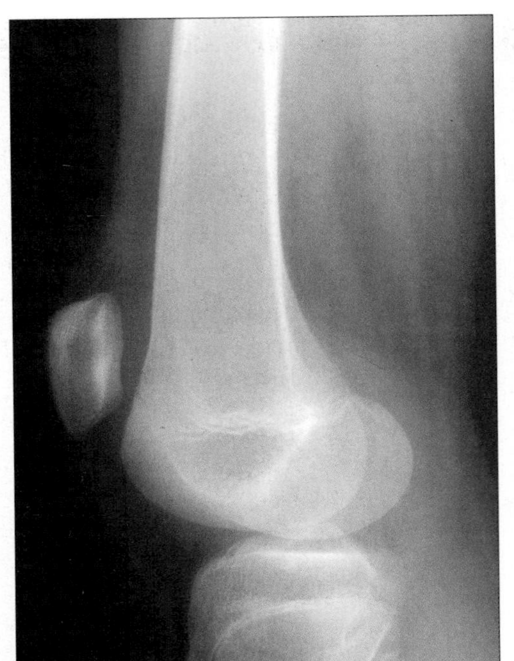

Fig. 11.7 Radiographic appearance of patella alta.

mechanism should be assessed by asking the patient to extend the knee against resistance. Rupture of the quadriceps or patellar tendons or fracture of the patella causes inability to extend the knee. The patient may still be able to straight leg raise due to the action of the iliotibial band and intact retinacular fibers; extension should therefore begin from a flexed position.

Sitting on the edge of the examining table the patient should actively flex and extend the knee. Crepitus may be felt during this movement. Tracking of the patella may be assessed by placing the thumb and forefinger on the patella. It may be seen to subluxate laterally on flexion in a patient with recurrent dislocation or subluxation. A small high patella (patella alta) (Fig. 11.7) may be noted and predisposes to recurrent dislocation.

The foot pulses should be palpated routinely, particularly in a patient under consideration for knee joint replacement. Finally every knee examination should finish with examination of the hip, as it is common, particularly in children, for hip pathology to present with knee pain.

THE DIFFERENTIAL DIAGNOSIS OF KNEE PAIN

Pain is the commonest presenting symptom of knee pathology. It may arise from within the knee joint itself, from periarticular structures or be referred from a distant site – usually the hip. Pain may also be referred from a femoral tumor or from the spine. The causes of knee pain tend to be age related and one convenient way to classify them is by age group and whether the pain is intra-articular, periarticular or referred (Fig. 11.8).

CHILDHOOD

Pain in the knee in this age group (2–10 years) is uncommon but is always significant. Intra-articular causes include a torn discoid lateral meniscus and osteochondritis dissecans. Inflammatory causes include pauciarticular juvenile chronic arthritis (see Chapter 5.18) and septic arthritis. Periarticular causes are osteomyelitis of the lower femur or upper tibia and, at the upper end of the age group, Osgood–Schlatter's disease and Sinding-Larsen–Johansson syndrome. Referred pain may come from the hip due to Perthe's disease.

ADOLESCENCE

Knee pain is common in adolescence (10–18 years). Intra-articular causes are usually related to osteochondritis dissecans or tears involving a discoid lateral meniscus. In girls the anterior knee pain syndrome

COMMON CAUSES OF KNEE PAIN IN DIFFERENT AGE GROUPS			
	Cause		
Age group	Intra-articular	Periarticular	Referred
Childhood (2–10 years)	Juvenile chronic arthritis Osteochondritis dissecans Septic arthritis Torn discoid lateral meniscus	Osteomyelitis	Perthe's disease Transient synovitis of the hip
Adolescence (10–18 years)	Osteochondritis dissecans Torn meniscus Anterior knee pain syndrome Patellar malalignment	Osgood–Schlatter's disease Sinding-Larsen–Johansson syndrome Osteomyelitis Tumors	Slipped upper femoral epiphysis
Early adulthood (18–30 years)	Torn meniscus Instability Anteroir knee pain syndrome Inflammatory conditions	Overuse syndromes Bursitis	Rare
Adulthood (30–50 years)	Degenerate meniscal tears Early degeneration following injury or meniscectomy Inflammatory arthropathies	Bursitis Tendinitis	Degenerative hip disease secondary to hip dysplasia or injury
Older age (>50 years)	Osteoarthritis Inflammatory arthropathies	Bursitis Tendinitis	Osteoarthritis of the hip

Fig. 11.8 Common causes of knee pain in different age groups.

and patellar maltracking are the most common causes of pain. Inflammatory causes are pauciarticular juvenile chronic arthritis and septic arthritis. Periarticular pain is usually due to traction apophysitis – Osgood–Schlatter's or Sinding-Larsen–Johansson syndrome. Tumors around the knee cause aching pain. Anteroposterior (AP) and lateral views of the femur and hip, and a bone scan, should be performed in cases of knee pain for which no cause can be found. Slipped upper femoral epiphysis in boys frequently presents with knee pain and a limp, and is common in this age group. The hip should be carefully examined as loss of internal rotation is an early sign of slipped upper femoral epiphysis. If this is suspected, AP and lateral radiographs of the hip should be performed.

EARLY ADULTHOOD

The most common cause of knee pain in this age group (18–30 years) is injury. Intra-articular causes include meniscal tears and pain associated with instability following a ligamentous injury. In females the anterior knee pain syndrome is still frequent. Inflammatory joint conditions such as reactive arthritis and ankylosing spondylitis (see Chapters 6.11 and 6.16) may occur. Periarticular causes include the overuse syndromes such as jumper's knee. Referred pain in this age group is relatively rare.

ADULTHOOD

In this age group (30–50 years) intra-articular causes of knee pain include degenerative meniscal lesions and post-traumatic degenerative change. Inflammatory conditions, such as rheumatoid arthritis and gout, are relatively common. Periarticular causes include bursitis and tendinitis. Referred pain may be secondary to early degenerative disease in the hip due to untreated congenital dislocation of the hip, Perthe's disease or fracture.

OLDER AGE

Degenerative disease is the most common cause of knee pain in those aged over 50 years. The knee is affected by osteoarthritis more commonly than any other joint (see Chapter 8.3). The pain is associated with stiffness and swelling especially after activity. Loose bodies secondary to the degeneration may cause episodes of sharp pain associated with locking of the joint. Periarticular causes include bursitis and tendinitis. Referred pain in this age group is usually secondary to osteoarthritis of the hip.

SPECIFIC DISORDERS

BURSITIS

Inflammation of the bursae around the knee is common and on occasion may cause diagnostic difficulty. An accurate knowledge of the anatomic sites of the bursae is helpful.

Prepatellar bursitis

Prepatellar bursitis is common. The condition is related to recurrent trauma and is seen most often in people who spend a lot of time kneeling, such as carpet fitters and, in earlier times, housemaids (hence the eponym, housemaid's knee). Diagnosis is usually obvious with a hot, red, well-circumscribed and fluctuant swelling over the front of the patella. The skin in the area is often thickened. Although the bursa may look infected, in most cases it is not. The inflammation may be caused by trauma or gout. Aspiration is necesary to prove infection and gout. Traumatic cases settle with rest and avoidance of kneeling. Gout responds to nonsteroidal anti-inflammatory drugs (NSAIDs). Septic bursitis is treated with rest, preferably with a posterior plaster splint, serial aspirations and parenteral followed by oral antibiotics. Surgical drainage is necessary in loculated or otherwise unimproved cases. Recurrent episodes of inflammation or infection may require surgical excision of the bursa.

Infrapatellar bursitis

The common term for this condition is Parson's knee. The presentation and treatment are the same as for prepatellar bursitis.

Anserine bursitis

The term anserine bursitis tends to be used loosely to describe pain over the medial aspect of the upper tibia in the region of the anserine bursa. While inflammation of the bursa may be the origin of the pain, it may also arise from the medial ligament or pes anserinus insertion, and the exact anatomic site may be impossible to identify. The conditions of anserine bursitis, medial ligament syndrome and pes anserinus tendinitis may therefore be impossible to separate. Treatment is initially by rest and NSAIDs. In persistent cases injection of a small amount of corticosteroid into the painful area is usually curative.

Bursae on the lateral side of the knee deep to the iliotibial band and the lateral ligament may occasionally become inflamed and cause symptoms.

TENDINITIS

The insertions of the tendons around the knee may become inflamed due to overuse or in association with an inflammatory arthropathy. It may be difficult to differentiate tendinitis from the medial ligament syndrome and bursal inflammation.

Patellar tendinitis (jumper's knee)

Patellar tendinitis[15] is a condition which most commonly affects young sportsmen but may also affect older patients. The symptoms are of pain at the inferior pole of the patella which is brought on by activity, particularly climbing stairs, running and jumping. The condition is due to mucoid degeneration of the patellar tendon at its insertion into the inferior pole of the patella. The majority of cases respond to rest and NSAIDs. For those that do not, injection of a small amount of corticosteroid (0.2ml) into the tender area is usually helpful. A larger volume should not be injected, since necrosis of the tendon can occur. Occasionally, operative treatment to excise the involved portion of tendon is necessary.

Pes anserinus tendinitis

The pes anserinus insertion may become inflamed but this may be indistinguishable clinically from anserine bursitis and the medial ligament syndrome. In cases of overuse, rest is usually curative but in persistent cases a small amount of corticosteroid injected into the point of maximum tenderness is usually curative.

Popliteus tendinitis

This is also an overuse injury which causes pain over the lateral aspect of the joint. It is caused by inflammation of the popliteus tendon and paratenon as it passes beneath the arcuate ligament complex. Symptoms usually settle with rest and NSAIDs.

ILIOTIBIAL BAND FRICTION SYNDROME (RUNNER'S KNEE)

This occurs in runners and is due to overuse[16]. It tends to occur in patients with genu varum and planus feet. The symptoms are of pain over the lateral epicondyle of the femur during running and are thought to be due to friction between the iliotibial band and the femur and may be due to an inflamed bursa. Tenderness is found over the lateral epicondyle. The symptoms usually settle with rest but in resistant cases a corticosteroid injection into the tender site may help.

MEDIAL LIGAMENT SYNDROME

This is an ill-defined syndrome in which the patient complains of pain at the site of insertion of the medial ligament. Examination reveals tenderness over the insertion of the ligament, and valgus stress may exacerbate the pain. It is more common in females than in males and is associated with valgus knees and the pain amplification syndrome. As stated previously it may be difficult to differentiate from anserine bursitis and pes anserinus tendinitis. The etiology is obscure but in some cases an inflammatory arthropathy, such as ankylosing spondylitis, is present. Treatment is initially conservative with rest and heat. Persistent symptoms usually settle following injection of a small amount of corticosteroid into the painful area.

PELLEGRINI–STIEDA DISEASE

Following an injury to the medial collateral ligament the patient presents with pain over the femoral insertion particularly on activity. The area is tender to palpation and pain is elicited on stressing the ligament. Radiographs reveal characteristic calcification at the ligament insertion[17] (Fig. 11.9). The condition is most likely due to calcification of a hematoma following injury to the femoral insertion of the medial collateral ligament. Treatment consists of rest and NSAIDs, since the condition is usually self-limiting. Occasionally a small amount of corticosteroid injected into the area will help resolve persistent cases.

POPLITEAL CYSTS AND SWELLING

Swellings occurring in the popliteal region are common and should be called popliteal cysts regardless of where they originate[13]. They may occur at any age from childhood onwards. The frequency of a communication between the knee joint and the gastrocnemius–semimembranosus bursa increases with age[18,19]. The communication occurs where the tendon of the medial head of gastrocnemius leaves the joint capsule. It is believed that, with increasing age, degeneration and loss of elasticity occurs in the capsule allowing a tear into the bursa to occur when the knee is extended. Fluid in the knee joint may then flow into the bursa causing it to distend.

The presenting complaint is usually of a swelling at the back of the knee. The swelling may be associated with aching and is more prominent when the knee is extended. In children there is usually no other abnormality found on examination of the knee but in adults the cysts are most commonly associated with rheumatoid arthritis and osteoarthritis. Plain radiographs may show a soft tissue swelling, and double contrast arthrography will confirm the diagnosis in those that communicate with the joint. Ultrasound is a reliable method of differentiating cysts from aneurysms and solid swellings. Computed tomographic (CT) scanning or magnetic resonance imaging (MRI) are useful, particularly where the diagnosis is in doubt and for preoperative planning. The differential diagnosis includes popliteal artery aneurysm, ganglia, nerve sheath tumors and sarcoma. Popliteal cysts may become very large due to a valve effect probably caused by inspissated debris, particularly in rheumatoid arthritis. If they burst they may simulate a deep vein thrombosis. The signs in the calf are similar but differentiation can usually be made due to a history of swelling in the popliteal fossa and the sudden onset of pain, often with a sensation of water running down the leg. Ultrasound in the early stages usually differentiates between the two. A phlebogram may be needed to conclusively rule out phlebitis.

Treatment in children should be conservative, as the cysts commonly decrease in size spontaneously and those which are operated on have a high recurrence rate. Treatment in adults should be aimed at the underlying pathology[20]. Knee aspiration and corticosteroid injection may be performed. Arthroscopic knee synovectomy often leads to spontaneous resorption of the cyst. With more effective medical and orthopedic therapies for rheumatoid arthritis, cyst removal is seldom indicated nowadays.

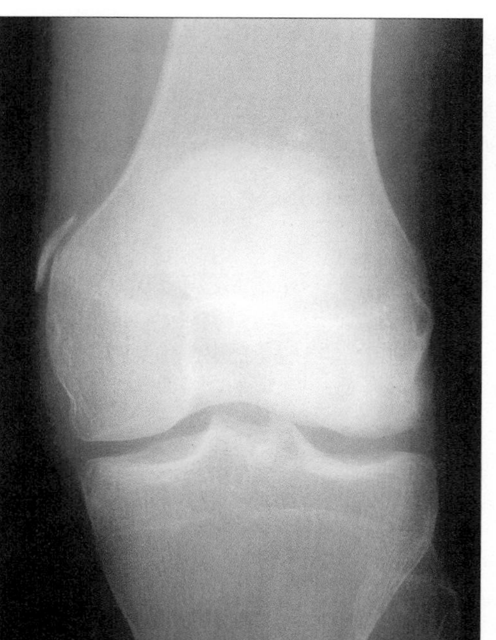

Fig. 11.9 Pellegrini–Stieda disease. Radiograph showing calcification of the insertion of the medial collateral ligament.

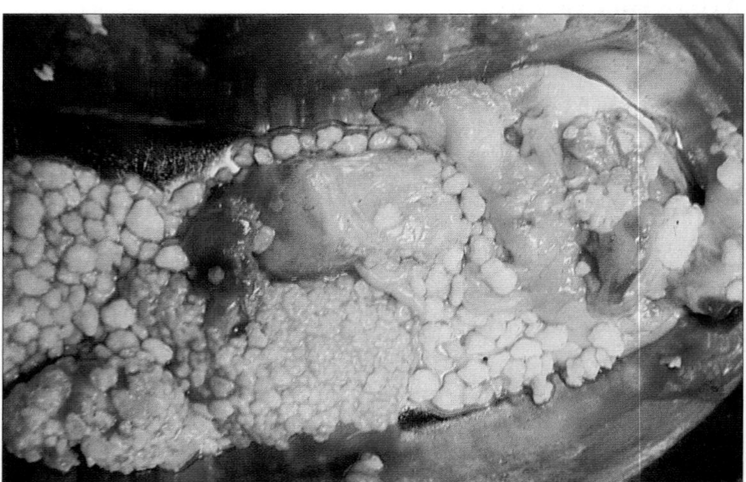

Fig. 11.10 Synovial chondromatosis. Cartilaginous bodies in the joint.

SYNOVIAL CHONDROMATOSIS

Synovial chondromatosis is a rare condition of unknown etiology in which multiple metaplastic foci of cartilage develop in joints, tendon sheaths and bursae. It occurs due to metaplasia in the subsynovial connective tissue. The cartilaginous bodies may become pedunculated or loose in the joint (Fig. 11.10). The knee is by far the most common joint affected by both intra-articular and extra-articular disease. Milgram[21] classified the disease into three phases: early, with active intrasynovial disease but no loose bodies; transitional, with active intrasynovial disease and loose bodies; and late, with multiple loose bodies but no synovial disease. The condition tends to occur in middle age but may present in the late teens. Pain is the usual presenting feature, commonly associated with swelling. Locking may be a feature when the lesions are loose or pedunculated. Examination reveals a swollen knee with thickened synovium, crepitus on movement and palpable loose bodies. In the later stages the range of motion may be decreased. Radiographs in the early stages may show multiple, stippled cartilaginous bodies. Double contrast arthrography is useful. In the later stages of the disease when the lesions have calcified they become more obvious on plain radiographs. Treatment of symptomatic disease involves arthroscopy or arthrotomy and removal of symptomatic loose bodies. In the first and second phases of disease the active synovium should be excised. Total synovectomy is impractical and unnecessary. Recurrence is only likely with generalized active disease, in which case a second arthrotomy may be necessary. The condition tends to resolve with time[21,22].

PIGMENTED VILLONODULAR SYNOVITIS

This condition, which tends to affect young adults, is characterized by a proliferative synovial reaction. The synovium becomes nodular and brown in color. The etiology of the condition is unknown. The knee joint is the most commonly affected joint. The presenting complaint is usually of pain and swelling. Locking may occur if the proliferative synovium becomes trapped between the joint surfaces. Examination reveals a swollen joint with thickened synovium and limitation of movement. Radiographs show lytic bone lesions and soft tissue swelling. Double contrast arthrography shows multiple filling defects in the synovium, which are diagnostic. MRI shows bone and synovial changes that are highly suggestive of the condition. Aspiration of brown synovial fluid in the absence of recent trauma is characteristic and may often be the first indication of the disease. On arthroscopy thickened nodular synovium which is reddish brown in color is seen. Histologic examination shows a stroma of reticulin and collagen fibers with multinucleated giant cells, foam cells and hemosiderin deposits. Treatment is by synovectomy, preferably arthroscopic. This may need to be repeated as the disease is liable to recur. Marked bone destruction can occur and may require radiation therapy in extreme cases[23].

THE KNEE JOINT IN CHILDHOOD AND ADOLESCENCE

Children and adolescents experience a different spectrum of knee problems than adults. Knee pain is common and must be differentiated from pain arising in the hip from Perthe's disease or from slipped upper femoral epiphysis. It is therefore mandatory to examine the hip in every child with knee pain. Occasionally tumors of the femur may present with knee pain. If doubt exists, radiographs of the hip and femur should be obtained.

OSTEOCHONDRITIS DISSECANS

Osteochondritis dissecans occurs most commonly in the knee joint. A fragment of cartilage with its underlying subchondral bone becomes detached and may become loose in the joint. Boys are affected more commonly than girls. The second decade is the usual time for presentation but it may occur earlier.

The symptoms are usually of an aching pain which occurs during and after activity. Clicking and giving way may occur. An antalgic gait may be present. There is often a mild effusion and tenderness over the site of the lesion. Wasting of the quadriceps is an early sign. If the fragment separates, symptoms of locking occur and a loose body may be palpable, usually in the suprapatellar pouch. Wilson's sign may be positive. The test involves straightening the internally rotated knee from a flexed position – pain at 30° of flexion which is relieved by externally rotating the tibia is said to be diagnostic of osteochondritis dissecans[24]. The etiology is unclear but the condition is associated with short stature, epiphyseal abnormalities and a positive family history. It is likely that vascular impairment, possibly associated with a traumatic initial event, is responsible for the lesions. Approximately 40% of patients give a history of injury[25,26]. The pathologic changes which occur are those of osteonecrosis and degenerative changes in the overlying cartilage, with softening, fibrillation and fissuring.

The lesions occur most commonly on the lateral aspect of the medial femoral condyle but may also affect the posterior aspect of the lateral condyle, the trochlea and the patella. Abnormalities of ossification also occur in these sites and may be mistaken for osteochondritis dissecans.

Osteochondritic lesions of the condyles can often be seen on AP and lateral radiographs but are best seen on a tunnel view. The radiographic appearance is diagnostic, showing a well circumscribed fragment of subchondral bone (Fig. 11.11). If the fragment has become detached an irregularity is seen at the site. CT scanning and MRI are useful to confirm the diagnosis and to define the extent of the lesion. In cases of doubt a bone scan may be useful to differentiate osteochondritis dissecans from abnormalities of ossification. A hot spot around the lesion confirms active disease; the uptake decreases with healing of the lesion[27].

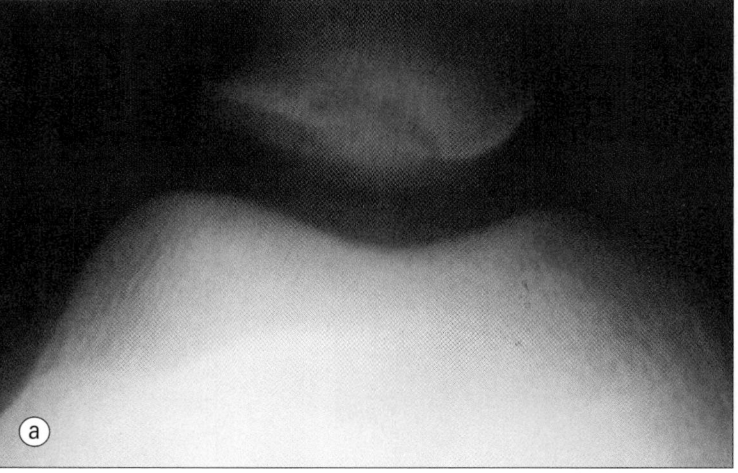

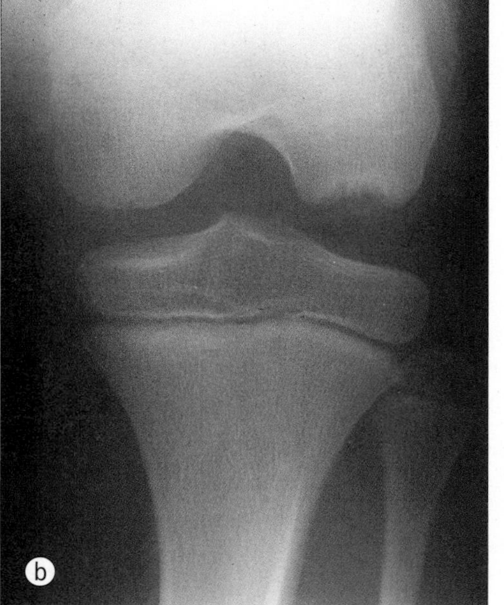

Fig. 11.11 Radiographic appearances of osteochondritic lesions of the patella (a) and lateral femoral condyle (b).

Treatment of the undisplaced fragment in the younger child is rest and avoidance of activities which may injure the knee until the lesion is healed. Long term immobilization should be avoided and isometric quadriceps and hamstring exercises should be performed to prevent muscle wasting. Treatment of the older child follows the same lines but if the symptoms persist or if the fragment generally does not separate, arthroscopic assessment should be undertaken and the fragment debrided and drilled if necessary. Loose fragments should be fixed if they are large. This may be performed open or arthroscopically using fine K-wires or Herbert screws. Smaller fragments loose in the joint should be removed arthroscopically. The defect which is left should be debrided and will fill with fibrocartilage. The prognosis is better in younger patients before skeletal maturity in whom the fragment does not separate.

OSGOOD–SCHLATTER'S DISEASE

Osgood–Schlatter's disease is a traction apophysitis of the tibial tuberosity[28,29]. It occurs most commonly in those aged 10–14 years and is associated with overuse. The patients present complaining of pain over the tibial tuberosity particularly on activity. The clinical findings are of tenderness over the tibial tuberosity which is often enlarged (Fig. 11.12).

Lateral radiographs show characteristic fragmentation of the tibial tubercle, and there may be a loose ossicle. The symptoms usually respond to rest and disappear at the time of fusion of the tibial tuberosity. Occasionally a loose ossicle may remain and cause symptoms which necessitate removal (Fig. 11.13).

SINDING-LARSEN–JOHANSSON SYNDROME

This is a condition similar to Osgood–Schlatter's disease occurring at the distal pole of the patella. It is a traction apophysitis and is related to overuse[30]. The patient complains of pain at the distal pole of the patella on activity. This area is tender and radiographs show fragmentation (Fig. 11.14). The condition responds to rest but may persist into adolescence as jumper's knee.

PATELLOFEMORAL DISORDERS

Disorders of the patellofemoral joint are common in children and adolescents.

Congenital dislocation

Congenital dislocation occurs in infancy and involves irreducible lateral displacement of the patella[31]. It is associated with genu valgum, a small patella, hypoplasia of the lateral femoral condyle and tethering of the lateral capsule. Treatment is surgical to release the tight lateral structures and realign the patella.

Habitual dislocation

In habitual dislocation lateral displacement of the patella occurs every time the knee is flexed. It is due to contracture of the vastus lateralis and iliotibial band with an abnormal insertion of the iliotibial band into the patella[32]. Because of this lateral contracture the patella must dislocate to allow the knee to flex. The constant physical sign is an inability to flex the knee when the patella is held reduced. Treatment is usually surgical and involves proximal realignment of the quadriceps mechanism by releasing the contracted lateral structures and if necessary lengthening the rectus femoris.

Recurrent dislocation and subluxation

Recurrent dislocation and subluxation of the patella are conditions in which intermittent episodes of dislocation or subluxation occur and may be grouped together under the heading of patella instability. This is common in adolescence, particularly in girls, but may also occur in younger children. It is associated with a variety of developmental abnormalities. These include generalized or localized joint laxity, patella alta and hypoplasia of the lateral femoral condyle. Genu valgum, external tibial torsion and persistent femoral anteversion increase the Q angle and predispose to patella instability.

In adolescence patella instability may follow an acute traumatic dislocation or occur spontaneously[33]. In acute dislocation the patient describes the patella dislocating laterally and may reduce it by pushing it back. Examination in the acute phase reveals a painful swollen knee with obvious lateral dislocation of the patella. If the patella has already been reduced the chief findings are of tenderness over the torn medial retinaculum associated with knee swelling. Acute dislocation may be associated with an osteochondral fracture of the lateral femoral condyle. Treatment in the acute phase is by immobilization in a plaster cast for

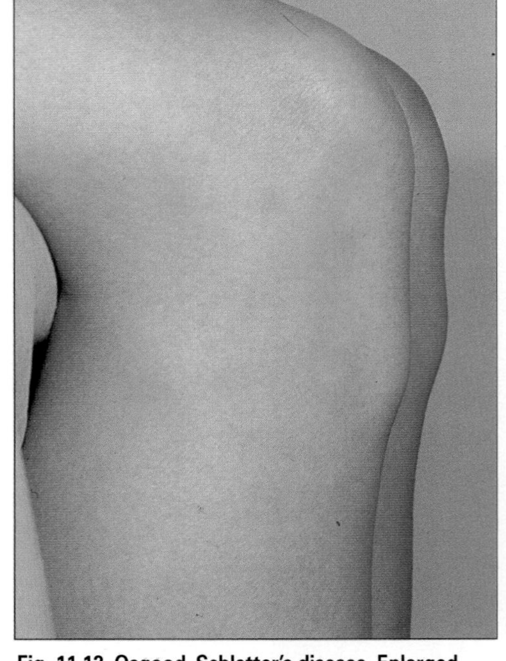

Fig. 11.12 Osgood–Schlatter's disease. Enlarged tibial tuberosity.

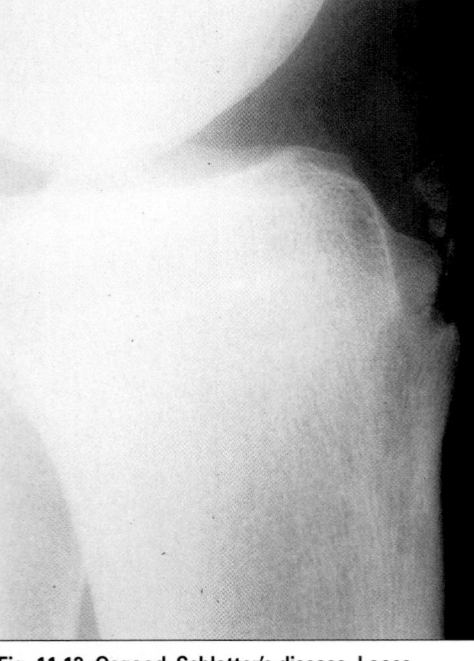

Fig. 11.13 Osgood–Schlatter's disease. Loose ossicles in the patella tendon.

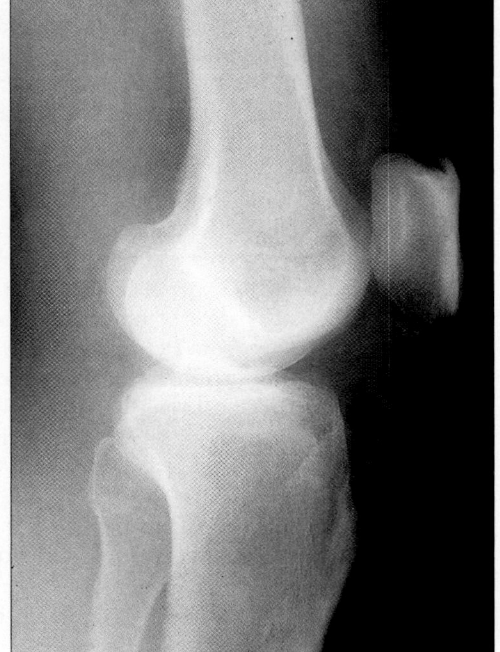

Fig. 11.14 Sinding-Larsen–Johansson syndrome. Radiograph showing fragmentation of the lower pole of the patella.

4 weeks, which allows the torn retinacular fibers to heal, followed by an isometric exercise program to restore the power of the quadriceps, particularly the vastus medialis obliquus.

In the chronic phase the diagnosis of recurrent dislocation is straightforward. The patient is usually an adolescent girl describing episodes of lateral dislocation of the patella, which either reduce spontaneously or which she pushes back. The episodes usually occur during activities which involve knee flexion but in severe cases may occur during everyday activities. Recurrent subluxation of the patella is more common than dislocation and is caused by the same factors, but the diagnosis may be more difficult to make. The patient often complains of a feeling of instability as the patella rides up on the lateral femoral condyle, and the knee may give way. Pain is due to compression of the lateral facet of the patella against the lateral femoral condyle. Pseudo-locking due to pain is common. The majority of cases are secondary to weakness of the vastus medialis obliquus associated with bony malalignment.

Examination may reveal any of the anatomic abnormalities mentioned above, and the patella may be found to track laterally on flexion of the knee. In the majority of adolescent girls with this condition there is poor muscle tone in the quadriceps, particularly the vastus medialis, and the Q angle may be increased due to the factors mentioned earlier[6]. Patellar tracking should be assessed clinically, as described in the section on examination. The apprehension test is usually positive in recurrent subluxation and dislocation. This is performed with the knee flexed to 30° and the examiner gently pushing the patella laterally. A positive test occurs when the patient feels as though the patella is going to dislocate and occasionally will push the examiner's hand away. In some girls with a small high patella it may be seen to sit laterally in full extension.

Lateral and AP views of the knee are useful to look for femorotibial malalignment, osteochondral fractures and patella alta. Patella alta is recognized on the lateral view by comparing the length of the patella to the length of the patella tendon. In normal knees the ratio is 1. In patella alta the patella is relatively short compared to the tendon and the ratio is less than 0.8[34]. Skyline views of the patella with the knee flexed at 30–40° may show it to be tilted laterally and to ride high on the lateral femoral condyle. A variety of special views and measurements have been described to quantify the degree of subluxation or tilting. The patella should sit centrally in the trochlea with an equal joint space medially and laterally. The skyline views may show it to be tilted laterally with a narrower joint space on the lateral side. Occasionally, sclerosis may be seen in the subchondral bone of the lateral facet indicating increased stress through it. The angle formed by the lateral facet of the patella and a line drawn across the femoral condyles is called the lateral patellofemoral angle and should be open laterally. If the lines are parallel or the angle is open medially this suggests patella malalignment[35]. CT scanning with the knee straight and flexed to 30° and 60° may show a laterally displaced patella and a deficient lateral femoral condyle. Unfortunately, radiographic findings such as these are common in the asymptomatic population and should only be taken as significant in conjunction with the clinical picture.

Recurrent dislocation or subluxation of the patella should initially be managed conservatively with isometric quadriceps and hamstring exercises[36]. Most patients will respond to conservative management provided they continue the exercises. Unfortunately many do not and the resultant weakening of the quadriceps may lead to recurrence. In the compliant patients who do not respond to conservative treatment, surgery is usually necessary as the condition can be disabling. An arthroscopic lateral release may be tried if there is a tight lateral tether but open surgery to realign the patella may be necessary.

ANTERIOR KNEE PAIN SYNDROME

Pain arising from the anterior aspect of the knee joint is common in adolescence. Specific conditions, such as patella malalignment, osteochondritis dissecans, Osgood–Schlatter's disease and trauma, may be responsible [37]. However, there is a group of patients in whom no cause for the pain can be found, despite careful investigation. It is this idiopathic condition which should be called anterior knee pain syndrome. It usually occurs in adolescent girls and is commonly bilateral. The patient complains of pain in the anterior aspect of the joint around the patella. It may be present during sporting activity and necessitate its cessation. The pain is often present at night and may wake the patient from sleep. In the past these patients have been wrongly labeled as having 'chondromalacia patellae'.

Many adolescent girls with anterior knee pain tend to have an increased Q angle and poor quadriceps strength but no demonstrable patella instability or malalignment. Wearing high-heeled shoes may be a cause as the patient walks with a crouched gait, putting increased load on the patellofemoral joint. Tight hamstrings have been implicated for the same reason and some of these patients have limitation of straight leg raising. The condition is self limiting in the majority of cases and usually settles in early adulthood. Treatment is conservative and should include reassurance that the condition is benign and that it will not lead to early degeneration. Isometric quadriceps strengthening exercises and hamstring strengthening and stretching exercises are also useful. Wearing high-heeled shoes should be avoided. Arthroscopy may occasionally be indicated to exclude intra-articular pathology but should be avoided unless there is a good indication. Empirical lateral release should be avoided.

CHONDROMALACIA PATELLAE

A diagnosis of chondromalacia patellae means softening of the articular cartilage of the patella and can only be made at arthroscopy or arthrotomy. It is a pathologic diagnosis and should not be used to describe the clinical syndrome of pain arising from the anterior knee joint. However, patients with anterior knee pain may be found to have chondromalacia patellae. It may be associated with patellar malalignment, in which case it is probably due to impact loading and shearing of the articular cartilage as the patella is compressed against the lateral femoral condyle. Articular cartilage is poor at resisting shear forces, and repetitive impact loading and shear may both be shown to produce cartilage softening. The majority of cases associated with malalignment respond to correction of the underlying abnormality provided cartilage loss has not occurred. Idiopathic chondromalacia patellae usually responds to the conservative measures of isometric quadriceps exercises and hamstring stretching.

BIPARTITE PATELLA

Bipartite patella occurs when the ossification centers of the patella fail to fuse. The defect is seen as a lucent line usually at the superolateral corner of the patella where it may be mistaken for a fracture. Occasionally the synchondrosis may fracture as a result of repetitive stress and cause pain and tenderness. Rest in a padded knee splint is usually curative.

PLICA SYNDROME

Embryologically, the knee is divided into three synovial compartments which break down in the fourth intrauterine month. Failure of complete breakdown leaves synovial shelves or plicae. Pain arising from these is termed the plica syndrome. The infrapatellar plica (ligamentum mucosum) is the most common but does not usually become inflamed or cause pain. The suprapatellar plica is a remnant of the membrane which separates the suprapatellar pouch from the rest of the knee. This may be virtually complete, with only a small foramen, or it may be seen as a crescentic fold[38]. It occasionally causes symptoms if it becomes inflamed. The medial patellar plica runs along the medial wall of the joint from the suprapatellar pouch to the infrapatellar fold. It is the most frequently symptomatic, becoming inflamed due to impingement as it passes over the medial femoral condyle. Occasionally it may be large and cover the medial femoral condyle. The medial patellar plica is the great imitator of symptoms in the knee and can be a diagnostic problem. It may present with pain, typically over the medial femoral condyle, but this may be generalized. A snapping sensation or giving way are also common. The diagnosis may be made clinically by palpating a tender thickened band over the medial femoral condyle. Commonly it is made at arthroscopy when a plica may be seen to impinge on the medial femoral condyle and there may be an associated impingement lesion. Treatment is initially rest but the plica may need to be resected arthroscopically if symptoms persist[39,40].

MENISCAL LESIONS AND DISCOID MENISCUS IN CHILDREN

Meniscal tears in children are uncommon due to the resilience of the fibrocartilage. When they occur they should be treated similarly to those in adults, leaving as much stable rim as possible. Cysts of the menisci usually arise from the lateral meniscus. Unlike cysts in adults they are rarely associated with a tear. They present as a swelling on the joint line and are of no functional consequence but may be removed for cosmetic reasons.

Discoid menisci usually occur on the lateral side of the joint and may affect both knees. They are normally asymptomatic unless they tear. However, a patient with an intact discoid meniscus can present with intermittent swelling over the lateral joint line or clicking in the knee. On examination the swelling may be palpated and a clunk felt on knee extension. The reasons for the formation of a discoid meniscus are unclear. It was initially thought to be due to persistence of the embryonic form but further studies have shown that this is unlikely, as the menisci are not discoid at any stage in development. No other theories satisfactorily explain their etiology. The diagnosis may be confirmed by double contrast arthrography or arthroscopy. Torn discoid menisci in children should be treated conservatively if possible, or by arthroscopic resection of the torn middle portion, leaving a stable rim. A discoid meniscus found coincidentally at arthroscopy should be left.

SEPTIC ARTHRITIS AND OSTEOMYELITIS

Septic arthritis of the knee in children is relatively common. The infection is usually blood-borne but may occur after a puncture wound. The patient complains of severe pain on even the slightest movement and is generally unwell with a tensely swollen knee and a pyrexia. Joint aspiration should be immediately performed forsynovial fluid cell count, differential, gram stain and culture. Thorough arthroscopic washout should be commenced as soon as the diagnosis is suspected. Arthroscopic washout is more efficient than arthrotomy and may need to be repeated. Arthrotomy is required if loculi have formed which cannot be broken down arthroscopically. Antibiotics should only be started after fluid has been sent for culture and sensitivity The differential diagnosis includes other inflammatory processes such as juvenile chronic arthritis and nonspecific synovitis.

Acute hematogenous osteomyelitis commonly affects the lower femoral and upper tibial metaphyses. The diagnosis is clinical with tenderness over the area and is supported by an increased white cell count and erythrocyte sedimentation rate (ESR). Radiographic changes may take a number of days to appear. A sympathetic effusion may be present in the knee joint.

KNEE INJURIES

MENISCAL INJURIES

The meniscus in the young is a resilient fibrocartilaginous structure. With age and degenerative change it loses this resilience and becomes stiffer. Thus, different types of meniscal injury are seen in different age groups.

Meniscal injuries are common in young adults, usually occurring secondary to sport injuries and often in combination with ligamentous injury (particularly ACL rupture). Meniscal injuries are also associated with chronic instability. The mechanism of the injury is usually a twisting force applied to the weight-bearing knee, causing entrapment of the meniscus between the tibial and femoral condyles. The resulting tear is usually longitudinal. If the tear is extensive the inner portion may displace into the joint causing the knee to lock (a bucket handle tear) (Fig. 11.15). This locking may be intermittent as the torn portion flips in and out of the joint. A tear may extend to the inner margin of the meniscus forming a 'parrot beak' tear. The flap formed can displace into the joint causing intermittent locking. Peripheral meniscal detachment may also occur.

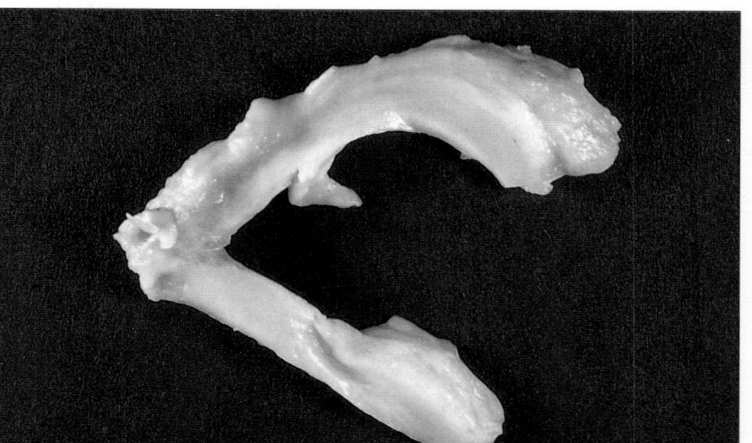

Fig. 11.15 Bucket handle tear of the meniscus. Reproduced with permission from Bullough PG. Orthopaedic Pathology, 3e. London: Mosby-Wolfe; 1997.

In the older age group, where the meniscus is less elastic, degenerative tears can occur[41]. These tears are usually horizontal cleavage tears or radial tears running into the substance of the meniscus.

The history of an acute meniscal tear in a young adult is often characteristic. A twisting injury occurs causing immediate severe pain. The patient is unable to weight bear and may be unable to fully extend the knee if a bucket handle tear has lodged in the joint. The knee swells within several hours. If a cruciate ligament rupture is also present a hemarthrosis will accumulate within an hour. The patient complains of pain well localized to the joint line. Examination reveals a painful knee with tenderness over the joint line adjacent to the tear. An effusion is virtually always present and if the torn portion has displaced into the joint, a springy block to full extension is felt.

In a chronic tear the patient may complain of pain over the joint line and a feeling of 'catching'. Joint line tenderness is usually present. True locking occurs when the torn portion of the meniscus displaces into the joint causing loss of full extension. Locking due to a meniscal tear always occurs with the knee flexed, although not necessarily weight bearing. Examination of a knee locked due to a meniscal tear reveals a springy block to extension; forced extension is painful. Flexion is usually full or only mildly reduced due to pain. Patients often confuse locking with stiffness and it is important to distinguish between the two. If the knee unlocks with a click or a clunk it is suggestive of a meniscal tear. McMurray's test[42] is widely used to diagnose meniscal tears. The test involves flexing and extending the knee while the tibia is first internally rotated and then externally rotated, with the thumb and fingers over the joint line. Pain and an associated click are said to be diagnostic of a meniscal tear. Apley's grinding test[43] is performed with the patient prone and the knee flexed. Downward pressure is exerted on the tibia while it is internally and externally rotated. Pain or a clicking sensation are said to be suggestive of a meniscal tear. However, these tests are not specific.

While the majority of acute and chronic meniscal injuries can be diagnosed on the history and examination, confirmation may be obtained by arthrography, MRI or arthroscopy (Fig. 11.16). MRI has been found to be accurate, but, if the tear is symptomatic, arthroscopy is preferable as the tear can be excised at the same time (Fig. 11.17).

The treatment of a symptomatic meniscal tear in a young adult depends on the site of the tear. If the tear is peripheral, in the outer one third, there is potential for healing and surgical repair should be considered. If the tear involves the avascular inner two thirds, arthroscopic partial meniscectomy is the treatment of choice. The recovery following this is much quicker than following arthrotomy and total meniscectomy.

It is well recognized that total meniscectomy increases the risk of degenerative change[44]. Jackson found a 21% incidence of degenera-

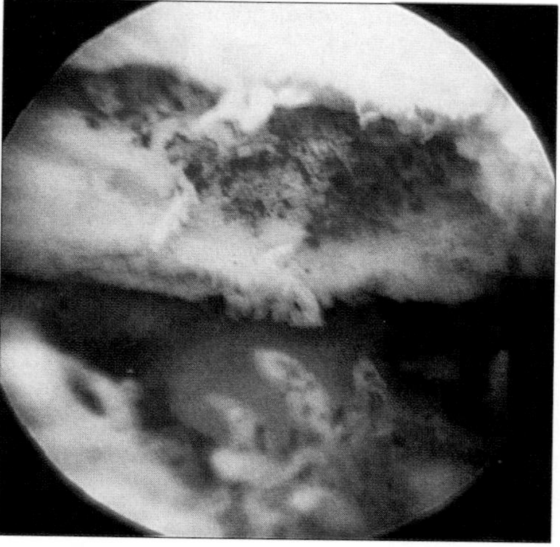

Fig. 11.16 Arthroscopic view of an osteochondritic lesion.

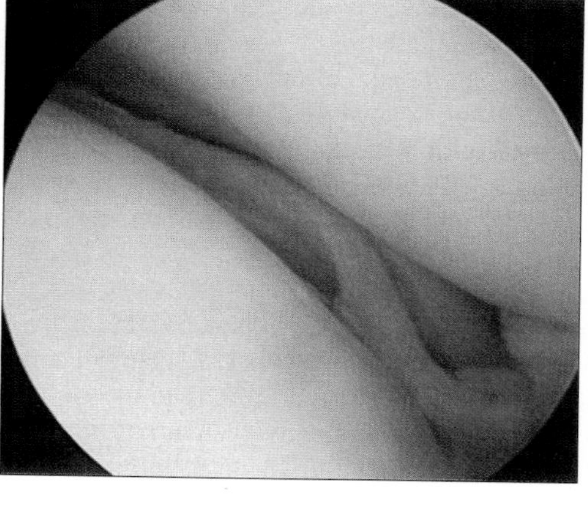

Fig. 11.17 Arthroscopic view of a meniscal tear.

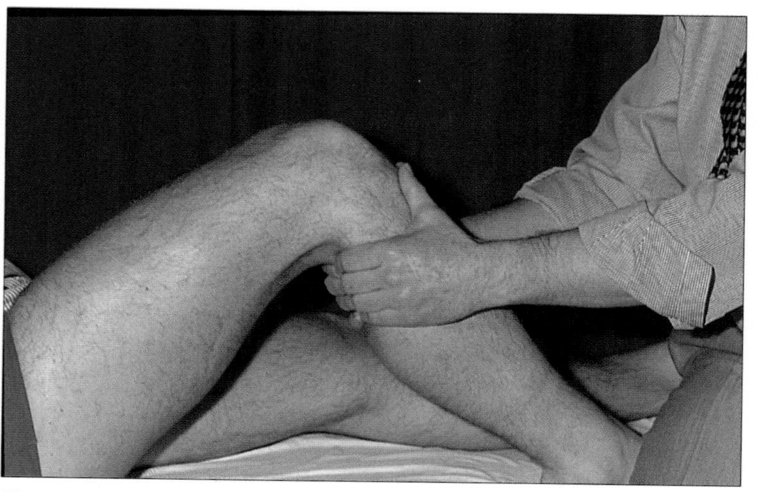

Fig. 11.18 The anterior drawer test.

tion following total meniscectomy compared with a 5% incidence on the other side[45]. The effect of partial meniscectomy has not been determined but it is likely that the rate of degeneration will be less than with total meniscectomy. As much of the meniscus as possible should be retained to leave a 'balanced' stable rim.

In older patients with degenerative tears an initiating injury may not be remembered. The patient usually complains of acute well-localized joint line pain which may wake him or her from sleep. Examination usually reveals joint line tenderness and a small effusion, although this is not a constant feature. Plain radiographs may reveal mild degenerative change and arthrography or MRI will confirm the diagnosis. Symptoms often settle with conservative treatment but arthroscopic resection of the torn portion of the meniscus may be required.

LIGAMENTOUS INJURIES

Ligamentous injuries are common in young athletes. The diagnosis and treatment of knee ligament injuries has improved over the past 15 years. In the past the majority of knee injuries were diagnosed as meniscal tears and the coexisting ligamentous injury was either not recognized or ignored. The recognition of rotatory instability as a result of ligamentous injury and its effect on knee function has been an important advance. Arthroscopy has enabled accurate diagnosis of intra-articular pathology and recognition of the association between instability, meniscal tears and degeneration. Most of the ligaments of the knee have dual roles; the loss of one ligament may initially be masked by the secondary restraining structures. Over a period of time these secondary restraints may stretch and the instability become evident.

Instability may be functional and cause symptoms, or it may be found at examination. Instability demonstrated at examination is of little significance unless functional instability is also present. This is because the muscles control the instability during activity. Many athletes have pathologically lax ligaments on examination, but no functional disability. The examination of the unstable knee is sometimes considered difficult. However, accurate diagnosis of ligamentous injury can be made clinically in the vast majority of cases.

A ligament sprain is an injury in which the fibers are torn. In a first degree sprain there are torn fibers but unimpaired function. In a second degree sprain more fibers are torn with stretching of the ligament causing abnormal joint movement. A third degree sprain implies complete tearing and loss of function with marked abnormal motion. This is used synonymously with the term 'rupture'[46]. The degree of instability following a ligament injury is described by the amount of abnormal tibial movement which occurs in relation to the femur during testing. Hence 1+ laxity is up to 5mm; 2+ is 5–10mm; and 3+ is 10–15mm. The pivot shift phenomenon is also scored on a 0–3 scale.

The examination of the unstable knee varies depending on the time from injury. In the acute phase, examination may be difficult due to pain and swelling. The knee should be examined for localized swelling, bruising and effusion or hemarthrosis. Of hemarthroses, 70% are associated with an anterior cruciate ligament (ACL) tear. Examination and arthroscopy under general anesthetic may be necessary to define the extent of the damage if pain precludes an adequate clinical assessment. Radiographs should always be obtained to rule out associated fractures.

In chronic lesions the examination should take the following form. The knee is inspected and palpated in the usual way. An effusion is suggestive of instability or a meniscal tear. The range of movement is tested but is usually normal unless there is a meniscal tear.

Tests for collateral ligament rupture

The integrity of the medial collateral ligament should be tested by applying a valgus stress with the knee held in 30° of flexion. Opening of the joint compared to the other side suggests laxity or rupture of the medial collateral ligament and posteromedial capsule. The test should be repeated with the knee in full extension. If laxity is present it suggests a tear of the medial collateral ligament, medial capsule, posteromedial corner and the posterior cruciate ligament[47]. This is because in full extension all these structures act as a check to valgus movement. The same test should be repeated using a varus stress with the knee in 30° of flexion to test the lateral collateral ligament and posterolateral capsule. The test should be repeated in full extension to test these and the posterior cruciate ligament[48].

Test for cruciate ligament laxity

With the knees flexed to 90° the profile of each knee should be examined. In posterior cruciate ligament (PCL) rupture the tibia sags back compared to the normal side, and when the tibia is pushed posteriorly no solid end point is felt. If this posterior sag is not recognized a PCL rupture may be mistaken for an ACL rupture as the tibia is reduced from its subluxated position during the anterior drawer test (Fig 11.18). In ACL rupture the knee may be seen to hyperextend slightly, as the ACL helps to limit extension. The anterior drawer test is performed with the knee flexed to 90° and the hamstrings relaxed. The tibia is pulled forwards on the femur. An increase in anterior translation of the tibia on the femur compared to the other side is suggestive of an ACL tear. If the PCL is intact, on internal rotation of the foot the amount of anterior drawer will be reduced. This is due to the PCL tightening and drawing the tibia onto the femur. With the foot in external rotation the anterior translation is often increased due to unwinding of the PCL.

The Lachman test is similar to the anterior drawer test but the knee is held in 20° of flexion and the tibia is pulled forward on the femur[49]. An increase in this anterior translation suggests an ACL tear (Fig. 11.19). It can sometimes be difficult to perform the Lachman test if the examiner's hands are small or the patient has a large leg. In this case, in order to perform the test it often helps to rest the patient's knee on the examiner's thigh.

Anterolateral rotatory instability is the most common type to occur with ACL rupture. The ACL is the primary restraint to anterior translation and internal rotation of the tibia on the femur. When it is ruptured the tibia is able to move forwards and internally rotate on the femur. This subluxation of the lateral tibial condyle occurs at between 15° and 20° of knee flexion, causing the pivot shift phenomenon [50]. The pivot shift is simply the term used to describe the phenomenon of subluxation or reduction of the tibia on the femur in a knee with anterolateral rotatory instability. This subluxation is what the patient describes as the knee 'giving way'. The secondary restraints of capsule, collateral ligaments and muscles may prevent subluxation during activity but if they have been damaged or become lax due to excessive loading and subsequent stretching, functional instability can occur.

A variety of tests have been described for the pivot shift phenomenon. The jerk test for anterolateral instability is performed with the examiner's upper hand over the tibia and the thumb behind the head of the fibula exerting a valgus force on the knee. The examiner's other hand internally rotates the foot (Fig. 11.20). As the knee is extended the lateral tibial condyle subluxates forwards, usually with a clunk, which the patient may recognize as the sensation experienced when the knee gives way. If the knee is then extended the tibial condyle will reduce again, often with a second clunk[51].

Anteromedial instability may also occur when the ACL is damaged in association with a lax medial collateral ligament and capsule. In this case the medial tibial condyle subluxates forwards. Anteromedial and anterolateral instability may coexist.

The reverse pivot shift is the opposite of the pivot shift phenomenon and is due to posterior subluxation of the lateral tibial condyle because of an injury to the posterolateral corner of the knee, and often the posterior cruciate ligament as well[52]. The reverse pivot shift test is essentially the reverse of the jerk test. The foot is held externally rotated while the upper hand applies a valgus force to the knee. As the knee is extended the lateral tibial condyle reduces at approximately 20° of flexion with a clunk.

Medial collateral ligament injuries

The medial collateral ligament is usually injured as a result of a valgus force, often associated with external rotation of the tibia. The classic example is a skiing injury where the ski moves laterally, causing a valgus external rotation force on the knee. In the acute phase the findings are of swelling and bruising over the course of the ligament with tenderness over the joint line or femoral insertion. Loss of full extension may be present in an incomplete tear due to pain as the ligament comes under tension in the last 20° of extension. Medial collateral ligament injuries may be associated with meniscal tears or peripheral detachment of the medial meniscus. An associated ACL injury may also be present. If doubt exists about the possibility of coexisting capsular or ACL damage an examination under anesthetic and arthroscopy should be performed. Treatment for isolated medial collateral ligament tears is conservative[53], consisting of 4 weeks in a cast brace with the range of motion set between 40° and 60° and then a further 4–6 weeks in a light brace to protect the ligament during rehabilitation.

Lateral collateral ligament injuries

The lateral collateral ligament is rarely injured in isolation but is usually torn in association with damage to the posterolateral ligament complex (lateral capsule, arcuate ligament and popliteus tendon). The cruciate ligaments may also be damaged. The mechanism of injury is usually a varus force on a flexed knee. The ligament usually ruptures at its fibular insertion or it may avulse the fibular styloid. A peroneal nerve palsy may be associated with a lateral collateral ligament tear and should be looked for at the time of the injury. Little functional instability arises from an isolated tear of the lateral collateral ligament, which therefore may be treated conservatively in a similar manner to the medial collateral ligament. Lesions of the lateral collateral ligament associated with capsular or cruciate ligament damage should be repaired acutely in active young athletes.

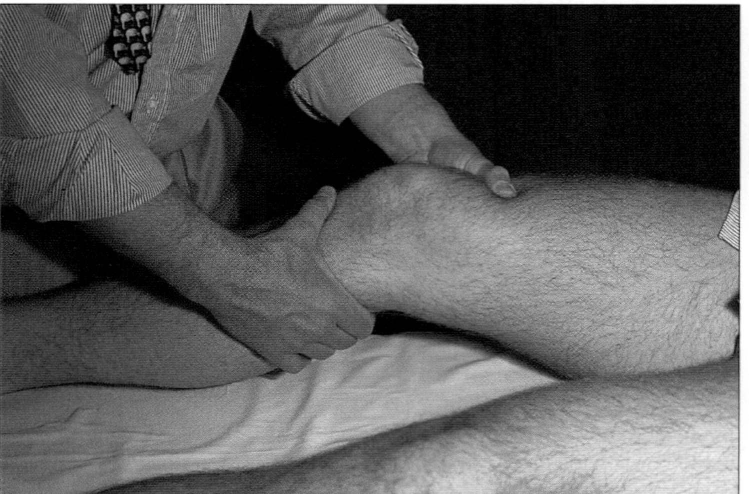

Fig. 11.19 The Lachman test for tears of the cruciate ligaments.

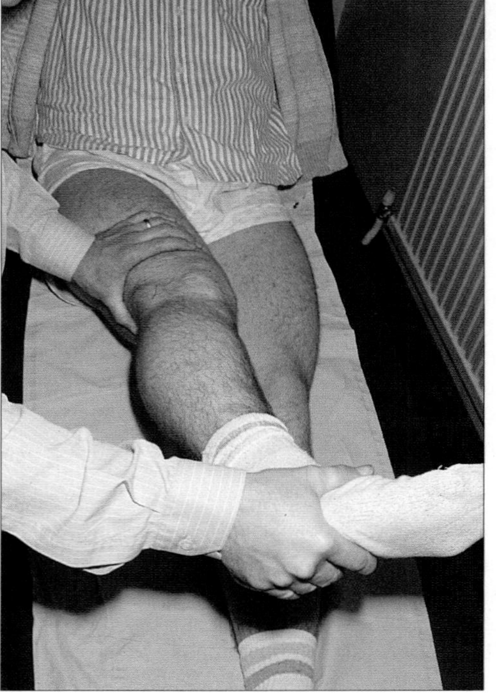

Fig. 11.20 The jerk test for anterolateral instability.

Anterior cruciate ligament injuries

The ACL is injured more frequently than previously thought, often with surprisingly little force. An acute tear of the ACL is usually associated with a hemarthrosis[54]. A pitfall occurs when an ACL tear is associated with capsular disruption when a tense hemarthrosis does not accumulate as the blood leaks out into the calf. Bruising and swelling in the calf is often an indication of serious knee disruption. The injury is usually a twisting injury. Two main mechanisms are recognized: a valgus external rotation injury to a flexed knee associated with damage to other structures; and a hyperextension internal rotation injury resulting in an isolated ACL tear. The patient usually feels the knee go out of joint and may hear a 'pop'. The ACL injury may be missed in the acute phase if other more obvious structures, such as the medial collateral ligament, are damaged. The Lachman test is a reliable indicator of ACL rupture and may be performed on an acutely injured knee without causing too much discomfort. In children, avulsion of the tibial spines tends to occur rather than a mid-substance tear.

Radiographs should be taken to look for avulsion injuries of the tibial spines and other associated fractures. A small flake of bone may be seen to be avulsed from the lateral aspect of the tibial condyle just above the fibula. This is called a Segond fracture and if present indicates a 60–70% chance of an ACL injury. If there is doubt about the diagnosis an examination under anesthesia and arthroscopy should be performed.

Approximately 60% of patients with an ACL rupture will have an associated meniscal tear and 20% will have an osteochondral fracture[55].

The symptoms of an ACL-deficient knee are giving way, swelling and pain. The patient experiences symptoms with twisting or jumping maneuvers. The symptoms are due to rotational instability rather than loss of anteroposterior stability. Symptoms of locking may occur, but these are usually due to a coexisting meniscal tear rather than to the ACL rupture itself. The incidence of meniscal tears in knees with functional anterolateral instability increases with time[56]. It is now generally agreed that recurrent episodes of subluxation will lead to early degeneration. The earliest degenerative changes occur on the medial femoral condyle in the area which is weight bearing when subluxation occurs. This area acts as the fulcrum for the pivot shift and, as articular cartilage is poor at withstanding shear stresses, breakdown occurs[57].

Treatment for acute ACL tears is controversial and beyond the scope of this chapter[58]. Most cases can be treated conservatively and any subsequent functional instability treated later. In athletes with ACL and associated ligamentous and meniscal damage, acute surgery is indicated.

Symptomatic chronic tears of the ACL in young patients which have not responded to conservative measures may be treated by intra-articular replacement of the ACL with autogenous tissue, such as patellar or semitendinosus tendon. In older patients extra-articular repair may control the instability.

Posterior cruciate ligament injury

This is much less common than ACL tears and usually occurs due to road traffic accidents, when a blow to the anterior aspect of the tibia in a flexed knee forces the tibia posteriorly, rupturing the PCL. Unless other structures have also been damaged the function of the knee following PCL rupture is usually good and reconstruction is not necessary[59]. Conservative treatment consists of a plaster cast for 6 weeks with the knee in 20° of flexion, followed by rehabilitation in a knee brace.

TENDON INJURIES

The most common tendon injury around the knee occurs in the elderly and affects the extensor mechanism. Catching a foot against the edge of a pavement, or tripping, with contraction of the quadriceps may be enough to cause rupture or avulsion of an already degenerate patellar or quadriceps tendon. On examination the patient is unable to extend the knee and there may be a high riding patella if the patella tendon has ruptured. If the quadriceps tendon has been avulsed a gap may be palpable above the patella. Fracture of the patella may be secondary to quadriceps contraction or a fall. It is associated with bruising, swelling and tenderness over the patella, and radiographs will confirm the diagnosis.

INJURIES IN DEGENERATIVE KNEES

An effusion is relatively common following minor trauma in degenerative knees, presumably due to synovitis. Hemarthrosis may also occur secondary to hyperemia. A lipohemarthrosis however indicates an intra-articular fracture and should be investigated further.

THE RELATIONSHIP OF INJURY TO DEGENERATION

It is well recognized that injury to the articular cartilage of a joint may lead to early degenerative changes. This relationship is important as it mainly affects young people. Prevention of joint degeneration following injury is therefore important, particularly in the knee. Intra-articular fractures of the femoral condyles or tibial plateau may cause extensive hyaline cartilage damage. The treatment of these fractures by internal fixation with accurate reduction of the articular surfaces and early joint movement may minimize degeneration.

As already mentioned, total meniscectomy increases the likelihood of degenerative change and should not be performed unless absolutely necessary[45]. It is now generally accepted that a patient with anterolateral instability of the knee leading to repeated episodes of subluxation is at increased risk of degeneration at an early age[58,60] (Fig. 11.21). This process is accelerated if the patient has had a total meniscectomy. Thus, patients with instability should be advised to avoid activities which result in repeated episodes of subluxation. Alternatively, they may undergo surgical stabilization of the joint, although at present there is no clear evidence that this decreases the risk of degenerative change and may actually accelerate it. Whether early changes in hyaline cartilage can be reversed by stabilizing the knee is also unclear. Both of these concepts are under investigation.

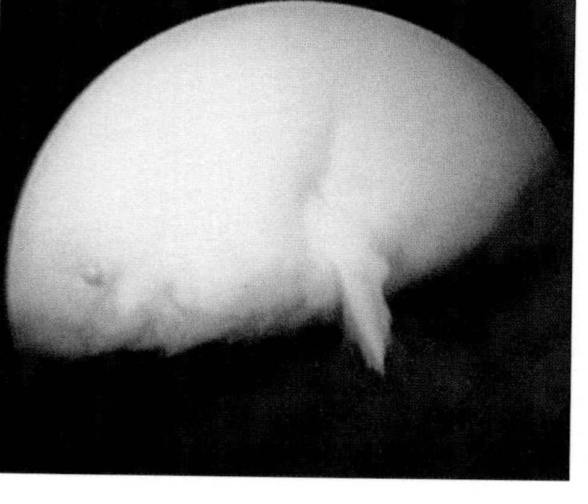

Fig. 11.21 Degeneration following repeated episodes of subluxation.

REFERENCES

1. Price CT, Allen WC. Ligament repair in the knee with preservation of the meniscus. J Bone Joint Surg. 1978;60(A):61–5.
2. Last RJ. Some anatomical details of the knee joint. J Bone Joint Surg. 1948;30(B):683–8.
3. Last RJ. The popliteus muscle and the lateral meniscus. J Bone Joint Surg. 1950;32(B):93–9.
4. Arnoczky SP, Warren RF. Microvasculature of the human meniscus. Am J Sports Med. 1982;10:90–5.
5. Goodfellow J, Hungerford DS, Zindel M. Patello-femoral mechanics and pathology I. Functional anatomy of the patello-femoral joint. J Bone Joint Surg. 1976;58(B):287–90.
6. Aglietti P, Insall JN, Cerulli G. Patellar pain and incongruence I: Measurements of incongruence. Clin Orthop. 1983;176:217–24.
7. Girgis FG, Marshall JL, Al Monajem ARS. The cruciate ligaments of the knee joint. Clin Orthop. 1975;106:216–31.
8. Brantigan OC, Voshell AF. The tibial collateral ligament: Its function, its bursae and its relation to the medial meniscus. J Bone Joint Surg. 1943;25:121–31.
9. Warren LF, Marshall JL, Girgis FG. The prime static stabiliser of the medial side of the knee. J Bone Joint Surg. 1974;56(A):665–74.
10. Fulkerson JP, Gossling HR. Anatomy of the knee joint lateral retinaculum. Clin Orthop. 1980;153:183–8.

11. Kaplan EB. The iliotibial tract. Clinical and morphological significance. J Bone Joint Surg. 1985;40(A):817–32.
12. Henigan SP, Schneck CD, Mesgarzadeh M, Clancy M. The semimembranosus–tibial collateral ligament bursa. J Bone Joint Surg. 1994:76(A):1322–7.
13. Burleson RJ, Bickel WH, Dahlin DC. Popliteal cyst. A clinico-pathological survey. J Bone Joint Surg. 1956;38(A):1265–74.
14. Apley AG, Solomon L. The knee joint. In: Apley's system of orthopaedics and fractures, 6E. London: Butterworth;1982:277–305.
15. James SL. Running injuries to the knee. J Am Acad Orthop Surg. 1995;3:309–18.
16. Renne JW. The iliotibial band friction syndrome. J Bone Joint Surg. 1975;57(A):1110–11.
17. Nachlas IW, Olpp JL. Para-articular calcification (Pellegrini–Stieda) in affectations of the knee. Surg Gynecol Obstet. 1945;81:206–12.
18. Lindgren PG, Willen R. Gastrocnemio-semimembranosus bursa and its relation to the knee joint. I. Anatomy and histology. Acta Radiol. 1977;18:497–512.
19. Lindgren PG. Gastrocnemio-semimembranosus bursa and its relation to the knee joint. IV. Clinical considerations. Acta Radiol. 1978;19:609–22.
20. Rauschning W, Lindgren PG. Popliteal cysts (Baker's cysts) in adults. I. Clinical and Roentgenological results of operative excision. Acta Orthop Scand. 1979;50:583–91.
21. Milgram JW. Synovial osteochondromatosis: a histo-pathological study of thirty cases. J Bone Joint Surg. 1977;59(A):792–801.
22. Maurice H, Crone M, Watt I. Synovial chondromatosis. J Bone Joint Surg. 1988;70(B):807–11.
23. Flandry F, Hughston JC. Pigmented villonodular synovitis. J Bone Joint Surg. 1987;69(A):942–9.
24. Wilson JN. A diagnostic sign in osteochondritis dissecans of the knee. J Bone Joint Surg. 1967;49(B):440–7.
25. Aichroth P. Osteochondritis dissecans of the knee. A clinical survey. J Bone Joint Surg. 1971;53(B):440–7.
26. Green JP. Osteochondritis dissecans of the knee. J Bone Joint Surg. 1966;48(B):82–91.
27. Cahill B. The treatment of juvenile osteochondritis dissecans and osteochondritis dissecans of the knee. Clin Sports Med. 1985;4:367.
28. Osgood RB. Lesions of the tibial tubercle occurring during adolescence. Boston Med Surg J. 1903;148:114.
29. Ogden JA, Southwick WO. Osgood–Schlatter's disease and tibial tuberosity development. Clin Orthop. 1976:116:180–9.
30. Sinding-Larsen C. A hitherto unknown affection of the patella in children. Acta Radiol. 1921;1:171.
31. Jones RD, Fisher RL, Curtis BH. Congenital dislocation of the patella. Clin Orthop. 1976;119:177–83.
32. Williams PF. Quadriceps contracture. J Bone Joint Surg. 1968;50(B):278–84.
33. Fulkerson JP. Patellofemoral pain disorders: evaluation and management. J Am Acad Orthop Surg. 1994;2:124–32.
34. Insall J, Salvati E. Patella position in the normal knee joint. Radiology. 1971;101:101–4.
35. Laurin CA, Levesque HP, Dussault R, Labelle H, Peides JP. The abnormal lateral patellofemoral angle: A diagnostic roentgenographic sign of recurrent patellar subluxation. J Bone Joint Surg. 1978;60(A):55–60.
36. Hungerford DS, Lennox DW. Rehabilitation of the knee in disorders of the patellofemoral joint: Relevant biomechanics. Orthop Clin North Am. 1983;14:397–402.
37. Stanitski CL. Anterior knee pain syndromes in the adolescent. J Bone Joint Surg. 1993;75(A):1407–16.
38. Hughston JC, Stone M, Andrews JR. The suprapatellar plica: Its role in internal derangement of the knee. J Bone Joint Surg. 1973;55(A):1318.
39. Johnson DP, Eastwood DM, Witherow PJ. Symptomatic synovial plicae of the knee. J Bone Joint Surg. 1993;75(A):1485–96.
40. Patel D. Arthroscopy of the plicae: Synovial folds and their significance. Am J Sports Med. 1978;6:217.
41. Noble J, Hamblen DL. The pathology of the degenerate meniscus lesions. J Bone Joint Surg. 1975:57(B):180–6.
42. McMurray TP. The semilunar cartilages. Br J Surg. 1941;29:407.
43. Apley AG. The diagnosis of meniscus injuries. Some new clinical methods. J Bone Joint Surg. 1947;29:78–84.
44. Fairbank TJ. Knee joint changes after meniscectomy. J Bone Joint Surg. 1948;30(B):664–70.
45. Jackson JP. Degenerative changes in the knee after meniscectomy. Br Med J. 1968;2:525–7.
46. Noyes FR, Grood ES, Torzilli PA. The definitions of terms for motion and position of the knee and injuries of the ligaments. J Bone Joint Surg. 1989;71(A):465–71.
47. Hugston JC, Andrews JR, Cross MJ, Moschi A. Classification of knee ligament instabilities. Part 1. The medial compartment and cruciate ligaments. J Bone Joint Surg. 1976;58(A):159–72.
48. Hughston JC, Andrews JR, Cross MJ, Moschi A. Classification of knee ligament instabilities. Part 2. The lateral compartment. J Bone Joint Surg. 1976;58(A):173–9.
49. Torg JS, Conrad W, Kalen V. Clinical diagnosis of anterior cruciate ligament instability in the athlete. Am J Sports Med. 1976;4:84–93.
50. Galway RD, Beaupre A, Macintosh DL. Pivot shift: a clinical sign of symptomatic anterior cruciate insufficiency. J Bone Joint Surg. 1972;54(B):763–4.
51. Ireland J, Trickey EL. Macintosh tenodesis for anterolateral instability of the knee. J Bone Joint Surg. 1980;62(B):340–5.
52. Jakob RP, Hassler H, Staeubli HU. Observations on rotatory instability in the lateral compartment of the knee. Acta Orthop Scand. 1981;191(Suppl):1–32.
53. Indelicato PA. Non operative treatment of complete tears of the medial collateral ligament of the knee. J Bone Joint Surg. 1983;65(A):323–9.
54. DeHaven KE. Diagnosis of acute knee injuries with hemarthrosis. Am J Sports Med. 1980;8:9–14.
55. Noyes FR, Basset RW, Grood ES, Butler DL. Arthroscopy in acute traumatic hemarthrosis of the knee. Incidence of anterior cruciate tears and other injuries. J Bone Joint Surg. 1980;62(A):687–95.
56. Indelicato PA, Bittar ES. A perspective of lesions associated with ACL insufficiency in the knee. A review of 100 cases. Clin Orthop. 1985;198:77–80.
57. Fairclough JA, Graham GP, Dent CM. Radiological sign of chronic anterior cruciate ligament deficiency. Injury. 190;21:401–2.
58. Noyes FR, McGinniss GH. Controversy about treatment of the knee with anterior cruciate laxity. Clin Orthop. 1985;198:61–76.
59. Cross MJ, Powell JF. The long term follow up of posterior cruciate ligament rupture: A study of 116 cases. Am J Sports Med. 1984;12:292–7.
60. Graham GP, Fairclough HA. Early osteoarthritis in young sportsmen with severe antero-lateral instability of the knee. Injury. 1988;19:247–8.

12

THE ANKLE AND FOOT

Adel G Fam

- Pain in the ankle and foot may arise from the bones and joints, periarticular soft tissues (cutaneous and subcutaneous tissues, plantar fascia, tendon sheaths and bursae), nerve roots and peripheral nerves, or vascular structures or be referred from the lumbar spine or knee joint.
- Static disorders, due to inappropriate footwear, foot deformities and/or weak intrinsic muscles, account for the vast majority of painful foot conditions.
- Precise diagnosis of ankle and foot pain rests upon a careful history, a thorough examination and a few rationally selected diagnostic studies.

FUNCTIONAL ANATOMY

The foot can be divided into three units: hind-, mid-, and forefoot (Fig. 12.1). The hindfoot comprises the calcaneus and talus[1–5]. The anterior two thirds of the calcaneus articulates with the talus, and the posterior third forms the heel. Medially the sustentaculum tali supports the talus and is joined to the navicular bone by the spring ligament. The talus articulates with the tibia and fibula above at the ankle joint, with the calcaneus below at the subtalar joint, and with the navicular in front at the talonavicular joint. Five tarsal bones make up the midfoot: navicular medially, cuboid laterally and the three cuneiforms distally. The midfoot is separated from the hindfoot by the mid- or transverse tarsal joint (talonavicular and calcaneocuboid articulations), and from the forefoot by the tarsometatarsal joints (Fig. 12.1). The forefoot comprises the metatarsals and phalanges. The great toe has two phalanges and two sesamoids embedded in the plantar ligament under the metatarsal head. Each of the other toes has three phalanges.

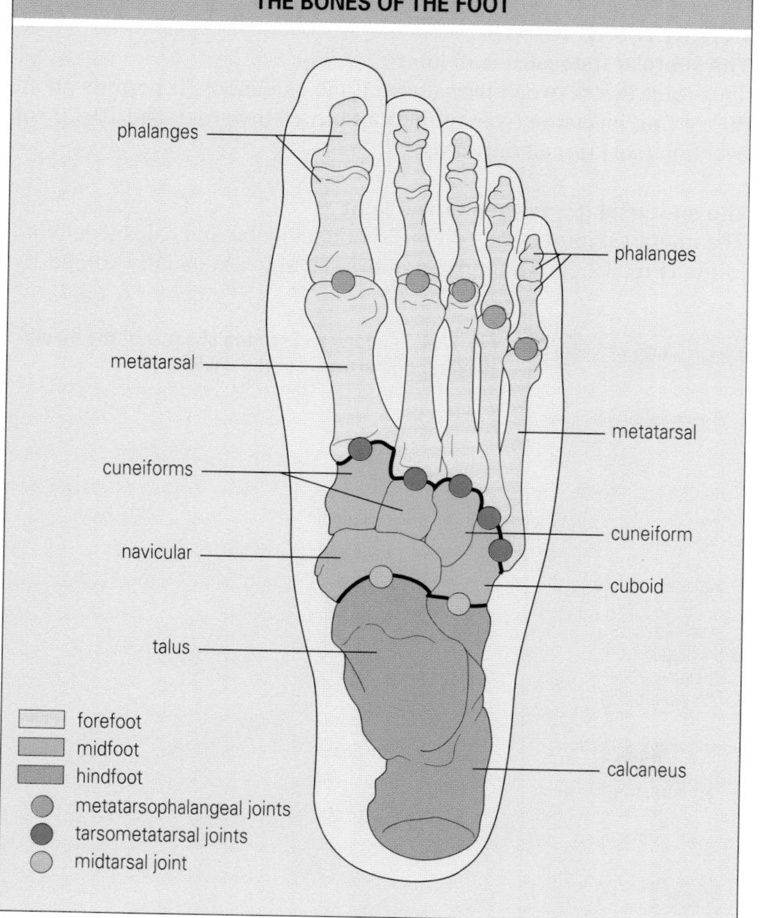

Fig. 12.1 The bones of the foot, superior view.

THE DISTAL TIBIOFIBULAR JOINT

The distal tibiofibular joint is a fibrous joint or syndesmosis between the distal ends of the tibia and fibula (Fig. 12.2). The joint only allows slight malleolar separation (<2mm) on full dorsiflexion of the ankle.

ANKLE (TALOCRURAL) JOINT

The talocrural joint is a hinge joint between the distal ends of the tibia and fibula and the trochlea of the talus[1–5] (Fig. 12.2). Most of the body weight is transmitted through the tibia to the talus. The tibial (medial) and fibular (lateral) malleoli extend distally to form the ankle mortise that stabilizes the talus and prevents rotation. The joint capsule is lax in front and behind but is strengthened medially by the powerful deltoid ligament and laterally by three distinct bands: the posterior talofibular, calcaneofibular and anterior talofibular ligaments. The synovial cavity does not normally communicate with other joints, adjacent tendon sheaths or bursae. Tendons crossing the ankle region are invested for part of their course in tenosynovial sheaths (see Figs 12.3 & 12.4). In the anterior or extensor compartment there are the tendons of tibialis anterior (most medial), extensor hallucis longus, extensor digitorum longus and peroneus tertius (most lateral). The dorsalis pedis artery runs between the extensor hallucis longus and extensor digitorum longus tendons. The superior and inferior extensor retinaculi bind down the extensor tendons as they cross at the ankle. The peroneus longus and brevis tendons are enclosed in a single synovial sheath

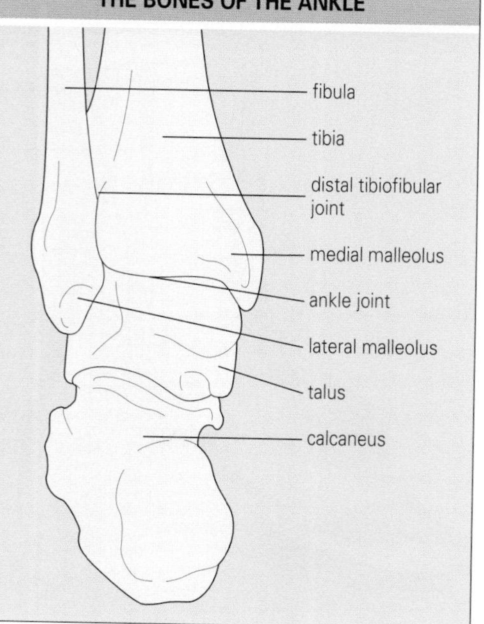

Fig. 12.2 The bones of the ankle, posterior view.

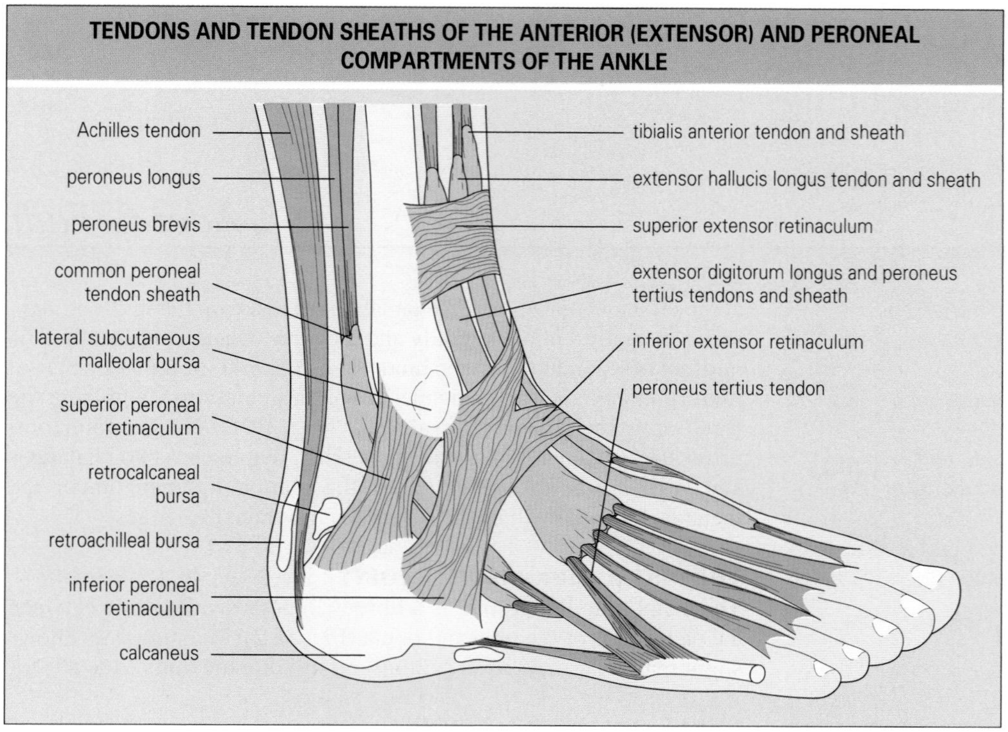

Fig. 12.3 Tendons and tendon sheaths of the anterior (extensor) and peroneal compartments of the ankle.

which runs behind and below the lateral malleolus in the lateral (peroneal) compartment (Fig. 12.3). The superior and inferior peroneal retinaculi strap down the peroneal tendons. The tendons of the tibialis posterior (most medial), flexor digitorum longus and flexor hallucis longus (most lateral) are located in the medial (flexor) compartment (Fig. 12.4). The posterior tibial artery and nerve lie between the tendons of the flexor digitorum longus and flexor hallucis longus. The flexor retinaculum bridges the interval between the medial malleolus and the calcaneus.

Posteriorly, the common tendon of the gastrocnemius and soleus (Achilles tendon or tendocalcaneus) is inserted into the posterior surface of the calcaneus. The tendon does not have a synovial sheath, but is surrounded by a loose connective tissue pseudosheath or peritenon. There are a number of bursae around the ankle (Figs 12.3–12.5). The retrocalcaneal bursa is located between the Achilles tendon insertion and the posterior surface of the calcaneus. The retroachillial bursa lies between the skin and the Achilles tendon and protects the tendon from external pressure. The subcalcaneal bursa is located beneath the skin over the plantar aspect of the calcaneus. Two bursae, the medial and lateral subcutaneous malleolar or 'last' bursae, are located near the medial and lateral malleoli respectively[5–7] (Figs 12.3–12.5).

Movements of the ankle include dorsiflexion and plantar flexion (Fig. 12.6). The axis of movement passes approximately through the malleoli. The gastrocnemius and soleus are the prime plantar flexors of the ankle. The tibialis anterior and extensor digitorum longus are the prime dorsiflexors.

INTERTARSAL JOINTS

The subtalar (talocalcaneal) joint

This joint lies between the talus and the calcaneus. It permits about 30° of foot inversion (sole of the foot turned inwards), and 10–20° of eversion (sole turned outwards)[1–4].

The midtarsal (transverse tarsal) joint

The midtarsal joint is the combined talonavicular and calcaneocuboid joints (Fig. 12.1). The cuboid and navicular are usually joined by

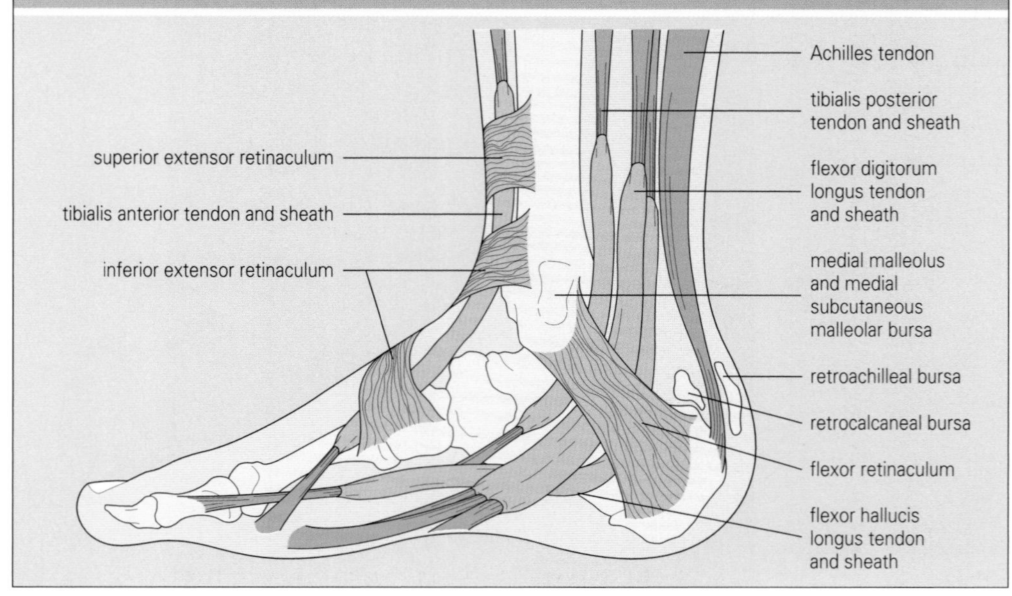

Fig. 12.4 Tendons and tendon sheaths of the medial (flexor) compartment of the ankle.

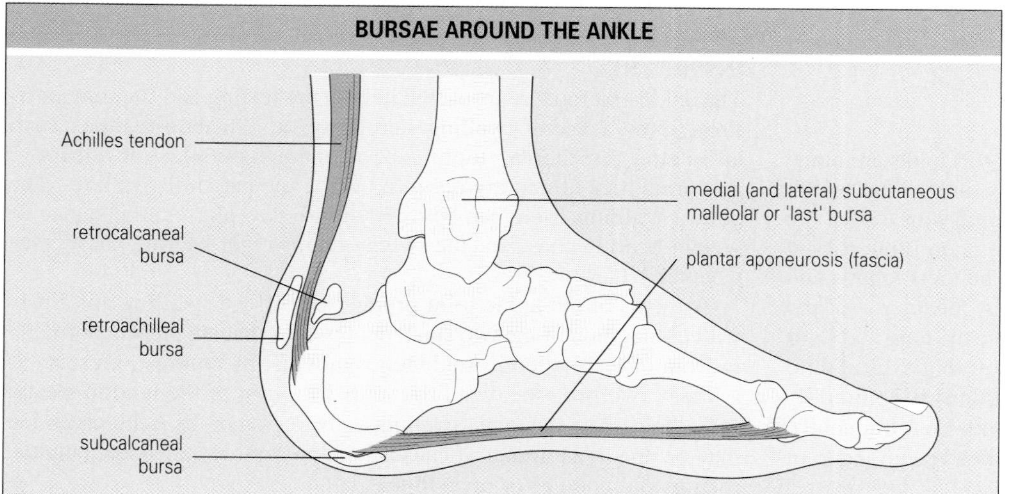

Fig. 12.5 Bursae around the ankle.

fibrous tissue, but a synovial cavity may exist between them. The midtarsal joint contributes to inversion (supination) and eversion (pronation) movements at the subtalar joint. It also allows 20° of adduction (foot turned toward the midline) and 10° of abduction (foot turned away from the midline)[1–4]. The axis of rotation of the subtalar and mid tarsal joints is such that inversion is invariably accompanied by adduction of the forefoot (called supination), and eversion with abduction of the forefoot (called pronation). The tibialis posterior and tibialis anterior, aided by the gastrocnemius, invert the foot. The peroneus longus, peroneus brevis and extensor digitorum longus, aided by the peroneus tertius, evert the foot. The intertarsal joints between the navicular, cuneiforms and cuboid are plane gliding joints which intercommunicate with one another and with the intermetatarsal and tarsometatarsal joints (Fig. 12.1).

THE METATARSOPHALANGEAL (MTP) JOINTS

These are ellipsoid joints lined by separate synovial cavities[1–5]. They lie about 2cm proximal to the webs of the toes. Their capsule is strengthened by the collateral ligaments on each side and by the plantar ligament (plate) on the plantar surface. The plantar ligaments are fused with the flexor tendon sheaths and are connected together by the transverse metatarsal ligament, which holds the metatarsal heads together preventing excessive splaying of the forefoot. Small bursae, the intermetatarsophalangeal bursae, are frequently present between the metatarsal heads[7] (Fig. 12.7). The long extensor tendons form the extensor expansions (aponeuroses) which overlay the dorsum of the MTP joints and digits. The intrinsic muscles of the foot, including flexor hallucis brevis, lumbricals, interossei and flexor digiti minimi brevis, are partly inserted into the extensor expansions and assist in plantar flexion of the MTP joints. The extensor hallucis longus, extensor digitorum longus and brevis dorsiflex the MTP joints. Movements at the first MTP joint consist of dorsiflexion to 70–90° and plantar flexion to about

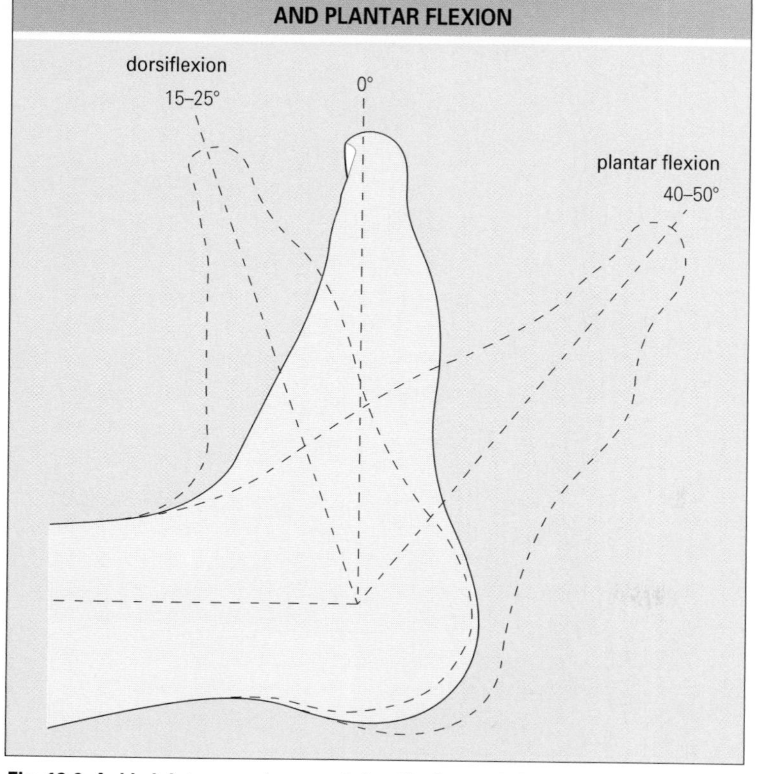

Fig. 12.6 Ankle joint: normal range of dorsiflexion and plantar flexion.

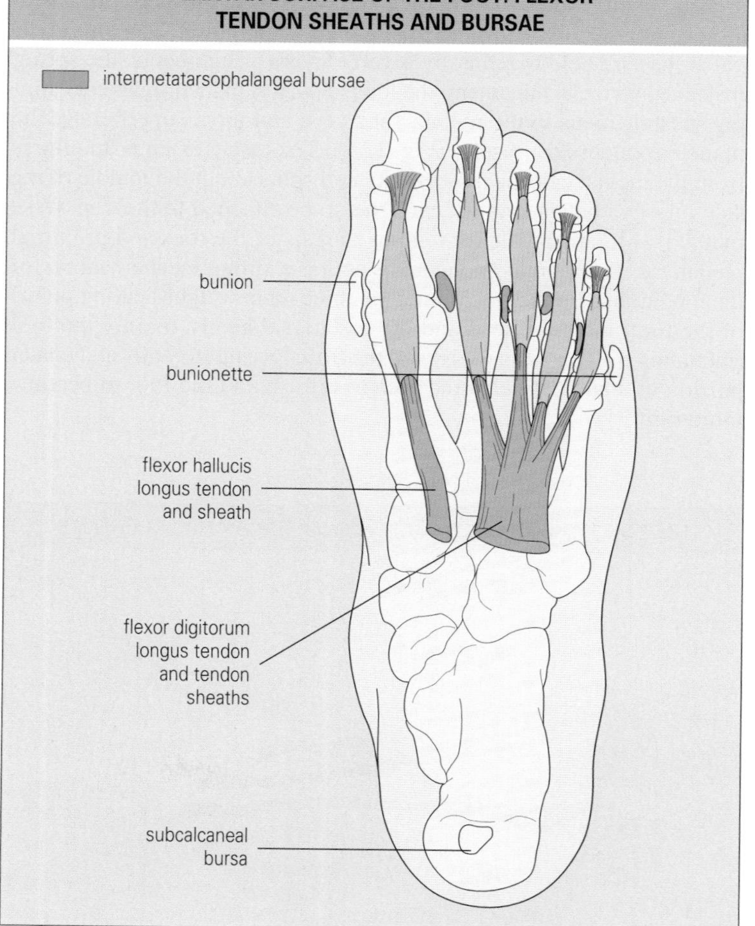

Fig. 12.7 Plantar surface of the foot: flexor tendon sheaths and bursae.

35–50°. The other MTP joints permit about 40° dorsiflexion and 40° plantar flexion. These joints also allow slight abduction and adduction movements.

INTERPHALANGEAL JOINTS

The proximal and distal interphalangeal (PIP and DIP) joints are hinge joints. The plantar flexors are the flexor hallucis longus and brevis (great toe), flexor digitorum longus (flexes the lateral four toes at the DIP joints) and flexor digitorum brevis (flexes the lateral four toes at the PIP joints). The dorsiflexors are the extensor hallucis longus and the extensor digitorum longus and brevis assisted by the interossei and lumbricals. The digital flexor tendon sheaths enclose the long and short flexor tendons extending along the length of the toes to the distal third of the sole proximally[7] (Fig. 12.7). A bursa (bunion) is commonly located over the medial aspect of the first MTP joint. Less frequently, a small bursa is present over the fifth metatarsal head (bunionette or tailor's bunion) (Fig. 12.7).

The PIP joints of the toes do not normally hyperextend. Plantar flexion is limited to approximately 50°. The DIP joints allow 10–30° dorsiflexion and 40–50° plantar flexion.

ARCHES

The arches of the foot are the result of the intrinsic mechanical arrangement of the bones supported by ligaments, intrinsic and extrinsic muscles, particularly the tibialis posterior and anterior muscles[3–5]. They act as shock absorbers during weight bearing. Each foot has two longitudinal and two transverse arches (Fig. 12.8). The medial longitudinal arch is high and flexible and comprises the medial three rays, cuneiforms, navicular, talus and calcaneus. It provides a resilient spring for weight bearing and forward propulsion in walking. The lateral two rays, cuboid and calcaneus constitute the low, more rigid lateral longitudinal arch. The anterior transverse metatarsal arch includes the second, third and fourth metatarsals and the heads of the first and fifth metatarsals. It becomes flattened on weight bearing but returns to its arched position when the weight is removed. The transverse midtarsal arch is more rigid and lies across the midtarsal region. The longitudinal arches are held together by several layers of ligaments: the spring (calcaneonavicular) ligament; the long and short plantar ligaments joining the calcaneus to the metatarsal bases; and most superficially the plantar aponeurosis (fascia) (Fig. 12.8). The fascia extends anteriorly from the medial calcaneal tuberosity and splits about the middle of the sole into five bands, one for each toe, to be attached to the transverse metatarsal ligament, flexor tendon sheaths of the toes and proximal phalanges. The plantar aponeurosis acts as a strong mechanical tie for the longitudinal arches by joining the three main weight-bearing points of the foot: the calcaneus and the metatarsal heads, mainly the first (including the two sesamoids) and the fifth. During 'toe-off' at the later portion of stance, it helps the arch to reform and the foot to become more rigid[3–5].

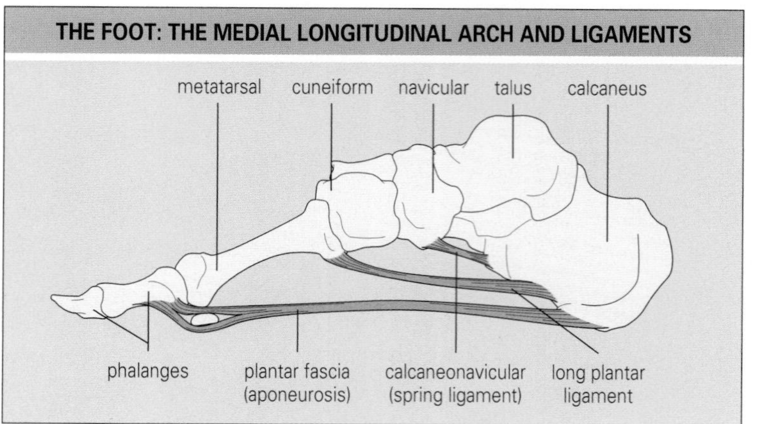

Fig. 12.8 The foot: the medial longitudinal arch and ligaments.

PHYSICAL EXAMINATION

INSPECTION

The ankle and foot are inspected in both the resting and standing positions for evidence of swelling, deformity, or skin abnormalities, such as edema, erythema, tophi, subcutaneous nodules or ulcers[1,2]. Abnormalities of gait are observed while the patient is walking. The gait or walking cycle can be divided into two phases: the stance or weight-bearing phase and the swing or nonweight-bearing phase[3] (see Chapter 1.12).

Arthritis of the ankle joint produces a diffuse swelling anteriorly with obliteration of the two small depressions that are present normally in front of the malleoli. Ankle tenosynovitis, by contrast, presents as a linear swelling, localized to the distribution of the tendon sheath extending across the joint. Swelling in the region of the Achilles tendon may be due to a number of causes: tendon rupture, calcaneal bursitis, rheumatoid nodules or urate tophi.

Arthritis of an intertarsal joint produces a diffuse swelling over the medial and dorsal surfaces of the foot. The exact location of the involved joint can only be determined by palpation. Synovitis of the MTP joints is associated with diffuse swelling on the dorsum of the forefoot that may obscure the extensor tendons. Digital flexor tenosynovitis produces a diffuse, tender swelling over the plantar aspect of the toe (sausage toe). Generalized swelling of the ankle and foot is common in edematous states. The fluid collects where the tissues are lax and most dependent, particularly below and behind the malleoli, obscuring the outline of the Achilles tendon.

In the standing position, the calcaneus normally maintains the line of the Achilles tendon. Deformities of the subtalar joint, resulting in eversion (calcaneovalgus) or inversion (calcaneovarus) of the heel are best observed from behind. Equinus and calcaneus refer to angulation of the ankle in plantar and dorsiflexion respectively. Inspection while the patient is standing may reveal lowering of the longitudinal arch (pes planus), or increased height of the arch (pes cavus). The toes are simple extensions of the metatarsals. The first and fifth toes are often slightly deviated toward the middle of the forefoot. Hallux valgus deformity refers to lateral deviation of the first (great) toe on the first metatarsal >10–15° (Fig. 12.9). Straightening or medial deviation of the great toe on the first

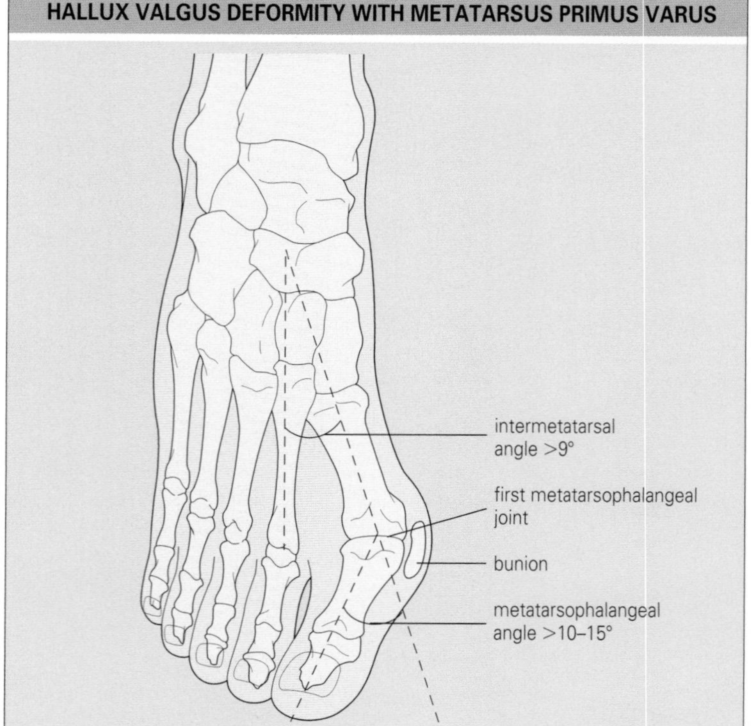

Fig. 12.9 Hallux valgus deformity.

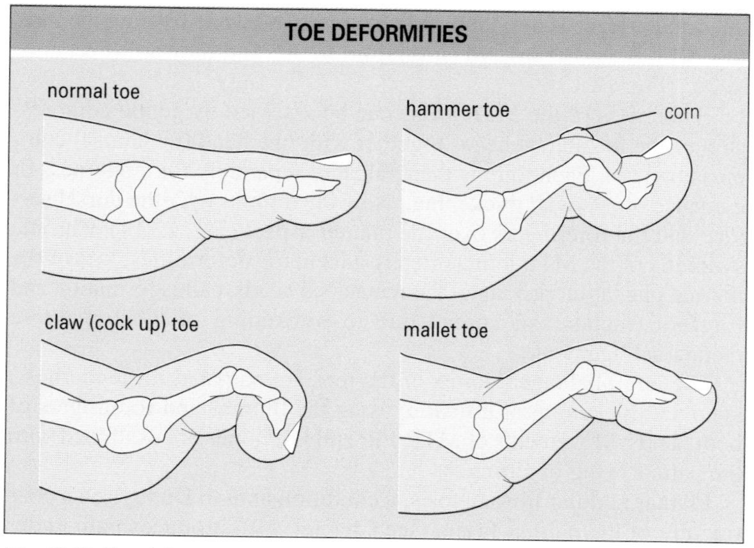

TOE DEFORMITIES

normal toe
hammer toe
corn
claw (cock up) toe
mallet toe

Fig. 12.10 Toe deformities.

metatarsal is hallux varus. Hallux rigidus refers to severe limitation of movement at the first MTP joint, usually from osteoarthritis.

Cock-up or claw toe deformity refers to dorsiflexion of the MTP joint and plantar flexion of both the PIP and DIP joints (Fig. 12.10). A hammer toe refers to plantar flexion deformity of the PIP joint, usually associated with dorsiflexion of the MTP and DIP joints (Fig. 12.10). In mallet toe deformity, the DIP joint is plantar flexed and PIP joint is neutral (or PIP joint is plantar flexed and DIP joint is neutral). It is usually associated with a dorsiflexed MTP joint (Fig. 12.10).

PALPATION

The ankle joint is palpated with the foot in slight plantar flexion. The joint is supported by the fingers of both hands while the thumbs firmly palpate the anterior aspect of the joint (Fig. 12.11). The capsule and synovial membrane are best palpated over the joint line just distal to the lower end of the tibia and medial to the tibialis anterior tendon. The margins of a swollen synovium in other locations may be difficult to outline owing to the presence of overlying tendons. A large ankle effusion may bulge both medial and lateral to the extensor tendons and produce fluctuation; pressure with one hand on one side of the joint produces a fluid wave transmitted to the second hand placed on the other side of the joint.

PALPATION OF THE ANKLE JOINT

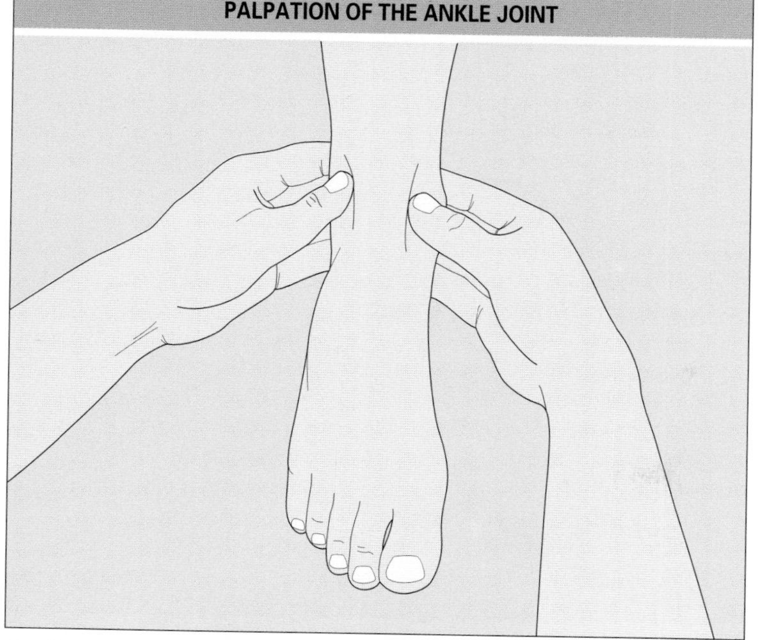

Fig. 12.11 Palpation of the ankle joint.

Ankle tenosynovitis produces a superficial, linear, tender swelling extending beyond the joint margins. Movements of the involved tendon often produce pain.

Distension of the lateral and medial 'last' bursae produces a localized, oval swelling over the anterolateral and anteromedial aspects of the joint respectively.

A painful tender heel may be due to a number of causes (see below). In plantar fasciitis, there is tenderness without swelling at the site of attachment of the plantar fascia to the inferomedial surface of the calcaneus. A painful calcaneal fat pad is associated with local tenderness in the center of the heel. In Achilles insertional tendonitis, tenderness is present over the tendon near its insertion into the os calcis. Subcalcaneal bursitis produces a tender swelling on the plantar surface of the calcaneus. Retroachillial bursitis is characterized by a tender subcutaneous cystic swelling overlying the Achilles tendon. Retrocalcaneal bursitis produces a more diffuse swelling anterior to the tendon and posterior to the ankle joint. Ankle movements are tested with the knee flexed. The normal range is 15–25° of dorsiflexion from the neutral position (foot at right angle to leg) and 40–50° of plantar flexion (Fig. 12.6).

The subtalar joint cannot be palpated. Subtalar movements are examined with the ankle in the neutral position. The calcaneus (heel) is grasped with one hand while the other stabilizes the distal leg (Fig. 12.12). The calcaneus is then turned inward (inversion) to 30°, and outward (eversion) to 20°.

The midtarsal, intertarsal and tarsometatarsal joints are palpated using the thumbs on the dorsal surface while the fingers support the plantar aspect of the foot. To test movements of the midtarsal joint, the

SUBTALAR JOINT: EXAMINATION AND RANGE OF MOVEMENTS

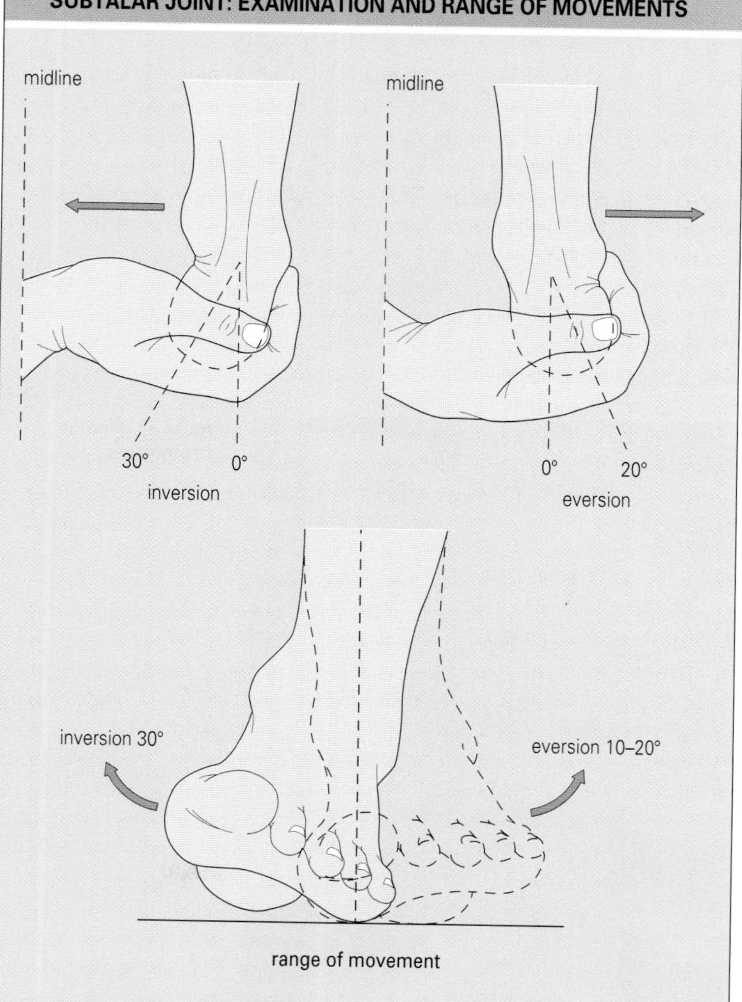

Fig. 12.12 Examination of the subtalar joint and range of movements.

talus and calcaneus are stabilized with one hand while rotating the forefoot with the other inward (inversion) to 30° and outward (eversion) to 20° (Fig. 12.13).

Tenderness of the MTP joints can be assessed by gentle compression of the metatarsal heads together with one hand (metatarsal compression test). Each joint is then palpated separately for tenderness or evidence of synovial thickening, using the thumbs over the dorsal surface and the forefingers over the plantar aspect (Fig. 12.14). Chronic synovitis of the MTP joints often results in toe deformities, loss of the normal plantar fat pad under the metatarsal heads, callus formation and forefoot (metatarsal) spread due to weakening of the transverse metatarsal ligament.

The interphalangeal joints of the toes are palpated for tenderness, synovial thickening or effusion, using the thumbs and forefingers of both hands. Movements of MTP, PIP and DIP joints are examined with the patient lying or sitting.

Plantar nodular fibromatosis, a condition akin to Dupuytren's contracture of the palmar fascia (see Chapter 4.9), produces pain under the midfoot associated with discrete palpable nodules in the plantar fascia[8] (Fig. 12.15).

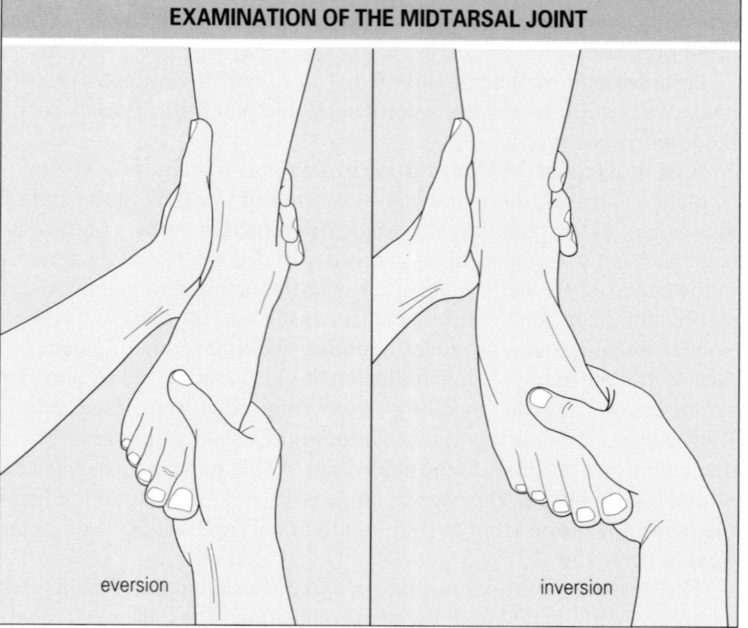

Fig. 12.13 Examination of the midtarsal joint.

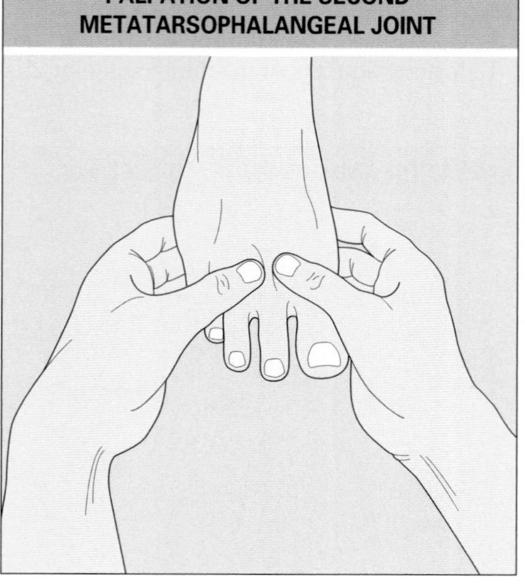

Fig. 12.14 Palpation of the second MTP joint.

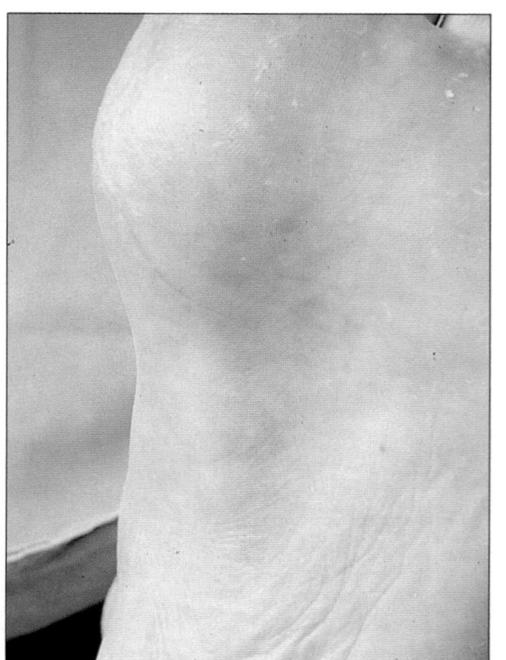

Fig. 12.15 Plantar fibromatosis.

SPECIAL MANEUVERS

In tarsal tunnel syndrome (see Chapter 4.16), percussion of the posterior tibial nerve at the flexor retinaculum behind the flexor digitorum longus tendon may produce paresthesia in the distribution of one or more of its two branches: medial and lateral plantar nerves (Tinel's sign). Similar symptoms can sometimes be induced by simple pressure on the nerve at the flexor retinaculum. In the tourniquet test, a sphygmomanometer cuff inflated around the leg to produce venous congestion may reproduce the paresthesia.

Inversion and eversion sprains of the ankle can result in tears of the lateral and medial ligaments respectively. Inversion sprains are more common and result in a tear of the lateral ligament, particularly its anterior talofibular band. In the anterior draw test, the distal tibia and fibula are held in one hand, while the calcaneus and talus are drawn forward by the other hand (Fig. 12.16). A major tear of the anterior talofibular ligament allows forward movement of the talus on the tibia (positive anterior draw sign).

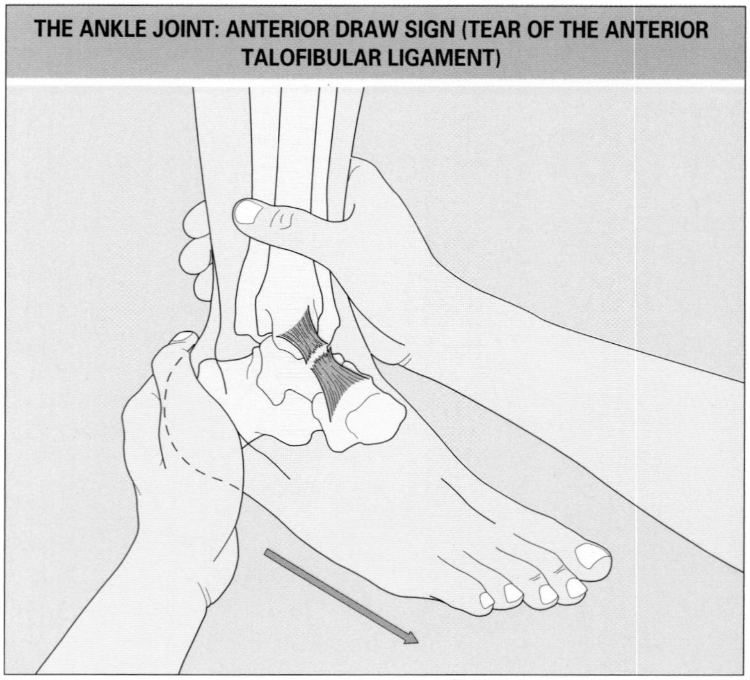

THE ANKLE JOINT: ANTERIOR DRAW SIGN (TEAR OF THE ANTERIOR TALOFIBULAR LIGAMENT)

Fig. 12.16 The ankle joint: anterior draw sign (tear of the anterior talofibular ligament).

DIFFERENTIAL DIAGNOSIS OF ANKLE AND FOOT PAIN

Painful disorders of the ankle and foot are a common presentation in both rheumatologic and orthopedic practices. The pain may arise from the bones and joints of the ankle and foot, periarticular soft tissue structures (cutaneous and subcutaneous tissues, plantar fascia, tendon sheaths and bursae), nerve roots and peripheral nerves, or peripheral vascular system, or be referred from the lumbar spine or knee joint[9]. A classification of painful disorders of the ankle and foot, based upon the site of origin and predominant location of the pain, is outlined in Figure 12.17. Static disorders, due to inappropriate footwear, foot deformities and/or weak intrinsic muscles, account for the vast majority of painful foot conditions.

Precise diagnosis of foot pain depends on a detailed history and a careful assessment of the joints, periarticular soft tissue structures, nerve and blood supply, and lumbar spine. Diagnostic studies may be required, including routine laboratory tests, synovial fluid analysis, plain radiographs[10], nerve conduction studies, noninvasive vascular (Doppler) studies, bone scintiscan, sonography, computed tomographic (CT) scans and magnetic resonance imaging (MRI)[11]. Other assessment methods, such as special radiographic views, xeroradiography, arthrography, arteriography, gait analysis and foot print studies, are occasionally needed.

SPECIFIC DISORDERS OF THE ANKLE AND FOOT REGION

DISORDERS OF THE ACHILLES TENDON REGION

Achilles tendinitis

Tendinitis of the Achilles tendon is characterized by pain, swelling, tenderness and sometimes crepitus, over the tendon near its insertion[12–20]. Thickening and irregularity of the tissues surrounding the tendon, and sometimes a palpable nodule, may be present. Passive dorsiflexion of the ankle intensifies the pain. It is usually caused by repetitive trauma and microscopic tears due to excessive use of the calf muscles in ballet dancing[12,13], distance running, basketball, jumping and other athletic activities, or from faulty footwear with a rigid shoe counter. Pain at the insertion of the Achilles tendon (enthesopathy) is frequently seen in the context of spondyloarthropathies. The tendon is also a common site for gouty tophi and rheumatoid nodules. An association between adult familial hypercholesterolemia, Achilles tendon xanthomas and Achilles tendinitis has also been described[17,18]. Abnormalities of the tendon and peritendinous tissues can be demonstrated by both sonography[19,20] and MRI[11,18].

Treatment consists of rest, avoiding the provocative occupational or athletic activity, shoe modification, a heel raise to reduce tendon stretching during walking, nonsteroidal anti-inflammatory drugs (NSAIDs) and physiotherapy, including local heat application, gentle stretching exercises and sometimes a temporary splint with slight plantar flexion[12–16]. Avoidance of hills and uneven running surfaces and diligent stretching before sport activities are often beneficial[16]. The Achilles tendon is vulnerable to rupture particularly in elderly individuals. Corticosteroid injections in or near the tendon are of questionable value[21]. They predispose to tendon rupture and should, therefore, be discouraged. Surgical excision of the inflamed peritendinous tissue is rarely required[12–16].

Achilles bursitis

Retrocalcaneal, sub-Achilles or subtendinous bursitis

This is associated with posterior heel pain made worse by passive dorsiflexion of the ankle. Bursal distension produces a tender swelling behind the ankle with bulging on both sides of the tendon. Known causes include rheumatoid arthritis (RA), psoriatic arthritis, ankylosing spondylitis and Reiter's syndrome[22]. It may also occur in association with Haglund's deformity[23] (abnormal prominence of the

DIFFERENTIAL DIAGNOSIS OF ANKLE AND FOOT PAIN
Articular
Trauma, sprain
Arthritis
Rheumatoid arthritis
Subtalar, midtarsal, MTP
Osteoarthritis
1st MTP>talonavicular>tarsometatarsal joint>intertarsal
Gout
1st MTP
Psoriatic arthritis
Sausage toe, MTP
Metatarsalgia
Toe disorders
Hallux valgus
Hallux rigidus
Hammer toe, claw toe
Arch disorders
Pes planus (flat feet)
Pes cavus (cavus feet)
Congenital disorders
e.g. clubfoot
Periarticular
Cutaneous and subcutaneous
Corns, calluses
RA nodules, tophi
Ingrowing toenail
Plantar fascia
Plantar fasciitis
Plantar nodular fibromatosis
Tendons and tendon sheaths
Achilles tendinitis
Achilles tendon rupture
Tibialis posterior tenosynovitis
Peroneal tenosynovitis
Bursitis
Retrocalcaneal and retroachillial bursitis
Lateral and medial last bursitis
Bunion
Bunionette
Acute calcific periarthritis
Hydroxyapatite pseudopodagra
Osseous
Fracture
Traumatic or stress (march) fracture
Epiphysitis (osteochondritis)
Second metatarsal head (Freiberg's disease)
Navicular (Köhler's disease)
Calcaneus (Sever's disease)
Bone neoplasms, infection
Painful accessory ossicles
Accessory navicular (near navicular)
Os trigonum (near talus)
Os intermetatarseum (between 1st and 2nd metatarsal bases)
Neurologic
Entrapment of lumbosacral nerve roots form herniated lumbar disc
Entrapment of the lateral popliteal nerve behind the neck of the fibula
Tarsal tunnel syndrome (posterior tibial nerve)
Interdigital (Morton's) neuroma
Peripheral neuropathy and insensitive foot
Vascular
Ischemic foot pain
Atherosclerosis, Buerger's disease, vasculitis
Vasospastic disorders with Raynaud's phenomenon
Cholesterol embolization with 'purple toes'
Referred pain from
Lumbar spine disorders
Knee disorders
Reflex sympathetic dystrophy syndrome

Fig. 12.17 Differential diagnosis of ankle and foot pain.

posterosuperior surface of the calcaneus) and with Achilles tendinitis as a result of repetitive trauma due to ballet dancing[12] and athletic overactivity, particularly in runners[22]. Haglund's deformity is often associated with a varus hindfoot[23]. When viewed from behind, it presents as a round bony swelling just lateral to the distal part of the Achilles tendon. The diagnosis of retrocalcaneal bursitis can be confirmed by radiography (showing obliteration of the retrocalcaneal recess), sonography[19,20], or MRI[12,24].

Rest, activity modification, moist heat application, a slight heel elevation using a felt heel pad and NSAIDs constitute sufficient therapy for most patients. A walking cast and/or a cautious corticosteroid injection into the bursa are sometimes required[25]. Surgical bursectomy and resection of the superior prominence of the calcaneal tuberosity are rarely indicated[12,21–23].

Retroachillial or subcutaneous calcaneal bursitis

Retroachillial or subcutaneous calcaneal bursitis, also known as 'pump bumps', produces a painful tender subcutaneous swelling overlying the Achilles tendon, usually at the level of the shoe counter (22). The overlying skin may be hyperkeratotic or reddened. It occurs predominantly in women, and is frequently caused and aggravated by improperly fitting shoes or pumps with a stiff, closely contoured heel counter. It may also occur in patients with Haglund's deformity and varus hindfoot[23]. Management consists of rest, heat application, NSAIDs, padding, and relief from shoe pressure by wearing a soft, nonrestrictive shoe without a counter. Local corticosteroid injections should be avoided. Surgical excision is rarely indicated[22,23].

Achilles tendon rupture

Rupture of the Achilles tendon typically occurs during a burst of unaccustomed physical activity involving forced ankle dorsiflexion[15,16,26]. The onset is often sudden, with pain in the region of the tendon and difficulty walking or standing on the toes. Swelling, ecchymosis, tenderness and sometimes a palpable gap are present at the site of the tear. In partial tendon rupture, active plantar flexion of the ankle may be preserved but painful. In those with complete rupture it is still possible to actively plantarflex the ankle by the adjacent intact flexor tendons. However, squeezing the calf muscles with the patient sitting or kneeling on a chair produces little or no passive ankle plantar flexion (positive Thompson calf squeeze test)[15,16]. The extent and orientation of the rupture can be accurately assessed by both sonography[19,20] and MRI[11,27].

Achilles tendon rupture may result from a sharp blow, a fall or from athletic injuries[15,16,26]. It also occurs in elderly patients with pre-existing Achilles tendinitis or retrocalcaneal bursitis, patients with systemic lupus erythematosus or RA receiving corticosteroids, in those on long-term hemodialysis, following local corticosteroid injections in the vicinity of the tendon, and in patients treated with fluoroquinolone antibiotics[28,29]. Orthopedic treatment with immobilization and/or surgery is required[15,16].

HEEL PAIN

Plantar fasciitis

Plantar fasciitis is the most common cause of subcalcaneal heel pain (Fig. 12.18). It results from repetitive microtrauma causing tearing and stretching of the fibers of the plantar fascia at its narrow proximal attachment into the medial calcaneal tuberosity[30–35]. Pain on the undersurface of the heel on weight bearing is the principal complaint. Often, the pain is worse when weight is borne after a period of rest (e.g., in the morning), and eases on walking. The pain worsens late in the day and can be quite severe on standing. Localized tenderness, without swelling, is present over the anteromedial portion of the plantar surface of the calcaneus. Passive dorsiflexion of the toes while everting the foot stretches the plantar fascia and often accentuates the discomfort.

Radiographic examination may show a plantar calcaneal spur which itself is not the cause of the pain. A relationship between pes planus, calcaneal spurs and plantar fasciitis has been observed[34]. Both MRI[35,36] and sonography[35] may provide an objective assessment of the morphologic changes associated with plantar fasciitis. Findings on MRI include thickening and signal intensity abnormalities of the plantar fascia origin[35,36].

Plantar fasciitis commonly occurs in obese[30–33], middle-aged and elderly patients as a result of repetitive trauma from athletic activities, occupations that entail excessive standing and walking (e.g. 'policeman's heel'[35]), changes in walking surfaces or from changes in shoewear. It may also occur in young individuals as a result of sport injuries, for example striking the heel with some force, or as an enthesopathy in association with ankylosing spondylitis, Reiter's syndrome or psoriatic arthritis[30–33] (see Chapter 6.13).

Subcalcaneal (infracalcaneal) bursitis may coexist with plantar fasciitis and distinguishing the two is sometimes difficult. Bursal distention produces a cystic swelling over the plantar aspect of the calcaneus[22,32]. Unlike plantar fasciitis, dorsiflexion of the MTP joints does not increase the discomfort. It usually occurs in older persons as a result of repetitive trauma from improperly fitting shoes, falls, pounding the heel with some force, prolonged walking or from recent weight gain.

A painful calcaneal fat pad (painful heel pad syndrome) is often confused with plantar fasciitis. The heel pad is normally composed of fibroelastic septa separating closely packed fat cells[4,32,33]. Rupture of the septa in elderly obese patients, under the influence of ordinary weight bearing or suddenly due to a severe impact, results in attrition of the heel pad, poor shock absorption and increased weight-bearing pressure on the calcaneus with reactive bony proliferation[30,32,33]. Pain is experienced beneath the heel with weight bearing, particularly on standing. Tenderness is present directly over the heel pad at the posterior weight-bearing portion of the calcaneal tuberosity. This is in contrast to the more anterior tenderness of plantar fasciitis. Soft tissue radiographs may show decreased density and volume of the calcaneal fat pad, and increased cortical density of the calcaneal tuberosity.

Bilateral plantar and calcaneal traction spurs are common in obese, middle-aged and elderly individuals (Fig. 12.19). They are frequently asymptomatic although heel pain may result from a coincidental plantar fasciitis, Achilles tendinitis or from a painful heel pad.

Treatment in all these conditions consists of weight reduction in obese patients, a period of rest, hot soaks, NSAIDs and reducing patient's weight-bearing pressure by using a soft rubber heel pad, cushion, mold

CAUSES OF PAIN ABOUT THE HEEL
Achilles tendinitis
Achilles bursitis: Retrocalcaneal Retroachillial
Subcalcaneal (infracalcaneal) bursitis
Plantar fasciitis
Enthesitis (enthesopathy) due to ankylosing spondylitis, Reiter's disease, psoriatic arthritis or sarcoidosis
Painful calcaneal fat pad
Painful plantar and dorsal calcaneal spurs
Bone (calcaneal) lesions: Exostosis Fracture Infection Neoplasm Calcaneal epiphysitis (Sever's disease)
Subtalar arthritis: e.g. RA, gout
Tarsal tunnel syndrome

Fig. 12.18 Causes of pain about the heel.

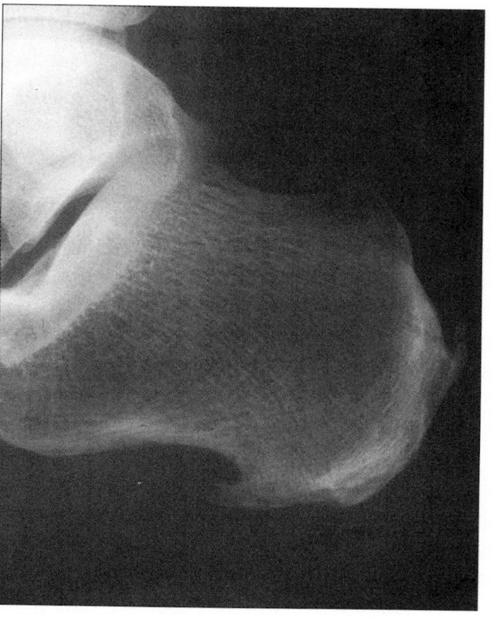

Fig. 12.19 Plantar calcaneal spur.

orthosis or heel cup, and wearing sponge-rubber heeled shoes[30–35]. Doughnut-hole heel pads cushion and unload the tender medial calcaneal tuberosity of the heel in plantar fasciitis. Heel cups are used in patients with painful subcalcaneal pad in order to cushion and contain the heel fat pad[33]. Orthoses are employed to correct pes planus and forefoot pronation, thus decreasing tension on the plantar fascia[33]. Stretching of the plantar fascia, by leaning forward against a wall while keeping the heel flat on the ground, is beneficial. Local injections of corticosteroids and an anesthetic are often helpful. Plantar fascia release and/or spur resection is rarely indicated in patients with refractory plantar fasciitis[32–35,37].

ARCH DISORDERS

Flat feet (pes planus)

Flattening of the longitudinal arch, or flat foot, is often asymptomatic but may result in muscle fatigue with aching and intolerance due to long hours of standing or walking[38,39]. The normal gait begins with the heel strike at the onset of stance followed by a supple period where the foot pronates (everts) and becomes more flat with weight bearing along its lateral border. As the weight gradually moves forward to the metatarsal heads, the foot supinates (inverts) during terminal stance heel rise, becomes more rigid and toe-off is completed[3,4]. If in the flat foot position the longitudinal arch is flat on standing, but reforms as the patient goes up on the toes, the foot is functioning relatively normally and there is often no pain. Pain usually results from unaccustomed physical activity, weight gain or from faulty footwear causing ligamentous strain.

Physical findings include loss of the medial longitudinal arch on weight bearing with medial and plantar displacement of the navicular and the talar head[38,39]. In severe cases, the calcaneus is everted (valgus) and the forefoot is abducted with ‘too many toes’ when viewed from behind. A callosity often develops over the prominent talar head. Marked wear of the soles of the shoes along the inner side is characteristic. In chronic pes planus deformity, secondary changes are common in the tarsal bones, spring and plantar ligaments and the Achilles and tibial tendons. Radiographic findings include flattening of the longitudinal arch on weight bearing (lateral view) with medial and downward displacement of the talar head.

Flat foot may be congenital or acquired. Congenital flat foot is more common and may be hypermobile or rigid. In the hypermobile or flaccid flat foot, the longitudinal arch is depressed with weight bearing and assumes a normal contour when the weight is removed. The subtalar and midtarsal joints are hypermobile and the Achilles tendon may be short. Other members of the same family may be affected. The deformity becomes manifest in childhood but pain and fatigue on walking or standing may not develop until adolescence or adulthood.

In the rigid flat foot, there is abnormal bridging between the talus and calcaneus or between the navicular and calcaneus (tarsal coalition). The union may be fibrous, cartilaginous or osseous. The medial longitudinal arch is absent in all positions, subtalar movement is limited and spasm of the peroneal muscles may be present. CT scans are particularly useful in delineating the location, extent and nature of the abnormal fusion[40]. Tarsal coalition usually becomes symptomatic in the second or third decade of life, and is often refractory to drugs and orthotics.

Acquired causes of flat foot include hypermobility syndromes, RA, neuropathic arthropathy and trauma. Excessive weight, faulty footwear, muscle fatigue and bad walking habits, superimposed on congenital hypermobile flat foot of a mild degree, may also result in static flat foot in adult life. The tibialis posterior tendon is one of the main dynamic stabilizers of the hindfoot against valgus (eversion) deformity. Chronic tenosynovitis and rupture of the tendon in obese, middle-aged women produces a painful, progressive asymmetric flat foot deformity or ‘collapsed foot’, often associated with hindfoot valgus (planovalgus deformity) and forefoot pronation[15,22,41–43]. Typically, the patient has difficulty standing on the tiptoes and ball of the afflicted foot while the contralateral foot is off the ground (positive single heel rise test).

Acquired flat foot may be classified as flexible, spastic or rigid. In the flexible (flaccid or mobile) type, the longitudinal arch is depressed only with weight bearing. If left untreated, peroneal muscle spasm may occur, producing a ‘spastic’ flat foot with spasm and tenderness of the peroneal muscles and tendons, and painful limitation of inversion. The rigid acquired flat foot is an end stage with the collapsed foot firmly fixed in eversion (hyperpronated foot).

No treatment is indicated for the asymptomatic flat foot. Pain and impaired function are indications for treatment. A soft orthotic, such as a polyethylene-foam-lined arch support, often produces symptomatic relief. If pain and deformity are severe, a hard plastic orthotic or Whitmans arch support is indicated but is often not well tolerated in the long term. Exercises to strengthen the intrinsic invertor muscles and properly fitting shoes with a Thomas heel or quarter inch wedge on the inner border of the heel to throw the weight on the outer border are often helpful. For the hyperpronated foot, a semirigid, well-molded orthotic device is often indicated. In patients with chronic tibialis posterior tenosynovitis, NSAIDs and longitudinal arch orthotic devices are often helpful, but cast immobilization or surgical decompression of the tendon sheath may be required[15,41]. If tendon rupture has occurred, early repair using a tendon transfer (flexor digitorum longus or flexor hallucis longus) may be possible[15,41,42]. In chronic pes planus deformity with collapse of the foot and advanced subtalar arthritis, a subtalar arthrodesis is the surgical treatment of choice. In tarsal coalition, resection of the bridging bar, with soft tissue interposition, is the preferred surgical treatment.

The cavus foot (pes cavus)

Pes cavus, or claw foot, is characterized by an unusually high medial arch[39]. In severe cases, there is shortening of the foot, plantar ligaments and extensor tendons, and clawing of the toes with calluses under the metatarsal heads.

Pes cavus is usually an hereditary condition, but may occur in patients with poliomyelitis, Friedreich’s ataxia, spina bifida or idiopathic scoliosis[44]. It is often asymptomatic but can cause foot fatigue and discomfort, particularly in runners and distance walkers. Talonavicular motion is impaired and the foot does not normally pronate (evert) after the heel strike, resulting in poor shock absorption and pain in the arch.

Shoe modification to accommodate the high instep and claw toes, metatarsal pads with cushioned high arch supports, and stretching exercises of the toe extensors are usually helpful[39]. In severe progressive deformity, surgical correction by tarsal and metatarsal osteotomies and plantar fasciotomy is indicated. An orthotic device is used postoperatively.

FOREFOOT DISORDERS

Metatarsalgia

During walking, weight is borne mainly on the first metatarsal head, secondarily on the fifth and to a lesser degree on the second, third and fourth. Each metatarsal head thus forms a fixed fulcrum about which the flexor tendon is angulated when the heel is raised off the ground and the toe dorsiflexed before the 'toe-off'[3–5]. During the 'toe-off' movement of a step, the intrinsic muscles flex the toes and help to elevate the central metatarsal heads off the ground, thus relieving them of pressure. Weakness of these muscles results in metatarsalgia with clawed toes, dropped metatarsal heads and the inevitable plantar calluses.

Metatarsalgia, or pain and tenderness in and about the metatarsal heads or MTP joints, may either be limited to a single joint or generalized across the ball of the foot[45–47]. Pain in the forefoot on standing and walking, and tenderness on palpation of the metatarsal heads and sometimes the MTP joints, are the main clinical findings. Prominent, dropped central metatarsal heads, plantar calluses and clawed toes are frequently present[45–47]. Metatarsalgia is a relatively common symptom of diverse causes. The condition often follows years of disuse and weakness of the intrinsic muscles due to chronic foot strain from improper foot wear with the toes cramped into tight or pointed shoes. Other causes include attrition of plantar fat pad in elderly individuals, plantar callosities, plantar plate rupture with secondary MTP joint (usually the second) instability[48], altered foot biomechanics due to flat, splay or cavus foot, hallux valgus, hallux rigidus, arthritis of the MTP joints, intermetatarsophalangeal bursitis, trauma, osteochrondritis of the second metatarsal head (Freiberg's disease), stress fractures, sesamoiditis, previous forefoot surgery, tarsal tunnel syndrome, interdigital (Morton's) neuroma, hemiplegia and arterial insufficiency including Buerger's disease[45–47].

Morton's interdigital neuroma

This is usually unilateral and is most common in middle-aged women (see Chapter 4.16). It often results from chronic foot strain and repetitive trauma caused by inappropriate fitting shoes, or from mechanical foot problems such as pronated flat foot and pes cavus[49,50]. It represents an entrapment neuropathy (rather than a true neuroma) of an interdigital nerve, typically between the third and fourth, and less frequently between the second and third metatarsal heads. The nerve is entrapped under the transverse metatarsal ligament causing perineurial fibrosis[49–51]. An intermetatarsophalangeal bursa or synovial cyst may also cause compression of the nerve. Typical symptoms include paroxysms of lancinating, burning or neuralgic pain in the affected interdigital clefts, and occasionally paresthesia or anesthesia of contiguous borders of adjacent toes[49–51]. Relief of pain when the shoe is removed and the foot is massaged is characteristic. Walking on hard surfaces or wearing tight or high-heeled shoes increases the discomfort. The metatarsal arch is often depressed and tenderness is present over the entrapped nerve between the third and fourth metatarsal heads. Altered sensation may be found on the lateral aspect of the third toe and the medial aspect of the fourth toe. A soft mass (neuroma) may be palpable between the metatarsal heads, and movements of the adjacent toes may produce a clicking sensation produced by extrusion of the neuroma from between the metatarsal heads[50]. The affected nerve may show slow sensory conduction velocity on electrophysiologic testing. The exact location and extent of the lesion can sometimes be determined by sonography or MRI[11].

Symptomatic treatment of metatarsalgia includes a soft or firm metatarsal pad placed proximal to the metatarsal heads, weight reduction in obese patients, strengthening of the intrinsic muscles by toe flexion exercises, and shoe alteration, including a wide toebox and, in patients with a pronated foot, an arch support[45–47]. If these measures fail, metatarsal osteotomy and/or metatarsal head resection are indicated. In Morton's neuroma, nonoperative measures, including proper footwear, metatarsal pad and local corticosteroid injections delivered from the dorsal aspect into the intermetatarsal space, are often helpful[49–52]. Surgical excision of the neuroma (interdigital neurectomy), epineurolysis or simple division of the transverse metatarsal ligament are required in refractory cases[49–52].

Sesamoiditis

The sesamoids provide an articulating surface under the first metatarsal head and a fulcrum that increases the strength of the muscle pull (3,4). If a runner runs entirely on the balls of the foot or a dancer jumps on the metatarsals without the smooth gliding heel-to-toe mechanism, the articular surface between the sesamoids and the first metatarsal head may be damaged resulting in chrondromalacia or osteoarthritis. The area becomes painful and inflamed, a condition referred to as sesamoiditis[12,45–47]. Treatment consists of shifting the weight elsewhere by means of a soft metatarsal support, rest, activity modification and NSAIDs. In patients with severe disability sesamoidectomy may be required[12,45–47].

Metatarsal stress fracture

Metatarsal stress (or march) fractures, commonly affect the neck or shaft of the second metatarsal[45–47]. There is often a history of prolonged use of the foot, such as a strenuous marching in recruits, hiking, distance running or dancing[12] (fatigue fractures). Fractures may also occur in patients with RA, osteoporosis or other metabolic bone disease (insufficiency fractures).

The patient complains of pain in the metatarsal area on weight bearing in the absence of a clear history of trauma. The dorsum of the foot is edematous, and tenderness is localized to the affected metatarsal. Stress fractures may not be visible on radiographs for 2–6 weeks, and bone scanning or CT are sometimes required for correct diagnosis. Management consists of rest, a stiff-soled shoe and avoidance of stress-provoking activities until healing occurs. Plantar padding and strapping of the foot, or cast immobilization, may occasionally be required[45–47].

Toe deformities

Hallus valgus

Hallux valgus is commonly associated with medial deviation and splaying of the first metatarsal (metatarsus primus varus) with an increased intermetatarsal angle >9° [53,54] (see Fig. 12.9). It is often asymptomatic but pain may arise from improper footwear, bursitis over the medial aspect of the first MTP joint (bunion) or secondary osteoarthritis. As the first metatarsal moves into varus at its joint with the first cuneiform, its head also moves dorsally resulting in a transfer of weight to the second metatarsal head. This is known as 'transfer lesion'. Altered weight bearing results in a callosity under the second metatarsal head with a hammer toe deformity, and a flattened transverse metatarsal arch. If the deformity is marked, the great toe may overlie or underlie the second toe and the sesamoids are displaced laterally[53,54].

Hallux valgus is more common in women and may be caused by a genetic predisposition aggravated by wearing short, narrow, high-heeled or pointed shoes. Other causes include congenital splay foot deformity, and arthritis of the first MTP joint due to RA or osteoarthritis. The severity of the deformity and its progression over time can be assessed radiographically by measuring the hallux valgus angle between the first metatarsal and first proximal phalanx[55]. Management consists of shoe correction to accommodate the bunion, a bunion pad and, in the presence of a transfer lesion, a metatarsal pad. Surgical correction (osteotomy of the first metatarsal base, resection of metatarsal head and/or base of proximal phalanx and realignment of the sesamoids) is indicated in patients with severe deformity and intractable pain[53,54].

Hallux rigidus

Hallux rigidus is characterized by intermittent aching pain and marked restriction of movement at the first MTP joint[45–47,56]. The joint may be tender and there is crepitus, osteophytic lipping, and painful limitation of movement, particularly toe dorsiflexion. It usually occurs in elderly patients with osteoarthritis. A primary type is seen in younger persons, and the condition may follow repetitive trauma as in ballet dancing[12]. The 'toe-off' is accomplished by the outer four toes and the distal phalanx of the great toe, thereby bypassing and protecting the first MTP joint from painful dorsiflexion[56]. Calluses often develop beneath the second, third and fourth metatarsal heads. In advanced stages, the first MTP joint becomes completely rigid in slight plantar flexion.

Management consists of a stiff-soled shoe with a wide toebox, and a bar across the metatarsal heads to allow walking with little movement at the first MTP joint. Intra-articular corticosteroid injections may produce temporary relief (see Chapter 2.12). In patients with severe pain and disability, arthrodesis or arthroplasty of the first MTP joint is indicated [56].

Bunionette

A bunionette (tailor's bunion) is an adventitious bursa developing over a prominent, laterally-deviated fifth metatarsal head (metatarsus quintus valgus) and a medially-deviated fifth toe[45–47,57,58]. It often occurs in conjunction with hallux valgus or splay foot deformity. Shoe modification and a bunion pad are often helpful but medial displacement fifth metatarsal osteotomy[57] or resection of the metatarsal prominence may be necessary[57,58].

Hammer toe

Hammer toe deformity most commonly affects the second toe. It is characterized by flexion deformity of the PIP joint, usually associated with dorsiflexion of the MTP and DIP joints[59] (see Fig. 12.10). A painful corn often develops over the dorsal prominence of the PIP joint. Ill-fitting footwear, particularly narrow high-heeled, pointed toed shoes is the leading mechanism. Other causes include congenital hammer toe deformity, trauma, RA or other forms of arthritis.

Nonoperative treatment includes a corn pad, and use of roomy shoes with a high, wide toebox and soft leather uppers. Surgical arthrodesis is indicated in patients with severe deformity[59].

REFERENCES

1. Fam AG. The ankle and foot. In: Little AH, ed. The rheumatological physical examination. Grune & Stratton: Orlando;1986:121–9.
2. Polley HF, Hunder GG. The ankle and foot. In: Polley HF, Hunder GG, eds. Physical examination of the joints, 2E. Philadelphia: WB Saunders; 1978:239–74.
3. Mann RA. Biomechanics of the foot. In: Gould JS, ed. The foot book. Baltimore: Williams & Wilkins; 1988:48–63.
4. Perry J. Anatomy and biomechanics of the hindfoot. Clin Orthop. 1983;177:9–15.
5. Sarrafian SK. Anatomy of the foot and ankle: descriptive, topographic, functional, 2E, Philadelphia: Lippincott. 1993:616 pages.
6. Gibbons RB. 'Last' bursitis: a second location. Arthritis Rheum.1980;23:872–3.
7. Hartmann. The tendon sheaths and synovial bursae of the foot. Foot Ankle. 1981;1(5):247–69.
8. Aviles E, Arlen M, Miller T. Plantar fibromatosis. Surgery 1971;69:117–120.
9. Raymakers R. The painful foot. Practitioner. 1975;215:61–8.
10. Ritchie GW, Keim HA. Major foot deformities. Their classification and x-ray analysis. J Can Assoc Radiol. 1968;19:155–66.
11. Roberts DK, Pomeranz SJ. Current status of magnetic resonance in radiologic diagnosis of foot and ankle injuries. Orthop Clin N Am. 1994;25(1):61–8.
12. Quirk R. Common foot and ankle injuries in dance. Orthop Clin N Am. 1994;25(1):123–33.
13. Fernandez-Palazzi F, Rivas S, Mujica P. Achilles tendinitis in ballet dancers. Clin Orthop. 1990;257:257–61.
14. Clement DB, Taunton JE, Smart GW. Achilles tendinitis and peritendinitis: etiology and treatment. Am J Sports Med. 1984;12(3):179–84.
15. Plattner PF. Tendon problems of the foot and ankle. Postgrad Med. 1989;86:155–70.
16. Scioli MW. Achilles tendinitis. Orthop Clin N Am. 1994;25(1):177–82.
17. Klemp P, Halland AM, Majoos FL, Steyn K. Musculoskeletal manifestations in hyperlipidaemia: a controlled study. Ann Rheum Dis. 1993;52:44–8.
18. Dussault RG, Kaplan PA, Roederer G. MR imaging of Achilles tendon in patients with familial hyperlipidemia: comparison with plain films, physical examination, and patients with traumatic tendon lesions. Am J Roentgenol. 1995;164:403–7.
19. Kainberger FM, Engel A, Barton P, Huebsch P, Neuhold A, Salomonowitz E. Injury of the Achilles tendon: diagnosis with sonography. Am J Roentgenol. 1990;155:1031–6.
20. O'Reilly MAR, Massouh H. Pictorial review: the sonographic diagnosis of pathology in the Achilles tendon. Clin Radiol. 1993;48:202–6.
21. DaCruz DJ, Geeson M, Allen MJ, Phair I. Achilles paratendinitis: an evaluation of steroid injection. Br J Sports Med. 1988;22(2):64–5.
22. Fleming LL. Tendinitis and bursitis. In: Gould JS, ed. The foot book. Baltimore: Williams & Wilkins; 1988:303–12.
23. Stephens MM. Haglund's deformity and retrocalcaneal bursitis. Orthop Clinic N Am. 1994;25(1):41–6.
24. Canoso JJ, Liu N, Traill MR, Runge VM. Physiology of the retrocalcaneal bursa. Ann Rheum Dis. 1988;47:910–12.
25. Canoso JJ, Wohlgethan JR, Newberg AH, Goldsmith MR. Aspiration of the retrocalcaneal bursa. Ann Rheum Dis. 1984;43:308–12.
26. Jozsa L, Kvist M, Balint BJ, Reffy A, *et al.* The role of recreational sport activity in Achilles tendon rupture. A clinical, pathoanatomical, and sociological study of 292 cases. Am J Sports Med. 1989;17(3):338–43.
27. Keene JS, Lash EG, Fisher DR, DeSmet AA. Magnetic resonance imaging of Achilles tendon rupture. Am J Sports Med. 1989;17(3):333–7
28. Ribard P, Andisio F, Kahn M-F, *et al.* Seven Achilles tendinitis including 3 complicated by rupture during fluoroquinolone therapy. J Rheumatol 1992;19:1479–81.
29. Szarfman A, Chen M, Blum MD. More on fluoroquinolone antibiotics and tendon rupture. N Engl J Med (Letter). 1995;332(3):193.
30. Furey JG. Plantar fasciitis. The painful heel

syndrome. J Bone Joint Surg. 1975;57(A):672–3
31. Hill Jr JJ, Cutting PJ. Heel pain and body weight. Foot Ankle 1989;9(5):254–6.
32. Karr SD. Subcalcaneal heel pain. Orthop Clinic N Am. 1994;25(1):161–75.
33. Schepsis AA, Leach RE, Gorzyca J. Plantar fasciitis: etiology, treatment, surgical results and review of the literature. Clin Orthop 1991;266:185–96.
34. Prichasuk S, Subhadrabandhu T. The relationship of pes planus and calcaneal spur to plantar heel pain. Clin Orthop. 1994;306:192–6.
35. Gibbon WW, Cassar-Pullicino VN. Heel pain. Ann Rheum Dis. 1994;53:344–8.
36. Berkowitz JF, Kier R, Rudicel S. Plantar fasciitis: MR imaging. Radiology. 1991;179:665–7.
37. Lester DK, Buchanan JR. Surgical treatment of plantar fasciitis. Clin Orthop. 1984;186:202–4.
38. Penneau K, Lutter L, Winter R. Pes planus: radiographic changes with foot orthoses and shoes. Foot Ankle. 1982;2:299–310.
39. The foot and the ankle. In: Turek SL, ed. Orthopedics: Principles and their application, 4E. JB Philadelphia: Lippincott; 1984;1407–82.
40. Deutsch AL, Resnick D, Campbell G. Computed tomography and bone scintigraphy in the evaluation of tarsal coalition. Radiology. 1982;144:137–40.
41. Johnson KA. Tibialis posterior tendon rupture. Clin Orthop. 1983;177:140–7.
42. Mann RA, Thompson FM. Rupture of the posterior tibial tendon causing flat foot. Surgical treatment. J Bone Joint Surg. 1985;67A:556–61.
43. Karasick D, Schweitzer ME. Tear of the posterior tibial tendon causing asymmetric flatfoot: radiographic findings. Am J Roentgenol. 1993;161:1237–40.
44. Carpintero P, Entrenas R, Gonzalez I, Garcia E, Mesa M. The relationship between pes cavus and idiopathic scoliosis. Spine. 1994;19:1260–3.
45. Mann RA. Metatarsalgia. Postgrad Med. 1984;75(5):150–67.
46. Scranton PE. Metatarsalgia: diagnosis and treatment. J Bone Joint Surg. 1980;62(A):723–32.
47. Gould JS. Metatarsalgia. Orthop Clin N Am. 1989;20:553–62.
48. Yao L, Do HM, Cracchiolo A, Farahani K. Plantar plate of the foot: findings on conventional arthrography and MR imaging. Am J Roentgenol. 1994;163:641–4.
49. Morris MA. Morton's metatarsalgia. Clin Orthop. 1977;127: 203–7.
50. Cameron B, Bennett G. Relieving the pain of Morton's neuroma. J Musculoskelet Med. 1995;12(6):14–23.
51. Ha'Eri GB, Fornasier VL, Schatzker J . Morton' s neuroma – pathogenesis and ultrastructure. Clin Orthop. 1979;141:256–9.
52. Greenfield J, Rea J, Ilfeld FW. Morton's interdigital neuroma. Indications for treatment by local injections versus surgery. Clin Orthop. 1984;185:142–4.
53. Inman VT . Hallux valgus: a review of etiologic factors. Orthop Clin N Am. 1974;5(1):59–66.
54. Coughlin MJ. Hallux valgus: causes, evaluation and treatment. Postgrad Med. 1984;75(5):174–87.
55. Budiman-Mak E, Roach KE, Stuck R, Spencer F, Polizos T, Conrad KJ. Radiographic measurement of hallux valgus in the rheumatoid arthritic foot. J Rheumatol. 1994;21:623–6.
56. Bingold AC, Collins DH. Hallux rigidus. J Bone Joint Surg. 1950;32(B):214–27.
57. Kitaoka HB, Leventen EO. Medical displacement metatarsal osteotomy for treatment of painful bunionette. Clin Orthop. 1989;243:172–9.
58. Karasick D. Preoperative assessment of symptomatic bunionette deformity: radiologic findings. Am J Roentgenol. 1995;164:147–9.
59. Coughlin MJ. Mallet toes, hammer toes, claw toes, and corns. Causes and treatment of lesser toe deformities. Postgrad Med.1984;75(5):191–8.

13

TEMPOROMANDIBULAR PAIN SYNDROME

David M Adlam

Definition

- Acute or chronic musculoskeletal pain with dysfunction of the masticatory system.
- Pain aggravated by jaw movements.
- Pain localized to temporomandibular joint and masticatory muscles, but may be associated with other joint pains.
- Independent of local oral and dental disease.

Clinical features

- Unilateral or bilateral joint pain with movement, worse when chewing.
- Joint stiffness and trismus.
- Joint may swing to the affected side on opening.
- Joint noises, clicking with dysfunction or internal derangement and crepitus with degenerative disease.
- Intermittent or persistent locking.
- Parafunctional habit, e.g. nail biting.
- Masticatory muscle tenderness.
- Headaches often present.

HISTORY

The temporomandibular pain syndrome (TMPS) is most commonly seen in young people, being one of the most frequently encountered types of pain in the head and neck, after headache and toothache. The syndrome of temporomandibular joint pain is associated with muscle tenderness, limited or deviated joint movement, joint noises and headache. It has been described by many names[1–11], alternative terminology including Costen's syndrome, temporomandibular pain dysfunction syndrome, craniomandibular dysfunction, psychogenic facial pain, myofascial pain and facial arthromyalgia. TMPS has many features of fibromyalgia (see Chapter 4.15, Fig. 15.1) where there is muscle pain with no obvious pathologic cause.

A distinction should be made between the different types of temporomandibular joint pain. Osteoarthritis presents in the fourth decade onwards with crepitus and pain localized to the joint. Internal derangement may present at any age, with a characteristic click of the joint if the meniscus is reducible and loss of the click with restricted opening when locked. Both osteoarthritis and internal derangement may be a result of chronic TMPS.

The first consultation is particularly important, not only to establish a thorough history and physical examination, but to gain a good rapport with the patient. It has been shown that a good doctor–patient relationship affects the success of treatment of facial pain[12,13]. It is not unusual for the patient to have been seen by several specialists with no cause found for the pain.

EPIDEMIOLOGY

Temporomandibular joint disorders are common, but not always reported by the patient [1–9]. The percentage of the population with signs is 50–75%, and the percentage with symptoms is only 20–25%. However, only 3–4% seek treatment.

The prevalence of symptoms between the sexes is similar, but 5:1 more females than males present for treatment.

CLINICAL FEATURES

Pain on mandibular movement is the main complaint in TMPS. The pain is usually chronic but may present acutely. The pain is described as a constant dull ache, which is worse on chewing, especially on chewing hard foods. When asked to localize the pain, the side of the face and cheek are often demonstrated, rarely the temporomandibular joint itself. The pain may radiate and this usually relates to the muscle groups affected by the associated muscle spasm. TMPS is more often seen unilaterally, the associated muscle spasm resulting in the deviation of the mandible to the affected side.

The patient is generally aware of a limitation of movement which is associated with the stiffness of the joint. This is often worse in the morning, especially if there is a history of nocturnal clenching of the teeth. Noises from the temporomandibular joint are common and described variously as clicking, popping or grinding. The noises may be easily audible to the examiner. Clicking may vary from day to day and even be absent at times. A loss of clicking and subsequent limitation of movement indicates displacement of the meniscus.

Locking may be a confusing term for the patient. It is a result of the disc displacement allowing only very limited opening. The patient may describe this as a jamming or dislocation of the joint. It usually occurs when the teeth are slightly apart during opening or closing of the mouth. This is very distressing to the patient should they be unable to overcome the lock. It may last a few seconds, spontaneously resolve or be overcome by the patient. Lateral movements of the jaw on opening with pressure over the joint may overcome the lock.

There are numerous associated problems seen in TMPS (Fig. 13.1) but the patient rarely volunteers the problems. They must be specifically enquired for. Habits such as bruxism, nail biting and cheek biting exacerbate both the pain and the muscle spasm. Stress-related problems are invariably present. Tension headaches with a pressure sensation

HISTORY AND CARDINAL FEATURES OF TMPS
History
Multiple specialist consultations for facial pain Stress-related problems Anxiety, depression Headache Pain in the neck, back and abdomen Disturbed sleep pattern Multiple previous treatments including alternative medicine Habits – nail biting, bruxism
Pain
Constant, dull, aching but can be severe with movement Masticatory muscle tenderness
Joint
Stiffness in the morning or end of the day Limitation of opening with deviation Locking Joint noises, clicking and popping

Fig. 13.1 History and cardinal features of TMPS.

over the top of the head and down the neck may be a daily occurrence. The headache may respond to simple analgesia but the dull ache in the jaw continues.

There is often a history of recent dental and ear, nose and throat (ENT) consultations, which will have revealed no abnormalities. The wisdom teeth may be suspected but are rarely a contributing factor in the pain. Many associated features are similar to those seen in fibromyalgia (see Chapter 4.15).

Emotional and stress-related problems may coincide with the onset of the pain. In the school-age group, problems of examinations, friendships and sibling rivalry are factors. Problems related to housing, work and marriage are seen in the older age group. Chronic ill health, post-traumatic stress disorder, bereavement and loneliness are other factors.

PHYSICAL EXAMINATION

The physical examination must be carefully recorded, since it is not only helpful in reaching a diagnosis and the formulation of a treatment plan but also invaluable in the monitoring of treatment success[1–12]. The physical examination of the joint and associated structures should aim to reproduce the symptoms.

EXTRA-ORAL EXAMINATION

First the joint itself must be examined. Look for any visible swelling. Palpation of the joint may reveal tenderness overlying the joint. A finger is placed in both the external auditory meati and the patient asked to open, close and protrude the mandible (Fig. 13.2). Clicking or joint noises during these movements should be noted, along with any deviation of movement. Biting on a wooden spatula or hard wax, either unilaterally or bilaterally, may stop the click or relieve the pain. Auscultation of the joint may confirm any clicking.

The muscles should then be examined. The masseter can be palpated bilaterally, with the fingers over the angle of the mandible (Fig. 13.3). Tenderness may be detected at rest or when the jaw is clenched. Additionally, a finger may be placed inside the mouth to bimanually palpate the muscle at rest or under tension (Fig. 13.4). Differences may be detected between the two sides.

The temporalis muscle covers a wide area over the temple. The whole area of the muscle should be palpated with the jaw relaxed and then clenched (Fig. 13.5). The patient may help to locate the area of tenderness.

The medial pterygoid is difficult to examine as it lies medial to the ramus of the mandible. The posterior border may be palpated extra-orally by placing the fingers around the posterior border of the ramus of the mandible. It can also be examined intra-orally by placing a finger on the medial ramus of the mandible (Fig. 13.6), but this often produces a gag-reflex, making interpretation difficult.

The lateral pterygoid is examined by standing behind the patient and placing the palm of the hand over the chin. The patient is then asked to open gently against resistance (Fig. 13.7) and then to move the jaw laterally. The lateral pterygoid can also be palpated intra-orally in a cooperative patient. The muscles of the neck and shoulder may require examination. The ear should be examined with an otoscope if indicated.

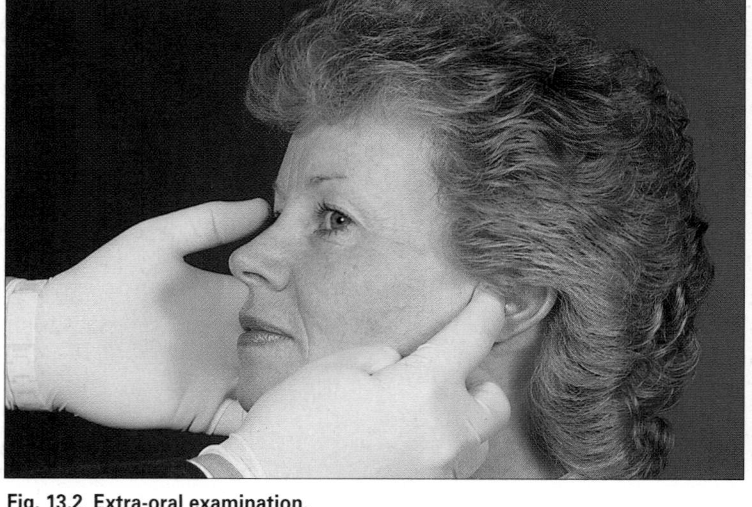

Fig. 13.2 Extra-oral examination.

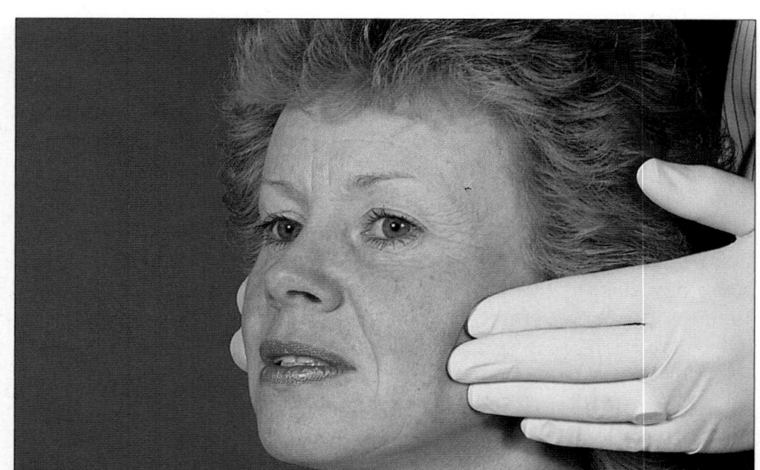

Fig. 13.3 Bilateral palpation of masseters.

Fig. 13.4 Bimanual palpation of masseter.

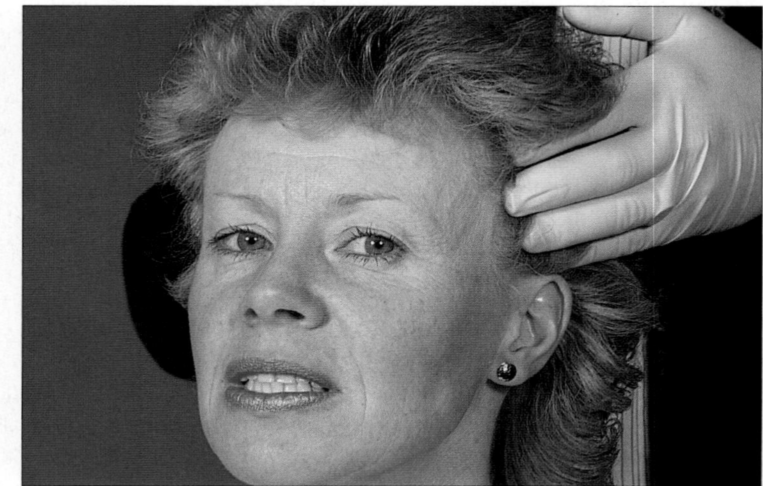

Fig. 13.5 Palpation of temporalis.

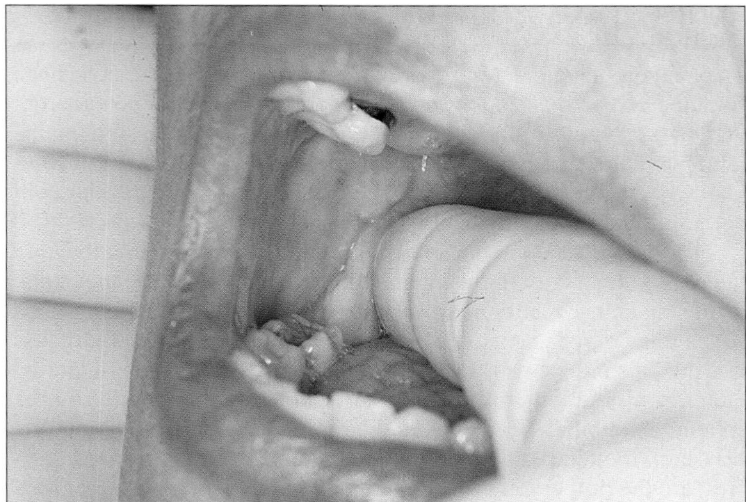

Fig. 13.6 Intra oral examination of medial pterygoid.

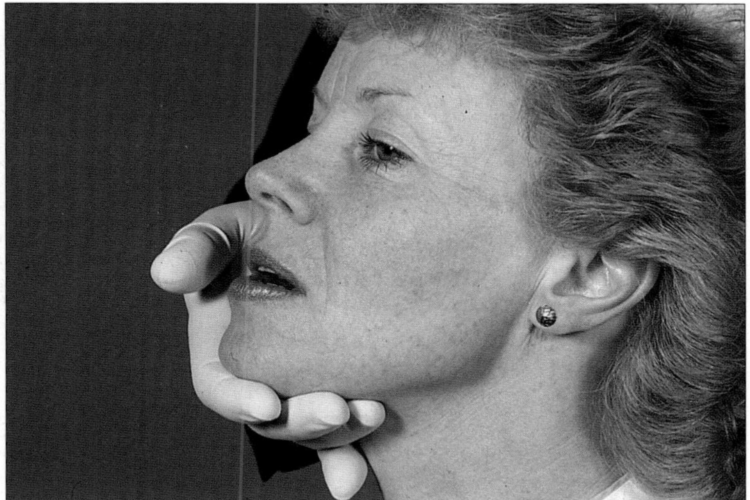

Fig. 13.7 Examination of lateral pterygoid.

INTRA-ORAL EXAMINATION

The movement of the jaw can be measured actively, with the patient opening the mouth, or passively, the jaw being manipulated by the examiner. The degree of opening is recorded for subsequent monitoring of treatment. The inter-incisor opening is measured which is normally 34–44mm.

Mouth opening should be straight. Any swing or deviations should be noted. The dental occlusion should be examined and recorded.

Active protrusion of the mandible should be measured and is normally up to 10mm. Lateral movements of the mandible should be equidistant from the midline and can be measured by asking the patient to move the jaw from side to side, with the teeth held lightly together. Lateral movement is normally in the region of 10mm to each side.

A simple examination of the teeth, noting any carious teeth, premature contacts, restorations and dentures, is required. The attrition of the teeth may be an indication of a grinding habit and a full occlusal analysis may be indicated. Cheek biting and scalloping of the lateral border of the tongue due to pressure against the teeth is often seen in TMPS.

INVESTIGATIONS

Investigations of the TMPS may be divided firstly into those aiming to exclude causes of pain outside the joint complex, and secondly into those specific investigations of the temporomandibular joint itself[11]. The majority of TMPS patients do not need complex investigation. The result of most investigations are negative in TMPS, but are helpful in osteoarthritis and with internal joint derangement. At the initial consultation an Orthopantogram (OPG) is useful to exclude pain which may be arising within the teeth and jaws. Periapical radiographs are needed if problems with specific teeth are suspected. The OPG allows a view of the temporomandibular joints but this should be interpreted with caution, as only gross changes may be seen.

Plain radiographs of the joints help to exclude osteoarthritis as a cause of the pain. In this respect transcranial views, open and closed, or transpharyngeal views (as described by Toller) are the most useful.

Tomography of the temporomandibular joints in two planes gives excellent detail of the joint surfaces but is rarely required in TMPS, in which the joint surfaces are usually normal. Sinus radiographs are useful to exclude sinus pathology as a cause of the pain.

Computer tomography (CT) and magnetic resonance imaging are the most sensitive noninvasive techniques available at present. Three-dimensional reconstruction allows detailed joint images to be produced. In a minority of patients, where internal derangement of the meniscus is suspected, this can be useful. Views of the joint, open and closed, clearly demonstrate the position and state of the meniscus.

Arthrography gives the best dynamic information on the temporomandibular joint, but is invasive. This is again useful where internal derangements are suspected, notably anterior displacement of the meniscus.

Arthroscopy of the temporomandibular joint has rapidly developed due to the availability of small diameter arthroscopes [14]. This procedure is best performed under general anesthesia, but may be performed under local anesthesia with sedation.

Electromyographic studies of the muscles of mastication are not widely available but demonstrate well the levels of muscular activity and the incoordination of muscle movements. Local anesthetic blocks of the temporomandibular joint are occasionally useful in confirming the source of the pain.

DIFFERENTIAL DIAGNOSIS

Facial pain is frequently complex and from more than one source. For example, TMPS and atypical facial pain may be seen together. The range of facial pains is large, some being very specific, such as giant cell arteritis and trigeminal neuralgia, others less so, such as TMPS and tension headache.

The following should be considered in the differential diagnosis of facial pain.

ATYPICAL FACIAL PAIN

This is a dull aching pain or, occasionally, a sharp pain, most commonly felt over the cheeks. It affects the nonmuscular parts of the face and may occur unilaterally or bilaterally. It is chronic in nature with no provoking or relieving factors. Analgesia has little effect. The pain may be worse at times of stress. A history of ENT and dental examinations with treatment is often found, with the latter resulting in no relief from the pain.

TRIGEMINAL NEURALGIA

Trigeminal neuralgia is a severe lancing pain in the face which lasts only a few seconds. It is characteristically provoked by stimulating a trigger zone. The pain is localized, most commonly in the mandibular or maxillary branches of the trigeminal nerve. Pain relief with carbamazepine may be considered diagnostic.

GIANT CELL ARTERITIS

Giant cell arteritis causes a severe throbbing pain, usually in the temporal region but which may involve any branch of the external carotid artery. The area is painful and tender to touch. Mastication may also be painful. There may be associated visual symptoms. The condition is more common in the elderly. A finding of raised erythrocyte sedimentation rate aids diagnosis (see Chapter 7.21).

OSTEOARTHRITIS

The pain in osteoarthritis is localized to the joint and is worse on movement with grinding noises. It is more commonly found after the fourth decade, but may affect any age group. The onset may be sudden, producing a constant dull aching pain with limitation in the range of jaw movements. However, unlike TMPS, the pain is localized to the joint that is tender and there is rarely associated muscle spasm.

Pain from degenerative joint disease of the cervical spine may also present as facial pain (see Chapter 4.4).

RHEUMATOID AND PSORIATIC ARTHRITIS

The temporomandibular joint although often affected by rheumatoid and psoriatic arthritis causes symptoms in only a minority of patients. Joint tenderness and stiffness are most frequently seen. But in severe disease there is destruction of the joint surface with pain, stiffness, crepitations and anterior open bite (AOB). An AOB is the inability to bite the front teeth together due to the loss of the height of the mandibular condyle.

STILL'S DISEASE

In Still's disease (see Chapter 5.22 and Prevention and Management of Developmental Abnormalities of the Lower Jaw in Chapter 5.16) the temporomandibular joint is affected in approximately 50% of cases. It is very destructive of the temporomandibular joints producing secondary effects in the dental occlusion such as anterior open bite.

FIBROMYALGIA

TMPS and fibromyalgia overlap (see Chapter 4.15) and present a similar constellation of signs and symptoms. There are many similar concomitant problems such as irritable bowel and depression. Management is also similar to TMPS (see Chapter 4.15).

SALIVARY GLANDS

The pain is localized to the affected salivary gland and is worse with eating, particularly if the gland is obstructed. Tenderness and swelling of the gland are normally evident but may have resolved by the time the patient is seen. Malignancy of the parotid gland may present as pain in the temporomandibular joint.

ENT CAUSES OF FACIAL PAIN

Pain from the sinuses may be unilateral or bilateral, and associated with infection or tumor. With maxillary sinus infections the maxillary teeth are often tender and hypersensitive. The pain may be exacerbated by changes in the position of the head. There is associated nasal congestion and discharge. The ear may be a source of pain and expert help is advised to differentiate this from joint pain.

CENTRAL AND VASCULAR CAUSES OF FACIAL PAIN

Cerebral tumors are a rare cause of facial pain but must be considered. CT scanning should be arranged when more common causes of pain have been excluded and no improvement of symptoms has been achieved with treatment. Psychogenic pain is particularly difficult to diagnose and psychiatric assessment is required. Headache is often associated with TMPS. Tension headache and migraine headache are the most frequent causes.

PAIN FROM THE ORAL CAVITY

Odontogenic causes of pain are generally specific but may be referred to the temporomandibular joint. Acute pulpitis is severe and throbbing, the pain being exacerbated by hot or cold but poorly localized. Chronic pulpitis and dental abscess produce a dull severe ache localized to a painful tender tooth.

FUNCTIONAL ANATOMY

The temporomandibular joints are formed from the membranous bone from the first branchial arch and cranium. The craniomandibular articulation is a synovial joint with an intracapsular meniscus dividing the joint into upper and lower joint compartments[15] (Fig. 13.8). The articulating joint surfaces are unusual in that they are lined by fibrous connective tissue and not by hyaline cartilage.

The temporomandibular joints are unique, firstly in that they are the only joints whose movement is limited and guided by the dental occlusion and secondly in that the mandible connects the two joints so that they move in unison. One joint cannot move alone. Tooth loss or dental restorative work may affect the joints. The joint is supported laterally by the temporomandibular ligament and medially by the sphenomandibular ligament. The main muscles of mastication, the masseter, the temporalis and the medial and lateral pterygoid muscles, are the primary muscles moving the joint, which allow opening and closing of the mouth as well as lateral and protrusive movements of the mandible. The temporalis muscle plays a major role in the limitation of joint loading, and the lateral pterygoid muscle helps to stabilize the joint by controlling both the meniscus (upper head of the lateral pterygoid) and the condylar position (lower head of the lateral pterygoid muscle).

The meniscus, which divides the joint, is closely adapted to the mandibular condyle and, hence, the lower joint compartment is small and more difficult to examine arthroscopically. The mandibular condylar head, which has rounded joint surfaces, rotates within the meniscus, which is firmly attached both medially and laterally (Fig. 13.9). The condyle is known to have great remodeling capacity. As the mouth opens more widely, there is a translatory movement in the upper joint

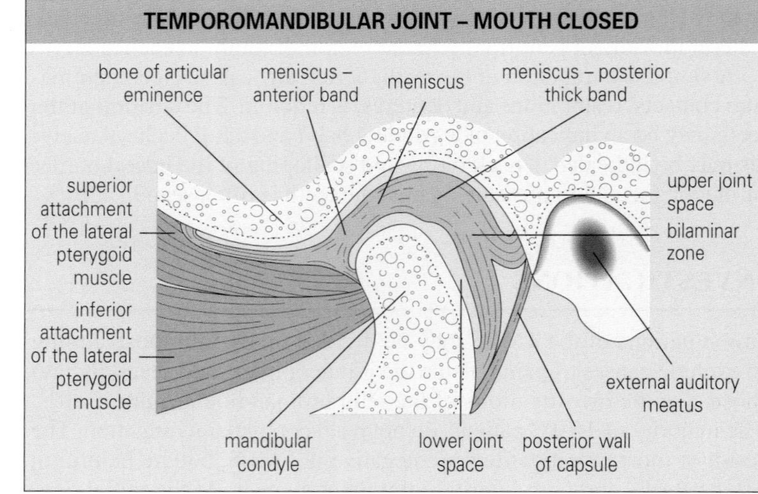

Fig 13.8 Sagittal section showing the anatomy of the temporomandiblar joint in the closed position.

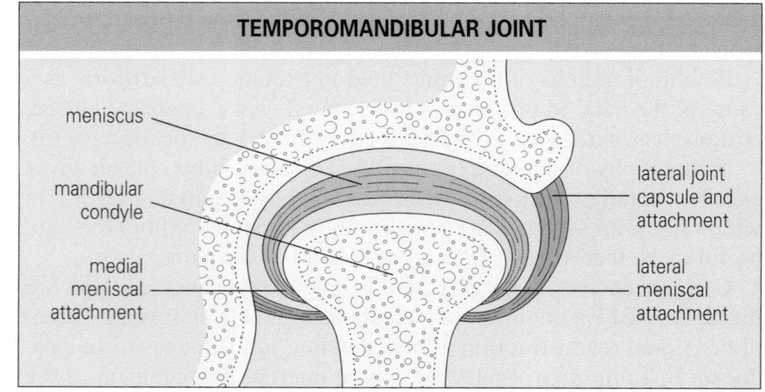

Fig 13.9 Coronal section of the anatomy of the temporomandibular joint.

space as the condyle moves forwards and down the articular eminence (Fig. 13.10). The upper joint space is easier to penetrate for arthrograms and arthrography.

The hinge movement of the lower joint space allows some 24mm of opening interincisorly and is rarely affected by joint dysfunction. Functional problems are usually related to the gliding or translatory movement of the upper joint space as the condyle moves forwards and down the articular eminence in wider mouth opening. Limited opening may be a result of muscle spasm or displacement of the meniscus which may or may not be reversible. Displacement of the meniscus anteriorly (Fig. 13.11) usually results in stretching of the bilaminar zone posteriorly. In normal active opening, there is a combination of hinge and gliding movement.

The meniscus is composed of avascular fibrous tissue and some cartilage. There is an anterior thick band and a thicker and larger posterior band, the narrowest area of the meniscus being between the condyle and the posterior surface of the articular eminence. Anteriorly, the meniscus is attached to the condyle and the upper head of the lateral pterygoid muscle. Posteriorly, the meniscus does not normally articulate and is attached to the bilaminar zone. In the bilaminar zone posteriorly, the superior surface is mostly composed of elastic tissue with vessels and nerves, the inferior portion being cartilaginous. The temporomandibular joint is innervated by the auriculotemporal nerve and also small components from the posterior deep temporal and masseteric nerves. The capsule, lateral ligament and posterior fat pads are innervated. However, the central part of the meniscus and the synovium does not appear to be innervated, an important consideration when diagnosing pain related to the joint.

There is much controversy as to whether the joint is load bearing. The joint is nonload bearing in the main but appears to be load bearing in some instances. This may be important in parafunction and a cause of pain. The horizontal fibers of the temporalis muscle limit joint loading. The aim of conservative management of the joint is to reduce joint loading and keep the meniscus in the correct relationship to the condyle. Hence, this restores the dental occlusion and corrects the closing pathway determined by the interdigitation of the teeth.

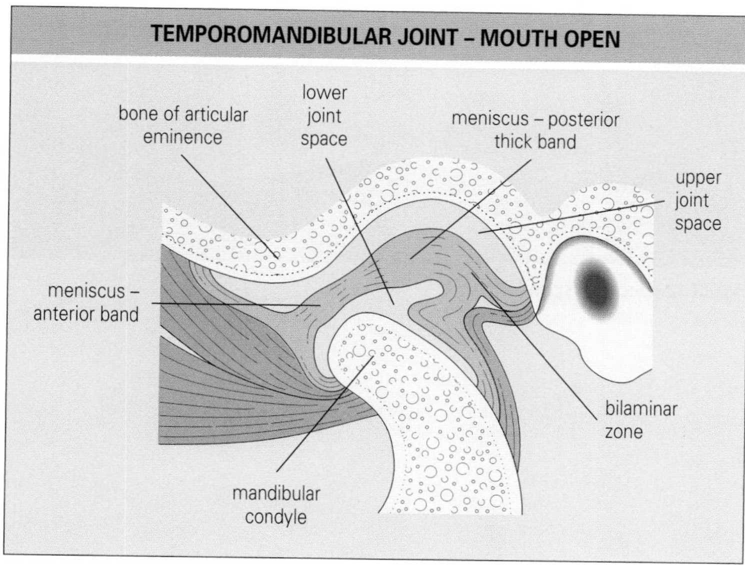

Fig. 13.10 The temporomandibular joint in the open position.

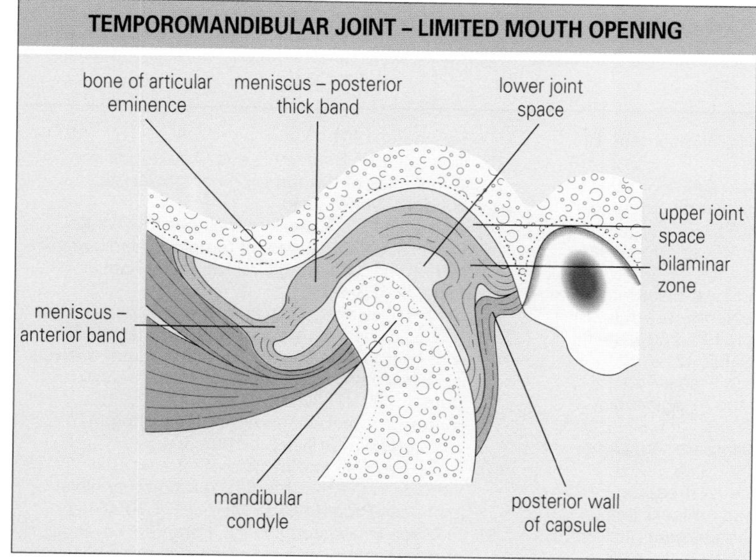

Fig. 13.11 Limited opening of the temporomandibular joint showing anterior displacement of the meniscus.

MANAGEMENT

TMPS represents a spectrum of facial pain and the treatment requirements vary to account for this. Failures in response to treatment require great perseverance and additional reassurance to the patient that the pain can be controlled. A reappraisal of the diagnosis may be necessary if, for example, the patient has progressed to true internal derangement of the joint. The management of all TMPS patients requires reassurance and an explanation of the pain and proposed treatment, including dental treatment.

The largest group of TMPS patients comprises those with an aching pain centered around the joint and the muscles of mastication and functional joint symptoms. There is muscle stiffness, muscle tenderness, clicking, locking on occasions and associated stress problems, such as headache. These patients respond to medical management and bite raising appliances such as occlusal splints.

There is a small refractory group of some 5% of patients who do not respond to medical management and occlusal appliances. These patients need further investigation, such as arthrograms and arthroscopy, since internal joint derangement should be suspected. Internal derangement, such as anterior displacement of the meniscus, probably represents the terminal stage of TMPS. This may respond to arthroscopic lysis and lavage or need open joint surgery to reposition the meniscus. The American Dental Association[12] has recommended only reversible therapy and stress the most important aspect of treatment includes a warm, positive and reassuring attitude by the clinician.

Finally, it is not unusual to see other types of facial pain, such as atypical facial pain or oral dysesthesia, in a patient with TMPS. Hence, medical management may need to be continued even after surgical intervention.

DENTAL PROBLEMS

Dental problems which may be contributing to the pain and joint dysfunction should be treated, including routine restorative treatment. Areas of unsupported occlusion may benefit from dentures or bridge work. Premature contacts should be relieved but no extensive occlusal equilibration undertaken. If dentures are worn, ensure that they are of the correct vertical dimension.

EXPLANATION REASSURANCE AND COUNSELLING

It is important to explain that TMPS is not a serious disease, as some patients are concerned about malignancy or degenerative joint disease. An explanation that the pain is from the cramped muscles, which have been under constant tension (from clenching for example), is helpful. This muscle spasm leads to stiffness of the muscles and to restricted jaw movements. The clicking in the joint is a result of the abnormal muscle spasm disrupting the normal meniscal movements. A diagram or model of the joint is helpful in explaining the problem.

Advice should also be given to stop habits such as clenching and parafunctional activities such as nail biting or pencil chewing. Simple measures may also be suggested, like avoiding wide opening when yawning or eating hard foods, such as crusty bread.

OCCLUSAL APPLIANCES

There are several types of occlusal appliances (bite guards, splints) available to treat TMPS. There are many theories[6] as to the mode of splint action. The splint disengages the occlusion, reduces joint loading, changes the vertical height and may allow the displaced meniscus to reposition. Splints also reduce muscle activity, possibly by a change in muscle length, and are helpful in the relief of pain in the masticatory muscles and headache. There is also a placebo effect in the use of the splint.

The soft occlusal splint (Fig 13.12) is similar to a gum shield for sport and is simple and cheap to make. It is a useful first splint to use with benefits being apparent in about 6 weeks. However a hard acrylic splint is recommended for use if splint therapy has proved beneficial and is required in the longer term. The full occlusal coverage acrylic splint[17] is the most widely used and is made to disengage the occlusion and may also be used to reposition the mandible.

ARTHROSCOPY

Patients who have not responded to medical management or occlusal appliances should be considered for arthroscopy[14], especially if internal joint derangement is suspected. Internal derangement such as anterior displacement of the meniscus may be relieved by lysis and lavage of the joint, even with a normal appearance at arthroscopy. Intra-articular injections may cause irreversible damage and are not recommended except with degenerative joint disease[19]. In the acute situation, where pain is severe, a local anesthetic block of the auricular temporal nerve may give immediate relief while more conventional splints and drugs are taking effect. There is a small group of patients who do not respond or who relapse and for whom additional counseling and psychiatric help may be required[18].

SURGERY

Surgery is reserved for internal joint derangements or degenerative joint disease failing to respond to more conservative management or arthroscopy. Careful case selection is essential since the long-term results from surgery are poor, particularly after 1–2 years. Continuing medical treatment after surgery should be considered.

Various types of temporomandibular joint surgery are advocated. Meniscal repositioning by plication in the bilaminar zone is the most commonly practiced. In this procedure, the joint is opened (or entered by arthroscopy) and the displaced meniscus (usually anterior or medial) mobilized and repositioned. A wedge of tissue in the stretched bilaminar zone is excised and repaired to hold the meniscus back in the correct position.

Meniscectomy is also advocated by some[20]. Surgery to the condylar surfaces is only recommended in degenerative conditions or for osteophytes. Total joint replacement with alloplastic materials has very poor long-term results. Overall the long term results for surgical intervention in the temporomandibular joint remain disappointing and conservative measures should be fully pursued in the first instance.

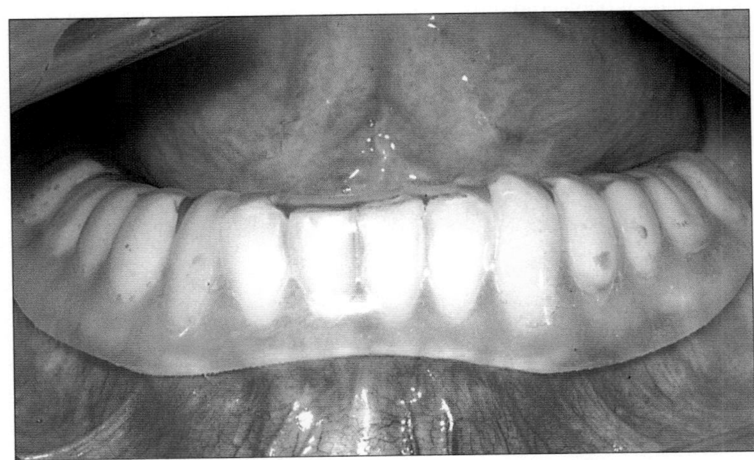

Fig. 13.12 Occlusal splint.

REFERENCES

1. Gray RJM, Davies SJ, Quayle AA. A clinical approach to temporomandibular disorders. Br Dent J. 1994;176(11):429–35.
2. Gray RJM, Davies SJ, Quayle AA. A clinical approach to temporomandibular disorders. Br Dent J. 1994;176(12):473–7.
3. Gray RJM, Davies SJ, Quayle AA. A clinical approach to temporomandibular disorders. Br Dent J. 1994;177(1):25–8.
4. Gray RJM, Davies SJ, Quayle AA. A clinical approach to temporomandibular disorders. Br Dent J. 1994;177(2):63–8.
5. Gray RJM, Davies SJ, Quayle AA. A clinical approach to temporomandibular disorders. Br Dent J. 1994;177(3):101–6.
6. Gray RJM, Davies SJ, Quayle AA. A clinical approach to temporomandibular disorders. Br Dent J. 1994;177(4):135–42.
7. Gray RJM, Davies SJ, Quayle AA. A clinical approach to temporomandibular disorders. Br Dent J. 1994;177(6):171–8.
8. Gray RJM, Davies SJ, Quayle AA. A clinical approach to temporomandibular disorders. Br Dent J. 1994;177(7):255–9.
9. Gray RJM, Davies SJ, Quayle AA. A clinical approach to temporomandibular disorders. Br Dent J. 1994;177(8):295–301.
10. Bull EE, ed. Orofacial pains, 4E. London: Year Book; 1989.
11. Solberg WK. Temporomandibular disorders: background and clinical problems. Teach In. Br Dent J. 1986;160(5):157–61, 195–200, 231–6, 273–7, 317–22, 351–6, 379–85, 421–8.
12. Laskin D, Greenfiled W, Gale F, eds. The president's conference on the examination, diagnosis and management of temporomandibular joint disorders. Am Dent Assoc. 1983;106:75.
13. Harris M, Feinmann C, Wise M, Treasure F. Temporomandibular joint and orofacial pain: clinical and medicolegal management problem. Br Dent J. 1993;174:129–36.
14. Thomas M, Bronstein S. Arthroscopy of the temporomandibular joint. Philadelphia: WB Saunders; 1991.
15. Norman JDP, Bramley P, eds. A textbook and colour atlas of the temporomandibular joint. London: Wolfe; 1990.
16. Takenoshita Y, Ikebe T, Yamamoto M, Oka M. Occlusal contact area and temporomandiblar joint symptoms. Oral Surg Oral Med Oral Path. 1991;72:388–94.
17. Gray R, Davies K, Quayle A. A comparison of two splints in the treatment of temporomandibular joint dysfunction syndrome. Can occlusal analysis be used to predict success of splint therapy? Br Dent J. 1991;170(2):55–60.
18. Hunter S. The management of 'psychogenic' orofacial pain. Br Med J. 1992;304:329.
19. Troller PA. Use and misuse of intra articular steroids in the treatment of temporomandiblar joint pain. Proc Roy Soc Med. 1977;70:461–3.
20. Eriksson R, Wastersson PL. Long term evaluation of menisectomy of the temporomandibular joint. J Oral Maxillofac Surg. 1985;43:263–9.

PRACTICAL PROBLEMS

ROTATOR CUFF TEARS AND CHRONIC IMPINGEMENT SYNDROME

Edward Craig

DEFINITION OF THE PROBLEM

Tearing of the rotator cuff is defined as the fiber failure of the musculotendinous cuff attachment to the greater tuberosity of the humerus. It is an extremely common clinical problem, and arguably the most common cause of painful shoulder in the adult patient. Tearing of the rotator cuff is multifactorial in origin. Among the potential etiologies are:

- intrinsic degeneration of the tendon secondary to aging,
- poor potential for healing,
- repetitive trauma, and
- lack of a predictable blood supply to a vulnerable area of the tendon.

However, the vast majority of cuff tears appear to be associated with extrinsic mechanical compression from the overlying coracoacromial arch, including the anterior acromion, coracohumeral ligament and undersurface of the distal clavicle (Fig. 14.1). This extrinsic mechanical compression, also known as impingement, produces a syndrome of painful shoulder aggravated by use of the arm above shoulder level. It is characterized by progressively severe mechanical wear on the rotator cuff tendon, initially producing partial thickness and finally full thickness tearing of the rotator cuff. The biceps tendon, also vulnerable to extrinsic compression, may undergo spontaneous tearing and rupture as well.

THE TYPICAL CASE

RW, a 57-year-old mother of three and an avid weekend tennis player, presented with 18 months of gradually progressive shoulder pain radiating down the lateral aspect of the arm and into the base of the neck. She had also noticed a cracking or clicking in the shoulder. While the rest of her review of systems was unremarkable, and she had no other joint complaints, she had been treated for some time by her family doctor for 'tendon strain' and 'bursitis'. She had been on anti-inflammatory medications, had undergone a program of rehabilitation and had been given two corticosteroid injections in the area of the shoulder girdle. While she did not notice much weakness in the arm, she had to give up her weekend tennis because of pain in the shoulder. She

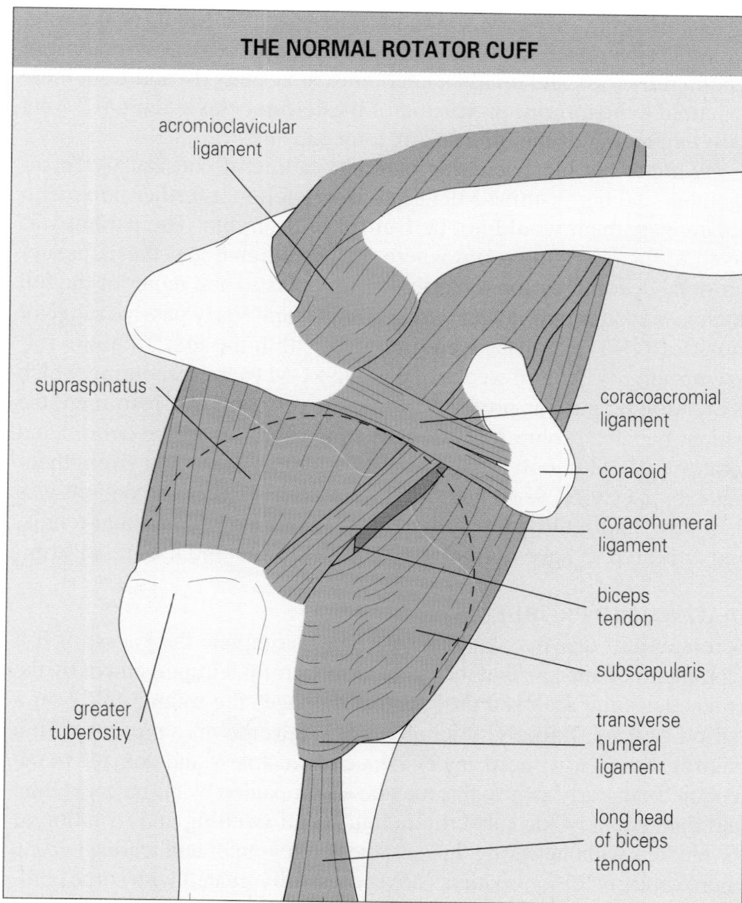

Fig. 14.1 The normal rotator cuff consists of the supraspinatus, infraspinatus, teres minor and subscapularis. The coracohumeral ligament often blends with the supraspinatus. The normal rotator cuff passes beneath the coracoacromial arch as the arm is moved through its usual arc of elevation. Adpated with permission from Master Techniques in Orthopedic Surgery.

was unable to sleep on the arm and was awakened from a sound sleep each night by pain. Her pain was clearly aggravated by using the arm above chest and shoulder level.

Physical examination revealed a normal range of motion of the neck without radicular symptoms or duplication of her shoulder pain. She had no atrophy of the shoulder girdle. She had a mild amount of right acromioclavicular joint tenderness and appeared to have a rupture of the long head of biceps. Palpation revealed subdeltoid crepitation, which was distinctly different from the contralateral shoulder. In lowering her arm from the fully elevated position to her side there was duplication of the pain along the lateral aspect of her arm as she reached the arc from 120° to 70°. She had duplication of her pain as her arm was forced into forward elevation against a fixed scapula (an impingement sign). She had pain as the arm was abducted and brought into slight internal rotation. Reaching up behind her back also reproduced the pain. Evaluation of passive motion showed that she had equal symmetric and normal forward flexion, abduction, external rotation and internal rotation. Her active motion equalled her passive motion, but she appeared to have 'give way' weakness when abduction was tested. This appeared to be secondary to a pain response. With her arms at her sides and her elbow flexed at 90°, as external rotation strength was tested, she clearly had weakness to external rotation in the involved extremity.

A series of plain radiographs were taken, including an anterio-posterior (AP), a scapular lateral and a supine axillary view. The AP view revealed some sclerosis on the undersurface of the acromion and a small projecting inferior acromial spur. She had cystic changes and bone-reactive changes in the area of the greater tuberosity. The acromiohumeral interval appeared normal. The glenohumeral joint also appeared normal and there was no evidence of osteopenia of either humerus or glenoid.

Because the patient had already received a considerable amount of nonoperative treatment without a satisfactory outcome magnetic resonance imaging (MRI) was requested to assess the status of the rotator cuff. This revealed a full thickness tear with a modest amount of tendon retraction and no associated muscle atrophy. In addition, there appeared to be inferior protrusion of the acromioclavicular (AC) joint with thickening of the inferior AC joint capsule.

Owing to her incapacitating pain, the failure of conservative management and her positive MRI scan, it was felt that further nonoperative management would not be fruitful or desirable. The patient was taken to the operating room where, under regional anesthesia, a subacromial decompression (anterior acromioplasty) and repair of the full thickness rotator cuff defect was accomplished. Early passive range of motion (ROM) exercises were initiated within the first 48 hours following surgery. After 6 weeks of passive ROM exercises, during which the tendon repair was protected while the program was instituted, the patient began a program of strengthening exercises of the deltoid and rotator cuff. Although rehabilitation including ROM and strengthening exercises took 8–10 months, 1 year after surgery the patient was pain free, had returned to full activity, including recreational tennis, and appeared to have normal strength, flexibility and use of her arm.

DIAGNOSTIC PROBLEMS

A rotator cuff tear may be either partial (incomplete thickness) or full (complete). It appears that mechanical subacromial impingement by the coracoacromial arch is a process that damages the rotator cuff over a period of time. Initially, impingement syndrome may present with a painful shoulder, without any evidence of weakness and damage to the tendon. In its early stages, this may be accompanied by chronic swelling and thickening of the subacromial bursa and swelling and irritation of the tendons without tearing. In the stage before rotator cuff tearing occurs, approximately 75% of patients are successfully treated with some combination of medication, subacromial injection and rehabilitation. Anti-inflammatory medications are intended to reduce the swelling of the rotator cuff and overlying bursa and thus help restore the space under the coracoacromial arch through which the rotator cuff passes. A subacromial corticosteroid injection may deliver a more concentrated anti-inflammatory medication directly to the area of tendon pathology. Exercises can also restore joint mobility and strengthen the head depressor activity of the rotator cuff and biceps tendon. In the early stages of rotator cuff disease, there may be diagnostic confusion between cervical spine-related pain, frozen shoulder syndrome, isolated acromioclavicular disease and early glenohumeral joint arthropathies. Acromioclavicular joint disease is characterized by point tenderness over the superior aspect of the AC joint. A frozen shoulder syndrome (adhesive capsulitis) is characterized by painful restriction of both passive and active ROM. Arthropathy of the glenohumeral joint is characterized by joint narrowing and evidence of cartilage loss radiographically. Cervical spine disease is characterized by reproduction of the shoulder pain by ROM and movement of the cervical spine.

As the disease process continues, further wear on the rotator cuff increases the chronicity of the pain; it often progresses to the point where pain may occur at rest and may interfere with sleep. Patients with a full thickness tear frequently report that as long as they are not using their arm, their shoulder is reasonably comfortable, but the more they try to do with the arm, the more discomfort they have. Patients may or may not notice weakness of the arm above shoulder level, but may complain more of fatigability. Active ROM of the arm above shoulder level may be maintained until the tendon tear is quite large, possibly because of the substitution by the biceps tendon and some of the other intact rotator cuff muscles for the torn supraspinatus. As the impingement process continues, wear on the supraspinatus and adjacent biceps tendon can progress to the point where these tendinous insertions are torn and the long head of biceps ruptures or a full thickness tear of the supraspinatus ensues (Fig. 14.2). As this process continues, the tendon tear can enlarge to include the adjacent infraspinatus

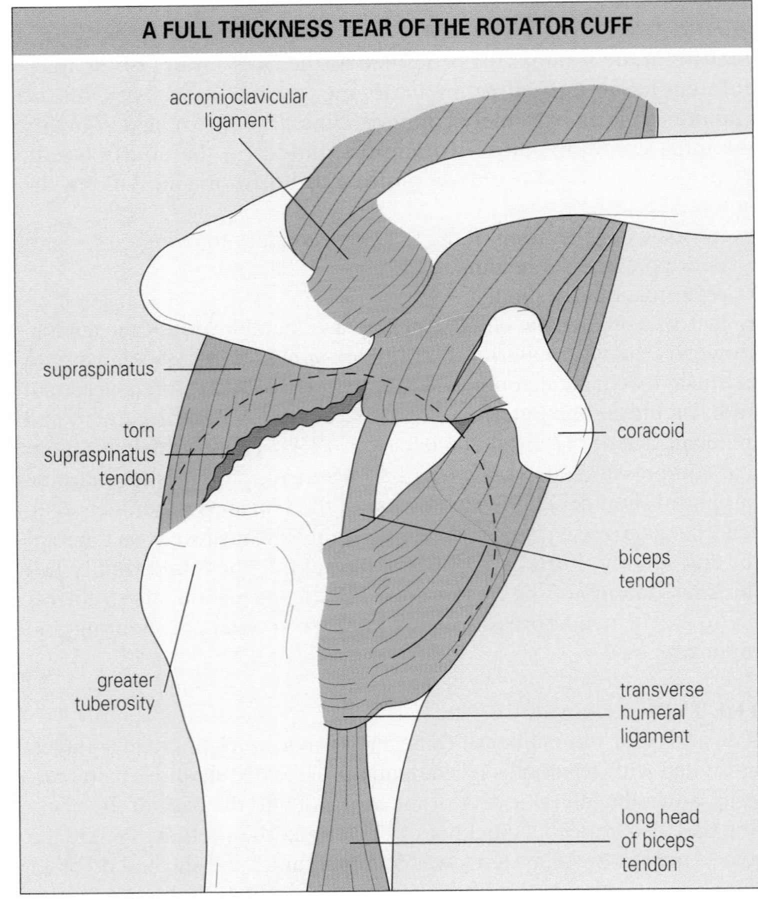

Fig. 14.2 A full thickness tear of the rotator cuff. The rotator cuff is torn from its attachment to the greater tuberosity. Most rotator cuff tears begin at the supraspinatus insertion and enlarge over a period of time to involve adjacent tendon structures. If the subacromial impingement involves the biceps as well, the biceps may be torn as part of the disease process. The coracoacromial ligament is not shown. Adpated with Permission from Master Techniques in Orthopedic Surgery.

and even the teres minor tendon. In the presence of a long-standing rotator cuff tear, atrophy of the supraspinatus and infraspinatus muscles frequently occurs. As the tear enlarges, radiographs often reveal diminution of the acromiohumeral interval (loss of the head depressor activity of the rotator cuff) and may eventually include glenohumeral arthrosis (cuff tear arthropathy).

THERAPEUTIC OPTIONS

Once the full thickness of the rotator cuff has torn, it does not have the capacity to heal itself. In fact the rotator cuff tear tends to enlarge over time, which may or may not be accompanied by worsening symptoms.

Diagnosis of a full thickness rotator cuff tear is usually by one of three radiographic studies. Single-contrast shoulder arthrography may show dye within the glenohumeral joint and leakage of dye out through the subacromial space. A diagnostic ultrasound may show a rotator cuff defect if it has reached a critical size. An MRI with a shoulder coil often accurately identifies the presence of either partial or full thickness tearing of the rotator cuff.

Once a full thickness rotator cuff tear is diagnosed, if the patient is sufficiently symptomatic to warrant treatment, and if a short course of nonoperative treatment has failed, surgical reconstruction is considered. As the process of rotator cuff tearing is usually brought on by mechanical wear from subacromial impingement, the surgery consists not only of a repair of the tendon defect itself, but also of a decompression of the coracoacromial arch via an anterior acromioplasty and removal of the coracohumeral ligament. This removes the offending structure contributing to the mechanical subacromial impingement. Rotator cuff repairs are ordinarily performed via an open operation, with direct reattachment of the tendon to the greater tuberosity. Following rotator cuff repair, the tendon must be protected for a period of time while it heals to the greater tuberosity. However, it is critical that the ROM of the shoulder be maintained as severe shoulder stiffness can occur if it is not rehabilitated during this phase.

CONCLUSIONS

Since the vast majority of rotator cuff tears occur in patients above 40 years of age, and occur via a progressive mechanical external impingement by the coracoacromial arch on the rotator cuff insertion, the treatment of this common condition is designed to reverse the pathologic process. Initially, in the early phases, conservative management can ‘reopen’ the subacromial space via diminution of swelling in the rotator cuff and overlying bursa, and exercises are intended to strengthen the muscles that depress the humeral head (and thus prevent superior migration of the humeral head). Eventually, if this process continues, direct fraying and wearing and eventually full thickness tearing of the rotator cuff (particularly the supraspinatus) may occur. At this point, nonoperative treatment is frequently inadequate to restore comfort to the shoulder. In the presence of full thickness tearing, it is often unwise to offer repeated injections of corticosteroids into the subacromial space. If the patient continues to be symptomatic, a surgical procedure aimed at decompressing the subacromial space and surgically repairing the tendon usually offers the patient the most predictable pain relief and restoration of shoulder function. The published evidence shows that approximately 85–90% of people will be pain free following a successful repair of a full thickness tear of the rotator cuff.

REFERENCES

Cofield RH. Current concepts review. Rotator cuff disease of the shoulder. J Bone Jt Surg. 1985;67A:974–979.

Craig EV. Open anterior acromioplasty for full thickness rotator cuff tears in master techniques in orthopedic surgery. In: Craig EV, ed. The shoulder. New York: Raven Press; 1995.

Neer CS. Anterior acromioplasty for the chronic impingement syndrome in the shoulder. J Bone Jt Surg. 1972;54A:41–50.

Shankwiler JA, Ciepiela MD, Burkhead WZ. The coracoacromial arch impingement syndromes in rotator cuff disorders. In: Burkhead WZ Jr, ed. Rotator Cuff Disorders. Philadelphia: Williams and Wilkins; 1996.

OLECRANON BURSITIS

Gerald D Groff

DEFINITION OF THE PROBLEM

The olecranon bursa is a subcutaneous synovial pouch which is located on the extensor aspect of the elbow. It allows the skin to glide freely over the olecranon process, preventing tissue tears. The space between bone and skin is narrow with minimal soft tissue padding. As a result, the olecranon bursa is vulnerable to trauma and infection through puncture wounds or cellulitis.

Olecranon bursitis occurs when the bursa swells due to trauma, inflammation or infection (Fig. 14.3). The swelling can be secondary to synovial tissue hypertrophy or fibrosis, fluid accumulation or nodular deposits (traumatic fibrosis, gouty tophi or rheumatoid nodules). Olecranon bursitis is a commonly seen outpatient problem (approximately 3 in 1000 outpatient visits) and occasionally requires hospitalization when septic (about 1 in 1000 hospitalizations). It occurs most often in young men with recurrent elbow trauma due to work (e.g. automobile mechanics, miners) or leisure activities (dart throwing, gymnastics, gardening).

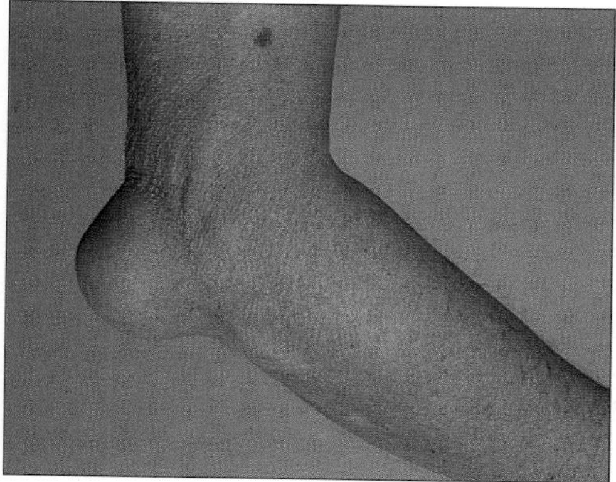

Fig. 14.3 Olecranon bursitis in early RA.

Olecranon bursitis can be classified clinically into three general categories (Fig. 14.4):

- traumatic (or idiopathic) noninflammatory,
- aseptic inflammatory or
- septic inflammatory.

Because appropriate therapy varies with bursitis category, it is important for the clinician to define the cause as soon as possible through examination and bursal aspiration. It is also necessary to recognize that the pathogenesis of bursitis can change over time. For example, a stable traumatic bursitis may become secondarily infected by a puncture wound or trivial abrasion.

THE TYPICAL CASE

OB is a 43-year-old automobile mechanic in good health except for mild obesity and diet-controlled hyperglycemia. He frequently plays darts at the local pub on his way home from work. While attempting to remove a muffler, he repeatedly struck and rubbed his elbows. As he pulled his shirt on the next day, he noted swelling the size of a ‘golf ball’ at the end of his right elbow. The arm was stiff but not painful.

Initial presentation at the clinic revealed a man of healthy appearance with olecranon bursal swelling. He was afebrile with firm thickening of the bursa and mild nontender fluctuance. No warmth, erythema or adenopathy was noted. The elbow ROM was normal and there was

DIFFERENTIAL DIAGNOSIS OF OLECRANON BURSITIS

	Traumatic (idiopathic) noninflammatory	Aseptic inflammatory			Septic inflammatory
		Rheumatoid arthritis	Crystalline	Uremia	
Clinical symptoms					
Trauma	+++	+	+	0/+	+++
Tenderness	+	+	++	+	+++
Skin breakage	+	0	0	0	+++
Clinical signs					
Fever	0	0	0	0	++
Warmth	+	+	++	+	+++
Erythema	+	+	++	+	+++
Cellulitis	0	0	+	+	+++
Lymphadenopathy	0	0/+	0/+	0	++
Edema	0/+	0/+	0/+	0	++
Bursal fluid					
Color	C, S, H	C, S	S, H	S	S, H, P
White blood cells per mm^3	50–10,000 (mean 1100)	1000–60,000 (mean 3000)	1000–20,000 (mean 2900)	1200	350–450,000 (mean 75,000)
Gram stain	Negative	Negative	Negative	Negative	Positive (70%)
Crystals	Negative	Rare cholesterol	Monosodium urate or pyrophosphate	Rare	Negative
Culture	Negative	Negative	Negative	Negative	Positive

Differential diagnosis: 0 usually absent, + rare, ++ occasional, +++ common. Bursal fluid color: C Clear, H Hemorrhagic, S Serosanguineous, P Purulent

Fig. 14.4 Differential diagnosis of olecranon bursitis.

no joint effusion. No additional tests were performed and the patient was given a diagnosis of traumatic olecranon bursitis. Therapy included ibuprofen 600mg p.o. t.i.d. for 7 days and an elastic elbow pad.

The patient responded well. The swelling gradually reduced, leaving thickened tissue at the olecranon prominence but no pain or limitation. He stopped wearing the elbow pad. Six weeks later he scraped the same elbow on a sharp metal edge and swelling recurred over 48 hours. He did not present to clinic until 5 days later, when he noted warmth, erythema and tenderness to touch.

Repeat examination revealed fluctuant bursal swelling with erythema over the bursa but not the adjoining skin. A small abrasion was still present. The patient was again afebrile and of nontoxic appearance. Bursal aspiration was performed with an 18-gauge sterile needle and produced 10ml of slightly yellow fluid. Gram stain demonstrated numerous white cells but no organisms. The patient was treated with dicloxacillin sodium 500mg p.o. q.i.d. and advised to call if fever or further skin redness developed. Subsequent synovial analysis revealed a white blood cell count of 63,000/mm^3. No crystals were noted. The culture was eventually positive for *Staphylococcus aureus*. Close follow up in the clinic with repeated aspiration demonstrated gradual improvement. Antibiotics were continued for 10 days, with resolution of erythema and swelling. He eventually gave up both car mechanics and darts to pursue a career in politics.

DIAGNOSTIC PROBLEMS

The differentiation between septic and nonseptic olecranon bursitis represents the main diagnostic challenge. Septic bursitis has the greatest potential for morbidity and must be diagnosed as soon as possible. In addition, the source of nonseptic bursitis should be clarified, since the presence or absence of inflammation can determine appropriate therapy and outcome. Finally, the clinician should be aware of the potential for rapid change in the cause of bursitis. As a result, a fresh diagnostic approach should be applied at each follow up visit.

The history should include questions regarding occupation, duration of symptoms and possible trauma or skin injury. Associated conditions such as rheumatoid arthritis (RA), gout or uremia may be primary causes of bursitis, while diabetes or immunosuppression may also increase the risk for sepsis. The physical examination should note the size, change in size and turgor of the bursa. The presence of nodules, lymphadenopathy, warmth and erythema of bursa or skin are important clues. Effusion occasionally occurs in the adjacent elbow joint, particularly with inflamatory conditions. Specific risk factors for bacterial infection include direct trauma, skin breakage and underlying illness (diabetes and immunosuppression) with the clinical findings of fever, erythema, tenderness or peribursal cellulitis which may actually represent bursal rupture.

Percutaneous diagnostic aspiration of the bursa should be performed whenever inflammation or infection is suspected. Patients with asymptomatic or obviously traumatic bursitis can be treated without aspiration but should be observed carefully. The aspiration technique is simple. A sterile 16- or 18-gauge needle with a syringe large enough to drain available fluid is used to enter the bursa from the side, through normally appearing skin, aiming the needle towards the center of the sac. Fluid color and volume should be noted, with specimens sent for gram stain, white blood cell count, crystal analysis and bacterial culture. The majority of bacterial infections are caused by *S. aureus* followed by group A β-hemolytic *Streptococcus*, *S. epidermidis*, *Haemophilus influenzae* and *Pseudomonas* species. Special cultures for mycobacterium, fungi or anaerobic bacteria may be necessary in immunocompromised patients. Elbow radiographs are rarely necessary and should only be used to rule out traumatic fracture or pre-existing joint injury. Diagnostic elements are summarized in Figure 14.4.

THERAPEUTIC OPTIONS

Appropriate treatment of olecranon bursitis depends on the cause and duration of symptoms. Noninflammatory, traumatic (or idiopathic) bursitis usually responds to conservative therapy. Patients with limited symptoms should receive rest, elbow protection and possibly nonsteroidal anti-inflammatory drugs (NSAIDs). Padded elbow supports serve to prevent further trauma and skin abrasion. Percutaneous needle aspiration without injection should be considered for patients having significant symptoms. Bursal aspiration reduces symptoms and serves to rule out inflammatory or infectious conditions. Intrabursal corticosteroid injection speeds recovery but can lead to complications (infection, skin atrophy, chronic pain) and should be used sparingly in traumatic bursitis.

Intrabursal corticosteroid injection is useful, however, in aseptic inflammatory olecranon bursitis related to RA or a crystalline process. The initial approach is similar to traumatic bursitis except that all symptomatic patients should receive bursal aspiration for decompression and diagnosis. If bacterial cultures are negative, and symptoms recur despite rest and NSAIDs, repeat aspiration with corticosteroid injection is useful. Injection with 20mg of methylprednisone acetate often leads to rapid recovery.

Septic inflammatory olecranon bursitis requires early recognition and immediate antibiotic therapy. Patients with clinical evidence for infection (fever, cellulitis, synovial fluid leukocytosis or positive gram stain) should receive coverage for penicillin-resistant *S. aureus* while cultures are pending. Antibiotic therapy is modified as soon as culture results are available.

Oral antibiotic therapy results in adequate intrabursal drug levels. Patients with good general health, minimal cellulitis and limited systemic symptoms can be treated successfully as outpatients. They require close, often daily, follow up.

Patients who fail to respond to outpatient therapy or who present with more severe initial infection should be hospitalized for intravenous antibiotic therapy. This would include patients with high fever, chills, prolonged duration of symptoms and cellulitis. Hospitalization is also preferred in patients with complicating medical conditions (diabetes, uremia, RA) and immunosuppression [malignancy, human immunodeficiency virus (HIV) positive status, or systemic corticosteroid therapy].

Drainage of the infected bursa is an essential part of therapy. This can be accomplished by daily percutaneous aspiration or percutaneous placement of a suction–irrigation system. Routine cell counts and culture of drainage fluid should be used to monitor response to therapy. The duration of therapy varies with the individual patient. Patients with symptoms for less than 1 week require an average of 4.4 days of antibiotic therapy to sterilize the bursa. Patients with symptoms lasting longer than 1 week require an average of 9.2 days. In general, antibiotic therapy should be continued for 10–14 days. Patients requiring initial intravenous antibiotic therapy can be switched to oral medication as soon as signs and symptoms show consistent improvement.

Surgical drainage or bursectomy is occasionally necessary in the management of olecranon bursitis. Recurrent traumatic olecranon bursitis can be approached by either arthroscopic or open resection. Persistent aseptic inflammatory bursitis may require open resection with careful dissection when symptoms result in dysfunction. Septic bursitis may require bursectomy if acute infection fails to resolve or repeated infection occurs in a fibrotic, chronically inflamed bursa.

CONCLUSIONS

Olecranon bursitis is a common condition that is easily recognized. Careful use of history, physical examination and percutaneous needle aspiration can enable differentiation of the main categories of olecranon bursitis: traumatic noninflammatory, aseptic inflammatory and septic inflammatory bursitis. Appropriate management requires an understanding of these diagnostic categories and the corresponding treatment regimens.

Septic olecranon bursitis is the most serious potential complication, and requires early diagnosis and immediate antibiotic therapy. Initial therapy should include antibiotic coverage for penicillin-resistant *S. aureus* and regular bursal drainage.

REFERENCES

Canoso JJ, Barza M. Soft tissue infections. Clin Rheum Dis. 1993;19:293–309.

Ho G Jr, Su EY. Antibiotic therapy of septic bursitis. Its implication in the treatment of septic arthritis. Arthritis Rheum. 1981;24:905–11.

McAfee JH, Smith DL. Olecranon and prepatellar bursitis – diagnosis and treatment. West J Med. 1988;149:607–10.

Raddatz DA, Hoffman GS, Franck WA. Septic bursitis: presentation, treatment and prognosis. J Rheumatol. 1987;14:1160–3.

Smith DL, McAfee JH, Lucas LM, Kumar KL, Romney DM. Treatment of nonseptic olecranon bursitis. A controlled, blinded prospective trial. Arch Intern Med. 1989;149:2527–30.

Weinstein PS, Canoso JJ, Wohlgethan JR. Long-term follow-up of corticosteroid injection for traumatic olecranon bursitis. Ann Rheum Dis. 1984;43:44–6.

REFRACTORY LATERAL EPICONDYLITIS

Robert Nirschl & Barry Kraushaar

DEFINITION OF THE PROBLEM

Lateral epicondylitis generally results from repetitive overuse of the wrist and forearm in patients over 35 years of age who have a high activity level or demanding activity technique and who sometimes have an inadequate fitness level. Although tenderness and swelling occur near the lateral epicondyle, histopathologic studies confirm that the lateral epicondyle of the humerus itself is not injured, and that acute inflammation is not the primary problem. Rather, a granulation tissue termed 'angiofibroblastic hyperplasia' (Fig. 14.5) occurs in the extensor carpi radialis brevis (ECRB) tendon origin as a result of eccentric overload in an area of poor vascularity. Hence, the term 'tendinosis' is perhaps more appropriate than 'tendinitis'. Although rest, bracing, nonsteroidal anti-inflammatory drugs (NSAIDs) and corticosteroid injections provide patients with symptomatic comfort, the promotion of healing requires proper rehabilitation and activity modification. When these efforts fail, surgical treatment becomes an option.

THE TYPICAL CASE

EF is a 51-year-old active tennis player who presented with 3 years of pain around the right elbow, which became worse with activity. Previous treatment included temporary rest, various types of elbow braces, NSAIDs and two injections of corticosteroid, which provided temporary relief. A physical therapy specialist administered a program of ultrasound, phonophoresis, stretching and strengthening. The patient also tried acupuncture, and she had a tennis professional modify her technique and equipment.

Physical examination revealed tenderness over the origin of her right ECRB tendon which was painful on resisted wrist extension and firm handshake. She was also tender over the rotator cuff, and weak in shoulder abduction and external rotation.

Surgical resection and repair of the lateral tennis elbow was performed, and a physical therapy protocol commenced. Therapy included electrical stimulation, hot packs and ice, as well as flexibility and strength exercises to the shoulder, elbow and wrist. She gradually returned to playing tennis at 3 months, without pain.

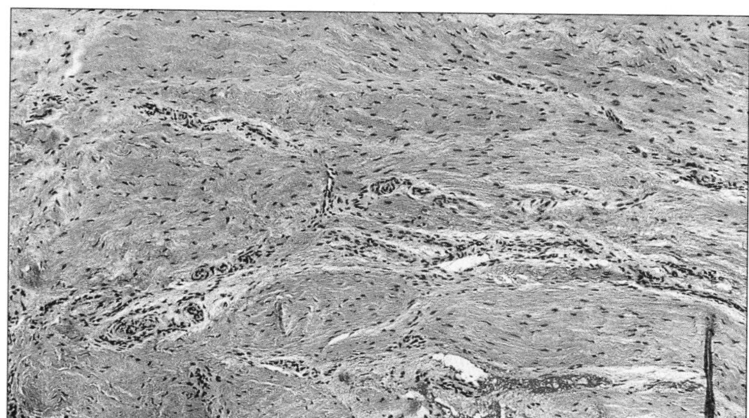

Fig. 14.5 Angiofibroblastic hyperplasia.

DIAGNOSTIC PROBLEMS

Various causes of lateral elbow pain are sometimes confused with tennis elbow. Although the radial nerve may be compressed under the brachioradialis muscle, this is a rare event and is painful more distally than tennis elbow. Synovial inflammation of the elbow and radio-capitellar articular disease are usually more responsive than lateral epicondylitis to medications and rest. A careful physical examination in the context of a characteristic history of overuse will help diagnose lateral epicondylitis. Specifically, pain just distal and medial to the lateral epicondyle after activity, that can be reproduced by resisted wrist extension and forceful grip, suggest the diagnosis. It is important to assess for carpal tunnel syndrome, medial elbow tendinosis, shoulder tendinosis and scapular and upper back weakness, as these problems are commonly found together. Radiographs should be taken routinely, as loose bodies, bone spurs and calcification of the ECRB tendon are found in 20% of cases. The diagnosis can be confirmed by MRI but this is reserved for subtle cases.

THERAPEUTIC OPTIONS FOR ANGIOFIBROBLASTIC HYPERPLASIA

- Relieve pain and inflammation
  - Protection, rest, ice, compression, elevation, medication, physical modalities
- Promote healing
  - Electrical stimulation
  - Exercises/conditioning
  - Protect from abuse
- General body conditioning
- Control force loads
  - Counterforce bracing
  - Improve sport technique/intensity
  - Modify equipment
- Surgery where indicated

Fig. 14.6 The management of elbow epicondylitis.

THERAPEUTIC OPTIONS

Initial treatment for lateral epicondylosis is the relief of pain and inflammation by measures such as protection, rest, ice, compression (i.e. counterforce bracing), elevation, NSAIDs, corticosteroid injections, and physical modalities (i.e. electrical stimulation).

Definitive treatment is aimed at healing of the injured tissues, in association with an overall restoration of strength, endurance and flexibility via rehabilitative exercise. Without the patient's active participation in the rehabilitation process, treatment commonly fails. Rehabilitation exercises of the entire region in a systematic fashion, however, results in recovery in better than 90% of patients. To prevent recurrence, modifications of the initiating overuse activities are made (i.e. improvement of the work or sport routine, technique and equipment).

Local corticosteroid injections is used in the unusual event that symptoms are so severe that they preclude rehabilitative exercise. A maximum of three injections are used, spread at least 1 month apart. If the combined medical and rehabilitative efforts fail and symptoms remain unacceptable to the patient, surgery may be considered.

Surgery for tennis elbow is an ambulatory procedure performed by incising over the common extensor origin, identifying the ECRB tendon and excising the grayish, edematous granulation tissue in the tendon. The lateral condylar cortical bone is drilled to invite fresh local bleeding and the edges of the tendon are freshened and sutured. The goal of surgery is resection of abnormal tissue and reconstruction of the tendon origin, not release of tendon tension. An elbow immobilizer is used for a few days in the immediate postoperative period, and exercises are started as soon as they are tolerated (usually within 1 week) (Fig. 14.6).

CONCLUSIONS

Lateral epicondylitis is not primarily an inflammatory process; it is a degenerative disorder due to repetitive overuse and failed tendon healing. Treatment includes not only medications and rest, but a simultaneous fitness program to all uninjured areas, and a rehabilitation program for the injured tissues. If these efforts fail, surgical treatment is an option with a good record of success. To prevent reinjury, it is beneficial to modify activities by adjusting intensity, technique and equipment. Most patients can return to full activity, including sports.

REFERENCES

Nirschl RP. Elbow tendinosis/tennis elbow. Clin Sports Med. 1992;4:851–70.

Nirschl RP. Muscle and tendon trauma. In: Morrey BF, ed. The elbow and its disorders. Philadelphia: WB Saunders; 1993:537–52.

Nirschl RP. Patterns of failed healing in tendon injury. In: Buckwalter J, Leadbetter W, Goodwin, eds. Sports-induced soft tissue inflammations. Chicago: American Academy of Orthopedic Surgeons; 1991:577–85.

Regan WD, Morrey BF. Physical examination of the elbow. In: Morrey BF, ed. The elbow and its disorders. Philadelphia: WB Saunders; 1993.

HIP PAIN DURING PREGNANCY

Emmanuel George

DEFINITION OF THE PROBLEM

Hip pain may develop at any time, in either sex and in any age group. Rarely, it may occur during pregnancy, adding to the diagnostic difficulties. Not only should the many causes of hip pain be considered (see Chapter 4.10), but also the possibility of a pregnancy-associated cause must also be taken into account. The situation is further complicated by the fact that the results of some investigations may be affected by the pregnancy itself, and what investigations to do and the subsequent management must be carefully considered because of the potential effects on the fetus.

THE TYPICAL CASE

CG, a 34-year-old in week 38 of her fourth pregnancy, presented with a 6-week history of left hip pain. She complained of a 'dull and toothache-like' pain in the front of the left hip and thigh. The pain had been gradual in onset and, although at first helped by rest, became almost constant, spreading down the back and side of her left leg as far as the knee. Her past medical history was unremarkable, and her previous pregnancies and deliveries had been uneventful.

Physical examination revealed that she walked with a slight left-sided antalgic gait, and there were no reflex, sensory or motor changes in either lower limb. She had a normal ROM of the left hip apart from some discomfort at extremes. There was slight tenderness in the trochanteric and gluteal areas of the left hip as compared with the right. Routine urine analysis was normal. Hemoglobin was 12.2g/dl, and the white cell count 5900/mm^3 with a normal differential. The erythrocyte sedimentation rate (ESR) was 57mm/h. Serum calcium, phosphate and alkaline phosphatase were normal. Ultrasound of the left hip revealed a small effusion which was aspirated, with symptomatic relief. Culture and microscopy of the fluid was negative. Limited radiographs of the hips, with fetal shielding, revealed marked localized osteopenia of the left femoral head and acetabulum.

A diagnosis of transient osteoporosis of pregnancy was made, and the patient mobilized with the aid of a cane and treated symptomatically with propoxyphene and acetaminophen [dextropropoxyphene HCl and paracetamol]. Her symptoms remained essentially unchanged until approximately 3 weeks after delivery, at which time they gradually subsided. Three months later the patient was completely free of pain, and radiographs revealed that the left hip density had returned to normal.

DIAGNOSTIC PROBLEMS

Problems in diagnosis fall into two categories: first, the exclusion, by pregnancy, of a number of diagnostic imaging tools; second, the differential diagnosis.

In pregnancy, radiographs should be avoided. If they are diagnostically essential, however, then limited views of the hip, with shielding of the fetus, are unlikely to cause problems in a fetus at this stage of development. Unless clinically considered to be absolutely necessary, MRI is contraindicated in pregnancy. Isotope scans are also contraindicated. Ultrasound can be carried out.

Hip disease can present as an isolated monoarthritis or as part of a generalized arthropathic condition. A careful history may reveal the possibility of a previous problem, now exacerbated by pregnancy, because of mechanical changes as a result of increasing weight, ligamentous laxity and changes in posture. Symptoms are often referred to the hip from the sacroiliac or lumbar joints. A thorough examination is essential, particularly to exclude soft tissue lesions such as tendinitis, fascia lata syndrome or a bursitis. Increasing intra-abdominal pressure may cause femoral and inguinal hernia and must be looked for. Nerve root irritation, in particular the obturator nerve (L3/L4), may cause pain to radiate over the upper anterior thigh, as a result of nerve compression at the pelvic brim during engagement of the fetal head.

Conditions of the proximal femur, acetabulum, articular surface and synovium must be considered and excluded as at any other time. Pregnancy-induced osteomalacia, particularly in Asians, can be excluded on the basis of a normal calcium and alkaline phosphatase. Infection is unlikely with a normal white cell count and absence of an effusion on ultrasound.

Aspiration of any fluid, if present, provides both therapeutic and diagnostic options. A good history should exclude traumatic causes and possible stress fractures.

Osteonecrosis is an uncommon condition in patients without an underlying predisposing cause and is even less likely to occur in pregnancy, but it must be considered. Radiographs may be taken if considered diagnostically necessary (limited views of the hip with shielding of the fetus). Radiographs in osteonecrosis are usually initially normal; although MRI is the investigation of choice in this condition, it is contraindicated in pregnancy unless clinically considered to be absolutely necessary. Isotope scans, even if they were not contraindicated in pregnancy, would provide no further information.

Transient osteoporosis is a rare but recognized condition of pregnancy. It may also affect children and young and middle-aged adults of both sexes. In pregnant women, typically the left hip is affected (Fig. 14.7), but involvement of the right hip and other joints has been described. Patients present with groin pain, sometimes referred to the anterior knee on weight bearing. The ESR or plasma viscosity is occasionally raised, but this may be difficult to distinguish from the normal elevation seen in pregnancy. There may be an associated effusion; synovial biopsies tend to be normal but occasionally show a nonspecific, mild, chronic inflammatory change.

Isotope scans may be positive much earlier than radiographic evidence of demineralization of the femoral head. Computed tomography (CT) can be used to demonstrate demineralization in idiopathic cases.

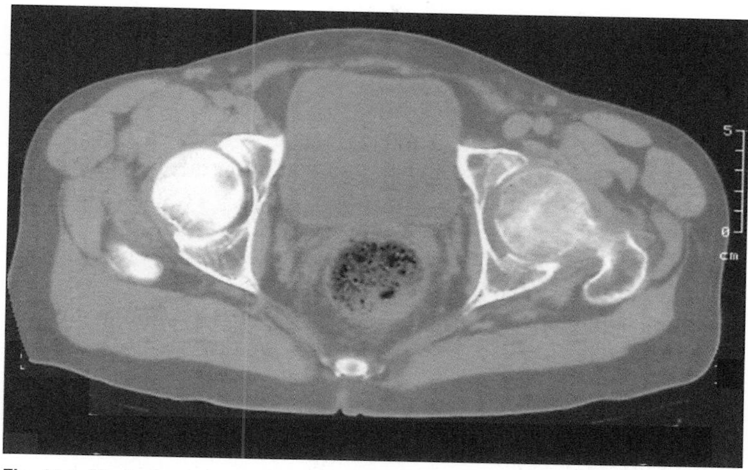

Fig. 14.7 Marked osteoporosis of the head of the left femur in a case of painful osteoporosis of the hip.

The cause of transient osteoporosis of pregnancy is unknown, but theories have implicated both endocrine changes and local compression of vessels or nerves resulting in a transient algodystrophy. These theories are unlikely to be correct, as these changes have also been seen in early pregnancy and nonpregnant states. Complete recovery in 2–6 months is the rule.

THERAPEUTIC OPTIONS

Conservative management is usually the rule unless otherwise clinically indicated. Radiographs should be avoided if possible. Ultrasound may reveal an effusion, which can be aspirated in order to provide therapeutic effect and allow microscopic and microbiological investigation. Investigations in most cases, unless clinically indicated, can usually be delayed until after delivery. Nonsteroidal anti-inflammatory agents should be avoided, particularly around the 3rd trimester, because of the potential effects on the fetal circulation. Acetaminophen (paracetamol) crosses the placenta easily, but with no effects on the fetus. Codeine and propoxyphene are also safe, but large amounts may result in fetal withdrawal symptoms.

CONCLUSIONS

Transient osteoporosis is a condition of unknown etiology. It is probably multifactorial, and more likely to be seen in pregnancy because of other contributory factors. Treatment is conservative, with complete recovery. Other causes of hip pain must be considered and excluded after a careful history and examination. Investigations and management must be tailored to fit the clinical situation.

REFERENCES

Bradwell JD, Burns JE, Kingbury GH. Transient osteoporosis of the hip of pregnancy. J Bone Jt Surg. 1989;71(A):1252–7.

Curtis PH, Kincaid WE. Transitory demineralization of the hip in pregnancy. J Bone Jt Surg. 1959;41A:1327–32.

Goldman GA, Friedman S, Hod M, Ovadia J. Idiopathic transient osteoporosis of the hip in pregnancy. Int J Gynaecol Obstet. 1994:46:317–20.

Lequesne M. Transient osteoporosis of the hip. A non traumatic variety of Sudeck's atrophy. Ann Rheum Dis. 1968;27:463–71.

Rhodes I, Matzinger F, Matzinger MA. Transient osteoporosis of the hip. Can Assoc Radiol J. 1993;44(5):399–402.

Schapira D. Transient osteoporosis of the hip. Semin Arthritis Rheum. 1992;22(2):98–105.

OSTEITIS PUBIS

Adrian J Crisp

DEFINITION OF THE PROBLEM

Osteitis pubis is a painful inflammatory condition involving all structures in the region of the symphysis pubis. It may be subdivided into three main groups:

- septic osteomyelitis of the os pubis, usually following pelvic surgery;
- osteitis pubis without focal bone infection. This often follows pelvic trauma or surgery and may be associated with infection in the urogenital tract;
- osteitis pubis associated with athletic trauma, seronegative spondyloarthopathy or unknown causes.

THE TYPICAL CASE

RL, a 50-year-old hospital porter, underwent circumcision under general anesthetic for paraphimosis. Three weeks later he developed severe pain in both groins exacerbated by walking and partially relieved by rest. This worsened over the next 2 months. About 3 months postcircumcision he was noted to be walking with a waddling gait. There was marked tenderness over the symphysis pubis and over the inferior pubic rami, painful and decreased bilateral hip joint abduction, painful hip joint adduction with muscle spasms and pain on lateral compression of the pelvis. Examination by a urologist revealed no scrotal, testicular or prostatic physical signs although a low grade epididymo-orchitis was considered possible. He had a pyrexia of 37.5°C.

Investigations included: hemoglobin 11.8g/dl; total leukocyte count 9.4×10^9/l (7.1×10^9/l granulocytes and 2.0×10^9/l lymphocytes); ESR 108mm/h; C-reactive protein (CRP) 39mg/l (normal range <6); alanine transferase 59U/l (<40); total alkaline phosphatase 433U/l (90–280). Repeated blood cultures and urine cultures (including for acid fast bacilli) were negative. Plain radiographs of the pelvis demonstrated widening and bony erosions of the symphysis pubis more severe on the right than on the left (Fig. 14.8). Bone scintigraphy revealed increased uptake over the symphysis pubis maximal on the right (Fig. 14.9) but an indium-labeled leukocyte scan showed no increased uptake. Computed tomography showed poorly defined tissue planes around the base of the bladder and seminal vesicles and anterior to the symphysis pubis compatible with widespread inflammatory change.

In spite of the failure to prove bacterial infection and the negative indium-labeled leukocyte scan, a usually reliable guide to infection, a diagnosis of osteitis pubis was made with a high index of suspicion of septic osteomyelitis. Oral ciprofloxacin 250mg q.i.d was started, but after a 4-week course he remained in some pain and his ESR was 65mm/h. Ciprofloxacin was continued and after a total of 8 weeks' treatment he was pain free and walking normally. His ESR had fallen to 6mm/h.

THE DIAGNOSTIC PROBLEM

Cases with frank osteomyelitis in the symphysis pubis or those associated with definite or possible infection in the urogenital tract typically occur 2 weeks to 3 months after a urogenital surgical procedure or event such as prostatectomy, bladder surgery, parturition or gynecologic surgery (especially vesicourethral suspension for prolapse). A complication is often associated, for example urinary or wound infection, or bladder or urethral perforation. Hematogenous spread of bacteria to the symphysis pubis from a distant site is very rare although this has been reported in intravenous drug abusers.

Some authors prefer to confine the use of the term osteitis pubis to the sterile symmetric condition without any evidence of true osteomyelitis of the os pubis. Confusingly this can also follow a urogenital surgical procedure and is more common than osteomyelitis. Erosive symmetric osteitis pubis may often be associated with seronegative spondyloarthropathy but is less painful and disabling than in postsurgical cases. It may be asymptomatic. Traumatic osteitis pubis also occurs in athletes undertaking running and kicking sports and an avulsion stress fracture at the origin of the gracilis muscle near the symphysis pubis has occasionally been implicated. Chondrocalcinosis of the symphysis pubis is a well-known radiologic finding in, for example, primary hyperparathyroidism but acute symphysitis in this context has not been reported.

RL exhibited most of the typical signs of osteitis pubis. Evidence of urogenital infection, e.g. prostatitis, epididymo-orchitis or sepsis elsewhere, may give a high probability of true osteomyelitis but may be misleading. Pyrexia may occur in both infective and noninfective cases.

The ESR and CRP may be raised in all cases. Normal values do not exclude osteomyelitis. Thorough investigation for bacterial infection is essential. Aspiration needle biopsy may be helpful and sometimes open biopsy to obtain adequate tissue samples for culture and histology may be indicated. Various organisms have been implicated in infective cases, e.g. *S. aureus*, *Pseudomonas aeruginosa* and *Escherichia coli*. Histology reveals thickened bone trabeculae, fibrous replacement of marrow by a nonspecific chronic inflammatory infiltrate of lymphocytes and plasma cells, an absence of acute inflammatory changes and typically negative cultures.

Plain radiographs may be normal for several weeks after onset of pain. Rarefaction and erosion of the os pubis then occurs with widening of the joint space. Healing with sclerotic changes and bone apposition then follows, usually within 6 months. Simple degenerative changes are also common, especially in women after childbirth. Bone scintigraphy is always positive and probably the single most useful test. It does not distinguish infective cases but a positive indium-labeled leukocyte scan would strongly indicate osteomyelitis.

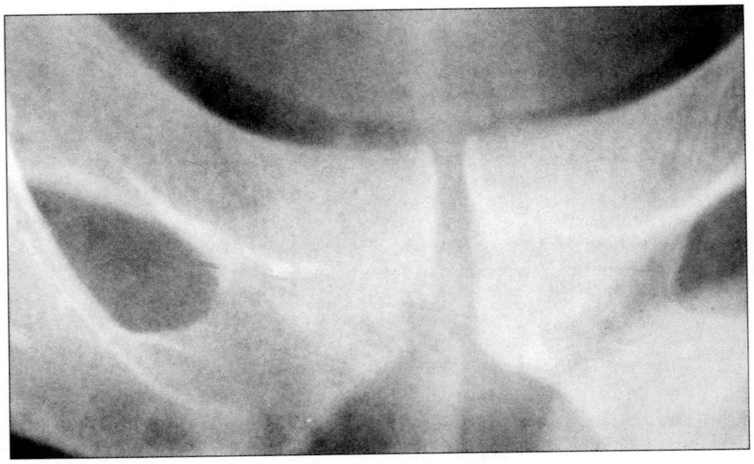

Fig. 14.8 Osteitis pubis. This anteroposterior radiograph of the pelvis shows widening of the symphysis pubis and erosion of bone in the inferior part of the right pubic ramus.

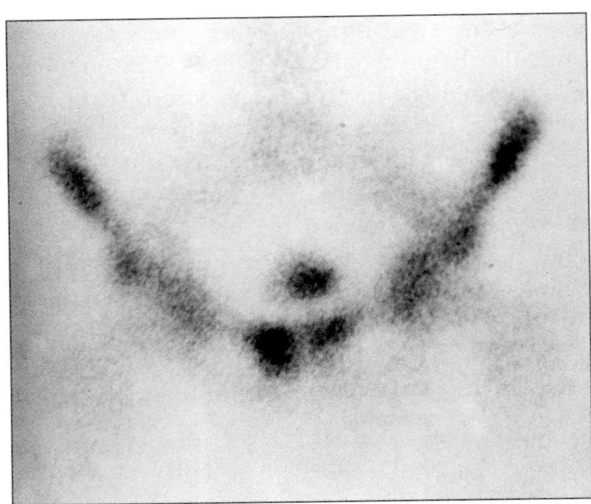

Fig. 14.9 Osteitis pubis. On this bone scan, taken 3 hours after injection of ^{99m}Tc-labeled diphosphonate, increased retention of isotope is seen at the symphysis pubis.

THERAPEUTIC OPTIONS

Osteitis pubis associated with osteomyelitis requires 6–12 weeks of appropriate antibodies, e.g. ofloxacin, ciprofloxacin or flucloxacillin.

Most other cases are self-limiting and settle with conservative therapy using, for example, NSAIDs, analgesics and physical therapy. Therapeutic trials of broad-spectrum antibiotics in the deteriorating patient may also be used even in the absence of proven infection, as in the case of RL. If severe pain continues for more than 6 months, and all conservative measures have been exhausted, it is worth considering a generous wedge resection of the symphysis pubis, which only rarely leads to pelvic instability as body weight is transmitted mainly through posterior pelvic structures.

The pathophysiology of osteitis pubis without osteomyelitis remains obscure. The posterior structures of the symphysis pubis drain into the veins of the lower urinary tract and incompetence of venous valves has been demonstrated. Retrograde venous flow in the retropubic area associated with urogenital infection or trauma might recur. This may lead to bone hyperemia and demineralization. Transient osteonocrosis is another possibility. Perhaps more convincingly, osteitis pubis with pain and reversible bone loss following trauma may be an example of algodystrophy (reflex sympathetic dystrophy).

CONCLUSIONS

Osteitis pubis is an uncommon condition of anterior pelvic pain. Most cases follow urogenital trauma. Many cases represent a focal osteomyelitis but some involve a sterile, inflammatory self-limiting condition of obscure pathophysiology.

REFERENCES

Coventry MB, Mitchell WC. Osteitis pubis. JAMA. 1961;178:898–905.

Grace JN, Sim FH, Shives TC, Coventry MB. Wedge resection of the symphysis pubis for the treatment of osteitis pubis. J Bone Jt Surg. 1989;71A:358–64.

Rosenthal RE, Spickard WA. Markham RD, Rhamy RK. Osteomyelitis of the symphysis pubis: a separate disease from osteitis pubis. Report of 3 cases and a review of the literature. J Bone Jt Surg. 1982;64A:123–8.

Sexton DJ, Heskestad L, Lambeth WR, *et al.* Postoperative pubic osteomyelitis misdiagnosed as osteitis pubis: report of 4 cases and review. Clin Infect Dis. 1993;17:695–700.

CHRONIC KNEE INSTABILITY

David S Tearse

DEFINITION OF THE PROBLEM

Joint, ligament and capsular injuries can lead to chronic instability, effusions and at least in some instances eventual development of osteoarthritis (OA). One of the most common and best understood examples of chronic joint instability following ligamentous and capsular injury is that associated with anterior cruciate ligament injuries (ACL). These injuries can occur with minor as well as major trauma. Diagnosis requires a high index of suspicion and careful examination.

THE TYPICAL CASE

MS, a 28-year-old nurse, suffered a knee injury while in-line skating 3 years previously. Her diagnosis at that time was 'knee sprain' and after several weeks of rest she was able to return to most of her usual activities, although she admitted her knee never returned to '100%'. Once or twice a year she noted that her knee would give out and swell. She presented complaining of pain and swelling after her knee buckled when she stepped off a curb several days before presentation. Examination revealed mild quadriceps atrophy and a 40ml knee effusion. Her ROM was limited in flexion by the effusion. She had tenderness over the medial joint line. Stability testing showed a positive Lachman test (anterior drawer test with the knee in 20° of flexion) and a pivot shift test confirmed moderate rotational pathologic laxity (grade II). McMurray's test was also positive. Plain radiographs of her knee were interpreted as normal (Fig. 14.10), but MRI showed a tear of the medial meniscus (Fig. 14.11) and absence of the ACL (Fig. 14.12). A diagnosis of chronic ACL-deficient knee with a medial meniscus tear was made. Treatment consisted of an arthroscopic-assisted meniscus repair and ACL reconstruction. Six months following surgery the patient was able to return to active sport without instability.

DIAGNOSTIC PROBLEMS

Although ACL injuries are frequently seen in competitive athletes subjected to significant trauma, they also occur following minimal joint injuries in individuals who are not participating in athletic activities. It is most important to make the diagnosis of an ACL tear early in order to initiate treatment (either operative or nonoperative) and avoid reinjury which will inevitably lead to a poor outcome. The first step is to maintain a high index of suspicion of an ACL injury for any twisting fall which causes a hemarthrosis. The reported incidence of ACL disruption with an acute hemarthrosis ranges from 62% to 81%. A meniscus tear occurs with an acute ACL injury approximately 50% of the time. This percentage increases over time with each reinjury. While there may be some disagreement about the long-term outcome of the ACL-deficient knee, there is clear evidence that loss of the meniscus inevitably leads to accelerated osteoarthritis.

The physical examination findings of an ACL tear may be very subtle – instrumental testing of a knee with a documented ACL tear may reveal anywhere from 2mm to 11mm of increased anterior laxity. In examining the knee a careful comparison should be made with the normal contralateral knee in order to pick up the more subtle cases. An experienced examiner may be more sensitive than a MRI study.

While a true natural history study of ACL-deficient knees is difficult to achieve, those studies which have followed nonoperatively treated patients over time have shown relatively poor results, especially in patients who attempt to remain athletically active. Complaints of pain, 'giving way' (instability) and recurrent injury causing meniscus tears, and ultimately OA, increase with time.

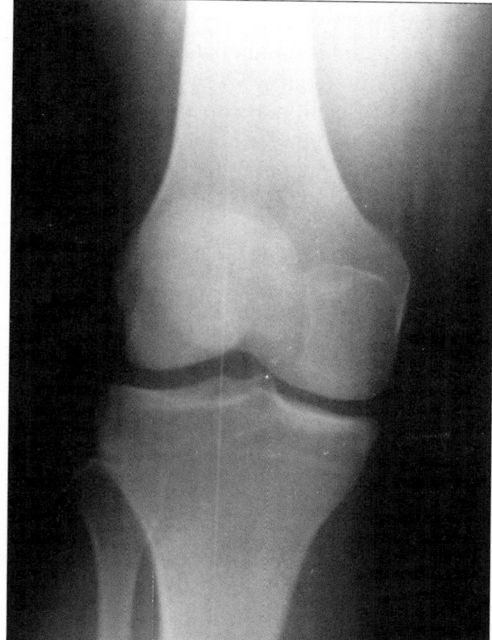

Fig. 14.10 AP radiograph of the knee shows no significant bony abnormalities.

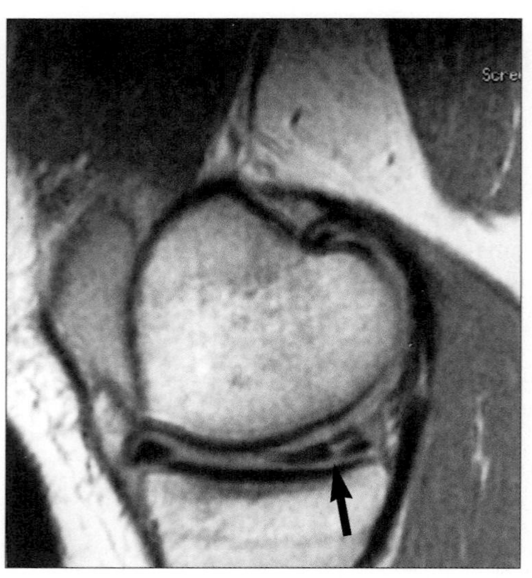

Fig. 14.11 Sagittal cut on MRI through the medial compartment shows the tear in the posterior horn of the medial meniscus (arrow). An effusion is also noted.

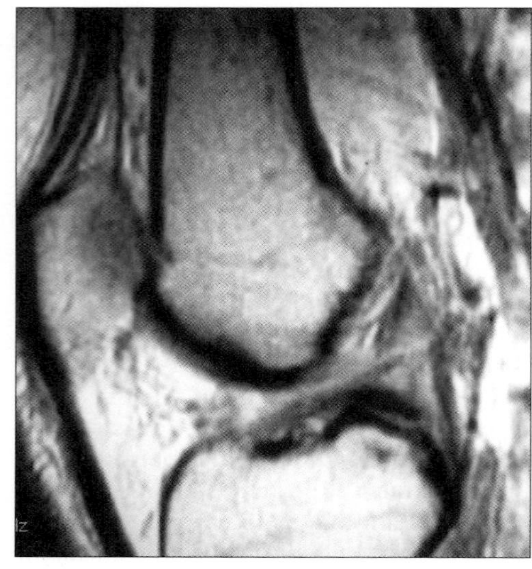

Fig. 14.12 Absence of the anterior cruciate ligament is shown on sagittal cut through the intercondylar notch.

THERAPEUTIC OPTIONS

In general, patients who are younger and more active and who have greater joint laxity should be considered for surgical reconstruction. However, an initial nonoperative approach emphasizing quadriceps and hamstring strengthening, proprioceptive training and bracing for high-demand activities is reasonable for all patients. It should be emphasized to the patient, however, that the goal of treatment is to avoid instability in order to preserve the menisci. Whether this can be achieved through surgery, exercise or activity modification is the patient's choice, unless instability is occurring with activities of daily living.

CONCLUSIONS

A chronic tear of the ACL may lead to unpredictable instability. Knee function often deteriorates in proportion to the frequency of episodes of 'giving way' of the knee. Meniscal tears and articular cartilage lesions significantly affect long-term outcome. Surgical reconstruction prior to development of OA may help preserve the menisci and allow participation in sport without the knee 'giving way'. Patients who function well with an ACL-deficient knee tend to have lower activity demands.

REFERENCES

Balkfors B. The course of knee ligament injuries. Acta Orthop Scand. 1982;53(Suppl):198:1–99.

Buss DD, Warren RF, Wrekewicz TL, *et al.* Arthroscopically assisted reconstruction of the ACL with the use of autogenous patellar ligament grafts. J Bone Jt Surg. 1993;75A:1346–55.

Daniel DM, Stone ML, Dobson BE, *et al.* Fate of the ACL-injured patient: a prospective outcome study. Am J Sports Med. 1994;22:632–44.

Hawkins RJ, Misamove GW, Merritt TR. Follow-up of the acute non-operated isolated anterior cruciate ligament tear. Am J Sports Med. 1986;14:205–10.

McDaniel WJ Jr, Dameron TB Jr. Untreated rupture of the anterior cruciate ligament: a follow-up study. J Bone Jt Surg. 1980;62A:696–705.

ANKLE SPRAIN

Gerald D Groff

DEFINITION OF THE PROBLEM

Ankle sprain results from the stretching or tearing of ankle ligaments following inversion or eversion foot injuries. It is the most common injury in athletics but can occur in any age group with trauma not related to sports. Fewer than 15% of ankle sprain patients have significant fractures. Although the injury is frequently self-limiting, recovery can be complicated by ankle dysfunction, recurrence and acute or chronic instability. As a result, it is important for clinicians to be familiar with clinical evaluation maneuvers, potential diagnostic problems and basic therapies.

THE TYPICAL CASE

MM is a 64-year-old woman in good health except for mild knee OA. While rushing to catch a bus, she stepped on the edge of a curb, 'twisting' her right ankle. She noted immediate sharp pain located inferior and anterior to the right lateral ankle. She developed rapid swelling with moderate pain and insecurity with standing.

Medical review of the injury suggested inversion of the ankle, supination of the foot and external rotation of the tibia. Examination revealed soft tissue swelling, mild ecchymoses and tenderness just inferior to the right lateral malleolus. Tests for instability, including the anterior drawer sign, were negative. Because of pain on weight bearing and bony palpation, a plain radiograph was performed. This was normal. She was treated with ankle elevation and ice for 24 hours, and then NSAIDs plus an air splint for an additional 5 days. Thereafter, gentle ROM and proprioceptive exercises, followed by muscle strengthening exercises, resulted in pain-free, stable ambulation after 3 weeks.

DIAGNOSTIC PROBLEMS

Although ankle sprain is common and often self-limiting, clinicians should be aware of potential problems. Areas of particular concern include concomitant fracture, instability due to ligamentous rupture and conditions that mimic or complicate ankle sprain.

Ankle sprain can be classified into three groups depending on clinical signs and functional loss:

- grade 1 – localized tenderness, minimal swelling or ecchymoses and normal ROM without instability;
- grade 2 – causes moderate to severe pain, swelling or ecchymoses and restricted ROM, potential mild instability and painful weight bearing;
- grade 3 – marked by severe pain, edema, hemorrhage, loss of motion and inability to ambulate; ankle instability is common, with complete functional loss.

The clinical grades reflect the degree of ligamentous injury, with stretching or minimal tearing in grade 1, partial tearing in grade 2 and complete tear in grade 3. Clinical classification is an important determinant of therapy and may require supportive radiographic studies.

The ankle ligaments are shown in Figures 14.13 and 14.14. Inversion ankle injury is much more common than eversion trauma. As a result, over 90% of sprains occur in the lateral complex, particularly the

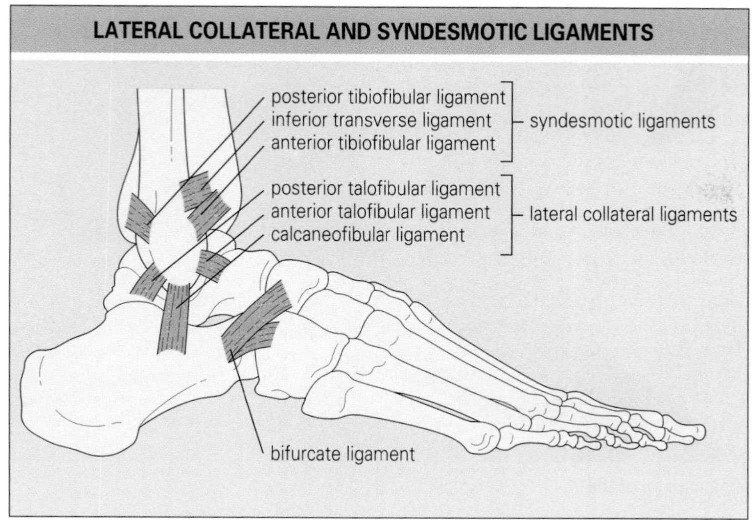

Fig. 14.13 Lateral collateral ligaments and syndesmotic ligaments of the ankle.

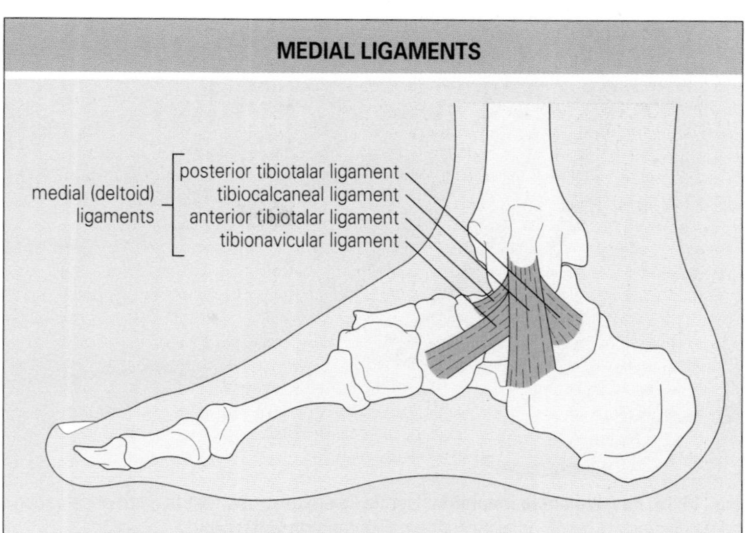

Fig. 14.14 Medial ligaments of the ankle.

anterior talofibular ligament. Rupture of the talofibular ligament alone can cause mild lateral and moderate anterior ankle instability, with pain and swelling inferior to the lateral malleolus. Additional rupture of the calcaneofibular ligament occurs in 25% of lateral complex sprains and results in greater lateral instability. The posterior talofibular ligament is rarely injured. The medial deltoid ligament is involved in 5% or less of all sprains and is frequently complicated by fracture. Inferior tibiofibular (syndesmotic) ligament injury can complicate ankle ligament damage during high-energy trauma. In this case, tenderness is present over the ligament, just above the line of the ankle joint.

The most common fractures during ankle sprain are avulsions of the malleoli or tarsal bones. Other sites include the anterior process of the calcaneus, the base of the 5th metatarsal (insertion of the peroneus brevis tendon), the talar neck, the cuboid and the bony epiphyses in children. The strength of the deltoid ligament makes it an uncommon site for injury, but when it occurs malleolar fracture or concomitant sprains of the syndesmosis are more likely. Standard radiographs should be obtained in patients fulfilling the Ottawa Ankle Rules (Fig. 14.15) which stress three sets of findings:

- the circumstances of the injury and whether the patient was able to bear weight on the sprained extremity within the first hour;
- the presence of bone tenderness at predetermined sites; and
- whether the patient is able to stand and bear weight.

Depending on the location of findings an ankle radiographic series or a foot radiographic series is obtained. In addition radiographs should be obtained for children with open epiphyses and elderly patients with osteoporosis risk factors.

Ankle instability due to lateral ligament rupture is an important condition which must be considered during the initial evaluation. Unrecognized and untreated acute instability can lead to functional insecurity and recurrent ankle sprain. Chronic ankle instability has been linked to the development of OA. Additional causes of persistent pain

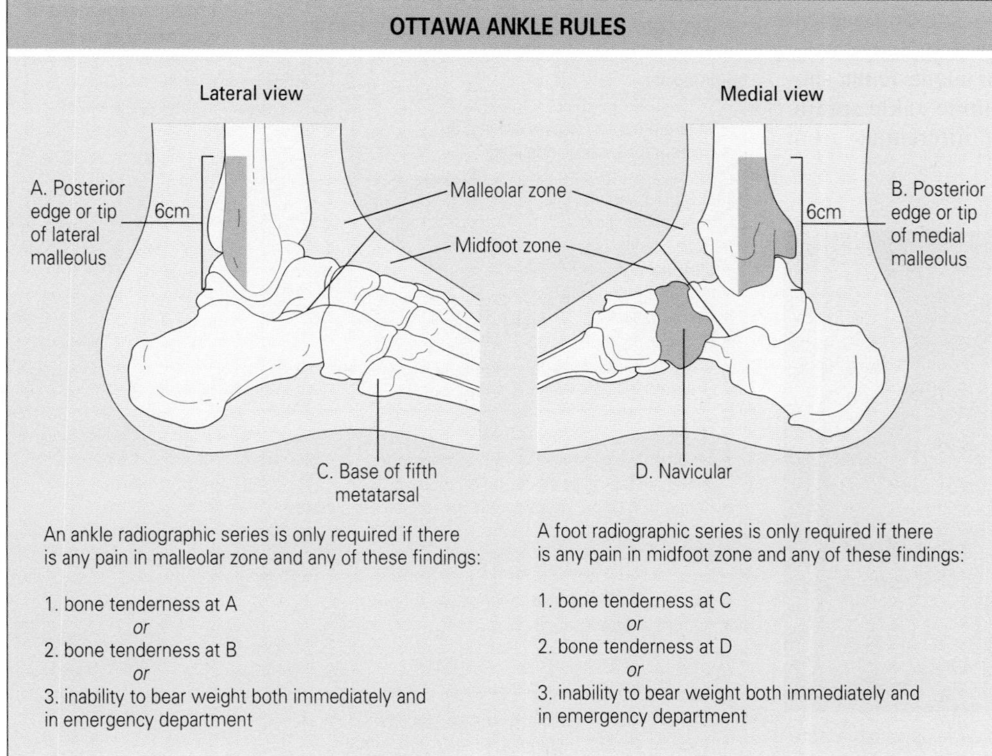

Fig. 14.15 Ottawa Ankle Rules for foot and ankle radiographic series in acute ankle injury patients. Adapted from Stiell *et al.* Implementation of the Ottowa Ankle Rules. JAMA. 1994:271;827–832.

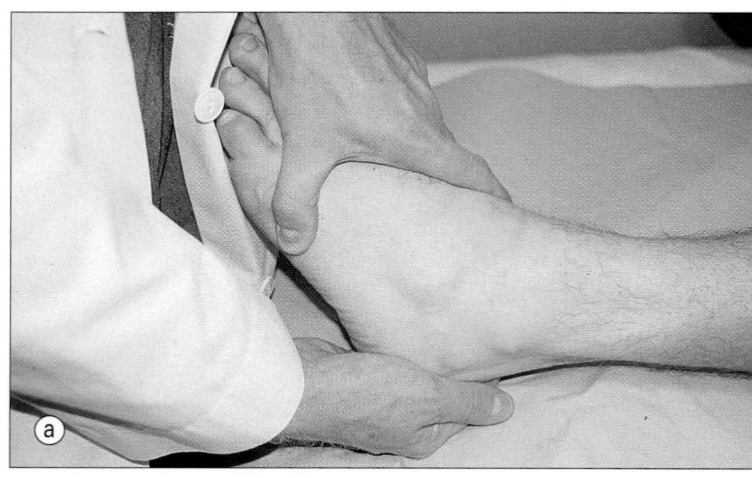

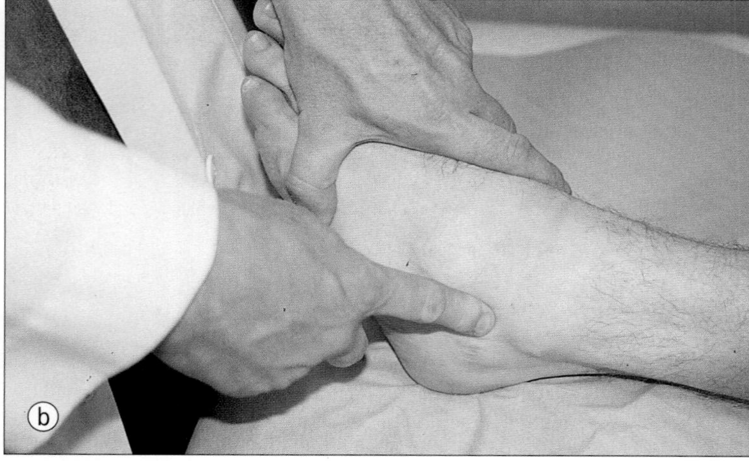

Fig. 14.16 Passive ankle inversion. Gentle inversion of the foot (a) with observation and palpations (b) of the talofibular joint. Motion or laxity suggests ligamentous instability.

after ankle sprain include incomplete rehabilitation, stress fractures, intra-articular lesions, subtalar sprain and instability, sinus tarsi syndrome (due to rupture of the talocalcaneal interosseous ligament), impingements, tendinitides, nerve injuries and reflex sympathetic dystrophy. The clinical assessment of stability includes passive ankle inversion (Fig. 14.16) and the anterior drawer test (Fig. 14.17). Instability can be estimated by comparing the degree of laxity with that of the uninjured ankle. The severity of sprain can usually be determined by physical examination. However, the examination may be limited by pain, swelling or muscle spasm. These patients, as well as those with demonstrable laxity, may require additional diagnostic studies. Stress radiography can be performed during the talar tilt and anterior drawer maneuvers. An opening of the posterior tibiotalar joint of 6mm or greater during the anterior drawer maneuver suggests anterior talofibular ligament rupture. However, the accuracy of these studies is limited by several factors, such as patient cooperation, the amount of force applied and the angle of ankle flexion. Arthrography is generally more accurate, although dye extravasation in as many as 25% of procedures can reduce the diagnostic value. Magnetic resonance imaging may prove to be the preferred procedure.

The differential diagnosis of 'ankle sprain' includes peroneal tendon subluxation or inflammation, Achilles tendon injury and sprain or rupture of the inferior tibiofibular syndesmosis. Syndesmotic ligament tears are unusual, but when involved can require prolonged recovery or cause chronic ankle instability. Rarely, subtalar or talonavicular subluxation and acute lateral ankle synovitis may mimic ankle sprain. Posterior tibial tendon rupture may be difficult to differentiate from the uncommon medial ankle sprain.

Fig. 14.17 The anterior drawer test. The distal leg is stabilized while upward pressure is applied to the heel. Anterior laxity of the ankle suggests ligamentous instability.

Systemic conditions may complicate recovery. Patients with peripheral neuropathy and poor proprioception (especially diabetics) can develop secondary reflex sympathetic dystrophy or destructive arthropathy. Patients with chronic hip or knee arthritis may have limitations to rehabilitation or may be at risk of recurrent sprain due to gait imbalance or chronic muscle weakness.

THERAPEUTIC OPTIONS

The goals of acute ankle sprain management are reduction of pain and swelling and the prevention of chronic instability. Grade 1 and 2 sprains respond well to conservative therapy as long as treatment is begun as soon as possible after injury (Fig. 14.18). Acute instability or fracture should be ruled out by examination and radiography when indicated. Therapy over the initial 24–48 hours includes rest, elevation and compression wrap. Cold packs may be applied for 15–20 minutes each hour as tolerated. Recovery may be accelerated if NSAIDs are started within the initial 24 hours of treatment. Early use of NSAIDs permits return to sports sooner than when ankle support alone is utilized.

AN APPROACH TO THE MANAGEMENT OF ACUTE ANKLE SPRAIN (GRADES 1 AND 2)
Immediate
• Rule out instability by examination • Radiography when indicated
Initial 24–48 hours
• Rest • Elevation • Ice • Compression • NSAIDs
2–7 days
• NSAIDs • Modified weight-bearing with ankle support (adhesive taping or air-stirrup support) • Range of motion, proprioceptive exercise as tolerated
7–28 days
• Progressive mobilization with ankle support • Additional strengthening exercises
Chronic
• Ankle support if insecurity or mild stability • Resume athletic training when pain is minimal

Fig. 14.18 An approach to the management of acute ankle sprain.

Depending on severity, healing may require 2–8 weeks. There is no precise information regarding the healing time of ligament injury. As a result, the guidelines for joint preservation and rehabilitation must be individualized. In general, patients with grade 1 sprains can begin careful rehabilitation after 48 hours. This would include plantar and dorsiflexion ROM exercises, Achilles tendon stretching and isometrics within the limits of discomfort.

After a few days, double- and single-leg toe raises with lateral ankle support helps to improve proprioception. Early mobilization with lateral ankle support is important. Grade 2 sprains may require a more prolonged period of immobilization during weight bearing, utilizing a cast brace or bivalved cast for 10–14 days. Rehabilitation may be more protracted with avoidance of ankle inversion. However, rehabilitation should be directed towards return to safe ambulation as soon as possible. The key to a successful outcome is a consistent, progressive rehabilitation program.

Ankle support with either adhesive taping or air stirrup is a useful adjunct to rehabilitation. Supports serve to limit the extremes of ankle motion and increase ankle proprioception. Acutely, this allows early weight-bearing while reducing the risk of reinjury during the initial 3–4 weeks of recovery. Patients with mild functional instability or athletes at risk for recurrent injury may benefit from more prolonged use of ankle support. However, the goal is to make supports unnecessary by ankle strengthening through exercise. Taping techniques are described by Balduini *et al.* (1987). The air stirrup consists of two segments of molded orthoplast with inflatable inner-lining air bags connected by a heel strap (Air Cast Inc., Summit NJ, USA). The air stirrup has the distinct advantages of being easy to remove for rehabilitation and allowing dorsi and plantar flexion while limiting inversion.

The treatment of grade 3 sprain (complete ligamentous rupture and instability) is controversial. Management with rigid casting or primary surgical repair depends on a variety of factors, including the degree of subjective and objective instability, the number and position of ruptured ligaments and the athletic goals of the patient. As a result, grade 3 sprains should be referred to an experienced orthopedic surgeon.

CONCLUSIONS

Ankle sprain is a common injury, occurring in the geriatric population as well as in athletes. Appropriate initial management is essential in preserving long-term ankle function and preventing instability or recurrent injury. It should include clinical assessment of instability with supportive plain or stress radiographs when indicated. Grades 1 and 2 sprains respond well to conservative treatment and careful rehabilitation. Grade 3 sprains should be referred to an orthopedic surgeon for consideration of casting or surgical intervention.

REFERENCES

Stiell IG, McKnight RD, Greenberg GH, *et al.* Implementation of the Ottawa Ankle Rules. JAMA. 1994;271:827–32.

Balduini F, Vesco J, Torg J, Torg E. Management and rehabilitation of ligamentous injuries to the ankle. Sports Med. 1987;4:364–80.

Cass J, Morrey B. Ankle instability: current concepts, diagnosis and treatment. Mayo Clin Proc. 1984:59;165–70.

Ouzounian T, Shereff M. Common ankle disorders of the elderly: diagnosis and management. Geriatrics. 1988;43:73–80.

Raatikainen T, Putkonen M, Puranen J. Arthrography, clinical examination and stress radiograph in the diagnosis of acute injury to the lateral ligaments of the ankle. Am J Sports Med. 1992;20:2–6.

Renström AFH. Persistently painful sprained ankle. J Am Acad Orthop Surg. 1994;2:270–80.

Stanley K. Ankle sprains are always more than 'just a sprain'. Postgrad Med. 1991;89:251–5.

PLANTAR HEEL PAIN

Shepard Hurwitz

DEFINITION OF THE PROBLEM

Plantar heel pain is common in the adult population at large and in seronegative arthropathy patients in particular. The most recalcitrant forms of plantar heel pain occur in those patients with radiographic enthesophyte formation and psoriatic arthritis, Reiter's syndrome and other spondyloarthropathies. These patients will commonly have posterior heel pain in addition to the plantar heel pain, a feature which is not commonly seen in plantar heel pain syndromes in the population at large.

THE TYPICAL CASE

HA, a 41-year-old woman, with a long-standing history of psoriatic arthritis presented with painful plantar heel discomfort. Her medications included hydrochloroquine 200mg b.i.d. and sulindac 200mg b.i.d. She had been wearing sneakers with cushioned insoles and was not able to walk with the assistance of a cane. Because of her extensive psoriasis hydrotherapy was not possible, nor could she use frequent ice packs. She presented after having been treated by her internist with several injections of corticosteroids into the fat pad under the right calcaneus. Physical examination revealed a stiff ankle and hindfoot without signs of posterior tibial nerve entrapment or posterior tibial tendinitis. She was tender on the plantar and plantar medial aspect of the heel near the prominence of the calcaneus. There were no skin lesions on the sole of her foot. A radiograph was obtained (Fig. 14.19).

THE DIAGNOSTIC PROBLEM

Evaluation of plantar heel pain should include careful physical examination which should differentiate between nerve pain, bone pain, soft tissue pain and the presence of any lesions such as tumor or infection (Fig. 14.16). Tendinitis of the posterior tibial or flexor digitorum longus tendons may mimic plantar heel pain or may indirectly cause pain by exerting compression on the contents of the tarsal tunnel. Nerve entrapment of the posterior tibial nerve or its major branches may be caused by inflamed synovium, a ganglion, varicose veins or soft tissue encroachment of swollen muscle or fascia. A syndrome involving entrapment of a specific nerve, the first branch of the lateral plantar nerve, has been described. Soft tissue pain may be the result of chronic or acute inflammation of the origin of the plantar fascia or any of the short muscles on the heel. Fibrosis of the plantar heel pad may lead to pain, as may disruption of the normal plantar

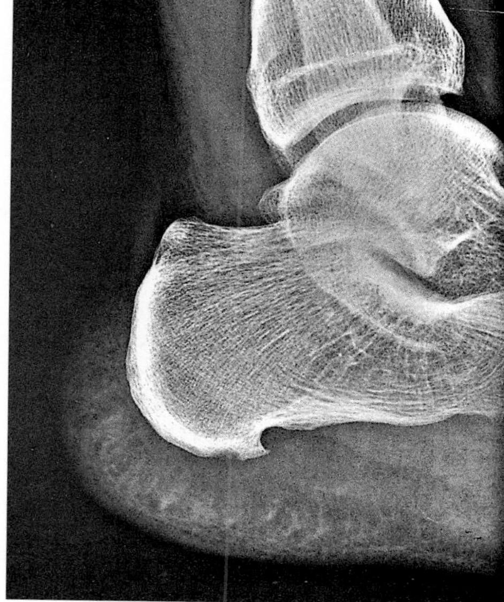

Fig. 14.19 Plantar heel pain in a patient with psoriasis. The radiograph shows erosive changes due to inflammation and proliferative bone change of the calcaneus.

DIFFERENTIAL DIAGNOSIS OF PLANTAR HEEL PAIN
Skin
Keratoses Verruca Ulcer Fissure
Connective tissue
Fat Atrophy Panniculitis
Dense connective tissue Inflammatory fasciitis Fibromatosis Enthesopathy Bursitis
Bone (calcaneus) Stress fracture Paget's disease Benign bone cyst/tumor Malignant bone tumor Metabolic bone disease (osteopenia)
Nerve
Tarsal tunnel Plantar nerve entrapment S1 nerve root radiculopathy Painful peripheral neuropathy
Infection
Dermatomycoses Acute osteomyelitis Plantar abscess
Miscellaneous
Foreign body Non union calcaneus fracture Psychogenic Idiopathic

Fig. 14.20 Differential diagnosis of plantar heel pain.

architecture following trauma. Infection of the soft tissues may be overt, such as in the case of a skin ulcer, or occult, such as with a plantar abscess or osteomyelitis of the calcaneus. Bone pain may be due to stress fracture, enthesopathy of the plantar fascia or short flexor muscles originating on the calcaneus.

Primary tumors of the calcaneus are possible; metastatic lesions to the calcaneus are exceedingly rare.

Lateral and axial radiographs are the appropriate views. The soft tissues may be evaluated with MRI; the bony architecture of the calcaneus is best evaluated with a CT scan. Radionuclide imaging of the calcaneus is a good screening examination when bone pain is suspected. However, this modality does not differentiate a periosteal process from an intraosseous process. Nerve conduction tests may detect slowing of transmission across the tarsal tunnel area and electrical studies may show denervation of a specific group of muscles, such as the abductor to the great toe for the medial plantar nerve and the abductor to the little toe for the lateral plantar nerve.

THERAPEUTIC OPTIONS

The painful plantar heel first needs a diagnosis. The pain of nerve entrapment may respond to a change in anti-inflammatory medication, including corticosteroids, but in all likelihood will require infiltration with corticosteroids at the point of entrapment. Physical therapy modalities such as iontophoresis with soluble corticosteroid preparations may work as well as infiltration via injection. Limitation of activity is helpful as an adjunct, primarily involving reduction in weight-bearing activity. Entrapment neuropathy does not respond to vitamin therapy or exercises.

Sources of bone pain respond to rest and immobilization in the case of stress fracture. Paget's disease of bone may require medical management while tumors will usually need surgical excision. The painful enthesopathy that is associated with proliferative bone change is a feature of the case presented above of a woman with seronegative arthritis. Optimum management of the inflammatory component of the disease is helpful. In these patients, indomethacin and phenylbutazone are often more effective than other NSAIDs. The results of surgery are highly controversial and surgical intervention is not one of the early treatment options. Physical modalities such as passive stretching of the plantar fascia and toe flexors in conjunction with a cushioned insole are also important. This orthosis should cushion the heel and provide medial arch support and supination of the foot. The orthosis is designed to reduce the stretch on the plantar fascia, the short muscles of the foot and the Achilles tendon. If the patient can tolerate pressure on the forefoot, then an elevation of the heel would be helpful to shunt some of the pressure to the forefoot and away from the painful heel. Other physical therapy modalities, including whirlpool, ultrasound, friction massage and assisted stretching exercises, have their place in nonsurgical management. Relief may be obtained under a tender area by preventing contact with that area of the orthotic insole.

Patients without nerve entrapment or large plantar osteophytes constitute the majority of cases. This problem is best managed nonoperatively with the same shoe modifications, footwear inserts, physical therapy and modalities, and judicious use of injected corticosteroids. A word of caution about corticosteroid injections is that there is an incidence of plantar fascia rupture, which in the case of a flexible foot will lead to pes planus. Surgery for soft tissue pain on the sole of the foot is not very rewarding and involves creating an iatrogenic disruption of the plantar fascia. Most recently, in North America, endoscopic plantar fascia incision with or without laser tools has become popular among podiatrists. There is great skepticism among orthopedic surgeons regarding the efficacy of this procedure. Patients with plantar fascia rupture or surgical excision should have an insole orthotic to try to control the hindfoot and support the arch, in an attempt to minimize mechanical collapse and pronation of the foot.

CONCLUSIONS

The patient with inflammatory seronegative arthritis and plantar heel pain presents a challenge to the clinician. The symptoms may be remarkably improved on a short-term basis by injection; however, this is probably not a long-term solution. Local radiotherapy may be helpful in selected patients (see Chapter 6.20). Surgery is not very successful.

Currently, treatment recommendations include the use of appropriate well-fitting shoes and orthotic devices, stretching and judicious use of local injections. Treatment is often needed for protracted periods of time. The patient should be counseled against jogging and court sports during the acute phase.

REFERENCES

Capen D, Scheck M. Seronegative inflammation of the ankle and foot. Clin Orthop Rel Res. 1981;155:147–52.

Resnick D, Niwayama K. On the nature of bony proliferation in 'rheumatoid variant' disorder. Am J Roentgenol. 1977;129:275–81.

Solomon G. Inflammatory arthritis. In: Jahss MH, ed. Disorders of the foot and ankle, 2 Ed. Philadelphia: WB Saunders; 1991:1681–1693.

DEFINITION OF THE PROBLEM

Physicians should consider the possibility of metastatic disease when evaluating patients with musculoskeletal pain, especially in individuals older than 40 years. Metastatic tumors are the most common neoplasms found in bone, and bone is the third most common site for metastatic disease after lung and liver. Delay in diagnosis and initiation of treatment may lead to unremitting pain, pathologic fracture, hypercalcemia and neurologic deficits. Although any malignant neoplasm can metastasize to bone, more than 80% of all patients with bone metastases have primary tumors of the breast, prostate or lung and about 50% of patients with these carcinomas develop skeletal disease. Many patients who present with skeletal pain due to metastatic disease have a known primary tumor. In these individuals the diagnosis is often readily apparent. However, in some patients, pain due to a metastatic lesion may be the first indication of the presence of malignancy, and in others musculoskeletal pain caused by metastatic disease may develop years after the diagnosis and apparently successful treatment of a primary malignant tumor. Making the correct diagnosis in these two groups of patients may be difficult, especially in patients who present with a solitary lesion; but in any patient with metastatic disease, early diagnosis is essential to initiate appropriate treatment and minimize the risk of complications.

THE TYPICAL CASE

JG, a 56-year-old man, presented with a 4-month history of left thigh and hip pain. He described the pain as a deep aching discomfort that has gradually increased in intensity and has not been relieved by rest. His past medical history included a myocardial infarction and carcinoma of the colon treated surgically 5 years previously. Examination revealed no limitations of joint motion and no reflex, sensory or motor changes in the limb. There were no palpable masses and no areas of tenderness. Laboratory studies, including hemoglobin, hematocrit, white cell count and serum calcium, phosphate and alkaline phosphatase, were normal. Radiographs of the thigh and hip were interpreted as normal. Initial treatment consisted of NSAIDs. Six weeks later the patient reported that his pain had increased to the extent that he could not sleep for more than an hour at a time despite regular use of medications including acetaminophen with codeine. New radiographs of the femur were initially interpreted as normal (Fig. 14.21), but a bone scan showed a small area of increased uptake in the proximal femur (Fig. 14.22) and a MRI study showed a marrow abnormality in the area of increased uptake (Fig. 14.23). Computed tomographic studies did not show evidence of neoplastic disease in the lungs or bowel, but they did demonstrate a lesion in the liver consistent with, but not diagnostic of, metastatic disease. A biopsy of the femoral lesion showed metastatic carcinoma of the colon and the femoral lesion was treated with radiation therapy.

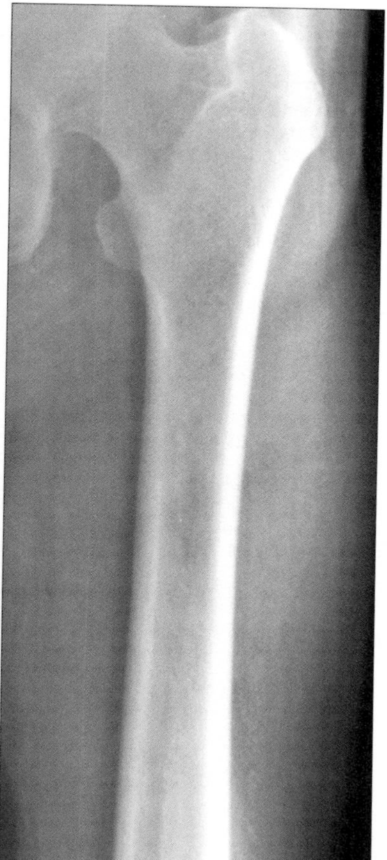

Fig. 14.21 Plain radiograph showing the left hip and femur. This study was initially interpreted as normal. After review of bone scintigraphy and MRI studies, an area of slightly decreased bone density was identified in the medullary cavity of the proximal femur.

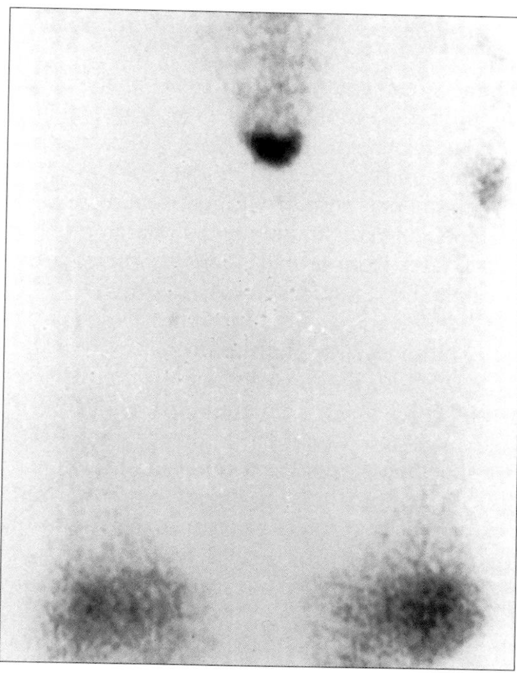

Fig. 14.22 Technetium bone scintigraphy study showing the pelvis and femurs. A small area of increased uptake is apparent in the proximal left femur.

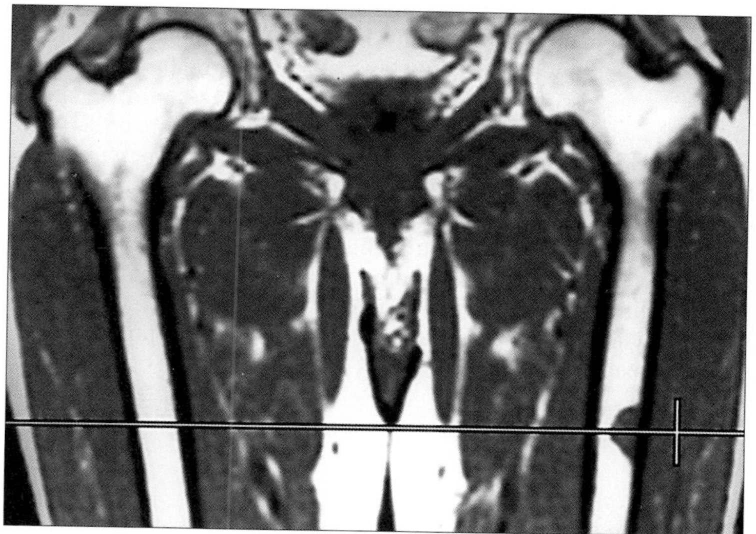

Fig. 14.23 MRI of the hips and femurs shows an area of marrow infiltration that matches the area of increased tracer uptake shown on bone scintigraphy (Fig.14.22).

DIAGNOSTIC PROBLEMS

Causes of musculoskeletal pain that may mimic metastatic disease include stress or insufficiency fractures, infections, primary benign and malignant neoplasms including myeloma, bone necrosis, hyperparathyroidism, degenerative joint disease, Paget's disease, neuropathies and herniated intervertebral disks. Metastatic disease of the skeleton can present as bone pain either in individuals with a previous history of malignancy or in individuals without history of cancer, and the pain can develop well before the appearance of physical findings, radiographic changes or laboratory abnormalities. In most patients rest does not relieve the pain; they may notice increased pain at night that disturbs their sleep. Nonnarcotic analgesics alone typically provide minimal relief. Acute onset of pain after minor trauma suggests the possibility of pathologic fracture. Physical examination may demonstrate bone tenderness or limited motion. If the lesion has penetrated the cortex, a soft tissue mass may be palpable. Some metastatic tumors, especially renal cell carcinomas with soft tissue extension, cause increased local vascularity and warmth, erythema and occasionally bruits. Plain radiographs may fail to demonstrate significant abnormalities early in the course of metastatic disease. This occurs because many metastatic lesions develop first in the medullary cavity, and while plain radiographs show changes in cortical bone as well, they do not show changes in cancellous bone until there has been extensive destruction or new bone formation.

Serum levels of the bone isoenzyme of alkaline phosphatase can be helpful in monitoring the progression of bone disease in patients with a known malignancy, but may not help distinguish skeletal metastases from other bone lesions and diseases. Combinations of serum tumor markers including tissue polypeptide antigen, squamous cell carcinoma antigen, carcinoembryonic antigen and alphafetoprotein may help distinguish metastases from primary bone lesions. Serum protein electrophoresis can help exclude myeloma.

Bone scintigraphy is a sensitive procedure for the early detection of skeletal metastases; combined with plain radiography it is the most frequently used approach to diagnosis of metastatic disease and monitoring of patients with a history of carcinoma. However, it is not specific for malignancy, and it may fail to detect some osteolytic lesions, in particular metastases from renal malignancies. Computed tomography can demonstrate the extent and pattern of bone destruction and may be useful in locating a primary tumor in the chest, abdomen or pelvis. Magnetic resonance imaging can demonstrate disruption of the bone cortex and soft tissue extension of metastatic lesions.

Patients who have bone pain and a bone lesion that has features consistent with metastatic disease, but who do not have a history of malignancy, present a difficult diagnostic problem. In addition to a thorough medical history and physical examination and laboratory studies, these individuals should have plain radiographs of the chest and any regions of the skeleton where they have pain. In most instances they should also have whole body technetium bone scintigraphy and CT examinations of the chest, abdomen and pelvis. After this evaluation, if biopsy is necessary, the optimal site and approach can be determined based on the imaging studies. Biopsies must be planned carefully to provide an adequate tissue sample and decrease the risks of complications including fracture, nerve damage, excessive bleeding and infection. The choice of the biopsy method and site should also be made carefully so as not to prevent optimal future surgical treatment.

THERAPEUTIC OPTIONS

Biopsy may not be necessary in patients with previously documented metastatic disease and characteristic findings on imaging studies. However, in those individuals where there is uncertainty concerning the presence of metastatic disease, biopsy is indicated. Confirmation of the presence of skeletal metastatic disease leaves the patient and physician with a number of therapeutic options even when it is not possible or appropriate to treat the primary malignancy. Patients with metastatic disease benefit from a systematic approach to pain management that includes education and counseling for the patient and family, analgesics and in some instances activity modification. The combination of a NSAID with a narcotic can decrease pain for many patients, but physicians should carefully monitor the efficacy of their approach to pain management and should not be hesitant to use different combinations of drugs, sufficient doses of drugs and nontraditional approaches to pain control. In some patients, chemotherapy, hormonal therapy or radiation therapy may be appropriate. Recent reports indicate that bisphosphonates may be helpful in patients with osteolytic metastases. In most individuals with persistent pain and lesions that are likely to fracture, either internal fixation or resection of the involved bone and prosthetic replacement should be performed. This is most often the case when the lesion has involved a significant portion of the bone cortex, is causing persistent increasing pain and pain with loading of the involved bone. A limited number of patients may benefit from amputation to control pain and improve mobility.

CONCLUSIONS

Metastatic disease of the skeleton can present a diagnostic dilemma in some patients. Plain radiographs may reveal the lesion but bone scans are usually more sensitive. In some individuals, CT or MRI may be helpful in detecting and defining the extent and precise location of a lesion. Biopsies of these lesions should be approached with caution and in some patients should be combined with internal fixation or resection of involved segments of the skeleton followed by prosthetic replacement. A systematic approach to pain management is a critical part of the treatment of patients with metastatic disease.

REFERENCES

Averbuch SD. New bisphosphonates in the treatment of bone metastases. Cancer. 1993;72:3443–52.

Chigira M, Shinozaki T. Diagnostic value of serum tumor markers in skeletal metastases of carcinomas. Arch Orthop Trauma Surg. 1990;109:247–51.

Dijstra S, Wiggers T, Geel BNV, Boxma H. Impending and actual pathological fractures in patients with bone metastases of the long bones. A retrospective study of 233 surgical treated fractures. Eur J Surg. 1994;160:535–42.

Gold RH, Bassett LW. Radionuclide evaluation of skeletal metastases: practical considerations. Skeletal Radiol. 1986;15:1–9.

Kanis JA, McCloskey EV, Taube T, O'Rourke N. Rationale for the use of bisphosphonates in bone metastases. Bone. 1991;12(suppl 1):13–18.

Rassmusson B, Vejborg I, Jensen AB, *et al*. Irradiation of bone metastases in breast cancer patients: a randomized study with one year follow-up. Radiother Oncol. 1995;34:179–84.

Reale MG, Santini D, Marchei GG, *et al*. Skeletal alkaline phosphatase as a serum marker of bone metastases in the follow-up of patients with breast cancer. Int J Biol Markers. 1995;10:42–6.

Rougraff BT, Kneisl JS, Simon MA. Skeletal metastases of unknown origin. A prospective study of a diagnostic strategy. J Bone Jt Surg. 1993;75:1276–81.

Sanal SM, Flickinger FW, Caudell HJ, Sherry RM. Detection of bone marrow involvement in breast cancer with magnetic resonance imaging. J Clin Oncol. 1994;12:1415–21.

Shih LY, Chen TH, Lo WH. Skeletal metastases from occult carcinoma. J Surg Oncol. 1992;51:109–13.

Twycross RG. Management of pain in skeletal metastases. Clin Orthop. 1995;312:187–96.

DEFINITION OF THE PROBLEM

It is not unusual for rheumatologists to encounter patients of either sex with synovitis confined to one knee and which has been present for longer than 3 months. These patients may have already received treatment with NSAIDs, oral antibiotics and intra-articular corticosteroid injections to no avail. Chronic monoarthritis of the knee occurs in persons of all ages and can result from any disease that, under other circumstances, causes polyarthritis. In younger patients the etiology often remains obscure despite intensive investigation. Treatment of such 'chronic monoarthritis of undetermined etiology' (CMUE) has to be empirical.

THE TYPICAL CASE

A 27-year-old male accountant developed monoarthritis of his left knee 6 months prior to consultation (Fig. 14.24). He was single, heterosexual and, despite being sexually active, he denied any recent sexual contact with anyone other than his regular girlfriend. Previously he had been fully fit and active, had not traveled abroad recently, nor had he or any other member of his family suffered from significant joint, skin, eye, gastrointestinal, genitourinary or back problems. Clinical examination was unhelpful and genitourinary investigation negative. Cultures of stool, throat swab and midstream urine. Tests for rheumatoid factor, antinuclear antibody (ANA) and HLA-B27 antigen were negative and uric acid and liver function tests were normal. Joint aspiration yielded 35ml of sterile straw-colored synovial fluid with 35,000/mm^3 leukocytes, which were predominantly lymphocytes. No crystals were visible under polarized light microscopy and cultures were negative.

Arthroscopy was performed and examination of a synovial biopsy confirmed nonspecific synovitis. Tissue stains and cultures were negative. The knee was washed out with saline to good effect. Synovitis persisted for the next 4 years, despite several subsequent intra-articular methylprednisolone injections, and active physiotherapy helped to minimize loss of quadriceps muscle bulk. He has been reluctant to start treatment with any drug other than NSAIDs.

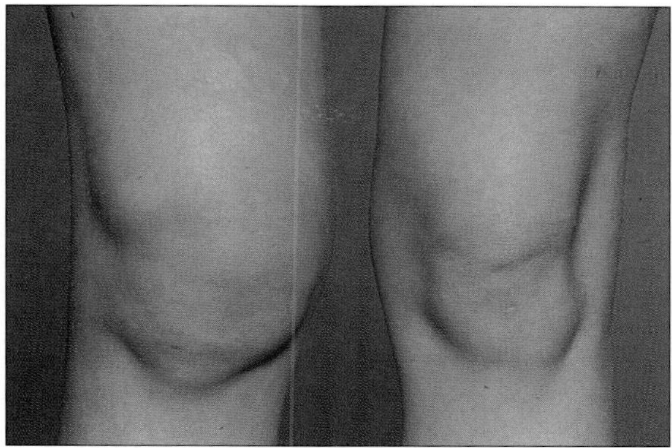

Fig. 14.24 Chronic monoarthritis of the right knee.

DIAGNOSTIC PROBLEMS AND INVESTIGATION

The differential diagnosis of a chronically inflamed knee is wide (Fig. 14.25). Infection must not be missed. Usually bacterial joint sepsis produces signs of severe inflammation, but these may be diminished or absent following antibiotic treatment or if the patient is immunosuppressed, elderly or has a joint prosthesis. Therefore joint aspiration and/or synovial biopsy are important investigations. Unusual organisms such as *Mycobacteria*, *Brucellae*, fungi, spirochetes and parasites may cause chronic monoarthritis and should be specifically looked for. Crystal arthritis may cause chronic synovitis as well as the more usual acutely inflamed joint. A foreign body synovitis is also an etiology to consider in a patient with chronic monoarthritis.

Chronic monoarthritis is a frequent mode of presentation of the spondyloarthropathies, especially in younger individuals. The family history is particularly important in this context, as well as a meticulous search for subtle ocular, cutaneous, gastrointestinal and genitourinary symptoms and signs (Fig. 14.26). Monoarthritis of the

MONOARTHRITIS: INVESTIGATION AND DIFFERENTIAL DIAGNOSIS

Investigation	Differential diagnosis
History **Examination** Clinical Microbiological **Radiology** CT Nuclear magnetic resonance	Trauma/foreign body 'Seronegative arthritis' Charcot's knee Osteonecrosis
Blood tests Complete blood count and differential Rheumatoid factor Antinuclear antibody Urate Microbial antibodies Tissue typing ? Testing for HIV	Connective tissue diseases including systemic lupus erythematosus Rheumatoid arthritis Reactive arthritis
Synovial fluid Microscopy Culture	Infection Crystal arthritis
Arthroscopy Macroscopic examination	Trauma/foreign body Osteoarthritis
Synovial biopsy Histology Culture	Crystal arthritis Infection (i.e. tuberculosis) Sarcoidosis/amyloidosis Neoplasia Villonodular synovitis Metabolic (i.e. ochronosis)

Fig. 14.25 Investigation and differential diagnosis of monoarthritis.

MONOARTHRITIS: HISTORY AND EXAMINATION

History taking: important history to elicit

- History of previous trauma to the knee
- Past or family history of arthritis/connective tissue disease
- History of past sexual contacts/genitourinary infections
- Gastrointestinal symptoms: bowel irregularity/diarrhea or recent food poisoning
- Symptoms of inflammation of the eyes/skin/spine or sacroiliac joints

Examination: important extra-articular signs that may evade detection

- Genital examination (i.e. balanitis) and microbiological examination of the urethra or cervix, even in asymptomatic patients if sexually active
- Psoriasis (including nails and scalp); hair loss (systemic lupus erythematosus) or other skin rash
- Tophi (ears, hands or feet)
- Tendonitis; seen typically with gonococcal sepsis
- Rheumatoid nodules over pressure points
- Spine and sacroiliac joints, for evidence of spondylitis
- Ophthalmologic examination: conjunctivitis, scleritis or uveitis
- Metabolic conditions such as ochronosis or Wilson's disease may rarely present as monoarthritis
- Microscopy and culture of stool, even when patients are asymptomatic

Fig. 14.26 History and examination in monoarthritis.

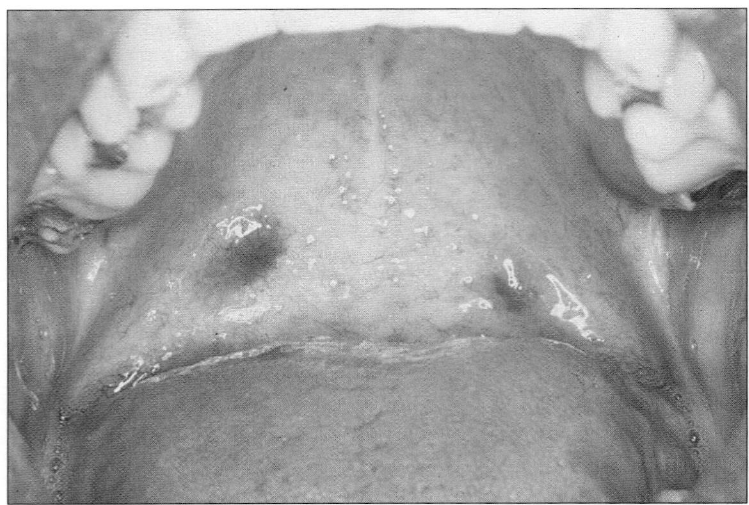

Fig. 14.27 Kaposi's sarcoma as the only other clinical feature of AIDS in a man presenting with sterile monoarthritis.

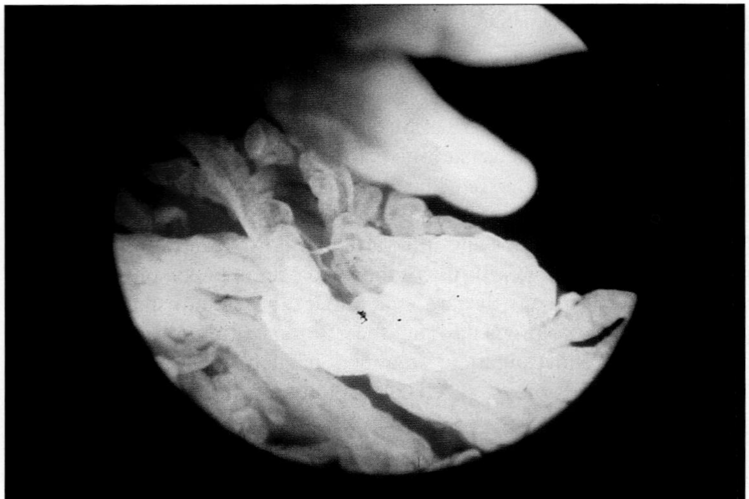

Fig. 14.28 Unsuspected pigmented villonodular synovitis seen in a patient with monoarthritis of the knee.

knee may be the presenting feature of HIV infection and tell-tale lesions elsewhere may not always be apparent (Fig. 14.27).

It is worthwhile performing certain blood tests. Chronic inflammation and infection may cause an anemia, neutrophilia and elevated ESR. A positive rheumatoid factor would strongly suggest the diagnosis of RA. Chronic, undifferentiated monoarthritis represents one of the rare clinical instances for which HLA-B27 typing may be helpful since an increased prevalence of positivity (30–40%) has been reported in this context and would strengthen a clinical suspicion of spondyloarthropathy. Other tests, for example for ANAs and serologies, are rarely helpful. Standing radiographs of the knee may reveal erosions, degenerative changes, areas of radiolucencies suggestive of osteoncrosis or radiographic or avascular necrosis or radiopaque foreign bodies.

Arthroscopy is safe and relatively easy to perform, allowing synovial biopsies to be obtained under direct visual control and the interior of the joint to be carefully examined. Cases of previously unsuspected neoplasia, pigmented villonodular synovitis (Fig. 14.28), amyloid, sarcoidosis and more unusual diseases such as ochronosis have been diagnosed as a result of histologic examination of synovial biopsies.

THERAPEUTIC OPTIONS

Treatment options are broadly similar to those available for patients with polyarthritis (Fig. 14.29). An intra-articular approach would appear to be the most logical treatment for monoarthritis of the knee.

THERAPEUTIC OPTIONS IN CHRONIC MONOARTHRITIS	
Local injections	Intra-articular corticosteroids Chemical synovectomy (yttrium, osmic acid) Radiation synovectomy (yttrium, samarium)
Drug treatment	Nonsteroidal anti-inflammatory drugs and analgesics Second-line drugs (sulfasalazine, methotrexate) Antibiotics
Physiotherapy	Quadriceps strengthening
Surgery	Arthroscopic washout Synovectomy (arthroscopic, surgical)

Fig. 14.29 Therapeutic options in chronic monoarthritis.

While intra-articular corticosteroids are sometimes adequate to control symptoms, chronic synovitis of the knee often proves refractory to this form of treatment. The use of second-line antirheumatic drugs will be determined by the patient's response to NSAIDs and by the degree of disability; they are not an attractive choice in the treatment of chronic monoarthritis. In this setting, gold and penicillamine are rarely helpful, daily sulfasalazine and weekly methotrexate being more commonly used. Antibiotics may also have a place over and above their value in the treatment of septic arthritis; tetracyclines, including minocycline, have been given with some benefit to patients with reactive arthritis and CMUE. This may reflect anti-inflammatory properties rather than antimicrobial activity.

The chronically swollen knee often responds well, albeit in the short term, to local saline washout performed at arthroscopy. Chemical or surgical synovectomy is still considered for refractory monoarthritis of the knee.

The regular performance of active quadriceps exercises is essential to minimize the muscle loss that always accompanies arthritis of the knee.

CONCLUSION

In many cases, chronic arthritis of the knee remains undifferentiated; CMUE should be a diagnosis of exclusion. Clinical history and examination alone can provide the most useful diagnostic information. It is vital to consider chronic infection or neoplasia as these may have drastic consequences. Remember that monoarthritis can be the presenting feature of acquired immunodeficiency syndrome (AIDS). Joint aspiration should be performed in all patients with a joint effusion, and the wearing of gloves and careful aseptic technique should minimize the risk of infection for both patient and clinician. Arthroscopy under local anesthetic is a safe and well-tolerated procedure that has a place in the investigation and treatment of patients with a chronically inflamed knee joint.

REFERENCES

Blocka KLN, Sibley JT. Undiagnosed chronic monoarthritis: clinical and evolutionary profile. Arthritis Rheum. 1987;30:1357–61.

Curry HLF. Acute monoarthritis – differential diagnosis and management. Reports on Rheumatic Diseases Series 2, vol 10. Arthritis and Rheumatism Council, London; 1988.

Revell PA. The synovial biopsy. Recent Adv Histopathol. 1987;13:79–93.

Rowe IF, Forster SM, Seifert MH, *et al.* Rheumatological lesions in individuals with human immunodeficiency virus infection. Q J Med. 1989;272:1167–84.

DEFINITION OF THE PROBLEM

Compartment syndromes result from increased pressure within confined anatomic compartments. The increased pressure causes muscle ischemia, which in turn causes pain and impaired muscle and nerve function. If unrelieved, excessive compartmental pressure leads to muscle necrosis, neurologic compromise and permanent muscle contractures. In some patients extensive myonecrosis results in the loss of a limb, sepsis or compromised renal function due to myoglobinuria.

Anatomic compartments contain muscles, blood vessels and nerves confined by stiff dense fascia, and in some locations bone and interosseous membranes. For example, the anterior compartment of the leg contains the tibialis anterior, extensor digitorum longus, extensor hallucis longus and peroneus tertius muscles, the anterior tibial artery and vein and the deep peroneal nerve. The lateral surface of the tibia, the anterior surfaces of the tibiofibular interosseous membrane and fibula, and the crural fascia form the boundaries of the compartment confining the muscles, nerve and blood vessels and creating an anatomic compartment which permits relatively little increase in volume. Compartment syndromes frequently occur in the anterior compartment of the leg, the other three compartments of the leg and volar compartment of the forearm, but they have been described in almost every muscle containing anatomic compartments, including the compartments of the hands and feet.

The precipitating causes and clinical presentations distinguish two types of compartment syndromes: acute and exertional (chronic or recurrent) compartment syndromes. Acute compartment syndromes most commonly follow trauma (primarily blunt soft tissue injuries and fractures), but also occur as a result of: intracompartmental bleeding; arterial injury and reconstruction; venous thrombosis; surgical procedures; external constriction of a compartment following injury or surgery, such as application of a cast or other restrictive dressing; prolonged external pressure applied to the surface of a compartment; infiltration of intravenous or surgical irrigation fluids; infections; tumors; intra-arterial injections; and seizures. Once established, untreated acute compartment syndromes typically progress to the point of causing muscle necrosis. Exertional compartment syndromes develop during or following exercise that increases muscle blood flow and volume, thereby increasing intracompartmental pressure. In most instances, exertional compartment syndromes resolve following cessation of activity, and then develop again during or following exercise. Poorly localized aching or cramping pain is usually the first symptom of a compartment syndrome. The initial physical findings include increased pain, with passive stretching of the muscles within the involved compartment and firm swelling of the compartment. Unfortunately, diagnosis of acute or exertional compartment syndromes in the early stages, before the development of muscle necrosis, can be difficult and almost always requires measurements of intracompartmental pressures.

THE TYPICAL CASE

LR, a 33-year-old woman, had experienced repeated episodes of diffuse anterior right leg pain, following jogging or hiking, for the previous 18 months. The pain occurred after running or while she was hiking in the mountains. She described the pain as a deep aching or cramping sensation that usually resolved within half-an-hour after cessation of activity. On physical examination there were no palpable masses, localized tenderness or fascial defects, and her neurologic and vascular exams were normal. She had a normal range of motion of the knee and ankle, and normal muscle tone and strength. Radiographs of her leg did not reveal any abnormalities. She was initially treated with anti-inflammatory agents and stretching exercises. She returned 6 weeks later and reported that the pain following running had increased slightly, and that on several occasions the pain had become so intense that she was not able to continue running and it had persisted for several hours after she had stopped. She also noted that on some occasions the pain was associated with paresthesias over the dorsum of her foot. Bone scan, MRI and nerve conduction studies did not reveal any abnormalities.

The patient was then evaluated for a possible exertional compartment syndrome. A catheter connected to a pressure monitor was inserted in the anterior compartment of her right leg and she began walking briskly on a treadmill at a slight incline. Initial measurement showed an anterior compartment pressure of 16mmHg. With exercise the pressure rapidly increased to greater than 65mmHg and the patient developed a severe, deeply aching, cramping sensation in her leg and decreased ability to dorsiflex her foot. One minute after completion of exercise, the anterior compartment pressure had declined to 39mmHg and five minutes after exercise it was 28mmHg. These measurements confirmed the diagnosis of exertional anterior compartment syndrome of the right leg. The patient initially tried modifying her running and hiking, but she still suffered considerable limitation of activity as a result of her exertional leg pain. Treatment with a fasciotomy relieved her symptoms and increased her exercise tolerance.

DIAGNOSTIC PROBLEMS

Poorly localized leg pain, associated with exercise, can be the result of multiple disorders including arthritis, tendonitis, stress fractures, acute and chronic soft tissue injuries and exertional compartment syndromes. The pain due to an exertional compartment syndrome usually begins during exercise, and may be delayed for hours after cessation of activity. Tenderness, muscle weakness and firm swelling of the compartment may be apparent and passive stretching of the affected muscles increases the pain. Elevation and ice packs provide little, if any, pain relief. Between episodes, the symptoms resolve, and physical examination at rest, imaging studies and nerve conduction studies are normal. The diagnosis is suggested by a history of exertion-related pain in the region of an anatomic compartment and can be confirmed by measurement of compartment pressures during and following exercise. The normal pressure in the anterior compartment of the leg at rest is less than 10mmHg and rises with exercise to as much as 50mmHg or more. After completion of exercise, the pressure normally drops quickly and returns to the resting value within 5 minutes. Many patients with exertional compartment syndromes have slightly elevated compartment pressures at rest and all of them have elevated compartmental pressures for an extended period of time following exercise. In these individuals,

COMPARTMENT SYNDROMES	
• Definition:	Increased pressure within a defined anatomic compartment causing painful muscle ischemia which may result in myonecrosis
• Classification:	• Acute: follows trauma, external pressure or other injury; typically progressive • Exertional (chronic/recurrent): related to exercise and something with rest
• Diagnosis:	Difficult: Suggestive history and physical exam; confirmation requires pressure recordings during and following exercise
• Treatment:	Urgent surgical release required for acute progressive types Mild exertional syndromes may be managed by activity modification

Fig. 14.30 Compartment syndromes.

compartmental pressures may rise to greater than 75mmHg during exercise and remain greater than 30mmHg for more than 5 minutes after exercise, with accompanying pain and paresthesias. Individuals with a history of exertional compartment syndrome can develop an acute progressive compartment syndrome during or following exercise, especially when they increase the duration and intensity of exercise above their accustomed level and continue exercise beyond the onset of compartment pain. Exertion-induced acute progressive compartment syndromes may also occur in individuals without a previous history of activity-related compartment pain.

Acute progressive compartment syndromes must be identified early in the course of the disorder and treated urgently. The initial signs and symptoms of progressive compartment syndrome include increasing pain (often the pain becomes so severe that the patient is incapacitated and analgesics provide little or no relief), firm swelling of the compartment and increased pain with passive stretching of the compartment muscles. Paresthesias and skin mottling, cyanosis or pallor may also occur relatively early in the course of a compartment syndrome. Paralysis and loss of pulses occur late in the course of compartment syndromes, and some patients may still have pulses after the development of extensive myonecrosis. A number of absolute values for compartment pressure have been suggested as criteria for the diagnosis of acute compartment syndromes (generally between 30–45mmHg), but physicians should not rely on compartment pressure alone in the diagnosis of compartment syndromes. Although development of muscle ischemia depends on the magnitude and duration of increased pressure, compartment pressure does not directly measure muscle ischemia – pressure may vary in different regions of the same compartment and the tolerance for a given compartment pressure level varies among patients, with the extent of muscle injury and probably between compartments. The difference between the compartmental pressure and the diastolic blood pressure appears to be the most important value in determining the risk of decreased muscle perfusion: a sustained compartmental pressure that is 30mmHg below the diastolic blood pressure or less is generally considered sufficient to cause impaired muscle perfusion and development of an acute progressive compartment syndrome.

As the syndrome progresses, patients develop pallor of the skin and paresthesias; late in the course they develop paralysis and loss of pulses. Patients with compartment syndromes that progress to the point of impaired vascular and neurologic function, which can be detected by physical examination, generally have at least some muscle necrosis.

TREATMENT OPTIONS

Individuals with chronic or exertional compartment syndrome may avoid symptoms by restricting their activity. However, the majority of individuals wish to continue to participate in moderate to vigorous physical activity, and are most effectively treated by surgical release of the fascia. This increases the potential volume of the compartment and usually decreases compartment pressure during and after exercise, improves exercise tolerance and relieves exertion-associated pain.

Acute progressive compartment syndromes must be diagnosed early in the development of the syndrome, when urgent surgical release of the compartment can restore muscle blood flow and avoid myonecrosis. Even when some muscle necrosis has occurred, restoration of blood flow can preserve the remaining viable muscle and allow for some muscle regeneration. However, the decision to perform a compartment release should not be based solely on the patient meeting the criteria for the diagnosis of a compartment syndrome. Some acute compartment syndromes do not progress and may resolve without extensive myonecrosis. For this reason, in selected patients with compartment pain, but normal pulses and neurologic function and relatively low compartment pressures on initial measurement, the appropriate course may be close observation, including continuous or repeated monitoring of compartmental pressures. If the compartmental pressures and pain decrease, surgery can be avoided. In people who have a late diagnosis of a compartment syndrome, it may be best to avoid surgical treatment since once the muscle has become completely necrotic surgical release does not restore muscle function, and increases the chances of infection in the necrotic muscle and septicemia. Even though the compartmental pressure can be high in these patients, it may be declining rather than increasing. If these patients are not treated surgically, the necrotic muscle will be replaced by a scar, containing scattered myofibers, and in most patients the limb will retain some function. Patients with extensive myonecrosis, for example patients with thigh compartment syndromes caused by severe crushing injuries, should have careful evaluation and monitoring of their renal function.

CONCLUSIONS

The clinical presentation of a compartment syndrome is often confusing, and even physicians with considerable experience may have difficulty making the diagnosis. The history and physical examination frequently do not provide sufficient information to determine if a compartment syndrome is present. Standard imaging techniques are not helpful and even defining a compartmental pressure level that is diagnostic for a compartment syndrome can be difficult. Patients with exertional compartment syndromes generally complain of repeated episodes of increasing pain and sometimes paresthesias, swelling and tenderness of the muscle compartment during or following physical activity. Physical examination between episodes, imaging studies and nerve conduction studies are generally normal, but the diagnosis can be confirmed by measurement of compartment pressures during and following exercise. Mild exertional compartment syndromes may be treated by activity modification, but patients with moderate or severe exertional compartment syndromes, and who want to participate in vigorous physical activity, usually benefit from surgical release of the compartment. Acute progressive compartment syndromes can have devastating consequences if the diagnosis is not made early in the course of the disorder, and followed by urgent surgical treatment. The first symptom of an acute progressive compartment syndrome is severe pain over the muscle compartment. Physical examination will usually reveal increased pain with passive stretch of the involved muscle, and pressure measurements will detect significant elevation of intracompartmental pressure. Fasciotomy performed before the development of myonecrosis usually results in restoration of normal function.

REFERENCES

Burnside J, Costello JM, Angelastro NJ, Blankenship J. Forearm compartment syndrome following thrombolytic therapy for acute myocardial infarction. Clin Cardiology. 1994;17(6):345–7.

Finkelstein JA, Hunter GA, Hu RW. Lower limb compartment syndrome: course after delayed fasciotomy. J Trauma. 1996;40:342–4.

Kahan JS, McClellan RT, Burton DS. Acute bilateral compartment syndrome of the thigh induced by exercise. J Bone J Surg. 1994;76A:1068–71.

Klondell CT, Pokorny R, Carrillo EH, Heniford BT. Exercise-induced compartment syndrome. Case report. Am Surg. 1996;62:469–71.

Robinson D, On E, Halperin N. Anterior compartment syndrome of the thigh in athletes – indications for conservative treatment. J Trauma. 1992;32(2):183–6.

Schepsis AA, Martini D, Corbett M. Surgical management of exertional compartment syndrome of the lower leg. Long term follow up. Am J Sports Med. 1993;21:811–17.

Schnall SB, Holtom PD, Silva E. Compartment syndrome associated with infection of the upper extremity. Clin Ortho Rel Res. 1994;306:128–31.

Seiler JG, Valadie AL, Drvaric DM, Frederick RW, Whitesides TE. Perioperative compartment syndrome. J Bone J Surg. 1996;78A:600–2.

Styf JR, Korner LM. Chronic anterior compartment syndrome of the leg. Results of treatment by fasciotomy. J Bone J Surg. 1986;68A:1338–47.

Tornetta P, Templeman D. Compartment syndrome associated with tibial fracture. J Bone J Surg. 1996;78A:1438–44.

15

FIBROMYALGIA AND RELATED SYNDROMES

Don L Goldenberg

Definition
- A chronic musculoskeletal syndrome characterized by diffuse pain and tender points.
- No evidence that synovitis or myositis are causes.
- Occurs in the context of unrevealing physical examination and laboratory and radiologic examination.
- Eighty to ninety percent of patients are women, and the peak age is 30–50 years.

Clinical features
- Generalized chronic musculoskeletal pain.
- Diffuse tenderness at discrete anatomic locations termed tender points.
- Other features, of diagnostic utility but not essential for classification of fibromyalgia, may include fatigue, sleep disturbances, headaches, irritable bowel syndrome, paresthesias, Raynaud's-like symptoms, depression and anxiety.

HISTORY AND DEVELOPMENT OF CRITERIA FOR CLASSIFICATION

Accurate accounts of fibromyalgia symptoms were reported in the mid-1800s. In 1850, Froriep reported that patients with 'rheumatism' had hard places in their muscles which were painful to pressure. Gowers coined the term fibrositis in 1904, although he actually described regional pain syndromes[1]. He emphasized the sensitivity to touch, the absence of systemic or localized inflammation and the presence of fatigue and sleep disturbances. Lewis and Kellgren, in the 1930s, provided eloquent descriptions of referred muscle pain following the injection of hypertonic saline into deep muscle tissue[2]. The distribution of pain referral patterns was uniform and differed from dermatomal patterns. During the next half-century, fibrositis, as it was then called, was considered by some to be a common cause of muscular pain, by others to be a manifestation of 'tension' or 'psychogenic rheumatism', and by the rheumatology community in general to be a nonentity.

The current concept of fibromyalgia was ushered in by studies from Smythe and Moldofsky in the mid-1970s[3]. They described that certain anatomic locations, termed tender points, were more tender in patients than in controls. These sites were often identical to those most tender in regional pain conditions such as 'tennis elbow', 'costochondritis' and cervical strain syndromes. They also reported that patients with fibromyalgia had a stage 4 sleep disturbance, and that experimental selective stage 4 disturbance produced the symptoms and muscle tenderness consistent with fibromyalgia.

The diagnostic utility of tender points was verified by a series of reports in the 1980s from different observers[4,5]. Various diagnostic criteria were suggested, each based on the exclusion of rheumatic or systemic diseases and the presence of certain symptoms and tender points. Authors debated the optimal number of tender points, as well as the relevance of the concept of primary and secondary fibromyalgia. Subsequently, a North American multicenter criteria committee determined the American College of Rheumatology (ACR) 1990 criteria for the classification of fibromyalgia[6]. Two hundred and ninety-three patients with fibromyalgia and 265 control patients were interviewed and examined by trained, blinded assessors. Controls were matched for age and sex and all had a rheumatic disorder that could be easily confused with fibromyalgia, such as 'possible' rheumatoid arthritis (RA) or neck and back pain syndromes. The combination of widespread pain, defined as bilateral, above and below the waist, and axial, and at least 11 of 18 specified tender points, yielded a sensitivity of 88.4% and a specificity of 81.1%. There were no significant differences in patients considered to have primary/concomitant versus secondary fibromyalgia, and for classification purposes such distinctions were to be discarded. No exclusions were made for laboratory or radiographic findings (Fig. 15.1).

EPIDEMIOLOGY

Estimates of the prevalence of fibromyalgia were first reported in the mid-1980s, utilizing modifications of currently accepted diagnostic criteria. These estimates varied from 2.1% in a family practice clinic[7], 5.7% in a general medical clinic[5], 5–8% in a hospital setting [8] and 14–20% in a rheumatology clinic[4,9] (Fig. 15.2). Initial population-based studies in Sweden and Norway reported that 1–2% of all randomly selected individuals had fibromyalgia[10,11]. In the most recent American study, the prevalence of fibromyalgia in the general population was 2%[12]. This prevalence increased with age, reaching 7% in women of age 60–80 years.

Eighty to ninety percent of patients have been female, and the mean patient age has varied from 30 to 60 years, depending on the patient populations[4,6,12,13]. In the ACR 1990 criteria study, the mean age was 49 years, 89% of patients were female, 93% were Caucasian, 5% Hispanic and 1% Black[6]. Educational level and family income have in general been higher than comparable US census figures.

Fibromyalgia may represent a continuum of pain and fatigue in the population at large, rather than a discrete disease[14]. However, the concept of fibromyalgia as a clinical syndrome has been useful both for epidemiologic and therapeutic studies[15]. Anecdotally, most physicians report that a diagnostic label provides reassurance to patients that their symptoms are real and that many other people have similar symptoms. Fibromyalgia is now the second or third most common disorder that rheumatolgists evaluate and treat[16,17]. Fibromyalgia is also common in children, although the exact prevalence has not been determined [18].

DIAGNOSTIC FEATURES OF FIBROMYALGIA
Cardinal features*
Chronic, widespread pain Tender points on examination
Characteristic features
Fatigue Sleep disturbances Stiffness Paresthesias Headaches Irritable bowel syndrome Raynaud's-like symptoms Depression Anxiety
*For classification criteria, patients must have pain for at least 3 months involving the upper and lower body, right and left sides, as well as axial skeleton, and pain in at least 11 of 18 tender points on digital examination.

Fig. 15.1 Diagnostic features of fibromyalgia.

PREVALENCE OF FIBROMYALGIA	
Population	Prevalance (%)
900 randomly selected individuals, aged 50–70 years [10]	1.0
3000 randomly selected community residents [12]	2.0
6000 randomly selected community residents [11]	0.6
Hospitalized patients [8]	7.5
General medical clinic [5]	5.7
Family practice clinic [7]	2.1
Rheumatology clinic [4]	14.0
Rheumatology clinic [9]	20.0

Fig. 15.2 Prevalence of fibromyalgia.

CLINICAL FEATURES

The cardinal symptom of fibromyalgia is diffuse, chronic pain. The pain often begins in one location, particularly the neck and shoulders, but then becomes more generalized[19]. Generally patients state that 'it hurts all over' and they have difficulty locating the site of pain arising from articular or non-articular tissues. Patients describe the muscle pain often as burning, radiating or gnawing and the intensity of the pain as modest or severe but varying greatly. In most studies utilizing pain intensity surveys, such as the McGill Pain Questionnaire and visual analog scales, fibromyalgia patients' self-rating of pain intensity has been greater than that of RA patients.

Most patients also report profound fatigue[20]. This is often notable when arising from sleep but also is marked in the mid-afternoon. Seemingly minor activities aggravate the pain and fatigue, although prolonged inactivity also heightens their symptoms. Patients are stiff in the morning and feel unrefreshed, even if they have slept 8–10 hours. Many patients do not report sleep disturbances, since they interpret

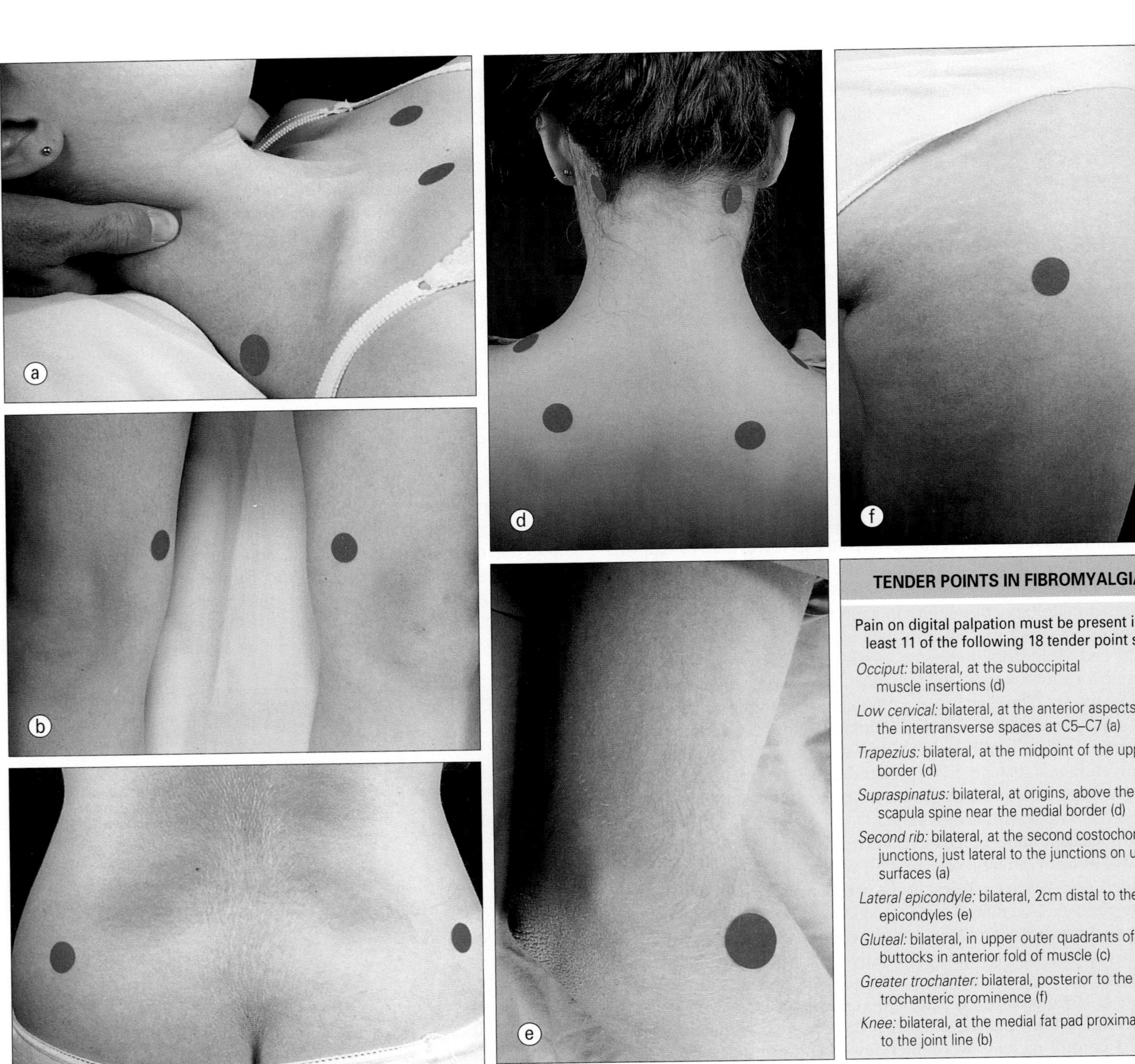

TENDER POINTS IN FIBROMYALGIA

Pain on digital palpation must be present in at least 11 of the following 18 tender point sites:

Occiput: bilateral, at the suboccipital muscle insertions (d)

Low cervical: bilateral, at the anterior aspects of the intertransverse spaces at C5–C7 (a)

Trapezius: bilateral, at the midpoint of the upper border (d)

Supraspinatus: bilateral, at origins, above the scapula spine near the medial border (d)

Second rib: bilateral, at the second costochondral junctions, just lateral to the junctions on upper surfaces (a)

Lateral epicondyle: bilateral, 2cm distal to the epicondyles (e)

Gluteal: bilateral, in upper outer quadrants of buttocks in anterior fold of muscle (c)

Greater trochanter: bilateral, posterior to the trochanteric prominence (f)

Knee: bilateral, at the medial fat pad proximal to the joint line (b)

Fig. 15.3 Locations of the nine pairs of tender points for diagnostic classification of fibromyalgia.

sleep problems in terms of insomnia. Nevertheless, they usually recognize that they sleep 'lightly', waking frequently during early morning and having difficulty getting back to sleep.

Headaches, either 'tension' or more typical migraine, and symptoms suggestive of irritable bowel syndrome are present in more than 50% of patients. True Raynaud's phenomenon or a Raynaud's-like excess sensitivity to cold have also been commonly reported. In many patients, multiple other seemingly unrelated somatic symptoms, such as dizziness, difficulty concentrating, dry eyes and dry mouth, palpitations, and sensitivity to foods, medications and allergens are common and may raise the suspicion of a somatoform disorder. About 25% of patients admit to recently or currently seeking mental health care, usually because of depression. Anxiety, particularly in regard to their diagnosis and future, is very common.

On examination, patients usually appear well with no obvious systemic illness or articular abnormalities. Many patients describe some joint or soft tissue swelling, but no obvious synovitis is present. Of course, fibromyalgia may complicate any systemic arthritis, so the presence of osteoarthritis (OA) or RA does not exclude coexistent fibromyalgia. Patients invariably complain of muscle weakness; however, formal muscle testing does not reveal significant weakness provided the pain does not prevent the patient from achieving maximal effort. Numbness and tingling, especially in the extremities, are present in more than 75% of patients, yet a neurologic examination usually does not demonstrate any significant abnormalities.

Thus, the only reliable finding on examination is the presence of multiple tender points. Although various sets of 'best' tender point discriminators in fibromyalgia have been proposed, the currently recommended nine pairs of tender points should be routinely examined since they were chosen for classification criteria (Fig. 15.3). The examiner must gain experience with the technique and in locating these sites. The patient should be seated comfortably on the examination table and queried as to the presence of pain following the palpation of each bilateral anatomic site. Palpation should be done with the thumb or forefinger, applying pressure approximately equal to a force of 4kg[6]. Excessive force may elicit pain in anyone. A systematic palpation of each site, beginning at the suboccipital muscle insertion at the posterior skull, progressing to the medial fat pad of the knee 2cm proximal to the joint line, should be followed (Fig. 15.3). 'Control' anatomic sites, such as over the thumbnail, mid forearm and forehead should also be palpated. These sites are not as painful on pressure as the selected anatomic sites, although most patients with fibromyalgia are more tender to palpation at many muscle and soft tissue sites than are normal controls. Patients are often not aware of the location of many of the tender points.

The diagnostic utility of a tender point evaluation has been objectively documented with the use of a dolorimeter or algometer, pressure-loaded gauges that accurately measure force per area, and by manual palpation (Fig. 15.4). Such instruments are useful in controlled studies but, in the clinic, digital palpation is usually adequate. The nine pairs of tender points are by no means inclusive, but they are representative. The criteria of at least 11 of 18 tender points are recommended for classification purposes, but should not be considered essential in individual patient diagnosis. Patients with less than 11 tender points certainly can be diagnosed with fibromyalgia provided other symptoms and signs are present. Other common findings on examination include muscle 'spasm' or taut bands of muscle, sometimes referred to by patients as nodules; skin sensitivity, in the form of skin roll tenderness or dermatographism (Fig. 15.5); or purplish mottling of the skin, especially of the legs following exposure to the cold, sometimes thought to be livedo reticularis but more accurately probably representing cutis marmorata.

INVESTIGATIONS

Laboratory and radiologic investigations in fibromyalgia are largely unrevealing and primarily useful for excluding other conditions[19]. At an initial evaluation, minimal baseline blood tests probably should include a complete blood count, an erythrocyte sedimentation rate, standard blood chemistries and thyroid function studies. These all are usually normal in fibromyalgia. Unless there is evidence of an associated arthritis or possible cervical or lumbar radiculopathy, plain radiographs, computed tomography (CT) scans, nuclear scans or MRI are not generally necessary. Serologic tests such as rheumatoid factor, antinuclear antibodies, or Lyme antibody assays, are of dubious diagnostic utility. Unless there is a clinical suspicion of a systemic connective tissue disease or Lyme disease, routine ordering of such tests will yield a large proportion of 'false positive' values, because each of these tests may be positive in healthy individuals. Approximately 10% of patients with fibromyalgia will have a positive antinuclear antibody test[21].

Complaints of paresthesias and minor cognitive dysfunction often lead to costly and invasive neurologic testing[22]. Unnecessary surgery, especially carpal tunnel release (which does not improve symptoms) or disc 'decompression', is common in patients with fibromyalgia. However, an informal or formal assessment of mood and functional impairment should be performed in all patients. Generally this can be performed with simple self-administered questions, but formal evaluation by a mental health professional should be obtained in patients with obvious mood disturbances. Muscle biopsies should not be performed unless there is clinical evidence suggesting inflammatory or metabolic myopathy. A careful sleep history should be obtained[23], including questions regarding possible sleep apnea, which is more common in males with fibromyalgia[24].

MANUAL AND DOLORIMETER TENDER POINT SCORES IN 293 FIBROMYALGIA PATIENTS AND 265 CONTROLS

Manual tender points	Fibromyalgia	Controls
Mean tenderness (0–4 scale)	1.5	0.5
Number of sites (maximum=24)		
Mild or more than mild tenderness	19.7	8.0
Moderate or more than moderate	12.5	3.6
Severe	5.0	1.3
Mean dolorimeter scores (0–6.5kg/cm scale)		
'Active' 18 sites (9 pairs)	3.4	4.9
Control 6 sites (3 pairs)	5.0	5.8

Fig. 15.4 Manual and dolorimeter tender point scores in 293 fibromyalgia patients and 265 controls.

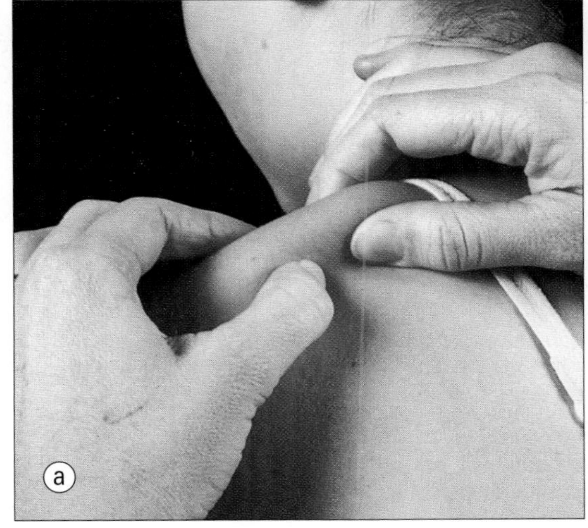

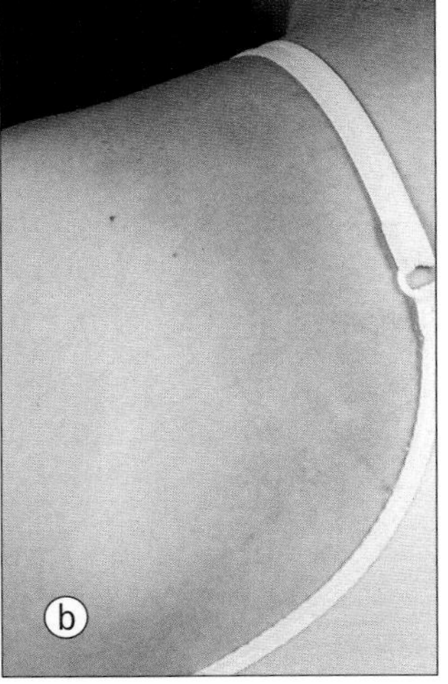

Fig. 15.5 Skin rolling tenderness(a) and reactive hyperemia (b) in fibromyalgia.

DIFFERENTIAL DIAGNOSIS AND ASSOCIATED CONDITIONS

The somewhat vague and nebulous symptoms of chronic, generalized pain and fatigue are present in many rheumatic and nonrheumatic diseases. These conditions should be initially considered in the differential diagnosis of fibromyalgia (Fig. 15.6). Certain rheumatic diseases such as RA, Sjögren's syndrome or systemic lupus erythematosus (SLE) may present initially with diffuse pain and fatigue. Furthermore, fibromyalgia may coexist with RA or SLE. In one study 12% of RA patients and 7% of OA patients had fibromyalgia[9]. In a recent report, 22% of patients with SLE had fibromyalgia[25]. Raynaud's phenomenon and dry eyes and dry mouth have been found in 20–35% and there is an association of fibromyalgia with primary Sjögren's syndrome[26]. Nevertheless, the characteristic synovitis and systemic features of connective tissue disorders are not features of fibromyalgia. Most other rheumatic diseases should not be difficult to distinguish from fibromyalgia (Fig. 15.6). Ankylosing spondylitis or other inflammatory back conditions may present with axial skeleton pain and stiffness, but characteristic radiologic features will be diagnostic. Polymyalgia rheumatica (PMR) may mimic fibromyalgia, although tender points have not been consistently reported. An elevated ESR is present in the vast majority of PMR patients and most respond extremely well to modest doses of corticosteroids. Inflammatory myositis and metabolic myopathies cause muscle weakness and muscle fatigue but usually are not associated with diffuse pain. Furthermore, patients with fibromyalgia do not have significant muscle weakness, other than that related to pain or disuse, and they have normal muscle enzyme tests and normal or nonspecific histopathologic findings on muscle biopsy.

Certain nonrheumatic systemic illnesses may initially mimic fibromyalgia, particularly hypothyroidism. In fact, there are some reports of fibromyalgia as a presenting manifestation of hypothyroidism[21]. However, there is no evidence that correcting the thyroid abnormality ameliorates the fibromyalgia nor that the majority of fibromyalgia patients have a history of thyroid dysfunction. As noted above, peripheral neuropathies, entrapment syndromes (such as carpal tunnel syndrome) and neurologic disorders (such as multiple sclerosis and myasthenia gravis) are sometimes considered in the differential diagnosis. However, the standard neurologic examination, as well as electromyography (EMG) and nerve conduction velocities, are usually normal in fibromyalgia.

DIFFERENTIAL DIAGNOSIS AND SYSTEMIC ILLNESSES THAT ARE ASSOCIATED WITH FIBROMYALGIA (FM)

Condition	Helpful differential features	% with FM
Rheumatoid arthritis	Synovitis, serologic tests, elevated erythrocyte sedimentation rate (ESR)	12
Systemic lupus erythematosus	Dermatitis, systemic vasculitis (renal, central nervous system, etc.)	22
Sjögren's syndrome	Lymphadenopathy, biopsy of salivary glands	11
Polymyalgia rheumatica	Elevated ESR, elderly, response to corticosteroids	?
Myositis	Increased muscle enzymes, weakness more than pain	?
Hypothyroidism	Abnormal thyroid function tests	?
Neuropathies	Clinical and electrophysiologic evidence of neuropathy	?

Fig. 15.6 Differential diagnosis and systemic illnesses that are associated with fibromyalgia.

The most confusing conditions in the differential diagnosis include a group of poorly understood disorders that may be best considered as part of the fibromyalgia concept or overlap with it (Fig. 15.7). Such conditions include depression, irritable bowel syndrome, migraine, chronic fatigue syndrome (CFS) and myofascial pain syndrome. Therefore, these associations will be explored in greater depth, particularly chronic fatigue and myofascial pain syndromes.

As discussed later, depression is more common in fibromyalgia than in normal controls or in RA patients[27]. Approximately 25% of fibromyalgia patients have current major depression and 50% have a lifetime history of major depression. Many of the symptoms of depression, such as fatigue, lack of energy and sleep disturbances, are identical to those in fibromyalgia, and some authors have proposed that fibromyalgia is a manifestation of depression. However, it would then be impossible to explain the finding that 75% of fibromyalgia patients do not have current psychopathology. Irritable bowel syndrome and migraine have been noted in more than 50% of patients and generally develop concurrently with fibromyalgia and we have suggested the term 'affective spectrum disorder' to account for the association of fibromyalgia, chronic fatigue syndrome, migraine, irritable bowel syndrome and depression[27].

CHRONIC FATIGUE SYNDROME

The history of CFS bears a striking resemblance to that of fibromyalgia[28]. The term neurasthenia was popularized by George Beard to account for patients with chronic unexplained fatigue. Beard wrote in 1869: 'The diagnosis of the neurasthenic condition is sometimes clear, and again is quite difficult. The diagnosis is obtained partly by positive symptoms, and partly by exclusion. Acute cases resulting from acute disease, usually recover rapidly, but sometimes become chronic, especially when the prior disease has been long and exhausting'[29]. The connection of chronic fatigue and infections, especially viral, was reported commonly during the polio epidemics of the 1930s and 1940s. Outbreaks of apparent postviral chronic fatigue were reported from Los Angeles County Hospital, the Royal Free Hospital, in Iceland, in Australia and in many other locations[28]. Some authors emphasized the chronic neuropsychiatric symptoms and the term 'benign myalgic encephalomyelitis' was used. Despite speculation that these conditions were related to a viral illness, extensive serologic, virologic and epidemiologic studies did not demonstrate an infectious etiology. Evaluation of patients who remained chronically fatigued after well-documented acute brucellosis demonstrated greater pre-existing psychopathology than those who recovered completely[28]. These same investigators noted that recovery time from the Asian influenza was longer in patients with pre-existing psychoneuroses, particularly depression.

During the mid 1980s, the concept of chronic Epstein–Barr viral (EBV) infection as a cause of what is now termed CFS became popular. However, despite elevated antibody titers to EBV antigens in many patients, there is no evidence that EBV is causally associated with the vast majority of patients with CFS. Therefore, a working case definition for CFS was suggested in 1988 based on clinical symptoms and signs and this definition has been recently revised[30] (Fig. 15.8). The

SYNDROMES THAT OVERLAP WITH FIBROMYALGIA

Syndrome	Relationship with fibromyalgia
Depression	Present in 25–60% of fibromyalgia cases
Irritable bowel	Present in 50–80% of fibromyalgia cases
Migraine	Present in 50% of fibromyalgia cases
Chronic fatigue syndrome (CFS)	70% of CFS cases meet criteria for fibromyalgia
Myofascial pain	May be a localized form of fibromyalgia

Fig. 15.7 Syndromes that overlap with fibromyalgia.

CLASSIFICATION SCHEMA FOR CHRONIC FATIGUE SYNDROME (CFS)
Classify as CFS or idiopathic chronic fatigue if:
Fatigue persists or relapses for ≥ 6 months History, physical examination and appropriate laboratory tests exclude any other cause for the chronic fatigue
Classify as CFS if, along with the fatigue, four or more of the following are present for > 6 months:
Impaired memory or concentration, sore throat, tender cervical or axillary lymph nodes, muscle pain, multijoint pain, new headaches, unrefreshing sleep, postexertion malaise.

Fig. 15.8 Classification schema for chronic fatigue syndrome. Modified from Fukuda *et al.*[30].

cardinal symptom is chronic, debilitating fatigue, and the evaluation discloses no other systemic illness. Fibromyalgia and major depression or anxiety do not exclude the diagnosis of CFS. The other symptoms that are characteristic are similar to symptoms associated with fibromyalgia (Fig. 15.8). In direct comparisons, 30–70% of patients with fibromyalgia have met the working case definition for CFS[31–33].

Demographic, immunologic and psychiatric studies as well as investigations of muscle fatigue have also demonstrated similarities with fibromyalgia. Chronic fatigue syndrome has been most often reported in previously healthy, young and middle-aged females. There has been a predominance of white middle-class patients, although selection bias may account for this. Laboratory findings reported in CFS have varied greatly, although many studies support the concept that patients with CFS differ immunologically from normal controls, although no one test is highly specific or sensitive for CFS[34]. Similar subtle neuroendocrine, psychiatric and neuroimaging findings have been demonstrated in CFS[27] and in fibromyalgia, as discussed below. One of the most intriguing issues has been the relationship of a prior infection to fibromyalgia and CFS (see etiology below)[31,33].

REGIONAL MYOFASCIAL PAIN SYNDROMES (REPETITIVE STRAIN SYNDROME)

Myofascial pain syndromes also overlap with fibromyalgia (Fig. 15.9). Many of the original reports of fibrositis describe what would now be termed myofascial pain syndrome. Myofascial pain is defined by the presence of trigger points, which include a localized area of deep muscle tenderness, located in a taut band in the muscle, and a characteristic reference zone of perceived pain that is aggravated by palpation of the trigger point [35]. Some authors also insist on the presence of a local twitch response.

The relationship of trigger points and tender points is not clear. Although trigger points may be latent, i.e. not associated with pain, trigger points are usually very tender. The location of the trigger point is deep within the muscle belly. Trigger points are said to result in decreased muscle stretch and pain with contraction. A 'twitch response', thought to be pathognomonic of an active trigger point, is a visible or palpable contraction of the muscle produced by a rapid snap of the examining finger of the taut band of muscle . There is a characteristic referred pain pattern (Fig. 15.10). However, recent reports have questioned the reliability of the trigger point evaluation and have found little difference in the symptoms and tender point examination in patients with fibromyalgia and those with myofascial pain syndrome[36,37]. Thus, myofascial pain may be just a localized or regional pain form of fibromyalgia.

Myofascial pain syndromes may include other common regional pain disorders such as tension headaches, idiopathic low back and cervical strain disorders, and temporomandibular joint syndrome. Therefore, myofascial pain syndrome may be one of the most common causes of pain and is often not recognized in general practice. The pathogenesis is not known, although mechanical, nociceptive and primary muscle pathology have been postulated. These potential pathophysiologic factors are similar to those described below in fibromyalgia. Futhermore, similar psychologic and sleep abnormalities have been reported in myofascial pain and fibromyalgia.

The term repetitive strain syndrome is often used when the myofascial pain occurs in the context of activities involving repetitious movement or postural constraint[38]. However, as with fibromyalgia, there is no evidence of persisting tissue damage or injury to the muscle–tendon unit. The term 'repetitive strain syndrome' derives from early observations of the epidemic of arm pain and disability which occurred in the mid-1980s in Australia[38]. It is likely the condition has been present for many decades. For instance, epidemics of 'writer's cramp' were first noted among mail clerks of the British Civil Service in the 1830s and were attributed by the workforce to the introduction of the steel nib. In 1908, 'telegraphist's cramp' was added to the schedule of diseases that was covered by the British Workman's Compensation Act of 1906. This was based on an unproven premise that the condition related to muscle damage caused by the rapid repetitive movements of telegraphy. Within 4 years, up to 60% of the workforce had reported symptoms and 30% had difficulties in manipulation. At the same time in the USA, only between 4 and 10% of telegraphic staff members reported 'cramp symptoms'. Cramp was known as 'losing the grip' in the

COMPARISON OF FIBROMYALGIA AND MYOFASCIAL PAIN SYNDROMES		
Variable	Fibromyalgia	Myofascial pain
Examination	Tender points	Trigger points
Location	Generalized	Regional
Response to local therapy	Not sustained	'Curative'
Sex	Females:males, 10:1	(?) Equal
Systemic features	Characteristic	(?)

Fig. 15.9 Comparison of fibromyalgia and myofascial pain syndromes.

EXAMPLES OF TRIGGER POINTS AND THEIR REFERRED PAIN PATTERNS IN MYOFASCIAL PAIN SYNDROME

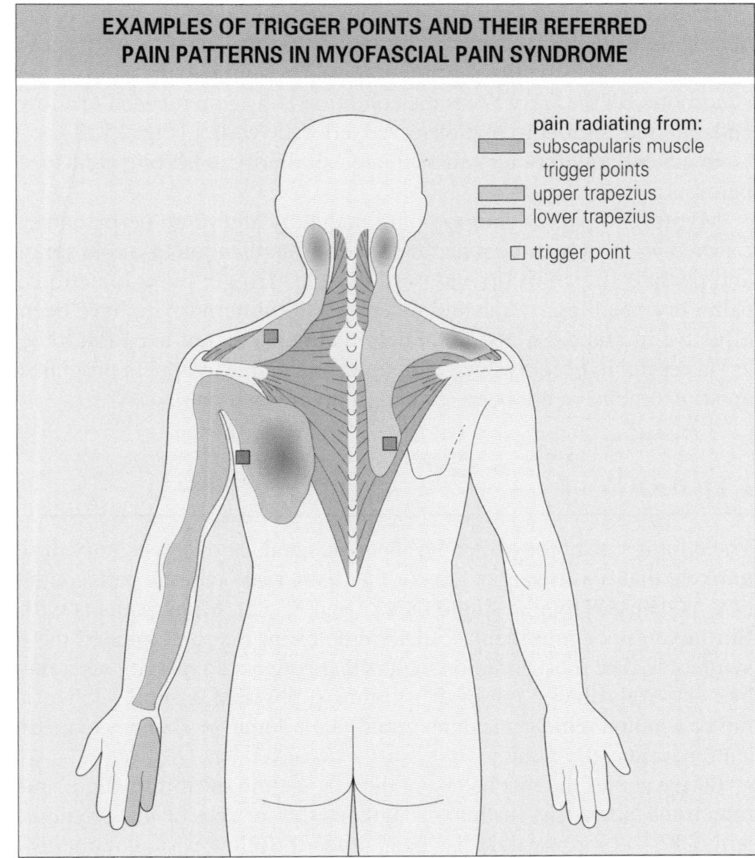

Fig. 15.10 Representative examples of myofascial pain syndrome trigger points and their referred pain patterns.

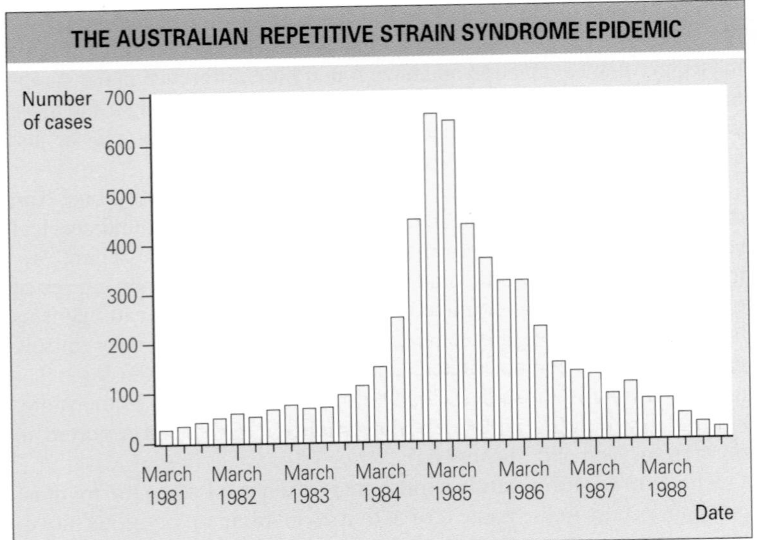

Fig. 15.11 The Australian repetitive strain syndrome epidemic. Cases of repetitive strain syndrome in a large Australian company during the 1980s.

USA. After exhaustive analysis of all possibilities, it was concluded that telegraphist's cramp was equivalent to a 'nervous breakdown' due to a combination of two factors: one related to personal susceptibility of the operator, and the other to ergonomic considerations. The principal symptoms were felt to have no relation to the 'amount of work performed'.

At the beginning of the 1980s the condition was uncommon in Australia, but by 1985 the prevalence of this condition, then known as repetitive strain injury (or RSI), was such that up to 30% of workers in some workplaces were suffering from pain and inability to continue to work (Fig. 15.11)[39,40]. The condition affected both blue- and white-collar workers, had a female predominance, was more prevalent in non-Australian-born workers and was not uniformly represented in workplaces, even in those with identical ergonomic and social backgrounds. Very few self-employed persons developed the problem. These demographic factors reflect psychosocial variables, rather than specific work activities, as being of prime importance in the expression of the syndrome. By the early 1990s the condition had again receded to a low endemic rate similar to that observed a decade earlier (Fig. 15.11).

In general, myofascial pain is treated similarily to fibromyalgia (see below).

Myofascial pain is said to be immediately and often permanently relieved by local treatment methods such as application of a cold spray and passive stretch of the involved muscle. Trigger point injections, using dry needling, saline and recently a botulinum toxin, have been effective in clinical trials[41–43]. Such treatment has not been felt to be as successful in fibromyalgia, although comparable treatment programs and outcome have not been studied in myofascial pain.

ETIOLOGY

The etiology of fibromyalgia has been debated for over a century. It is unlikely that fibromyalgia, nor for that matter any chronic pain condition, is 'caused' by one single factor (Fig. 15.12). Many patients with fibromyalgia cannot identify any single event that precipitated their symptoms. The most common factors that patients do identify are a flu-like or 'viral' illness; minor or substantial physical trauma, such as a fall or a motor vehicle accident; emotional trauma; or changes in medication, especially withdrawing corticosteroids[19,44].

Of particular interest has been the association of fibromyalgia and infections, since this further strengthens the overlap of fibromyalgia with CFS[45]. Fibromyalgia has been noted to follow various viral diseases, including human immunodeficiency virus (HIV) infection and Lyme disease[45–47]. About 25–40% of patients with documented Lyme disease who were treated appropriately with antibiotics developed persistent pain and fatigue, consistent with fibromyalgia/chronic fatigue syndrome. In these reports, there is no evidence of persistent microbial infection. The infection may act similarily to other stressors and initiate both neurohormone and psychosocial dysfunction[45].

MOST COMMON PRECIPITATING FACTORS IN FIBROMYALGIA

- Flu-like viral illness
  - Usually unspecified
  - Chronic fatigue syndrome
  - HIV infection
  - Lyme disease
- Physical trauma
- Emotional trauma
- Medications, especially steroid withdrawal

Fig. 15.12 Most common precipitating factors in fibromyalgia.

PATHOGENESIS

ABNORMALITIES OF MUSCLE AND MECHANICAL FACTORS

The search for possible abnormalities in muscle structure and function have been largely unrewarding[48–50]. Light microscopic and electron microscopic muscle examinations have demonstrated type II fiber atrophy, abnormal 'rubber band-like' or reticular fibers, focal edema, changes in lipids and glycogen and mitochondrial alterations in fibromyalgia[48]. The trapezius muscle (tender point) of fibromyalgia patients had significantly lower ATP, ADP, phosphocreatine and energy charge potential and increased AMP and creatine than in normals[51,52]. However, when controls were matched for levels of exercise and activity, there were no significant differences either in muscle structure or metabolism. For example, using phosphorus magnetic resonance spectroscopy, there were no differences in the levels of phosphocreatine, inorganic phosphate and intracellular pH of the upper trapezius and tibialis anterior muscles after exercise in 13 women with fibromyalgia and 13 sedentary control females[49].

Most investigators now believe that the muscle abnormalities are secondary to inactivity and pain. However, these may also reflect a generalized change in the peripheral[53] and autonomic nervous system[54]. This may also relate to the increased skin hyperreactivity and cold sensitivity and Raynaud's-like phenomenon noted in fibromyalgia. Twelve of 29 fibromyalgia patients had a decrease in finger systolic pressure of more than 20% after cooling, representing a positive Nielsen test for digital vasospasm[54]. There was also a relationship between an abnormal Nielsen test and an increased level of platelet α_2-adrenergic receptors. Increased levels of platelet α_2-receptors have also been noted in primary Raynaud's phenomenon and in major depression. Thus, both skin and muscle blood-flow vasospasm may be important in fibromyalgia and may be related to both environment and psychologic stress and to exercise, and may be partially genetically predetermined, for example via the α_2-adrenergic receptor density. Increased sympathetic nervous system activity or enhanced responsiveness to sympathetic activity would enhance the symptoms (see Fig. 15.13).

CENTRAL NERVOUS SYSTEM

Psychiatric conditons

It is not surprising that many authors have concluded that fibromyalgia is a psychiatric illness or a manifestation of psychophysiologic abnormalities[27]. Patients look well and there are no objective findings to account for the chronic symptoms based on the physical examination, laboratory or radiologic findings. Furthermore, many patients do report depression, anxiety and high levels of stress. Thus, fibromyalgia was often considered to be a form of 'masked' depression or a somatisation disorder, termed psychogenic rheumatism.

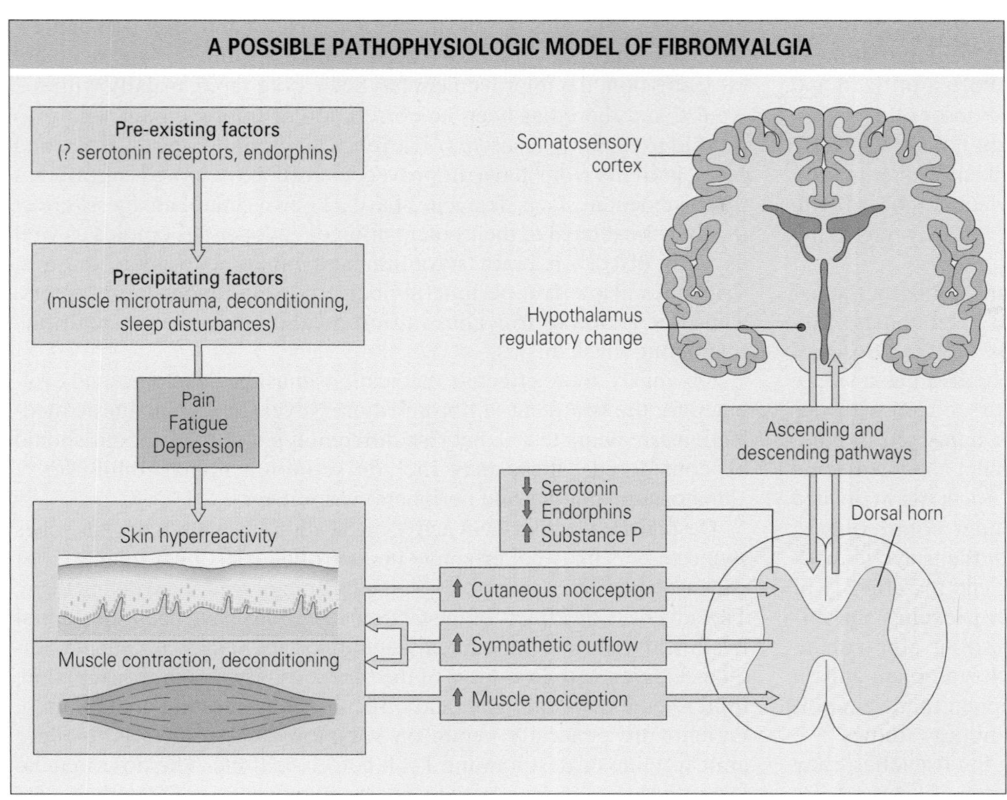

Fig. 15.13 A possible pathophysiologic model of fibromyalgia.

Controlled studies using standard psychologic instruments and applying validated operational diagnostic criteria have concluded the following:

- There are greater psychologic symptoms in fibromyalgia patients than controls, but elevated scores on tests such as the Minnesota Multiphasic Personality Inventory (MMPI) are related to pain and do not differentiate a physical from a psychologic symptom.
- The majority of patients do not have an active psychiatric illness, although major depression is found in 25% of patients and a lifetime history of major depression in 50% of patients. There is also a greater prevalence of a family history of depression in fibromyalgia compared with RA patients and normal controls.
- There is no evidence for a specific personality type, such as obsessive–compulsive disorder, and somatoform disorders are unusual .

Nevertheless, fibromyalgia is not only associated with depression, but also with anxiety disorders, migraine, CFS and irritable bowel syndrome[32]. Such disorders, which we have termed affective spectrum disorders, may share an as yet undetermined psychophysiologic abnormality[27]. Recent reports have also found increased physical and emotional trauma in fibromyalgia. This was especially true for a history of sexual abuse in childhood[55,56]. Such chronic stress also fits the hypothesis regarding various traumatic events being associated with fibromyalgia (Fig. 15.13).

Sleep disturbances

The first 'laboratory' or 'objective' abnormality found in fibromyalgia was the report that patients had an abnormal slow-wave sleep pattern, termed alpha-delta sleep[3]. Moldofsky and coworkers also experimentally induced the same nonrestorative sleep in normal controls, and the controls developed symptoms of fibromyalgia as well as tender points in their muscles. Unfortunately, the significance of these findings has been debated because of the absence of large, well-controlled studies. Although a number of different laboratories have confirmed the finding by electroencephalography of an alpha sleep anomaly in fibromyalgia, such sleep patterns are common in RA and CFS, and can be seen in healthy people. Furthermore, many fibromyalgia patients do not have the alpha-delta sleep abnormality[57] and other sleep disturbances, such as nocturnal myoclonus and obstructive sleep apnea, have been reported in fibromyalgia[24].

NEUROHORMONES AND PAIN

Fibromyalgia represents a disorder of generalized heightened pain sensitivity. Primary or secondary alterations in substances such as serotonin, endorphins or substance P may integrate the changes in sleep, pain and mood. For example, the level of substance P in the cerebrospinal fluid was three fold higher in fibromyalgia patients than in normal controls[58]. Substance P release is influenced by serotonin, and serotonin deficiency, in either the peripheral or central nervous system, could cause an exaggerated perception of normal sensory stimuli. Fibromyalgia patients have reduced pain tolerance to pressure, heat and electrical pulse, both at classic tender points and control points[59,60]. The regional cerebral blood flow, as detected by single photon emission computed tomography, was reduced in the left and right hemithalami and the right heads of the caudate nuclei in fibromyalgia compared to controls[61]. These areas of the brain are important in pain perception.

There is also evidence to suggest neurohormonal abnormalities in fibromyalgia. Two studies have demonstrated reduced levels of growth hormone in some patients with fibromyalgia[62,63]. Growth hormone is important in muscle homeostasis and excreted primarily during stage 4 sleep. Fibromyalgia patients were noted to have low urinary free cortisol and a decreased cortisol response to corticotropin releasing hormone (CRH)[64,65]. Plasma neuropeptide Y levels were also low in fibromyalgia. These studies all suggest a relative adrenal hyporesponsiveness, which could be the result of a chronic stress reaction (Fig. 15.13).

MANAGEMENT

During the past 10 years, there have been a number of controlled therapeutic trials in patients with fibromyalgia. These have included medications and nonmedicinal therapies. Although the choice of specific therapeutic approaches has in some situations been largely empirical, the proposed pathophysiologic abnormalities just reviewed have provided a rational basis for treatment. Such approaches might include:

- enhance peripheral and central analgesia,
- improve sleep disturbances,
- diminish mood disturbances,
- increase blood flow to muscle and superficial tissues.

MEDICATION

Despite the fact that there is no evidence of tissue inflammation in fibromyalgia, anti-inflammatory medications are often utilized and have been studied in controlled trials. 'Therapeutic' doses of naproxen and ibuprofen and 20mg daily of prednisone were not significantly better than placebo in clinical trials[66]. Nonsteroidal anti-inflammatory drugs (NSAIDs) may have a synergystic effect when combined with central nervous system (CNS) active medications, but they may be no more effective than simple analgesics.

In contrast, certain CNS active medications, most notably the tricyclics amitriptyline and cyclobenzaprine, have been consistently found to be better than placebo in controlled trials[67–70]. The doses of amitriptyline studied have been 25–50mg, usually given as a single dose at bedtime. In one report, amitriptyline was associated with significant improvement compared with placebo or naproxen in pain, sleep, fatigue, patient and physician global assessment and the manual tender point score[67] (Fig. 15.14). Cyclobenzaprine, 10–40mg in divided dose, also improved pain, fatigue, sleep and tender point count[69]. However, clinically meaningful improvement with the tricyclic medications has occurred in only 25–45% of patients and the efficacy of these medications may level-off over time[70]. Other tricyclics and different classes of CNS active medications, including alprazolam, temazepam, and fluoxetine, as well as 5-hydroxytryptophan and an analgesic containing carisoprodol and acetaminophen (paracetamol) have been found to be somewhat effective in preliminary studies[66,71].

The efficacy of CNS medications, particularly the tricyclics, may provide further insights into the pathophysiology of fibromyalgia. However, the possible mechanisms of action of these medications in fibromyalgia is extremely varied (Fig. 15.15). It is unlikely that the efficacy of tricyclics in fibromyalgia relates to their effect on depression, since the doses used have been 'subtherapeutic' for the treatment of depression, the improvement has been more rapid, usually within 2 weeks, and there has been no correlation of improvement with premorbid psychiatric disorders. Tricyclics do promote stage 4 sleep, and most patients who have improved overall have noted significant improvement in sleep. Tricyclics have a known central analgesic effect that may be related to their potentiation of endogenous opioids as well as their effect on brain serotonin and other neurogenic amines. Tricyclics also effect peripheral nociceptors and mechanoreceptors. Thus, the action of tricyclics in fibromyalgia may involve multiple, interacting mechanisms.

Obviously, more effective medications must be developed and evaluated for the treatment of fibromyalgia. Novel CNS or analgesic medications are being tested, but also different types of medications should be considered. These may include serotonin uptake inhibitors[71], somatostatin analogs and peripheral vasodilators.

Despite the fact that CNS active medications have been the only ones found to be somewhat effective in controlled trials, less than 50% of patients with fibromyalgia seen in rheumatology clinics are taking them. The adverse side effects of the CNS medications have been substantial in clinical trials and undoubtedly are important in lack of patient compliance. Even with low doses of the tricyclics, dry mouth, constipation, fluid retention, weight gain and difficulty concentrating are common. Patients are generally begun on very low doses, such as 5–10mg amitriptyline or desipramine 1–3h before bedtime. The dose may be increased after 2 weeks, with increases of 5mg at 2-week intervals. The final dose should be set by the patient, based on efficacy and side effects, always keeping the dose as low as possible. Just as switching from one

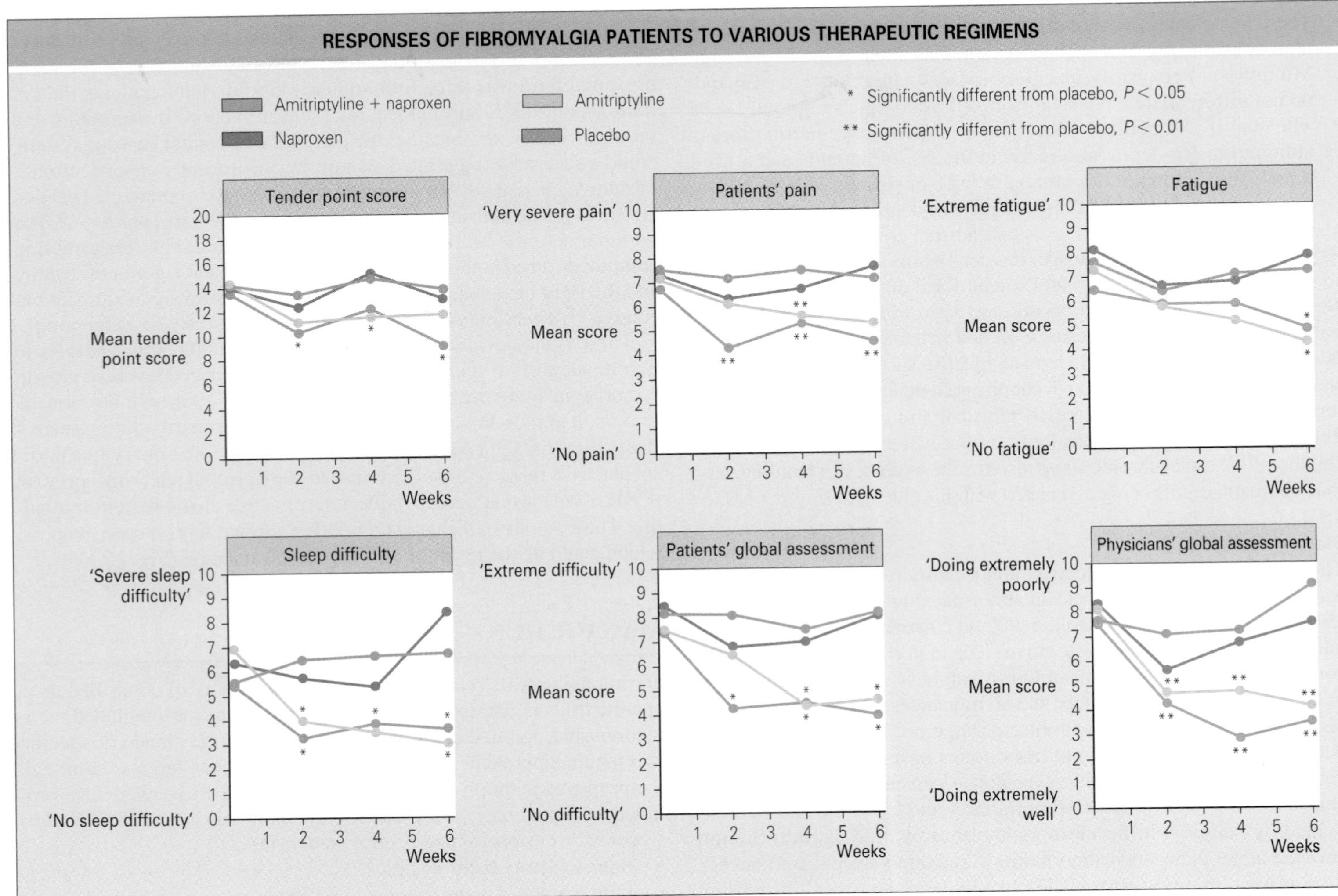

Fig. 15.14 Responses of fibromyaglia patients to various therapeutic regimens[67].

POSSIBLE MODES OF ACTION OF TRICYCLIC MEDICATIONS IN FIBROMYALGIA	
Mode of action	Evidence in fibromyalgia
They may increase brain serotonin or other amines	Plasma tryptophan and platelet receptor studies suggest seratonin release
Endogenous opioids are increased	Elevated substance P in spinal fluid in fibromyalgia
Promotes stage 4 sleep	Not proven with sleep EEG studies
Central nervous system (brainstem) reduction of motor activity (muscle spasm)	Electromyelography evidence that tricyclics reduce spasm
Anticholinergic action	Neurogenic 'flare' in fibromyalgia may be blunted
Relief of depression	Anecdotal evidence that pain and depression correlate

Fig. 15.15 Possible modes of action of tricyclics in fibromyalgia. Reproduced with permission[66].

NSAID to another may be worthwhile in the treatment of inflammatory arthritis, a trial of different tricyclics or different classes of CNS active medications or combinations of such medications should be considered[71]. Simple analgesics may be of limited help, but chronic use of narcotics should be avoided and 'therapeutic' doses of NSAIDs may not be more effective than analgesic doses.

NONMEDICINAL TREATMENT

Although widely utilized in the treatment of fibromyalgia, nonmedicinal therapy has been rarely studied in a controlled fashion. Those few treatments evaluated in controlled studies include cardiovascular fitness training (CFT)[72], EMG biofeedback[73], hypnotherapy[74] and cognitive behavioral therapy[75,76]. Forty-two fibromyalgia patients were randomly assigned to a 20-week program of CFT or a flexibility exercise program[72]. Eighty-three percent of those patients assigned to the CFT program improved their physical fitness by incremental stationary bicycle riding. There was significant improvement in tender point pain threshold and in patient and physician global assessment in the CFT group but no significant differences in pain intensity or sleep disturbances in the two groups.

The possible ameliorative effects of CFT on fibromyalgia may involve mechanisms as diverse as improved muscle blood flow or CNS-induced hypoalgesia, felt to be related to activation of endogenous opioids. Vigorous exercise also induces increases in adrenocorticotropic hormone (ACTH) and cortisol, which may also promote analgesia. Unfortunately, despite this report demonstrating the beneficial effect of CFT and the widely accepted virtues of cardiovascular exercise, it is difficult to start and maintain fibromyalgia patients in a structured cardiovascular exercise program. Patients generally perceive that their pain and fatigue worsen as they begin to exercise. The majority of patients are physically unfit. Therefore, it is important to instruct patients in the principles and methods of gradual incremental cardiovascular fitness programs. Low impact aerobic activities such as fast walking, biking, swimming or water aerobics are most successful. However, the type and intensity of the program should be individualized, and physical therapists or exercise physiologists can provide helpful instruction. A minimum of 30 minutes of aerobic exercise three times per week in a range near target heart rate is recommended for optimal CFT.

The only controlled report of EMG biofeedback training randomized 12 fibromyalgia patients to EMG biofeedback or sham biofeedback[73]. The EMG biofeedback group had a significant improvement in pain, morning stiffness and tender points. Hypnotherapy was found to be better than physical therapy in 40 patients with refractory fibromyalgia[74]. The hypnotherapy group demonstrated better outcome in pain, fatigue, sleep and global assessment, but not in tender points. We have found that a mindfullness meditation-based relaxation response program is helpful in fibromyalgia[75]. Other less well studied non-medical treatments include transcutaneous electrical nerve stimulation (TENS), acupuncture, laser treatment and tender point injections.

EDUCATING THE PATIENT

A key aspect of treatment is to first educate the patient and his or her family in regard to fibromyalgia and similar disorders such as CFS. This first involves reassuring the patient that the illness is real, not imagined, but also that it is not likely to be caused by an infection or other illness over which the patient has no control. Patients must be told that this is not a deforming or deteriorating condition, it is never life-threatening nor a cosmetic problem. Analogies with conditions such as migraine can be useful. The complicated psychosocial and physiological interactive pathway (see Fig. 15.13) should be discussed as a basis for treatment. At the initial visit, it would be helpful to discuss the role of sleep disturbances and also the potential relationship of neurohormones with pain, fatigue, abnormal sleep and mood disturbances. Such a discussion reassures the patient that even though we do not know the cause of the condition, we are not totally ignorant about the physiologic changes responsible for the symptoms. This is a natural springboard to a discussion of tricyclic medications.

A discussion of muscle 'spasm' and low muscle blood flow would then lay the groundwork for exercise recommendations. The patient must be convinced that the pain is not related to an inflammatory or structural process, and that a gradual cardiovascular and physical therapy program is not only possible but will eventually be beneficial. The patient can then also be encouraged to learn simple relaxation techniques or to enroll in a structured cognitive behavior program that emphasizes stress and its role in aggravating chronic pain. Simple analgesics, such as acetaminophen (paracetamol), may be prescribed.

The discussion of fibromyalgia and its management should be as extensive as possible. Providing patients with educational material which discuss various aspects of the disorder is often helpful. It is impossible to complete a patient examination and adequate discussion and treatment plan in less than 60–90 minutes, and it is important that family members are involved. Without a correct diagnosis and a thorough sympathetic explanation, patients may resort to alternative therapies (holistic 'medicine', allergy fads, megavitamin therapy, etc.), which leads to a delay in effective managment and involves the patient in unnecessary expense and further worry.

Patients need to be followed at regular intervals until they have achieved some significant improvement and stability in their symptoms. A team, employing nurse educators, psychiatrists or other mental health workers, physiatrists and physical therapists will be especially useful in more difficult cases[77].

PROGNOSIS OUTCOME AND DISABILITY

There have been few longitudinal studies in fibromyalgia and they have demonstrated persistent pain and significant impact on function. Thirty-nine patients were surveyed for 3 consecutive years in regard to their symptoms[78]. Although more than 80% of patients continued to take medications for fibromyalgia, 67% reported feeling poor or fair and having moderate or severe pain with no significant change in symptoms over the 3 years. Factors associated with improved outcome were a younger age and lower global and pain scores at the time of the initial survey. A recent follow-up of the majority of those patients 8 years later found that although all still had fibromyalgia symptoms, 65% felt better than when they were initially diagnosed[79]. Only 9% had to leave their job because of fibromyalgia. Pain is the most important determinant of 'severity', but psychologic status and functional disability contribute independently to severity.

With regard to function in fibromyalgia, studies have reported varying disability rates from 9–44%[79–81]. Using a computer-assisted work simulator, fibromyalgia patients and RA patients had comparable ability to perform standardized work tasks, and both were only 60% of that done by normal controls[81]. The Stanford Health Assessment Questionnaire (HAQ) was the best predictor of work ability in both groups of patients. Disability has been most strongly associated with functional and work status, pain, mood disturbances, coping ability and depression[44]. Patients in tertiary referral practices with a special interest in fibromyalgia may represent the 'tip of the iceberg' in terms of severity and functional disability. Community-based fibromyalgia patients have fared much better in outcome[82]. Nearly one half of community fibromyalgia patients no longer met criteria for the diagnosis 2 years after conservative treatment had begun[82].

The variable severity of fibromyalgia must be considered in any discussion of prognosis and outcome. The somewhat bleak outcome reported from tertiary referral clinics with a specialty interest in fibromyalgia may not be representative of the general community. Less problematic patients may often do well with simple reassurance, education and attention to physical fitness and ergonomic issues. Many patients respond well to very low doses of tricyclics or other CNS medications, and particularly as their sleep improves, they cope well and find fibromyalgia to be a nuisance condition. Nevertheless, most patients do continue to report chronic symptoms and a complete and permanent remission is rather unusual. Thus, a foundation of patient and family education, explaining in detail and repeatedly what fibromyalgia is and just as importantly what it isn't, is crucial.

MEDICOLEGAL ASPECTS

As might be expected from the disability numbers given above, fibromyalgia has become an important medicolegal condition[66]. Fibromyalgia was responsible for disability payments in 9% of cases at a major Canadian life insurance company, which would translate to $200 million per year paid out in Canada in long-term disability claims for fibromyalgia. Public education, standardized diagnostic criteria and emphasis on rehabilitation, not compensation, will be necessary to interrupt the expanding area of disability in fibromyalgia.

Many patients with fibromyalgia and repetitive strain syndrome are involved in disputes about compensation, litigation or disability assessment. The issue of whether compensation is appropriate is one that has to be worked out by each individual country and community. Many argue that countries with compensation schemes which encompass any symptom that occurs at work actually encourage, inadvertently, such chronic pain syndromes to occur. The medicolegal aspects of fibromyalgia and myofascial pain are anxiety-provoking for both the patient and physician. However, in our litigious society, such issues have become common and rheumatologists will by necessity have to render opinions in legal cases.

One simple way to deal with such questions is to state that fibromyalgia is never related to injury and is never disabling. Of course, such responses are contrary to what patients tell us. Physical trauma is, in fact, one of the most common precipitating factors in fibromyalgia. It is reported that 10–30% of patients with fibromyalgia are disabled because of their symptoms. A more reasonable approach to the questions posed would be the following:

- The diagnosis of fibromyalgia should be specified and confirmed according to current classification criteria. It is helpful to note that the locations of tender and control points are usually not known to patients, making it difficult to fake a tender point evaluation.
- The prognosis is impossible to predict in any chronic condition. However, it should be stressed that the majority of patients are working full time.
- The relationship of the 'injury' to fibromyalgia is best approached by using the terms 'precipitating factor' or temporal relationship of the 'injury' to the onset of symptoms. We certainly do not know the 'cause' of fibromyalgia and it would be inappropriate to tackle issues of causation.
- Reports do now describe significant work loss, work modifications and work disability in fibromyalgia. What is such disability related to, since there are no objective measures of physical impairment? Pain is more prominent than in many disabling conditions such as RA. Fatigue may also cause disability. However, according to some countries' social security guidelines, pain, without objective physical or laboratory abnormalities, is not a sufficient factor in disability determinations. Tender points might then be utilized as an objective measure of pain and dysfunction.

Our more important role is to convince the patient that the medicolegal issues may be a negative influence on the condition and to steer employers and lawyers to a course of rehabilitation rather than confrontation. A finite time away from work, devoted to a team approach to chronic pain rehabilitation, should be recommended. Formal evaluation of the patient by the rheumatologist, a physiatrist or physical therapist, and a mental health professional should provide a treatment plan. Evaluation of the patient's specific job and possible job modification, as well as workplace 'hardening', will be helpful. The goal of everyone must be to restore the patient's confidence and desire to return to work, with the knowledge that the team of professionals as well as the employer are 'on the patient's side' rather than being adversaries.

CONCLUSION

In conclusion, fibromyalgia is a common condition that, despite being well described 150 years ago, is just beginning to be accepted as a discrete syndrome. Controversy regarding the presence of inflammation, and confusion regarding terminology and overlap with other pain syndromes, has resulted in a healthy skepticism about its existence. However, recent epidemiologic studies conclude that fibromyalgia is a discrete syndrome with a uniform set of symptoms and signs that can be readily distinguished from other causes of chronic musculoskeletal pain. This recognition will undoubtedly lead to a better understanding of the complicated pathophysiologic mechanisms involved, and ultimately will lead to a better treatment for this perplexing syndrome.

REFERENCES

1. Gowers WR. Lumbago: Its lessons and analogues. Br Med. 1904;1:117–21.
2. Kellgren JH. Observations on referred pain arising from muscle. Clin Sci. 1938;3:175–90.
3. Smythe HA, Moldofsky H. Two contributions to understanding the 'fibrositis syndrome'. Bull Rheum Dis. 1978;26:928–31.
4. Yunus M, Masi AT, Calabro JJ, Miller KA, Feigenbaum SL. Primary fibromyalgia (fibrositis): clinical study of 50 patients with matched normal controls. Semin Arthritis Rheum. 1981;11:151–71.
5. Campbell SM, Clark S, Tindall EA, Forehand ME, Bennett RM. Clinical characteristics of fibrositis. I. A 'blinded', controlled study of symptoms and tender points. Arthritis Rheum. 1983;26:817–824
6. Wolfe F, Smythe HA, Yunus MB, *et al.* The American College of Rheumatology 1990 criteria for the classification of fibromyalgia: Report of the Multicenter Criteria Committee. Arthritis Rheum. 1990;33:160–72.
7. Hartz A, Kirchdoerfer E. Undetected fibrositis in

primary care practice. J Family Prac. 1987;25:365–9.
8. Doherty M, Abawi J, Pattrick M. Audit of medical inpatient examination: a cry from the joint. J R Coll Physicians Lond. 1990;24:115–8.
9. Wolfe F, Cathey MA. Prevalence of primary and secondary fibrositis [brief communication]. J Rheumatol. 1983;10:965–8.
10. Jacobsson L, Lindgärde F, Manthorpe R. The commonest rheumatic complaints of over six weeks' duration in a twelve-month period in a defined Swedish population. Prevalences and relationships. Scand J Rheumatol. 1989;18:353–60.
11. Prescott E, Kjøller M, Jacobsen S, Bülow PM, Danneskiold-Samsøe B, Kamper-Jørgensen F. Fibromyalgia in the adult Danish population: I. A prevalence study. Scand J Rheumatol. 1993;22:233–7.
12. Wolfe F, Ross K, Anderson J, Russell IJ, Hebert L. The prevalence and characteristics of fibromyalgia in the general population. Arthritis Rheum. 1995;38:19–28.
13. Yunus MB, Masi AT, Aldag JC. Preliminary criteria for primary fibromyalgia syndrome (PFS): multivariate analysis of a consecutive series of PFS, other pain patients, and normal subjects. Clin Exp Rheumatol. 1989;7:63–9.
14. Croft P, Schollum J, Silman A. Population study of tender point counts and pain as evidence of fibromyalgia. Br Med J. 1994;309:696–9.
15. Goldenberg DL. Fibromyalgia: why such controversy? Ann Rheum Dis. 1995;54:3–5
16. Marder WD, Meenan RF, Felson DT, *et al.* Editorial: The present and future adequacy of rheumatology manpower: A study of health care needs and physician supply. Arthritis Rheum. 1991;34:1209–17.
17. White KP, Speechley M, Harth M, Østbye T. Fibromyalgia in rheumatology practice: A survey of Canadian rheumatologists. J Rheumatol. 1995;22:722–6.
18. Buskila D, Neumann L, Hershman E, Gedalia A, Press J, Sukenik S. Fibromyalgia syndrome in children – an outcome study. J Rheumatol. 1995;22:525–8.
19. Goldenberg DL. Fibromyalgia syndrome. An emerging but controversial condition. JAMA. 1987;257:2782–2787
20. Goldenberg DL. Fatigue in rheumatic disease. Bull Rheum Dis. 1995;44:4–8.
21. Dinerman H, Goldenberg DL, Felson DT. A prospective evaluation of 118 patients with the fibromyalgia syndrome: prevalence of Raynaud's phenomenon, sicca symptoms, ANA, low complement, and Ig deposition at the dermal–epidermal junction. J Rheumatol. 1986;13:368–73.
22. Simms RW, Goldenberg DL. Symptoms mimicking neurologic disorders in fibromyalgia syndrome. J Rheumatol. 1988;15:1271–3.
23. Moldofsky H. Chronobiological influences on fibromyalgia syndrome: Theoretical and therapeutic implications. Baillière's Clin Rheumatol. 1994;8:801–10.
24. May KP, West SG, Baker MR, Everett DW. Sleep apnea in male patients with the fibromyalgia syndrome. Am J Med. 1993;94:505–8.
25. Middleton GD, McFarlin JE, Lipsky PE. The prevalence and clinical impact of fibromyalgia in systemic lupus erythematosus. Arthritis Rheum. 1994;37:1181–8.
26. Bonafede RP, Downey DC, Bennett RM. An association of fibromyalgia with primary Sjögren's syndrome: A prospective study of 72 patients. J Rheumatol. 1995;22:133–6.
27. Hudson JI, Pope HG. The concept of affective spectrum disorder: Relationship to fibromyalgia and other syndromes of chronic fatigue and chronic muscle pain. Baillière's Clin Rheumatol. 1994;8:839–56.
28. Briggs NC, Levine PH. A comparative review of systemic and neurological symptomatology in 12 outbreaks collectively described as chronic fatigue syndrome, epidemic neuromyasthenia, and myalgic encephalomyelitis. Clin Infect Dis. 1994;18:S32–S42.
29. Beard GM. Neurasthenia, or nervous exhaustion. Boston Med Surg J. 1869;3:217–21.
30. Fukuda K, Straus SE, Hickie I, Sharpe MC, Dobbins JG, Komaroff A. The chronic fatigue syndrome: A comprehensive approach to its definition and study. Ann Intern Med. 1994;121:953–9.
31. Goldenberg DL, Simms RW, Geiger A, Komaroff AL. High frequency of fibromyalgia in patients with chronic fatigue seen in a primary care practice. Arthritis Rheum. 1990;33:381–7.
32. Hudson JI, Goldenberg DL, Pope HG, Jr., Keck PE,Jr., Schlesinger L. Comorbidity of fibromyalgia with medical and psychiatric disorders. Am J Med. 1992;92:363–7.
33. Buchwald D, Garrity D. Comparison of patients with chronic fatigue syndrome, fibromyalgia, and multiple chemical sensitivities. Arch Intern Med. 1994;154:2049–53.
34. Bates DW, Buchwald D, Lee J, *et al.* Clinical laboratory test findings in patients with chronic fatigue syndrome. Arch Intern Med. 1995;155:97–103.
35. Fricton JR. Myofascial pain. Baillière's Clin Rheumatol. 1994;8:857–80.
36. Wolfe F, Simons DG, Fricton J, *et al.* The fibromyalgia and myofascial pain syndromes: a preliminary study of tender points and trigger points in persons with fibromyalgia, myofascial pain syndrome and no disease. J Rheumatol. 1992;19:944–51.
37. Tunks E, McCain GA, Hart LE,*et al.* The reliability of examination for tenderness in patients with myofascial pain, chronic fibromyalgia and controls. J Rheumatol. 1995;22:944–52
38. Littlejohn GO. Fibrositis/fibromyalgia syndrome in the workplace. Rheum Dis Clin N Am. 1989;15:45–60.
39. Littlejohn G. Medicolegal aspects of fibrositis syndrome. J Rheumatol. 1989;16 Suppl. 19:169–73.
40. Reilly PA, Littlejohn GO. Fibrositis/fibromyalgia syndrome: The key to the puzzle of chronic pain. Med J Australia. 1990;152:226–8.
41. Hong C-Z. Lidocaine injection versus dry needling to myofascial trigger point. The importance of the local twitch response. Am J Phys Med Rehab. 1994;73:256–63.
42. Hopwood MB, Abram SE. Factors associated with failure of trigger point injections. Clin J Pain. 1994;10:227–34
43. Cheshire WP, Abashian SW, Mann JD. Botulinum toxin in the treatment of myofascial pain syndrome. Pain. 1994;59:65–9.
44. Goldenberg DL, Mossey CJ, Schmid CH. A model to assess severity and impact of fibromyalgia. J Rheumatol. 1995;22:2313–8.
45. Goldenberg DL. Do infections trigger fibromyalgia? Arthritis Rheum. 1993;36:1489–92.
46. Steere AC, Taylor E, McHugh GL, Logigian EL. The overdiagnosis of lyme disease. JAMA. 1993;269:1812–6.
47. Hsu VM, Patella SJ, Sigal LH. 'Chronic lyme disease' as the incorrect diagnosis in patients with fibromyalgia. Arthritis Rheum. 1993;36:1493–500.
48. Jacobsen S. Chronic widespread musculoskeletal pain – the fibromyalgia syndrome. Dan Med Bull. 1994;41:541–64.
49. Simms RW, Roy SH, Hrovat M, *et al.* Lack of association between fibromyalgia syndrome and abnormalities in muscle energy metabolism. Arthritis Rheum. 1994;37:794–800.
50. Jubrias SA, Bennett RM, Klug GA. Increased incidence of a resonance in the phosphodiester region of ^{31}P nuclear magnetic resonance spectra in the skeletal muscle of fibromyalgia patients. Arthritis Rheum. 1994;37:801–7.
51. Bengtsson A, Henriksson KG, Larsson J. Reduced high-energy phosphate levels in the painful muscles of patients with primary fibromyalgia. Arthritis Rheum. 1986;29:817–21.
52. Lund N, Bengtsson A, Thorborg P. Muscle tissue oxygen pressure in primary fibromyalgia. Scand J Rheumatol. 1986;15:165–73.
53. Arroyo JF, Cohen ML. Abnormal responses to electrocutaneous stimulation in fibromyalgia. J Rheumatol. 1993;20:1925–31.
54. Bennett RM, Clark SR, Campbell SM, Ingram SB, Burckhardt CS, Nelson DL, Porter JM. Symptoms of Raynaud's syndrome in patients with fibromyalgia. A study utilizing the Nielsen test, digital photoplethysmography, and measurements of platelet alpha-2-adrenergic receptors. Arthritis Rheum. 1991;34:264–9.
55. Boisset-Pioro MH, Esdaile JM, Fitzcharles M-A. Sexual and physical abuse in women with fibromyalgia syndrome. Arthritis Rheum. 1995;38:235–41.
56. Taylor ML, Trotter DR, Csuka ME. The prevalence of sexual abuse in women with fibromyalgia. Arthritis Rheum. 1995;38:229–34.
57. Carette S, Oakson G, Guimont C, Steriade M. Sleep electroencephalography and the clinical response to amitriptyline in patients with fibromyalgia. Arthritis Rheum. 1995;38:1211–7.
58. Russell IJ, Orr MD, Littman B, *et al.* Elevated cerebrospinal fluid levels of substance P in patients with the fibromyalgia syndrome. Arthritis Rheum. 1994;37:1593–601.
59. Gibson SJ, Littlejohn GO, Gorman MM, Helme RD, Granges G. Altered heat pain thresholds and cerebral event-related potentials following painful CO_2 laser stimulation in subjects with fibromyalgia syndrome. Pain. 1994;58:185–93.
60. Lautenbacher S, Rollman GB, McCain GA. Multi-method assessment of experimental and clinical pain in patients with fibromyalgia. Pain. 1994;59:45–53.
61. Mountz JM, Bradley LA, Modell JG,*et al.* Fibromyalgia in women. Abnormalities of regional cerebral blood flow in the thalamus and the caudate nucleus are associated with low pain threshold levels. Arthritis Rheum. 1995;38:926–38.
62. Bennett RM, Clark SR, Campbell SM, Burckhardt CS. Somatomedin-C levels in patients with the fibromyalgia syndrome: a possible link between sleep and muscle pain. Arthritis Rheum. 1992;35:1113–6.
63. Griep EN, Boersma JW, de Kloet ER. Pituitary release of growth hormone and prolactin in primary FS. J Rheumatol. 1994;21:2125–30.
64. Crofford LJ, Pillemer SR, Kalogeras KT, *et al.* Hypothalamic–pituitary–adrenal axis perturbations in patients with fibromyalgia. Arthritis Rheum. 1994;37:1583–92.
65. Griep EN, Boersma JW, de Kloet ER. Evidence for neuroendocrine disturbance following physical exercise in primary fibromyalgia syndrome. J Musculoskel Pain. 1993;1:217–22.
66. Goldenberg DL. Treatment of fibromyalgia syndrome. Rheum Dis Clin N Am. 1989;15:61–71
67. Goldenberg DL, Felson DT, Dinerman H. A randomized, controlled trial of amitriptyline and naproxen in the treatment of patients with fibromyalgia. Arthritis Rheum. 1986;29:1371–7.
68. Carette S, McCain GA, Bell DA, Fam AG. Evaluation of amitriptyline in primary fibrositis. A double-blind, placebo-controlled study. Arthritis Rheum. 1986;29:655–9.
69. Bennett RM, Gatter RA, Campbell SM, Andrews RP, Clark SR, Scarola JA. A comparison of cyclobenzaprine and placebo in the management of fibrositis. A double-blind controlled study. Arthritis Rheum. 1988;31:1535–42.
70. Carette J, Bell MJ, Reynolds WJ, *et al.* Comparison of amitriptyline, cyclobenzaprine, and placebo in the treatment of fibromyalgia. A randomized, double-blind clinical trial. Arthritis Rheum. 1994;37:32–40.
71. Goldenberg DL, Mayskiy M, Mossey CJ, Ruthazer R, Schmid C. The independent and combined efficacy of fluoxetine and amitriptyline in the treatment of fibromyalgia [Abstract]. Arthritis Rheum. 1995;38(Suppl.):S229.
72. McCain GA, Bell DA, Mai FM, Halliday PD. A controlled study of the effects of a supervised cardiovascular fitness training program on the manifestations of primary fibromyalgia. Arthritis Rheum. 1988;31:1135–41.
73. Ferraccioli G, Ghirelli L, Scita F, *et al.* EMG-biofeedback training in fibromyalgia syndrome. J Rheumatol. 1987;14:820–5.
74. Haanen HCM, Hoenderdos HTW, van Romunde LKJ, *et al.* Controlled trial of hypnotherapy in the treatment of refractory fibromyalgia. J Rheumatol. 1991;18:72–5.
75. Goldenberg DL, Kaplan KH, Nadeau MG, Brodeur C, Smith S, Schmid CH. A controlled study of a stress-reduction, cognitive-behavioral treatment program in fibromyalgia. J Musculoskel Pain. 1994;2:53–66.

76. White KP, Nielson WR. Cognitive behavioral treatment of fibromyalgia syndrome: A follow-up assessement. J Rheumatol. 1995;22:717–21.
77. Bennett RM, Campbell S, Burckhardt C, Clark SR, O'Reilly C, Wiens A. A multidisciplinary approach to fibromyalgia treatment. J Musculoskel Med. 1991;8:21–32.
78. Felson DT, Goldenberg DL. The natural history of fibromyalgia. Arthritis Rheum. 1986;29:1522–6.
79. Kennedy MJ, Goldenberg DL, Felson DT. A prospective long-term study of fibromyalgia (abstract). Arthritis Rheum. 1994;37(suppl):S213.
80. Hawley DJ, Wolfe F, Cathey MA. Pain, functional disability, and psychological status: a 12-month study of severity in fibromyalgia. J Rheumatol. 1988;15:1551–6.
81. Cathey MA, Wolfe F, Kleinheksel SM, *et al.* Functional ability and work status in patients with fibromyalgia. Arthritis Care Res. 1988;1:85–98.
82. Granges G, Zilko P, Littlejohn GO. Fibromyalgia syndrome: assessment of the severity of the condition 2 years after diagnosis. J Rheumatol. 1994;21:523–9.

16

ENTRAPMENT NEUROPATHIES

David J Nashel

- An entrapment neuropathy results from increased pressure on a nerve as it passes through an enclosed space.
- Knowledge of the anatomy of each potential site of entrapment is essential for an understanding of the clinical manifestations of these syndromes.
- Conservative measures such as splinting, NSAIDs and local corticosteroid injections usually suffice when symptoms are mild and of short duration. Surgical procedures to decompress the nerve are indicated in more severe cases.

INTRODUCTION

Entrapment neuropathy results from increased pressure on a nerve as it passes through an enclosed space. A nerve is most vulnerable to compression as it traverses a fibro-osseous canal, where there is a disproportion of contents and capacity. Nerves that have previously been affected by a neuropathic process, as with diabetes or alcoholism, appear to be even more vulnerable to entrapment. For the clinician to fully fathom the manifestations of each syndrome, familiarity with the anatomy of each site is essential.

Mechanisms for nerve injury by compression are not fully understood. Mild amounts of pressure can lead to physiologic dysfunction, while friction and ischemia may also play a role in this process[1]. Surgical exposure often reveals nerve swelling proximal to the site of entrapment.

The signs and symptoms that accompany nerve entrapment may at times be subtle and easily confused with rheumatic disorders. In addition, rheumatic diseases that manifest synovitis or tenosynovitis are capable of causing compression neuropathy. Because entrapment neuropathies produce focal neurologic deficits, other conditions that can present with similar patterns (e.g. vasculitis, radiculopathy, reflex sympathetic dystrophy) must be included in the differential diagnosis.

The number of recognized sites of neural entrapment is considerable (Fig. 16.1). This chapter deals with those compressive neuropathies that are most often encountered in clinical practice.

THORACIC OUTLET SYNDROME

Thoracic outlet syndrome (TOS) is a term that encompasses a number of clinical entities. The syndrome results from compression of one or more of the neurovascular elements that pass through the superior thoracic aperture. In the majority of cases, it is neurogenic entrapment that accounts for the symptoms and rarely is there an isolated vascular lesion (see Chapter 4.18).

Anatomy

The thoracic outlet consists of several narrow channels through which the subclavian vessels and the lower trunk of the brachial plexus (eighth cervical and first thoracic fibers) pass from the thoracocervical region to the axilla (Fig. 16.2). The first area of narrowing, and potential entrapment, is between the scalenus anterior and scalenus medius muscles as they attach to the first rib. Next is the costoclavicular space, which is bordered by the clavicle anteriorly, the first rib posteromedially and the superior margin of the scapula posterolaterally. Lastly, the neurovascular bundle travels under the coracoid process and beneath the pectoralis minor tendon.

Causes

Because the thoracic outlet has the three well-defined areas of narrowing (described above), traditional teaching has ascribed specific clinical syndromes to each area. Thus, a fairly rigid classification has evolved which includes the anterior scalene, costoclavicular and hyperabduction syndromes. However, it is more likely that anatomic abnormalities

ENTRAPMENT NEUROPATHIES

	Nerve	Location/syndrome
Upper extremity and thorax	Brachial plexus	Thoracic outlet
	Dorsal scapular	Scalenus medius
	Suprascapular	Scapular notch
	Musculocutaneous	Elbow
	Radial	Posterior interosseous nerve syndrome
	Median	
	At elbow	Ligament of Struthers
	At forearm	Pronator teres
	At wrist	Carpal tunnel syndrome
	Anterior interosseous	Forearm
	Ulnar	
	At elbow	Cubital tunnel syndrome
	At wrist	Ulnar tunnel syndrome
Lower extremity	Obturator	Pelvis
	Sciatic	Piriformis syndrome
	Ilioinguinal	Lower abdomen
	Lateral femoral cutaneous	Meralgia paresthetica
	Femoral	Hip
	Peroneal	Fibular tunnel
	Saphenous	Hunter's canal
	Sural	Lower leg
	Posterior tibial	Tarsal tunnel syndrome
	Interdigital plantar	Morton's metatarsalgia

Fig. 16.1 Peripheral entrapment neuropathies.

THE THORACIC OUTLET

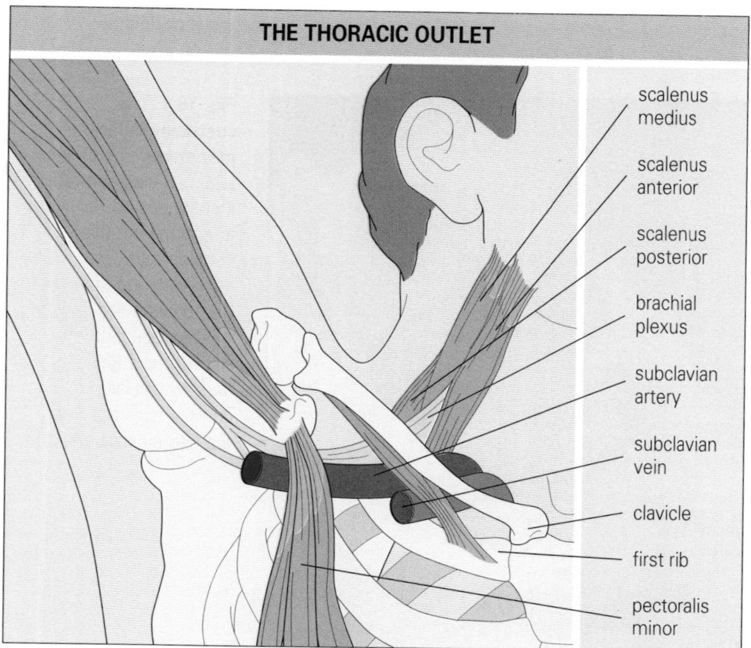

Fig. 16.2 The thoracic outlet. Three narrow channels of the outlet include the scalene triangle, costoclavicular passage and pectoralis minor attachment at the coracoid process.

and trauma to the shoulder girdle region play a far more pivotal role in causing this syndrome.

Cervical ribs, some incomplete and having fibrous attachments to the first rib, are an anomaly often associated with TOS (see Chapter 4.18c). Some have suggested that too much significance has been placed on this finding, since cervical ribs may be noted in up to 0.5% of routine radiographs. Furthermore, abnormal anatomy of the thoracic outlet, and in particular the presence of fibrous bands, is a common finding in the general population[2]. The congenital bands may arise from a cervical rib, from the transverse process of the seventh cervical vertebra or they may be associated with the scalene muscles. These cervical bands and certain scalene muscle abnormalities appear to play an important role in the pathogenesis of neurogenic TOS[3].

Signs and symptoms

Patients usually experience sensory symptoms as the first manifestation of TOS. Paresthesias are common, which follow the ulnar nerve distribution along the medial aspect of the arm and forearm and then to the fourth and fifth fingers. Aching pain, radiating to the neck, shoulder and arm, is a frequent complaint, often being more diffuse than the paresthesias. Carrying heavy objects, persistent abduction of the shoulder and work that requires using the arms over the head may exacerbate these symptoms. TOS is also more likely to occur in individuals with poor posture and drooping shoulders.

Signs of motor weakness, if they appear, usually follow the sensory complaints. The patients may describe a feeling of weakness or clumsiness in using the hand. Wasting of the thenar, hypothenar and intrinsic muscles of the hand may be noted.

A small number of patients have vasomotor disturbances. These may take the form of coldness, blanching or cyanosis. In more extreme cases, trophic changes and even infarction of tissues at the fingertips may appear[4].

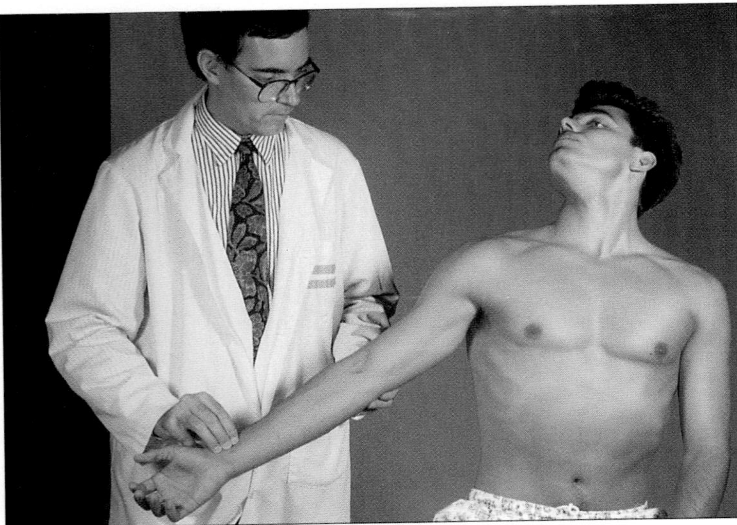

Fig. 16.3 The Adson maneuver. The patient inhales deeply, extends the neck fully and turns the head to the side being examined. This tests for compression in the scalene triangle and is positive if there is a diminution in the radial pulse and reproduction of the patient's symptoms.

Diagnosis

The most useful diagnostic approach to TOS is a careful neurologic examination, which may reveal tenderness over the brachial plexus, sensory deficits, motor weakness or signs of muscle atrophy. Certain clinical stress tests have traditionally been used to diagnose TOS. The Adson, costoclavicular and hyperabduction maneuvers (Figs 16.3–16.5) are used. However, because these maneuvers are positive in the majority of normal individuals (there is a reduction in the radial pulse), they have diagnostic utility only when the patient's sensory symptoms are reproduced.

A radiograph of the cervicothoracic region may reveal a cervical rib or an elongated transverse process of C7, a clue to the presence of a fibrous band. Nerve conduction studies in TOS are often difficult to interpret and may be most useful in diagnosing other conditions that might be confused with TOS, such as cervical radiculopathy, cubital tunnel syndrome or carpal tunnel syndrome.

The differential diagnosis of TOS should include cervical lesions (tumors, disc disease, spondylosis), reflex sympathetic dystrophy and carpal tunnel syndrome. In patients with vascular signs, other disorders of vessels should be considered (e.g. vasculitis and atherosclerosis).

Treatment

Conservative management of TOS is the course that should be pursued initially. This consists of appropriate exercises designed to improve posture by strengthening the rhomboid and trapezius muscles. Avoidance of hyperabduction is important, and patients may have to consider changing occupation if their job requires prolonged use of the arms above the head.

The concurrence of TOS and carpal tunnel syndrome (double crush syndrome) has been reported in up to 44% of patients with TOS[5]. It must be remembered, however, that carpal tunnel syndrome may present as

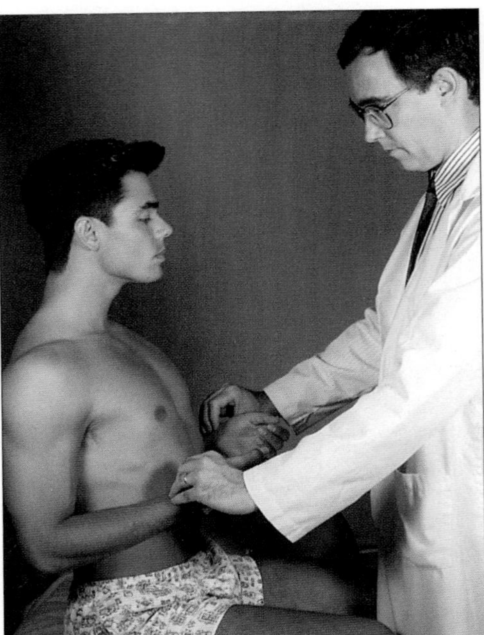

Fig. 16.4 The costoclavicular maneuver. The patient takes an exaggerated military position of attention with the shoulders thrust backward and downward. Decreased radial pulse and reproduction of symptoms suggest neuro-vascular compression between the clavicle and first rib.

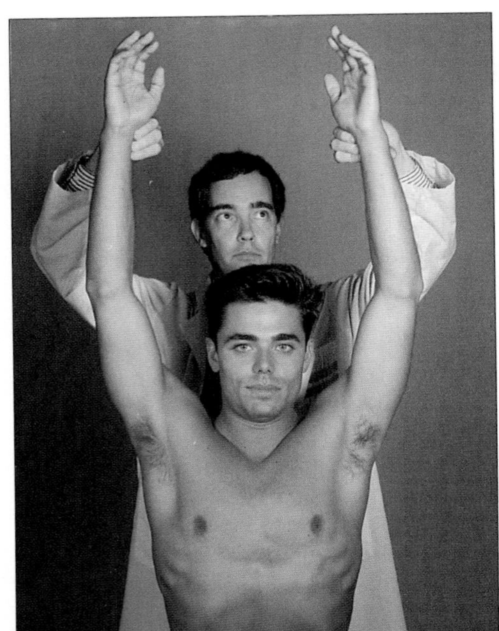

Fig. 16.5 The hyperabduction maneuver. The patient lifts his hands above his head with the elbows somewhat flexed and extending out laterally from the body, testing compression by the pectoralis minor at the coracoid process.

pain radiating to the shoulder region and may thus be confused with TOS[6]. Accordingly, distal nerve entrapment should be excluded before definitive therapy for TOS is considered.

Caution must be the watchword when considering surgical treatment of TOS. The large number of treatment failures reported by some authors makes careful screening of patients mandatory prior to surgery. Additionally, there is considerable risk of injury to the brachial plexus during surgery[7]. Conservative therapy should be continued as long as the neurologic symptoms are only subjective. Surgical intervention is considered if there are signs of the following: signs of muscle wasting, intermittent fleeting paresthesias replaced by continuous sensory loss, incapacitating pain or worsening circulatory impairment (if present)[4].

Since it is often difficult to define an exact anatomic area of compression preoperatively, success rates of particular surgical procedures are, not surprisingly, quite variable. The transaxillary approach with first rib resection has many proponents. This method is useful for costoclavicular compression. Others prefer supraclavicular exploration with removal of the scalenus anterior muscle. In either case, the surgeon must also search for constricting fibrous bands.

ULNAR NERVE COMPRESSION SYNDROMES

CUBITAL TUNNEL SYNDROME

Compression neuropathy of the ulnar nerve as it traverses the elbow has long been recognized as a complication of local trauma, particularly as a result of fractures of the humerus. Only in recent years has the concept of constriction of the nerve in a fibro-osseous tunnel been proffered [8].

Anatomy

The osseous portion of the cubital tunnel is formed anteriorly by the medial epicondyle, the fibrous portion by the ulnohumeral ligaments laterally and the aponeurosis of the two heads of the flexor carpi ulnaris posteromedially (Fig. 16.6). The size of the tunnel is reduced when the elbow is placed in flexion.

Causes

Without a history of trauma it may be difficult to give a precise cause for cubital tunnel syndrome (CUTS). However, chronic pressure over the ulnar groove, which may be exerted by occupational stress or from unusual elbow positioning, appears to play an etiologic role. Arthritic conditions that result in synovitis at the elbow, or osteophyte production, may also cause compression of the nerve.

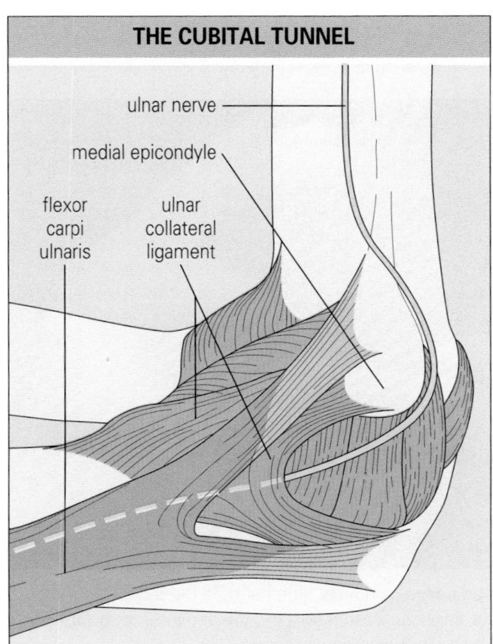

Fig. 16.6 The cubital tunnel. The fibro-osseous canal is formed by the medial epicondyle, ulnar collateral ligament and flexor carpi ulnaris muscle. Elbow flexion decreases the volume of the channel.

Signs and symptoms

Paresthesias are noted in the distribution of the ulnar nerve and, in many instances, the neuropathy is bilateral. Symptoms are often aggravated by prolonged use of the elbow in flexed position. Tinel's sign may be positive over the ulnar groove, and pain may be provoked by putting pressure directly on the nerve which may be noticeably swollen. A majority of patients will demonstrate atrophy of intrinsic muscles and weakness in pinch and grasp. There may be wasting of the hypothenar muscles and slight clawing of the fourth and fifth fingers. A positive Wartenberg's sign indicates weakness in adduction of the fifth finger.

Diagnosis

Consideration must be given to compression of the ulnar nerve at other locations, including the cervical spine, thoracic outlet and in Guyon's canal (see later). Also, CUTS must be differentiated from tardy ulnar palsy where neuropathy develops years after an injury.

Radiographs may be helpful in defining the cubital tunnel area, and may reveal lesions such as osteophytes, which may impinge on the nerve. Electrodiagnosis is useful in establishing that the site of ulnar compression is indeed the elbow and in following recovery after treatment. The readily accessible location of the entrapment area allows for direct testing of sensory and motor conduction across the cubital tunnel.

Treatment

When the symptoms are primarily sensory and motor weakness is not marked, avoidance of prolonged elbow flexion may be sufficient treatment. Compression due to inflammatory lesions, such as rheumatoid synovitis, may respond to local corticosteroid injection along the ulnar groove, paying particular attention to avoid direct needle contact with the nerve.

In more advance cases of CUTS a number of surgical procedures to decompress the nerve have been employed. These include simple release of flexor carpi ulnaris aponeurosis, medial epicondylectomy and anterior transposition of the nerve, the latter operation being the most demanding[9]. Because reinnervation of the nerve occurs slowly, postsurgical recovery in severe cases may take up to a year following a decompression procedure.

ULNAR TUNNEL SYNDROME

Ulnar tunnel syndrome (UTS) results from entrapment of the ulnar nerve in Guyon's canal at the wrist[10]. Many factors that affect the carpal tunnel can also influence the ulnar tunnel, which is in close proximity, at times both areas being simultaneously involved.

Anatomy

The ulnar tunnel is bounded on the sides by the hook of the hamate and the pisiform bone. Above and below the tunnel are the volar and transverse carpal ligaments, respectively (Fig. 16.7). While inside the tunnel, the ulnar nerve divides into sensory and motor branches.

Causes

The most common cause of nerve compression in Guyon's canal is due to ganglia. Aberrant muscles, Dupuytren's disease, rheumatoid arthritis (RA) and osteoarthritis may also cause impingement. Chronic trauma from use of certain tools and occupations that require blows to the palm also predispose to UTS.

Signs and symptoms

When compression of the nerve occurs in the proximal portion of the ulnar tunnel, the patient will have combined sensory and motor deficits, hypoesthesia in the hypothenar region and fourth and fifth fingers (see Fig. 16.12) as well as weakness of the intrinsic muscles of the hand. More distal lesions may present with either motor or sensory impairment.

Diagnosis

Electrodiagnostic studies are helpful in determining the site of entrapment and in defining which branches are involved. Ulnar

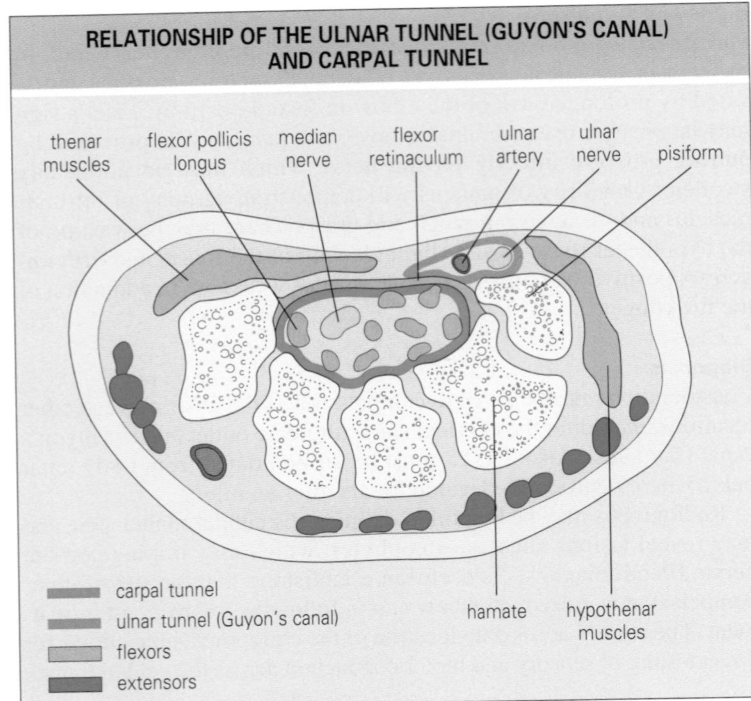

Fig. 16.7 The ulnar tunnel (Guyon's canal). Because of the close relationship of the ulnar tunnel to the carpal tunnel, pathology affecting one may simultaneously affect the other.

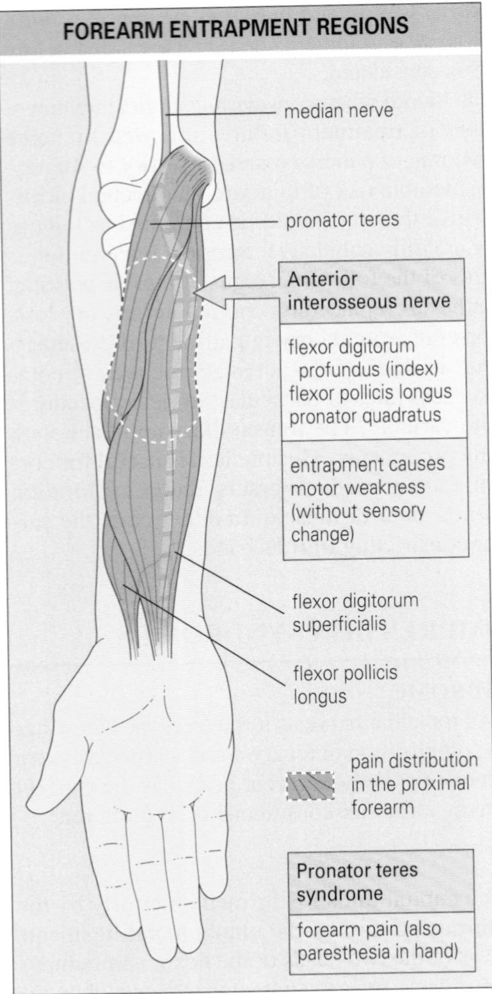

Fig. 16.8 Forearm entrapment regions. The median nerve may be compressed at several locations in the forearm, most commonly as it traverses the pronator teres muscle. The anterior interosseous branch of the median nerve is solely motor, thus entrapment produces no sensory deficit.

tunnel syndrome must be differentiated from TOS and CUTS.

Treatment

If conservative measures, such as avoidance of trauma to the palm, do not result in improvement then surgical decompression may be necessary. When entrapment is due to ganglia, synovitis or fibrosis, offending tissue is excised.

MEDIAN NERVE COMPRESSION SYNDROMES

FOREARM ENTRAPMENTS

Anterior interosseous nerve syndrome

The anterior interosseous nerve is a purely motor branch of the median nerve (Fig. 16.8). It innervates the pronator quadratus, the flexor pollicis longus and the flexor digitorum profundus to the index finger. The nerve branches off from the median nerve about 6cm below the lateral epicondyle. Entrapment may result from compression by aberrant or accessory muscles, fibrous bands beneath the pronator teres or by pressure from an enlarged bicipital bursa.

Because there are no sensory fibers in the nerve, the patient has no sensory complaints and experiences only motor weakness. The typical pattern is loss of distal flexion of the thumb and index finger giving a characteristic pinch sign (Fig. 16.9). The pronator quadratus is tested with the elbow fully flexed. There will be decreased resistance to forced supination of the forearm. The patient may also note a dull, aching pain in the volar aspect of the proximal forearm.

Confirmation of anterior interosseous nerve entrapment depends on electromyography of the forearm muscles. Differential diagnosis for this syndrome should include rupture of the flexor pollicis longus tendon, which may occur in RA and more proximal lesions such as brachial neuritis.

Because most patients improve with time, initial management is conservative unless the condition has been brought about by a wound. The patient is advised to avoid repetitive forearm motions (pronation–supination). If the weakness does not resolve after 2 or 3 months, surgery is usually recommended[11].

Pronator teres syndrome

There are several potential sites of median nerve entrapment in the forearm (Fig. 16.8). It may occur at the lacertus fibrosus, at the proximal edge of the flexor digitorum superficialis or most commonly by the pronator teres muscle itself or fibrous bands at the superficial head of this muscle.

The most consistent symptom in pronator teres syndrome (PTS) is an aching pain in the proximal forearm which often begins insidiously. This may be exacerbated by activities which are elbow-intensive and require pronation and grasping. Paresthesias are common and follow the median nerve distribution into the hand (see Fig. 16.12). As sensory findings are

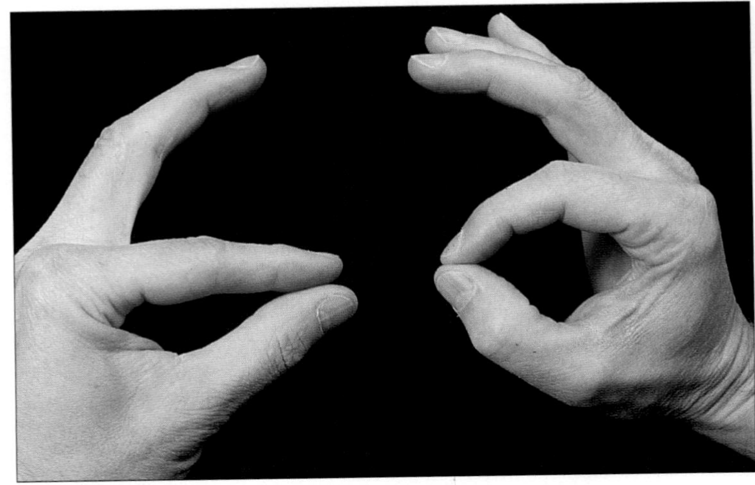

Fig. 16.9 Anterior interosseous nerve paralysis. The hand on the left demonstrates loss of function of flexor pollicis longus and flexor digitorum profundus muscles, resulting in a characteristic flattened pinch pattern.

similar to carpal tunnel syndrome (CTS), the two conditions may be confused. However, unlike CTS, nocturnal paresthesias are less frequent.

Physical examination may reveal local tenderness on palpation over the pronator teres muscle. In addition, percussion in this area may elicit a positive Tinel's sign with radiation of pain into the hand. A provocation test that may reproduce the pain consists of pronation of the forearm and flexion of the wrist performed against resistance. Some thenar atrophy may be noted, but profound muscle weakness is rare.

In a study by Hartz *et al.*[12], electrophysiologic testing was often inconclusive and could not be relied on to exclude PTS. Differential diagnosis of PTS should include CTS and more proximal nerve lesions at the cervical spine or thoracic outlet. However, with thoracic outlet lesions the pain usually radiates into the ulnar rather than radial portion of the hand.

For some patients, sufficient treatment may be abstention from activities that aggravate the condition. Surgical decompression is performed when symptoms become chronic.

CARPAL TUNNEL SYNDROME

Carpal tunnel syndrome is the most common entrapment neuropathy. The syndrome has gained increased recognition in recent years because of the prominent attention it has received in certain industrial settings, and it is now one of the most commonly reported occupational illnesses.

Anatomy

The carpal tunnel is bound on its dorsal and lateral surfaces by the carpal bones with their connecting ligaments and on the volar or anterior aspect by the transverse carpal ligament (Fig. 16.10). Nine flexor tendons and the median nerve pass through the tunnel. There are two ways in which the median nerve may be entrapped. Pressure may be exerted on the nerve due to reduction in capacity of the carpal tunnel, as with swelling or lesions of surrounding tissues, or there may be an increase in volume of the contents of the tunnel, an example being flexor tenosynovitis. Increased intracarpal canal pressures in patients with CTS have been confirmed by use of a wick catheter measuring device[13].

Causes

There are many causes of CTS (Fig. 16.11), but in some patients an underlying disease process cannot be identified and the designation idiopathic CTS is used. Because there is an increased awareness that certain occupational activities predispose to this disorder, and since more sophisticated diagnostic techniques have been developed, an attributable cause for CTS can now often be found.

Carpal tunnel is noted most commonly in persons whose occupation or avocation requires substantial use of the hands. The fact that CTS is found to occur more often in the dominant hand of both right-

THE CARPAL TUNNEL AND COURSE OF THE MEDIAN NERVE

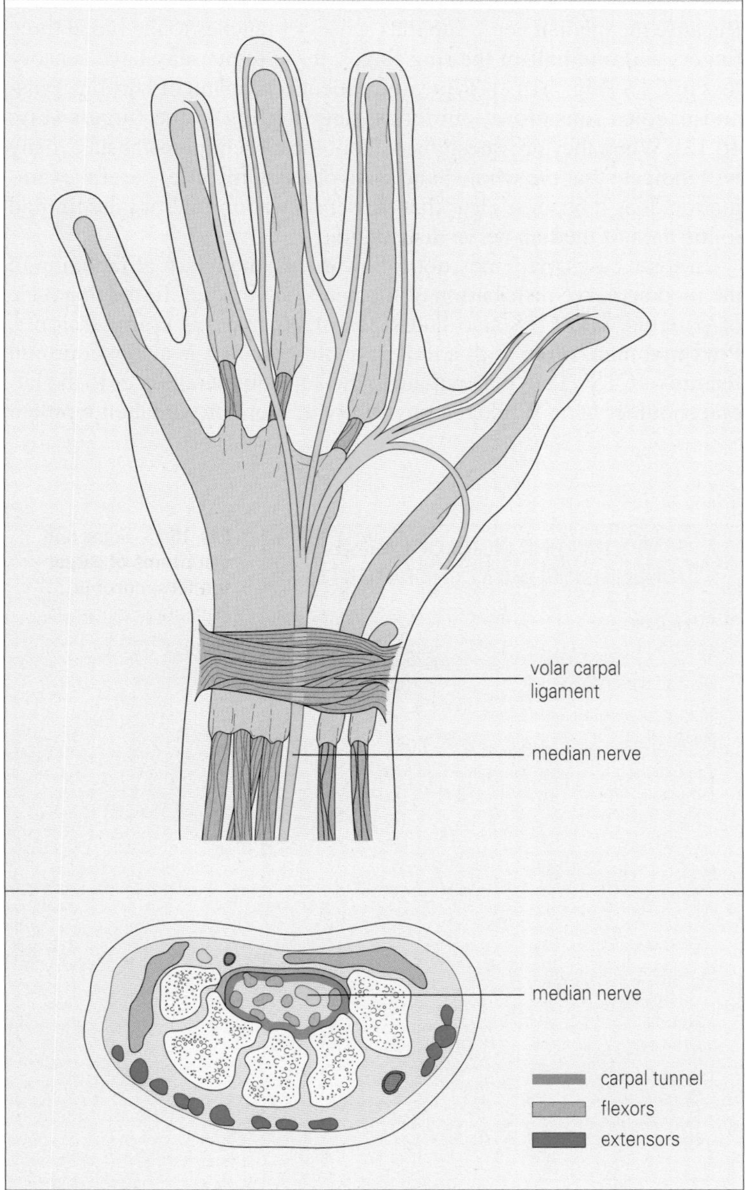

Fig. 16.10 The carpal tunnel and course of the median nerve. The space for the median nerve and flexor tendons is very confined. The median nerve courses under the region occupied by the palmaris longus and flexor carpi radialis tendons.

CONDITIONS ASSOCIATED WITH CARPAL TUNNEL SYNDROME	
Space-occupying lesions	Ganglia Hemangioma Osteoid osteoma Lipoma Thickened transverse carpal ligament (familial) Anomalous muscles Tenosynovitis (nonspecific)
Connective tissue disease	Rheumatoid arthritis Osteoarthritis Progressive systemic sclerosis Polymyositis Polymyalgia rheumatica
Crystal-induced rheumatic disease	Gout Calcium pyrophosphate dihydrate disease Hydroxyapatite disease
Occupational disease (repetitive motion disorders)	Meat cutters Musicians Keyboard workers
Metabolic and endocrine disease	Diabetes Thyroid (myxedema) Acromegaly Mucopolysaccharidosis
Infection	Osteomyelitis (carpal bones) Tenosynovitis *Mycobacterium tuberculosis* Atypical mycobacteria Histoplasmosis Coccidioidomycosis
Iatrogenic	Hematoma Phlebitis
Miscellaneous conditions	Pregnancy Amyloidosis Dialysis Fractures

Fig. 16.11 Conditions associated with carpal tunnel syndrome.

and left-handed individuals supports the concept that aggregate activity of the hand plays an important role in the genesis of this disorder.

Crystal-induced rheumatic disorders have been known to cause CTS. In the case of gout, tophaceous deposits or tenosynovitis may result in nerve entrapment. Both calcium pyrophosphate dihydrate and apatite crystals have been found in biopsy material taken from tendon sheaths during surgery for CTS.

Carpal tunnel syndrome is reported as a complication of several connective tissue diseases including scleroderma, polymyositis, polymyalgia rheumatica and, most commonly, RA (see Chapter 5.16). There are widely varying estimations of CTS frequency in RA, but that it occurs commonly is the experience of many practitioners. Indeed, prolonged median nerve sensory conduction velocities have been noted in up to half of all rheumatoid patients tested[14]. Generally, CTS is a result of rheumatoid flexor tenosynovitis. When the symptoms are mild, it may be difficult to differentiate the muscle atrophy noted in CTS from that associated with severe rheumatoid disease. Interestingly, when CTS complicates juvenile chronic arthritis, sensory abnormalities are rare whereas thenar atrophy is more commonly noted than in adult CTS[15].

Uremia, which is often complicated by peripheral neuropathy, also predisposes patients to entrapment neuropathy. CTS is particularly common in patients on hemodialysis[16] and in many of these cases it is the result of beta$_2$-microglobulin amyloid deposition. The erosive arthropathy associated with this variety of amyloid may also cause CTS when the wrist is affected[17].

A number of metabolic and endocrine diseases may have CTS as one of their manifestations. These include diabetes, myxedema, mucopolysaccharidosis and acromegaly. There is also an interesting, but as yet unexplained, association between idiopathic CTS and lateral humeral epicondylitis.

Infections involving carpal bones or flexor tendons at the wrist may result in CTS. These include chronic granulomatous infections caused by coccidioidomycosis, histoplasmosis, *Mycobacterium tuberculosis* and atypical mycobacteria.

Familial occurrence of CTS has also been reported. Amyloid deposition has not been identified in these individuals, but in some cases thickening of the transverse carpal ligament has been noted at surgery. This condition might be an important factor in compression of the median nerve. In one family, the mean age of onset of CTS was 24 years and flexor tenosynovitis was the dominant finding[18]. The onset of symptoms in familial CTS may even occur in early childhood.

All varieties of amyloidosis, primary, secondary, hereditary and associated with myeloma, may cause CTS. Some hereditary forms of amyloidosis predispose to development of peripheral neuropathy, while others are more likely to cause CTS. Lambird and Hartmann have shown that the transverse carpal ligament may appear grossly normal at the time of surgery but, unless histologic stains for amyloid are performed, the diagnosis of hereditary amyloidosis may be missed[19]. In myelomatosis, there may be significant amyloid deposition along the flexor tendons resulting in tethering of the tendons in the carpal tunnel.

While the occurrence of CTS in pregnancy has been well documented, the high incidence of this disorder has not been appreciated. It has been attributed, by some, to fluid retention. In one series, fully 21% of pregnant women described paresthesias or hypesthesia quite typical of CTS[20]. For the majority of patients, symptoms begin in the third trimester, usually resolve spontaneously after delivery and do not require surgery.

Also CTS may be a manifestation of repetitive strain syndrome. Workers who spend long hours using a keyboard, musicians who keep the wrist in a flexed position and meat cutters are all especially prone to developing CTS.

A number of local space-occupying lesions may impinge on the contents of the carpal tunnel. These include an anomalous median artery, ganglia, hemangiomas, osteoid osteomas and lipomas. Anomalous muscles may also compromise the carpal tunnel space. Most often this is caused by abnormalities of the palmaris longus, an extremely variable muscle, which inserts on the transverse carpal ligament.

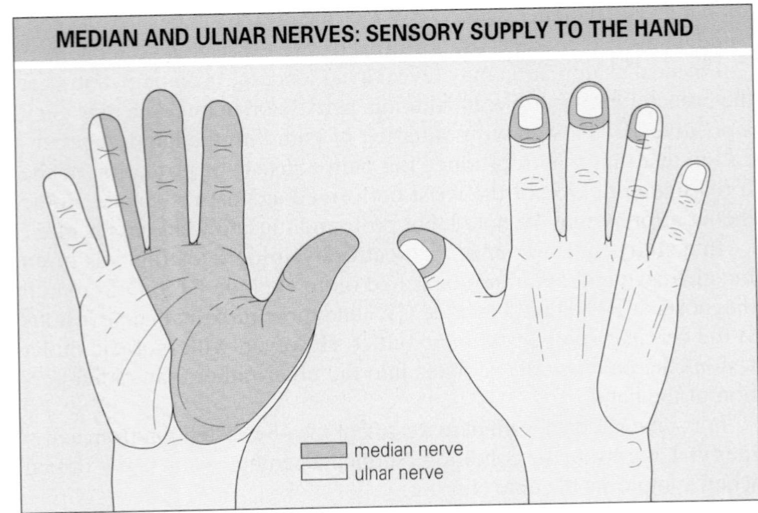

Fig. 16.12 Median and ulnar nerve innervation of the hand. The radial three digits and half of the ring finger are supplied by sensory branches of the median nerve. The fifth finger and half of the ring finger are supplied by sensory branches of the ulnar nerve.

Symptoms

Because the median nerve supplies sensory branches to the radial three fingers and one-half of the ring finger, these digits may have sensory loss in CTS (Fig. 16.12). Typically, patients complain of burning, pins-and-needles sensations, numbness and tingling in the fingers (Fig. 16.13). When they are questioned about location of paresthesias, many will indicate that the whole hand is involved. Only after careful examination does it become clear that the sensory abnormalities are limited to the area of median nerve distribution.

In some cases, pain may not follow the usual pattern of radiation in the median nerve distribution of the hand. Silver et al. found that 34% of patients with CTS also had signs of ulnar nerve compression[22]. Proximal pain, often with a dull or aching quality, is also a common feature of CTS[6]. Pain may radiate to the antecubital region or to the lateral shoulder area. While the possibility of more proximal entrapment

SYMPTOMS AND SIGNS OF CARPAL TUNNEL SYNDROME IN 1016 PATIENTS

Symptom or sign	Percentage of patients
Median parethesias	100
Nocturnal parethesias	71
Proximal extension of pain	38
Tinel's sign	
Positive	55
Negative	29
Unknown	17
Phalen's test	
Positive	53
Negative	23
Unknown	24
Sensation on sensory examination	
Decreased	28
Normal	36
Unknown	36
Thenar muscle strength	
Decreased	18
Normal	42
Unknown	41
Thenar muscle bulk	
Wasted	18
Normal	31
Unknown	50

Fig. 16.13 Signs and symptoms of carpal tunnel syndrome. Data from Spinner *et al.*[21]

should be kept in mind, the majority of patients improve following nerve decompression at the carpal tunnel.

Perhaps the archetypal complaint of patients with CTS is that they are awakened at night by abnormal sensations. Often it is this interruption of sleep that is the most troublesome aspect of CTS. Commonly, the patient will shake the hand in an attempt to relieve the numbness and may run it under warm water to improve the circulation.

Activities that result in persistent or repeated flexion or extension of the wrists are more likely to intensify symptoms. These include holding a newspaper or book, grasping a steering wheel and occupations such as meat cutting in which a utensil is grasped with the wrist in flexion. Some patients report that they are more prone to drop objects, and they attribute this to hand weakness. However, these individuals rarely have profound weakness on grip testing, and it is more likely that the problem stems from sensory deficit at the finger tips.

Signs

Tinel's sign consists of tapping lightly over the median nerve and is positive if the patient perceives paresthesia which radiates distally. The diagnostic value depends largely on how the test is conducted. Mossman and Blau found that to be effective percussion must be done with the wrist in extension so that the carpal tunnel is compressed[23]. They also noted that using a fingertip or small neurologic hammer is less effective than using a broad-head hammer that can percuss over the whole transverse carpal ligament and somewhat more proximally (Fig. 16.14). The wrist flexion test or Phalen's test (Fig. 16.15) is performed by having the patient hold the wrists in extreme but unforced flexion for one minute. It is positive if paresthesias are reproduced. As with Tinel's sign, the wrist flexion test in CTS is not invariably positive, but when it is, it helps substantiate the diagnosis.

Dorwart has described a new sign in CTS, which she called the 'volar hot dog'[24]. Sixty-one of 63 patients with CTS of various etiologies had a firm 'hot-dog shaped' swelling at the wrist. This sausage-shaped structure (1cm wide and 2.5cm long) was located on the ulnar side of the palmaris longus tendon and extended proximally from the wrist crease. The swelling disappeared with effective treatment of the CTS.

To determine motor loss, the strength of the thenar muscles should be tested. The easiest muscle to test is the abductor pollicis brevis. With the thumb first adducted toward the fifth finger, the patient is then asked to abduct against resistance to the distal phalanx. The opponens pollicis muscle is tested by having the patient touch the tip of the thumb to the tip of the fifth finger, then the examiner attempts to break the pinch. Inspection of the hand may reveal atrophy of the thenar muscles (Fig. 16.16).

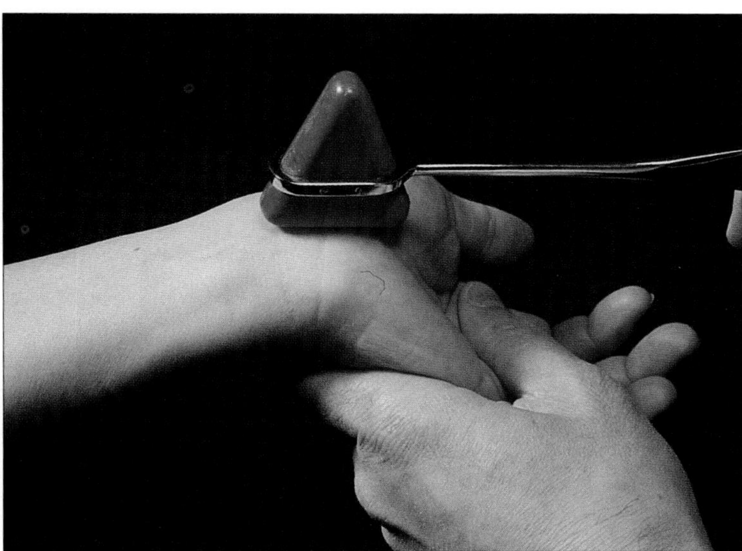

Fig. 16.14 Tinel's sign. The wrist is held in extension while gentle percussion is performed over and just proximal to the transverse carpal ligament.

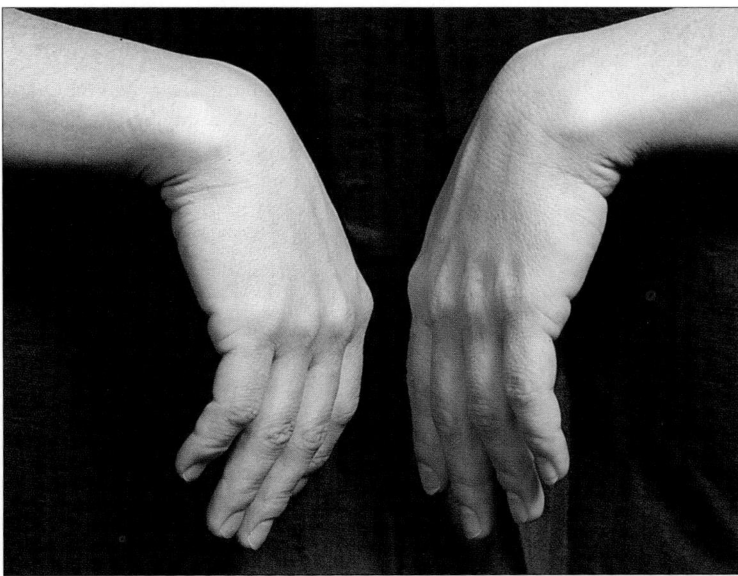

Fig. 16.15 Phalen's (wrist flexion) test. With the wrists held in unforced flexion for 30–60s, a positive test reproduces or worsens the patient's symptoms.

Diagnosis

While CTS is diagnosed on the basis of the patient's history and clinical examination, imaging and electrodiagnostic studies may be useful in confirming the diagnostic impression. Conventional radiographs using a carpal tunnel projection can help to delineate the soft tissues and the carpal bones. However, the anatomy of the carpal tunnel, including swelling or distortion of the median nerve, thickening of flexor tendon sheaths or presence of space occupying lesions or aberrant muscle can be better visualized by magnetic resonance imaging[25].

The most important electrodiagnostic study is the measurement of sensory nerve conduction velocity across the carpal tunnel. A slowed conduction velocity, along with prolongation of distal motor latency, lends support to the diagnosis of CTS.

In about 15% of the population, fibers from the median nerve travel via the ulnar nerve to the thenar muscles: the Martin Gruber anastomosis. It is important to recognize this entity since it may result in the sparing of the thenar muscles in CTS. A clue to the presence of this anatomic variation is the finding of normal proximal latency but a prolonged distal latency.

Differential diagnosis of CTS must include median nerve entrapment proximal to the carpal tunnel[5]. The double crush syndrome refers to dual compression of a nerve along its course. It has been postulated that a proximal lesion renders a nerve more vulnerable to distal compression. In the case of CTS, this syndrome may be manifested by more proximal lesions such as pronator teres syndrome, thoracic outlet

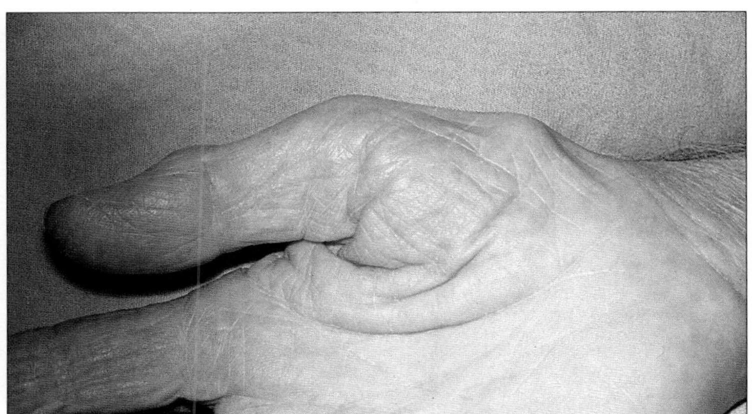

Fig. 16.16 Thenar muscle atrophy. Chronic entrapment of the median nerve in the carpal tunnel or more proximally may produce thenar atrophy as seen in this patient.

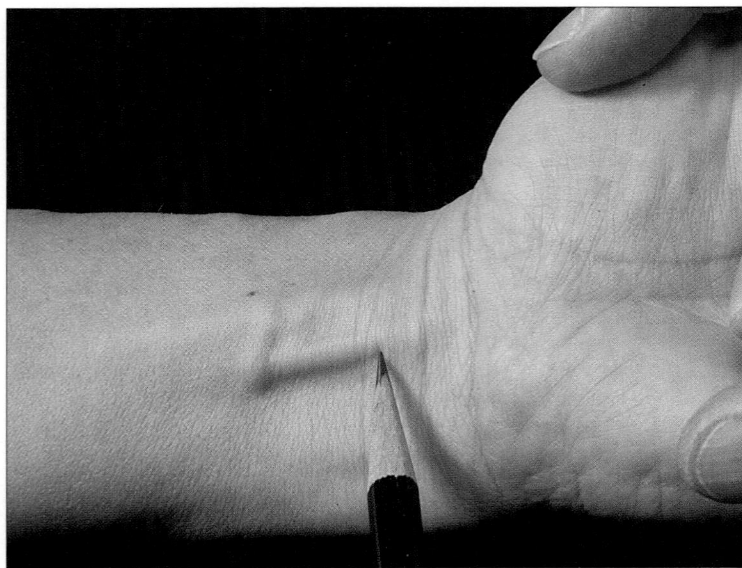

Fig. 16.17 Palmaris longus tendon. The pencil point identifies the tendon of the palmaris longus muscle, an important landmark in determining the injection site for carpal tunnel syndrome. The tendon of the flexor carpi radialis can be seen just to the radial side of the palmaris longus tendon.

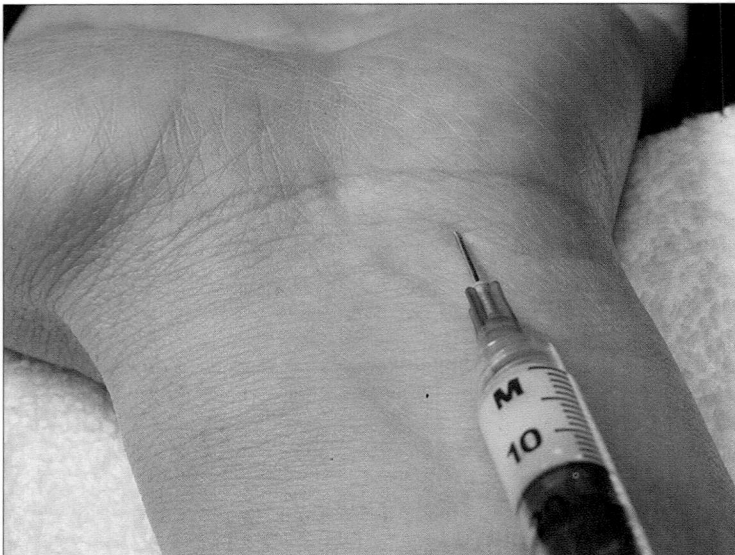

Fig. 16.18 Carpal tunnel injection. The needle is inserted just proximal to the wrist crease and to the ulnar side of the palmaris longus tendon.

syndrome and cervical radiculopathy (usually C6/C7). Therefore, for older patients with CTS and proximal pain symptoms, studies of the cervical region should be done as well.

Treatment

The specific treatment of CTS depends, to a large degree, on whether there is an identifiable cause of the entrapment. Conservative measures may suffice when symptoms are of short duration. Repeated electromyographic determinations, done over time, may help the clinician determine the correct therapeutic approach. Patients with progressive increases in distal motor latency times should be considered for surgery.

Splinting

Splinting is a simple and cost-effective modality which, if successful in relieving symptoms, helps to confirm the diagnosis of CTS. Since wrist motion often worsens CTS, splinting is an important treatment element. A volar wrist splint which keeps the wrist in a neutral position is particularly helpful during the night when the wrist often falls into a position of flexion. Splinting alone may be sufficient to relieve CTS, primarily in cases where symptoms are of recent onset.

Local corticosteroid injection

Injection of the carpal tunnel is another effective therapy in individuals whose disease is of shorter duration and where there is no significant muscle wasting. The best response to injection is in patients whose symptoms have been present for less than a year and in whom there is no significant muscle atrophy or weakness. Girlanda *et al.* studied the short- and long-term benefits of local corticosteroid injection in idiopathic CTS. They found that while most patients improved initially, 50% of patients had worsening of their symptoms by 6 months[26].

Before injection is attempted, certain landmarks should be identified, including the tendons of the palmaris longus and flexor carpi radialis muscles (Fig. 16.17). This is most easily accomplished by asking the patient to flex against resistance. Injection can be facilitated if the wrist is placed in slight extension (the wrist draped over a small rolled-up towel). The needle is inserted ulnar (medial) to the palmaris longus tendon and proximal to the wrist crease (Fig. 16.18). Local anesthetic may be used, but deep infiltration is unwise, since the patient will not be responsive to needle contact with the median nerve and a neuritis might result. If the patient notes median nerve paresthesia during injection, the needle should be withdrawn and repositioned. Methylprednisolone or triamcinolone may be used to treat CTS and, if improvement is not complete, consideration may be given to a second injection. Frequent injections are proscribed because there is danger of tendon rupture.

Nonsteroidal anti-inflammatory drugs and other agents

Use of nonsteroidal anti-inflammatory drugs (NSAIDs) is generally limited to instances where there is an underlying inflammatory lesion, such as tenosynovitis. There are several reports of CTS improvement with pyridoxine supplements, usually in doses of 100–200mg/day. However, pyridoxine must be used with caution because sensory neuropathy may be a complication of excess pyridoxine intake.

Surgery

Surgical release of the transverse carpal ligament is the definitive treatment for CTS. The traditional surgical approach of ligament sectioning using a palmar incision is increasingly being replaced by endoscopic release. The latter technique, while equally effective, must be performed with great care to avoid injury to the superficial palmar arterial arch or to the median or ulnar nerves[27]. Surgical intervention in CTS is indicated when response to conservative measures is inadequate, when there are progressive or persistent neurologic changes or where there is muscle atrophy. In those circumstances where there is marked tenosynovitis, as with RA or granulomatous disease, simple decompression of the carpal tunnel may not be sufficient. Additional tenosynovectomy with lysis of adhesions may be necessary. Furthermore, when there are infiltrating processes, such as amyloid deposits, attached to tendons, the more complicated procedure of tenolysis may be necessary. Because tuberculosis and fungal infections are sometimes a cause of CTS, appropriate cultures and histologic studies should be done at the time of surgery, particularly if tenosynovitis is noted.

Failure of surgery to relieve symptoms is often the result of incomplete release of the ligament. In addition, the response to surgery of patients with median nerve double-crush injury appears to be less successful than patients with isolated CTS. Postoperative improvement depends in part on the severity of initial nerve deficit. While most patients' symptoms are ameliorated by surgery, those individuals whose occupations require repetitive motions may need to be retrained for less hand-intensive work.

MERALGIA PARESTHETICA

The term meralgia has it roots in the Greek words for thigh (meros) and a painful condition (algia). Meralgia paresthetica (MP) is caused by entrapment of the lateral femoral cutaneous nerve. One of the earliest descriptions of this entity was by Sigmund Freud, in which he related the typical MP symptoms that he experienced[28]. While MP occurs primarily in adults, children may be affected and often there is a significant delay in diagnosis[29].

Anatomy

The lateral femoral cutaneous nerve is entirely sensory and arises from the second and third lumbar roots. It proceeds from the lateral border of the psoas muscle, along the ilium to pass under or through the lateral aspect of the inguinal ligament just medial to the anterior superior iliac spine, the most common site of entrapment (Fig. 16.19). The nerve travels down the anterior thigh, where it divides into anterior and posterior branches. These supply sensation to the anterolateral portion of the thigh.

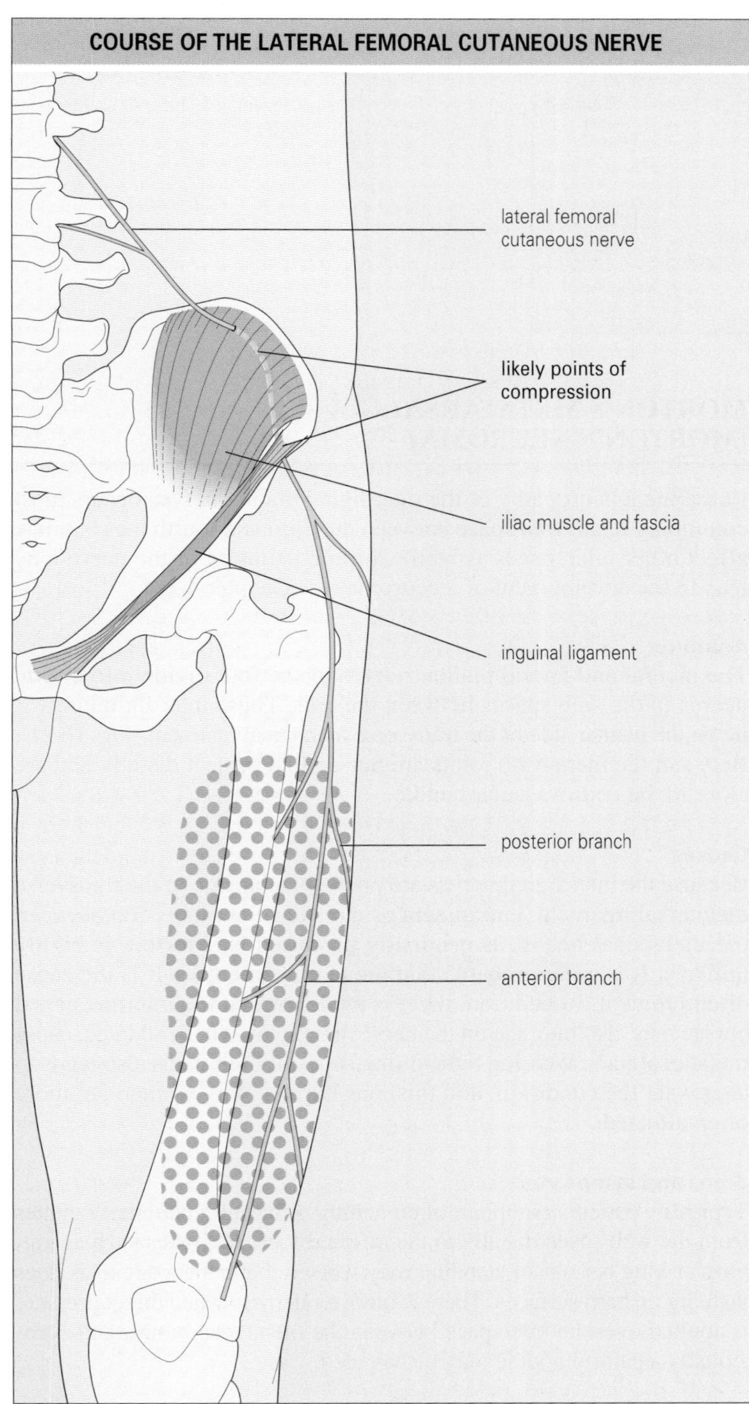

Fig. 16.19 Course of the lateral femoral cutaneous nerve. The potential for entrapment of the lateral femoral cutaneous nerve can be seen by its course just under the inguinal ligament and medial to the anterior superior iliac spine.

Causes

Direct pressure from belts and other tight-fitting garments may contribute to the entrapment of the lateral femoral cutaneous nerve as it passes under the inguinal ligament. Workers who support heavy bundles on their thigh are also at risk. Several clinical conditions have been associated with the development of MP, including obesity, pregnancy, diabetes, ascites and trauma to the thigh or inguinal region. The neuropathy may also occur as a consequence of direct injury to the nerve during surgery in the pelvic region (e.g. appendectomy, inguinal herniorrhaphy, iliac bone procurement).

Signs and symptoms

Patients with MP typically complain of burning pain and dysesthesia in the sensory distribution of the nerve. However, a smaller area of sensory deficit is common[29]. The patient may volunteer that certain positions seem to exacerbate the discomfort, for example sitting with the legs crossed, prolonged standing or extending the leg posteriorly.

Diagnosis

In the differential diagnosis of MP it is important to consider the possibility that there may be radiculopathy of the L2 or L3 roots or a spinal stenosis causing the symptoms[30]. Some patients will report direct tenderness over the inguinal ligament.

Electrodiagnosis, using superficial electrodes to measure conduction velocity of the nerve, may be useful in confirming the diagnosis[31]. Nerve block may also affirm the diagnosis as well as offer pain relief.

Treatment

Since MP is often self-limiting, conservative measures should be used. These might include weight reduction, elimination of occupational trauma and avoidance of external mechanical pressure over the inguinal ligament. Local injection of anesthetic and corticosteroids may be useful, as may be NSAIDs.

If MP becomes chronic and the pain unremitting, surgical decompression (neurolysis) may be considered, although results have been disappointing in many instances. A recently described suprainguinal approach for release of the entrapped nerve may offer improved operative results[32]. When MP is of spinal origin, epidural injection of corticosteroid may be helpful.

TARSAL TUNNEL SYNDROME

The occurrence of tarsal tunnel syndrome (TTS) is undoubtedly more frequent than is suggested by isolated reports in the literature[33]. It is often mistaken for other foot disorders and clinicians are less apt to include this entrapment neuropathy in the differential diagnosis of foot pain.

Anatomy

The tarsal tunnel is a fibro-osseous canal formed by the flexor retinaculum (laciniate ligament) as it extends from the medial malleolus down onto the calcaneus (see Fig. 16.20). The posterior tibial nerve passes through the tunnel, along with vascular structures, tendons of the flexor hallucis longus and the flexor digitorum longus muscles. Along its course, the tibial nerve gives off calcaneal branches and then lateral and medial plantar branches (see Fig. 16.20). While the calcaneal branches are solely sensory, the plantar nerves have mixed motor and sensory functions. Because the narrowest aspect of the tunnel is the distal or anterior–inferior portion, this is where the plantar nerve branches are most likely to be entrapped.

Causes

A number of abnormalities have been described as causing TTS. These include bone deformity after fractures, pressure from casts, hypertrophy of the laciniate ligament or of the abductor hallucis muscle,

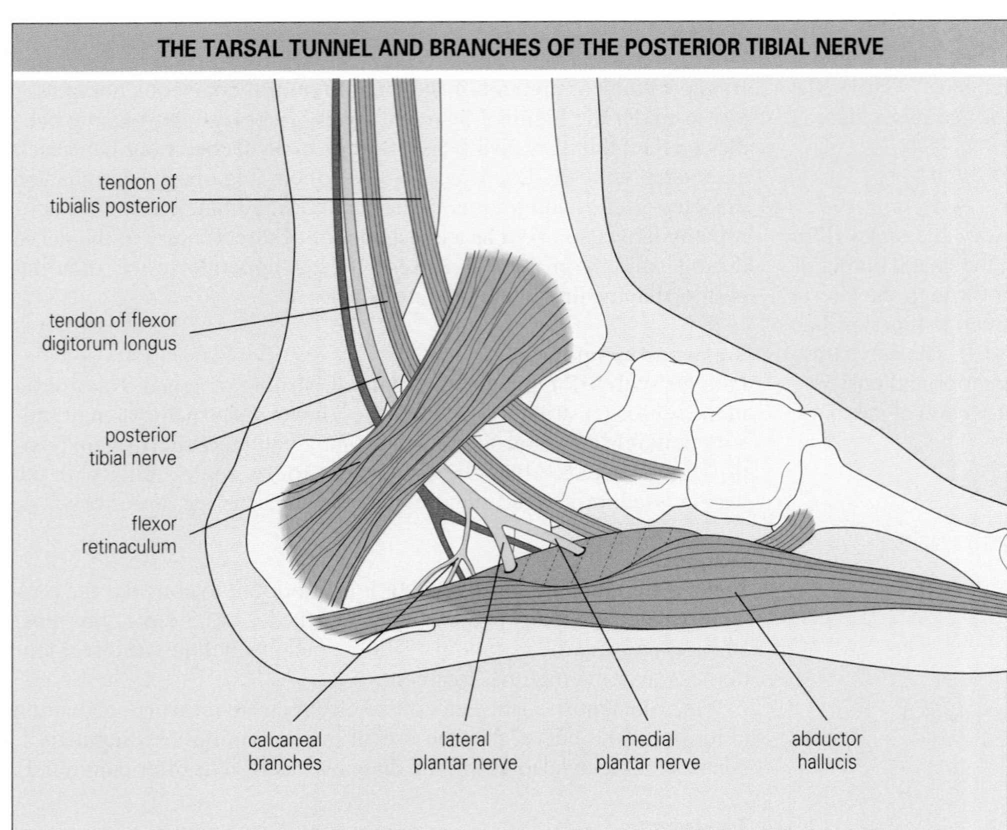

Fig. 16.20 The tarsal tunnel. Entrapment of branches of the posterior tibial nerve occurs under the flexor retinaculum, which attaches to the medial malleolus. As there are calcaneal as well as medial and lateral plantar branches of the posterior tibial nerve, symptoms of entrapment will depend on which branches are affected.

flexor tenosynovitis, synovial cysts, ganglia and diabetes mellitus. Proliferative synovitis accompanying RA is also a cause of TTS.

Signs and symptoms

Symptoms of TTS depend on the level of stenosis and consequently on which branches of the posterior tibial nerve are involved. The patient usually complains of burning pain or paresthesias in the toes, sole or heel of the foot. As in CTS, pain may awaken the patient at night and may move in a retrograde fashion to the calf. Relief may be obtained by walking about. Commonly, there is tenderness to direct palpation over the nerve posterior to the medial malleolus, and there may be a fusiform swelling in this region. Other findings can include a positive Tinel's sign over the tarsal tunnel, vasomotor changes and weakness of toe flexion and of the intrinsic muscles of the foot.

Diagnosis

In the differential diagnosis of TTS one must consider arthritis of the tarsal bones, plantar fasciitis, vascular insufficiency and systemic peripheral neuropathy. TTS may also be confused with lumbosacral nerve root radiculopathy. Another condition which must be kept in mind, particularly in runners, is hypertrophy of the abductor hallucis muscle. But in this case, the compression of the plantar nerve occurs distal to the laciniate ligament.

Electrodiagnostic studies are useful in confirming the diagnosis of TTS. Nerve conduction velocities are often diminished, and there may be abnormalities of distal motor latencies. Prolonged distal motor latencies of plantar nerves have been reported in 25% of rheumatoid patients[34].

Treatment

A number of conservative therapies have been used in TTS, including local corticosteroid injection, NSAIDs and orthotics. None of these has been consistently effective. The standard treatment is surgical decompression, which gives excellent results in the majority of patients. If the patient's symptoms are the result of pressure on the nerve from the abductor hallucis muscle, release of the muscle at its origin is performed rather than sectioning of the flexor retinaculum.

MORTON'S METATARSALGIA (MORTON'S NEUROMA)

Entrapment neuropathy of the interdigital plantar nerves occurs most commonly in the web space between the third and fourth toes but may affect other interspaces as well. Chronic irritation of the nerve may lead to the development of a neuroma (see Chapter 4.12).

Anatomy

The medial and lateral plantar nerves of the foot divide into digital nerves in the web spaces between the toes. These interdigital nerves lie on the plantar side of the transverse metatarsal ligament (Fig. 16.21). Between the metatarsal joints are bursae that project distally and are close to the neurovascular bundle.

Causes

Because the interdigital nerves are on the plantar side of the transverse metatarsal ligament, entrapment as a result of compression between the metatarsal heads, as originally proposed by Morton, is highly unlikely. It is more probable that the taut ligament itself is the cause of entrapment. In addition, there is evidence that the intermetatarsal bursae may also impinge on the nerve directly or, when inflamed, cause metatarsalgia[35]. Wearing tight-fitting shoes or high-heels also tends to aggravate the condition, and this may explain why women are more often affected.

Signs and symptoms

Typically, patients complain of an aching or burning pain that radiates from the web space distally to the affected toes. Activities such as jogging or long periods of standing may worsen the metatarsalgia, as does walking on hard surfaces. There is often tenderness when direct pressure is applied over the interspace between the metatarsal bones, and occasionally a painful nodule may be palpated.

Diagnosis

Morton's metatarsalgia must be differentiated from inflammatory conditions affecting the forefoot. Rheumatoid arthritis may present as

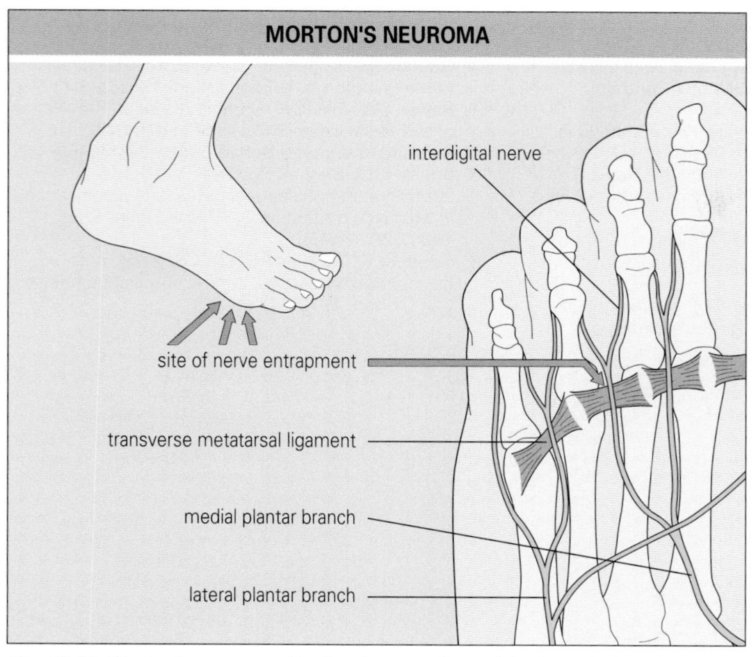

Fig. 16.21 Morton's neuroma. On the plantar surface of the foot, the interdigital nerve is compressed below the transverse metatarsal ligament and not between the metatarsal heads (plantar view).

metatarsalgia, but in most cases examination reveals synovitis and neuritic pain is uncommon. Conventional radiographs are of little value in diagnosing Morton's neuroma. Sonography can identify neuromas, which appear as ovoid, hypoechoic lesions. Magnetic resonance imaging has also been successfully employed in localizing the neuroma.

Treatment

Initial treatment should include conservative measures such as padding the metatarsal area and use of broad-toed shoes. There are also reports of benefit derived from injection of local anesthetic and corticosteroids.

When conservative therapy fails, the traditional approach has been surgical resection of the neuroma. The clear drawback to this procedure is that the patient is left with a sensory deficit. Another strategy is release of the transverse metatarsal ligament and epineural neurolysis of the interdigital nerve[36]. This method avoids neurectomy while decompressing the nerve.

REFERENCES

1. Dawson DM, Hallett M, Millender LH. Pathology of nerve entrapment. In: Entrapment neuropathies, 2E. Boston: Little & Brown; 1990:5–23.
2. Juvonen T, Satta J, Laitala P, *et al.* Anomalies at the thoracic outlet are frequent in the general population. Am J Surg. 1995;170:33–7.
3. Liu JE, Tahmoush AJ, Roos DB, Schwartzman. Shoulder–arm pain from cervical bands and scalene muscle anomalies. J Neurol Sci. 1995;128:175–80.
4. Sunderland S. In: Nerve and nerve injuries, 2E. Edinburgh: Churchill Livingstone; 1978:905–19.
5. Wood VE, Biondi J. Double-crush nerve compression in thoracic-outlet syndrome. J Bone Joint Surg. 1990;72A:85–7.
6. Cherington M. Proximal pain in carpal tunnel syndrome. Arch Surg. 1974;108:69.
7. Dale WA. Thoracic outlet compression syndrome. Arch Surg. 1982;117:1437–45.
8. Folberg CR, Weiss AP, Akelman E. Cubital tunnel syndrome. Part 1: Presentation and diagnosis. Orthop Rev. 1994;23:136–44.
9. Watchmaker GP, Lee G, Mackinnon SE. Intraneural topography of the ulnar nerve in the cubital tunnel facilitates anterior transposition. J Hand Surg Am. 1994;19:915–22.
10. Moneim MS. Ulnar nerve compression at the wrist. Ulnar tunnel syndrome. Hand Clin. 1992;8:337–44.
11. Chan KM, Lamb DW. The anterior interosseous nerve syndrome. J R Coll Surg (Edin). 1984;29:350–53.
12. Hartz CR, Linscheid RL, Gramse RR, Daube JR. The pronator teres syndrome: compressive neuropathy of the median nerve. J Bone Joint Surg. 1981;63A:885–90.
13. Gelberman RH, Hergenroeder PT, Hargens AR, *et al.* The carpal tunnel syndrome. A study of carpal canal pressures. J Bone Joint Surg. 1981;63A:380–3.
14. Barnes CG, Currey HLF. Carpal tunnel syndrome in rheumatoid arthritis. 1967;26:226–33.
15. Ishikawa K, Patiala H, Raunio P, Vainio K. Carpal tunnel syndrome in juvenile rheumatoid arthritis. Arch Orthop Trauma Surg. 1975;82:85–91.
16. Halter SK, DeLisa JA, Stolov WC, *et al.* Carpal tunnel syndrome in chronic renal dialysis patients. Arch Phys Med Rehabil. 1981;62:197–201.
17. Kessler M, Hestin D, Aymard B, Mainard D, *et al.* Carpal-tunnel syndrome with beta$_2$-microglobulin amyloid deposits and erosive arthropathy of the wrist and spine in a uraemic patient before chronic haemodialysis. Nephrol Dial Transplant. 1995;10:298–9.
18. Gray RG, Poppo MJ, Gottlieb NL. Primary familial bilateral carpal tunnel syndrome. 1979;91:37–40.
19. Lambird PA, Hartmann WH. Hereditary amyloidosis, the flexor retinaculum, and the carpal tunnel syndrome. Am J Clin Pathol. 1969;52:714–19.
20. Gould JS, Wissinger A. Carpal tunnel syndrome in pregnancy. South Med J. 1978;71:144–6.
21. Spinner RJ, Bachman JW, Amadio PC. The many faces of carpal tunnel syndrome. Mayo Clin Proc. 1989;64:829–36.
22. Silver MA, Gelberman RH, Gellman H, Rhoades CE. Carpal tunnel syndrome: Associated abnormalities in ulnar nerve function and the

effect of carpal tunnel release on these abnormalities. J Hand Surg. 1985;10A:710–13.
23. Mossman SS, Blau JN. Tinel's sign and the carpal tunnel syndrome. 1987;294:680.
24. Dorwart BB. Volar 'hot dog' at the wrist: A new sign in carpal tunnel syndrome. Clin Res. 1983;31:649A.
25. Mesgarzadeh M, Triolo J, Schneck CD. Carpal tunnel syndrome. MR imaging diagnosis. Magn Reson Imaging Clin N Am. 1995;3:249–64.
26. Girlanda P, Dattola R, Venuto C, *et al*. Local steroid treatment in idiopathic carpal tunnel syndrome: short- and long-term efficacy. J Neurol. 1993;240:187-90.
27. Shinya K, Lanzetta M, Connolly WB. Risk and complications in endoscopic carpal tunnel release. J Hand Surg [Br]. 1995;20:222–7.
28. Freud S. Uber die Bernhardt sche Sensibilitats-storungam Oberschenkel. Neurol Centralbl. 1985;14:491–2.
29. Edelson R, Stevens P. Meralgia paresthetica in children. J Bone Joint Surg [Am]. 1994;76:993–9.
30. Guo-Xiang J, Wei-Dong X, Ai-Hao W. Spinal stenosis with meralgia paresthetica. J Bone Joint Surg. 1988;70B:272–3.
31. Spevak MK, Prevec TS. A noninvasive method of neurography in meralgia paresthetica. Muscle Nerve 1995;18:601–5.
32. Aldrich EF, van den Heever CM. Suprainguinal ligament approach for surgical treatment of meralgia paresthetica. J Neurosurg. 1989;70:492–4.
33. Goodgold J, Kopell HP, Spielholz NI. The tarsal-tunnel syndrome. N Engl J Med. 1965;273:742–5.
34. Baylan SW, Paik SW, Barnert AL, *et al*. Prevalence of the tarsal tunnel syndrome in rheumatoid arthritis. Rheumatol Rehabil. 1981;20:148–50.
35. Bossley CJ, Cairney PC. The intermetatarsophalangeal bursa – its significance in Morton's metatarsalgia. J Bone Joint Surg. 1980;62B:184–7.
36. Gauthier G. Thomas Morton's disease. A nerve entrapment syndrome. A new surgical technique. Clin Orthop. 1979;142:90–92.

17

SPORTS MEDICINE: THE CLINICAL SPECTRUM OF INJURY

J David Perry

- Sports medicine encompasses the science and medicine of exercise and sport.
- Age, body habitus and anatomical variants contribute significantly to the risk of injury.
- Immediate swelling of a joint implies hemarthrosis.
- Hemarthrosis generally indicates significant intra-articular injury (fracture, ligamentous tears).
- Chronic overuse injuries affect mainly the soft tissues. About one tenth of these injuries involve stress fractures (fatigue failure of bone).
- Stress fractures are suggested by 'crescendo' activity–related pain and localized tenderness. Initial X-rays are often normal.
- An underlying spondylarthropathy should not be missed in a youngster with 'overuse' tendinitis or 'internal derangement' of a joint.

INTRODUCTION

Sports medicine is the medicine and science of exercise and sport. Athletic endeavor, both elite and recreational, has advanced and expanded steadily, but medical practice has often been slow to respond to the changing needs of a more fitness- conscious society. However, there is now developing an increasing awareness of the benefits of active exercise in health promotion[1], so that physical exercise has become an important part of many people's daily routine. The Surgeon General's Report (1979) in the US and the Health of the Nation (1992) strategy[2] in the UK highlighted the importance of regular exercise as a means of improving the general fitness of the population with the aim of reducing mortality rates from the cardiovascular diseases. Unfortunately, the increase in exercise consciousness has led to an epidemic of injury, much of it attributable to inappropriate or poorly advised activity. The term 'athlete' is used loosely to describe any individual engaged in sport or regular exercise.

SCOPE OF CLINICAL PROBLEMS

The purpose of this chapter is to highlight the mechanisms and risks of injury with particular reference to soft tissue problems. Some musculoskeletal problems are found almost exclusively in sportspeople, but the common conditions covered in previous chapters occur frequently in this group as well, although their presentation, severity and management may differ. Chronic overuse injuries mainly affect soft tissues, but about a tenth of these involve fatigue failure of bone.The nature of the injury is dependent on the type of sport and repetitive loading forces involved, the age and body habitus of the individual, as well as the training environment (e.g. properties of the training surface) and equipment, including footwear. All these factors must be taken into account, both in diagnosis and management, which should therefore aim to restore function and prevent reinjury.

Major trauma causing fracture, ligamentous disruption or hemarthrosis requires immediate orthopedic opinion. Most of the patients presenting with acute traumatic hemarthosis may have a significant intra-articular injury, such as anterior cruciate ligament rupture, osteochondral or chondral fracture, or meniscal tear. Frequently, however, because the significance of the presenting history is ignored, the diagnosis is not made until the patient presents with symptoms of instability or meniscal damage. Late diagnosis may therefore lead to increased risk of degenerative hyaline cartilage damage.

INTERRELATIONSHIP BETWEEN EXERCISE, INJURY AND MUSCULOSKELETAL DISEASE

It is equally important, when assessing patients with apparent injury through sport, to confirm that the 'injury' can be explained by the history of the forces or overuse described. Where it cannot, a primary rheumatologic disorder, possibly modified by the sporting activity, must be considered (Fig. 17.1). In adolescents and young adults, the most common inflammatory condition causing confusion is the enthesopathic or monoarticular presentation of the spondyloarthropathies (see Chapters 6.13 and 6.16). The predominantly lower limb involvement of the entheses by these conditions has many factors in common with the overuse injuries. Several studies[3,4] have shown that enthesitis is the most common initial presentation of seronegative spondyloarthritis, and that children are frequently misdiagnosed and inappropriately investigated. Recognition of the importance of either a personal or a family history of associated problems is often crucial in separating this group from children with traumatic enthesitis. Furthermore, confusion may arise from the effects of injury on attachment sites, producing radiologic erosions indistinguishable from primary inflammatory involvement. An example of this is symphysitis or instability of the symphysis pubis through sport with frank radiologic evidence of erosive change (see Fig. 17.2). This is in keeping with the view that there are a limited number of ways in which a bone or joint can react to a variety of pathologic processes. Furthermore, these radiologic changes may be seen in asymptomatic sportspeople and must be interpreted with full consideration of the presenting history and physical examination.

THE SIMILARITIES BETWEEN SOFT TISSUE INJURY AND THE PERIPHERAL INVOLVEMENT OF SPONDYLOARTHROPATHY

Common soft tissue injuries of the lower limb		Soft tissue involvement in spondyloarthritis
Hip girdle	Groin strains Adductor, hamstring Tendinitis Symphysis instability	Pelvic enthesopathies (especially adductor) Symphysitis
Knee	Sinding–Larsen–Johansson disease Patellar ligament tendinitis Osgood–Schlatter apophysitis	Enthesopathies of tibial tubercle and patellar poles
Hindfoot	Plantar fasciitis Achilles Paratendinitis Tendinitis Deep tears Sever's apophysitis (os calcis) Periosteal reaction due to stress fracture	Plantar fasciitis Achilles Tendinitis Enthesopathy Bursitis Periostitis at or close to enthesis

Fig. 17.1 The similarities between soft tissue injury and peripheral involvement of spondyloarthropathy.

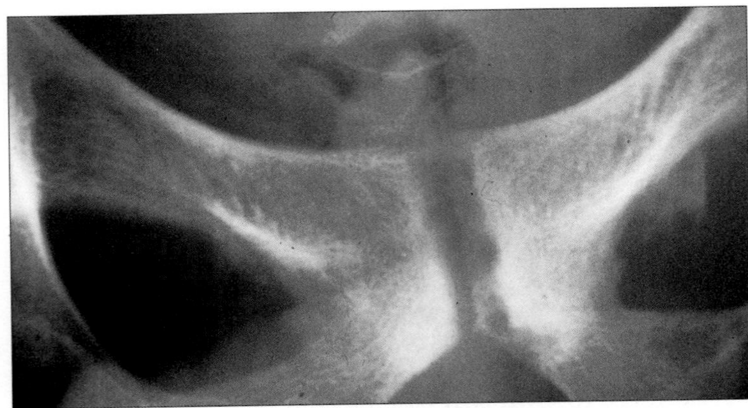

Fig. 17.2 **Radiograph showing erosion of the symphysis pubis in a marathon runner.**

SPORT AND EXERCISE IN SOCIETY

Many factors, including labor-saving devices and motorized transport, have led to an overall decrease in the level of population fitness, in Western societies particularly. A simultaneous rise in the incidence of cardiovascular disease suggests that change to a more sedentary lifestyle may be detrimental to the individual and potentially costly for society, although no clear cause-and-effect relationship has yet been shown. Nevertheless, epidemiologic evidence strongly suggests the beneficial effect of physical exercise in reducing the morbidity and mortality levels due to the cardiovascular diseases, with active individuals also less likely to indulge in other potentially cardiotoxic pursuits, such as smoking. Physical activity can now also be considered a valuable component in the management of systemic hypertension, obesity and some forms of obstructive airway disease and musculoskeletal disease, such as osteoporosis. The International Federation of Sports Medicine has recommended[5] in normal healthy individuals a regular program of three to five fairly vigorous aerobic exercise sessions each week, but with a prior screening examination by a doctor if the subject is over 35 years of age or has known 'risk' factors. Figure 17.3 provides some indication of the epidemiology of the 'fitness craze'[6-8].

EFFECTS OF EXERCISE ON BLOOD PARAMETERS

Parameter	Effect	Reference
Hemoglobin Hematocrit	Chronic endurance training may increase plasma volume diluting hemoglobin	9
MCH/MCHC	Progressive rise during marathon run probably due to loss of red cell water	9
WBC	Immediate leukocytosis during exercise, settling rapidly, delayed prolonged leukocytosis peaking some hours after exercise	10
	Immunomodulation through exercise	11
CPK	Chronic elevation in endurance exercise up to 19-fold increase, with peak 6–24 hours post marathon	12
CRP	Peak elevation 24 hours after intense endurance exercise	13
Cortisol	Increase by high intensity aerobic and heavy resistance exercise and overtraining; less marked in well-conditioned athlete	14–16
Ferritin Antitrypsin	Marked rise after intense load in overtrained	17

CPK – creatine phosphokinase
CRP – C-reactive protein
MCH – mean corpuscular hemoglobin
MCHC – MCH concentration
WBC – white blood cells

Fig. 17.4 **Effects of exercise on blood parameters.**

FREQUENCY OF REGULAR EXERCISE IN THE GENERAL POPULATION

15% of Americans jog regularly
59% of American adults exercise regularly
16% of American adults exercise >5 hours weekly
11% of American adults are joggers
50% of boys aged 8–16 years take part in competitive sport
25% of girls aged 8–16 years take part in competitive sport

Fig. 17.3 **Frequency of regular exercise in the general population.**

THE PHYSIOLOGIC EFFECTS OF EXERCISE

This is a complex subject beyond the scope of this chapter, but it is worth stressing that clinicians need to be aware, when examining patients for whatever reason, that some of the physiologic effects of exercise may cause apparent or real abnormalities of examination or investigation indices (Fig. 17.4). Vigorous exercise leading to increased adrenocorticotropic hormone (ACTH) output and subsequent elevation of cortisol, as well as an endorphin response particularly to anaerobic exercise, may modify the symptomatology of established inflammatory conditions such as ankylosing spondylitis[18]. It is important, therefore, in any patient presenting with musculoskeletal symptoms to assess the level of exercise that the individual maintains. Changes in their activity level may affect symptomatology, including the duration of early morning stiffness.

THE EPIDEMIOLOGY OF INJURY

The frequency of injury is not always easy to assess because of the variability of reporting and attendance[19,20]. However, there is no doubt that the increased fitness awareness of Western society has led to a great increase in injuries (Fig. 17.5).

The issue of sport and osteoarthritis (OA) is a more complex relationship, but there seems to be little evidence of increased OA risk as a result of repetitive loading, unless there is significant biomechanical derangement or underlying traumatic or pre-existing hyaline cartilage change[27].

Osteoporosis can be improved by regular exercise[27]. However, it can also be caused by the amenorrhea that can be induced by high-intensity training in female athletes[28].

THE EPIDEMIOLOGY OF INJURY

Frequency	Example	Reference
9%	Of casualty attendances are due to sport in Finland	21
3%	Of casualty and routine outpatient attendances in Sweden are due to sport	22
21%	Of childhood accidents seen in casualty are sport related	23
16%	Of sample of 50 men referred to a rheumatology clinic with back pain appeared to have a sport-related problem	24
57%	Of world class swimmers troubled by shoulder pain	25
30–50%	Of sports injuries are overuse type	26
	3.7 injuries occur per 1000 skier days	19
	9.4 injuries occur per 1000 player hours of ice hockey	20

Fig. 17.5 **The epidemiology of injury.**

COMMON SITES OF TRACTION APOPHYSITIS			
Eponym	Site	Specific clinical features	Specific management features
Osgood–Schlatter	Tibial tubercle (patellar tendon)	Boys, esp. age 13–14 years Girls, esp. age 10–11 years Chronic condition may develop	Reduce activity initially Quadriceps strengthening and progressive stretching
Larsen–Johansson	Inferior patellar pole (patellar tendon)	Tender inferior patellar pole and radiographic evidence of small inferior patellar avulsion	If acute usually requires immobilizing in cylinder cast
Sever's	Os calcis (Achilles)	Relative increase in tightness of gastrocnemius/soleus, and weakness of dorsiflexors	Supervised flexibilty Dorsiflexion strengthening Orthotics if indicated
(Prominent) Accessory navicular syndrome	Navicular (at tibialis posterior attachment)	Due to apophyseal separation, often associated with pes planus and secondary pain due to irritation of soft tissues by prominent navicular	Orthotic Modify footwear
Thrower's elbow	Medial Epicondyle Elbow	Medial epicondyle is last elbow growth plate to close Often due to poor technique in tennis players, and round arm throw in javelin	Modify technique

Fig. 17.6 Common sites of traction apophysitis.

STRUCTURE AND FUNCTION

In discussing the mechanisms of overuse injury it is necessary to understand the structure and function of soft tissues[29,30].

TENDONS AND LIGAMENTS

Tendons comprise clusters of collagen fibrils interspersed with occasional fibrocytes. Larger tendons are made up of multiple fascicles separated by loose connective tissue, containing nerve fibers and blood vessels. Tendons passing through constricted areas or acting as a pulley across a sharp joint angle are invested with a tendon sheath, whereas the larger heavily loaded tendons, such as Achilles' and patellar, have a paratenon.The enthesis is particularly susceptible to injury in young adolescents, tendons and ligaments effectively being stronger than bone at this age. If overloading occurs to tendons and ligaments attaching to an epiphysis (apophysis), the resulting condition is an apophysitis, such as Osgood–Schlatter's disease (Fig. 17.6). Paradoxically, adult tendons are more susceptible to intrasubstance tears, vascular insufficiency probably being a major factor in the localization of such injuries in the Achilles at the watershed 4–6cm above the insertion. Structure therefore determines, in part, the type of response to injury, particularly as tendons must provide flexibility and resistance to tension. They allow concentration of force from a muscle, which may be large, to a relatively small attachment area. Others, for example in the hand, permit fine concentration of pull to provide precision.

In contrast, ligaments function passively, being superior for constant tension. They usually show a less regular orientation of collagen and contain elastin.

The collagen in tendons unaffected by injury is almost all type I, but in Achilles' tendon rupture there may be an increase in type III, probably as part of repair of previous partial tear, rather than an intrinsic abnormality[31]. Nevertheless, this increase in type III collagen may lead to decreased resistance to tensile forces and therefore reinjury, supporting the view that Achilles' tendon rupture frequently follows previous minor or asymptomatic degeneration[32].

Tendon loading

Tendon or ligament loading causes a brief alignment of fibers, as at rest they are slightly misaligned from parallel. Following this 'toe-in' period, there is linear extension to the limit of elasticity (according to Hooke's Law of Elasticity), at which point individual fiber failure and eventually complete rupture will occur (Fig. 17.7).

Healthy heavily loaded tendons such as the patellar have been estimated as capable of coping with loads of up to four times the usual maximum load of everyday activity. Failure will however occur at lower loading if there is predisposing weakness due to:

- previous injury,
- age changes,
- abnormal collagen, or
- loss of strength due to inactivity.

Immobilization particularly decreases the strength of the bone–ligament complex, with changes both in the ligament substance and attachment (enthesis). Noyes *et al.* demonstrated a 39% decrease in maximum failure load of primate anterior cruciate ligament after 8 weeks' immobilization[33]. Histologically, there is ligament atrophy with increased collagen degradation and osteoclastic periosteal resorption around ligament insertion sites[34]. In the explosive loading of jumping or repetitive loading of endurance sports, there may therefore be microtearing of collagen fibers, followed by a cellular reaction with vascular proliferation, edema and increased tendon volume[35].

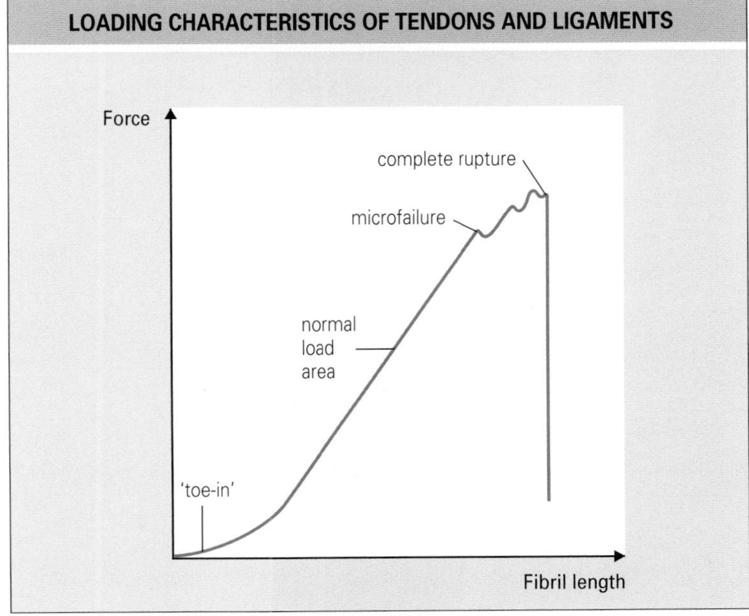

Fig. 17.7 Loading characteristics of tendons and ligaments.

The other major factor in chronic soft tissue injury is the length of recovery time of tendon strength. Paratendinitis or tenosynovitis may further reduce tendon vascularization, due to increased diffusion distance. Healing is therefore often incomplete, leaving a weakened tendon, subject to the risk of further tearing.

MUSCLE

Muscle injury

Muscles provide the power for movement, with a balanced control between agonists and antagonists, but injury is common in both trained and untrained individuals. Muscle contusions frequently result from direct blows to muscle. Partial and complete tears of the muscle tendon junctions occur primarily as a result of eccentric contractions, that is, forceful contraction of the muscle as the muscle tendon unit is being lengthened. The muscle tendon junctions extend for a substantial length of muscle in the hamstrings and rectus femoris muscles, and these muscles are common sites of muscle tendon junction tears.

Partial tears ('pulled muscle') can be deep (central) or superficial (peripheral), with the degree of tearing and bleeding influencing recovery. The latter can lead to major hematoma or, by later fibrosis, a deep intramuscular cyst.

Myositis ossificans

Myositis ossificans, the formation of bone within skeletal muscle, may also develop 6–8 weeks after muscle injury (Fig. 17.8). The exact mechanisms responsible for myositis ossificans are unknown. It is most commonly seen in the thigh, but also occurs with relatively high frequency in the arm muscles.

Symptoms are continuing and excessive pain following injury, with loss of movement and muscular swelling with a deep woody feel. Active stretching and massage must be avoided as they aggravate the changes. Radiographic change may take 6 weeks to develop, with consolidation over the following months. Resorption may occur and surgery, which should only be considered if functional disability continues, must be delayed until active turnover (as judged by technetium scan) has stopped, usually over a year after injury.

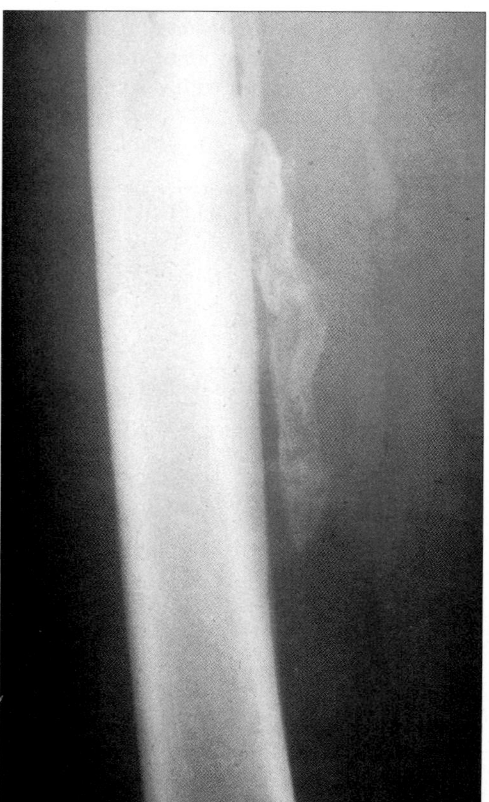

Fig. 17.8 Radiograph of the thigh showing myositis ossificans.

Muscle soreness

More diffuse muscle symptoms after exercise are very common and can be broadly divided into three types:

- Acute: occurring during sustained isometric contractions at near tetanus levels.
- Delayed: occurring 12–48 hours after exercise, particularly after eccentric work. This is probably due to ischemia during sustained contractions, with release of factors irritating pain receptors.
- Injury to muscle fibrils: this can be caused by rapid repetitive movement with load, disturbing the normal control system of agonist and antagonist, with the risk of muscle and joint hyperextension. The rapid reversals of direction of stretch taxes the elastic component of muscle.

Creatine phosphokinase (CPK) levels in plasma rise in individuals undergoing intensive training, and high levels are found for several days after marathon running, especially downhill running, so such indices must be interpreted with great caution in athletes[12].

Muscular hypertrophy can cause compartmental syndrome (see later).

CHRONIC OVERUSE AND BONE

Stress fractures

Stress fractures in bone occur in athletes due to fatigue failure in normal bone, secondary to overloading through intensive exercise or biomechanically abnormal loading[36]. They should be considered as distinct from the fatigue failure in the bones of the elderly, where bone strength is either reduced through aging or markedly reduced because of major osteoporosis. Amenorrhoeic athletes commonly suffer stress fractures.

The typical history is of localized increasing (crescendo) pain on exercise, easing with rest. With increasing severity, the pain occurs earlier on exercise and in some cases will eventually occur in everyday activities. Localized swelling may be seen, particularly in children and the elderly, with tenderness and, at some sites such as the fibula, pain on stressing by springing the bone at a more proximal site. Radiographs are frequently normal, although callus may become evident after about 6 weeks. Technetium scan will show localized increased uptake (Fig. 17.25). Pain induced by testing the site with high-frequency ultrasound can be helpful in supporting the diagnosis, before specific investigation.

The most common site involved is the junction of the lower third of the medial tibia, followed by the tarsal bones, metatarsals, femur and fibula.

Early recognition and treatment is important as the athlete must not be advised to 'run it off', which at a few sites, particularly the mid tibia, risks complete fracture. Early immobilization, or surgery if severe, is advised by some in stress fractures of the mid tibia, femoral neck, and proximal diaphysis of the 5th metatarsal and navicular; but, in general, rest from the loading of sport is sufficient for other sites. It is important to maintain general fitness, and water training may be very helpful. Rest for 6 weeks' is usually sufficient in mild cases, but up to 12 weeks or longer may occasionally be necessary, and very graduated reloading is crucial thereafter.

Stress fracture of the pars interarticularis of one of the lower lumbar vertebrae can occur due to repetitive hyperextension stress, in sports such as gymnastics and high-jumping. Single photon emission computed tomography (SPECT) now appears to be the investigation of choice. If there is a spondylolysis on standard lateral or oblique spinal radiographs, but no increased uptake on SPECT, the pars defect can be defined as longstanding, with no bony healing potential. If radiographs are normal but SPECT positive, CT scan should be performed to grade the pars lesion.

Stress fracture of the tarsal navicular is not infrequently a chronic problem and is particularly seen in the running and jumping sports. Positive uptake on technetium bone scan (Fig. 17.25) should be followed up, in cases that do not settle rapidly, by CT scan to assess the extent of fracture. In some series, recovery has been shown to take up to 6 months for undisplaced fractures. For the more serious displaced lesion for which surgery is necessary, recovery times have been reported to be as long as 18–24 months.

PROFILE OF COMMON STRESS FRACTURES IN INDIVIDUAL SPORTS	
Sport	Site of stress fracture
Basketball	Patella, calcaneum, hallux sesamoid femur and pubis
Cricket (fast bowlers)	Pars interarticularis, patella and tibia
Diving	Tibia
Fencing	Pelvis
Golf	Ribs (posterolateral, esp. 4th–6th)
Gymnastics	Upper limb and pars interarticularis
High jumping	Hallux sesamoid, patella and pars interarticularis (Fosbury flop)
Ice skating	Fibula
Javelin throwing	Olecranon or shaft of ulna
Long/triple jumping	Navicular, hallux sesamoid and pelvis
Rowing	Ribs
Running	Tibia, tarsal (especially navicular), metatarsal, femur, fibula and pelvis
Tennis	Humerus and ulna
Volleyball	Pisiform

Fig. 17.9 Profile of common stress fractures in individual sports.

It is vital that abnormal biomechanical factors are recognized and modified. Rigid pes cavus appears to increase the risk of metatarsal and femoral neck fracture. Excessive foot pronation increases tibial torsion and is found more commonly in stress fractures of the tibia and fibula. Female athletes should be screened for amenorrhoeic osteopenia.

Several important etiological factors can be considered as part of the underlying cause of stress fractures. Muscle weakness reduces the shock absorption of the lower extremity and causes redistribution of forces to bone, increasing the stress at focal points. This probably is a factor in femoral neck stress fracture[28].

Stress fractures seen in nonweight-bearing bones of the upper extremity (e.g. the humerus in baseball pitchers) lend support to the view that muscle pull across a bone can produce sufficient repetitive force to produce fatigue failure. This is also likely to be the major component in lower medial tibial stress fractures, particularly where there is altered biomechanical loading through gait abnormalities, such as hyperpronation in the stance phase.

Compression stress fractures through direct loading force occur particularly in the calcaneum. Stress fractures can therefore be considered as focal structural weaknesses in bone that occur during remodeling (early osteoclastic resorption followed by osteoblastic activity) in response to the repeated application of subthreshold stresses. Increased uptake on technetium scanning at asymptomatic sites in athletes suggests that painless remodeling of bone is common in relation to stress – this can be considered as bone strain, representing a continuum of response to physical stress, similar to that seen with muscles, ligaments and tendons.

Individual sports are associated with quite specific stress fracture profiles summarized in Figure 17.9.

Amenorrhea and reduced bone density

In female athletes, the beneficial effects of physical training may be offset by intensive exercise-induced amenorrhea. Although this change in reproductive physiology may appear to the athlete a 'pleasant convenience', secondary amenorrhea is known to be associated with reduced bone mass. Drinkwater showed decreased trabecular (spinal) density but normal cortical (radius) density, whereas Lindberg reported reduced cortical and trabecular density and a marked increase in stress fracture rate in amenorrheic athletes compared with a eumenorrheic group[37].

Intensive physical training before puberty can delay menarche and if commenced soon after menarche is associated with oligo- or amenorrhea and reduced levels of circulating estrogen. Since this can be seen in swimmers and gymnasts, as well as runners, the type of physical activity appears unimportant, but the intensity is crucial. Marcus showed very low levels of body fat in amenorrheic athletes and Firsch suggested that a critical level of body fat is essential for normal estrogen status, although this is likely to be too simplistic a view[37].

In practical terms, physicians seeing amenorrheic female athletes should exclude an organic cause for the amenorrhea; the athlete should be counseled about the risk in terms of reduced bone strength and modified training schedules should be discussed.

INJURY IN RELATION TO BODY HABITUS

Generalized joint laxity or hypermobility (Fig. 17.10) is usually inherited as a benign multisystem disorder of connective tissue (see Chapter 8.51). More serious causes such as Ehlers–Danlos syndrome are rare, but even the benign condition is associated with an increased risk of soft tissue injuries. Selection for some activities, such as gymnastics and dance, may favor the hypermobile but thus result in a higher incidence of injury. However, it is worth noting that measures of hypermobility, such as the Beighton index[38], may miss important localized laxity, which may be a major factor in some joint injuries, such as those of the shoulder.

Fig. 17.10 Generalized hypermobility associated with anterior cruciate rupture of the right knee.

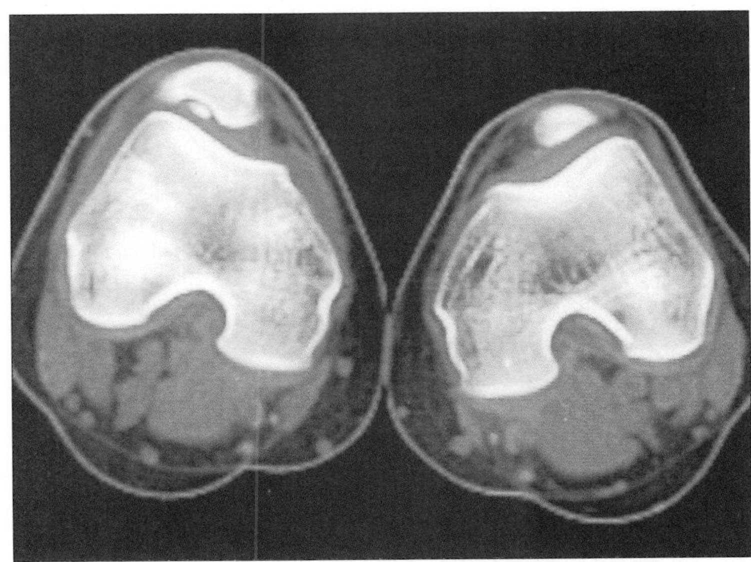

Fig. 17.11 Osteochondritis dissecans of the right patella, due to traumatic dislocation, demonstrated by CT scan.

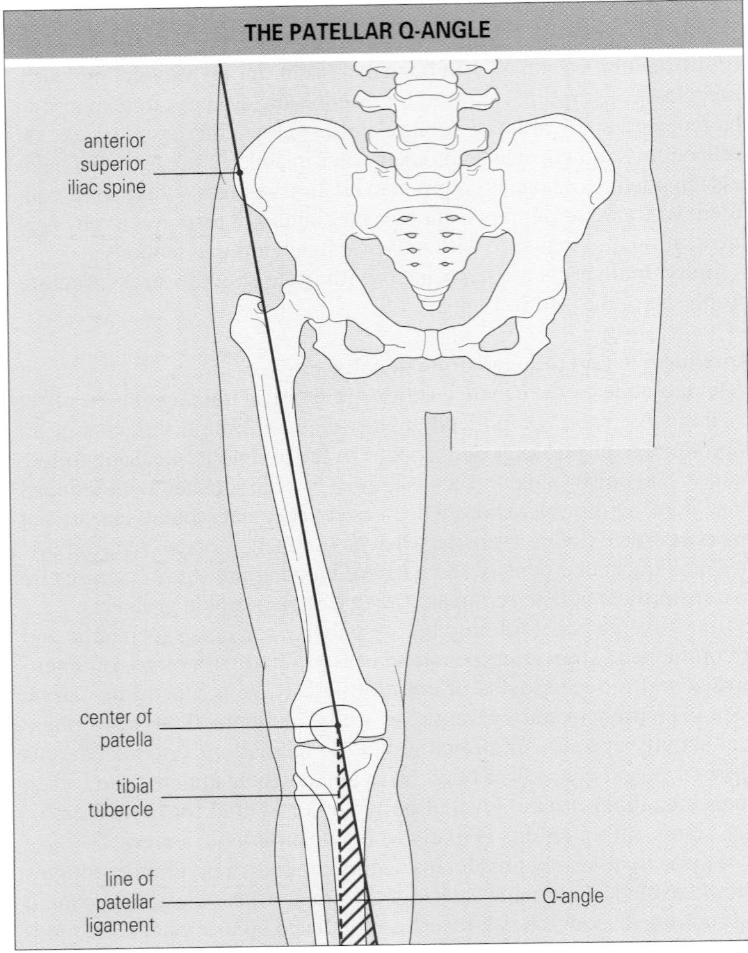

Fig. 17.12 The patellar Q-angle. The Q-angle is the angle between the line from the anterior superior iliac spine through the center of the patella and the line of the patellar ligament (i.e. patellar center to tibial tubercle).

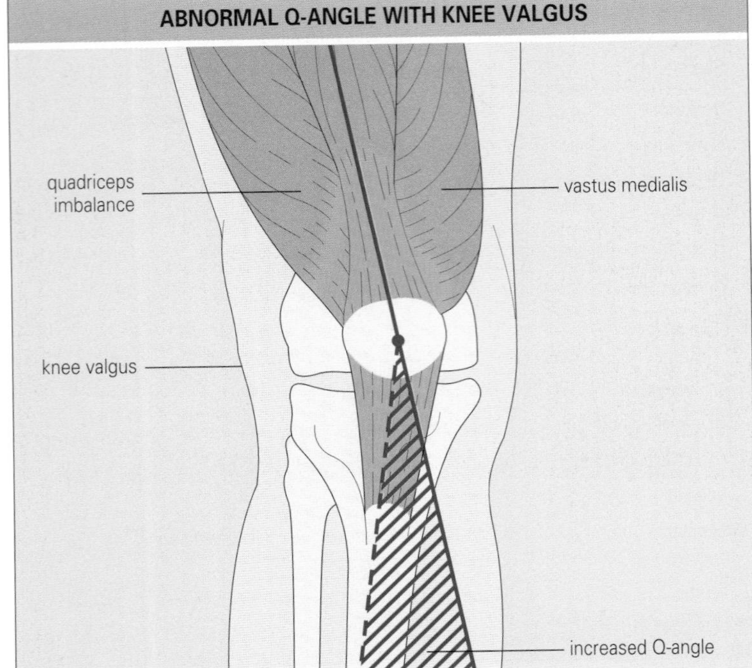

Fig. 17.13 Abnormal Q-angle seen in knee valgus.

INJURY FACTORS IN CHILDREN

Children are included in the epidemic of overuse injuries, but several factors in the growing child modify the type of injury seen:

- Ligaments and tendons are comparatively stronger in relation to bone than in adult structures; injuries therefore most commonly occur at the attachment site (enthesis).
- Growth spurts may lead to rapid lengthening of bone with measurable increase in muscle–tendon tightness, causing loss of flexibility which adds to the risk of overuse injury.
- Growth cartilage is located not only at the epiphyses and joint surfaces but also at the apophyseal attachments of major muscle–tendon complexes. Apophysitis (e.g. Osgood–Schlatter) is an unfortunate term implying primary inflammation, whereas lesions of the apophyseal attachment in growing children are usually primarily traumatic in origin. They need, however, to be differentiated from the enthesitis of inflammatory arthritis (see Fig. 17.1).
- Asymmetric traction loads or partial separation through sudden trauma to a growth plate (epiphysis), if not recognized, will lead to uneven growth, with risk of long bone asymmetry. This will alter the loading through joints, and the altered biomechanics carries the risk of premature OA in adult life.
- Excessive use of weight training can lead to marked asymmetry of muscle growth and joint laxity (e.g. 'tennis shoulder'). As a general rule, growing children should only use their own body weight for muscle strengthening.
- Osteochondritis dissecans (Fig. 17.11) is usually considered to be predominantly a condition of the immature skeleton, possibly related to trauma or ischemia or a combination of these factors.

ANATOMIC VARIANTS

Minor anatomic variants, which in the nonathlete may have no significance, may lead to specific injury problems when major stress or recurrent overuse affects these sites. Common examples are the os trigonum leading to posterior impingement at the ankle, minor leg length inequality and the anatomy of the patellar mechanism, although abnormalities in the latter are commonly associated with symptoms in nonathletic teenage girls as well.

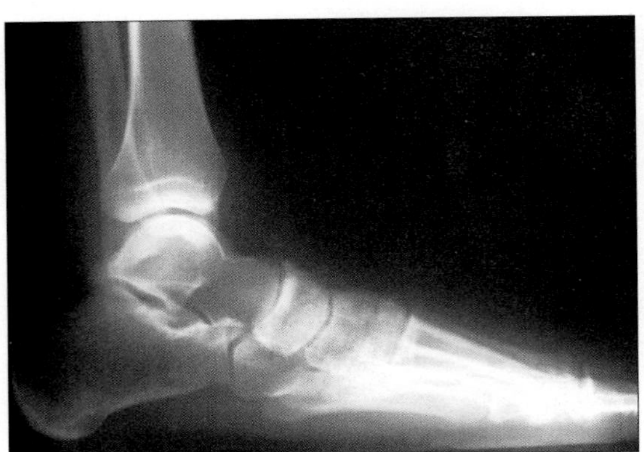

Fig. 17.14 Radiograph of large os trigonum associated with posterior heel pain in a runner.

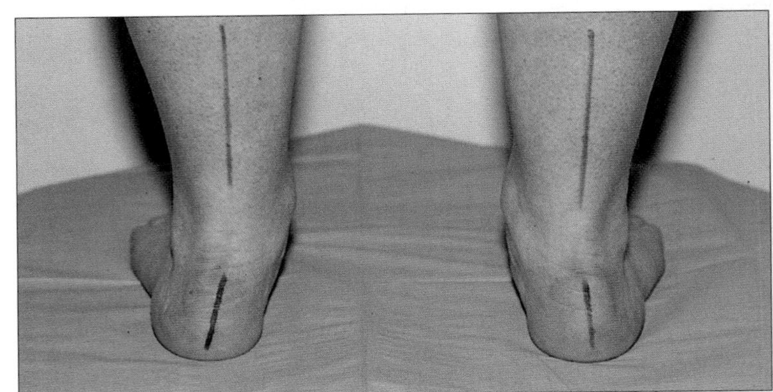

Fig. 17.15 Hyperpronation of the feet with hind foot valgus.

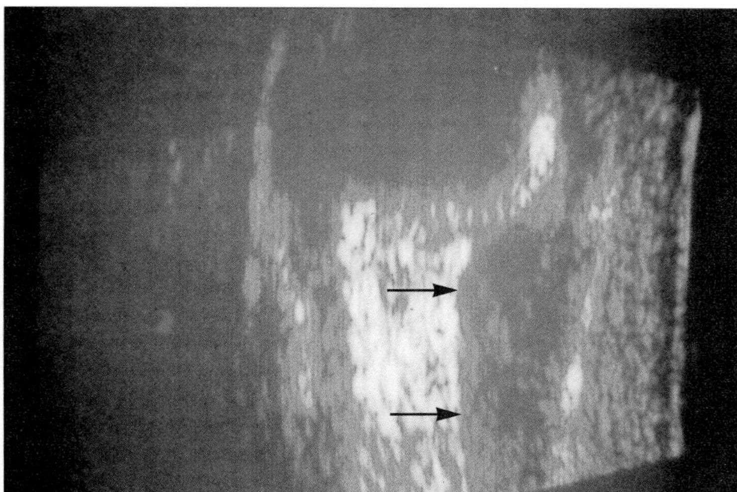

Fig. 17.16 Ultrasound of an abnormal patellar tendon with enlargement and reduced echogenicity of the tendon (arrows).

Relationship of the patella to the femur and tibia (Q-angle)

The position of the patella is assessed by measurement of the Q-angle, between a line drawn from the anterior superior iliac spine to the center of the patella and the line of the patellar tendon to the tibial tubercle (see Fig. 17.12 and Chapter 4.11). The ratio of the patellar tendon length to patellar length should be less than 1.2:1. The patella tends to be displaced laterally during forced extension of the knee, but this is counteracted by the buttress of the prominent lateral surface of the lower femur and by the retaining action of the lower fibers of vastus medialis obliquus, which insert into the medial patellar border.

An increased Q-angle (Fig. 17.13) and/or hyperextension (genu recurvatum) increases the risk of patellar subluxation and anterior knee pain, with or without true chondromalacia patellae found at arthroscopy. Patella alta with recurvatum increases the risk of anterior horn meniscal injury, medial collateral ligament injury and anterior or posterior ligament rupture. Such individuals should be counseled about the need to change to lower risk noncontact sports.

Management of anterior knee pain must include a period of reduced activity, vastus medialis strengthening and correction of foot hyperpronation if present, as this also effectively increases the Q-angle.

Os trigonum

The presence of an os trigonum (an unfused epiphysis of the posterior tubercle of the talus; Fig. 17.14) may lead to posterior heel pain, particularly in sports involving maximal plantar flexion, such as long jumping and dancing *en pointe*. The os trigonum impinges between the tibia and the calcaneum, as the foot plantar flexes. There may also be a pre-Achilles, bursitis.

Abnormalities of gait

Walking and running are coordinated processes of extraordinary complexity, in which individual movements occur at many body sites simultaneously in three planes. The six major components of gait are pelvic rotation and tilt, lateral pelvic displacement, knee extension and flexion and ankle joint movement. If there is a fault in this coordinated system, altered function will also occur at other sites. If this is amplified by repetitive loading through sport, soft tissue injury and, in some cases, cartilage damage may result.

Anatomic asymmetry, joint laxity and gait must therefore be carefully assessed in patients with chronic lower limb symptoms and with backache in particular. Gait abnormalities may require a treadmill assessment, as abnormal patterns may not be apparent until the athlete runs or becomes fatigued.

Hyperpronation of the feet (Fig. 17.15) in the stance phase of running increases the risk of such disorders as shin splints, medial tibial stress fractures and Achilles' tendon injury when repetitive loading occurs.

CLINICAL CONDITIONS

TENDON INJURY

The type of injury depends upon the levels of loading and the site of injury; where there is a tendon sheath, frictional tenosynovitis can occur, particularly at the wrist and ankle.

Overuse tenosynovitis

The sites commonly involved through sport are the flexor and extensor tendons in the hands, wrists and ankles and also in the shoulder. The following features are particularly important: tendinitis, deformity and triggering.

Tendinitis must still be excluded and may be difficult to distinguish in the presence of tenosynovitis. It usually causes more pain and restriction of movement across a joint, such as the ankle. A history of a sudden snap must be taken very seriously if complete rupture is to be avoided.

Tendinosis is a term used to describe the degenerative, often cystic change seen due to repetitive microtearing within tendons and is best assessed by magnetic resonance imaging (MRI).

Deformity, indicating rupture, must be noted. At the ankle, tibialis posterior rupture will cause flattening of the medial arch. In the fingers, extensor tendon rupture is particularly seen in catching sports such as cricket, and may occur at two common sites:

- dorsum of the base of the middle phalanx, causing boutonnière deformity;

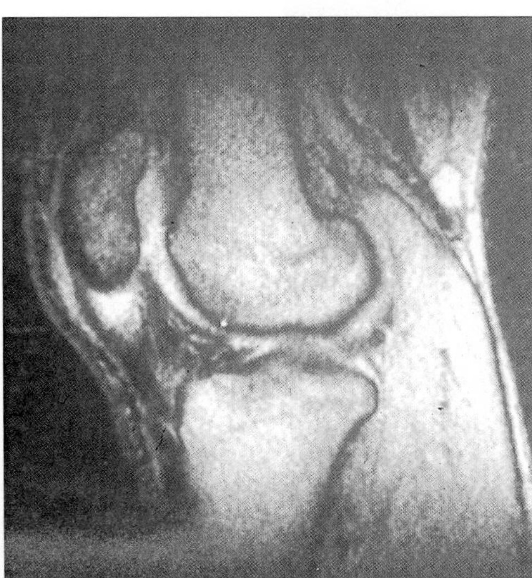

Fig. 17.17 Sagittal MRI in patellar pole tendinitis.

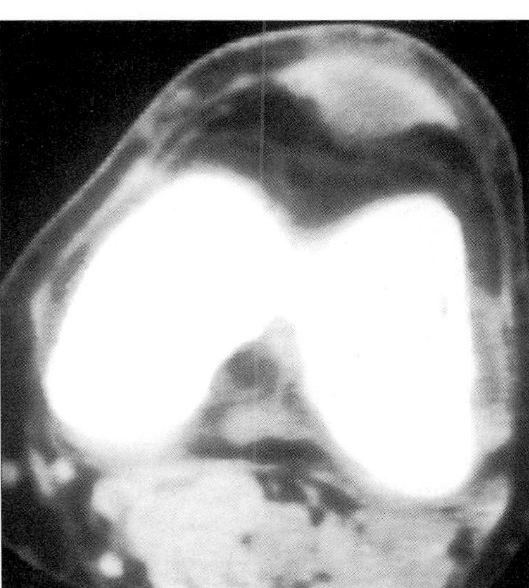

Fig. 17.18 CT scan showing large cystic lesion in mid patellar ligament.

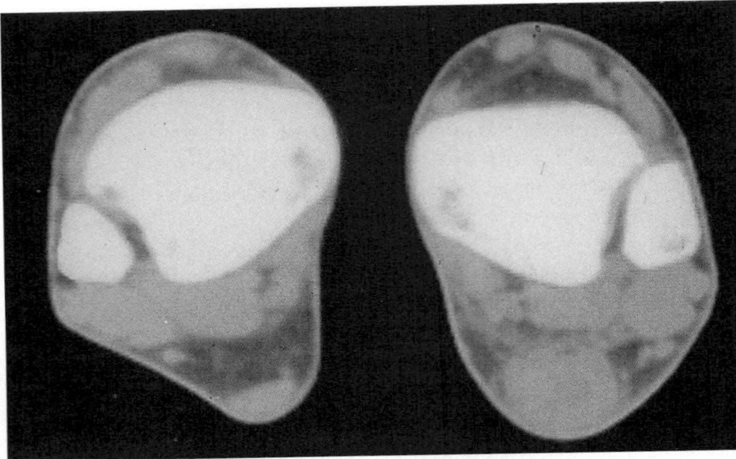

Fig. 17.19 Cross-sectional CT view of both lower legs showing a thickened left Achilles' tendon with central necrosis.

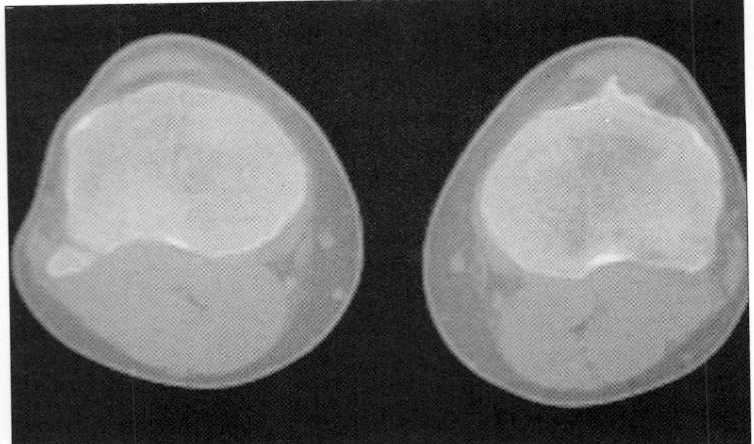

Fig. 17.20 CT scan showing tibial tubercle prominence due to previous Osgood–Schlatter disease causing patellar tendinitis.

- dorsum of the base of the terminal phalanx, causing mallet deformity.

Triggering in the hand flexors of sportspeople may require surgery, as it implies either repeated synovitis, causing flexor tendon thickening, usually at the metacarpophalangeal (MCP) joint, or a nodule caused by superficial rupture of the spiral tendon fibers.

Management

In early uncomplicated tenosynovitis, rest in a support is frequently sufficient. If not, a corticosteroid injection, avoiding direct intratendinous injection, is usually successful provided recurrence is not induced by too rapid a return to sport. However, in certain conditions, for example extensor tendon tenosynovitis due to repetitive rapid wrist movement in rowers and flexor tendon triggering, constriction of the tendon may be so marked that urgent decompression is essential, to avoid further tendon-substance damage.

Ankle tenosynovitis will frequently reflect an abnormal running gait, for example tibialis posterior involvement and flattening of the medial longitudinal arch. Suitable orthotic advice is an important part of management.

Tibialis anterior tenosynovitis, on the other hand, is rare even in sportspeople. However, if present, it usually exemplifies the role of specific repetitive action in etiology, being seen particularly after long periods of downhill activity in hikers, long-distance runners and skiers.

Paratendinitis and tendinosis

At heavily loaded tendons without a tendon sheath, such as the patellar and Achilles' tendons, there may be an associated inflammation in the paratenon (paratendinitis). 'Jumper's knee' is due to microtearing at the inferior patellar pole attachment and corresponds with Sinding–Larsen–Johansson syndrome in children (see Fig. 17.6). Lesions can extend down the patellar tendon or can sometimes be localized to the mid tendon region. They are best assessed by ultrasound scan (Fig. 17.16) or MRI (Fig. 17.17), although computerized tomography (CT) scanning (Fig 17.18) may still be utilized if MRI is not available.

Achilles tendinopathy

There are many types of Achilles' injury, and only the most common are described here.

Superficial injury: paratendinitis

The most treatable cause is due to chronic frictional irritation by the heel tab of the shoe, which can be avoided by better shoes or cutting the heel tab. Paratendinitis or paratenon effusion can occur due to simple overuse.

Deep tendinosis

This is clinically likely with a history of recurrent achillodynia and, on examination, swelling with local tenderness at rest, which decreases when the tendon is put under stretch by dorsiflexion (London Hospital sign).

In this condition microtearing occurs due to accumulated impact loading, aggravated by the whipping action of the Achilles' tendon as the foot pronates, or due to eccentric loading when the fatigued runner alters his or her gait.

Management includes a reduction of training level, especially on hills, use of a heel lift to decrease strain and supervised stretching. Nonsteroidal anti-inflammatory drugs (NSAIDs) may facilitate rehabilitation, but in deep lesions corticosteroids should be avoided. Deep lesions frequently require surgery and can be assessed by CT scanning (Fig. 17.19) or other imaging.

If there is an abnormal running pattern an orthotic may be indicated, particularly for excessive pronation, and tibialis posterior should be strengthened.

Bursitis

A pre-Achilles' bursitis produces tenderness which is anterior to the tendon. Other patterns of heel bursitis are discussed in Chapter 4.12.

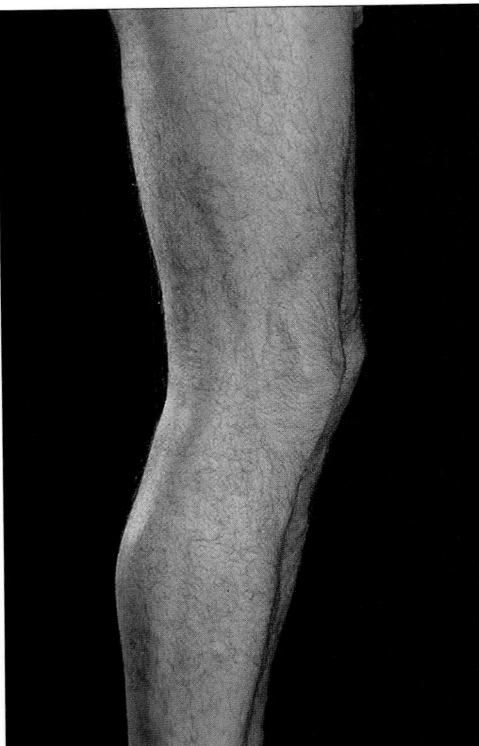

Fig. 17.21 Lateral view of the right leg showing the iliotibial band.

Complete rupture
This is uncommon in young athletes, with a mean age at which rupture occurs of about 35 years, and it appears more frequently in sports involving explosive forwards movement. Kaalund *et al.*[39] showed that of 96 ruptures seen in Denmark over a 2.5 year period, 40% were due to badminton and only 18%[17] due to the UK's most popular sport, soccer. Supporting the view that poor muscle coordination in tired players is an important risk factor, 87% occurred in the middle or last period of the game. Following surgery, 46% resumed sport within 6 months and 82% by 1 year, but seven individuals did not return to sport.

Tendon injury in children
Traction apophysitis

Children are particularly prone to attachment injury (traction apophysitis) of which Osgood–Schlatter apophysitis of the tibial tubercle is the best known. The other common conditions and clinical features are set out in Figure 17.6. Attachment injuries may be seen at any heavily loaded apophysis, for example ischial hamstring attachments in sprinters and dancers.

Osgood–Schlatter apophysitis

This was previously typically seen in athletically active boys of 13–14 years of age. Now, with the increase in sporting activity, it is being seen also in young girls aged 10–11 years (equivalent in skeletal maturity to boys of 13–14 years).

Pain is felt at the tibial tubercle, aggravated by heavy activity. The main signs are local tibial tubercle tenderness and swelling, with quadriceps tightness part of the underlying cause.

Chronic symptoms of pain on activity continuing into adult life are usually due to separated ossific bodies irritating the patellar tendon. Surgery is then often necessary and may need to include modification of any tubercle prominence, which may be much more obvious using CT scanning (Fig. 17.20).

ILIOTIBIAL BAND SYNDROME
The iliotibial tract (ITT) or band (Fig. 17.21) is thickened fascia connecting the ilium with the lateral tibia, and it receives part of the insertion of tensor fasciae latae and gluteus maximus. When the hip is flexed the tensor fasciae latae pull the iliotibial tract forwards, but when extended the gluteus maximus pulls it backwards. Therefore, repetitive flexion and extension can lead to irritation of either the iliotibial tract or its associated bursa over the lateral femoral condyle, usually due to high-intensity training, particularly if camber running (running on a sloping surface).

Pain usually takes some miles of running before building up and is localized to 2cm above the joint line. A stiff-legged gait may be adopted as this relieves pain.

The signs include:

- Local tenderness at the lateral femoral condyle.
- Pain on standing on the flexed (30–40%) knee.
- Tight iliotibial tract detected by Ober's test: with the patient lying on the unaffected side with hip flexed, the affected knee is flexed and the hip abducted and extended to line up with the trunk. In now attempting to adduct the hip, it will be found that this is limited because the short iliotibial tract will be caught on the greater trochanter.

Excess forefoot pronation may play a part in etiology and should be controlled with an orthotic. Reduction of mileage and avoidance of camber running may resolve the condition, but local corticosteroid injection may be required.

BURSITIS
Bursae are commonly affected by injury, but deeper lesions are frequently overlooked. Bursae have an indistinct synovial cell lining, with underlying fibrovascular tissue and are situated between fascial planes or subcutaneously. They improve the gliding motion of two adjoining structures by reducing friction. Direct trauma causes a hemobursa and chronic irritation an inflammatory bursitis, often leading to chronic bursal thickening with calcium deposition. A septic bursitis should be suspected and excluded by aspiration culture if the bursa is acutely inflamed, particularly if there is an overlying skin abrasion (e.g. prepatellar). Gouty bursitis may also be exacerbated by trauma, so fluid must be sent for crystal examination by polarizing light microscopy.

In sportspeople, subacromial bursitis is usually due to repetitive overhead throwing, hitting or lifting, especially in tennis, swimming and weightlifting. Osteophytosis of the inferior aspect of the acromioclavicular joint may contribute to the impingement. Olecranon bursitis usually follows a fall onto a firm surface, but may be due to repetitive bending, as in gymnastics.

Iliopsoas bursitis, with pain on hip extension, is an important condition in the differential diagnosis of groin pain.

The pes anserinus bursa, lying between the medial collateral ligament and the overlying pes anserinus (comprising the tendons of sartorius, gracilis and semitendinosus) is typically affected in swimmers ('breaststroker's knee') and runners.

Retrocalcaneal or pre-Achilles' bursitis may be associated with a prominent os trigonum (see Fig. 17.14) and is particularly seen in hill running.

Superficial Achilles' bursitis ('pump bump') is frequently secondary to frictional irritation by inadequate footwear. Haglund's disease refers to pain in the posterior heel, characterized by a painful 'pump-bump' and a typical radiographic configuration of the posterior border of the os calcis with convexity of the posterior soft tissues due to the bursitis.

COMPARTMENTAL SYNDROMES
These can be defined as an increase in tissue pressure, within a confined space or muscle compartment, that compromises local circulation and function.

Acute compartment syndrome
Acute compartment syndrome may result from a direct blow to the muscle from the trauma associated with a fracture or from prolonged pressure over a muscle compartment. It also occurs more rarely following prolonged exertion. Acute compartment syndromes can lead to a rapid and complete muscle necrosis. Early surgical decompression of the compartment may allow restoration of circulation to the muscle and preserve function. The clinical diagnosis of acute compartment syndrome is based on patients who have pain which is out of proportion to the injury or history of injury, swelling or firmness of muscle compartment and pain with passive stretch. Later in the evolution of acute compartment syndrome, patients develop signs of decreased perfusion including decreased pulses, decreased capillary refill and skin

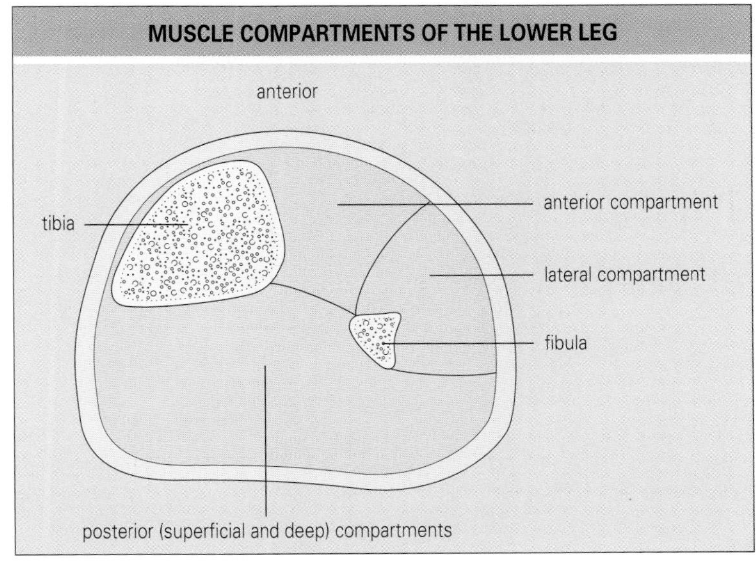

Fig. 17.22 The muscle compartments of the lower leg.

pallor. Neurologic symptoms may also appear. With appropriate history and physical findings the diagnosis may be readily apparent. In cases where there is uncertainty measurement of compartment pressures will make it possible to determine if an acute compartment syndrome exists.

Chronic compartment syndrome

This is the typical form seen in athletes and is characterized by a return to normal function between episodes of exercise-induced pain. It is most commonly seen in the lower leg. The muscles of the leg are contained within four compartments separated by deep transverse fascia (Fig. 17.22). The athlete describes aching or cramping of the leg, roughly in the distribution of the involved compartment. The period from commencement of exercise to the onset of symptoms is variable and depends upon the type and intensity of exercise but is usually within 10–30 minutes. Return to normal is also variable, taking minutes in most cases, but in more severe cases occasionally taking hours for complete resolution. Neurologic symptoms may occur due to ischemia of nerves, particularly in the anterior tibial syndrome.

There are no diagnostic signs at rest, although fascial defects may be found in up to 40%. After sufficient exercise, tenderness and fullness will be found in the muscle compartment involved, most commonly the anterolateral.

Slit catheter measurement of intracompartmental pressure before and after exercise can be used to select patients suitable for surgical decompression, provided it is performed in a specialist center with reliable standardization. It is likely that nuclear magnetic resonance will prove of increasing importance in diagnosis, with the development of more sophisticated imaging techniques looking at biochemical shifts or pH changes.

Compartmental syndrome of the forearm is much less common, but may be seen in weightlifters and rowers particularly. The deep fascia of the forearm encloses both the flexor and extensor muscles, which are separated by the radius, ulna and interosseus membrane. The deep flexor compartment of the forearm is most susceptible.

SHIN SPLINTS

The term 'shin splints' has been used to cover a variety of conditions causing lower medial tibial pain, but the American Medical Association's definition limits the use of the term to musculotendinous inflammation, causing pain or discomfort in the leg from repetitive running on hard surfaces or forcible excessive use of the foot dorsiflexors. It is therefore also referred to as 'medial tibial stress syndrome' and excludes stress fractures or ischemic disorders.

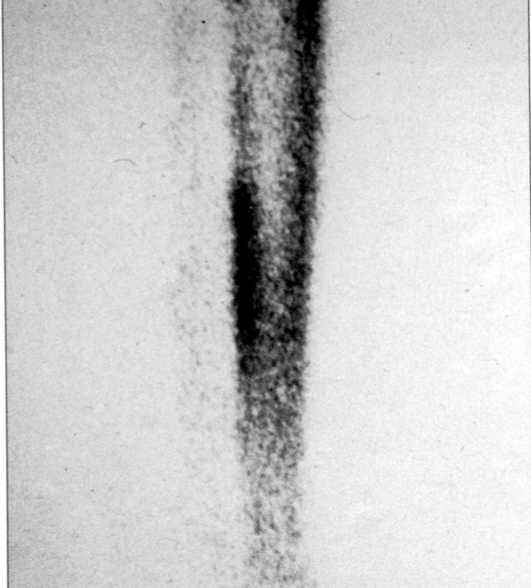

Fig. 17.23 Technetium scan showing diffuse medial tibial periosteal uptake.

The history is initially of medial tibial pain at the beginning of a workout, but later pain may become persistent and in severe cases may even develop in some everyday activities. On examination, there is a 3–6cm area of tenderness on the posteromedial border of the distal third of the tibia which is much less localized than a stress fracture. The pain can only infrequently be aggravated by active plantar flexion and inversion of the foot against resistance. Radiographs are normal, but technetium bone scan may show increased longitudinal uptake involving the posteromedial tibia cortex (Fig. 17.23), unlike the more pisiform shape of the increased uptake of a stress fracture (Fig. 17.24).

GROIN INJURY

Groin problems are particularly common in soccer and jumping sports. The term 'groin strain' is best avoided and specific localizing signs sought. The sites of pain and local tenderness, as well as pain on resisted stress or stretching, are important in defining injury to rectus femoris, iliopsoas and adductors. Limitation of hip movement, due to hip disease, and referred pain, due to spinal disorders, must be defined.

Adductor tendon injury

This is characterized by pain when sprinting, pivoting or kicking. Symptoms may spread through compensation mechanisms to the opposite side. On examination there is tenderness in gracilis and adductor brevis, close to the insertion, with pain on resisted adduction and on abduction stretch. The risk of injury to the adductors appears to be increased by spinal problems, hip disorders and abdominal muscle insufficiency. Leg length inequality or foot deformity may also be important factors in injury to the adductors and symphysis.

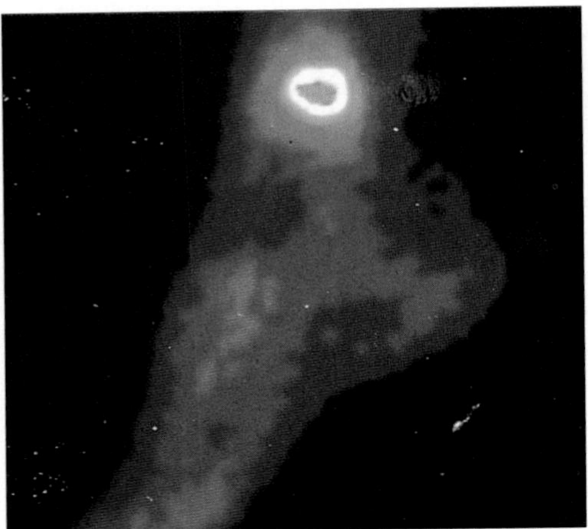

Fig. 17.24 Technetium scan showing focal uptake of a stress fracture of the lower tibia.

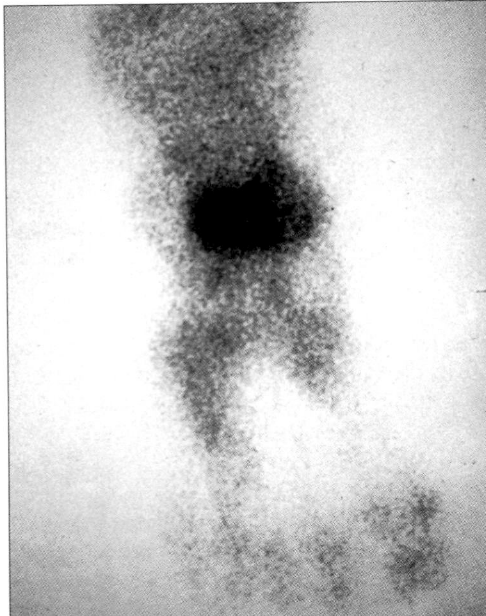

Fig. 17.25 Technetium scan showing localized uptake in navicular stress fracture.

Symphysitis

Symphysitis, or symphysis instability, must be excluded, particularly if there are bilateral groin and lower abdominal symptoms. However, plain radiographs frequently show symphysis irregularity in footballers without clinical signs of instability (see Fig. 17.2). True instability can be demonstrated by flamingo views, with movement of the pubic rami in relation to each other when the patient stands on one leg, then on the other. Technetium isotope scan, with squat views following bladder emptying, may confirm symphysitis if there is focally increased uptake at the symphysis.

A long period of withdrawal from sport is essential. In one series, time to recovery was 9.5 months in men and 7 months in women, with a 25% relapse rate in men.

Conjoint tendon injury of the inguinal ring

This should be considered, even in the absence of a defined hernia, when there is localized tenderness with cough-induced pain, at the external ring and internal ring, which usually feels dilated, and an absence of localizing features of adductor tendon injury or symphysitis. The term 'groin strain' is inadequate because, at surgical exploration, conjoint tendon injury is frequently found and appropriate repair may allow return to full sporting activity relatively quickly. Herniogram is no longer generally recommended, but direct scopic visualization and repair appears to offer the best chance of return to full sporting activity quickly. However, follow up studies of this technique are needed to fully assess its value and the risk of recurrence.

Neuropathies

Compression neuropathies may occur due to direct trauma or chronic repetitive loading, resulting in either a traction or compressive entrapment, including muscular hypertrophy affecting the nerve. The common sites of compression are described in Chapter 4.16. Less common compression sites and the sports involved are summarized in Figures 17.26 and 17.27.

The ulnar nerve illustrates best some of these injury risks. At the elbow, it is particularly vulnerable in racquet and throwing sports. These produce a valgus stress on the elbow in flexion such that a valgus laxity of the ulnar collateral ligament may develop, which alters the biomechanics of the elbow joint. In adolescents, before fusion of

SPORT-INDUCED UPPER LIMB COMPRESSION NEUROPATHIES

Site	Nerve	Symptoms	Signs	Sport
Shoulder				
Erb's point Scapular notch	Suprascapular	Traction injury Direct or repetitive injury	Infraspinatus Supraspinatus weakness Pain (sensory supply to posterior joint capsule)	Rugby
Spinoglenoid notch		Often pain free (if compression distal to sensory branch to shoulder)	Infraspinatus only	Volleyball
Quadrilateral space	Axillary	Acute with shoulder dislocation Chronic	Deltoid weakness with sensory loss over deltoid	Throwing sports
	Long thoracic nerve of Bell	Acute more common than chronic	Serratus anterior weakness	
	Musculocutaneous	Weak elbow flexion	Biceps and/or brachialis weakness Sensation loss: lateral cutaneous nerve of forearm	
	Spinal accessory	Weak shoulder elevation	Trapezius and sternocleidomastoid weakness	
Elbow				
Pronator syndrome	Median	Forearm pain on activity Sensory symptoms but rarely at night Negative Tinel's sign	Weakness of flexor digitorum profundus and pronation Entrapment by muscular hypertrophy	Weightlifting
Radial tunnel syndrome	Radial	Pain, paresthesias and weakness	Weakness of wrist extension	
Posterior interosseus syndrome	Posterior interosseus	Motor symptoms only	Extensor carpi ulnaris weak: wrist dorsiflexes radially Weak extension at MCPs Normal extension at PIPs (intrinsics)	
Medial elbow	Ulnar	Pain Paresthesias of 4th and 5th digits	Local tenderness Positive Tinel's sign Elbow flexion test (3 min of full flexion of elbow with wrist fully extended)	Throwing Racquet sports Weightlifting Gymnastics
Wrist/hand				
Carpal tunnel	Median	Carpal tunnel syndrome Paresthesia at night or on use	Weakness of abductor pollicis brevis Sensory loss, especially in index and middle fingers	
Canal of Guyon Type I (proximal or 1st part of canal)	Ulnar	Weakness and paresthesias	Paresthesias; spares dorsal cutaneous branch to ulnar aspect of hand	Cycling Racket sports
Type II (distal canal and hook of hamate)	Ulnar	Pure motor symptoms	Reduced grip Froment's paper sign	Ball handling sports
Type III (distal canal, beyond hamate)	Ulnar	Pure sensory symptoms	Palmar loss of sensation in 4th and 5th digits	
Thumb Ulnar digital nerve to thumb, beyond hamate	Ulnar	Pure sensory symptoms Pain and paresthesias	Local tenderness Positive Tinel's sign	Bowling

Fig. 17.26 Upper limb compression neuropathies due to sport.

SPORT-INDUCED LOWER LIMB COMPRESSION NEUROPATHIES				
Site	Nerve	Symptoms	Signs	Sport
Hindfoot Between deep fascia of abductor hallucis brevis and medial margin of quadratus plantae	1st branch of lateral plantar	Chronic heel pain increased by walking, greatly increased by running	Tenderness deep to abductor hallucis brevis Foot may be hypermobile	Running Jogging
Tarsal tunnel (flexor retinaculum, medial calcaneum, talus and medial malleolus)	Posterior tibial	Burning paresthesias in sole of foot, spreading to toes Increased by standing/running and at night	Ankle injury prior to onset often recorded. Positive Tinel's sign; eversion may increase (exclude spinal)	Running
Medial arch and navicular tuberosity	Medial plantar	Medial arch pain	Foot eversion increased (excessive heel valgus on running – may be precipitated by use of arch support)	Jogging
At exit from deep fascia (local compartment)	Superficial peroneal	Pain in distal calf and lateral foot, increased by running	Tenderness at deep fascial exit Palpable fascial defect in 60% of cases History of chronic ankle sprains common	Running Hockey Tennis
Forefoot Microtrauma against distal edge of intermetatarsal ligament especially if pronation increased	Interdigital (neuromas) Plantar digital nerves especially in 3rd (or 2nd) web space	Plantar or forefoot pain on activity, often radiating to toes	Point tenderness between metatarsal heads Relief by removal of shoe, rest and massage	Running Ballet dancing

Fig. 17.27 Lower limb compression neuropathies due to sport.

the secondary ossification center occurs, the growth plate of the medial epicondyle represents the weakest attachment of the flexor pronator muscle group, so repetitive stress may produce a traction lesion. This valgus laxity, or in older participants osteophytes, may be a cause of ulnar impingement and it has been reported that 16% of the population demonstrated recurrent dislocation of the ulnar nerve in flexion, which increases the traction risk to the nerve.

GENERAL MANAGEMENT PRINCIPLES

It is crucial in dealing with individuals engaged in active sport who develop an injury to define:

- the exact anatomic site and type of injury;
- the forces and training load involved in injury, and to modify these following recovery to prevent recurrence;
- abnormalities of running gait or sports technique that will require adjustment.

MANAGEMENT OF ACUTE INJURY

The team doctor, coach or physical therapist may be able to help in clarifying the likely injury, by describing the 'event' and the observed forces of injury. If the injured athlete is seen immediately and has a joint injury, it is important to examine the joint before protective muscle spasm makes this impossible.

Immediate swelling of a joint at the time of injury implies hemarthrosis. In the knee this will usually be due to osteochondral damage or cruciate ligament tear. Urgent arthroscopy is important, followed by appropriate intensive rehabilitation where anterior cruciate ligament rupture has occurred and cannot be repaired immediately. The anterior cruciate deficient knee requires a program of balanced hamstring and quadriceps muscle strengthening, with later secondary repair only if instability is a functional problem. Meniscal injury is frequently the cause of symptoms in an anterior cruciate deficient knee and should be treated first. Anterior cruciate tear is best assessed by the Lachman test and the pivot shift test (see Chapter 4.11).

Having excluded severe injuries, such as fracture, dislocation and ligament rupture, the medical attendant should advise in the less severe injuries without skin breakage the application of the principles of 'RICE':

- Rest: short-term immediate rest reduces bleeding and inflammation. It is essential to reintroduce activity after injury in a graduated way, and to avoid any training errors that may have contributed to the problem.
- Ice: application of an ice pack (covered with a towel to prevent skin burning), decreases vascularity and inflammation and has an analgesic effect.
- Compression: reduces bleeding and tissue swelling.
- Elevation: reduces swelling.

Management after this early period is dependent on the type and severity of injury. Controlled stretching is important, particularly in hamstring and Achilles' injury. Early return to activity is advisable in mild ankle ligament injury, but the individual should not return to sport until he or she is pain free and full ankle control has been achieved. This involves a program of exercises to re-educate ankle proprioceptive muscle control, progressing through use of the wobble board.

MANAGEMENT OF CHRONIC INJURY

Local corticosteroid injections in chronic soft tissue injury

The use of local corticosteroid injections in chronic soft tissue injury in sportspeople has become a somewhat unnecessarily emotive issue. This seems generally to be based on inappropriate administration of corticosteroids by some clinicians, and misinterpretation of the available literature on the effects of corticosteroids on collagenous structures.

There is clear evidence from animal experiments that injection of some corticosteroid preparations into tendons or ligaments may cause alteration in their structure and behaviour. The injudicious use of corticosteroid injections, allowing too rapid a return to heavy loading, will almost inevitably lead to further microfailure in tendons weakened by injury; it is important to reduce activity in the period after injury. Where corticosteroids have been allowed to enter the tendon substance, complete rupture may occur if the tendon is subjected to very heavy loading. Although very rare, this complication is usually only reported in athletes, particularly in the Achilles' tendon, and the elderly.

Experimental effects of corticosteroids on tendons and ligaments

Carstram[40] and Wrenn *et al.*[41] showed that intramuscular cortisone inhibits the formation of adhesions in the healing process after tendon injury with some weakening of the tendon structure. Direct injection of corticosteroid into healthy tendons at doses comparable with those used therapeutically has produced variable experimental data, possibly partly reflecting differences in length of follow-up. Mackie *et al.*[42] and Phelps *et al.*[43] concluded that there were no significant changes in the mechanical properties of rabbit tendons injected in this way. Noyes *et al.*[44], however, showed clear evidence of decreases in monkey anterior cruciate ligament stiffness, failure load and energy absorption following direct intracollagenous injection of methylprednisolone acetate, the changes persisting for up to 52 weeks. Kapetanos[45] confirmed that a long-acting corticosteroid (triamcinolone acetonide) injected into artifically injured rabbit Achilles' tendons significantly decreased tendon weight, adhesion response, load to failure and energy to failure. Wesley McWhorter *et al*[46] failed to show any difference, compared with controls, in rat Achilles' tendon strength or consistent reduction of cell types recognized as components of the healing process after peritendinous hydrocortisone acetate injection.

Rational use of corticosteroid injections

When an inflammatory response in chronically injured tendons is unresponsive to local treatment and is inhibiting rehabilitation, with inevitable loss of strength in the entire muscle–tendon complex, local corticosteroid injection is justified, providing the following precautions are observed:

- Short-acting preparations should be used.
- Great care must be taken to avoid injecting directly into tendon tissue. This can be ensured by careful siting of the needle and recognition that injection must never be forced in under pressure.
- Injection should be followed by a period of graduated restrengthening, on the basis that recovery of tendon strength takes considerably longer than generally recognized.
- Heavily loaded tendons should be adequately assessed because, in the apparently peritendinous injection, corticosteroid may travel into the tendon substance where there is a significant destructive lesion.

It is recommended that peritendinous injection of the Achilles' tendon in athletes is not performed without a soft tissue scan to exclude deeper Achilles' injury. Only in simple paratendinitis chronically resistant to treatment should peritendinous injection be considered.

Intra-articular corticosteroid injections should not be given to athletes, unless a fully investigated primary rheumatologic condition, such as synovitis due to spondyloarthritis, has been defined.

Localized injection of deep frictional bursitis is less contentious, but chronic superficial bursitis around the knee is usually poorly responsive to corticosteroid injection.

Nonsteroidal anti-inflammatory drugs

These are of value in the active inflammatory phase, particularly where major pain and swelling inhibit muscle function and therefore adequate rehabilitation. Attention must always be paid to previous dyspeptic history, as NSAIDs may potentiate stress-induced gastric changes after endurance events.

Experimental evidence from studies of wound healing points to the importance for adequate healing of the initial, marked, polymorphonuclear leukocyte infiltration. As experimental removal of the polymorphonuclear phase reduces fibroblastic proliferation and angiogenesis, medication inhibiting this process could be suspected of resulting in poorly healed soft tissue structures, with risk of further failure. (For this reason, corticosteroids should never be given in the acute phase of injury response.)

Local NSAID application by gel formulation or patch merits further analysis, particularly as combination with ultrasound may promote delivery to soft tissue sites. The occasional report of exacerbation of asthma by such preparations illustrates that their use should be initiated and supervised by a medical practitioner who has fully assessed the athlete.

SURGICAL TREATMENT: GENERAL PRINCIPLES

Urgent surgical intervention is generally necessary for injuries causing complete tendon or ligament rupture, and sometimes for muscle rupture with extensive bleeding. It has already been emphasized that a history of immediate joint swelling after trauma usually indicates hemarthrosis, an indication of major injury, for example in knee anterior cruciate ligament rupture, requiring immediate orthopedic referral. Intensive postoperative rehabilitation must be coordinated between the surgeon, therapist and patient.

Similarly, surgical intervention in chronic injury, after conservative treatment has failed, should only be undertaken as part of a defined program designed to restore as near normal coordinated musculoskeletal function as is possible. The aims and limitations of surgery must therefore be discussed with the athlete and a carefully planned rehabilitation program, commencing as soon after surgery as the procedure allows, must be defined by the therapist and patient. No guarantee of return to full athletic prowess should be given to the patient. Surgical intervention in chronic injury can be defined as:

- Diagnostic: for example, arthroscopy.
- Decompressive: for example, exploration and release of tendon, muscle or nerve constricted through injury.
- Reconstructive: involving secondary procedures designed to restore function, for example in anterior cruciate ligament (ACL) rupture.
- Corrective: where modification is attempted of normal variants or abnormalities of skeletal anatomy, which through the repetitive stresses of sport are causing pain and/or loss of function, for example in os trigonum impingement.

Diagnostic arthroscopy

The development of arthroscopy, particularly as a day-case facility, has revolutionized the management of intra-articular knee pathology (see Chapter 4.11). It provides not only an accurate diagnostic assessment but also therapeutic intervention at the same time. This allows early treatment of symptomatic meniscal tears and other intra-articular pathology, without the frequently rapid loss of muscle function and risk of further, often more complex, injury. A locked knee, where there is a block to full extension of the knee due to a meniscal tear, is a surgical emergency requiring urgent arthroscopy. Now, ACL repair is frequently performed with arthroscopic techniques and long-term follow-up results are awaited with interest.

Although the knee has been the focus for arthroscopic intervention over the past 10 years, the technique is playing an increasingly important role in the management of shoulder pathology, particularly in the treatment of resistant subacromial impingement and rotator cuff injury. Ankle arthroscopy has an important role in diagnosis of osteochondral injury of the talus.

Decompressive surgery

Decompressive surgery should be performed when injury has resulted in major constriction or compression of soft tissues, for example in tenosynovitis of the hands, wrists or ankles. Removal of necrotic tissue, inhibiting function in large tendons without tendon sheaths, allows the residual normal tendon tissue to return to more normal function and thus permits recovery of tendon strength through appropriate rehabilitation. Removal of bony projections caused by previous injury may be indicated where frictional irritation of overlying soft tissue structures is occurring.

Reconstructive surgery

Reconstructive surgery involves more major intervention and should only be considered when, for example, it is clear that a chronically deficient ligament is the cause of symptoms and cannot be compensated for by improvement in muscle function. Many sportspeople have been shown to be playing often top-class sport with unsuspected ACL injury. Frequently, knee symptoms in the ACL-deficient knee are due to meniscal tear, and the latter should be treated surgically before consideration of surgery for the ligament rupture. Indeed, many authors recommend up to 9 months' rehabilitation of balanced hamstring and quadriceps function before considering surgery in the chronically symptomatic ACL-deficient knee. Similarly, adequate recovery of proprioceptive function in the ankle by intensive rehabilitation usually precludes the need for surgery after ankle ligament injury, unless there is associated osteochondral injury.

Recurrent dislocation of the shoulder must be defined clearly as a real problem and nonresponsive to compensatory restrengthening, before further investigation, such as CT arthrography or MRI with a view to surgery, is discussed with the patient.

Corrective surgery

Corrective surgery is carried out to modify anatomic variants associated with symptoms through the repetitive stresses of sport. In the case of os trigonum impingement, the problem is relatively straightforward and the need for surgery is usually clearly defined. However, in other situations this can be a form of intervention fraught with potential problems. Only patients with severe and chronic symptoms unresponsive to conservative treatment, including physical therapy and, if appropriate, orthotic advice, should be considered for this type of surgery.

The problems of patellofemoral pain and patellar malalignment exemplify the risks of intervening in this type of condition. Long-term results should be analyzed as part of the overall problem of the management of anterior knee or patellofemoral knee pain.

Management of anterior knee pain in sportspeople

Patellofemoral pain is a common complaint of athletes, representing a quarter of all knee problems treated at one injury clinic. Chondromalacia patellae should not be used as a synonym for patellofemoral pain. Arthroscopy has shown that in patients with symptoms and signs thought to be clinically consistent with a diagnosis of chondromalacia patellae, up to 50% show no macroscopic abnormalities. Much attention has focused on the possibility that a great deal of patellofemoral pain, in athletes particularly, reflects extensor mechanism dysfunction (vastus medialis deficiency).

Conservative management must be given adequate time and should include modification of activity, with avoidance of repetitive knee loading in flexion, an NSAID if required, to permit adequate rehabilitation of vastus medialis obliquus, patellar strapping and, in patients in whom foot abnormalities are a factor, orthotics. However, many studies have shown that up to 20% of athletes fail to improve adequately with such regimens, and surgery should be considered in these cases.

Surgical intervention has produced variable results, for example in lateral release of the patella[47]. The majority of studies show that over 80% of patients with chronic patellofemoral pain respond initially to this procedure, but with increasing time there is diminishing long-term benefit. Recent analysis by Kolowich *et al.*[48] suggests that the ideal candidates for this procedure are patients with chronic anterior pain who on examination show tight lateral patellar soft tissues but a normal Q-angle (see Fig. 17.12). Conversely, patients with excessive laxity of the patellar retinaculum and an abnormal Q-angle showed poor results. However, it is the patients who fall between these two extremes who present difficulty in prediction of response to surgery. This excellent study of the risk–benefit ratio of surgery in a broad group of patients is the type of critical analysis that should be applied to surgical intervention of this kind in the management of chronic sports injuries.

Sportspeople may opt for any intervention offered in a search for athletic success, but it is essential that the clinician provides realistic goals.

REFERENCES

1. Morris JN, Everitt MG, Pollard R, Chave SPW, Semmence AM. Vigorous exercise in leisure-time: Protection against coronary heart disease. Lancet. 1980;2:1207–10.
2. The health of the nation: a strategy for health in England :1992, HMSO.
3. Jacobs JC, Berdon E, Johnson AD. LA-B27 associated spondyloarthritis and enthesopathy in childhood: Clinical, pathological and radiographic observations in 58 patients. Pediatrics. 1982;100:521–8.
4. Jacobs JC. Spondyloarthritis and enthesopathy. Arch Intern Med. 1983;143:103–7.
5. International Federation of Sports Medicine. Physical exercise – an important factor for health. Br J Sports Med. 1990;24(2):82.
6. Mack RP, ed. Biomechanics of running. In: American Academy of Orthopedics symposium on the foot and leg in running sports. St. Louis: Mosby; 1982.
7. Lehman WL. Overuse syndromes in runners. AFP. 1984;29(1):157–64.
8. Stanitski CL. Common injuries in preadolescent and adolescent athletes: Recommendations for prevention. Sports Med. 1989;7:32–41.
9. Davidson RJL, Robertson JD, Galea G, Maughan RJ. Haematological changes associated with marathon running. Int J Sports Med. 1987;8:19–25.
10. McCarthy DA, Dale MM. The leucocytosis of exercise – A review and model. Sports Med. 1988;6:333–6.
11. Pedersen BK. Influence of physical activity on the cellular immune system: Mechanisms of action. Int J Sports Med. 1991;12:23–9.
12. Young A. Plasma creatinine kinase after the marathon – A diagnosic dilemma. Br J Sports Med. 1984;18(4):269–7
13. Strachan AF, Noakes TD, Kotzenberg G, Nel AE, De Beer FC. C-Reactive protein concentrations during long distance running. Br Med J. 1984;289:1249–51.
14. Farrell PA, Garthwaite TL, Gustafson AB. Plasma adrenocorticotropin and cortisol responses to submaximal and exhaustive exercise. J Appl Physiol. 1983;55:1441–4.
15. Bloom S, Johnson R, Park D, Rennie M, Sulaiman W. Differences in the metabolic and hormonal response to exercise between racing cyclists and untrained individuals. J Physiol. 1976;258:1–18.
16. O'Connor PJ, Morgan WP, Raglin JS, Barksdale CM, Kalin NK. Mood state and salivary cortisol levels following overtraining in female swimmers. Psychol Neurol Endocrinol. 1989;14:303–10.
17. Roberts D, Smith DJ. Effects of high intensity exercise on serum ferritin and antitrypsin in trained and untrained men. Clin Sports Med. 1989;1:63–71.
18. Carbon RJ, Macey MG, McCarthy DA, Pereira FP, Perry JD, Wade AJ. The effect of 30 min cycle ergometry on ankylosing spondylitis. Br J Rheumatol 1996;35:167–77
19. Warme WJ, Feagin JA, Paul King PA, Lambert KL, Cunningham RR. Injury statistics,1982–1993 Jackson Hole Ski Resort Am J Sports Med. 1995;23(5):597–600.
20. Stuart MJ, Aynsley Smith RN. Injuries in Junior A ice hockey: A three-year prospective study. Am J Sports Med. 1995;23(4):458–61.
21. Sandelin J, Kiviluoto O, Santavirta S, Honkanen R. Outcome of sports injuries treated in a casualty department. Br J Sports Med. 1985;19:103–6.
22. De Loës M. Medical treatment and costs of sports-related injuries in a total population. Int J Sports Med. 1990;11:66–72.
23. Kvist M, Kujala UM, Heinonen OJ, *et al.* Sports-related injuries in children. Int J Sports Med. 1989;10:81–6.
24. Gibson T. Sports injuries. Bailliére's Clin Rheumatol. 1987;13:583–600.
25. Richardson AB, Jobe FW, Collins HR. The shoulder in competitive sports. Am J Sports Med. 1980;8:159–63.
26. Dalton SE. Overuse injuries in adolescent athletes. Sports Med. 1992;13(1):58–70.
27. Lane NE, Bloch DA, Jones HM, Marshall WH, Wood P, Fries JF. Long-distance running, bone density and osteoarthritis. JAMA. 1986;255(9):1147–51.
28. McBryde AM. Stress fractures in athletes. J Sports Med. 1975;3:212–17.
29. Renstrom PAFH, Leadbetter WB. Tendinitis 1: basic concepts. Clin Sports Med 1992;II:533–77.
30. Archambault JM, Wiley JP, Bray RC. Exercise loading of tendons and the development of overuse injuries. Sports Med. 1995;20(2):77–89.
31. Coombs RRH, Klenerman L, Narcisi P. Collagen typing in Achilles tendon rupture. J Bone J Surg. 1980;62(B):258.
32. De Stefano V. Pathogenesis and diagnosis of ruptured Achilles tendon. Orthop Rev. 1975;4:17.
33. Noyes F, Trovik PJ, Hyde WB. Biomechanics of ligament failure (II) : An analysis of immobilization, exercise and reconditioning effects in primates. J Bone J Surg. 1974;56(A):1406–18.
34. Butler DL, Grood ES, Noyes FR, Zernkka RF. Biomechanics of ligaments and tendons. Exerc Sport Sci Rev. 1978;6:125–81.
35. Kvist M, Järvinen M. Clinical, histochemical and biomechanical features in repair of muscle and tendon injuries. Int J Sports Med. 1982;3:12–14.
36. Matheson GO, Clement DB, McKenzie DC, Taunton JE, Lloyd Smith DR, MacIntyre JG. Stress fractures in athletes: A study of 320 cases. Am J Sports Med. 1987;15(1):46–58.
37. Editorial: Athletic women, amenorrhoea and skeletal integrity. Ann Int Med. 1985;102(2):258–9.
38. Beighton P, Grahame R, Bird H. Hypermobility of joints. Springer Verlag; 1983.
39. Kaalund S, Lass P, Hogsaa B, Nøhr M. Achilles tendon rupture in badminton. Br J Sports Med. 1989;23(2):102–4.
40. Carstram N. Prevention of experimental tendon adhesions by cortisone. Acta Orthop Scand. 1952;22:15.
41. Wrenn RN, Goldner JL, Markee JL. An experimental study of the effect of cortisone on the healing process and tensile strength of tendons. J Bone J Surg. 1954;36(A):588–601.
42. Mackie JW, Goldin B, Foss M, Cockrill JL. Mechanical properties of rabbit tendons after repeated anti-inflammatory steroid injections. Med Sci Sports. 1974;6:198–202.
43. Phelps D, Soustegard DA, Matthews LS. Corticosteroid injection effects on the biomechanical properties of rabbit patellar tendons. Clin Orthop. 1974;100:345–8.
44. Noyes FA, Nussbaum NS, Tomk PJ, Cooper SM. Biomechanical and ultrastructural changes in ligaments and tendons after local corticosteroid injections. Proc Orthop Res Sociol J Bone J Surg. 1975;57(A):876.
45. Kapetanos G. The effect of the local corticosteroids on the healing and biomechanical properties of the partially injured tendon. Clin Orthop Res. 1982;163:170–9.
46. Wesley McWhorter J, Francis RS, Heckmann RA. Influence of local steroid injections of traumatized tendon properties: A biomechanical and histological study. Am J Sports Med. 1991;19(5):435–9.
47. Ogilvie-Harris DJ, Jackson RW. The arthroscopic treatment of chondromalacia patellae. J Bone J Surg. 1984;66(B)(5):660–5.
48. Kolowich PA, Paulos LE, Rosenberg TD, Farnsworth S. Lateral release of the patella: indications and contradictions. Am J Sports Med. 1990;18(4):359–65.

SOFT TISSUE

18

PRACTICAL PROBLEMS

DIFFICULT FIBROMYALGIA

Geoffrey Littlejohn

DEFINITION OF THE PROBLEM

Fibromyalgia syndrome (FMS) is a common cause of musculoskeletal symptoms, in both its generalized and localized forms. Generalized FMS may be mild and intermittent or severe and persistent, the latter presenting a difficult management problem.

THE TYPICAL CASE

RP is a 40-year-old mother of three who presented with a 10-year history of variable musculoskeletal aching, pain, stiffness and fatigue. Her symptoms fluctuated according to activity, weather change or stress. While at times she was comfortable and without complaint, more usually she had episodes of distressing symptoms lasting weeks to months. These led to significant diminution in her enjoyment of life and her ability to carry out a number of otherwise routine household, work-related and recreational activities. Her persisting symptoms have led to concern among her family members and have resulted in many investigations and treatments over a number of years.

She recalled episodes, at the age of 13 years of nocturnal myalgia, usually in the thigh and calf regions, which were often relieved by rubbing and simple analgesia. A jarring injury while playing volleyball at age 15 resulted in 6 months of significant low back pain, which gradually subsided with modification of activity. Radiologic investigations at the time were unremarkable. In her early 20s she was a very active person, working full time as a teacher, marrying at the age of 23 and subsequently having three children over the next 7 years. During these years she played tennis regularly, entertained friends, continued to work on a part-time basis and was busy 'always doing something'.

Without obvious reason, although she did have an upper respiratory tract infection that took longer than usual to throw off, she developed aching and discomfort around the neck and shoulder-girdle regions. This problem persisted and muscular aching was later prominent in thoracic, lumbar, buttock and leg regions. She noted that her sleep pattern, which had previously been good, had become disturbed, with fragmented shallow sleep. She would wake up feeling unrefreshed in the mornings. Morning stiffness became prominent and nocturnal dysesthesia in the hands was noted.

She continued to do part-time work but had to reduce it in order to be able to cope with her domestic responsibilities. Even in the home she required help to do all the day's jobs.

The persistent distressing symptoms and disability led to a review by medical practitioners, who found that routine investigations for inflammatory disease, hormone dysfunction, biochemical disturbance and radiologic abnormality were all unremarkable. Various diagnostic labels had been attached to the symptoms as they persisted over the years, including 'postviral myalgia,' 'seronegative arthritis' and similar nonspecific titles. Her local doctor became frustrated by the lack of resolution of the symptoms, having prescribed simple analgesics and, later, anti-inflammatory medication. Opinions followed from other health professionals, including specialists in neurology, orthopedics and rheumatology, as well as other family physicians. She became upset when told 'there is nothing wrong with you.' Help from non-medical sources included courses of acupuncture, naturopathy and physical treatments. Short-term help was obtained from some of these approaches, but expense precluded their continuation.

A thorough physical examination showed no abnormality in major organ systems. There was clearly defined abnormal tenderness to palpation in the tender points that characterize FMS. In addition, abnormal sensitivity to palpation of a fold of skin of the upper back, held between the thumb and forefinger, was prominent, together with exaggerated cutaneous wheal and flare on light stimulation of the same region with the finger nail. There was prominent paravertebral tightness and tenderness in the low cervical, mid-thoracic and low lumbar region. Her grip strengths were below the expected range for her body size and rings were tight at the time of examination.

DIAGNOSTIC PROBLEMS

In retrospect, such a history is typical of the difficult FMS patient, and anyone familiar with the syndrome will quickly predict the diagnosis prior to examination (see Chapter 4.15). However, as a syndrome may evolve over a long period of time, when there is no obvious precipitating cause, it may be necessary to consider a number of possibilities, depending on the presenting symptoms and signs. The experienced clinician also recognizes that this is a syndrome and not all features are present at one point in time. Important clues to the possibility of FMS are detailed in Figure 18.1. A recurring history of protracted painful episodes during adolescence may be noted. This is by no means invariable, and many have sudden onset of fibromyalgia more clearly associated with a triggering event. This might include an injury, usually 'soft tissue' in nature but often involving spinal regions such as 'whiplash' or a jarring low back injury.

Many patients develop FMS in the context of significant stress which is not perceived as such by themselves at the time. A history of coping extremely well with an extraordinarily large number of tasks only to begin, for no apparent reason, to cope poorly is also often seen.

CLUES TO THE POSSIBILITY OF FIBROMYALGIA SYNDROME

- Past/present prolonged localized pain complaint – important tests negative
- Often prior nonspecific label – 'lumbago', 'chronic fatigue' syndrome, 'restless legs' syndrome, 'whiplash', 'growing pains'
- Past/present tension headache, irritable bowel, fluid retention or similar syndromes
- Widespread joint/muscle pain
- Poor-quality sleep
- Background stress factors (may be subtle)

Fig. 18.1 Clues to the possibility of fibromyalgia syndrome.

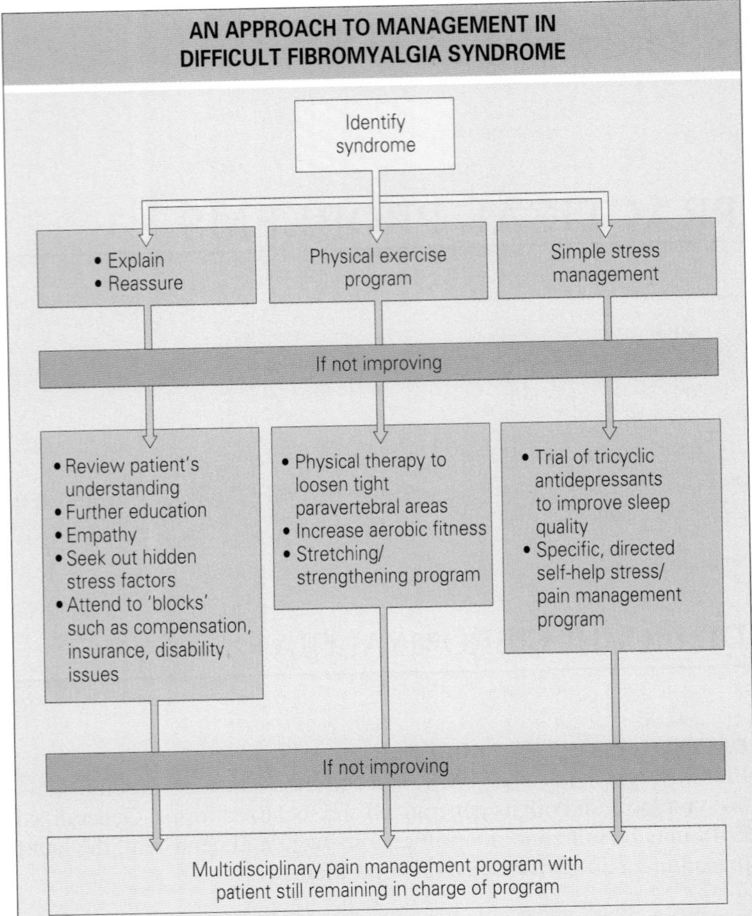

Fig. 18.2 An approach to management in difficult fibromyalgia syndrome.

Many patients have seen numerous physical therapists for mild and reasonably transient symptoms relating to neck, shoulder, back or buttocks. Initially there is reasonable improvement in symptoms with physical therapy approaches, such as massage, mobilization, manipulation or similar treatments.

It is important to note that inflammatory joint diseases, such as rheumatoid arthritis (RA) or systemic lupus erythematosus (SLE), may present with myalgia. Objective signs of inflammatory joint disease and markers of inflammation and serologic abnormality need to be sought out. In contrast, it is common for patients with FMS to be extensively investigated and those younger females with low-titer, nonspecific antinuclear antibody (ANA) levels are often mislabeled as having 'mild lupus'.

Other conditions that occur in the context of FMS include irritable bowel syndrome, 'tension' headaches, menstrual abnormality, fluid retention, pelvic pain problems, irritable bladder syndromes and chronic anxiety. A history of these conditions will also make the likelihood of FMS more apparent.

THERAPEUTIC OPTIONS

Clearly, accurate diagnosis is the essential initial ingredient for the appropriate management of even the most difficult case. Careful clinical examination and appropriate selected investigations will eliminate most of the common problems that might mimic the condition. The clinical features are usually straightforward, and the most useful ones are the abnormal pain threshold, most prominent in the tender point regions, paravertebral muscular tightness, limb–girdle muscle co-contraction, dermatographia and allodynia. With accurate diagnosis comes appropriate explanation as to the nature of the syndrome and reassurance on the absence of other causes that may be worrying the patient, such as arthritis, cancer or other poorly perceived conditions like multiple sclerosis. In milder cases, simple reassurance, explanation, a physical exercise program and attention to simple life stresses is usually most efficacious. If sleep disturbance is prominent, use of low-dose tricyclic medication in the mid-evening may be useful.

Where there have been persisting and significant symptoms, and where life disruption is prominent, much more attention needs to be placed on the psychological background of the patient, both from the point of view of chronic background stresses and from the reaction of the patient to the chronic painful problem. This entails a careful clinical history, empathy and understanding on the part of the doctor, and often some time and return visits to identify the key factors that seem relevant. In many instances, this role can be better played by a clinical psychologist or someone particularly skilled in chronic pain management. Uncommonly, there is a defined psychiatric illness in such patients; if present, this will need to be treated appropriately. For instance, depression would require higher dose antidepressant medication and a severe chronic anxiety syndrome might require appropriate counseling.

More commonly seen are simple everyday background stresses building up in normal people in a subtle and additive fashion to the degree where some change in the central pain control pathways is effected. It is very helpful and appropriate to explain the nature of the condition in terms of a pain amplification syndrome that alters pain threshold. The patient then realizes how physical activity initiates pain. The syndrome is expressed in terms of an abnormality of control of the pain pathways and the patient is reassured that there is no abnormality in the tissues within the body. This allows him or her to have confidence in participating in an exercise program to stretch tight areas, particularly in paraspinal regions which seem to be prominent in causing referred pain into more peripheral regions. It is also emphasized to the patient that any lively exercise program will by itself induce relaxation and hence better control of the amplified pain system.

Self-help is the key to management and this means aerobic exercise (pushing into the pain), stretching and strengthening paraspinal and abdominal musculature, as well as developing skills in stress and pain management, such as relaxation, meditation, yoga, tai-chi or similar activities. Each person will have to choose the modality that is best for them, and often several methods will need to be examined over time.

Patients such as the case described may need guidance in regard to time management. Finding 'space' in the day's activities for themselves is important. It allows for relaxation, renewal of energy and better management of pain and fatigue. Exercise programs create time away from life stresses. In addition, allocation of the day's tasks can be improved with advice, further diminishing everyday stresses. Stress management tactics are essential for pain management and need to be built into all everyday life activities.

Clinical psychologic programs are usually straightforward, practical, nonthreatening and helpful to the patient. The patient with FMS is treated in the context of their total life, family and personal situation, and strategies to deal with the FMS are based on the premise that the patient does not have to 'learn to live with it' but that the pain syndrome will usually improve significantly with this understanding and approach.

Where there are blocks to this process through anger, resentment or other forces, which may often be of a medicolegal nature, such approaches will not work. The 'blocks' need specific and insightful attention. Finally, any new symptoms in such patients require careful independent assessment as other illnesses can coexist with this syndrome. Figure 18.2 outlines the key management strategies in difficult FMS.

REFERENCES

Goldenberg DL. Treatment of fibromyalgia syndrome. Rheum Dis Clin North Am. 1989;15:61–72.

McCain GA. Nonmedicinal treatments in primary fibromyalgia. Rheum Dis Clin North Am. 1989;15:73–90.

THE MANAGEMENT OF CHRONIC FATIGUE SYNDROME

Don L Goldenberg

DEFINITION OF THE PROBLEM

Chronic fatigue lasting longer than 3 months affects 5–20% of the general population. Two thirds of these cases arise from a medical or psychiatric illness but one third are idiopathic. Many of these patients with idiopathic chronic fatigue will meet current classification criteria for chronic fatigue syndrome (CFS) and/or fibromyalgia. These classification criteria are based on patients' symptoms of debilitating fatigue, myalgia, headache, sleep disturbances and neuropsychiatric symptoms. Most patients have normal physical findings, although 30–70% of patients classified as having CFS will meet tender point criteria for fibromyalgia. Chronic fatigue syndrome and fibromyalgia are poorly understood, overlapping disorders that should be considered in patients with idiopathic chronic fatigue and chronic myalgias.

THE TYPICAL CASE

MP is a 45-year-old woman who presents with a 2-year history of severe fatigue and generalized muscle soreness. She was well until she developed a flu-like illness, from which she 'never recovered'. Her sleep is light and she feels unrefreshed in the morning. She reports aching in all her muscles and joints, but there is no history of joint swelling or signs or symptoms of a connective tissue disease. She has seen many different specialists but no one has given her a diagnosis. Some of them felt that she was depressed; however, a consulting psychiatrist told her that she was not depressed. During the past year she stopped all exercise, even though she used to exercise regularly and enjoyed it. In the past 4 months she has had daily 'muscular' headaches and noted alternating constipation and diarrhea. During the past 6 weeks she took leave of absence from her job as a secretary because her fatigue was so overwhelming.

The physical examination demonstrated no significant abnormalities except for muscle tenderness around the elbows, neck, upper back and thighs. There was no lymphadenopathy or organomegaly. The neurologic examination was unremarkable.

Recent extensive radiographs, imaging studies of the brain, and blood tests were all essentially normal. She did have a positive ANA test, but it was at a low titer and more specific serologic tests were normal. Her thyroid tests and erythrocyte sedimentation rate (ESR) were normal.

THERAPEUTIC OPTIONS

The most important treatment for this patient is reassuring her that her illness is not fatal or progressive, and also that it is not 'all in her head' as she has been told by some. MP was particularly concerned that she might have SLE, but once the nonspecificity of the ANA test was explained to her, she was greatly relieved. A detailed explanation of the interaction of sleep, pain, muscle spasm and lack of activity set the groundwork for a treatment program.

She was started on 10mg of amitriptyline at bedtime. Within 2 weeks, she slept deeper, felt more energy and was less achy. However, she still felt too exhausted to return to full-time employment. She then began to attend a formal group relaxation program and started some gentle stretching and water exercises. A psychiatric evaluation found evidence for a reactive depression. Low doses of fluoxetine (10mg) were given in the morning along with the amitriptyline at bedtime.

Gradually, over the next 6 months, her fatigue improved significantly and she felt much better. She returned to her former levels of work and recreation although she continues to have bouts of modest fatigue and myalgias.

CONCLUSIONS

Many medications have been suggested for CFS, some based on the hypothesis that an infection and/or immune dysfunction are responsible for the symptoms. Most of these suggested treatments have not been subjected to appropriate clinical trials. Currently, the most prudent approach to treatment should be modeled on the treatment of overlapping disorders, including fibromyalgia, irritable bowel syndrome and mood disturbances. This includes judicious use of medications to help restore sleep and decrease fatigue, treatment of any coexisting mood disturbances and avoidance of inactivity. Currently, there is no evidence that antimicrobial agents, immune modulators or anti-inflammatory medications are effective in the treatment of CFS.

REFERENCES

Fukuda K, Straus SE, Hickie I, *et al.* The chronic fatigue syndrome: a comprehensive approach to its definition and study. Ann Intern Med. 1994;121:953–9.

Goldenberg DL, Simms RW, Geiger A, Komaroff AL. High frequency of fibromyalgia in patients with chronic fatigue seen in a primary care practice. Arthritis Rheum. 1990;33:381–7.

Shafran ST. The chronic fatigue syndrome. Am J Med 1991;90:730–9.

Wilson A, Hickie I, Lloyd A, Wakefield D. The treatment of chronic fatigue syndrome: science and speculation. Am J Med. 1994;96:544–50.

THORACIC OUTLET SYNDROME

David J Nashel

DEFINITION OF THE PROBLEM

Of all the entrapment neuropathies, the diagnosis and management of thoracic outlet syndrome (TOS) is by far the most controversial. Some authors deny its very existence while others present data describing successful treatment of large numbers of patients with this condition. A number of syndromes fall under this rubric, so it is little wonder that there are no well-established criteria for its identification and management . Undoubtedly, there are cases of TOS that fit a distinctive pattern but these are indeed rare.

THE TYPICAL CASE

CV, a 45-year-old woman, had been experiencing intermittent discomfort in the right shoulder, forearm and hand over a 7-month period. She reported an aching pain and a tingling sensation that radiated down

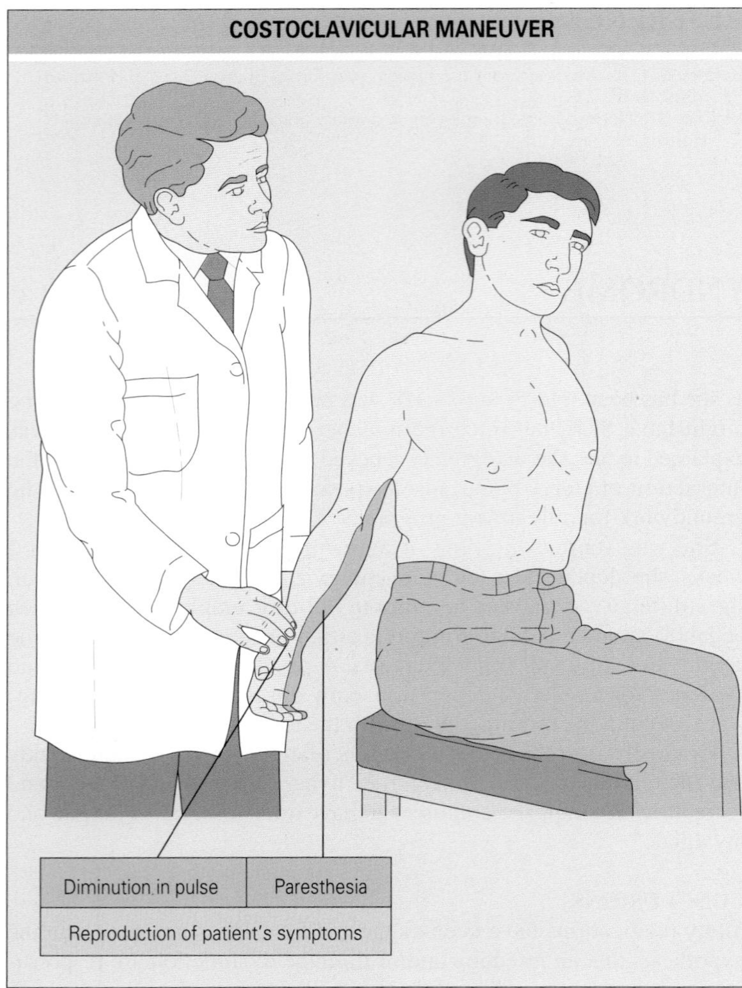

Fig. 18.3 The costoclavicular maneuver. A positive response to the maneuver may cause these findings.

her arm. Carrying a heavy object such as a piece of luggage worsened the discomfort. She was not bothered by hand weakness and was unaware of any episodic color changes in the hand. She was somewhat obese and had a noticeable shoulder droop. There was no discernible weakness on muscle strength testing nor was there muscle atrophy. Costoclavicular maneuver (Fig. 18.3) caused increased paresthesia in the affected arm, and there was hypoesthesia along the inner aspect of the forearm. Tinel's test at the wrist was negative. Radiographs of the thorax and cervical spine were unremarkable. Motor and sensory nerve conduction studies, as well as electromyography (EMG), were normal. A slight reduction in sensory action potential from the fifth finger was reported. Initial treatment with ibuprofen 600mg q.i.d provided no relief. A neurosurgeon felt that the patient had TOS and suggested that she consider surgical intervention if the symptoms persist. The patient undertook an intensive physical therapy program that emphasized strengthening of the shoulder-girdle muscles. Over the next 2 months her symptoms gradually abated.

DIAGNOSTIC PROBLEMS

Unfortunately, there is no single test which identifies the presence of neurogenic TOS and stress maneuvers have limited utility (see below). Nonetheless, certain sensory and motor abnormalities are frequently noted (Fig. 18.4). The finding of a cervical rib, while supportive of the diagnosis, is by no means pathognomonic for this disorder. It is not uncommon to find this anomaly on routine radiography.

In point of fact, TOS is more appropriately a diagnosis of exclusion. Such entities as carpal tunnel syndrome with a proximal pain radiation pattern, cervical disc disease, reflex sympathetic dystrophy, cervical radiculopathy and tumor may be mistaken for TOS.

The usefulness of electrodiagnostic studies in TOS has been challenged. Sensory and motor conduction studies are invariably normal while nerve conduction across the thoracic outlet itself is quite variable, even in unaffected persons. There are data to suggest that quantitative EMG and measurement of sensory action potentials may provide more reliable diagnostic information.

In performing Adson's maneuver, the hyperabduction maneuver or the costoclavicular maneuver, the examiner looks for alteration or obliteration of the radial pulse. However, the validity of these tests is a matter of debate because they are often positive in asymptomatic, normal individuals. The diagnostic utility of these maneuvers is limited to those situations in which the maneuver reproduces the patient's original symptoms.

For patients with signs or symptoms of arterial or venous compression at the thoracic outlet (Fig. 18.5), vascular patency must be assessed without delay. For acute or chronic venous obstruction, venography is the essential diagnostic study, while Doppler sonography may be a useful adjunct. If complete arterial occlusion is suspected, subclavian arteriography is useful, whereas monitoring of the arterial Doppler waveform during stress maneuvers may be helpful in determining subclavian compression.

CLINICAL FEATURES OF NEUROGENIC THORACIC OUTLET SYNDROME
Sensory disturbances
Pain, often as a dull ache Diffuse pain distribution from shoulder to hand Paresthesias, usually of the medial aspect of the arm and ulnar aspect of the hand (may not follow C8–T1 dermatome) Worsening of paresthesias may occur when carrying objects or positioning arm overhead Coolness of the hand (subjective feeling only)
Motor disturbances
Weakness of the hand with diminished pinch or grasp Easy fatigability with repetitive motions of the hand Wasting of intrinsic muscles of the hand, may affect interosseous, hypothenar and thenar muscles Dyscoordination of hand movements
Patients may have only one or may have several of the signs and symptoms listed; they are not invariably present

Fig. 18.4 Clinical features of neurogenic thoracic outlet syndrome.

CLINICAL FEATURES OF VASCULAR- INDUCED THORACIC OUTLET SYNDROME
Arterial
Pallor; may have cyanosis with dependency and be mistaken for Raynaud's phenomenon Coldness Muscle ache Claudication Supraclavicular bruit Trophic skin changes Digital ulceration
Venous
Edema of the extremity Pain and swelling made worse with exercise Cyanotic discoloration Venous engorgement Collateral vessel development across shoulder and chest
Patients may have only one or may have several of the signs and symptoms listed; they are not invariably present

Fig. 18.5 Clinical features of vascular-induced thoracic outlet syndrome.

THERAPEUTIC OPTIONS

Early operation is indicated for patients with evidence of vascular occlusion. However, it is compression of the trunks of the brachial plexus and not vascular compromise that accounts for TOS symptoms in the majority of patients. The initial management approach for patients with neurogenic TOS should focus on conservative treatment measures, and these should be pursued for weeks to months before operative measures are undertaken. When possible, factors should be identified that might be contributing to TOS and these should be ameliorated. This might consist of avoidance of heavy lifting or even a change in occupational activities, such as limiting those work situations that entail prolonged use of the hands above the head. Patients should avoid sleeping with an arm in a hyperabducted position.

Postural problems are often noted in patients with symptoms consistent with TOS. Thus, the initiation of a physical therapy program is an important treatment element. This should include specific shoulder-girdle strengthening exercises.

In recent years, enthusiasm for operative correction of TOS has waned, and some have even suggested that there be a moratorium on surgical correction. Too often patients have undergone surgery for presumed TOS when the diagnosis had not been adequately established and before more conservative treatment modalities had been pursued. A minority of patients are found to have progressive hand weakness, lack of coordination and muscle atrophy, indicating a more advanced stage of TOS. In this setting, consideration of surgical intervention is appropriate.

It is increasingly evident that too many patients have been operated on for presumed TOS, when in fact the symptoms may have been due to a concomitant disorder such as carpal tunnel syndrome. Also militating against surgical intervention are data that indicate that a number of patients will have continuing symptoms no matter which of several surgical approaches is taken to correct the disorder. And, finally, injury to the brachial plexus at the time of operation is a potentially serious complication of this surgery.

CONCLUSIONS

A diagnosis of TOS should be made only after other causes of upper extremity pain have been excluded. In those uncommon circumstances in which conservative treatment measures fail to provide adequate pain relief, or when there is convincing evidence of nerve entrapment (e.g. weakness, dysfunction of the hand, muscle atrophy), operative intervention may be necessary. Surgery may also be an appropriate option in the rare instance in which there is evidence of vascular obstruction.

REFERENCES

Baxter BT, Blackburn D, Payne K, Pearce WH, Yao JST. Noninvasive evaluation of the upper extremity. Surg Clin North Am. 1990;70:87–97.

Lindgren K-A, Oksala I. Long-term outcome of surgery for thoracic outlet syndrome. Am J Surg. 1995; 169: 358–60.

Juvonen T, Satta J, Laitala P, Luukkonen K, Nissinen J. Anomalies at the thoracic outlet are frequent in the general population. Am J Surg. 1995;170:33–7.

Pang D, Wessel HB. Thoracic outlet syndrome. Neurosurgery 1988;22:105–21.

Peet RM, Henriksen JD, Anderson TP, Martin GM. Thoracic-outlet syndrome: evaluation of therapeutic exercise program. Proc Staff Meet Mayo Clin. 1956;31:281–7.

TARSAL TUNNEL SYNDROME

Charles G Peterfy

DEFINITION OF THE PROBLEM

Evaluating patients with foot pain is often challenging from both a diagnostic and a therapeutic standpoint. One important surgical consideration, tarsal tunnel syndrome (TTS), usually presents with characteristic clinical findings, but may nevertheless be overlooked by clinicians or mistaken for other causes of tarsal pain.

THE TYPICAL CASE

JS is a 36-year-old man who developed progressive burning sensation and paresthesia along the plantar surface of the left foot over a period of several months. He gave no history of prior injury, diabetes mellitus, other paresthesias, joint pain or any constitutional symptoms. A trial of nonsteroidal anti-inflammatory drugs (NSAIDs) did not improve his symptoms. On physical examination, the patient revealed mild tenderness beneath the medial malleolus of his left ankle, but no mass was palpable. He had no plantar tenderness, but showed decreased sensation along the plantar aspect of the foot and weak flexion of the big toe. Electromyography was not done. Radiographs of the foot and ankle showed no abnormalities. A small, well-circumscribed fluid collection between the flexor digitorum longus and flexor hallucis longus tendons at the level of the sustentaculum tali was seen on magnetic resonance imaging (MRI) of the left ankle (Fig. 18.6). The patient was referred for surgery, and a small ganglion cyst was excised from the tarsal tunnel of the left ankle. His pain resolved completely following surgery, but a mild degree of hypoesthesia remained.

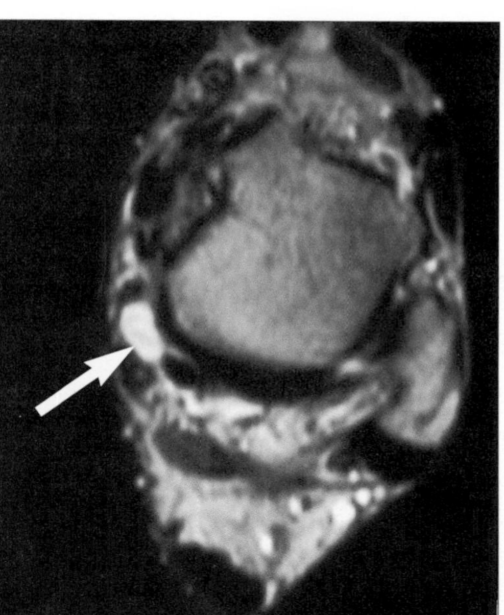

Fig. 18.6 Ganglion cyst causing TTS. Transverse T2-weighted spin-echo MRI shows a small ganglion cyst (arrow) between the tendons of the flexor digitorum longus and the flexor hallucis longus in the tarsal tunnel.

DIAGNOSTIC PROBLEMS

Tarsal tunnel syndrome is a compression neuropathy of the posterior tibial nerve or its branches resulting from impingement in a fibro-osseous compartment called the tarsal tunnel in the posteromedial ankle (see Chapter 4.16). The tarsal tunnel extends from above the medial malleolus to the abductor hallucis muscle in the foot. It is bounded laterally by the calcaneus and talus and superficially by the flexor retinaculum (Fig. 18.7). The tibialis posterior, flexor digitorum longus and flexor hallucis longus tendons, as well as the posterior tibial nerve, course through the tarsal tunnel as they curve beneath the medial malleolus to enter the foot. The posterior tibial nerve runs between the flexor digitorum longus and flexor hallucis longus tendons and divides distally into medial and lateral plantar branches, which, along with small calcaneal branches, provide sensory innervation to the plantar surface of the foot.

As in other compartment syndromes, any process that decreases the volume of the compartment or increases the volume of its contents can produce a compression neuropathy. Entrapment of the posterior tibial

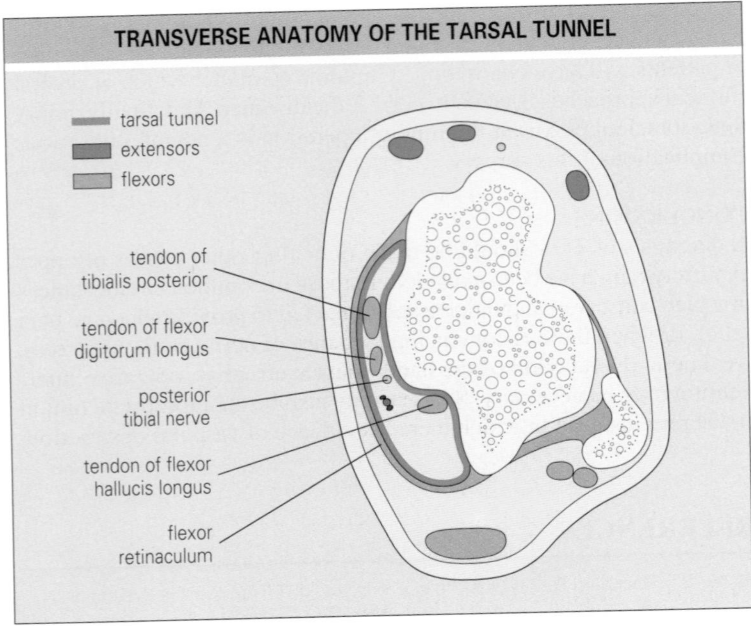

Fig. 18.7 Transverse anatomy of the tarsal tunnel.

nerve typically results in pain and paresthesia radiating along the sole of the foot to the toes. Palpation posterior to the medial malleolus may elicit pain or reveal fullness in this region. Electromyography can be helpful in establishing the diagnosis of TTS.

The most common cause of TTS is a space-occupying lesion, such as a ganglion cyst, between the tendons of the flexor digitorum longus and flexor hallucis longus. As illustrated by the present case, even small lesions in this location can produce severe symptoms. Ganglion cysts are particularly easy to detect with MRI, as they usually exhibit very high signal intensity on T2-weighted images (Fig. 18.6). Other less common mass lesions in the tarsal tunnel include anomalous muscles (Fig. 18.8), aberrant vessels, or neoplasms such as lipomas or peripheral nerve sheath tumors. Fractures of the calcaneus involving the sustentaculum tali also can cause TTS. In the acute setting, this is usually because of local hematoma or direct entrapment in the fracture. As the fracture heals, the nerve can become incorporated in local callus or encased by retracting scar tissue. Tarsal coalition can also be responsible for TTS because of progressive deformity of the sustentaculum tali. Tenosynovitis of the posteromedial flexors of the ankle occasionally causes TTS in patients with RA. Each of these causes is easily differentiated by MRI.

Plantar fasciitis can mimic TTS clinically but is easily differentiated on MRI by the presence of fluid tracking along the plantar aponeurosis (Fig. 18.9). Other differential considerations include vascular insufficiency and systemic peripheral neuropathy. However, these are usually distinguishable on clinical grounds.

THERAPEUTIC OPTIONS

As with other compartment syndromes, surgical decompression is the principal therapeutic approach to TTS. Simple division of the flexor retinaculum is usually successful in relieving symptoms, particularly when the cause is a space-occupying lesion. Occasionally, an enlarged or irregular sustentaculum tali must be shaved down, or an infiltrative intracompartmental mass must be resected. With more extensive surgery, however, there is increased risk of recurrent symptoms due to postoperative scarring. Certain causes of TTS may be managed conservatively, particularly cases related to acute trauma such as calcaneal fracture or strain and swelling of anomalous muscles in the tarsal tunnel.

CONCLUSIONS

Despite its relatively characteristic presentation, TTS is often not considered in the differential diagnosis of foot pain. Plantar burning pain associated with compression neuropathy of the posterior tibial nerve is most commonly caused by a ganglion cyst within the tarsal tunnel, but can also result from other mass lesions, tenosynovitis, tarsal coalition or fractures of the sustentaculum tali. Differential considerations include tarsal arthritis, plantar fasciitis, vascular insufficiency and systemic peripheral neuropathy. Magnetic resonance imaging can differentiate between many of these conditions and help exclude other causes of foot pain.

REFERENCES

Ho V, Peterfy C, Helms C. Tarsal tunnel syndrome caused by strain of the flexor digitorum longus accessorus: an MRI-specific diagnosis. J Comput Assist Tomogr. 1993;71:822–3.

Kerr R, Frey C. MRI in tarsal tunnel syndrome. J Comput Assist Tomogr. 1991;15:280–6.

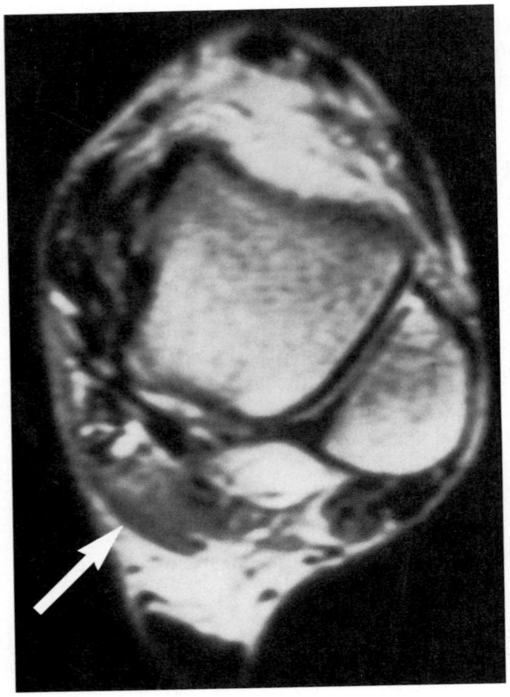

Fig. 18.8 Strained accessory muscle causing TTS. Transverse T2-weighted spin-echo MRI showing a swollen and edematous accessory muscle (flexor digitorum longus accessorus) (arrow) in the tarsal tunnel of a patient who developed TTS following an inversion injury of his ankle. With permission from Ho V, Peterfy C, Helms C, Tarsal tunnel syndrome caused by strain of the flexor digitorum longus accessorus: an MRI-specific diagnosis. J Comput Assist Tomogr. 1993;71:822–3.

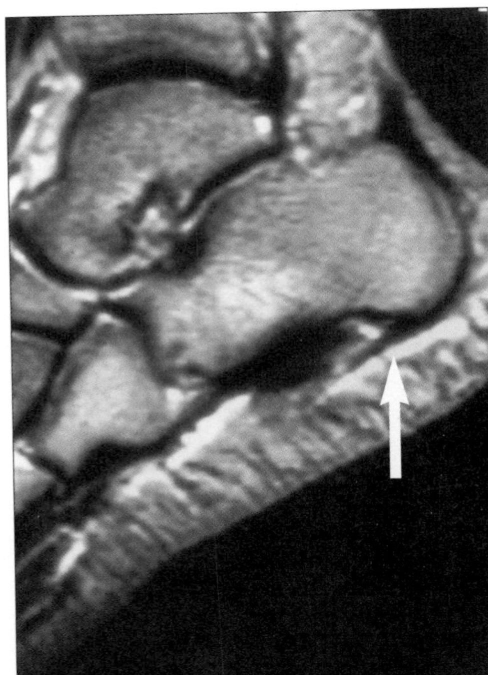

Fig. 18.9 Plantar fasciitis. Sagittal, fat-suppressed T2-weighted spin-echo image showing high signal intensity fluid tracking along the low signal intensity plantar aponeurosis (arrow).

PHYSICAL TECHNIQUES FOR THE PREVENTION AND THERAPY OF ARM PAIN IN THE WORKPLACE

Joanne Borg Stein

DEFINITION OF THE PROBLEM

Arm pain in the workplace, often termed 'cumulative trauma disorder' or 'repetitive strain injury', is a highly prevalent syndrome and has become more widely recognized recently. These industrial injuries account for 51% of occupational illnesses in US workplaces. Employees can experience substantial pain and functional impairment which, in severe cases, may require a change of occupation. In addition to the personal toll suffered by those with this disorder, there are substantial costs to industry in lost productivity, higher medical expenses and disability payments. Commonly, symptoms are not related to a discrete trauma. Rather, they develop insidiously after sustained performance of repetitive tasks over weeks, months or years.

THE TYPICAL CASE

EP is a 47-year-old right-handed checkout cashier for a large supermarket who was referred for treatment of right elbow region pain of 4 months' duration, with inability to work for that period of time. She related the insidious onset of right lateral epicondylar region pain which was exacerbated by lifting items from the basket and pulling them through the checkout counter and using the cash register. She had already been given a splint to immobilize the wrist as well as a course of physical therapy, which included phonophoresis, stretching and gentle right upper extremity strengthening, over the previous 2 months. She reported that prior treatment had resulted in an overall improvement of '80%'. She denied any other neurologic or rheumatologic symptoms and there was no sleep disorder present. Of note, she was using a resting hand splint at night only on the left hand for symptoms of carpal tunnel syndrome. She had minimal pain with vacuuming and emptying the garbage at home. The physical examination was notable for mild tenderness on the right forearm at the insertion of the wrist extensors and mild tenderness 3cm distal to this. There was no pain with resisted wrist, finger or elbow extension or forearm pronation and supination. Neurologic examination of the right upper extremity was within normal limits. A gradual return to work after this 4-month leave was then recommended along with continued strengthening.

She did well until 2 months later when she presented with a further exacerbation of symptoms. She then had a right lateral epicondylar corticosteroid injection and 'modified' work duty. Over the next 2 months the acute right lateral epicondyle region pain resolved and she returned with a more widespread right forearm burning sensation and sleep disturbance secondary to pain, without neurologic deficits on repeat physical exam. Amitriptyline (10mg at bedtime) and subsequently clonazepam (0.25mg b.i.d.) were begun, with improvement of sleep and burning pain. She underwent further strengthening, a worksite evaluation, ergonomic modification and fabrication of a new splint. She was able to return to her position as a cashier and was stably functioning in that position at a 16-month follow-up.

DIAGNOSTIC PROBLEMS

The differential diagnosis of arm pain in the workplace includes tendinitis or tenosynovitis of the shoulder, elbow or wrist regions. Common sites include the rotator cuff, biceps, wrist flexors and extensors, and thumb tendons in the first dorsal compartment (de Quervain's tenosynovitis). Lateral and medial epicondylitis are also common. Entrapment neuropathies should be considered, and may include ulnar nerve entrapment at the elbow (cubital tunnel syndrome) or wrist (Guyon's canal), median nerve entrapment at the pronator teres or carpal tunnel, or radial nerve entrapment at the elbow (posterior interosseous nerve). Cervical radiculopathy may also present as arm pain. Regional myofascial pain syndrome may also cause arm pain.

Localized muscle fatigue may result in discomfort and fatigue and can occur without underlying inflammation or nerve entrapment. Workers who use vibrating tools for extended periods of time may develop episodic numbness, pain, tingling and cold-induced finger blanching labeled the 'hand–arm vibration syndrome.' Nerve conduction and EMG studies may be helpful to differentiate among the various neurogenic possibilities.

THERAPEUTIC OPTIONS

Treatment can be challenging since the predominant symptom is often pain (Fig. 18.10). This pain may persist even when no clinical evidence of inflammation remains. Nonsteroidal anti-inflammatory drugs have a role on initial presentation for the treatment of inflammation from tendinitis or tenosynovitis. For neuropathic symptoms such as burning dysesthesias or for sleep disturbances low-dose tricyclic antidepressants are helpful. Benzodiazepines may reduce both muscle spasm through a central mechanism and anxiety occurring as a secondary event.

Adjunctive early phase treatment with physical modalities such as ice, heat, phonophoresis, iontophoresis and electric stimulation may be useful. Cooling reduces edema and inflammation and provides analgesia. Heating modalities induce muscle relaxation, reduce pain and enhance stretching and mobilization. Superficial heat can be applied via conduction through hydrocollator packs and paraffin. Whirlpool and fluidotherapy utilize convection to transmit heat. Deep heating is obtained with the use of ultrasound, which converts acoustic vibration into 'deep' heat. Penetration to a depth of 4–5cm can be attained. Phonophoresis uses ultrasound with a corticosteroid cream as the coupling medium. This provides a variable amount of transdermal penetration of the corticosteroid. Electric stimulation may be used in conjunction with a topical corticosteroid solution for iontophoresis, in which the electric current facilitates the penetration of the corticosteroid into the underlying tissue. This technique may be helpful in the treatment of tendinitis, contusions and epicondylitis. Since the depth of penetration is approximately 1cm, this technique is only useful for superficial structures. Transcutaneous electrical nerve stimulation (TENS) has been used for pain control in more severe regional chronic pain syndromes, though its efficacy remains disputed. Certain electrical stimulation programs, such as 'acupuncture-like TENS', have been advocated as a treatment for myofascial trigger points.

Static splints are useful as a means of protecting an injured extremity in the workplace. These may be prefabricated or custom made. They

PHYSICAL TECHNIQUES FOR THE PREVENTION AND THERAPY OF ARM PAIN IN THE WORKPLACE
Primary and secondary prevention
Worksite ergonomic analysis Careful design of job tasks, tools Risk factor reduction: repetition, high force, awkward posture, vibration, cold or prolonged posture
Initial management: control of pain inflammation
NSAIDs Splint rest or modified duty Local corticosteroid injection Modalities: ice, heat, phonophoresis, iontophoresis
Subsequent management: rehabilitation
Tricyclic antidepressants if neuropathic symptoms, or sleep disturbance Stretching Progressive strengthening Aerobic conditioning Secondary prevention

Fig. 18.10 Physical techniques for the prevention and therapy of arm pain in the workplace.

offer support and decrease repetitive forceful exertions, resulting in rest of the injured area. In an acutely inflamed joint or tendon, this rest reduces inflammation. In chronic cases with soft tissue or pericapsular restrictions to active motion, a dynamic splint may improve range of motion.

Therapeutic exercise remains the cornerstone of treatment. Stretching of the involved area, as well as other nearby postural muscle groups such as the neck, upper back and shoulders, should be performed several times a day. Stretching should be slow, sustained and held for several seconds. Isometric strengthening (which results in no change in muscle length) is indicated when joint range of motion is limited or painful. In most cases, this should progress to isotonic or isokinetic strengthening. Progressively increasing both the number of repetitions and the amount of resistance should further increase strength. Upper extremity muscular endurance may be promoted by aerobic conditioning on an upper body ergometer.

Job modifications are critical to prevent the risk of recurrence. The goal is to decrease the work-related risk factors which predispose to the development of these injuries. These include:

- repetition,
- high force,
- awkward posture or joint position,
- environmental factors such as vibration or cold and
- prolonged time in one position.

To accomplish this, ideally an onsite ergonomic evaluation should be performed. Posture, seat height, lighting, tool design and biomechanics of task performance are examples of factors that can be evaluated and adjusted. Further retraining in a setting supervised by an experienced occupational therapist can be accomplished in an occupational rehabilitation program. At all stages, close communication with the employer is imperative.

CONCLUSIONS

The prevention and management of arm pain in the workplace is complex. Medication, judicious use of injection, physical modalities, splinting, exercise, functional retraining, job analysis, risk factor reduction and good communication between physician, therapist and employer are crucial. Early intervention may prevent progression to more severe disability. Ultimately, prevention through proper ergonomic analysis and design of job tasks is the most effective means of reducing the prevalence of these disorders.

REFERENCES

Falkenburg SA, Schultz DJ. Ergonomics for the upper extremity. Hand Clin. 1993;9:263–71.

Guidotti TL. Occupational repetitive strain injury. Am Fam Physician. 1992;45:585–92.

Johnson SJ. Therapy of the occupationally injured hand and upper extremity. Hand Clin. 1993;9:289–98.

Johnson SJ. Ergonomic hand tool design. Hand Clin. 1993;9:299–311.

Rempel DM, Harrison RJ, Barnhart S. Work-related cumulative trauma disorders of the upper extremity. JAMA. 1992;267: 838–42.

5

RHEUMATOID ARTHRITIS AND OTHER SYNOVIAL DISORDERS

Ravinder N Maini & Nathan J Zvaifler

RHEUMATOID ARTHRITIS

1

HISTORY

Poul Halberg

Definition

- A common, severe inflammatory disorder, affecting men and women of all ages, with a peak incidence in young adults and premenopausal women.
- A disease of multifactorial origin, including a genetic predisposition, and characterized by immune-driven, chronic inflammation.
- Marked by a variable course, involving exacerbations and remissions of disease activity. Many cases are chronic and progressive, resulting in severe disability and sometimes death.

Clinical features

- Rheumatoid factors are detectable in the serum in most cases.
- Main target organ is the synovial lining of joints, bursae and tendon sheaths.
- Synovitis results in erosion of articular cartilage and marginal bone, with subsequent joint destruction.
- Extra-articular features are common, numerous and sometimes serious. Most are due to serositis, nodule (granuloma) formation or vasculitis.

INTRODUCTION

The name rheumatoid arthritis (RA) was coined in 1859 by Garrod [1]. However, compared with today's use of the word it was a misnomer since it included not only inflammatory polyarthritis but also polyarticular osteoarthritis. In 1922 the term covered only inflammatory polyarthritis [2], and in 1958 the seronegative arthritides, for example psoriatic arthritis, were excluded from the term [3]. The concept of a disease entity changes continuously, influenced by advances in knowledge and by 'splitters' and 'lumpers' of syndromes. Many clinicians feel that even the modern classification of RA includes more than one disease entity.

Since the name RA is relatively new and since the content of the word has already changed a great deal during its existence it is difficult to know for sure whether or not RA has been in existence in the past under different names. On the other hand, few diseases are truly new, and usually some evidence will show that even newly described diseases actually have been in existence for a long time, although they were included in other entities. However, Snorrason [4] and other authors [5,6] have argued that RA may, after all, be a new disease since no convincing descriptions of the disease dating from before the year 1800 or, possibly, before the end of the 17th century, have been found. However, the issue remains controversial. During the past few years the discussion has been renewed as a consequence of American skeletal findings indicating that RA may have existed in the New World 3000–5000 years ago. It has been suggested that, like syphilis, RA may have crossed the Atlantic Ocean after 1492 [7]. This possibility is not only of historical, but also of epidemiologic interest since it raises the possibility of an environmental factor in the etiology of RA.
Several attempts have been made to estimate the age of RA, mainly by scrutinizing medical and nonmedical literature, visual arts and paleopathologic findings. Using such methods it has been established, beyond doubt, that ankylosing spondylitis, gout and osteoarthritis have existed for several thousand years.

EVIDENCE OF THE HISTORY OF RHEUMATOID ARTHRITIS

MEDICAL LITERATURE

The first entirely convincing description of RA was published in the year 1800 by Landré-Beauvais. He named the disease 'la goutte asthénique primitive', and he felt that it had not been described previously. His thesis has been reviewed and commented by Snorrason [5] and Short [6]. It describes nine patients all of whom were women, which the authors considered significant because of the male predominance among the sufferers of gout, the most important differential diagnosis. It has been suggested that gout was common in former times as a result of lead intoxication originating from the use of lead-containing cooking pots and water pipes [9] and from drinking wine contaminated with lead salts, which were used at the time to stop the fermentation. The patients described by Landré-Beauvais were asthenic persons, unlike the robust and wealthy persons who were mostly afflicted with gout. Furthermore the 'new disease' started as a polyarthritis, not as an episodic monarthritis the way gout usually does. According to Landré-Beauvais the new disease caused permanent swelling of the joints and deformities, and, after several years, some patients became severely disabled. Autopsy showed ulcers of the cartilage, bone destructions and osteopenia, but no tophi. It was known at the time that tophi contained sodium urate. Shortly after the thesis of Landré-Beauvais several other convincing descriptions of RA were published (Fig. 1.1), one of them by Brodie who also, unequivocally, described Reiter's disease in several patients almost 100 years before Reiter's case history. It is possible that RA was recognized in 1676 by Sydenham [6,9] who mentioned a joint disease characterized by chronicity and deformities, possibly including swan neck deformities, suggestive of RA. In 1703 Musgrave [9] described a chronic polyarthritis which, he felt, was different from gout and rheumatic fever, and Heberden may have known the disease near the end of the 18th century [9]. Snorrason [4] and Short [6] referred to various types of joint disorders described by a number of classical Greek and Roman authors without finding a convincing description of RA. Galen, for example, refers to 'rheumatism', a generalized arthritis with deformities and disability suggestive of RA [10]. However, he also stated that everybody affected by this illness had previously suffered from gout [11], and his description of 'rheumatism' is compatible with chronic, polyarticular gout.

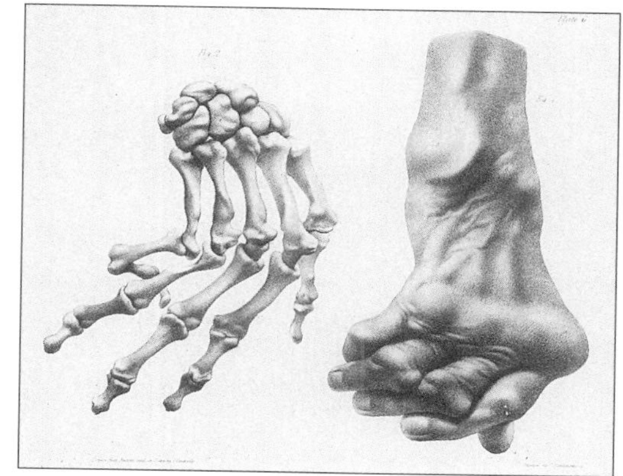

Fig. 1.1 A drawing from the atlas of Robert Adams, published in 1857, showing changes typical of rheumatoid arthritis.

NONMEDICAL LITERATURE

The nonmedical literature before 1800 includes a number of descriptions of arthritis most of which are suggestive of gout. However, a few exceptions have been highlighted in recent papers about the antiquity of RA. Madame de Sevigne, who died in 1696, has described her own joint disorder in her letters [12]. The disease had several features suggestive of RA, and according to the reviewers it satisfied the criteria of the American Rheumatism Association for the classification of RA. The Byzantine emperor Constantine IX who died in 1055 was severely affected by a chronic, polyarticular, deforming and increasingly disabling joint disorder [13]. The disease, which was described by a courtier, started in the feet, and the condition was subject to bouts of severe aggravation. The reviewer felt that the emperor probably had RA. However, chronic polyarticular gout cannot be excluded.

VISUAL ARTS

Several authors have emphasized the lack of evidence of RA in the visual arts dating from before 1800 [4,6], which they felt argued in favor of the concept that the disease might be of recent origin. This has stimulated other authors to search for pictures showing abnormalities indicative of RA. Flemish paintings from 1400–1700 turned out to be a particularly fertile field for such investigations because the Flemish painters made many portraits and had a keen feeling for details, which they reproduced in a seemingly very realistic manner [14]. Once the search had been started several new examples were found in a number of European countries. The issue was reviewed in 1987 [15]. One of the first examples found was a picture by Justus van Gent showing Federico da Montefeltro who died in 1482. The condottiere from Urbino is shown wearing his armour and reading a book. His hands are distinctly shown and reveal swelling of the metacarpophalangeal (MCP) joints of his left hand. Botticello in 1483 painted a young man with his right hand on his chest. The fingers are deformed in a way which is very suggestive of RA. Erasmus from Rotterdam, who died in 1536, was painted by Quinten Metsys. Erasmus is shown writing, with swelling of three MCP joints clearly visible on his right hand. Written sources also relate that Erasmus suffered from joint disease. Jacob Jordaen, who died in 1678, painted his own family and included the maid servant whose hands show symmetrical swelling of MCP and proximal interphalangeal (PIP) joints very suggestive of RA (see Chapter 1.1). Rubens was much troubled by a joint disease which is usually interpreted as gout. However, several of his paintings show hand deformities compatible with RA, possibly reflecting his own disease which may have been RA rather than gout [16]. These are only a few of a considerable number of examples of changes compatible with RA in the visual arts described in recent literature. The changes often look very convincing to the rheumatologist, but some art historians caution against overinterpretation [17]. Although the works of art mentioned seemingly show realistic features, such representations differ profoundly from accurate scientific illustrations made for the purpose of showing particular details. In contrast to the latter, artistic representations are subject to artistic conventions and individual interpretations, which may easily cause distortions of normal anatomy. Consequently, the risk of overdiagnosing rheumatic changes is a very real one. When looking at the paintings with this warning in mind the evidence in favor of RA seems somewhat doubtful.

PALEOPATHOLOGY

Until recently it was accepted by most workers that even though spondylitis, osteoarthritis and gout could be identified in skeletons dated as far back as 4000 years or more, unequivocal evidence of RA had not been found in material from before the 18th century. This impression may have to be modified because new information has been forthcoming within the past few years. The skeletal remains of archaic Indians found in Alabama date back to precolumbian time and indicate symmetrical, erosive polyarthritis in small and large back joints. Such changes were found in 36 of more than 8000 skeletons in 8 of 72 sites examined [7,18]. The joint erosions described were distributed to the margins of bones, symmetrically involving diarthrodial joints, especially the MCP, metatarsophalangeal (MTP) and PIP joints, the carpus, and the ulna styloid, which was occasionally completely destroyed. Similar erosions were found in the shoulders and in some other large joints, but the distal interphalangeal (DIP) joints were not involved. The lesions were found to be similar to the changes of contemporary rheumatoid skeletons. Radiologic examinations were performed with the bones positioned in routine anatomic views. Periarticular osteopenia and marginal erosions indistinguishable from the abnormalities noted in routine rheumatology practice were demonstrated. The radiologic examination was less sensitive than the gross examination, especially when applied to the large joints. The erosive changes were more common in women than in men. The sacroiliac joints were normal, and no syndesmophytes, enthesopathies or periostitis were found. Consequently, it was

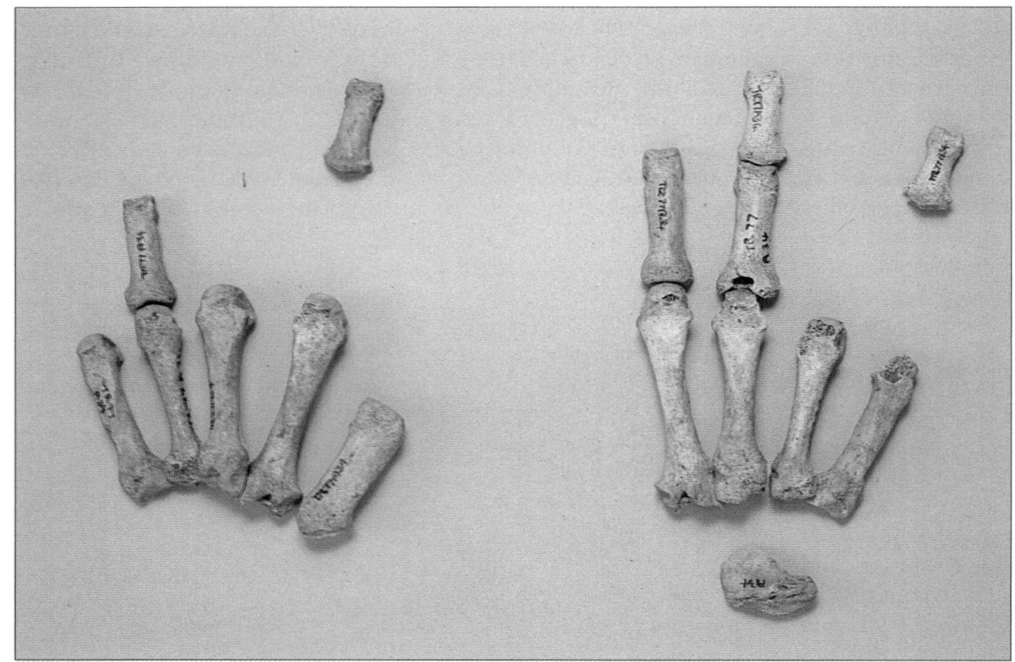

Fig. 1.2 Bones of the hand recovered from a Saxon burial site in England. Erosive changes are present in the right middle finger MCP joint. This skeleton illustrates some of the problems encountered in making diagnoses from old bones; only 30% of the skeleton was recovered and some of the bones were badly damaged during excavation, making it impossible to obtain a clear idea of the pattern of distribution of the arthropathy. Courtesy of Dr J Rogers.

felt that the lesions demonstrated represented RA, and that seronegative arthropathy was an unlikely interpretation.

Bone changes felt to be compatible with RA were found in two neolithic skeletons from Gotland, Sweden [19]. Both were males, the changes were asymmetric in one skeleton and the abnormalities included ankylosed joints and periostitis. Consequently, seronegative arthritis may be another possible interpretation of the findings. An English study involving 800 skeletons from an archeological excavation showed very few erosive changes, and lesions compatible with RA were found in only one skeleton [20]. The interpretation of such findings has not remained unchallenged. The diagnosis of RA based on examination of ancient skeletons remains controversial (Figs 1.2 & 1.3). The most important controversy concerns the nature of the cortical defects; these are interpreted as erosions by some investigators and this is disputed by others [21].

CONCLUSION

The hypothesis that RA may have originated in the 19th century has been refuted by evidence for the existence of the disease before the first generally accepted description of the disease in the year 1800. However, no completely convincing observations make it necessary to give up the idea that RA is a new disease, at any rate as far as the Old World is concerned. The recent American paleopathological observations may indicate a different situation in the New World. However, the discussion of how to interpret these findings is not yet over. The hypothesis that RA is a new disease rests exclusively on negative evidence, which is less convincing than positive evidence. The failure to produce convincing proof that RA existed before the year 1800 may well be caused by inadequate material for examination rather than the absence of the disease. On the other hand, if it could be proved that RA is really a new disease the situation would be an almost unique one in human pathology. If it is eventually possible to interpret the paleopathological observations, this may be the most fruitful field for further research.

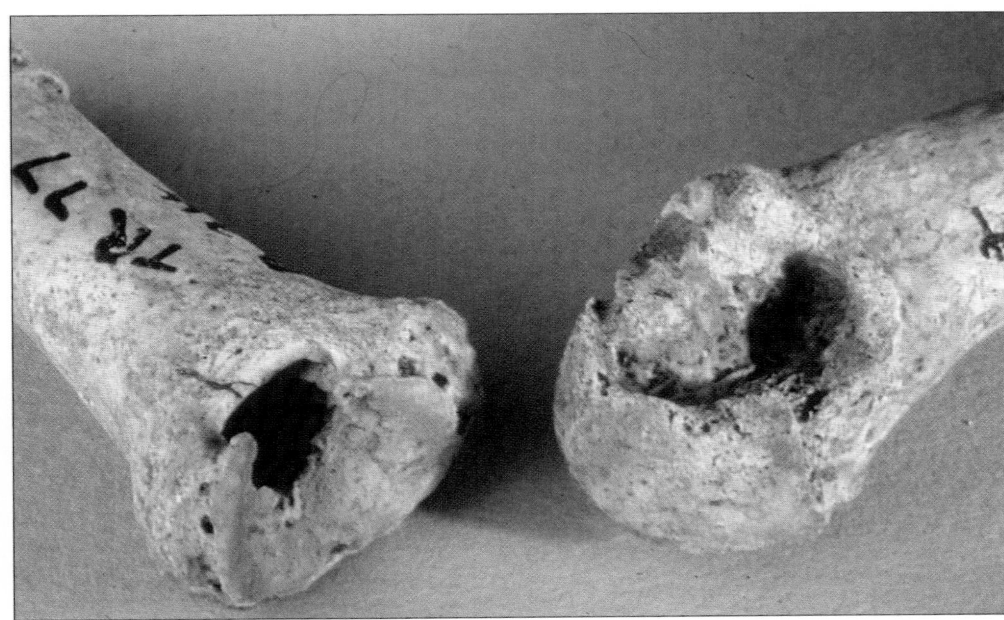

Fig. 1.3 The typical appearances of erosive changes in old skeletal material. The remodeling of the bone in and around the defect indicates long-standing antemortem changes, clearly distinguishing these lesions from postmortem bone damage. Although the erosion is compatible with RA, no diagnosis was possible in this case since no other skeletal lesions were identified. Courtesy of Dr J Rogers.

REFERENCES

1. Garrod AB. The nature and treatment of gout and rheumatoid gout. London: Walton and Maberley;1859.
2. Parish LC. A historical approach to the nomenclature of rheumatoid arthritis. Arthritis Rheum. 1963;6:138–58.
3. Ropes MW, Bennett GA, Cobb S, *et al.* 1958 revision of the diagnostic criteria for rheumatoid arthritis. Bull Rheum Dis. 1958;9:175–6.
4. Snorrason E. Landré-Beauvais and his goutte asthenique primitive. Acta Med Scand. 1952;142 (suppl. 266):115–8.
5. Boyle JA, Buchanan WW. In: FA Davis, ed. Clinical rheumatology. Philadelphia: Lippincott; 1971:71–2.
6. Short CL. The antiquity of rheumatoid arthritis. Arthritis Rheum. 1974;17:193–205.
7. Rothschild BM, Woods RJ. Symmetrical erosive disease in archaic indians: The origin of rheumatoid in the New World. Semin Arthritis Rheum. 1990;19:278–84.
8. Wedeen RP. Poison in the pot. The legacy of lead. Carbondale and Edwardsville: Southern Illinois University Press; 1984.
9. Fraser KJ. Anglo-French contributions to the recognition of rheumatoid arthritis. Ann Rheum Dis. 1982;41:335–43.
10. Dieppe PA. Did Galen describe rheumatoid arthritis? Ann Rheum Dis. 1988;47:84–5.
11. Lopes Ferez JA. Rheumatism, arthritis and gout in Galen. In: Appelboom T, ed. Art, history and antiquity of rheumatic diseases. Elsevier: Brussels; 1987;84.
12. Tamisier JN, Thomas P, Brury B. Retrospective diagnosis of Mme De Sevigne's rheumatoid condition. In: Appelboom T, ed. Art, history and antiquity of rheumatic diseases. Elsevier: Brussels; 1987:78.
13. Caughey DE. The arthritis of Constantin IX. Ann Rheum Dis. 1974;33:77–80.
14. Dequeker J. Arthritis in Flemish paintings (1400–1700). Br Med J. 1977:1:1203–5.

15. Dequeker J. Rheumatic diseases in visual arts. General review. In: Appelboom T, ed. Art, history and antiquity of rheumatic diseases. Elsevier: Brussels;1987:84.
16. Appelboom T, de Boelpaepe C, Eherlich GE, *et al.* Rubens and the question of antiquity of rheumatoid arthritis. JAMA. 1981:245:483–6.
17. Philippot P. Stylistic and documentary understanding of fine arts. In: Appelboom T, ed. Art, history and antiquity of rheumatoid diseases. Elsevier: Brussels; 1987:12.
18. Rothschild BM, Woods RJ, Rothschild C, Sebes JI. Geographic distribution of rheumatoid arthritis in ancient North America: Implications for pathogenesis. Sem. Arthritis Rheum. 1992;22:181–7.
19. Leden I, Persson E, Persson O. Aspects of the history of rheumatoid arthritis in the light of recent osteoarcheological finds. Scand J Rheumatol. 1988;17:341–52.
20. Dieppe PA, Heywood A, Rogers J, Waldron T, Watt I. The paleopathology of rheumatic diseases. In: Appelboom, T, ed. Art, history and antiquity of rheumatic diseases. Elsevier: Brussels;1987:109.
21. Rogers J, Dieppe PA. Skeletal paleopathology and the rheumatic diseases: Where are we now? Ann Rheum Dis. 1990;49:885–6.

CLASSIFICATION AND EPIDEMIOLOGY

Alex J MacGregor & Alan J Silman

- Rheumatoid arthritis has an annual incidence of approximately 0.1–0.2/1000 in males and 0.2–0.4/1000 in females.
- A prevalence of 0.5–1% is reported in diverse populations worldwide, though a higher prevalence has been reported in certain Native Americans and the disease is reported to be absent in parts of rural Africa.
- A genetic influence is suggested by a fourfold increase in concordance in monozygotic compared with dizygotic twins; genes encoding HLA molecules have an important contribution this genetic risk.
- Hormonal and reproductive factors contribute to the female excess and parity, breast feeding and exogenous hormones have been implicated in determining susceptibility.
- No other single factor in the external environment shows a clear or consistent association with the disease.

CLASSIFICATION OF RHEUMATOID ARTHRITIS

The currently accepted classification scheme for rheumatoid arthritis (RA) is the 1987 American College of Rheumatology (ACR) criteria set. The scheme is published in two formats: as a 'traditional' list (Fig. 2.1) and as a classification tree (Fig. 2.2)[1]. The 1987 criteria set was developed to replace the existing classification schemes which had not been revised since the 1960s. Earlier criteria sets defined RA with various degrees of certainty as 'classic', 'definite', 'probable' and 'possible' disease. This ambiguity was removed in the new criteria set in which only the single disease 'rheumatoid arthritis' is now designated. Earlier schemes also had a number of impractical features, including the need for invasive procedures such as synovial biopsy.

The 1987 ACR criteria set was developed using data from patients who attended hospital outpatient clinics and is most efficient at distinguishing active RA from other inflammatory arthritides. In such settings, validation studies have shown both the traditional and classification tree formats to be accurate in classifying disease against the 'gold standard' of physician diagnosis, with a sensitivity in the range 77–95% and specificity in the range 85–98%[2].

In contrast to studies based in hospital clinic settings, epidemiologic studies of RA have additional requirements for case definition[3]. Population surveys require criteria that have the ability to ascertain currently inactive disease. Prospective studies require classification criteria sets that are sensitive to the presence of early disease. Evidence suggests that the 1987 ACR criteria set has important limitations when used for case recognition in both these circumstances. Its limitations in cross-sectional studies stem from the failure to include features of inactive but established RA in the criteria set as it is formulated in Figure 2.1. There are no accepted criteria for 'early RA'.

An early attempt to define criteria for epidemiologic studies which included inactive RA (the 'New York' criteria) failed to gain widespread acceptance because the criteria were too complex and failed to specify a cut-off to indicate the presence of disease[3]. An adapted

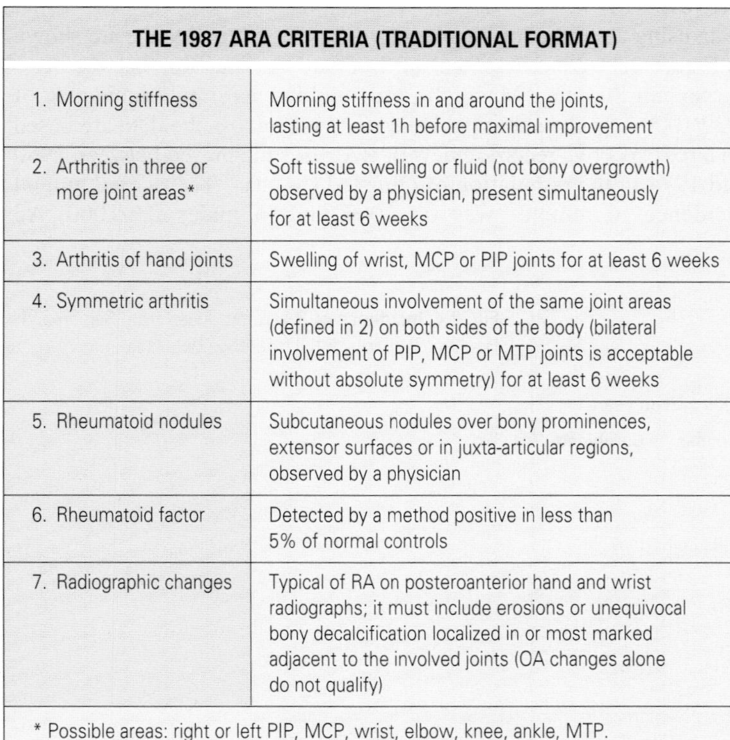

THE 1987 ARA CRITERIA (TRADITIONAL FORMAT)	
1. Morning stiffness	Morning stiffness in and around the joints, lasting at least 1h before maximal improvement
2. Arthritis in three or more joint areas*	Soft tissue swelling or fluid (not bony overgrowth) observed by a physician, present simultaneously for at least 6 weeks
3. Arthritis of hand joints	Swelling of wrist, MCP or PIP joints for at least 6 weeks
4. Symmetric arthritis	Simultaneous involvement of the same joint areas (defined in 2) on both sides of the body (bilateral involvement of PIP, MCP or MTP joints is acceptable without absolute symmetry) for at least 6 weeks
5. Rheumatoid nodules	Subcutaneous nodules over bony prominences, extensor surfaces or in juxta-articular regions, observed by a physician
6. Rheumatoid factor	Detected by a method positive in less than 5% of normal controls
7. Radiographic changes	Typical of RA on posteroanterior hand and wrist radiographs; it must include erosions or unequivocal bony decalcification localized in or most marked adjacent to the involved joints (OA changes alone do not qualify)

* Possible areas: right or left PIP, MCP, wrist, elbow, knee, ankle, MTP.

Fig. 2.1 The 1987 ARA criteria (traditional format). At least four criteria must be fulfilled for classification as RA; patients with two clinical diagnoses are not excluded. Reproduced from Arnett *et al.*[1].

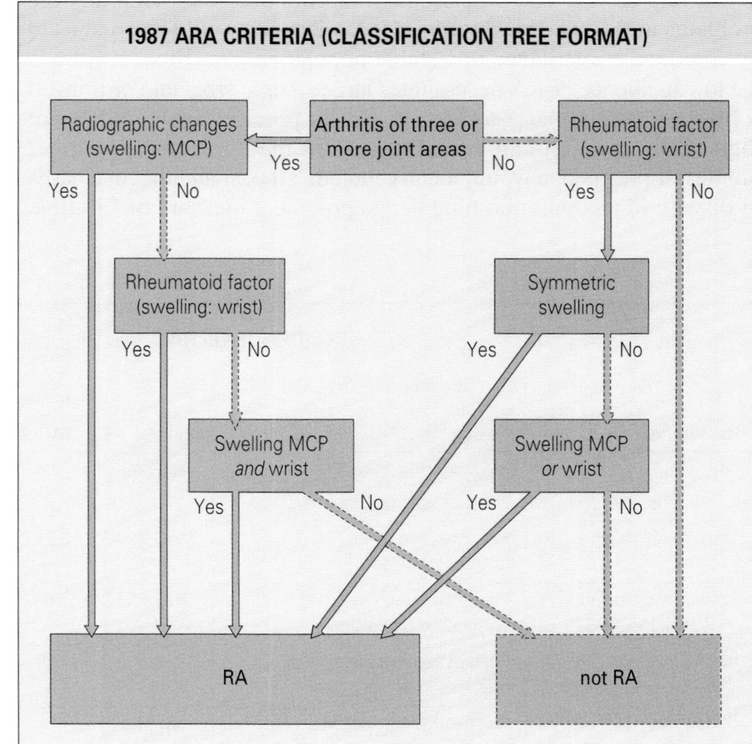

Fig. 2.2 1987 ARA criteria (classification tree format). Variables in parentheses can be used when data on the first listed variable is unavailable. Reproduced from Arnett *et al.*[1] and MacGregor[3].

FORMAT FOR APPLICATION OF THE 1987 ARA CRITERIA TO POPULATION AND FAMILY STUDIES	
1 Morning stiffness	Morning stiffness in and around the joints lasting at least 1h before maximal improvement at any time in the disease course
2 Arthritis in at least three joint areas*	Soft tissue swelling or fluid observed by a physician, with swelling at current examination or deformity and a documented history of swelling
3 Arthritis of hands	Swelling of wrist, MCP or PIP joints with swelling at current examination or deformity and a documented history of swelling
4 Symmetric arthritis	Simultaneous involvement of the same joint areas (defined in 2) on both sides of the body (bilateral involvement of PIP, MCP or MTP joints is acceptable without absolute symmetry) with swelling at current examination or deformity and a documented history of swelling
5 Rheumatoid nodules	Over bony prominences, extensor surfaces or in juxta-articular regions, observed by a physician and present at current examination or documented in the past
6 Rheumatoid factor	By a method positive in less than 5% of normal controls at current examination or documented to have been positive in the past by any assay method
7 Radiograph changes	Typical of RA on posteroanterior hand and wrist radiographs; it must include erosions or unequivocal bony decalcification localized in or most marked adjacent to the involved joints (OA changes alone do not qualify)
*Possible areas: right or left PIP, MCP, wrist, elbow, knee. ankle, MTP.	

Fig. 2.3 Format for application of the 1987 ARA criteria to population and family studies. At least four criteria must be fulfilled for classification as RA. Reproduced from Arnett *et al.*[1] and MacGregor[3].

version of the current 1987 criteria set is, however, an effective alternative (see Fig. 2.3). These adapted criteria additionally ascertain inactive RA by allowing joint deformity to substitute for joint swelling and by accepting historical data on the past occurrence of rheumatoid factor (RF) and rheumatoid nodules. The criteria in this format are sufficiently sensitive to allow their use in population studies of RA[3].

DISEASE OCCURRENCE

Disease occurrence is assessed through two measures: incidence (the rate of new cases arising in a given period) and prevalence (the number of existing cases). The measurement of both presents methodologic problems in RA. The ideal study of RA incidence would be conducted by continual surveillance of a stable population over time. However, the low incidence of RA necessitates large sample sizes and prolonged follow-up for estimates to be statistically precise. Such studies are logistically difficult and are infrequent in the published literature. Studies of prevalence would ideally include all past and inactive cases of disease in a population (and hence provide a measure of 'lifetime cumulative prevalence'). As discussed earlier, for a study to recognize remitted disease requires the use of criteria specifically designed for this purpose. In practice it is frequently difficult to establish the extent to which remitted disease has been included in published reports.

Direct comparisons of published data of RA occurrence are problematic because of the need to take into account differences in the sensitivity and specificity of criteria sets used at the time of the study. In addition, the incidence and severity of RA may be declining and the disease may be entering remission earlier after treatment. Hence older prevalence estimates may be less relevant to the contemporary pattern of occurrence of the disease.

INCIDENCE

Data using a number of approaches to assess RA incidence are shown in Figure 2.4[4]. An assessment of 'interval' cases arising between two surveys in Sudbury, Massachusetts, yielded an annual incidence of 0.29/1000 [5]. In the study published by Linos *et al.*, the data are based on a retrospective record review of RA cases diagnosed between 1950 and 1974 in the population of Olmsted County[6]. The overall annual incidence in females was 0.5/1000 and in males 0.2/1000. An

INCIDENCE OF RA

Researcher	Design	Year	Incidence/1000 person years: Males	Females	Combined
O'Sullivan *et al.*, 1968	Interval cases developing between two cross-sectional surveys	1964–1965	–	0.29	–
Linos *et al.*, 1980	Retrospective review of hospital attendants	1950–1974	0.22	0.48	0.37
Royal College of General Practitioners, 1979	Prospective recording of new episodes in primary care	1970–1972	1.63	4.20	2.99
Royal College of General Practitioners, 1986	Prospective recording of new episodes in primary care	1981–1982	1.50	3.34	2.47
Dugowson, 1991	Prospective notification of new referrals	1987–1989	–	0.24	
Symmons *et al.*, 1992	Prospective monitoring of community ascertained cases	1990	0.15	0.36	

Fig. 2.4 Incidence of RA. Reproduced from Silman and Hochberg[4] (in which full reference details are given).

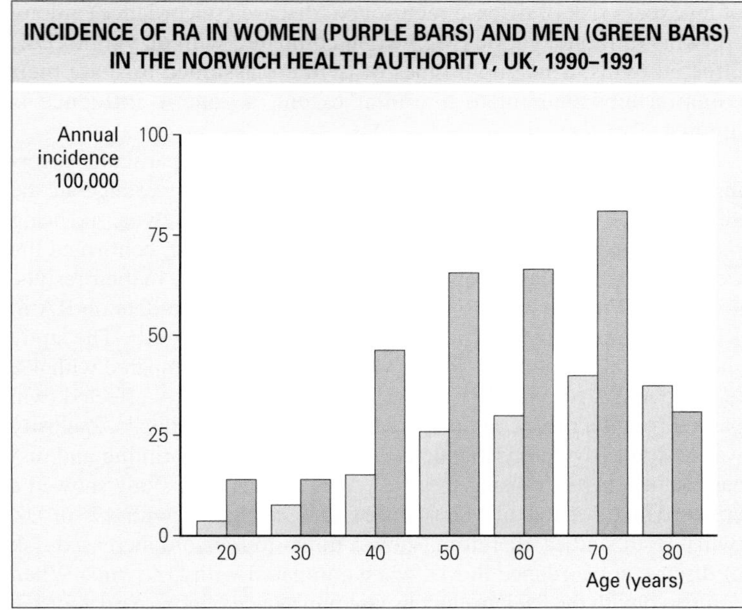

Fig. 2.5 Incidence of RA in women (green bars) and men (purple bars) in the Norwich Health Authority, UK, 1990–1991. Adapted from Symmons *et al.*[8].

There have been two recent prospective studies of RA incidence. Dugowson *et al.* identified new cases of RA that occurred in women attending a health maintenance organization in Seattle, Washington, between 1987 and 1989[7]. The overall annual RA incidence (adjusted to the 1980 US population) was 0.24/1000. The incidence was shown to increase with increasing age. Symmons *et al.* derived incidence figures from data collected from a population register in Norfolk, UK[8]. This study is unique among incidence studies in RA in that all the cases of inflammatory polyarthritis that presented to general and hospital practitioners were ascertained. RA was classified using the 1987 criteria. In the first year of the register (1990) the annual incidence of RA in females was 0.36/1000, compared with 0.14/1000 in males. The incidence in males rose sharply with age. In contrast to the Rochester and Seattle data, the incidence in females reached a plateau between the ages of 45 and 75 years and declined at older ages (Fig. 2.5).

PREVALENCE

There have been a number of large contemporary studies of RA prevalence based on cross-sectional population samples (Fig. 2.6)[4]. In caucasian, European and North American populations RA prevalence ranges from 0.5 to 2% in those aged over 15 years. Most studies show a female to male excess of between 2 and 4 times. In all studies, age-specific prevalence rates rise with age, which reflects that these studies have measured the cumulative lifetime risk of disease for individuals in the population.

increasing incidence rate with age was observed which continued into the seventh decade. The female rate was higher than the male rate at all ages, with the greatest female excess occurring in those under 50 years.

GEOGRAPHIC VARIATION

Remarkably similar estimates of RA prevalence have been obtained from diverse population groups worldwide (Fig. 2.6)[4]. Several estimates of

PREVALENCE OF RA

Researcher	Population	*N*	Prevalence of definite RA (%)		
			Males	Females	Combined
African					
Beighton *et al.*, 1975	Rural Tswana, South Africa	801	–	0.1	–
Solomon *et al.*, 1975	Urban Soweto, South Africa	964	nil	1.4	0.9
Moolenburgh *et al.*, 1986	Lesotho	1070	nil	0.4	0.3
Silman *et al.*, 1986	Igbo-ora, Nigeria	2000	nil	nil	nil
Asian and Far Eastern					
Schichikawa *et al.*, 1981	Kamitonda, Japan	2276	–	0.3	–
Beasley *et al.*, 1983	Kinmet, China	5629	0.2	0.4	0.3
Darmawan, 1988	Java, Indonesia	4683	–	0.2	–
Symmons *et al.*, 1986	Hong Kong	2002	–	–	0.3
European and North American Caucasian					
Lawrence, 1961	Leigh and Wensleydale, UK	2324	0.5	1.6	1.1
Engel and Burch, 1968	US adults	6672	0.5	1.7	1.0
Cathcart and O'Sullivan, 1970	US whites	4552	–	–	0.9
Sorenson, 1973	National sample, Denmark	19,100	0.3	1.2	0.8
Recht *et al.*, 1989	Sjobo, Sweden	5262	–	0.6	–
Aho *et al.*, 1989	Heinola, Finland	8000	–	5.3	–
Mau *et al.*, 1991	Hanover, Germany	11,534	–	–	0.5
Native American					
Oen *et al.*, 1986	Inuit Eskimo, Canada	2055	–	0.6	–
Boyer *et al.*, 1988	Yupik Eskimo	4600	0.2	1.0	0.6
Del Puente, 1989	Pima Indians, USA	1449	–	5.3	–
Boyer *et al.*, 1988	Southeast Alaskan Indians	5169	1.3	3.5	2.4
Middle Eastern					
Al-Rawi *et al.*, 1978	Iraq	6999	–	–	1.0
Pountain, 1991	Oman	1925	–	–	0.8

Fig. 2.6 Prevalence of RA. Reproduced from Silman and Hochberg[4] (in which full reference details are given).

between 0.5–1% have been obtained in studies across Europe, North America, Asia and South Africa. There are, however, notable exceptions. Certain native North American Indians, including the Pima, Yakima and Chippewa, have a high prevalence of disease at approximately 5%. This excess is not seen in other North American Indians, such as the Blackfeet and Haida[4]. By contrast, RA appears to be exceptionally rare in rural African black populations, and in both rural and urban Chinese groups. The relative influences of genetic and environmental factors on this geographic variation in prevalence are discussed later.

TIME TRENDS

A number of studies have examined whether the incidence of RA has changed over time[4,9]. Data from a population register in Finland showed that the incidence of registered seropositive RA remained static in that country between the years 1970 and 1980. In other populations the incidence of RA appears to be declining. In the Rochester Epidemiology Program, data relating to disease incidence between 1950 and 1975 showed a declining incidence in females from approximately 1960 onwards[6]. During that time the incidence in males remained stable. A similar trend in females was seen in the UK Royal College of General Practitioners Morbidity Study (Fig. 2.7)[9]. More recently, in a study of Pima Indians Jacobsson *et al.* observed a halving of the incidence of RA in both males and females in the 25 years between 1965 and 1990[10].

The severity of RA may also be declining over time, although the available evidence suggests that the nature of this change is complex. In an analysis of the features of disease severity in successive birth cohorts of patients, Silman *et al.* showed that there was a peak in erosive, seropositive and nodular disease in individuals presenting with RA in the 1960s, but a decline in the severity of disease in generations presenting subsequently[11].

GENETIC FACTORS

TWIN AND FAMILY STUDIES

Several studies have demonstrated a small but consistently increased risk of disease in siblings of individuals affected with RA[4]. Such data indicate that either shared genetic or shared environmental factors contribute to disease. Compelling evidence to support a genetic influence comes from twin studies in which there are a number of reports of an excess risk of disease recurrence (disease concordance) among co-twins of monozygotic (MZ) when compared with dizygotic (DZ) affected twins. Since both types of twin are assumed to share their common environment to a similar extent, a genetic influence is implied.

Twin studies are prone to biased ascertainment, in particular favoring inclusion of disease concordant MZ pairs, which may exaggerate the genetic risk. Two recent studies based on large groups of twins and using rigorous methods of case ascertainment have, however, confirmed the excess MZ concordance for RA with striking similarity in their results. A study in Finland by Aho *et al.* examined population data on RA in 13,299 twin pairs using a national record linkage system[12]. The study showed a concordance for RA in MZ twins of 12% compared with 4% in DZ pairs. A recent study in the UK recruited 203 RA-affected twin pairs through a media campaign and from hospital clinics[13]. Zygosity was assigned by deoxyribonucleic acid (DNA) fingerprinting and disease status classified using the 1987 ACR criteria. The study showed a concordance for RA in MZ twins of 15% compared with 4% in DZ twins. Both studies, therefore, show a three- to fourfold increased risk of disease concordance in MZ when compared with DZ twins. When compared with the background disease prevalence of approximately 1% in nonrelatives, these twin concordance data indicate that genetic factors have a substantial contribution to the disease risk.

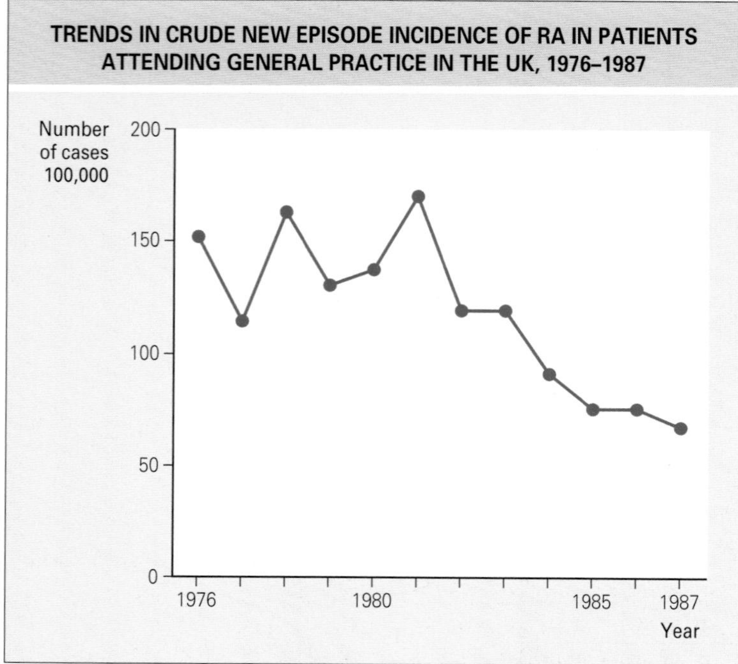

Fig. 2.7 Trends in crude new episode incidence of RA in patients attending general practice in the UK, 1976–1987. Adapted from Silman[9].

GENETIC MARKERS

Evidence that suggests familial and twin clustering is at least in part genetic in origin is strongly supported by the finding that genetic markers are associated with the disease. Stastny's report of an increased frequency of HLA-DR4 among patients with severe RA provided the first evidence of such an association[14]. The association between RA and HLA has since been refined to alleles coding for a 'shared epitope' on the HLA-DRB1 molecule. The nature of the human leukocyte antigen (HLA) association is discussed in detail in Chapter 5.7. The epidemiologic significance of these findings is that the variation in the population prevalence of 'shared epitope'-encoding alleles can, to some extent, explain the heterogeneity in the geographic distribution of RA and suggests a genetic basis for this variation. The role of any non-HLA genes revealed through linkage studies in multicase families will also need to be tested in population association studies.

INFLUENCE ON DISEASE SUSCEPTIBILITY AND SEVERITY

There remains a question over the extent to which genetic factors determine an individual's susceptibility to RA *per se* or to the severity of the disease once it develops. While there is a clear association with HLA in individuals with established disease who attend hospital clinics, a similar association has failed to be seen in data from two community-based studies. This suggests that HLA may have a greater influence on disease severity. It is of interest that recently published data from the Norfolk Arthritis Register, UK, have failed to show significant familial clustering of RA among first-degree relatives of cases of established RA ascertained in the community[15]. Several studies of RA patients also show that HLA alleles are more strongly associated with features of severe disease, such as seropositivity for RF, erosions and nodules[16]. The genetic influence on disease features is, however, not clear cut. Monozygotic twins and sibling pairs concordant for RA show enormous diversity in features of disease severity such as joint erosions and degree of disability[17].

HOST FACTORS

REPRODUCTIVE AND ENDOCRINE FACTORS

The greater female incidence of RA, which is apparent before the menopause (see Fig. 2.5), suggests an influence of reproductive and hormonal factors in conferring risk. Epidemiologic interest has focused on the influence of pregnancy itself, on risk factors such as breastfeeding in the postpartum period and on the role of endogenous and exogenous hormones.

Nulliparity has been suggested as a risk factor for RA from the results of several case-control studies. This association, however, is inconsistent and continues to be disputed: no association with nulliparity was found in recently published data from a large prospective cohort in Finland[18]. If there is an association with nulliparity, it is difficult to determine epidemiologically whether this reflects an increased risk of infertility prior to the development of RA or a protective effect of pregnancy itself. The observations that RA risk is no greater in unmarried than in married women and that family size is similar for patients with RA compared with controls suggest that pregnancy does not have a protective influence overall[4,19].

The relationship between RA and pregnancy is likely to prove complex. There is evidence to suggest that pregnancy influences the timing of onset of disease. One study showed that the risk of newly developing RA is reduced during pregnancy itself, but increased in the 12 months after delivery[20]. This effect was most apparent after the first pregnancy. Breastfeeding has been proposed as an explanation of the increased risk of RA postpartum. Such an influence is supported by one case-control study of 187 women who developed RA in the first 12 months after pregnancy; exposure to breastfeeding after the first pregnancy increased the risk of RA fivefold[21].

The importance of the timing of pregnancy to susceptibility to RA suggests an influence of endogenous hormones. The available data are, however, limited. Some studies indicate that women with RA have a relative androgen deficiency, with lower levels of testosterone and dehydroepiandrosterone. Males with RA have also been found to have low testosterone levels. It is unclear whether these observations represent a causal relationship or an effect of the disease itself[4].

The influence of exogenous hormones has also been examined, with interest focusing on the use of the oral contraceptive pill (OCP) and hormone replacement therapy. A possible protective influence of OCP use first emerged from a prospective study of 23,000 UK women in whom current pill use was associated with halving of the risk of developing RA[22]. Subsequent studies have, however, produced conflicting results. An attempt to resolve the issue through meta-analysis concluded that OCP use had no influence on RA risk overall, but may postpone the onset of disease[23]. There have been fewer studies of the effect of hormone replacement, but a similarly conflicting picture has emerged.

HOST IMMUNE FUNCTION

Host factors may contribute to disease by altering immune function. A number of autoimmune diseases are recognized to occur more commonly in individuals with RA, including thyroid disease and insulin dependent diabetes. Impairment of host immune defenses was initially proposed as a mechanism to explain two reports of an association between prior lymphoid surgery and RA. These studies, however, had methodologic limitations and a recent carefully designed longitudinal study of RA cases in female patients using community controls failed to confirm the association[4].

EXTERNAL ENVIRONMENT

INFECTIOUS AGENTS

Classic epidemiologic evidence of an infectious etiology for RA has not been forthcoming. Cases of RA do not cluster in space or time. Concordant MZ twins, sibling pairs and spouse couples show very little similarity in the timing of disease onset – similarity would be expected if an infectious agent were the cause. Overcrowding as assessed by sibship size is also not found to be a risk factor.

These observations cannot, however, rule out infection as a potential cause of RA – it is conceivable that an ubiquitous infectious agent may be responsible for the disease in a genetically susceptible host. Plausible biological mechanisms for the action of several specific infectious agents in inducing RA have been suggested by the results of animal models, from the isolation of specific agents from human synovium, and from the existence of homology between the antigenic components of infectious organisms, synovium and cartilage[24].

Attempts to confirm these observations epidemiologically have focused on examining the serologic evidence for past infection. A number of potential associations with infectious agents have been found. Raised titers of antibodies to the Epstein–Barr virus (EBV) have been demonstrated in RA; titers were also shown to be raised prior to disease onset in a small group of patients in one longitudinal study[25]. Antibodies to human parvovirus B19 were also found to be elevated in females with RA in one case-control study[26]. The association with EBV has, however, not been reported consistently across studies and it is conceivable that elevated antibody levels may be a reflection of the disease process itself. Similarly with parvovirus, the observations are not reported consistently and the agent is unlikely to cause disease in the majority. Serologic data have yielded no conclusive evidence of association with a number of other putative infectious triggers, including proteus, cytomegalovirus (CMV), retroviruses, mycoplasma and mycobacteria[23,27]. A reasonable conclusion overall is that there is no current epidemiologic evidence to implicate a single infectious cause.

SOCIOECONOMIC STATUS AND OCCUPATION

Although a number of studies have suggested that adverse socioeconomic status is associated with worse disease outcome in RA, few have examined the influence on disease susceptibility. The available data are conflicting. A US population survey found a lower frequency of RA in males in the highest social groups, whereas a UK study showed a lower frequency in females in the lower social groups[28,29]. Recent data gathered prospectively from the Norfolk Arthritis Register, UK, using more rigorous methods of case definition, have shown no association with social class or other indicators of socioeconomic status[30].

Specific occupations have been implicated as risk factors; however, adequate epidemiologic proof of reported associations is lacking. Early observations of an increased frequency of RA in coal miners were not confirmed in a subsequent formal epidemiologic study. There have been single reports of an increased risk among granite workers and in those working in the fish industry. A recent Swedish survey indicated an increased risk of RA in occupations that involve handling organic solvents[4].

URBAN AND INDUSTRIALIZED ENVIRONMENTS

A more general association between RA and urban industrialized environments has been suggested. In the 1970s, Lawrence proposed that the declining incidence of RF in successive birth cohorts may be related to the decline in atmospheric pollution following the Clean Air Acts in 1956[29]. An influence of urbanization was also suggested in two studies by Solomon *et al.* and Beighton *et al.* which showed the prevalence of RA among Bantu living in urban Johannesburg to be similar to that found in Whites in the industrialized West, but higher than in Bantu living in rural Western Transvaal[31,32].

An association with urbanization has, however, not been confirmed in other population groups. In the Chinese, a similar low prevalence was observed in urban Hong Kong when compared with that in found in rural Kinmet[4]. A recent study of RA prevalence in inner-city Manchester showed a lower prevalence among blacks when compared with whites living in the same area[33].

LIFESTYLE FACTORS

Data on lifestyle factors in RA are limited, provide conflicting information and are difficult to interpret. In case control studies, in particular, it is frequently hard to separate the influence of risk factors on disease activity from their effect on susceptibility. Studies of the influence of diet have shown olive oil consumption to be protective in one retrospective analysis; there is also weak evidence that copper deficiency and selenium deficiency are linked with RA[4]. An increased risk of RA associated with smoking was shown in two prospective studies. The association was also confirmed in a study of twins with RA[34]. As with other potential risk factors, the association with smoking is not consistent with at least one case-control study suggesting a protective effect.

CONCLUSIONS

The currently accepted classification scheme for RA is the 1987 ACR criteria set which may be applied in a traditional or classification tree format. These criteria are both sensitive and specific for recognizing active disease in the setting of hospital clinics, but require modification to recognize past and inactive disease in studies of the epidemiology of RA.

Estimates of RA occurrence suggest the annual incidence is approximately 0.1–0.2/1000 in males and 0.2–0.4/1000 in females. The female excess in incidence is most marked in the premenopausal years. The prevalence of RA is remarkably similar worldwide, with many estimates in diverse populations of between 0.5 and 1%. There are, however, notable exceptions with frequencies of 5% reported in certain native American Indians and an absence of RA reported in rural Nigeria. Both the incidence and severity of RA may be declining with time.

Twin concordance data in RA suggest the disease has a multifactorial etiology with a significant contribution from both genetic and environmental factors. Also, HLA genes have been identified as having an important contribution to the genetic risk, although the extent to which HLA determines disease severity rather than disease susceptibility is still being debated. The HLA association may, to an extent, explain the geographic variation in the prevalence of disease.

The female excess of RA indicates an influence of hormonal and reproductive factors. Parity, breastfeeding and the use of exogenous hormones have been implicated in determining susceptibility to the disease. Studies of a range of other potential environmental influences have, however, been unrevealing. Although it is evident that an environmental influence exists in RA, its precise nature remains elusive.

REFERENCES

1. Arnett FC, Edworthy SM, Bloch DA, *et al.* The American Rheumatism Association 1987 revised criteria for the classification of rheumatoid arthritis. Arthritis Rheum. 1988;31:315–24.
2. Moens HJB, Mart AFJ, van der Laar MAFJ, van der Korst JK. Comparison of the sensitivity and specificity of the 1958 and 1987 criteria for rheumatoid arthritis. J Rheumatol. 1992;19:198–203.
3. MacGregor AJ. Classification criteria for rheumatoid arthritis. Baillière's Clin Rheumatol. 1995;9:287–304.
4. Silman AJ, Hochberg MC. Epidemiology of the rheumatic diseases. Oxford: Oxford University Press; 1993.
5. O'Sullivan JB, Cathcart ES, Bolzan JA. Diagnostic criteria and the incidence of rheumatoid arthritis in Sudbury, Massachusetts. In: Bennett PH, Wood PHN. Population studies of the rheumatic diseases. Amsterdam: Exerpta Medica Foundation; 1968:109–13.
6. Linos A, Worthington JW, O'Fallon WM, Kurland LT. The epidemiology of rheumatoid arthritis in Rochester, Minnesota: a study of the incidence, prevalence and mortality. Am J Epidemiol. 1980;111:87–98.
7. Dugowson CE, Koepsell TD, Voigt LF, Bley L, Nelson JL, Daling JR. Rheumatoid arthritis in women: incidence rates in a group health co-operative, Seattle, Washington 1987–1989. Arthritis Rheum. 1991;34:1502–7.
8. Symmons DPM, Barrett EM, Bankhead CR, Scott DGI, Silman AJ. The occurrence of rheumatoid arthritis in the United Kingdom: results from the Norfolk Arthritis Register. Br J Rheumatol. 1994;33:735–9.
9. Silman AJ. Has the incidence of rheumatoid arthritis declined in the United Kingdom? Br J Rheumatol. 1988;27:77–8.
10. Jacobsson LT, Hanson RL, Knowler WC, *et al.* Decreasing incidence and prevalence of rheumatoid arthritis in Pima Indians over a twenty-five year period. Arthritis Rheum. 1994;37:1158–65.
11. Silman AJ, Davies P, Currey HLF, Evans SJW. Is rheumatoid arthritis becoming less severe? J Chron Dis. 1983;36:891–7.
12. Aho K, Koskenvuo M, Tuominen J, Kaprio J. Occurrence of rheumatoid arthritis in a nationwide series of twins. J Rheumatol. 1986;13:899–902.
13. Silman AJ, MacGregor AJ, Thomson W, *et al.* Twin concordance rates for rheumatoid arthritis: results from a nationwide study. Br J Rheumatol. 1993;32:903–7.
14. Stastny P. Association of the B-cell alloantigen DRw4 with rheumatoid arthritis. N Engl J Med. 1978;298:869–71.
15. Jones MA, Silman AJ, Whiting S, Barrett EM, Symmons DPM. Occurrence of rheumatoid arthritis is not increased in the first degree relatives of a population based inception cohort of inflammatory polyarthritis. Ann Rheum Dis. 1996;55:89–93.
16. Ollier WE, MacGregor A. Genetic epidemiology of rheumatoid arthritis. Br Med Bull. 1995;51:267–85.
17. MacGregor AJ, Bamber S, Carthy D, *et al.* Heterogeneity of disease phenotype in monozygotic twins concordant for rheumatoid arthritis. Br J Rheumatol. 1995;34:215–20.
18 Heliovaara M, Aho K, Reunanen A, Knekt P, Aromaa A. Parity and risk of rheumatoid arthritis in Finnish women. Br J Rheumatol. 1995;34:625–8.
19. Hazes JMW. Pregnancy and its effect on the risk of developing rheumatoid arthritis. Ann Rheum Dis. 1991;50:71–2.
20. Silman AJ, Kay A, Brennan P. Timing of pregnancy in relation to the onset of rheumatoid arthritis. Arthritis Rheum. 1992;35:152–5.
21. Brennan P, Silman A. Breast-feeding and the onset of rheumatoid arthritis. Arthritis Rheum. 1994;37:808–13.
22. Wingrave SJ, Kay CR. Royal College of General Practitioners Study. Reduction in incidence of rheumatoid arthritis associated with oral contraceptives. Lancet. 1978;i:569–71.
23. Spector TD, Hochberg MC. The protective effect of the oral contraceptive pill on rheumatoid arthritis. An overview of the analytic epidemiological studies using meta-analysis. J Clin Epidemiol. 1990;43:1221–30.
24. Phillips PE. Evidence implicating infectious agents in rheumatoid arthritis and juvenile rheumatoid arthritis. Clin Exp Rheumatol. 1988;6:87–94.
25. Kouri T, Peterson J, Rhodes G, *et al.* Antibodies to synthetic peptides from Epstein–Barr nuclear antigen-1 in sera of patients with early rheumatoid arthritis and in preillness sera. J Rheumatol. 1990;17:1442–9.
26. Hajeer AH, MacGregor AJ, Rigby AS, Ollier WER, Carthy D, Silman AJ. Influence of previous exposure to human parvovirus B19 in explaining susceptibility to rheumatoid arthritis: an analysis of disease discordant twin pairs. Ann Rheum Dis. 1994;53:137–9.
27. Walker DJ, Griffiths ID, Madeley R. Autoantibodies and antibodies to microorganisms in rheumatoid arthritis: comparison of histocompatible siblings. J Rheumatol. 1987;14:426–8.
28. Engel A. Rheumatoid arthritis in US adults 1960–2. In: Bennett PH, Wood PHN. Population studies of the rheumatic diseases. Amsterdam: Exerpta Medica; 1968:83–9.
29. Lawrence JS. Rheumatism in populations. London: Heinemann; 1977.
30. Bankhead C, Silman AJ, Barrett B, Scott D, Symmons D. The incidence of rheumatoid arthritis is not related to indicators of socio-economic deprivation. J Rheumatol. 1996;23:2039–42.
31. Solomon L, Robin G, Valkenburg HA. Rheumatoid arthritis in an urban South African Negro population. Ann Rheum Dis. 1975;34:128–35.
32. Beighton P, Solomon L, Valkenburg HA. Rheumatoid arthritis in a rural South African Negro population. Ann Rheum Dis. 1975;34:136–41.
33. MacGregor AJ, Riste LK, Hazes JMW, Silman AJ. Low prevalence of rheumatoid arthritis in Black-Caribbean compared with Whites in inner-city Manchester. Ann Rheum Dis. 1994;53:293–7.
34. Silman AJ, Newman J, MacGregor AJ. Cigarette smoking increases the risk of rheumatoid arthritis: results from a nationwide study of disease discordant twins. Arthritis Rheum. 1996;39:732–5.

CLINICAL FEATURES OF EARLY, PROGRESSIVE AND LATE DISEASE

Duncan A Gordon & David E Hastings

- The 1987 ARA criteria for the classification of RA highlight symmetric polyarthritis, nodules, radiographically evident erosions and rheumatoid factor.
- Early on these may not be definitive criteria, since the subsequent course may indicate other diagnoses.

Inflammation
- Clinical evaluation is fundamental to the management of RA and includes examination for joint inflammation.
- Unchecked RA inflammation may lead to clinical and radiologic evidence of damage and destruction.
- In RA, inflammation primarily affects synovium, but bursae, tendon and other extra-articular features may evolve.

Course
- RA may be categorized as early, progressive or late.
- Onset may be acute, gradual or insidious.
- Subsequent course may be self-limited, episodic or progressive.
- Health status self-report questions may be helpful for assessing the ongoing progress or prognosis of disease.

INTRODUCTION

Rheumatoid arthritis (RA) is a disease that affects at least twice as many women as men. Although it may begin at any age its peak onset is in the fourth and fifth decades of life, rising sharply with age thereafter. The onset of RA appears to be more frequent in the winter than the summer months [1,2]. Its diagnosis is compatible with a variety of presentations and a clinical course that can last from a few weeks or months of discomfort to many years of profound disability. Although diagnostic criteria [3] may be helpful in diagnosis, in a given case they may not be definitive since the diagnosis may only become obvious with the passage of time.

Although we know a good deal about the epidemiology and immunologic and genetic aspects of RA, it is a sporadic condition of unknown cause and we have no idea what initiates or perpetuates the process (see Chapters 5.7–5.13). Until the cause of RA becomes known it cannot be precisely defined. A heterogeneous model for RA seems best because it may be one disease with more than one cause or more than one disease with a single cause [4]. At present, RA is best defined by a clinical description such as the 1987 criteria of the American Rheumatism Association (ARA) (Fig. 3.1) [3].

These criteria were presented in two forms, a traditional one (Fig. 3.1) and a classification tree (Fig. 3.2). In the first, a patient fulfilling

AMERICAN RHEUMATISM ASSOCIATION REVISED CRITERIA FOR RHEUMATOID ARTHRITIS CLASSIFICATION

Criterion	Definition
1. Morning stiffness	Morning stiffness in and around the joints, lasting at least 1 hour before maximal improvement
2. Arthritis of three or more joint areas	At least three joint areas (out of 14 possible areas: right or left PIP, MCP, wrist, elbow, knee, ankle, MTP joints) simultaneously have had soft-tissue swelling or fluid (not bony overgrowth alone) as observed by a physician
3. Arthritis of hand joints	At least one area swollen (as defined above) in a wrist, MCP or PIP joint
4. Symmetric arthritis	Simultaneous involvement of the same joint areas (as defined in 2) on both sides of the body (bilateral involvement of PIPs, MCPs or MTPs without absolute symmetry is acceptable)
5. Rheumatoid nodules	Subcutaneous nodules over bony prominences or extensor surfaces, or in juxta-articular regions as observed by a physician
6. Serum rheumatoid factor	Demonstration of abnormal amounts of serum rheumatoid factor by any method for which the result has been positive in less than 5% of normal control subjects
7. Radiographic changes	Radiographic changes typical of rheumatoid arthritis on posteroanterior hand and wrist radiographs, which must include erosions or unequivocal bony decalcification localized in, or most marked adjacent to, the involved joints (osteoarthritis changes alone do not qualify)

Note: For classification purposes, a patient has RA if at least 4 of these criteria are satisfied (criteria 1–4 must have been present for at least 6 weeks)

Fig. 3.1 The 1987 American Rheumatism Association revised criteria for the classification of RA [3]. If at least four of these criteria are satisfied (1–4 for at least 6 weeks), the patient has RA. Patients should not be designated as having classic, definite or probable RA.

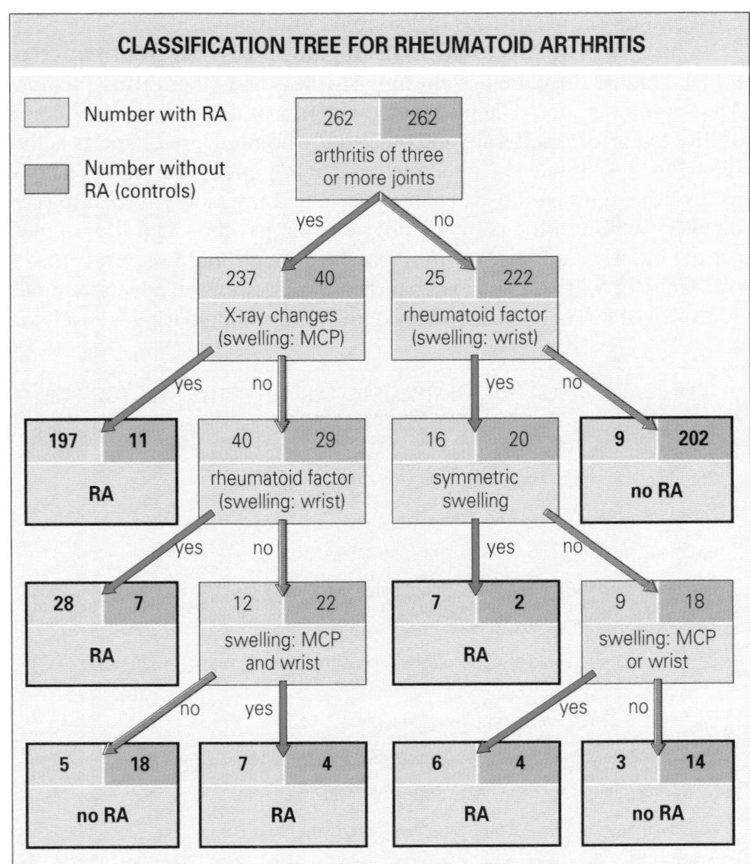

Fig. 3.2 A modified classification tree for RA [3]. The clinical criteria must have been observed by a physician and been present for at least 6 weeks. Subjects can be classified as having or as not having RA (no RA). In parentheses are indicated surrogate variables that can be used when another variable (radiograph or rheumatoid factor test result) is not available.

four of seven criteria is said to have RA. In the second scheme criteria 1 and 5 were deleted so that arthritis of three or more joints for 6 weeks or more with radiographic joint erosions or the presence of rheumatoid factor meets criteria for the diagnosis of RA. The entire criteria set strongly separates patients with RA from those with other conditions. Moreover, unlike the previous 1958 criteria the classification tree format shows better accuracy in patients with disease duration of one year or less [3,4]. These new criteria include objective features seen in a majority of patients with RA, but unlike the former set there are no exclusions [3].

The natural history of persons who meet criteria for classification of RA may also vary greatly from self-limited, to mild, to severe outcomes. For this reason Pincus and Callahan have suggested the need for subclassification according to different types of courses [5].

When faced with a patient with polyarthritis, many other conditions resembling RA must be kept in mind. It is important to distinguish such disorders from RA as soon as possible, because the correct diagnosis of RA is fundamental to the application of good management (see Chapters 5.14 and 5.15).

CLINICAL EVALUATION

A careful clinical evaluation is the first step towards winning the patient's confidence and cooperation. And it is the most important step in the successful management of RA.

HISTORY

Making a diagnosis of RA depends on an accurate description of the patient's illness, obtained from a careful history (Fig. 3.3). Success in this endeavor requires effective communication with the patient and family, and this takes time. Diffuse symmetric joint pain and swelling affecting the small peripheral joints are the commonest presenting symptoms. These symptoms are often associated with difficulty making a fist and morning stiffness of variable duration.

A history of nonrestorative sleep pattern may be informative in understanding the patient's morning stiffness and other diffuse aching. The symptoms should be interpreted in terms of the patient's functional ability to perform self-care and other daily home, work or sports activities (Fig. 3.4). It must be remembered that RA affects the patient's body as a whole, not just the articular system, and invariably has an impact on every aspect of the patient's physical and psychosocial life. In men (or the elderly), the disease may pursue a much more severe course [6] (see Chapter 5.4). RA in teenage girls may also show an adverse course. A history of RA in other members of the family should trigger suspicion of hereditary influences and heighten suspicion that the patient's symptoms could be an expression of early RA (see Chapter 5.7). It can be the case, however, that this knowledge has heightened the patient's anxiety about the symptoms, regardless of whether RA is the correct diagnosis.

It might be assumed that anxiety and depression would correlate with continuing disease activity, but it appears that socioeconomic factors may be greater determinants of depression than physical factors [7,8]. In other instances, patients who exhibit increased diffuse pain at a time when they exhibit decreased joint activity may show features of fibromyalgia, which explains this paradoxical reaction [9,10]. The role of physical trauma as a cause of RA is uncertain, but physical trauma in someone with RA may be a significant aggravating factor delaying recovery. A history of psychologic trauma or stress preceding the onset of RA should be sought, although the relevance of psychological factors in the cause of RA is unproven. A retrospective study of a group of twins discordant for RA examined this aspect of their disease [11]. In each case the twin affected by arthritis had a background of psychologic entrapment not seen in the unaffected twin. Moreover, the role of environmental factors in the causation of RA is highlighted in twin studies, where in monozygotic twins discordant for RA the genetic contribution to disease was only 15% [12] (see Chapter 5.8).

Hormones have an important influence in women with RA [13]. The manifestations of RA subside in about 70% of women during pregnancy and recur in the early postpartum period. A decreased risk of RA has been reported in women with previous pregnancies [14] and low androgen concentrations have been implicated as an explanation for a reduced incidence of RA in women taking oral contraceptives [13]. Interestingly, the proinflammatory effect of prolactin may explain why breast-feeding after the first pregnancy may increase the risk of the development of RA [15].

The patient's educational background and occupation may affect management and outcome and should be carefully documented. Notwithstanding genetic and sex factors, patients with more years of education seem to develop less severe disease [16]. Young men who are cigarette smokers may be at increased risk of RA [17]. However, evidence is much stronger that miners exposed to mineral dusts may be at risk not only of RA, but also, once it has developed, at increased risk of developing associated pneumoconiosis, Caplan's syndrome [18]. Persons whose occupations are associated with less physical stress, however, show a better functional outcome.

FUNCTIONAL DISABILITY INDICES

A number of self-report questionnaires, such as the Stanford Health Assessment Questionnaire (HAQ), Functional Disability Index (FDI), Arthritis Impact Measurement Scales (AIMS) and modifications of these, have been developed for the ongoing evaluation of patients with

CLINICAL EVALUATION OF RHEUMATOID ARTHRITIS – HISTORY OF PRESENT ILLNESS
Chronological account of illness from the onset
Onset: acute or gradual, with details
Location of pain (local or referred): precise anatomy, presence/absence of swelling
Pattern of joint involvement: axial, peripheral, symmetric
Type of pain: quality and character
Severity: pain threshold effects, interference with activities of daily living, range of joint movement
Radiation of pain: local or deep referred type
Clinical course: duration, frequency, periodicity, persistence
Modifying factors: aggravating, relieving, medication effects
Associated symptoms: fatigue, other systemic symptoms
Duration of morning stiffness: nonrestorative sleep pattern
Present status: regional review of joints, extra-articular features, functional class, activities of daily living, psychologic state

Fig. 3.3 Clinical evaluation of RA: details required from the history of present illness.

CLINICAL EVALUATION OF RHEUMATOID ARTHRITIS – FUNCTIONAL CAPACITY AND ACTIVITIES OF DAILY LIVING
Classification of functional capacity
Normal function without or despite symptoms
Some disability, but adequate for normal activity without special devices or assistance
Activities restricted, requires special devices or personal assistance
Totally dependent
Classification of activities of daily living
Mobility: walking, climbing, use of transport, bed–chair transfers
Personal care: eating, dressing, washing, grooming, use of toilet
Special hand functions: door handles, keys, coins, jar tops, carrying, pen, scissors
Work and play activities: work outside home, light and heavy work in house, hobbies, sports

Fig. 3.4 Clinical evaluation: functional capacity and activities of daily living.

SELF-REPORT QUESTIONNAIRE FOR RHEUMATOID ARTHRITIS				
Please check (✓) the ONE best answer for your abilities.				
At this moment, are you able to:	Without any difficulty	With some difficulty	With much difficulty	Unable to do
a. Dress yourself, including tying shoelaces and doing buttons?				
b. Get in and out of bed?				
c. Lift a full cup or glass to your mouth?				
d. Walk outdoors on flat ground?				
e. Wash and dry your entire body?				
f. Bend down to pick up clothing from the floor?				
g. Turn regular faucets (taps) on and off?				
h. Get in and out of a car?				

Fig. 3.5 Self-report questionnaire for RA. The questionnaire is used to assess quantitatively the functional capacity of the patient to carry out the tasks of daily living [21].

RA (Fig. 3.5) [18–22]. These provide clinically useful information not available by conventional means. They can be used to document the patient's functional status, with results similar to many traditional measures of RA activity, including joint-count score, radiographic score, sedimentation rate and walking time. It is questionable, however, whether they can reliably assess problems of anxiety or depression in the patient with RA [22]. The value of these scales is attested by many rheumatologists who have incorporated them into their practice routines. Basic demographic variables are also part of this documentation.

EXAMINATION

As RA is a systemic condition, the clinical evaluation should include a complete physical examination that also documents the presence or absence of a number of extra-articular features. These include subcutaneous nodules, digital vasculitis and the other systemic features described in Chapter 5.4. Any one of these may be mistaken for a non-rheumatoid condition and their presence indicates a more ominous form of the disease. Various systemic features may also be the result of an adverse drug reaction. The joints shown in Figure 3.6 should be examined systematically, as described in the next three sections of this chapter, to determine which ones are inflamed or damaged. The pattern of joint involvement, whether symmetrical, axial or peripheral, should be recorded.

JOINT INFLAMMATION

The key signs of joint inflammation in RA are those of tenderness and swelling. These may be associated with local heat, but erythema is not a feature of rheumatoid inflammation. Heat and erythema may be seen with coincidental septic or gouty arthritis, however.

A joint is considered 'active' if it is tender on pressure or painful on passive movement with stress and/or swelling other than bony proliferation. The presence or absence of pain and swelling are recorded separately. Joint swelling may be periarticular or intra-articular. Intra-articular swelling is associated with the detection of a joint effusion, described below.

A diagram depicting the joints (Fig. 3.6) may be used at each assessment to record signs of disease activity or tender joint count. Joint effusions are recorded separately, because although the presence of an effusion usually indicates inflammation, this is not always the case. In any event, if fluid is detected the matter can be settled by aspirating and examining it to see whether leukocytosis or other signs of rheumatoid joint inflammation are present. At this juncture it is useful to mention the distinction between a tender 'joint count' and a tender 'point count'. Patients with RA or fibromyalgia may have widespread pain, and sometimes both conditions coexist (see Chapter 4.15). In the case of RA, however, tenderness is related to one or more joints specifically, whereas fibromyalgia is defined as present in a patient if 11 or more of 18 specific tender point sites are found that are not articular. It is also helpful to use a diagram to record tender points. The number of minutes of morning stiffness and measurements of grip strength using a blood-pressure cuff manometer are other commonly used indices of disease activity.

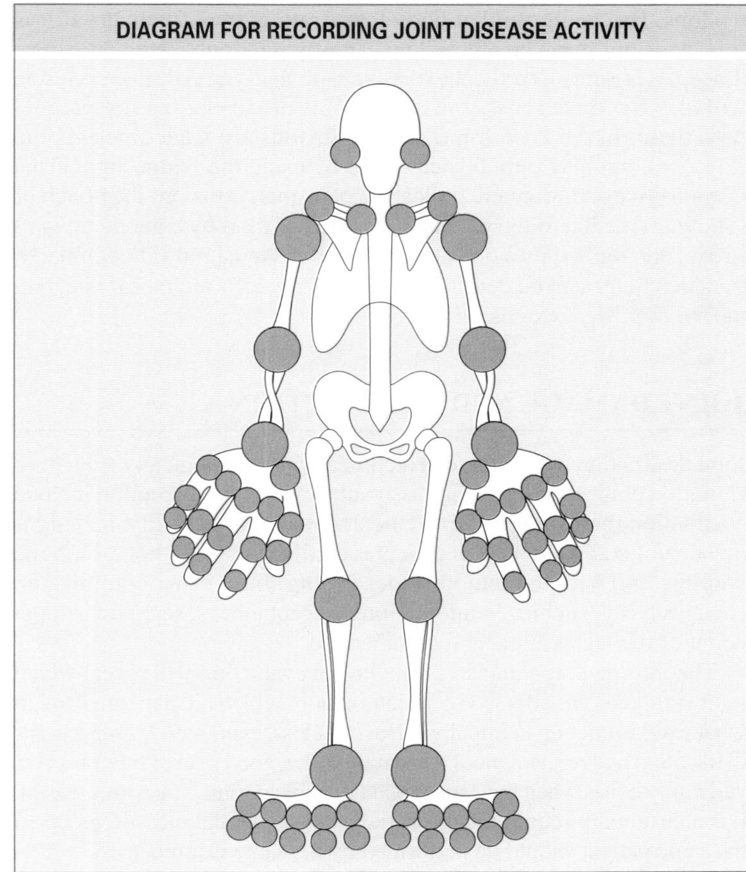

Fig. 3.6 Pictorial method for indicating joint disease activity or destruction. The cartoon may be used on a printed form or rubber stamp to chart which joints are active or deformed at the time of each assessment. The joints circled here should always be assessed.

TENDERNESS

This is elicited by direct palpation pressure over the joint. Firmer pressure on the tissues between or remote from the joints should not be tender with the exception of the fibrositic tender points (see above). Testing for joint tenderness is particularly useful for detecting disease activity in the wrist, finger and toe joints. Pain during the arc of movement, however, may be due to bare bone rubbing on bare bone from loss of articular cartilage, and is not a reliable indication of the presence of inflammation. For this reason, the hips should be excluded from the routine simple joint count.

STRESS PAIN

Stress pain is produced when a joint at the limit of its range of movement is nudged a little further. It is an especially useful symptom in the shoulder (limit of internal and external rotation), wrists, metacarpophalangeals, and joints in the ankle region. To determine how hard to press in testing for stress pain, the general level of tenderness can be assessed by squeezing control sites in the midtrapezius and lower calf, and by pressing over the manubrium, metacarpals and proximal phalanges. Pressure on joints should be about 20% less than that required to reach the pain threshold over the control sites. When in doubt, it is best to record the joint as inactive.

SYNOVIAL EFFUSION

The most reliable general sign of a synovial effusion is the demonstration of fluctuation: the hydraulic effect of an increase in fluid tension produced by pressure in one direction is transmitted equally in all three planes (Fig. 3.7). This is the four-finger technique – relatively easy to learn, but applicable only when the joint can be surrounded. For most joints, a two-finger or two-thumb technique must be used, one pressing downward, the other feeling an upward lift. These techniques can be practiced on a slightly softened grape. In the latter technique, the direction of pressure should differ slightly from the sensor finger to prevent false-positive scorings due to lateral shifts of fat or tendons. Fat, being fluid at body temperature, may fluctuate. If it is subcutaneous, it can be pinched up in a way impossible with effusions; if deep, it is rarely exactly coextensive with the synovial space. Muscle will also fluctuate across the direction of the fibers, but not parallel with them. In the knee joint, small effusions are sometimes visible (Fig. 3.8), but may only be detectable by using the 'bulge sign'. This is a sensitive and dramatic indication of a small effusion: the pouch of synovium medial to the patella is emptied of fluid by a gentle upward stroke, and refilled by a downward stroke on the lateral side. Similarly, a sudden bulge can be detected when a mildly affected elbow is gently moved to 90% of extension.

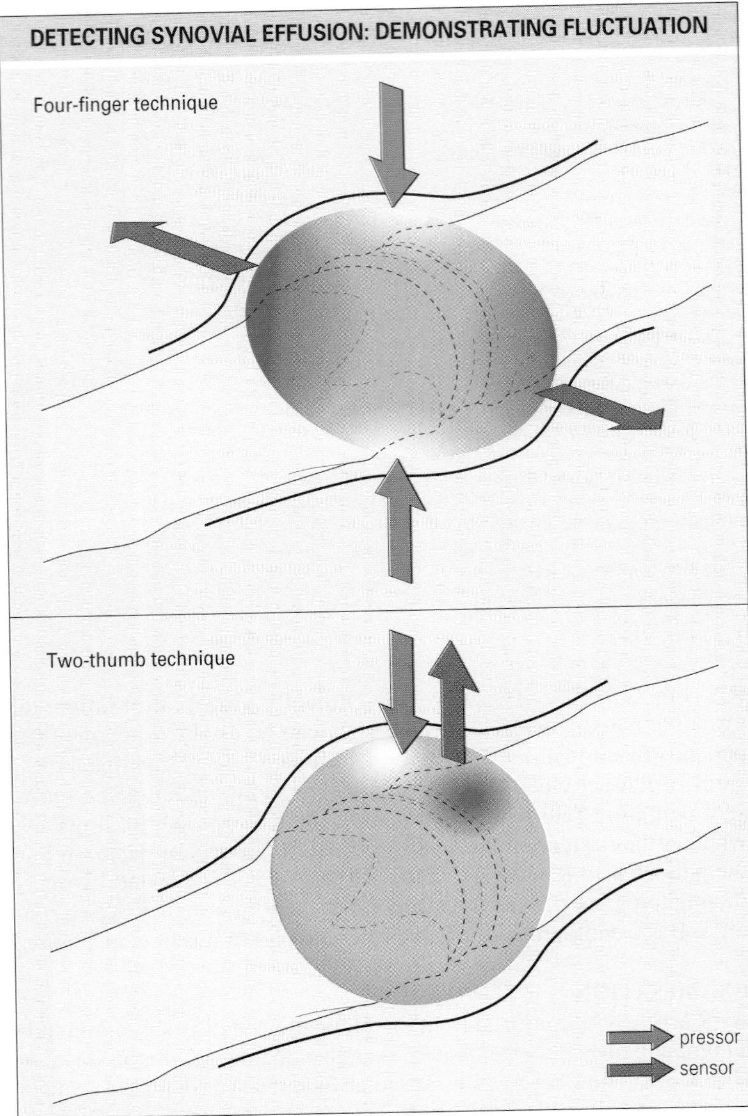

Fig. 3.7 Demonstration of fluctuation for the detection of a synovial effusion. An increase in fluid tension induced by finger pressure in one area is transmitted so that the sensor finger(s) can detect it elsewhere. In the two-thumb (or two-finger) technique the pressure should be in a slightly different direction to the sensor finger, to avoid false-positive results.

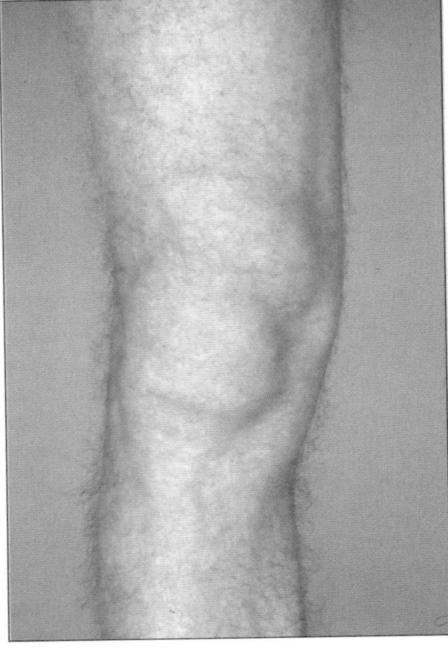

Fig. 3.8 Early rheumatoid arthritis of the knee showing extension of a small effusion into the suprapatellar pouch.

JOINT DAMAGE AND DESTRUCTION

Joint destruction may be assessed clinically or radiologically (Fig. 3.9). Common clinical observations associated with joint disruption include a reduction in the range of movement, collateral instability, malalignment, subluxation or loss of articular cartilage causing bone-on-bone crepitus. No simple method of describing these often complicated changes has yet achieved international acceptance. A separate, simple count of damaged joints is recommended.

The information obtained from clinical evaluation will reveal which joint structures are affected by inflammation, which are damaged and to what extent function is impaired. Nevertheless, even with training, standardization and refinement of these methods, a good deal of interobserver variability exists when they are applied to clinical trials [23]. For this reason, it is a customary requirement for trials that sequential measurements in the same patient should be performed by the same examiner.

After the foregoing baseline evaluations have been accomplished, the diagnosis of RA can usually be confirmed and the patient can be categorized as having early, progressive or late disease.

CLINICAL EVALUATION OF RHEUMATOID ARTHRITIS – EXAMINATION
Extra-articular features
Record presence of nodules, Raynaud's phenomenon, digital infarcts, episcleritis, peripheral neuropathy, palmar erythema, leg ulcers
Note tendon sheath involvement, or tendon nodules, subluxation or rupture
Check for anemia, splenomegaly, leukopenia, pleuritis or pericarditis, the sicca syndrome or renal involvement
Articular: measures of inflammatory activity
Check for tenderness, stress pain, synovial effusion, grip strength and duration of morning stiffness
Articular: measures of destruction and deformity
Check for lax collaterals, subluxation, malalignment, metatarsal prolapse, hammer toes and bone-on-bone crepitus

Fig. 3.9 Clinical evaluation of RA – examination.

EARLY DISEASE

This describes patients who as yet exhibit no clinical evidence of joint damage or radiologic signs of cartilage loss or bone erosion. Our use of the term 'early disease' is synonymous with 'mild disease' activity. It is not meant to have any particular prognostic significance. Although it is unpredictable whether patients with early disease will eventually run a benign or malignant course, most exhibit an intermediate, smoldering activity [2]. Spontaneous remission may occur, especially where the onset of polyarthritis has been quite sudden [1]. Even though patients are categorized as having 'early disease', a number of prognostic factors should be sought (Fig. 3.10). These factors when present suggest a more unfavorable outlook and may indicate a need for more aggressive therapy.

Often the diagnosis of RA is obvious, but frequently there are too few definite features and the diagnosis can only be tentative, in which case the patient may be placed in this early category. The ARA criteria for classification of RA may not always be helpful in diagnosis of patients at the earliest stage of disease. Over time, developments may show that a presumptive diagnosis of early RA was incorrect and features of another diffuse connective tissue disorder – such as systemic lupus erythematosus (SLE), scleroderma, or psoriatic arthritis – may evolve. Thus, it may be a mistake to apply the RA 'label' to a patient too soon, because when new symptoms arise other diagnostic possibilities or unrelated complications may not be considered soon enough to effect better treatment.

PROGRESSIVE DISEASE

Some patients show a more progressive course from the outset. They have unrelenting, continuous disease activity despite treatment. In addition to persistent polyarthritis, these individuals usually have an elevated erythrocyte sedimentation rate (ESR), positive rheumatoid factor test and early radiographic evidence of joint erosions. They may also have one or more of the systemic features of RA.

LATE DISEASE

This category is used to describe patients whose disease has led to definite joint damage with all its attendant complications. In most cases, the disease is of many years' duration and its damaging effects are a reflection of its severity. Typically these patients have been resistant to various disease-suppressive medications, though in some patients the disease may have 'burned itself out', leaving only residual joint damage.

INDIVIDUAL JOINTS – A REGIONAL APPROACH

Joint involvement in RA is symmetrical, and while wrists, fingers, knees and feet are the most commonly affected joints, severe disease is associated with larger joints that contain more synovium, such as the shoulders, elbows and knees. In fact, articular indices weighted for size and amount of synovium, such as the historical Lansbury index [24], have been found to correlate better with the amount of inflammation than simple joint counts [25]. The simultaneous presence of joint tenderness and swelling also shows a higher correlation with joint inflammation than either variable alone [25]. Eventually, if unchecked, persistent inflammation leads to destruction of soft tissue with ligamentous laxity and deformity.

THE HANDS

Examination of the hands is important because the features they exhibit are frequently a reflection of the patient's overall disease, whether early, late or progressive. Symmetric swelling of the metacarpophalangeal (MCP) and proximal interphalangeal (PIP) joints, with fusiform swelling of the latter, are typical of RA (Fig. 3.11). Distal interphalangeal (DIP) involvement may be seen, but should be distinguished from coincidental osteoarthritis. Tenderness on palpation will determine which of these joints are to be noted as 'active'. Effusion should be sought using the four-finger technique (see Fig. 3.7). Hand assessment is incomplete without recording grip strength, but it is worth noting that poor grip strength may be as much a reflection of tendon involvement as of joint disease affecting wrists and fingers.

Although local swellings of the MCP and PIP joints are characteristic of RA, massive diffuse swelling of both hands with a 'flipper' or

FACTORS IN RHEUMATOID ARTHRITIS INDICATING AN UNFAVORABLE PROGNOSIS
Accumulated joint damage rate Uncontrolled polyarthritis Structural damage and deformity Functional disability
Presence of extra-articular features Local and/or systemic
Psychosocial problems
Rheumatoid factor seropositivity Presence of immune complexes
Immunogenetic testing for ≥1 HLA-DR4 cluster of RA susceptibility genes (DRB1* 0401, 0404, 0405) ≥

Fig. 3.10 Clinical evaluation of RA – prognostic factors. The presence of these factors suggests a more unfavorable outlook.

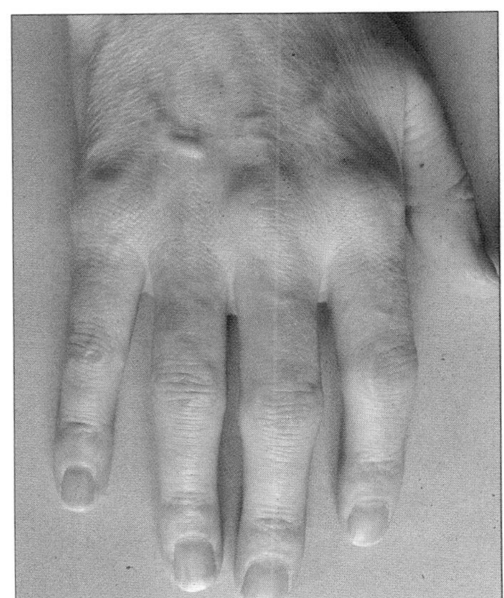

Fig. 3.11 The hand in early RA. View of the right hand, showing swelling of the MCP and PIP joints. Fusiform swelling of the PIP joints is typical of RA and associated with morning stiffness, difficulty making a fist, reduced grip strength and tenderness of the affected joints. The left hand showed similar changes. Reproduced with permission from Dieppe *et al.* [26].

'boxing glove' appearance may be associated with an acute onset. Pitting edema is characteristic of this swelling, and if a seronegative elderly person is affected, a more likely diagnosis is that of benign polyarthritis of the aged [27]. If diffuse swelling of one or both hands is associated with signs of sympathetic overactivity and shoulder stiffness, then reflex dystrophy may be a better explanation than RA. However, reflex dystrophy may coexist with RA or contribute to its disease expression. Interestingly, articular signs may be absent when RA develops in a patient with pre-existing hemiparesis [28]. The greater the paralysis the less the degree of joint inflammation.

Inspection of the hands may reveal other extra-articular features. Raynaud's phenomenon may be seen in a minority of patients, and palmar erythema in more. Digital and nail-fold infarcts indicate rheumatoid vasculitis and a more severe form of arthritis.

A more detailed examination of joints and tendons is required to monitor progressive hand deformity in RA. Hasting's classification and description is helpful in identifying these problems (Fig. 3.12).

Metacarpophalangeal joints

MCP involvement, with the development of volar subluxation and ulnar drift, is a characteristic deformity of RA. A number of factors favor its occurrence and progression [29]. Synovitis within the MCP joints tends to weaken the dorsal and radial structures and relatively lengthen the collateral ligaments. Inherent mechanical factors then favor ulnar drift of the fingers. The power of hand grip pulls the tendons ulnar-wards as the fifth metacarpal descends. The ulnar collateral ligaments are shorter and less oblique than the radial counterparts, and thus the elongation is greater on the radial than the ulnar side. The firm attachment of the volar plate also fixes the pull of the long flexors to the proximal phalanx and tends to displace the proximal phalanx in both an ulnar and volar direction. The transverse linkage of the extensor tendons functions much like a clothesline, so that anything pulling the extensor tendon of the fifth finger in an ulnar direction will pull the other fingers the same way. An effect of radial deviation of the wrist must also be considered. In the presence of ulnar drift, a normal wrist will tend to radially deviate to compensate for that deformity. Moreover, any wrist involvement that produces radial deviation will tend to aggravate the tendency to ulnar drift of the fingers.

HASTING'S CLASSIFICATION OF RHEUMATOID HAND

Joint involvement	MCP joints	Synovitis Passively correctable ulnar drift Fixed volar subluxation, ulnar drift
	PIP joints	Synovitis Boutonnière deformity Swan-neck deformity Flail IP joint
	Thumb	Flail IP joint Boutonnière deformity Duckbill thumb (CMC) dislocation
	Wrist	Synovitis Carpal supination–subluxation Radiocarpal dislocation
Tendon involvement	Flexor tendon disease	Loss of active flexion Triggering Tendon rupture Median nerve involvement
	Extensor tendon disease	Synovitis – dorsal mass Extensor tendon rupture Extensor tendon dislocation

Fig. 3.12 Hasting's classification of rheumatoid hand deformities. Data from Hastings [30].

Proximal interphalangeal joints

Three deformities due to lack of collateral ligament support characterize PIP joint involvement – the boutonnière, the swan-neck (Fig. 3.13) and the unstable PIP joint. Synovitis in the PIP joint can produce any of these deformities. As noted, synovitis with joint effusion in early RA causes fusiform swelling. Synovitis may appear as a bulge on the dorsal aspect, often on each side of the extensor tendon.

A boutonnière deformity develops when there is relative laxity or attenuation of the central slip and the lateral bands move in a volar direction. This destroys the extensor balance of the fingers and extension is concentrated on the terminal phalanx while the lateral bands actually become flexors of the PIP joints. The lack of passive flexion of the terminal IP joint with the PIP joint in extension is the earliest sign of this complication. It may be rapidly progressive. A swan-neck deformity represents the reverse of the boutonnière deformity and exists when the main extensor forces focus on the base of the proximal phalanx and the lateral bands sublux to a dorsal position. It may be a physiological deformity, the result of trauma, secondary to PIP joint disease or a result of MCP joint disease with secondary intrinsic contracture. In the early stages, the deformity seems relatively reversible, but as the lateral bands displace to the dorsal position, flexion becomes increasingly difficult. Often the movement is only accomplished by a snap as the lateral bands move from the dorsal to the normal dorsal–lateral position. Once the lateral bands become fixed in a dorsal position, then flexion of the PIP joint is no longer possible.

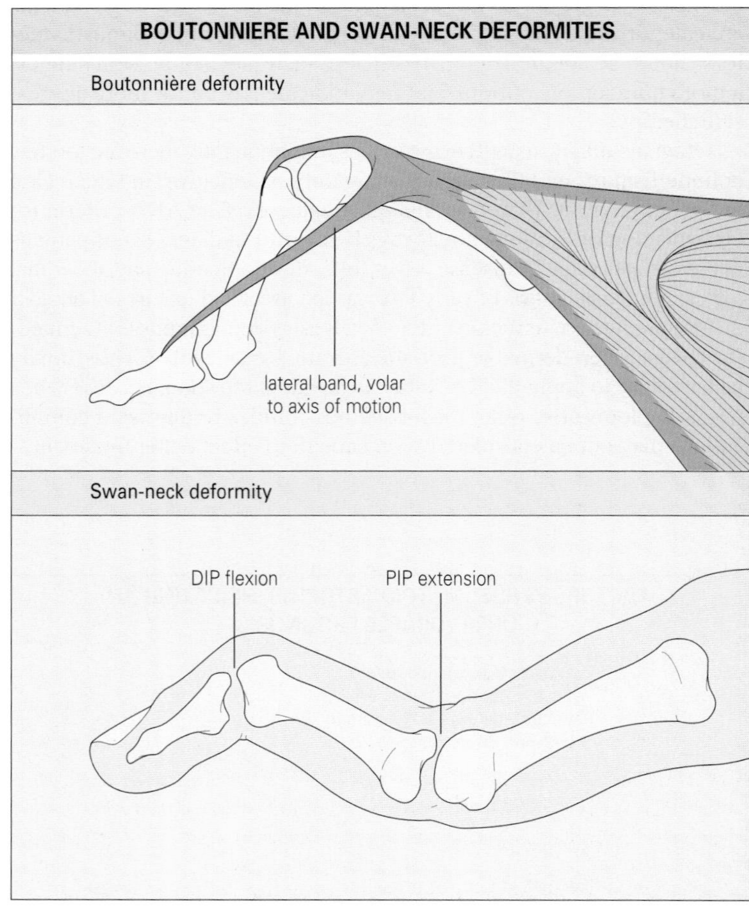

Fig. 3.13 PIP joints deformities in RA. The boutonnière deformity – PIP flexion and dorsal interphalangeal (DIP) hyperextension – results from relaxation of the central slip, with 'button-holing' of the PIP joint between the lateral bands. The swan-neck deformity – MCP flexion, PIP hyperextension and DIP flexion – may be mobile, snapping or fixed. Its pathogenesis may be related primarily to PIP or MCP involvement. Combinations of MCP and PIP involvement are less frequent. Adapted with permission from Hastings and Welsh [31].

Distal interphalangeal joints

Involvement of the DIP joint is not characteristic of RA but probably occurs more frequently than appreciated [32]. It is never an initial or isolated manifestation of RA, and it is usually episodic and more likely to occur in seropositive RA. DIP disease must be distinguished from coincidental osteoarthritis that at times may also show inflammatory features.

The rheumatoid thumb

Three deformities affect the thumb: the flail IP joint, the boutonnière thumb and the relatively rare duckbill thumb. The flail IP joint results from synovitis leading to the destruction of the collateral ligaments. Pinching pushes the terminal phalanx away and the patient begins to pinch against the proximal phalanx. The boutonnière thumb is the same deformity as that described earlier for the other fingers. MCP synovitis weakens the insertion of the extensor pollicis brevis to the base of the proximal phalanx and results in an MCP flexion deformity and a secondary IP hyperextension due to the unbalanced action of extensor pollicis longus. The duckbill thumb develops when the primary pathology is at the first carpometacarpal joint. This is a dislocation accompanied by an adduction deformity of the first metacarpal. The MCP joint is hyperextended and the IP joint flexed; the deformity is similar to a swan-neck deformity of the finger.

Flexor tendon involvement

Tendons, as well as joints, are sheathed with synovium and when inflamed the condition is known as tenosynovitis. Flexor tenosynovitis can take many different forms.

Loss of active flexion

If passive flexion of a finger exceeds active flexion, tenosynovitis is present. Crepitus can be felt in the palm as the fingers are extended and flexed. Adhesions between the superficial and deep tendons may limit the excursion of the profundus tendon and the patient will not be able to make a full fist. A trigger finger is a frequent feature of flexor tenosynovitis. The pathology is a thickening of the tendon (often by a rheumatoid nodule within the tendon) rather than stenosis of the tendon sheath.

Ruptures of flexor tendons occur but are much less common than extensor rupture. The tendon most likely to rupture is the flexor pollicis longus. The cause is usually synovitis in the carpal tunnel and wrist disease, with encroachment of a spicule of carpal bone from the floor of the carpal tunnel.

Florid flexor tenosynovitis of the carpal tunnel leads to compression of the median nerve. Volar wrist pain may be confused with articular disease, but the weakness, finger tingling and thenar wasting point to nerve involvement that can be confirmed by electromyographic studies. RA can actually present with a carpal tunnel syndrome as the sole feature before polyarthritis becomes apparent [33]. Occasionally, triggering may develop in the carpal tunnel.

Extensor tendon involvement

Extensor tenosynovitis is evident by swelling over the dorsum of the wrist, below the extensor retinaculum. Asking the patient to extend the fingers will accentuate the swelling – the 'tuck' sign (Fig. 3.14). This mass on the back of the wrist is usually only a painless cosmetic deformity. Painful finger extension, however, may indicate active tendon erosion. There may be a triggering effect, and with further erosion tendon rupture follows. This is usually the result of carpal supination–subluxation and attrition of the tendons over the distal ulna. It is important to differentiate an extensor tendon rupture from an extensor tendon dislocation at the MCP joints. At first, the latter is passively correctable, but it soon becomes fixed. Examination will reveal the intact extensor tendon over the dorsum of the hand. Another rare complication is the loss of finger extension caused by an entrapment neuropathy of the posterior interosseous branch of the radial nerve, due to rheumatoid synovitis about the elbow [34].

THE WRIST

Symmetrical disease of the wrists is almost invariably present in RA [30]. Ulnar styloid swelling and loss of wrist extension indicate early involvement. Synovitis commonly affects the weakest support of the wrist on the ulnar side. Attenuation of the weak triangular ligament allows displacement of the wrist in a volar direction. The wrist also tends to rotate around the stronger radial dorsal ligament, promoting a deformity known as carpal supination–subluxation. This subluxation is responsible for the prominence of the distal ulna, causing erosion of the floor of the extensor compartments and extensor tendon rupture. As the wrist rotates into supination, subluxation of the extensor carpi ulnaris occurs so that this tendon no longer functions as a dorsiflexor. Contracture of the extensor carpi radialis longus and brevis leads to unopposed radial dorsiflexion with ulnar translocation of the carpus. With disease progression, the volar and ulnar aspect of the radius erodes, with the carpus moving in a volar and ulnar direction. This strains the extensor carpi radialis brevis and if this tendon ruptures, the wrist goes on to volar dislocation. The intercarpal ligaments may also be affected, with wrist collapse. This accentuates the instability. Rarely, synovitis appears to promote fibrous and then bony ankylosis of the carpal bones. Then stiffness, rather than instability, becomes the problem.

THE ELBOW

This joint is frequently involved in RA, with loss of extension as an early sign. Even with extensive involvement, elbow function is usually well maintained. When loss of flexion occurs, however, this can become a great problem as it interferes with the patient's self-care activities. Elbow effusions are visible and palpable in the dimple between the tip of the olecranon and the head of the radius. When small effusions are not visible, gentle extension to 90% may show a sudden bulge. Periarticular cysts may be associated with elbow effusion and, as in the knee, may rupture (into the forearm) with inflammatory swelling. With persistent synovitis, erosive changes first develop in the humeroulnar joint. Because the radius is linked to the ulna by an interosseous membrane, the two move as a unit. When the cartilage between the humerus and the ulna is lost, the head of the radius moves proximal to the capitellum, blocking flexion and extension. Loss of elbow extension precedes loss of flexion. Constant abutment of the radial head produces typical lateral pain, limited supination and crepitus with pronation and supination. Medial swelling of the elbow joint with damage and destruction may be associated with an ulnar entrapment neuropathy. As well, synovitis of the lateral elbow joint may cause entrapment of the posterior interosseous branch of the radial nerve [34].

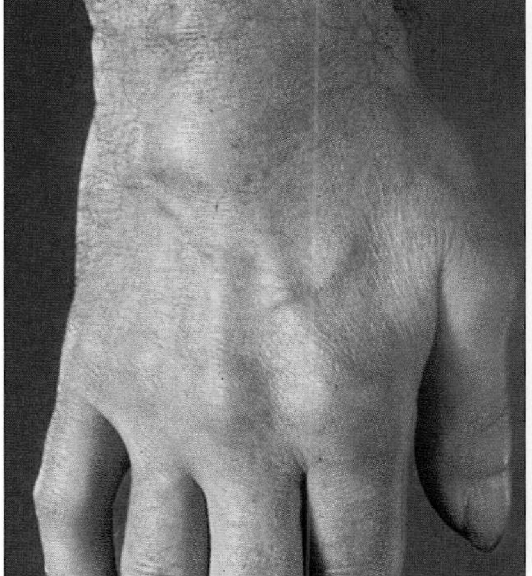

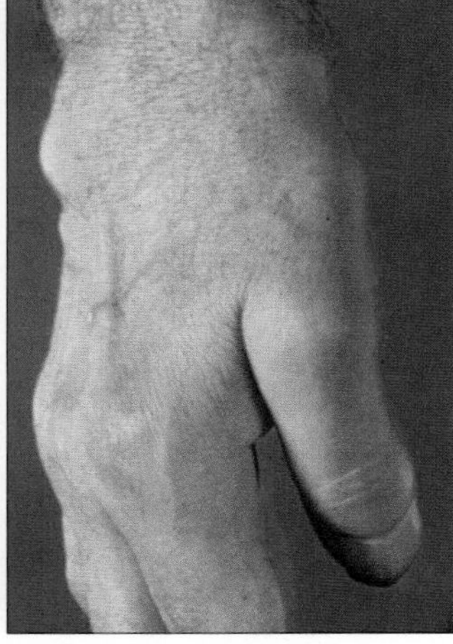

Fig. 3.14 Tenosynovial swelling from tenosynovitis – the 'tuck' sign. Tenosynovial swelling overlies the metacarpals of the right hand. Bulging becomes accentuated with full extension of all the fingers of the hand. Persistent tenosynovitis over the dorsal wrist may lead to extensor tendon erosion and rupture, particularly of the tendons of the fourth and fifth fingers.

Subcutaneous nodules

Subcutaneous nodules overlying the extensor aspect of the proximal ulna are present in about 30% of patients with RA. Not only is the nodule a cardinal diagnostic feature of RA, but it may break down, forming a cyst and serving as a site for local infection (Fig. 3.15) or as a portal for complicating systemic infection causing septic arthritis. Vasculitis of the skin overlying the nodule may also contribute to these complications. Subcutaneous nodules or rheumatoid nodulosis may form over other pressure locations, such as the occiput, palms of the hands, sacrum or Achilles tendon, and may become infected (see Chapters 5.4 and 5.16). They should be sought in any RA patient who has septic complications.

The olecranon bursa

Bursae should not be overlooked in the evaluation of any joint region since they may be a site of rheumatoid activity [35]. There are about 80 bursae on each side of the body and they are lined by a synovial membrane that secretes synovial fluid and may develop rheumatoid synovitis. Only occasionally do they communicate with an adjacent joint space. Involvement of the olecranon bursa by RA is an obvious example of bursitis. Pain and swelling may be manifestations of synovitis or infection (Fig. 3.15). While septic arthritis is almost invariably the result of hematogenous spread of bacteria, septic olecranon bursitis is always a consequence of a skin break with direct entry from outside. Skin vasculitis overlying bursal swelling can contribute to this septic complication. Occasionally the bursa ruptures and causes diffuse forearm edema.

Other bursae that may be similarly affected include the subacromial, trochanteric, iliopsoas, gastrocnemius, semimembranosus, subachilles and posterior calcaneal. Sometimes multiple bursae may be affected by rheumatoid granulomas [36].

THE SHOULDER

Involvement of the shoulder joint in RA is variable but is usually only a feature in patients who have progressive disease. Often shoulder symptoms do not arise until joint destruction has become advanced. This is because adaptive mechanisms – the hands, wrists and elbows – are sufficiently good for daily self-care activities to be maintained for a long time.

Synovitis leads to erosion and damage of both the humeral head and the glenoid fossa. When shoulder effusions develop they appear anteriorally below the acromion. Subacromial bursal swelling may also appear as a pouch independent of the glenohumeral joint. The bursa may also rupture. The long head of the biceps may also rupture in patients with RA. This can be detected as a biceps bulge when the patient flexes the elbow against resistance.

The rotator cuff is also lined with synovium and may show inflammation and destruction, with monoarticular pain and limitation sufficiently acute to mimic septic arthritis. Frequently, there is weakening and loss of attachment of the rotator cuff, with secondary upward migration of the humeral head.

Acromioclavicular joint disease is frequently found in RA and may be the prime source of shoulder pain. Acromioclavicular involvement also correlates with the degree of glenohumeral disease.

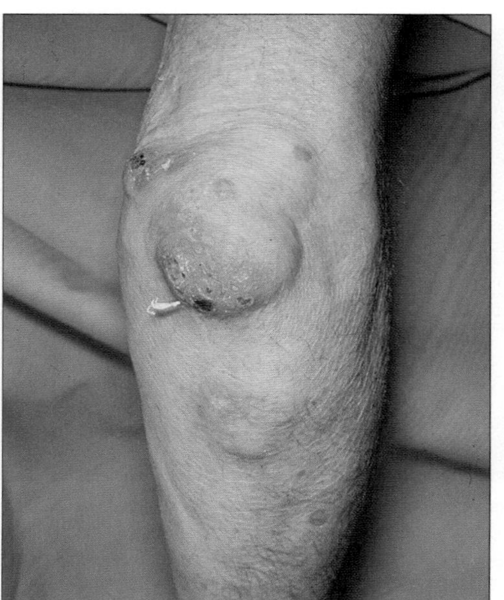

Fig. 3.15 Olecranon bursitis and subcutaneous nodule. Olecranon swelling with erythema from septic bursitis after incision and drainage. A subcutaneous nodule appears distal to the olecranon bursa. Either of these lesions may serve as a portal for systemic infection.

THE TEMPOROMANDIBULAR JOINT

This joint is commonly involved, with tenderness and painful limitation of mouth opening. It may eventually become associated with a receding or 'gump jaw' deformity.

THE CRICOARYTENOID JOINT

Involvement of this joint is commonly associated with hoarseness. Superimposed upper respiratory infections may lead to upper airway obstruction with respiratory stridor requiring life-saving tracheostomy [37]. Limitation of cricoarytenoid movement may also be associated with lung aspiration and attendant complications.

OSSICLES OF THE EAR

Ankylosis of these joints may be associated with hearing loss independent of a medication-induced effect.

STERNOCLAVICULAR AND MANUBRIOSTERNAL JOINTS

These joints possess synovial and cartilage portions and are more commonly affected than appreciated. Subluxation and actual dislocation of the manubriosternal joint may occur [38].

THE CERVICAL SPINE

The neck is an important target in RA, particularly at the C1–C2 level. The space between the odontoid process and the arch of the atlas normally measures 3mm or less. If this space exceeds 3mm this is defined as atlantoaxial subluxation (AAS). It can often exceed 10mm. Cervical subluxation at any level is common in severe erosive RA and may be found in 30% of patients in this category [39]. Although neck stiffness is common in RA, the majority of patients with AAS are not much affected by severe neck pain. When neck pain occurs it is usually high in the cervical spine, with radiation into the occiput or occasionally into temporal and retro-orbital regions. Sometimes AAS is associated with a frightening 'clunking' sensation on neck extension.

When considering the cervical spine at the C1–C2 level, it is helpful to divide the space through the arch of the atlas into thirds; one-third for the odontoid process, one-third for the spinal cord and one-third free. If a C1–C2 slip exceeds 10mm, the free third is lost and cervical cord damage becomes a risk (Fig. 3.16 and see Chapter 5.16). There is a synovial articulation between the transverse ligament of the atlas and the posterior aspect of the odontoid. This transverse ligament prevents a forward slip of C1 on C2, and continuing synovitis in this articulation compromises the ligament and may produce erosions of the dens. Synovial involvement may also affect the apophyseal joints in the occipitoatlantal area. If this causes loss of bone and change in shape, the odontoid may move up through the foramen magnum, producing basilar invagination and threatening the upper cervical cord and medulla. In these patients sudden death may occur after unexpected vomiting or physical trauma. Basilar–vertebral vascular insufficiency may also occur in these cases, with syncope after downward gaze. The usual indication for neurosurgical intervention in these cases is either intractable neck pain or pyramidal tract weakness of the arms and legs. RA of the apophyseal joints and disk spaces may cause subluxation at other levels, which may slowly lead to quadriparesis [40]. Fortunately, these complications are rare.

In patients with cervical symptoms despite negative radiographic findings contrast enhanced magnetic resonance imaging may be of value in characterization of the craniocervical region [41].

When a patient with RA requires surgery, the presence of cervical subluxation presents a general anesthetic risk. Preoperative assessment by lateral flexion cervical radiographs is essential to exclude this possibility. If cervical involvement is detected, then special precautions are required perioperatively to prevent cervical cord damage.

THE THORACIC AND LUMBAR SPINE

Involvement of these regions is very uncommon in RA. Apophyseal synovitis may rarely present as an epidural mass, and lumbar spinal stenosis has been reported. Compression fractures secondary to the osteoporosis of RA aggravated by corticosteroids are common in the thoracic region. Compression fractures in the lumbar region are not characteristic of RA and suggest that other underlying causes, such as osteomyelitis or cancer, should be considered and excluded.

THE SACROILIAC JOINTS

Radiographic changes of the sacroiliac joints may be seen in advanced RA; usually they consist of erosions and osteopenia. However, ankylosing spondylitis and RA may occasionally coexist, usually in men, just as RA may be seen in patients with psoriasis, gout or osteoarthritis [42].

THE HIP

Early symptoms of hip involvement may be an abnormal gait or groin discomfort. Even with progressive RA, however, the hips are often spared. Moreover, the onset of hip disease in patients with RA is subtle, because patients maintain a pain-free range of hip movement until synovitis causes a progressive loss of cartilage space. Once this symmetric erosive process becomes established, bilateral protrusion of the acetabulae is inevitable [43]. Alternatively, with collapse of the femoral head from osteonecrosis, the deformity is lateral migration rather than protrusion into the pelvis. Once these complications arise, stiffness and pain interfere with the patient's ability to walk. A previous history of glucocorticosteroid use is often noted in these cases.

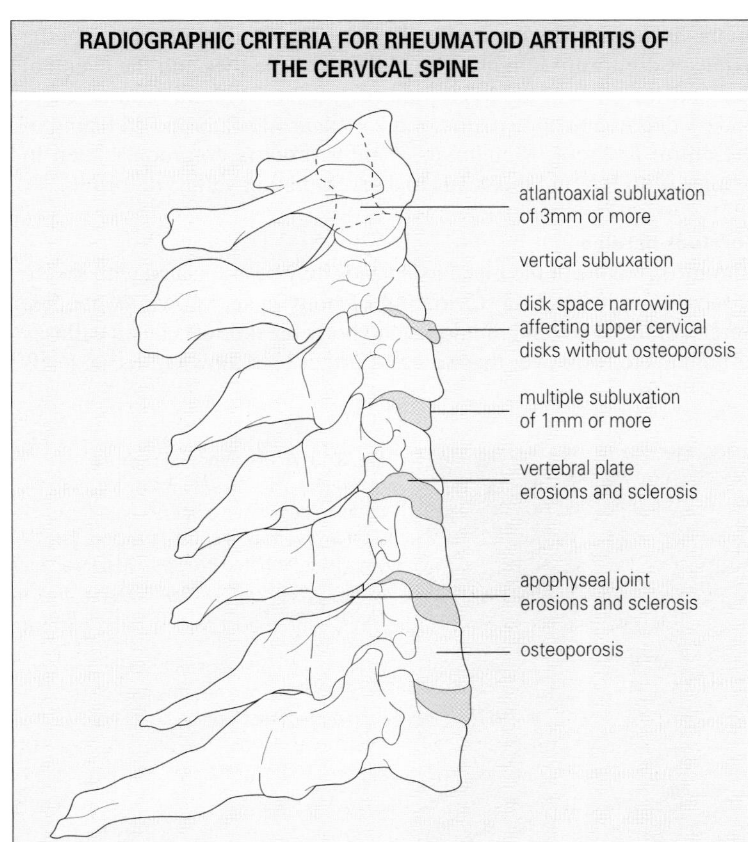

Fig. 3.16 The cervical spine in RA. These radiographic criteria for RA of the cervical spine are modified after Winfield *et al.* [39].

Iliopsoas bursa

Synovitis and effusion of the iliopsoas bursa (Fig. 3.17) may present with a unilateral or bilateral inguinal mass, or with lower extremity swelling without obvious relationship to the hip [44]. The bursa lies between the capsule of the hip and the iliopsoas muscle lateral to the femoral vessels. It rarely communicates with the hip joint and it is the largest bursa around the hip. Symptoms that may be mistaken for a hernia, lymphadenopathy or aneurysm arise from the inguinal mass. Femoral vein compression may lead to lower limb edema and a picture resembling deep-vein thrombosis.

Trochanteric and ischial bursae

Bursitis of the trochanteric bursa is more common than that of the ischial bursa. Either may be mistaken for true hip joint involvement (Fig. 3.17).

THE KNEE

Involvement of the knee is common in RA and usually is obvious. Sometimes, however, meniscal surgery has been performed in patients before the diagnosis of RA became apparent. Small effusions of the knee joint are detectable in early disease by means of the 'bulge' sign (*see* Fig. 3.8). Although this sign is useful for detecting small amounts of fluid, it does not necessarily confirm an inflammatory process unless the results of synovial fluid analysis show changes consistent with RA. The normal skin temperature of the knee is significantly lower than that of the thigh or tibia. This is the basis of the 'cool patella' sign [45]. In the case of knee inflammation, palpation over the thigh, patella and calf with the back of the hand shows the temperature over the patella to be equal to the heat over the thigh and tibia (i.e. a loss of the cool patella sign).

With an increase in the amount of the knee effusion, the fluid bulge sign disappears and positive ballottement or the patellar tap sign develops. The patient tends to assume a more comfortable position with the knee flexed and, if this becomes a habit, a loss of full knee extension eventually results. In full extension, the recumbent patient will be unable to push the popliteal surface of the knee into the examiner's hand.

Popliteal (Baker's) cysts

Knee extension lag may be associated with popliteal fullness caused by a Baker's cyst. The cyst can extend from its location in the gastrocnemius bursa down into the medial aspect of the calf. This is seen best by observing the standing patient from behind (*see* Fig. 3.18). Sometimes these cysts extend into the medial ankle region. The Baker's popliteal cyst arises as an extension from the joint cavity; synovial tissue acts as a ball-valve allowing fluid accumulation without means for decompression [46]. Exertion sufficient to raise the intra-articular knee joint pressure can lead to rupture of the synovial cyst, with extravasation of inflam-

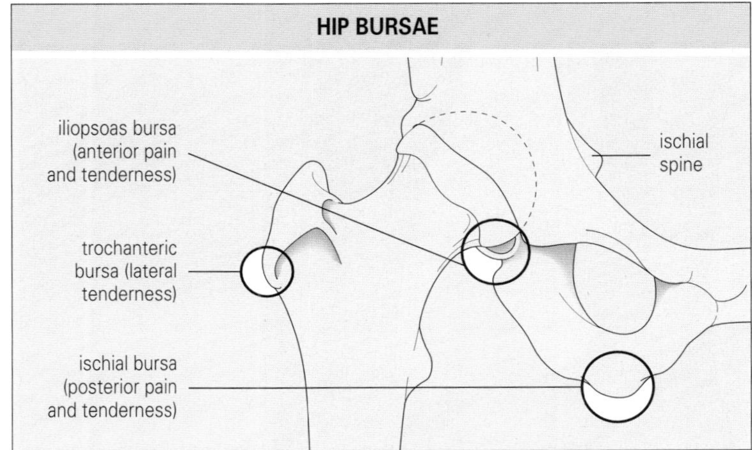

Fig. 3.17 Hip bursae that may be affected by rheumatoid granuloma. Involvement of the iliopsoas bursa is associated with an inguinal mass that may be mistaken for a hernia, lymphadenopathy or aneurysm [44].

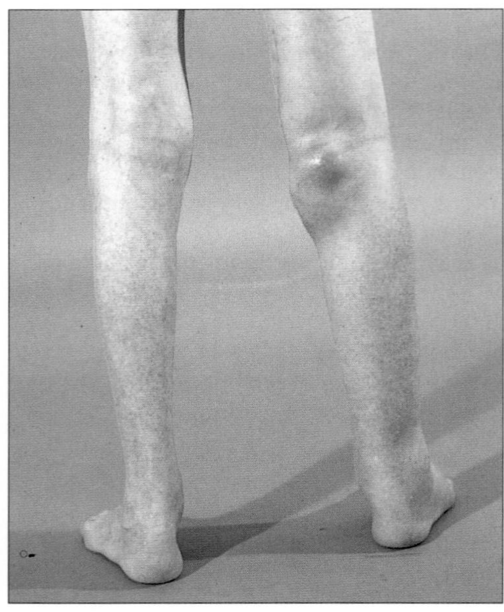

Fig. 3.18 Baker's popliteal cyst. Posterior view showing rheumatoid swelling behind the right knee. Swelling of the lower limb was related to venous compression by popliteal synovitis.

matory synovial fluid into the calf presenting a picture that mimics acute thrombophlebitis [46] (see Chapter 5.16). A hemorrhagic 'crescent' sign in the skin about the ankle below the malleoli is characteristic of synovial rupture and is not a feature of thrombophlebitis [47].

Rarely, after inflammation from a rupture into the calf has subsided, another rupture may cause posterior thigh extravasation and hemorrhage (Fig. 3.19). Anterolateral joint cysts may also extend below the knee, but this is a very rare occurrence [48].

Later disease

Eventually destruction of the knee by RA leads to limitation in walking similar to the disability seen with the rheumatoid hip. With loss of cartilage comes laxity of the collateral and cruciate ligaments. This is detected by stressing the knee joint for lateral and medial collateral stability with the knee cradled in the arms of the examiner at 15% of flexion. Cruciate anterior–posterior instability is detectable by means of the 'drawer' sign. A special problem arises in women with physiologic valgus. This produces increasing loading on the lateral compartment of the knee joint with erosion of the tibial plateau and progressive valgus deformity. As the valgus increases so does the loading, so that a vicious cycle is produced. Less common is the same set of circumstances in a varus position. With varus there is often collapse or fracture of the medial plateau and even more severe deformity.

Occasionally, inflammation results in binding of the collateral ligaments to the side of the femoral condyle. This destroys the normal anteroposterior gliding motion of the tibia on the femur and leads to a relative posterior subluxation of the tibia. The resultant deformity is usually associated with fixed flexion of the knee, and as the tibia tries to extend it digs into the femoral condyle producing a bony block anteriorly.

THE ANKLE

The ankle joint (tibial–talar articulation) is not as frequently involved as the subtalar and midtarsal joints of the hind foot. Persistent synovitis of the ankle joint leads to loss of cartilage and bone-on-bone contact. However, ankle involvement is not usually a cause of great disability because the joint remains quite stable. Sometimes a stress fracture of the distal fibula may masquerade as a flare of ankle arthritis [49].

THE FOOT

Hindfoot involvement

The subtalar and talonavicular joints are commonly affected in RA, but this is not always appreciated. Synovitis of these joints causes pain and stiffness and sometimes subtalar dislocation. Secondary peroneal muscle spasm develops and tends to immobilize the subtalar joint. The spasm promotes a valgus deformity and causes a peroneal spastic flat foot. As cartilage loss and bone erosion develop, valgus deformity increases, with progressive flattening of the longitudinal arch. Eventually the os calcis abuts against the lateral malleolus with collapse through the midfoot, producing pressure points over the head of the talus. At this stage the joint may spontaneously fuse without further progression.

Although heel pain is a characteristic of the spondyloarthropathies it can be a particular problem in RA. It can arise with development of a subachilles or retrocalcaneal bursitis that may be associated with nodule formation in the Achilles tendon. Rupture of the Achilles tendon may also complicate the picture [50]. Persistent heel pain caused by a calcaneal stress fracture is sometimes misinterpreted as subtalar or ankle synovitis.

The forefoot

Disease of the metatarsal heads is common in RA, causing much pain and disability. Forefoot deformity usually starts with synovitis of the metatarsophalangeal (MTP) joints and involvement of the flexor tendons within their sheath. Because of volar pain, the patient tends to walk on the heels with maximum dorsiflexion. This leads to reactivity of the extensor digitorum longus, with clawing of the toes and the eventual dorsal dislocation of the MTP joint (Fig. 3.20). With this comes a secondary depression and erosion of the metatarsal heads and widening of the entire forefoot. Metatarsus primus varus is commonly seen in women with RA and this leads to a severe hallux valgus deformity.

Forefoot fistulae

Chronic synovitis of the metatarsal heads may be associated with severe erosive changes and the formation of bony cysts known as geodes. Spread of the synovial granuloma and bony breakdown causes calluses or bunions to form over these areas. Further breakdown of tissue leads

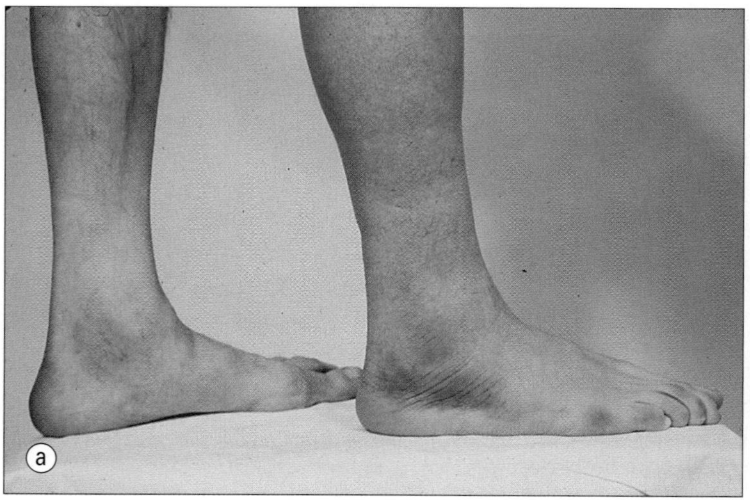

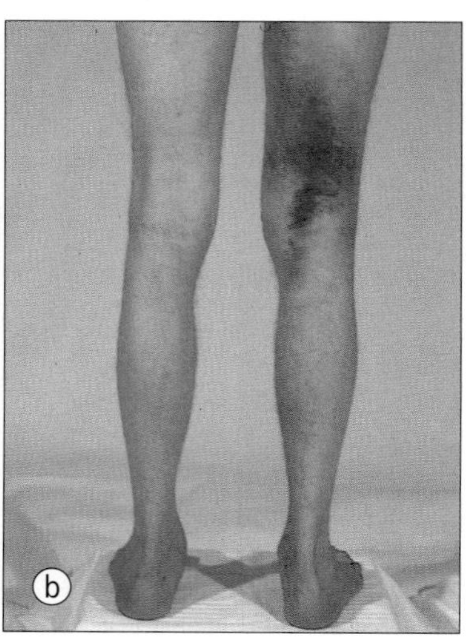

Fig. 3.19 Acute synovial rupture. A 51-year-old man with RA of 3 years' duration developed a right knee effusion after an evening of square dancing. Two days later he noted progressive pain and swelling of the right calf and 6 days later bluish discoloration of both sides of the ankle (a). A few weeks later, after more dancing, he noted posterior thigh pain and swelling that soon became associated with purple discoloration of his right posterior thigh (b) [47].

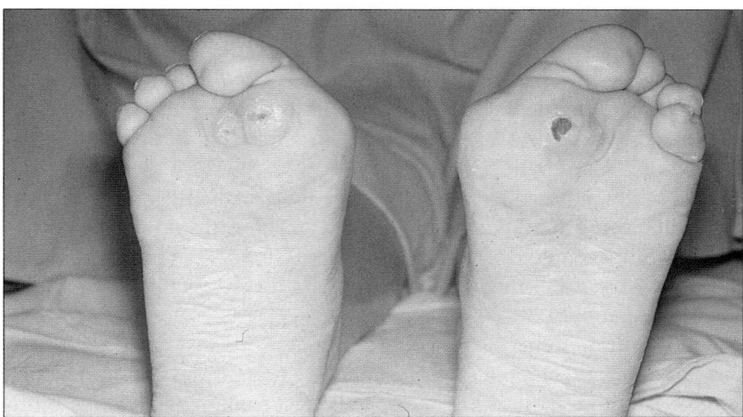

Fig. 3.20 Rheumatoid forefoot. Plantar view of the feet in a patient with RA. Hallux valgus, MTP subluxation and bursal swelling under weight-bearing areas are seen. Subluxation of the metatarsal head is associated with clawing of the toes, cock-up digital deformities and over-riding of the toes. The ulcerated bursae under the left metatarsal head may become associated with a chronic synovial fistula and secondary infection [51].

to a chronic cutaneous fistula as synovial fluid tracks from the MTP joint to the dorsal or plantar surface of the foot [51]. Secondary infection along this fistulous track is a hazard that may require surgery extending back into the MTP joint. Although chronic fistulous rheumatism is seen most often with metatarsal synovitis, chronic cutaneous fistulae may develop in relation to any rheumatoid joint. Diffuse pitting edema of the feet may be due to local venous insufficiency, obstruction of lymphatics or veins from a swollen ankle, knee or hip, or it may even relate to cardiac disease, sometimes associated with RA, such as pericarditis. Numbness of the medial aspect of the forefoot may result from a tarsal tunnel entrapment neuropathy of the medial peroneal nerve.

NATURAL HISTORY

DISEASE ONSET

The clinical course of RA follows an onset of disease that may be either abrupt and acute, or gradual and insidious, or subacute between these extremes [1,2]. For this reason the measurement of disease activity in RA is not easily defined [52]. A gradual onset is most common (at least 50% of cases), whereas a sudden onset is much less common (10–25%) [1,2]. RA begins predominantly as an articular disease and one or many joints may be affected. It may also start with an extra-articular or nonarticular presentation, such as a local bursitis or tenosynovitis, or as a systemic presentation with diffuse polyarthralgia or polymyalgia. Although the onset is predominantly articular, it is frequently associated with a variety of extra-articular features, including generalized weakness, anorexia, weight loss or fever. In some cases, fatigue alone or diffuse nonspecific aching with other extra-articular features, such as pulmonary disease, may herald by weeks or months the onset of polyarthritis [2].

PATTERN OF PRESENTATION

Gradual onset

The commonest presentation at onset is a gradual or insidious one affecting small peripheral joints such as the wrists, MCP, PIP, ankles or MTPs. A gradual onset is defined as one that the patient can only date to the nearest month. This gradual onset is usually symmetric with considerable morning stiffness and the patient complaining of difficulty making a fist and poor grip strength. The morning stiffness may last minutes to hours.

Slow, monoarticular presentation

Less common is a slow monoarticular presentation affecting larger joints such as shoulders or knees. The symptoms may remain confined to one or two joints, but frequently spread over the ensuing days and weeks additively to affect wrists, fingers, ankles or feet in a widespread fashion.

Abrupt, acute polyarthritis

Less frequently RA presents as an abrupt acute polyarthritis of the shoulders, elbows, wrists, fingers, hips, knees, ankles and feet, with intense joint pain, diffuse swelling and limitation leading to incapacitation. A sudden onset is defined as one for which the patient can give a specific date. This type of onset may affect patients at any age but has particular significance in the elderly. Aged males especially may develop a syndrome of 'remitting, seronegative, symmetric, synovitis with pitting edema (RS3PE syndrome)' [28] that may be confused with RA. A similar subgroup of elderly British males showed an acute 'stormy' onset with resolution usually within a year – 'benign RA of the aged' [53]. However, a prospective controlled study of 71 Dutch patients over 60 years of age, mostly with an acute onset, showed after 2 years a more progressive course than their younger counterparts [6].

Acute monoarthritis

An acute monoarthritis of a knee, shoulder or hip can present a picture suggesting a septic, pseudogout or gouty process, though this presentation is rare. Joint pain more severe than that found in RA is characteristic of the latter conditions, which may resemble or even complicate RA. The results of synovial fluid analysis should settle any diagnostic confusion in these cases. An acute monoarticular presentation may proceed to more widespread involvement with any of the preceding patterns.

Tenosynovitis or bursitis may also be associated with mono- or polyarthritis and subcutaneous nodules over extensor surfaces, such as the elbow, sacrum or Achilles tendon, may appear.

Palindromic rheumatism

Another variation of the abrupt onset of polyarthritis is known as palindromic rheumatism [54]. Here, variable episodes of polyarthritis suddenly affect one or more large and/or peripheral joints, last a few hours or a few days, and then spontaneously subside, with complete clearing of all rheumatic signs between attacks. These short-lived episodes may recur over weeks or months, with increasing frequency and severity, and may herald the onset of persistent polyarthritis. At least one-third of these palindromic cases evolve into typical RA.

Local extra-articular features

As noted, bursitis and tenosynovitis may be associated with RA. Sometimes, however, the earliest manifestation and presentation of RA may be a median nerve compression (carpal tunnel syndrome) from volar wrist tenosynovitis [33]. Similarly, other local extra-articular features may be the presenting feature.

Systemic extra-articular features

Elderly patients, in particular, may present with polyarthralgias and polymyalgias affecting the neck and shoulders or hips and knees, with associated profound fatigue. Although these features, especially in association with fever and high ESR lasting several weeks, suggest a diagnosis of polymyalgia rheumatica, this picture may be a forerunner of full-blown RA. Moreover, some investigators have advanced the notion that seronegative RA in the elderly has more in common with polymyalgia rheumatica than typical seropositive erosive RA [55].

PATTERN OF PROGRESSION

No matter what the onset or presentation, the patient's subsequent progress may follow several different patterns. It may be a course that is brief or episodic, prolonged and progressive, or something intermediate. The severity may vary from mild to intense. Attacks may be prolonged and smoldering or prolonged and progressive. With continuing disease activity, the patient's daily activities and functional capacity are affected to a greater or lesser extent. Although disability is usually proportional to the amount of painful joint involvement, in men who do physically hard work there is sometimes progressive joint dysfunction and disability without much pain. The physical abilities of patients who have this 'neuropathic' picture may dwindle insidiously before the seriousness of the situation becomes apparent. This highlights the importance of careful evaluation and re-evaluation of the patient's condition. For this reason, good records are essential to document the patient's progress and response to therapy, and these records should incorporate the features contained in the American Rheumatism Association (ACR) criteria for clinical remission in RA (Fig. 3.21) [56]. The criteria include features thought to predict a favorable outcome and are mostly inflammatory articular characteristics of RA. Unlike the self-report questionnaires these criteria do not take into account the patient's present functional state. The latter is frequently a better predictor of the patient's future condition [19]. Moreover, when a patient is not responding to therapy as expected, it is important to be aware of all the factors that may adversely affect outcome. The patient's systemic reaction and extra-articular features and serologic status may in fact be more important than the articular features and their complications (see Chapter 5.4). Alternatively, the patient may be showing an adverse reaction to one or more medications. Contrary to many patients' belief, weather conditions do not appear to influence symptoms of arthritis.

ACR CRITERIA FOR CLINICAL REMISSION OF RHEUMATOID ARTHRITIS

A minimum of five of the following for at least 2 consecutive months:

1. Morning stiffness not to exceed 15 minutes
2. No fatigue
3. No joint pain
4. No joint tenderness or pain on motion
5. No soft tissue swelling in joints or tendon sheaths
6. ESR (Westergren's method) less than 30mm/h (females) or 20mm/h (males)

Exclusions prohibiting a designation of complete clinical remission:

- Clinical manifestations of active vasculitis
- Pericarditis
- Pleuritis
- Myositis
- And/or unexplained recent weight loss or fever secondary to RA

Fig. 3.21 The ACR preliminary criteria for complete clinical remission of RA. In a patient with a definite or classic RA, at least five of these must be fulfilled for at least 2 consecutive months [56].

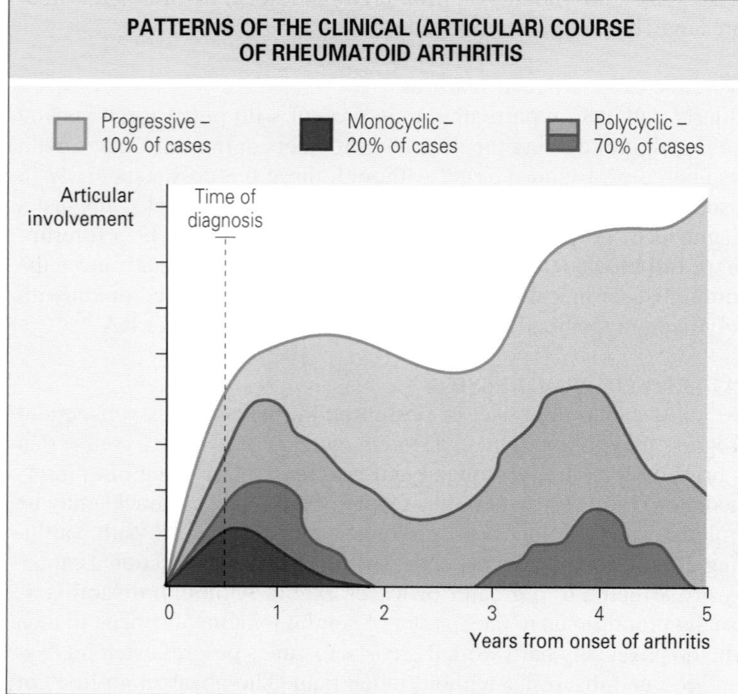

Fig. 3.22 Clinical (articular) course patterns in RA: articular patterns in 50 patients with RA. Data from Masi *et al.* [57].

Few studies have examined the natural history of a group of patients with a well-defined RA over a long period of time. One such representative study is that by Masi *et al.* who followed 50 patients with early RA for almost 6 years and described three articular patterns (Fig. 3.22) [57].

- Monocyclic pattern: a single cycle with remission for at least 1 year, seen in 20% of patients.
- Polycyclic pattern: seen in 70% of patients with either intermittent or continuing subtypes. The latter group showed smoldering activity with incomplete remission or progression.
- Progressive pattern: with increasing joint involvement seen in about 10% of patients.

Patients with malignant RA would fall under this last category. Most authorities would agree with these general observations, but many current ideas on the natural history of RA must remain speculative until the results of modern, long-term clinical population studies become available.

CLINICAL COURSE – MORBIDITY AND MORTALITY

Studies of the natural history of RA could provide insights into outcome variables and prognosis. Understanding prognosis helps us to evaluate better the medicolegal or psychosocial implications for estimating work disability in RA, and social implications, such as health-service planning and costs. It is worthwhile considering whether the type of disease onset and patterns of presentation previously outlined can be used to predict the subsequent course of RA. A generally held view is that an acute onset forecasts a favorable prognosis whereas an insidious onset heralds a worse outlook.

ACUTE ONSET PATTERN

In a series of 102 early cases of adult RA, Fleming *et al.* reported that 11 cases with sudden onset showed after 5 years a better functional outcome than 69 patients with a slow onset of disease [1]. However, in a later series of 100 patients, Jacoby *et al.* observed that after an 11-year follow up, there was no difference in functional class whether disease onset was acute, subacute or gradual [2]. In the past, a favorable prognosis may have been ascribed to cases of acute onset RA because they had not yet evolved into a different, more benign condition. For example, cases with acute onset due to a reactive or viral polyarthritis may have been mistaken for RA. Another explanation of why patients with acute onset may have had a better outcome is that they were more likely to seek prompt medical attention than were patients with a gradual onset of disease. The favorable course of mild or transient RA, however, has not attracted much attention, because rheumatologists are mostly concerned with progressive RA.

GRADUAL ONSET PATTERN

In Fleming's report a worse prognosis was found in patients with disease that was gradual in onset and associated with large joint involvement (shoulders, elbows, wrists, knees) as well as involvement of the first and second MTPs [1]. In the Jacoby series [2], the type of onset was not predictive of functional status after 11 years; moreover, in a later Finnish study of 235 RA patients, radiographically evident damage after 7 years was the same whether the onset had been acute (69), subacute (55) or gradual (111) [58].

GENERAL VARIABLES

A number of variables are thought to have prognostic implications (see Fig. 3.10). In a large Finnish population survey of 7217 adults, the detection of rheumatoid factor in 15 of 21 patients with seropositive RA antedated the onset of RA usually by 5 years [59]. Thus, in spite of the validity of the factors listed in Figure 3.10, better markers are needed for detecting early disease and identifying at an early stage patients who are likely to pursue a progressive course. Ideally, some of the newer immunogenetic, synovial or imaging methods may fulfill these needs.

HEALTH STATUS QUESTIONNAIRE ASSESSMENTS

In assessing prognosis, a number of health status self-report questionnaires have been developed and found valuable for routine and research use [19–22]. Data obtained by rheumatologists using these suggest that the overall prognosis in patients with RA may be much worse than previously estimated. Wolfe and Cathey assessed functional disability using the Stanford HAQ and FDI in 1274 patients with RA followed up longitudinally for up to 12 years [60]. Half of the patients showed loss of function that was moderate within 1–2 years, severe in 2–6 years and very severe in 10 years. The progression of disability was most rapid in the early years and then tapered off. Simple demographic and clinical assessment showed that disease worsened more quickly in women and was associated with a longer duration of disease, decreased grip strength, and worse pain, global severity and psychologic scores. Older patients also showed more systemic features associated with greater functional loss [6].

In another longitudinal study, from Santa Clara County, California, patients with disease for more than 20 years deteriorated more rapidly than those with disease of a shorter duration [61]. The Stanford HAQ disability index also showed more rapid deterioration in women, in patients with fewer years of education and with increased age. The same investigators showed that the Stanford HAQ disability index is a useful prognosticator of length of survival [62]. Patients with more severe disease are more likely to receive prednisone, and its long-term use was a risk factor associated with greater disability and premature death [62].

Severity measured by these prognostic factors may predict not only morbidity but also a two-fold increase in mortality rate that is comparable to malignant conditions such as Hodgkin's disease or chronic heart disease [63]. Moreover, these prognostic analyses confirm that RA is a marker for the development of many comorbid chronic conditions, such as bacterial infections and renal disease. Estimates of functional status using these questionnaires also appear to provide a better estimate of long-term prognosis than radiographic or serologic measures [64].

Although self-report questionnaires have proved valuable, patients with limited education find them difficult to use and rheumatologists are reluctant to rely on questionnaire data alone. Pincus *et al.* studied three simple measures of functional status – grip strength, walking time and a button test [65]. Their results were comparable to laboratory measures, showed reliable reproducibility and were similar to self-report questionnaires in their capacity to predict outcome [66] (Fig. 3.23). While patients with poor long-term outlook have attracted the attention of hospital-based rheumatologists, these severely affected patients may not be representative of RA as a whole. This is because RA may currently be a milder disease than thought in the past [67-69].

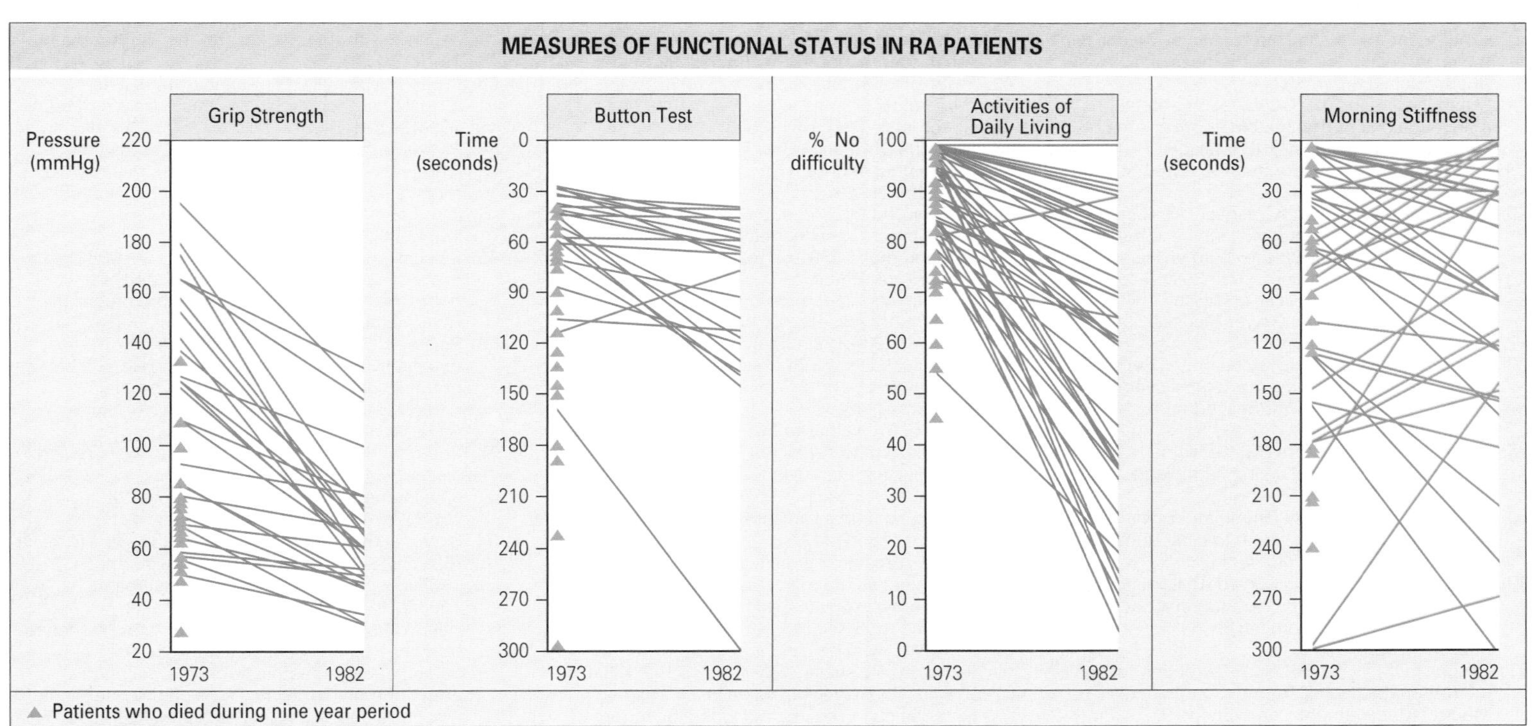

Fig. 3.23 Morbidity in RA patients. Data from Pincus *et al.* [65] and Pincus and Callahan [66].

REFERENCES

1. Fleming A, Crown JM, Corbett M. Early rheumatoid disease. I. Onset. II. Patterns of joint involvement. Ann Rheum Dis. 1976;35:357–63.
2. Jacoby RK, Jayson MIV, Cosh JA. Onset, early stages and prognosis of rheumatoid arthritis: a clinical study of 100 patients with 11 year follow-up. Br Med J. 1973;2:96–100.
3. Arnett FC, Edworthy SM, Bloch DA, *et al.* The American Rheumatism Association 1987 revised criteria for the classification of rheumatoid arthritis. Arthritis Rheum. 1988;31:315–24.
4. Weyand CM, Goronzy JJ. Inherited and noninherited risk factors in rheumatoid arthritis. [Review] Curr Opin Rheumatol. 1995;53:206–13.
5. Pincus T, Callahan LF. How many types of patients meet classification criteria for rheumatoid arthritis? [editorial] J Rheumatol. 1994;21:1385–9.
6. Desiree MFM, van der Heijde, Piet LCM, *et al.* Older versus younger onset rheumatoid arthritis: results at onset and after 2 years of a prospective follow-up study of early rheumatoid arthritis. J Rheumatol. 1991;18:1285–9.
7. Hawley DJ, Wolfe F. Anxiety and depression in patients with rheumatoid arthritis: a prospective study of 400 patients. J Rheumatol. 1988;15:932–41.
8. McFarlane AC, Brooks PM. Determinants of disability in rheumatoid arthritis. Br J Rheumatol. 1988;27:7–14.
9. Moldofsky H, Chester WJ. Pain and mood patterns in patients with rheumatoid arthritis. Psychosom Med. 1970;32:309–18.
10. Wolfe F, Cathey, MA, Kleinkeksel SM, *et al.* Psychological status in primary fibrositis and fibrositis associated with rheumatoid arthritis. J Rheumatol. 1984;11:500–6.
11. Meyerowitz S, Jacox RF, Hess DW. Monozygotic twins discordant for rheumatoid arthritis. Arthritis Rheum. 1968;11:1–21.
12. Silman AJ, MacGregor AJ, Thomson W, *et al.* Twin concordance rates for rheumatoid arthritis: results from a nationwide study. Br J Rheumatol. 1993;32:903–7.
13. Masi AT. Sex hormones and rheumatoid arthritis: cause or effect relationships in a complex pathophysiology? [Review] Clin Exp Rheumatol. 1995;13:227–40.
14. Hazes JMW, Dijkmans AC, Vandenbroucke JP, *et al.* Pregnancy and the risk of developing rheumatoid arthritis. Arthritis Rheum. 1990;33:1770–5.

15. Brennan P, Silman AJ. Breast-feeding and the onset of rheumatoid arthritis. Arthritis Rheum. 1994;37:808–13.
16. Leigh JP, Fries JF. Education level and rheumatoid arthritis: evidence from five data centers. J Rheumatol. 1991;18:24–34.
17. Heliovaara M, Aho K, Aromaa A, *et al.* Smoking and risk of rheumatoid arthritis. J Rheumatol. 1993;20:1830–5.
18. Gordon DA, Hyland RH, Broder I. Rheumatoid arthritis. In: Cannon GW, Zimmerman GA, eds. The lung in rheumatic diseases. New York: Marcel Dekker; 1990;229–59.
19. Wolfe F, Kleinheksel SM, Cathey MA, *et al.* The clinical value of the Stanford Health Assessment Questionnaire Functional Disability Index in patients with rheumatoid arthritis. J Rheumatol. 1988;15:1480–8.
20. Anderson JJ, Felson DT, Meenan RF, Williams HJ. Which traditional measures should be used in rheumatoid arthritis clinical trials? Arthritis Rheum. 1989;32:1093–9.
21. Pincus T, Callahan LF, Brooks RH, *et al.* Self-report questionnaire scores in rheumatoid arthritis compared with traditional physical, radiographic, and laboratory measures. Ann Intern Med. 1989;110:259–66.
22. Hagglund KJ, Roth DL, Haley WE, Alarcon GS. Discriminant and convergent validity of self-report measures of affective distress in patients with rheumatoid arthritis. J Rheumatol. 1989;16:1428–32.
23. Klinkhoff AV, Bellamy N, Bombardier C, *et al.* An experiment in reducing interobserver variability of the examination for joint tenderness. J Rheumatol. 1988;15:492–4.
24. Lansbury J, Haut DD. Quantitation of the manifestations of rheumatoid arthritis. Area of joint surfaces as an index to total joint inflammation and deformity. Am J Med Sci. 1956;232:150–5.
25. Thompson PW, Silman AJ, Kirwan JR, Currey HLF. Articular indices of joint inflammation in rheumatoid arthritis. Correlation with the acute phase response. Arthritis Rheum. 1987;30:618–23.
26. Dieppe PA, *et al.* Slide atlas of clinical rheumatology. London: Gower Medical Publishing;1983.
27. McCarty DJ, O'Duffy JD, Pearson L, Hunter JB. Remitting seronegative symmetrical synovitis with pitting edema. (RS3PE) syndrome. JAMA. 1985;2545:2763–7.
28. Thompson M, Bywaters EGL. Unilateral rheumatoid arthritis following hemiplegia. Ann Rheum Dis. 1961;21:370–7.
29. Hastings DE, Evans JA. Rheumatoid wrist deformities and their relation to ulnar drift. J Bone Joint Surg. 1975;57A:930–4.
30. Hastings DE. In Gordon DA, ed. Rheumatoid arthritis – contemporary management series, 2E. New York: Medical Examination Publishing;1985:147–9.
31. Hastings DE, Walsh RP. Surgical reconstruction of the rheumatoid hand. Toronto: Orthopaedic Medical Management Corporation;1979.
32. Jacob J, Sartorius D, Kursunoglu S, *et al.* Distal interphalangeal joint involvement in rheumatoid arthritis. Arthritis Rheum. 1986;29:10–15.
33. Chamberlain A, Corbett M. Carpal tunnel syndrome in early rheumatoid arthritis. Ann Rheum Dis. 1970;29:149–52.
34. Chang LW, Gowans JDC, Granger CV, *et al.* Entrapment neuropathy of the posterior interosseous nerve. Arthritis Rheum. 1972;15:350–2.
35. Bywaters EGL. The bursae of the body. Ann Rheum Dis. 1965;24:215–18.
36. Yasuda M, Ono M, Naono T, Nobunaga M. Multiple rheumatoid bursal cysts. J Rheumatol. 1989;16:1986–8.
37. Polisar I, Burbank B, Levitt LM, *et al.* Bilateral midline fixation of cricoarytenoid joints as a serious medical emergency. JAMA. 1960;172:901–6.
38. Khong TK, Rooney PJ. Manubriosternal joint subluxation in rheumatoid arthritis. J Rheumatol. 1982;9:712–15.
39. Winfield J, Young A, Williams P, *et al.* A prospective study of the radiological changes in the cervical spine in early rheumatoid disease. Ann Rheum Dis. 1981;40:109–14.
40. Nakano KK, Schoene WC, Baker RA, Dawson DM. The cervical myelopathy associated with rheumatoid arthritis: an analysis of 32 patients, with 2 postmortem cases. Ann Neurol. 1978;3:144-51.
41. Stiskal MA, Neuhold A, Szolar DH, *et al.* Rheumatoid arthritis of the craniocervical region by MR imaging: detection and characterization. Am J Roentgenol. 1995;165:582–92.
42. Fallet GH, Barnes CG, Berry H, *et al.* Coexisting rheumatoid arthritis and ankylosing spondylitis. J Rheumatol. 1987;14:1135–8.
43. Hastings DE, Parker SM. Protrusio acetabuli in rheumatoid arthritis. Clin Orthop. 1975;108:76–83.
44. Underwood PL, McLeod RA, Ginsburg WW. The varied clinical manifestations of iliopsoas bursitis. J Rheumatol. 1988;15:1683–5.
45. Menard HA, Paquette D. Skin temperature of the knee: an unrecognized physical sign of inflammatory disease of the knee. Can Med Assoc J. 1980;122:439–40.
46. Gerber NJ, Dixon AStJ. Synovial cysts and juxta-articular bone cysts. Semin Arthritis Rheum. 1974;3:323–48.
47. Kraag G, Thevathasan EM, Gordon DA, Walker IH. The hemorrhage crescent sign of acute synovial rupture. Ann Intern Med. 1976;85:477–8.
48. Thevenon A, Hardouin P, Duquesnoy B. Popliteal cyst presenting as an anterior tibial mass. Arthritis Rheum. 1985;28:477–8.
49. Wei N. Stress fractures of the distal fibula presenting as monoarticular flares in patients with rheumatoid arthritis. Arthrits Rheum. 1994;37:1555–6.
50. Rask MR. Achilles tendon rupture owing to rheumatoid disease. JAMA. 1978;239:435–6.
51. Shapiro RF, Resnick D, Castles JJ, *et al.* Fistulization of rheumatoid joints. Spectrum of identifiable syndromes. Ann Rheum Dis. 1975;34:489–98.
52. Boers M, van Riel PL, Felson DT, Tugwell P. Assessing the activity of rheumatoid arthritis. [Review] Baillieres Clin Rheumat. 1995;9(2):305–17.
53. Corrigan AB, Robinson RG, Terenty TR, *et al.* Benign rheumatoid arthritis of the aged. Br Med J. 1974;1:444–6.
54. Schumacher HR. Palindromic onset of rheumatoid arthritis. Clinical, synovial fluid and biopsy studies. Arthritis Rheum. 1982;25:361–9.
55. Healey LA, Sheets PK. Polymyalgia rheumatica and seronegative rheumatoid arthritis may be the same entity. J Rheumatol. 1992;19:270–2.
56. Pinals RS, Masi AF, Larsen RA, et al. Preliminary criteria for clinical remission in rheumatoid arthritis. Bull Rheum Dis. 1982;32:7–10.
57. Masi AT, Feigenbaum SL, Kaplan SB. Articular patterns in the early course of rheumatoid arthritis. Am J Med. 1983;75(suppl 6A):16–26.
58. Luukkainen R, Isomaki H, Kajander A: Prognostic value of the type of onset of rheumatoid arthritis. Ann Rheum Dis. 1983;42:274–5.
59. Aho K, Heliovaara M, Maatela J, *et al.* Rheumatoid factors antedating clinical rheumatoid arthritis. J Rheumatol. 1991;18:1282–4.
60. Wolfe F, Cathey MA. The assessment and prediction of functional disability in rheumatoid arthritis. J Rheumatol. 1991;18:1298–1306.
61. Leigh JP, Fries JF, Parikh N. Severity of disability and duration of disease in rheumatoid arthritis. J Rheumatol. 1992;19:1906–11.
62. Leigh JP, Fries J. Mortality predictors among 263 patients with rheumatoid arthritis. J. Rheumatol. 1991;18:1307–12.
63. Wolfe F, Mitchell DM, Sibley JT, *et al.* The mortality of rheumatoid arthritis. Arthritis Rheum. 1994:37:481–94.
64. Pincus T, Brooks RH, Callahan LF. Prediction of long-term mortality in patients with rheumatoid arthritis according to simple questionnaire and joint count measures. Ann Intern Med. 1994;120:26-34.
65. Pincus T, Brooks RH, Callahan LF. Reliability of grip strength, walking time and button test performed according to a standard protocol. J Rheumatol. 1991;18:997–1000.
66. Pincus T, Callahan LF. Predictive value of quantitative physical and questionnaire measures of functional status for 9-year morbidity in rheumatoid arthritis. J Rheumatol. 1992;19:1051–7.
67. Eberhardt KB, Fex E. Functional impairment and disability in early rheumatoid arthritis – development over 5 years. J Rheumatol. 1995;22:1037–42.
68 Suarez-Almazor ME, Soskolne I, Saunders D, Russell AS. Outcome in rheumatoid arthritis. A 1985 inception cohort study. J Rheumatol. 1994;21:1438-46.
69. Hakala P, Nieminen O, Koivisto O. More evidence from a community based series of better outcome in rheumatoid arthritis. Data on the effect of multidisciplinary care on the retention of functional ability. J Rheumatol. 1994;21:1432–7.

CLINICAL FEATURES AND SYSTEMIC INVOLVEMENT

Eric L Matteson, Marc D Cohen & Doyt L Conn

Definition
- Extraarticular involvement affecting multiple organ systems
- Systemic features may be associated with a poor prognosis, especially vasculitis, amyloidosis and pulmonary fibrosis

Clinical features
- The major clinical features reflecting systemic involvement in rheumatoid arthritis include: fevers, malaise and weight loss.

INTRODUCTION

Constitutional features of rheumatoid arthritis (RA), such as fatigue and weight loss, may occur early in the course of the disease and may predominate, overshadowing the joint manifestations. At times inflammation may extend beyond the joints and involve other organs. Patients with seropositive RA with extra-articular features have a diminished life span compared with patients without RA[1]. Influencing the poor outcome is the presence of vasculitis, amyloidosis and pulmonary fibrosis[2]. Laboratory abnormalities that accompany systemic involvement include elevated erythrocyte sedimentation rate (ESR), anemia, thrombocytosis and elevation of certain liver function tests (Fig. 4.1). In some populations, HLA-DR1 and DR4 genes are associated with a higher frequency of extra-articular disease[3,4].

NODULES

Subcutaneous nodules occur in 20% of RA patients with positive tests for blood rheumatoid factors and rarely in seronegative patients. The nodules reflect the level of rheumatoid disease activity and accompany severe disease. Rheumatoid nodulosis (multiple, widespread nodules) occasionally presents as a separate condition, usually in men, with a low grade and sometimes barely detectable synovitis[5].

Nodules develop most commonly on pressure areas, including the elbows, finger joints, ischial and sacral prominences, occipital scalp and Achilles tendon. Rheumatoid nodules are firm and frequently adherent to the underlying periosteum. Histologically there is a focal central fibrinoid necrosis with surrounding fibroblasts. This is thought to occur as a result of small vessel vasculitis with fibrinoid necrosis which forms the center of the nodule, and surrounding fibroblastic proliferation (see Chapter 5.6).

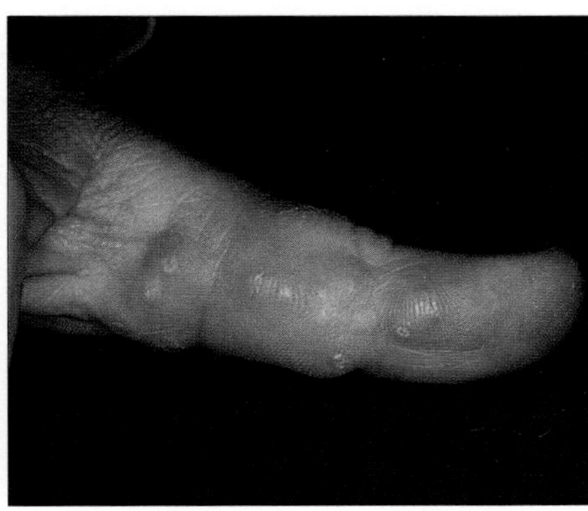

Fig. 4.1 Finger nodules developing in patient with RA treated with low-dose weekly methotrexate.

Subcutaneous nodules may regress during treatment with disease-modifying drugs, usually as the RA improves. Methotrexate treatment paradoxically may result in an increase in nodules, particularly over finger tendons (Fig. 4.1), despite improvement in the overall disease activity[6,7].

HEMATOLOGIC ABNORMALITIES

The cause of anemia in RA is multifactorial. Iron utilization is impaired, as reflected by decreased serum iron and transferrin concentrations. As with other forms of chronic inflammation, there is an increased synthesis of ferritin and hemosiderin, abnormal retention of iron from senescent red blood cells by the reticuloendothelial system, and increased lactoferrin which contributes to the binding and lowering of serum iron. Also contributing to the anemia of RA are reduced erythropoietin levels and a slightly depressed response of the bone marrow to erythropoietin. Ineffective erythropoiesis occurs with premature destruction of red blood cells and inhibition of production of red blood cell precursors. Red blood cell life span may be reduced. Additional factors include an increased phagocytosis of red blood cells by lymph nodes and even the synovium.

The degree of anemia in RA correlates with the activity of the underlying disease, particularly the degree of articular inflammation. It is commonly normochromic and normocytic unless complicated by concomitant conditions, such as blood loss, poor nutrition, hemodilution, intercurrent infections, or drug-induced hemolytic anemia or bone marrow suppression.

While various medications used to treat RA can contribute to the anemia, that caused by rheumatoid inflammation can improve with therapy that treats the disease successfully. The administration of erythropoietin to patients with RA has been shown to improve red blood cell counts without influencing disease activity[8]. Iron deficiency may complicate the anemia associated with RA, but repletion of iron may fail since the anemia is due to inhibition of hemoglobin synthesis caused by inflammation.

Thrombocytosis is a frequent finding in active RA. The degree of thrombocytosis may correlate with the number of joints involved with active synovitis, and may be associated with extra-articular features. The mechanism of thrombocytosis is uncertain. Increased intravascular coagulation with a compensatory increase in platelet production has been suggested. The thrombocytosis does not predispose to an increase in thrombotic events and is not correlated with bone marrow neoplastic changes.

Thrombocytopenia is rare in RA, except when related to drug treatment or Felty's syndrome. Drug-induced platelet dysfunction may be seen. Coagulation inhibitors may be produced and hyperviscosity has rarely been reported. It occurs in association with high titers of rheumatoid factor and may cause neurologic and vascular occlusive symptoms.

Eosinophilia accompanying RA is sometimes associated with extra-articular manifestations. The pathogenesis is not known. Immune complexes may be chemotactic for eosinophils, and cytokines known to stimulate eosinophil production could be important. Eosinophilia has been associated with high titers of blood rheumatoid factor, elevated of serum gamma globulins, and diminished serum complement levels. Pulmonary complications may be associated with eosinophilia[9]. A number of drugs used to treat RA, especially gold, may cause eosinophilia.

Lymphadenopathy is frequent in patients with active RA. Palpable lymph nodes are generally detected in the axillary, inguinal, and epitrochlear areas. These lymph nodes are usually mobile and non-tender. The presence of lymphadenopathy has no bearing on the outcome of the disease. As the RA is controlled, the lymphadenopathy will decrease. Histologic examination reveals follicular hyperplasia occasionally prominent enough to suggest lymphoma. Concomitant Sjögren's syndrome may confer an increased risk of lymphoma[10].

FELTY'S SYNDROME

Felty's syndrome is defined as RA in combination with splenomegaly and leukopenia. The syndrome characteristically occurs in patients with long-standing, seropositive, nodular, deforming RA. Approximately one-third of this group of patients have no active synovitis at the time Felty's syndrome develops. Many of these patients have lower extremity ulcerations, hyperpigmentation, and antinuclear antibodies.

Bacterial infections are common in Felty's syndrome, correlate with a polymorphonuclear leukocyte count of less than 1000/mm^3, and account for most deaths in this syndrome[11]. Other factors associated with an increased incidence of infections are skin ulcers, glucocorticoid dose, hypocomplementemia and high levels of immune complexes. Immune complexes coat granulocytes, which results in their sequestration and reduced survival, and specific antibodies directed against white blood cell surface antigens (granulocyte-specific antinuclear antibodies) may contribute to the leukopenia. In some patients, the bone marrow does not respond appropriately to the degree of leukopenia, perhaps because of inhibitors which suppress myelopoiesis. Thrombocytopenia also occurs in Felty's syndrome.

Treatment of the rheumatoid disease with disease-modifying drugs, such as parenteral gold, frequently improves the cytopenias, cutaneous vasculitis, and may decrease susceptibility to infection[12]. Splenectomy may improve the hematologic abnormalities and may be indicated for recurrent serious infections caused by the neutropenia which has been unresponsive to disease-modifying drugs. Splenectomy rarely helps the underlying disease process, although it might improve leg ulcers. Despite splenectomy, granulocytopenia may recur and persist. Glucocorticoids transiently improve the granulocytopenia but may predispose to infections. Parenteral testosterone, lithium and other treatments such as granulocyte colony stimulating factor have been used with success in selected patients, but large studies using such agents are not available.

There is an increased risk for the development of lymphoproliferative malignancies in patients with Felty's syndrome[13]. A variant of Felty's syndrome has been described in which patients have neutropenia and an increase in the number of large granular lymphocytes (LGL) in blood and bone marrow[14] (Fig. 4.2). The actual white blood count may be normal or increased. The LGL in these patients represents *in vivo* activated cytotoxic T-cells and clonality is present. However, clonality does not necessarily mean malignancy or decreased survival. In a recent study of 68 patients, 90% were alive at a median follow up of 44 months[15]. Such patients may also have thrombocytopenia, anemia and splenomegaly. This syndrome occurs in older patients and early in the course of the arthritis. In patients with symptoms related to neutropenia, improvement may occur with treatment with glucocorticoids and/or immunosuppressive agents[14], but splenectomy is contraindicated.

HEPATIC

Active RA may be associated with an elevation of liver enzymes (especially serum glutamic oxaloacetic transaminase and alkaline phosphatase)[16]. Liver function abnormalities may parallel the anemia, thrombocytosis and increased ESR. With control of the rheumatoid inflammation the liver function abnormalities return to normal. Examination of liver histology at the time of liver function abnormality

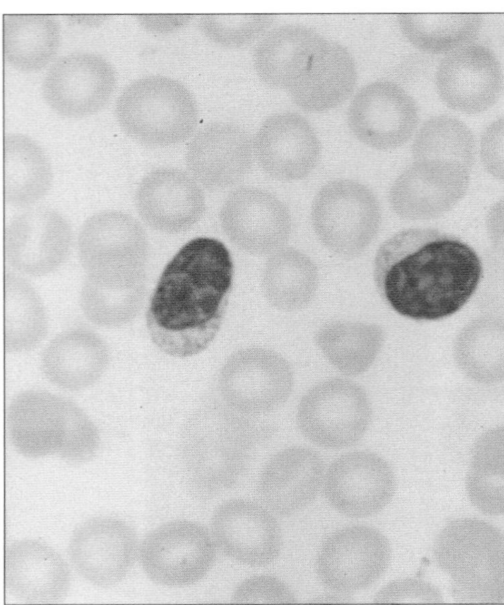

Fig. 4.2 Large granular lymphocyte.

reveals only minimal non-specific changes with some periportal mononuclear cell infiltration.

Nonsteroidal anti-inflammatory drugs (NSAIDs) may induce liver enzyme abnormalities and it may be difficult to differentiate between drug effects and disease activity. However, if the liver function abnormalities are due to NSAIDs, enzyme levels will improve with their discontinuation. NSAIDs seldom cause serious liver deterioration.

Liver involvement may be present in up to 65% of patients with Felty's syndrome[17]. There may be histologic abnormalities, even when liver function tests are normal. The liver pathology varies from portal fibrosis and abnormal lobular architecture to nodular regenerative hyperplasia. The nodular regenerative hyperplasia may be secondary to inflammation of small portal veins, possibly immune-complex induced. Frequently a liver wedge biopsy (an open biopsy) is necessary to establish the diagnosis. These patients can develop portal hypertension, esophageal varices and variceal bleeding.

PULMONARY

Pulmonary involvement in RA is frequent, although the clinical features may be subtle. In autopsy studies, involvement of the pleura is reported in up to 50% of patients with RA[18]. Pleural involvement is usually asymptomatic. Rheumatoid pleural effusions are transudates with low cell counts, predominately lymphocytes. Glucose levels are often less than 25mg/dl (1.4mmol/l). The low glucose in rheumatoid pleural effusions is a result of impaired transport across an inflamed pleura. Pleural fluid hemolytic complement levels are low, rheumatoid factor is present, and the leukocytes have inclusions containing rheumatoid factor. Pleurisy and pleural effusions may improve spontaneously or may require treatment. Persistent effusions can lead to fibrosis.

Parenchymal pulmonary nodules (Fig. 4.3) are generally asymptomatic and are found in seropositive RA patients who have widespread synovitis and usually nodules elsewhere. The pulmonary nodules tend to be peripheral in location, and can measure less than 1cm or up to 6–8cm in diameter. They can cavitate and cause pleural effusions and bronchopleural fistulas. Pathologic examination of the nodules reveals a central necrotic zone surrounded by a cellular area of proliferating fibroblasts. The pathogenesis of nodular formation is unknown, although vasculitis has been implicated. The differential diagnosis of pulmonary rheumatoid nodules includes neoplasms, tuberculosis and fungal infections. In the case of a solitary rheumatoid nodule in the lung, an excisional biopsy may be necessary to confirm the diagnosis. Treatment of the underlying rheumatoid disease frequently results in improvement of the pulmonary nodules.

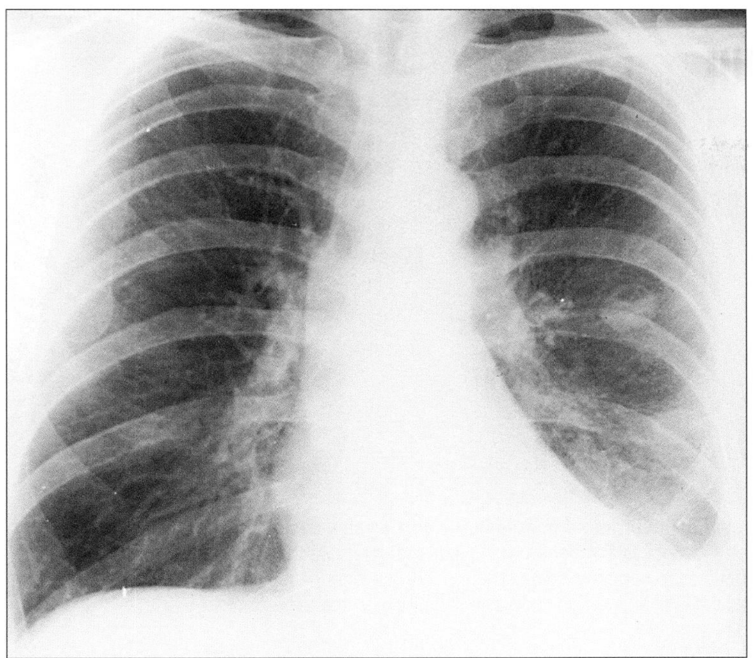

Fig. 4.3 Pleural effusion and rheumatoid nodule in RA.

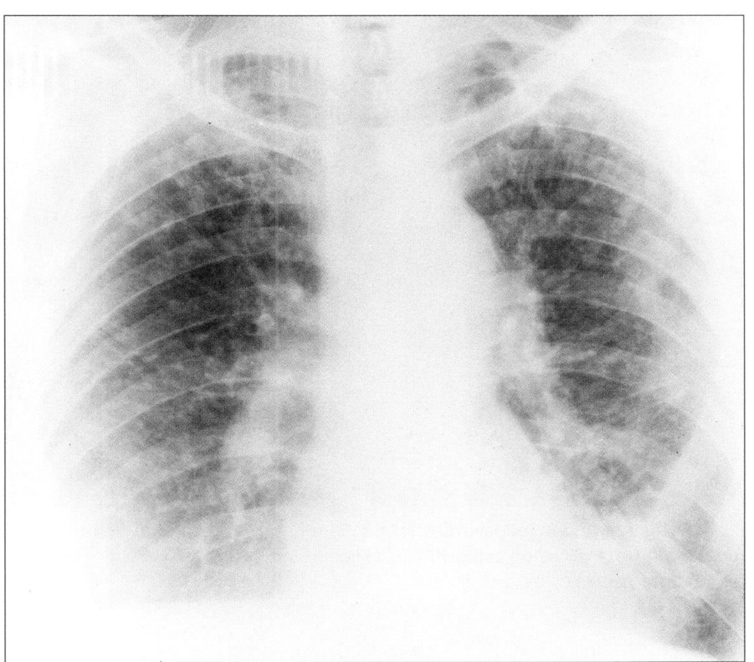

Fig. 4.4 Caplan's syndrome.

Pulmonary nodulosis and pneumoconiosis in patients with RA (Caplan's syndrome) is characterized by multiple nodules greater than 1cm in diameter scattered throughout the peripheral lung field (Fig. 4.4)[19]. Caplan's syndrome is seen in individuals with extensive exposure to coal dust, although exposure to silica and asbestos may also lead to pulmonary nodulosis in these patients.

Diffuse interstitial pulmonary fibrosis was first described in RA in 1948. An incidence of 28% has been reported. The prevalence of diffuse interstitial pulmonary fibrosis varies depending on diagnostic methodology and other factors. High resolution computerized tomography (CT) increases the likelihood of discovering interstitial disease[20–22]. Joint disease precedes the interstitial lung involvement in most cases. The clinical presentation and course of pulmonary fibrosis in RA are similar to those of idiopathic pulmonary fibrosis. Rheumatoid interstitial pulmonary disease is seen more frequently in men than women, particularly those who have long-standing, nodular, seropositive disease[23]. Histologic findings and results of bronchoalveolar lavage can be variable, ranging from lymphocytic alveolitis to neutrophilic inflammation to pulmonary fibrosis. The pathogenesis of rheumatoid pulmonary fibrosis has been related to production of inflammatory mediators, the presence of certain HLA genes, such as HLA-DRB1 and perhaps HLA-B40, and non-RA-associated factors such as tobacco usage and α_1-antitrypsin phenotype[24]. Treatment of interstitial pulmonary fibrosis in RA remains controversial, although a certain subset of patients may respond to aggressive immunosupressive therapy.

Broncholitis obliterans organizing pneumonia (BOOP) can be associated with RA. This type of pulmonary involvement responds to glucocorticoid therapy and has a generally good prognosis[24]. Another distinct type of pulmonary disease in RA, obliterative or constrictive bronchiolitis, responds poorly to treatment and has a poor prognosis[25]. Pulmonary biopsy should be performed if there is progressive pulmonary disease despite appropriate treatment to confirm the underlying pathology and to aid in therapeutic decisions.

Airway obstruction may develop in patients with RA. It may not necessarily be caused by the disease itself, but rather by other factors known to predispose to obstructive pulmonary disease.

Isolated pulmonary arteritis is a rare complication of RA. It is frequently associated with other manifestations of rheumatoid lung disease, such as interstitial fibrosis and nodulosis.

Several of the drugs used to treat RA may cause pulmonary complications including methotrexate, D-penicillamine and intramuscular gold compounds[26].

Pulmonary involvement in RA increases the morbidity and mortality of the underlying disease. Therapy for these conditions remains empirical.

CARDIAC

The acute and chronic inflammatory disease of RA may lead to cardiac disease by mechanisms of vasculitis, nodule formation, amyloidosis, serositis, valvulitis and fibrosis[27]. Pericarditis is the most common cardiac manifestation of RA. Although symptomatic pericarditis is relatively uncommon, both random electrocardiographic evaluation of RA patients and autopsy studies reveal evidence of pericardial inflammation in 50% of patients[28]. Pericarditis occurs in seropositive patients with nodules[29]. An analysis of pericardial fluid reveals changes similar to those found in rheumatoid pleural effusions, including a variable white blood cell count, high protein levels, decreased complement, decreased glucose concentrations, the presence of rheumatoid factor and immune complexes. Commonly the pericarditis resolves as the rheumatoid disease is controlled. Symptomatic patients generally respond to NSAIDs. Occasionally glucocorticoids are required if the symptoms are severe and recalcitrant to the usual management. Chronic, constrictive pericarditis is an infrequent sequela. In these cases, pericardiectomy may be required.

Myocardial disease resulting from nodular granulomatous lesions or more diffuse fibrosing lesions has been seen in RA (Fig. 4.5). Nonspecific myocarditis is usually asymptomatic and rarely effects cardiac size or function. Male patients with RA may suffer a higher frequency of congestive heart failure than persons without RA, and even in asymptomatic patients left ventricular diastolic function is more often impaired than in those without RA in spite of normal left ventricular systolic function[30]. Abnormalities in the conduction pathways have also been described. Endocardial involvement may be diffuse, but is rarely clinically significant.

Echocardiographic evidence for some degree of valve involvement can be detected in about 30% of patients, but is usually hemodynamically insignificant. Lesions typical of RA in the absence of symptomatic cardiac

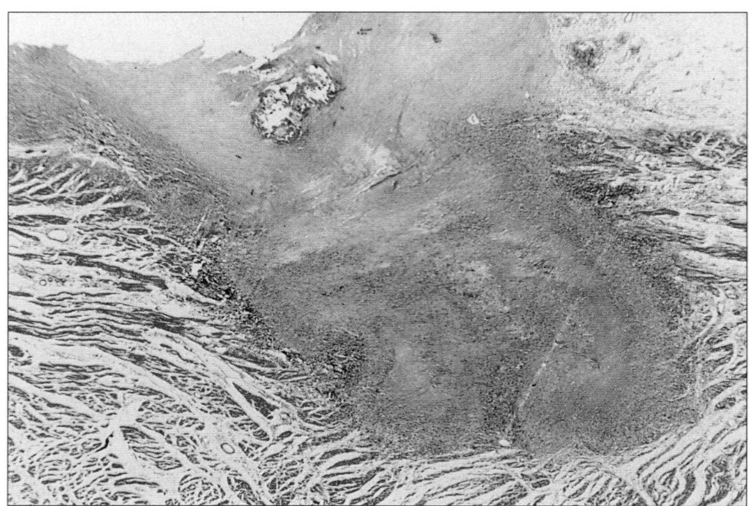

Fig. 4.5 Rheumatoid myoepicarditis with inflammatory cellular and rheumatoid nodular infiltrate of the epicardium and myocardium. (Hematoxylin and eosin stain, original magnification ×5.)

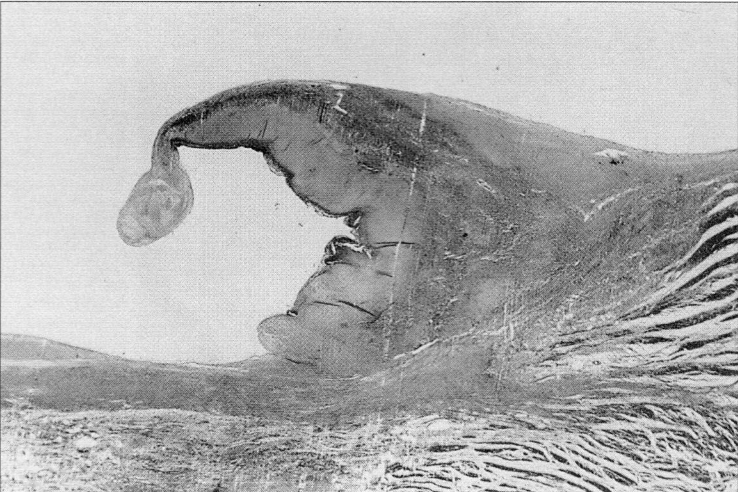

Fig. 4.6 Rheumatoid nodule in the aortic valve cusp in a 54-year-old woman. The cusp is seen as a finger-like projection to the left. At the base of the cusp, a rheumatoid nodule is noted. The muscle tissue in the lower right corner is of the left ventricle. (Hematoxylin and eosin stain, original magnification ×2.5.)

disease include posterior pericardial effusion, aortic root abnormalities and valvular thickening[31]. However, a few patients develop valvular incompetence (Fig. 4.6). Coronary arteritis can occur as part of systemic rheumatoid vasculitis (Fig. 4.7). Because myocardial and endocardial diseases associated with RA are usually a result of vasculitis and nodule formation, appropriate treatment of the underlying disease is necessary.

OCULAR

The most common ocular involvement in RA is keratoconjunctivitis sicca (KCS) which affects between 10 and 35% of patients (see Chapter 7.32). The severity of the symptoms may not be correlated with that of the arthritis. Symptoms range from dry eyes to burning, foreign body sensation and a mucoid discharge. Tear production may be assessed by Schirmer's test or by corneal staining with fluorescein or rose-bengal dye. Treatment of KCS is symptomatic.

Episcleritis usually correlates with the activity of RA (Fig. 4.8; see also The Red Eye in Rheumatoid Arthritis in Chapter 5.16). This process, which may be either nodular or diffuse, appears acutely and causes eye redness and pain, but only rarely changes in visual acuity. Scleritis is less common than episcleritis but is more obviously correlated with vasculitis, long-standing arthritis and active joint inflammation. Untreated scleritis may progress to scleromalacia (Fig. 4.9). Control of the RA may not improve the episcleritis or scleritis. The avascular nature of the sclera contributes to its resistance to treatment. Other rare ocular findings in RA include uveitis, episcleral nodulosis, corneal melt and peripheral ulcerative keratitis (PUK) (see Diagnosis and Management of Corneal Melt in Chapter 5.16). These conditions may require topical or systemic cytotoxic and glucocorticosteroid therapy; some (such as PUK) can herald impending vasculitis[32].

Drugs used to treat RA can also affect the eyes. Glucocorticoids may cause cataracts and glaucoma, gold may result in conjunctival and corneal deposition, and chloroquine derivatives cause both a keratopathy and a retinopathy.

An uncommon ocular complication of RA is Brown's syndrome, which is defined as diplopia upon upward and inward gaze and is thought to be due to inflammation and thickening of the superior oblique tendons[33].

NEUROLOGIC

Nerve compression is a common cause of neurologic impairment in RA. Peripheral entrapment neuropathies tend to correlate with the degree and severity of local synovitis, but are not related to duration, level of activity or severity of extra-articular manifestations of RA. They generally occur when the nerve is compressed by the inflamed synovium against a fixed structure. The median, ulnar, posterior tibial and the posterior interosseous branch of the radial nerve are the most commonly involved nerves. The diagnosis is suggested by clinical symptoms and neurologic findings. Percussion over the carpal tunnel and tarsal tunnel may elicit symptoms (Tinel's sign). The pain and paresthesias from the affected nerves often have a nocturnal accentuation and may radiate from the site of compression. Medical treatment may be effective, particularly if the synovitis can be controlled, but surgical release may be necessary to prevent permanent muscle atrophy.

Atlantoaxial subluxation (AAS) caused by erosion of the odontoid process and/or the transverse ligament of Cl may allow the odontoid process to slip posteriorly and cause a cervical myelopathy (Fig. 4.10)[34]. Basilar invagination, with upward impingement of the odontoid process into the foramen magnum, can also result in cord compression (Fig. 4.11)[35]. The presence of cord compression is indicated by a positive Babinski sign, hyper-reflexia and weakness. This may require surgical stabilization. These complications are seen in association with severe progressive, destructive, long-standing rheumatoid disease. This is discussed further in Instability of the Cervical Spine in Chapter 5.16.

Subaxial cervical spine involvement, including subluxation, spondylodiskitis and apophyseal joint changes, may occur at multiple levels, leading to pain and neurologic compromise. Neurologic sequelae may be more common in subaxial subluxation than AAS because of the

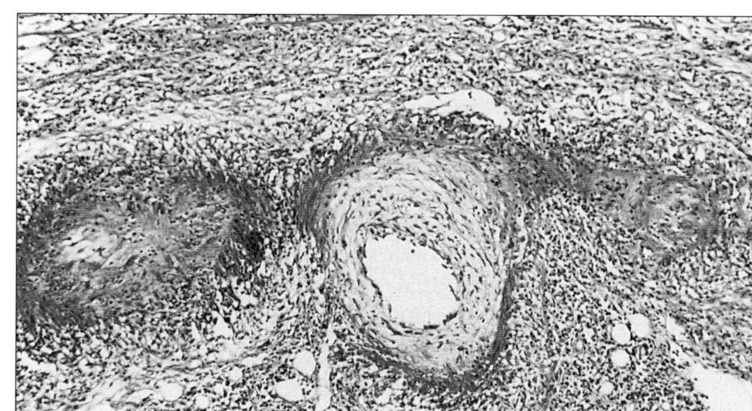

Fig. 4.7 Coronary arteritis. Two arteries are seen. There is a dense inflammatory infiltrate in the adventitia with some intimal luminal narrowing and destruction of the media of one artery. (Hematoxylin and eosin stain, original magnification ×25.)

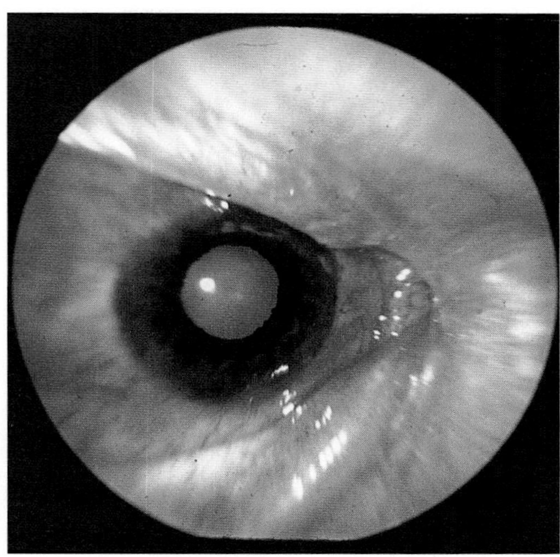

Fig. 4.8 Episcleritis in a patient with RA.

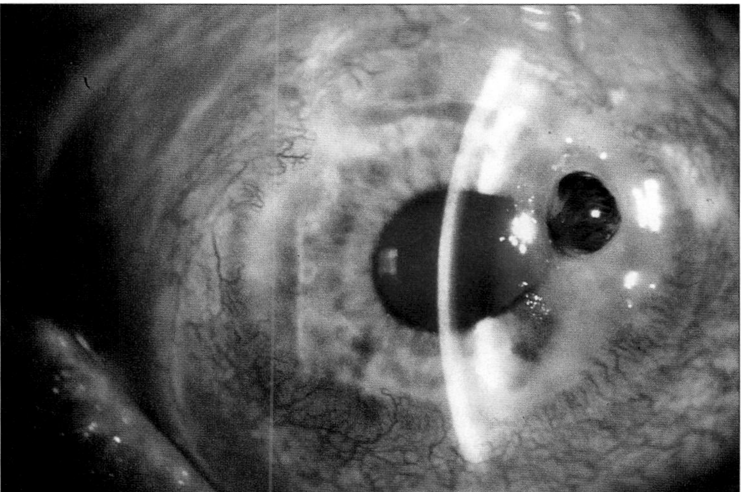

Fig. 4.9 Scleromalacia in a patient with RA.

more accommodating spinal canal in the upper cervical spine and odontoid erosions, which create more space in the C1–C2 area.

Central nervous system disease may manifest as stroke, seizure, hemorrhage, encephalopathy and meningitis due to cerebral vasculitis, amyloidosis and/or rheumatoid nodules in the dura and choroid plexus of the brain[36,37]. Extradural nodules may lead to nerve root compression and myelopathy. Most patients have long-standing RA with other extra-articular disease.

MUSCULAR

Muscle weakness in RA is usually due to muscle atrophy secondary to joint inflammation. Isometric, isokinetic and aerobic capacity are markedly reduced compared with healthy persons[38]. Occasionally nutritional problems, medication and neurologic dysfunction also contribute. A rare inflammatory myopathy has been described in RA with a patchy cellular infiltration in muscle fibers resulting in some fiber degeneration. Similar changes have been seen in other systemic inflammatory conditions. Usually, such patients have normal or only modestly elevated levels of serum creatine phosphokinase. Peripheral neuropathies on the basis of arteritis may result in muscle atrophy.

Other forms of secondary muscle involvement in RA include a diffuse polymyositis caused by D-penicillamine and a neuromyopathy with hydroxychloroquine. The muscle atrophy of chronic corticosteroid use is common and leads to further debility.

RENAL

The kidneys are usually spared in RA, although a low-grade membranous nephropathy, glomerulitis, vasculitis and secondary amyloidosis have all been described. In a study of 110 patients with RA undergoing renal biopsy, mesangial glomerulonephritis was the most common histopathologic finding (n=40), while amyloidosis (n=33) was the most common finding among patients with nephrotic syndrome[39]. Renal abnormalities frequently result from the agents used in treating RA, notably gold, D-penicillamine, cyclosporin and NSAIDs. Disease- and treatment-related microalbuminuria have been noted in up to one-quarter of patients with RA, and may be a marker of disease activity[40].

AMYLOIDOSIS

Amyloidosis may rarely complicate long-standing RA. Its true incidence varies widely. Amyloidosis may be primary, associated with myeloma and related disorders, or secondary, as in RA, and develops as a result of long-standing active inflammation[41]. In patients with active RA, serum amyloid-A protein levels are elevated, stimulated by increased cytokine production associated with the inflammatory state[42,43]. Proteinuria is a frequent finding in the amyloidosis associated with RA. Virtually every organ system may be involved in secondary amyloidosis that complicates RA, including the heart, kidney, liver, spleen, intestines and skin. The diagnosis of amyloidosis is con-

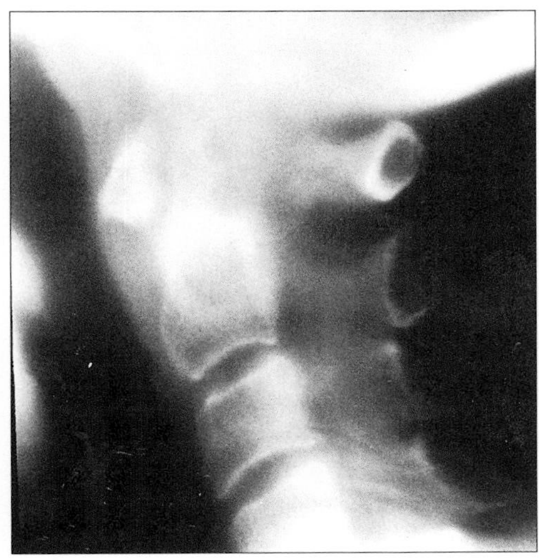

Fig. 4.10 CT of cervical spine showing erosion of the odontoid.

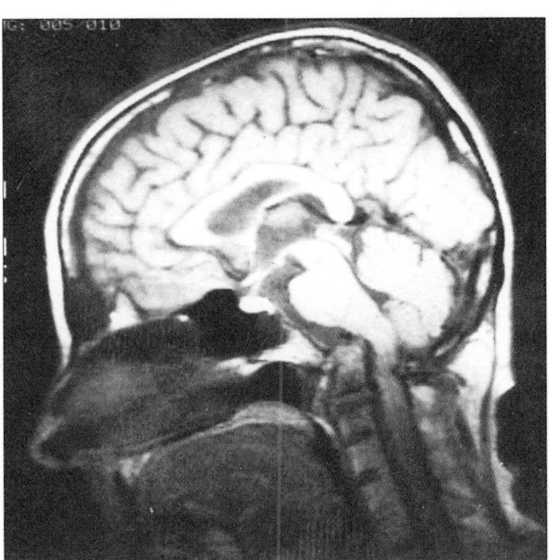

Fig. 4. 11 MRI of the cervical spine showing basilar invagination.

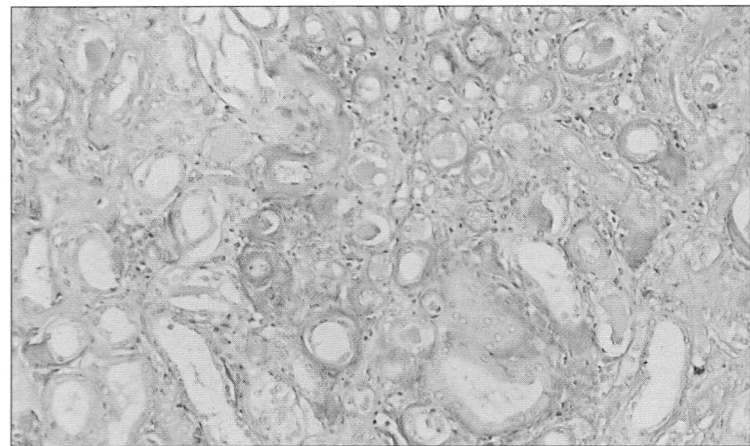

Fig. 4.12 Renal amyloidosis in RA (secondary AA). There is diffuse amyloid deposition throughout the renal parenchyma, with deposition in blood vessel walls. Amyloid deposits are green colored. (Sulfated Alcian blue stain ×40.)

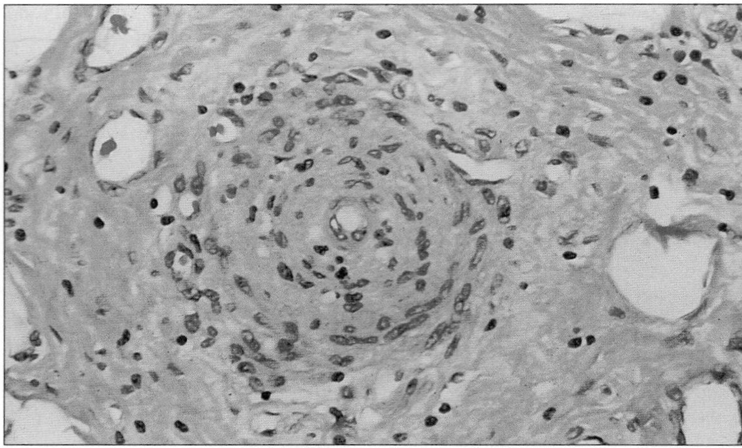

Fig. 4.13 Artery with intimal proliferation and luminal occlusion. (Hematoxylin and eosin stain, original magnification ×312.)

firmed by biopsy of involved tissue (Fig. 4.12). The presence of secondary amyloidosis in patients with RA portends a poor outcome and there is no satisfactory treatment.

RHEUMATOID VASCULITIS

A small vessel vasculitis is intimately associated with many of the clinical manifestations seen in RA. Subclinical vasculitis is probably common in patients with seropositive RA, and immune deposits have been demonstrated in clinically uninvolved skin and labial salivary glands[44]. The long-term effect of subclinical vasculitis on outcome is unknown.

The earliest events in the development of the rheumatoid nodule are a small-vessel vasculitis. Inflammation of the small- and medium-sized arteries in the extremities, peripheral nerves and, occasionally, other organs may complicate RA. There is a higher frequency of HLA-DRB1 alleles and particularly B1 0401 homozygotes in patients with rheumatoid vasculitis than in uncomplicated RA[45].

Study of involved vessels from patients with rheumatoid vasculitis reveals a pathologic picture and distribution similar to that seen in polyarteritis, but renal involvement is rare. Early lesions show fibrinoid necrosis of the vessel wall with an inflammatory cell infiltrate. Chronic changes with artery wall fibrosis, occlusion and recanalization may be seen (Fig. 4.13). One pathologic difference from polyarteritis is the finding of small- and medium-sized arteries involved with an occlusive intimal proliferation and little inflammation. The acute arterial lesions are immune-complex mediated, as indicated by the finding of immunoglobulins and complement in the involved arteries (Fig. 4.14). Immune deposits are not detected in the more chronic lesions, rather, fibrinogen is found (Fig. 4.15). Elevated levels of adhesion molecules ICAM-1 and ICAM-3 are found in the circulation of patients with rheumatoid vasculitis[46].

The systemic vasculitis that complicates RA is uncommon. It usually occurs in rheumatoid patients who have long-standing disease, usually of 10 years or more. Rarely, a systemic vasculitis is present at the onset of RA, and in such cases the outcome is poor[47]. Men are afflicted as commonly as women. These patients have more severe RA with destructive joint disease, rheumatoid nodules and high titers of blood rheumatoid factor 1. Patients with Felty's syndrome are more likely to develop vasculitic complications. Rheumatoid synovitis may not be active when the features of the systemic vasculitis are present. Small vessel vasculitis commonly involves the skin and causes nail-fold infarcts (Fig. 4.16), digital gangrene (Fig. 4.17) and leg ulcers (see Leg Ulcers in Chapter 5.16). Patients with nail-fold infarcts and leg ulcers usually do not develop more widespread vascular involvement. Distal sensory neuropathy is another manifestation seen in small vessel vasculitis that also may occur alone without progressing to widespread vascular involvement.

The more ominous manifestations of vasculitis are the appearance of infarcts of the fingertips and a sensorimotor neuropathy. Rapid, progressive and widespread appearance of new areas of involvement, including clinical cutaneous vasculitis and multiple neuropathies, indicates systemic arterial disease and a poorer outcome[48]. In some patients, the vasculitis may extend to involve mesenteric, coronary and cerebral arteries.

It is likely that other factors, in addition to the vasculitis, influence the final vascular outcome. In the pathogenesis of leg ulcers there is usually an underlying vasculitis which initiates the lesions, but ulcer

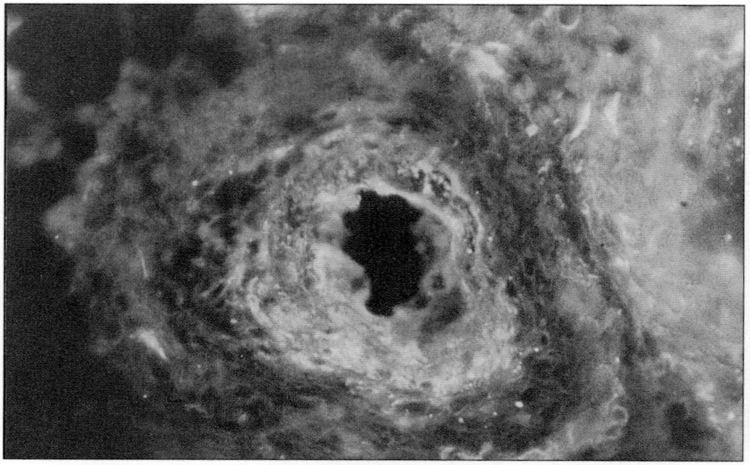

Fig. 4.14 IgM in artery with fibrinoid necrosis. (IgM by immunofluorescence, original magnification ×312.)

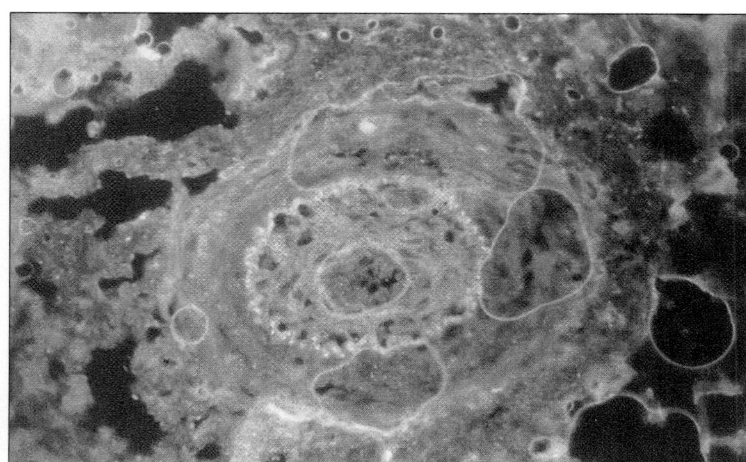

Fig. 4.15 Fibrinogen in artery with intimal proliferation. (Fibrinogen by immunofluorescence in artery with intimal proliferation ×312.)

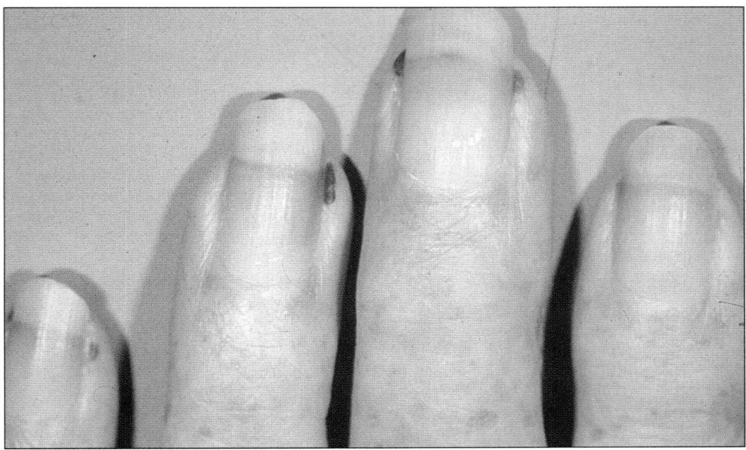

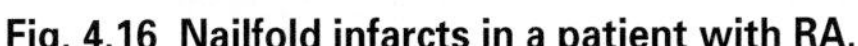

Fig. 4.16 Nailfold infarcts in a patient with RA.

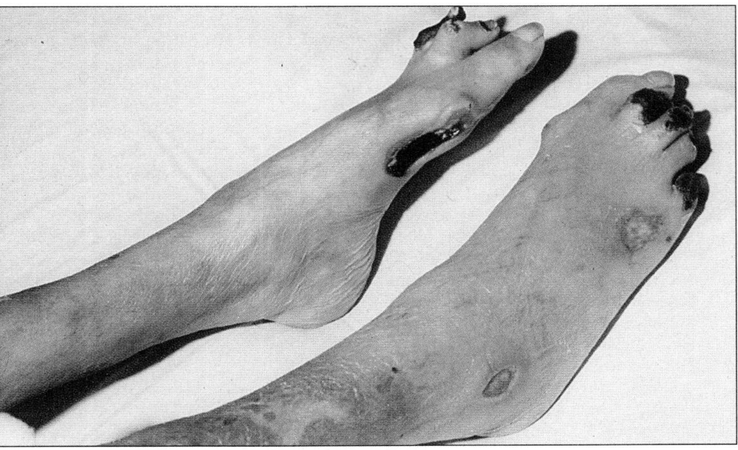

Fig. 4.17 Digital tip infarcts in a patient with RA.

expansion and its chronicity may be influenced by other features, including concomitant venous insufficiency, arterial insufficiency, dependent edema, trauma and chronic glucocorticoid use.

Patients with rheumatoid vasculitis have high serum titers of rheumatoid factor, low serum complement, cryoglobulins and circulatory immune complexes[49]. In addition, they will usually have an elevated ESR, anemia, thrombocytosis, and a diminished serum albumin.

Despite the belief that the widespread vasculitis which complicates RA is caused by glucocorticoids, patients who have never taken glucocorticoids may develop vasculitis. However, wide fluctuations in glucocorticoid dose, such as those caused by abruptly stopping the drug, seem to allow an underlying vasculitis to blossom.

The chronic use of glucocorticoids to treat RA predisposes to atherosclerosis and may permit the transformation from vasculitis to an occlusive vasculopathy. Conversely, NSAIDs may modify and lessen the vasculopathic changes. A poor prognosis is influenced by older age, concomitant atherosclerosis and the severity of vascular involvement.

The treatment of rheumatoid vasculitis must be individualized. In patients with progressive widespread systemic vasculitis involving peripheral nerves, digits, viscera and/or the central nervous system, the inflammation must be treated and the resulting vasculopathy anticipated. High doses of prednisone may be needed initially to control the inflammation[50]. Cytotoxic drugs, including cyclophosphamide, given possibly in pulses, may be necessary to allow long-term control and reduction of the corticosteroid dose. Low doses of aspirin as an antiplatelet agent and pentoxylline as an inhibitor of tumor necrosis factor should also be considered. In limited vasculitis, manifested as nailfold infarcts and leg ulcers, the management should be directed towards control of the RA generally, local wound care and reducing trauma to involved areas. Smoking should be stopped.

REFERENCES

1. Vollertsen RS, Conn DL, Ballard DJ, *et al.* Rheumatoid vasculitis: Survival and associated risk factors. Medicine. 1986;65:365–75.
2. Suzuki A, Ohosone Y, Obana M, *et al.* Cause of death in 81 autopsied patients with RA. J Rheumatol. 1994;21:33–6.
3. Weyand CM, Hicok KC, Conn DL, Goronzy JJ. The influence of HLA-DR beta-1 genes on disease severity in RA. Ann Intern Med .1992;117:801–6.
4. Agrawal S, Aggrarwal A, Dabadghao S, et al. Compound heterozygosity of HLA-DR4 and DR1 antigens in Asian indians increases the risk of extra-articular features in RA. Br J Rheum. 1995;34:41–4.
5. Wisnieski JJ, Askari AD. Rheumatoid nodulosis: a relatively benign rheumatoid variant. Arch Intern Med. 1981;141:615–9.
6. Segal R, Caspi D, Tisher M, et al. Accelerated nodulosis and vasculitis during methotrexate therapy for RA. Arthritis Rheum. 1988;31:1182–5.
7. Combe B, Didry C, Gutierrez M, *et al.* Accelerated nodulosis and systemic manifestations during methotrexate therapy for RA. *Eur J Med.* 1993;2:153–6.
8. Pincus T, Olsen NJ, Russell JI, *et al.* Multicenter study of recombinant human erythropoietin in correction of anemia in RA. Am J Med. 1990;89:161–8.
9. Crisp AJ, Armstrong RD, Grahame R, *et al.* Rheumatoid lung disease, pneumothorax, and eosinophilia. Ann Rheum Dis. 1982;41;137–40.
10. Kassan SS, Chused TL, Moutsopoulos HM, *et al.* Increased risk of lymphoma in Sicca syndrome. Ann Intern Med. 1978;89:888–92.
11. Breedveld FC, Fibbe WE, Hermans, *et al.* Factors influencing the incidence of infections in Felty's syndrome. Arch Intern Med. 1987;147:915–20.
12. Dillon AM, Luthra HS, Conn DL, *et al.* Parenteral gold therapy in the Felty syndrome: Experience with 20 patients. Medicine. 1986;65:112.
13. Gridley G, Klippel JH, Hoover RN, Fraumeni JF Jr. Incidence of cancer among men with the Felty syndrome. Ann Intern Med 1994;120:35–9.
14. Barton JC, Prasthofer EF, Egan ML. Rheumatoid arthritis associated with expanded populations of granular lymphocytes. Ann Intern Med. 1986:104:314–23.
15. Dhodapkar MV, Li CY, Lust JA, *et al.* Clinical spectrum of clonal proliferations of T-large granular lymphocytes: a T-cell clonopathy of undetermined significance? Blood. 1994;84:1620–7.

16. Fernandes L, Sullivan S, McFarlane JG, *et al.* Studies on the frequency and pathogenesis of liver involvement in RA. Ann Rheum Dis. 1979;38:501–6.
17. Thorne C, Urowitz MB, Wanless I, *et al.* Liver disease in Felty's syndrome. Am J Med. 1982;73:35–40.
18. Walker WC, Wright V. Pulmonary lesions and RA. Medicine. 1968;47:501–20.
19. Caplan A. Certain unusual radiological appearances in the chest of coal-miners suffering from RA. Thorax. 1953;8:29–37.
20. McDonagh J, Concaves M, Wright AR, *et al.* High resolution computerized tomography of the lungs in patients with RA and interstitial lung disease. Br J Rheum. 1994;33:118–22.
21. Remy-Jardin M, Remy J, Cortet B, *et al.* Lung changes in RA: Computerized tomography findings. Radiology. 1994;193:375–82.
22. Hassan WU, Keaney NP, Hollerd CD, *et al.* High resolution computerized tomography of the lung in lifelong non-smoking patients with RA. Ann Rhem Dis. 1995;54:308–10.
23. Shadick NA, Fanta CH, Wierblatt ME, *et al.* Bronchiectasis: a late feature of RA. Medicine. 1994;73:161–70.
24. Anaya JM, Dicthelm L,Ortiz LA, *et al.* Pulmonary involvement in RA. Sem Arthritis Rheum.1995;24:242–54.
25. Penny WJ, Knight RK, Rees AM, *et al.* Obliterative bronchiolitis in RA. Ann Rheum Dis. 1982;41:469–72.
26. Hacking JC, Flower CDR. Causes and investigation of increasing dyspnoea in RA. Ann Rheum Dis. 1995;54:17–19.
27. Bely M, Apathy A, Beke-Martos E. Cardiac changes in RA. Acta Morphol Hun. 1992;40:149–86.
28. Bonfiglio T, Atwater EC. Heart disease in patients with seropositive RA. Arch Intern Med. 1969;124:714–9.
29. Hara KS, Ballard DJ, Ilstrum DM, *et al.* Rheumatoid pericarditis: Clinical features and survival. Medicine. 1990;69:81–91.
30. Mustonen J, Laakso M, Hirvonen T, *et al.* Abnormalities in left ventricular diastolic function in male patients with RA without clinically evident cardiovascular disease. Eur J Clin Invest. 1993;23:246–53.
31. Corrao S, Salli L, Arnonne S, *et al.* Cardiac involvement in RA: evidence of silent heart disease. Eur Heart J. 1995;16:253–6.
32. Jifi-Bahlool H, Saadeh C, O'Conner J. Peripheral ulcerative keratitis in the setting of RA: Treatment with immunosuppressive therapy. Sem Arthritis Rheum. 1995;25:67–73.
33. Cooper C, Kirwan JR, McGill NW, *et al.* Brown's syndrome: an unusual ocular complication of RA. Rheum Dis. 1990;49:188–9.
34. Lipson SJ. Rheumatoid arthritis of the cervical spine. Clin Orthop. 1984;182:143–9.
35. Menezes AH, Van Gilder JC, Clark CR, *et al.* Odontoid upward migration in RA. J Neurosurg. 1985;63:500–9.
36. Matsuki Y, Suzuki K, Tanaka N, *et al.* Amyloidosis secondary to RA associated with plexiform change in bilateral temporal lobes. Int Med. 1994;33:764–7.
37. Markenson JA, McDougal JS, Tsairis P, *et al.* Rheumatoid meningitis:a localized immune process. Ann Intern Med. 1979;90:786–9.
38. Ekdahl C, Broman G. Muscle strength, endurance, and aerobic capacity in RA: a comparative study with healthy subjects. Ann Rheum Dis. 1992;51:35–40.
39. Helin HJ, Korpela MM, Mustonen JT, Pasternack AI. Renal biopsy findings and clincopathologic correlations in RA. Arthritis Rheum 1995;38:242–7.
40. Pedersen LM, Nordin H, Svensson B, Bliddal H. Microalbuminuria in patients with RA. Ann Rheum Dis. 1995;54:189–92.
41. Tiitinen S, Kaarela K, Helin H, *et al.* Amyloidosis: incidence and early risk factors in patients with RA. Scand J Rheumatol. 1993;22:158–61.
42. Chambers RE, MacFarlane CG, Whicher JT, Dieppe PA. Serum amyloid-A protein concentration in RA and its role in monitoring disease activity. Ann Rheum Dis. 1983;42:665–7.
43. McNiff PA, Stewart C, Sullivan J, *et al.* Synovial fluid from RA patients contains sufficient levels of IL-1beta and IL-6 to promote production of serum amyloid A by Hep3B cells. Cytokine 1995;7:209–19.
44. Flipo RM, Janin A, Hachulla E, *et al.* Labial salivary gland biopsy assessment in rheumatoid vasculitis. Ann Rheum Dis. 1994;53:648–52.
45. Weyand CM, Hickok KC, Conn DL, Goronzy JJ. The influence of HLA-DRB1 genes on disease severity in RA. Ann Intern Med. 1992;117:801–6.
46. Voskuyl AE, Martin S, Melchers I, *et al.* Levels of circulating intercellular adhesion molecule-1 and -3 but not circulating endothelial leucocyte adhesion molecule are increased in patients with rheumatoid vasculitis. Br J Rheumatol. 1995;34:311–5.
47. Lakhanpal S, Conn DL, Lie JT. Clinical and prognostic significance of vasculitis as an early manifestation of connective tissue disease syndromes. Ann Intern Med. 1984;101:743–8.
48. Puechal X, Said G, Hilliquin P, *et al.* Peripheral neuropathy with necrotizing vasculitis in RA. Arthritis Rheum. 1995;38:1618–29.
49. Scott DGI, Bacon PA, Allen C, *et al.* IgG rheumatoid factor, complement, and immune complexes in rheumatoid synovitis and vasculitis: Comparative and serial studies during cytotoxic therapy. Clin Exp Immunol. 1981;43:54–63.
50. Luqmani RA, Watts RA, Scott DGI, Bacon PA. Treatment of vasculitis in RA. Ann Intern Med. 1994;145:566–76.

RHEUMATOID ARTHRITIS 5

IMAGING

Anne C Brower

Summary

- Imaging serves an important role in diagnosis and objective assessment of the progression of rheumatoid arthritis.

Key radiographic features of RA

- Symmetrical soft tissue swelling.
- Juxta-articular osteoporosis.
- Erosions of subchondral bone.
- Absence of bone repair.

INTRODUCTION

Rheumatoid arthritis (RA) is a symmetric polyarticular disease of the appendicular skeleton, sparing the axial skeleton except for the cervical spine. The common radiographic findings are periarticular soft-tissue swelling, osteoporosis, marginal erosions progressing to severe erosions of subchondral bone, synovial cyst formation and lack of bone repair. The distribution of the disease is the hands, feet, knees, hips, cervical spine, shoulders and elbows, in decreasing order of frequency[1,2].

It is important that the joints involved be imaged with the appropriate modality. The modalities used for imaging patients with RA include conventional radiography, specialized film radiography, bone scintigraphy, arthrography, computed tomography (CT) and magnetic resonance imaging (MRI). The role played by each of these modalities in the evaluation of individual joints in RA is discussed in this chapter.

CONVENTIONAL RADIOGRAPHY

The evaluation of any patient with RA should begin with the conventional radiograph. With high-quality radiographs of properly positioned joints, sufficiently accurate evaluation can often be made to avoid the need for further imaging.

THE HAND AND WRIST

Technique

All patients with RA will have involvement of their hands and/or wrists. The conventional radiograph of the hand and wrist is used to determine state and/or progression of disease[3,4] and to measure the therapeutic effect of various drugs on the outcome of disease. Therefore, quality films must be produced. This requires appropriate film, appropriate exposure of film and appropriate positioning of the joint.

High-resolution images are necessary to detect early erosive disease. High resolution is obtained through a film–screen combination of low-system speed. The routine two-screen–film combination cassettes used in most radiology departments do not provide the low-system speed needed. New single screen–film combinations should be used instead. Appropriate exposure of the film is extremely important. Erosive disease is lost in both underexposed and overexposed films.

As with any bone disorder, appropriate evaluation includes at least two views of the bone involved. Therefore, radiographic assessment of the arthritic hand should not be performed on the posterior–anterior (PA) view only. The second view obtained should be a Nørgaard view or supinated-oblique view. Nørgaard demonstrated that erosive disease can be identified earlier on this view than on the PA view[5]. The Nørgaard view images the radial aspect of the base of the proximal phalanges, the radial aspect of the base of the fourth metacarpal and the triquetral–pisiform joint, where the first erosive changes will often be observed (Fig. 5.1). While the use of this view has been questioned in the literature, most nevertheless agree that erosive disease is seen in the triquetral–pisiform joint before it is seen in the ulnar styloid.

Early radiographic changes

The earliest radiographic changes seen in the hand are soft-tissue swelling symmetrically around the joints involved, juxta-articular osteoporosis and erosions of the 'bare' areas of bone (i.e. areas lacking articular cartilage)[5–8]. Soft-tissue swelling and juxta-articular osteoporosis are nonspecific changes but help to confirm the presence of an inflammatory problem.

Erosive disease indicates the aggressiveness of the arthropathy. The first erosive changes are in the 'bare' areas of bone, or 'bare' bone within the joint-space capsule. These erosions occur before there is joint-space loss. They may be very subtle, imaging as a loss of continuity of the white cortical line (Fig. 5.2). On the PA view, erosive disease is best observed on the radial aspect of the metacarpal heads and in the thumb on the ulnar–volar aspect of the base of the distal phalanx

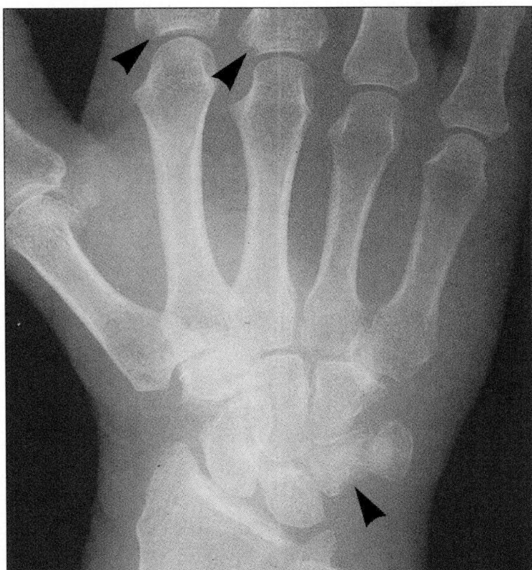

Fig. 5.1 Nørgaard view of the MCP joints and wrist in RA. Early erosive changes are demonstrated between the triquetrum and pisiform and at the radial aspect of the base of the proximal phalanges of the second and third MCP joints (arrows).

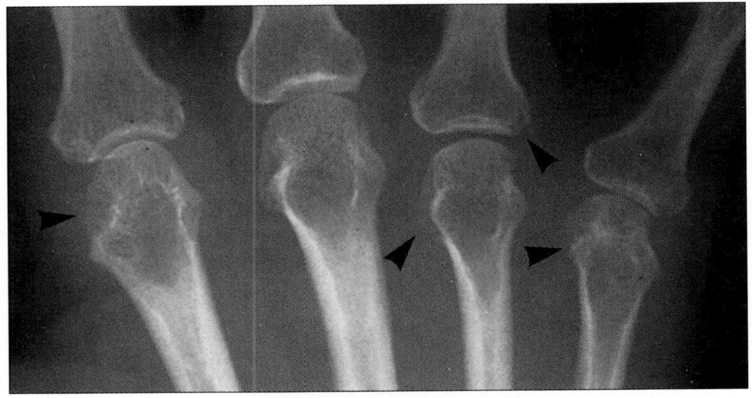

Fig. 5.2 Early erosions in the 'bare' areas of the second and fourth metacarpal heads in RA. The erosions are the disruption of continuity of the white cortical line (arrows).

and the radial–ulnar aspect of the metacarpal head. On the Nørgaard view, erosive disease is best seen on the radial aspect of the base of the proximal phalanges.

Early changes observed in the wrist are soft-tissue swelling and juxta-articular osteoporosis. Early erosions are seen on the PA view in the ulnar styloid, the radial styloid, the midportion of the scaphoid, the lateral portion of the hamate as it articulates with the fifth metacarpal, the distal radial aspect of the trapezium and the waist of the capitate (Fig. 5.3).

Late radiographic changes

Later changes in the fingers show joint-space loss, with a decrease in soft-tissue swelling. Juxta-articular osteoporosis progresses to diffuse osteoporosis. The subtle marginal erosions progress to become large subchondral erosions. Subluxations occur, producing either boutonnière or swan-neck deformities of the phalanges. At the metacarpophalangeal joints (MCPs) there is ulnar drift of the proximal phalanges. There is fairly uniform involvement of the MCP and/or proximal interphalangeal joints (PIPs) with relative sparing of the distal interphalangeal joints (Fig. 5.4). There may be fibrous ankylosis of the digits, but no bone ankylosis.

Later changes in the wrist produce pancompartmental loss of the joint spaces[7]. The erosions progress to become large subchondral erosions[9]. There will be erosion of the radial–ulnar joint, producing diastasis of this joint, with dorsal subluxation of the ulna and ulnar migration of the wrist in relation to the radius. In the wrist, bone ankylosis may occur. Eventually, the radiographic image may be one of 'arthritis mutilans'.

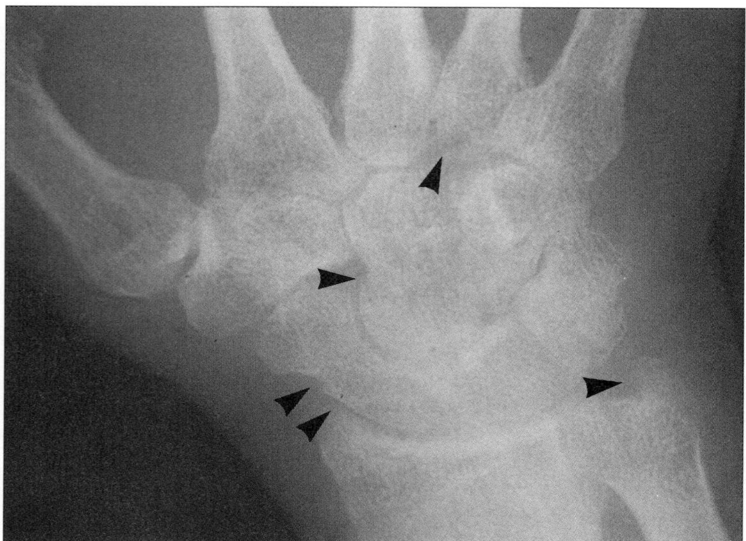

Fig. 5.3 PA view of the wrist demonstrating early erosive changes in RA. There are erosions at the waist of the scaphoid, the waist of the capitate, the ulnar styloid, the radial styloid and the base of the fourth metacarpal (arrows).

THE FOOT

Technique

The foot is involved in 80–90% of RA patients. Some studies indicate that 10–20% of the patients will have foot involvement before hand involvement[10]. However, in these studies, Nørgaard views were not performed on the hands. In general, changes in the feet accompany or lag somewhat behind changes in the hands. The radiographic changes are evaluated on anteroposterior (AP) and lateral views of the foot. As for the hand, high-resolution films are needed to evaluate the metatarsophalangeal joints of the foot. Similarly, high-resolution films should be obtained for evaluation of the calcaneus on the lateral view. Attention should be paid to the attachments of the plantar aponeurosis and Achilles tendon on the lateral view.

Early radiographic changes

Early radiographic changes in the feet are juxta-articular osteoporosis and erosion of the 'bare' areas on the heads of the metatarsals (Fig. 5.5). The first erosive change is usually seen on the lateral aspect of the head of the fifth metatarsal, as a loss of continuity of the white cortical line. The other metatarsals are eroded first medially and then laterally. Early erosive changes will also be seen in the interphalangeal joint of the big toe. A hallux valgus may be present.

Late radiographic changes

Later changes show progression of the marginal erosions to large subchondral erosions. There is loss of the joint space. There is fibular subluxation of the proximal phalanges in relation to the metatarsals (Fig. 5.6). There may be dorsiflexion deformities of the PIP joints. The tarsal bones will be affected in a uniform fashion (Fig. 5.7). There may be bone ankylosis of the tarsals, but only fibrous ankylosis will occur distal to the tarsals. Close observation may show erosive change at the attachment of the plantar aponeurosis and/or the attachment of the Achilles tendon.

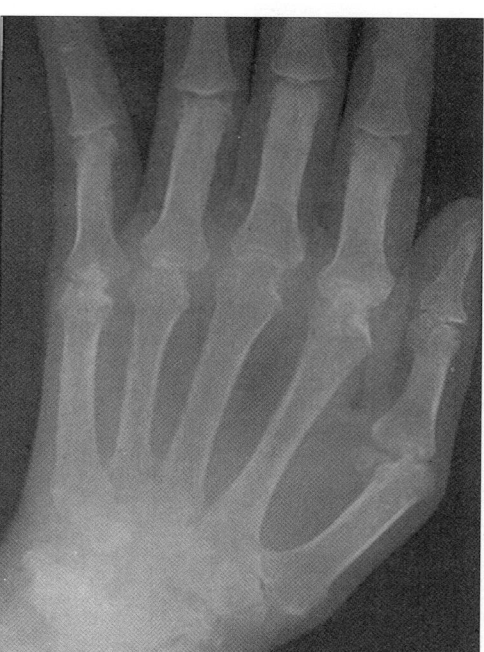

Fig. 5.4 PA view of the hand in advanced stages of RA. Diffuse osteoporosis is present. There is cartilage loss and erosion in the MCP and pancarpal joints as well as in several PIP joints.

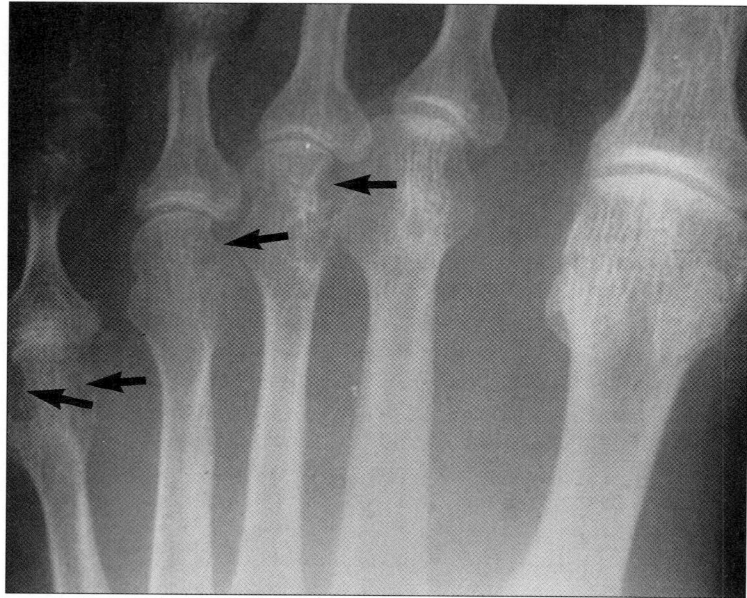

Fig. 5.5 AP view of the forefoot in early RA. Erosions of the 'bare' areas of bone (areas not covered by cartilage) in the metatarsal heads are demonstrated (arrows).

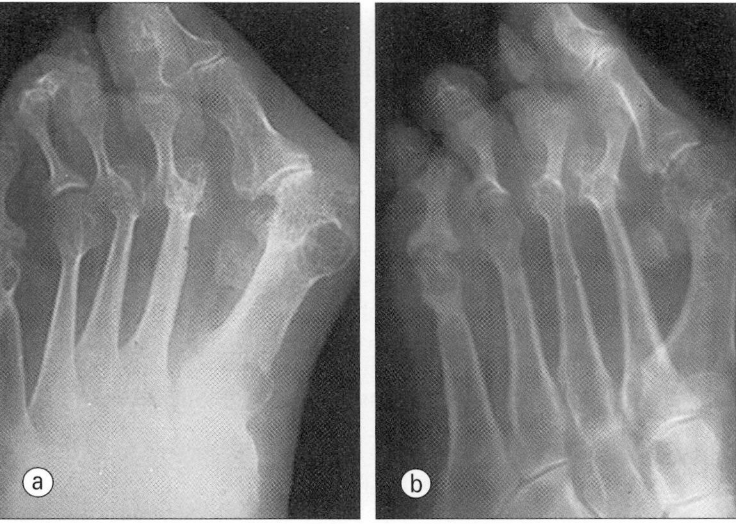

Fig. 5.6 AP (a) and oblique (b) view of the forefoot showing late changes of RA. There is osteoporosis, dramatic erosive changes and subluxation involving the metatarsal heads. There is also fibular subluxation of the proximal phalanges in relationship to the metatarsal heads.

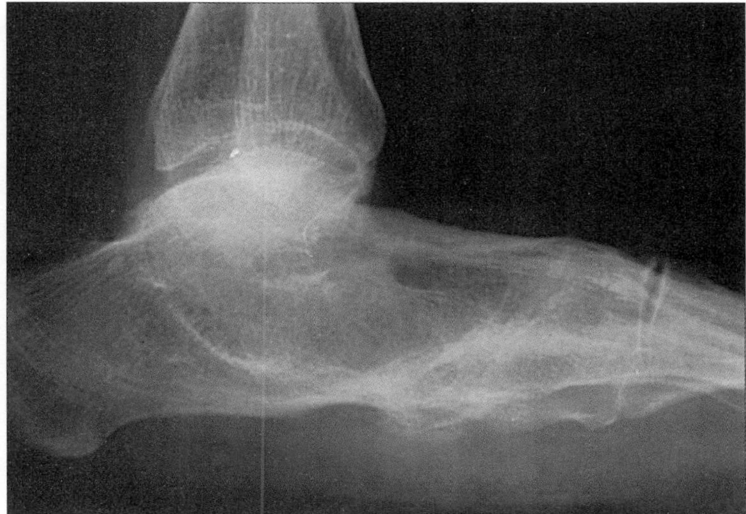

Fig. 5.7 Lateral view of the mid- and hindfoot in advanced stages of RA. The tarsal joints are involved in a uniform fashion, with bone ankylosis.

THE KNEE

Technique

The knees are involved in 80% of patients with RA. Evaluation of the knee should be performed on a standing AP view and a flexed lateral view. An abnormally narrowed knee joint may appear normal on a routine radiograph taken tabletop. A standing view must be used to accurately assess actual cartilage loss and subluxations[11]. A flexed lateral view allows accurate assessment of the patella and its relationship to the functioning joint.

Radiographic changes

In RA, the knees are involved bilaterally and symmetrically. There is uniform loss of the cartilage in all three compartments: the medial, lateral and patellofemoral. Despite the knee being a weight-bearing joint, there is little to no reparative response in the presence of even severe loss of cartilage. Marginal erosions may be present. In this joint, there is a propensity to develop intraosseous synovial cysts (Fig. 5.8)[12]. The synovium breaks through the cartilage and protrudes into the bone. A ball-valve effect of the synovial fluid within the cyst causes enlargement; such large synovial cysts are described as geodes. A geode should not be mistaken for a neoplasm.

THE HIPS

Technique

The hip is affected in 50% of patients with RA. The radiograph should be performed in AP and frog-leg lateral position. On the AP view, the hip should be internally rotated in order to image the femoral neck to its fullest advantage. The frog-leg lateral view is imaged with the hip in abduction and allows viewing of the anterior and posterior portions of the femoral head. Occasionally, on the frog-leg lateral view, a vacuum phenomenon will be introduced into the joint, allowing the exclusion of the presence of synovial fluid and aiding determination of cartilage thickness.

Radiographic changes

The hip will migrate in an axial (superomedial) direction within the acetabulum, consistent with uniform loss of cartilage (Fig. 5.9)[13]. As the cartilage is lost, the femoral head will begin to erode the acetabulum, and bone will be laid down on the acetabular side. This eventually

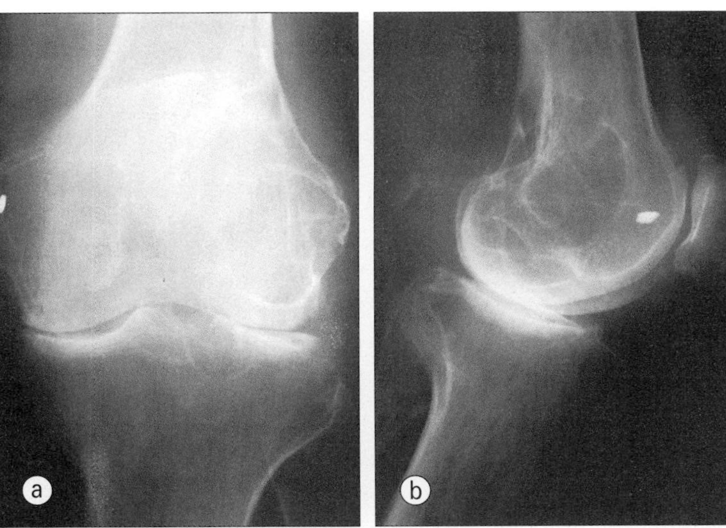

Fig. 5.8 AP (a) and lateral (b) views of the knee in RA. There is narrowing of the medial, lateral and patellofemoral compartments. There is generalized osteoporosis. Synovial cysts (geodes) are present in the tibial plateau and the lateral femoral condyle. (Reproduced with permission from Kantor S, Brower AC, In: Rothermich N, Whisler R, Rheumatoid arthritis. Orlando: Grune & Stratton; 1985.)

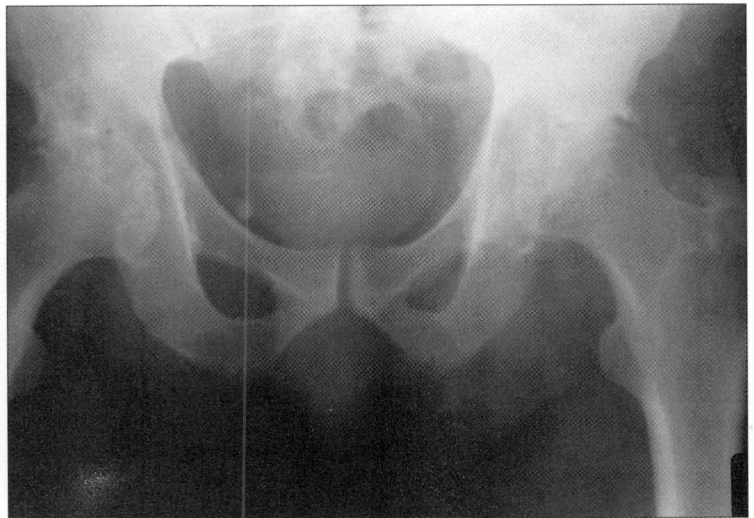

Fig. 5.9 AP view of the hips in RA. There is bilateral, symmetric, uniform narrowing of the hip joints. Both femoral heads have moved in an axial direction. Erosive disease is present.

leads to acetabular protrusion[14]. Protrusion is defined as being present when the acetabular line is medial to the ilioischial line by 3mm in males and by 6mm in females. This occurs in 15% of patients with rheumatoid hip disease.

Erosive change is first seen at the chondro-osseous margin of the femoral head where it joins the neck. Synovial cyst formation may also occur. There is little, if any, reparative response in the form of osteophytes or subchondral bone formation.

The typical rheumatoid pelvis shows bilateral symmetric involvement of the hips, with acetabuli protrusio, osteoporosis and a noticeable absence of reparative bone and osteophyte formation (Fig. 5.10). Occasionally, osteonecrosis may occur in the femoral head secondary to corticosteroid therapy.

THE SHOULDER

Technique

Of RA patients, 60% will ultimately have involvement of the shoulders. The shoulder is imaged in an AP direction, with the humeral head positioned in internal and external rotation[15]. This allows visualization of all surfaces of the humeral head. The internal rotation view shows the anterior and posterior portion of the head.

Radiographic changes

When evaluating the shoulder, three compartments need to be assessed: the glenohumeral joint, the acromioclavicular joint and the acromiohumeral space. In RA, there is usually involvement of all three compartments (Fig. 5.11). With narrowing of the glenohumeral joint space, there is medial migration of the humeral head. With loss of the acromiohumeral space, there is upward migration of the humeral head. This narrowing between the humerus and acromion is the result of an associated rotator-cuff tear. Erosive changes will occur at the distal end of the clavicle, at the superior lateral aspect of the humeral head adjacent to the greater tuberosity and at the attachment of the coracoclavicular ligament to the clavicle[15]. Synovial cysts may form in the humeral head. Again, these should not be mistaken for neoplasms.

OTHER APPENDICULAR JOINTS

The elbow, the ankle, the sacroiliac joint, the sternoclavicular joint and the temporomandibular joints may all be involved[1,2], with joint-space loss and erosive changes. Early disease in the elbow may cause a positive fat-pad sign secondary to the presence of synovial fluid, osteoporosis, joint-space narrowing and small erosions. As the cartilage is destroyed in the elbow, there may be apparent widening of the elbow joint (Fig. 5.12). Observation of a positive fat-pad sign at this stage would indicate the pus of infection rather than the synovial fluid of RA.

Changes around the ankle are often accompanied by a single layer of periosteal reaction. In the ankle, periostitis is a radiographic manifestation of RA; it should be distinguished from periostitis accompanying stress fracture or an osteomyelitis.

THE CERVICAL SPINE

Technique

The cervical spine becomes involved in 60–70% of RA patients. The two most important views to be obtained in examining the cervical spine are a flexed lateral view of the cervical spine and an open-mouth frontal view demonstrating the odontoid. The flexed lateral view allows evaluation of ligamentous laxity and apophyseal joint disease.

Radiographic changes

The cervical spine can be involved anywhere from the occiput to T1. The synovial joints, cartilaginous joints, joints of Luschka, tendons and ligaments are the sites involved. The radiographic changes divide into those related to the occipitoatlantoaxial joints and those in the subaxial portion of the spine.

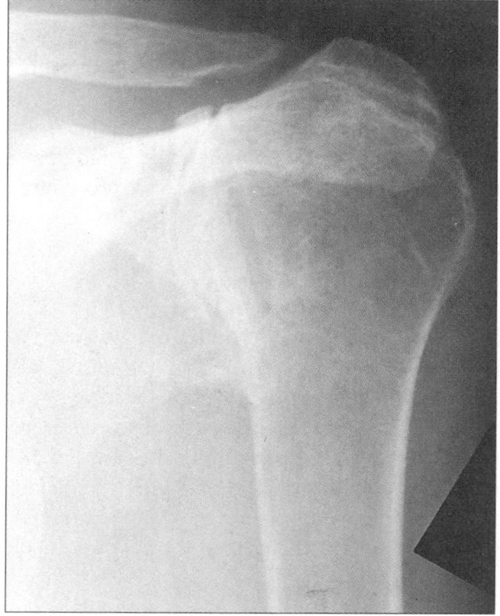

Fig. 5.11 AP view of the shoulder in RA. There is generalized osteoporosis. The humeral head has migrated proximally and superiorly, secondary to loss of cartilage in the glenohumeral joint and the acromiohumeral space. There is erosion of the distal end of the clavicle. (Reproduced with permission from Brower AC. Arthritis in black and white. Philadelphia: WB Saunders, 1988.)

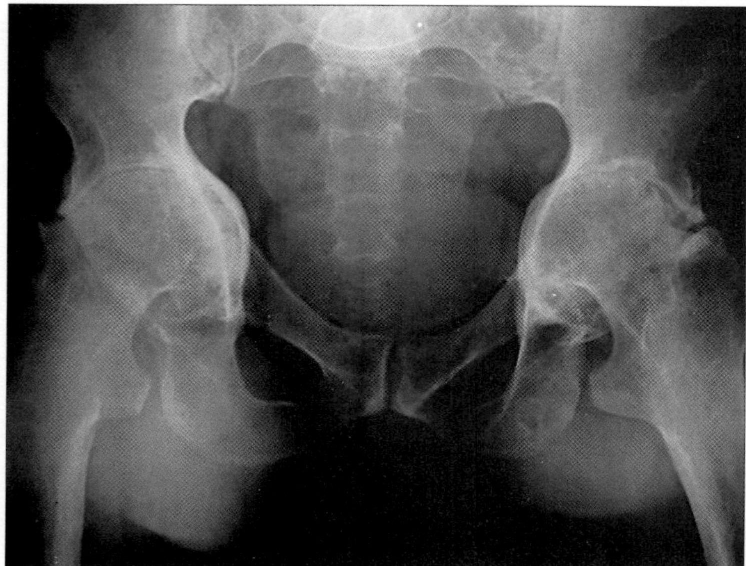

Fig. 5.10 AP view of hips in severe RA. There is severe bilateral acetabuli protrusio in a superomedial direction. Extensive osteoporosis is evident and there is little evidence of bone repair.

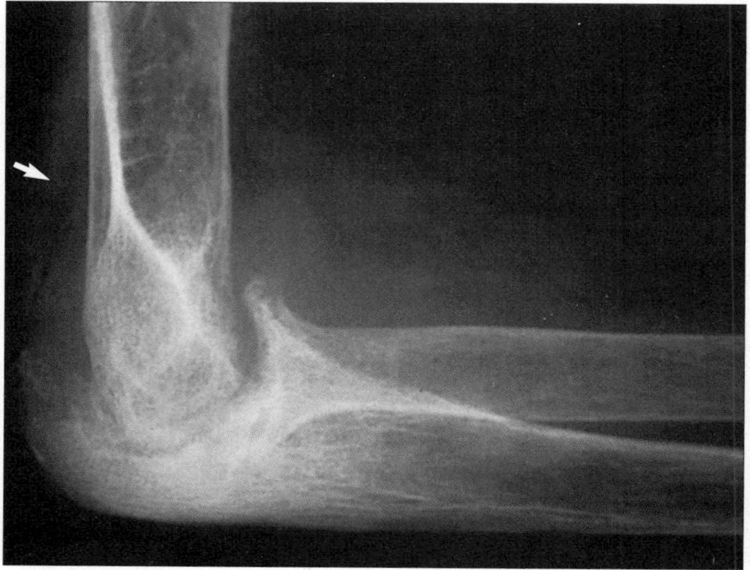

Fig. 5.12 Lateral view of the elbow in RA. Extensive erosion has created an apparent widening of the elbow joint. Note positive fat pads indicating the presence of fluid (arrow).

At the occipitoatlantoaxial joints, various subluxations with or without erosions may occur. The most common finding is atlantoaxial subluxation, occurring in 50% of individuals with RA. This is primarily due to laxity of the transverse ligament that holds the odontoid to the atlas. This can be demonstrated only on the flexed lateral view of the cervical spine (Fig. 5.13). In other patients the laxity is so severe as to be demonstrable in the neutral position. It is accepted that when a gap of 8mm or more exists between the odontoid and the atlas, surgical intervention should be considered[16] (see Practical Problem 5.16, Instability of the cervical spine).

Vertical subluxation or cranial settling going on to vertical translocation can occur at Cl–2[17]. With vertical translocation, there is usually disruption and collapse of the osseous and/or articular structures. Lateral subluxation of the atlantoaxial joints may also occur. Any and all of the above may produce mild to severe neurologic abnormalities. Actual odontoid erosion is observed less frequently than ligamentous laxity.

Subaxial radiographic changes observed are subluxation, diskovertebral destruction[18] and/or apophyseal involvement. The first subluxation will usually occur at C3–4, then C4–5 and then eventually stair-step down the spine (Fig. 5.14). A disk space may become narrowed or even destroyed secondary to either trauma from apophyseal joint instability or extension of a synovitis from the joint of Luschka (Fig. 5.15). Apophyseal joint changes consist primarily of erosion leading to instability. In some cases, fibrous ankylosis of the apophyseal joints can occur.

COMPLICATIONS

The main bone and joint complications of RA are secondary infection, stress fracture and osteonecrosis. Infection[19] should be considered when there is rapid deterioration of a joint in the presence of an effusion (see Practical Problem 5.16, Tendon rupture in the hand with RA). If the cartilage of a joint has been destroyed by RA, a synovial effusion should not be present; if it is present, it is usually pus (Fig. 5.16).

Stress fractures occur as insufficiency fractures in osteoporotic bone. They most commonly occur in the proximal portion of the tibia just beneath the tibial plateau, and in the distal portion of the tibia just above the ankle joint (see Fig. 5.17). Osteonecrosis as a result of corticosteroid therapy is seen most commonly in the hip.

SPECIALIZED TECHNIQUES

Three specialized techniques applying conventional radiography have been used in the past in an effort to obtain more information regarding erosive disease and soft-tissue changes[20].

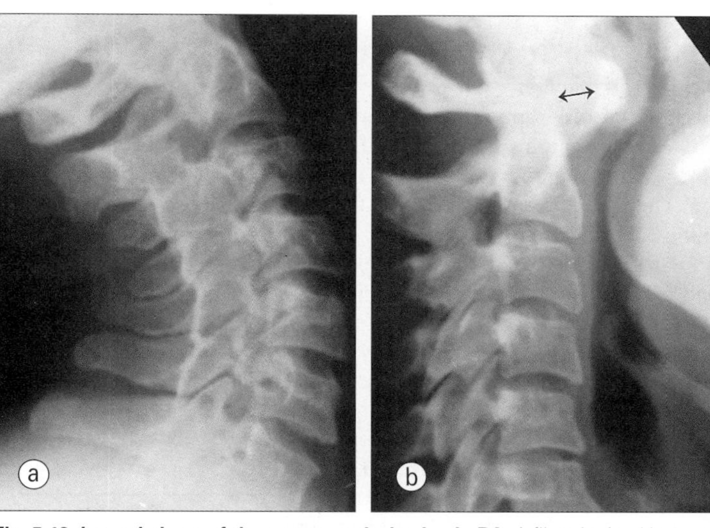

Fig. 5.13 Lateral views of the upper cervical spine in RA. A film obtained in neutral position showed no significant abnormality (a). Another film was taken in the flexed position (b) and showed increased distance between the atlas and odontoid (arrows). This demonstrates laxity of the transverse ligament.

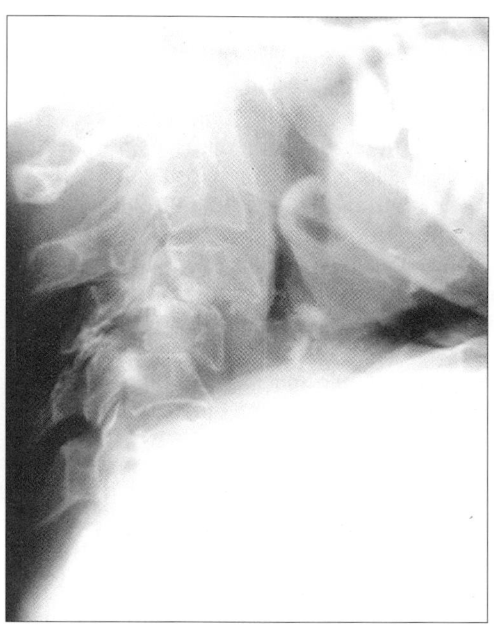

Fig. 5.14 Lateral view of the cervical spine in advanced RA. Severe osteoporosis and subaxial subluxations with loss of disk spaces are seen (Reproduced with permission from Kantor S, Brower AC, in: Rothermich N, Whistler R, Rheumatoid arthritis. Orlando: Grune & Stratton; 1985.)

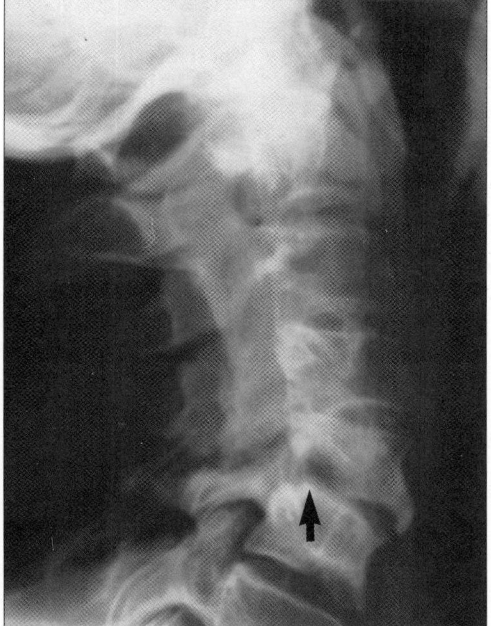

Fig. 5.15 Lateral view of the cervical spine in advanced RA. Disk destruction (arrow) secondary to extension of a synovitis from the joint of Luschka has occurred.

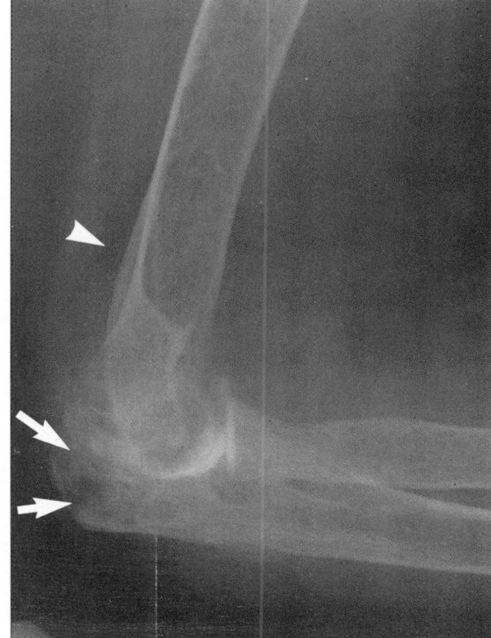

Fig. 5.16 Lateral view of the elbow in RA with infection. The joint space is completely destroyed. A posterior fat pad is demonstrated (arrowhead). This is due to the presence of pus. There is extensive erosion of the olecranon (arrows).

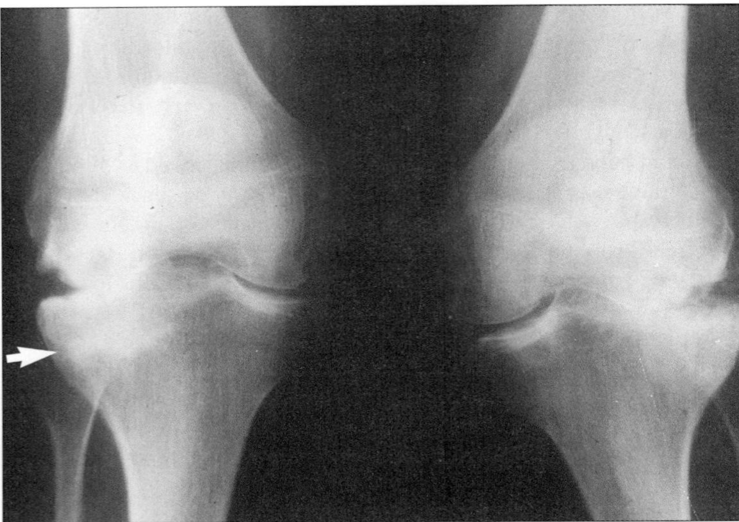

Fig. 5.17 AP view of rheumatoid knee with stress fracture. There is narrowing of medial and total loss of the lateral compartments. The line of sclerosis just distal to the lateral tibial plateau of the right knee (arrow) represents the stress fracture.

Magnification techniques

Magnification techniques are said to be more sensitive in detecting erosive disease and soft-tissue changes than is conventional radiography. Erosive disease is easier to see on magnification films only because the area imaged is larger. However, higher radiation doses are received by the patient and the examination is technically more difficult to obtain. There are two methods of magnification: optical and radiographic. Using the optical technique, the films are viewed with a magnifier. Kodak industrial M-film is used and must be developed manually. A 100cm focus film distance and a focal spot of 1.2mm are essential.

Radiographic magnification is obtained by the use of a special machine with a microfocus X-ray tube. The radiation dose is less than that used in the optical technique and no special magnifier is required for viewing. However, positioning is difficult and only a small area can be imaged on one film.

Low-kilovolt radiography

Low-kilovolt radiography is used to give greater contrast between the soft tissues. A special molybdenum target and filter are used. Again, there is increased radiation exposure, and films should be read with a magnifying glass. This technique allows visualization of thickening of tendons, ligaments and joint capsules, as well as of inflammation of the soft tissues and of increased vascularity.

Xeroradiography

Xeroradiography was used to give greater detail of both osseous and periarticular soft-tissue structures on the same image. It has superior edge-enhancement properties and broad latitude in recording different densities of thickness. However, due to the high radiation dose, this modality is no longer readily available.

SCINTIGRAPHY

After conventional radiography, bone scintigraphy is probably the most helpful imaging modality available in RA[21]. It is useful in three ways: it confirms the presence of disease, it demonstrates the distribution of disease and it evaluates the activity of disease. Bone scintigraphy is the most sensitive indicator of active disease. It will confirm the presence of hyperemia and inflammation that may not be apparent on the conventional radiograph. An area that demonstrates increased activity on the bone scan should be observed carefully for anatomic distribution. On a high-resolution image of a joint, it is possible to distinguish a tendinitis from a synovitis or a synovitis from a primary bone lesion.

As well as confirming abnormality in one joint, observation by scintigraphy of increased activity in other joints will help make the clinician aware of all problem joints. Observed differences in intensity of uptake in the various joints involved usually correlates with differences in clinical activity of disease in the various joints. Serial bone scintigraphy of a particular joint is helpful in evaluating the activity of the disease over time. It may also help to differentiate active disease from disease in remission.

ARTHROGRAPHY

Arthrography plays a minor role in the evaluation of patients with RA. It has been used to demonstrate rotator-cuff disruption in the shoulder. It may also be used to demonstrate the presence of a Baker's cyst[22], a synovial cyst extending into the soft tissues around the knee, and the status of that cyst (Fig. 5.18). Ultrasound, a noninvasive procedure, may also be used for the same purposes. However, the Baker's cyst that causes symptoms of thrombophlebitis is one that has ruptured and extravasated material into the soft tissues[22]. In this instance, to demonstrate the extravasation of contrast material from the cyst, the arthrogram is preferable to ultrasound.

COMPUTED TOMOGRAPHY

Computed tomography plays a minor role in evaluation of RA[4]. The two areas in which it may be useful are the pelvis and the cervical spine[20]. In the pelvis, it is used in the patient with acetabular protrusion. The degree of protrusion and the thickness of the acetabular roof can be better evaluated on axial CT images, giving information important in total hip replacement. The extent of osteonecrosis of a femoral head is better appreciated on an axial CT image.

Imaging with CT is frequently used in evaluation of the cervical spine, especially at the craniocervical junction and the atlantoaxial region. Transaxial images better define the anatomy of this area.

MAGNETIC RESONANCE IMAGING

The use of MRI in evaluating RA is currently in a period of development. Although MRI offers less spatial resolution than radiography, because MRI is a tomographic technique it shows greater sensitivity

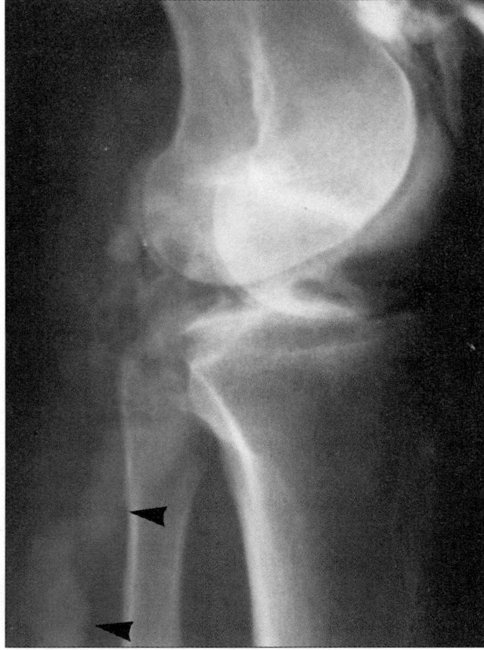

Fig. 5.18 Arthography of the soft tissues posterior to the knee and the tibia. Contrast material fills a huge Baker's cyst.

for detecting bone erosions that may be obscured by overlapping structures on projectional radiographs. Moreover, MRI is uniquely capable of imaging the medullary contents of the bone, articular cartilage, fibrocartilage, muscles, tendons and fat[23,24]. Each of these can be separated from the others by differences in signal intensity, thus allowing excellent image contrast.

The most sensitive modality for detecting osteonecrosis is MRI (see Chapter 8.47). When osteonecrosis secondary to corticosteroid therapy is suspected in a patient with RA and is not visualized by conventional radiography, MRI should be employed. However, while MRI is very sensitive it is also nonspecific; therefore, signal change must be interpreted with caution. Also, MRI is the most sensitive technique for detecting insufficiency fractures, which typically show linear or diffuse water signals in the marrow space.

Cartilage can be imaged by MRI. Hyaline cartilage can be distinguished from fibrous cartilage and adjacent synovial fluid and fat. How and in which cases this information will be useful in RA depends on the needs of the clinician.

Magnetic resonance imaging visualizes ligaments and tendons and is becoming the modality of choice in evaluation of rotator-cuff tears (see Practical Problem 4.14, Rotator cuff tears and chronic impingement syndrome). Exciting work has been done on delineating synovial fluid from synovial hypertrophy using MRI with gadolinium administration[25]. The applicability of this combination in demonstrating effectiveness of therapy in the acutely inflamed joint is presently being assessed.

Since MRI has replaced most other modalities for imaging spine disorders, it should be used to evaluate the cervical spine in rheumatoid patients with neurologic symptoms. On one image the spinal cord, disks, ligaments, synovium around the odontoid and the odontoid itself can be visualized, and the problems delineated (Fig. 5.19). Also, MRI is becoming the modality of choice in the evaluation of temporomandibular joint arthritis.

In the future, MRI will probably play an important role in the evaluation of the patient with RA. However, further improvements in image resolution, acquisition time and imaging costs, as well as increased experience in image interpretation, are needed.

EVALUATION OF DISEASE PROGRESSION

Accurate assessment of the progression of disease is a significant problem in RA[3]. It is believed that the radiograph images the true biological end point of inflammation and enzymatic degradation of cartilage and subchondral bone. It is well known that the treated patient often becomes asymptomatic while the radiograph demonstrates continuing progression of disease. As long as there is radiographic progression of disease, the patient is considered to be treated inadequately. There is continuing controversy over what role conventional radiography should play in the assessment of disease[26]. The problems in using radiographic images center around technical, clinical, interpretational and pathophysiologic variables.

The need to have quality images for interpretation has already been discussed. At present, radiographs of the hands and wrists are employed to assess progression of disease. However, RA has such a variable course, with different joint groups having different time-courses of involvement[27], that it is probably inappropriate to evaluate only the hands and the wrist.

Currently, the radiographic changes observed to determine progression of disease are the number of erosions and degree of joint-space loss[28]. There are problems with both of these parameters. First, these two changes occur independently of each other. Second, there is a tremendous variability in erosive disease: some patients never develop erosions; some go into spontaneous remission of their erosive disease and some progress relentlessly with erosion. Third, joint-space or cartilage loss may be caused by either the disease itself or by mechanical stress. Present scoring methods require that any degree of joint-space loss be recorded as progressive change due to RA. However, if sclerosis and osteophyte formation accompany joint-space loss, osteoarthritis has been superimposed on RA (Fig. 5.20); this

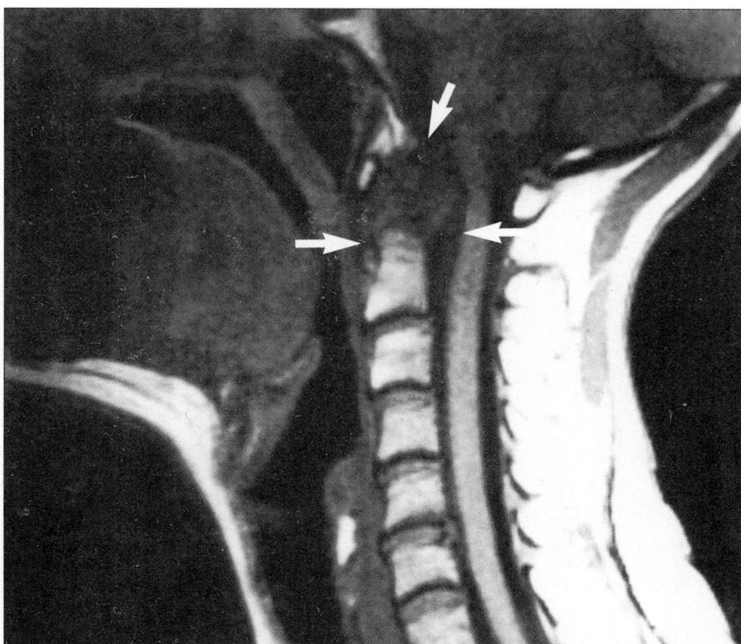

Fig. 5.19 A T1-weighted sagittal MRI of the cervical spine. There is replacement of the odontoid process by abnormal decreased soft tissue intensity, compatible with rheumatoid pannus (arrows). Stenosis of the canal and compression of the spinal cord can be seen. (Courtesy of John L Sherman, Washington Imaging Center, Washington DC.)

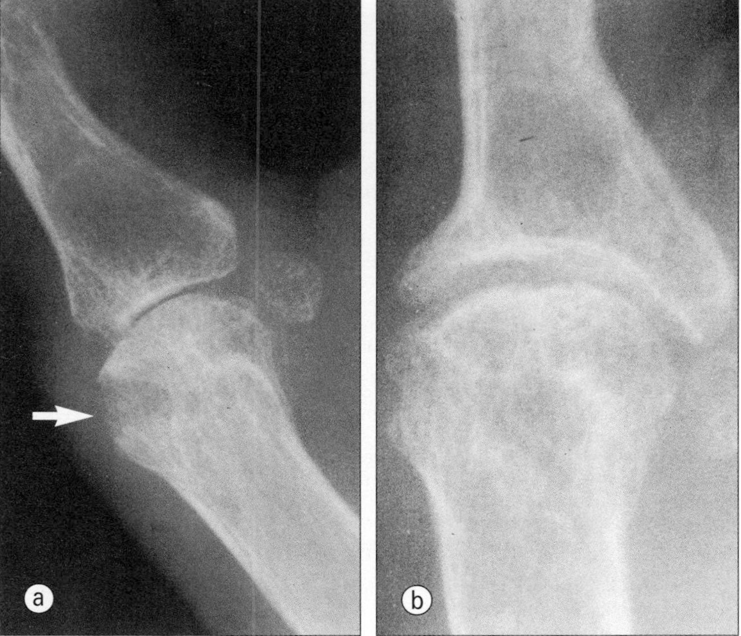

Fig. 5.20 Lateral views of the MCP joint of the thumb in untreated and treated RA. The untreated thumb (a) shows erosive disease (arrow). Radiography of the treated thumb (b) shows not only progressive loss of the base of the proximal phalanx, but also cortication and osteophyte formation. The erosion of the metacarpal head has filled in and developed an adjacent osteophyte. This represents osteoarthritis superimposed on healed RA. (Reproduced with permission from Weinblatt ME, *et al.* Arthritis Rheum. 1988;31:167–75).

indicates healing rather than progression of disease. Other radiographic parameters could be assessed in evaluating progression of disease, such as increasing osteoporosis, increasing subluxation and presence of rheumatoid nodules.

Perhaps other imaging modalities may give more useful and accurate evaluation of the true pathologic change. Bone scintigraphy physiologically demonstrates the actively inflamed joints. Serial bone scintigraphy might help in evaluating changed state of activity. Magnetic resonace imaging may be useful in imaging early changes in the tendons and the synovium. However, RA appears to have two phases, acute and chronic, of inflammation. The phase being imaged must correspond with the phase being treated. The radiologist and rheumatologist must always work together to understand what images mean with respect to the clinical picture and treatment plan.

REFERENCES

1. Brower AC. Rheumatoid arthritis. In: Brower AC, ed. Arthritis in black and white. Philadelphia: WB Saunders; 1988:137–65.
2. Resnick D. Rheumatoid arthritis. In: Resnick D, ed. Bone and joint imaging, 2E. Philadelphia: WB Saunders; 1996:195–209.
3. Brower AC. Use of the radiograph to measure the course of rheumatoid arthritis disease: the gold standard vs. fool's gold. Arthritis Rheum. 1990;33:316–24.
4. Brower AC. Imaging techniques and modalities. In: Brower AC, ed. Arthritis in black and white. Philadelphia: WB Saunders; 1988:1–20.
5. Nørgaard F. Earliest roentgenological changes in polyarthritis of the rheumatoid type: rheumatoid arthritis. Radiology. 1965;85:325–29.
6. Martel W, Hayes JT, Duff IF. The pattern of bone erosion in the hand and wrist in rheumatoid arthritis. Radiology. 1965;84:204–14.
7. Resnick D. Rheumatoid arthritis of the wrist: The compartmental approach. Med Radiogr Photogr. 1976;52:50–88.
8. Brower AC. Arthritis in black and white. Philadelphia: WB Saunders; 1988.
9. Monsees B, Destouet JM, Murphy WA, Resnick D. Pressure erosions of bone in rheumatoid arthritis: a subject review. Radiology. 1985;155:53.
10. Calabro JJ. A critical evaluation of the diagnostic features of the feet in rheumatoid arthritis. Arthritis Rheum. 1962;5:19–29.
11. Leach RE, Gregg T, Ferris JS. Weight-bearing radiography in osteoarthritis of the knee. Radiology. 1970;97:265–8.
12. Magyar E, Talerman A, Feher M, Wouters HW. The pathogenesis of the subchondral pseudocyst in rheumatoid arthritis. Clin Orthop. 1974;100:341–8.
13. Hastings DE, Parker SM. Protrusio acetabuli in rheumatoid arthritis. Clin Orthop Rel Res. 1975;108:76–83.
14. Resnick D. Patterns of migration of the femoral head in osteoarthritis of the hip: roentgenographic–pathologic correlation and comparison with rheumatoid arthritis. AJR. 1975;124:62–74.
15. Sbarbaro JL. The rheumatoid shoulder. Orthop Clin N Am. 1975;6:593–6.
16. Weissman BNW, Aliabadi P, Weinfield LS. Prognostic features of atlanto-axial subluxation in rheumatoid arthritis patients. Radiology. 1982;144:745–51.
17. El-Khoury GY, Wener MH, Menezes AH, Dolan KD, Kathol MEH. Cranial settling in rheumatoid arthritis. Radiology. 1980;137:637–42.
18. Martel W. Pathogenesis of cervical discovertebral destruction in rheumatoid arthritis. Arthritis Rheum. 1977;20:1217–25.
19. Gelman MI, Ward JR. Septic arthritis: a complication of rheumatoid arthritis. Radiology. 1977;122:17–23.
20. Resnick D. Diagnostic techniques. In: Resnick D, ed. Bone and joint imaging, 2E. Philadelphia: WB Saunders; 1996:19–164.
21. Weissberg DL, Resnick D, Taylor A, *et al.* Rheumatoid arthritis and its variants: analysis of scintiphotographic, radiographic, and clinical examinations. AJR. 1978;131:665–73.
22. Good AE. Rheumatoid arthritis, Baker's cyst and thrombophlebitis. Arthritis Rheum. 1964;7:56–64.
23. Adams ME, Li DKB. Magnetic resonance imaging in rheumatology. J Rheumatol. 1985;12:1038–40.
24. Berquist TH. Articular disorders. Top Magn Reson Imaging. 1989;1:1–84.
25. Weissman BN, Hussain S. Magnetic resonance imaging of the knee. Rheum Dis Clin N Amer. 1991;17930:637–68.
26. Weisman MH. Use of radiographs to measure outcome in rheumatoid arthritis. Am J Med. 1987;83:96–100.
27. Scott DL, Coulton BL, Bacon PJ, *et al.* Methods of X-ray assessment in rheumatoid arthritis: a re-evaluation. Br J Rheumatol. 1985;24:31–9.
28. Sharp JT, Lidsky MD, Collins LS, *et al.* Methods of scoring the progression of radiologic changes in rheumatoid arthritis. Arthritis Rheum. 1971;24:706–29.

THE SYNOVIUM

Jo CW Edwards

Summary

- Synovium lines diarthrodial joints, tendon sheaths and bursae.
- Intimal layer macrophages carry receptors for immune complexes. Intimal fibroblasts synthesize hyaluronan, adhesion molecules and complement decay-accelerating factor.
- In RA, binding of immune complexes to intimal macrophages may, via cytokine release, induce synovial fibroblasts to support B lymphocyte survival and maturation.

INTRODUCTION

Normal synovium is a rather unremarkable looking soft connective tissue. The specialized properties of the tissue relate largely to the intimal layer, which probably forms less than 1/10,000th of body mass. However, this layer appears to be the target of inflammatory disease capable of producing extensive disabilty. There is increasing evidence to indicate that synovial intimal cells are specialized, not only in their ability to synthesize synovial fluid and matrix components, but also in their ability to interact with elements of the immune response, including antigen–antibody complexes, complement proteins and B lymphocytes. In this chapter the basic properties of synovial tissue are described and the possible roles of these properties in the genesis of rheumatoid arthritis (RA) discussed.

DEFINITIONS

Synovium may be defined as the soft tissue lining the spaces of diarthrodial joints, tendon sheaths and bursae. These spaces contain a small amount of fluid which is usually rich in hyaluronan (syn. hyaluronic acid). Hyaluronan gives the fluid the consistency of egg white. The word synovium comes from *syn* = with, *ovium* = egg.

Synovial spaces are distinguished from other ill-defined interconnecting spaces in loose connective tissue by a continuous lining layer of compact connective tissue with a nonadherent surface[1]. It is the continuous nature of this layer which allows synovium to retain its fluid contents. The nonadherent surface allows movement between, rather than within, connective tissue elements. Synovial surfaces are populated by a mixture of specialized macrophages and fibroblasts. This is in contrast to serosal surfaces which derive from extra-embryonic coelom and carry a mesothelium with a basal lamina.

The definition of synovium includes both the surface layer of cells and the specialized matrix known as the intima, as well as the underlying tissue, known as subintima. The subintima must be included in the concept of synovium because it carries the synovial vascular plexus and may also carry a reservoir of specialized fibroblasts. The orthopedic surgeon has a concept of a 'synovial membrane' which can be dissected out, picked up with forceps and passed to the pathologist or laboratory scientist. This structure consists of both intima, which is a mere 20–40μm thick, and areolar subintima, which can be up to 5mm thick. At some sites there is no discrete membrane, as where subintima consists of fat pad or fibrous tissue.

Synovium is not always typical. The surface layer of cells may be absent. Superficial bursae may contain little or no detectable hyaluronan-rich fluid[2]. Ganglia are distended sacs which contain hyaluronan-rich fluid. They do not occur at the sites of shearing associated with bursae, do not have a typical surface layer of cells and may not be considered truly synovial. Diseased synovial tissue may lose any recognizable structure. These exceptions to the definition of synovium probably reflect the interplay of several different factors in synovial histogenesis.

STRUCTURE

The microscopic anatomy of synovial tissue was first fully described by Key[3] whose lack of preconceptions makes his account still worth reading. Key divided synovium into three main types on the basis of subintimal structure: fibrous, areolar and adipose (Fig. 6.1). He also pointed out that subintima may be continuous with periosteum, perimysium or even hyaline or fibrocartilage.

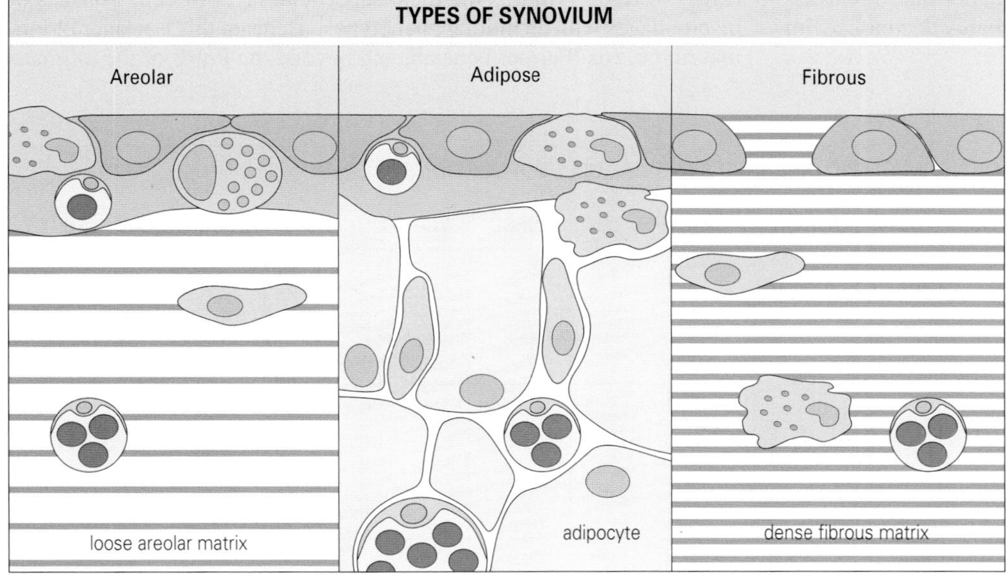

Fig. 6.1 Adipose, areolar and fibrous forms of synovium.

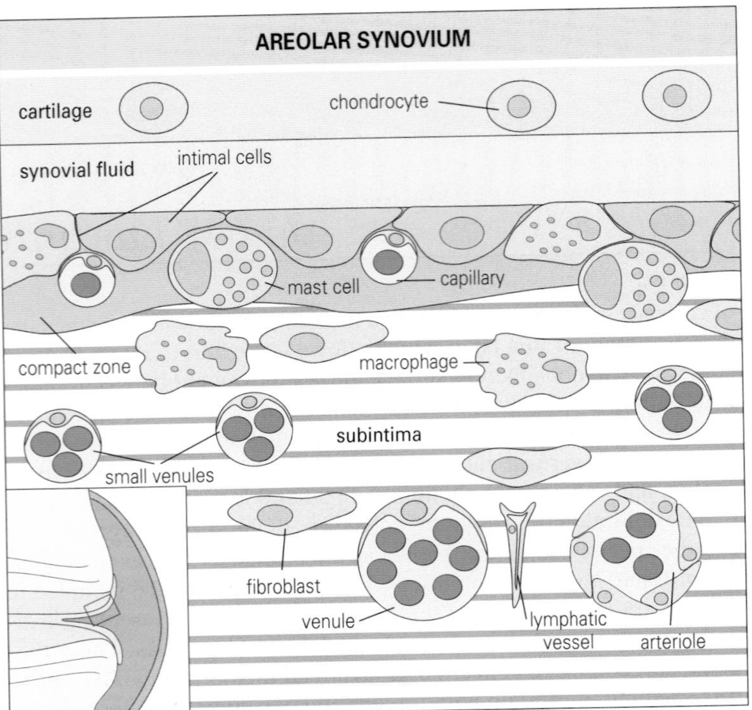

Fig. 6.2 Diagrammatic representation of typical areolar synovium.

Areolar synovium is the most specialized form. It is often thrown into folds, which may disappear as the tissue is stretched. Less often it may carry projections or villi. A more or less continuous layer of cells lies one or two deep on the tissue surface (Fig. 6.2). Immediately beneath these cells are capillaries. Further into the tissue there is a plexus of small venules[4,5]. Both types of small vessel are associated with mast cells. Nerve fibers are present, chiefly in association with blood vessels[6].

Three layers of tissue matrix may be distinguished. The intima is associated with a fine fibrillar or amorphous matrix with intermittent or absent collagen fibers[7]. Beneath this is a layer relatively rich in collagen which forms the basis of the physical membrane. It is often extremely extensible. Beneath this is a loose layer which allows the membrane to move freely. Beyond the loose layer will lie ligament, tendon, periosteum or some other fibrous structure.

Adipose synovium occurs as fat pads and also as complex projections or villi. It bears a complete intimal layer of cells and a superficial net of capillaries with associated mast cells close to the intima. The intima may lie directly on adipocytes but is usually associated with a thin band of collagen-rich substratum, particularly in the case of villi. The deeper tissue is fat, with an unremarkable vascular pattern. Villi usually have a central arteriole and venule but smaller ones are avascular. The amount of fat in villi is variable and probably decreases with age, with a relative increase in fibrous tissue.

Fibrous synovium is hardly a distinct structure, consisting of fibrous tissue such as ligament or tendon on which lies a very variable and intermittent layer of cells, with a similarly variable number of blood vessels. Fibrous synovium may be very difficult to distinguish from fibrocartilage, especially in the annular pads found in finger joints.

THE INTIMAL CELLS

The earliest observers noted that intimal cells are heterogeneous. In 1962 Barland *et al.* defined two distinct types by electron microscopy, one consistent with a macrophage (type A) and the other a fibroblast (type B)[8]. During the 1970s and 1980s there was an active debate about the relationship between these two cell types and the existence of intermediate forms. This debate has been resolved with the general acceptance that the macrophages, like macrophages elsewhere, are derived from bone marrow precursors and the fibroblastic cells are locally derived (see below; cell origins).

Ultrastructural classification of intimal cells has two disadvantages. Firstly, electron microscopy is cumbersome and, secondly, macrophages and fibroblasts are known to show major ultrastructural overlap in inflammation. Cytochemical techniques for the demonstration of individual gene products or messenger RNAs have largely superseded the electron microscope as tools for cell identification. It is now possible to identify the two major intimal cell populations very satisfactorily by light microscopy. Intimal macrophages show high activity of nonspecific esterase (NSE). Intimal fibroblasts show intense activity of the enzyme uridine diphospho-glucose dehydrogenase (UDPGD) and prominent expression of a number of cell-surface related molecules, including vascular cell adhesion molecule-1 (VCAM-1) and complement decay-accelerating factor (DAF). In most disease states the cells of the intima increase in size and number. This is not 'hyperplasia' but rather a complex change in cell populations, both in terms of origin and function[9]. Thus, it is essential to identify the two cell types in any analysis of intimal changes in disease.

Synovial macrophages

Macrophages are present both in the intima and subintima. Synovial intimal macrophages carry the markers expected of the macrophage lineage. In normal tissue they show prominent NSE activity and CD68 content, and express modest amounts of CD14 (Fig. 6.3). Notably, they express the immunoglobulin receptor FcγRIIIa. Recent studies indicate that FcγRIIIa is restricted to intimal macrophages in normal synovium, and, at 12 weeks gestation, present on no other cells throughout the entire fetal limb[10]. Macrophages make up a minority of intimal cells and tend not to lie exposed on the surface, being covered by fibroblast cell processes. In diseased tissue both the number and proportion of macrophages increases, accounting for up to 80% of intimal cells. Detailed distribution varies but a particular pattern commonly occurs (Figs 6.4 & 6.5). In this the most superficial layer of cells consists of macrophages with an intimal phenotype[11]. Beneath this is a layer of intimal fibroblasts. Further beneath, and beyond the limits of the intima is

PROPERTIES OF NORMAL AND DISEASED SYNOVIAL CELL POPULATIONS

			CD68	NSE	CD14	HLA-DR	FcγRI	FcγRIII	UDPGD	VCAM-1	DAF	ICAM-1	CR2	BST-1
Normal	Macrophage	intimal	+++	+++	+	++	+	++	–	–/?+	+	++	–	–
		subintimal	+++	+	++	++	++	+	–	–	+	+	–	–
	Fibroblast	intimal	–	–	–	–	–	–	+++	+++	+++	++	–	–
		subintimal	–	–	–	–	–	–	–	–	–	?–	–	–
Inflamed	Macrophage	intimal	+++	+++	+	++	+	++	–	–/?+	+	++	–	?–
		subintimal	+++	+	++	++	++	+	–	–	+	+	–	–
	Fibroblast	intimal	+	–	–	+	–	–	++	+++	+++	++	–	+
		subintimal	–	–	–	?	–	–	+	–/++	–/+	–/++	–/+	–
		FDC	–	–	–	?–	?	?–	–	+++	+++	+/++	+++	?

Fig. 6.3 Properties of normal and diseased synovial cell populations.

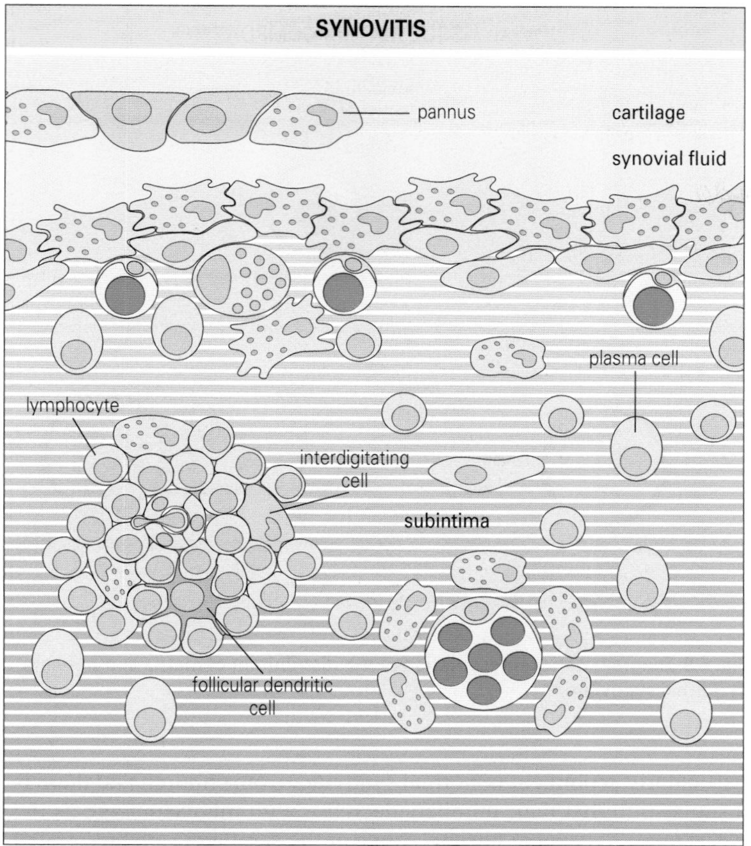

Fig. 6.4 Diagrammatic representation of inflamed synovium.

a zone of NSE-weak, strongly CD14 and FcγRI positive macrophages, closely associated with small vessels. It seems likely that the deep, strongly CD14 positive cells are freshly recruited cells and the superficial cells are more mature.

CD68 is often considered to be the most reliable panmacrophage marker. However, unlike other fibroblasts, synovial intimal fibroblasts express moderate amounts of CD68 in diseased tissue and NSE activity is a better marker for macrophages in the intima. In the subintima CD68 may be reliable[12].

In addition to true macrophages, there is evidence for a small number of antigen presenting interdigitating dendritic cells in normal synovial intima. Interdigitating dendritic cells carry abundant stainable surface class II and may preferentially express HLA-DQ (Fig. 6.3), although this remains open to debate. CD68 negative, DQ positive cells can be found sparsely scattered in the intima of normal synovium. Such cells are much more frequent in diseased tissue, but overlap of markers is much greater in disease making interpretation difficult[13–15].

Synovial fibroblasts

There has been a long-standing view that the intima contains cells specifically adapted to the production of hyaluronan, although direct evidence has been hard to obtain. The development of cytochemical techniques has led to the demonstration that synovial intimal fibroblasts are indeed specialized in terms of their machinery for hyaluronan synthesis, and of a number of other functions besides.

In 1992, Wilkinson *et al.*[16] showed that the CD68-negative lining cells alone demonstrate high activity of the enzyme UDPGD in normal tissue (Fig. 6.6). After tissue disaggregation these cells can be identified as large mononuclear or, more rarely, multinucleate cells with long branching processes (Figs 6.7 & 6.8). UDPGD converts UDP-glucose

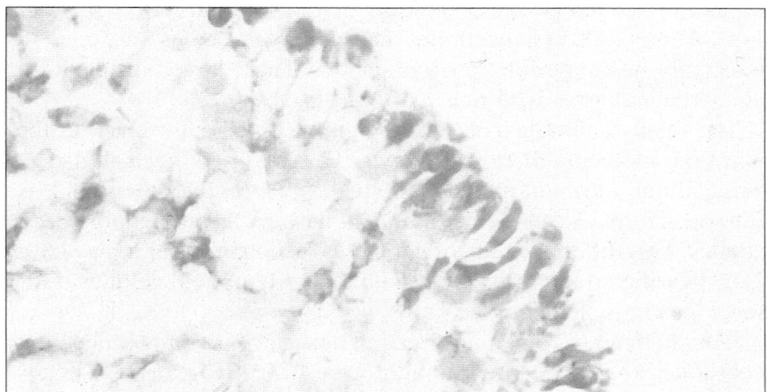

Fig. 6.5 Photomicrograph of inflamed synovium showing esterase positive macrophages on the surface and weakly UDPGD positive fibroblastic cells beneath.

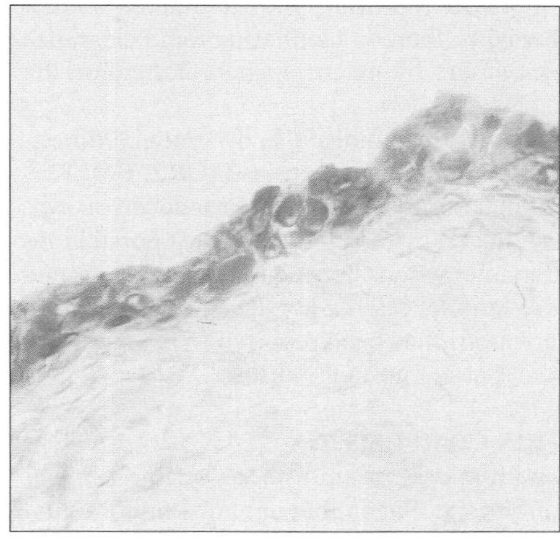

Fig. 6.6 Photomicrograph of normal synovium showing intense UDPGD activity confined to the surface layer.

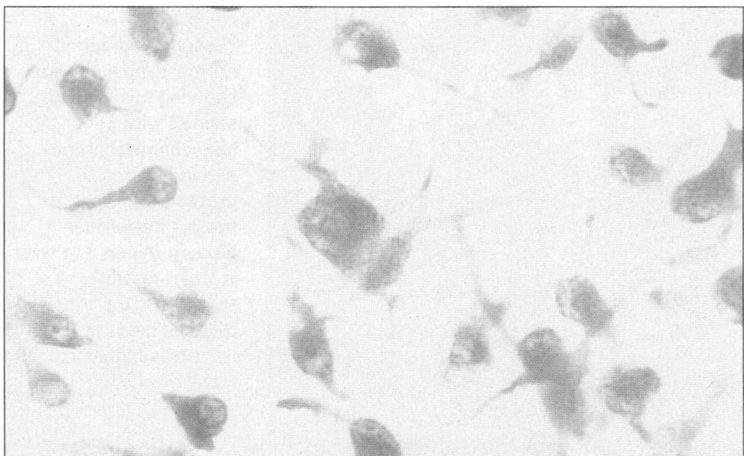

Fig. 6.7 Photomicrograph of cells disaggregated from osteoarthritic synovium showing the branching morphology of the UDPGD-rich cells.

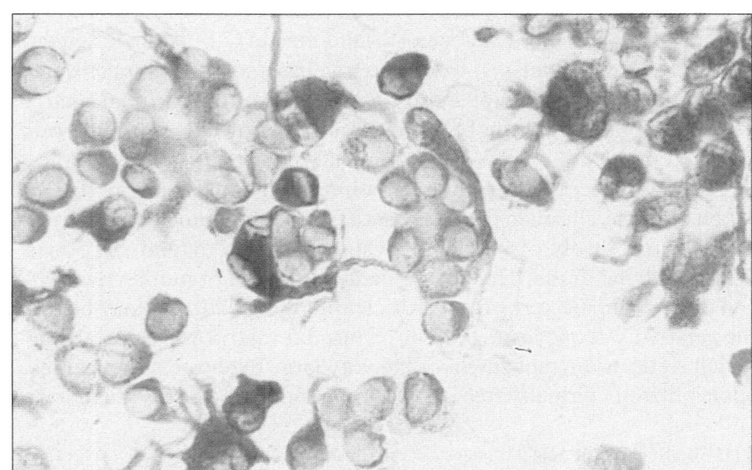

Fig. 6.8 Photomicrograph of cells disaggregated from osteoarthritic synovium double labeled for CD68 (red) and UDPGD (blue) showing the two distinct cell types.

into UDP-glucuronate, which is one of the two substrates required by hyaluronan synthase for assembly of the hyaluronan polymer. Unlike many other enzymes, UDPGD activity in intimal fibroblasts tends to be reduced rather than enhanced in diseased tissue.

Cells with fibroblast culture characteristics from inflamed synovium have been shown to produce high levels of metalloproteinases[17]. These cells have particularly abundant broad ramifying processes. It is not known whether they derive from intimal or subintimal cells. In tissue sections immunoreactivity for collagenase and gelatinase is patchy and not confined to the intima.

In 1983 Palmer and colleagues reported the detection of an unknown molecule on synovial intimal cells recognized by a monoclonal antibody coded mab67. This epitope has subsequently proven to be complement DAF (CD55) and has been shown to be present on intimal fibroblasts rather than macrophages[18,19]. It is present at high levels on internal body cavity surfaces, follicular dendritic cells (FDC) and cells in bone marrow, and at much lower levels on leukocytes and endothelium. The function of DAF on synovial intimal fibroblasts is not clear, although it may be that by protecting internal surfaces from the effects of complement activation it reduces the risk of subsequent scarring and loss of function.

Synovial intimal fibroblasts also show prominent expression of a number of surface ligands involved in binding to other cells or extracellular matrix[20]. These include VCAM-1, intercellular adhesion molecule-1 (ICAM-1), CD44 and β_1 integrins. The expression of VCAM-1 is particularly unusual, since it is completely absent from most other normal fibroblast populations, whereas CD44 and β_1 integrins are present, but at lower levels. The role of VCAM-1 on intimal fibroblasts is puzzling, but may, like DAF, modulate the way synovium responds to injury. The ligand for VCAM-1, $\alpha_4\beta_1$ integrin, is present on mononuclear leukocytes, but not polymorphs. Thus, intimal fibroblasts may allow the transmigration of polymorphs into synovial fluid but inhibit the passage of mononuclear cells, thereby facilitating rapid clearance of debris from the synovial cavity by macrophages retained on the tissue surface.

The expression of two other surface molecules by synovial fibroblasts is worthy of mention. Complement receptor 2 (CR2, CD21) is not expressed by normal intimal fibroblasts but can be induced on synovial fibroblasts in culture[21], in contrast to other fibroblast populations analyzed. CR2 is involved in interactions between B lymphocytes and stromal cells. A bone marrow stromal cell marker, BST-1, also involved in B cell–stromal cell interactions, has been reported to be expressed on fibroblasts in rheumatoid, but not normal, intima[22].

SYNOVIAL TISSUE MATRIX COMPOSITION

The intima is associated with matrix of amorphous or fine fibrillar ultrastructure. It is poor in type I collagen, but contains minor collagens, including types III, IV, V and VI (Fig. 6.9)[20,23,24]. The intimal matrix also contains laminin, fibronectin and chondroitin-6-sulfate rich proteoglycan (C-6-SP). Collagen IV, laminin and C-6-SP are basement membrane components. However, no true basement membrane is present in the intima. The apparently looser structure of intimal matrix may be explained on the basis of an absence of entactin, which is involved in the linking of other components in basement membrane.

Intimal matrix contains large amounts of hyaluronan (Fig. 6.10). Much of the hyaluronan is closely associated with lining cells, but relatively high levels of stainable hyaluronan also extend 20–50μm deeper into the tissue. This may indicate diffusion of mobile hyaluronan down from the surface towards clearing lymphatics. It may be that the relatively loose arrangement of intimal matrix provides a filter which restricts the movement of the very large hyaluronan molecules, while allowing virtually free passage of proteins (see below; function).

THE VASCULAR NET

A rich microvascular net is present beneath the surface of synovium[4,5]. Capillaries are present in close proximity to the intimal cells and may lie within the intima (Fig. 6.11). These capillaries appear to be

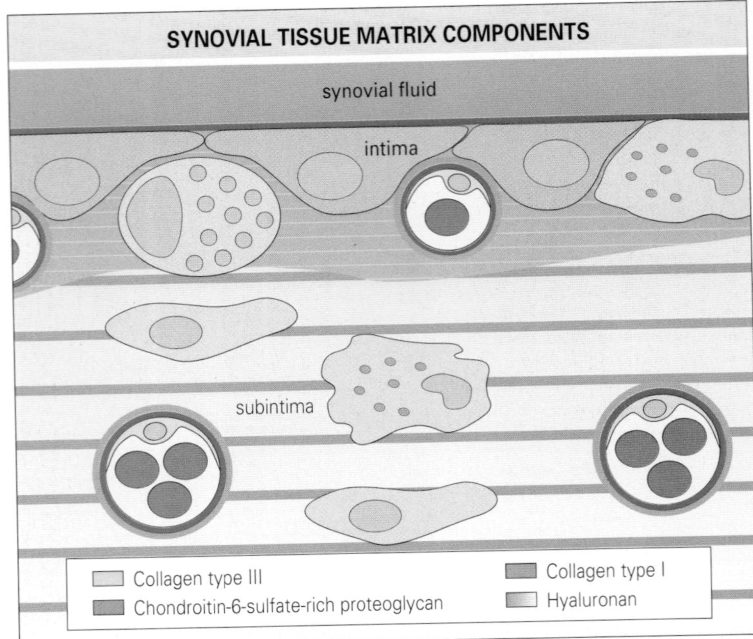

Fig. 6.9 Diagrammatic representation of the distribution of matrix components in normal synovium.

particularly prominent in normal synovium from children and there is a suggestion that their numbers decrease with increasing age as the tissue tends to become fibrotic. Some of the capillaries are fenestrated and the fenestrae tend to face towards the tissue surface[25]. About 50–100 μm beneath the surface small venules are prominent, the number of venular profiles exceeding that of capillaries in tissue sections. About 200μm beneath the surface larger venules are found in association with arterioles and lymphatics. These larger vessels form a quadrilateral array with rich anastomosis.

The small venules just beneath the intima express low levels of the adhesion molecule E-selectin (syn. ELAM-1) in normal tissue. Intracellular adhesion molecule-1 (ICAM-1), on the other hand, is more generally expressed but at the highest levels on the large deep venules. This differential distribution of adhesion molecules may have some bearing on the pattern of myeloid and lymphoid cellular infiltrates seen in inflamed tissue.

Lymphatics can be demonstrated in normal synovium by injection techniques and by double immunofluorescence (Fig. 6.11). Vessels with lymphatic staining characteristics are difficult to find in rheumatoid synovium, suggesting that small lymphatics are either destroyed by the inflammatory process or change their cell surface chemistry.

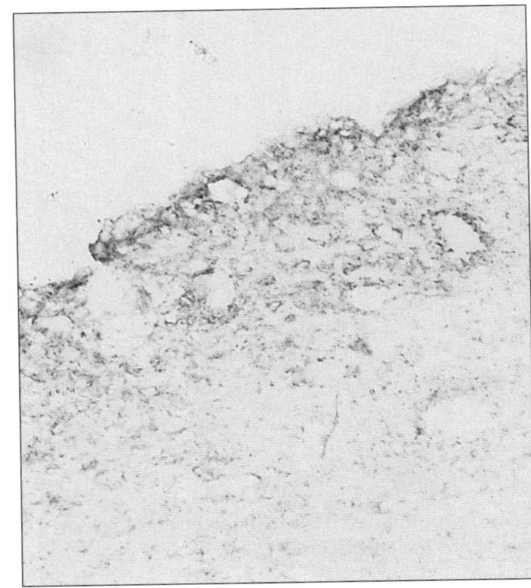

Fig. 6.10 Photomicrograph of normal synovial tissue showing hyaluronan stained with a histochemical probe derived from proteoglycan core protein hyaluronan binding region. Staining is most intense surrounding the lining cells and gradually decreases further into the tissue.

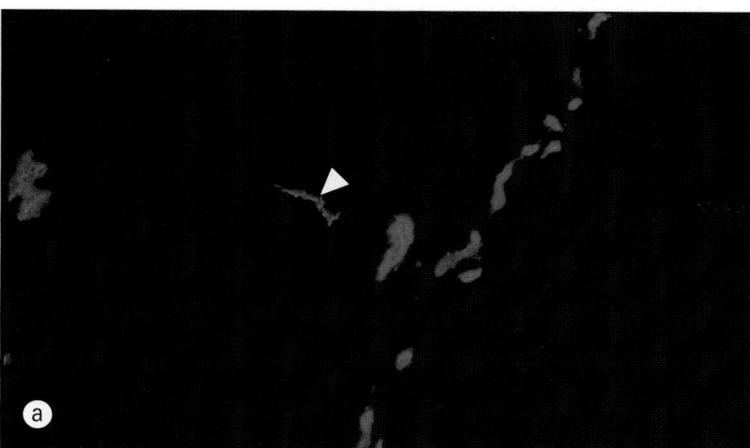

Fig. 6.11 Photomicrograph of normal synovium showing vessels stained (a) with *Ulex europeaus* lectin and (b) with a PAL-E/antidesmin cocktail. The surface capillary net is seen running from top to botton on the right. The lymphatic vessel (arrowed) fails to stain in (b).

DEVELOPMENTAL BIOLOGY

Early in the development of the embryonic limb bud, a central core of tissue, or blastema, appears, which will form the skeletal tissues. Within this core, foci of cartilage appear, each destined to become an individual bone. The tissue remaining between cartilage foci is known as interzone, and it is from this interzone that synovium forms. From the stage of early cartilage focus formation, the interzone appears continuous with perichondrium and both show strong immunohistochemical staining for CD44. The entire interzone is CD44 positive. Shortly before the joint cavity forms, DAF expression appears and is strictly limited to the cells destined to become synovial intimal fibroblasts, along the line where the cavity will form[26]. Expression of VCAM-1 does not appear until after the cavity has formed. After cavity formation the intimal layer also takes on a relatively high level of expression of CD44 and β_1 integrins in comparison to subintima.

The mechanism of cavity formation is not fully understood, but a working hypothesis implicates interactions between interzone cells bearing CD44 (a hyaluronan receptor) and hyaluronan itself[27,28]. Shortly before cavity formation, the cells of the potential joint line show high UDPGD activity, suggesting an increase in local hyaluronan synthesis. At the time of cavity formation high levels of hyaluronan appear along the joint line (see Fig. 6.12). Hyaluronan has a bimodal effect on intercellular adhesion. At low concentration extracellular hyaluronan cross links CD44 molecules on adjacent cells, inducing cell aggregation. At high levels, hyaluronan saturates CD44 and disaggregation occurs. Thus, before joint cavity formation CD44 and low levels of hyaluronan may keep the interzone cells together, but when hyaluronan levels rise at the joint line a cavity forms.

Although cavity formation might be expected to require lysis of fibrous matrix components such as collagen, recent evidence indicates that in human synovial joints cavity formation is not associated with increased local levels of matrix metalloproteinases at the joint line. Apoptotic cells can be identified in the interzone prior to cavity formation, but, unlike UDPGD activity and DAF expression, are not restricted to the cells of the potential joint line and their significance is unclear.

CELL ORIGINS AND RECRUITMENT

Evidence to date indicates that both intimal and subintimal macrophages are bone marrow derived cells arriving via the circulation as monocytes[29]. Most of these monocytes may arrive via subintimal postcapillary venules and migrate to the intima.

Intimal fibroblasts are thought to arise by division within synovium but the exact site remains open to speculation. It may be that intimal fibroblasts are a discrete self-replicating population, distinct from subintimal fibroblasts. Several pieces of evidence are against this. Rates of cell division within the intima are very low, even in disease. Following arthroplasty or synovectomy an intimal layer regenerates and carries DAF, UDPGD and VCAM-1 positive cells. These may arise from intimal rests left at surgery, but it seems more likely that they are replaced from the subintimal fibroblast pool. If synovial fibroblasts are disaggregated and cultured *in vitro*, they lose VCAM-1 and DAF expression, but the majority, apparently including cells of subintimal origin, will express these markers following cytokine stimulation. Fibroblasts of dermal or subcutaneous origin express no DAF and little, if any, VCAM-1 either following the formation of an internal surface in vivo or following cytokine stimulation *in vitro*. These findings suggest that synovial fibroblasts, both in the intima and subintima, belong to a specialized population with a propensity to express VCAM-1 and DAF. These two molecules are normally only expressed when cells are within the intima, but in disease subintimal cells may also express them.

FUNCTION

The functions of synovial tissue are often taken as self evident, but are remarkably difficult to define[30]. This may be because the tissue is a connective tissue, but being at a surface has become adapted to functions associated with epithelia. It also relates to the difficulty in assessing synovial function experimentally. If other tissues (e.g. kidney) are removed, loss of function is readily appreciated. If synovium is removed no major problems necessarily arise.

Like other soft connective tissue, synovium provides a deformable packing which allows movement of adjacent, relatively nondeformable tissues. The difference between synovium and other soft connective tissue is that it allows most of the movement to occur between rather than within tissues. The matrix of areolar synovium may also have unusual viscoplastic properties for coping with the stretching, rolling and folding it undergoes during joint movement, but these have yet to be defined. The functions of the tissue relating to the presence of a cavity may be considered in terms of:

- maintenance of an intact nonadherent tissue surface;
- control of volume and composition of synovial fluid;
- lubrication of cartilage and nutrition of chondrocytes within joints.

MAINTENANCE OF THE TISSUE SURFACE

Synovial surfaces must be nonadherent to allow continued movement. The production of free hyaluronan by intimal fibroblasts may be important in inhibiting adhesion. Plasminogen activator produced by intimal cells and DAF on intimal fibroblasts may also be important in preventing fibrin adhesions and scarring after injury. In order to retain synovial fluid, the intimal matrix must consist of a fibrous mat of a particular porosity that allows free exchange of crystalloids and proteins but inhibits rapid convective transit of the viscous hyaluronan solution which makes up the fluid. These functions presumably reflect the combined activities of the intimal macrophages and fibroblasts. The

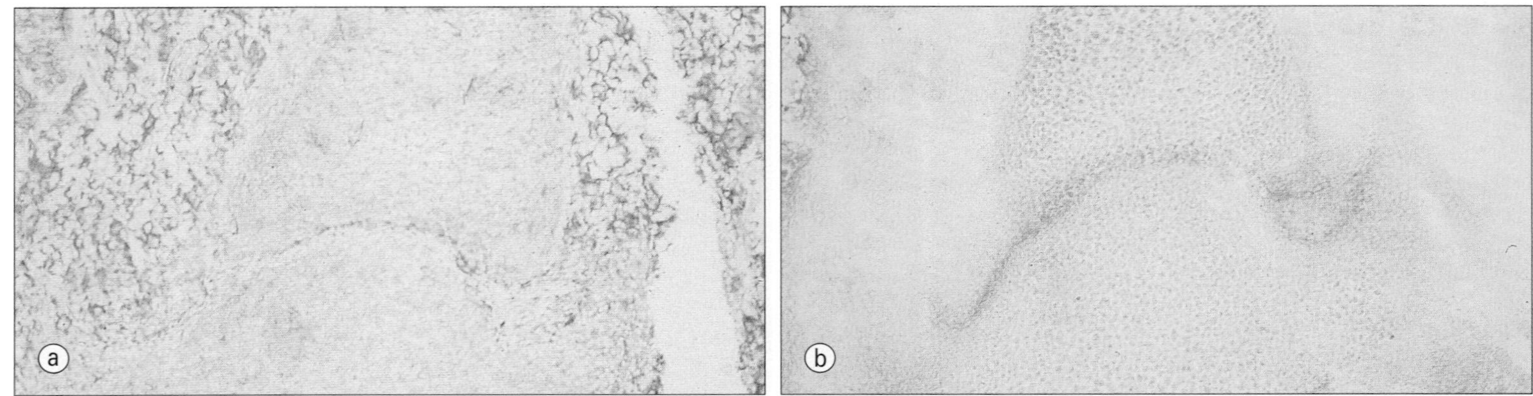

Fig. 6.12 Photomicrographs of adjacent sections of fetal mouse ankle showing the band of (a) hyaluronan-rich matrix and (b) UDPGD activity which develops just before joint cavitation.

vascular plexus is likely to be important not only in intimal cell nutrition but also in the recruitment of new cells. New macrophages will enter the tissue through venules and perivascular fibroblasts may well provide the main pool of intimal fibroblast precursors.

LUBRICATION

It is likely that the lubricating solutes in synovial fluid are synthesized by cells of the synovial intima, and probably specifically by intimal fibroblasts. The ability of synovial fluid to lubricate cartilage surfaces is dependent on the presence of glycoproteins[31]. One particular protein, lubricin, has been implicated. Hyaluronan does not appear to contribute to the ability of synovial fluid to lubricate cartilage in *ex vivo* systems. However, the glairy quality imparted to the fluid by hyaluronan may be important in maintaining a film of lubricant on the cartilage surfaces *in vivo*.

CONTROL OF SYNOVIAL FLUID VOLUME AND COMPOSITION

Synovial fluid consists of a dialysate of plasma to which has been added hyaluronan. Synovial fluid is unlike a secretion in that there is no net directional flow over time. Everything that enters the synovial space from the synovial intima leaves the space via the intima. Solvent and solutes may eventually leave the joint via the lymphatics but they have to cross the intima and penetrate the subintima to do so.

The chief means of exchange of water molecules is by diffusion, but during rest and exercise there is probably a convective shift of water in and out of the cavity. There may also be simultaneous bidirectional flow across the intima at a microscopic level. The control of the volume of water in the cavity is not fully understood. It is likely to be dependent on a balance between, on the one hand, tensile forces generated by the recoil of the surrounding synovial tissue and oncotic forces due to the swelling pressure generated by the hyaluronan in the fluid tending to increase volume, and, on the other, negative hydrostatic pressure in the synovial interstitium tending to reduce volume. Hyaluronan may have a polarizing effect on the movement of fluid by a molecular process analogous to clogging of a filter. The details of possible mechanisms are discussed elsewhere[32]. Briefly, plasma ultrafiltrate may pass relatively unimpeded to the synovial cavity, but may be inhibited from returning to the tissue lymphatics by the clogging effect of hyaluronan in the superficial layers of the tissue (see above under intimal matrix). Such mechanisms have been explored algebraically by Levick[32] and are under active investigation.

Whatever the precise forces interacting to alter fluid volume it is likely that the presence of hyaluronan in synovial fluid is the main factor responsible for retaining a reasonably constant volume of fluid during exercise. This constant volume is probably important as a cushion for synovial tissue and as a reservoir of lubricant for cartilage. It is likely that the rate of synthesis of hyaluronan and its exportation into the synovial fluid compartment are dependent on the mechanical stimulation of intimal fibroblasts and are influenced by the effectiveness of the synovial fluid cushion. Thus when synovial fluid volume is high it reduces mechanical stresses on intimal fibroblasts with a resultant reduction in the rate of hyaluronan production and vice versa, providing a negative feedback control system. This may be important in the management of effusions, particularly if excessive drainage leads to increased mechanical stimulation of inflamed synovial tissue.

Joint effusions represent a failure of synovial fluid volume control. Two quite distinct mechanisms operate. In joint disease in which synovium is mechanically irritated by worn bone and cartilage the composition of the fluid remains reasonably normal. The implication is that an excessive production of hyaluronan by intimal fibroblasts is stimulated by frictional forces and this excess of hyaluronan retains plasma dialysate in the synovial cavity. In inflammatory disease the effusion is simply an accumulation of inflammatory exudate akin to pleural effusion, i.e. an overspill from the inflammatory edema in synovial tissue created by increased vascular permeability.

CHONDROCYTE NUTRITION

There is little doubt that synovium provides the major route of nutrition for chondrocytes. In normal joints a large proportion of hyaline cartilage lies within 50μm of a synovial surface. In any one position only a small proportion of cartilage is apposed to the other articular surface and synovium packs most of the space between less congruent areas. In immature joints the subchondral plate is incomplete and may contribute to nutrition, but in adult joints this route is unlikely to be significant.

Nutrition of areas of cartilage which do not come into close contact with synovium must take an indirect route. This is likely to be particularly relevant to concave articular surfaces. Nutrition may occur by smearing of a thin film of fluid over these surfaces during movement. However, the amount of nutrient carried by the fluid film is probably small. It may be that indirect routes through cartilage matrix, and also the apposed articular cartilage matrix, are as important[30]. In areas where synovium is closely apposed to cartilage the synovial fluid film is usually so thin that it will have little effect on the rate of flux of small molecules.

Despite the fact that the vessels in synovium provide the most direct route for cartilage nutrition there is no evidence that they are structurally adapted to this function. The fenestrae seen in superficial capillaries are present in tendon sheath synovium at sites where there is no cartilage (or in fact tendon) dependent on their supply of small molecules. Surgical removal of synovium does not lead to rapid necrosis of cartilage. However, synovial vascularity may be very important in the control of cartilage growth. This may explain the relatively rich capillary net seen in juvenile synovium and the overgrowth of epiphyses seen with the hypervascular synovium of juvenile chronic arthritis.

LOCALIZATION OF PATHOLOGICAL PROCESSES

The central feature of RA is chronic synovitis. An understanding of the factors which determine the localization of inflammation to synovium would be a major step forward in the effort to control the clinical manifestations of the disease. Such an understanding has been lacking but a number of possible mechanisms have been proposed and recent evidence suggests that the answer may lie in a combination of factors including mechanical stimuli, cell surface ligand expression and immune complex handling (see Chapters 5.11 & 5.13).

REQUIREMENTS OF A LOCALIZATION HYPOTHESIS

A hypothesis addressing the distribution of inflammatory lesions in RA needs to explain not only joint disease but tenosynovitis, bursitis and, in a subset of cases, subcutaneous nodules. The first three sites are all synovial, indicating that the target tissue within the joint is synovium rather than cartilage. Autoreactivity to cartilage-specific antigens in animals does produce an arthritis, but also a severe endostitis at the cartilage growth plate. Inflammation around cartilaginous structures distant from joints is not a feature of RA.

The pattern of synovial disease varies markedly from case to case and only a minority of patients have nodules. These features suggest that localization of inflammation depends on at least two independent factors, which carry a different degree of weight in each case. One factor may be a universal characteristic of synovial tissue and the second factor an aspect of local tissue environment irrespective of tissue type. Mechanical stress has been the most popular candidate for this second type of factor.

SYNOVIAL ANTIGENS

No antigens specific to synovial tissue have been defined despite detailed studies using two-dimensional sodium dodecyl sulfate–polyacrylamide gel electrophoresis and differential display of messenger RNA. Several observations weigh against the implication of a synovial-specific antigen. No autoantibodies against synovium have been demonstrated using traditional immunochemical techniques. No synovial antigen has been retrieved from immune complexes obtained from joint fluid. Autoimmunity to a synovial antigen might be expected to affect all synovial sites. Moreover, implication of a synovial antigen does not explain the genesis of nodules.

ADHESION MOLECULES AND OTHER CELL SURFACE LIGANDS

An alternative to the concept of synovium as an antigenic target is that of synovium as a 'lymphocyte trap'. Synovitis may reflect an ability of synovial cells to encourage cellular immigration or persistence within the tissue. This idea initially arose in the context of adhesion molecules and leukocyte–endothelial interactions. However, the general pattern of synovial vasculature is similar to that of skin, an organ only occasionally involved in RA, and, despite a continued search, no synovium-specific endothelial adhesion molecules have been identified.

What is more unusual about the adhesion molecule profile of synovial cells is the presence of VCAM-1 on intimal fibroblasts. This might be expected to promote interactions between intimal fibroblasts and mononuclear leukocytes. Within both normal lymphoid tissue and ectopic lymphoid foci in synovial subintima, VCAM-1 expressing stromal cells are most strikingly associated with B lymphocytes[12]. The association between B lymphocytes and cells co-expressing VCAM-1 and DAF is even stronger. The only other fibroblast-like cells in the body to co-express VCAM-1 and DAF are the FDC of germinal centers and, perhaps, bone marrow stromal cells. This raises the possibility that VCAM-1 and DAF on synovial fibroblasts are involved in promoting interactions with B lymphocytes[33]. The idea is further supported by the expression on synovial fibroblasts of ICAM-1, CR2 and BST-1, under conditions which are not associated with expression of these molecules on other fibroblasts (see above). The expression of all these molecules on stromal cells is essential to survival and maturation of B cells at several stages of their life history. The potential significance of this fact is borne out by recent experiments showing that synovial fibroblasts are superior to all other fibroblast populations tested in the promotion of B cell survival and terminal differentiation into plasma cells[34].

A number of unanswered questions relate to the relationship between intimal and subintimal synovial fibroblasts in this respect. Intimal fibroblasts are rarely, if ever, seen in contact with healthy B cells, but subintimal fibroblasts appear to be able to support B cell survival and function if they are induced to express VCAM-1, with or without co-expression of DAF and CR2. For this reason, a better understanding of the ontologic relationship between intimal and subintimal fibroblasts would be of great value.

The implication of the above is that synovial fibroblasts, through facilitated expression of B cell survival cofactors, may allow the development of ectopic lymphoid tissue within synovium in response to proinflammatory events which might be self-limiting in other tissues.

This makes it possible to see synovitis and nodules as responses to the same initiating stimulus, one involving extensive lymphocyte and plasma cell accumulation and the other not, as observed. Histochemical studies confirm the absence of VCAM-1 or DAF on nodular palisade fibroblasts.

MECHANICAL STRESS

Both rheumatoid nodules and synovitis occur at sites of mechanical stress. The palisading cell layer of rheumatoid nodules has features in common with inflamed synovial intima, being a layer of macrophages and fibroblasts which divides vascular tissue containing mononuclear cells from an avascular compartment containing necrotic debris and polymorphs. These observations support the idea that the two types of lesion have a common initiation. Mechanical forces could promote an inflammatory response via several routes. Vascular flow may be altered, as may the flux of fluid and macromolecules within extracellular matrix. Alternatively, forces acting on cells may lead to production of cytokines, growth factors, adhesion molecules or matrix components.

CHANGES IN VASCULAR FLOW

During movement it is likely that, even in normal joints, microvascular perfusion is repeatedly interrupted. The same applies to common nodule sites, such as the skin over the olecranon. Nail-fold vasculitic lesions also occur chiefly at sites of blanching during grip[35]. Vascular compression may lead to stasis and hypoxia. Blake and colleagues have suggested that episodes of hypoxia cause modulation of the xanthine dehydrogenase enzyme to an oxidase form, capable of generating oxidative radicals[36]. Hypoxic changes can be documented in the established rheumatoid joint and may well contribute to local chronicity, but it is difficult to know whether they could be involved in the initial events in normal tissue.

IMMUNE COMPLEXES, FcγRIIIA AND TGFβ

The existence of immune complexes, and rheumatoid factor-based complexes in particular, is well recognized in RA (see Chapters 5.11 & 5.13). Immune complexes are implicated in the genesis of other autoimmune syndromes with very different patterns of organ involvement. This suggests that immune complexes in RA exert their effects in a specific way. The existence of FcγRIIIa on synovial intimal macrophages and the way in which FcγRIIIa expression is regulated suggest a mechanism. Immune complexes can interact with FcγRIIIa, leading to the generation of macrophage products such as reactive oxygen species and tumor necrosis factor alpha (TNF-α). FcγRIIIa is inducible on macrophages by transforming growth factor beta (TGF-β), which, in turn is likely to be produced locally under the influence of mechanical stress. A number of cells could be responsible for TGF-β secretion, including mast cells, and secretion may occur as a direct response to stress or in response to neuropeptides generated by C fibers as part of an axon reflex. Thus a direct link between mechanical stress and the generation of macrophage products by immune complexes can be envisaged. This process may be seen as a distinct variant of the type III hypersensitivity reaction, and because of the production of cytokines such as TNF-α, may generate a prominent acute-phase response, including a rise in serum C-reactive protein.

The reasons why the immune complexes encountered in RA should interact with FcγRIIIa may be several. As indicated above, synovial intima has the potential to act as an asymmetric macromolecular filter which may encourage the accumulation of complexes if both antibody and antigen are plasma derived. This would include complexes formed from self-associating IgG rheumatoid factors. Perhaps more significantly, IgG rheumatoid factor-based complexes may have unusual dissociation kinetics, because of the presence of excess soluble antigen, and may be able to interact with both FcγRIIIa and complement in an aberrant fashion because the 'antigen' as well as the 'antibody' carries an Fc domain.

CONCLUSION

The preceding discussion leads to the possibility that both the fibroblasts and macrophages of the synovial lining are involved in the genesis of rheumatoid disease through the local expression of surface ligands such as VCAM-1, DAF and FcγRIIIa. This may provide insight into the reasons why synovial fibroblasts have evolved to express VCAM-1 and DAF. The former probably inhibits macrophage efflux into synovial fluid and DAF probably protects against complement-mediated damage. The requirement for these protective mechanisms may relate directly to the coexistence of macrophages which express FcγRIIIa in response to the effects of continual mechanical stimulation. Immune complexes and even rheumatoid factors are generated normally during an immune response. Also, DAF may protect synovium against interactions between such immune complexes and the FcγRIIIa-positive macrophages. Of note, both DAF and FcγRIIIa expression are dependent on mast cell products; histamine and TGF-β respectively. Unfortunately, the ability to express VCAM-1 and DAF appears to be a double-edged sword: in the presence of inflammation it may encourage the genesis of ectopic lymphoid tissue.

This model implies that RA is an almost predictable failure of a complex immune response involving immune complexes, complement and cell surface receptors in which compromises are struck between the need for a rapid response to infection and the need to protect self against damage. A wide range of genetic and environmental factors might be expected to tip the balance, including hormonal environment and the modulatory effect of MHC Class II allotype on interactions between T and B lymphocytes. Rheumatoid factor containing immune complexes are implicated specifically in seropositive nodular RA, but other types of immune complex or shifts in the regulation of either B or T lymphocyte migration may lead to indistinguishable changes in synovium. This may be relevant to seronegative RA and other syndromes such as psoriatic arthropathy and Reiter's disease.

REFERENCES

1. Edwards JCW. Structure of synovial lining. In: Henderson B, Edwards JCW, eds. The synovial lining in health and disease. London: Chapman and Hall; 1987:17–40.
2. Canoso JJ, Stack MT, Brandt K. Hyaluronic acid content of deep and superficial subcutaneous bursae of man. Ann Rheum Dis. 1983;42:171–5.
3. Key JA: The synovial membrane of joints and bursae. In: Special cytology, vol. 2. New York: PB Hoeber Inc; 1932:1055–76.
4. Davies DV, Edwards DAW. The blood supply of the synovial membrane and intra-articular structures. Ann R Coll Surg 1948;142–56.
5. Wilkinson LS, Edwards JCW. Microvascular distribution in normal human synovium. J Anat. 1989;167:129–36.
6. Mapp PI. Innervation of synovium. Ann Rheum Dis. 1995;54:398–403.
7. Ghadially FN. Fine structure of joints. In: Sokoloff L, ed. The joints and synovial fluid. New York: Academic Press 1978:105–76.
8. Barland P, Novikoff AB, Hamerman D. Electron microscopy of the human synovial membrane. J Cell Biol. 1962;14:207–16.
9. Henderson B, Revell P, Edwards JCW. Synovial lining cell hyperplasia in rheumatoid arthritis : dogma and fact. Ann Rheum Dis. 1988;47:348–9.
10. Blades *S*, Edwards JCW, Cambridge G. The relationship between FcγRIIIa, VCAM-1 and DAF expression explains both synovitis and nodules in rheumatoid arthritis. Arth Rheum. 1996;Abst (suppl.):in press.
11. Bröker B, Edwards JCW, Fanger M, Lydyard P. The prevalence and distribution of macrophages bearing FcRI, FcRII and FcRIII in synovium. Scand J Rheumatol. 1990;19:123–35.
12. Edwards JCW, Wilkinson LS. Immunohistochemistry of synovium. In: Henderson B, Edwards JCW, Pettifer ER, eds. Mechanisms and models in rheumatoid arthritis. New York: Academic Press; 1995:133–50.
13. Poulter LW, Janossy G. The involvement of dendritic cells in chronic inflammatory disease. Scand J Immunol. 1985;21:401–7.
14. Harding B, Knight SC. The distribution of dendritic cells in the synovial fluid of patients with arthritis. Clin Exp Immunol. 1986;63:594–602.
15. Wilkinson LS, Worrall JG, Sinclair HS, Edwards JCW. Immunohistochemical reassessment of accessory cell populations in normal and diseased human synovium. Br J Rheumatol. 1990;29:259–63.
16. Wilkinson LS, Pitsillides AA, Worrall JG, Edwards JCW. Light microscopic characterisation of the fibroblastic synovial lining cell (synoviocyte). Arthritis Rheum. 1992;35:1179–84.
17. Krane SM, Goldring SR, Dayer JM. Interactions among lymphocytes, monocytes and other synovial cells in the rheumatoid synovium. Lymphokines. 1982;7:75–87.
18. Stevens CR, Mapp PI, Revell PA. A monoclonal antibody (Mab 67) marks type B synoviocytes. Rheumatol Int. 1990;10:103–6.
19. Medof ME, Walter EI, Rutgers JL, Knowles DM, Nussenzweig V. Identification of the complement decay accelerating factor on epithelium and glandular cells and in body fluids. J Exp Med. 1987;165:848–64.
20. Edwards JCW. Synovial intimal fibroblasts. Ann Rheum Dis 1995;54:395–7.
21. Leigh RD, Cambridge G, Edwards JCW. Epression of B cell survival cofactors on synovial fibroblasts. Br J Rheumatol. 1996;Abst (suppl. I):110.
22. Lee BO, Ishihara K, Denno K, *et al.* Elevated levels of the soluble form of bone marrow stromal cell antigen 1 in the sera of patients with severe rheumatoid arthritis. Arthritis Rheum. 1996;39:629–37.
23. Revell PA, Al-Saffar N, Fish S, Osei D. Extracellular matrix of the synovial intimal cell layer. Ann Rheum Dis. 1995;54:404–7.
24. Ashhurst DE, Bland YS, Levick JR. An immunohistochemical study of the collagens of rabbit synovial interstitium. J Rheumatol. 1991;18:1669–72.
25. Suter ER, Majno G. Ulstrastructure of the joint capsule in the rat: presence of two kinds of capillaries. Nature. 1964;202:920–1.
26. Edwards JCW, Wilkinson LS. Distribution in human tissues of the synovial lining associated epitope recognised by monoclonal antibody 67. J Anat. 1996;188:119–27..
27. Craig FM, Bayliss MT Bentley G, Archer CW. A role for hyaluronan in joint development. J Anat. 1990;171:17–23.
28. Edwards JCW, Wilkinson LS, Jones HM, *et al.* The formation of human synovial joint cavities: a possible role for hyaluronan and CD44 in altered interzone cohesion. J Anat. 1994;185:355–67.
29. Athanasou N. Synovial macrophages. Ann Rheum Dis. 1995;54:392–4.
30. Edwards JCW. Functions of synovial lining. In: Henderson B, Edwards JCW, eds. The synovial lining in health and disease. London: Chapman and Hall; 1987:41–74.
31. Unsworth A. Lubrication of human joints. Mechanics of human joints. In: Wright V, Radin EL, eds. New York: Marcel Dekker; 1993:137–62.
32. Levick JR. Fluid movement across synovium in healthy joints: role of synovial fluid macromolecules. Ann Rheum Dis. 1995;54:417–23.
33. Edwards JCW, Cambridge G. Is rheumatoid arthritis a failure of B cell death in synovium?. Ann Rheum Dis. 1995;54:696–700.
34. Dechanet J, Merville P, Durand I, Banchereau J, Miossec P. The ability of synoviocytes to support terminal differentiation of activated B cells may explain plasma cell accumulation in rheumatoid synovium. J Clin Invest. 1995;95:456–63.
35. Edwards JCW. Relationship between pressure and digital vasculitis in rheumatoid disease. Ann Rheum Dis. 1980;39:138–40.
36. Henderson EB, Grootveld M, Farrell A, Smith EC, Thompson PW, Blake DR. A pathological role for damaged hyaluronan in synovitis. Ann Rheum Dis. 1991;50;196–200.

7

GENETICS OF THE MAJOR HISTOCOMPATIBILITY COMPLEX IN RHEUMATOID ARTHRITIS

Gerald T Nepom
& Barbara Nepom

- The major histocompatibility complex (MHC) in human chromosome 6 encodes the class I and class II histocompatibility antigens that form the human leukocyte antigen (HLA) 'types'.
- The extremely high degree of allele diversity of the MHC is the genetic cornerstone underlying the cellular interaction required for immune activation in normal and autoimmune states.
- The interaction between an antigenic peptide and the peptide-binding groove of the HLA molecule is a primary structural determinant for the genetic control of the immune response. A proper 'fit' leads to permissive binding and antigen presentation; lack of a structural 'fit' obviates this interaction.
- The class II molecules associated with rheumatoid arthritis (RA) have in common HLA-DRB1 genes that encode a sequence of amino acids from codons 67 to 74 of the DRB molecules. The sequences LLEQRRAA or LLEQKRAA constitute the shared RA epitope.
- The DRB1*04 (DR4) alleles which carry the shared RA epitope are markers for susceptibility for more severe, erosive RA; the prospective use of these genes as prognostic indicators requires additional validation.

THE HLA COMPLEX

The human major histocompatibility complex on chromosome six (6p21.3) encodes histocompatibility antigens which form the traditional HLA 'types'. Strong genetic associations between specific genes in this complex and clinical features of RA provide a direct and useful way to improve our understanding of disease susceptibility and immunologic events in RA.

CLASS I AND CLASS II GENES

The HLA class I genes are located in a 2000 kilobase (kb) stretch of DNA at the telomeric end of the human MHC. As shown in Figure 7.1, there are six well-characterized HLA class I loci. The HLA-A, B and C loci encode the principle transplantation antigens in humans and are expressed on all nucleated cells. The HLA-E gene has a more restricted distribution of tissue expression[1], while expression of the HLA-F and G genes, which are truncated relative to the other class I genes, is less well understood. Transcription, but not a protein product, of the HLA-F gene has been detected in some tissues[2], while expression of the HLA-G gene has been noted only in the placental trophoblast, a finding with intriguing functional implications[3].

Each of the class I transplantation antigens HLA-A, B, and C is highly polymorphic in the population. This polymorphism is created by a high degree of allelic variation at each of these three loci (Fig. 7.1). Each of the class I genes encodes a single polypeptide, the HLA class I heavy chain. This polypeptide complexes with β2-microglobulin, a protein encoded outside of the MHC region, to form the mature HLA class I molecule.

The HLA class II complex is also illustrated in Figure 7.1. Individual haplotypes contain up to 14 different class II loci, clustered into three major subregions, termed HLA-DR, DQ and DP. Each of these subregions contains at least one functional beta (B) locus and one functional alpha (A) locus, as well as additional pseudogenes or genes of unknown function. The HLA-DRA and DRBl loci encode the α and β polypeptides, respectively, which form a mature class II HLA-DR molecule. Similarly, products of the DQAl and DQBl loci form the DQ molecule, and the DPAl and DPBl loci encode the DP molecule. A second expressed DR molecule is encoded on most haplotypes by the DRA and DRB3 (or related DRB4 or DRB5) loci. Thus, in spite of the genetic complexity, most haplotypes encode only four distinct expressed class II molecules.

The HLA class II loci are extremely polymorphic. A partial listing of allelic variation in the population for each of the major class II loci is shown in Figure 7.1. Since the HLA genes are physically linked to one another, there is a high degree of linkage disequilibrium among HLA loci; i.e., different alleles at the different HLA loci do not randomly assort in each generation but rather exist on haplotypes which are relatively fixed in the population. Therefore, inheritance of a specific allele at one locus is often accompanied by the inheritance of a specific allele at a nearby linked locus. For example, the DRBl*0404 allele, which encodes one of the DR4-positive class II β chains, is almost always linked to DQAl*0301 and DQBl*0302 alleles at the DQ locus, and is often linked to the HLA-B*4001 allele at the HLA-B locus. This linkage phenomenon imparts some constraints on the overall diversity of HLA haplotypes commonly found in the population. This means that when a polymorphic HLA marker is noted to be associated with a particular disease, the actual susceptibility gene may be that HLA marker itself, a gene closely linked to that marker or a gene at some distance from that marker, but present on the same haplotype.

Since most individuals in the population are heterozygotes, an individual's HLA phenotype is determined by two HLA haplotypes. Thus, most individuals express six class I molecules and at least eight class II molecules. In addition, transcomplementation provides a further source of diversity in heterozygotes. Since HLA class II molecules are α–β heterodimers encoded by two HLA genes, it is possible for an α chain encoded on one haplotype to complement with a β chain encoded on the other haplotype, creating novel dimers in heterozygotes. Thus, for example, an individual heterozygous for the DQAl*0501 and DQBl*0201 genes on one haplotype, and the DQAl*0301 and DQBl*0302 genes on the other haplotype, actually expresses four, not two, different DQ heterodimers resulting from the combinatorial association of each of the α and β chains. However, not all combinations of α and β chains in the class II complex can form these transcomplementing dimers[4], so that the extent of the additional diversity depends on the specific haplotypes in each individual.

OTHER GENES IN THE MHC

The six class I genes and 14 class II genes mentioned above represent only about half of the known genes lying within the 4 megabase (Mb) human MHC[5,6]. Several of the remaining genes have interesting immunologic functions which could be of critical importance for participating in pathogenic events relating to HLA-associated autoimmune disease. Particularly enigmatic are a collagen gene centromeric of the class II region, an hsp (heat-shock protein) 70 gene near the HLA class I complex and cytokine genes for lymphotoxin (TNF-β) and tumor necrosis factor(TNF)-α centromeric of the HLA-B locus[7–9].

Two other areas are particularly notable. The HLA class III region is a name given to a cluster of genes between the class I and class II complexes. Although no known transplantation antigens are encoded here, a number of active genes are located in this region, including the

GENE ORGANIZATION OF THE MHC ON CHROMOSOME 6

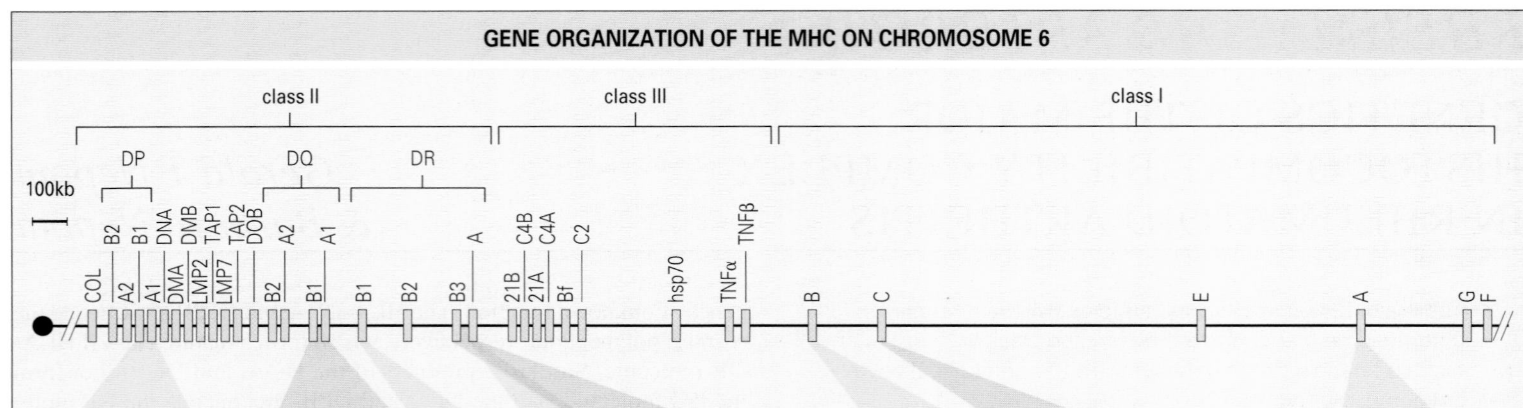

DP		DQ		DRB1		Other DRB		HLA-B		HLA-C		HLA-A	
Allele	Specificity	Allele	Specificity	Allele	Specificity	Allele	Specificity	Allele	Specificity	Allele	Specificity	Allele	Specificity
DPA1*0101	–	DQA1*0101	–	DRB1*0101	DR1	DRB3*0101	DRw52a	B*0701	B7	Cw*0101	Cw1	A*0101	A1
DPA1*0102	–	DQA1*0102	–	DRB1*0102	DR1	DRB3*0201	DRw52b	B*0702	B7	Cw*0201	Cw2	A*0201	A2
DPA1*0103	–	DQA1*0103	–	DRB1*0103	DR"BR"	DRB3*0202	DRw52b	B*0801	B8	Cw*0202	Cw2	A*0202	A2
DPA1*0201	–	DQA1*0201	–	DRB1*1501	DRw15(2)	DRB3*0301	DRw52c	B*1301	B13	Cw*0301	Cw3	A*0203	A2
		DQA1*0301	–	DRB1*1502	DRw15(2)			B*1302	B13	Cw*0501	Cw5	A*0204	A2
DPB1*0101	DPw1	DQA1*0401	–	DRB1*1601	DRw16(2)	DRB4*0101	DRw53	B*1401	B14	Cw*0601	Cw6	A*0205	A2
DPB1*0201	DPw2	DQA1*0501	–	DRB1*1602	DRw16(2)			B*1402	Bw65(14)	Cw*0701	Cw7	A*0206	A2
DPB1*0202	DPw2	DQA1*0601	–	DRB1*0301	DRw17(3)	DRB5*0101	DRw15(2)	B*1501	Bw62(15)	Cw*1101	Cw11	A*0207	A2
DPB1*0301	DPw3			DRB1*0302	DRw18(3)	DRB5*0102	DRw15(2)	B*1801	B18	Cw*1201	–	A*0208	A2
DPB1*0401	DPw4	DQB1*0501	DQw5(w1)	DRB1*0401	DR4, Dw4	DRB5*0201	DRw16(2)	B*2701	B27	Cw*1301	–	A*0209	A2
DPB1*0402	DPw4	DQB1*0502	DQw5(w1)	DRB1*0402	DR4, Dw10	DRB5*0202	DRw16(2)	B*2702	B27	Cw*1401	–	A*0210	A2
DPB1*0501	DPw5	DQB1*0503	DQw5(w1)	DRB1*0403	DR4, Dw13			B*2703	B27			A*0301	A3
DPB1*0601	DPw6	DQB1*0601	DQw6(w1)	DRB1*0404	DR4, Dw14			B*2704	B27			A*0302	A3
DPB1*0801	–	DQB1*0602	DQw6(w1)	DRB1*0405	DR4, Dw15			B*2705	B27			A*1101	A11
DPB1*0901	DP"Cp63"	DQB1*0603	DQw6(w1)	DRB1*0406	DR4, Dw'KT2'			B*2706	B27			A*2401	A24(9)
DPB1*1001	–	DQB1*0604	DQw6(w1)	DRB1*0407	DR4, Dw13			B*3501	B35			A*2501	A25(10)
DPB1*1101	–	DQB1*0201	DQw2	DRB1*0408	DR4, Dw14			B*3701	B37			A*2601	A26(10)
DPB1*1301	–	DQB1*0301	DQw7(w3)	DRB1*1101	DRw11(5)			B*3801	B38(16)			A*2901	A29(w19)
DPB1*1401	–	DQB1*0302	DQw8(w3)	DRB1*1102	DRw11(5)			B*3901	B39(16)			A*3001	A30(w19)
DPB1*1501	–	DQB1*0303	DQw9(w3)	DRB1*1103	DRw11(5)			B*4001	Bw60(40)			A*3101	A31(w19)
DPB1*1601	–	DQB1*0401	DQw4	DRB1*1104	DRw11(5)			B*4002	Bw40			A*3201	A32(w19)
DPB1*1701	–	DQB1*0402	DQw4	DRB1*1201	DRw12(5)			B*4101	Bw41			A*3301	Aw33(w19)
DPB1*1801	–			DRB1*1301	DRw13(w6)			B*4201	Bw42			A*6801	Aw68(28)
DPB1*1901	–			DRB1*1302	DRw13(w6)			B*4401	B44(12)			A*6802	Aw68(28)
				DRB1*1303	DRw13(w6)			B*4402	B44(12)			A*6901	Aw69(28)
				DRB1*1401	DRw14(w6)			B*4601	Bw46				
				DRB1*1402	DRw14(w6)			B*4701	Bw47				
				DRB1*0701	DR7			B*4901	B49(21)				
				DRB1*0702	DR7			B*5101	B51(5)				
				DRB1*0801	DRw8			B*5202	Bw52(5)				
				DRB1*0802	DRw8			B*5701	Bw57(17)				
				DRB1*0803	DRw8			B*5801	Bw58(17)				
				DRB1*0901	DR9								
				DRB1*1001	DR1w10								

Fig. 7.1 Gene organization of the major histocompatibility complex. The MHC is located on the short arm of chromosome 6 with the centromere symbolized to the left. HLA genes cluster into two regions, the class I and class II regions. Some of the class II genes are pseudogenes or are not known to be expressed; those transcribed and translated into α and β chains which dimerize to form the classic class II proteins are designated with shading (DP, DQ, DRB1, DRB3). The non-HLA class III cluster includes the genes for certain complement components [C4B, C4A, properdin factor B (Bf)], 21-hydroxylase (21B, 21A), a heat shock protein (hsp70), and tumor necrosis factors (TNF-α, TNF-β). Other non-HLA genes encoded in the MHC which are known or suspected to be relevant for immune function and/or autoimmune disease include a gene for collagen (COL), peptide transporter molecules (TAP1 and TAP2), HLA-DMA and DMB, and two proteasome components (LMP2 and LMP7). The expressed HLA genes are highly polymorphic. The lower portion of the figure is a partial listing of current nomenclature for many of the polymorphic class I and class II alleles, along with previously used designations.

genes for complement components C2, C4 and Bf, as well as the structural genes for 21-hydroxylase[10,11]. Another interesting part of the MHC lies in the class II complex between the DQ and DP clusters. The TAP and LMP genes within this region encode polypeptides which are implicated in HLA class I antigen processing and peptide transport[12–15]. Cells defective for the DMA and DMB genes in this region are lacking in the ability to properly complex HLA class II molecules with antigen (see below).

DETECTION OF HLA POLYMORPHISM

The extremely high degree of allelic diversity described above and illustrated in Figure 7.1 is the principle genetic cornerstone which underlies the basic functions of the MHC. This allelic polymorphism has important functional consequences which dictate cellular interactions required for immune activation in normal and autoimmune states. Detection of this genetic polymorphism, then, is extremely important for understanding the basis of the genetic contributions to disease.

Until very recently, analysis of genetic polymorphisms within the MHC was somewhat confusing. Now, however, with the advent of elegant but simple molecular technologies, such as polymerase chain reaction amplification, HLA genotyping is a more precise and straightforward matter[16]. Different methods of HLA typing and their interrelationships are summarized in Figure 7.2. Historically, HLA typing was performed by serologic methodology, in which sera from multiparous women were used as reagents to identify alloantigens on lymphocytes from unrelated individuals. Such sera occasionally contained alloantibodies, resulting from sensitization during pregnancy or delivery, which cross-reacted on similar alloepitopes from unrelated individuals, and formed the basis for a complex HLA 'typing' taxonomy based on these serologic specificities. The nomenclature from this serologic typing includes the commonly identified HLA specificities HLA-DRl, DR2, DR3, DR4, etc. For the most part, the relationship between the HLA serologic nomenclature and the subsequently defined genetic loci has been maintained, so that the DR specificities refer to products of the HLA-DR subregion, DQ specificities to products of the DQ subregion and HLA-A, B and C specificities to products of the HLA-A, B and C loci, respectively. Unfortunately, however, the relationships of individual specificities within each loci have not always been precisely preserved so that, for instance, HLA-DR2$^+$ molecules may be encoded by the DRB1*15 or *16 alleles, the DR5 specificities by the DRB1*11 or *12 alleles, etc. These relationships are illustrated for the DR4 specificity in Figure 7.2.

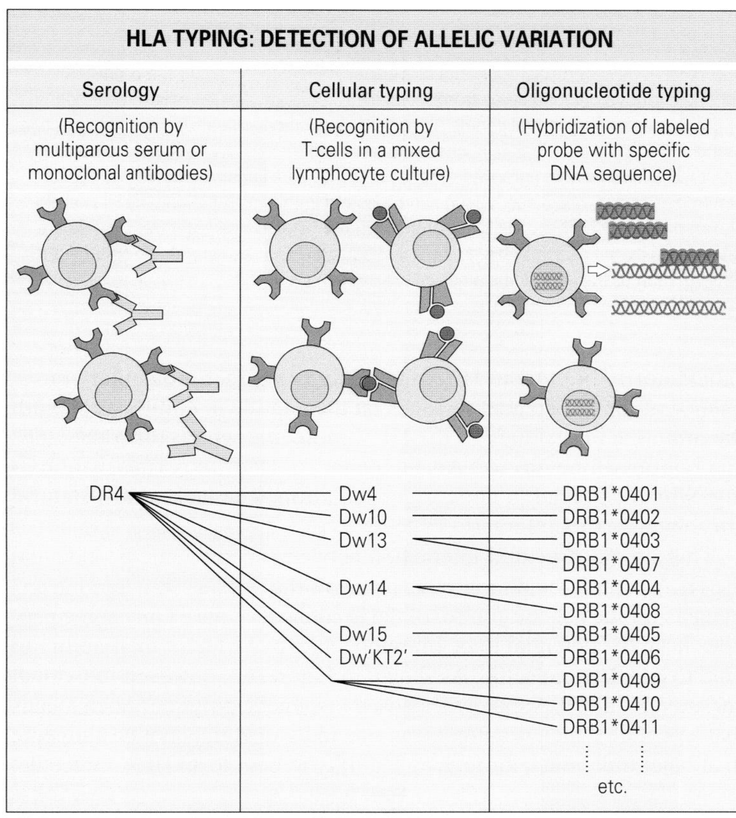

Fig. 7.2 HLA typing: detection of allelic variation. The left panel illustrates serologically-based HLA typing, using sera from multiparous females (or monoclonal antibodies) that recognize alloantigens. Traditionally, the antisera are used in a complement-dependent cytotoxicity assay, such that cells carrying the alloantigen recognized by the sera are lysed. These sera often recognize 'public' serologic specificities, such as DR4, which are epitopes present on a number of different alleles. Finer discrimination is frequently obtained through cellular typing, as schematized in the second panel. In this case, well-characterized irradiated lymphoid cells act as stimulator cells in mixed lymphocyte culture for responder T-cells of unknown HLA type; if proliferation does not occur it indicates that the responder cells share the HLA type of the stimulator cells. In this way, six 'subtypes' of DR4 were defined: Dw4, Dw10, Dw14, etc. Currently, many laboratories utilize oligonucleotide typing, as outlined in the third panel. Based on the known nucleotide sequence of different alleles, synthetic labeled oligonucleotide probes are designed which hybridize specifically to the DNA sequence unique to the gene of interest. In some cases, a series of oligonucleotide probes is required to distinguish among the different alleles, and a 'matrix' approach can be utilized[16]. In this way even minor differences among alleles can be recognized; for example, this has led to the identification of over 20 different DR4$^+$ alleles.

Structural studies in the early and mid-1980s identified one of the major difficulties with HLA serologic typing, namely that some of the HLA serologic specificities were present on multiple different HLA molecules. One of the first and clearest examples was the HLA-DR4 specificity, now known to be a serologic determinant on the products of at least 20 different HLA class II molecules encoded by 20 different DRB1 alleles (see Fig. 7.2). These different DR4-positive molecules all share a similar serologic epitope reacting with the DR4 alloantisera, which accounts for their similar serologic typing. However, they differ in other determinants, some of which can be recognized immunologically, such as by T-cells in mixed lymphocyte culture. This T-cell recognition of HLA class II molecules forms the basis for another HLA typing taxonomy, known as the HLA-D system, which in some cases is more discriminating than the serologic system. Instead of sera, T-cell recognition in mixed lymphocyte proliferative assays is used to define some of the specificities present on class II molecules. Within the HLA-DR4 family of alleles, for example, six of these cellularly defined specificities are well described, and are given the arbitrary names Dw4, Dw10, Dw13, Dw14, Dw15 and Dw 'KT2'. Thus, the cellular specificities form one system for 'subtyping' within a single serologic specificity, since class II molecules which carry any of these six Dw specificities also type as HLA-DR4. However, the cellularly defined specificities are also incomplete and fail to detect some relevant allelic polymorphism. As illustrated in Figure 7.2, some of the HLA-D specificities are themselves present on the products of two or more class II molecules encoded by different alleles.

To make the field of HLA typing more precise in light of our current understanding of allelic variation, HLA laboratories are now using oligonucleotide-based typing for the detection of specific alleles. This typing methodology, which detects nucleotide variation, provides a satisfactory method for specific genetic detection accurately reflecting the high degree of allelic polymorphism within the HLA complex. Oligonucleotide typing is based on the principle that under proper conditions a synthetic oligonucleotide probe can specifically hybridize with an exact complementary sequence of DNA from the genome, permitting detection of individual genes based on the nucleotide substitutions which vary between alleles.

THE NATURE OF POLYMORPHIC VARIATION

Most HLA alleles within a single locus are highly related. The variations which distinguish one allele from another can be quite small, as little as one nucleotide difference encoding one amino acid replacement. The variation among alleles is not randomly distributed across the length of the genes. Rather, allelic differences cluster in the 5′ proximal exons, that is, the portions of the genes which encode the amino terminal segments of the HLA molecules which are situated farthest from the cell membrane. Within each HLA locus, nucleotide sequence is highly conserved, with variation determining allelic polymorphism confined to one or two specific sites of diversity. This clustering of polymorphic sites within the HLA genes has direct implications for the structure and function of the HLA molecules, as described in the next section.

HLA MOLECULAR STRUCTURE

Several HLA molecules have been purified and studied by detailed X-ray crystallographic analysis to determine their structure[17–20]. They all share some very important structural motifs, which can be seen in the analysis of the class II molecule depicted in Figure 7.3. In its native state on the surface of a cell, the HLA molecule is presumed to extend from the membrane into the extracellular space. The 'side' view is depicted as a supporting scaffold underlying the key recognition domains of the molecule, which extend towards the external

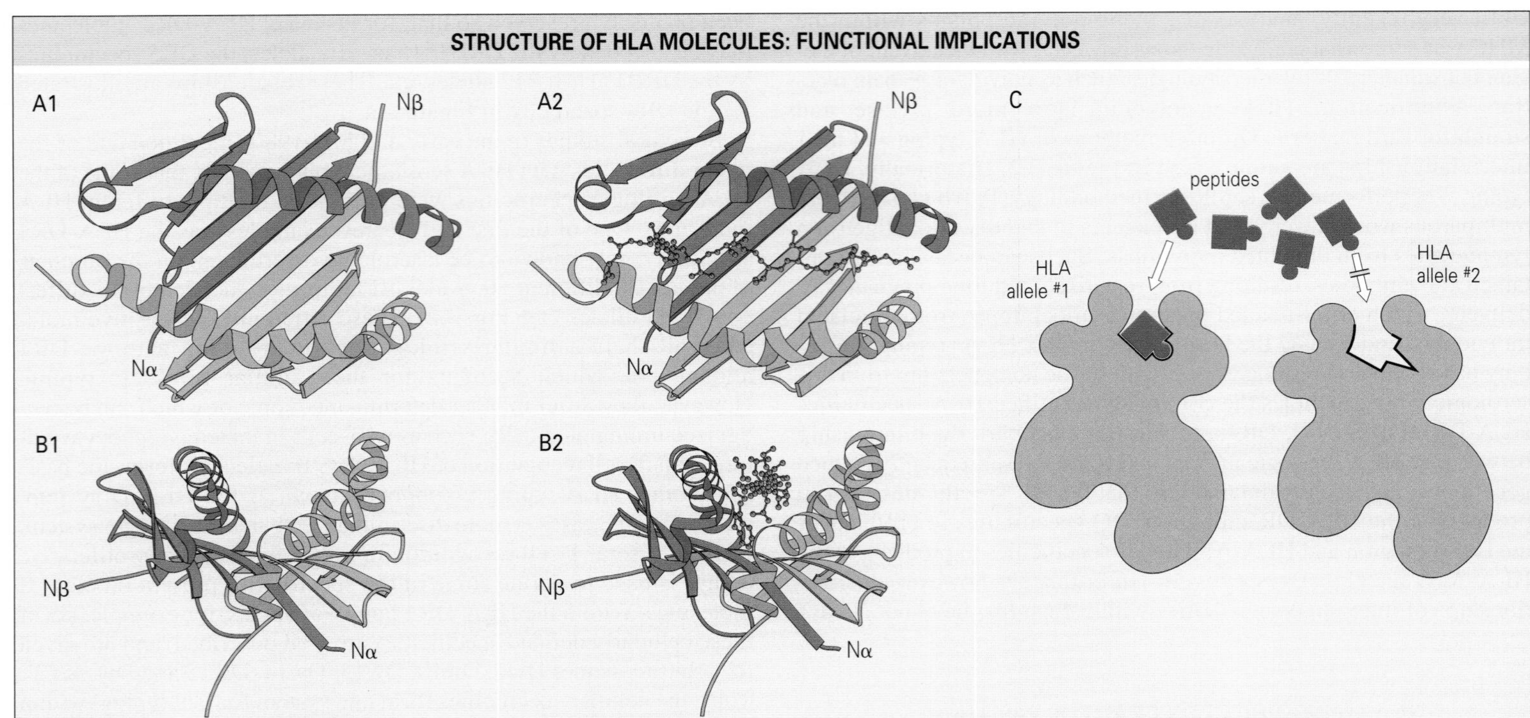

Fig. 7.3 Structure of HLA molecules: functional implications. Schematic representation of the HLA-DRB1*04 molecule. (A1) These ribbon diagrams are viewed from above, as a T-cell might visualize the recognition structure. Parallel α helices form the 'walls' of a presumed antigen-binding groove, whose floor is formed by β-pleated sheets. In class I molecules, two α helices and β-pleated sheet structures are encoded by the α_1 and α_2 domains of the class I heavy chain polypeptide. In the comparable class II structure, the α chain (darker color) provides one α helix and part of the β-pleated sheet (from the α_1 domain); the class II β chain (lighter color) provides the other α helix and the rest of the β-pleated sheet (from the β_1 domain). Adapted from Stern *et al.*[20]. (B1) View from the open end of a class I molecule, showing the α helices forming a groove opening away from the cell into the extracellular milieu, and resting on the β sheets. The central panels A2 and B2 show the same structures with peptide bound in the groove (in red). (C) Schematic representation of two distinct HLA alleles, with their antigen-binding grooves emphasized with dark lines. Antigenic peptide is symbolized as a puzzle piece, which can be bound in this example only by HLA allele #1, not by allele #2. These allelic differences in the binding of a particular peptide are determined by the polymorphic amino acid sequence and resulting three-dimensional conformation of the antigen-binding groove of each molecule.

cellular environment. The recognition domains of the HLA molecule consist of an interesting structural motif forming a distinct deep groove within a partially unroofed tube-like structure. This deep groove, or pocket, is bordered on either side by extended α-helical loops, and the floor of the groove consists of a series of β-pleated sheets forming a platform. The schematic view of this groove shown in Figure 7.3 is presumably the view presented by the HLA molecule to the external environment of the cell.

Comparison of this structure with the nucleotide variation encoding HLA molecules immediately provides insights into the function of polymorphic variation among HLA molecules important for immune activation. As already noted, most of the amino acid variation which distinguishes different HLA alleles is clustered in the amino terminal domains of the molecule. These are the same domains which form the recognition structure illustrated in Figure 7.3. Furthermore, the specific sites of allelic variation cluster within small segments of these domains which, when superimposed on the structural model, form the floor and walls of the deep HLA molecular groove[19,21]. Most of the rest of the structure is relatively conserved among alleles at a given locus. In other words, the important allelic variation is localized specifically to sites which create a genetically unique conformation of amino acids lining the boundaries of the groove on the surface of the HLA molecule.

The importance of this structural variability is also illustrated in Figure 7.3. The primary function of HLA molecules is to bind antigenic peptides, as a requisite part of the immune activation pathway leading to presentation of the antigen to a T-cell. The ability of an antigenic peptide to be bound by an HLA molecule is a primary determinant of whether or not an immune response to that peptide can be generated. The importance of amino acid variation in the HLA molecule, localized at the boundaries of the groove-like structure, becomes clear: this groove is the site of binding for these antigenic peptides. The determination of whether or not a peptide will satisfactorily bind to an HLA molecule is a direct molecular consequence of the amino acid residues on the peptide in combination with the amino acid residues of the HLA molecule which form the sides and bottom of the groove. An adequate 'fit' leads to permissive binding, which can lead to antigen presentation. The lack of a structural 'fit' obviates this interaction[22–25].

This simple structural interaction between an antigenic peptide and the HLA peptide-binding groove is one of the primary structural determinants for the genetic control of the immune response. Only some peptides have the potential to be immunogenic, by virtue of their ability to bind to an HLA molecule. As shown in Figure 7.3, however, individual variation in the HLA molecule caused by genetic polymorphism means that a peptide which is antigenic in one individual may not be antigenic in another individual, through an inability to bind to an HLA molecule.

THE CLASS I PATHWAY FOR ANTIGEN PRESENTATION

HLA molecules are compartmentalized in the cell after the polypeptides are translated on ribosomes. This compartmentalization forms a pathway for class I molecules to assemble, bind peptide and move to the cell surface where they are capable of preferential interactions with selected T-cells[26,27]. Several of the structural features of class I molecules, as summarized above, are critical for important aspects of this compartmentalized pathway (Fig. 7.4).

After synthesis, the class I heavy chain is transported to the endoplasmic reticulum (ER). Studies of mutant antigen-presenting cells show that this compartment is a preferred site for early critical interactions between class I molecules and antigenic peptides[28]. Cytosolic proteins, both of self and non-self (i.e., viral polypeptides) genetic origin, are partially degraded by proteasomes (which utilize the MHC-encoded LMP genes), and make their way as proteolytically cleaved peptides into the ER in a form suitable for binding to class I molecules[29]. This movement of antigenic peptides into the ER is

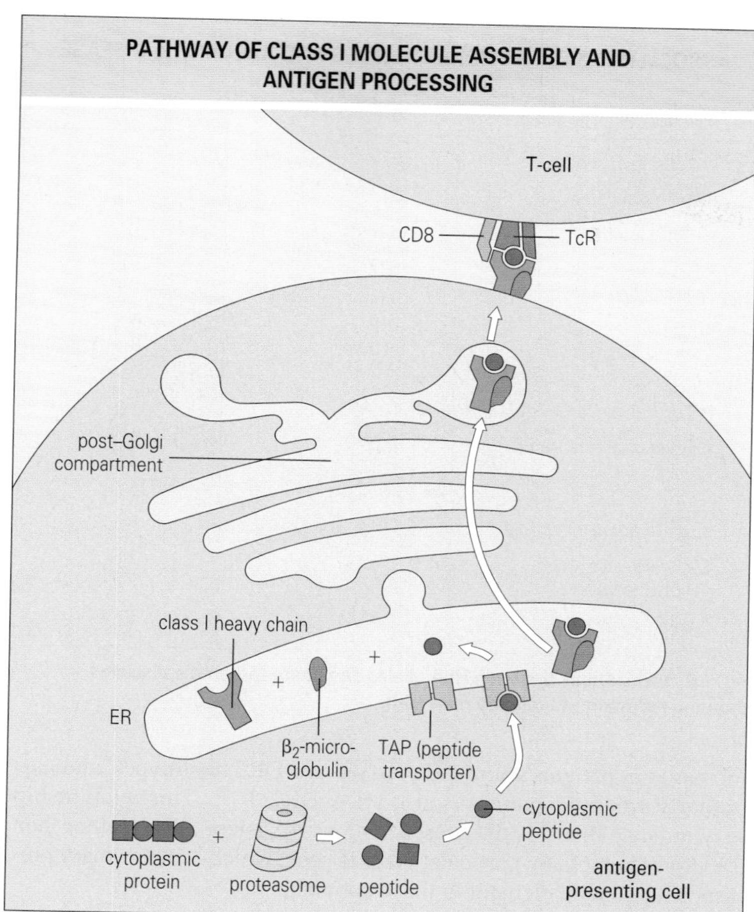

Fig. 7.4 Pathway of HLA class I molecule assembly and antigen processing: showing the preferential compartmentalization of class I molecules during their synthesis and transport within the cell. Cytoplasmic proteins are processed by a proteasome complex. Peptide is then transported into the ER by TAP molecules, which reside in the ER membrane and move peptide from the cytosol into the ER. The class I heavy chain and β_2-microglobulin combine to form the class I molecule, also in the ER. This dimer binds the processed peptide; binding of the peptide may occur as the class I molecule is being assembled. The class I–peptide complex then traffics through the Golgi and post-Golgi compartments and moves to the cell surface. At the surface, it is available to interact with T-cells, facilitated by interaction with the CD8 molecule, which is thought to bind to the α_3 domain of the class I molecule. This compartmentalized pathway apparently restricts the binding of class I molecules primarily to cytoplasmic peptides; the binding interaction between the class I heavy chain and the CD8 molecule directs class I cytoplasmic peptide complexes to interact with CD8⁺ T-cells.

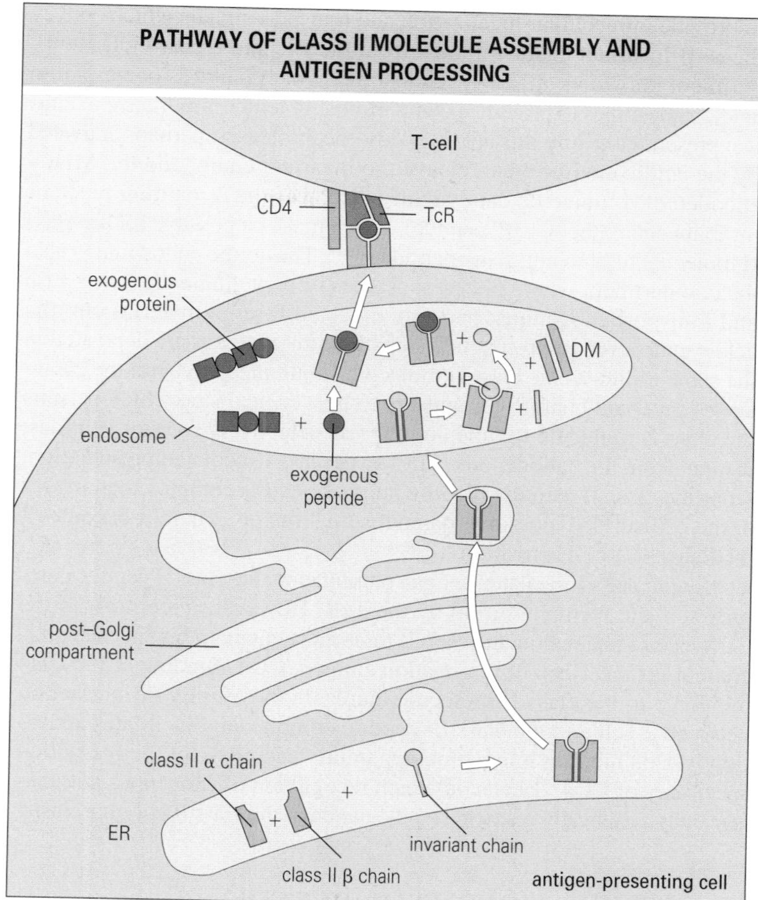

Fig. 7.5 Pathway of HLA class II molecule assembly, antigen processing and cell surface interactions. In the class II pathway, class II α and β chains are assembled in the ER along with the invariant chain, which is thought to interact in such a way that peptide cannot bind to the antigen-binding groove. Thus most cytoplasmic peptides, which are transported to the ER (see Fig. 7.4), are unable to bind class II molecules. After transport through the Golgi and post-Golgi compartments, the class II α–β-invariant chain complex moves to an acidic endosome, where the invariant chain is proteolytically cleaved into fragments, including CLIP. The DMA–DMB heterodimer (labelled DM in illustration) induces dissociation of CLIP from class II molecules. Exogenously derived peptides which have been brought to the endosome through fusion of phagolysosomes or recycling endosomes may now bind to the class II molecule. This class II molecule–peptide complex then is transported to the cell surface, where it is available to interact with an appropriate T-cell. The structure of the class II molecule allows preferential interaction with the CD4 molecule, which facilitates recognition between the class II–peptide complex and an appropriate TcR.

accomplished by a transporter molecule encoded by the TAP genes within the MHC complex between DQ and DP[30]. The interaction of the class I heavy chain and an antigenic peptide occurs at this point and results in transport of the class I-peptide complex into the Golgi and post-Golgi compartments on the way to the plasma membrane. Although somewhat controversial, it appears that most class I molecules use this trafficking pathway and consequently bind endogenously synthesized polypeptides from within the cell preferentially. In addition, there is some evidence that peptide and β_2-microglobulin exchange may occur at the cell surface on class I molecules so that there is also potential for binding of exogenous peptide[31]. In general, however, the features of the class I pathway imply that this is the preferred pathway for presentation of self-peptides and viral or other endogenously synthesized antigens.

Once present on the cell surface, the class I peptide complex forms a recognition signal for T-cell receptor (TcR) interactions. Both the HLA molecule and the bound peptide are essential for the binding and activation of an antigen-specific T-cell. The HLA class I molecule also contains a binding site for recognition by the T-cell coreceptor known as CD8[32]. Binding of CD8 to the class I molecule does at least two things: it increases the affinity of interaction between T-cell and antigen-presenting cell, thus facilitating activation, and secondly it provides an element of specificity in that it focuses the attention of CD8⁺ T cells on antigens presented via the class I pathway. It is this coreceptor function of CD8 interaction with HLA class I which accounts for the apparent 'restriction' of cytotoxic CD8⁺ T-cells for MHC class I-associated antigens.

THE CLASS II PATHWAY OF ANTIGEN PRESENTATION

The maturation and transport of the class II molecule within an antigen-presenting cell is also highly compartmentalized, but is distinct from the class I pathway[26,33]. As illustrated in Figure 7.5, the class II α and β polypeptides are synthesized on ribosomes and localized in the ER in association with a third polypeptide chain, known as the invariant chain. The presence of the invariant chain here has at least two critical functions: first, it stabilizes the formation of the α–β dimer and, second, it appears to block the peptide-binding groove of the class II molecule, thus preventing the association of peptide with the molecule in this compartment[34]. The ability of the invariant chain to bind selectively to class II, but not class I, molecules is thought to provide the essential mechanism whereby class I molecules present endogenous peptides, but class II molecules generally do not. A third function of the invariant chain is to provide intracellular localization and transport signals which convey the α–β-invariant chain complex from the ER into a post-Golgi compartment known as an 'early' endosome, which matures or fuses into acidic endosomes to provide a compartment of major importance to antigen presentation[35]. In this acidic endosome, proteases, perhaps activated by the acidic environment, cleave the invariant chain, and the MHC-encoded DM molecule catalytically displaces the remaining piece of invariant chain (the 'CLIP' peptide), which makes it possible for the class II molecule to bind antigenic peptides[36,37]. The acidic endosome is also the compartment where phagolysosomes or recycling endosomes fuse and transport exogenous, partially digested foreign material into the acidic endosome environment. Thus, 'foreign' antigens are deposited in the same milieu as the class II molecule simultaneously with the cleavage of invariant chain. This appears to be a critical step which permits the class II molecule to bind and present selectively foreign peptides, distinct from the endogenous pathway of class I-mediated presentation. After the class II–peptide binding interaction, this complex then moves to the cell surface, possibly via endosomal fusion, where it becomes a mediator of T-cell activation.

As with class I-mediated antigen presentation, the class II peptide complex is a site for recognition by the TcR. However, in contrast to the CD8–class I interaction, the class II molecule contains a binding site preferential for the T-cell differentiation antigen, CD4. Binding of the CD4 molecule to the class II molecule increases the affinity of interaction between T-cell and the class II–peptide complex and facilitates activation[38]. This binding interaction apparently accounts for the restriction specificity of $CD4^+$ T-cells, in which recognition of exogenous antigens is usually genetically restricted by the nature of the class II polymorphism.

HLA ASSOCIATIONS WITH DISEASE

The association of specific HLA polymorphisms with several of the rheumatic diseases has been well recognized for over a decade[39]. Up until the mid-1980s, most studies of HLA and disease correlated the presence of serologic specificities associated with HLA polymorphisms which were more prevalent in patients than in controls. More recent studies have used molecular techniques to identify specific haplotypes and, in some cases, specific genes which account for these associations. Figure 7.6 lists the best characterized examples of rheumatic disorders associated with HLA genes. The strength of genetic association is reflected in the term 'relative risk', which is a statistical odds ratio representing the risk of disease in an individual carrying a particular genetic marker compared to the risk in individuals in that population without that marker.

Four of the diseases listed are associated with an HLA class I marker, in each case the HLA-B27 specificity. This is, to date, the only HLA class I marker clearly implicated in rheumatic disease and likely reflects the direct involvement of the HLA-B27 gene product in the pathogenesis of spondylitis and arthritis. The other rheumatic diseases listed are associated with different markers from the HLA class II complex. It now appears that several of these different HLA associations may actually represent differing genetic mechanisms reflecting, in some cases, the role of genes linked to the class II complex; in other cases, a combination of more than one class II gene; and in others, the function of a specific allele, or even the function of a specific amino acid sequence embedded within the HLA class II molecule. Examples of rheumatic diseases whose HLA associations may arise through each of these mechanisms are discussed below.

Some forms of SLE may represent diseases associated with HLA class II molecules because of linkage with nearby non-HLA genes[40,41]. Both HLA-DR2 and DR3 haplotypes are associated with systemic lupus erythematosus (SLE) in Caucasians[40]. The predominant HLA-$DR3^+$ haplotype in Caucasians has very tight linkage with other genes within the MHC, notably HLA-A1, B8, Cw7 and C4A. This last gene, a structural gene for the C4 complement component, is a silent allele on this DR3 haplotype. Notably, C4A 'null' alleles are significantly

ASSOCIATIONS BETWEEN HLA ALLELES AND RHEUMATIC DISEASE

Disease	HLA marker	RR
Ankylosing spondylitis	B27	90
Reiter's syndrome	B27	41
Psoriatic arthritis	B27	10
Inflammatory bowel disease with spondylitis	B27	10
Adult RA	DR4	6
	Dw4	6
	Dw14	5
Polyarticular juvenile RA	DR4	7
Pauciarticular juvenile RA	DR8	5
	DR5	4.5
	DP2.1	4
Juvenile dermatomyositis	DR3	4
Systemic lupus erythematosus	DR2	3
	DR3	3
Sjögren's syndrome	DR3	6

Fig. 7.6 Associations between HLA alleles and some rheumatic diseases showing approximate relative risks (RR).

increased in patients with SLE even on non-DR3 haplotypes, and particularly when the patient is also HLA-$DR2^+$[42–44]. This relationship may indicate that it is the presence of a C4A silent allele, rather than the expression of any particular class II gene, which is the primary predisposing genetic element in these patients.

A different example of the complexity of interpreting HLA associations with disease is seen in disorders associated with more than one HLA gene or haplotype. This appears to be the case in patients with Sjögren's syndrome or some forms of SLE, in which high levels of the autoantibody anti-Ro(SS-A) are found. Patients with this autoantibody profile have an unexpectedly high frequency of heterozygosity for DR2, DQw1 and DR3, DQw2 haplotypes, suggesting some synergy or interaction between two distinct susceptibility genes[45].

A similar phenomenon has been reported for pauciarticular juvenile chronic arthritis (JRA), in which the disease is associated with genes at the DRB1 locus and also with genes at the DPB1 locus[46,47]. Interestingly, patients with both a DP2.1 allele and a DRB1 susceptibility allele (DR8, DR5 or DR6), either in *cis* or in *trans*, have a higher relative risk than expected from the additive effect of these genes alone[48].

Perhaps the most dramatic example of an HLA genetic synergism in the rheumatic diseases is in another subset of JRA patients, those with rheumatoid factor-positive polyarticular disease. Like adult RA, polyarticular JRA is associated with both the Dw4 and the Dw14 genes. However, heterozygotes carrying both Dw4 and Dw14 have a relative risk greater than 100, reflecting an apparent synergy in individuals inheriting both of the known susceptibility markers[49,50].

In contrast to these fairly complicated examples of HLA associations with disease, some of the better-known examples appear to be more straightforward. The B27 association with disease, for example, has undergone intense scrutiny. There are at least six different alleles at the HLA-B locus which encode class I heavy chains positive for HLA-B27 which, in different populations, are all associated with similar B27-associated spondyloarthropathies[51,52]. This has given rise to the notion that it is the HLA-$B27^+$ molecule itself, rather than any linked gene, and rather than any unique B27 subtype, which is associated with disease. Support for this notion has recently come from animal studies in which rats were genetically engineered to carry human HLA-B27 and β_2-microglobulin transgenes[53]. Offspring of these rats expressing the B27 molecule displayed a clinical syndrome with many features similar to human spondylitis and psoriatic arthritis. Since the only human molecule expressed in these rats was B27 itself, these studies strongly support the notion that this molecule is directly implicated in pathogenesis.

COMPARISON OF AMINO ACID SEQUENCES CONFERRING RA SUSCEPTIBILITY

Allele	Sequence (positions 20, 40, 60, 80 marked on reference)
RA susceptibility DRB1 genes:	
*0101 (DR1, Dw1)	GDTRPRFLWQLKFECHFFNGTERVRLLERCIYNQEESVRFDSDVGEYRAVTELGRPDAEYWNSQKDLLEQRRAAVDTYCRHNYGVGESFTVQRR
*0401 (DR4, Dw4)	E V H F D YF H Y K
*0404 (DR4, Dw14)	E V H F D YF H Y V
*0405 (DR4, Dw15)	E V H F D YF H Y S
*1402 (DR6, Dw16)	E YSTS F YFH N
Closely related DRB1 genes not conferring RA susceptibility:	
*0402 (DR4, Dw10)	E V H F D YF H Y I DE V
*0403 (DR4, Dw13)	E V H F D YF H Y E V
*1301 (DR6a)	E YSTS F D YFH N F I DE V
*1401 (DR6b)	E YSTS F D YFH F A H R E V
Other more distantly related DRB1 genes not conferring RA susceptiblity:	
*1501 (DR2, Dw2)	Q D Y F H D DL F D
*1502 (DR2, Dw12)	Q D Y F H G N F D
*0301 (DR3, Dw3)	E YSTS Y D YFH N F K GR N V
*0406 (DR4, Dw'KT2')	E V H F D YF H E V
*1101 (DR5, Dw5)	E YSTS F D YF Y F E F D
*1102 (DR5, Dw'JVM')	E YSTS F D YF Y F E I DE V
*1201 (DR5, Dw'DB6')	E YSTG Y HFH LL F V S I D AV
*0701 (DR7, Dw17)	Q G YK QF LF F V S I D GQ V
*0801 (DR8, Dw8.1)	E YSTG Y F D YF Y S F D L
*08031 (DR8, Dw8.3)	E YSTG Y F D YF Y S I D L
*09011 (DR9, Dw23)	Q K D Y H G N V S F R E V
*1001 (DRw10)	E EV RVH YA Y R

(1)

(2)

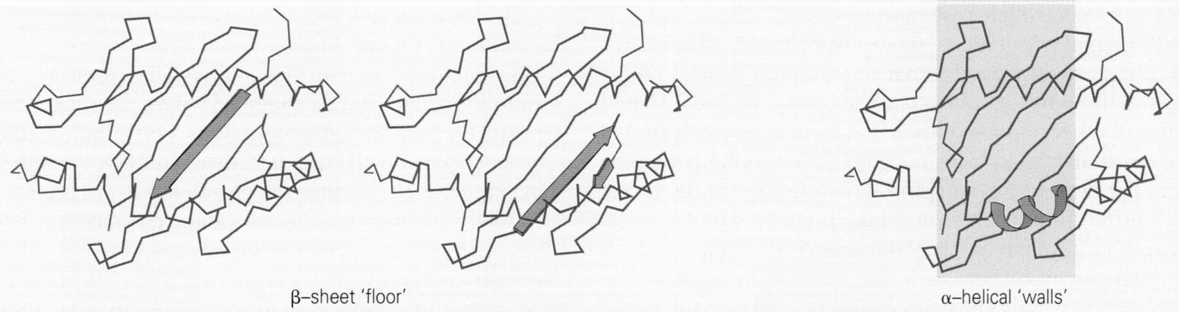

β–sheet 'floor'   α–helical 'walls'

Amino acid code (single letter): A, alanine; R, arginine; N, asparagine; D, aspartic acid; C, cysteine; Q, glutamine; E, glutamic acid; G, glycine; H, histidine; I, isoleucine; L, leucine; K, lysine; M, methionine; F, phenylalanine; P, proline; S, serine; T, threonine; W, trytophan; Y, tyrosine; V, valine

Fig. 7.7 Comparison of amino acid sequences for HLA-DRB1 genes which do or do not confer susceptibility to RA in different populations. (1) At the top are listed the sequences (using the single letter amino acid code) of the DRB1 genes known to confer susceptibility to RA, with the Dw14 epitope highlighted. Under these sequences are listed very similar sequences from closely related DRB1 genes which do not confer RA susceptibility. Finally, the lower portion of panel 1 contrasts the sequences of other more distantly related DRB1 genes which are not known to confer RA susceptibility. In each case the Dw14 epitope region is highlighted, demonstrating that the epitope occurs only in susceptibility genes and does not occur in nonsusceptibility genes, even when their 'background' sequence is very similar or identical to the susceptibility alleles. (2) Schematic representation of how the amino acid sequence of the first domain of DRB1 relates to the three-dimensional conformation of the final molecule. Red highlighted arrows correspond to clustered hypervariable sequences in the DRBI regions shown above, illustrating that the Dw14 epitope constitutes part of the α helical 'wall' of the antigen-binding groove.

There is one prominent example in the rheumatic diseases in which the primary HLA association with disease has been mapped to a specific nucleotide sequence which lies within several different class II alleles. This is an extreme example of 'genetic reductionism', at the other end of the genetic spectrum from multiple gene effects or linked genes. In this example, a small sequence of nucleotides within a gene encodes a stretch of amino acids which appears to be the primary genetic element associated with disease. The disease is RA, and the stretch of important amino acids has been called the Dw14 epitope or the shared epitope[54,55].

SUSCEPTIBILITY TO RHEUMATOID ARTHRITIS

The HLA DR4 molecules associated with RA are the Dw4 and Dw14 molecules (Fig. 7.6) encoded by the DRB1*0401 and DRB1*0404 alleles, respectively[56–59]. There are a few specific structural and genetic differences between these genes and other closely related DR4-positive alleles which characterize genes associated with RA. The molecular characteristics specific for the DRB1*0401 and *0404 alleles are the sequence of amino acids from codons 67 to 74 of the DRβ molecule. The RA-associated DR4 molecules carry the sequence LLEQRRAA or LLEQKRAA in this region (see footnote to Figure 7.7 for amino acid code) while the non-RA-associated genes carry one or more differences in this region, usually including a negatively charged amino acid such as D (Asp) or E (Glu). This is illustrated in Figure 7.7, which represents the amino terminal domain of the most prevalent DRB1 alleles. This is the same domain which, as discussed previously, folds into a recognition structure containing a peptide binding groove. Directly below the linear sequence in Figure 7.7 is an illustration of the location of the polymorphic sites for each linear segment in the three dimensional model of the class II molecule.

RA: HLA-DRB1 SUSCEPTIBILITY

	DRB1 suscep-tibility gene	Epitope sequence	Prevalence in RA	Relative risk
Caucasians	*0401 (DR4, Dw4) *0404 (DR4, Dw14) *0101 (DR1, Dw1)	LLEQKRAA LLEQRRAA LLEQRRAA	50% 30% 24%	6 5 1
Japanese	*0405 (DR4, Dw15)	LLEQRRAA	71%	3.5
Yakima	*1402 (DR6, Dw16)	LLEQRRAA	83%	3.3
Israeli Jews	*0101 (DR1, Dw1)	LLEQRRAA	28%	6

Fig. 7.8 Summary of the important HLA-DRB1 genes conferring susceptibility to RA in different ethnic populations. Their approximate prevalences in RA patients in each population, along with relative risks are listed. Each of these genes includes the Dw14 epitope (or a close variation), even though the sequence of the rest of the DRB1 gene may be quite varied among these alleles.

The sequences representing the shared epitope are highlighted in Figure 7.7. They form a portion of the molecule which lies in the middle of the alpha helical portion of the DRB1 encoded class II molecule. In addition to DRB1*0401 and *0404, DRB1*0101, DRB1*0405 and DRB1*1402 carry the same sequence in this region. Remarkably, each of these HLA alleles is also associated with RA. These latter alleles are predominantly associated with RA in populations with a low prevalence of the DRB1*0401 and DRB1*0404 genes. Examples are shown in Figure 7.8: in Japan, the most highly associated HLA allele is DRB1*0405; in Israel DRB1*0101. In Native Americans, as first described in studies of the Yakima Nation[60], the RA-associated DRB1 allele is *1402. Thus, although the DR4-associated alleles are most highly associated with RA in Caucasian and Oriental populations, other DRB1 genes which carry the same shared epitope sequence are associated with RA in other ethnic groups. Although all these RA-associated alleles carry the same shared epitope, they differ in other regions of the HLA molecule, as illustrated in Figure 7.7. In particular, sequences corresponding to the β-pleated sheet structures in the floor of the antigen-binding groove of the molecule are radically different in each case. Thus, it appears that it is the shared epitope itself, rather than any specific single HLA allele, which is the principle determinant of genetic susceptibility. In some ethnic groups with a low prevalence of DR4 susceptibility alleles in the population and a low prevalence of RA, there are no clear HLA associations with the shared epitope[61,62]. Even in these studies, however, DR4-positive susceptibility alleles, when present, are associated with increased risk, but their low overall frequency in the populations studied makes this clinically insignificant.

In Caucasians, DRB1*0401, *0404 and *0101 are all associated with RA, and there have been extensive studies to determine whether differences between these alleles, or whether differences in gene dosage, influence the degree of susceptibility or clinical course. Although there are some differences in reports on these topics, it is clear that the DR4-positive RA-associated alleles are most frequent among patients with more severe, erosive disease. The DR1-associated susceptibility alleles, on the other hand, are often associated with milder or seronegative disease. These different correlations with clinical course suggest as yet unknown differences in disease mechanism among different susceptibility alleles. They also support the practical and useful conclusion that the DR4-positive disease associated alleles confer susceptibility to severe disease.

This point is illustrated in Figure 7.9, which summarizes the distribution of each of these RA-associated alleles in a series of Caucasian patients with different forms of RA. Patients with polyarticular rheumatoid factor (RF)-positive juvenile RA had the highest frequency of both DRB1*0401 and *0404, and the lowest of DRB1*0101. Adults with severe RF positive RA had high levels of DRB1*0401 and *0404, as well. Levels of these DR4-positive alleles were somewhat reduced in RF-negative patients with RA, as well as in patients with nonerosive

DISTRIBUTION OF THREE RA-ASSOCIATED DRB1 ALLELES AMONG PATIENTS WITH DIFFERENT FORMS OF RA

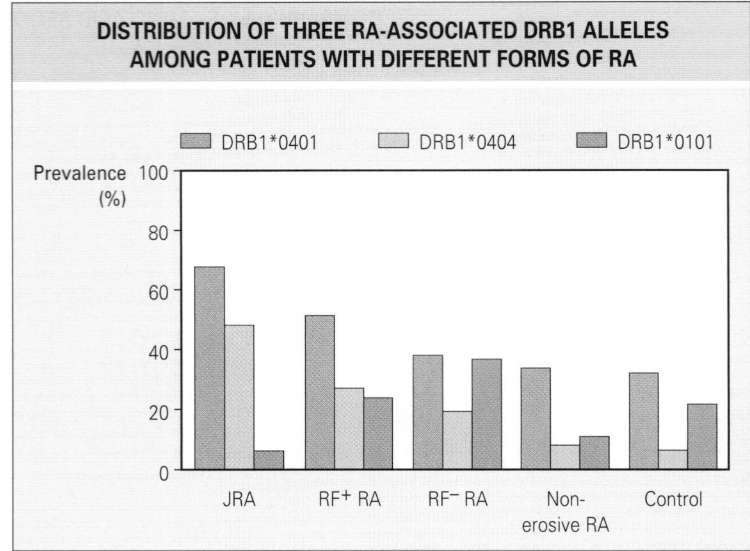

Fig. 7.9 Distribution of three RA-associated DRB1 alleles among patients with different forms of RA (JRA, rheumatoid factor positive juvenile rheumatoid arthritis; RF+ RA, rheumatoid factor positive rheumatoid arthritis; RF− RA, rheumatoid factor negative rheumatoid arthritis; nonerosive RA, rheumatoid factor negative nonerosive arthritis). The frequency of DRB1*0401 and DRB1*0404 roughly parallels the degree of disease severity seen among the patient groups, whereas the frequency of DRB1*0101 does not. Adapted with permission from Nepom G. Prediction of susceptibility to rheumatoid arthritis by HLA genotyping. Rheumatic Disease Clinics of North America. 1992; 18:785–92.

forms of the disease. The DR4-positive alleles correlate with more severe forms of disease, but this was not evident for the DRB1*0101 association (Figure 7.9)[50,57,63].

It is important to note that, although the frequency of these DRB1 susceptibility alleles in RA patients is high, the same genes are also prevalent in the unaffected population. This characteristic has important consequences for the use of genetic analysis to predict susceptibility to RA. Figure 7.10 summarizes prevalence estimates for the three RA susceptibility alleles in Caucasians. These estimates are based on a projected disease frequency of approximately 1% in the population; since each of these susceptibility alleles is present in 5–15% of the unaffected population, most individuals with the susceptibility alleles will not get disease. For example, for every 50 individuals with DRB1*0401 who have RA, approximately 1800 with the same gene are unaffected, for an absolute risk ratio of 1 in 35. Thus, although DR4 is associated with a high relative risk because most patients with RA have the DR4 susceptibility alleles, the absolute risk for an individual in the population with this gene is still fairly low. The highest absolute risk for susceptibility to RA comes

RISK ESTIMATES FOR RA IN CAUCASIANS

	Frequency/10,000 population		
HLA Class II gene	+ RA	No RA	Approximate risk ratio
DRB1 *0401	50	1800	1 in 35
DRB1 *0404	25	500	1 in 20
DRB1 *0101	25	2000	1 in 80
0401 or 0404	65	2300	1 in 35
0401, 0404 or 0101	90	4200	1 in 46
0401 and 0404	15	100	1 in 7
Other	10	5800	1 in 580

Fig. 7.10 Risk estimates for HLA genes associated with RA in Caucasians. These numbers represent the 'absolute risk' of developing clinical RA among Caucasians. They are based on a disease frequency of 7–10/1000 population, and as such represent an upper limit of predictive value. Adapted with permission from Nepom G. (details as in fig. 7.9)

in individuals who carry both a DRB1*0401 and a DRB1*0404 gene. These compound heterozygotes are rare, but have an absolute risk of RA of approximately 1 in 7. In addition to this increased risk in individuals with multiple susceptibility genes, some studies suggest that gene dosage also correlates with a degree of disease severity[64–66]. Patients with RF-s positive erosive disease, often with associated extra-articular manifestations including rheumatoid vasculitis or Felty's syndrome, are more likely to carry two DRB1 susceptibility alleles than are patients with milder forms of disease.

Recognition that the specific DRB1 susceptibility genes are present in patients with severe erosive forms of RA provides an opportunity to use HLA genotyping as a tool for disease prediction. However, as noted above, the prevalence of the same DRB1 alleles in the unaffected population is sufficiently high that use of genetic typing to predict RA in the general population is not practicable. Thus, while the accuracy of DRB1 genotyping for RA diagnosis is low, the accuracy and utility for disease prognosis in patients with RA is quite high[67]. At the present time, it appears that a combination of RF and DRB1 testing as part of the early assessment of patients with RA can be a useful adjunct to early identification of patients likely to have a poor disease course[68,69]. The most likely clinical benefit from use of DRB1 typing in early assessment protocols will be to help identify patients who could benefit from aggressive types of therapies. Although combination drug therapies are more efficacious in preventing morbidity in patients with RA[70], the selection of patients needing such aggressive therapy is often a management dilemma. The use of DRB1 stratification in such patients may provide a useful adjunct to clinical decision making[71].

GENETIC MECHANISMS OF DISEASE SUSCEPTIBILITY

As emphasized above, the primary characteristic of HLA genes associated with disease is the discrete structural polymorphism which identifies a disease-associated allele. When an HLA class I or class II gene is itself directly implicated in disease susceptibility, it appears that a limited number of specific amino acid polymorphisms in residues contributing to peptide binding and T-cell recognition are the key determinants for the disease association. What are the likely immunologic mechanisms by which such limited polymorphism has such a major effect? We briefly outline three principle models for this genetic control of disease susceptibility, using as an example the strong association of the shared Dw14 epitope with RA.

As discussed above, the polymorphic residues of the HLA molecule are the essential structural determinants of specific interactions with peptide and with the variable portions of the TcR. Figure 7.11 presents a model of the HLA-DR4 molecules associated with RA, highlighting the role of the key polymorphic residues within the shared epitope region. Changes in these specific amino acids, at codons 67, 70, 71 and 74, are sufficient to alter the disease susceptibility associated with the DR4 molecule. Therefore, it is likely that direct structural interactions involving these four sites provide the mechanistic basis for disease susceptibility. As indicated in Figure 7.11, these amino acid residues form an important molecular contact surface associated with the β-chain α helix of the class II molecule. One of the amino acids, residue 71, is positioned to contact the bound peptide. The others are positioned predominantly to contact the TcR which recognizes the composite surface along the 'top' of the molecule formed by the combination of peptide and MHC contact sites.

The molecular insights provided by this structural model for RA disease susceptibility imply that the shared epitope sequence controls the nature of the trimolecular interaction between TcR, peptide and MHC molecule. It may do this by influencing the specific sequence of the peptide bound within the class II groove, by influencing the direct recognition of the MHC peptide complex by the TcR or by a combination of these two events. Evidence in favor of the peptide selection hypothesis comes from a detailed analysis of the types of peptides which can be bound by DR4 molecules. Many such studies have been performed[72–79], which indicate that peptides are most

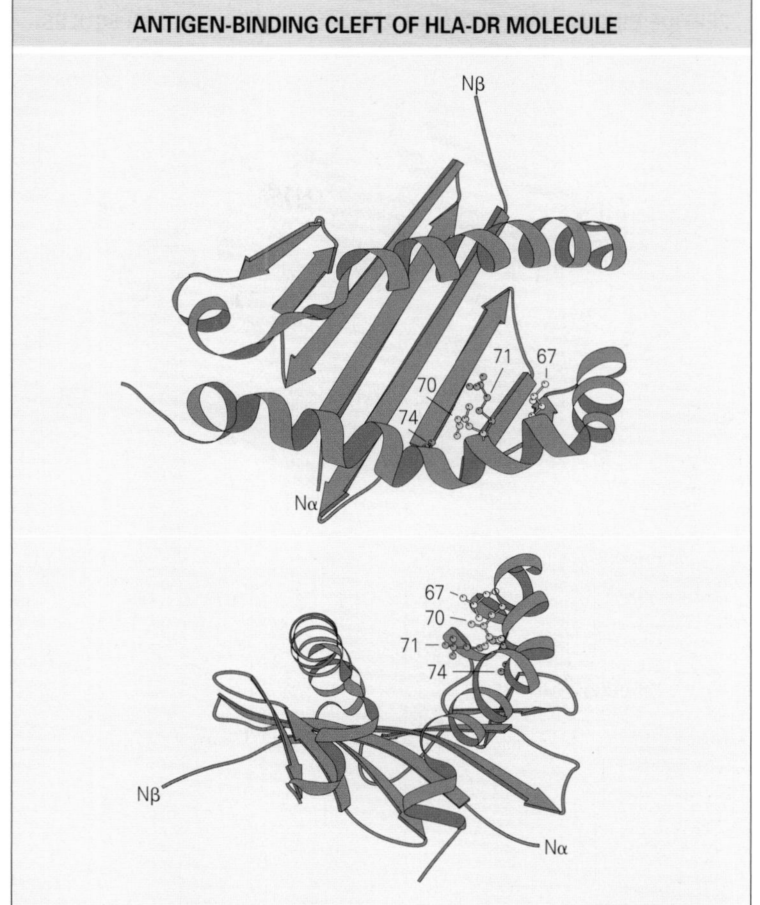

Fig. 7.11. Presumed location of important polymorphic residues within the RA-associated 'shared epitope'. Ribbon diagram of a DRA/DRB1*0401 molecule, showing view looking down from above (top panel) and side view (bottom panel). Amino acids 67, 70, 71 and 74, the residues noted from sequence comparisons and from site-directed mutagenesis analysis to be critical in the function of the 'shared epitope', are shown pointing into or out of the peptide binding groove as predicted from the three-dimensional structure. The residues pointing into the groove would presumably be important in binding peptide, while those pointing out of the a helix would be hypothesized to interact directly with TcR.

successful in binding within the groove of the DR4 molecule if they contain a particular motif of amino acid side chains. This is summarized in Figure 7.12. Although a peptide which binds a class II molecule may be from 8 to 20 amino acids, or even longer, whether such a peptide will efficiently bind a DR4 molecule is primarily determined by four amino acid side chains contained within the peptide, at relative positions 1, 4, 6 and 9. Peptides which efficiently bind the RA susceptibility alleles encoded by DRB1*0401 and DRB1*0404 carry the motif identified in Figure 7.12. Peptide side chain residue 1 must be hydrophobic (usually W, Y, F, L, V or I), the side chain at residue 4 cannot carry a positive charge and the side chain at pocket 6, in common for all the DR4 molecules, prefers a somewhat polar residue. For the DRB1*0401 and *0404 alleles the amino acid residue at peptide position 9 cannot have a negative charge; this is not the case with the Asian RA-associated DRB1*0405 allele, where a negative charge is permitted at residue 9. Thus, the significance of the preferred motif for residue 9 in RA is not clear.

This detailed outline of the peptide motif preferred for binding to RA-associated class II molecules may have some utility in identifying specific arthritogenic peptides which, in concert with DR4, play a mechanistic role in severe RA. On the other hand, it is possible that the principle disease-associated role of the shared epitope is to influence directly the TcR contact sites in the trimolecular complex, relatively independent of the specific peptide bound. Molecular modeling of the trimolecular complex associated with shared epitope recognition

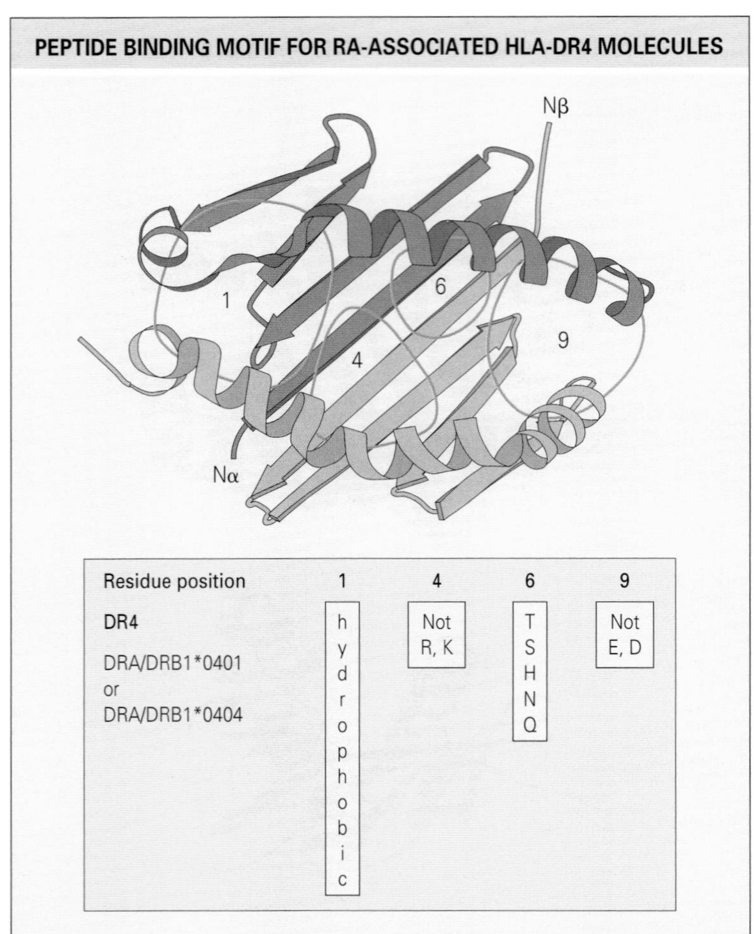

Fig. 7.12 Peptide binding motif for RA-associated HLA-DR4 molecules. Upper panel shows a ribbon diagram of the class II molecule with its antigen binding groove. Side chains of the amino acids from the bound peptide fit into 'pockets' formed in the groove by the class II molecule. Pockets for the major anchor residues (relative positions 1, 4, 6, and 9) of the peptides are outlined. The lower panel summarizes the preferred residues which can be accommodated in these pockets by the RA-associated allele DRB1*0401. Polymorphic differences in the amino acids lining the fourth pocket dictate that certain charged residues in that position in the peptide are not permitted in 'shared epitope' positive alleles.

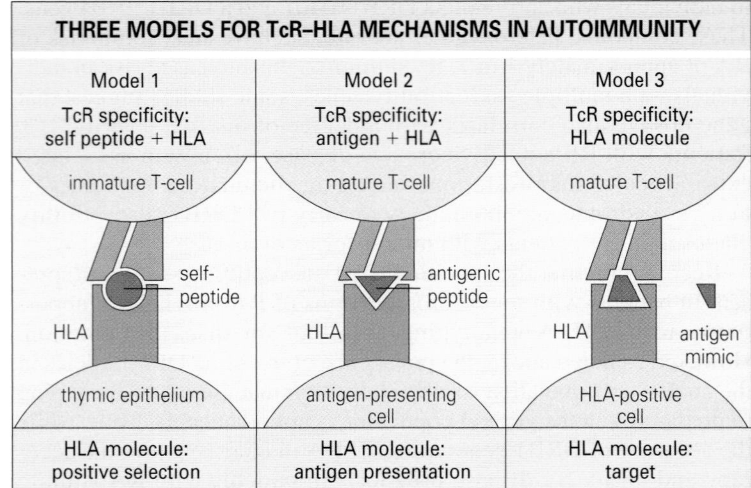

Fig. 7.13 Three models for postulated TcR–HLA mechanisms in autoimmunity. The key role of polymorphic amino acid residues in the HLA molecules associated with disease indicates that intimate contacts between these amino acids and antigenic peptides and/or TcR are important genetically regulated triggering events in autoimmunity. In Model 1, the polymorphic HLA molecule, in combination with a bound self-peptide, plays a key selection role, presumably during the thymic development of maturing T-cells. An immature T-cell 'tests' its receptor specificity before exiting the thymus; a suitable recognition and stimulation by the HLA molecule at this point is postulated to lead to the maturation and expansion of this T-cell specificity which, in an appropriate context, may be potentially autoreactive. In Model 2, a similar recognition event occurs in the peripheral immune system between a mature T-cell and an HLA-expressing antigen-presenting cell. The polymorphic determinants on the HLA molecule determine the binding and presentation of an antigenic peptide related to the target tissue, such as the joint. In Model 3, the T-cell specificity is directed towards the polymorphic amino acid residues of the HLA molecule itself by molecular mimicry. The immune response is postulated to focus on an HLA-positive target by virtue of cross-reaction with an antigen mimic which has successfully bypassed normal tolerance mechanisms and stimulated the reactive T-cell. A variation of the mimicry hypothesis which partly reconciles all three models postulates that the polymorphic sequence on the HLA molecule is the primary antigenic target, but that this is seen by the TcR or as a processed self-peptide, bound and presented by another intact HLA molecule.

suggests that at least three crucial contact sites are likely in which shared epitope residues directly interact with specific TcR β-chain recognition loops[80]. Notably, in such a model the specific peptide bound by the disease-associated class II molecule may be either allele specific or allele nonspecific in its binding, based on the notion that the disease-associated structural interactions are predominantly bimolecular between MHC and TcR directly.

Figure 7.13 summarizes three different models for how such specific polymorphisms could potentially lead to antigen-specific T-cell-mediated autoimmunity. Model 1 (Fig. 7.13) emphasizes the role of the polymorphic HLA molecule in the selection and establishment of the antigen-specific T-cell repertoire. After T-cells rearrange and express their α–β receptor, they undergo a series of selection events in which interactions with HLA molecules are responsible for instructing the T-cell to discriminate self from nonself[81,82]. T-cells are both negatively selected (deleted or inactivated to avoid self-reactivity), and positively selected to establish a repertoire of cells capable of recognizing foreign antigen in the context of self-MHC. Most of these selection events happen during T-cell development in the thymus, although peripheral mechanisms have also been suggested. In the example illustrated, it is possible that expression of the shared epitope serves to select positively for a set of potentially autoreactive T-cells. This lack of immunologic tolerance could then be a predisposing factor for the subsequent triggering of these autoreactive clones in disease-associated pathogenic events.

At the time of onset of an immune response, the primary role of the HLA molecule is to bind peptide and present it to antigen-specific T-cells. Thus, as in Model 2 (Fig. 7.13), another suitable model for the role of HLA in disease pathogenesis predicts that HLA polymorphisms such as the Dw14 epitope control the structural architecture of the class II–peptide–TcR interaction. Amino acid residues within the shared epitope are likely to be directly responsible for creating a precise fit between the members of this trimolecular complex leading to subsequent T-cell activation. Indeed, site-directed mutagenesis experiments which change amino acid residues within the Dw14 epitope sequence directly demonstrate this critical recognition function[83]. In this model, the primary genetic determinants of triggering events in autoimmunity are presumed to occur during the induction phase of disease. This model offers some promising prospects for therapeutic intervention, since it may be possible to interfere with the formation of the trimolecular complex, either through the administration of peptide analogs, which would disrupt the class II–peptide binding, or with reagents which would directly interfere with specific TcR or HLA residues.

A third model to account for the specific association of polymorphic HLA residues in disease (Model 3 in Fig. 7.13) is often called the molecular mimicry hypothesis. It is a speculative model based on the homology of specific amino acid polymorphisms within some HLA molecules when compared with amino acid sequences of potentially antigenic proteins derived from infectious agents[84]. For example, portions of the Dw14 epitope sequence also occur within one of the

Epstein–Barr virus glycoproteins, and it has been hypothesized that immunity to the virus may be a sufficient stimulus to 'break tolerance' and generate autoreactive T-cell clones with potentially pathogenic consequences leading to the triggering of RA[85]. Similar mimicry mechanisms have been proposed to account for the B27-associated spondyloarthropathies, although direct evidence for immunologic mimicry with an HLA molecule in disease has yet to be demonstrated.

A variation of the molecular mimicry hypothesis has been suggested specifically for the shared epitope associated with RA. Based on sequence homology between the shared epitope and the heat shock binding dna j protein from *E. coli*, it has been suggested that mammalian hsp proteins may have peculiar avidity for shared epitope positive DR4 molecules, resulting in some aberrant hsp-associated pathogenic event[86].

When considering mechanisms of HLA associations with disease it is well to remember that just as HLA genetics are complex, so are the mechanisms likely to be heterogeneous. While the HLA contribution in one rheumatic disease may be due principally to specific peptide binding and activation of the trimolecular complex, in another rheumatic disorder it may be due primarily to T-cell repertoire selection. As noted above, several of the rheumatic diseases are associated with two different HLA class II molecules, often with a synergistic risk in heterozygous individuals. This suggests the intriguing possibility that disease susceptibility may be a multi-step process in which one of the HLA-associated functions is to establish a repertoire of potentially autoreactive T-cells, while another HLA-associated function is to provide the essential peptide-binding specificity for TcR recognition. In this scenario involving two distinct HLA molecules, either HLA molecule alone would contribute to disease susceptibility, but the presence of both would synergize mechanistically to facilitate an accelerated pathway of disease.

Finally, it should be emphasized that the genetic contributions in disease predisposition are not sufficient by themselves for disease expression. Other environmental, infectious or developmental triggering factors also must play key roles in a genetically susceptible host in the final pathways leading to disease.

MHC structural models for the figures in this chapter were constructed using molecular homology modeling techniques by Carol DeWeese, Department of Bioengineering, University of Washington School of Medicine.

REFERENCES

1. Shimuzu Y, Geraghty DE, Koller BH, *et al.* Transfer and expression of three cloned human non-HLA-A,B,C class I major histocompatibility complex genes in mutant lymphoblastoid cells. Proc Natl Acad Sci USA. 1988;85:227–31.
2. Koller BH, Geraghty DE, DeMars R, *et al.* Chromosomal organization of the human major histocompatibility complex class I gene family. J Exp Med. 1989;169:469–80.
3. Geraghty DE, Koller BH, Orr HT. A human major histocompatibility complex class I gene that encodes a protein with a shortened cytoplasmic segment. Proc Natl Acad Sci USA. 1987; 84:9145–9.
4. Kwok WW, Schwarz D, Nepom BS, *et al.* HLA-DQ molecules form α-β heterodimers of mixed allotype. J Immunol. 1988;141:3123–7.
5. Ragoussis J, Monaco A, Mockridge I, *et al.* Cloning of the HLA class II region in yeast artificial chromosomes. Proc Natl Acad Sci USA. 1991;88:3753–7.
6. Kelly A, Trowsdale J. Novel genes in the human major histocompatibility complex class II region. Int Arch Allergy Immunol. 1994;103:11–15.
7. Hanson IM, Gorman P, Lui VCH, *et al.* The human α_2(XI) collagen gene (COL11A2) maps to the centromeric border of the major histocompatibility complex on chromosome 6. Genomics. 1989;5:925–31.
8. Carroll MC, Katzman P, Alicot EM, *et al.* Linkage map of the human major histocompatibility complex including the tumor necrosis factor genes. Proc Natl Acad Sci USA. 1987;84:8535–9.
9. Sargent CA, Dunham I, Trowsdale J, *et al.* Human major histocompatibility complex contains genes for the major heat shock protein HSP70. Proc Natl Acad Sci USA. 1989;86:1968–72.
10. Carroll MC, Campbell RD, Bentley DR, *et al.* A molecular map of the human major histocompatibility complex class III region linking complement genes C4, C2, and factor B. Nature. 1984;307:237–41.
11. White PC. Molecular genietics of the class III region of the HLA complex. In: Dupont B, ed. Immunobiology of HLA. Immunogenetics and Histocompatibility. New York: Springer-Verlag; 198: 62–69.
12. Spies T, Blanck G, Bresnahan M, *et al.* A new cluster of genes within the human major histocompatibility complex. Science. 1989;243:214–17.
13. Deverson EV, Gow IR, Coadwell WJ, *et al.* MHC class II region encoding proteins related to multidrug resistance family of transmembrane transporters. Nature. 1990;348:738–741.
14. Trowsdale J, Hanson I, Mockridge I, *et al.* Sequences encoded in the class II region of the MHC related to the 'ABC' superfamily of transporters. Nature. 1990;348:741–4.
15. Spies T, Bresnahan M, Bahram S, *et al.* A gene in the human major histocompatibility complex class II region controlling the class I antigen presentation pathway. Nature. 1990;348:744–747.
16. Scharf SJ, Griffith RL, Erlich HA. Rapid typing of DNA sequence polymorphism at the HLA-DRB1 locus using the polymerase chain reaction and nonradioactive oligonucleotide probes. Hum Immunol. 1991;30:190–201.
17. Bjorkman PJ, Saper MA, Samraoui B, *et al.* Structure of the human class I histocompatibility antigen, HLA-A2. Nature. 1987;329:506–12.
18. Garrett TP, Saper MA, Bjorkman PJ, *et al.* Specificity pockets for the side chains of peptide antigens in HLA-Aw68. Nature. 1989;342:692–6.
19. Bjorkman PJ, Saper MA, Samraoui B, *et al.* The foreign antigen binding site and T cell recognition regions of class I histocompatibility antigens. Nature 1987;329:512–18.
20. Stern LJ, Brown JH, Jardetzky TS, *et al.* Crystal structure of the human class II MHC protein HLA-DR1 complexed with an influenza virus peptide. Nature. 1994;368:215–21.
21. Brown JH, Jardetzky T, Saper MA, *et al.* A hypothetical model of the foreign antigen binding site of class II histocompatibility molecules. Nature. 1988;332:845–50.
22. Buus S, Sette A, Colon SM, *et al.* The relation between major histocompatibility complex (MHC) restriction and the capacity of Ia to bind

immunogenic peptides. Science. 1987;235:1353–8.
23. Sette A, Buus S, Appella E, *et al.* Prediction of major histocompatibility complex binding regions of protein antigens by sequence pattern analysis. Proc Natl Acad Sci USA. 1989;86:3296–300.
24. Allen PM, Matsueda GR, Evans RJ, *et al.* Identification of the T-cell and Ia contact residues of a T-cell antigenic epitope. Nature. 1987;317:359.
25. Falk K, Rötzschke O, Stevanovic S, *et al.* Allele-specific motifs revealed by sequencing of self-peptides eluted from MHC molecules. Nature. 1987;327:713–5.
26. Brachiale TJ, Brachiale VL. Antigen presentation: structural themes and functional variations. Immunol Today. 1991;12:124–9.
27. Carbone FR, Bevan MJ. Class I-restricted processing and presentation of exogenous cell-associated antigen *in vivo*. J Exp Med. 1990;171:377–87.
28. Cerundolo V, Alexander J, Anderson K, *et al.* Presentation of viral antigen controlled by a gene in the major histocompatibility complex. Nature. 1990;345:449–52.
29. Belich MP, Trowsdale J. Proteasome and class I antigen processing and presentation (review). Molec Biol Reports. 1995;21:53–6.
30. Spies T, DeMars R. Restored expression of major histocompatibility class I molecules by gene transfer of a putative peptide transporter. Nature. 1991;351:323–4.
31. Rock KL, Rothstein LE, Gamble SR, *et al.* Reassociation with beta 2-microglobulin is necessary for Db class I major histocompatibility complex binding of an exogenous influenza peptide. Proc Natl Acad Sci USA. 1991;88:301–4.
32. Rosenstein Y, Ratnofsky S, Burakoff SJ, *et al.* Direct evidence for binding of CD8 to HLA class I antigens. J Exp Med. 1989;169:149–60.
33. Cresswell P, Blum JS, Kelner DN, Marks MS (ed. Atassi, MZ). Biosynthesis and processing of class II histocompatibility antigens. In CRC critical reviews in immunology. Boca Raton: CRC; 1987: 31–53.
34. Roche PA, Cresswell P. Invariant chain association with HLA-DR molecules inhibits immunogenic peptide binding. Nature. 1990;345:615–8.
35. Lotteau V, Teyton L, Peleraux A, *et al.* Intracellular transport of class II MHC molecules directed by invariant chain. Nature. 1990;348:600–5.
36. Blum JS, Cresswell P. Role for intracellular proteases in the processing and transport of class II HLA antigens. Proc Natl Acad Sci USA. 1988;85:3975–9.
37. Busch R, Mellins ED. Developing and shedding inhibitions: how the MHC class II molecules reach maturity. Curr Opin Immunol. 1996;8:51–8.
38. Mittler RS, Goldman SJ, Spitalny GL, *et al.* T-cell receptor-CD4 physical association in a murine T-cell hybridoma: induction by antigen receptor ligation. Proc Natl Acad Sci USA. 1989;86:8531–5.
39. Tiwari J, Terasaki P. HLA and disease associations. New York: Springer-Verlag; 1985.
40. Arnett FC, Reveille JD, Wilson RW, *et al.* Systemic lupus erythematosus: current state of the genetic hypothesis. Semin Arthritis Rheum. 1984;14:24–35.
41. Schur PH. Complement and lupus erythematosus. Arthritis Rheum. 1982;25:793–8.
42. Fielder AH, Walport MJ, Batchelor JR, *et al.* Family study of the major histocompatibility complex in patients with systemic lupus erythematosus: importance of null alleles of C4A and C4B in determining disease susceptibility. Br Med J. 1983;286:425–8.
43. Howard PF, *et al.* Relationships between C4 null genes, HLA-D region antigens, and genetic suscetibility to systemic lupus erythematosus in Caucasian and black Americans. Am J Med. 1985;81:187–295.
44. Christiansen FT, Zhang WJ, Griffiths M, *et al.* Major histocompatibility complex (MHC) complement deficiency, ancestral haplotypes and systemic lupus erythematosus (SLE): C4 deficiency explains some but not all the influence of the MHC. J Rheumatol. 1991;18:1350–8.
45. Arnett FC, Bias WB, Reveille JD. Genetic studies in Sj'øgren's syndrome and systemic lupus erythematosus. J Autoimmun. 1989;2:403–13.
46. Maksymowych WP, Glass DN. Population genetics and molecular biology of the childhood chronic arthropathies. Bailliere's Clin Rheumatol. 1988;2:649–71.
47. Nepom BS. The immunogenetics of juvenile rheumatoid arthritis. In: Athreya BH, ed. Rheumatic disease clinics of North America. Philadelphia: WB Saunders Company; 1991: 825–42.
48. Nepom BS, Malhotra U, Schwarz DA, *et al.* HLA and T cell receptor polymorphisms in pauciarticular juvenile rheumatoid arthritis. Arthritis Rheum. 1991;34:1260–7.
49. Nepom B, Nepom GT, Schaller J, *et al.* Characterization of specific HLA-DR4-associated histocompatiblity molecules in patients with juvenile rheumatoid arthritis. J Clin Invest. 1984;74:287–91.
50. Vehe RK, Begovich AB, Nepom BS. HLA susceptibility genes in rheumatoid factor positive juvenile rheumatoid arthritis. J Rheumatol. 1990;17(suppl.):11–15.
51. Khan MA. Ankylosing spondylitis and heterogenaeity of HLA-B27. Semin Arthritis Rheum. 1988;18:134–41.
52. Breur-Vriesendorp BS, Dekker-Saeys AJ, Ivany P. Distribution of HLA-B27 subtypes in patients with ankylosing spondylitis: the disease is associated with a common determinant of the various B27 molecules. Annals Rheum Dis. 1987;46:353–6.
53. Hammer RE, Maika SD, Richardson JA, *et al.* Spontaneous inflammatory disease in transgenic rats expressing HLA-B27 and human β2m: an animal model of HLA-B27-associated human disorders. Cell. 1990;63:1099–112.
54. Gregersen PK, Silver J, Winchester RJ. The shared epitope hypothesis: An approach to understanding the molecular genetics of susceptibility to rheumatoid arthritis. Arthritis Rheum. 1987;30:1205–13.
55. Seyfried CE, Mickelson E, Hansen JA, *et al.* A specific nucleotide sequence defines a functional T cell recognition epitope shared by diverse HLA-DR specificities. Hum Immunol. 1988;21:289–99.
56. Wordsworth B, Lanchbury JSS, Sakkas LI, *et al.* HLA-DR4 subtype frequencies in rheumatoid arthritis indicate that DRB1 is the major susceptibility locus within the HLA class II region. Proc Natl Acad Sci USA. 1989;86:10049–53.
57. Nepom GT, Byers P, Seyfried C, *et al.* HLA genes associated with rheumatoid arthritis. Arthritis Rheum. 1989;32:15–21.
58. Ronningen KA, Spurkland A, Egeland T, *et al.* Rheumatoid arthritis may be primarily associated with HLA-DR4 molecules sharing a particular sequence at residues 67–74. Tissue Antigens 1990;36:235–40.
59. Nepom GT. In: Wolfe F, Pincus T, eds. Prognosis and treatment of rheumatic diseases. New York: Marcel Dekker; 1994: 115–29.
60. Willkens RF, Nepom GT, Marks CR, *et al.* The association of HLA-Dw16 with rheumatoid arthritis in Yakima Indians: Further evidence for the 'shared epitope' hypothesis. Arthritis Rheum. 1991;34:43–7.
61. McDaniel DO, Alarcon GS, Pratt PW, *et al.* Most African-American patients with rheumatoid arthritis do not have the rheumatoid antigenic determinant (epitope). Ann Intern Med. 1995;123:181–7.
62. Boki KA, Panayi GS, Vaughan RW, *et al.* HLA class II sequence polymorphisms and susceptibility to rheumatoid arthritis in Greeks. The HLA-DR beta shared-epitope hypothesis accounts for the disease in only a minority of Greek patients. Arthritis Rheum. 1992;37:749–55.
63. Nepom GT, Seyfried CE, Holbeck SL, *et al.* Identification of HLA-Dw14 genes in DR4+ rheumatoid arthritis. Lancet. 1986;ii:1002–5.
64. Combe B, Eliaou J-F, Daures J-P, *et al.* Prognostic factors in rheumatoid arthritis. Comparative study of two subsets of patients according to severity of articular damage. Br J Rheum. 1995;34:529–34.
65. Weyand CM, Hicok KC, Conn DL, *et al.* The influence of HLA-DRB1 genes on disease severity in rheumatoid arthritis. Ann Intern Med. 1992;117:801–6.
66. Wordsworth P, Pile KD, Buckley JD, *et al.* HLA heterozygosity contributes to susceptibility to rheumatoid arthritis. Am J Hum Genet. 1992;51:585–91.
67. Nepom GT, Gersuk V, Nepom BS. Prognostic implications of HLA genotyping in the early assessment of patients with rheumatoid arthritis. J Rheumatol. 1996;23:5–9.
68. Gough A, Faint J, Salmon M, *et al.* Genetic typing of patients with inflammatory arthritis at presentation can be used to predict outcome. Arthritis Rheum. 1994;37:1166–70.
69. Wilske KR, Yocum DE. RA: The status and future of combination therapy. J Rheumatol. 1996;23:110.
70. O'Dell JR, Haire CE, Erikson N, *et al.* Treatment of rheumatoid arthritis with methotrexate alone, sulfasalazine and hydroxychloroquine, or a combination of all three medications. N Engl J Med. 1996;334:1287–91.
71. O'Dell J, Nepom B, Haire C, *et al.* DRB1 typing in rheumatoid arthritis (RA) is useful in predicting response to specific therapy. Arthritis Rheum. 1997; (in press).
72. Friede T, Gnau V, Jung G, *et al.* Natural ligand motifs of closely related HLA-DR4 molecules predict features of rheumatoid arthritis associated peptides. Biochim Biophys Acta. 1996;1316:85–101.
73. Rothbard JB, Marshall K, Wilson KJ, *et al.* Prediction of peptide affinity to HLA DRB1*0401. Int Arch Allergy Immunol. 1994;105:1–7.
74. Fu X, Bono CP, Woulfe SL, *et al.* Pocket 4 of the HLA-DR(α,β1*0401) molecule is a major determinant of T cell recognition of peptide. J Exp Med. 1995;181:915–26.
75. Sette A, Sidney J, Oseroff C, *et al.* HLA-DR4 Dw4-binding motifs illustrate the biochemical basis of degeneracy and specificity in peptide–DR interactions. J Immunol. 1993;151:3163–70.
76. Hammer J, Bono E, Gallazzi F, *et al.* Precise prediction of major histocompatibility complex class II-peptide interaction based on peptide side chain scanning. J Exp Med. 1994;180:2353–8.
77. Kirschmann DA, Duffin KL, Smith CE, *et al.* Naturally processed peptides from rheumatoid arthritis associated and non-associated HLA-DR alleles. J Immunol. 1995;155:5655–62.
78. McNicholl JM, Whitworth WC, Oftung F, *et al.* Structural requirements of peptide and MHC for DR(α,β 1*0401)-restricted T cell antigen recognition. J Immunol. 1995;155:1951–63.
79. Woulfe SL, Bono CP, Zacheis ML, *et al.* Negatively charged residues interacting with the p4 pocket confer binding specificity to DRB1*0401. Arthritis Rheum. 1995;38:1744–53.
80. Penzotti JE, Doherty D, Lybrand TP, *et al.* A structural model for TcR recognition of the HLA class II shared epitope sequence implicated in susceptibility to rheumatoid arthritis. J Autoimmun. 1996;9:287–93.
81. Marrack P, Lo D, Brinster R, *et al.* The effect of thymus environment on T cell development and tolerance. Cell. 1988;53:627–34.
82. Kisielow P, Teh HS, Blüthmann H, *et al.* Positive selection of antigen-specific T cells in thymus by restricting MHC molecules. Nature. 1988;335:730–3.
83. Hiraiwa A, Yamanaka K, Kwok WW, *et al.* Structural requirements for recognition of the HLA-Dw14 class II epitope: A key HLA determinant associated with rheumatoid arthritis. Proc Natl Acad Sci USA. 1990;87:8051–5.
84. Oldstone MBA (ed. Oldstone, MBA). Molecular mimicry as a mechanism for the cause and as a probe uncovering etiologic agents of autoimmune disease. In: Current topics in microbiology and immunology, Vol. 145. Berlin-Heidelberg: Springer-Verlag; 1989: 127–35.
85. Roudier J, Rhodes G, Petersen J, *et al.* Hypothesis: The Epstein–Barr virus glycoprotein gp110, a molecular link between HLA DR4, HLA DR1, and rheumatoid arthritis. Scand J Immunol. 1988;27:367–71.
86. Auger I, Escola JM, Gorvel JP, *et al.* HLA-DR4 and HLA-DR10 motifs that carry susceptibility to rheumatoid arthritis bind 70-kD heat shock proteins. Nature Med. 1996;2:306–10.

ANIMAL MODELS OF ARTHRITIS

Paul H Wooley

- Arthritis may be induced in animals by immunization with cartilage components, nonspecific immune stimuli, infectious agents or transgenic manipulation of genetic information.
- Genes that regulate the immune system, including MHC and T-cell genes, influence animal models of arthritis.
- Experimentally induced arthritis suggests that an interaction exists between the immune system, the endocrine networks and the nervous system.
- Animal models serve an important role in the evaluation of antirheumatic therapies.

INTRODUCTION

Experimental animal models of arthritis have contributed to the understanding of the basic mechanisms of joint disease. A marked diversity is seen among the numerous models, with arthritis induced by:
- immunization with cartilage components,
- injection of nonspecific immune stimuli,
- infectious agents or their components and
- the manipulation of genetic information in transgenic animals.

This diversity may suggest that disparate etiological pathways may exist in rheumatoid arthritis (RA). As no single model provides a definitive archetype of human disease, the interpretation of data generated in all experimental models must be made with caution. However, models provide valuable preclinical data for the development of therapies, both pharmacologic and biological, and insights into relevant mechanisms common to experimental arthritis and RA, and may ultimately lead to the development of effective antiarthritic agents.

MECHANISMS OF EXPERIMENTAL ARTHRITIS INDUCTION

AUTOIMMUNITY TO CARTILAGE COMPONENTS

Immunization with either of the two major components of hyaline cartilage (type II collagen and aggrecan proteoglycans) may elicit an autoimmune response and the subsequent development of arthritis. Collagen-induced arthritis (CIA) occurs in mice, rats and primates, while proteoglycan-induced arthritis (PGIA) has only been successfully established in BALB/c mice. Both models require a vigorous immune response directed initially against the immunizing (heterologous) cartilage antigen, which subsequently reacts with autologous cartilage antigens. A hypothetical mechanism for the development of collagen-induced and proteoglycan-induced experimental arthritides is shown in Figure 8.1. Susceptible strains of animals immunized with either type II collagen or high-density aggrecan proteoglycans in adjuvant recognize specific epitopes presented in the context of major histocompatibility complex (MHC) class II antigens, the equivalent of HLA-D region antigens. Autoreactive $CD4^+$ T-cells respond against either cross-reactive epitopes (antigens common to both the heterologous and autologous cartilage components) or cryptic epitopes (immunologically privileged antigens normally concealed from immunologic surveillance), and elicit connective tissue antigen-specific TH1 cells and autoantibodies (via TH2 mechanisms). Adoptive and passive transfer experiments suggest that both immunologic elements may be required for the generation of chronic arthritis. The localization of antibody and reactive cells in synovial joints causes immune-mediated cartilage damage, and the immune response may be perpetuated by the release of cartilage antigens. The pathologies of CIA and PGIA appear similar and resemble the features of RA[1,2]. Synovial hypertrophy and hyperplasia give rise to pannus formation, cartilage erosion and destruction. In severe cases, cartilage may be completely destroyed, and joint ankylosis follows. In general, CIA is a more relentless erosive disease, with a higher incidence of joint ankylosis, compared with PGIA.

THE RESPONSE TO NONSPECIFIC IMMUNOLOGIC STIMULI

The injection of nonspecific agents with adjuvant activity (the capacity to provoke an indirect immunologic response) can provoke experimental arthritis in certain species[3]. The classic example is of adjuvant-induced arthritis (AA) in the rat. The precise contributions of the oil and mycobacterial components of complete Freund's adjuvant (CFA) in the pathologic pathway of this experimental disease remain unclear. Recent observations that incomplete Freund's adjuvant (IFA) and the mineral oil pristane may induce arthritis in rats and

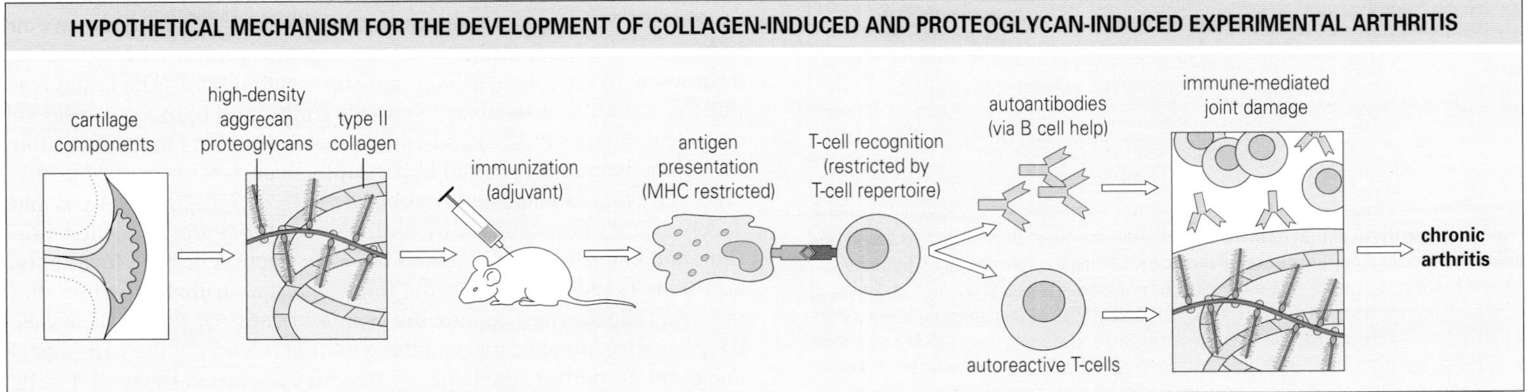

Fig. 8.1 Hypothetical mechanism for the development of collagen-induced and proteoglycan-induced experimental arthritides. Animals are immunized with type II collagen or high-density aggrecan proteoglycans, and an autoimmune response results when specific epitopes are presented in the context of MHC class II antigens and recognized by autoreactive $CD4^+$ T-cell populations. Autoantibodies and T-effector cells reactive against cartilage components localize in the synovial joints and cause an immune-mediated inflammatory response. The immune response is perpetuated by the release of cartilage antigens within the damaged joint, and chronic arthritis develops.

mice[4,5] suggest that oil may be the critical component, but the arthritogenic consequences appear ultimately to depend upon a reaction against either exogenous or autologous antigens. Heat shock proteins (HSP) may be the autoimmune target in AA[6]. A hypothetic mechanism for the development of AA and pristane-induced arthritis (PIA) is shown in Figure 8.2. In susceptible strains of animals, macrophages phagocytose nondegradable oil components, become intensely activated, produce high levels of proinflammatory cytokines [interleukin (IL)-1, tumor necrosis factor (TNF)-α, IL-6 and γ-interferon (IFN)], and may polyclonally activate T-cells and B cells. This is particularly apparent in PIA, where lymphadenopathy and hypergammaglobulinemia precede the onset of disease. The expansion of autoreactive T-cell and B cell populations occurs as a consequence of the activation process, resulting in autoantibodies against a spectrum of antibodies against cartilage antigens (PIA) and HSP (PIA and AA). Autoreactive T-cells migrate to the joint and contribute to immune-mediated joint damage. Production of rheumatoid factors in PIA may amplify the process. Macrophage-derived cytokines may also act directly upon synovial cells and chondrocytes, resulting in synovial hypertrophy, abnormal expression of MHC class II antigens and adhesion molecules, and atypical production of matrix components. Arthritis appears as a consequence of the chronic inflammatory stimulation, although disease onset is rapid in AA (16–19 days) and slow in PIA (3–6 months). Mycobacterial components may serve to accelerate the pathology of AA, although the evolution of the two diseases is markedly different, with AA presenting as an acute inflammatory arthritis, leading to rapid and extensive bone loss, whereas PIA is characterized by chronic synovitis and marginal and periosteal bone erosions and rarely culminating in joint ankylosis.

Antigen-induced arthritis (AIA) has been produced in rabbits and most rodent species by the injection of a soluble protein antigen (typically methylated bovine serum albumin) into the knee joint of an animal previously hypersensitized by immunization with antigen in FCA. The arthritis that develops is confined to the injected joint[7]. The histology of AIA resembles that of RA, with a joint infiltrate consisting of T-lymphocytes (mostly CD4+), B lymphocytes, mast cells and macrophages. The lack for a requirement of a joint-associated antigen suggests that AIA may occur simply as a consequence of an intra-articular immune response, but this may be an oversimplification. The antigen must persist within the synovial joint, and the immunogenetic requirements of this model suggest that specific immune mechanisms may contribute to susceptibility[8].

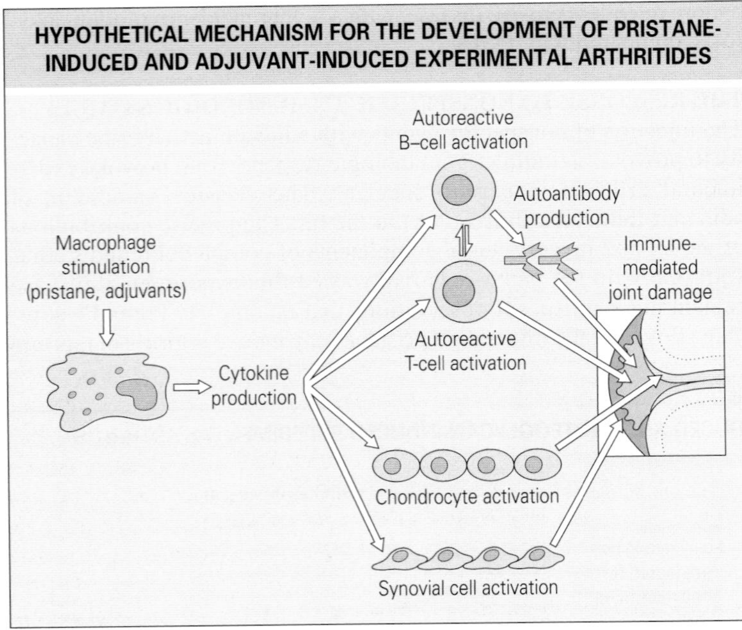

Fig. 8.2 Hypothetical mechanism for the development of pristane-induced and adjuvant-induced experimental arthritides. Circulating macrophages become intensely activated by the nondegradable oil components and produce high levels of proinflammatory cytokines (IL-1, TNF-α, IL-6 and γ-IFN). In susceptible rodent strains, autoreactive T-cells and B cells become activated and clonally expand. Autoantibodies to cartilage antigens and heat shock proteins may develop, and joint-reactive T-cells migrate to the joint, resulting in immune-mediated joint damage. Cytokines may also act directly upon both synovial cells and chondrocytes, resulting in synovial hypertrophy, abnormal expression of MHC class II antigens and adhesin molecules, and atypical production of matrix components. Arthritis develops due to the chronic nature of the inflammatory stimulation.

INFECTIOUS AGENTS

The development of arthritis as a consequence of infection is apparent in both natural and induced animal models. A wide variety of organisms may induce joint disease in a broad range of animal species, including rabbits, dogs, pigs, goats, rats, mice and hamsters. Although some models employ intra-articular inoculation to establish disease, many infectious agents may be administered intravenously or via other extra-articular routes to induce joint-based disease. The infectious agent may be trophic for the joint due to expression of adhesins or other molecules that promote sequestration within synovial tissues[9]. Staphylococcal species produce a range of receptors for connective tissue components, including collagen and fibronectin. Chronic, persistent infection of the joint can generate excessive local antigenic stimulation, resulting in an inflammatory and immune complex-mediated reactions. Bacterial cell wall and mycoplasma membrane components may also provide nonspecific immune activation through mitogenic activity. Viral infection of synovial cells may elicit novel cell surface antigens or abnormal expression of activation antigens and the overproduction of potential autoantigens such as HSPs. Alternatively, viral infection may disrupt normal immune regulation, induce production of proinflammatory cytokines and promote increased immune activity against the normally immunologically privileged components of the joint.

Lentivirus-induced arthritis in goats is an example of a viral disease that closely resembles RA[10]. Caprine arthritis encephalitis virus (CAEV) infects macrophages and monocytes and leads to an inflammatory synovitis with a marked mononuclear cell infiltrate. A hypothetical mechanism for the induction of disease is represented in Figure 8.3. The histologic and radiologic features of this disease are characterized by progressive lesions consisting of membrane villus hypertrophy with extensive angiogenesis and mononuclear cell infiltration, and a progression to marked erosive changes. Joint disease is accompanied by an immune response to viral glycoproteins, chronic B cell activation, and the accumulation of activated macrophages and CD8+ T-cells within the synovium. The precise sequence of events that leads from viral infection to erosive joint disease remains to be characterized. Susceptibility to CAEV arthritis is subject to genetic regulation. However, it is unclear which loci play a dominant role in the disease.

Several hypothetical mechanisms for arthritis induced by bacteria are represented in Figure 8.4. Experimental *Staphylococcus aureus* arthritis is a model in mice, rats and rabbits that illustrates a number of relevant pathways in infectious joint disease[11]. This organism can induce an exudative arthritis in one or more joints, with extensive destruction of articular cartilage and subchondral bone. The initial features of *S. aureus* arthritis are synovial infiltration by polymorphonuclear leukocytes (PMNs) and endothelial-like cells. One month after infection, extensive synovial hypertrophy occurs, with marked proliferation by macrophage and fibroblastic cells and infiltration by B and T-cells. Granulomatous tissue with bacterial foci are frequently present, and extensive cartilage and bone destruction occurs. Invariably, *S. aureus* is recovered from the joint, and the virulence factors that mediate arthritis may include the profile of capsular polysaccharides, the production of adhesins and the secretion of endotoxins with superantigenic properties (the capacity to activate a broad range of T-cells by direct binding to the Vβ portion of the T-cell receptor rather than by conventional antigen presentation)[12]. However, the persistence of bacterial antigens within the joint appears to be critical for the induction of arthritis.

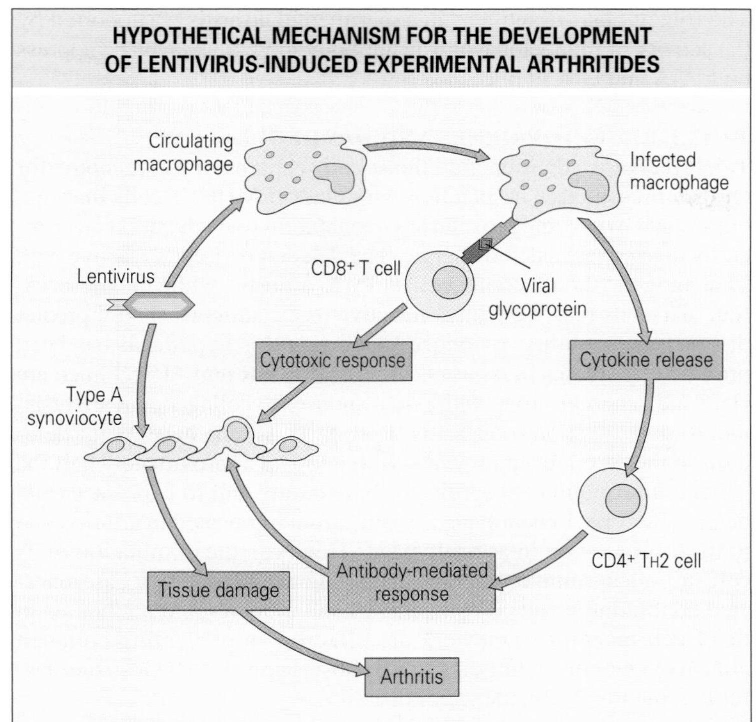

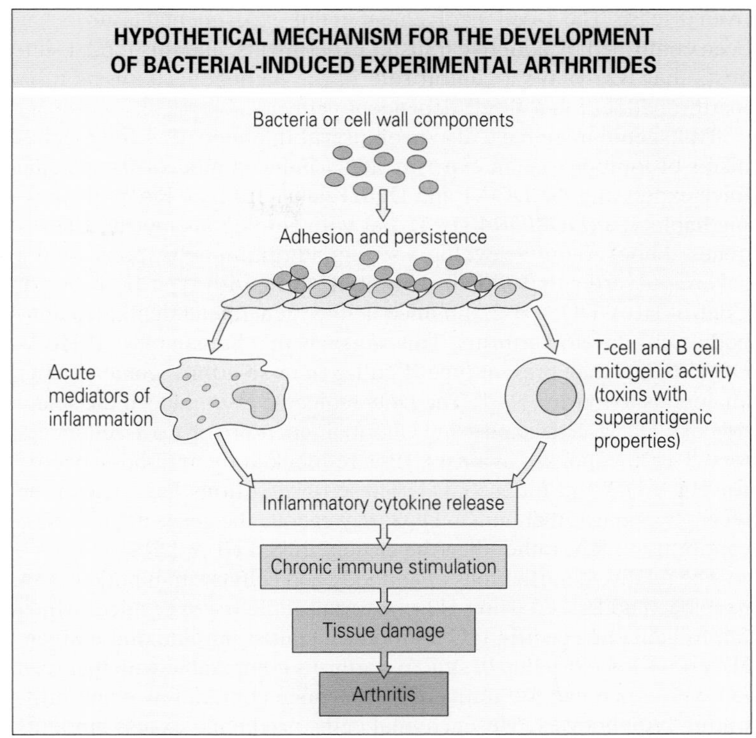

Fig. 8.3 Hypothetical mechanism for the development of lentivirus-induced experimental arthritis. The infection of macrophages and monocytes induces both the expression of cell surface viral antigens and cytokine release. The macrophage activation appears to promote both CD4+ TH2 cell expansion and the development of activated CD8+ T cells. T-cell cytotoxicity directed against infected type A (macrophage lineage) synovial cells may result in a local inflammatory reaction within the joint, and cartilage may be damaged concomitantly. The increased TH2 activity may contribute to local immune complex formation, eventually leading to chronic inflammatory activity within the joint and the development of arthritis.

Fig. 8.4 Hypothetical mechanism for the development of bacterial-associated experimental arthritis. Arthritis may be induced by infectious microorganisms (*Mycoplasma arthritidis*, *S. aureus*, *Yersinia enterocolitica*) or cell wall components (*Streptococcus* spp., *Escherichia coli*, *Eubacterium aerofaciens*). Infectious agents may colonize the joint due to the expression of cell adhesins, and may disrupt the regulation of the normal immune response by the production of superantigenic toxins. The immune response to the microorganisms may either cross-react with joint components (molecular mimicry) or react with immunologically privileged antigens (cryptic epitopes), leading to chronic cytokine production, immune-mediated joint damage and arthritis.

This point is emphasized by streptococcal cell wall (SCW) experimental arthritis in rats, where viable bacteria are unnecessary for disease induction[13]. An aqueous suspension of cell wall fragments injected intraperitoneally in susceptible rat strains evokes a chronic, erosive polyarthritis that has a course of remissions and exacerbations, a feature rarely observed in other animal models. The initial arthritis occurs rapidly, with acute inflammation in rear paws peaking approximately 4 days postimmunization. This inflammation recedes, but chronic arthritis recurs between 2–4 weeks, with synovitis, pannus formation and erosion of cartilage and bone. Cycles of remission and exacerbation may persist over several months and culminate in joint fibrosis and ankylosis. The severity of the disease appears to correlate with the level and persistence of SCW antigen within the synovium. The disease can be consistently reproduced by the direct injection of SCW suspension into synovial joints, with flare reactions subsequently elicited by intravenous SCW antigen or bacterial superantigen injection. The initial acute arthritis is T-cell independent, but requires an intact alternative complement pathway. In contrast, the chronic phase is complement independent, but mediated by T-cell-dependent mechanisms. Disease exacerbations in SCW arthritis may be provoked by the use of several proinflammatory cytokines (IL-1β, TNF-α, and γ-IFN), although IL-2 alone does not mediate a flare reaction.

GENE MANIPULATION AND TRANSGENIC ANIMALS

Transgenic animals, defined as novel strains generated by the insertion, deletion or manipulation of particular genes, have resulted in several models of joint disease. In addition, genetic modifications may alter susceptibility to the induction of experimental arthritis in transgenic rodents.

Mice transgenic for the env-pX region of the human T-cell leukemia virus (HTLV) type 1 genome develop a spontaneous chronic arthritis[14]. Onset occurs at 2–3 months of age in female mice, but is delayed several months in male animals. Ankle joints are most frequently affected, and pannus formation leading to severe erosions of cartilage and bone is observed in transgenic mice after several months of disease. In affected joints of these mice, cytokine genes (IL-1α, IL-1β, IL-6, TNF-α, TGF-β1, γ-IFN and IL-2) are activated, leading to elevated serum cytokine levels. Circulating antibody levels (IgG) are also elevated, and the mice produce rheumatoid factors and antibodies against type II collagen and HSPs. Abnormal cellular responses include the increased expression of class II MHC antigens, and reactivity against type II collagen and HSP. These observations have added to the speculation that a retrovirus such as HTLV-1 may be involved in the pathogenesis of RA.

Mice carrying 3′-modified hTNF-α transgenes exhibit deregulated TNF-α expression and develop chronic inflammatory polyarthritis[15]. At 2 weeks of age in TNF-α transgenics, moderate synovitis is present in rear paws. Cartilage changes may also occur in the absence of synovial infiltrate, with chondrocyte hyperproliferation, cartilage malformation and marked proteoglycan loss. Clinical disease is visible in rear paws at 3–4 weeks of age, with swelling of the ankle joints, while front paws become involved later. Synovitis, bony erosions and periosteal inflammation continue to worsen, and the ankle and wrist joints fuse leading to impaired mobility. No clinical or histologic signs of arthritis are observed in nontransgenic litter mates at any age.

Rats and mice transgenic for the human HLA-B27 gene have shown striking similarities with some of the features of human B27-associated diseases[16]. One B27 transgenic rat strain develops spontaneous inflammatory disease involving the gastrointestinal tract, peripheral and vertebral joints, male genital tract, skin, nails and heart. Disease susceptibility appears to correlate with the B27 gene copy number and the level of expression of B27 by lymphoid cells. The disease can be adoptively transferred to nontransgenic rats using either bone marrow or fetal liver cells, but athymic B27 transgenic (nude) rats are protected from disease. The T-cell involvement in this experimental arthritis has been confirmed by adoptive transfer experiments, and this model suggests that B27 plays a central role in the pathogenesis of spondyloarthropathies via a T-cell-dependent pathway.

Transgenic mice have also been useful in elucidating the mechanisms of joint disease in experimentally induced models. Transgenic mice expressing the DQA1 and DQB1 genes from an RA-predisposing haplotype (DQ8/DR4/Dw4), but with autologous murine class II genes 'knocked out', develop a strong autoimmune response and a severe polyarthritis following immunization with type II collagen. Control HLA-DQ8-,H-2Ab0 mice neither generate anticollagen antibodies nor develop arthritis. This suggests that human class II HLA-DQ antigens may present type II collagen in an arthritogenic manner analogous to murine H-2^q. The DQ8 molecule also induced the selection of $CD4^+$ T-cells expressing a normal repertoire of Vβ T-cell receptors. T-cell responses against CII were blocked by antibody specific for HLA-DQ and mouse CD4. These observations have led to the recent hypothesis that human DQ8 may encode the genes defining susceptibility to RA, rather than the closely linked HLA-DR4[17].

The relative contributions of antibody and cellular immunity to AIA have been addressed using H2-c-*fos* transgenic (c-*fos*+) mice, which fail to generate specific IgG antibodies against immunizing antigen. H2-c-*fos*+ mice develop destructive arthritis comparable with that seen in c-*fos*– mice, but the joints of c-*fos*+ mice contain few or no infiltrating lymphocytes. Mesenchymal cells, producing excess amounts of c-fos protein, participate extensively in the joint destruction in c-*fos*+ mice[18]. This observation calls into question the central role of lymphocytes in experimental arthritis.

IMMUNOREGULATION OF EXPERIMENTAL ARTHRITIS

CLASS II MHC GENES

A variety of gene loci are involved in the regulation of arthritis susceptibility among the different experimental models (Fig. 8.5). Research has focused on the MHC class II genes and the T-cell receptor genes, because of the close parallels with the immunogenetics of RA. The cell surface structures involved in antigen presentation and immune recognition – MHC antigens and T-cell receptors – and the trimolecular complex of antigen, MHC class II and the T-cell receptor appear to be central to the immunogenetic regulation of autoimmune disease[19]. Collagen-induced arthritis has provided a definitive model for the recognition and response to a cartilage autoantigen subject to strict regulation by MHC class II genes. Gene regulation of MHC class II in rat CIA bears a strong resemblance to the mouse CIA model. The RT1 locus is associated with the arthritogenic response to type II collagen, presumably via the selection of arthritogenic versus nonarthritogenic epitopes for presentation to the immune response system.

The immunogenetic regulation of pristane-induced arthritis in mice exhibits considerable homology with collagen-induced arthritis[4]. However, the production of autoantibodies in this model cannot be associated with the MHC phenotype with precision, and the role of MHC class II in the presentation of autoantigens in PIA remains unresolved. The role of class II antigens in experimental arthritis is supported by the activity of monoclonal anti-Ia antibody in vivo [4,20], which suppress both AIA and CIA in mice.

T-CELL RECEPTOR GENES AND *MLS* REGULATION

T-cell receptor genes encode the α and β chains of the receptor for antigen presented in association with class II MHC. T-cells that recognize self *Mls-1* antigens during neonatal thymic education are generally deleted or rendered anergic. The deletion of T-cells reactive with joint antigens should confer resistance to arthritis, while the preservation of T-cells reactive with connective tissue antigens should predict disease susceptibility. Evidence supporting this hypothesis has been provided by studies in mouse CIA[21]. Both SWR and AUss/J mice are H-2^q and generate strong antibody responses to collagen, but are resistant to the induction of arthritis. Both these strains have major deletions in the T-cell receptor genes, with a loss of approximately half the genetic information. Accordingly, both strains fail to express T-cells bearing the Vβ8.1 phenotype, a T-cell subset implicated in arthritis due to its accumulation in arthritic paws. However, the elimination of T-cell subsets by immunotherapy with Vβ-specific antisera has generated conflicting results. While anti-CD4 antibodies and antibodies to the T-cell receptor framework are effective in preventing collagen arthritis induction, antibodies to Vβ subsets appear to be less successful in reducing the incidence of disease.

NEUROENDOCRINE FACTORS IN EXPERIMENTAL MODELS OF ARTHRITIS

Recent studies indicate an additional role for neuroendocrine factors in joint disease[22]. Inflammatory cytokines, particularly IL-1, TNF-α, and IL-6, act at the level of the hypothalamus to increase the production of corticotropin-releasing hormone (CRH) (Fig. 8.6), which stimulates the production of adrenocorticotropin (ACTH) by the pituitary gland. This results in the production of glucocorticosteroids by the adrenal cortex. Hence the communication between the immune system and hypothalamic–pituitary–adrenocortical (HPA) axis serves as a feedback mechanism to downregulate inflammation via the action of endogenous corticosteroids. Adjuvant arthritic rats have elevated ACTH and corticosterone levels[23]. The transfer of spleen cells from AA rats to syngeneic recipients causes pituitary pro-opiomelanocortin (POMC; ACTH precursor), mRNA accumulation and increased circulating ACTH to levels similar to those seen in arthritic donors. This transfer of immune cells is not associated with disease transfer, but, on the contrary, protects recipients from the subsequent induction of AA. These data support the concept of a direct interaction between immune mediators (presumably cytokines) and the mediators of the neuroendocrine system.

The high level of susceptibility of the Lewis rat strain to the induction of several experimental arthritides (adjuvant arthritis, collagen arthritis and SCW-induced arthritis) may be related to a neuroendocrine defect[24]. Lewis rats secrete diminished levels of CRH in response to cytokine stimulation, and produce elevated levels of arginine vasopressin (AVP). This results in inadequate corticosteroid

THE GENETIC REGULATION OF EXPERIMENTAL MODELS OF ARTHRITIS

Disease model	MHC class I	MHC class II	Complement genes	*Mls*	T-cell genes	Immunoglobulin genes
Collagen-induced arthritis	–	+++	++	+++	+++	++
Proteoglycan-induced arthritis	?	?	?	++	++	++
Pristane-induced arthritis	?	++	+	+++	+++	+
Adjuvant-induced arthritis	–	+	?	?	++	?
Bacterial cell wall arthritis	–	++	++	?	++	+

Fig. 8.5 The genetic regulation of experimental models of arthritis

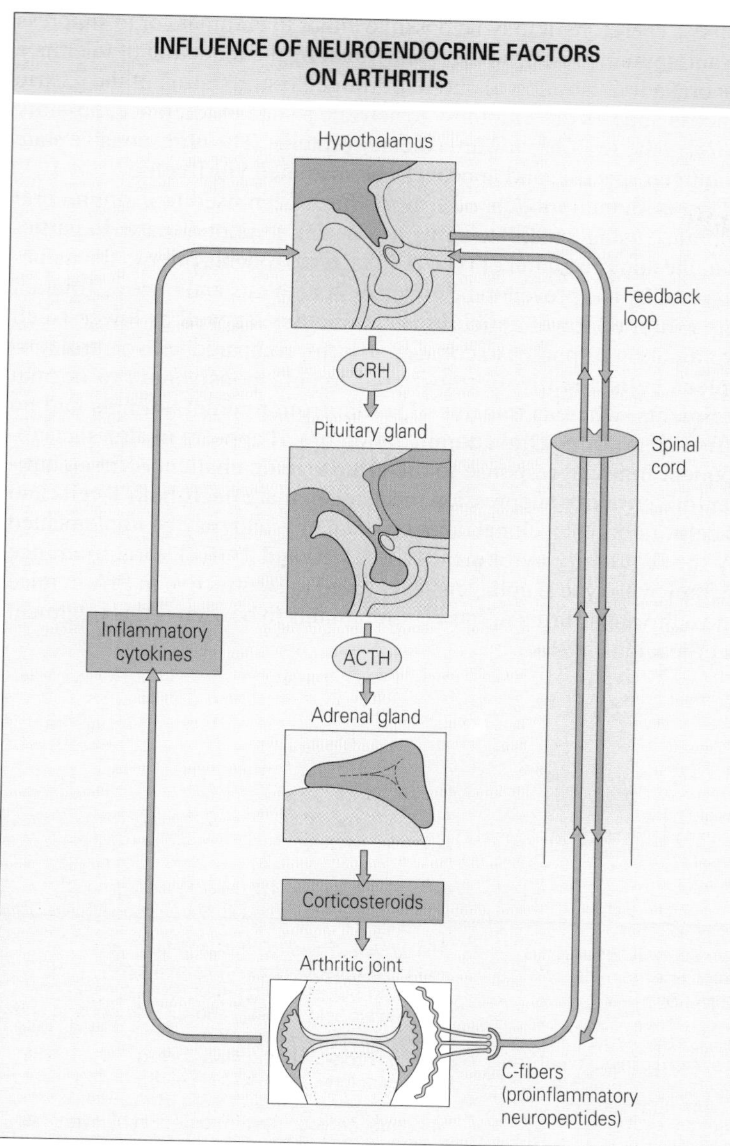

Fig. 8. 6 The influence of neuroendocrine factors on arthritis. Inflammatory cytokines act at the level of the hypothalamus to increase the production of CRH, which stimulates the production of ACTH by the pituitary gland. This subsequently results in the production of corticosteroids by the adrenal cortex, and functions as a feedback mechanism to suppress inflammation. However, neuron-derived CRH, in combination with other proinflammatory neuropeptides derived from the sensory afferent unmyelinated C-fibers which innervate the synovium, augments the chronic inflammation of the joint. The activation of C-fiber afferent nerves within the arthritic joint transmits an ascending signal via the spinal cord that results in an inhibitory feedback of the inflammatory process.

production, and this failure of the feedback pathway may be a permissive factor in the development of chronic inflammatory disease. The histocompatible Fisher rat strain, with abnormally high CRH responses, exhibits resistance to the induction of chronic experimental arthritis. However, Fisher rats treated with the corticosteroid receptor inhibitor RU896 develop chronic SCW-induced arthritis.

Neuroendocrine regulation of inflammatory disease is complicated by differences between the central and peripheral actions of the mediators. In the joint, both CRH and AVP appear to promote experimental synovitis. CRH has been detected in the spinal cord, and is depleted by capsaicin treatment in a similar manner to the neuropeptide substance P (SP)[25]. It is therefore hypothesized that neuron-derived CRH, in combination with SP and other neuropeptides derived from the sensory afferent unmyelinated C-fibers which innervate the synovium, augments the chronic inflammation of the joint. The activation of C-fiber afferent nerves within the adjuvant arthritic joint transmits an ascending signal via the spinal cord that results in an inhibitory feedback of the inflammatory process at a second joint. This feedback is dependent upon an intact HPA axis, and appears to be mediated via endogenous corticosteroids[26].

The neuroendocrine network is influenced by the activities of the sex and pituitary hormones on immune function[27]. Estrogen and testosterone modulate B cell functions, while the hormone prolactin, follicle stimulating hormone and luteinizing hormone may have effects on T-cell activation. Hypophysectomized rats are resistant to the induction of experimental arthritis, and the administration of prolactin has been shown to restore diminished immune responses caused by hypophysectomy. In adjuvant arthritis, increased pituitary prolactin activity and elevated prolactin plasma levels have been demonstrated before the onset of disease. At the same time, decreased pituitary POMC and plasma corticosteroid levels are observed. In collagen arthritis, pregnancy suppresses the onset of disease, but a postpartum flare, which is frequently observed, has been attributed to increases in prolactin. However, the treatment of collagen arthritic mice with bromocriptine or haloperidol (to inhibit or enhance prolactin levels, respectively) showed that elevated prolactin levels increased the severity of arthritis only during the induction of experimental disease, whereas bromocriptine treatment could not prevent arthritis onset, and actually exacerbated the development of disease[28]. Overall, the data suggest that an imbalance between the proinflammatory effects of prolactin and the anti-inflammatory effects of corticosteroids may be central to the development and regulation of chronic disease.

EXPERIMENTAL MODELS IN THE DEVELOPMENT OF ANTIARTHRITIS THERAPIES

Animal models have been critical to the development of most antiarthritis drugs in use today, and are currently denoting novel areas for therapeutic intervention in inflammatory and autoimmune disease. Adjuvant arthritis has been used as a benchmark for the evaluation of nonsteroidal anti-inflammatory drugs (NSAIDs) since the early 1960s[3], although the contrast between the effective 'cure' of AA by typical NSAIDs and their less efficacious results in RA apparently weakens the resemblance of the pathogenesis of this model to that of RA. Collagen-induced arthritis is only weakly responsive to NSAIDs or methotrexate, and is essentially unaffected by gold salts, chloroquine, colchicine or levamisole[29]. Antigen-induced arthritis models are responsive to NSAIDs during the chronic phase of the disease, but do not exhibit the 'cure' phenomenon observed in AA. Hydrocortisone, cyclophosphamide and sulfasalazine are effective in the prevention and treatment of CIA, but the discovery that cyclosporin prevented the onset of arthritis and slowed the progression of established disease in both CIA and AIA ushered in an era of therapies targeted at T-cells in RA. Anti-CD4 antibody therapy proved highly effective in CIA[30], an observation supported by findings in AIA, PIA and SCW arthritis. Anti-CD4 therapy in RA has proved less exciting. Although this approach still remains viable, the dramatic reductions in circulating T-cell levels achieved in the experimental models (around 2% of the normal blood count) are not considered desirable in human trials. Thus the lack of efficacy of anti-CD4 therapy in RA may reflect a failure to effectively target autoimmune T-cells (particularly synovial resident T cells) rather than the failure of the conceptual approach.

Two current areas of potential antiarthritis therapies indicated by successful outcomes in arthritis models are inflammatory cytokine inhibition and oral tolerance[29]. Inflammatory cytokines clearly influence several experimental arthritis models. IL-1 administered intra-articularly causes acute arthritis in several species, although this cytokine alone does not appear to provoke chronic joint disease. Strategies to inhibit the activity of IL-1β using IL-1 receptor antagonist protein (IRAP), soluble IL-1 receptors or antibodies to IL-1β have proved successful in experimental arthritis. Analogous findings have been described using strategies to inhibit TNF-α activity. Anti-TNF-α immunotherapy, or the administration of soluble TNF receptor or recombinant TNF receptor: human Fc fusion protein have potent antiarthritic activity in CIA[31]. The results suggest that the TNF receptor may have both immunosuppressive and antiarthritic properties. Antibodies to TNF-α may be even more efficacious, since both the development of arthritis and the premature death of mice carrying 3′-modified hTNF transgenes have been ameliorated by continuous infusion of anti-TNF-α antisera. Transforming growth factor (TGF)-β has also been implicated as an antiarthritic cytokine in arthritis models. However, reports that TGF-β exerts an antiarthritic effect, particularly in CIA, are tempered by contradictory findings on the effects of this regulatory cytokine on experimental arthritis, with some reports suggesting that TGF-β may accelerate disease. It may prove problematic to utilize TGF-β effectively in arthritis, since the effects of this cytokine on chondrocytes, as well as on immune cells, may make the outcome unpredictable.

As autoimmune diseases are characterized by an abnormal level of immune reactivity to autoantigens, influencing the balance between the level and specificity of the anti-self response could represent a key to the therapy of autoimmune disease. Tolerance induction may be achieved by exposure to antigens under certain conditions, either by clonal deletion, clonal anergy or clonal suppression of responsive cells[32]. Therefore, it may be possible either to eliminate or to suppress an autoimmune response in an individual by the induction of tolerance via oral administration of antigen. Antigenic stimulation of the gastric mucosa appears preferentially to activate a state of tolerance, possibly to avoid the response towards dietary proteins. The unresponsive state is antigen specific, and appears to be mediated via T-cells.

Experimental models of arthritis have been used to examine oral tolerance using candidate antigens relevant to joint disease. In particular, the administration of type II collagen to rodents prior to the induction of CIA has proved to be effective in both rats and mice[29]. Tolerant rats exhibited lower anticollagen antibodies, as well as lower T-cell proliferation responses to collagen *in vitro*, compared with control rats. Spleen cells adoptively transferred hyporesponsiveness to normal recipients, whereas transfer of serum from tolerant animals had no effect on arthritis. Oral administration of CII appears to alter the subsequent immune response to the arthritogenic challenge via an antigen-driven active suppression mechanism that affects both T-cells and B cells, rather than clonal deletion or anergy, and may be implemented by the regulatory cytokines IL-4, IL-10 and TGF-β. Oral tolerance therapy with type II collagen also proved to be effective in PIA in mice and adjuvant arthritis in rats[33,34]. It remains to be seen if this treatment is efficacious in RA.

REFERENCES

1. Wooley PH, Luthra HS, Stuart JM, David CS. Type II collagen-induced arthritis in mice. I. Major histocompatibility complex (I region) linkage and antibody correlates. J Exp Med. 1981;154:688–700.
2. Glant TT, Mikecz K, Arzoumanian A, Poole AR. Proteoglycan-induced arthritis in BALB/c mice. Clinical features and histopathology. Arthritis Rheum. 1987;30:201–12.
3. Billingham MEJ. Adjuvant arthritis: the first model. In: Henderson, B, Edwards, JCW, Pettipher, ER, eds. Mechanisms and models in rheumatoid arthritis. London: Academic Press; 1995:389–410.
4. Wooley PH, Seibold JR, Whalen JD, Chapdelaine JM. Pristane-induced arthritis. The immunological and genetic features of an experimental murine model of autoimmune disease. Arthritis Rheum. 1989;32:1022–30.
5. Kleinau S, Erlandsson H, Holmdahl R, Klareskog L. Adjuvant oils induce arthritis in the DA rat. I. Characterization of the disease and evidence for an immunological involvement. J Autoimmun. 1991;4:871–80.
6. van Eden W, Hogervorst EJ, Hensen EJ, *et al.* A cartilage-mimicking T-cell epitope on a 65K mycobacterial heat-shock protein: adjuvant arthritis as a model for human rheumatoid arthritis. Curr Topics Microbiol Immunol. 1989;145:27–43.
7. Howson P, Shepard N, Mitchell N. The antigen-induced arthritis model: the relevance of the method of induction to its use as a model of human disease. J Rheumatol. 1986;13:379–90.
8. Brackertz D, Mitchell GF, Mackay IR. Antigen-induced arthritis in mice. I. Induction of arthritis in various strains of mice. Arthritis Rheum. 1977;20:841–50.
9. Patti JM, Bremell T, Krajewska-Pietrasik D, *et al.* The *Staphylococcus aureus* collagen adhesin is a virulence determinant in experimental septic arthritis. Infect Immun. 1994;62:152–61.
10. Wilkerson MJ, Davis WC, Baszler TV, Cheevers WP. Immunopathology of chronic lentivirus-induced arthritis. Am J Pathol. 1995;146:1433–43.
11. Bremell T, Lange S, Yacoub A, Rydén C, Tarkowski A. Experimental *Staphylococcus aureus* arthritis in mice. Infect Immun. 1991;59:2615–23.
12. Herman A, Kappler JW, Marrack P, Pullen AM. Superantigens: mechanism of T-cell stimulation and role in immune responses. Ann Rev Immunol. 1991;9:745–72.
13. Koga T, Kakimoto K, Hirofuji T, *et al.* Acute joint inflammation in mice after systemic injection of the cell wall, its peptidoglycan, and chemically defined peptidoglycan subunits from various bacteria. Infect Immun. 1985;50:27–34.
14. Iwakura Y, Tosu M, Yoshida E, *et al.* Induction of inflammatory arthropathy resembling rheumatoid arthritis in mice transgenic for HTLV-I. Science. 1991;253:1026–8.
15. Keffer J, Probert L, Cazlaris H, *et al.* Transgenic mice expressing human tumour necrosis factor: a predictive genetic model of arthritis. EMBO J. 1991;10:4025–31.
16. Hammer RE, Maika SD, Richardson JA, Tang JP, Taurog JD. Spontaneous inflammatory disease in transgenic rats expressing HLA-B27 and human beta 2m: an animal model of HLA-B27-associated human disorders. Cell. 1990;63:1099–112.
17. Zanelli E, Gonzalez-Gay MA, David CS. Could HLA-DRB1 be the protective locus in rheumatoid arthritis? Immunol Today. 1995;16:274–8.
18. Shiozawa S, Tanaka Y, Fujita T, Tokuhisa T. Destructive arthritis without lymphocyte infiltration in H2-c-fos transgenic mice. J Immunol. 1992;148:3100–4.
19. Wooley PH. Immunogenetics of animal models of rheumatoid arthritis. In: Henderson, B, Edwards, JCW, Pettipher, ER, eds. Mechanisms and models in rheumatoid arthritis. London: Academic Press; 1995:373–87.
20. van den Broek MF, van den Berg WB, van de Putte LB. Monoclonal anti-Ia antibodies suppress the flare up reaction of antigen induced arthritis in mice. Clin Exp Immunol. 1986;66:320–30.
21. David CS. Genes for MHC, TCR and MIs determine susceptibility to collagen induced arthritis. Acta Pathol Microbiol Immunol Scand. 1990;98:575–84.
22. Chikanza IC, Chrousos G, Panayi GS. Abnormal neuroendocrine immune communications in patients with rheumatoid arthritis. Eur J Clin Invest. 1992;22:635–7.
23. Harbuz MS, Rees RG, Eckland D, *et al.* Paradoxical responses of hypothalamic corticotropin-releasing factor (CRF) messenger ribonucleic acid (mRNA) and CRF-41 peptide and adenohypophysial proopiomelanocortin mRNA during chronic inflammatory stress. Endocrinology. 1992;130:1394–400.
24. Sternberg EM, Young WS 3rd, Bernardini R, *et al.* A central nervous system defect in biosynthesis of corticotropin-releasing hormone is associated with susceptibility to streptococcal cell wall-induced arthritis in Lewis rats. Proc Nat Acad Sci. 1989;86:4771–5.
25. Crofford LJ, Sano H, Karalis K, *et al.* Local secretion of corticotropin-releasing hormone in the joints of Lewis rats with inflammatory arthritis. J Clin Invest. 1992;90:2555–64.
26. Green PG, Miao FJ, Janig W, Levine JD. Negative feedback neuroendocrine control of the inflammatory response in rats. J Neurosci. 1995;15:4678–686.
27. Wilder RL. Neuroendocrine–immune system interactions and autoimmunity. Ann Rev Immunol. 1995;13:307–38.
28. Mattsson R, Mattsson A, Hansson I, *et al.* Increased levels of prolactin during, but not after, the immunisation with rat collagen II enhances the course of arthritis in DBA/1 mice. Autoimmunity. 1992;11:163–70.
29. Staines NA, Wooley PH. Collagen arthritis – what can it teach us? Br J Rheumatol. 1994;33:798–807.
30. Ranges GE, Fortin S, Barger MT, Sriram S, Cooper SM. *In vivo* modulation of murine collagen induced arthritis. Int Rev Immunol. 1988;4:83–90.
31. Brennan FM, Maini RN, Feldmann M. TNF alpha – a pivotal role in rheumatoid arthritis? Br J Rheumatol. 1992;31:293–8.
32. Gammon G, Sercarz E. How some T cells escape tolerance induction. Nature. 1989;342:183–5.
33. Thompson SJ, Thompson HS, Harper N, *et al.* Prevention of pristane-induced arthritis by the oral administration of type II collagen. Immunology. 1993;79:152–7.
34. Zhang ZJ, Lee CSY, Lider O, Weiner HL. Suppression of adjuvant arthritis in Lewis rats by oral administration of type II collagen. J Immunol. 1990;145:2489–93.

RHEUMATOID ARTHRITIS

9

AUTOANTIBODIES IN RHEUMATOID ARTHRITIS

David G Williams

- Antibodies of diagnostic significance occuring in the serum of patients with rheumatoid arthritis include rheumatoid factor, anti-keratin and anti-perinuclear factor.
- Additional autoantibody specificities that occur in rheumatoid arthritis include antibodies to collagen, chondroctye, heat shock protein, HLA, endothelial cell and histone antigens.
- Autoantibodies have been studied for their relationship to disease and disease activity, pathological potential, etiologic importance and effects on synovial physiology.

INTRODUCTION

Waaler's observation of high levels of serum rheumatoid factor (RF) in patients with rheumatoid arthritis (RA)[1] revolutionized earlier concepts of RA as a disease of abnormal connective tissue metabolism and suggested that the immune system is also involved. Autoimmune phenomena distinguish RA from other common arthritides. This concept is further reinforced by the association of increased risk of RA, with inheritance of particular alleles of the class II major histocompatibility complex, the molecules presenting exogenous antigens to T lymphocytes.

Patients with RA are autoimmune to a set of ubiquitous antigens and to antigens restricted to articular joints. Steffen hypothesized that RA is a collagen autoimmune disease. Animal models of collagen type II-induced arthritis support this possibility[2]. The particular autoantigens that are critical in RA remains unclear. Persistent autoimmunity in RA may be significant as:

- a marker of disease, prognosis or therapeutic effectiveness;
- indicators of antigens driving the disease-triggering immunity;
- indicators of immune responses secondary to joint damage, driving disease chronicity.

A characteristic of RA is infiltration of the joint lining by immune and inflammatory cells together with cartilage and bone erosions. Sublining and deeper layers of rheumatoid synovium contain abundant lymphocytes and plasma cells (Fig. 9.1) distributed diffusely or as follicles around small blood vessels. These follicles may have immune function. Thus, rheumatoid synovial infiltrates are enriched in activated dendritic cells (DC) which synergize with phagocytic cells to present processed antigen to $CD4^+$ T cells. Most rheumatoid synovial T cells are fully differentiated memory cells which can stimulate B lymphocyte differentiation. Clonal lymphocyte proliferation in these follicles[3] suggests that immune responses similar to those of the lymph node germinal center are occurring.

IMMUNOGLOBULIN GENE EXPRESSION IN RA SYNOVIUM

An antigen-specific immune response will drive selective lymphocyte expansion which can be identified by analyzing immunoglobulin mRNA expression (as cDNA). Study of cDNA libraries prepared from RA synovium has demonstrated somatic mutation in V_H and V_L genes and a clonal relationship amongst κ light chains and γ heavy chains. There was also preferential usage of genes associated with fetal development or autoreactivity e.g. over-representation of the V_H1 51P1 gene.

Selective clonal expansion in rheumatoid synovium is also indicated by both the synovial fluid antibody and lymphocyte populations. Synovial plasma cells produce immunoglobulin more restricted than blood, as shown by:

- an immunoglobulin κ/λ ratio reduced from 3 in serum to below 1;
- an increased proportion of IgG3 in synovial cells;
- enrichment of IgM RF activity in synovial cells;
- reduced clonal heterogeneity of synovial fluid IgG protein.

Taken together, these data suggest that synovial lymphocytes are selectively activated and clonally expanded by local antigens, whose nature remains enigmatic. An infectious etiology for RA is postulated, but evidence for its persistent involvement in a significant proportion of RA patients is lacking. A current hypothesis is that an unknown transient exogenous trigger, at some time prior to disease, activates a set of autoimmune cross-reactive lymphocytes which can be chronically stimulated by autoantigen.

RHEUMATOID FACTOR

Presence of IgM rheumatoid factor (IgM-RF) in RA is the sole serologic indicator included in the ARA disease criteria. Rheumatoid factor (RF)[1] is a subset of antiglobulin antibodies directed against the Fc region of IgG. Antibodies to the IgG Fab and pepsin agglutinators are not included. Most antiglobulin activity in normal serum may be Fab-specific, whereas that in RA serum is mostly Fc-specific. RF is detected in 75–80% of RA patients. However, serum RF is also found in other conditions of B-cell hyperactivity, e.g. infectious and autoimmune diseases, hyperglobulinemias, B-cell lymphoproliferative disorders and also in the aged.

MEASUREMENT OF RHEUMATOID FACTOR

Rheumatoid factor is measured classically by agglutination methods, (Fig. 9.2) which are most sensitive to IgM RF. The latex fixation test

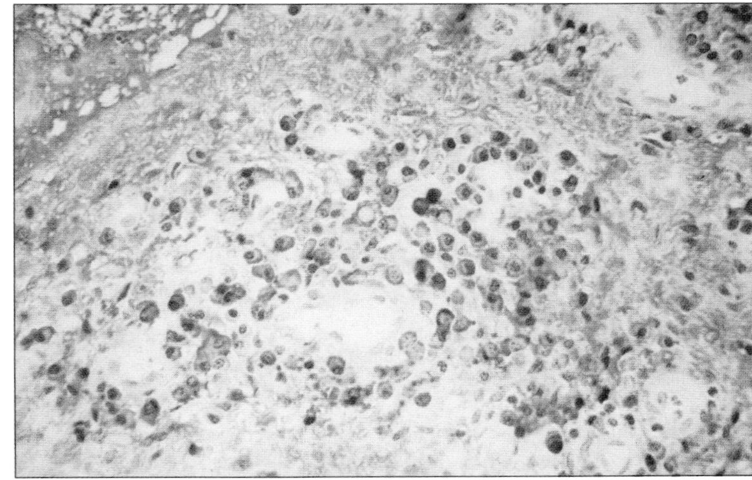

Fig. 9.1 Synovial cells making immunoglobulin. Section of a synovial villus immunostained brown with anti-immunoglobulin light chain to visualize B cells making antibody. (Courtesy of the Department of Histopathology, Charing Cross & Westminster Medical School).

(LFT) uses particles, coated with aggregated human IgG, which are visibly agglutinated by IgM RF. The titer is the highest serum dilution causing agglutination. A titer greater than 1:80 is visually considered positive. The LFT is more sensitive than the bentonite flocculation test (BFT) or the sheep cell agglutination test (SCAT), which uses sheep erythrocytes coated with rabbit IgG. The SCAT is more specific for RFs in RA because firstly anti-allotype binds human but not rabbit IgG, and secondly RFs from RA, but not non-RA patients, more frequently cross react with rabbit IgG.

Binding sites for RF

These include:

- genetically inherited variants of the Gm type associated with particular IgG subclasses and restricted to particular animal species;
- subclass-specific antigens;
- species-specific antigens;
- neoantigens on altered IgG.

IgG contains three constant domains. Many RF-binding sites, including Ga determinants, lie within the Cγ2 and Cγ3 domains (Fig. 9.3). Ga is a common specificity of RF from Waldenström's macroglobulinemias and is expressed on IgG1, 2, and 4. Histidine 435, in Cγ3, necessary for binding Ga-specific RFs is absent from unreactive IgG3. Residues 252–254 and 309–311 in the Cγ2 domain are also part of this determinant. Up to half of RFs, including Gm and Ga specificity, bind conformational determinants on the Fc surface, whilst the rest bind linear polypeptide determinants scattered in eight regions of Cγ2 and 12 regions of Cγ3.

RF from RA patients binds all subclasses of IgG. Lymphocytes from RA synovium produce RF *in vitro* with increased binding avidity for human versus rabbit IgG, and a selectivity for IgG3. On the other hand, RA blood lymphocytes secrete RF which binds human and rabbit IgG equally and is selective for IgG1 and IgG2. This selectivity of synovial RF for IgG3 may relate to the enhanced production of IgG3 by synovial lymphocytes.

ROLE OF CARBOHYDRATE IN RHEUMATOID FACTOR BINDING

Both constant and variable regions of IgG are glycosylated. N-linked oligosaccharides are situated on asparagine (Asn)297 in the Cγ2 domain and at sequence-dependent positions in the V domain. Fully galactosylated oligosaccharides on Asn297 are decreased in RA. This oligosaccharide normally fits into a cleft in the adjacent IgG surface. Some self-associating IgG-RF activity may be a lectin-like activity of the Fc region. IgG molecules lacking the Asn297 galactose have a cleft available to bind the oligosaccharide from a different, galactosylated IgG. In support of this, the frequency of agalactosylated Cγ2 oligosaccharides is raised in patients with RA, tuberculosis and Crohn's disease[4]. In one–third of monoclonal synovial RFs, IgG binding is inversely related to the galactosylation of IgG Fc. Glycosylation of Asn 297 inhibits IgG3-reactive IgM-RF binding to IgG3 but does not affect the binding of IgM RF to other IgG subclasses.

MEASUREMENT OF RHEUMATOID FACTOR
Human IgG-sensitized particle agglutination latex fixation test (LFT) or bentonite floculation test (BFT)
Rabbit IgG-sensitized erythrocyte agglutination e.g. sensitized sheep cell agglutination assay (SSCA), (SCAT), rheumatoid arthritis hemagglutination assay: (RAHA or Rose–Waaler test)
Radioimmunoassay (RIA)
Indirect immunofluoresence
Enzyme-linked immunoadsorbent assay (ELISA)
Laser nephelometry

Fig. 9.2 Measurement of rheumatoid factor[8].

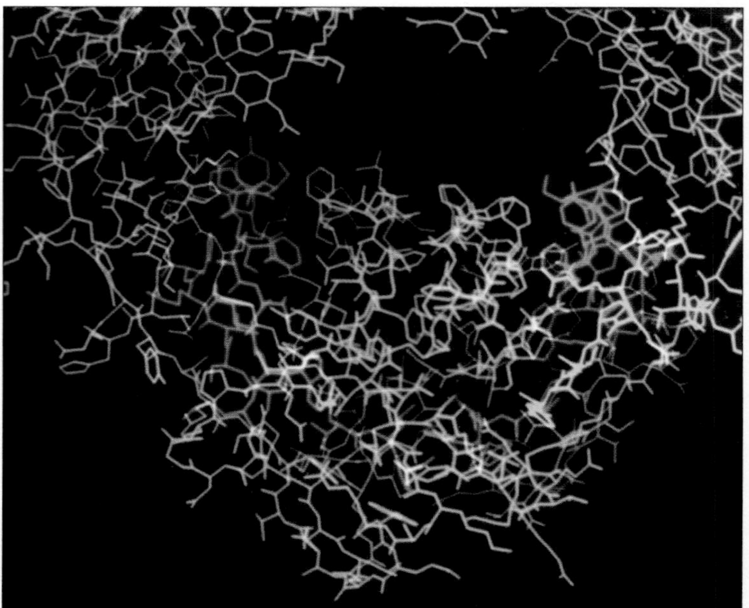

Fig. 9.3 RF Epitopes on IgG Fc. Molecular model of the CH2 and CH3 domains of IgG showing (in yellow) the antigenic sequence around the His 435, which can be seen to protrude from the surface (With permission of Elsevier Science Ltd, reprinted from Peterson C, Malone CC, Williams RC Jr. Rheumatoid–factor–reactive sites on CH3 established by overlapping 7–mer peptide epitope analysis. Molecular Immunology 1995;32:57–75).

CROSS REACTIVITY OF RHEUMATOID FACTOR

Some RF cross react with the cell nucleus, peptidoglycans or bromelain-treated erythrocytes. An idiotypic similarity between antibacterial peptidoglycan antibody and RF suggests that RFs are an internal-image anti-idiotype to anti-microbial antibodies. Thus, mice immunized with RF develop both anti-RF idiotype and anti-streptococcal peptidoglycan antibody.

IgM RFs from most RA patients but not from mixed cryoglobulinemia or Waldenström's paraproteinemia patients bind the invariant chain of MHC class I antigen, β_2-microglobulin. It appears to stem from structural homology between β_2-microglobulin and IgG CH3.

CD5$^+$B LYMPHOCYTES

There exists in the serum of healthy individuals a common population of 'natural' low affinity, multispecific autoantibodies binding DNA, cytoskeleton, thyroglobulin and so on. These may function in clearance of breakdown products. CD5$^+$B lymphocytes produce such natural autoantibodies including RF in addition to antibacterial antibodies. These cells characteristically produce low affinity, polyreactive IgM encoded by unmutated V_H genes, and represent a more primitive lineage than conventional CD5$^-$ B lymphocytes.

The CD5$^+$ B-cell subset normally accounts for 20% of circulating B cells; this figure rises to 45% in patients with RA[5], polyarticular JRA and Sjögren's syndrome. Correlation between blood CD5$^+$B cells and RF suggests that a high frequency expression of CD5$^+$B lymphocytes may predispose to IgM-RF production. CD5$^+$B lymphocytes from RA patients produce both low affinity polyreactive RF with K_d in the range of 10^{-3}–10^{-5} M; and high affinity monoreactive RF with K_d up to 10^{-7} M[6]. High affinity RF may derive from clonal expansion of somatically mutatated RF-specific lymphocytes. Despite earlier conclusions that CD5$^+$B cells produce unmutated IgM, they do express somatically mutated RF in RA. Compared with serum RF in SLE, Sjögren's syndrome or healthy individuals, serum RF in RA has a higher titer but a lower functional affinity[7].

RHEUMATOID FACTOR BINDING AFFINITY TO NATIVE AND AGGREGATED IGG

Rheumatoid factor binds with equal affinity to both native IgG and aggregated IgG. Despite this, nanograms of IgG in the form of immune complexes preferentially bind IgM RF in the presence of milligrams of free IgG. Increased avidity for aggregated IgG is due to multivalency. Valency of IgG is usually increased by complexation with antigen but in RA synovial fluid, IgG aggregation may be induced by free radicals liberated by activated neutrophils and macrophages.

RHEUMATOID FACTORS ARE SYNTHESIZED IN THE SYNOVIUM

Although the blood RF-specific B-cell precursor frequency is no higher in seropositive than in seronegative RA patients, the frequency of synovial RF-specific B cells is four times higher than blood, and only detectable in seropositive RA suggesting that serum IgM-RF is produced in joints. The majority of synovial immunoglobulin synthesis is IgG, with 10% IgA and 10% IgM (Fig. 9.4)[8]. Although only 2.6% of this IgG has demonstrable RF activity, this may be low due to self-association.

STIMULI FOR RHEUMATOID FACTOR PRODUCTION

Two types of stimuli regularly induce IgM RF synthesis in man and mouse: immune complexes and polyclonal B cell activators. Transient synthesis of IgM RF accompanies secondary immune responses and is probably part of the immunoregulatory process. Optimal RF production requires the presence of both antibodies and T cells specific for the immunizing antigen. RF is produced during bacterial endocarditis, probably in response to immune complexes containing bacterial antigens. Sustained RF production depends on antigen, and ceases after antibiotic treatment. A distinguishing feature of RF in RA is its persistence for many years. This can be related at least in part to the persistence of the individual RF-secreting B cell clone which may survive for at least 5 years. Immune complexes are also continually present in the serum and synovial fluid of RA patients. These complexes can stimulate IgM-RF production *in vitro*, suggesting their role in the chronic RF response.

A minor proportion of RFs from RA patients cross react with a variety of antigens which may stimulate production. A new hypothesis has recently emerged, based on the presence of an amino-acid sequence, QKRAA, within the polymorphic region of the β1 chain of HLA-Dw4, -Dw14 or -DR1 haplotypes. This sequence is reproduced in the gp110 protein of the Epstein–Barr virus, a common, chronic infection. It is a potent stimulus for T-cell proliferation[9] and may drive abundant production of antibodies to gp110. The gp110, as an immune complex, will bind to RF-specific B cells, which will present it to, and gain T-cell help from, QKRAA-reactive T cells.

High concentrations of conventional recall antigens stimulate IgM-RF production by peripheral lymphocytes. This appears to be due to antigen-induced polyclonal B-cell activation. Epstein–Barr virus stimulates RF synthesis by peripheral lymphocytes equally from healthy donors or RA patients[10] by stimulating resting lymphocytes. In contrast, RF production is induced by pokeweed mitogen stimulation of peripheral lymphocytes (preactivated subset) from RA patients, but not from healthy donors.

THE PATTERN OF IN VITRO IMMUNOGLOBULIN SYNTHESIS IN SYNOVIUM, SPLEEN AND LYMPH NODE

	IgG	IgA	IgM
Synovium	79	12	10
Lymph node-1	81	11	8
Lymph node-2	49	23	28
Spleen	85	6	9

Fig. 9.4 Pattern of in vitro immunoglobulin synthesis in RA synovium, spleen and lymph node. Percentage of ^{14}C-labeled Ig in each class synthesized in vitro by tissue lymphocytes.

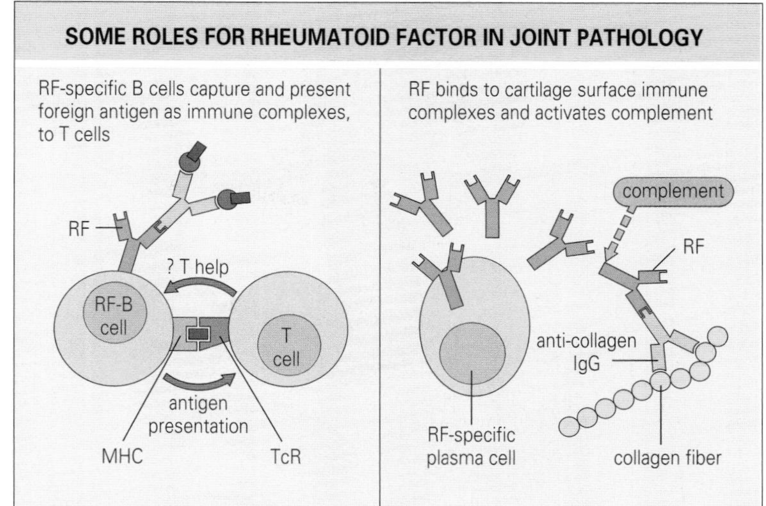

Fig. 9.5 Some roles for RF in joint pathology.

ASSOCIATION OF RF WITH PATHOGENESIS

High titer RF is associated with more severe disease and the presence of extra-articular features and rheumatoid nodules in later disease. In the first 2 years of RA (early RA), serum RF does not correlate with disease activity. In fact, serum IgM RF may precede the onset of RA by several years[11]. In established RA, serum IgM- and IgG-RF tends to correlate with the presence of articular disease, rheumatoid vasculitis and nodules. The presence of either IgG- or IgA-RF in patients with long-standing RA may be a good prognostic indicator of systemic manifestations[12]. IgA-RF may be a marker of inflammation of the mucosal membranes or secretory organs in RA and of bone erosions[12].

PATHOGENIC MECHANISM /NORMAL FUNCTION OF RF

A pathogenic role for RF in RA remains unclear but has been demonstrated in a mouse system. Monoclonal IgG2a-specific IgG-RF, from the MRL/lpr mouse, is a cryoglobulin and induces skin and renal lesions. The vasculitis depends absolutely on the RF activity and its ability to form immune complexes *in vivo*[13]. An important function of IgM is efficient complement fixation. Complement fixation by IgG-containing immune complexes is enhanced by IgM-RF binding. These immune complexes will also include the anti-cartilage antibodies and will be further discussed in the next section.

Natural killer cells have multiple potential regulatory functions including cytokine induction and the control of hematopoiesis and antibody production. RF-IgG complexes activate NK cells via the low affinity IgG receptor on NK cells (CD16) to stimulate TNF-α and IFN-γ synthesis. RF-specific B cells may be important antigen-presenting cells in certain situations (Fig. 9.5). Antigen presentation by B cells is of general importance in memory responses, when their surface antigen receptors bind specific antigen prior to its presentation to T cells[14]. Surface RF facilitates the uptake of IgG-complexes and presentation of the antigenic component to antigen-specific T lymphocytes. Hence antigen may be presented to synovial T cells, and vice versa, the RF-specific B cells may obtain T-cell help.

IMMUNE RESPONSES TO ANTIGENS IN JOINTS

CARTILAGE

Of the 25% dry weight of articular cartilage, 70% is collagen, 20% proteoglycans and 10% other cartilage matrix proteins.

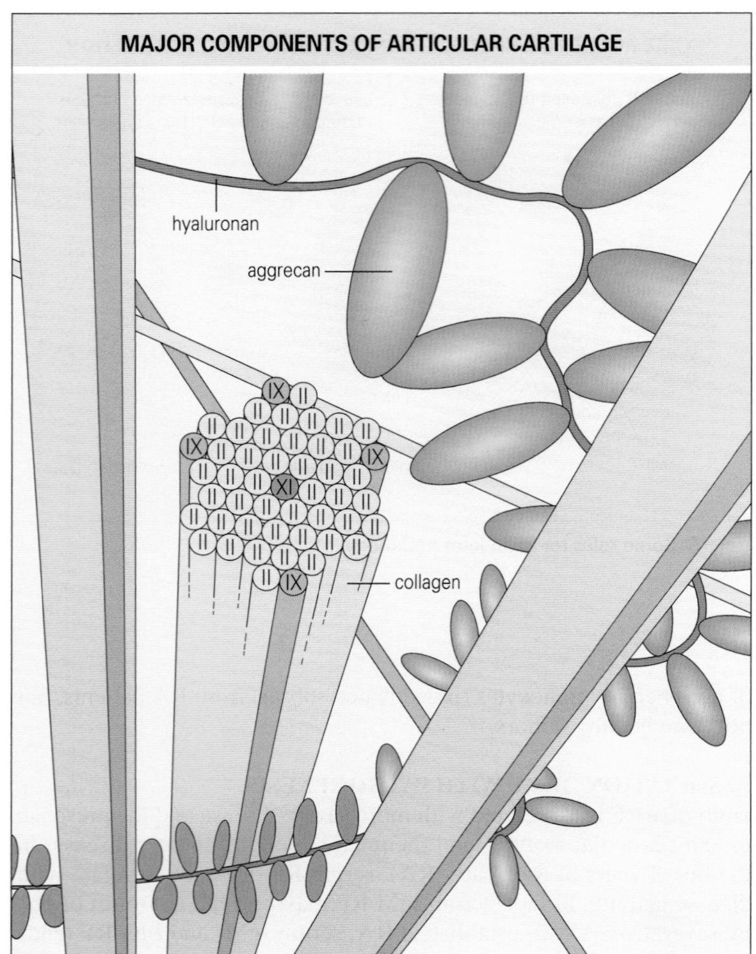

Fig. 9.6 **Major components of articular cartilage.**

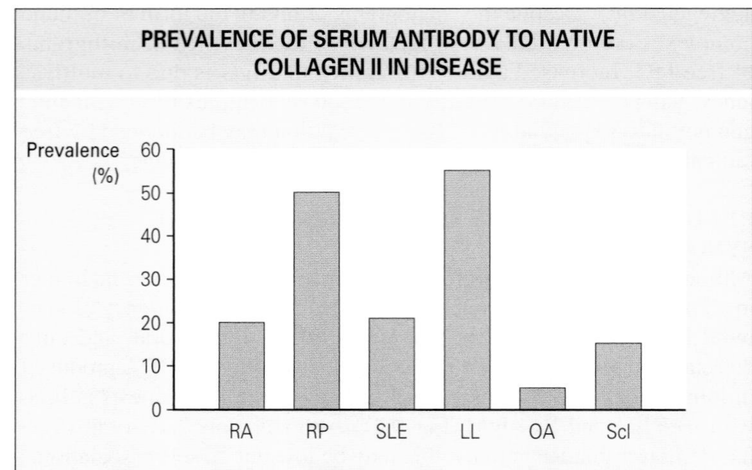

Fig. 9.7 Prevalence of serum antibody to native collagen II in disease. (RA: rheumatoid arthritis; RP: relapsing polychondritis; SLE: systemic lupus erythematosus; LL: lepromatous leprosy; OA: osteoarthritis; Scl: scleroderma.)

Proteoglycans

The most abundant type of proteoglycan in cartilage is the high molecular weight aggregating species, aggrecan, which attaches, together with link protein, to the high molecular weight polysaccharide, hyaluronan. Aggrecan consists of a 230kD polypeptide core to which are attached 80–100 chondroitin sulphate chains, 30 keratan sulfate chains, 50 O-linked oligosaccharides and 5–10 N-linked oligosaccharides. Antibodies to proteoglycans are rarely detectable in RA.

Collagens

Collagen is the most abundant animal protein and a structural component of every tissue, forming a matrix to support tissue cells, a framework for calcification in bone or a high-tensile-strength fiber in tendon. The collagen family is composed of at least 27 different gene products, α-chains, which combine to form 14 unique collagens. Five collagens are found in cartilage: CII, CIX, CX and CXI are mostly restricted to cartilage alone; CVI is also present elsewhere.

Cartilage collagen fibrils consist of a bundle of type II collagen surrounding a type XI core and bearing peripheral type IX, in a ratio of 8:1:1 (Fig. 9.6). The extremely slow turnover rate of collagen ($t_{1/2}$=100 years) compared to proteoglycans may lead to a relative absence of collagen catabolites in normal synovial fluid and reduced positive immune tolerance towards collagen compared with proteoglycan. Thus trauma to cartilage, leading to a release of collagen fibrils, may assist the induction of collagen immunity.

Collagen is secreted as a procollagen polypeptide, which is cleaved at each end and cross-linked to stabilize the higher order association of individual molecules within the triple helical collagen molecule and the collagen fiber. The repeating $(\text{Gly-X-Y})_n$ motif occupies much of the collagen sequence and is essential to the triple helical conformation of all collagens. IgG antibodies to collagen type II were detected with low sensitivity (they occur in 3.3% of patients with RA) by indirect immunofluorescent staining of xenogeneic cartilage sections in early studies. Cross-linking results in a resistance to solubilization, and the necessity to extract cartilage collagen by pepsin digestion, which liberates the central helical region freed from intermolecular cross links. This soluble material was used in later studies on collagen autoimmunology.

Measurement of anti-collagen antibodies

Anti-collagen antibodies have been detected or measured by:

- indirect immunofluorescence (IDIF) on rat trachea;
- radio immunoassay (RIA) using labelled anti-collagen antibody;
- radio labelled antigen immunosorbent assay (RLISA);
- enzyme-linked immunosorbent assay (ELISA);
- passive hemagglutination (PH) assay using collagen-sensitized erythrocytes.

Radio immunoassays are more sensitive than either the passive hemagglutination or immunofluorescent techniques[15]. Serum proteins (e.g. fibronectin) or DNA bind collagen, producing false positive hemagglutination reactions and discrepancies in the early literature. Antibodies to native collagen type II are by no means restricted to RA but found at high levels in relapsing polychondritis (RP), lepromatous leprosy (LL) as well as in SLE, scleroderma (Scl) and OA (Fig. 9.7).

Collagen-type specificity of collagen epitopes

Unique dominant epitopes on native collagen II are not expressed on collagens I, III, IV or V. These epitopes are lost after denaturation. Antibodies to native collagen II from patients with RA or lepromatous leprosy do not cross react with collagens I, III, IV or V. On the other hand, denatured collagen expresses new epitopes, absent in the native molecule, which are common to collagen types I, III, IV and V (Fig. 9.8). RA serum antibodies to the collagen II α1 chain also bind the α3 chain of collagen XI. These cross reactive proteins are very similar in primary sequence. Synovial membrane contains collagen types III and V whereas bone contains predominantly type I. Their erosion in RA will lead to release of collagens I, II, III, V, IX and XI and presentation to the immune system, and may lead to the spectrum of anti-collagen antibodies observed in RA (Fig. 9.8).

Antibodies to collagen IX differ from those to types II and XI in

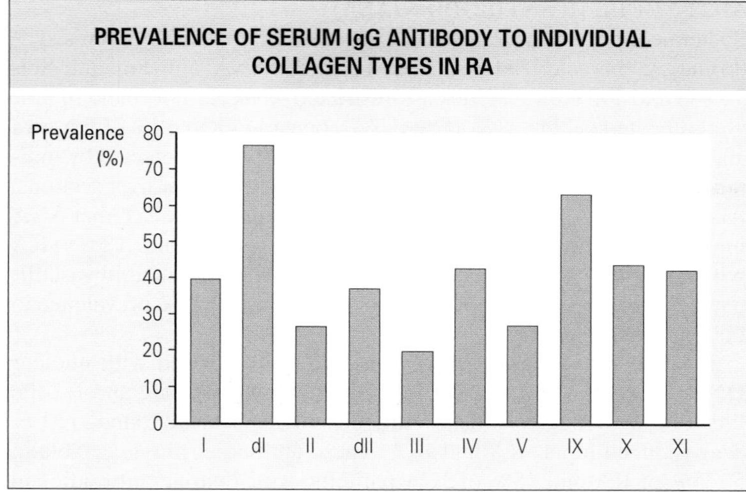

Fig. 9.8 Prevalence of serum IgG antibody to individual collagen types in RA. (d: denatured form.)

PREVALENCE AND PROPORTION OF IgG ISOTYPES IN SERUM ANTI-NATIVE COLLAGEN TYPE II ANTIBODIES FROM RA PATIENTS

IgG subclass	Prevalence of IgG subclass (%)	Proportions of IgG as subclass (%)
1	86	6
2	23	0
3	86	92
4	6	2

Fig. 9.9 Prevalence and proportion of each IgG subclass of anti-native collagen type II in serum of RA patients.

that they are more prevalent in RA (44%) compared with osteoporosis (17%) or Paget's disease (14%), whereas the prevalence of anti-type II and type XI in all three diseases is 30% and 42–52% respectively.

Species specificity of collagen epitopes

Much data on collagen II immunity arises from the use of bovine or chicken collagen, which, although sharing human sequences, also have unique conformational epitopes. RA serum antibody has a higher affinity for denatured, but a lower affinity for native, human collagen II compared to bovine collagen. Antibodies from a significant proportion of healthy and some RA individuals only bind to xenogeneic collagen, raising the possibility of collagen-immunization via dietary intake.

Synovium is a site of collagen antibody synthesis

Antibodies to native and denatured collagen exist in most RA synovial fluids. Antibodies to denatured collagen II are higher in synovial fluid than serum[16] suggesting local immunoglobulin synthesis. Synovial B lymphocytes secreting antibodies to native collagen I or II have been demonstrated in 21 of 27 patients with RA but not in other joint diseases. These cells were detectable in patients lacking serum antibodies to collagen, suggesting that these antibodies are adsorbed by cartilage. Synovial B lymphocytes producing anti-collagen II are only detectable in RA patients expressing the MHC DR4 allele[17], which suggests that this immune response depends on the T cell repertoire, which is shaped through interaction with HLA class II antigen.

Cartilage absorbs antigens and antibodies

Cartilage is a large, exposed matrix containing negatively-charged glycosaminoglycans ready to absorb mobile molecules including antigens, antibody and immune complexes. The superficial layer of cartilage in most RA and a few OA patients contains immunoglobulin, IgG- and IgM-RF, and complement components[18]. Cartilage from 69% of RA patients contains extractable antibodies to native collagen II, even when serum antibody is undetectable. Some is disulfide-bonded to cartilage proteoglycan. Antibodies penetrate normal cartilage to 400μm, but up to 1400μm in RA cartilage. Increased cartilage permeability in RA is due to inflammatory processes such as neutrophil elastase digestion. The consequent presence of immobilized IgG within cartilage matrix may contribute to local macrophage activation and pannus persistence in RA[19].

Pathogenicity of anti-collagen antibody

Immune complexes containing IgG, IgM and collagen are present in both sera and synovial fluids from RA patients[20]. Collagen immune complexes in RA synovial fluid also contain C1q, from complement activation. IgG1 and IgG3 are the most prevalent subclasses of anti-collagen II antibodies in RA (Fig. 9.9) and are highly efficient at fixing complement. IgG3 accounts for the majority, up to 90%, of serum IgG anti-collagen II in RA. Complement activation is an important pathological event mediated by collagen-specific antibodies in the rheumatoid joint and may contribute to pathogenesis of active disease.

Associations of anti-collagen immunity and disease

High levels of serum antibodies to native collagen II are restricted to a subset of patients with RA, leprosy and the rare disease, relapsing polychondritis, whereas low titer antibodies and those to denatured collagen II are found more generally (Fig. 9.7).

Most studies do not find a significant correlation between autoimmunity to collagen II and disease duration, disease activity, ARA functional class, age, sex, race, erythrocyte sedimentation rate (ESR), or the levels of IgG RF or circulating immune complexes (CIC) in RA. Negative data on anti-collagen II antibodies in pre-RA individuals[21] led to proposals that collagen immunization is secondary to cartilage erosion. Positive association with anti-nuclear antibody and with IgM RF has been described. Antibodies to native collagen I have been associated with extra-articular symptoms.

Chondrocyte antigens

Cartilage matrix is synthesized and catabolized by the chondrocyte, a potent source of cartilage autoantigens. MHC class II antigens are inducible on the chondrocyte surface by interferon-γ, facilitating efficient stimulation of memory T cells. On the other hand, chondrocyte membranes themselves, when presented by autologous monocytes, induce vigorous proliferation of T lymphocytes from RA patients. The frequency of chondrocyte-specific peripheral T cells is 10-fold higher in RA than in healthy individuals[22]. This T cell proliferation correlated with the ESR and the presence of ANA but not with the level of IgM RF or disease activity. Although chondrocyte autoantigens cause peripheral T cell activation, it has yet to be shown that synovial lymphocytes also respond.

Serum IgG antibodies to chondrocyte membranes are also elevated in RA[23]. These antibodies do not appear to be synthesized in the joint. As immune complexes, they stimulate chondrocytes *in vitro* to release metalloproteinases, generate superoxide anion and reduce aggrecan synthesis thereby potentially contributing to cartilage erosion.

ANTIGENS IN SYNOVIUM

A set of proteins expressed in both normal and RA synovium bind antibodies in RA synovial fluid. The largest proteins: 140, 160 and 182 kD respectively, are found in synovium, skin, muscle and liver. Antibodies to the smallest proteins: 28, 29 and 30 kD (probably closely related to the RA33 antigen discussed below) are also found in 30% of early RA patients[24]. Antibodies to a soluble 43kD protein found only in RA synovium and an insoluble 53 kD protein are also found in some RA synovial fluids and sera from early RA patients.

The lung and serosa, in addition to synovium, are often inflamed in RA. One common feature is that mesothelial cells in all these tissues contain lamellar bodies which are storage organelles for surfactants and lubricants. The major protein associated with these organelles is surfactant protein A (SP-A) which is highly expressed in RA synovial intima and which shares antigenic determinants with the mycobacterial 65kD heat shock protein.

BACTERIAL IMMUNITY AND RA

Mycobacteria

Heat shock proteins (HSPs) are families of proteins with diverse functions, which are produced on exposure to environmental insults, such as a sudden change in temperature, anoxia, reactive oxygen metabolites or altered glucose level (glucose-regulated proteins: grp).

Heat shock protein antigens in mycobacterial infection and RA

Heat shock protein antigens (HSPs) are dominant immunogens in bacterial, mycobacterial, protozoal and helminthic infections. Mice immunized with *Mycobacterium tuberculosis* (MTb) produce antibodies to HSPs 70, 60, 18 and 12. Human HSP60 and mycobacterial HSP70 have similar sequences (60% homology) raising the possibility of induction of autoimmunity during infection. T lymphocytes to self HSP are detectable in healthy individuals, leading to the conclusion that, despite the risk of autoimmunity, immune recognition of HSP is important to anti-bacterial immunity. High levels of HSP58 epitopes are detectable in the cytoplasm of cells in the synovial lining layer, cartilage/pannus junction and subcutaneous nodules of patients with RA but not in normal tissues. HSP58, 70 and 90 are expressed in the cytoplasm of synovial membrane and fluid cells from RA patients. Levels of IgG and IgA anti-MTb HSP60 and HSP70 are raised in RA and SLE[25], compared with healthy individuals. A reduced level of detectable anti-MTb HSP60 antibodies in synovial fluid suggests they may form complexes with human HSP58 in the joint.

Proteus mirabilis and *Escherichia coli* heat shock proteins and the 'shared epitope'

Proteus mirabilis is associated with upper urinary tract infection. Elevated levels of anti-proteus IgM and IgA antibodies are found in RA, and antiserum to the RA-associated HLA class II allele, DR4, cross reacts with proteus[26]. Anti-proteus antibodies are not raised in other autoimmune states, suggesting a specific association with RA. IgM antibodies to *E. coli* are also raised in RA. Interestingly, the HLA class IIβ chain hypervariable sequence (70–74) QKRAA / RRRAA associated with RA, also known as the shared epitope, binds the *E. coli* 70kD heat shock protein, dnaK[27]. The natural ligand of dnaK is another *E. coli* heat shock protein, dnaJ (40kD), which contains a QKRAA sequence in the dnaK-binding region. Although, unsurprisingly, RA patients have a normal antibody level to dnaJ, antibodies to dnaJ fragments encompassing the shared epitope sequence are significantly raised[28]. Anti-dnaJ immunity is cross reactive with HLA class II, and may give rise to the anti-HLA class IIβ chain antibodies found in RA. Anti-HLA II antibody titers in RA correlate with disease activity and may be immunoregulatory.

ANTI-NUCLEAR ANTIBODIES (ANA)

Systemic lupus erythematosus (SLE), scleroderma and Sjögren's syndrome are characterized by disease-restricted ANA: anti-Sm; anti-Scl-70 and anti-La. However, disease-restricted ANA are not found in RA. Granulocyte-specific ANA (GSANA), appear in up to 68% of RA sera and 20% of juvenile chronic polyarthritis sera[29] when detected by indirect immunofluorescence on human granulocytes and rat liver sections. About half of the GSANA sera are specific for eosinophils. Other ANA include anti-extractable nuclear antigen (ENA) (prevalence 18% in RA with vasculitis); anti-histone, (77% prevalence in rheumatoid vasculitis; 40% in non-vasculitic RA) and anti-chromatin (45% prevalence in both groups).

Histones are found in all tissues tightly associated with nuclear DNA: H2a, H2b, H3 and H4 form the nucleosome core and H1 the linker between nucleosomes. Antibodies to histones are found in SLE, drug-induced lupus, RA and JRA. These antibodies are detectable in 5–75% of RA and 45% of JCA patients. Anti-histone antibodies in SLE patients may recognize all histones, the H2A–H2B or the H3–H4 complexes. The strongest responses are directed against H1 and H2b. Antibodies to H1 predominate in RA patients**.** The incidence of antibodies to the core histones is greater in JCA than in RA and an association of anti-H3 with anterior uveitis has been observed. Anti-histone antibody is associated with rheumatoid vasculitis but not with disease activity or IgM-RF.

Antibodies to HnRNP Proteins A1 and A2 (RA33)

The heterogeneous nuclear RNA products of RNA polymerase II are processed in the nucleus in association with HnRNP (ribonucleoprotein) particles, which contain a core of 6 polypeptides: A1, A2, B1, B2, C1 and C2. These are distinct from the small nuclear ribonucleoproteins (snRNPs), Sm and nRNP, which are recognized by antibodies from SLE patients. Anti-HnRNP A1 antibody, found in 47% of RA patients, cross-reacts with a homologous sequence in keratin. Further antibody cross-reactivity between HnRNP A1 and HnRNP A2 may be due to N terminal homology.

Serum antibodies to HnRNP A2, (RA33), are detected in one–third of RA patients[30]. They may be prognostic of RA in early arthritis (prevalence 23%). Although these antibodies are not found in healthy sera, they are also found in mixed connective tissue disease (MCTD) (38%) and SLE (23%), but in Finland their prevalence in RA is only 7%, limiting their utility. This antibody is infrequently found in JCA. No correlation has been observed between anti HnRNP A2 and either RF, AKA or APF antibody.

ANTI-CYTOPLASMIC ANTIBODIES

Anti-endothelial cell

Rheumatoid vasculitis (RV) is a rare (1% of RA) but serious complication including skin rash, cutaneous ulceration, gangrene, neuropathy and abnormalities of visceral organs (see Chapter 5.4). Patients with RV have higher levels of serum immune complexes, and IgG anti-endothelial cell antibodies (AECA) are common[31]. These antibodies may reflect vascular damage. AECA in SLE include anti-cardiolipin antibody, but their specificity in RA is unclear.

Anti-cardiolipin antibody

Anticardiolipin antibodies in SLE are associated with arterial and venous thromboses, thrombocytopenia, recurrent fetal loss, circulating anticoagulant, cutaneous vasculitis and migraines, features of the 'antiphospholipid syndrome' (see Chapter 7.35). Anticardiolipin antibodies in RA are not associated with antiphospholipid syndrome nor do they produce a positive VDRL or lupus anticoagulant assay. This indicates a qualitative difference in epitope specificity of these antibodies in RA and SLE.

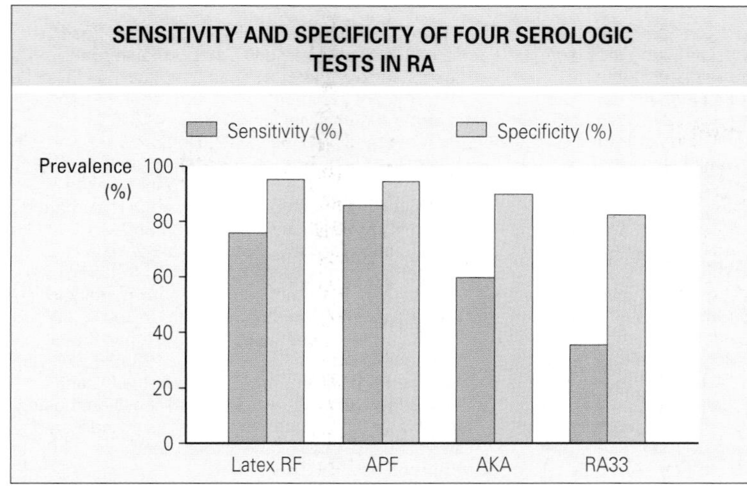

Fig. 9.10 **Sensitivity and specificity of four serologic tests in RA.**

PREVELENCE OF RA-ASSOCIATED AUTOANTIBIODIES IN HEALTHY INDIVIDUALS BEFORE THE ONSET OF RA

AKA−,APF− AKA−,APF+ AKA+,APF+ AKA+,APF−

Prevalence (%) 60 50 40 30 20 10 0

RF+ RF−

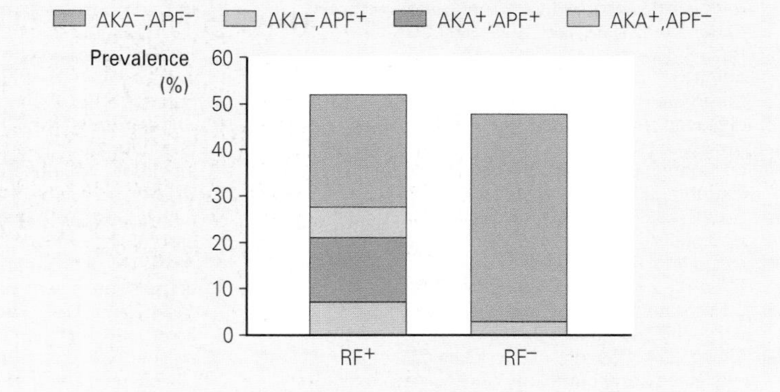

Fig. 9.11 **Antikeratin antibody (AKA) and antiperinuclear factor (APF) prevalencies (%) within RF seropositive and seronegative groups of healthy individuals before the onset of RA.**

Anti-neutrophil cytoplasmic antibody (ANCA)

ANCA are characteristic of vasculitides including Wegener's granulomatosis and are directed against three major antigens: myeloperoxidase, proteinase 3 and lactoferrin (see Chapter 7.19).

However, in RA, the dominant target antigen appears to be different. This antibody is found in 38% of RA patients without vasculitis and is not associated with disease activity, or ANA.

Anti-Ro (SS-A) antibody

Antibodies to the cytoplasmic ribonucleoprotein, Ro, are present in Sjögren's syndrome, scleroderma, polymyositis, MCTD and SLE. This antibody is found in RA, associated with more severe extra-articular but not articular disease, sicca features or disease duration. Anti-Ro may be a marker of patients with RA who respond less well to remission inducing drugs or have a high incidence of side effects to D-penicillamine[32].

OTHER DIAGNOSTIC ANTIBODIES

In addition to RF anti-perinuclear factor (APF) and anti-keratinized epithelial antibody (AKA) may be useful diagnostic markers of RA, being relatively disease-restricted and positive in seronegative RA. The sensitivity and specificity of these three tests compared with the RA33 assay[33–35] is shown in Figure 9.10.

Anti-keratinized epithelium antibody (AKA)

AKA produces a smooth lamellar staining of stratum corneum in the rat mid-esophagus. AKA recognizes three proteins (A: 210kD; B:120–90kD; C130–60kD) related to filaggrin, an intermediate filament aggregating, histidine-rich protein. AKA binds a 40kD neutral/acidic isoform of basic filaggrin in human epidermis[36]. They do not, however, recognize keratohyaline granules, which contain profilaggrin. Although the assay sensitivity is low, specificity for RA is high (95–100%) (Fig. 9.10). AKA is associated with raised CRP, ESR, IgM-RF, subcutaneous nodules and functional criteria such as Steinbrocker's index but not with age, sex, disease duration or other laboratory parameters. In JCA, levels of AKA are lower, the prevalence is 27%, though raised to 42% in seronegative patients with polyarticular onset, and is not associated with disease activity. Up to 30% of pre-RA sera contain IgG-AKA or APF or both (Fig. 9.11), but they are all RF seropositive. This shows that immunological abnormalities precede RA, often by many years, and that there is significant overlap between AKA and APF.

Anti-perinuclear factor (APF)

The perinuclear factor antigen is found in keratohyaline granules of the stratum granulosum layer of epithelium. Only epithelial cells synthesizing soft keratin, such as those of the buccal mucosa and esophageal mucosa, express this antigen whose identity remains unknown. APF is adsorbed on purified epidermal filaggrin and binds to a protein, which also binds AKA[37], suggesting that APF and AKA are overlapping specificities. The antigen source for the APF assay remains human buccal mucosa epithelial cells. The antigen is labile during storage, leading to a variation in assay sensitivity between laboratories. The problem is compounded by variability in antigen expression between donors. APF occurs at titers from 1:5 in healthy individuals to 1:800 in autoimmune patients. The antibody is present in RA, SLE, systemic sclerosis and infectious mononucleosis. The sensitivity of the APF assay, using 1:5 diluted serum, is 86% in RA and its specificity is 96% (Fig. 9.10)[34]. It is usefully present in 40% of RF seronegative RA, associated with more severe disease, higher ARA functional class, more extra-articular features per patient and more rapid radiologic change. The prevalence of APF in JCA patients is only 2%.

REFERENCES

1. Waaler E. On the occurrence of a factor in human serum activating the specific agglutination of sheep blood corpuscles. Acta Pathologica Et Microbiologica Scandinavica 1940;17:172–88.
2. Holmdahl R, Malmstrom V, Vuorio E. Autoimmune recognition of cartilage collagens. Ann Med. 1993;25:251–64.
3. Schroder AE, Greiner A, Seyfert C, Berek C. Differentiation Of B-Cells In the Nonlymphoid Tissue Of the Synovial-Membrane Of Patients With Rheumatoid-Arthritis. Proc Nat Acad Sci. (USA) 1996;93:221–5
4. Parekh RB, Dwek RA, Sutton BJ, et al. Association of rheumatoid arthritis and primary osteoarthritis with changes in the glycosylation pattern of total serum IgG. Nature 1985;316:452–7.
5. Plater-Zyberk C, Maini RN, Lam K, Kennedy TD, Janossy G. A rheumatoid arthritis B cell subset expresses a phenotype similar to that in chronic lymphocytic leukemia. Arthritis Rheum.

1985;28:971–6.
6. Burastero SE, Casali P, Wilder RL, Notkins AL. Monoreactive high affinity and polyreactive low affinity rheumatoid factors are produced by CD5+ B cells from patients with rheumatoid arthritis. J Exper Med. 1988;168:1979–92.
7. Rath S, Hogben DN, Devey ME. Functional affinity of IgM rheumatoid factor in patients with rheumatoid arthritis and other autoimmune diseases. Ann Rheum Dis. 1988;47:291–4.
8. Smiley JD, Sachs C, Ziff M. In vitro synthesis of immunoglobulin by rheumatoid synovial membrane. J Clin Invest. 1968;47:624–32.
9. Roudier J, Petersen J, Rhodes GH, Luka J, Carson DA. Susceptibility to rheumatoid arthritis maps to a T-cell epitope shared by the HLA-Dw4 DR beta-1 chain and the Epstein-Barr virus glycoprotein gp110. Proc Nat Acad Sci (USA).1989;86:5104–8.
10. Carson DA, Pasquali JL, Tsoukas CD, et al. Physiology and pathology of rheumatoid factors. Springer Seminars In Immunopathology 1981;4:161–79.
11. Aho K, Palosuo T, Raunio V, Puska P, Aromaa A, Salonen JT. When does rheumatoid disease start?. Arthritis Rheum. 1985;28:485–9.
12. Jonsson T, Valdimarsson H. Is measurement of rheumatoid factor isotypes clinically useful?. [Review]. Ann Rheum Dis. 1993;52:161–4.
13. Reininger L, Berney T, Shibata T, Spertini F, Merino R, Izui S. Cryoglobulinemia induced by a murine IgG3 rheumatoid factor: skin vasculitis and glomerulonephritis arise from distinct pathogenic mechanisms. Proc Nat Acad Sci (USA). 1990;87:10038–42.
14. Kurt-Jones EA, Liano D, HayGlass KA, Benacerraf B, Sy MS, Abbas AK. The role of antigen-presenting B cells in T cell priming in vivo. Studies of B cell-deficient mice. J Immunol. 1988;140:3773–8.
15. Clague RB, Firth SA, Holt PJ, Skingle J, Greenbury CL, Webley M. Serum antibodies to type II collagen in rheumatoid arthritis: comparison of 6 immunological methods and clinical features. Ann Rheum Dis. 1983;42:537–44.
16. Rowley MJ, Williamson DJ, Mackay IR. Evidence for local synthesis of antibodies to denatured collagen in the synovium in rheumatoid arthritis. Arthritis and Rheumatism 1987;30:1420–5.
17. Ronnelid J, Lysholm J, Engstrom-Laurent A, Klareskog L, Heyman B. Local anti-type II collagen antibody production in rheumatoid arthritis synovial fluid. Evidence for an HLA-DR4-restricted IgG response. Arthritis Rheum. 1994;37:1023–9.
18. Jasin HE. Autoantibody specificities of immune complexes sequestered in articular cartilage of patients with rheumatoid arthritis and osteoarthritis. Arthritis Rheum. 1985;28:241–8.
19. Shiozawa S, Jasin HE, Ziff M. Absence of immunoglobulins in rheumatoid cartilage-pannus junctions. Arthritis Rheum. 1980;23:816–21.
20. Clague RB, Moore LJ. IgG and IgM antibody to native type II collagen in rheumatoid arthritis serum and synovial fluid. Evidence for the presence of collagen-anticollagen immune complexes in synovial fluid. Arthritis Rheum. 1984;27:1370–7.
21. Mottonen T, Hannonen P, Oka M. Antibodies against native type II collagen do not precede the clinical onset of rheumatoid arthritis.. Arthritis Rheum. 1988;31:776–9.
22. Alsalameh S, Mollenhauer J, Hain N, Stock KP, Kalden JR, BurmesterGR. Cellular immune response toward human articular chondrocytes. T cell reactivities against chondrocyte and fibroblast membranes in destructive joint diseases. Arthritis Rheum. 1990;33:1477–86.
23. Mollenhauer J, von der Mark K, Burmester G, Glückert K, Lütjen-Drecoll E, Brune K. Serum antibodies against chondrocyte cell surface proteins in osteoarthritis and rheumatoid arthritis. J Rheum. 1988;15:1811–7.
24. McColl GJ, Cram DS, Harrison LC. Antibodies to Synovial Antigens In Recent-Onset Rheumatoid-Arthritis. Arthritis Rheum. 1995;38:1418–1428
25. Tsoulfa G, Rook GA, Bahr GM, et al. Elevated IgG antibody levels to the mycobacterial 65-kDa heat shock protein are characteristic of patients with rheumatoid arthritis. Scand J Immunol. 1989;30:519–27.
26. Ebringer A, Khalafpour S, Wilson C. Rheumatoid arthritis and Proteus: a possible aetiological association. Rheumatology International 1989;9:223–8.
27. Auger I, Escola JM, Gorvel JP, Roudier J. HLA-DR4 and HLA-DR10 motifs that carry susceptibility to rheumatoid arthritis bind 70-kD heat shock proteins.. Nature Medicine 1996;2:306–10.
28. Albani S, Keystone EC, Nelson JL, et al. Positive selection in autoimmunity: Abnormal immune response to a bacterilal dnaJ antigenic determinant in patients with early rheumatoid arthritis. Nature Medicine 1995;1:448–52.
29. Rosenberg JN, Johnson GD, Holborow EJ, Bywaters EG. Eosinophil-specific and other granulocyte-specific antinuclear antibodies in juvenile chronic polyarthritis and adult rheumatoid arthritis. Ann Rheum Dis. 1975;34:350–3.
30. Hassfeld W, Steiner G, Studnicka-Benke A, Skriner K, Graninger W, Smolen JS. Autoimmune response to the spliceosome. An immunologic link between rheumatoid arthritis, mixed connective tissue disease, and systemic lupus erythematosus. Arthritis Rheum. 1995;38:777–85.
31. Heurkens AH, Hiemstra PS, Lafeber GJ, Daha MR, Breedveld FC. Anti-endothelial cell antibodies in patients with rheumatoid arthritis complicated by vasculitis. Clinical and Experimental Immunology 1989;78:7–12.
32. Drosos AA, Lanchbury JS, Panayi GS, Moutsopoulos HM. Rheumatoid arthritis in Greek and British patients. A comparative clinical, radiologic, and serologic study [see comments]. Arthritis Rheum. 1992;35:745–8.
33. Wolfe F, Cathey MA, Roberts FK. The latex test revisited. Rheumatoid factor testing in 8,287 rheumatic disease patients. Arthritis Rheum. 1991;34:951–60.
34. Janssens X, Veys E, Verbruggen G, Declerq L. The diagnostic significance of the antiperinuclear factor for rheumatoid arthritis. J Rheumatol. 1988;15:1346–50.
35. Vincent C, Serre G, Lapeyre F, Fournie B, Ayrolles CF, Soleilhavoup JP. High diagnostic value in rheumatoid arthritis of antibodies to the stratum corneum of rat oesophagus epithelium, so-called 'anti-keratin antibodies'. Ann Rheum Dis. 1989;48:712–22.
36. Simon M, Girbal E, Sebbag M, Gomes-Daudrix V, Vincent C, Salama G. The cytokeratin filament-aggregating protein filaggrin is the target of the so-called 'antikeratin antibodies,' autoantibodies specific for rheumatoid arthritis. J Clin Invest. 1993;92:1387–93.
37. Sebbag M, Simon M, Vincent C, et al. The antiperinuclear factor and the so-called antikeratin antibodies are the same rheumatoid arthritis-specific autoantibodies. J Clin Invest. 1995;95:2672–9.

10

CELLULAR IMMUNITY IN RA

JS Hill Gaston

- There is no clear candidate autoantigen or foreign antigen that drives the inflammatory process in RA.
- Human leukocyte antigens shape the T-cell repertoire but the effects of HLA-DR4 are not clear in RA patients.
- Joint T-cells are polyclonal; a disease-specific subset has not been identified.
- T-cell cytokines are not abundant in RA joints, but T-cells can drive monokine [interleukin-1 (IL-1), tumor necrosis factor (TNF)] production in RA.
- The TH1 subset [which makes interferon-gamma (IFN-γ)] is more prominent in synovium than the TH2 subset (which makes IL-4) in RA.

INTRODUCTION

The immune system is generally considered to be central to the pathogenesis of rheumatoid arthritis (RA), so the disease is often classified as autoimmune. There are several reasons for this view:

- Components of the immune system are prominent within affected synovial membrane, which can eventually resemble an ectopic lymph node.
- Susceptibility to disease correlates strongly with major histocompatibility complex (MHC) antigens whose function is to control immune responses.
- Finally, various therapies directed against the immune system (cyclosporin A, total lymphoid irradiation) have had some measure of success.

Despite much research effort, so far it has not been possible to determine exactly what aspect of the immune system's function (or malfunction) is responsible for rheumatoid disease. However, given the relatively recent discovery of many important components of the *normal* immune system (e.g. cytokines, lymphocyte co-stimulatory molecules), it is perhaps not surprising that a full immunologic description of RA is still not available.

POSSIBLE TARGETS OF THE IMMUNE RESPONSE IN RA

The immune system's function is the recognition of antigens, so it is natural to ask which are the critical antigens that drive the pathologic immune response in RA. There are two main categories of antigen to be considered – autoantigens and foreign antigens.

AUTOANTIGENS

The immune system is designed to avoid recognition of self, using central (thymus and bone marrow) mechanisms to edit out autoreactive T- and B cells, with back-up peripheral mechanisms to ensure self-tolerance. Nevertheless, it is impossible to construct an immune system with no potential to recognize self, because the set of epitopes ('shapes' recognized by T-cells or antibodies) which makes up 'self' overlaps considerably (possibly completely) with the set of epitopes contained in foreign antigens, particularly those of pathogens. This is particularly the case for proteins which are conserved in function between all living organisms and therefore show structural and sequence similarity, e.g. heat shock proteins (see below). Therefore there is always a potential for autoreactivity. The question in RA is whether the disease is truly autoimmune and, if so, whether any of the proposed candidate autoantigens (Fig. 10.1) play a central role.

Type II collagen

Arthritis can readily be induced in rodents and primates by immunization with heterologous or homologous native type II collagen[1]. Extensive studies of this model have shown that the arthritis requires both collagen-specific B and T-cells, susceptibility depends on MHC antigens[2] and the disease can be modulated by interventions such as depletion of specific T-cells, vaccination against T-cells and induction of tolerance by oral administration of type II collagen[3]. This last observation has led to therapeutic trials of oral collagen in RA, but only some of these have shown positive results[4,5]. Despite the attractiveness of the model and the undoubted lessons learned from it, the importance of immune responses to type II collagen in RA remains unclear. Collagen-specific T- and B cells can be isolated from RA patients[6], but only from a minority; these cells may be easier to find in synovial tissue, but even here they are not invariable. The possibility that they arise secondary to joint destruction and exposure of type II collagen to the immune system has not been entirely discounted, although in a recent study there was no correlation between degree of destruction and presence of collagen-specific B cells in synovial fluid[7]. It can be argued that autoimmunity to type II collagen might occur in humans, but that it would produce polychondritis rather than RA, since the distribution of affected tissues in polychondritis more closely follows the known distribution of type II collagen.

Proteoglycans

There has been much less work on immunity to proteoglycans (PG) in arthritis; mice immunized with human cartilage PG do develop erosive arthritis, but also marked spondylitis[8,9]. This may therefore be a model of ankylosing spondylitis (AS) rather than of RA; indeed, PG-specific T-cells have been identified in AS patients[10]. It is necessary to use fetal PG, since it lacks keratan sulfate, and to digest it to remove chondroitin sulfate; such maneuvers probably help to expose the PG polypeptide to the immune system. These experiments have involved the most abundant PG, aggrecan, but there are many other components of cartilage which could be targets of autoimmunity in RA, particularly the smaller PG molecules such as biglycan and decorin, but these have yet to be tested.

Chondrocyte antigens

It has been suggested that the chondrocyte must be the critical source of autoantigens in RA because joint inflammation subsides when cartilage is completely removed (e.g. at joint replacement), whereas

Fig. 10.1 Candidate antigens for driving the immune response in RA.

CANDIDATE ANTIGENS FOR DRIVING THE IMMUNE RESPONSE IN RA	
A. Autoantigens	B. Foreign Antigens
Type II collagen	Bacteria
Proteoglycans	Viruses
Chondrocyte antigens	Superantigens
Heat shock proteins	
Immunoglobulins	

synovectomy only affords temporary relief. T-cell responses to chondrocyte antigens have been reported in RA and AS, but none of the proteins involved has yet been fully characterized.

Heat shock protein 60

Heat shock protein 60 (hsp60) occurs in all cells; it has an important role in controlling the correct folding of cellular proteins. Thus autoimmune responses to hsp60 would only be expected to cause arthritis if its expression was unusually prominent in the joint – there is some evidence that this is so, but it may be a consequence of inflammation rather than a cause. Interest in this antigen stemmed again from animal studies when mycobacterial hsp60 was shown to be an important T-cell target in adjuvant arthritis[11]. Extensive sequence identity between bacterial and human hsp60 lead to the proposal that T-cells initially triggered to recognize hsp60 in the course of infection might cross-react with the human protein[12]. Although such cross-reactive T-cells have been described they are not confined to RA patients, and their frequency as compared with noncross-reactive T-cells is not known. In adjuvant arthritis it was thought that the mycobacterial hsp60-specific T-cells caused arthritis because they cross-reacted with a component of PG[13], but this has not been shown conclusively. No cross-reactive cells of this kind have been found in human RA.

Paradoxically, when tested using highly purified antigens, RA patients' T-cells are rather *less* responsive to mycobacterial hsp60 than are controls, although they readily recognize other mycobacterial antigens. The significance of this is unclear, but there is evidence that some immune responses to hsp60 may be protective against the development of arthritis, so that a decreased response to hsp60 could reflect an immunoregulatory defect. Thus, in rats arthritis can be prevented by prior immunization with mycobacterial hsp60 – they are no longer susceptible to induction of adjuvant arthritis. The immunization is thought to alter the response to hsp60 from the arthritogenic one, seen when the antigen is presented in the context of killed mycobacteria and oil ('adjuvant'), to recognition which is nonarthritogenic. The change may well reflect the pattern of cytokines produced by T-cells activated in these different ways. It has also been suggested that immunization with bacterial hsp60 produces T-cells which cross-react with human hsp60, but that instead of such cells being mediators of autoimmune disease, they may be able to downregulate inflammatory responses[14]. The idea is that, since hsp60 is generally overexpressed during inflammatory responses, it might be a useful target for immunoregulation by T-cells. Failure to generate these T-cells could lead to a decreased ability to control inflammatory responses.

Immunoglobulins

Rheumatoid factors are autoantibodies directed against the Fc portion of IgG molecules (Chapter 5.09). The affinity maturation characteristic of rheumatoid factors in RA strongly suggests involvement of T-cells in their generation, but it is not clear that this necessarily requires T-cells that also recognize IgG – B cells which make rheumatoid factors can internalize antibody–antigen complexes and present the foreign antigen to T-cells, thereby receiving help for the manufacture and maturation of rheumatoid factor[15] (Fig. 10.2). However, T-cells which recognize immunoglobulin itself have also been identified by investigating T-cell clones reactive with a component in autologous synovial fluid[16].

Conclusion

No definitive autoantigen has been identified in RA. If parallels with insulin-dependent diabetes mellitus and multiple sclerosis hold true, a *number* of different joint antigens may be involved at various stages in the autoimmune process[17,18]. Some of the responses to autoantigens which have been documented may arise as a consequence of joint destruction, and subsequent display to the immune system of joint components not normally accessible to it (e.g. chondrocyte antigens). Currently the amino acid sequences of known joint components are being scanned for peptide sequences which predict binding to HLA-DR4, the HLA antigen conferring susceptibility to RA. This binding

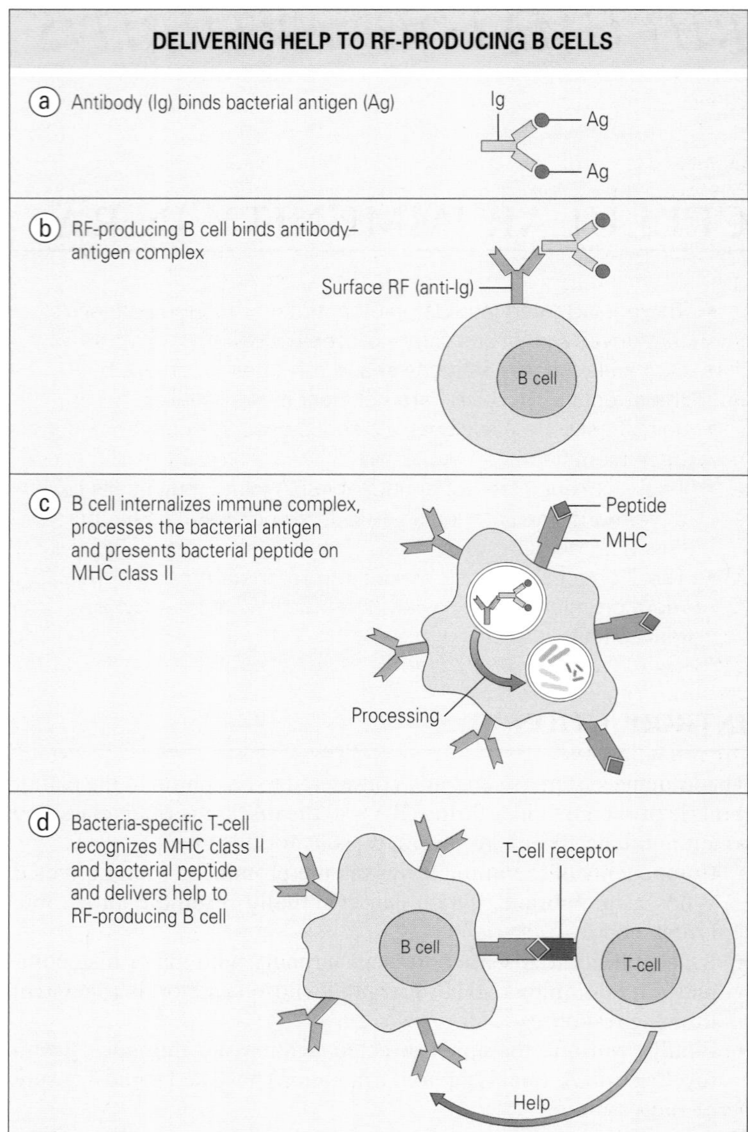

Fig. 10.2 Possible mechanism for delivering help to rheumatoid factor (RF)-producing B cells without requiring autoreactive T-cells.

will then be checked experimentally, and responses to the peptides sought in RA patients and controls. This strategy may allow additional potential autoantigens to be discovered.

FOREIGN ANTIGENS

An infective etiology for RA has often been postulated, but as yet no organism has been implicated.

Bacteria

Bacteria are attractive possibilities; mycobacterial and streptococcal antigens are good inducers of inflammatory arthritis in experimental animals, as are organisms derived from normal gut flora. Whipple's disease is an example of an arthritis caused by an unculturable bacterium now positively identified by sequencing its ribosomal ribonucleic acid (RNA) genes[19]. Since RA does not show the epidemiologic features of a classic infectious disease, a candidate etiologic agent should be ubiquitous and well tolerated by the majority of those infected, with disease only occurring in those with susceptibility genes, such as HLA-DR4 and others as yet unidentified[20]. The relationship between peptic ulcer disease and Helicobacter infection might be taken as a useful model – there is a high incidence of infection in the population, but disease is mainly associated with particular risk factors (smoking, secretor status, etc.).

One such ubiquitous organism is *Escherichia coli*; it has been noted that an *E. coli* heat shock protein, dnaJ, contains a 5 amino acid sequence identical to amino acids 70–74 of HLA-DRB1*0401, the sequence associated with susceptibility to RA, the so-called 'shared epitope'. Patients with early RA have been found to have enhanced responses to dnaJ, especially in synovial fluid. The normal function of dnaJ is to bind to the *E. coli* 70 kDa heat shock protein, dnaK; presumably because of their sequence similarity, some (but not all) DR alleles associated with RA bind to the homologous human hsp, hsp73. It has been suggested that binding to hsp73 in the endoplasmic reticulum may affect the ability of DR molecules to take part in efficient antigen presentation[21], but how such a defect might predispose to RA is not known.

Another bacterial protein which contains a region with some sequence similarity to the shared epitope is the hemolysin of *Proteus mirabilis* [22]. There is evidence which suggests that RA patients have higher titers of antibody to Proteus antigens, but no other convincing data to implicate Proteus infection[23]. As is discussed below (see 'molecular mimicry'), better understanding of the mechanism of T-cell recognition means that less emphasis is now attached to finding short stretches of identical amino acid sequence in bacterial and human proteins.

Viruses

Viruses are known to cause joint inflammation in humans (e.g. rubella, parvovirus B19, arboviruses); also caprine arthritis–encephalomyelitis virus is a retrovirus which causes a chronic rheumatoid-like disease in goats, although only a small number of synoviocytes are infected. Thus considerable effort has gone into the detection of viruses in the synovium, but has produced either negative results or occasional positive results that have not been confirmed. Herpesviruses, such as the Epstein–Barr virus (EBV), cause ubiquitous lifelong infection, so that an abnormal immune response to EBV could be associated with a disease such as RA. Abnormal antibody responses to certain EBV-encoded antigens have been described in RA, particularly an area of glycine repeats in the EBNA-1 antigen[24]. Such glycine repeats appear in several autoantigens (e.g. keratin, fibrillarin) so that the anti-EBNA-1 antibodies can cross-react with self. However, the significance of this cross-reactivity for the pathogenesis of RA remains unknown.

Molecular mimicry

Although bacterial or viral infection might be a direct cause of arthritis, it has often been suggested that disease would occur when foreign antigens 'mimic' autoantigens present in the joint because of similarity in the amino acid sequence (Fig. 10.3). Thus immune responses properly directed against the pathogen could cross-react with self and lead to autoimmunity. When first formulated the idea was thought of in terms of antibody cross-reactivity, which can be demonstrated by showing antibodies that bind to short linear peptides derived from a bacterial or viral protein and an autoantigen (see Fig. 10.3 and, for an example, Schwimmbeck *et al.*[25]). Mimicry is also possible in respect of shared conformational epitopes (those not determined by simple similarity between linear peptides), but is harder to demonstrate.

However, when molecular mimicry at T-cell level is considered the situation is more complex. T-cells recognize short linear peptides bound to MHC, but it is now known that only a small number of amino acids within an antigen are actually necessary for T-cell recognition (Fig. 10.3). The critical amino acids are those which allow binding to MHC and those which make contact with the T-cell receptor. This means that two peptides with a very low level of overall sequence identity can both stimulate T-cells as long as the few critical residues are conserved. For binding to MHC there is usually a choice of preferred amino acids, so the main determinants of specificity are those small number of amino acids which influence interaction with the T-cell receptor, and these need not be contiguous. Thus, while searching protein databases for peptides which share a high degree of sequence identity with a self protein can reveal epitopes which are candidate mimics as far as antibody recognition is concerned, for molecular mimicry at the T-cell level it is necessary to identify the critical residues and then look for peptides which have these features, even if their overall sequence identity is not striking. Such an exercise was recently described with respect to myelin basic protein and certain viral antigens that might be relevant to the pathogenesis of multiple sclerosis (Fig. 10.3 and Wucherpfennig and Strominger[26]).

Superantigens

Superantigens are bacterial or viral proteins which are able to activate large subsets of T-cells because they bind to all T-cell receptors which use certain variable region genes (e.g. Vβ5, Vβ8, etc.); (Fig. 10.4). Acute activation of all T-cells with receptors using, for example, $V\beta8^+$ has been shown to result in the clinical picture seen in toxic shock syndrome caused by staphylococcal superantigens[27]. Early analyses of Vβ gene usage by synovial T-cells indicated a predominance of certain Vβ families, raising the possibility that this represented activation by local superantigens, particularly when the same Vβ families seemed to be depleted from peripheral blood T-cells[28]. However, more recent analyses have not confirmed these initial speculations and a role for superantigens has not been demonstrated clearly. One group of organisms which produce superantigens and have been studied in animal models of arthritis are the mycoplasmas; their possible involvement in RA has long been the subject of speculation.

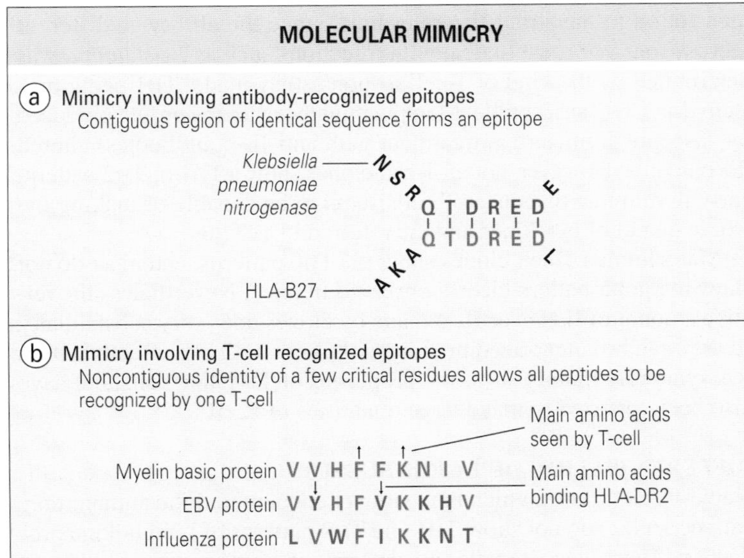

Fig. 10.3 Molecular mimicry of self peptides by foreign peptides has different requirements for antibody and T-cell recognition.

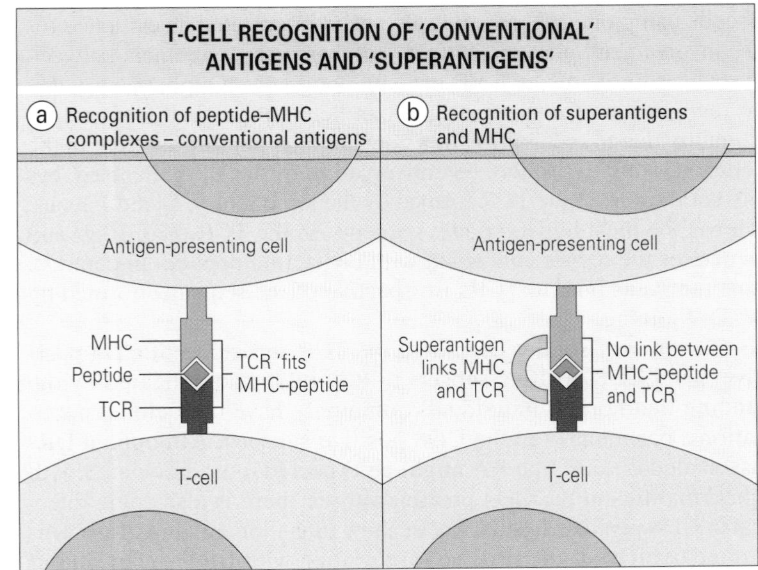

Fig. 10.4 Comparison of T-cell recognition of (TCR) 'conventional' antigens and 'superantigens'.

THE T-CELL RECEPTOR REPERTOIRE IN RA

The uncertainty surrounding the antigens which drive the cellular immune response in RA has led to studies of T-cell receptors (TCRs), since this approach might give clues to pathogenesis. Both the total set of TCR available to RA patients' immune systems ('global repertoire') and those expressed in the joint have been examined.

GLOBAL REPERTOIRE

Rheumatoid arthritis is associated with HLA-DR4; as well as presenting foreign antigens to T-cells, DR4 molecules in the thymus play a role in the selection of the T-cells released to populate the periphery. Those with a high affinity for self peptides bound to DR4 are deleted ('negative selection'), but T-cells which can interact to some extent only with DR4–self peptide are allowed to mature ('positive selection')[29]. Therefore the total set of T-cell receptors available to recognize antigen will be different in DR4 positive and DR4 negative individuals, and so their ability to respond to certain antigens will differ. It can be argued that DR4 positive patients might lack the T-cells needed to respond efficiently to an important pathogen – i.e. they would have a 'hole' in their repertoire. Such 'holes' have been hard to demonstrate in humans; since DR4 has been maintained at a relatively high frequency in the population (ca. 20%), it is more likely that the T-cell repertoire with which it is associated is beneficial to human survival. However, a repertoire which was efficient at dealing with, say, mycobacteria might be maintained even if it carried a higher chance of responding inappropriately to joint antigens.

Monozygotic twins discordant for RA have been studied in the search for associations between repertoire and disease. Differences are seen but there is no consistent feature common to affected twins[30]. However, it has to be remembered that monozygotic twins do not have identical T-cell repertoires since T-cell receptors are generated by chance recombinations, rather than by inheritance.

TCR REPERTOIRE IN THE JOINT

The use of TCRs by synovial T-cells has been studied to see whether there is a disease-specific population of T-cells with similar receptors, referred to as 'oligoclonality'. In experimental autoimmune diseases, autoantigen-specific T-cells commonly use a very restricted number of TCR genes, so diseases can be treated by depleting all T-cells using one family of TCR genes (e.g. Vβ8 in murine collagen-induced arthritis). Although oligoclonality was found in early studies of synovium[31], the results are difficult to interpret because in these studies the synovial T-cell population was commonly expanded *in vitro* so that the 'oligoclonality' observed was almost certainly generated *in vitro* by unequal rates of growth from the starting population. Dominance of T-cells using one Vβ gene has also been interpreted as evidence for the involvement of a superantigen, but there is no agreement between investigators as to which Vβ gene predominates. Oligoclonality due to recognition of a superantigen can be distinguished from oligoclonality due to recognition of a conventional peptide antigen; in the latter, not only will there be conservation of the Vβ gene used, but also of the part of the TCR formed by the joining of V, D and J genes. This is the most hypervariable sequence in the TCR (Fig. 10.5) and generates the region concerned with contacting peptide. In contrast, superantigens bind to TCRs irrespective of the sequence formed by V–D–J joining.

More recent studies examined the TCR repertoire of CD4 positive[32] and CD8 positive subsets in RA; this is complicated by the finding that normal individuals commonly have oligoclonal populations, particularly in the CD8 positive subset[33]. Although a DR-associated disease like RA might be expected to be associated with abnormalities in the CD4 positive subset, there is also some interest in CD8 positive T-cells. These show oligoclonality in Felty's syndrome (which has the strongest association with DR4)[34], but similar oligoclonality of this subset has been described in RA without Felty's syndrome[35].

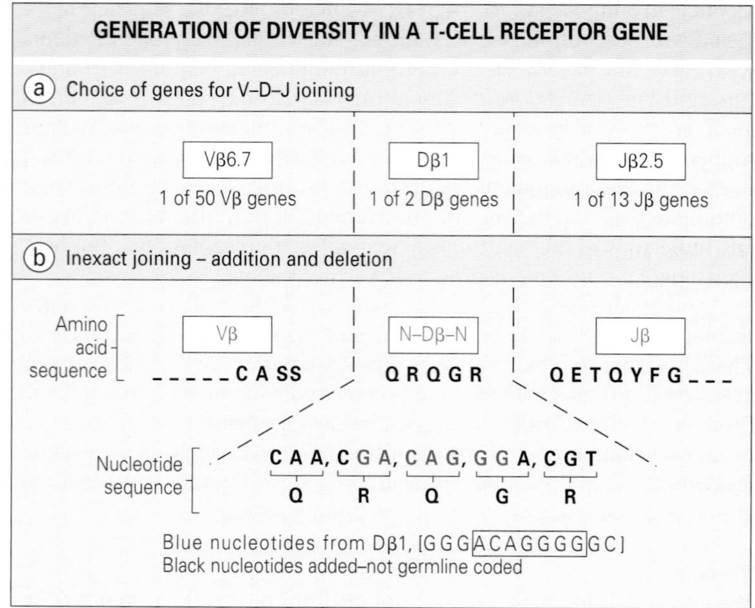

Fig. 10.5 Generation of diversity in a T-cell receptor gene.

CHARACTERISTICS OF THE IMMUNE RESPONSE IN RA

The consequences of an immune response do not depend primarily on the kind of antigen recognized, but on the cytokines which are produced, which reflects the properties of the activated T-cells, particularly their differentiation state.

T-CELL SUBSETS

The nature of a cell-mediated response is determined by the subset of T-cells involved. In addition to the early subdivision of T-cells into helper and cytotoxic, it has been possible to recognize subsets which produce different sets of cytokines[36]. This was first demonstrated in the mouse where established T-cell clones show two polar patterns of cytokine production: TH1 cells produce IFN-γ, lymphotoxin and IL-2, whereas TH2 cells produce IL-4, -5, -6, -9 and -10; IFN-γ and IL-4 are the two cytokines used to classify T-cells as TH1 and TH2. Both subsets can make IL-3, granulocyte–macrophage colony-stimulating factor (GMCSF), TNF and chemokines. The TH1 subset is important in mediating delayed type hypersensitivity responses, whereas TH2 cells induce IgE synthesis and eosinophil recruitment, and thus mediate allergic responses. These subdivisions based on *in vitro* testing of clones were then found to have real-life relevance, since the ability of different inbred strains of mice to deal with infections such as *Leishmania* was determined by the kind of T-cell response they made, TH1 being protective and TH2 susceptible. Manipulating the cytokine profile produced by susceptible mice (e.g. treatment with anti-IL-4 antibodies) altered the outcome. However, not all T-cell clones show a TH1 or TH2 pattern; early in immune responses T-cells seem to be capable of making the whole gamut of cytokines and are referred to as TH0.

Many human T-cell clones show the TH0 patterns, and most do not show the polar pattern clearly observed in mice. Nevertheless the relative amount of IFN-γ or IL-4 made by clones does vary substantially so they can be categorized broadly as TH1- or TH2 like. T-cells within RA synovium mainly show the properties of TH1-like cells, but have also been reported to make large quantities of IL-10 [37].

DIFFERENTIATION OF T-CELL SUBSETS

Naive T-cells (those which have not yet encountered the antigen they can recognize) do not show TH1 and TH2 patterns of lymphokine production. These characteristics are determined after activation with antigen and subsequent differentiation. They are influenced by the presence of cytokines during differentiation: IL-4 favors the production of TH2 cells whereas IL-12, IFN-γ and transforming growth factor beta (TGF-β) favor TH1 cell development. In addition IL-10 inhibits cytokine production by TH1 cells whereas IFN-γ inhibits TH2 cell proliferation. Thus the two T-cell subsets interact with each other by production of IL-4, IFN-γ and IL-10; IL-12 is derived from macrophages, and the IL-4 required early in immune responses may come from a newly defined CD4 negative, CD8 negative T-cell subset, or from mast cells.

It would be very convenient if T-cells in different subsets could be readily distinguished by their expression of surface markers; unfortunately this is not the case and has given rise to some confusion. As cells change from naive to experienced (or memory) they alter their expression of different isoforms of the CD45 surface marker (termed RA, RB, RC, RO). Naive cells are CD45-RA$^+$, RO$^-$, RB^{bright}, whereas memory cells are CD45-RA$^-$, RO$^+$, RB^{dull}. Since naive and memory cells differ in their cytokine production (naive mainly make IL-2 alone) at one time CD45-RA$^+$ and CD45-RO$^+$ cells were thought to represent sub-divisions equivalent to the TH1 and TH2 subsets described in mice. CD45-RO$^+$ cells were described as 'helper-inducer' and CD45-RA$^+$ as 'suppressor-inducer' because of their effects on *in vitro* antibody synthesis. However, it is now clear that these divisions bear no relationship to the TH1 and TH2 subsets, all of which are antigen-experienced and therefore CD45-RO$^+$.

T-CELL SUBSETS IN THE JOINT

The joint contains a preponderance of memory T-cells, which inevitably produces differences in functional tests between synovial fluid-derived T-cells and those of peripheral blood, which contains equal proportions of naive and memory cells. This preponderance of memory T-cells in the joint reflects recruitment to the synovium since, by virtue of their expression of adhesion molecules, memory cells have preferential access to inflamed tissues. This has been elegantly demonstrated by experiments that raise skin blisters over intradermal challenges with a recall antigen such as PPD, and examination of the phenotype of the cells entering the blister[38].

What is the activation state of synovial T-cells? If joint inflammation is driven by T-cell recognition of antigen, it might be predicted that a population of T-cells in the joint would be actively dividing, secreting cytokines and showing surface markers associated with activation such as the IL-2 receptor. However, this is only true to a limited extent. Only a small proportion of synovial T-cells are actively dividing and, while they do express certain activation markers such as CD69 and HLA-DR, others, particularly the IL-2 receptor, are absent[39,40]. The T-cell specific cytokine IFN-γ can be detected in the joint, particularly by using sensitive techniques such as polymerase chain reaction or intracellular staining, but positively stained T-cells are present in small numbers[41] and free cytokine is scarcely detectable in comparison with the readily detected monokines IL-1 and TNF-α. However, it is noteworthy that a similar proportion of IFN-γ secreting T-cells is seen in the murine type II collagen-induced arthritis, a model which is known to be completely T-cell dependent. There is general agreement that IL-4 is not usually demonstrable in the RA joint and so the T-cell response can be classified as TH1-like. Indeed, TH2 cytokines such as IL-4 and IL-13 modulate monokine and enzyme production by RA synovial tissue *ex vivo*, and can decrease joint inflammation and cartilage destruction when administered in animal models of arthritis. This has not yet been tried in human studies.

One curious feature of the surface phenotype of synovial T-cells is that it is characteristic of neither resting cells nor those activated in conventional ways. As noted, levels of IL-2 receptor are low, but both the early marker of activation CD69 and the late appearing HLA-DR are both prominent. 'Early' and 'late' are defined by *in vitro* studies of T-cell activation by antigens and mitogens, but such definitions may not apply to T-cell activation *in vivo*. As judged by their expression of the CD45-RB isoform, synovial T-cells appear to be highly differentiated since they have very low levels which only occur *in vitro* after multiple rounds of cell division (Fig. 10.6)[42]. Normally such cells have a high likelihood of undergoing apoptosis because they express high levels of the apoptosis-promoting molecule *Fas* and low levels of the apoptosis-protecting molecule *bcl-2*. Despite this phenotype few of the synovial T-cells can be shown to have undergone apoptosis (in contrast to the marked levels of apoptosis shown by synovial lining cells in the rheumatoid joint). It seems that they are protected from dying by factors within the synovial environment, including IL-15, a recently described product of macrophages and fibroblasts[43].

Studies of the phenotype of synovial T-cells have been conducted in the context of established and often chronic disease so that they probably tell us nothing about the role of these cells in the initiation of rheumatoid synovitis. Nevertheless, even in established disease certain T-cell modulating therapies (e.g. total lymphoid irradiation) are effective in diminishing synovitis, suggesting a continuing role for cell-mediated immune processes, although their role may be different in disease maintenance compared with initiation.

The activation phenotype of synovial T-cells may be important for their role in joint destruction since recent experiments have shown that activated T-cells can induce the production of collagenase from synoviocytes by cell–cell contact rather than by secretion of cytokines[44]. Thus persistence of the activated phenotype in the joint might be an important factor in chronic synovitis.

CONCLUSIONS

- It has not yet been established whether the cellular immune response which drives joint inflammation in RA is directed against autoantigens or exogenous antigens.
- CD4 positive T-cells in the joint are not oligoclonal, nor does usage of one TCR variable gene family predominate, as would be expected if superantigens were important in the etiology. The findings are consistent with the hypothesis that inflammation is driven by a small number of antigen-specific T-cells. Oligoclonal CD8 positive populations have been described, but their function is still mysterious.
- Synovial T-cells are enriched for memory cells and are maintained in a highly differentiated state, possibly by factors in the local environment. Antigen presentation and costimulatory activities of synoviocytes are greatly enhanced compared with those in peripheral blood. Many of the T-cells show features associated with activation but only a few make lymphokines, mainly those associated with the TH1 subset.
- The monokine production which is responsible for the features of inflammation and joint destruction may be due to a combination of antigen-specific T-cells producing small but important quantities of lymphokines and cell-surface effects of nonspecifically activated T-cells.

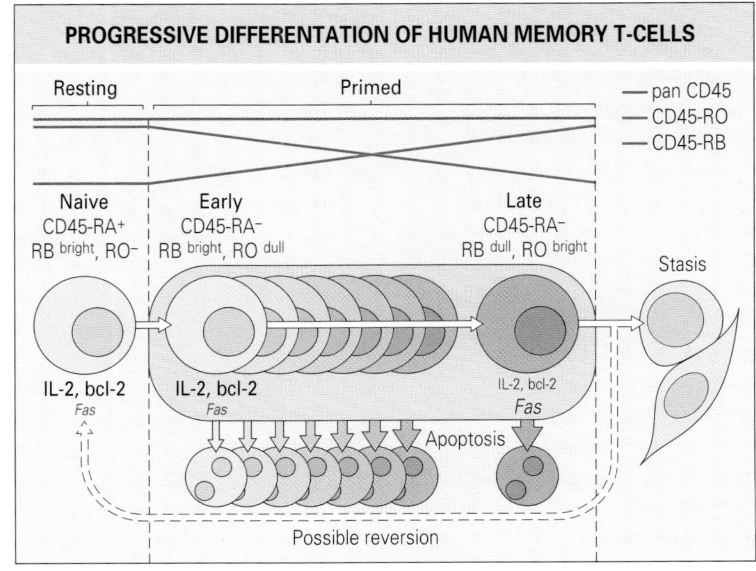

Fig. 10.6 The progressive differentiation of human memory T-cells. (With permission from Salmon and Gaston[42]).

REFERENCES

1. Holmdahl R, Klareskog L, Rubin K, *et al.* Role of T lymphocytes in murine collagen induced arthritis. Agents Actions. 1986;19:295–305.
2. Brunsberg U, Gustafsson K, Jansson L, *et al.* Expression of a transgenic class II Ab gene confers susceptibility to collagen-induced arthritis. Eur J Immunol. 1994;24:1698–702.
3. Yoshino S, Quattrocchi E, Weiner HL. Suppression of antigen-induced arthritis in Lewis rats by oral administration of type II collagen. Arthritis Rheum. 1995;38:1092–6.
4. Trentham DE, Dynesius-Trentham RA, Orav EJ, *et al.* Effects of oral administration of type-II collagen on rheumatoid arthritis. Science. 1993;261:1727–30.
5. Sieper J, Kary S, Sorensen H, Alten R, Eggens U, Huge W, *et al.* Oral Type II collagen treatment of early rheumatoid arthritis: a double-blind, placebo-controlled, randomized trial. Arthritis Rheum. 1996;39:41–51.
6. Londei M, Savill C, Verhoef A, *et al.* Persistence of collagen type II specific T-cell clones in the synovial membrane of a patient with rheumatoid arthritis. Proc Natl Acad Sci USA. 1989;86:636–40.
7. Ronnelid J, Lysholm J, Engstrom Laurent A, Klareskog L, Heyman B. Local anti-type II collagen antibody production in rheumatoid arthritis synovial fluid – evidence for an HLA-DR4-restricted IgG response. Arthritis Rheum. 1994;37:1023–9.
8. Glant T, Mikecz K, Arzoumanian A, Poole A. Proteoglycan induced arthritis in BALB/c mice. Clinical features and histopathology. Arthritis Rheum. 1987;30:201–12.
9. Goodacre JA, Pearson JP. Human cartilage proteoglycans as T-cell autoantigens. Ann Rheum Dis. 1992;51:1094–7.
10. Mikecz K, Glant T, Baron M, Poole A. Isolation of proteoglycan specific T lymphocytes from patients with ankylosing spondylitis. Cell Immunol. 1988;112:55–63.
11. Van Eden W, Thole J, Van der Zee R, *et al.* Cloning of the mycobacterial epitope recognized by T lymphocytes in adjuvant arthritis. Nature. 1988;331:171–3.
12. Life PF, Bassey EOE, Gaston JSH. T-cell recognition of bacterial heat-shock proteins in inflammatory arthritis. Immunol Rev. 1991;121:113–35.
13. Van Eden W, Hogervorst E, Hensen E, Van der Zee R, Van Embden J, Cohen I. A cartilage mimicking T-cell epitope on a 65K mycobacterial heat shock protein: adjuvant arthritis as a model for human rheumatoid arthritis. Curr Top Microbiol Immunol. 1989;145:27–43.
14. Anderton SM, Van der Zee R, Prakken B, Noordzij A, Van Eden W. Activation of T-cells recognizing self 60-kD heat shock protein can protect against experimental arthritis. J Exp Med. 1995;181:943–52.
15. Roosnek E, Lanzavecchia A. Efficient and selective presentation of antigen–antibody complexes by rheumatoid factor B cells. J Exp Med. 1991;173:487–9.
16. Van Schooten WCA, Devereux D, Ho CH, Quan J, Aguilar BA, Rust CJJ. Joint-derived T-cells in rheumatoid arthritis react with self-immunoglobulin heavy chains or immunoglobulin-binding proteins that copurify with immunoglobulin. Eur J Immunol. 1994;24:93–8.
17. Steinman L. Multiple sclerosis: a co-ordinated immunological attack against myelin in the central nervous system. Cell. 1996;85:291–7.
18. Tisch R, McDevitt H. Insulin-dependent diabetes mellitus. Cell. 1996;85:291–7.
19. Relman DA, Schmidt TM, MacDermott RP, Falkow S. Identification of the uncultured bacillus of Whipple's disease. New Engl J Med. 1992;327:293–301.
20. Silman AJ. Is rheumatoid arthritis an infectious disease? Br Med J. 1991;303:200–1.
21. Auger I, Escola J, Gorvel J, Roudier J. HLA-DR4 and HLA-DR10 motifs that carry susceptibility to rheumatoid arthritis bind 70-kD heat shock proteins. Nature Med. 1996;2:306–10.
22. Ebringer A, Cunningham P, Ahmadi K, Wrigglesworth J, Hosseini R, Wilson C. Sequence similarity between HLA-DR1 and DR4 subtypes associated with rheumatoid arthritis and Proteus/Serratia membrane haemolysins. Ann Rheum Dis. 1992;51:1245–6.
23. Gaston H. Proteus – is it a likely aetiological factor in chronic polyarthritis? Ann Rheum Dis. 1995;54:157–8.
24. Vaughan JH. The Epstein–Barr virus in autoimmunity. Springer Semin Immunopath. 1995;17:203–30.
25. Schwimmbeck P, Yu D, Oldstone M. Autoantibodies to HLA-B27 in the sera of HLA-B27 patients with ankylosing spondylitis and Reiter's syndrome. J Exp Med. 1987;166:173–81.
26. Wucherpfennig KW, Strominger JL. Molecular mimicry in T-cell-mediated autoimmunity: Viral peptides activate human T-cell clones specific for myelin basic protein. Cell. 1995;80:695–705.
27. Choi Y, Kotzin B, Herron L, Callahan J, Marrack P, Kappler J. Interaction of *Staphylococcus aureus* toxin 'superantigens' with human T-cells. Proc Natl Acad Sci USA. 1989;86:8941–5.
28. Paillard X, West S, Lafferty J, *et al.* Evidence for the effects of a superantigen in rheumatoid arthritis. Science. 1991;253:325–9.
29. Allen PM. Peptides in positive and negative selection – a delicate balance. Cell. 1994;76:593–6.
30. Kohsaka H, Taniguchi A, Chen PP, Ollier WER, Carson DA. The expressed T-cell receptor V-gene repertoire of rheumatoid arthritis monozygotic twins – rapid analysis by anchored polymerase chain reaction and enzyme-linked immunosorbent assay. Eur. J Immunol. 1993;23:1895–901.
31. Stamenkovic I, Stegagno M, Wright K, *et al.* Clonal dominance among T lymphocyte infiltrates in arthritis. Proc Natl Acad Sci USA. 1988;85:1179–83.
32. Khazaei HA, Lunardi C, So AK. CD4 T-cells in the rheumatoid joint are oligoclonally activated and change during the course of disease. Ann Rheum Dis. 1995;54:314–17.
33. Morley JK, Batliwalla FM, Hingorani R, Gregersen PK. Oligoclonal CD8(+) T-cells are preferentially expanded in the CD57(+) subset. J Immunol. 1995;154:6182–90.
34. Bowman SJ, Sivakumaran M, Snowden N, *et al.* The large granular lymphocyte syndrome with rheumatoid arthritis – immunogenetic evidence for a broader definition of Felty's syndrome. Arthritis Rheum. 1994;37:1326–30.
35. Hingorani R, Monteiro J, Furie R, *et al.* Oligoclonality of V beta 3 TCR chains in the CD8(+) T-cell population of rheumatoid arthritis patients. J Immunol. 1996;156:852–8.
36. Mosmann T, Sad S. The expanding universe of T-cell subsets: TH1, TH2 and more. Immunol. Today. 1996;17:138–46.
37. Cohen SBA, Katsikis PD, Chu CQ, *et al.* High level of interleukin-10 production by the activated T-cell population within the rheumatoid synovial membrane. Arthritis Rheum. 1995;38:946–52.
38. Pitzalis C, Kingsley G, Covelli M, Meliconi R, Markey A, Panayi G. Selective migration of the human helper-induced memory T cell subset – confirmation by in vivo cellular kinetic studies. Eur J Immunol. 1991;21:369–76.
39. Pitzalis C, Kingsley G, Lanchbury J, Murphy J, Panayi G. Expression of HLA–DR, DQ, and DP antigens and interleukin-2 receptor on synovial-fluid T-lymphocyte subsets in rheumatoid arthritis – evidence for frustrated activation. J Rheumatol. 1987;14:662–6.
40. Afeltra A, Galeazzi M, Ferri G, *et al.* Expression of CD69 antigen on synovial fluid T cells in patients with rheumatoid arthritis and other chronic synovitis. Ann Rheum Dis. 1993;52:457–60.
41. Ulfgren AK, Lindblad S, Klareskog L, Andersson J, Andersson U. Detection of cytokine producing cells in the synovial membrane from patients with rheumatoid arthritis. Ann Rheum Dis. 1995;54:654–61.
42. Salmon M, Gaston JSH. The role of T-lymphocytes in rheumatoid arthritis. Br Med Bull. 1995;51:332–45.
43. Akbar AN, Borthwick NJ, Wickremasinghe RG, *et al.* Interleukin-2 receptor common gamma-chain signaling cytokines regulate activated T-cell apoptosis in response to growth factor withdrawal: selective induction of anti-apoptotic (*bcl*-2, *bcl*-x(L)) but not pro-apoptotic (*bax, bcl*-x(S)) gene expression. Eur J Immunol. 1996;26:294–9.
44. Miltenburg AMM, Lacraz S, Welgus HG, Dayer JM. Immobilized anti-CD3 antibody activates T-cell clones to induce the production of interstitial collagenase, but not tissue inhibitor of metalloproteinases, in monocytic THP-1 cells and dermal fibroblasts. J Immunol. 1995;154:2655–67.

NEUROPEPTIDES AND FREE RADICALS IN RA

Martin Lotz

- Neuropeptides and oxygen-derived free radicals are important in the pathogenesis of RA.
- Neuropeptides such as substance P increase vascular permeability and activate leukocytes and mesenchymal cells.
- Superoxide anion is responsible for oxygen-radical mediated damage through mechanisms of cytotoxicity, degradation of extracellular matrix, and production of inflammatory mediators.
- Nitric oxide derived from cytokine-activated chondrocytes and cells within the synovium causes chondrocyte apoptosis and modules matrix turnover.

INTRODUCTION

Tissue injury caused by the inflammatory process in rheumatoid arthritis (RA) predominantly occurs in the synovium, articular cartilage and bone. Other organs, most commonly lungs and pericardium, can also be affected. Rheumatoid vasculitis is associated with the development of digital infarcts and sensory neuropathy, but this is pathogenetically distinct from the mechanisms leading to cartilage and bone destruction. However, vasculitis may also contribute to extra-articular manifestations in lungs and heart. Tissue injury (Fig. 11.1) is the result of an interplay between cellular and humoral immune and inflammatory systems (see also Chapters 1.7 & 1.8). Activation of endothelial cells is required for the attachment and subsequent migration of leukocytes into the joint. The complement and contact systems are the sources of preformed soluble mediators of inflammation that can be activated rapidly by specific proteases. Neuropeptides function as preformed cellular mediators of inflammation and their immediate release following injury is an important component in the initiation of an inflammatory response. Neuropeptides and humoral mediators of inflammation activate the endothelium and increase vascular permeability. Leukocytes infiltrate the synovial tissue and fluid. Resident cells in synovium, cartilage and bone also become part of the pathogenetic process (see also Chapter 5.13). They are activated to produce inflammatory mediators and proteases. Synoviocytes undergo pathologic proliferation while cell death of articular chondrocytes is part of cartilage injury. Cell-derived mediators of inflammation and tissue damage include cytokines, autoantibodies, lipid metabolites, oxygen radicals and proteases. The interactions of the different cell types and mediator systems trigger cell death and degradation of extracellular matrix, the final common events in the generation of tissue damage in cartilage and bone. The first part of this chapter reviews the role of neuropeptides in pathogenesis. The second part discusses the contribution of oxygen-derived free radicals in the induction of tissue damage.

INFLAMMATORY SYSTEMS AND TISSUE DAMAGE
Activation of neurovascular inflammatory pathways
Neuropeptide release Mast cell activation Vasodilation Plasma extravasation Endothelial cell activation
Activation of humoral inflammatory system
Complement Contact system
Leukocyte infiltration and activation in synovium and synovial fluid
Monocytes Release of cytokines, prostaglandins, oxygen radicals, antigen presentation Lymphocytes T-helper function for autoantibody production Cytokine production Neutrophils Degranulation, radical production
Activation of resident connective tissue cells
Synoviocytes Abnormal proliferation, cytokine and protease release Chondrocytes Cytokine, protease release; cell death Osteoclasts Bone resorption

Fig. 11.1 Inflammatory systems and tissue damage.

THE CONTRIBUTION OF NEUROPEPTIDES TO JOINT INFLAMMATION AND TISSUE DAMAGE

Certain clinical findings suggest an involvement of the nervous system in the pathogenesis of RA. The distribution of synovitis is usually symmetric. Joints in the paretic side of hemiplegic patients who later develop RA are spared from the inflammatory process and the development of erosions. Similarly, gout or Heberden's nodes are less common on paralyzed limbs. In the rat, adjuvant-induced arthritis (which is also a symmetric arthropathy) is less severe in limbs that have been denervated prior to the induction of arthritis. Furthermore, joints that are more severely affected have a higher density of innervation by nociceptive primary afferents.

The nervous system can influence immune and inflammatory responses in arthritis by at least four different mechanisms (Fig. 11.2). First, are the well characterized effects of neuropeptides, such as substance P (SP) or calcitonin gene-related peptide (CGRP), that are released from sensory neurons. Second, a contribution of the autonomic nervous system is suggested by effects of sympathectomy on experimentally induced arthritis and in patients with RA. Third, interactions between the central nervous system (CNS) and the immune and inflammatory response are also important. Cytokines that are produced in the

NEURAL INFLUENCES ON IMMUNE AND INFLAMMATORY RESPONSES
Neuropeptide release from sensory neurons at sites of inflammation
Effects of autonomic nervous system on lymphoid organs
Release of pituitary hormones; effects on leukocytes
Production of neuropeptides by leukocytes and mesenchymal cells

Fig. 11.2 Neural influences on immune and inflammatory responses.

inflamed joints enter the circulation and induce changes in the CNS. Conversely, CNS-derived hormones have effects on the cells that initiate and maintain the inflammatory response in the joint. A fourth level at which neuropeptides may contribute to synovitis is through their production by leukocytes and mesenchymal cells in the joint. These four mechanisms are discussed below, after a review of joint innervation.

NORMAL JOINT INNERVATION AND CHANGES IN ARTHRITIS

Cutaneous afferents and branches of adjacent muscle afferents innervate the joints (Fig. 11.3). Sensory innervation extends into joint capsule, ligaments, subchondral bone, periosteum and synovium. Cartilage is aneural[1]. Unmyelinated Group IV or C sensory nerve fibers containing neuropeptides, such as SP or CGRP, are present in the synovial lining and sublining tissue and in the vascularized peripheral parts of the joint menisci. Furthermore, periosteum, bone marrow and epiphyseal growth plates are innervated, whereas innervation of the diaphyseal and metaphyseal bone is more sparse[2]. Normal synovial tissue is richly innervated with both sensory and sympathetic nerves[3,4]. Sympathetic fibers are exclusively located around blood vessels. Mast cells and afferent nerve terminals are frequently observed in all parts of the normal synovium and densities of mast cells appear to be greatest at sites proximal to the nerve terminals[5]. Some of the pro-inflammatory effects of neuropeptides from sensory fibers are mediated by the activation of mast cells (see below).

Several structural and functional changes occur in joint innervation during the course of arthritis. Electrophysiologic studies have demonstrated that within the range of normal joint movement there is little afferent traffic. Intense deformation or inflammation-induced expansion within the joint will evoke activity in the Group III or A delta fibers[6,7]. During acute experimentally induced synovial inflammation a marked sensitivity to modest movement of the affected joint or a hyperalgesia is observed[8]. Similarly, the acute phases of human arthritis are almost invariably associated with an exquisite hyperalgesia.

Joint pain in arthritis is predominantly a consequence of inflammation.Other mechanisms that can induce joint pain are changes in blood flow in subchondral bone, activation of nerve fibers in the periosteum during bone resorption and by osteophytes, inflammation of ligaments or distention of the joint capsule. Activation of sensory nerve fibers induces nociceptive responses that result in the subjective experience of pain. However, in chronic or long-standing arthritis, even in cases with pronounced synovial thickening and cartilage destruction, often only a relatively low level of pain is reported. This appears to be related to changes in synovial innervation that result from the chronic inflammation. Inflamed synovium from adjuvant arthritic rats shows an absence of SP and CGRP nerves in heavily infiltrated villous synovial tissue, whereas healthy synovial tissue and noninflammatory areas are innervated by SP and CGRP nerves close to normal synovial tissue resident cells[9]. With the lower density of nerve fibers in arthritic synovium, there is also a decrease or absence of nerve-associated mast cells[5]. A similar loss in nerve fibers is seen in human RA synovium. This shows innervation typical of that seen in normal human synovium in the deep tissue layers, but fibers immunoreactive for SP are absent in the more superficial layers. In addition, immunostaining of neuropeptides in the deep tissue is weaker in the arthritic synovium than in normal controls[10,11]. These findings suggest either that neuropeptides are depleted from the nerves or that formation of new nerve fibers may occur at a slower rate than proliferation of rheumatoid synovium. Nerve fibers may also be destroyed by locally produced proteolytic enzymes and various reactive oxygen species in the vicinity of inflammatory cells. Collectively, these findings raise the possibility that the discrepancy between the prominent synovial thickening and the relatively low degree of tenderness in some patients with chronic arthritis may be at least in part due to changes in the density of sensory fibers.

JOINT INNERVATION			
Receptor type	Morphology	Location	Function
Type I	Thinly encapsulated globular corpuscles	Joint capsule (superficial)	Static and dynamic mechanoreceptors
Type II	Thickly encapsulated conical corpuscles	Joint capsule (deep layer)	Dynamic mechanoreceptors
Type III	Thinly encapsulated fusiform corpuscles	Surfaces of ligaments	Dynamic mechanoreceptors
Type IVa	Tridimensional plexus of unmyelinated fibers	Joint capsule fat pads	Nociceptive receptors
Type IVb	Free unmyelinated nerve endings	Joint capsule ligaments, Subchondral bone, Periosteum, Synovium	Nociceptive receptors

Fig. 11.3 Joint innervation. Adapted from Wyke[1].

NEUROPEPTIDES RELEASED FROM PRIMARY SENSORY AFFERENTS

Several observations from experimentally induced arthritis suggest a pro-inflammatory role of neuropeptides that are released from sensory neurons. In adjuvant-induced arthritis the ankle joints are more severely involved and more densely innervated by SP-containing fibers than are the knee joints. Slow infusion of SP into a knee increased the severity of the adjuvant-induced swelling, bone loss and cartilage degradation. Selective destruction of SP-containing neurons by treatment with the neurotoxin capsaicin reduced the inflammatory response in this model[12]. Substance P is the best studied neuropeptide from the unmyelinated primary afferents. In addition to SP, other neuropeptides are released from the peripheral terminals. Somatostatin, vasoactive intestinal peptide and CGRP are regulators of smooth muscle tone, secretion of exocrine glands and leukocyte function.

Substance P was discovered in the 1930s as a peptide that stimulated salivary gland secretion and its role in nociception is now clearly established[13]. It is a member of the tachykinin family of structurally related peptides that share the common C-terminal sequence Phe-Xaa-Gly-Leu-Met-NH_2 where the terminal residue contains an amide group. Substance P is generated from two preprotachykinin genes. Alpha-preprotachykinin contains a single SP sequence while beta-preprotachykinin contains SP and sequences that encode other tachykinins. The primary translation products are prohormones that are processed proteolytically into mature peptides. Preprotachykinin gene expression and peptide processing are functions of sensory neurons in the dorsal horn and dorsal root ganglia. In these neurons chronic nociceptive stimuli cause adaptation of gene expression, which may be mediated by nerve growth factor. Mature peptides are released at the peripheral terminals and also into the spinal cord. In both body fluids and at the surface of cells, SP is degraded by different proteinases. Synovial fibroblasts express on their cell surface neutral endopeptidase 24.11 and dipeptidyl(amino)peptidase IV that are capable of cleaving SP[14].

The tachykinins act mainly by activating three neurokinin (NK) receptors, NK-1, NK-2 and NK-3; SP has highest affinity for the NK-1 receptor. These three receptors have been molecularly characterized by complementary deoxyribonucleic acid (cDNA) cloning and functional expression, and all are members of the superfamily of receptors coupled to regulatory G proteins. Second messenger systems known to be activated by tachykinin receptor stimulation include the hydrolysis of inositol-containing phospholipids by a phospholipase C mechanism[15]. In some cell types, such as mast cells and keratinocytes, SP regulates secretory function or proliferation, but NK-1 receptors are apparently not expressed, suggesting interaction with other receptor molecules. Expression of NK receptors undergoes adaptive changes during inflammation. Very high concentrations of SP receptor binding sites were expressed in colon tissue and within the germinal center of lymph nodules from ulcerative colitis and Crohn's disease patients. Expression of a variety of other neuropeptide receptors did not differ between inflamed and normal colon tissue[16]. Specific, high-affinity binding sites for SP were localized to vascular endothelial cells in human synovial tissue. These binding sites had characteristics of the NK-1 receptor subtype[17].

The interaction of SP with cellular receptors triggers a cascade of events which results in characteristic biological responses.

PRO-INFLAMMATORY EFFECTS OF SUBSTANCE P

Substance P has been studied extensively as a mediator of pain and inflammation. Studies in cell culture and experimental models of joint disease support a role of SP in the pathogenesis of arthritis. The wheal and flare response in the skin is the classic example of a neurogenic inflammatory response. Activation of the peripheral terminals of the unmyelinated type IV or C fibers initiates signals that reach central terminals in the spinal cord (orthodromic) and trigger release of SP. These signals also reach branching points of axon collaterals and are conducted antidromically to other peripheral terminals in the innervated tissues. This causes release of SP and CGRP and results in the wheal and flare response, mainly due the effect of these peptides on blood vessels. Many of the vascular changes associated with acute inflammation, including vasodilation, increased vascular permeability and margination of polymorphonuclear neutrophil leukocytes (PMN), can be induced by the direct application of SP[18].

During joint inflammation neuropeptides are released from the peripheral terminals after activation by bradykinin, serotonin, K^+, H^+, histamine and movement. The primary afferent fibers are sensitized by prostaglandins (PGs), bradykinin or adenosine[13]. Synovial fluid SP levels exceed plasma levels in most types of arthritis and are elevated in RA, osteoarthritis (OA), Reiter's syndrome and post-traumatic arthritis[19].

Substance P promotes pro-inflammatory responses by acting on different cell types in the extravascular space (Fig. 11.4). In mononuclear phagocytes, SP induces directly or in combination with other stimuli the production of PGE_2 and a large number of cytokines[20]. Monocytes of patients with RA released a significantly higher amount of oxygen-radical intermediates than did those of normal controls after treatment with SP[21]. In human neutrophils, SP induced the activation of respiratory burst, and the secretion of specific and azurophilic granules[22]. This required high concentrations of the peptide. However, potent synergistic effects of nanomolar doses of SP were observed on the migratory and cytotoxic functions of human PMNs stimulated by the chemotactic peptide fMLP and complement C5a. This synergism between SP and chemotactic peptides suggests that neurogenic stimuli may prepare neutrophils for an exaggerated inflammatory response to other phlogistic mediators[23].

In lymphocytes, SP can alter proliferation and induce phenotypic changes. These effects are mediated by specific high-affinity SP receptors which have been characterized both kinetically and biochemically[24]. Lymphocytes from RA patients may be more sensitive to the effects of SP than similar cells from normal donors[25]. Mast cells are intermediates in some of the pro-inflammatory effects of SP. SP causes degranulation of mast cells[26,27]; also wheal and flare responses induced by intradermal injection of SP are inhibited by antihistamines. Fibroblast proliferation is an important component in the formation of rheumatoid pannus. Substance P enhances proliferation of human skin and lung fibroblasts[28,29] and rheumatoid synoviocytes[30]. In fibroblast-like cells from rheumatoid synovium, SP also induces the synthesis and release of collagenase[30].

PRO-INFLAMMATORY EFFECTS OF SUBSTANCE P	
Target	Effect
Blood vessels	Vasodilatation and plasma extravasation
Mast cells	Histamine release
Monocytes	Cytokine synthesis
Synoviocytes	PGE_2 release, collagenase production, proliferation
PMN	Granule release, oxygen radical production
T-lymphocytes	Proliferation

Fig. 11.4 Pro-inflammatory effects of substance P.

INTERACTIONS OF SUBSTANCE P WITH OTHER MEDIATOR SYSTEMS

Substance P is part of a network of inflammatory mediators. It can stimulate the production of other regulatory factors, such as cytokines from monocytes or histamine from mast cells, which in turn modulate the function of other cell types. Interactions between SP and other factors can be additive, synergistic or antagonistic. Intra-articular injection of interleukin-1 (IL-1) or tumor necrosis factor (TNF) in rabbit knees increases the number of leukocytes in the joint fluid and causes cartilage degradation. Both cytokines also increase SP levels in the joint fluid[31]. Treatment with indomethacin or dexamethasone reduced leukocyte counts, and PGE_2 and SP concentrations, but not IL-1-induced proteoglycan loss. Elevated SP and PGE_2 in the joint may thus amplify or sustain an initial receptor-mediated inflammatory response to IL-1 and is a stimulus for the continued production of IL-1 and other cytokines.

Similar interactions occur between kinins and SP. Kinins belong to the group of inflammatory mediators that stimulate SP release. In a blister model in the rat footpad, perfusion of bradykinin elicited both vasodilation and plasma extravasation responses. In rats pretreated as neonates with capsaicin to destroy primary sensory afferents, the inflammatory response to bradykinin was significantly smaller. Nitric oxide (NO), a potent endothelial cell-derived vasorelaxation factor, was suggested as an additional intermediate since the selective inhibitor of NO synthase, N^G-nitro-L-arginine, attenuated the inflammatory response to bradykinin in normal rats. Vasodilation and plasma extravasation induced by direct application of SP were reduced by an inhibitor of nitric oxide formation[32].

The interaction with CGRP, which is usually colocalized and coreleased with SP, is additive or synergistic. Vasoactive intestinal peptide (VIP) has qualitatively opposing effects to SP in the regulation of inflammation and smooth muscle contraction. A comparative study addressed the effects of the different peptides from the sensory nerve fibers using knee perfusion with capsaicin as an experimental model of neurogenic inflammation. Perfusion of capsaicin into the knee joint increased plasma extravasation. In contrast, perfusion of SP or CGRP, which are released by acute capsaicin administration, had no significant effect on plasma extravasation. Coperfusion of these two neuropeptides, however, evoked an increase in plasma extravasation that was greater and of longer duration than that produced by capsaicin alone[33].

Antagonistic interactions in both the induction of pain and in inflammatory responses occur between SP and opioid peptides. Receptor-selective opioid agonists inhibited extravasation induced in the rat knee joint by continuous perfusion of either bradykinin or capsaicin. Selective delta- or kappa-opioid agonists attenuated the bradykinin effects. In contrast, coperfusion of a selective mu-opioid agonist did not reduce bradykinin-induced plasma extravasation, but was able to completely inhibit the plasma extravasation produced by capsaicin. Inhibition of neurogenic plasma extravasation by receptor-selective opioids may thus depend on the relative contribution to plasma extravasation of unmyelinated afferent and sympathetic postganglionic neuron terminals[34].

THE AUTONOMIC NERVOUS SYSTEM IN ARTHRITIS

Sympathetic efferent neurons can affect inflammatory and immune responses through several mechanisms. Sympathetic nerve stimulation increases vascular permeability and plasma extravasation. This is reduced after sympathectomy[35]. Neuropeptide Y-containing postganglionic nerves are present in the synovium and are thought to mediate the reflex neurogenic inflammation in the limb contralateral to the affected limb. An interaction with nociceptive neurons has also been demonstrated. Activation of the nociceptive afferents increases the activity of the postganglionic sympathetic efferents. Rats that have been treated with guanethidine monosulfate, which depletes catecholamines by selectively destroying the sympathetic postganglionic neurons, show a decreased severity of joint erosions during adjuvant-induced arthritis[36]. In spontaneously hypertensive rats, the experimentally induced arthritis was also more severe as compared with nonhypertensive rats. Furthermore, adrenalin and β_2-adrenergic receptor agonists exacerbate arthritis[37].

Lymphoid tissues are innervated by sympathetic neurons and direct contacts between lymphocytes and noradrenergic nerve fibers have been demonstrated in the spleen[38]. Postganglionic sympathetic efferents are activated by local stimuli via a spinal reflex and release noradrenalin, adenosine triphosphate (ATP), adenosine, PGI_2, PGE_2, IL-1 and neuropeptide Y. Beta-adrenergic receptors are present on lymphocytes and effects of the sympathetic nervous system on immune responses have been demonstrated *in vitro* and *in vivo*.

There is also some clinical evidence that supports a role for the sympathetic nervous system in synovitis. Regional sympathetic blockade with guanethidine monosulfate resulted in clinical improvement in RA[39]. Adult RA patients have high sympathetic activity. Severe autonomic dysfunction has been observed in patients with juvenile RA and patients with reflex sympathetic dystrophy may have synovitis.

INTERACTIONS BETWEEN CNS AND THE INFLAMMATORY RESPONSE

The CNS induces adaptive changes in response to stress. This occurs through the release of corticotropin-releasing hormone (CRH) in the hypothalamus and noradrenergic neurons in the brainstem. The peripheral limbs involved with the stress response are the hypothalamic–pituitary–adrenal (HPA) axis and the autonomic (sympathetic) system (Fig. 11.5). Dysregulation of the stress system has been implicated in the development of experimentally induced inflammation. The susceptibility of female Lewis (LEW/N) rats to the development of streptococcal cell wall-induced arthritis and other autoimmune phenomena is associated with the inability of their HPA axis to adequately respond to inflammatory stimuli. In contrast, the relative resistance to inflammatory disease in Fischer (F344/N) rats is related to their potent HPA axis response to the same stimuli[40]. *In vivo* studies also showed that LEW/N pituitary adrenocorticotropic (ACTH) responses to exogenous CRH were blunted compared to those in F344/N.

Immune cytokines not only activate immune function, but also recruit central stress-responsive neurotransmitter systems in the modulation of the immune response and in adaptive behaviors during injury or inflammation. Peripherally generated cytokines, such as IL-1, signal hypothalamic CRH neurons to activate pituitary–adrenal counter-regulation of inflammation through the anti-inflammatory effects of glucocorticoids. Corticotropin-releasing hormone not only activates the pituitary–adrenal axis, but also sets in motion a coordinated series of behavioral and physiologic responses, suggesting that the CNS may coordinate both behavioral and immunologic adaptation during stressful situations. Pathophysiologic perturbation of this feedback loop may contribute to the development of inflammatory syndromes, such as RA.

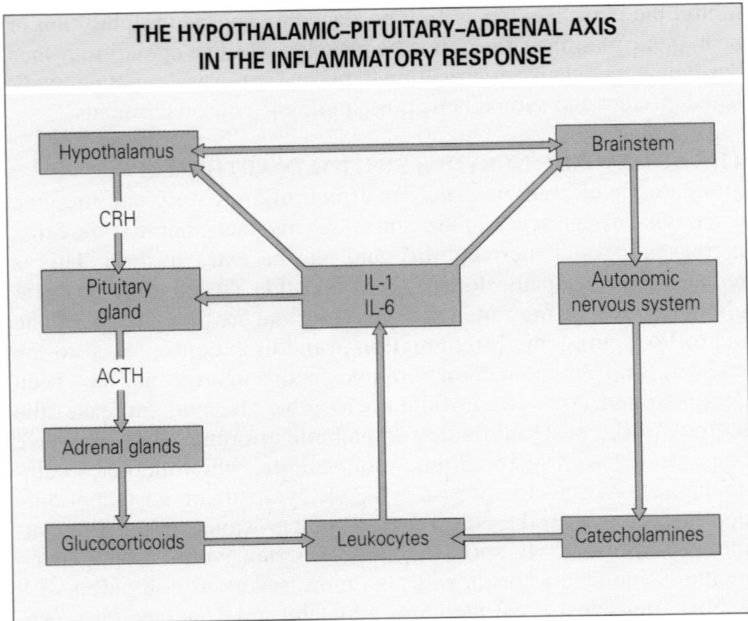

Fig. 11.5 The hypothalamic–pituitary–adrenal axis in the inflammatory response.

One study examined the HPA axis in RA patients and found mildly deficient adrenocortical responsiveness with a compensatory elevation in basal evening ACTH concentrations. However, it was not clear whether this was related to a pre-existing abnormality, active disease or drug therapy[41].

NEUROPEPTIDES PRODUCED OUTSIDE THE NERVOUS SYSTEM

A phenomenon that has clearly been established and is beginning to be understood in its biological and pathogenetic significance is the production of certain neuropeptides by cells outside the nervous system. Recent findings indicate that neuropeptides from non-neuronal sources may play a role in activating receptors on neurons; a second function of these peptides may be in the regulation of non-neuronal cell function (Fig. 11.6).

Cells of the immune system contain receptors for neuroendocrine hormones and are also a source of pituitary and hypothalamic peptides. The pro-opiomelanocortin (POMC) gene encodes a family of peptides originally identified in the pituitary gland. An important POMC-derived peptide hormone, ACTH, is also produced by leukocytes and modulates *in vitro* immune functions. The structure and pattern of synthesis of these peptides by leukocytes appear similar to those of neuroendocrine hormones, although some differences exist. POMC messenger ribonucleic acid (mRNA) expressed in the pituitary utilizes all three exons, while a majority of POMC mRNA expressed in lymphocytes lacks exons 1 and 2. Once secreted, these peptide hormones may function as endogenous regulators of the immune system, as well as messengers from the immune to the neuroendocrine system.

Mitogen-activated lymphocytes release ACTH with an antigenic specificity identical to pituitary-derived ACTH. The material is biologically active and stimulates the *in vitro* release of corticosterone from cocultured rat adrenal cells[41]. The plasma hormone concentrations contributed by lymphocytes usually do not reach these levels when the pituitary gland is the source, but because immune cells are mobile they have the potential to locally deposit the hormone at the target site. Likewise, other studies show that cells of the neuroendocrine system contain receptors for cytokines and can also be considered a source of cytokines, particularly IL-1 and IL-6. The cytokines, including IL-1, IL-2, IL-6, interferon-gamma (IFN-γ), and TNF, exert profound effects on the hypothalamic–pituitary axis[42].

The high level expression of the preproenkephalin gene by murine lymphocytes was an unexpected observation[43]. During a screen for induction-specific cDNAs, preproenkephalin mRNA was found to represent up to 0.5% of the total mRNA in activated cells, but was absent in resting cells. Induced T-helper cell culture supernatants had met-enkephalin-immunoreactive material. Similar activation-dependent expression of this gene was found in normal human peripheral blood mononuclear cells. Monocytes, but not T-cells, secreted completely processed met-enkephalin peptides[44]. Human articular chondrocytes also express high levels of preproenkephalin mRNA. Chondrocytes store met-enkephalin intracellularly and secrete this neuropeptide in both mature and precursor forms. Gene expression is inducible by

PERIPHERAL PRODUCTION AND EFFECTS OF NEUROPEPTIDES

Peptide	Cell source	Function
ACTH	Lymphocytes	Immunosuppression
Enkephalins	Lymphocytes Monocytes Fibroblasts Chondrocytes	Regulation of cell proliferation Peripheral analgesia
Opioids	Lymphocytes Macrophages	Peripheral analgesia

Fig. 11.6 Peripheral production and effects of neuropeptides.

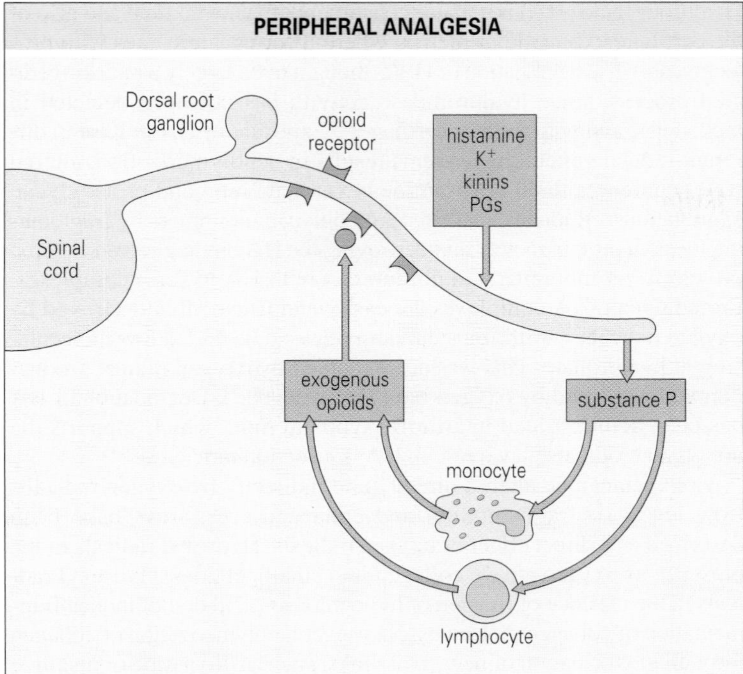

Fig. 11.7 Peripheral analgesia.

serum factors. High levels of preproenkephalin mRNA are detected in proliferating chondrocytes, but not in confluent, contact-inhibited cells. Furthermore, transforming growth factor beta (TGF-β) and platelet derived growth factor (PDGF) upregulate gene expression while IL-1, an inhibitor of chondrocyte proliferation, suppresses expression of this gene. Proliferating, but not resting, cells express preproenkephalin mRNA, suggesting a dependence on and potentially a role in the regulation of cell proliferation[45]. This notion was supported by the finding of nuclear localization of the enkephalin precursor, proenkephalin, in fibroblasts and myoblasts. In fibroblast cell populations that are in transitional to growth arrest, proenkephalin responds promptly to mitogen withdrawal and cell–cell contact by transient changes in nuclear distribution. A similar phenomenon is observed in myoblasts undergoing differentiation. The recognition of growth arrest and differentiation signals by nuclear proenkephalin suggests its integration with transduction pathways mediating these signals[46].

A second effect of peripherally produced opioid peptides, which has received much attention recently, is in the regulation of pain (Fig. 11.7). The antinociceptive effects of opioids were initially ascribed to events within the CNS. However, recent studies indicate that opioids can inhibit pain by binding to specific receptors at the peripheral sensory nerve endings[47]. The opioid receptors are produced by the neuronal cell body in the dorsal root ganglion and transported to both the peripheral and central terminals. An abundance of opioid-containing cells is present in inflamed synovial tissues[48] and the immune cell-derived opioid peptides can activate opioid receptors on peripheral sensory nerves to inhibit inflammatory pain. Opioid release from lymphocytes and macrophages within inflamed tissue is stimulated by corticotropin-releasing hormone or IL-1[49]. This mechanism is likely to be activated in inflammation since leukocytes and joint tissue cells produce opioid active peptides. Enkephalin immunoreactivity can be detected in synovial fluids from arthritis patients, is also present in rheumatoid synovium and is produced by cultured synoviocytes and chondrocytes. A role for locally produced opioids in the regulation of pain in arthritis has been demonstrated. Patients undergoing arthroscopic knee surgery received naloxone intra-articularly or intravenously. All pain scores were higher in the group where the intra-articular opioid receptors were blocked with naloxone[49].

FREE RADICALS AND TISSUE DAMAGE

A large body of information supports a role for free radicals in the pathogenesis of arthritis; studies on experimental models of arthritis suggest that inhibitors of free radical production or radical scavengers are of potential therapeutic value. The most important free radical species in biological systems are derivatives of molecular oxygen, sulfhydryl or nitrogen compounds, polyunsaturated fatty acids, quinones and quinone-like compounds. Previously this field was predominantly concerned with the oxygen-derived free radicals, superoxide and hydroxyl. The production of superoxide by intact cells was first demonstrated by Babior *et al.* in 1973[50], who showed that leukocytes incubated with latex particles produced an activity that reduced cytochrome C and had the characteristics of superoxide. Since the demonstration in 1987 that NO can be produced by mammalian cells, interest in this area of research has rapidly expanded. First, because of the diverse physiologic and pathogenetic effects of NO and, second, because of the interactions of NO and superoxide to form peroxynitrite, a highly reactive species which may account for much free-radical induced toxicity.

Free radicals are chemical species that possess one or more unpaired electrons. In contrast, stable compounds have even numbers of electrons, paired in orbitals with opposite spins whose magnetic fields neutralize each other. A free radical has either an odd number of orbital electrons, with one unpaired, or pairs of electrons of the same spin isolated singly in separate orbitals. The presence of one or more unpaired electrons causes the species to be attracted to a magnetic field. Molecular oxygen (O_2) is a biradical, having two unpaired electrons of parallel spin in its outer orbitals. The reactivity of O_2 is reduced because of the parallel directions of spin of the unpaired electrons.

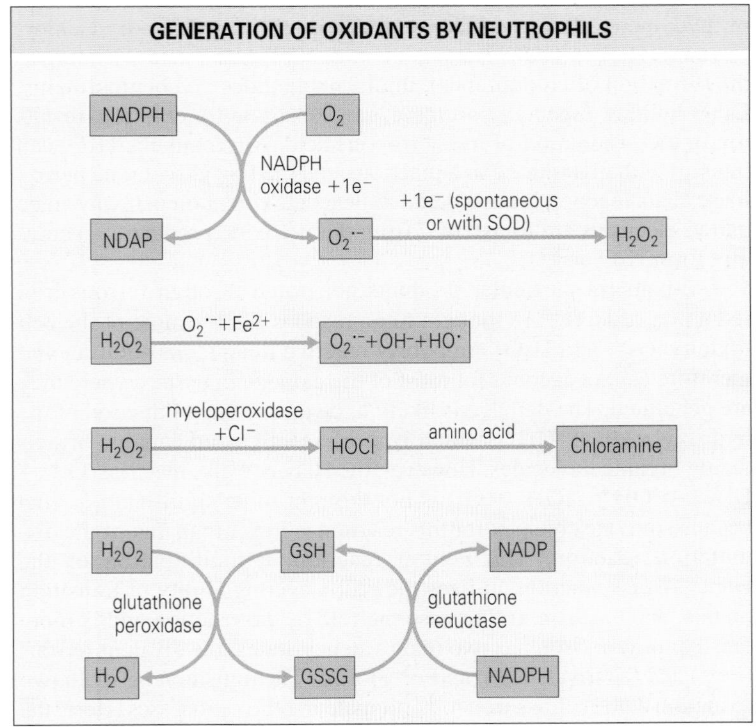

Fig. 11.8 Oxygen radical production. Activation of the neutrophil membrane NADPH oxidase is a consequence of neutrophil stimulation. Single electrons are transferred to O_2 to generate the superoxide anion ($O_2^{\bullet-}$). Hydrogen peroxide (H_2O_2) is generated by transfer of a second electron. This occurs spontaneously at a slow rate and at a much more rapid rate in the presence of the enzyme superoxide dismutase (SOD). In the presence of ferous iron (Fe^{2+}) and $O_2^{\bullet-}$, H_2O_2 can be further reduced to the hydroxyl radical ($HO^\bullet$). Alternatively, in the presence of the enzyme myeloperoxidase and a source of halide, e.g. Cl^-, H_2O_2 can be converted to hypochlorous acid (HOCl) and subsequently, in the presence of an amino acid source, to chloramine. Finally, H_2O_2 can be metabolized via glutathione peroxidase into H_2O with the concomitant oxidation of reduced glutathione (GSH). This last pathway probably serves to detoxify H_2O_2 under most conditions.

When O_2 reacts with an atom or molecule with the more usual unpaired electron configuration, it has a tendency to take one electron at a time, resulting in the formation of superoxide ($O_2^{\bullet-}$) (Fig. 11. 8). This exists in equilibrium with a protonated form, the perhydroxyl radical ($HO_2^{\bullet}$). More reactive forms of O_2, known as singlet oxygens, can be formed with the input of energy.

The single covalent bond between two molecules or atoms can be considered as sharing of a pair of electrons. Fission of this bond in the presence of sufficient energy leads to the formation of a free radical. Asymmetric dissociation is termed heterolysis, symmetric dissociation is termed homolysis. Each of the species produced is a radical and can initiate further chain reactions. The rate of propagation of radical chain reactions depends upon the reactivity of the radicals with the substrates available.

Free radicals are produced during many biological processes by mitochondria, and enzymatic reactions of xanthine oxidase, aldehyde oxidase, flavin dehydrogenase generate superoxide. All cell types produce small amounts of oxygen radicals within their cytoplasm. However, phagocytes, including neutrophils, mononuclear phagocytes and eosinophils, have the nicotinamide–adenine dinucleotide diphosphate (NADPH) oxidase system. When these cells are stimulated by particulate materials, such as immune complexes, crystals or bacteria, or by nonparticulate materials, such as cytokines, neuropeptides, complement C5a, Fc fragments of immunoglobulins, leukotriene B4, platelet activating factor or fMLP, they undergo a respiratory burst with a marked increase in oxygen consumption. This is associated with increased glucose metabolism via the hexose monophosphate shunt whereby NADPH production increases and the NADPH oxidase cytochrome B system is activated, leading to the production of superoxide. Spontaneous breakdown of $O_2^{\bullet-}$ is slow, but more rapid in the presence of superoxide dismutase to form hydrogen peroxide (H_2O_2). H_2O_2 can be metabolized through various pathways. In the presence of myeloperoxidase and chloride it can be converted into hypochlorous acid (HOCl). HOCl is a potent oxidant of amino acids (leading to the formation of chloramines), thiols, nucleotides and hemoproteins. Other halides, especially bromide, can substitute for chloride, resulting in the production of hypobromous acid. Alternatively, H_2O_2 can interact with glutathione in a reaction catalyzed by glutathione peroxidase. This reaction is considered to be a detoxification pathway since paired electrons are transferred from the peroxide product to eventually form H_2O and O_2.

Oxidants, in particular products generated through ferrous iron reduction of H_2O_2, are thought to be responsible for most of the cell toxicity. $O_2^{\bullet-}$ and H_2O_2 are poorly reactive in aqueous solution and therefore cannot account for most of the damage in tissues where they are generated. The damage is likely to be due to the production of the hydroxyl radical ($OH^{\bullet}$), which is more reactive and capable of oxidizing organic molecules. However, the Haber–Weiss reaction ($O_2^{\bullet-} + H_2O_2 \rightarrow OH^{\bullet} + OH^- + O_2$) is not thought to be significant *in vivo* because the rate constant for this reaction is lower than that of the dismutation reaction. The Fenton reaction, a modification of the Haber–Weiss reaction, utilizes the redox cycling ability of transition metals, such as iron, to increase the rate of the reaction and is more feasible *in vivo*. Iron has two main valency states, the divalent ferrous (Fe^{2+}) and the trivalent ferric (Fe^{3+}) forms. The transition between two oxidation states allows iron to participate in redox processes. Here, the $O_2^{\bullet-}$ radical both dismutates to form H_2O_2 and reduces iron complexes to the ferrous form ($O_2^{\bullet-} + Fe^{3+} \leftrightarrow O_2 + Fe^{2+}$). Fe^{2+} ions and H_2O_2 then react to form hydroxyl radicals ($OH^{\bullet}$), which react with almost every molecule found in living cells.

OXYGEN RADICALS AND EXTRACELLULAR MATRIX DEGRADATION

Oxygen radicals can cause joint tissue damage through several mechanisms. They lead directly and indirectly to the degradation of extracellular matrix, affect cell proliferation and survival, and modulate the production of pro-inflammatory mediators (Fig. 11.9).

Hyaluronic acid (HA) is a major constituent of synovial fluid and also of the cartilage extracellular matrix, where it forms aggregates with proteoglycans. The degradation of HA is thought to be largely a radical-mediated process, since hyaluronidase activity has not been detected in leukocytes, synovial fluid or cartilage[51]. Exposure of HA *in vitro* to different radical generating systems results in depolymerization, altered water content, altered hexosamine:hexuronate ratio and proteoglycan aggregation[52]. Radicals also alter proteoglycan monomers by fragmenting the core protein moiety and destroying the HA binding region. Altered proteoglycan monomers do not interact with HA to form complexes. Proteoglycan–HA complexes are easily and irreversibly destroyed by oxygen radicals[53]. Arthritic synovium released degraded low molecular weight hyaluronate. This was accompanied by oxygen radical production and prevented by oxygen radical scavengers[54]. Degradation of HA has been demonstrated in arthritic synovial fluid, which supports the notion that radicals play a role in HA destruction *in vivo*.

Collagen can be altered directly and indirectly by oxygen radicals. Low levels of fragmentation and enhanced cross-links have been described as a direct effect of oxygen radicals. Hydroxyl radicals in the presence of oxygen cleave collagen into small peptides. Hydroxyl radicals in the absence of oxygen or hypochlorous acid do not induce fragmentation of collagen molecules, but trigger a polymerization of collagen through the formation of new cross-links, such as dityrosine or disulfide bridges[55]. The significance of radical-mediated initial cleavages could be in making collagen more susceptible to subsequent enzymatic cleavage. Even more important may be indirect radical effects via activation of latent collagenase and neutralization of protease inhibitor activity. Neutrophils release and activate the latent enzymes gelatinase and collagenase. The ability of neutrophils to activate these enzymes depends on myeloperoxidase, HOCl and H_2O_2. A further mechanism for radicals to promote matrix degradation is through neutralization of the inhibitor activity of α_1-antiprotease against elastase[56].

RADICALS AND IMMUNOGLOBULINS

At least two aspects of the interaction between radicals and immunoglobulins are of significance in RA. Radical-induced alteration of immunoglobulin molecules may play a role in autoantibody formation and immune complexes can induce radical production. When human IgG is exposed to free-radical generating systems, such as ultraviolet irradiation, peroxidizing lipids or activated human neutrophils, polymeric IgG is formed through inter- and intramolecular cross-links involving tyrosine and histidine residues. The radical-induced IgG complexes can stimulate the release of superoxide from normal human neutrophils similar to identical complexes that are present in RA sera and synovial fluid. Radical-exposed IgG is able to bind rheumatoid factor (RF) to the same extent as aggregated IgG and results in the

OXYGEN RADICAL EFFECTS RELEVANT TO ARTHRITIS
Extracellular matrix
Depolymerization of hyaluronic acid Destruction of hyaluronic acid–proteoglycan complexes Low level of collagen fragmentation Enhanced collagen cross-links Activation of latent metalloproteinases Neutralization of protease inhibitors
Immunoglobulins
IgG complex formation, leading to oxygen radical production and complement activation Autoantigenicity of Ig and stimulation of rheumatoid factor production
Cells
Cytotoxicity Activation of transcription factors NF κB and AP-1, resulting in expression of inflammatory mediators

Fig. 11.9 Oxygen radical effects relevant to arthritis.

generation of C3a. This has led to the suggestion that aggregated IgG may be formed by free radicals derived from neutrophils, and that this reaction may be self-perpetuating within the rheumatoid joint[57]. Alteration of IgG by oxygen-derived free radicals may also render IgG autoantigenic and lead to the production of RF. These results support the hypothesis that free radical damage to gammaglobulins plays a role in the chronicity of the inflammatory reaction in RA[58].

EFFECTS OF FREE RADICALS ON CELLS

Radicals can affect cell replication, survival and biosynthetic functions. Chondrocyte proliferation is inhibited by oxygen radicals[59], while in fibroblasts oxygen-derived free radicals at low concentrations increase cell density and thymidine incorporation[60]. At higher doses cell damage and death by necrosis occur. In chondrocytes, oxygen radicals inhibit glycosaminoglycan and protein synthesis[61]. Exposure to H_2O_2 leads to a decrease in ATP concentrations as a result of inactivation of glyceraldehyde-3-phosphate dehydrogenase[62]. Free radicals may attack polyunsaturated fatty acids of membrane phospholipids and thus initiate lipid peroxidation and damage to cell membranes.

Reactive oxygen species can also function as signaling messengers to activate transcription factors and induce gene expression. The nuclear factor κB (NF κB) is responsive to diverse pathogenic signals and mediates activation of a multitude of genes that are involved in host defense and inflammation. Cell stimulation leads to activation of a pre-existing cytoplasmic form of NF κB that, after translocation into the nucleus, initiates transcription of genes in synergy with other factors. The activation of transcription factor NF κB by TNF or IL-1 was inhibited by antioxidants, suggesting a role of oxygen radicals as intermediates. Furthermore, with cell lines that overexpress catalase or superoxide dismutase it was shown that H_2O_2 acts as a messenger of TNF-induced activation of NF κB[63]. Transcription factor AP-1 is an ubiquitous regulatory protein complex that interacts with the AP-1 binding sites of target genes to regulate transcription in response to a broad spectrum of stimuli. Activation of AP-1 was shown to be regulated by a hydroxyl radical-mediated change of the intracellular redox equilibrium towards a more oxidizing environment[64].

Several investigators had previously observed oxygen radical-dependent production of a neutrophil chemotactic activity. At least one molecular mechanism that can explain this has now been identified. Interleukin-8 is a cytokine that functions as a potent neutrophil chemoattractant and activator. In lipopolysaccharide (LPS)-stimulated human whole blood, radical scavengers inhibit IL-8 production and direct exposure to reactive oxygen intermediates stimulates IL-8 production[65]. The induction of monocyte chemoattractant protein-1 and colony-stimulating factor-1 by TNF, or aggregated IgG, in monocytes was also at least in part dependent on free radicals. Addition of NADPH to activate a membrane-bound NADPH-oxidase increased cytokine mRNA levels and further enhanced the stimulation by TNF or aggregated IgG[66].

REGULATION OF NITRIC OXIDE PRODUCTION

The first demonstration of NO release from mammalian cells was in the vascular endothelium, where it was established as the endothelium-derived factor that causes smooth muscle relaxation. Since then NO has been shown to be produced in many tissues and to regulate diverse cell functions. The production of NO by leukocytes is associated with nonspecific defense against certain microorganisms; it acts as a neurotransmitter in the CNS and in nonadrenergic noncholinergic (NANC) peripheral neurons[67]. The role of NO in the pathogenesis of inflammatory diseases varies with the type of inflammatory stimulus and the organ involved. A significant function of NO in cartilage and bone is suggested by the high levels of NO production in these tissues.

NO and equal amounts of citrulline are enzymatically formed from L-arginine and molecular oxygen (O_2) by nitric oxide synthases (NOS) which require NADPH, tetrahydrobiopterin (BH_4), flavin adenine dinucleotide (FAD) and flavin adenine mononucleotide (FMN) as cofactors (Fig. 11.10). Two classes of enzymes are known, the constitutive

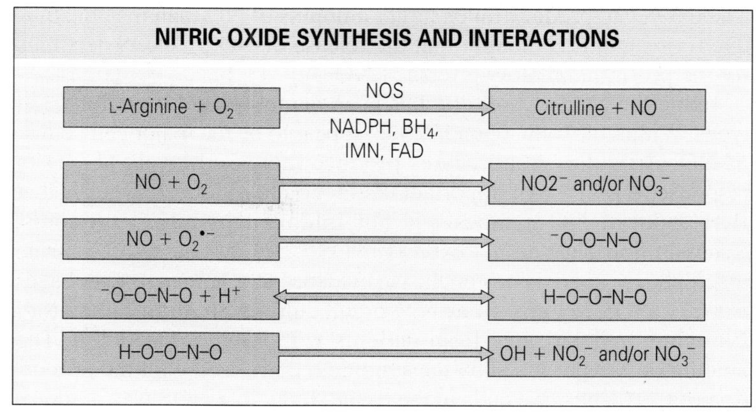

Fig. 11.10 NO synthesis and interactions. The generation of NO is catalyzed by NOS which require L-arginine, NADPH and molecular oxygen as substrates. L-Arginine is oxidized at a terminal nitrogen on the guanidino group, resulting in the formation of citrulline. NO is unstable and highly reactive, while nitrite (NO_2^-) and nitrate (NO_3^-) are stable and measurable end products. In the presence of NO and superoxide ($O_2^{\bullet -}$) the formation of peroxynitrite occurs (⁻O-O-N-O). Peroxynitrite can protonate to produce peroxynitrous acid (H-O-O-N-O), which decays rapidly to form the OH• and NO_2^- or NO_3^-.

NOS (cNOS) and inducible NOS (iNOS). Tissue-specific subtypes have been described for cNOS, notably the neuronal and the endothelial cell cNOS[67]. Neuronal and endothelial cell cNOS are encoded by distinct genes, but can also be expressed in other cell types. The activities of cNOS are regulated by the intracellular free calcium concentration and the Ca^{2+} binding protein calmodulin. At resting Ca^{2+}, both isozymes are inactive; they become fully active after an increase in intracellular levels of Ca^{2+}. Besides the conversion of L-arginine, cNOS generates H_2O_2 and reduces cytochrome p450, activities that are Ca^{2+} and calmodulin-dependent. Other redox activities, such as the reduction of nitroblue tetrazolium to diformazan (NADPH–diaphorase activity) or of quinoid dihydrobiopterin to tetrahydrobiopterin, by cNOS appear to be Ca^{2+} and calmodulin-independent.

A second class of NOS is represented by iNOS, originally isolated from mouse macrophages. Only a single gene for iNOS has been identified. cDNA sequences cloned from human hepatocytes, articular chondrocytes and bone cells are identical[67,68]. The inducible enzyme from murine macrophages displays only 50% sequence identity to the neuronal enzyme. Like neuronal cNOS, macrophage iNOS has recognition sites for FAD, FMN and NADPH; it also has a consensus calmodulin binding site. In contrast to cNOS, iNOS binds calmodulin tightly with no requirement for elevated Ca^{2+}. This may explain why iNOS is independent of both Ca^{2+} and elevated calmodulin, and appears to be activated simply by being synthesized. Inducible NOS activity appears slowly after exposure of cells to cytokines, such as IL-1, TNF or IFN-γ, and bacterial products; its expression is sustained.

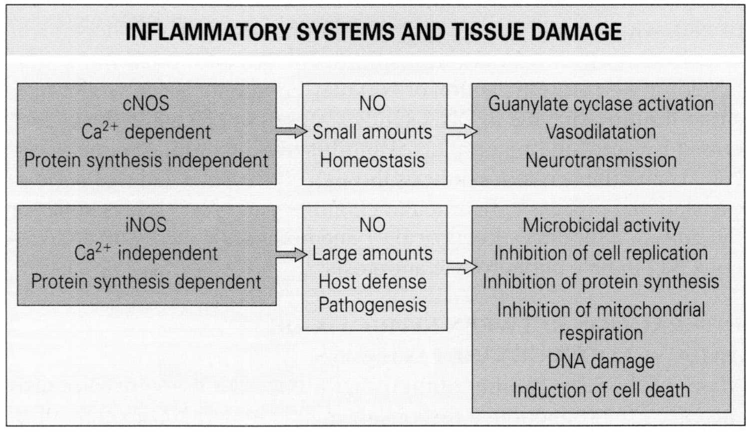

Fig. 11.11 Distinct biological roles of low versus high levels of NO produced by cNOS versus iNOS.

The iNOS can produce much larger amounts of NO than the constitutive forms and it is thought that the release of NO by iNOS accounts for the pro-inflammatory effects of NO (Fig. 11.11).

Inducible NOS expression has been demonstrated in various cell types. Within the joint, chondrocytes appear to be the major cell source of NO. Articular chondrocytes produce increased levels of NO in response to IL-1[69]. An important distinction to other cell types is that IL-1 induced NO synthesis is not inhibited by glucocorticoids. Synovial fibroblast do not express iNOS[70] and, in contrast to murine macrophages, there is no conclusive evidence that human macrophages express iNOS *in vitro*. In *ex vivo* organ cultures, both inflammatory synovium and cartilage from patients with RA produced NO. The amount of NO produced by the synovium correlated with the proportion of CD14-positive cells in the tissue. Inducible NOS was predominantly expressed in synovial lining cells, endothelial cells and chondrocytes. The synovial cells expressing iNOS were CD14 positive, suggesting that they are type A synoviocytes[71].

MOLECULAR NITRIC OXIDE EFFECTS

NO reacts with other radicals, with carbohydrates, proteins, lipids and nucleic acids. It can bind iron and thus regulate the activity of a large number of enzymes. Well characterized is NO binding to the heme iron in guanylate cyclase, which is at the active site of the enzyme. This results in a conformational change and activation of the enzyme. NO stimulates the mono-ADP-ribosylation of the glycolytic enzyme glyceraldehyde-3-phosphate dehydrogenase. Associated with ADP-ribosylation is a loss of enzymatic activity. This may be relevant as a cytotoxic effect of NO complementary to its inhibitory actions on iron–sulfur enzymes, like aconitase and electron transport proteins of the respiratory chain[72]. N-terminal groups of some proteins can be modified by nitric oxide, perhaps by deamination[73]. Nitric oxide can also cause genomic alterations. *In vitro*, NO deaminated deoxynucleosides, deoxynucleotides and intact DNA, and caused DNA strand breakage[74]. Similar DNA damage can also occur *in vivo* and observed DNA sequence changes were consistent with a cytosine-deamination mechanism[75]. NO reacts in the presence of specific protein thiols to form *S*-nitrosoprotein derivatives that have endothelium-derived relaxing factor-like properties. Human plasma contains substantial levels of *S*-nitrosothiols, most of which is accounted for by *S*-nitroso-serum albumin[76]. By contrast, plasma levels of free NO are very low.

NITRIC OXIDE EFFECTS ON CELL GROWTH AND SURVIVAL

NO donors inhibit cell proliferation and endogenous NO production is at least in part responsible for the growth inhibition induced by cytokines or other agents. Conversely, factors that stimulate cell proliferation often inhibit NO formation[77,78]. NO is at least in part responsible for cytotoxicity induced by monocytes or cytokines, such as IFN-γ, IL-2, TNF or LPS. In the CNS, NO is involved with the neurotoxicity of glutamate[79]. Interleukin-1 toxicity for islet cells occurs via inducing the synthesis and release of NO, which is highly toxic for islet cells[80]. Several mechanisms may account for the cytotoxic effects of NO, which could be due to an L-arginine or glycolysis-dependent impairment of mitochondrial respiration[81]. An additional molecular target for the cytostatic action of NO may be ribonucleotide reductase, a rate-limiting enzyme in DNA synthesis, as both NO gas and NO generated by activated macrophages inhibit ribonucleotide reductase[81]. NO also inhibits protein synthesis through either a translational or post-translational process[82]. In articular chondrocytes NO is responsible for the growth inhibitory effects of IL-1 and both NO donors and endogenous NO induce chondrocyte apoptosis[83].

INTERACTION BETWEEN NITRIC OXIDE AND CYCLOOXYGENASE PATHWAYS

Many of the extracellular stimuli that induce iNOS expression also increase PG production, a response which is in part NO-mediated. In mouse macrophages LPS causes an increase in the release of NO and PGE_2. Production of both NO_2 and PGE_2 was blocked by NOS inhibitors, which was thought to be a direct NO interaction with cyclooxygenase (COX) to cause an increase in the enzymatic activity[84]. NO donors also increased COX activity in endothelial cells and intravenous infusion of NO donors *in vivo* released 6-keto-$PGF_{2\alpha}$, the stable metabolite of PGI_2[85]. Besides the activation of COX function, NO donors also amplified IL-1β-induced PGE_2 production and potentiated IL-1β -induced mRNA and protein expression of COX-2 in macrophages and mesangial cells[86].

PEROXYNITRITE

Many cell types produce both NO and superoxide. The generation of these two radicals can lead to the formation of peroxynitrite[87] (see Fig. 11.10). The formation of this relatively long lived, strong oxidant from the reaction of nitric oxide and superoxide may contribute to inflammatory cell-mediated tissue injury[88]. Because superoxide and nitric oxide can react with each other to form peroxynitrite, they modulate each other's half life and the quality of their biological effects. Superoxide can limit the effects of NO by directing it to peroxynitrite and some NO effects, such as vasodilation, are prolonged in the presence of superoxide scavengers[89]. Conversely, NO can be regarded as a scavenger of the superoxide anion, which suggests that NO may provide a chemical barrier to cytotoxic free radicals. Some effects of these radicals are clearly dependent on the formation of peroxynitrite. The inhibition of aconitases is only observed in the presence of peroxynitrite, but not by NO in the absence of superoxide. Peroxynitrite is capable of oxidizing a variety of molecules, including sulfides, thiols, deoxyribose, lipids, ascorbate and α_1-protease inhibitor. In the case of α_1-protease inhibitor peroxynitrite oxidizes the methionine residue to sulfoxide and inactivates the protein. Peroxynitrite also inactivates the tissue inhibitor of metalloproteinase-1 (TIMP-1) activity towards gelatinase-A. High concentrations of peroxynitrite cause protein fragmentation, while lower concentrations inactivate TIMP-1 without altering the molecular weight[90]. Peroxynitrite initiates lipid peroxidation and this mechanism contributes to O_2- and NO-mediated cytotoxicity[85]. Reactive peroxynitrite anion may also exert cytotoxic effects in part by oxidizing tissue sulfhydryls[91].

Peroxynitrite can decompose to products that nitrate aromatic amino acids. Such nitro-aromatics may be 'markers' of NO-dependent oxidative damage. Nitrotyrosine residues were first demonstrated in atherosclerotic plaques and subsequently in synovial fluids. Serum and synovial fluid from patients with the RA contain 3-nitrotyrosine. By contrast, body fluids from normal subjects and patients with OA contain no detectable 3-nitrotyrosine. The demonstration of nitrotyrosine formation represents evidence for the production of peroxynitrite *in vivo* since tyrosine is nitrated by peroxynitrite but not by nitric oxide[92].

THE ROLE OF NITRIC OXIDE IN ARTHRITIS
NO production *in vivo*
Demonstrated in experimentally induced arthritis Presence of nitrite, nitrate and nitrotyrosine in arthritic synovial fluid iNOS expression in RA synovium and cartilage
NO production *in vitro*
Chondrocytes, cartilage, RA synovium
NO effects
Chondrocyte apoptosis Inhibition of proteoglycan synthesis Activation of latent metalloproteinases Activation of cyclooxygenase Inhibition of osteoblast function
NO-directed therapy
Experimentally induced joint inflammation and cartilage degradation is attenuated by NO synthesis inhibitors

Fig. 11.12 The role of NO in arthritis.

NITRIC OXIDE AND ARTHRITIS

Separate lines of research support a role for NO in the pathogenesis of arthritis (Fig. 11.12). NO is produced in inflamed joints, studies in experimental models of arthritis have indicated a therapeutically beneficial effect of NO synthesis inhibitors and, with *in vitro* experiments, NO has been demonstrated to affect cartilage and bone.

In Lewis rats, adjuvant arthritis was exacerbated by L-arginine. The NO synthesis inhibitor N^G-nitro-L-arginine-methylester (L-NAME) suppressed paw swelling of adjuvant-injected rats when given intraperitoneally and orally. L-NAME was also suppressive when given after adjuvant inoculation, suggesting that NO is involved in the development and maintenance of joint swelling[93]. MRL-lpr/lpr mice which spontaneously develop various manifestations of autoimmunity, including an inflammatory arthropathy and immune complex glomerulonephritis, excreted more urinary nitrite and nitrate. Peritoneal macrophages for these mice had an enhanced capacity to produce nitric oxide *in vitro* and oral administration of N^G-monomethylarginine (NMA) prevented the development of glomerulonephritis[94]. In streptococcal cell wall (SCW) fragment induced arthritis, NO was elevated in the inflamed joints. Administration of NMA reduced synovial inflammation and tissue damage[95].

Collectively, these studies implicate the NO pathway in the pathogenesis of inflammatory arthritis and demonstrate the ability of NOS inhibitors to modulate the disease. A role of NO in human arthritis is supported by findings that serum nitrite concentrations in patients with RA and OA were significantly elevated above those in controls. In both disease groups synovial fluid nitrite was significantly higher than serum nitrite. Synovial fluid nitrite concentrations in RA exceeded those in OA[96]. Urinary nitrate and/or nitrite levels were also higher in RA patients than in healthy controls. Findings on the serum levels in RA vary among the different studies[96–98].

Most of the currently available data suggest that NO promotes cartilage extracellular matrix degradation. Some discrepancies in the NO effects appear to relate to species differences. Studies with human[99], rat[100] and rabbit cartilage[101] indicate that NO donors and IL-1 induced endogenous NO inhibits proteoglycan synthesis. This was not observed with bovine cartilage[102]. NO also activates matrix metalloproteinases[103] and depolymerizes hyaluronan[104].

Human and rat osteoblasts express iNOS and produce NO after cytokine stimulation. Cytokine-induced increases in NO production are associated with an inhibition of osteoblast proliferation, alkaline phosphatase activity and osteocalcin production. The data suggest that osteoblast-derived NO may have an important role in mediating localized bone destruction associated with inflammatory bone diseases such as RA[105,106].

REFERENCES

1. Wyke B. The neurology of joints: a review of general principles. Clin Rheum Dis. 1981;7:223–39.
2. Hukkanen M, Konttinen YT, Rees RG, Gibson SJ, Santavirta S, Polak JM. Innervation of bone from healthy and arthritic rats by substance P and calcitonin gene related peptide containing sensory fibers. J Rheumatol. 1992;19:1252–9.
3. Hukkanen M, Konttinen YT, Rees RG, Santavirta S, Terenghi G, Polak JM. Distribution of nerve endings and sensory neuropeptides in rat synovium, meniscus and bone. Int J Tissue React. 1992;14:1–10.
4. Heppelmann B, Schaible HG. Origin of sympathetic innervation of the knee joint in the cat. Neurosci Lett. 1990;108:71–5.
5. Hukkanen M, Gronblad M, Rees R, *et al.* Regional distribution of mast cells and peptide containing nerves in normal and adjuvant arthritic rat synovium. J Rheumatol. 1991;18:177–83.
6. Clark FJ. Information signaled by sensory fibers in medial articular nerve. J Neurophysiol. 1975;38:1464–72.
7. Schaible HG, Schmidt RF. Time course of mechanosensitivity changes in articular afferents during a developing experimental arthritis. J Neurophysiol. 1988;60:2180–95.
8. Schepelmann K, Messlinger K, Schaible HG, Schmidt RF. Inflammatory mediators and nociception in the joint: excitation and sensitization of slowly conducting afferent fibers of the cat's knee by prostaglandin I_2. Neuroscience. 1992;50:237–47.
9. Konttinen YT, Hukkanen M, Segferberg M, *et al.* Relationship between neuropeptide immunoreactive cells in adjuvant arthritic rats. Scand J Rheumatol. 1992;21:55–9.
10. Pereira da Silva JA, Carmo-Fonseca M. Peptide containing nerves in human synovium: immunohistochemical evidence for decreased innervation in rheumatoid arthritis. J Rheumatol. 1990;17:1592–9.
11. Mapp PI, Kidd BL, Gibson SJ, *et al.* Substance P-, calcitonin gene-related peptide- and C-flanking peptide of neuropeptide Y-immunoreactivity fibres are present in normal synovium but depleted in patients with rheumatoid arthritis. Neuroscience. 1990;37:143–53.
12. Levine JD, Clark R, Devor M, Helms C, Moskowitz MA, Basbaum AI. Intraneuronal substance P contributes to the severity of experimental arthritis. Science. 1984;226:547–9.
13. Pernow B. Substance P. Pharmacol Rev. 1983;35:85–141.
14. Bathon JM, Proud D, Mizutani S, Ward PE. Cultured human synovial fibroblasts rapidly metabolize kinins and neuropeptides. J Clin Invest. 1992;90:981–91.
15. Krause JE, Takeda Y, Hershey AD. Structure, functions, and mechanisms of substance P receptor action. J Invest Dermatol. 1992;98:2–7.
16. Mantyh PW, Catton MD, Boehmer CG, *et al.* Receptors for sensory neuropeptides in human inflammatory diseases: implications for the effector role of sensory neurons. Peptides. 1989;10:627–45.
17. Walsh DA, Mapp PI, Wharton J, *et al.* Localisation and characterisation of substance P binding to human synovial tissue in rheumatoid arthritis. Ann Rheum Dis. 1992;51:313–17.
18. Payan DG. Neuropeptides and inflammation: the role of substance P. Ann Rev Med. 1989;40:341–52.
19. Marshall KW, Chiu B, Inman RD. Substance P and arthritis: analysis of plasma and synovial fluid levels. Arthritis Rheum. 1990;33:87–90.
20. Lotz M, Vaughan JH, Carson DA. Effect of neuropeptides on production of inflammatory cytokines by human monocytes. Science. 1988;241:1218–21.
21. Laurenzi MA, Persson MA, Dalsgasard CJ, Haegerstrand A. The neuropeptide substance P stimulates production of interleukin-1 in human monocytes: activated cells are preferentially influenced by the neuropeptide. Scand J Immunol. 1990;31:529–33.
22. Serra MC, Bazzoni F, Della Bianca V, Greskowiak M, Rossi F. Activation of human neutrophils by substance P. Effect on oxidative metabolism, exocytosis, cystolic Ca^{2+} concentration and inositol phosphate formation. J Immunol. 1988;141:2118–24.
23. Perianin A, Snyderman R, Malfroy B. Substance P primes human neutrophil activation: a mechanism for neurological regulation of inflammation. Biochem Biophys Res Commun. 1989;161:520–4.
24. McGillis JP, Mitsuhashi M, Payan DG. Immunomodulation by tachykinin neuropeptides. Ann NY Acad Sci. 1990;594:85–94.
25. Yokoyama MM, Fujimoto K. Role of lymphocyte activation by substance P in rheumatoid arthritis. Int J Tissue React. 1990;12:1–9.
26. Cross LJ, Heaney LG, Ennis M. Further characterization of substance P induced histamine release. Inflamm Res. 1996;45:11–21.
27. de Paulis A, Marino I, Ciccarelli A, *et al.* Human synovial mast cells. I. Ultrastructural *in situ* and *in vitro* immunologic characterization. Arthritis Rheum. 1996;39:1222–33.
28. Harrison NK, Dawes KE, Kwon OJ, Barnes PJ, Laurent GJ, Chung KF. Effects of neuropeptides on human lung fibroblast proliferation and chemotaxis. Am J Physiol. 1995;268:278–83.
29. Kahler CM, Herold M, Reinisch N, Wiedermann CJ. Interactions of substance P with epidermal growth factor and fibroblast growth factor in cyclooxygenase-dependent proliferation of human skin fibroblasts. J Cell Physiol. 1996;166:601–8.
30. Lotz M, Carson DA, Vaughan JH. Substance P activation of rheumatoid synoviocytes: neural pathway in pathogenesis of arthritis. Science. 1987;235:893–5.
31. Green PG, Basbaum AI, Levine JD. Sensory neuropeptide interactions in the production of plasma extravasation in the rat. Neuroscience. 1992;50:745–9.
32. Ralevic V, Khalil Z, Helme RD, Dusting GJ. Role of nitric oxide in the actions of substance P and other mediators of inflammation in the rat skin microvasculature. Eur J Pharmacol. 1995;284:231–9.
33. Green PG, Basbaum AI, Levine JD. Sensory neuropeptide interactions in the production of plasma extravasation in the rat. Neuroscience. 1992;50:745–9.
34. Green PG, Levine JD. Delta and kappa opioid agonists inhibit plasma extravasation induced by bradykinin in the rat. Neuroscience. 1992;49:129–33.
35. Engel D. The influence of the sympathetic nervous system on capillary permeability. Res Exp Med. 1978;173:1–8.
36. Levine JD, Taiwo YO, Collins SD, Tam JK. Contribution of sensory afferents and sympathetic efferents to joint injury in experimental arthritis. J Neurosci. 1986;6:3423–9.
37. Basbaum AI, Levine JD. The contribution of the nervous system to inflammation and inflammatory disease. Can J Physiol Pharmacol. 1991;69:647–51.
38. Felten SY, Felten DL. Innervation of lymphoid tissue. In: Ader R, Felten DL, Cohen N, eds. Psychoneuroimmunology. San Diego: Academic Press; 1991:28–69.
39. Levine JD, Fye K, Heller P, Basbaum AI, Whiting-O'Keefe Q. Clinical response to regional intravenous guanethidine in patients with rheumatoid arthritis. J Rheumatol. 1986;13:1040–3.
40. Wilder RL. Neuroendocrine–immune system interactions and autoimmunity. Ann Rev Immunol. 1995;13:307–38.
41. Clarke BL, Gebhardt BM, Blalock JE. Mitogen-

stimulated lymphocytes release biologically active corticotropin. Endocrinology. 1993;132:983–8.
42. Weigent DA, Blalock JE. Associations between the neuroendocrine and immune systems. J Leukocyte Biol. 1995;58:137–50.
43. Zurawski G, Benedik M, Kamb BJ, Abrams JS, Zurawski SM, Lee FD. Activation of mouse helper T cells induces abundant preproenkephalin mRNA. Science. 1986;232:772–5.
44. Kuis W, Villiger PM, Leser HG, Lotz M. Differential processing of proenkephalin-A by human peripheral blood monocytes and T lymphocytes. J Clin Invest. 1991;88:817–24.
45. Villiger PM, Lotz M. Expression of the preproenkephalin gene in human articular chondrocytes is linked to cell proliferation. EMBO J. 1992;11:135–43.
46. Bottger A, Spruce BA. Proenkephalin is a nuclear protein responsive to growth arrest and differentiation signals. J Cell Biol. 1995;130:1251–62.
47. Stein C, Comisel K, Haimerl E. Analgesic effect of intra-articular morphine after arthroscopic knee surgery. N Engl J Med. 1991;325:1123–6.
48. Stein C, Pfluger M, Yassouridis A, *et al.* No tolerance to peripheral morphine analgesia in presence of opioid expression in inflamed synovia. J Clin Invest. 1996;98:793–9.
49. Stein C. The control of pain in peripheral tissues by opioids. N Engl J Med. 1995;332:1685–90.
50. Babior BM, Kipnes RS, Curnutte JT. Biological defense mechanisms. The production by leukocytes of superoxide, a potential bactericidal agent. J Clin Invest. 1973;52:741–4.
51. Kresse H, Glossl J. Glycosaminoglycan degradation. Adv Enzymol. 1987;60:217–311.
52. McNeil JD, Wiebkin OW, Betts WH, Cleland LG. Depolymerization products of hyaluronic acid after exposure to oxygen-derived free radicals. Ann Rheum Dis. 1985;44:780–9.
53. Panasyuk A, Frati E, Ribault D, Mitrovic D. Effect of reactive oxygen species on the biosynthesis and structure of newly synthesized proteoglycans. Free Radical Biol Med. 1994;16:157–67.
54. Schenck P, Schneider S, Miehlke R, Prehm P. Synthesis and degradation of hyaluronate by synovia from patients with rheumatoid arthritis. J Rheumatol. 1995;22:400–5.
55. Monboisse JC, Borel JP. Oxidative damage to collagen. Exs. 1992;62:323–7.
56. Carp H, Janoff A. Potential mediator of inflammation: phagocyte-derived oxidants suppress the elastase inhibitor capacity of alpha$_1$-proteinase inhibitor *in vivo*. J Clin Invest. 1980;66:987–95.
57. Lunec J, Blake DR, McCleary SJ. Self-perpetuating mechanisms of immunoglobulin G aggregation in rheumatoid arthritis. J Clin Invest. 1985;76:2084–90.
58. Swaak AJ, Kleinveld HA, Kloster JF, Hack CE. Possible role of free radical altered IgG in the etiopathogenesis of rheumatoid arthritis. Rheumatol Int. 1989;9:1–6.
59. Vincent F, Brun H, Clain E, Ronot X, Adolphe M. Effects of oxygen-free radicals on proliferation kinetics of cultured rabbit articular chondrocytes. J Cell Physiol. 1989;141:262–6.
60. Murrell GA, Francis MJ, Bromley L. Modulation of fibroblast proliferation by oxygen free radicals. Biochem J. 1990;265:659–65.
61. Larsen NE, Lombard KM, Parent EG, Balzas EA. Effect of hylan on cartilage and chondrocyte cultures. J Orthop Res. 1992;10:23–32.
62. Baker MS, Feigan J, Lowther DA. The mechanism of chondrocyte hydrogen peroxide damage. J Rheumatol. 1989;16:7–14.
63. Schreck R, Meier B, Mannel DN, Droge W, Baeuerle PA. Dithiocarbamates as potent inhibitors of nuclear factor κB activation in intact cells. J Exp Med. 1992;175:1181–94.
64. Pinkus R, Weiner LM, Daniel V. Role of oxidants and antioxidants in the induction of AP-1, NF-kappaB, and glutathione S-transferase gene expression. J Biol Chem. 1996;271:13422–9.
65. DeForge LE, Preston AM, Takeuchi E, Kenney J, Boxer LA, Remick DG. Regulation of interleukin-8 gene expression by oxidant stress. J Biol Chem. 1993;268:25568–76.
66. Satriano JA, Shuldiner M, Hora K, Xing Y, Shan Z, Schlondorff D. Oxygen radicals as second messengers for expression of the monocyte chemoattractant protein, JE/MCP-1, and the monocyte colony-stimulating factor, CSF-1, in response to tumor necrosis factor-alpha and immunoglobulin G. Evidence for involvement of reduced nicotinamide adenine dinucleotide phosphate (NADPH)-dependent oxidase. J Clin Invest. 1993;92:1564–71.
67. Bredt DS, Snyder SH. Nitric oxide: a physiologic messenger molecule. Ann Rev Biochem. 1994;63:175–95.
68. Maier R, Bilbe G, Rediske J, Lotz M. Inducible nitric oxide synthase from human articular chondrocytes: cDNA cloning and analysis of mRNA expression. Biochim Biophys Acta. 1994;1208:145–50.
69. Stadler J, Stefanovic-Racic M, Billiar TR, *et al.* Articular chondrocytes synthesize nitric oxide in response to cytokines and lipopolysaccharide. J Immunol. 1991;147:3915–20.
70. Rediske J, Koehne CF, Zhang B, Lotz M. The inducible production of nitric oxide by articular cell types. Osteoarthritis Cartilage. 1994;2:199–206.
71. Sakurai H, Kohsaka H, Liu MF, *et al.* Nitric oxide production and inducible nitric oxide synthase expression in inflammatory arthritis. J Clin Invest. 1995;96:2357–63.
72. Dimmelker SFL, Brune B. NO causes ADP-ribosylation and inhibition of glyceraldehyde-3-phosphate dehydrogenase. J Biol Chem. 1992;267:16771–4.
73. Moriguchi M, Manning LR, Manning JM. Nitric oxide can modify amino acid residues in proteins. Biochem Biophys Res Commun. 1992;183:598–604.
74. Nguyen T, Brunson T, Crespi CL, Penman BW, Wishnok JS, Tannenbaum SR. DNA damage and mutation in human cells exposed to nitric oxide. Proc Natl Acad Sci USA. 1992;80:3030–4.
75. Wink DA, Kasprzak KS, Margos CM, *et al.* DNA deaminating ability and genotoxicity of nitric oxide and its progenitors. Science. 1991;254:1001–3.
76. Stamler JS, Jaraki O, Osborne JA, *et al.* Nitric oxide circulates in mammalian plasma primarily as an *S*-nitroso adduct of serum albumin. Proc Natl. Acad Sci USA. 1992;89:7674–7.
77. Garg UC, Hassid A. Inhibition of rat mesangial cell mitogenesis by nitric oxide-generating vasodilators. Am J Physiol. 1989;257:60–6.
78. Blanco FJ, Geng Y, Lotz M. Differentiation-dependent effects of IL-1 and TGFβ on human articular chondrocyte proliferation are related to inducible nitric oxide synthase expression. J Immunol. 1995;154:4018–26.
79. Dawson VL, Dawson TM, London ED, Bredt DS, Snyder SN. Nitric oxide mediates glutamate neurotoxicity in primary cortical cultures. Proc Natl Acad Sci USA. 1991;88:6368–71.
80. Kolb H, Kolb-Bachofen V. Nitric oxide: a pathogenetic factor in autoimmunity. Immunol Today. 1992;13:157–60.
81. Dijkmans R, Billiau A. Interferon-gamma/lipopolysaccharide-treated mouse embryonic fibroblasts are killed by a glycolysis/L-arginine dependent process accompanied by depression of mitochondrial respiration. Eur J Biochem. 1991;202:151–9.
82. Curran RD, Ferrari FK, Kispert PH, *et al.* Nitric oxide and nitric oxide generating compounds inhibit hepatocyte protein synthesis. FASEB J. 1991;5:2085–92.
83. Blanco FJ, Ochs RL, Schwarz H, Lotz M. Chondrocyte apoptosis induced by nitric oxide. Am J Pathol. 1995;146:75–85.
84. Salvemini D, Misko TP, Masferrer JL, Seibert K, Currie MG, Needleman P. Nitric oxide activates cyclooxygenase enzymes. Proc Natl Acad Sci USA. 1993;90:7240–4.
85. Radi R, Beckman JS, Bush KM, Freeman BA. Peroxynitrite-induced membrane lipid peroxidation: the cytotoxic potential of nitric oxide and superoxide. Arch Biochem Biophys. 1991;288:481–7.
86. Tetsuka T, Daphna-Iken D, Miller BW, Guan Z, Baier LD, Morrison AR. Nitric oxide amplifies IL-1 induced cyclooxygenase-2 expression in rat mesangial cells. J Clin Invest. 1996;97:2051–6.
87. Beckman JS, Beckman TW, Chen J, Marshall PA, Freeman BA. Apparent hydroxyl radical production by peroxynitrite: implications for endothelial injury from nitric oxide and superoxide. Proc Natl Acad Sci USA. 1990;87:1620–4.
88. Pryor WA, Squadrito GL. The chemistry of peroxynitrite: a product from the reaction of nitric oxide with superoxide. Am J Physiol. 1995;268:L699–722.
89. Murphy ME, Sies H. Reversible conversion of nitroxyl anion to nitric oxide by superoxide dismutase. Proc Natl Acad Sci USA. 1991;88:10860–4.
90. Frears ER, Zhang Z, Blake DR, O'Connell JP, Winyard PG. Inactivation of tissue inhibitor of metalloproteinase-1 by peroxynitrite. FEBS Lett. 1996;381:21–4.
91. Radi R, Beckman JS, Bush KM, Freeman BA. Peroxynitrite oxidation of sulfhydryls. The cytotoxic potential of superoxide and NO. J Biol Chem. 1991;266:4244–50.
92. Kaur H, Halliwell B. Evidence for nitric oxide-mediated oxidative damage in chronic inflammation. Nitrotyrosine in serum and synovial fluid from rheumatoid patients. FEBS Lett. 1994;350:9–12.
93. Ialenti A, Moncada S, Di Rosa M. Modulation of adjuvant arthritis by endogenous nitric oxide. Br J Pharmacol. 1993;110:701–6.
94. Weinberg JB, Granger DL, Pisetsky DS, *et al.* The role of nitric oxide in the pathogenesis of spontaneous murine autoimmune disease: increased nitric oxide production and nitric oxide synthase expression in MRL-lpr/lpr mice, and reduction of spontaneous glomerulonephritis and arthritis by orally administered N^G-monomethyl-L-arginine. J Exp Med. 1994;179:651–60.
95. McCartney-Francis N, Allen JB, Mizel DE, *et al.* Suppression of arthritis by an inhibitor of nitric oxide synthase. J Exp Med. 1993;178:749–54.
96. Farrell AJ, Blake DR, Palmer RJ, Moncada S. Increased concentrations of nitrite in synovial fluid and serum samples suggest increased nitric oxide synthesis in rheumatic diseases. Ann Rheum Dis. 1992;51:1219–22.
97. Stichtenroth DO, Fauler J, Zeidler H, Frolich JC. Urinary nitrate excretion is increased in patients with rheumatoid arthritis. Ann Rheum Dis. 1995;54:820–4.
98. Grabowski PS, England AJ, Duykhuizen R, *et al.* Elevated nitric oxide production in rheumatoid arthritis. Detection using the fasting urinary nitrate:creatinine ratio. Arthritis Rheum. 1996; 39:643–7.
99. Hauselmann HG, Opplinger L, Michel BA, Stefanovic-Racic M, Evans CH. Nitric oxide and proteoglycan biosynthesis by human articular chondrocytes in alginate cultures. FEBS Lett. 1994; 352:361–4.
100. Jarvinen TAH, Miolanen T, Jarvinen TLN, Miolanen E. Nitric oxide mediates interleukin-1 inhibition of glycosaminoglycan synthesis in rat articular cartilage. Med Inflamm. 1995;4:107–11.
101. Taskiran D, Stefanovic-Racic M, Georgescu H, Evans CH. Nitric oxide mediates suppression of cartilage proteoglycan synthesis by interleukin-1. Biochem Biophys Res Commun. 1994;200:142–8.
102. Stefanovic-Racic M, Morales TI, Taskiran D, McIntyre LA, Evans CH. The role of nitric oxide in proteoglycan turnover by bovine articular cartilage organ cultures. J Immunol. 1996;156:75–88.
103. Murrell GAC, Jang D, Williams RJ. Nitric oxide activates metalloproteinase enzymes in articular cartilage. Biochem Biophys Res Commun. 1995;206:15–21.
104. Stefanovic-Racic M, Stadler J, Evans CH. Nitric oxide and arthritis. Arthritis Rheum. 1993;36:1036–44.
105. Ralston SH, Todd D, Helfrich M, Benjamin M, Grabowski PS. Human osteoblast-like cells produce nitric oxide and express inducible nitric oxide synthase. Endocrinology. 1994;135:330–6.
106. Hukkanen M, Hughes FJ, Buttery LD, *et al.* Cytokine-stimulated expression of inducible nitric oxide synthase by mouse, rat and human osteoblast-like cells and its functional role in osteoblast metabolic activity. Endocrinology. 1995;136:5445–53.

ANGIOGENESIS IN RA

Leslie Schrieber & Christopher J Jackson

Summary

- Angiogenesis is the formation of new capillary blood vessels and occurs in rheumatoid synovium. It is an essential component of the destructive process.
- Angiogenesis is promoted by several cell types and their secreted products, such as fibroblast growth factors, vascular endothelial cell growth factor and certain soluble adhesion molecules, all of which occur in abundance in RA joints and are regulated by hypoxia and proinflammatory cytokines.
- Anti-angiogenic therapy may prove beneficial.

INTRODUCTION

Until recently the endothelium was thought to be a passive bystander in the inflammatory process. However, it is now known to play an active and pivotal role in a variety of inflammatory and immunologic processes, including coagulation, mediator and cytokine production, antigen presentation and the tissue recruitment of leukocytes and angiogenesis.

In rheumatoid arthritis (RA) the synovial microvasculature undergoes two distinct morphologic changes: high endothelial venule (HEV) formation, which may facilitate the trafficking of lymphocytes to the synovium; and new blood vessel formation (angiogenesis, or neovascularization), which is believed to contribute to cartilage destruction. This chapter focuses on the roles of the endothelium in angiogenesis, particularly as it pertains to the rheumatoid synovial membrane.

ROLE OF ANGIOGENESIS IN RHEUMATOID ARTHRITIS

Angiogenesis is the formation of new capillary blood vessels from existing capillaries. It is of broad significance throughout embryonic development and adult life. It plays an essential role in the physiologic processes of growth, reproduction and wound healing and in a variety of neoplastic and inflammatory disorders (Fig. 12.1). Solid tumors secrete angiogenic factors which direct the growth of new blood vessels. In fact, solid tumor growth is limited by the rate of new blood vessel formation. The inflammatory joint in RA can be regarded as being analogous to a localized tumor. Similarities between the two disorders include the presence of high levels of tissue oncoproteins, the secretion of metalloproteinases and tissue invasion by highly proliferative cell types. However, a major difference between arthritis and tumors is that the inflammatory pannus contains no malignant cells.

Histologic examination of rheumatoid synovium reveals synovial cell hyperplasia, infiltration by plasma cells, lymphocytes, macrophages and mast cells, and the overgrowth of a fibrovascular granulation tissue, known as pannus. The last progressively covers and erodes articular cartilage, leading to irreversible joint destruction. As in the case with tumors, angiogenesis is an essential component of pannus formation (Fig. 12.2). Normal articular cartilage is avascular and resistant to invasion by new vessel growth. In RA, this barrier is broken and blood vessels grow into the articular cartilage[1], contributing to its destruction. The new blood vessels also provide a vehicle to allow inflammatory cells to enter the joint cavity. Folkman *et al.*[2] have proposed that pannus formation and cartilage destruction cannot occur in the absence of angiogenesis. Angiogenesis is also thought to play a role in the production of the cartilaginous and bony lesions in osteoarthritis (OA)[3]. The mechanisms that control the development of synovial angiogenesis in RA are poorly understood.

BIOLOGY OF NEW BLOOD VESSEL FORMATION

Angiogenesis is a complex process in which new blood vessels develop from the existing microvascular bed. New capillaries develop by a series of sequential steps (see Fig. 12.3). The first step involves degradation of the basement membrane mediated by the action of matrix degrading enzymes, the matrix metalloproteinases (MMPs) and the serine proteases. The latter include the plasminogen activators (PA), urokinase-type PA and tissue-type PA, which convert plasminogen into the active enzyme plasmin – a serine protease with very broad specificity. The MMPs are a group of matrix-degrading enzymes which require divalent

THE ROLES OF ANGIOGENESIS IN PHYSIOLOGY AND PATHOLOGY
Physiologic
Wound healing Female reproductive system ovary endometrium placental development
Pathologic
Solid tumors and metastases Rheumatoid arthritis Psoriasis Diabetic retinopathy Atherosclerotic plaques Hemangioma

Fig. 12.1 The roles of angiogenesis in physiology and pathology.

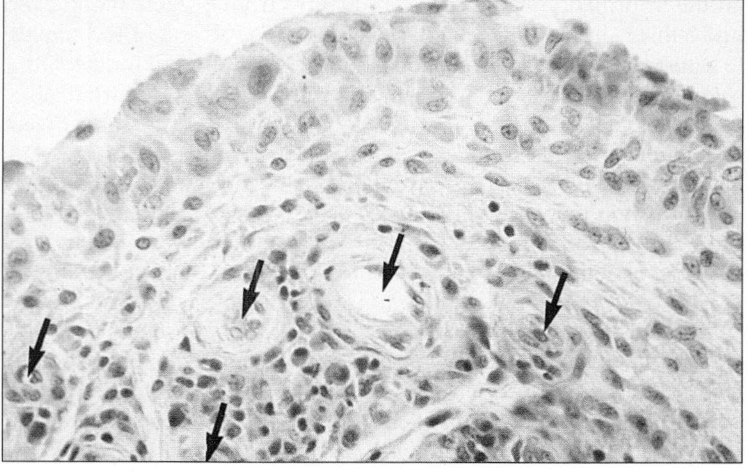

Fig. 12.2 Synovial angiogenesis. Tissue section of rheumatoid synovial pannus showing prominent new blood vessel formation (arrows).

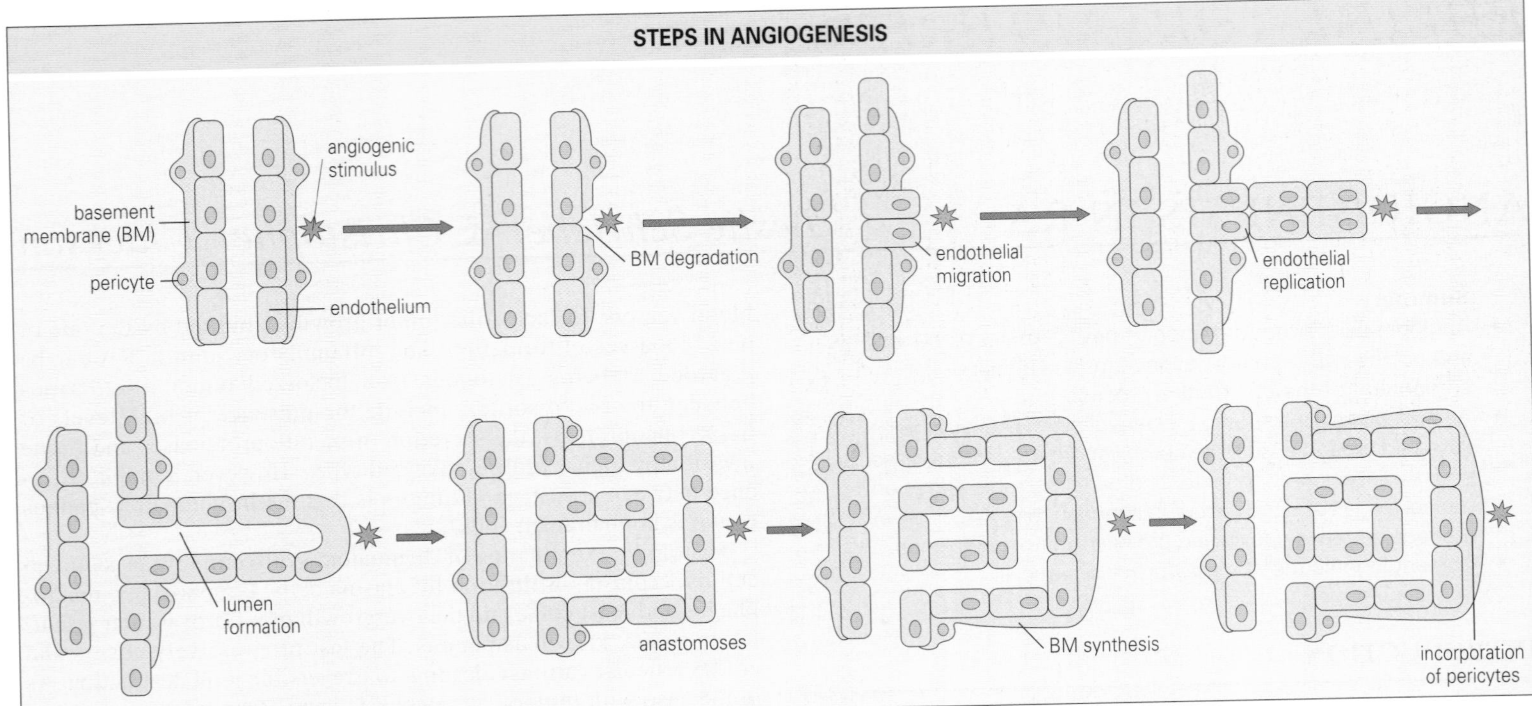

Fig. 12.3 Steps in angiogenesis.

metal ions for their biological activity and can break down all the components of the extracellular matrix. They are secreted by numerous cell types, including stimulated endothelial cells. Endothelial cells then migrate through the hole created in the basement membrane towards the angiogenic stimulus forming a sprout. Endothelial cells in the midsection of the sprout begin to undergo mitosis, while those at the tip of the sprout continue to migrate but do not divide. The endothelial cells are initially aligned in a solid sprout which subsequently becomes luminated. Individual sprouts anastamose with each other and existing vessels to form capillary loops. A new basement membrane is then synthesized by the endothelial cells and finally, pericytes develop along the length of the new capillaries and blood begins to flow.

METHODS TO STUDY ANGIOGENESIS

A number of methods to study angiogenesis have been developed which involve *in vivo* animal models or *in vitro* assays. The two most commonly used *in vivo* bioassays are the chick chorioallantoic membrane (CAM) and the corneal micropocket models. In these systems the potential angiogenic modulator to be tested is implanted in the cornea or the CAM and new blood vessel growth or inhibition is assessed.

Folkman and Haudenschild[4] have shown that endothelial cells have all the information necessary to transform from a stable monolayer into a three-dimensional capillary network. The advent of techniques to isolate and culture human endothelial cells has allowed for the direct study of angiogenesis and its regulation without interference from other cell types. The study of angiogenesis *in vitro* has mostly utilized endothelium derived from large vessels, such as human umbilical vein endothelium. However, the vasculature is heterogeneous, and ultrastructural and functional differences exist not only between endothelium derived from large as opposed to small blood vessels, but also between endothelium from different microvascular beds. Jackson *et al.*[5] have developed a technique to isolate microvascular endothelial cells from synovium. This depends on their ability to selectively bind to superparamagnetic polystyrene beads coated with the glycoprotein lectin *Ulex europaeus* I (UEAI) via l-fucose residues expressed on the endothelial cell surface (Fig. 12.4). These cells are von Willebrand factor positive, grow to confluence as a cobblestone-like monolayer and can be propagated in culture. Furthermore, they retain their *in vivo* expression of the adhesion molecules, E-selectin and intercellular adhesion molecule-1(ICAM-1), in culture[6].

A number of assays have been developed which correlate with the stages of angiogenesis (Fig. 12.3). These cell culture experiments measure endothelial cell MMP and PA synthesis, migration, proliferation and tube formation. The latter assays are commonly performed in the presence of an extracellular matrix component. When exposed to commercially available basement membrane material (Matrigel®), fibrin or type I collagen cultured endothelial cells are capable of morphologic transition into vascular tube-like structures. For example, Jackson and Jenkins[7] have reported that fibrillar type I collagen induces vascular tube formation when it contacts the apical side of cultured endothelium (Fig. 12.5), a process which is dependent on heparin.

REGULATION OF ANGIOGENESIS IN ARTHRITIS

Angiogenesis is a highly regulated process. One or more of a myriad of soluble and/or insoluble agents may regulate angiogenesis in

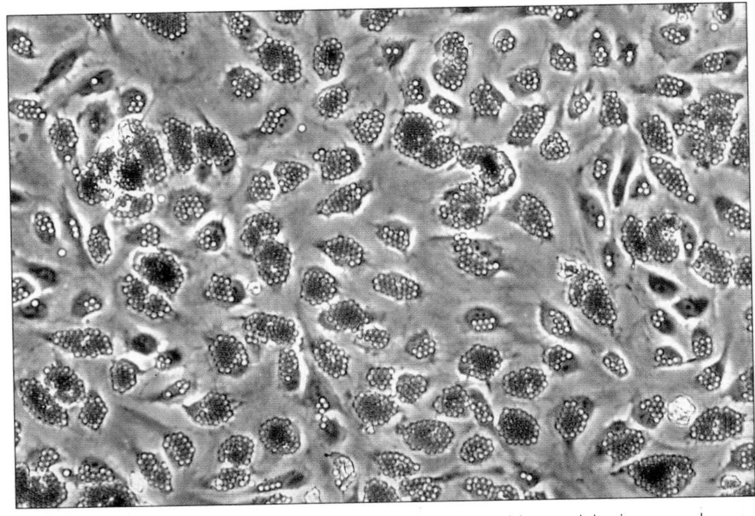

Fig. 12.4 Isolation of synovial endothelium. Rheumatoid synovial microvascular endothelial cells isolated by and bound to UEAI coated superparamagnetic beads. The latter appear as refractile spheres bound to individual endothelial cells (Reproduced with permission from Jackson *et al.*[5]).

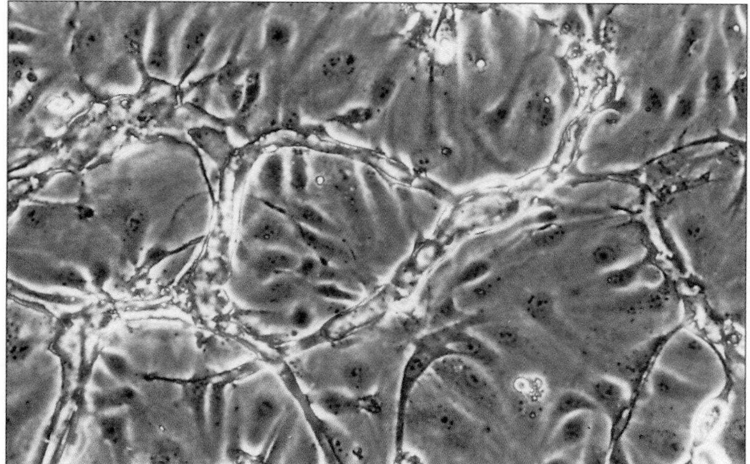

Fig. 12.5 Collagen *in vitro* model of angiogenesis. Vascular network formation after applying soluble type I collagen to a monolayer of human neonatal microvascular endothelial cells (phase contrast microscopy).

SOLUBLE ANGIOGENESIS PROMOTERS IN RA
Direct
Fibroblast growth factors (acidic FGF, basic FGF) Vascular endothelial growth factor/vascular permeability factor (VEGF/VPF) Platelet-derived endothelial cell growth factor (PD-ECGF) E-selectin and vascular cell adhesion molecule-1 (VCAM-1)
Indirect
Angiogenin Platelet-derived growth factor (PDGF) Prostaglandins (PGE_1, PGE_2) Heparin and sulfated polysaccharides Interleukin-1, -8 Platelet-activating factor (PAF) Transforming growth factor-β (TGF-β) Tumour necrosis factor-α (TNF-α) Granulocyte–macrophage–colony stimulating factor (GM-CSF)

Fig. 12.6 Soluble angiogenesis promoters in RA.

arthritis, including the influx of inflammatory cells, such as macrophages or mast cells, into inflamed synovium. In addition, physical factors such as oxygen tension affect angiogenesis. Both stimulators and inhibitors of angiogenesis have been described in arthritic synovium and synovial fluid. Synovial angiogenesis may be viewed as resulting from an imbalance between the levels and/or production of stimulators and inhibitors which favors the former.

FACTORS THAT PROMOTE ANGIOGENESIS IN ARTHRITIS

Inflammatory cells and synovial fluid

Several cell types, including macrophages, lymphocytes, polymorphonuclear leukocytes, mast cells and fibroblasts, as well as their secreted products, can stimulate angiogenesis. Many of these cell types are present in increased numbers within the rheumatoid joint, and any combination of them may be responsible for the development of new blood vessels during pannus formation. Macrophages isolated from rheumatoid synovial membrane stimulate angiogenesis in the rat cornea[8]. The angiogenic activity of synovial fluid from arthritic joints, both rheumatoid and osteoarthritic[9], may be attritutable to the presence of increased levels of soluble angiogenic promoters found in these fluids. In general, RA synovial fluid contains higher levels of angiogenic agents than OA synovial fluid.

Soluble factors

A variety of soluble molecules are able to stimulate angiogenesis, either directly by interacting with endothelial cell receptors or by an indirect mechanism (Fig. 12.6). Direct angiogenic agents present at increased levels in arthritic synovial fluid and/or synovium which may account for this activity include fibroblast growth factors (FGFs), vascular endothelial cell growth factor (VEGF), platelet-derived endothelial cell growth factor (PD-ECGF) and certain soluble forms of adhesion molecules. Of these, VEGF and PD-ECGF are the only promoters specifically mitogenic for endothelial cells. Anti-VEGF antibodies neutralize the endothelial chemotactic and mitogenic activity induced by RA synovial fluid and synovial tissue extracts[10]. In addition, the VEGF receptors, flt-1 and flk-1, are strongly expressed in endothelial cells in the rheumatoid synovium. Koch *et al.*[11] have shown that soluble forms of the endothelial cell adhesion molecules, E-selectin and vascular cell adhesion molecule-1 (VCAM-1), induce chemotaxis of human endothelial cells and are angiogenic in the rat corneal assay. The angiogenic activity of RA synovial fluid is blocked by antibodies to either soluble E-selectin or soluble VCAM-1. Thus, endothelial adhesion molecules may be important not only in facilitating leukocyte migration but also in promoting angiogenesis in the inflamed joint.

Indirect angiogenic promoters stimulate angiogenesis *in vivo* without stimulating endothelial cells directly[12]. These agents may work by activating secondary cells, such as macrophages, to release direct angiogenic mediators. Indirect angiogenic promoters include peptides, such as tumor necrosis factor-α (TNF-α), transforming growth factor-β and low molecular mass nonpeptide factors including prostaglandin E_1 and prostaglandin E_2. Elliot *et al.*[13] have reported that chimeric antibodies to TNF-α produce significant clinical and laboratory improvement in patients with RA. Although TNF-α has a number of different actions, including the modulation of endothelial and leukocyte binding, the blocking of its potent angiogenic activity may be at least partially responsible for its efficacy.

Insoluble factors

The rheumatoid synovium and cartilage harbors cellular infiltrates within various extracellular matrix components including proteoglycans and collagens. In addition the basement membrane of capillaries comprises matrix proteins including type IV collagen, glycosaminoglycans, elastin and laminin. Collagens, especially type I collagen, and laminin promote vascular tube formation *in vitro*[7]. The endothelial cell integrin receptors, $\alpha_v\beta_3$ which binds to vitronectin and laminin, and $\alpha_2\beta_1$ which binds to collagen, are also important during angiogenesis. Antibodies to $\alpha_2\beta_1$ regulate endothelial cell tube formation *in vitro*[14,15]. Antibodies to $\alpha_v\beta_3$ block human breast cancer cell growth and angiogenesis in human skin[16]. The high molecular weight proteoglycan, hyaluronic acid, inhibits angiogenesis, whereas partial degradation products of hyaluronic acid, which are present in the rheumatoid joint, induce angiogenesis.

Hypoxia

Low oxygen tension is a feature of the rheumatoid joint. In rheumatoid synovitis, the joint pressure is greater than the capillary perfusion

ANGIOGENESIS INHIBITORS IN RA
SAARDs
Angiostatin
Thrombospondin
Platelet factor 4
Cartilage-derived inhibitor

Fig. 12.7 Angiogenesis inhibitors in RA.

pressure, leading to hypoxic-perfusion injury[17]. Hypoxia is also a feature of other angiogenic-dependent processes including wound healing and the development of atherosclerotic plaques. In all these situations decreased oxygen levels induces the synthesis of soluble angiogenic factors, particularly VEGF, and may lead to angiogenesis[18].

FACTORS THAT INHIBIT ANGIOGENESIS (ANTI-ANGIOGENESIS) IN ARTHRITIS

Several cell types, tissues and soluble molecules (Fig. 12.7) have the ability to inhibit angiogenesis in the RA joint. Pericytes which are intimately associated with vascular endothelial cells exert an inhibitory influence on endothelial cell growth. Hyaline articular cartilage is a highly specialized tissue which is normally avascular and resistant to angiogenesis. Cartilage extracts or whole tissue fragments inhibit tumor-angiogenesis-factor-induced neovascularization *in vivo* and isolated chondrocytes inhibit lymphocyte-induced angiogenesis. Moses *et al.*[19] purified a protein from cartilage which inhibits both mammalian collagenase and angiogenesis *in vivo*. In RA, the balance between promoters and inhibitors is disturbed and new blood vessels invade the articular cartilage.

Thrombospondin, platelet factor 4 and angiostatin are naturally occurring angiogenic inhibitors. Thrombospondin, a 450kDa disulfide-linked trimer, is produced by normal cells but not by angiogenic tumor cells. It is localized in the vasculature of RA joints. Interestingly, the expression of thrombospondin is under the control of the p53 tumor-suppressor gene. Platelet factor 4 is a specific inhibitor of endothelial cells and is released from activated platelets. Angiostatin is a 38kDa protein which specifically inhibits endothelial proliferation. It is found in the serum of patients with primary tumors and disappears rapidly after the removal of the tumor, suggesting that it is derived from the primary tumor. Thus, ironically, removal of the primary tumor can result in angiogenic-dependent metastases. Whether angiostatin is present in the RA joint is unknown.

Many of the slow acting anti-arthritic drugs (SAARDs) (see Chapter 3.8) have anti-angiogenic activity. Gold compounds (sodium aurothiomalate and auranofin), D-penicillamine and sulfasalazine inhibit endothelial cell proliferation[20,21]. In addition, D-penicillamine (plus copper), auranofin, gold sodium thiomalate, indomethacin and methotrexate inhibit endothelial proliferation and angiogenesis in the rabbit cornea. Although these drugs have numerous other actions they may act, in part, by inhibiting synovial angiogenesis.

ANTI-ANGIOGENESIS AS THERAPY FOR RHEUMATOID ARTHRITIS

The development of agents that selectively inhibit synovial angiogenesis should prevent cartilage degradation. Two inhibitors likely to be important in arthritis include angiostatic corticosteroid–heparin moieties and AGM-1470. Corticosteroid–heparin moeities suppress tumor-associated angiogenesis but have a number of potential side-effects such as, immunosuppression. Angiostatic corticosteroids which have no mineralo- or corticosteroid activity, and thus fewer side effects, inhibit the degradation of cartilage in an *in vivo* granuloma-mediated cartilage destruction model[22]. AGM-1470 is a synthetic derivative of fumagillan, a naturally occurring product of *Aspergillus fumigatus fresenius*. This compound has marked anti-angiogenic activity in tumor models. It also suppresses rat adjuvant arthritis and type II collagen-induced arthritis in rats[23]. No adverse effects have been observed with its use. Other agents currently being tested for potential use as therapeutic angiogenesis inhibitors include antibodies to VEGF, antagonists to the VEGF receptors and inhibitors of MMPs.

Anti-angiogenic treatment has low toxicity – it is directed at proliferating capillaries and does not appear to have side-effects. Furthermore, endothelial cells do not develop resistance to the drugs. Such therapy is likely to be most beneficial if treatment is sustained for long periods of time, as demonstrated for animal tumor models. A combination of currently used anti-rheumatic agents and anti-angiogenic therapy may prove to be more effective than either treatment alone[24].

REFERENCES

1. Kobayashi I, Ziff M. Electron microscopic studies of the cartilage–pannus junction in rheumatoid arthritis. Arthritis Rheum. 1975;18:475–83.
2. Folkman J, Ausprunk DH, Langer R Connective tissue, small blood vessels and capillaries. In: Kelly WN et al. eds. Textbook of Rheumatology, 2E. Philadelphia: WB Saunders; 1985:197–210.
3. Brown RA, Weiss JB. Neovascularisation and its role in the osteoarthritic process. Ann Rheum Dis. 1988;47:881–5.
4. Folkman J, Haudenschild C. Angiogenesis *in vitro*: implications for tumour biology. In: Pathobiology of the endothelial cell. Nossel H, Vogel L, Vogel HJ, eds. New York: Academic Press; 1982:79–93.
5. Jackson CJ, Garbett PK, Nissen B, Schrieber L. Binding of human endothelium to *Ulex europaeus* I-coated dynabeads: application to the isolation of microvascular endothelium. J Cell Sci. 1990;96:257–62.
6. To SST, Newman PM, Hyland VJ, Robinson BG, Schrieber L. Regulation of adhesion molecule expression by human synovial microvascular endothelial cells *in vitro*. Arthritis Rheum. 1996;39:467–77.
7. Jackson CJ, Jenkins KL. Type 1 collagen fibrils promote rapid vascular tube formation upon contact with the apical side of cultured endothelium. Exp Cell Res. 1991;192:319–23.
8. Koch AE, Polverini PJ, Leibovich SJ. Stimulation of neovascularisation by human rheumatoid synovial tissue macrophages. Arthritis Rheum. 1986;29:471–9.
9. Brown RA, Weiss JB, Tomlinson IW. Angiogenic factor from synovial fluid resembling that from tumours. Lancet. 1980;i:682–5.
10. Koch AE, Harlow LA, Haines GK, *et al.* Vascular endothelial growth factor – a cytokine modulating endothelial function in rheumatoid arthritis. J Immunol. 1994;152:4149–56.
11. Koch AE, Halloran MM, Haskell CJ, Shah MR, Polverini PJ. Angiogenesis mediated by soluble forms of E-selectin and vascular cell adhesion molecule-1. Nature. 1995;376:517–19.
12. Folkman J, Klagsbrun M. A family of angiogenic peptides. Nature 1987;329:671–2.
13. Elliott M, Maini RN, Feldmann MA *et al.* Treatment of rheumatoid arthritis with chimeric monoclonal antibodies to tumour necrosis factor alpha. Arthritis Rheum. 1993;12:1681–90.
14. Jackson CJ, Jenkins KL, Schrieber L. Possible mechanisms of type I collagen-induced vascular tube formation. In: Angiogenesis: Key principles–Science–Technology–Medicine. Steiner J, Weisz PB, Langer R, eds. Basel: Birkhauser Verlag; 1992:198–204.
15. Gamble JR, Matthias LJ, Meyer G *et al.* Regulation of invitro capillary tube formation by anti-integrin antibodies. J Cell Biol. 1993;121:931–43.
16. Brooks PC, Clark RAF, Cheresh DA. Requirement of vascular integrin alpha(V)beta(3) for angiogenesis. Science. 1994;264:569–71.
17. Mapp PI, Grootveld MC, Blake DR. Hypoxia, oxidative stress and rheumatoid arthritis. Br Med Bull. 1995;51:419–36.
18. Shweiki D, Itin A, Soffer D, Keshet E. Vascular endothelial growth factor induced by hypoxia may mediate hypoxia-initiated angiogenesis. Nature. 1992;359:843–5.
19. Moses MA, Sudhalter J, Langer R. Identification of an inhibitor of neovascularization from cartilage. Science. 1990;248:1408–10.
20. Matsubara T, Ziff M. Inhibition of human endothelial cell proliferation by gold compounds. J Clin Invest. 1987;79:1440–6.
21. Matsubara T, Saura R, Hirohata K, Ziff M. Inhibition of human endothelial cell proliferation *in vitro* and neovascularization *in vivo* by D-penicillamine. J Clin Invest. 1989;83:158–67.
22. Colville Nash PR, Ghazaly M, Willoughby DA. The use of angiostatic steroids to inhibit cartilage destruction in an *in vivo* model of granuloma-mediated cartilage degradation. Agents Actions 1993;38:126–34.
23. Peacock DJ, Banquerigo ML, Brahn E. A novel angiogenesis inhibitor suppresses rat adjuvant arthritis. Cell Immunol. 1995;160:178–84.
24. Folkman J. Angiogenesis in cancer, vascular, rheumatoid and other disease. Nature Med. 1995;1:27–31.

RHEUMATOID SYNOVITIS AND PANNUS

Gary S Firestein

Definition

- The synovium in RA is marked by expansion of the intimal lining cell population and massive infiltration of the sublining by T-cells, macrophages and B-cells.
- Products of macrophages and fibroblasts are abundant in the rheumatoid joint, while T-cell products are absent or present in low concentrations.
- Cytokines regulate and perpetuate many aspects of RA, including production of metalloproteinases, recruitment of new cells to the joint, expression of small molecule mediators of inflammation, and cell proliferation.
- The initiation and perpetuation of RA are distinct events and might be regulated by different cell types.
- Chronicity appears to involve complex interactions between fibroblasts, macrophages and T-cells.

INTRODUCTION

Although rheumatoid arthritis (RA) possesses many clinical features of a systemic disease, abnormalities in synovial structure and function are the primary manifestations. Over the past two decades, there has been an explosion of information on the pathogenesis of synovitis (i.e. inflammation of the synovium) based on *in vitro* and *in vivo* studies, and it is hoped that a detailed understanding of the mechanisms of inflammation will provide a rational basis for novel therapeutic interventions.

In this chapter, an extensive review of the functional and phenotypic changes that occur in the rheumatoid synovium will be presented. These observations will be put into context by discussing current paradigms that attempt to integrate this information into a unified hypothesis.

THE NORMAL SYNOVIUM

Histopathologic examination of normal adult synovium usually reveals a relatively acellular structure with two distinct layers (Fig. 13.1). The first, called the synovial lining or the intima, is in direct contact with the intra-articular cavity. The lining is a loosely organized, avascular layer of cells that is only one or two cells deep. Although the intima superficially appears to be a barrier that lines and protects the joint, the intimal cells of the synovium are only loosely associated and are not supported by a true basement membrane. Occasionally, the lining is discontinuous and there can be large sections where the sublining is in direct contact with the synovial fluid. Ultrastuctural studies of the synovial lining show at least two cell types of cell, usually called type A and type B cells (Fig. 13.2). The former possess many features of tissue macrophages, including a prominent Golgi apparatus, abundant digestive vacuoles and scanty rough endoplasmic reticulum. These cells also contain nonspecific-esterase activity and express macrophage surface differentiation markers (such as CD68 and CD14), class II major histocompatability proteins (such as HLA-DR) and Fc receptors. This phenotype is also characteristic of bone marrow derived macrophages, and it has been demonstrated that type A synoviocytes are likely derived from this lineage[1].

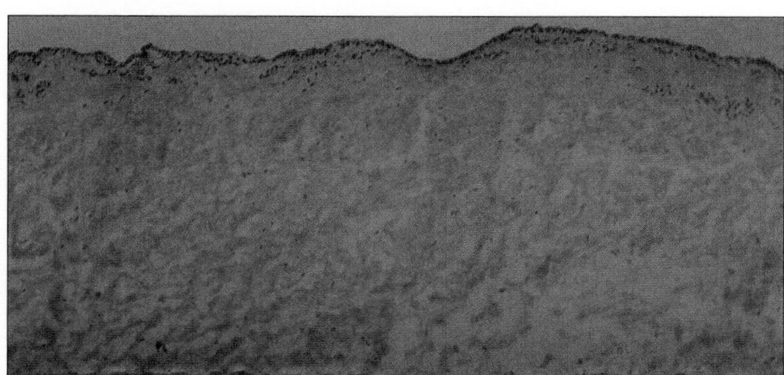

Fig. 13.1 Normal synovium. Low-power view of a normal synovial tissue. The intimal lining shown at the top of this section is only 1–2 cell layers deep and sublining blood vessels and mononuclear cells are sparse.

In contrast, type B cells appear to be of mesenchymal origin. Light microscopy reveals a bipolar fibroblast-like morphology and prominent secretory machinery, including a rough endoplasmic reticulum and regular ribosomal arrays. Immunohistochemistry has also demonstrated the presence of the enzyme uridine diphosphoglucose dehydrogenase (UDPGD) in type B synoviocytes[2]. This enzyme participates in the synthesis of hyaluronic acid, which, in addition to being a major component of synovial fluid, is also deposited in the synovial tissue. The presence of large intracellular pools of UDPGD in type B synoviocytes distinguishes them from stromal fibroblasts that are present deep in the subsynovium.

The second layer of the normal synovium is the subsynovium, also called the sublining or subintima. Normally, this region is relatively acellular, containing scattered blood vessels, fat cells and fibroblasts. Small capillaries or venules usually predominate immediately below the lining, while larger caliber vessels, including arterioles, are seen in the deep sublining tissues. Occasional mononuclear cells, including lymphocytes and macrophages, can be seen. The acellular extracellular matrix contains a variety of macromolecules, including collagen, fibronectin and proteoglycans. As one moves outwards from the articular cavity, the subsynovium is gradually replaced by loosely organized connective tissue. A more complete description of the cells of the normal synovium is presented in Chapter 5.6.

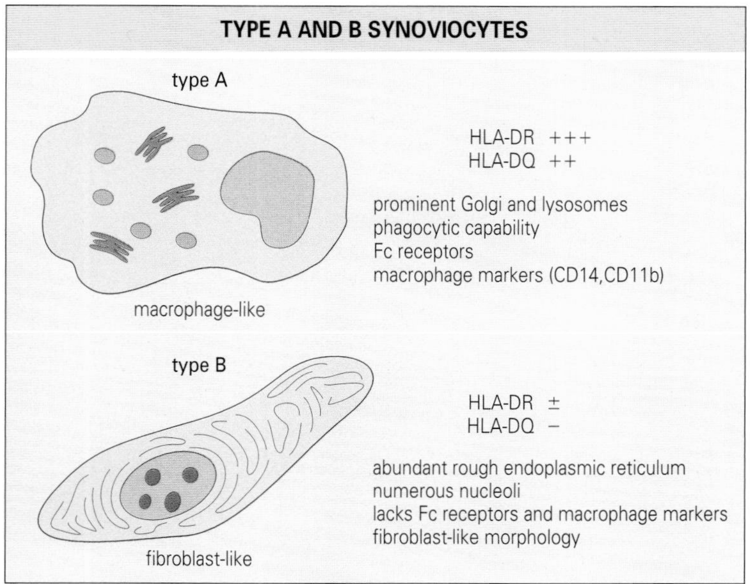

Fig. 13.2 Type A and B synoviocytes. Features of type A (macrophage-like) and type B (fibroblast-like) synoviocytes.

THE SYNOVIUM IN RHEUMATOID ARTHRITIS

HISTOLOGY

In RA as well as in other inflammatory arthritides, the synovium changes dramatically. On gross examination, the mass of synovial tissue is increased because of edema, multiple redundant folds and villae. The histopathologic appearance of the synovium is also altered, although the changes vary with the chronicity of the disease. In the first weeks to months of disease, tissue edema is prominent. Striking proliferation of blood vessels is also observed. Synovial lining hyperplasia can occur in this phase, while the sublining inflammatory infiltrate is usually mild and consists of scattered lymphocytes and neutrophils.

As the disease enters the chronic phase, the histologic appearance of the tissue also evolves (Fig. 13.3). Synovial lining hyperplasia becomes quite prominent, sometimes extending to a depth of over ten cells. While the increase is due to greater numbers of both type A and type B cells, most of the expansion occurs in the former. It is not certain whether this is caused by *in situ* replication or by migration of new cells into the lining. Evidence of active cell division in the lining of tissues from patients with chronic RA is scant, and only a very small number (<1%) of cells incorporate tritiated thymidine. Occasional cells express the cell cycle specific nuclear antigen Ki67, but the percentage is also very low[3]. In animal models of arthritis, proliferation of synovial lining cells (as measured by tritiated thymidine uptake) is prominent very early in the disease (i.e. in the first few weeks), after which time DNA synthesis rapidly decreases to basal levels. It is possible that a similar situation occurs in RA, with much of the lining hyperplasia resulting from synoviocyte proliferation in the first weeks of the process. In a more recent study, cells expressing the cell cycle specific antigen PCNA and the nuclear rearrangement apparatus (which are expressed during cell division) were localized to the intimal lining in RA but not osteoarthritis. These antigens were associated with high levels of the proto-oncogene c-myc, which is also associated with cell division[4,5]. Taken together, these data suggest either that intimal lining cells can actively proliferate or that their growth cycle is arrested.

The sublining also experiences dramatic alterations in both the degree and content of the cellular infiltrate. The most prominent change is an exuberant infiltration with mononuclear cells, including T-cells, B cells, macrophages and plasma cells. Multinucleate giant cells (likely resulting from the coalescence of macrophages) can be seen in granuloma-like lesions in the synovium. Hemosiderin-laden macrophages are present and are indicative of previous local microscopic hemorrhages. Lymphocytes often organize into discrete aggregates similar to those seen in lymph nodes, or in extralymphatic sites, such as Peyer's patches in the colonic mucosa. In some patients, there is diffuse infiltration of the subsynovium with sheets of mononuclear cells that lack obvious organization. A minority of patients have only a bland fibrous reaction, with very few mononuclear cells.

Increased numbers of blood vessels remain a prominent finding in the chronic phase of RA. In some cases, the number of venules is so great that histologic sections have a 'Swiss cheese' appearance (Fig. 13.4). However, capillary morphometry suggests that expansion of the synovium outstrips the proliferation of blood vessels, perhaps contributing to the relatively ischemic environment of the rheumatoid joint. Both the relative density and the distribution of blood vessels in the rheumatoid synovium are abnormal. Capillaries and postcapillary venules are abundant, especially in the region immediately below the lining. Frozen sections of synovial tissue sometimes demonstrate mononuclear and polymorphonuclear (PMN) leukocytes within these vessels. The cells are frequently in close apposition to the vascular endothelium and are probably in the process of margination and adhesion, before migration into the tissue.

Three basic regions within the sublining of rheumatoid synovial tissue have been described. First, plasma-cell-rich zones, which comprise nearly 75% plasma cells, can frequently be identified. Second, a lymphocyte-enriched region, which is usually perivenular and contains about 80% lymphocytes, is observed. Cells in this area are surprisingly quiescent in appearance, with scant cytoplasm and small round nuclei. Blasts are uncommon in this region, although many of the T-lymphocytes express surface markers that suggest prior activation, such as HLA-DR and VLA-1 (very late antigen). The third region of the sublining is called the 'transitional' zone. A higher percentage of the cells in this area appear to be blasts compared to the lymphocyte-enriched region, and, on ultrastructural studies, T-cells appear to interdigitate with HLA-DR-bearing antigen-presenting cells. A substantial number of plasma cells, small lymphocytes, macrophages and macrophage-like cells that are HLA-DR$^+$, but devoid of the macrophage marker CD14 are also present in the transitional zone[6]. Although the latter appear similar to a distinct lineage of potent antigen-presenting cells known as dendritic cells, the same phenotype is recapitulated in interferon-γ (IFN-γ) or granulocyte–macrophage colony-stimulating factor (GM-CSF) treated macrophages[7]. A monoclonal antibody that recognizes a subpopulation of dendritic cells (RFD1) binds to cells in transitional zones as well as in the periphery of lymphoid aggregates and confirms their presence in synovial tissue[8].

The synovium of RA often shows features similar to lymph nodes, particularly in areas with lymphoid follicles or a germinal center. There are some differences, however. In lymph nodes, for example, suppressor/cytotoxic lymphocytes are usually interspersed among the interdigitating antigen-presenting cells and CD4$^+$ T-lymphocytes. This is

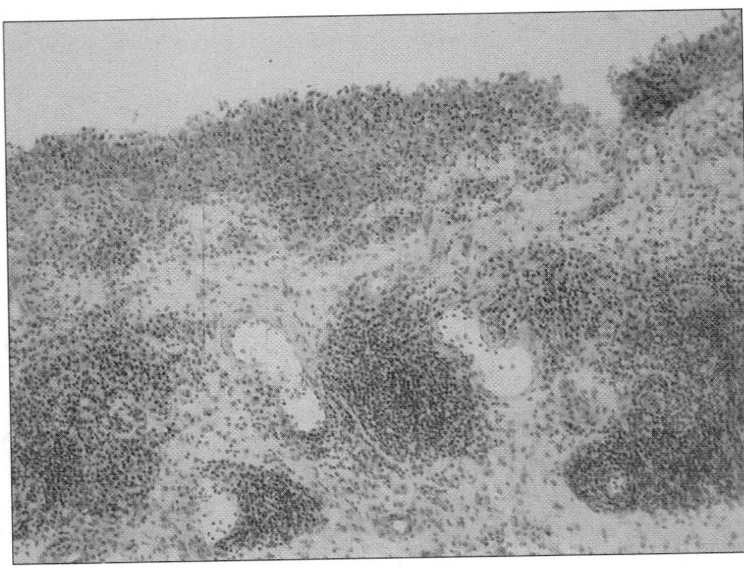

Fig. 13.3 RA synovium. Typical chronic RA synovitis with synovial lining hyperplasia, increased numbers of blood vessels and infiltration of the sublining with mononuclear cells.

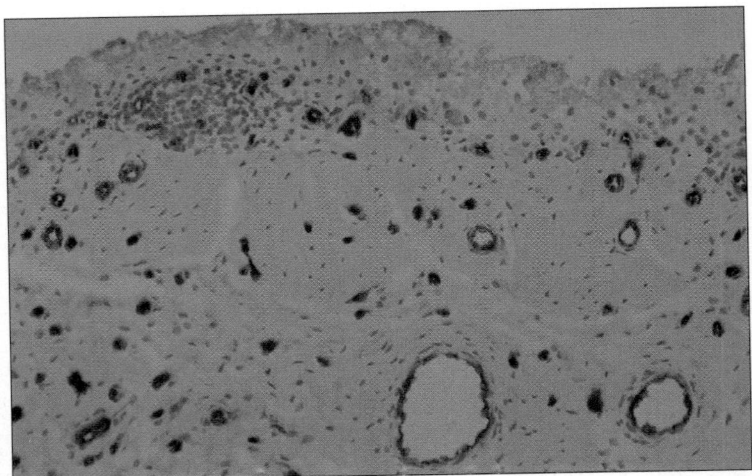

Fig. 13.4 Blood vessels in RA synovium. A dramatic increase in the number of blood vessels is characteristic of RA. This photomicrograph shows a frozen section of RA synovial tissue stained with a monoclonal antibody that binds to endothelial cells (brown pigment). The intimal lining is devoid of blood vessels and, immediately below the lining layer, there is a network of capillaries and venules.

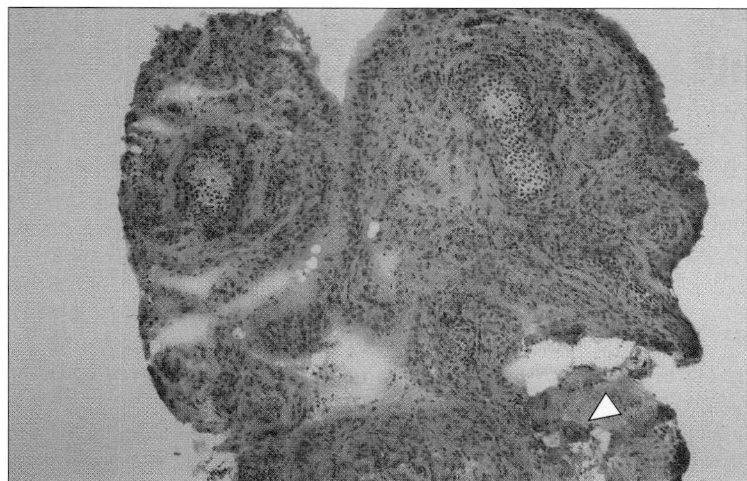

Fig. 13.5 Gout synovium. Non-rheumatoid forms of arthritis that are clearly not mediated by an autoimmune response can mimic the histopathologic features of RA. This is an example of chronic tophaceous gout in which synovial lining hyperplasia, angiogenesis and sublining infiltration with mononuclear cells are prominent.

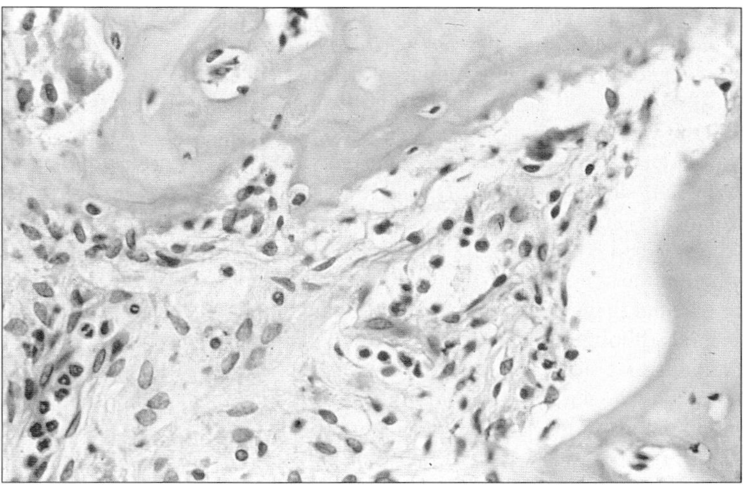

Fig. 13.6 Synovial pannus in RA. Photomicrograph of the pannus at the synovium–bone interface in RA, with synoviocytes invading bone. (Courtesy of Dr R. Wilder.)

not the case in rheumatoid synovitis, where the CD8$^+$ T-cells are usually present in small numbers and are located at the periphery of aggregates. This has led to speculation that macrophages or dendritic cells in the synovium present antigen to T-helper cells in the immunoreactive transitional zone. The paucity of CD8-bearing lymphocytes and resultant lack of T-cell suppressor activity might contribute to local B cell hyperreactivity and increased synthesis of immunoglobulins, thus accounting for the plasma cells and the large amounts of antibodies produced by the rheumatoid synovium. That paradigm is supported by the fact that the relatively small synovial fluid helper/inducer CD4$^+$ population is also highly enriched for 'pure' helper cells (Leu3a$^+$/Leu8$^-$). The lack of suppressor cells would also support unrestrained expansion of T-helper cell populations. However, significant proliferation of helper cells is not observed in the synovium; DNA synthesis occurs in only a very small percentage of synovial T-cells, and the rare mitoses are usually observed in the CD8$^+$ population.

In RA, histologic examination of synovium is of limited value as a diagnostic tool. This is in part because of the high degree of variability in the histologic picture between RA patients. There are also differences in the degree of inflammation seen in the synovium within a single joint, since some regions can demonstrate typical rheumatoid characteristics while others can appear more benign. Also, there is significant overlap with other diseases, since virtually any chronic inflammatory arthritis can have the same histology. This includes arthritides that are probably driven by specific antigens, like Lyme disease and reactive arthritis, as well as diseases that are clearly not mediated by T-cells, like chronic tophaceous gout (Fig. 13.5). Synovial biopsies might provide some prognostic information, since the extent of macrophage infiltration appears to correlate with erosive disease[9]. Although osteoarthritis (OA) synovium tends to be less inflammatory than RA, there is considerable overlap.

One feature of RA that distinguishes it from other inflammatory arthropathies is the propensity for synovium to become locally invasive at the synovial interface with cartilage and bone. This destructive mass of tissue is sometimes referred to as 'pannus' and is responsible for the characteristic marginal erosions observed in RA. Pannus has histologic characteristics that distinguish it from other regions of the synovium (Fig. 13.6). It comprises primarily invasive lining cells with very little sublining lymphocytic infiltration. The lining cells have the appearance of transformed mesenchymal cells with open, pleomorphic nuclei, high expression of oncogenes, and large amounts of mRNA encoding destructive metalloproteinases. The invasive properties of pannus in the absence of T-lymphocyte cells suggest that the RA synoviocytes express some qualities attributed to transformation. Pannus is unique to RA; other inflammatory arthropathies can be locally destructive but do not possess this characteristic histologic appearance.

CELLS OF THE RHEUMATOID SYNOVIUM

MACROPHAGE-LIKE CELLS

Rheumatoid synovial tissue can be dispersed into single cells *in vitro* using enzymes like collagenase to digest the extracellular matrix. About 20% of these cells express macrophage surface markers, such as CD14, CD68, or CD11b[10]. This population presumably represent a mixture of macrophage-like type A synoviocytes and true tissue macrophages that were present in the sublining. The macrophage lineage cells characteristically express very high levels of surface HLA-DR (Fig. 13.7). Since processed antigen is presented to CD4$^+$ T-cells in the groove of HLA-DR on antigen-presenting cells, it is thought that increased class II MHC expression enhances the antigen-presenting capacity of synovial macrophages. HLA-DR expression is maximal on synovial macrophages, and exposure to exogenous cytokines like IFN-γ (a potent DR-inducer) *in vitro* does not increase expression further. These cells maintain an activated phenotype *in vitro* for at least a month, suggesting that the macrophages either secrete factors that help maintain DR expression or that the cells are altered in a way that results in constitutive expression of the major histocompatibility (MHC) antigen. *In situ* hybridization and immunoperoxidase studies on intact synovial tissues also demonstrate intense HLA-DR gene expression and surface antigen expression in the lining where the type A synoviocytes are located. Sublining DR is also abundant in RA tissues and is expressed on synovial macrophages, T-cells and B cells. Synovial macrophages appear to be the source of many

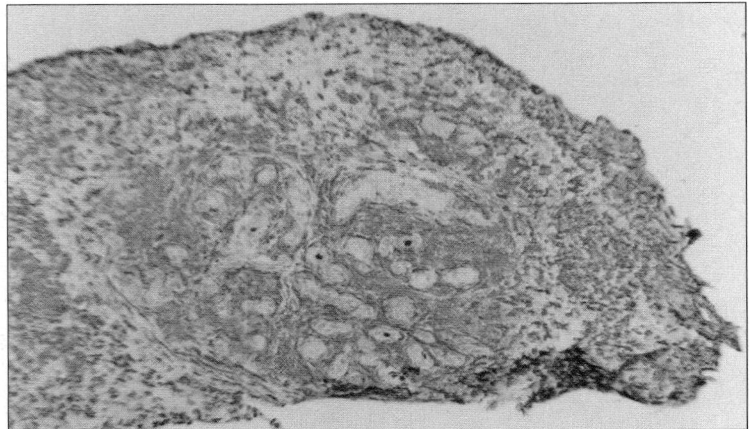

Fig. 13.7 HLA-DR expression in synovium. RA synovial tissue stained with a monoclonal antibody directed against HLA-DR. HLA-DR$^+$ regions stain with a brown color. Note prominent staining of the intimal lining as well as of sublining mononuclear cells.

of the cytokines produced by the synovium (see page 13.9).

Cells of macrophage lineage can also be isolated from synovial effusions of patients with inflammatory arthritis. Synovial fluid monocytes presumably reach the joint through the circulation, traverse the tissue, and migrate through the lining to enter the joint space. These cells, like their counterparts in synovial tissue, express a highly activated phenotype, and surface density of class II MHC antigens on synovial fluid monocytes is significantly greater than on peripheral blood monocytes from the same patient[11]. As with synovial lining cells, it is not known whether the synovial fluid cells are activated prior to entry into the joint or whether they receive this signal during their passage through the synovium. Although the cytokine milieu of inflamed synovial tissue is more than adequate to account for the activated phenotype of synovial fluid monocytes/macrophages, there is also evidence that peripheral blood monocytes are not entirely quiescent. For instance, HLA-DR expression is normal in RA peripheral blood cells, but blood monocytes cultured under serum-free conditions show increased spontaneous production of angiotensin-converting enzyme and interleukin 1β (IL-1β) compared to cells from normal individuals or OA patients[12]. Also, spontaneous production of prostaglandins and leukotrienes is increased in RA monocytes. These abnormalities are particularly pronounced in patients with elevated erythrocyte sedimentation rates or early disease.

FIBROBLAST-LIKE CELLS

A second major population of cells isolated from enzymatically dispersed synovium has the appearance of fibroblasts. These cells are non-phagocytic and lack demonstrable surface HLA-DR or macrophage differentiation antigens. Unlike fibroblasts isolated from the skin, synovial fibroblasts constitutively express vascular cell adhesion molecule (VCAM-1) and stain positively for the enzyme UDPGD[13]. Some have long, branched cytoplasmic extensions and a dendritic or stellate morphology (Fig. 13.8). However, they should be distinguished from the antigen-presenting cells known as dendritic cells, which are much smaller and rich in class II MHC surface antigen. The stellate morphology likely represents a phenotype of fibroblasts transformed by the inflammatory products of the synovium, including IL-1 and prostaglandin E_2. Synovial fibroblasts can also act as accessory cells for T-cell stimulation by superantigens, especially after they have been treated with IFN-γ[14].

When enzymatically dispersed adherent synovial tissue cells are cultivated *in vitro* for several weeks, the percentage of macrophage-like cells gradually decreases, ultimately leaving a relatively homogeneous population of fibroblast-like cells. These cells proliferate *in vitro* and can be maintained for many months. During the first few passages after isolation from the intact synovium, they spontaneously secrete large amounts of hyaluronic acid, cytokines and arachidonic acid metabolites; hence the culture supernatant has many characteristics of synovial fluid. The low level of class II MHC molecules sometimes expressed on their surface *in vivo* completely disappears within days and there is a decline in the production of inflammatory mediators and effectors of matrix degradation-like collagenase. After several weeks, however, the fibroblast-like cells become quiescent and proliferate more slowly. These functions can be rapidly restored by the addition of cytokines such as IL-1 or TNF-α to the culture[15,16]. However, even without stimulation, they continue to secrete cytokines and growth factors such as IL-6, TGF-β and fibroblast growth factor, as well as high levels of tissue inhibitor of metalloproteinases (TIMP) for many months. Late passage OA and RA synoviocytes are often functionally and phenotypically indistinguishable, although some data suggest that the latter spontaneously secrete significantly greater amounts of cytokines and growth factors.

The origin of the fibroblast-like cells that overgrow synovial cell cultures is not certain, but it is often assumed (or at least hoped) that they are derived from the type B synoviocytes identified in the lining. It can be difficult to distinguish this population from sublining synovial fibroblasts that might proliferate in the cultures, although the presence of VCAM-1 is a valuable clue. Elevated production of proteoglycans by early passage cells suggests that many originate from the lining. Although fibroblast-like synoviocytes appear and behave like fibroblasts from other organs (for example, skin and lung), they also possess some characteristics that are associated with transformed cells. For instance, normal cultured fibroblasts proliferate in culture until they reach confluence. At this point, DNA synthesis stops and the cells form a monolayer in the culture dish. Malignant or transformed fibroblasts lose this control mechanism (known as contact inhibition), and continue to divide and pile up on each other. Under some conditions (particularly in the presence of platelet-derived growth factor (PDGF)), cultured fibroblast-like synoviocytes also escape contact inhibition. Normal fibroblasts require adherence to a surface in order to proliferate, while transformed cells can grow in suspension or in semi-solid medium. Cultured synoviocytes, like the transformed cell lines, grow in an anchorage-independent manner and express several oncogenes that are characteristic of rapidly dividing cells that have escaped normal growth-regulatory mechanisms. Loss of growth control in fibroblast-like synoviocytes might contribute to synovial lining hyperplasia and the locally invasive properties of pannus. The notion of a 'transformed' synoviocyte has recently been supported by experiments using severe combined immunodeficiency (SCID) mice (which lack an intact immune system and cannot reject xenotransplants) as a model for *in vivo* invasiveness. Cartilage explants can survive for prolonged periods of time in these animals. When either synovial cells or purified fibroblast-like synoviocytes from RA patients are implanted at the site of the explant, they migrate into the cartilage matrix and spontaneously produce proteases[17]. Control synoviocytes from OA patients and dermal fibroblasts do not invade the cartilage implants. Therefore, RA fibroblast-like synoviocytes maintain their ability to invade cartilage, even in the absence of other synovial cells.

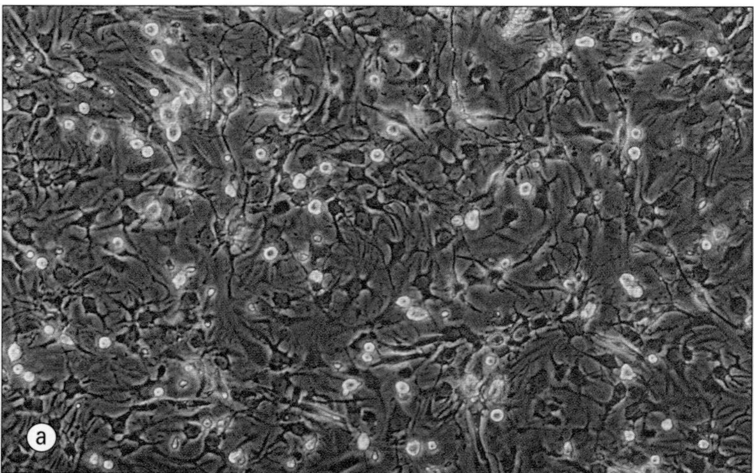

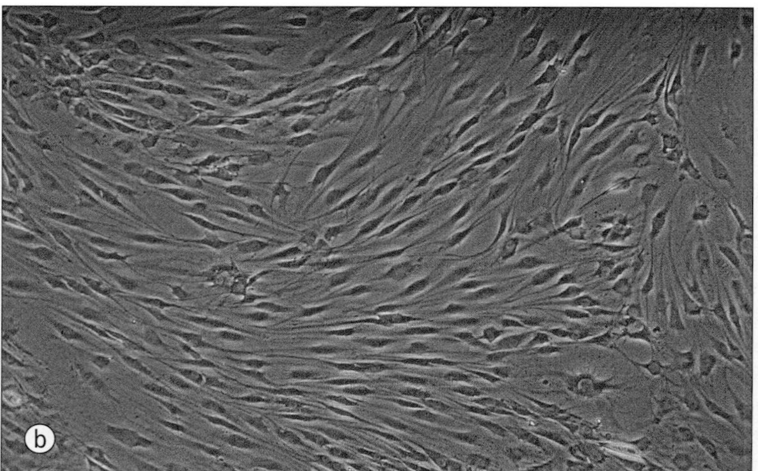

Fig. 13.8 Primary and late passage synoviocytes. Photomicrographs of primary (a) and late (b) cultured synoviocytes. The primary culture contains a mixed population of fibroblast-like and macrophage-like cells with variable morphology. After several weeks, the cultures contain a homogeneous population of quiescent fibroblast-like cells.

'PANNOCYTES'

While fibroblast-like synoviocytes isolated from synovium have some characteristics reminiscent of transformation, it is also possible that another cell type is primarily responsible for tissue destruction at the cartilage–pannus junction. Such a cell could digest and invade the extracellular matrix despite the absence of lymphocytes in pannus. Several groups have identified candidates isolated directly from enzymatically dispersed pannus[18]. These primitive cells can express phenotypic and functional features of both fibroblast-like synoviocytes and chondrocytes. The cells, sometimes referred to as 'pannocytes', have the ability to grow in culture for a prolonged time without becoming senescent, express very high amounts of the adhesion molecule VCAM-1, and produce proteoglycans and matrix metalloproteinases (MMPs). It is uncertain whether they represent a separate lineage of cells or merely dedifferentiated synoviocytes or chondrocytes.

T-CELLS

Phenotype and distribution

T-cells comprise about 30–50% of synovial tissue cells. The predominant T-cell subset in the sublining of RA patients is the $CD4^+$ helper/inducer lymphocyte, and the CD4/CD8 ratio ranges from 4:1 to 14:1. This value is generally greater than the ratio found in peripheral blood. The majority of the CD4 cells also express surface antigens characteristic of mature memory cells, such as CD45RO[19], which suggests previous exposure to antigen followed by a postactivation 'resting' or primed state. Although naive $CD45RA^+/CD45RO^-$ T-cells are also seen, they represent a distinct minority. Some of the memory T-cells in the synovium express HLA-DR antigens on their surface, but the amounts observed are significantly less than those on articular macrophages. This, along with expression of other activation antigens like VLA-1, is a non-specific finding in many forms of chronic arthritis.

There are two basic histologic patterns of T-cell infiltration in the rheumatoid synovium. First, aggregates of lymphocytes which contain up to several hundred T-cells collect in the sublining, particularly near blood vessels. The number of aggregates present in this region varies widely among patients. In some individuals, the sublining is completely replaced by many organized lymphoid collections, while in others only a few small scattered aggregates are seen. A second pattern is a diffuse T-cell infiltration without obvious organization. In this case, the T-cells are usually located immediately below the lining and extend 1–2mm into the sublining tissue. The lining itself is usually devoid of T-cells.

Although T-cells are abundant in synovial fluid, they are not a random sampling of cells from synovium. The numbers of CD4 and $CD8^+$ cells are approximately equal in synovial fluid in contrast to the vast excess of CD4 cells in the tissue. The reason for this reversal of T-cell subsets is not clear, but could represent shunting of $CD8^+$ cells from the synovium into the synovial fluid. Furthermore, since IL-6 preferentially induces $CD8^+$ T-cell proliferation, it is possible that high synovial fluid levels of IL-6 favor local expansion of this population. However, the very low rate of division of synovial fluid T-cells makes this explanation less likely.

Oligoclonality of synovial T-cells

Oligoclonality of infiltrating synovial T-cells in RA has been the focus of intense investigation in recent years. The data on T-cell receptor (TcR) rearrangements in RA are far from conclusive. Several reports have been published describing over-representation of various combinations of TcR genes. There is no general agreement, but some studies have suggested a preponderance of $V_\beta3$, 14 and 17 T-cells in RA[20–23]. These specific V_β genes are of particular interest because they have related sequences and are able to bind to some superantigens (which activate T-cells in an antigen-independent fashion). This could cause oligoclonal expansion of certain T-cells and cytokine production as well as account for blunted antigen and mitogen responses of articular T-cells. However, it is important to note that many other studies have not found any evidence of oligoclonality or have identified different V_β or V_α chains[24,25]. Methodologic and epidemiologic differences in study design account for some of these differences, and insufficient control populations often make data interpretation difficult. It is also important to remember that expansion of specific TcR-bearing cells might be due to secondary antigens in the joint, like proteoglycans or type II collagen, rather than to an etiologic agent.

T-cell responsiveness and antigen specificity

Lymphocytes in both synovial fluid and synovial tissue tend to have blunted proliferative responses after challenge by mitogens, cytokines, or anti-CD3 antibodies. T-cells in RA synovial fluid also do not respond normally when exposed to autologous stimulators, as in the autologous mixed leukocyte reaction (AMLR)[26]. There are several possible reasons for these suboptimal responses, including the fact that synovial cells are bathed in a variety of immunosuppressive factors. Inhibitors of several cytokines, including IL-1, IL-2, and IFN-γ, have been identified in synovial fluid. When normal peripheral blood cells are stimulated in the presence of synovial fluid, proliferation and cytokine production are markedly decreased. TGF-β also appears to be an important suppressive factor in synovial fluid since antibodies to TGF-β neutralize much of the inhibitory activity[27].

Studies of articular T-cell responses to specific antigens to determine the nature of a potential etiologic agent have, in general, been disappointing (reviewed in Chapter 5.10). Several putative antigens have been investigated over the years, including heat shock proteins (HSP), proteoglycans and type II collagen. For instance, synovial fluid T-cells from patients with RA demonstrate a brisk proliferative response to both the acetone-precipitable fraction of *Mycobacterium tuberculosis* and recombinant 65kDa HSP[28,29]. The response to mycobacterial antigen is not specific to RA, however, and also occurs in synovial fluid T-cells from patients with reactive arthritis. In adjuvant arthritis (AA), rats immunized with complete Freund's adjuvant (CFA) develop a T-cell dependent symmetric polyarticular arthritis that shares some histopathologic features of RA. The epitopes in CFA that cause arthritis appear to reside on the 65kDa mycobacterial HSP[30]. Some epitopes on proteoglycan molecules cross-react with HSP, and HSP-responsive T-cell clones derived from animals with AA also proliferate if exposed to proteoglycans[31], Hence, a process causing immunity to HSP could lead to an inflammatory response directed at the cartilage matrix[32].

Type II collagen is another major component of cartilage that can potentially induce antigen-specific responses in the synovium. When susceptible strains of mice and rats are immunized with native type II collagen, a symmetric inflammatory arthritis ensues that is known as collagen-induced arthritis (CIA). The relevance of type II collagen immunity to RA is not established. Serum antibodies that bind to collagen occur in RA as well as in many other forms of inflammatory arthritis. There is also active synthesis of antibodies to type II collagen by synovial tissue cells from most patients with RA[33]. The synovial antibody response to type II collagen is relatively specific, since production of type I collagen antibodies is infrequent. However, there is little correlation between the production of antibodies in the synovium and serum titers.

The importance of T-cell specific responses directed against these and other local antigens is not known. The lack of specificity for any particular disease suggests that they are general properties of chronic synovial inflammation and are probably a secondary phenomenon. Hence, any stimulus that initiates inflammatory arthritis (e.g., reactive arthritis or RA) could cause release of local antigens from normally restricted sites as a result of matrix destruction. This would lead to local immunity directed against articular antigens. While such a process certainly could contribute to disease severity and perpetuation, it might not be the primary driving force.

DENDRITIC CELLS

Dendritic cells (DC) are potent antigen-presenting cells that express large amounts of surface class II MHC antigens (particularly HLA-DQ), lack macrophage differentiation antigens like CD14 and FcRs, and are non-phagocytic. These cells are distinct from the stellate cells derived from enzymatically digested synovial tissue, whose phenotype is the result of exposure to inflammatory mediators. GM-CSF, which is produced by RA synovial fibroblasts and macrophages, is required for full differentiation and activation of DCs[34]. Methods of distinguishing DCs from macrophages are often indirect and rely on identification of the above features, as well as characteristic morphologic and ultrastructural features, such as long processes on DCs that can contact and envelop T-cells. This interaction results in characteristic immunoreactive clusters that contain one DC and several T-cells. Large numbers of DCs are found in synovial effusions of patients with RA, and comprise up to 5% synovial fluid mononuclear cells (compared to <1% of peripheral blood cells)[35]. They are found in the synovial fluid of patients with other forms of inflammatory arthritis, but the number is significantly less than in RA. Early data suggested that RA articular DCs present antigen more efficiently that those isolated from other sites. However, some data indicate that synovial fluid DCs in RA are functionally similar to other DCs, since the response of normal peripheral blood T-cells to allogeneic stimulation is the same regardless of the source (RA synovial fluid, non-RA synovial fluid, or normal peripheral blood). Immunostaining of RA synovial tissue with antibodies that detect surface markers relatively specific to DCs (like RFD1) detect DC-like cells in several locations of the inflamed synovium. These cells also express the co-stimulatory molecule B7-2 and are located near dense lymphoid aggregates and high endothelial venules. Synovial DCs migrate from the peripheral blood, presumably under the influence of a chemotactic gradient. Once in the joint, they can serve as potent antigen-presenting cells for either an etiologic agent or local antigens released by ongoing synovial inflammation.

B CELLS AND RHEUMATOID FACTORS

B cells constitute a relatively small fraction of synovial cells (1–5%) but contribute significantly to the local inflammatory process through the production of autoantibodies that form immune complexes *in situ*. Plasma cells, which are terminally differentiated B cells, also infiltrate the subintima of most patients with RA. The antigen specificities of some synovial B cells have been defined. For example, rheumatoid factors are readily detected and are secreted in large amounts. B cells that synthesize and secrete type II collagen antibodies are also abundant. The location of antibody-producing B cells within the synovium varies, but they tend to occur in transitional and plasma-cell-rich zones described earlier. Some characteristics of B cells in RA distinguish them from other B cells. For instance, a significant percentage express the surface antigen CD5, which is normally displayed by T-cells. It is also expressed on a small number of immature B cells in adults but on most B cells in the fetus. Circulating $CD5^+$ B cells are elevated in a variety of autoimmune diseases and are associated with the production of autoantibodies, including rheumatoid factors. There is some evidence of oligoclonal expansion of B cells in RA. When one looks at the surface phenotype of circulating lymphocytes, there is an abnormal κ chain to λ chain ratio compared with normal controls. There are two likely explanations for this observation: 1) an inciting antigen preferentially stimulates only specific subsets of B cells; or 2) only specific subsets of B cells are capable of producing rheumatoid factor.

Rheumatoid factors are produced by peripheral blood and synovial B cells in RA and can comprise any of the major immunoglobulin classes (IgM, IgG, IgA, and IgE). The percentage of patients that are seropositive depends on the type of assay used, with the greatest sensitivity observed using an enzyme-linked immunosorbent assay (ELISA) for IgM rheumatoid factor. While over 90% are positive for IgM rheumatoid factor, about two thirds of patients are positive for IgA, IgE and IgG rheumatoid factor. Disease activity and levels of circulating immune complexes seem to correlate best with IgM and IgA.

The rheumatoid factors produced by RA B cells differ from those produced by B cells in normal individuals[36]. Genes that encode rheumatoid factors are present in the human germ line, and anti-idiotype antibodies have been developed that can identify these proteins. The germline derived rheumatoid factors are produced by immature $CD5^+$ B cells as well as by about a quarter of B lymphocytes in fetal spleen germinal centers. Many paraproteins produced by malignant B cells (such as Waldenstrom's macroglobulinemia) also reflect the germ line sequences. Finally, normal B cells in adult human tonsil tissue express and synthesize germ line encoded rheumatoid factors. These cells are prevalent in the mantle zones of lymphoid tissues even though circulating rheumatoid factor is not detected; it is likely that they do not secrete the protein even though it is expressed on the surface. It has been suggested that these cells can trap immune complexes very efficiently by virtue of their ability to bind to immunoglobulins. The antigens in the complexes could then be processed and presented to local T-cells in the context of surface class II MHC molecules expressed on the surface of the B lymphocyte. However, recent experiments using B cell knock out mice do not demonstrate a significant alteration of T-cell function[37].

The situation is very different with rheumatoid-factor-producing B cells in RA synovium and lymphoid tissues[38]. These proteins are not encoded by germ line sequences and are not recognized by the aforementioned antibodies. Instead, their sequence appears to be derived through rearrangements and somatic mutations that occur during life. In contrast to 'normal' rheumatoid-factor-producing cells, RA B cells secrete large amounts of the autoantibody. In fact, the rheumatoid synovium is a potent antibody-producing organ in which 10–20% of its total immunoglobulin production possesses rheumatoid factor activity. These antibodies are polyclonal and can form large immune complexes in the joint, with resultant complement fixation, neutrophil activation and acute inflammation.

NEUTROPHILS

One surprising aspect of rheumatoid synovitis is the paucity of neutrophils in the synovium compared to synovial effusions. Although some granulocytes can be observed in synovial tissue in early disease, it is uncommon to find significant numbers in chronically inflamed synovium, even during acute flares. Like monocytes, neutrophils presumably reach the joint space via the circulation and migrate into the tissue. Since tissue neutrophils are relatively short-lived cells, there is likely to be a continuous flux through the synovium in order to maintain a constant number of neutrophils in the synovial fluid, possibly under the influence of immune complexes, chemotactic factors like C5a, or cytokines like IL-8. A possible explanation for the relative ease with which neutrophils pass from synovial fluid to synovial tissue is that they lack the adhesion molecule VLA-4 on their surface. This molecule comprises the α_4/β_1 subunits of the integrin family of adhesions molecules and participates in cellular binding to matrix proteins, such as alternatively spliced fibronectin and the adhesion molecules VCAM-1 (see page 13.17). Of particular interest is VCAM-1, which is highly expressed by the synovial intimal lining. Because of the lack of VLA-4 on neutrophils, they might be able to follow chemotactic factor gradients into the synovial fluid without hindrance. This contrasts with lymphocytes and macrophages, which express VLA-4 and are selectively retained in the synovium.

Although neutrophils do not appear to play a major role in the synovium, they are prominent effectors of cartilage damage and inflammation in the synovial fluid. The relative abundance of granulocytes in synovial fluid is variable, with anywhere from <1000 to over 100,000 neutrophils/mm^3 in synovial fluid. Neutrophils can be activated by several factors in the synovial fluid milieu, including IL-8, GM-CSF and immune complexes. After ingestion of the latter, the cells can release their contents of lysozomal enzymes (such as myeloperoxidase, lysozyme, elastase, collagenase and gelatinase) and generate destructive oxygen radicals that can damage cartilage and supportive joint structures. In addition, PMNs from synovial fluid in RA secrete a variety of newly synthesized proteins, including fibronectin, neutral proteinases, and IL-1. Synovial fluid neutrophils also produce the IL-1 receptor antagonist (IL-1ra) as a major product[39]. The absolute quantity of IL-1ra produced by each neutrophil is much lower than by individual macrophages. However, the large number of neutrophils in effusions suggests that their quantitative contribution to total synovial effusion IL-1ra can be substantial.

MAST CELLS

Small numbers of mast cells are present in the rheumatoid synovium, but there are significantly more in joint samples from patients with RA compared to those of normal individuals[40]. It is not known whether the increase in mast cells in RA is a cause or an effect of the inflammatory process. Given their ability to secrete proteinases, vasoactive materials and chemotactic factors, it is possible that mast cells are actively involved in synovitis. The presence of mast cell growth factors in RA synovial fluid could contribute to local accumulation of mast cells[41].

NATURAL KILLER CELLS

Natural killer (NK) cells mediate non-MHC restricted cytotoxicity. These cells display surface FcRs (CD16) and the C3bi receptor (CD11b) as well as CD57. NK cells primarily damage target cells with an activated phenotype, such as high surface expression of transferrin receptors, or cells coated with IgG antibodies (i.e. antibody dependent cellular cytotoxicity). Less than 1% of mononuclear cells in rheumatoid synovial tissue are NK cells and thoracic duct lymph from RA patients contains very few of these cells. Lysis of NK-sensitive targets by cells enzymatically dispersed from synovial tissue is less than with paired peripheral blood mononuclear cells. NK cells suppress a number of immune responses, including immunoglobulin production and the autologous mixed leukocyte reaction. Hence, the absence of effective NK cells could contribute to the chronic lymphoid stimulation in the rheumatoid joint. There is a significant percentage of cells in the synovial fluid that co-express CD57 and CD8 (usually found on suppressor T-cells) compared to normal or RA peripheral blood. Morphologically, these cells have the appearance of large granular lymphocytes. Their role in RA is unknown, but similar cells isolated from peripheral blood suppress cell differentiation induced by pokeweed mitogen and cellular cytotoxicity dependent on lectin.

CYTOKINES, GROWTH FACTORS, AND OTHER SOLUBLE MEDIATORS

CYTOKINE ASSAYS AND ARTIFACTS

Cells communicate with one another either through direct contact, as with membrane-bound cytokines, or through the release of soluble mediators. The latter, which include cytokines and low molecular weight mediators like prostaglandins and leukotrienes, diffuse away from cells and ultimately interact with specific receptors. Because quantifying cell-cell interactions is quite difficult, most studies on the role of cytokines in RA have been directed towards elucidation of the soluble cytokine milieu.

There are two basic methods for assaying soluble cytokines. The first and most sensitive is usually a biological assay in which a factor induces a functional or phenotypic change in a target cell (e.g. cell proliferation). Although this technique is quite sensitive, it often suffers from lack of specificity. Immunoassays are the second major method for measuring cytokines. Although there are many possible techniques, one of the most common uses a two antibody 'sandwich' assay (Fig. 13.9). Immunoassays are usually simpler and more specific than biological assays. When analyzing synovial fluid, it is also important to remember that the high viscosity can prevent proteins from diffusing freely and interacting with an immobilized antibody; this can usually be prevented by preincubating the sample with hyaluronidase to digest proteoglycans. Another limitation of immunoassays in RA is interference by rheumatoid factors. This problem arises because of the ability of rheumatoid factors to link the Fc portions of primary and secondary antibodies, thereby causing a false positive result (Fig. 13.9).

In addition to the difficulties inherent in assaying RA synovial fluid and other biological samples for cytokines, there are theoretic problems that need to be considered. Degradation of cytokines by proteases and absorption of factors by activated cells or soluble receptors are two other potential pitfalls. The concentrations of free cytokine might also be decreased due to interactions with the matrix proteins like glycosaminoglycans. The steady state levels of a protein in synovial fluid represent a balance between local production, ingress from the blood and egress from the synovial fluid via the lymphatics. This last consideration is probably of secondary importance because proteins tend to leave the synovial fluid slowly.

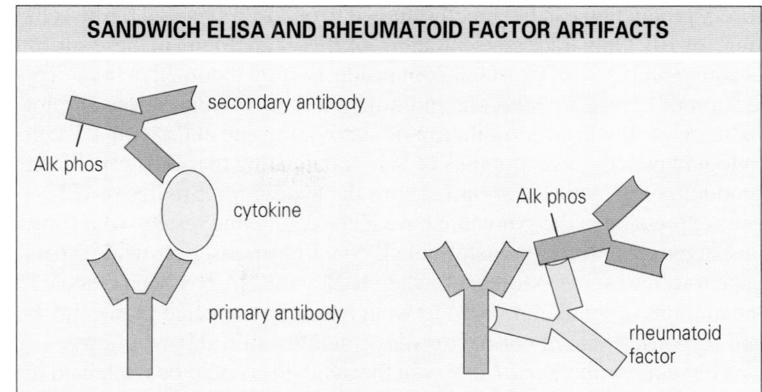

Fig. 13.9 Sandwich assay and effect of rheumatoid factor. Sandwich-type immunoassays (left) and a proposed mechanism for rheumatoid factor interference (right). Rheumatoid factors can bind to the Fc portions of the primary antibody and conjugated secondary antibody, which results in a false positive signal.

T-CELL PRODUCTS

Interferon-γ

The first studies of cytokines in rheumatic disease were reported in the late 1970s when IFN bioassays were performed on serum and synovial effusions of patients with RA. Using viral cytopathic protection assays, high titers of IFN-like activity were identified. Because the activity was acid labile, it was tentatively identified as immune IFN (i.e. IFN-γ). The presence of IFN-γ activity in these samples appeared to confirm its putative role in inflammatory synovitis. At the time, IFN-γ was the only cytokine known to induce HLA-DR expression on cells, and high expression of this marker on many kinds of synovial cells is a cardinal finding of RA. The detection of IFN in joint samples was not surprising and seemed to explain the elevated class II MHC antigen expression.

However, later experiments raised questions regarding the amount of IFN-γ in the joint. First, the biological assays used in these studies lacked specificity, and non-IFN factors (like tumor necrosis factor (TNF) and IL-6) were later identified in synovial fluid that could give false positive results[42]. Second, RA synovial fluid T-cells and peripheral blood T-cells stimulated by IL-2 or by autologous antigen-presenting cells – i.e. the autologous mixed leukocyte reaction (AMLR) – have defective production of IFN-γ. The defect in the AMLR appears to be due to increased sensitivity of RA T-cells to the effects of prostaglandins. Subsequently, studies of immunoreactive IFN-γ protein in frozen sections of synovial tissue demonstrated only trace amounts of the cytokine[43]. Finally, although synovial fluid and supernatants of cultured synovial tissue cells contain a factor that can induce HLA-DR expression on monocytes, it is not neutralized by antibodies to IFN-γ.

Because of the potential problems with biological assays, sensitive and specific immunoassays were performed to help clarify the question of how much IFN-γ is in the inflamed joint. Only trace amounts of immunoreactive IFN-γ (usually <0.5 U/ml) were detected in the joint effusions of patients with RA. Similar amounts were found in other seronegative inflammatory arthritides. Artifactual explanations for the lack of IFN-γ in RA synovial fluid, such as the effects of rheumatoid factors, enzymatic degradation and absorption by synovial fluid cells, have been excluded. For comparison, peripheral blood mononuclear cells can produce over 100 U/ml *in vitro* when stimulated by mitogens or by allogeneic cells, and 10–20 U/ml are needed to induce HLA-DR surface expression on monocytes comparable to those found in the joint. Of course, it is difficult to be certain of the effect of very low concentrations of IFN-γ alone or in combination with other cytokines on cells for a prolonged period of time *in vivo*. It is also not clear whether small amounts of IFN-γ produced in the microenvironment could have a more potent effect. However, it is worth noting that other T-cell mediated disease in humans, such as tuberculous pleuritis, result in the production of high levels of IFN-γ, with levels of about 80 U/ml achieved in pleural fluid[44].

IFN-γ production can be directly studied in cultured synovial tissue cells (Fig. 13.10). Only trace concentrations of IFN-γ are found in these supernatants; inhibition of prostaglandin production by indomethacin or separation of cells into adherent and nonadherent subpopulations do not increase production. Stimulation of synovial tissue cells with a T-cell mitogen induces large amounts of IFN-γ indicating that cells capable of producing the cytokine are present in the synovium. Studies of IFN-γ gene expression in the synovium have given conflicting results, with some investigators reporting no detectable IFN-γ RNA transcripts while others appear to find some. Moreover, when IFN-γ mRNA has been detected, the amount is small compared to what might be expected in normal T-cell responses (e.g. in normal tonsils or in tuberculin skin reactions).

The relative absence of IFN-γ in the synovium could be explained in several ways. First, as described earlier, patients with RA have a specific defect in IFN-γ production that could contribute to this phenomenon. Second, endogenous production of immunosuppressive factors, like IL-10 and TGF-β, inhibits cytokine production. This possibility is supported by studies showning that neutralizing anti-IL-10 antibodies sometimes increase endogenous IFN-γ production by cultured synovial cells[45]. A third possibility is that the T-cells in the synovium have not received the appropriate activation signal. Finally, small amounts of IFN-γ delivered in the microenvironment might be sufficient to stimulate target cells. The last scenario is known to occur in other situations, such as the nonobese diabetic (NOD) mouse. In that case, islet cells isolated from NOD mice produce little IFN-γ *in vitro*, although systemic administration of anti-IFN-γ antibodies to the animals ameliorates glucose intolerance[46].

Interleukin-2

IL-2 is another T-cell derived cytokine that plays a central role in immune responses. A primary function is to serve as a T-cell growth factor in either an autocrine or paracrine manner, but IL-2 also activates and differentiates B cells into immunoglobulin-secreting cells. Macrophages express surface IL-2 receptors and IL-2 causes significant functional and phenotypic alterations. Although originally identified as a T-cell stimulating factor in RA synovial tissue, data on IL-2 production in the rheumatoid joint are conflicting. As with IFN-γ, some studies using biological assays have suggested that IL-2 is present in abundance. Synovial fluid can induce IL-2 responsive T-cell lines to proliferate in a standard IL-2 bioassay, but specific monoclonal antibodies that block the IL-2 receptor do not interfere with this activity[41]. Therefore, other non-IL-2 factors must be responsible. Immunoassays support this conclusion, since synovial fluid from only a minority of patients contains IL-2 and, when present, the concentrations are very low[47]. Immunofluorescence of RA synovium only demonstrates trace amounts of immunoreactive protein.

Tumor necrosis factor-α and -β

TNF-α is a pleotropic cytokine that is expressed by a variety of cells, including T-cells, macrophages and mast cells. It is produced as a homotrimer that can be expressed on the cell surface and ultimately released after cleavage by a matrix metalloproteinase. TNF-α is a major regulator of normal immune function as well as a primary mediator of inflammatory diseases like septic shock. Although large amounts of TNF-α are present in RA synovial fluid, macrophages and fibroblasts, not T-cells, are the primary source (see below). Synovial fluid contains little or no detectable TNF-β, a homologue of TNF-α that is usually derived from activated T-cells and binds to TNF surface receptors[48].

Other T-cell cytokines (IL-3, IL-4, IL-6, GM-CSF)

Several laboratories have measured the levels of other T-cell products in synovial fluid or in the supernatants of cultured synovial tissue cells. In each case, the concentrations have been low. For instance, mRNA encoding IL-3, a cytokine that supports bone marrow stem cell differentiation and also has some immunostimulatory properties (such as induction of class II MHC antigens on macrophages), has not been detected in RA synovial tissue. IL-4, a T-cell derived factor that possesses T-cell, B cell and macrophage stimulating activities, is also essentially absent from RA synovial fluid. IL-6 and GM-CSF (which are described in more detail below), like TNF-α, can be made by T-cells under some circumstances and are present in synovial fluid. However, the source of these cytokines in the rheumatoid joint is not T-cells. It is interesting to contrast the cytokine profile of RA tissues with other *in vivo* reactions known to involve T-cells. As with IFN-γ in tuberculous pleuritis, T-lymphocyte products are present in other immune-mediated diseases. For instance, IL-4 mRNA is abundant in cutaneous allergic reactions[49], and T-cells in the airway make large amounts of GM-CSF in allergen-induced asthma[50]. These studies are very useful for comparison with RA, since they validate the methods used and indicate that T-cell lymphokines are often easily detected in active T-cell mediated processes.

Helper T-cell subsets: TH0, TH1, and TH2

Cultured helper T cell clones from mice can be divided into distinct subsets based on the types of cytokines that they produce (Fig. 13.11)[51]. TH1 cells, for instance, produce IFN-γ and IL-2 but not IL-4, while TH2 cells produce IL-4 and IL-10 but not IL-2 or IFN-γ. Both subsets produce IL-3 and TNF-α. A third type, called TH0, has an unrestricted cytokine profile and might be a precursor for TH1 and/or TH2 cells. T-cell subsets modulate different aspects of immunity, with TH1 cells mediating delayed type hypersensitivity reactions and TH2 cells regulating allergic and antibody responses. The T-cell subsets can regulate each other, and IFN-γ or IL-12 produced by TH1 cells suppresses TH2 development while IL-4 and IL-10 produced by TH2 cells suppresses TH1 cells. The situation in humans is somewhat more complex in that T-cell clones do not segregate as cleanly into these specific groups. However, TH0, TH1 and TH2 cytokine patterns have been described.

IFN-γ PRODUCTION BY RHEUMATOID SYNOVIAL TISSUE CELLS

Synovial tissue (ST) samples	IFN-γ (U/ml)
ST cells	0.10 ± 0.09
ST + 1μg/ml indomethacin	0.20 ± 0.10
ST adherent cells	0.20 ± 0.05
ST nonadherent cells	0.10 ± 0.06
ST + 1μg/ml phytohemagglutinin	52 ± 34

Fig. 13.10 IFN-γ in RA ST supernatants. Isolated RA synovial tissue cells do not spontaneously produce IFN-γ nor do adherent (macrophages and fibroblasts) or nonadherent (lymphocyte) cells. However, if stimulated with a mitogen (phytohemagglutinin), large amounts of the cytokine are secreted. Synovial tissue supernatants were harvested after 3 days.

CYTOKINE PROFILES OF HELPER T-CELL SUBSETS

	TH1	TH2
IL-2	+	–
IL-3	+	+
IL-4	–	+
IL-5	–	+
IL-6	–	+
IL-10	–	+
IL-13	–	+
IFN-γ	+	–
TNF-α	+	+
TNF-β	+	–
GM-CSF	+	+

Fig. 13.11 Cytokine profiles of TH1 and TH2 subsets of T-cells. A TH0 subset has an unrestricted cytokine profile. In humans, many T-cells do not fit precisely into any of these categories.

Analyses of T-cell clones from RA synovium suggest that the infiltrating T-cells are biased towards a TH1 phenotype[52]. Very sensitive RT-PCR studies of synovial mRNA support this notion *in vivo*, with a similar bias towards small amounts of TH1 cytokine mRNA-like IFN-γ but essentially no IL-4 expression (or other TH2 cytokines)[53]. It is important to remember, however, that the vast majority of T-cells in the synovium do not actively express cytokine genes. A pertinent question is whether shifting the bias from TH1 to TH2 would be beneficial in RA. Providing exogenous TH2 cytokines, like IL-4 or IL-13, suppresses joint inflammation in murine collagen induced arthritis[54]. Also, enhanced TH2 activity is one proposed mechanism for inducing oral tolerance to type II collagen in patients with RA[55].

MACROPHAGE/FIBROBLAST PRODUCTS

In contrast to T-cells, the soluble products of macrophages and fibroblasts are abundant in synovium and synovial fluid. The multitude of products from these cells supports the notion that macrophages and fibroblasts are highly activated in the rheumatoid synovium and that they play an intimate role in the perpetuation and destructive properties of synovitis.

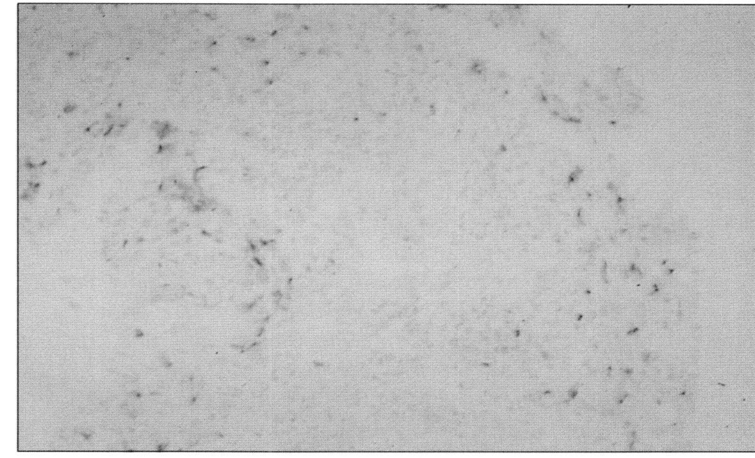

Fig. 13.12 IL-1 in RA synovial tissue. Distribution of IL-1 protein in RA synovial tissue using an immunoperoxidase technique on a noncounterstained section. Prominent staining (brown pigment) is seen in perivascular regions, with smaller amounts in the intimal lining. (Courtesy of Dr M. Field.)

Interleukin-1 and TNF-α

These two cytokines are often considered together because they possess similar activities on synovial cells even though they bind to distinct surface receptors. IL-1 is a 17kDa protein produced during antigen presentation that was originally identified as a product of macrophages. However, a variety of other cells also possess the capacity to produce IL-1, including fibroblasts, endothelial cells and T- and B-lymphocytes. Two forms of IL-1 have been demonstrated (α and β). Although these two molecules bind to the same high affinity receptor and possess essentially identical activities *in vitro*, they share only 26% amino acid sequence homology.

Both IL-1 and TNF-α are arthritogenic in animals[56,57]. Injections of either cytokine directly into the joint results in transient synovitis, and coadministration has a synergistic effect. The degree of arthritis is variable and depends on the dosing schedule and the location of the joint injected. IL-1 also can serve as an adjuvant in an antigen-induced arthritis model in which animals are immunized systemically against methylated bovine serum albumin followed by injection of the antigen into the joints. In this system, parenteral injections of IL-1 greatly enhance the synovial inflammatory response.

IL-1 and TNF-α are both present in RA synovial fluid and synovial cell supernatants as measured with biologic and immunologic assays. Enzymatically dispersed synovial cells spontaneously produce large amounts of both cytokines *in vitro*. The location and identification of their cellular sources in tissue has been determined by immunostaining techniques which detect protein and *in situ* hybridization which detects mRNA[10]. Immunoperoxidase studies identify immunoreactive TNF-α in 40% of lining cells and 5–10% of the sublining cells. The data for IL-1α are similar, with about 20% of lining cells and 25% of sublining mononuclear cells containing the protein (Fig. 13.12). Double staining experiments demonstrate that these two cytokines are produced almost exclusively by cells expressing macrophage surface markers like CD14. Only about 1% of T-cells stain with the anti-TNF-α antibody, although it is not known whether these cells produced TNF-α or if it was only bound to surface receptors. The phenotype of the cytokine producing cells has also been studied using *in-situ* hybridization on isolated enzymatically dispersed synovial cells. Using this method, 5–15% of the total population of synovial cells hybridize to the IL-1 or TNF-α probes. When subpopulations of cells are examined for cytokine gene expression, macrophages are identified as the responsible cells.

In addition to participating in the activation of T-cells during antigen presentation, both TNF-α and IL-1 are potent stimulators of synoviocytes[15,16]. Upon exposure to either cytokine, cultured fibroblast-like synoviocytes proliferate, produce metalloproteinases (such as collagenase and stromelysin), express adhesion molecules and secrete cytokines (such as GM-CSF). Prostaglandin production also increases dramatically. IL-1 and TNF-α are usually synergistic, since addition of both factors results in even higher amounts of effector production by synoviocytes. IL-1 can also serve as an autocrine growth factor for synoviocytes, since it induces expression of its own gene.

IFN-γ and TNF-α have opposing actions on many functions of cultured synoviocytes[15]. For instance, IFN-γ inhibits TNF-α mediated synoviocyte proliferation, collagenase production and GM-CSF secretion, while TNF-α inhibits IFN-γ mediated HLA-DR induction on fibroblast-like synoviocytes (Fig. 13.13). Therefore, TNF-α and IFN-γ can be mutually antagonistic, i.e. each inhibit the individual stimulating effects of the other. More recent data demonstrate that the antagonism occurs only with specific actions, and IFN-γ and TNF-α can sometimes be additive, such as with induction of intercellular adhesion molecule 1 (ICAM-1) expression. Nevertheless, mutual antagonism between IFN-γ and TNF-α suggests a novel homeostatic control mechanism in synovitis since their combined presence may serve to attenuate some aspects of articular inflammation. This is especially important in RA, where T–cells are unable to produce normal amounts of IFN-γ after stimulation and levels are quite low in the joint. The relative absence of IFN-γ could result in unopposed stimulation of type B (fibroblast-like) synoviocytes by TNF-α and could contribute to the perpetuation of synovitis. This model would predict that administration of IFN-γ would be

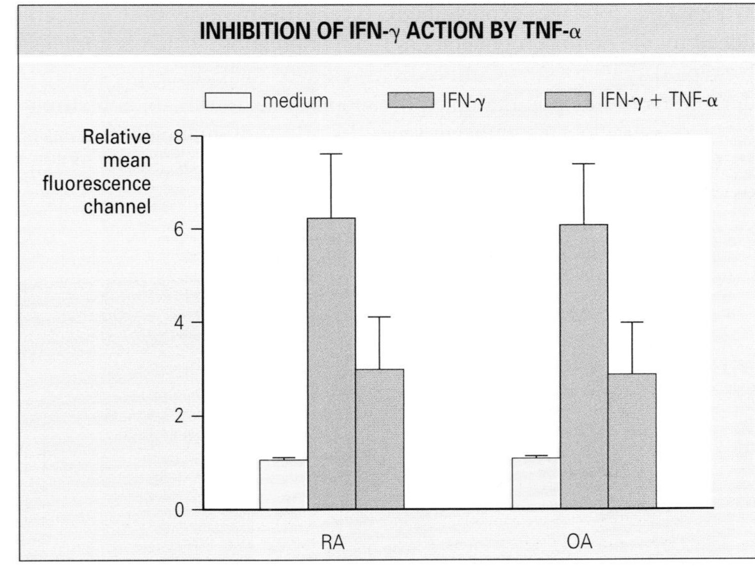

Fig. 13.13 TNF-α inhibits IFN-γ action on synoviocytes. IFN-γ induces HLA-DR expression on both OA and RA synoviocytes as determined by flow cytometry and immunofluorescence. This effect is inhibited by TNF-α. (From Alvaro-Gracia *et al.*[15], reproduced by copyright permission of The American Society for Clinical Investigation

beneficial in RA. Clinical trials with IFN-γ (both systemic and intra-articular) have met with only limited success, perhaps because the redundancy of the cytokine loops requires blockade at several sites.

Most investigators would agree that IL-1 and TNF-α are pivotal cytokines in the pathogenesis of RA. The relative contributions of each are, of course, difficult to assess in humans. Animal models of arthritis can be used to distinguish their specific actions. For instance, in murine antigen-induced arthritis, antagonists to IL-1 or TNF-α have been used as therapeutic agents[58]. These studies indicate that IL-1 is primarily responsible for the destructive phase of the disease, especially damage to proteoglycans in cartilage. TNF-α appears to cause the proliferative phase and inflammatory aspects since neutralization of this cytokine decreases swelling but not proteoglycan loss.

In humans, there is also a suggestion that TNF-α can serve as a critical cytokine. This hypothesis was supported by early studies suggesting that anti-TNF-α antibodies decrease the production of cytokines by cultured synovial tissue cells. However, recent data using sensitive and specific ELISAs indicate that anti-TNF-α antibody only modestly decreases IL-1β and has no effect on IL-1α in these cultures. Moreover, neutralization of either IL-1 or TNF-α activity alone can decrease production of some cytokines; neutralization of both cytokines is often additive[59]. The notion that TNF-α is the single critical cytokine in RA probably is an oversimplification of the complex cytokine networks. Recent data showing that anti-TNF-α antibody treatment decreases circulating IL-1 and IL-6 levels are intriguing in light of the putative importance of TNF-α. Even if TNF-α is not paramount, however, its importance is certainly demonstrated by the clinical efficacy of anti-TNF-α antibody in RA[60]. It remains to be seen if this approach will have disease modifying activity also.

Interleukin-6

IL-6 has many activities that have potential importance in rheumatic diseases, particularly B cell stimulating effects that could contribute to the local production of antibodies and rheumatoid factors. It is also a T-cell growth factor and could participate in the systemic features of the disease by inducing acute phase protein production at a distant site, such as the liver. IL-6 levels are extremely high in both RA synovial fluid and in the supernatants of cultured synovial cells. The sources of IL-6 in the synovium have been identified using the same techniques as for IL-1 and TNF-α. As with these two cytokines, most of the cells containing IL-6 protein are located in the synovial lining. *In situ* hybridization of frozen sections of synovial tissue also show IL-6 mRNA in the lining (Fig. 13.14). However, the phenotype of the cells responsible for IL-6 production is different from the cells producing IL-1 and TNF-α. While some synovial macrophages express the IL-6 gene, the majority of IL-6 is produced by the nonmacrophage/non-T-cell population, which is enriched for type B synoviocytes. Cultured synoviocytes, which are presumably derived from this population, spontaneously secrete IL-6, and stimulation of synoviocytes with cytokines, like IL-1, dramatically increases IL-6 gene expression and secretion. The contribution of T-cells to synovial IL-6 production appears to be very small.

Granulocyte–macrophage colony-stimulating factor

GM-CSF was originally defined by virtue of its ability to induce bone marrow precursor cells to mature into granulocytes and macrophages. In common with other major colony-stimulating factors (macrophage-CSF, granulocyte-CSF, and IL-3), GM-CSF also possesses a broad range of immunoregulatory activities. For instance, it is a potent macrophage activator and induces tumoricidal activity, intracellular parasite-killing, IL-1 secretion, and priming for enhanced release of TNF-α and prostaglandin E_2. GM-CSF also activates dendritic cells and enhances neutrophil effector functions, like antibody-dependent cytotoxicity, phagocytosis, chemotaxis and the production of oxygen radicals.

GM-CSF is present in RA synovial fluid and is produced by RA synovial tissue cells. The ability of GM-CSF to induce HLA-DR expression on the surface of macrophage lineage cells has stimulated interest in its role in the pathogenesis of RA. GM-CSF synergizes with TNF-α and is additive with IFN-γ in HLA-DR induction assays on human monocytes. The importance of this factor as an endogenous regulator of class II MHC induction is supported by the observation that antibodies to GM-CSF neutralize the HLA-DR inducing activity in supernatants of cultured synovial tissue cells. Therefore, GM-CSF might be a factor in the joint that supports the high level of DR expression, particularly in combination with TNF-α. As with TNF-α and IL-6, lymphocytes can produce GM-CSF under some circumstances, but studies of the cellular origin of GM-CSF show little, if any, of its RNA transcript in synovial T-cells. Synovial macrophages spontaneously produce GM-CSF and cultured synoviocytes express the gene and secrete the protein after stimulation with IL-1 or TNF-α.

Interleukin-8 and the chemokine family

A family of related chemoattractant peptides known as chemokines has recently been identified and characterized. These factors provide chemotactic signals that attract and activate specific cell types. Chemokines are divided into two families based on an unusual juxtaposition of characteristic cysteine residues. These families are sometimes called C-C or C-X-C, depending on whether two cysteines are adjacent to each other or separated by an amino acid. As one might expect from the exuberant inflammatory infiltrate, many chemokines are present in the rheumatoid joint. The concentrations of chemokines are higher in RA synovial effusions compared with noninflammatory joint disease. The chemokines are also found in serum, albeit at lower levels, suggesting that they are produced in the joint and provide a gradient for inflammatory cells.

Of the chemokine family, IL-8 (which is a member of the C-X-C family and was originally characterized as a neutrophil chemoattractant) was the first identified in RA and contributes to the large number of neutrophils that migrate into the joint. Large concentrations of IL-8 have been detected in RA synovial fluid and smaller amounts in RA serum. IL-8 protein has been localized in synovium, using immunohistochemistry, to sublining perivascular macrophages and occasional intimal lining cells. Northern blot analysis shows that the gene is expressed by the tissue *in situ*[61]. Synovial tissue macrophages constitutively produce IL-8

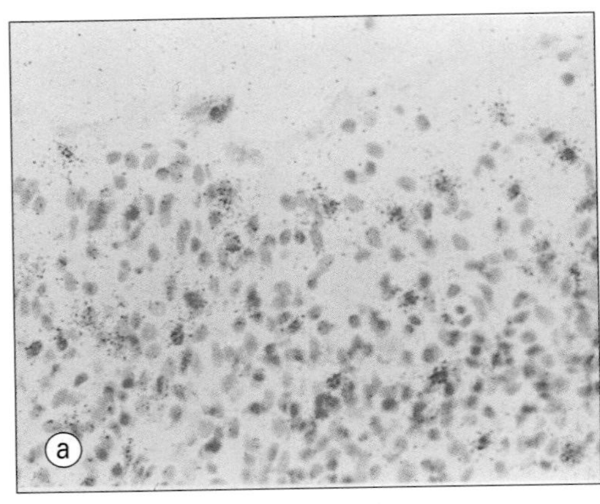

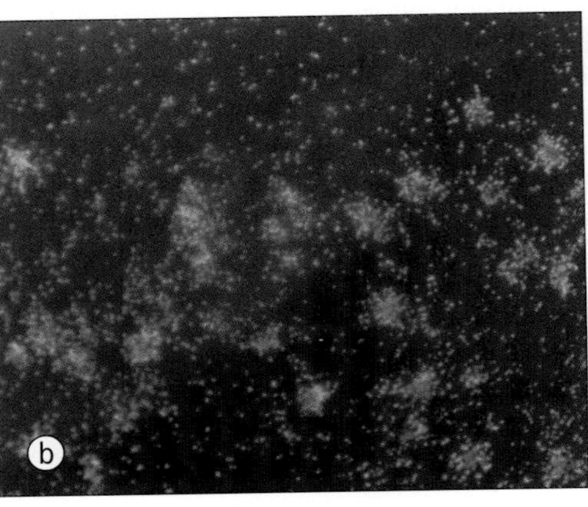

Fig. 13.14 IL-6 mRNA in RA synovial tissue. *In situ* hybridization demonstrates IL-6 mRNA (silver grains) in the intimal lining of an RA synovial tissue (dark field view). Bright-field and dark-field views of the same field show the location of cells and the mRNA. (From Firestein *et al.*[10], with permission. Copyright 1990, The American Association of Immunologists.

in tissue culture, while cultured fibroblast-like synoviocytes require stimulation by IL-1 and TNF-α to produce IL-8.

Many other chemokines have also been identified in synovial fluid and synovial tissue, each of which appears to be derived from macrophages or fibroblasts. Macrophage-inhibitory protein-1α (MIP-1α), MIP-1β, macrophage chemoattractant protein-1 (MCP-1), and RANTES, all of which are C-C chemokines, are produced by RA synovium[62,63]. Other C-X-C chemokines, like epithelial neutrophil activating peptide-78 (ENA-78), are also present[64]. About 40% of neutrophil chemotactic activity in RA synovial fluid can be eliminated with anti-ENA-78 antibody (Fig. 13.15). Regulation of individual chemokines in fibroblast-like synoviocytes is controlled by cytokines like IL-1 and TNF-α. Cytokines can alter the pattern of chemoattractants seen by circulating cells. RANTES production by synoviocytes, for example, is decreased by IL-4 and increased by IFN-γ, while the reverse occurs with IL-8[65].

Macrophage colony-stimulating factor (M-CSF)

M-CSF (sometimes called CSF-1) is a macrophage-derived protein that supports macrophage proliferation in normal bone marrow. Surprisingly, the human protein, while a potent CSF on mouse marrow, is only marginally effective on human cells (although costimulation with very small amounts of GM-CSF significantly increases its potency). M-CSF also stimulates monocyte TNF-α production. M-CSF was the first CSF identified in rheumatoid joints, and was discovered based on its ability to stimulate mouse bone marrow colony formation. It is present in high concentrations in synovial fluid and is constitutively produced by synovial tissue cells.

Growth factors

The distinction between a cytokine and a 'growth factor' is artificial and is more a reflection of history than science. The latter were defined as growth factors because of their ability to induce certain cells to proliferate in culture. Obviously, many cytokines also possess this activity. There are several factors traditionally included in this category that are present in abundance in the inflamed synovium, including TGF-β, platelet-derived growth factor (PDGF) and fibroblast growth factor (FGF). TGF-β is one of the most important factors because of its suppressive effects on T-cell function. It is ubiquitous in synovial tissue; immunoreactive protein is detected throughout the synovium, including synovial lining cells and many interstitial mononuclear cells (probably macrophages). In contrast, only a small percentage of cells in lymphoid aggregates contain the protein. TGF-β mRNA is readily detected in RNA extracts of whole synovial tissue, and *in situ* hybridization demonstrates the mRNA in synovial cells. TGF-β is found in very high concentrations in both inflammatory and noninflammatory synovial fluid and is constitutively produced by macrophages in synovial fluid. It is normally secreted in a latent form, which can be activated *in vitro* with acid. 70–90% of the TGF-β in synovial fluid is in the latent form.

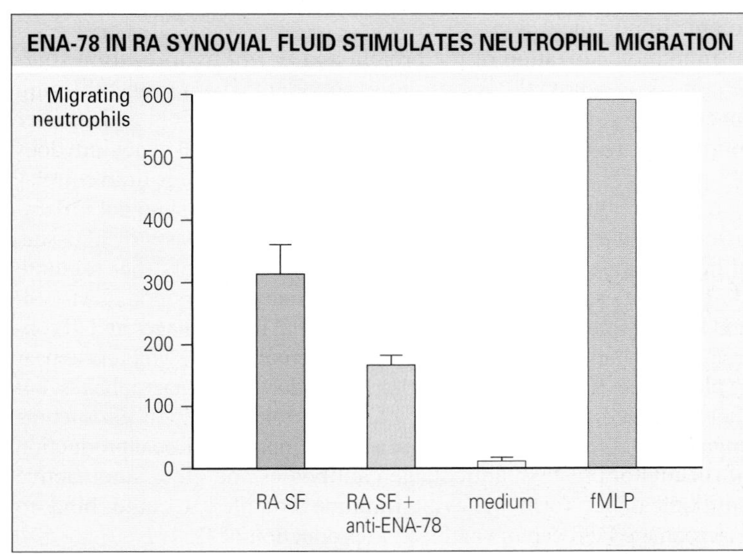

Fig. 13.15 ENA-78 is a chemokine that accounts for about 40% of neutrophil chemoattractant activity in RA synovial fluid (SF), as determined by the addition of neutralizing antibodies. fMLP (which is a chemotactic peptide) is a positive control. (Adapted from Koch *et al.*[79], with permission.)

TGF-β has potent effects on a variety of cell types, although these activities can vary depending on its concentration, the culture conditions, and the state of the target cell. It is a potent inducer of collagen production by fibroblasts. Because it also decreases collagenase production, the net effect is to increase the amount of collagen in the extracellular matrix. This property is thought to be important in wound healing and could also contribute to the remodeling of synovial tissue in pannus. The suppressive effects of TGF-β on immune function are impressive. TGF-β can downregulate IL-1 receptor expression and is a potent inhibitor of T-cell proliferation and cytokine production, possibly contributing to the lack of T-cell activation in the joint. TGF-β also binds to the core protein of the matrix proteoglycan decorin. This interaction inhibits its biological activity, probably due to competition with TGF-β cell surface receptors. However, the binding is reversible, so decorin might serve as a tissue reservoir for the growth factor.

TGF-β can exacerbate or suppress arthritis in animal models: when it is injected into the knees of animals, cellular infiltration and massive synovial lining hyperplasia develops[66]. The histologic picture that evolves is different from true synovitis, since the degree of lining hyperplasia far exceeds the mononuclear infiltration. The role of TGF-β as an immune suppressant has been investigated in streptococcal cell wall arthritis, where parenteral administration of the protein ameliorates the disease[67]. Since large amounts of TGF-β are already present in the inflamed synovium, it is not known if administration of additional recombinant protein would be beneficial to patients with RA. Although most of the TGF-β in the RA joint is latent, the concentrations of the active protein generally exceed those required to induce a physiologic reaction *in vitro*.

Another growth factor that probably plays a role in fibroblast and synoviocyte proliferation in arthritis is PDGF. Its two chains (A and B) are about 60% homologous and can combine in any of three combinations (AA, AB and BB). The B chain seems to be made preferentially by macrophages, while the A chain is expressed by endothelial cells. Two types of PDGF receptors have also been identified: an α-receptor binds all three forms of PDGF, while the β-receptor binds primarily to BB. PDGF is produced by RA synovium and is the most potent stimulator of cultured synoviocyte proliferation in serum-free conditions. *In situ* hybridization demonstrates PDGF B-chain mRNA in vascular endothelial cells and some stromal elements in rheumatoid but not normal synovium[68]. The PDGF receptors also localize to the adjacent cells in RA synovium, suggesting the presence of a paracrine system.

Fibroblast growth factor (FGF) can function as an autocrine signal for synoviocyte growth. Basic FGF (bFGF) is a 16kDa polypeptide that is found in many tissues, including cartilage, retina and brain. Proteoglycans, with a strong negative charge, can avidly bind FGF as well as other cytokines and growth factors. This interaction appears to be essential for FGF biological activity, since free bFGF does not bind to the FGF receptors (see Fig. 13.16). bFGF binding to heparan likely causes a change in conformation and permits engagement of the FGF receptor. Hence, proteoglycans can serve as a reservoir for a variety of 'soluble' mediators by holding them in the matrix and perhaps presenting them to the target cell in an activated form. FGF is present in synovial fluid and is produced spontaneously by cultured synovial fibroblasts. Cultured synoviocytes express specific FGF receptors and proliferate after exposure to the growth factor. Hence, FGF can serve as an autocrine factor that contributes to synovial fibroblast hyperplasia.
In addition to stimulating division of synoviocytes, FGF can also function as an angiogenesis factor and can induce proliferation of blood vessels in RA synovium. A variety of other factors in the inflamed joint contribute to the angiogenic activity in synovium, including chemokines like IL-8. Perhaps the most important one is vascular endothelium growth factor (VEGF). Hypoxia is a key stimulus for VEGF

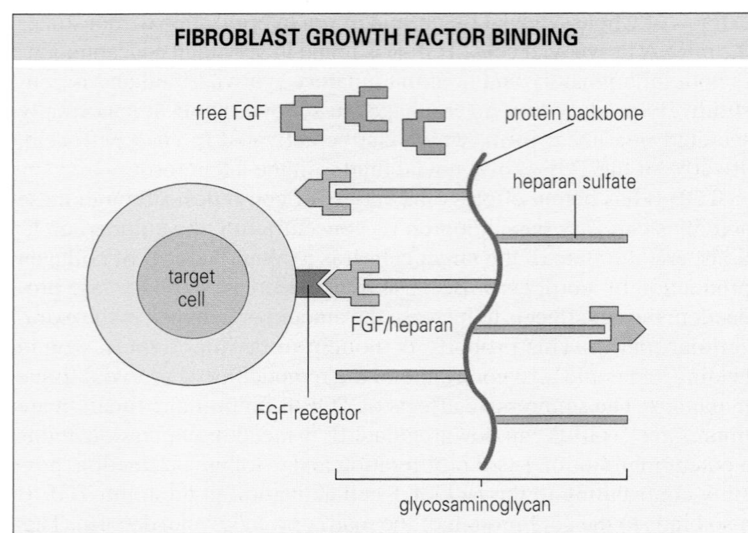

Fig. 13.16 Fibroblast growth factor binding. FGF binds to its receptor after it associates with heparan sulfate.

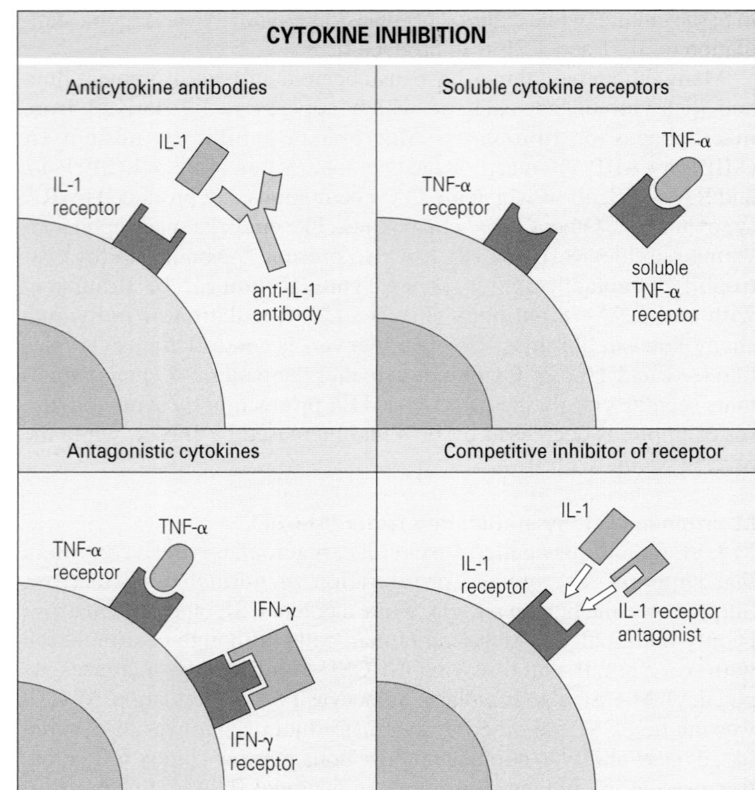

Fig. 13.17 Cytokine inhibition. Four mechanisms for the inhibition of cytokine function.

expression and, given the low oxygen tension in the rheumatoid joint, might account for VEGF production by the intimal lining[69]. The local cytokine network, including IL-1 and TNF-α, might also increase VEGF expression. VEGF protein levels are increased in RA synovial fluid compared to noninflammatory fluids[70]. *In situ* hybridization shows that the intimal lining is the major source of VEGF, and VEGF receptors are expressed on synovial blood vessels.

NEUROPEPTIDES

A role for the nervous system in the pathogenesis of immune-mediated disease has long been suspected. The association of clinical flares with psychologic stress suggests a link between immunity and the central nervous system, and the relative sparing of joints in paretic limbs of patients with RA offers further proof. There is evidence to suggest that these effects are expressed through peptide mediators produced by neurons known as neuropeptides. For instance, substance P likely participates in synovitis through of its ability to increase monocyte production of cytokines, such as IL-1 and IL-6. It is also a potent activator of cultured fibroblast-like synoviocytes and is able to increase both proliferation and collagenase production by these cells. Another neuropeptide, met-enkephalin, enhances B cell antibody production and macrophage oxygen radical generation and serves as a potent macrophage and lymphocyte chemotactic factor. Both met-enkephalin and substance P have been detected in synovial fluid. A more complete discussion of the role of these peptide mediators in RA is presented elsewhere in Section 5.

CYTOKINE INHIBITORS

Inhibitors of cytokine function play a major role in normal immunity and homeostasis by interrupting positive feedback loops and unrestrained cellular activation. Indeed, it is possible that defective negative interactions could play a role in the perpetuation of synovitis. There are at least four basic mechanisms of cytokine inhibition, including receptor-binding proteins, soluble receptors, antagonistic cytokines, and anticytokine antibodies (Fig. 13.17).

Cytokine receptor binding proteins

Because of the importance of IL-1 in RA, intensive efforts have been directed towards developing methods of blocking its inflammatory effects. A natural IL-1 inhibitory activity was originally described in the urine of febrile patients and in the supernatants of adherent macrophages. The gene encoding an IL-1 inhibitor was cloned and the recombinant protein studied. This factor, IL-1ra, is a glycosylated protein that binds to the high affinity surface IL-1 receptor. Despite engaging the receptor and competing with IL-1 for the binding site, IL-1ra possesses no agonist activity. IL-1ra can be produced by a variety of cells, including macrophages, keratinocytes and fibroblasts. The kinetics of macrophage IL-1 and IL-1ra production suggest that IL-1 is produced early in the differentiation of a monocyte/macrophage, while IL-1ra predominates in the mature tissue macrophage. This suggests a mechanism for turning off inflammation by interrupting a positive feedback loop.

Surprisingly, IL-1ra levels are high in the rheumatoid joint. Up to 50 ng/ml have been measured in RA synovial fluid[71], and studies of synovial tissue mRNA show that the IL-1ra gene is expressed in both RA and OA synovium[72]. Concentrations of IL-1ra in the synovial fluid correlate with the number of neutrophils in the fluid, and granulocytes have been suggested as one possible source. Immunoreactive IL-1ra is more difficult to detect in noninflammatory fluids from patients with OA. Since IL-1 concentrations in synovial fluid are frequently less than 1ng/ml, low levels of IL-1ra in OA synovial fluid could still have physiologic importance.

Immunolocalization of the protein and *in situ* hybridization studies on RA synovial tissue show abundant IL-1ra in sublining macrophages, particularly in a perivascular distribution, and smaller amounts of IL-1ra in the lining (Fig. 13.18)[72]. Normal synovium does not produce significant amounts of the inhibitor. There is little correlation between the amount of IL-1ra and the degree of synovial inflammation. Of interest, IL-1ra is found in the lining in OA synovial tissue, although the sublining contains very little. The factors that regulate IL-1ra gene expression in the joint are partially understood. GM-CSF and IL-10, which are produced by RA synovial macrophages and fibroblasts, can stimulate IL-1ra production by macrophages *in vitro* and appear to play a role. IL-4 also increases IL-1ra production in macrophages, but there is very little IL-4 in the joint. Noncytokine influences, such as engagement of Fc receptors, might also be important. Local production of rheumatoid factors, anticollagen antibodies and other autoreactive antibodies that form synovial immune complexes could bind to macrophage Fc receptors and lead to production of IL-1ra.

The degree of active synovial inflammation observed in RA despite the presence IL-1ra is in part due to the fact that IL-1ra is a relatively weak inhibitor of IL-1 biological activity. It must be present in great excess to function effectively because cells are activated by IL-1 even

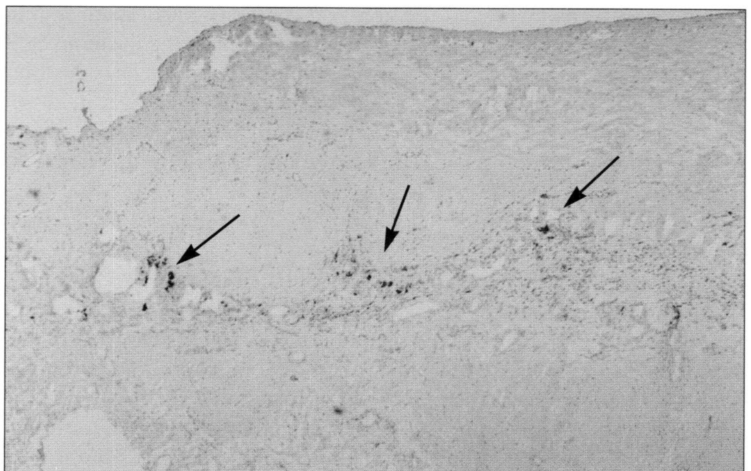

Fig. 13.18 IL-1ra protein in RA synovial tissue. Immunoreactive IL- 1 ra is demonstrated in perivascular sublining mononuclear cells, particularly macrophages. The brown pigmentation in the sublining region identifies synovial IL-1ra in this hematoxylin-stained section. In other tissues, synovial lining cells also contain the inhibitor.

if only a small percentage of IL-1 receptors are occupied. However, the IL-1ra:IL-1 ratio in supernatants of cultured synovial tissue cells is only about about 3:1, compared to the hundred-fold excess of IL-1ra required for effective IL-1 antagonism[73]. This is due, in part, to the fact that the IL-1ra gene is preferentially expressed by fibroblast-like synoviocytes as an alternatively spliced form that lacks a leader sequence and is not secreted[73]. Therefore, even though the protein is produced, it remains inside cells. Continued disease activity despite the presence of synovial IL-1ra could also be due to the great redundancy of cytokine loops in arthritis, since inhibition of only one cytokine might not significantly impact the disease. In this regard, the use of pharmacologic doses of IL-1ra in animal models of arthritis have been mixed; when massive amounts of the protein are injected prior to induction of arthritis, synovitis is attenuated but not eliminated. Human studies with IL-1ra reportedly demonstrate some clinical efficacy in RA, although the pharmacokinetics of the recombinant protein could, in combination with its limited efficacy as an IL-1 antagonist, limit its utility.

Soluble receptors

Cytokine receptors can be released from cells as soluble proteins either by proteolytic cleavage or through the production of an alternatively spliced form that lacks a transmembrane region. The soluble receptors can bind cytokines in the milieu and prevent them from activating neighboring cells. Alternatively, soluble receptors sometimes prolong the half-life of circulating cytokines and, in the case of the soluble IL-6R:IL-6 complex, even transduce signals to bystander cells.

The soluble IL-2 receptor (IL-2R) was the first soluble cytokine receptor characterized in RA. The intact receptor has at least several components, and high affinity IL-2 binding occurs only when all are present. The soluble IL-2R contains only one of these polypeptides and binds IL-2 with very low affinity. Hence, it is an inefficient inhibitor of IL-2 biological activity and has only limited capacity for removing excess IL-2 from the circulation or from a body fluid.

The percentage of cells in the synovium that express IL-2R is actually similar to that of resting peripheral blood lymphocytes (about 1–2%). Yet, elevated concentrations of soluble IL-2R have been reported in serum and synovial effusions of patients with RA and the levels seem to correlate with disease activity. In OA, synovial fluid generally has lower levels of soluble IL-2R compared to RA. An IL-2 inhibitory activity in synovial fluid has been attributed to soluble IL-2R. However, soluble IL-2R does not prevent IL-2 from binding to high affinity IL-2 receptors or interfere with the IL-2-mediated activation of T-cells. Hence, other inhibitors of IL-2 must be present and account for the activity detected in bioassays.

Soluble receptors to IL-1 (IL-1R) and TNF (TNF-R) probably play a more important physiologic role in downregulating inflammatory responses since they bind much more avidly to their ligands. TNF-R is part of a superfamily of receptors that include TNF-R (type I and II), ILA and binding proteins for nerve growth factor. Unlike soluble IL-2R, TNF-R can effectively remove its ligand from circulation and neutralize TNF biological activity. Soluble forms of both TNF receptors are present in blood and synovial fluid of patients with RA[74]. The concentrations of soluble TNF-R in RA effusions are up to 10–50ng/ml, which is many fold higher than the levels of TNF-α. This probably accounts for the lack of TNF biological activity in synovial fluid despite the presence of immunoreactive protein.

Two types of IL-1 receptors have also been characterized. Type I receptor is more important for signal transduction while type II receptor (which is expressed on macrophages) has only a small cytoplasmic domain and appears to act as a 'decoy'. The decoy receptor is released by activated cells and can neutralize IL-1 biological activity. This receptor has been detected in RA synovial fluid, and it can interfere with both bioassays and immunoassays for IL-1[75]. Its anti-inflammatory effects could be mitigated by the fact that it binds IL-1ra and interferes with the biological activity of the inhibitor as well.

Anticytokine antibodies

Autoantibodies that bind to and neutralize cytokines also occur in RA. Little is known about natural anticytokine antibodies *in vivo*, although one might anticipate their presence in diseases with marked B cell hyperreactivity. Anti-IL-1α antibodies are found in the blood of about 16% of RA patients and 5% of normal individuals[76]. Similar studies have not been performed on synovial fluid, although it would be surprising if it were devoid of anti-IL-1α activity since plasma proteins generally are detected in synovial effusions.

Inhibitory or antagonistic cytokines

Interleukin-10

IL-10 is an immunosuppressive cytokine produced mainly by T-cells (TH2 cells) and macrophages. It was originally identified by virtue of its ability to inhibit cytokine production by T-cells. This activity is mediated through the suppression of antigen-presenting cells and TH1 cell development. A physiologic role for IL-10 has been established in pregnancy, where it inhibits immune responses directed against paternal MHC antigens, and in susceptibility to some parasitic infections. An Epstein–Barr virus (EBV) protein with structural homology to human IL-10 has been identified and might meditate EBV-induced immunosuppression[77]. IL-10 can block cytokine production by cultured synovial tissue explants, albeit not as efficiently as IL-4[78]. IL-10 protein is present in RA synovial fluid and the gene is expressed by synovial tissue cells[79,80]. Synovial macrophages are the major source of IL-10 in RA. As noted earlier, IL-10 serves as an endogenous inhibitor of cytokine production by cultured RA synovial cells. Anti-IL-10 antibodies also increase the severity of collagen-induced arthritis in mice, indicating that it acts as a physiologic anti-inflammatory cytokine[81]. One interesting question is why rheumatoid synovial inflammation is not suppressed by rather high concentrations of IL-10 in the tissues and effusions. One possibility is that IL-10 possesses other activities that could contribute to synovitis, such as B cell stimulating activity or the ability to enhance collagenase gene expression by fibroblasts.

Other antagonistic or suppressive cytokines

The effects of one cytokine sometimes can be inhibited by another cytokine. The mutual antagonism between IFN-γ and TNF-α, which was described earlier in this chapter, is one example of this type of interaction, and the absence of IFN-γ could contribute to perpetuation of synovitis. TGF-β is another cytokine that can suppress the immune response in synovitis. In animal models of arthritis, systemic administration of TGF-β downregulates T-cell responses in the synovium and suppresses disease. Synovial fluid is known to inhibit IL-1-mediated thymocyte production. This activity is neutralized in part by anti-TGF-β antibody. TGF-β also downregulates IL-1 receptor expression on chondrocytes. Another cytokine with potential anti-inflammatory properties is IL-4. This factor is a potent antagonist of cytokine and rheumatoid factor production by cultured RA synovial explants. As with IFN-γ, the absence of IL-4 could contribute to synovitis.

JOINT DESTRUCTION: METALLOPROTEINASES AND METALLOPROTEINASE INHIBITORS

The metalloproteinases are a family of enzymes that are responsible for matrix degradation and remodeling. Control of metalloproteinase production is obviously of great interest in diseases like RA where matrix degradation plays such a prominent role. Metalloproteinase inhibitors in animal models of arthritis markedly decrease bone destruction and suggest that they represent a potential therapeutic target[82]. Their efficacy could be due to a direct effect on matrix degradation as well as an indirect effect inhibiting the proteolytic release of TNF-α from cell membranes. Although the ligand specificities of individual members of the family differ, they possess a number of structural similarities suggesting that they are derived from a common gene. Metalloproteinases are generally secreted as inactive proenzymes that require proteolytic cleavage for activation (Fig. 13.19). Their proteolytic activity depends on the presence of a zinc cation (hence the name 'metalloproteinases'). In the latent forms, the zinc ion is chelated to a cysteine residue, and this bond must be broken in order for the molecule to express proteolytic activity. Activation of the latent enzyme is usually initiated by limited proteolysis. This can be accomplished by many enzymes, including trypsin, plasmin, tryptase and other proteases. In general, after cleavage the chelating cysteine in the released fragment diffuses away and the zinc ion is free to participate in the enzymatic reaction. In some cases (as with plasmin), the cysteine can still remain in the activated enzyme after activation of the enzyme, but enough of the peptide is removed that the residue is no longer in close apposition to the metal cation. Metalloproteinases share other structural features, including a catalytic domain and, in some cases, a matrix-like region that resembles fibronectin.

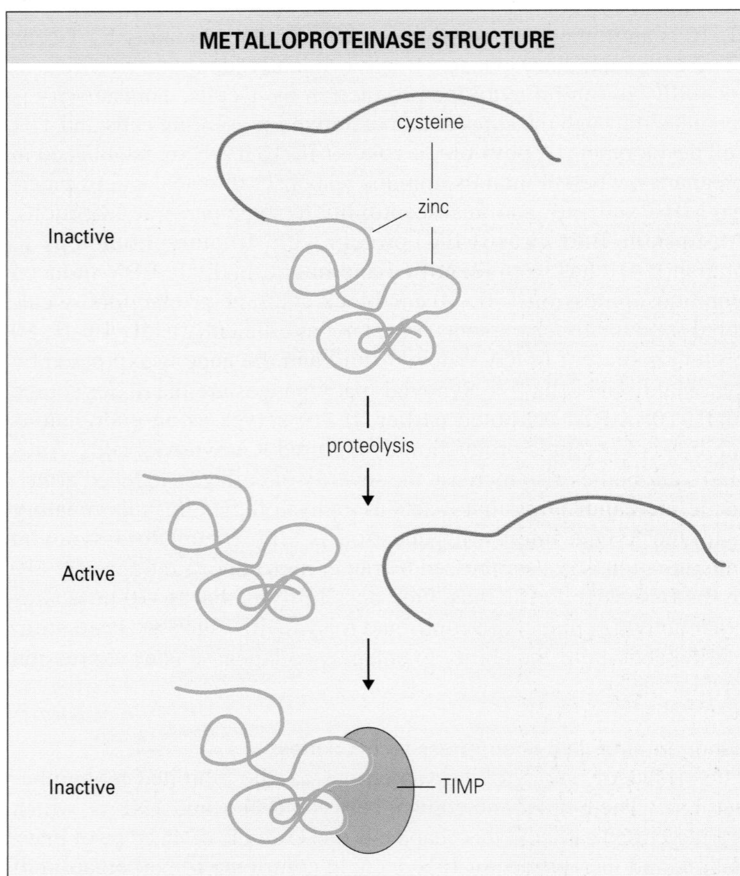

Fig. 13.19 Metalloproteinase structure. Schematic representation of metalloproteinase activation by limited proteolysis. After cleavage, the zinc cation is no longer complexed with the cysteine and is available to catalyze the enzymatic reaction. TIMP can bind to the active enzyme and inhibit metalloproteinase activity.

STROMELYSIN

The stromelysin gene was originally identified and cloned in transformed fibroblasts from rats (where it was called 'transin'). Initial studies on the role of transin/stromelysin in arthritis were performed in the streptococcal cell wall (SCW) arthritis model in Lewis rats, which is a destructive form of arthritis marked by significant matrix degradation. Transin mRNA is present in synovial tissues isolated from arthritic animals, and immunohistochemical staining of synovia with chronic SCW arthritis shows transin protein in the cells of the lining layer, the underlying stroma, chondrocytes, and subchondral osteoclasts[83]. The large amounts of metalloproteinases are accompanied by intense nuclear staining for the c-*Myc* oncogene product. Transin expression occurs very early in the disease (even before the influx of mononuclear cells) and, along with proto-oncogene expression, has been cited as evidence of the synoviocyte transformation. Stromelysin/transin has fairly broad substrate specificity. In addition to digesting interstitial collagen that has been previously nicked by collagenase, it cleaves proteoglycans, laminin and fibronectin. Stromelysin is also able to activate latent collagenase, thereby providing a positive feedback signal for matrix destruction.

Stromelysin protein has also been detected in the lining and sublining regions of RA synovium, and significantly more is found in RA synovial tissue compared to OA. Interestingly, *in situ* hybridization of synovial tissue with stromelysin probes demonstrates a somewhat different distribution, since large amounts of mRNA are present in the lining but not in the sublining. Although it is possible that the insensitivity of *in situ* hybridization technique prevents detection of stromelysin mRNA in sublining endothelium and other cells that stain positively with the protein, it is clear that the vast majority of gene expression occurs in the lining. Protein produced in the lining probably diffuses into the sublining and is absorbed by other cells, accounting for the immunohistochemistry observations. In addition to stromelysin, homologous metalloproteinases called stromelysin-2 and stromelysin-3 have been cloned from rheumatoid arthritis synoviocytes and other cells.

Only small amounts of stromelysin are constitutively produced by resting synoviocytes. The gene is rapidly induced after exposure to inflammatory cytokines like IL-1 or TNF-α. Matrix molecules like fibronectin can also regulate MMP expression. For instance, engagement of the fibronectin receptor (FnR) on fibroblast-like synoviocytes results in expression of a variety of genes involved with matrix remodeling. This process, which requires crosslinking of FnR and can be accomplished with anti-FnR antibodies, causes a dramatic increase in expression of the stromelysin and collagenase genes. Within 2 hours, these two proteins can account for up to 5% of the protein secreted by cultured synoviocytes. The response is carefully regulated and specific, since other metalloproteinases, like gelatinase, are not increased. Interestingly, TIMP production actually decreases slightly after stimulation by anti-FnR, tipping the balance towards matrix degradation. Treatment of fibroblasts with peptide fragments of fibronectin also increases metalloproteinase secretion. Multimeric peptides containing the Arg-Gly-Asp sequence are the most effective, while monomeric forms that cannot crosslink the receptors are inactive.

COLLAGENASE

Collagenase is a second critical metalloproteinase that mediates tissue destruction in RA. It digests native triple helical collagen at a single glycine–isoleucine bond near the amino terminus of the molecule. Collagenase can degrade the interstitial helical collagens (e.g. types I, II, III, and X collagens) but not types IV, V, IX, other non-helical collagens, or denatured collagens. The combination of collagenase and stromelysin is a potent matrix remodeling force since it can degrade virtually all the important structural proteins within joints. As for stromelysin, activated rheumatoid synoviocytes secrete large amounts of collagenase. The collagenase gene is expressed almost exclusively by the lining (Fig. 13.20). Quantitative *in situ* hybridization studies have demonstrated significantly more collagenase mRNA in RA synovial tissue compared to OA synovium[84,85]. Furthermore, there is a correlation between the amount of its RNA transcript in the lining and the degree of sublining inflammation.

Although stromelysin and collagenase are both produced by synovial lining cells in patients with chronic RA, less is known about their regulation in early disease. Synovial tissue from animals with collagen-induced arthritis contains immunoreactive stromelysin in both the synovium and in cartilage cells within a few days after the onset of disease. In contrast, collagenase is detected in the synovium but not in the cartilage. Staining for both enzymes is particularly intense in the pannus–cartilage junction[86]. These studies suggest that metalloproteinases are produced very early in inflammatory arthritis and that chondrocytes can participate in this process. Recently, a synovial biopsy study of patients with early RA (1 to 3 months of disease) demonstrated significant metalloproteinase gene expression, suggesting that aggressive therapy in early disease to prevent joint destruction has some justification[87].

As with other effectors, the control of collagenase secretion is likely mediated by the cytokine milieu. Collagenase production and gene expression have been extensively studied in cultured fibroblast-like synoviocytes, where IL-1 and TNF-α are the most potent inducers. Collagenase mRNA begins to accumulate within hours of cytokine stimulation and increases for several days. IFN-γ decreases the collagenase activity in the supernatant of IL-1 and TNF-α stimulated synoviocytes. The mechanism of the interaction between IL-1 and IFN-γ does not appear to be by a decrease in collagenase gene expression or an increase in TIMP production. Instead, IFN-γ specifically inhibits IL-1-mediated induction of stromelysin production[88]. Since stromelysin is a potent activator of latent collagenase, decreased amounts of stromelysin in supernatants might interfere with the activation of collagenase. IFN-γ also inhibits TNF-α-mediated induction of collagenase[15].

The molecular mechanism of collagenase gene activation affords a unique opportunity to combine the study of oncogenes and metalloproteinases. Collagenase gene expression can be initiated by the activation of protein kinase C and src–related tyrosine kinases by cytokines, which subsequently induce production of the oncogenes[89]. The c-*jun* and c-*fos* genes are expressed within 30 minutes of cytokine stimulation; c-*Jun* protein then binds with c-*Fos*, and this complex interacts with the AP-1 binding site in the collagenase gene, resulting in collagenase gene transcription. Hence, the abundant oncogene expression observed in the RA synovium has direct implications with regard to matrix degradation, and interfering with proto-oncogene production or action could have important clinical benefits.

OTHER METALLOPROTEINASES AND PROTEASES IN RA

In addition to collagenase and stromelysin, several other metalloproteinases participate in degradation of articular structures. Preformed neutrophil collagenase (MMP8) can be released by synovial fluid neutrophils and mediate cartilage destruction. This enzyme is thought to be important primarily when the neutrophil count in effusions is extremely high. A newly described collagenase, MMP13, is also capable of digesting native type II collagen. Preliminary data suggest that this gene is expressed mainly by chondrocytes[90]. Gelatinases (72kD and 92kD forms) are also produced and can degrade denatured collagen. The 92kD gelatinase is constitutively expressed by early passage RA synoviocytes but not by OA synoviocytes[91].

Metalloproteinases are responsible for much of the destruction of cartilage and bone, but other classes of proteases may play a role in joint destruction. For instance, cysteine proteases like the cathepsins may also be active both inside and outside of cells. Cathepsin L and D gene expression has been confirmed in RA synovium using *in situ* hybridization[92]. The distribution differs from metalloproteinases since enzyme production occurs both in the lining and the sublining. Moreover, a cathepsin B inhibitor decreased both inflammation and bone destruction in animal models of arthritis[93]. Serine proteinases (e.g. elastase and plasmin) are probably involved as well, both as direct mediators of tissue destruction and as activators of latent metalloproteinases.

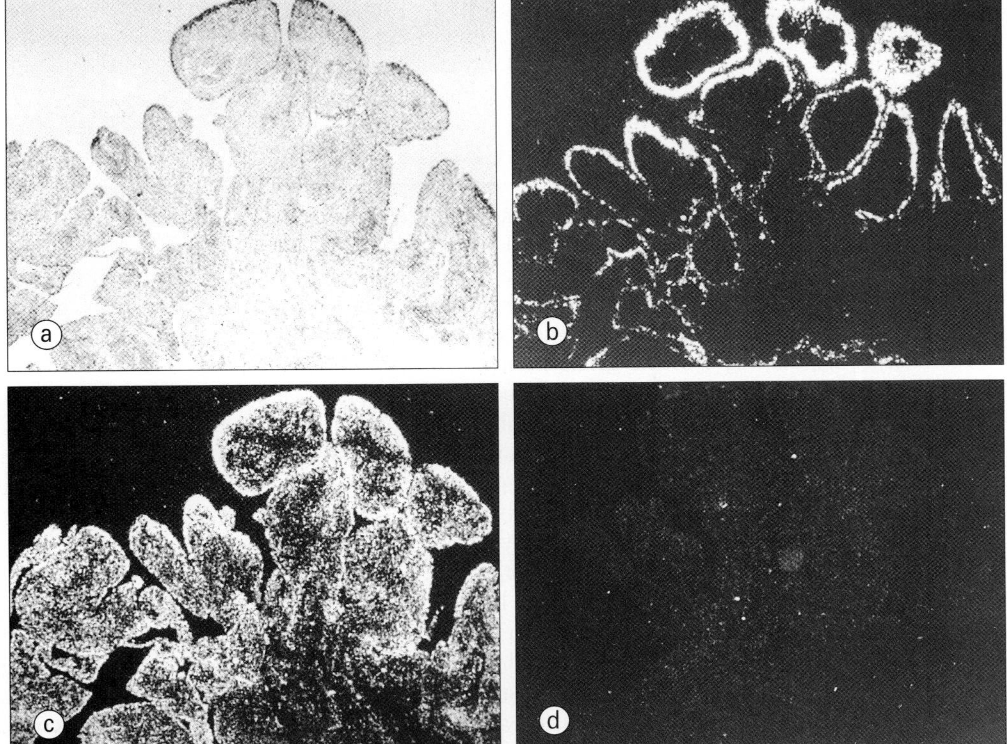

Fig. 13.20 Collagenase and HLA-DR mRNA in RA synovium. Localization of collagenase (b), HLA-DR (c) and negative control probe (d) hybridization to inflammatory synovium. Collagenase mRNA is found only in the synovial intimal lining while the distribution of HLA-DR is more diffuse. Bright-field view is also shown (a). (From Firestein *et al.*[84], with permission.)

TISSUE INHIBITOR OF METALLOPROTEINASE (TIMP) AND OTHER PROTEASE INHIBITORS

One of the key inhibitors of metalloproteinases in the joint is TIMP. The TIMPs are now known to be a family of metalloproteinase inhibitors that include at least three members (TIMP-1, -2 and -3). These proteins block enzyme activity by binding with extremely high avidity to metalloproteinases in a stoichiometric fashion (1:1)[94]. Although the latent enzymes will sometimes bind to some TIMPs, this is generally a property of activated metalloproteinases.

In situ hybridization studies of frozen sections of synovial tissue demonstrate large amounts of TIMP-1 mRNA in the synovial lining of patients with RA[84]. In contrast to collagenase, TIMP gene expression is similar in RA and OA. Hence, the ratio of TIMP to collagenase is greater in noninflammatory arthritis than in RA. This has important implications for the pathogenesis of cartilage destruction in RA and raises the possibility that the TIMP system is overwhelmed by massive amounts of metalloproteinase production in RA.

Two-color immunofluoresence staining of synovial tissue with specific antibodies to collagenase or TIMP shows that intimal lining cells synthesize both proteins[95]. Using *in situ* hybridization, discoordinate expression of stromelysin and TIMP has also been shown. TIMP and metalloproteinase genes also have unique transcriptional controls in cultured fibroblast-like synoviocytes. The TIMP-1 gene is constitutively expressed, while only small amounts of stromelysin and collagenase are produced. Cytokines like IL-1 and TNF-α dramatically increase stromelysin production but have little impact on TIMP gene expression, while IL-6 increases TIMP-1 but not stromelysin. Therefore, the cytokine milieu can fine tune the ratio of metalloproteinases and inhibitors and control the rate of matrix destruction.

In addition to the TIMP family, other protease inhibitors are present in RA. Most of the collagenase inhibitory activity in serum is due to α_2-macroglobulin (α_2M). Unlike TIMP, which blocks metalloproteinases without forming new covalent bonds, α_2M inactivates proteases by offering a hydrolyzable 'bait' with subsequent covalent linkage to the protease. Neutrophils, when present in high numbers in synovial fluid, inactivate significant amounts of α_2M by releasing elastase and serine proteinases that subseqently bind to the inhibitor. SERPINs, or serine protease inhibitors, are also abundant in synovial effusions and plasma. They directly protect the extracellular matrix by blocking serine protease function and can act indirectly by preventing serine protease-mediated activation of metalloproteinases. One SERPIN, α_1-antitrypsin, has been detected in RA synovial fluid but is inactivated after oxidation by reactive oxygen species in inflammatory effusions.

MODULATION OF METALLOPROTEINASE GENE EXPRESSION *IN VIVO*

Since metalloproteinases are responsible for much of the damage that occurs in the inflamed joint, one key objective of therapy is to decrease their production. Recent studies have used synovial biopsies to examine the effect of various treatments on synovial gene expression. In one protocol, synovial biopsies were obtained before and after an intra-articular glucocorticosteroid injection and metalloproteinase gene expression was determined using quantitative *in situ* hybridization[84]. Precorticosteroid synovial biopsies in patients with active RA showed abundant collagenase mRNA, as expected. However, 1–2 weeks after injection of a potent glucocorticoid, collagenase RNA transcripts were no longer detected. The decrease in synovial collagenase gene expression was probably a direct effect of the corticosteroid by virtue of its inhibition of collagenase gene transcription by interfereing with transcription factor AP-1. Corticosteroids might also inhibit production of cytokines like IL-1 and TNF-α that induce synoviocyte collagenase production. In a second study of synovial gene expression, the novel anti-inflammatory agent tenidap significantly decreased synovial stromelysin gene expression in patients with RA[97]. Piroxicam, a traditional nonsteroidal anti-inflammatory (NSAID), had no effect on metalloproteinase production.

In a longer term study, the effect of chronic low dose methotrexate therapy on synovial gene expression was examined (Fig. 13.21).

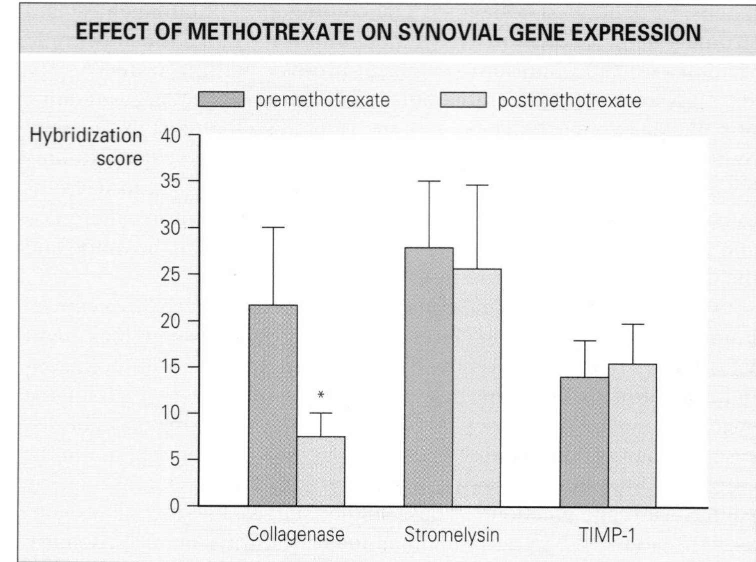

Fig. 13.21 Effect of methotrexate on synovial gene expression. Percutaneous synovial biopsies were performed on patients with RA before treatment and after 3 months of methotrexate therapy. Collagenase gene expression was significantly decreased, while TIMP-1 and stromelysin were unchanged. Gene expression was quantified using computer-assisted image analysis. (* $p<0.05$ compared with pre-methotrexate.)(Adapted from Firestein *et al.*[98], with permission.)

Methotrexate decreased collagenase mRNA by nearly 70% but did not change stromelysin or TIMP-1 expression[98]. The decrease in collagenase gene expression suggests that a lower collagenase: TIMP ratio might be responsible for decreased bone destruction in some patients. The selectivity of the effect for collagenase was surprising, but other studies have shown discoordinate expression of stromelysin and collagenase. The mechanism of collagenase suppression is not due to a direct effect of methotrexate on synoviocytes. Recent studies, however, indicate that at least a portion of the acute anti-inflammatory effects of methotrexate are mediated by enhanced production of endogenous adenosine[99]. This raises the possibility that inhibition of collagenase by methotrexate *in vivo* might also be related to adenosine. *In vitro* experiments using cultured fibroblast-like synoviocytes show that adenosine receptor stimulation mimics the effect of methotrexate by decreasing collagenase, but not stromelysin or TIMP-1 expression[100]. This is mediated through the A_{2b} adenosine receptor and increased intracellular cyclic AMP (cAMP) production.

ARACHIDONIC ACID METABOLITES

Prostaglandins (PG) and leukotrienes are low molecular weight inflammatory molecules that are synthesized by synovial fluid cells and by synovium. The initial step in synthesis is mediated by the activation of phospholipase A_2 which cleaves arachidonic acid from membrane phospholipids. The released arachidonic acid is further metabolized to PGG_2 by cyclooxygenase. The bulk of PG production in the rheumatoid synovium appears to be produced by the inducible cyclooxygenase (COX2) instead of COX1, which is constitutively expressed. COX2 expression in synoviocytes can be induced by IL-1 and suppressed by corticosteroids (see Fig. 13.22)[101]. Subsequent enzymatic steps result in the synthesis of a broad variety of prostaglandins, including PGE_1, PGE_2 and $PGF_{2\alpha}$. Alternatively, the lipoxygenase enzymes metabolize arachidonic acid to 5-HPTE as the initial step in leukotriene synthesis. Prostaglandins and leukotrienes are potent immunomodulators that are probably important feedback regulators in synovitis. For instance, PGE_2 potentiates the vasodilating effects and vascular permeability changes induced by complement fragments, histamine and the leukotriene LTB4. PGEs also serve as negative feedback elements in immune responses: a physiologic concentration (e.g. 10^{-8}mol/l) inhibits IFN-γ production by T-cells, HLA-DR expression by macrophages and T-cell proliferation. The importance of prostaglandins in synovitis is supported by the clinical benefits observed using agents that block cyclooxygenase activity (i.e. NSAIDs). The specific cells that synthesize arachidonic acid metabolites in the synovium have not been established. However, it is likely that neutrophils, macrophages and fibroblast-like synovial lining cells participate. *In vitro* production of prostaglandins by synoviocytes is greatly increased by IL-1 and TNF-α, and this activity is blocked by IFN-γ[102].

COMPLEMENT ACTIVATION

Immune complexes in the rheumatoid joint provide ample substrate for complement activation and participate in the local inflammatory process. The content of the complexes is varied, although rheumatoid factors are one consistent component. Serum rheumatoid factor (RF) levels correlate positively with complement consumption in RA. IgM RF is a potent stimulus for complement fixation compared to other classes of rheumatoid factor in both sera and synovial fluids. A role for *in vivo* complement activation in RA is supported by the observation of accelerated C4 consumption. Furthermore, the presence of C4 fragments in the plasma of rheumatoid patients correlates with titers of IgM RF.

Complement fragments like C5a act as chemoattractants to neutrophils and induce local degranulation. Damage to cartilage mediated by the release of neutrophil-derived enzymes can result in the increased levels of additional antigens (such as type II collagen or proteoglycan) that can contribute to local autoantibody production, immune complex formation and additional complement fixation. Inflammatory products can then accumulate in synovial fluid during acute inflammation. Neutrophils can also feedback and enhance local complement activation. Neutrophil lysosomal lysates are capable of generating chemotactic activity (probably C5a) from fresh serum. As noted above, C5a is then able to induce further lysosomal release, establishing yet another amplification loop in inflammatory joint disease.

The liver is the major source of complement synthesis in humans and passive transfer of serum proteins into synovial fluid can account for some of the complement proteins found there. However, these proteins are also produced locally in the joint. Biosynthesis of complement proteins by synovial tissue was first demonstrated in the 1970s. Macrophages and/or fibroblasts are the likely sources, and *in vitro* studies show that both can produce many complement proteins, depending on the cytokine milieu. For instance, IFN-γ induces C2 and C3[103] while IL-1 and TNF-α induce C3[104]. IFN-γ represents about half of the C2-inducing activity in the supernatants of stimulated mononuclear cells and IFN-γ stimulation of C2 production is amplified by IL-4.

Complement gene expression occurs in distinct regions of the synovium. C2 mRNA is detected primarily in the lining (and to a much lesser extent in the sublining) while C3 mRNA is found primarily in sublining macrophages interspersed among lymphoid aggregates[84]. Factor B also appears to be localized to the lining. The cells in the lining that express complement genes have not been identified, and both type A and B synoviocytes might participate.

ENDOTHELIUM AND ADHESION MOLECULES IN RA

Vascular adhesion molecules play a critical role in the migration of inflammatory cells into the synovium. One of the best characterized, ICAM-1 (a ligand for the β_2 integrin family on leukocytes), is readily detected in RA synovium blood vessels and helps recruit lymphocytes, monocytes and neutrophils to the joint. This observation was one rationale behind clinical trials of anti-ICAM-1 antibodies in RA. Immunohistochemistry of synovial tissue also localizes ICAM-1 to sublining macrophages, macrophage-like synovial lining cells, and intimal lining fibroblasts. Other members of the ICAM family can also be detected in the rheumatoid synovium using similar techniques. ICAM-2 is expressed in RA blood vessels, although no more than in normal vessels, while ICAM-3 is preferentially expressed in the RA intimal lining and sublining macrophages[105].

ICAM-1 is expressed constitutively by cultured fibroblast-like synoviocytes. Addition of TNF-α, IL-1 or IFN-γ to synoviocyte cultures dramatically increases ICAM-1 expression[106,107] (Fig. 13.23). The inducing effect requires continuous cytokine exposure, and ICAM-1 levels decrease to baseline within a couple of days if the cytokine is removed. Hence, the very high level of this protein on the surface of synoviocytes *in vivo* probably reflects continuous exposure to the inflammatory milieu. One ligand for ICAM-1, α_L/β_2 (LFA-1), is also present on synovial T cells and could play a role in both the ingress and retention of T lymphocytes.

α_4/β_1 (also called VLA-4) is another leukocyte integrin that helps recruit and retain cells in inflamed tissues. VLA-4 is expressed by lymphocytes, monocytes, and eosinophils, but not neutrophils. It has a number of counter-receptors, most notably VCAM-1 and a 25 amino acid sequence in an alternatively spliced region of fibronectin known as CS1[108,109]. The former is a member of the IgG supergene family and is expressed by activated endothelial cells and the intimal lining. The binding sites for CS1 and VCAM-1 on VLA-4 are either very close to each other or overlap.

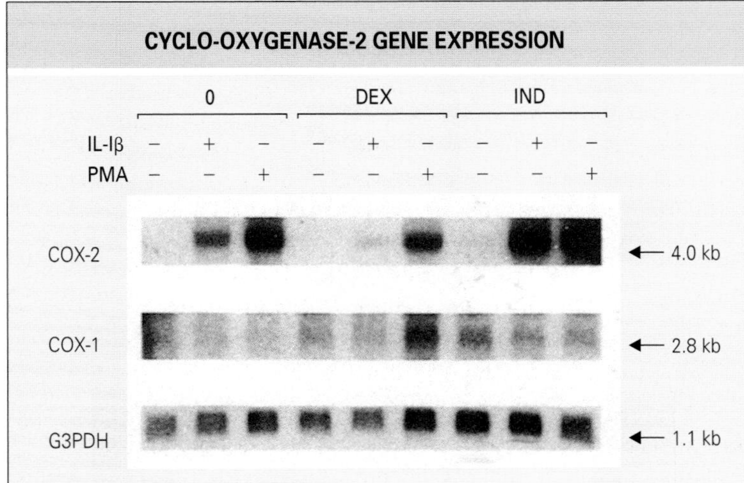

Fig. 13.22 Cyclo-oxygenase-2 (COX2) gene expression. COX2 gene expression by cultured synoviocytes is induced by IL-1 and PMA and suppressed by dexamethasone. The constitutively produced COX1 is unchanged (DEX: dexamethasone; IND: indomethacin; PMA: phorbolester). (From Crofford *et al.*[101], by copyright permission of The American College for Clinical Investigation.

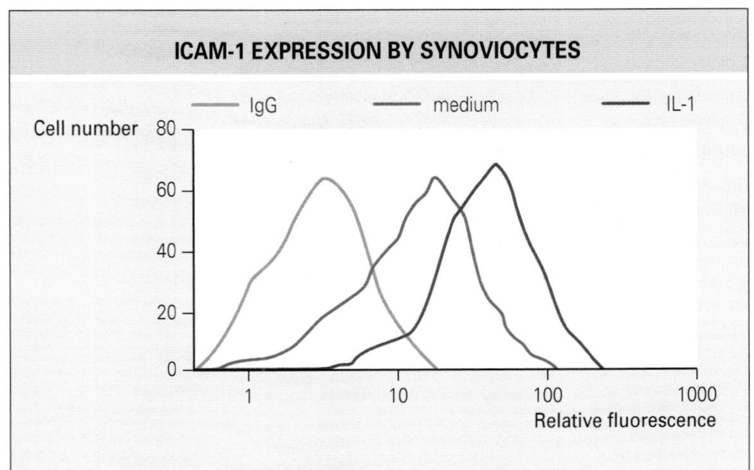

Fig. 13.23 ICAM-1 expression by synoviocytes. Synoviocytes constitutively express low levels of ICAM-1 as determined by flow cytometry and immunofluorescence (compare unstimulated cells stained with the ICAM-1 antibody (medium) to unstimulated cells stained with a negative control antibody (IgG)). If the cells are incubated with IL-1, then ICAM-1 expression significantly increases.

VCAM-1 is expressed by RA synovial endothelium, although the level of expression is surprisingly modest. The synovial intimal lining actually has been identified as the region of the joint expressing the most VCAM-1 (Fig. 13.24). Normal synovial lining expresses VCAM-1, albeit less than RA tissue. Type B synoviocytes are probably responsible for this observation in RA, and cultured fibroblast-like synoviocytes constitutively express VCAM-1[107]. Various cytokines, including IL-1, TNF-α, IFN-γ and IL-4, enhance VCAM-1 display by synoviocytes. VCAM-1 on cultured synoviocytes is functional and can bind T-cells. High endothelial venules in RA synovium can bind T cells, in part through the interaction between VLA-4 and VCAM-1[110].

The expression and functional significance of CS1-containing forms of fibronectin generated by alternative splicing has also been studied in RA[111]. Unlike most molecular forms of fibronectin typically found in the extracellular matrix, CS1 expression is restricted to inflamed RA vascular endothelium and the synovial intimal lining. Normal synovial tissue contains little, if any, CS1 fibronectin. Ultrastructural studies show that CS1-expressing fibronectin molecules decorate the lumen of RA endothelial cells but not the abluminal side of the endothelium. Local expression of the gene by endothelial cells has been confirmed by *in situ* hybridization[112]. T-cell adhesion to RA synovial microvasculature can be blocked by anti-α_4 antibody or synthetic CS1 peptide suggesting that the CS1/VLA-4 interaction is critical to lymphocyte homing to the joint. Immunoelectron microscopy also showed that CS1 fibronectin is expressed on the surface of fibroblast-like synoviocytes in the synovial intimal lining. A portion of VLA-4 mediated T-cell adhesion to cultured synoviocytes is blocked by CS1 peptides indicating that the surface CS1 is functional.

A role for VLA-4 in arthritis has been suggested by a number of experimental observations. In adjuvant arthritis in rats, anti-α_4 antibody decreased lymphocyte accumulation in the joint[113]. In SCW arthritis, systemic administration of CS1 peptide decreased the severity of acute and chronic arthritis[114]. T-lymphocytes isolated from the synovial fluid and synovial membrane of RA patients exhibit increased VLA-4 mediated adherence to both CS1 and VCAM-1 compared to autologous peripheral blood lymphocytes[115]. Therefore, leukocytes expressing functionally activated VLA-4 are selectively recruited to inflammatory sites in RA.

Another integrin that can bind to VCAM-1, α_4/β_7, is a specific adhesion molecule involved in lymphocyte homing to Peyer's patches. Nearly all intraepithelial and 40% of lamina propria lymphocytes express α_4/β_7; this molecule is rarely identified in other lymphoid tissues. α_4/β_7 expression on peripheral blood lymphocytes of patients with RA is similar to controls (less than 10%), while over 25% of synovial fluid lymphocytes express this adhesion molecule[116]. This is yet another potential linkage between the gastrointestinal epithelium and the joint.

E-selectin is also expressed in RA synovium, although the levels are much less than those of integrins. This might be due, in part, to the fact that E-selectin is only transiently expressed on endothelial cells after cytokine stimulation (only about 6h). This occurs even in the continued presence of cytokine, perhaps explaining the relatively low amounts in chronically inflamed tissue. In one study, E-selectin expression was decreased in synovial biopsies after patients were treated with injectable gold and corticosteroids[117].

MODELS FOR THE PATHOGENESIS OF RA

Elucidation of the cytokine profile of inflammatory arthritis, along with studies of TcRs and macrophage/fibroblast function, have led to revisions of conventional models for RA. More recent paradigms attempt to integrate the observation of blunted T-cell response in RA synovial tissue with the highly activated macrophage/fibroblast system. There is general agreement that the initiation of RA is probably a T-cell mediated, antigen-specific process. The arthrotropic agent is not yet defined, but could be a retrovirus (as in the goat–derived arthritis/encephalitis model), a bacterial product, or an organism, such as a spirochete, chlamydia, or mycobacterium. In a susceptible host (i.e. one with the appropriate HLA haplotype as well as other genetic influences), there is an early T-cell response that results in the elaboration of T-cell cytokines with resultant recruitment of inflammatory cells, including neutrophils, macrophages, B cells, and memory T-cells that possess a broad array of antigen specificities. When the disease becomes established, several basic models of RA diverge (Fig. 13.25). However, when interpreting these models, it is important to recognize that these theories attempt to explain the perpetuation of chronic synovitis, not the initiation of the disease. It is equally important to appreciate the fact that the models are not mutually exclusive.

T-CELL DRIVEN IMMUNE RESPONSE

If an arthrotropic antigen persists in the synovial tissue, an antigen-specific T-cell mediated immune response would presumably ensue. Much evidence has been advanced to support this sequence of events. For instance, the joint lesions of Lyme arthritis, in which spirochetal antigens are likely to be pathogenic, are similar to those of RA. HLA-DR surface density is high on synovial lining cells, interdigitating macrophages and dendritic cells and suggests active antigen presentation. Also, the T cells from synovial effusions and subintimal tissues often express cell surface activation markers, including class II MHC antigens and transferrin receptors. Lymphocytes in 'transitional areas' are

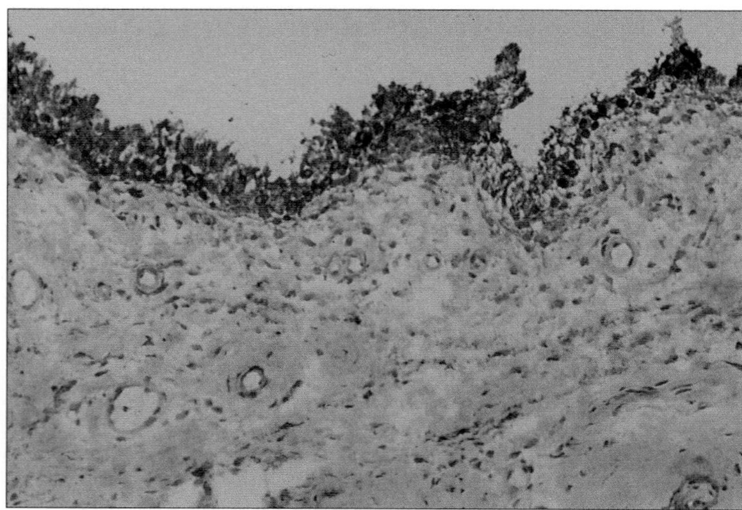

Fig. 13.24 VCAM expression in the synovial lining. Immunoperoxidase experiment demonstrating that VCAM-1 (brown pigment) is expressed in the synovial lining. In other sections, blood vessels and sublining mononuclear cells also stain positively.

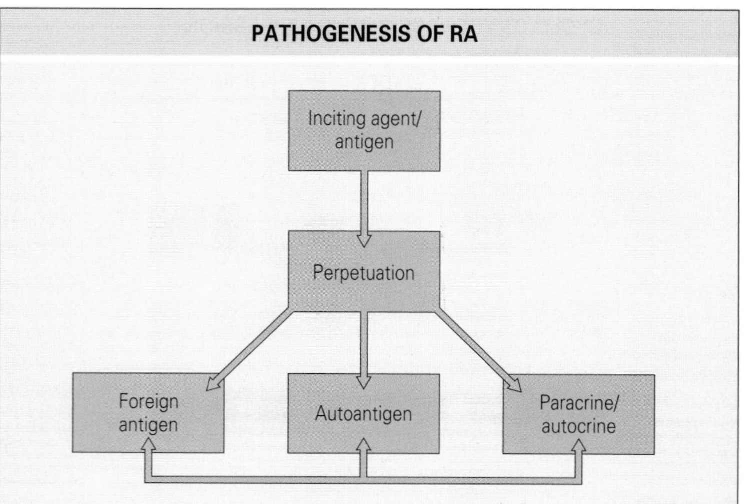

Fig. 13.25 Models for RA. During the chronic phase of RA, the disease can potentially be perpetuated by T-cell dependent and independent mechanisms. These mechanisms are not mutually exclusive and can interact with each other.

intimately associated with HLA-DR-rich accessory cells and can have a blast-like appearance. Products of these activated cells could, along with macrophage-derived factors, potentially induce class II MHC expression, promote synovial lining cell proliferation and support the growth and differentiation of B lymphocytes. The fact that T-cell 'specific' therapies, such as thoracic duct drainage, total nodal irradiation and cyclosporin A, are modestly effective in RA supports this model.

Thus the notion that RA synovitis results from a T-cell driven immune response could theoretically explain many of features of RA, including 1) the accumulation of T lymphocytes; 2) synovial lining cell hyperplasia and increased cell surface HLA-DR expression; 3) B cell hyperactivity resulting in local antibody production and 4) the HLA-OR haplotype associations. However, as noted above, not all of the data are consistent with this hypothesis. In particular, the soluble mediators (i.e. cytokines) produced in the joint are primarily of non-T-cell origin, and T-cell lymphokines are only detected in small quantities. Although suppressive factors (such as IL-10, TGF-β or IL-1ra) could contribute to the relative lack of T-cell products, it is difficult to invoke a causal relationship between T-cell activation and the very high degree of lining cell activation if these products are so difficult to identify. There are other potential explanations for this paradox. For instance, it is possible that even very small numbers of T-cells can activate cells in their microenvironment by secreting limited amounts of cytokines, or that the matrix masks the detection of T-cell products. Absorption or degradation of lymphokines is possible, but cannot account for the lack of some products in which this problem has been directly addressed, like IFN-γ. Some studies at the level of gene expression suggest that TH1 type cytokines can be produced, albeit in limited quantities, while the lack of TH2 cytokines could exacerbate disease. The possibility that direct T-cell contact could be a mechanism of macrophage or fibroblast activation also should be considered. However, it is clear that T-cell derived factors are much more easily detected in other T-cell mediated responses in humans, like tuberculous pleuritis, delayed-type hypersensitivity in the skin, allergen-induced asthma in the airway or inflamed tonsils. These questions have led to alternative hypotheses to explain the perpetuation of rheumatoid synovitis, i.e. the autoreactive T-cell and a paracrine/autocrine model of synovitis.

THE AUTOREACTIVE T-CELL

It is sometimes assumed that the initiating agent in RA is responsible for both the early changes and the perpetuation of chronic arthritis. However, this is not necessarily the case. The chronic rheumatoid lesion might just as well be the result of responses to antigens quite distinct from those responsible for starting the process. A similar scheme has been proposed in other autoimmune diseases, such as autoimmune thyroiditis where an appropriate response to a presumed viral insult results in the local elaboration of IFN-γ. This cytokine induces HLA-DR expression on thyrocytes, which then become the target of immune attack or serve as antigen-presenting cells. The reaction between HLA-DR-bearing stimulator cells and autologous T-lymphocytes is known as the autologous mixed leukocyte reaction (AMLR). A localized AMLR may occur in the synovium of patients with RA, although the data are largely circumstantial. First, the cytokine profile of RA synovitis is very similar to that of AMLR, where only small amounts of T-cell derived factors like IL-2 and IFN-γ are present and non-IL-2 T-cell growth factors might participate. Also, the cytotoxic T-cells present in RA joint effusions are similar to the NK-like cells produced in AMLR. Finally, the articular cavity and synovium contain a variety of potential stimulator cells in close apposition with responder cells. These include type A synoviocytes and dendritic cells; the latter are the most potent stimulators of mixed leukocyte reactions and constitute about 5% of the mononuclear cells in synovial effusions.

In addition to class II MHC antigens, synovial T-cells in chronic synovitis could respond directly to other autologous antigens in the joint released into the T-cell rich milieu. One example of this type of response is immunity to type II collagen. Autoreactive T-cells could also be stimulated through molecular mimicry. Examples of this have been discussed in this chapter, such as HSPs and proteoglycans. Another possible example of molecular mimicry involves EBV, which can infect B lymphocytes and induce proliferation and rheumatoid factors production. T cells from patients with RA do not effectively control EBV infection *in vitro*. The abnormality is due to defective IFN-γ production by RA T-cells and a monocyte-derived IL-1 inhibitor.

Computer analysis of EBV-encoded proteins has revealed sequence homology between the EBV glycoprotein gp110 and human HLA-DW4/DW14/DR1[118]. Disease susceptibility and/or severity in RA has been mapped to a five amino-acid sequence in the third hypervariable region of the DRβ_1 chain; this epitope is shared by both gp110 and the RA-associated HLA-DR haplotypes. Hence, an appropriate T-cell response directed against gp110 could inadvertently result in damage to normal cells that express these surface MHC molecules. One mechanism for the role of HSPs in autoimmunity is reminiscent of EBV molecular mimicry. A 65kDa mycobacterium lepra-specific helper T-cell clone has been isolated that reacts with a synthetic peptide found in the third hypervariable region of the HLA-DR 2 β chain. This raises the possibility that HSP and the RA-associated DR haplotypes could share epitopes. In fact, the *Escherichia coli* J protein (which is also a heat shock protein) also shares the EBV gp110 epitope.

PARACRINE/AUTOCRINE MODEL

The perpetuation of rheumatoid synovitis in the two previously mentioned models is orchestrated solely by T-lymphocytes. In these schemes, the products of T-cells diffuse throughout the tissue and directly stimulate sublining macrophages and synoviocytes, induce adhesion molecule expression in postcapillary high endothelial venules and stimulate local immunoglobulin production through the proliferation and differentiation of B cells. However, as discussed in detail earlier, studies that specifically measure T-cell activation in the joint have had difficulty demonstrating products of the putative activation (Fig. 13.26).

In contrast, products secreted by activated macrophage-like and fibroblast-like cells in the synovium, such as IL-1, TNF-α, IL-6, IL-8, GM-CSF, M-CSF, TGF-β, prostaglandins, complement proteins, TIMP, stromelysin, and collagenase, are abundant in synovial fluids and synovial tissues. These cells also possess an activated phenotype based on ultrastructural analysis and surface HLA-DR expression. This suggests

CELLULAR SOURCES OF SYNOVIAL CYTOKINES IN RA

Cytokines	Detected in RA synovium/synovial fluid
Products of T-cells	
IL-2	–
IL-3	–
IL-4	–
IL-6	±
IFN-γ	–
TNF-α	–
TNF-β	–
GM-CSF	–
Products of macrophages/ type A synoviocytes	
IL-1	+++
IL-6	+
IL-8	+++
TNF-α	++
M-CSF (CSF-1)	+
GM-CSF	+
TGF-β	++
MCP-1	++
Products of fibroblasts/ type B synoviocytes	
IL-6	+++
GM-CSF	+
MCP-1	+

Fig. 13.26 T-cell and macrophage/fibroblast cytokine production. Comparison of cytokines produced by T-cells and macrophages/fibroblasts in the RA synovium. A dash in the right-hand column indicates negligible or no detection. (MCP-1 = monocyte chemoattractant protein-1.)

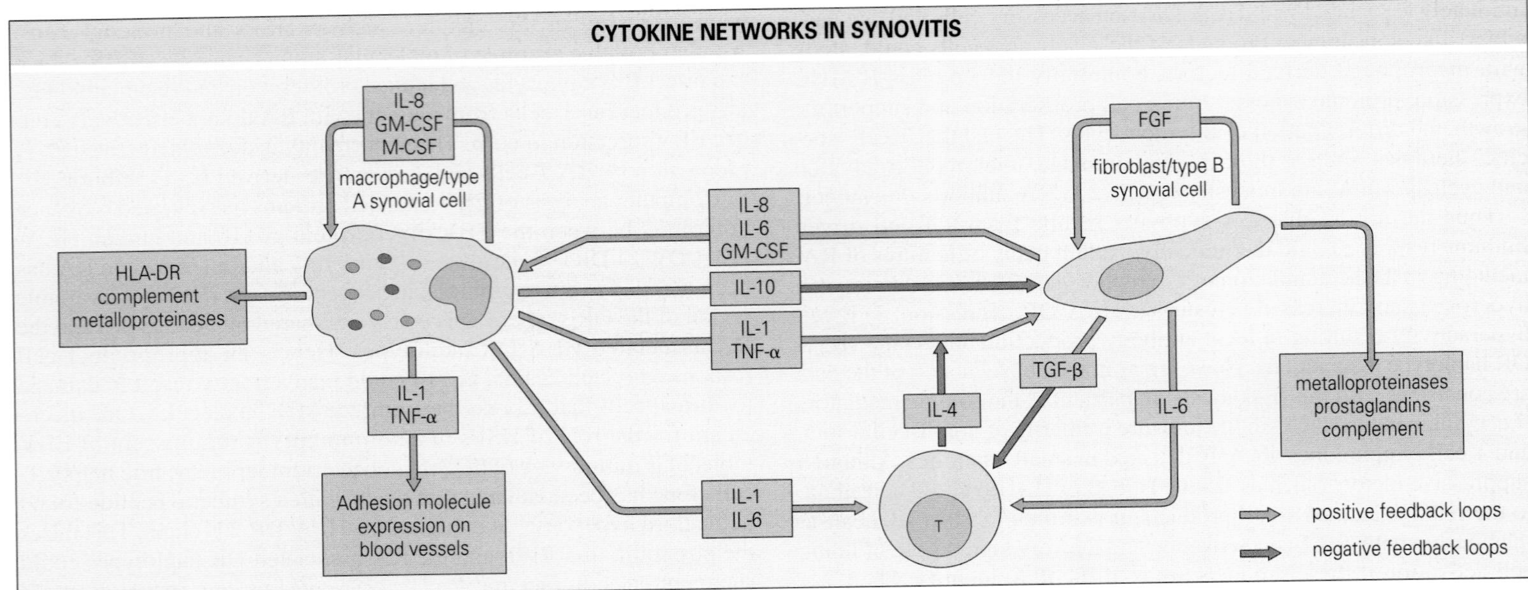

Fig. 13.27 Cytokine networks. Simplified version of the complex cytokine network in RA involving macrophages and fibroblasts. The precise T-cell cytokines that might participate are not clear because they are very difficult to detect.

an alternative to the traditional T-cell driven paradigms for the perpetuation of synovitis, i.e. that synovial inflammation is sustained by factors produced by neighboring macrophages and synovial fibroblasts in the joint lining in a paracrine or autocrine fashion. Many factors already identified in the joint could participate in such a system and explain lining cell hyperplasia, HLA-DR induction and synovial angiogenesis.

Figure 13.27 shows a simplified schematic diagram of the complex cytokine circuits that exist between synovial cells. IL-1 and TNF-α, both of which are produced by synovial cells of macrophage lineage, stimulate fibroblast proliferation and increase secretion of IL-6, IL-8, GM-CSF and effector molecules like stromelysin and collagenase. GM-CSF, which is produced by synovial macrophages and IL-1β or TNF-α-stimulated fibroblast-like synoviocytes, is a potent inducer of IL-1, TNF-α and IL-8 secretion. GM-CSF, particularly in combination with TNF-α, also increases HLA-DR expression on macrophages and monocytes, possibly obviating the need for IFN-γ. Fibroblast-like cells also possess an autocrine loop and can contribute to their own dysregulation through the elaboration of growth factors like FGF. The local production of cytokines by macrophages and fibroblasts could induce angiogenesis (e.g. FGF, TNF-α, VEGF and IL-8), increase adhesion molecule expression (e.g. IL-1 and TNF-α), and provide chemotactic stimulation to other cells (e.g, IL-8 and the other chemokines). Cytokines could also contribute to the modest degree of T-cell activation. B-cell activation and rheumatoid factor production might result from T-cell independent mechanisms or as yet undefined T-cell products. The notion of the transformed synoviocyte also fits into the paracrine/autocrine schema since the transformation phenotype likely relies on autocrine stimulation from factors like FGF and PDGF. Moreover, recent data indicating that fibroblast-like cells can retain an invasive phenotype even when free of macrophages suggests that an irreversible change might occur in this lineage.

One prediction of this alternative model is that the cytokine milieu attracts T-cells into the synovium in a non-antigen specific fashion. As discussed earlier, molecules such as IL-1 and TNF-α are potent inducers of adhesion molecules like ICAM-1, E-selectin and VCAM on endothelial cells. T-cells expressing the counter-receptors would preferentially bind to synovial vessels and migrate into the tissue. However, this is not an antigen-specific process; rather, a broad mix of memory T-cells accumulates preferentially because they express more adhesion molecules like VLA-4 (α_4/β_1) compared to the naive subset. In very early disease, preferential expression of certain TcR-bearing cells might occur. As the inflammatory process becomes chronic, nonspecific stimuli attract all T-cells with the appropriate chemokine receptors and adhesion molecules, thereby diluting out a putative pathogenic clone (Fig. 13.28). A significant over-representation of a particular subset of T-cells expressing a specific TcR in the synovium could have a variety of explanations. First, the cells could proliferate locally due to interaction with a specific antigen or a superantigen. However, as previously discussed, there is little evidence for aggressive *in situ* proliferation of CD4$^+$ T-cells. Alternatively, exposure either to the 'RA antigen' or to an irrelevant antigen (like a recent vaccine) outside the joint could skew the population of circulating memory T-cells and result in an increase in that particular V_β rearrangement in the joint. The HLA genotype of individuals also can shape the TcR repertoire

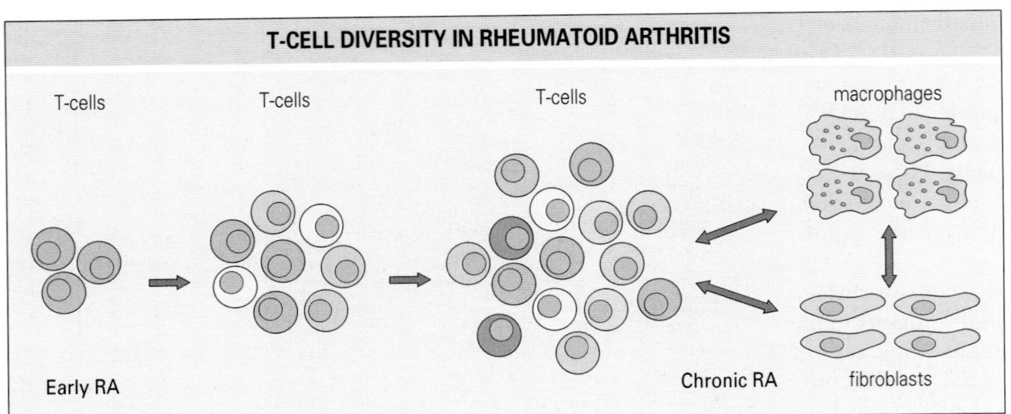

Fig. 13.28 T-cell diversity in RA. Early in RA, there might be a homogeneous population of antigen-specific T-cells. As the disease progresses, nonspecific recruitment results in the ingress of a broad array of T-cells. Macrophages, fibroblasts and T-cells communicate in paracrine networks during the perpetuation phase.

and the bias towards specific HLA molecules in RA can determine the TcR chains that accumulate in the joint. Obviously, if the etiologic agent in RA is distributed systemically, this population could also enter the joint preferentially.

Cytokine inhibitors also play a role in the autocrine/paracrine model, since negative feedback loops probably are important normal homeostatic mechanisms for controlling synovial inflammation. However, these inhibitors appear to be ineffective methods of interrupting the proinflammatory cytokines in RA. One example is IL-1ra, which theoretically should be beneficial in RA. Yet, synovial inflammation persists despite the presence of this inhibitor in the joint, most likely because of the low concentrations relative to IL-1. The lack of IFN-γ and IL-4 could also contribute to the inflammatory process, since the former antagonizes the proinflammatory effects of TNF-α and the latter has general suppressive effects on synovial metalloproteinase and cytokine production. Paradoxically, the absence of IFN-γ might be due, in part, to an overproduction of TGF-β, another potent inhibitor of immune responses. IL-10 production by synovium clearly dampens the local cytokine response. However, it appears to be insufficient to downregulate inflammation and destruction.

A UNIFYING HYPOTHESIS: T-CELL/MACROPHAGE/FIBROBLAST AXIS.

These basic models encompass a broad spectrum of philosophies and theories on the pathogenesis of RA. In reality the perpetuation of synovitis in RA likely results from a combination of all three, with interplay between T-cells, fibroblast-like cells and macrophage-like cells. The relative contribution of each probably depends on the degree of chronicity, the extent of therapeutic interventions and other poorly defined factors. Because of the highly complex inter-relationship between these cells, it is possible that therapies aimed at only one aspect will succeed in chronic disease. Hence, although T-cell specific therapies (e.g. anti-CD4, anti-CD5 and anti-CD52 antibodies and cyclosporin) in chronic RA have some success, in general the percentage of patients that respond and the degree of improvement are disappointing. Perhaps treating early RA, which is closer to the initial T-cell mediated injury, with these methods would be more helpful. Similarly, attempts to interrupt the cytokine loops are only modestly successful. Even though IFN-γ is an inhibitor of some TNF-α actions and should have benefit based on *in vitro* data, it is certainly not the magic bullet for RA. The advent of more potent TNF-α inhibitors has produced striking clinical improvement. However, it is not known if this will alter the destructive phase of the disease in addition to ameliorating symptoms due to inflammation. Other therapies with narrow scope, such as NSAIDs, are relegated to adjunct roles. Prevention of chronic synovial inflammation will require a comprehensive approach to the entire T-cell/macrophage/fibroblast axis implying a need for novel combination therapies (Fig. 13.28).

ALTERNATIVE MECHANISMS OF SYNOVIAL HYPERPLASIA: EXCESSIVE CELL RECRUITMENT AND DEFECTIVE CELL DEATH

The accumulation of cells in tissue can be expressed by the following formula:

$$\text{cell number} = [\text{cell ingress} - \text{cell egress}] + [\text{cell proliferation} - \text{cell death}]$$

Hence, there are two major components to synovial intimal lining expansion. The first involves cell trafficking, which can account for accumulation of various cell types if recruitment exceeds the rate that the cells exit the joint. This probably accounts for increased numbers of macrophage-like synoviocytes, which arise from the bone marrow and migrate to the synovium through the blood. The expansion of the fibroblast-like synoviocyte population might be due, in part, to cell division, although the actual extent of proliferation is marginal. A second way to increase the cell number involves changes in the balance between cell division and cell death. Because of the limited amount of DNA synthesis and mitosis in both cell populations, a defect in cell death could contribute to cell accumulation. Cell death can occur through two basic mechanisms: 1) necrosis, which causes disruption of cell membranes and release of cellular contents in a hostile environment; and 2) apoptosis, or programmed cell death, which is a normal stereotypic mechanism of removing cells by enzymatic degradation of DNA molecules into 180-200 base fragments and meticulous packaging of the intracellular contents without disturbing the environment.

Rheumatoid synovial tissues have been examined to determine if and where apoptosis occurs[119]. Surgical specimens of RA synovium demonstrate DNA ladders characteristic of apoptosis. Cells with fragmented DNA are found primarily in the synovial lining (Fig. 13.29) and could be localized to both macrophage-like and fibroblast-like cells. DNA fragmentation can be induced in cultured fibroblast-like synoviocytes by IL-1 and TNF-α and prevented by IFN-γ. Anti-*Fas* (cD95) antibody also induces apoptosis, and the *Fas* protein is constitutively expressed by cultured synoviocytes. The role of *Fas* as a natural mediator of programmed cell death is well known, and it might play a role in other autoimmune diseases like systemic lupus erythematosus (SLE)[120]. These data suggest a potential link between the cytokines produced in RA and the propensity for apoptosis: macrophage and fibroblast products like TNF-α (and possibly *Fas* ligand) are abundant in the joint while IFN-γ is very low. Therefore, the cytokine profile of the rheumatoid synovitis, along with exposure to noxious stimuli like oxygen radicals, tends to favor apoptosis in synovial lining cells.

Although DNA fragmentation is readily detected in RA synovium, the number of cells that actually progress to the late stages of apoptosis is limited. Using electron microscopy, less than 1% of cells exhibit the ultrastructural features of programmed cell death[121]. This suggests that the final pathway might be defective and that cells with DNA strand breaks can either recover or persist for prolonged periods of time. A mechanism of abnormal apoptosis in RA (if it exists) could involve defects in a variety of proteins known to be involved in the regulation of cell proliferation and death, including the oncogene c-*myc* or the p53 tumor suppressor gene. Figure 13.30 shows one possible schema for this model. DNA fragmentation can be induced by either cytokines or local oxygen radicals. Both of these can subsequently induce oncogene expression, which under some circumstances activate p53. The p53 protein then directs the cell towards apoptosis as a type of 'fail-safe' mechanism to prevent excessive cell accumulation or transformation. A defect in these pathways, either due to somatic mutations or other functional alterations, can potentially lead to arrested apoptosis and increased cell number.

In contrast to those in the intimal lining, sublining lymphocytes seem to be more resistant to DNA fragmentation. This could be due to *Bcl2* expression by lymphocytes, especially in lymphoid aggregates. *Bcl2* is a

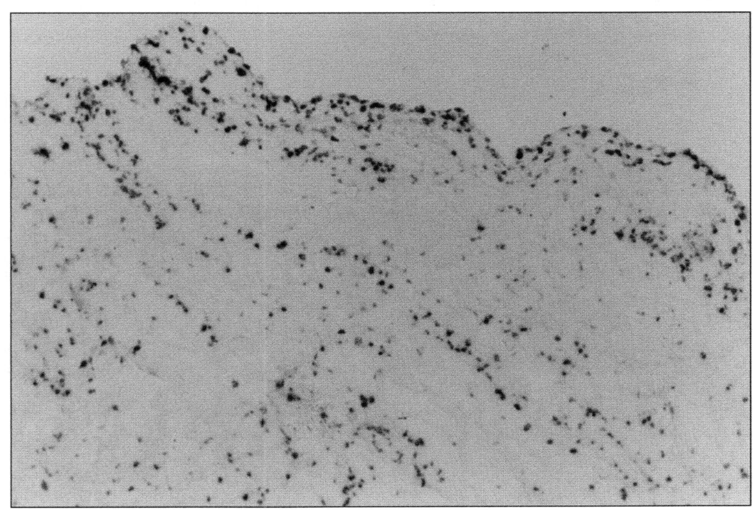

Fig. 13.29 Cells with fragmented DNA are present in the rheumatoid synovial intimal lining. Nuclei with damaged DNA are purple in this eosin-counterstained section.

proto-oncogene that was first identified in follicular B cell lymphomas and is known to block apoptosis. The overexpression of *Bcl2* in synovial lymphocytes could inhibit programmed cell death and lead to prolonged survival of synovial T-cells. This might contribute to the accumulation of quiescent memory lymphocytes in rheumatoid synovium.

These data suggest the following paradigm: synovial lining expansion occurs in the rheumatoid joint because of increased recruitment of macrophage-like and fibroblast-like cells in combination with deficient apoptosis. While some cells in the latter population might have progressed beyond G_0 (the resting phase in the cell cycle), it is very difficult to detect DNA synthesis or mitosis to support the notion that unbridled proliferation is primarily responsible for synovial lining expansion. Cell recruitment and nominal cell division are opposed by two forces. On the one hand, a certain number of cells are shed from the lining into the synovial fluid. The precise rate of cell egress is unknown for RA, so it is difficult to assess its contribution. On the other hand, apoptosis appears on first blush to be an active process that involves both macrophage-like and fibroblast-like cells and is enhanced by the local cytokine milieu, regional production of reactive oxygen species and intermittent ischemia and reperfusion in the joint. Despite the evidence for abundant DNA fragmentation consistent with apoptosis, this process is not sufficient to prevent the synovial lining from becoming hyperplastic.

If apoptosis is, indeed, defective, then this could contribute to synovial lining 'hyperplasia'. The mechanism of this process offers a novel therapeutic target for interfering with chronic inflammatory processes. Management of programmed cell death, in combination with the myriad of approaches suggested by the previous models, is a fertile fields for the discovery of new treatment approaches to RA.

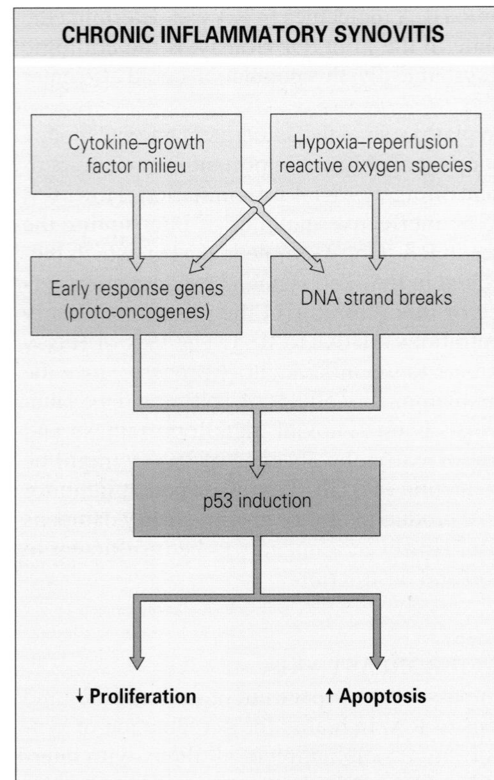

Fig. 13.30 Proposed relationship between DNA damage, cytokines and cell survival in the synovium.

REFERENCES

1. Edwards JCW, Willoughby DA. Demonstration of bone marrow derived cells in synovial lining by means of giant intracellular granules as genetic markers. Ann Rheum Dis. 1982;4:177–82.
2. Pitsillides AA, Wilkinson LS, Mehdiadeh S, Bayliss MT, Edwards JCW. Uridine diphosphonate dehydrogenase activity in normal and rheumatoid synovium: the description of a specialized synovial lining cell. Int J Exp Pathol. 1993;74:27–34.
3. Lalor PA, Mapp PI, Hall PA, Revell PA. Proliferative activity of cells in the synovium as demonstrated by a monoclonal antibody, Ki67. Rheumatol Int. 1987;7:183–6.
4. Ritchlin C, Dwyer E, Bucala R, Winchester R: Sustained and distinctive patterns of gene activation in synovial fibroblasts and whole synovial tissue obtained from inflammatory synovitis. Scan J Immunol. 1994;40:292–8.
5. Qu Z, Garcia CH, O'Rourke LM, Planck SR, Kohl M, Rosenbaum JT. Local proliferation of fibroblast-like synoviocytes contributes to synovial hyperplasia. Results of proliferating cell nuclear antigen/cyclin, c-*myc*, and nucleolar organizer region staining. Arthritis Rheum. 1994;37:212–20.
6. Iguchi T, Kurosaka M, Ziff M. Electron microscopic study of HLA-DR in monocyte/macrophage staining cells in the rheumatoid synovial membrane. Arthritis Rheum. 1986;29:600–13.
7. Firestein GS, Zvaifler NJ. Down regulation of human monocyte differentiation antigens by interferon gamma. Cell Immunol. 1987;104:343–54.
8. Van Dinther-Janssen ACHM, Pals ST, Scheper R, Breedveld F, Meijer CJLM. Dendritic cells and high endothelial venules in the rheumatoid synovial membrane. J Rheumatol. 1990;17:11–17.
9. Yanni G, Whelan A, Feighery C, Bresnihan B. Synovial tissue macrophages and joint erosion in rheumatoid arthritis. Ann Rheumatic Dis. 1994;53:39–44.
10. Firestein GS, Alvaro-Gracia JM, Maki R. Quantitative analysis of cytokine gene expression in rheumatoid arthritis. J Immunol. 1990;144:3347–53.
11. Ridley MG, Kingsley G, Pitzalis C, Panayi GS. Monocyte activation in rheumatoid arthritis: Evidence for *in situ* activation and differentiation in joints. Br J Rheumatol. 1990;29:84–8.
12. Goto M, Fujisawa M, Yamada A, *et al.* Spontaneous release of angiotensin converting enzyme and interleukin-1β peripheral blood monocytes from patients with rheumatoid arthritis under serum-free condition. Ann Rheum Dis. 1990;49:172–6.
13. Edwards JC, Wilkinson LS, Pitsillides AA. Palisading cells of rheumatoid nodules: comparison with synovial intimal cells. Ann. Rheum. Dis. 1993;52:801–5.
14. Tsai D, Diaz LA Jr, Singer NG, *et al.* Responsiveness of human T lymphocytes to bacterial superantigens presented by cultured rheumatoid arthritis synoviocytes. Arthritis Rheum. 1996;39:125–36.
15. Alvaro-Gracia JM, Zvaifler NJ, Firestein GS. Cytokines in chronic inflammatory arthritis. V. Mutual antagonism between interferon-gamma and tumor necrosis factor-alpha on HLA-DR expression, proliferation, collagenase production, and granulocyte macrophage colony-stimulating factor production by rheumatoid arthritis synoviocytes. J Clin Invest. 1990;86:1790–8.
16. Dayer JM, de Rochemonteix B, Burrus B, Demczuk S, Dinarello A. Human recombinant interleukin-1 stimulates collagenase and prostaglandin E_2 production by human synovial cells. J Clin Invest. 1986;77:645–8.
17. Geiler T, Kriegsmann J, Keyszer GM, Gay RE, Gay S. A new model for rheumatoid arthritis generated by engraftment of rheumatoid synovial tissue and normal human cartilage into SCID mice. Arthritis Rheum. 1994;37:1664–71.
18. Zvaifler NJ, Firestein GS. Pannus and pannocytes. Alternative models of joint destruction in rheumatoid arthritis. Arthritis Rheum. 1994;37(6):783–9.
19. Kidd BL, Moore K, Walters MT, Smith JL, Cawley MI. Immunohistological features of synovitis in ankylosing spondylitis: A comparison with rheumatoid arthritis. Ann Rheum Dis. 1989;48:92–8.
20. Grom AA, Thompson SD, Luyrink L, Passo M, Choi E, Glass DN. Dominant T-cell-receptor beta chain variable region V beta 14+ clones in juvenile rheumatoid arthritis. Proc Natl Acad Sci USA. 1993;90:11104–8.
21. Paliard X, West SG, Lafferty JA, *et al.* Evidence for the effects of a superantigen in rheumatoid arthritis. Science 1991;253:325–9.
22. Howell MD, Diveley JP, Lundeen KA, *et al.* Limited T-cell receptor beta-chain heterogeneity among interleukin 2 receptor-positive synovial T cells suggests a role for superantigen in rheumatoid arthritis. Proc Natl Acad Sci USA. 1991;88:10921–5.
23. Jenkins RN, Nikaein A, Zimmermann A, Meek K, Lipsky PE. T cell receptor V beta gene bias in rheumatoid arthritis. J Clin Invest. 1993;92:2688–70.
24. Uematsu Y, Wege H, Straus A, *et al.* The T-cell-receptor repertoire in the synovial fluid of a patient with rheumatoid arthritis is polyclonal. Proc Natl. Acad Sci USA. 1991;88:8534–8.
25. Olive C, Gatenby PA, Serjeantson SW. Analysis of T cell receptor V alpha and V beta gene usage in synovia of patients with rheumatoid arthritis. Immunol Cell Biol. 1991;69:349–54.
26. Bergroth V, Tsai V, Zvaifler NJ. Differences in responses of normal and rheumatoid arthritis peripheral blood T cells to synovial fluid and peripheral blood dendritic cells in allogeneic mixed leukocyte reactions. Arthritis Rheum. 1989;32:1381–9.
27. Wahl SM, Allen JB, Wong HL, Dougherty SF, Ellingsworth LR. Antagonistic and agonistic effects of transforming growth factor-beta and IL-1 in rheumatoid synovitis. J Immunol. 1990;145:2514–19.
28. Gaston JSH, Life PF, Bailey LC, Bacon PA. *In vitro* responses to a 65-kilodalton mycobacterial protein by synovial T cells from inflammatory arthritis patients. J Immunol. 1989;143:2494–500.
29. Gaston JSH, Life PF, Jenner PJ, Colston MJ, Bacon PA. Recognition of a mycobacteria-specific epitope in the 65-kDa heat-shock protein by

synovial fluid-derived T cell clones. J Exp Med. 1990;171:831–41.
30. Van Eden W, Thole JER, van der Zee R, *et al.* Cloning of the mycobacterial epitope recognized by T lymphocytes in adjuvant arthritis. Nature. 1988;331:171–3.
31. van Eden W, Holoshitz J, Nevo Z, Frenkel A, Klajman A, Cohen IR. Arthritis induced by a T lymphocyte clone that responds to mycobacterium tuberculosis and to cartilage proteoglycans. Proc Natl Acad Sci USA. 1985;82:5117–20.
32. Holoshitz J, Klajman A, Druker I, *et al.* T lymphocytes of rheumatoid arthritis patients show augmented reactivity to a fraction of mycobacteria cross reactive with cartilage. Lancet. 1986;2:305–9.
33. Tarkowski A, Klareskog L, Carlsten H, Herberts P, Koopman WJ. Secretion of antibodies to types I and II collagen by synovial tissue cells in patients with rheumatoid arthritis. Arthritis Rheum. 1989;32:1087–92.
34. Larsen CP, Ritchie SC, Hendrix R, *et al.* Regulation of immunostimulatory function and costimulatory molecule (B7-1 and B7-2) expression on murine dendritic cells. J Immunol. 1994;152:5208–19.
35. Tsai V, Zvaifler NJ. Dendritic cell–lymphocyte clusters that form spontaneously in rheumatoid arthritis synovial effusions differ from clusters formed in human mixed leukocyte reactions. J Clin Invest. 1988;82:1731–45.
36. Carson DA, Chen PP, Kipps TJ. New roles for rheumatoid factor. J Clin Invest. 1991;87:379–83.
37. Phillips, JA, Hobbs MV, Romball CG, Ernst DN, Shultz, L, Weigle WO. CD4$^+$ T cell activation and tolerance induction in B cell knockout mice. J Exp Med. 1996;183:1339–44.
38. Victor KD, Randen I, Thompson K, *et al.* Rheumatoid factors isolated from patients with autoimmune disorders are derived from germline genes distinct from those encoding the Wa, Po, and Bla crossreactive idiotypes. J Clin Invest. 1991;87:1603–13.
39. McColl SR, Paquin R, Menard C, and Beaulieu AD. Human neutrophils produce high levels of the interleukin 1 receptor antagonist in response to granulocyte/macrophage colony-stimulating factor and tumor necrosis factor alpha. J Exper Med. 1992;176:593–8.
40. Okada Y. The mast cells in synovial membrane of patients with joint disease. J J Ortho Surg. 1973;47:657–74.
41. Firestein GS, Xu WD, Townsend K, *et al.* Cytokines in chronic inflammatory arthritis. I. Failure to detect T cell lymphokines (IL-2 and IL-3) and presence of macrophage colony-stimulating factor (CSF-1) and a novel mast cell growth factor in rheumatoid synovitis. J Exp Med. 1988;168:1573–86.
42. Kohase M, Henriksen-deStefano D, May LT, Vilcek J, Sehgal PB. Induction of β_2 interferon by tumor necrosis factor: a homeostatic mechanism in the control of cell proliferation. Cell. 1986;45:659–66.
43. Husby G, Williams RC Jr. Immunohistochemical studies of interleukin-2 and interferon-2 in rheumatoid arthritis. Arthritis Rheum. 1985;28:174–81.
44. Barnes PF, Fong SJ, Brennan PJ, Twomey PE, Mazumder A, Modin RL. Local production of tumor necrosis factor and IFN-γ in tuberculous pleuritis. J Immnunol. 1990;145:149–54.
45. Katsikis PD, Chu CQ, Brennan FM, Maini RN, Feldmann M. Immunoregulatory role of interleukin 10 in rheumatoid arthritis. J Exp Med. 1994;179:1517–27.
46. Cambell IL, Kay TWH, Oxbrow L, Harrison LC. Essential role for interferon-gamma and interleukin 6 in autoimmune insulin-dependent diabetes in NOD/WEHI mice. J Clin Invest. 1991;87:739–42.
47. Miossec P, Naviliat M, Dupuy d'Angeac A, Sany J, Banchereau J. Low levels of interleukin-4 and high levels of transforming growth factor beta in rheumatoid arthritis. Arthritis Rheum. 1990;145:2514–19.
48. Saxne T, Palladino MA Jr, Heinegard D, Talal N, Wollheim FA. Detection of tumor necrosis factor alpha but not tumor necrosis factor beta in rheumatoid arthritis synovial fluid and serum. Arthritis Rheum. 1988;31:1041–5.
49. Kay AB, Yiing S, Varney V, *et al.* Messenger RNA expression of the cytokine gene cluster, interleukin 3 (IL-3), IL-4, IL-5, and granulocyte/macrophage colony-stimulating factor, in allergen-induced late-phase cutaneous reactions in atopic subjects. J Exp Med. 1991;173:775–8.
50. Broide DH, Firestein GS. Endobronchial allergen challenge in asthma. Demonstration of cellular source of GM-CSF by *in situ* hybridization. J Clin Invest. 1991;88:1048–53.
51. Mosmann TR, Coffman RL. TH1 and TH2 cells: different patterns of lymphokine secretion lead to different functional properties. Ann Rev Immunol. 1989;7:145–73.
52. Miltenburg AM, van Laar JM, de Kuiper R, Daha MR, Breedveld FC. T cells cloned from human rheumatoid synovial membrane functionally represent the TH1 subset. Scan J Immunol. 1992;35:603–10.
53. Simon AK, Seipelt E, Sieper J. Divergent T-cell cytokine patterns in inflammatory arthritis. Proc. Natl Acad Sci USA. 1994;91:8562–6.
54. Bessis N, Boissier M-C, Caput D, Fradelizi D, Fournier C. IL-4 or IL-13 transfected xenogenic fibroblasts in the treatment of collagen induced arthritis in mice. Clin Rheumatol. 1995;12:261.
55. Weiner HL, Friedman A, Miller A, *et al.* Oral tolerance: immunologic mechanisms and treatment of animal and human organ-specific autoimmune diseases by oral administration of autoantigens. Ann Rev Immunol. 1994;12:809–37.
56. Chandrasekhar S, Harvey AK, Hrubey PS, Bendele AM. Arthritis induced by interleukin-1 is dependent on the site and frequency of intraarticular injection. Clin Immunol Immunopathol. 1990;55:382–400.
57. Henderson B, Pettipher ER. Arthritogenic actions of recombinant IL-1 and tumour necrosis factor alpha in the rabbit: evidence for synergistic interactions between cytokines *in vivo*. Clin Exp Immunol. 1989;75:306–10.
58. van de Loo FAJ, Arntz OJ, van Lent PLEM, van den Berg WB. Enhanced degradation of articular cartilage in flares of antigen-induced arthritis: Direct effect of IL-1 on chondrocytes. Arthritis Rheum. 1995;38:S400.
59. Brennan FM, Butler DM, Maini RN, Feldmann M. Modulation of proinflammatory cytokine release in rheumatoid synovial membrane cell cultures with an anti-TNF-alpha monoclonal antibody: Comparison with blockade of IL-1 using the recombinant IL-1 receptor antagonist. Arthritis Rheum. 38:S400, 1995.
60. Elliott MJ, Maini RN, Feldmann M, *et al.* Randomised double-blind comparison of chimeric monoclonal antibody to tumour necrosis factor alpha (cA2) versus placebo in rheumatoid arthritis. Lancet. 1994;344:1105–10.
61. Koch AE, Kunkel SL, Burrows JC, *et al.* Synovial tissue macrophage as a source of the chemotactic cytokine IL-8. J Immunol. 1991;147:2187–95.
62. Koch AE, Kunkel SL, Harlow LA, *et al.* Enhanced production of monocyte chemoattractant protein-1 in rheumatoid arthritis. J Clin Invest. 1992;90:772–9.
63. Hosaka S, Akahoshi T, Wada C, and Kondo H. Expression of the chemokine superfamily in rheumatoid arthritis. Clin Exper Immunol. 1994;97:451–7.
64. Koch AE, Kunkel SL, Harlow LA, *et al.* Epithelial neutrophil activating peptide-78: a novel chemotactic cytokine for neutrophils in arthritis. J Clin Invest 1994;94:1012–8.
65. Rathanaswami P, Hachicha M, Sadick M, Schall TJ, McColl SR. Expression of the cytokine RANTES in human rheumatoid synovial fibroblasts. Differential regulation of RANTES and interleukin-8 genes by inflammatory cytokines. J Biol Chem. 1993;268:5834–9.
66. Allen JB, Manthey CL, Hand AR, Ohura K, Ellingsworth L, Wahl SM. Rapid onset synovial inflammation and hyperplasia induced by transforming growth factor beta. J Exp Med. 1990;171:231–47.
67. Brandes ME, Allen JB, Ogawa Y, Wahl SM. Transforming growth factor beta-1 suppresses acute and chronic arthritis in experimental animals. J Clin Invest. 1991;87:1108–13.
68. Reuterdahl C, Tingstrom A, Terracio L, Funa K, Heldin CH, Rubin K. Characterization of platelet-derived growth factor beta-receptor expressing cells in the vasculature of human rheumatoid synovium. Lab Invest. 1991;64:321–9.
69. Mukhopadhyay D, Tsiokas L, Zhou XM, Foster D, Brugge JS, Sukhatme VP. Hypoxic induction of human vascular endothelial growth factor expression through c-*src* activation. Nature. 1995;375:577–81.
70. Fava RA, Olsen NJ, Spncer-Green G et al. Vascular permeability factor/endothelial growth factor (VPF/VEGF): accumulation and expression in human synovial fluids and rheumatoid synovial tissue. Journal of Experimental Medicine 1994;180:341–6.
71. Malyak M, Swaney RE, Arend WP. Levels of synovial fluid interleukin-1 receptor antagonist in rheumatoid arthritis and other arthropathies. Potential contribution from synovial fluid neutrophils. Arthritis Rheum. 1993, 36:781–9.
72. Firestein GS, Berger AE, Tracey DE, *et al.* IL-1 receptor antagonist protein production and gene expression in rheumatoid arthritis and osteoarthritis synovium. J Immunol. 1992;149:1054–62.
73. Firestein GS, Boyle DL, Yu C, *et al.*Synovial interleukin-1 receptor antagonist and interleukin-1 balance in rheumatoid arthritis. Arthritis Rheum. 1994;37:644–52.
74. Steiner G, Studnicka-Benke A, Witzmann G, Hofler E, Smolen J. Soluble receptors for tumor necrosis factor and interleukin-2 in serum and synovial fluid of patients with rheumatoid arthritis, reactive arthritis and osteoarthritis. J Rheum. 1995;22:406–12.
75. Arend WP, Malyak M, Smith MF Jr, *et al.* Binding of IL-1 alpha, IL-1 beta, and IL-1 receptor antagonist by soluble IL-1 receptors and levels of soluble IL-1 receptors in synovial fluids. J Immunol. 1994;153:4766–74.
76. Suzuki H, Kamimura J, Ayabe T, Kashiwagi H. Demonstration of neutralizing autoantibodies against IL-1α in sera from patients with rheumatoid arthritis. J Immunol. 1990;145:2140–6.
77. Vieira P, de Waal-Malefyt R, Dang MN, *et al.* Isolation and expression of human cytokine synthesis inhibitory factor cDNA clones: homology to Epstein–Barr virus open reading frame BCRFI. Proc Natl Acad Sci USA. 1991;88:1172–6.
78. Chomarat P, Vannier E, Dechanet J, *et al.* Balance of IL-1 receptor antagonist/IL-1 beta in rheumatoid synovium and its regulation by IL-4 and IL-10. J Immunol. 1995;154:1432–9
79. Katsikis KD, Chu CQ, Brennan FM, Maini RN, Feldmann M. Immunoregulatory role of interleukin 10 in rheumatoid arthritis. J Exp Med. 1994;179:1517–27.
80. Cush JJ, Splawski JB, Ranjeny T, *et al.* Elevated interleukin-10 levels in patients with rheumatoid arthritis. Arthritis Rheum. 1995;38:96–104.
81. Kasama T, Strieter RM, Lukacs NW, Lincoln PM, Burdick MD, Kunkel SL. Interleukin-10 expression and chemokine regulation during the evolution of murine type II collagen-induced arthritis. J Clin Invest. 1995;95:2868–76.
82. Conway JG, Wakefield JA, Brown RH, *et al.* Inhibition of cartilage and bone destruction in adjuvant arthritis in the rat by a matrix metalloproteinase inhibitor. J Exp Med. 1995;182:449–57.
83. Case JP, Sano H, Lafyatis R, Remmers EF, Kumkumian GK, Wilder RL. Transin/stromelysin expression in the synovium of rats with experimental erosive arthritis. *In situ* localization and kinetics of expression of the transformation-associated metalloproteinase in euthymic and athymic Lewis rats. J Clin Invest. 1989;84:1731–40.
84. Firestein GS, Paine MM, Littman BH. Gene expression (collagenase, tissue inhibitor of metalloproteinases, complement, and HLA-DR) in rheumatoid arthritis and osteoarthritis synovium: Quantitative analysis and effect of intraarticular corticosteroids. Arthritis Rheum. 1991;34:1094–105.
85. McCachren SS, Haynes BF, Niedel JE.

Localization of collagenase mRNA in rheumatoid arthritis synovium by *in situ* hybridization histochemistry. J Clin Immunol. 1990;10:19–27.
86. Hasty KA, Reife RA, Kang AH, Stuart JM. The role of stromelysin in the cartilage destruction that accompanies inflammatory arthritis. Arthritis Rheum. 1990;33:388–97.
87. .Zvaifler NJ, Boyle D, Firestein GS. Early synovitis—synoviocytes and mononuclear cells. Semin Arthritis Rheum. 1994;23(Suppl 2):11–16.
88. Unemori EN, Bair MJ, Bauer EA, Amento EP. Stromelysin expression regulates collagenase activation in human fibroblasts. Dissociable control of two metalloproteinases by interferon-gamma. J Biol Chem. 1991;266:23477–82.
89. Yang-Yen HF, Chambard JC, Sun YL, *et al.* Transcriptional interference between c-Jun and the glucocorticoid receptor: mutual inhibition of DNA binding due to direct protein–protein interaction. Cell. 1990;62:1205–15.
90. Shlopov BV, CL Mainardi, KA Hasty. Neutrophil collagenase (MMP-3) and collagenase 3 (MMP-13) are expressed in osteoarthritic and stimulated chondrocytes. Arth Rheum. 1995;38: S313 (abstract).
91. Unemori EN, Hibbs MS, Amento EP. Constitutive expression of a 92-kDa gelatinase (type V collagenase) by rheumatoid synovial fibroblasts and its induction in normal human fibroblasts by inflammatory cytokines. J Clin Invest. 1991;88:1656–62.
92. Keyszer GM, Heer AH, Kriegsmann J, *et al.* Comparative analysis of cathepsin L, cathepsin D, and collagenase messenger RNA expression in synovial tissues of patients with rheumatoid arthritis and osteoarthritis, by *in situ* hybridization. Arthritis Rheum. 1995;38:976–84.
93. .Buttle DJ, Handley CJ, Ilic MZ, *et al.* Inhibition of cartilage proteoglycan release by a specific inactivator of cathepsin B and an inhibitor of matrix metalloproteinases. Evidence for two converging pathways of chondrocyte-mediated proteoglycan degradation. Arthritis Rheum.1993;36:1709–17.
94. Crawston TE. Protein inhibitors of metalloproteinases. In: Barrett AJ, Salvesen G, eds. Proteinase Inhibitors. Amsterdam:Elsevier; 1986;589–610.
95. Okada Y, Gonoji Y, Nakanishi I, Nagase H, Hayakawa T. Immunohistochemical demonstration of collagenase and tissue inhibitor of metalloproteinases (TIMP) in synovial lining cells of rheumatoid synovium. Virchows Archiv B Cell Pathology. 1990;59:305–12.
96. Abbink JJ, Kamp AM, Nuijens JH, Swaak TJ, Hack CE. Proteolytic inactivation of alpha-1 antitrypsin and alpha-1 antichymotrypsin by neutrophils in arthritic joints. Arthritis Rheum. 1993;36:168–80.
97. Littman BH, Drury CE, Schumacher R, Boyle D, Weisman M, Firestein GS. *In vivo* reduction of RA synovial tissue metalloproteinase mRNA levels by tenidap. Arthritis Rheum. 1994;37:S420.
98. Firestein GS, Paine MM, Boyle DL. Mechanisms of methotrexate action in rheumatoid arthritis. Selective decrease in synovial collagenase gene expression. Arthritis Rheum. 1994;37:193–200.
99. Cronstein BN, Naime D, Ostad E. The anti-inflammatory mechanism of low-dose methotrexate: increased adenosine release at inflamed sites diminishes leukocyte accumulation in an *in vivo* model of inflammation. J Clin Invest., 1993;92:2675–82.
100. Boyle DL, Sajjadi FG, Firestein GS. Adenosine receptor stimulation inhibits synoviocyte collagenase gene expression. Arthritis Rheum. in press.
101. Crofford LJ, Wilder RL, Ristimaki AP, *et al.* Cyclo-oxygenase-1 and -2 expression in rheumatoid synovial tissues. Effects of interleukin-1 beta, phorbol ester, and corticosteroids. J Clin Invest. 1994;93:1095–101.
102. Nakajima H, Hiyama Y, Tsukada W, Warabi H, Uchida S, Hirose S. Effects of interferon gamma on cultured synovial cells from patients with rheumatoid arthritis: inhibition of cell growth, prostaglandin E2, and collagenase release. Ann Rheum Dis. 1990;49:312–6.
103. Strunk RC, Sessions Cole F, Perlmutter DH, Colten HR. Gamma-interferon increases expression of class III complement genes C2 and factor B in human monocytes and in murine fibroblasts transfected with human C2 and factor B genes. J Biol Chem. 1985;260:1280–5.
104. Perlmutter DH, Goldberger G, Dinarello CA, Mizel SB, Colten HR. Regulation of class III major histocompatibility complex gene products by interleukin-1. Science. 1986;232:850–2.
105. Szekanecz Z, Haines GK, Lin TR, *et al.* Differential distribution of intercellular adhesion molecules (ICAM-1, ICAM-2, and ICAM-3) and the MS-1 antigen in normal and diseased human synovia. Their possible pathogenetic and clinical significance in rheumatoid arthritis. Arthritis Rheum. 1994;37:221–31.
106. Chin JE, Winterrowd GE, Krzesicki RF, Sanders ME. Role of cytokines in inflammatory synovitis. The coordinate regulation of intercellular adhesion molecule 1 and HLA class I and class II antigens in rheumatoid synovial fibroblasts. Arthritis Rheum. 1990;33:1776–86.
107. Morales-Ducret J, Wayner E, Elices MJ, *et al.* Alpha 4/beta 1 integrin (VLA-4) ligands in arthritis. Vascular cell adhesion molecule expression in synovium and on fibroblast-like synoviocytes. J Immunol. 1992;149:1424–31.
108. Elices MJ, Osborn L, Takada Y, *et al.* VCAM-1 on activated endothelium interacts with the leukocyte integrin VLA-4 at a site distinct from the VLA-4/fibronectin binding site. Cell. 1990;60:577–84.
109. Guan JL, Hynes RO. Lymphoid cells recognize an alternatively spliced segment of fibronectin via the integrin receptor $\alpha 4\beta 1$. Cell 1990;60:53–61.
110. van Dinther-Janssen AC, Pals ST, Scheper RJ, Meijer CJ. Role of the CS1 adhesion motif of fibronectin in T cell adhesion to synovial membrane and peripheral lymph node endothelium. Ann Rheum Dis. 1993;52:672–6.
111. Elices MJ, Tsai V, Strahl D, *et al.* Expression and functional significance of alternatively spliced CS1 fibronectin in rheumatoid arthritis microvasculature. J Clin Invest. 1994;93:405–16.
112. Muller-Ladner U, Elices M, Kriegsmann JB, *et al.* Expression of the alternatively spliced CS-1 fibronectin isoform and its counter-receptor VLA-4 in rheumatoid arthritis synovium. Submitted for publication.
113. Issekutz TB, Issekutz AC. T lymphocyte migration to arthritic joints and dermal inflammation in the rat: differing migration patterns and the involvement of VLA-4. Clin Immunol Immunopathol. 1991;61:436–47.
114. Wahl SM, Allen JB, Hines KL, *et al.* Synthetic fibronectin peptides suppress arthritis in rats by interrupting leukocyte adhesion and recruitment. J Clin Invest. 1994;94:655–62.
115. Laffon A, Garcia-Vicuna R, Humbria A, *et al.* Upregulated expression and function of VLA-4 fibronectin receptors on human activated T cells in rheumatoid arthritis. J Clin Invest. 1992;88:546–52.
116. Jorgensen C, Travaglio-Encinoza A, Bologna C. Human mucosal lymphocyte marker expression in synovial fluid lymphocytes of patients with rheumatoid arthritis. J Rheumatol. 1994;21:1602–7.
117. Corkill MM, Kirkham BW, Haskard DO, Barbatis C, Gibson T, Panayi GS. Gold treatment of rheumatoid arthritis decreases synovial expression of the endothelial leukocyte adhesion receptor ELAM-1. J Rheumatol. 1991;18:1453–60.
118. Roudier J, Rhodes G, Petersen J, Vaughan JH, Carson DA. The Epstein Barr virus glycoprotein gp110, a molecular link between HLA-DR4, HLA-DR1, and rheumatoid arthritis. Scand J Immunol. 1988;27:367–72.
119. Firestein GS, Yeo M, Zvaifler NJ. Apoptosis in rheumatoid arthritis synovium. J Clin Invest. 1995;96:1631–8.
120. Mountz JD, Wu J, Cheng J, Zhou T. Autoimmune disease. A problem of defective apoptosis. Arthritis Rheum. 1994;37:1415–20.
121. Nakajima T, Aono H, Hasunuma T, *et al.* Apoptosis and functional *fas* antigen in rheumatoid arthritis synoviocytes. Arthritis Rheum. 1995;38:485–91.

EVALUATION AND MANAGEMENT OF ACTIVE INFLAMMATORY DISEASE

14

Piet LCM van Riel, Math JH Wijnands & Leo BA van de Putte

- Internationally accepted core set variables are used for disease assessment.
- Treatment goals have shifted from the control of symptoms to the control of the disease process.
- Pharmacotherapy with NSAIDs and second line agents is the cornerstone of treatment of active inflammatory synovitis.
- Pharmacotherapy with second line agents is started early in the disease.
- A multidisciplinary approach is mandatory for those patients with inadequately controlled disease.

INTRODUCTION

The management of rheumatoid arthritis (RA) has changed substantially in the past 15 years as a result of new insights into the course of the disease and the proliferation of therapeutic agents for its treatment. Attitudes to therapeutic intervention have been influenced by several studies that demonstrate radiographic evidence of damage early in the disease and that severe RA may shorten survival. Increasing numbers of slow acting anti-rheumatic drugs (SAARDs) are becoming available, and some of these drugs have a fast mode of action. Exciting data are also emerging that show a potential role for biological agents; some of these, especially agents which block tumor necrosis factor-α (TNF-α), have been seen to suppress inflammation rapidly, although long-term results are not yet available (see Chapter 3.10). These developments have changed the management of RA: a strategy based on long-term treatment with nonsteroidal anti-inflammatory drugs (NSAIDs) and the addition of SAARDs only in a later phase of the disease (pyramid strategy) has evolved to a more aggressive approach with the early introduction of SAARDs in most patients with RA. Furthermore, in common with the current practice in oncologic medicine, combination therapy is becoming increasingly used. Recent studies have shown that some SAARDs combinations are superior to monotherapy. This new strategy stresses the need for accurate disease assessment in order to monitor treatment. In recent years a consensus has emerged as to useful process variables and outcome measures. Standardization of measurements has also improved. Another important step forward is a refined definition of treatment goals, progressing from the concept of control of symptom modification to the control of disease[1]. Finally, factors which determine the course of the disease are increasingly being recognized, although the practical use of these prognostic markers for the individual patient is still limited.

Despite impressive improvements in treatment in recent years, a considerable number of patients has disease which is inadequately controlled by pharmacotherapy. Against this background there is a clear need for a multidisciplinary approach to the management of patients with RA.

This chapter outlines disease assessment and the management of patients with an established active inflammatory RA. Problems related to the later phase of the disease, where irreversible destruction is a major problem, will be dealt with in Chapter 5.15.

ASSESSMENTS IN RHEUMATOID ARTHRITIS

Disease assessment in RA continues to be of prime importance both in daily practice and in clinical trials. Disease expression varies considerably between patients as well as within the same individual. This has led to the use of an increasing number of variables to measure different aspects of the disease process, including joint counts, laboratory measurements, measures of pain and physical disability and health status measures. This 'divergence' in measurement is necessary to cover the whole spectrum of the disease process. However, there is also a need for 'convergence' in the material used to achieve uniformity among assessors for comparison and simplicity. Recent efforts have been aimed at reaching a consensus on a minimum set of disease activity variables which should be measured in clinical trials. Indices have also been developed which combine several of the disease activity variables into a single score. The different measurements can be classified as either process variables, which indicate what happens along the way, or as outcome variables, defined as the end result of the disease process[2]. Process variables measure a disease state at a certain point in time and therefore reflect actual disease activity. However, to evaluate the efficacy of treatment, disease activity variables need to be expressed over a timespan. This can be done by accumulating disease activity measurements or by calculating a change in disease activity over time. Response criteria have been developed for this purpose[3,4]. Finally, the ultimate goal of the treatment of RA is to achieve 'remission', defined as the absence of disease symptoms during a certain period.

Reproducibility and validity are of the utmost importance in developing or choosing variables or indices to measure disease activity. Reproducibility (precision) means that repeated measurements under the same circumstances give the same results. Validity means that a measure really measures what it is supposed to:

- it represents the true state (criterion validity),
- it fits with the theory about the process (construct validity),
- the measure is reasonable (face validity),
- it includes all aspects of the feature to be measured (content validity) and
- it can detect the smallest important difference between groups or within a group over time (discriminant validity or sensitivity to change)[5].

In the following section we discuss prognostic markers, core sets of measures, indices, response definitions and remission criteria.

PROGNOSTIC MARKERS

With the increasing potential for early intervention, for longer-term treatment and with aggressive drugs, it would be very useful to be able to predict the disease course in order to assess the risk/benefit ratio of pharmacotherapy. Prognostic factors for progressive joint damage and disability have been extensively reviewed[6]. Probably most useful are those factors that are independent of disease activity, such as the presence of rheumatoid factor (RF) and the so-called shared epitope of HLA-DR[7]. The early presence of bony erosions is another important prognostic marker[8]. In addition, clinical indicators, e.g. many affected joints, the presence of extra-articular features and a considerable degree of physical disability at onset, are associated with a poor prognosis, as are sociodemographic markers such as older age at onset and a lower level of formal education. It should be noted the prognostic markers

CORE SETS OF VARIABLES TO ASSESS DISEASE ACTIVITY IN RA

Disease activity measure	Core sets		
	EULAR	OMERACT	ACR
Tender joint count	✓(28)*	?	✓(68)*
Swollen joint count	✓(28)*	?	✓(66)*
Pain on visual analog scale	✓	✓	✓
Patient's global on disease activity	✓	✓	✓
Assessor's global on disease activity		✓	✓
Physical function	✓	✓	✓
Radiographic analysis	✓	✓	✓
Acute-phase reactant	✓	✓	✓

* Numbers in brackets indicate the number of joints assessed.
✓ = included.

Fig. 14.1 Core sets of variables to assess disease activity in RA. With permission from van Riel PLCM, van de Putte LBA. Clinical assessment and clinical trials in rheumatoid arthritis. Curr Opin Rheumatol. 1994:6;132–9.

have been identified in cohort studies and are currently of limited use in individual patients in clinical practice (see also Practical Problem 5.16, Assessing the activity and outcome of RA).

CORE SETS

Different approaches by different groups have been undertaken to identify core sets of valid variables to assess disease activity in patients with RA. In the spring of 1992 the Outcome Measures in Rheumatoid Arthritis Clinical Trials (OMERACT) conference was held to select a core set of measurements to be included in clinical trials, to determine clinically relevant improvement of the disease activity variables and to explore whether indices of disease activity are applicable in clinical trials[9]. Eight variables were chosen for inclusion in the preliminary core set (see Fig. 14.1). A core set of variables for assessing disease activity in RA was selected by statistical analysis and published on behalf of the European League Against Rheumatism (EULAR)[10]. In addition to five process variables [number of tender joints, number of swollen joints, pain score on a visual analog scale, patient global score on a visual analog scale and erythrocyte sedimentation rate (ESR)] two outcome variables – functional capacity and a radiographic assessment of the joints of the hands and feet – were selected. In June 1993 the American College of Rheumatology (ACR) also adopted a modified core set of variables of response to therapy[11] (Fig. 14.1).

It remains a matter of dispute whether the physician's assessment of disease activity should be included in the core sets as it seems to depend on the results of the other core set variables. During the fifth International League of Associations for Rheumatology/ World Health Organization (ILAR/WHO) task force meeting on rheumatic diseases in Geneva in 1993, it was decided, pending a further validation procedure, to include the assessor global score into the core set of variables.

Joint counts

The most important clinical sign of RA is joint inflammation which results in swelling, tenderness, decreased range of motion and sometimes deformity.

Many different systems of counting joints are available to measure one or more of these signs. They vary according to the number of joints, whether the joints are assessed separately or collectively, graded for severity or weighted for size. In the ACR core set, for example, the initial recommendation was to assess the 68 joint count, which includes the distal interphalangeal (DIP) joints of the hands and the proximal interphalangeal (PIP) joints of the feet. As the DIP joints of the hand are often affected by osteoarthritic changes as well, this may disturb or influence the validity of the joint score. In a prospective longitudinal study of patients with early RA to evaluate more than 60 different possible joint scores[13], no major differences were found except for reduced validity of weighted joint scores. As the simplicity of an assessment has been found to improve its reliability, the 28 joint score has been recommended for assessing both tenderness and swelling of the joints [10 PIP joints, 10 metacarpophalangeal (MCP) joints, 2 wrists, 2 elbows, 2 shoulders and 2 knees]. Both the ACR Committee on Outcome Measures in Rheumatoid Arthritis Clinical Trials[12] and the EULAR Standing Committee on International Clinical Studies Including Therapeutic Trials[13] have adapted the use of reduced joint counts for clinical trials. The joints not included in reduced joint counts, however, may still be of clinical importance in the management of individual patients[12].

In their recent review Thompson and Kirwan concluded that tenderness and swelling provide different information[14]. Joint tenderness is more sensitive to change and correlates with pain, whereas swollen joint counts predict joint damage. They also concluded that grading for severity improves sensitivity and weighting for joint size improves correlation with the acute phase response, but that these latter factors increase interobserver variation[14].

Acute phase reactants

The most frequently used laboratory measures for disease activity are the ESR and C-reactive protein (CRP). These variables correlate with other measures of disease activity[15], and have been found to be sensitive to change in trials comparing second line agents (SLA)[16–18]. There is some evidence to show that these measures predict radiographic progression[15,19]. Both ESR and CRP are nonspecific measures of inflammation. However, CRP correlates more closely with the inflammatory process and is less susceptible to disturbing factors such as renal function, food intake and immunoglobulin levels[20]. In some centers plasma viscosity, as another indirect indicator of the acute phase reaction, is being used in place of ESR[17].

Pain

The major problem for patients with active RA is pain. Several measurement techniques have been developed to assess pain levels, including: numerical rating scales, verbal rating scales, visual analog scales (VAS), questionnaires[21,22] and behavioral observation methods[23]. In choosing a particular instrument, ease of use, reliability and sensitivity should be considered. The VAS, one of the most frequently used instruments, has been shown to be sensitive to change[16,24], but was more difficult for elderly and illiterate patients to complete[25]. Bosi Ferraz *et al.* concluded that a numerical rating scale (10 possible scores) was more reliable than a VAS or a verbal rating scale (5 possible scores) for both literate and illiterate patients[25]. The Arthritis Impact Measurement Scales (AIMS) pain questions were also sensitive to change in pain levels[16,24]. The ACR recommends the use of a 10cm horizontal VAS with 'no pain' at one end and 'worst possible pain' at the other, without intermediate categories, or the Likert scale (1 = asymptomatic, 2 = mild, 3 = moderate, 4 = severe, 5 = very severe), to assess current pain in clinical trials[3].

Global disease activity

Patients' assessments of global disease activity are generally measured on a VAS using the AIMS question: 'Considering all the ways your arthritis affects you, mark "X" on the scale for how well you are doing', even though it has not been subjected to any validation studies. According to the ACR, the Likert scale response is also an acceptable instrument for patients' global assessment. The same instruments are considered valid for physicians' (or an assessor's) global assessments of disease activity[3]. Some of the participants at the OMERACT consensus meeting on assessment end points felt that the physician's assessment should be included in the core set, whereas others felt that it was a superfluous instrument which should only be used as an overall criterion against which to compare others[26].

Physical/functional disability

The available tools to assess disability can be classified as:

- measures based on clinical judgment,
- measures based on observed patient performance and
- self-reported assessments[27].

Clinical judgment regarding function is subject to considerable inter-observer variation, and observation of performances is very time-consuming. Self-reporting questionnaires are the most popular instrument, although there may be discrepancies between actual performance and reported performance of patients. Both generic and disease-specific health status questionnaires have been developed[22,28–33]. These are often multidimensional, assessing physical as well as psychological and social disability. The two most frequently used self-reported questionnaires in arthritis patients, AIMS and the Health Assessment Questionnaire (HAQ), are sensitive to clinical changes[2,34–36]. Buchbinder *et al.* compared three quality-of-life measures: a modified McMaster–Toronto Arthritis Patient Preference Disability Questionnaire (MAC–TAR), HAQ and AIMS[24]. The AIMS physical function score appeared to be the least sensitive to a treatment effect. The MAC–TAR questionnaire could detect small clinically important changes in function[32]. Liang *et al.* compared efficiency and sensitivity of five health status instruments [HAQ, AIMS, Functional Status Index (FSI), Index of Well Being (IWB), Sickness Impact Profile (SIP)] and concluded that no single instrument consistently outperformed the others[37]. The ACR recommends that: 'any patient self-assessment instrument which has been validated, has reliability, has been proven in RA trials to be sensitive to change, and which measures physical function in RA patients is acceptable. Instruments which have been demonstrated to be sensitive in RA trials include the AIMS, the HAQ, the Quality (or Index) of Well Being, the McMaster Health Index Questionnaire (MHIQ), and the MAC–TAR[3]. Therefore, to improve uniformity among trials one of these instruments should be chosen as the core set measure for physical function.

Imaging modalities

In the evaluation of SAARDs, the assessment of radiographic damage has always been a gold standard. Recently a new classification scheme for antirheumatic drugs has been proposed which further stresses the importance of the radiographic assessment. A drug which has been shown to delay or stop radiographic progression, as well as preserve functional capacity, may be called a disease-controlling antirheumatic treatment (DCART). An agent which relieves symptoms but does not halt the progression of disease is termed a symptom-modifying antirheumatic drug (SMARD)[1]. The two most frequently used validated radiographic scoring methods were developed by Sharp *et al.*and Larsen[38,39]. Both methods have been modified several times[40,41]. Pincus *et al.* compared the Steinbrocker radiographic stage, modified Sharp method and the Larsen method and concluded that they correlate with each other and show similar correlations with other clinical measures[42]. One drawback to using the Sharp or Larsen methods is the so-called 'ceiling effect': when the maximum score in a joint is reached, further damage cannot be quantified. According to Sharp *et al.* better methods are needed which use direct measurements of damage in standard units (mm^2)[38]. Newer imaging techniques, e.g. magnetic resonance imaging (MRI) and dual X-ray absorptiometry (DXA), are promising tools both for clinical evaluation and to test new therapies[43–45].

INDICES OF DISEASE ACTIVITY

Indices of disease activity combine multiple disease activity measures into a single measure. Advantages of an index are:

- unambiguous interpretation of disease activity,
- comparability of trial results and
- more power in clinical trials.

Several indices have been developed using statistical, pseudostatistical or heuristic approaches. The disadvantages of an index are that it cannot easily be reconverted to its components and that the calculations involved are fairly complex. The indices differ in terms of what they measure, i.e. current disease activity or change, and of their scales, e.g. continuous or ordinal (Fig. 14.2)[46].

INDICES OF DISEASE ACTIVITY		
	Continuous scale	Ordinal scale (no. of classes)
Current disease activity	Lansbury systemic index Disease activity score	Mallya/Mace index (4) Stoke index (4) ARA remission (2)
Improvement criteria		
Change in disease activity	Pooled index	Paulus improvement (2) ACR improvement (2)
Combination of change and current disease activity	—	Simple index (6) EULAR response (3)
ARA = American Rheumatism Association; EULAR = European League Against Rheumatism; ACR = American College of Rheumatology		

Fig. 14.2 Indices of disease activity. Reproduced with permission from[46] by courtesy of Marcel Dekker, Inc.

Current disease activity

When following the course of the disease or assessing disease activity at a certain moment in time a measure should be chosen which assesses current disease activity. The advantage of a continuous scale is that no information is lost, thus increasing sensitivity. The Lansbury systemic index is the oldest measure[46], although it has not been thoroughly validated. The Disease Activity Score (DAS)[47,48], a statistically derived index combining tender joints, swollen joints, ESR and general health, has been validated in several studies[15,48,49]. The Mallya/Mace index and its modifications[50–52] is a valid[15,53] ordinal measure of current disease activity. The Stoke index[53] requires further validation. The American Rheumatism Association (ARA) remission criteria are a special kind of disease activity measure which groups patients in only two categories: remission or no remission[54] (discussed below).

Improvement criteria

For treatment evaluation a time component should be included in the measure, i.e. change in disease activity within a certain period. Response to treatment can be defined using, for example, the pooled index developed by Smythe *et al.*[55] for groups, or, for individual patients, the Paulus improvement criteria[56], the preliminary ACR improvement criteria[3], the EULAR response criteria[4], and a simple index proposed by Scott[57] to assess disease activity. Individual response criteria quantify the number of patients who respond and the degree of improvement, which is an important addition to mean group values as endpoint variables in clinical trials.

Improvement criteria based on change in disease activity

The pooled index developed by Smythe *et al.* is a linear sum of the weighted mean changes in single measures[55]. The change in a variable is divided by the standard deviation of the difference of that variable. The transformed changes of all variables are summated. Drawbacks to this method are:

- no predefined single variables are included,
- no weights are assigned to the relative contribution of single variables and
- it can only be used to compare groups because the group standard deviation of the difference has to be calculated.

Ordinal measures for treatment evaluation are the Paulus improvement criteria[56], the preliminary ACR improvement criteria[3], the EULAR response criteria[4] and a simple index to assess disease activity proposed by Scott *et al.*[57]. These measures are developed to measure individual treatment response. Paulus *et al.*[56] arbitrarily selected a group of variables (duration of morning stiffness, ESR, joint tenderness score,

RESPONSE CRITERIA BASED ON CHANGE IN DISEASE ACTIVITY

Improvement in:	Paulus (4 out of 6)	ACR (5 out of 7 including first 2)
Joint tenderness	≥20%	≥20%
Joint swelling	≥20%	≥20%
ESR	≥20%	≥20%
Physician global disease activity	≥40%	≥20%
Patient global disease activity	≥40 %	≥20%
Morning stiffness	≥20%	
Pain		≥20%
Disability		≥20%

ACR = American College of Rheumatology

Fig. 14.3 Response criteria based on change in disease activity. Reproduced with permission from[46] by courtesy of Marcel Dekker Inc.

joint swelling score, physician global disease activity and patient global disease activity assessments) and studied how many variables had to improve and to what extent to discriminate between active drug and placebo. The preliminary ACR improvement criteria are a modification of the Paulus criteria (see Fig. 14.3). They derive from a study which investigated ease of use, credibility and discriminant validity (versus placebo) of improvement criteria[3].

Improvement criteria based on change and current disease activity

The simple index[57] and the EULAR response criteria[4] are different because they include not only change in disease activity but also current disease activity. The simple index proposed by Scott *et al.* shares some features with the ARA criteria for remission in RA[54]. It comprises six variables – four variables reflecting current disease activity (morning stiffness ≤15min, ≤3 tender joints, ≤3 swollen joints, ESR ≤30mm/h) and two variables reflecting change from baseline (≥50% pain reduction, ≥40 functional improvement). One point is awarded for every criterion that is met after 6 months' therapy. The total score ranges from 0 to 6, with patients spread fairly evenly between each of the seven classes of response. Before this simple index can be recommended further validation is required. The EULAR response criteria are based upon an index of disease activity (DAS). To be classified as responders patients should have a significant change in DAS and low current disease activity. Three categories are defined: good, moderate and nonresponders (Fig. 14.4).

So far the EULAR response criteria have been compared with the ACR and the WHO/ILAR response criteria in one double-blind comparative study of two SAARDs and showed better construct and discriminant validity[4]. The performance of these criteria needs further study in clinical trials before a uniform measure can be selected to define individual treatment response.

Remission criteria

Complete remission of RA means the disappearance of disease activity either spontaneously or with antirheumatic therapy, without subsequent relapse. Although it occurs infrequently, remission is the ultimate goal of therapy and should therefore be defined. Any usable criterion should include a time component as follow-up for an indefinite period is unrealistic in most clinical settings. The ARA developed preliminary criteria for clinical remission in RA[54] (Fig. 14.5) based on optimum discrimination between patients with and without remission as assessed by their rheumatologists.

A duration of longer than 2 months was chosen arbitrarily because 90% of patients fulfilled this criterion. There are also several features of the definition that limit its clinical usefulness. No specifications are given as to which measurement technique should be used for the different clinical variables; two out of the six variables used are not included in the core set data and the outcome is dichotomous, which implies that a small change in disease activity may have a disproportionate impact on the allocated class. An alternative approach would be to define remission with a continuous variable of disease activity such as DAS and add the time during which the patient was at a certain level or simply calculate cumulative disease activity over a certain time period. A DAS was calculated for patients who were classified according to the ARA criteria as either in remission or not. At an arbitrarily chosen DAS cutoff value of 1.6, the percentage of misclassification for both groups was 10%[58]. The advantage of this method is that the cutoff value for remission can be adjusted according to new data from validation procedures.

THE MULTIDISCIPLINARY APPROACH

Traditionally the multidisciplinary treatment of the patient with RA has been provided during hospitalization. Especially before antirheumatic agents were available – up to 15 years ago – other nonpharmacologic interventions such as bedrest, assistive devices and physical therapy were very important aspects of therapy. This approach is less relevant today. The ideal situation is to suppress the inflammatory process completely by pharmacotherapeutic means. However, despite the improvements in the pharmacologic treatment of RA in recent decades, this goal is seldom achieved. In most cases the disease still has significant physical, psychologic and socioeconomic consequences for the patient. All in all the increased complexity of current pharmacotherapy, the rise in the number of surgical interventions, the increased awareness of patients and the reduced opportunities for hospitalization make the multidisciplinary approach much more necessary now than previously. In contrast with earlier practice multidisciplinary treatment should not be limited to inpatients as outpatients can benefit as well. It is important for the rheumatologist to identify patients who would benefit from a multidisciplinary approach: the few who are fortunate enough to achieve a complete remission early in the disease course may not require it.

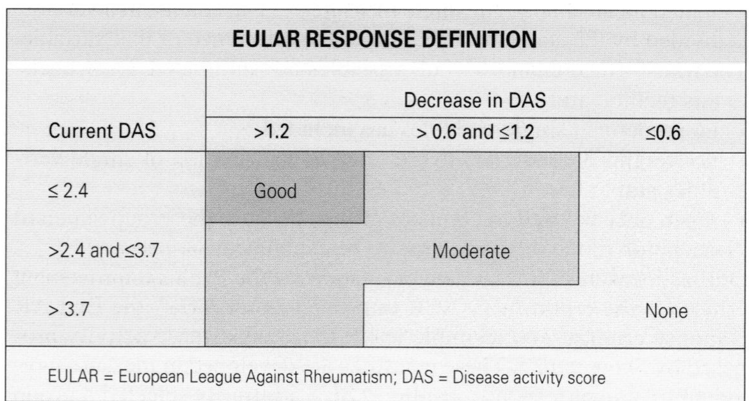

EULAR RESPONSE DEFINITION

Current DAS	Decrease in DAS >1.2	> 0.6 and ≤1.2	≤0.6
≤ 2.4	Good	Moderate	None
>2.4 and ≤3.7	Moderate	Moderate	None
> 3.7	Moderate	None	None

EULAR = European League Against Rheumatism; DAS = Disease activity score

Fig. 14.4 EULAR response definition. Reproduced with permission from[46] by courtesy of Marcel Dekker Inc.

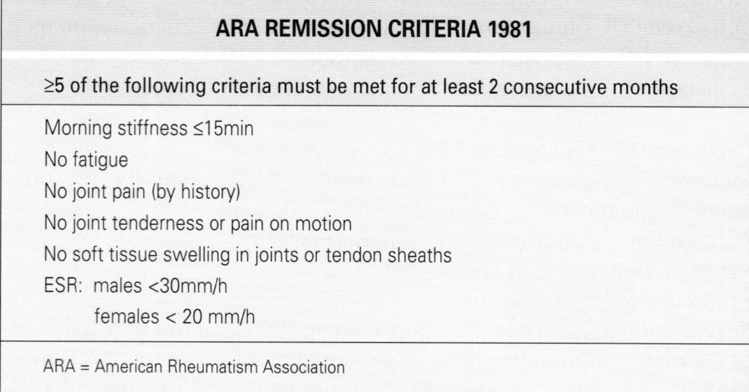

ARA REMISSION CRITERIA 1981

≥5 of the following criteria must be met for at least 2 consecutive months

- Morning stiffness ≤15min
- No fatigue
- No joint pain (by history)
- No joint tenderness or pain on motion
- No soft tissue swelling in joints or tendon sheaths
- ESR: males <30mm/h
  females < 20 mm/h

ARA = American Rheumatism Association

Fig. 14.5 ARA remission criteria 1981. Reproduced with permission from[46] by courtesy of Marcel Dekker Inc.

The multiple and complex problems of RA may require a multidisciplinary team including a rheumatologist, specialist nurse, social worker, occupational therapist, physical therapist and orthopedic surgeon (Fig. 14.6). Although the benefits of and the need for a multidisciplinary approach in the treatment of the RA patient are not disputed, it is only recently that a controlled study has shown a direct and long-lasting (2 years) effect for a short period (11 days) of inpatient multidisciplinary care for patients with active disease[59]. As inpatient resources are limited, further studies are needed to investigate whether the same results can be achieved on an outpatient basis. These issues are discussed further in Chapter 5.15.

COORDINATING PERSON

In most cases the rheumatologist coordinates contributions made by the different disciplines. There is a need to communicate in the language of the patient and to discuss aspects of the disease, prognosis and treatments in the broadest sense. Involvement of other members of the team depends on the stage of the disease and the needs of the patient. In order to appropriately refer the patient to other team members, the rheumatologist should become familiar with the principles of the different modalities. Team members should meet at regular intervals to discuss the various problems and therapeutic plan for individual patients.

PATIENT EDUCATION AND VOCATIONAL COUNSELING

Soon after receiving a diagnosis of RA, the patient will seek information about the disease, its course, the different treatment modalities and their (side) effects, the consequences of the disease and how to cope with it. This information is provided by the rheumatologist and other members of the team as part of the routine care. However, these problems are often complex. To address them adequately, several educational programs have been developed to enhance the patients' psychological well-being and understanding and to improve outcome of the various interventions by facilitating voluntary changes in behaviour. As several studies have shown, these programs do have a small effect on, for instance, pain, depressive symptoms and the utilization of health-care services, and are thus an important additional modality in the management of patients with RA[60].

Patients are often limited in their choice of work; therefore counseling about employment, for instance by a social worker or vocational counselor, is an important aspect of care which should be included in the multidisciplinary approach.

OCCUPATIONAL THERAPY

Overuse of joints can increase inflammation and thus pain and loss of function; it may also contribute to further joint destruction. Therefore patients are advised how to use their joints with the minimum amount of stress when performing daily activities.

It is important to integrate such advice with the patient's lifestyle and to teach the patient to monitor his or her activities, and stop when discomfort occurs. Splints can be used to reduce inflammation in the acute phase of the disease. Splinting of an actively inflamed wrist joint, for instance, supports the joint, protects it from excessive and painful motion and consequently makes functional activities possible that would otherwise not be. In addition, splints are also used to correct or prevent joint deformity. There are, however, conflicting views especially about the use of splints for the latter indication. This underlines the need for a good working relationship between the rheumatologist, orthopedic surgeon and occupational therapist before these devices are recommended for patient use (see also Practical Problem 5.16, Preventing and treating contractures: joint protection and splinting).

MEMBERS OF THE MULTIDISCIPLINARY TEAM
Rheumatologist
Nurse
Occupational therapist
Physical therapist
Social worker
Psychologist/Psychiatrist
Neurologist
Orthopedic surgeon
General physician
Podiatrist

Fig. 14.6 Members of the multidisciplinary team.

PHYSICAL THERAPY

A variety of techniques can be used to help decrease inflammation and pain, including the application of heat or cold, transcutaneous nerve stimulation (TENS) and iontophoresis (see Chapter 3.11). Physical therapy may also help maintain range of motion as well as prevent muscle atrophy by exercise. Patients may benefit from hydrotherapy which enables muscle strength to be increased without joint overuse.

The joints of the feet are almost always involved in the disease process. Often the patient with RA first experience problems in the feet. Small alterations to shoes can reduce the stress, for instance, on the metatarsophalangeal (MTP) joints, thus reducing the pain and increasing walking distance. In more severe cases these alterations are not sufficient for symptom relief and surgical procedure and/or orthopedic footwear are needed.

PHARMACOTHERAPY OF RHEUMATOID ARTHRITIS

The drugs used in the treatment of RA are conventionally divided into first- and second-line drugs. First-line drugs include NSAIDs, which have a rapid suppressive effect on signs of inflammation, including pain and stiffness. Unfortunately they do not influence the progression of radiographic joint damage. In contrast, SAARDss are assumed to influence the disease process by decreasing disease activity, slowing down the progression of joint damage and preserving functional capacity. Drugs used in the pharmacotherapy of rheumatoid arthritis may be classified according to their therapeutic effects [e.g. disease modifying antirheumatic drugs (DMARDs), remission-inducing drugs (RIDs)], their onset or duration of action (SAARDs), or their presumed mode of action (cytotoxic, immunosuppressive or antiproliferative drugs). A new classification of antirheumatic agents divides drugs according to their effects into symptom modifying antirheumatic drugs (SM-ARDs) and disease controlling antirheumatic therapies (DC-ARTs)[1], depending on their effect on disease symptoms and signs, progression of radiographic joint damage and functional outcome. Glucocorticosteroids are usually considered as a separate category and still are indispensable in the treatment of at least some patients with RA.

NSAIDs

Nonsteroidal anti-inflammatory drugs (NSAIDs) are frequently used for the symptomatic treatment of RA and many other rheumatic diseases (see Chapter 3.5). The traditional 'pyramid' treatment approach, starting with NSAIDs for a prolonged period followed by the least toxic (i.e. least effective) SAARDs and progressing to more effective (toxic) agents, has now been abandoned. However, drug treatment early in RA always commences with NSAIDs. As responses vary substantially among individuals, it is sometimes necessary to try several different NSAIDs. In contrast to earlier practice, NSAIDs should be given in combination with one of the SAARDss after a few weeks' treatment in cases of persistent disease activity. Corticosteroids, administered either intra-articular, or systemically (as chronic low-dose or pulse high-dose) can be added or used to 'bridge' over a period of high disease activity after starting an SAARDs (Fig. 14.7).

SECOND-LINE AGENTS

It has been generally recognized that SAARDss have effects on process and outcome variables, at least in short-term studies. However, their long-term efficacy has been disputed by a number of rheumatologists[61,62]. Although shortcomings in the design of previous studies may have contributed to this negative view, this is probably not the only or even the main reason for the controversy.

It should be remembered that few SAARDs were available before 1980, and this influenced the timing of treatment. At the time it was customary in many institutions to treat patients with early active RA with NSAIDs for at least for 6–12 months before adding a SAARDs. In addition, in cases of marginal efficacy, treatment with a SAARDs was continued as long as possible for want of anything better. In general, the underlying principle was 'go low, go slow'. Moreover, without a sufficient number of SAARDs available, it was practically impossible to suppress disease activity effectively over longer time periods. As every study evaluating the long-term efficacy of SAARDs began at this time, it is not surprising that conclusions about their long-term efficacy were negative. However, in the past decade the armamentarium of SAARDs has increased considerably (Fig.14.8), making it possible to treat patients for longer periods. Some of these agents, such as sulfasalazine and methotrexate, have a faster mode of action and. moreover, a greater proportion of patients continue to benefit for longer periods than with other drugs.

Importance of early treatment

There is an increasing tendency to initiate SAARDs therapy in patients with RA earlier in the disease course. A number of arguments have led to this change in strategy. First, it has been shown that a considerable degree of radiographically detectable joint damage in RA occurs in the first years of the disease[63]. Second, recent studies have indicated that, especially in the early phase of the disease, radiographically detectable articular damage (which usually underrepresents actual damage in the joint), can be favorably influenced by early treatment with SAARDs[64]. Another important argument for early treatment comes from studies by Pincus and Callahan[65], who demonstrated that RA is not a benign disease and that, apart from morbidity, there is considerable mortality associated with the disease. The number of swollen joints was one of the important risk factors for mortality. It is therefore possible that early adequate treatment of joint inflammation may ultimately improve patient survival. Probably the most important advantage of both early treatment and the availability of an extending range of SAARDs is that 'early and aggressive' therapy increases the total number of years during which patients receive adequate treatment and therefore enjoy a better quality of life.

A PHARMACOLOGIC APPROACH TO ACTIVE INFLAMMATORY RA
Active inflammatory RA
NSAIDs
Often more than one has to be tried before the right NSAID is found for the individual patient
If disease activity is insufficiently suppressed consider adding SLA
SLA
First choice – fast mode of action, e.g. sulfasalazine or methotrexate
In case of adverse reactions or inefficacy, second choice of SLA (in alphabetical order) depends on disease severity
Antimalarial
Azathioprine
Gold (oral, intramuscular)
D-Penicillamine
If response is inadequate or absent, try combining SLAs instead of substitution.
Low-dose oral corticosteroids can be combined with a NSAID and SLA
Treatment of flares or bridge therapy
Intramuscular methylprednisolone injections (120mg every month) or bolus infusions (500–1000mg)
Acute inflammation of a single joint
Intra-articular non-absorbable corticosteroid injections
If response is inadequate – synoviorthesis, arthroscopic or surgical synovectomy
SLA = Second-line agent

Fig. 14.7 A pharmacologic approach to active inflammatory RA.

Importance of fast mode of action

The traditional SAARDs, including hydroxychloroquine, parenteral gold and D-penicillamine, usually become effective 3–6 months after initiation of therapy. In contrast the 'new' drugs, sulfasalazine and methotrexate, may show clinical efficacy after 3–6 weeks. Apart from patient's and doctor's satisfaction, this faster mode of action has the great advantage of more precise titration of pharmacotherapy. However, discontinuation of fast-acting SAARDs may rapidly provoke a flare. This may also have an unexpected beneficial effect, motivating the patient to resume and continue treatment.

Treatment strategy

Treatment strategies are increasingly based on the assumption that early, fast and effective pharmacotherapy is important for controlling disease. This means that, soon after the diagnosis of RA is established, a SAARDs is prescribed. Sometimes, depending in part on the severity of the disease, the interval between initiation of therapy with a particular SAARDs and onset of clinical effect is 'bridged' by low-dose corticosteroids. The rank order in which SAARDs should be prescribed is still a matter for debate. In a meta-analysis of trials of SAARDs, Felson *et al.*[65] classified drugs currently available according to their efficacy/toxicity ratios. In this study methotrexate and sulfazalazine were shown to have the most favorable ratios. Since these are also the fastest SAARDs and have the best drug survival curve[67], they are increasingly chosen as initial treatment. In the US methotrexate is usually the drug of first choice whereas in Europe sulfasalazine is frequently preferred. It should be noted that, at present, it is impossible to predict which of the SAARDs will be effective or toxic in an individual patient.

Effects on disease activity

After weeks or months of SAARDs treatment, a reduction in the number of painful and swollen joints can be observed. Usually in parallel, pain, stiffness and fatigue diminish. So far there have been no clearcut effects of SAARDs on extra-articular manifestations. In terms of laboratory variables, the effects of treatment with SAARDs include suppression of the acute phase response, reflected, for example, by a decrease in ESR or CRP, improvement in hemoglobin and a (slow) decrease of RF titer. An exception seems to be azathioprine – and probably cyclosporin – which can influence clinical disease activity without affecting variables such as ESR.

Effects on progression of radiographic damage

Whether or not SAARDs actually slow down progression of radiographic evidence of damage in the long term is still a matter for debate. In 1983 Iannuzzi *et al.*[61] reviewed 17 controlled studies, including radiographic assessment of both 'second-line treated' and control groups. They concluded that, of the drugs used at the time, only parenteral gold and cyclophosphamide showed some evidence of being effective in slowing down progression of joint destruction as determined by radiography. Since then many related studies have been published. Probably due to differences in study design, patient selection (e.g. with regard to disease duration, pre-existing radiographic damage, earlier second-line treatment, etc.), duration of treatment and differences in methods of assessment of radiographic abnormalities, the results of these studies are equivocal. However, the data seem to

SECOND-LINE AGENTS FOR RA
Azathioprine
Cyclophosphamide
Hydroxycholoroquine
Methotrexate
Oral gold (auranofin)
Parenteral gold (aurothioglucose or sodium aurothiomalate)
D-Penicillamine
Sulfasalazine
Cyclosporine

Fig. 14.8 Second-line agents for RA. With permission from van de Putte & van Riel[62].

indicate that the long-term clinical response is usually associated with slowing of the progression of radiographic joint damage, confirming the relationship between persisting joint inflammation and joint destruction. However, this relationship is certainly not a simple one and is still open to debate. No direct significant correlation between changes in inflammatory indices and radiographic progression was reported by Scott *et al.*[68,69] and Pullar *et al.*[70], although subgroups of patients in both studies who had persistently low ESR had a related reduction in progression of radiographic damage in the 2nd, 6th and 12th months of treatment. More recently several studies have been published which show an association of clinical (synovial) swelling and laboratory parameters (ESR, CRP) with radiographic progression[71,72]. Prolonged control of the inflammatory process seems to be of particular importance in producing radiographic evidence of slowed progression of damage.

Certain SAARDs, such as sulfasalazine and methotrexate, have been shown to delay radiographically detectable progression of joint destruction[64,73]. The beneficial effect of sulfasalazine can be sustained for at least a period of 12–36 months[74].

Toxicity and monitoring

Unfortunately SAARDs frequently provoke adverse drug reactions, i.e. unintended events caused by drugs in therapeutic doses. These can be divided into two groups: the more or less predictable 'toxic' reactions and the unpredictable 'idiosyncratic' ones. The former are often dose-dependent and are related to the known intrinsic action of the drug. The latter are mostly immune-mediated and unrelated to the dose or pharmacologic action of the SAARDs, and may be related to the patient's (immunologic, genetic) susceptibility.

Prevention of adverse events is of great importance. Before starting SAARDs treatment, contraindications such as pre-existing diseases, renal or hepatic impairment, drug interaction, pregnancy or known intolerance to the medication should be excluded, as far as possible. The next preventive measure is to detect a drug reaction as early as possible, and thus probably in a less severe phase. Since adverse events due to SAARDs usually (but certainly not always) occur during the first few months of treatment, monitoring should be carried out most intensively and frequently in this initial treatment phase. For some SAARDs a test dose or gradual increase in dosage has been advocated. Neither serum nor urine drug concentrations are routinely used to monitor SAARDs treatment. Drug concentrations can be measured to estimate compliance or check for gross overdosage. The authors' approach to baseline assessment and monitoring of SAARDs treatment is presented in Figure 14.9[75].

The relationship between (cumulative) dose and the occurrence of adverse events in SAARDs use is indicated in Figure 14.10[81]. It should be noted that almost all the side effects are reversible when dosage is reduced or treatment discontinued. Exceptions are (hydroxy)chloroquine-induced retinopathy, methotrexate-induced liver cirrhosis and rare blood dyscrasia. Further information on side effects and their management is found in Chapter 3.8 and in a recent review[75].

Combination therapy

Despite the demonstrated beneficial effects of SAARDs, treatment with a single SAARDs often fails to induce true disease remission. Since combining two or more drugs has been shown to be effective in areas such as transplantation and oncology, many attempts have been made to treat RA with combinations of SAARDs. Rationales for this approach have included the following: combining SAARDs that may influence different pathophysiologic mechanisms operative in RA; combining SAARDs of different toxicities to minimize risks; combining lower doses to reduce toxicity; or combining higher doses of toxic drugs in combination to eradicate RA[76].

Unfortunately, until recently the results of these studies have been disappointing[77]. This may be due, in part, to the many problems inherent in designing such studies. A few recently published studies indicate that combining SAARDs may in fact be successful. Tugwell *et al.*[78] conducted a 6-month randomized, double-blind trial to compare combination therapy with cyclosporin and methotrexate with methotrexate and placebo in 148 patients with RA. The subjects had residual inflammation and disability despite partial but substantial response to prior methotrexate treatment, and the primary outcome was the change in the number of tender joints. The authors found that patients with severe RA and only partial response to methotrexate had clinically significant improvement after combining methotrexate with cyclosporin. Interestingly, side effects did not increase substantially. Another study by O'Dell *et al.*[79] investigated combination therapy with methotrexate, sulfasalazine and hydroxychloroquine and compared it with either methotrexate alone or with a combination of sulfasalazine and hydroxychloroquine. This 2-year trial indicated that patients receiving the triple therapy regimen showed better results than those receiving either methotrexate alone or sulfasalazine and hydroxychloroquine. Although additional long-term studies are needed for further confirmation, it appears that some combinations have at least an additive effect compared with monotherapy.

CORTICOSTEROIDS

Enthusiasm for the use of corticosteroids in rheumatology has waxed and waned. Despite this, they are often used either systemically or locally in everyday rheumatologic practice. A recent study has suggested that systemic low-dose corticosteroids may have a beneficial effect on radiographically detectable progression of joint damage[80]. The following offers a brief review of the systemic and local use of corticosteroids.

Systemic use

In the 1940s Hench studied the beneficial effect of pregnancy on disease activity in patients with RA. This amelioration was attributed to hormones, such as adrenocorticotropic hormone (ACTH) and hydrocortisone, produced in pregnancy. In 1949 enough synthetic cortisone became available to treat RA patients[81]. Initially there was a great enthusiasm for this treatment due to the significant and rapid relief of symptoms, and Kendall and Hench were awarded a Nobel prize for their work. However, recognition of the considerable side effects of corticosteroids, especially at higher doses, rapidly tempered the initial enthusiasm and physicians became more reluctant to prescribe these drugs. Interest in systemic corticosteroids was renewed when treatment with lower doses was proposed as so-called 'bridge therapy'[82], which aims to relieve symptoms of RA during the period between initiation of SAARDs and onset of effects.

Effects on disease activity

Prompt relief of the symptoms of inflammation, such as swelling and duration of early morning stiffness, usually results from corticosteroid treatment. More 'systemic' complaints, e.g. fatigue and loss of appetite, may also improve. Decreases in laboratory parameters such as ESR and CRP, as well as an increase in hemoglobin levels, are often noticed. Early studies compared corticosteroids with high-dose salicylates, the standard treatment at the time. More recently, placebo-controlled trials have generally shown[80,82,83] beneficial effects on disease activity, particularly, if not exclusively, in the initial phase of treatment.

Effects on radiographic progression

A few studies have been published on the protective effect of corticosteroids against progression of radiographic damage. All these trials showed equal, and in some cases superior, results for radiographic progression of joint damage in corticosteroid-treated patients, compared with various control groups. Statistically significant differences were shown in only three studies[80,84,85]. One study primarily compared a regimen of anti-inflammatory and antirheumatic drugs with one consisting of maintenance of activity, anti-inflammatory and antirheumatic drugs and systemic corticosteroids as necessary. After 10 years, the radiographic changes in individual joints were broadly similar for the two groups, but the 'activity–corticosteroid' group showed fewer erosions in the wrist, MCP and PIP joints[84]. In the published study of the UK Joint Committee of the Medical Research Council and Nuffield Foundation, a statistically significant difference in favor of the corticosteroid-treated patients was only observed for the first 2 years of follow up[85]. The recently published study by Kirwan and the Arthritis and Rheumatism Council's low-dose glucocorticoid study group[80] showed a reduction in the rate of radiographic progression of disease in 128 patients with active RA of less than 2 years' duration in a multicenter, randomized, double-blind trial comparing oral prednisolone 7.5mg versus placebo. Patients were maintained on other SAARDs. After 2 years, radiographic progression of joint damage was minimal in the prednisone group, whereas the placebo group showed substantial joint destruction. Because of the increased morbidity and mortality associated with oral corticosteroids found in prospective long-term observations, this study has prompted an interesting and vigorous debate.

Corticosteroids and toxicity

The adverse effects of long-term corticosteroid treatment are well recognized, but exact figures on their prevalence and severity are lacking. The risk of complications caused by corticosteroid treatment are in general dose- and time-dependent (see also Chapter 3.6).

There are no precise guidelines for prescribing oral glucocorticoids in RA. Long-term therapy with prednisone in excess of 10mg daily should be avoided because of the side effects, especially as

ALGORITHM MONITORING DISEASE-MODIFYING ANTIRHEUMATIC DRUG TREATMENT

Drug	Contraindications	Clinically relevant drug interactions	Monitoring before treatment				Monitoring during treatment					
			Blood count[a]	Liver[b]	Kidney[c]	Other	Interval	Blood count[a]	Liver[b]	Kidney[c]	Urine[d]	Other
Sulfasalazine	G6PD deficiency Acute intermittent porphyria Allergy to sulfonamides or salicylates		✓	✓	✓		3 months: 2-weekly 3 months: 4-weekly then: 12-weekly	✓ ✓ ✓	✓ ✓ ✓			
Methotrexate	Hepatitis B Hepatitis C	Folic acid antagonists (trimethoprim) Plasma protein-binding drugs (sulfamethoxazole) Weakly acid drugs (probenecid, high-dose salicylates)	✓	✓	✓	CXR	3 months: 2-weekly 3 months: 4-weekly then: 12-weekly	✓ ✓ ✓	✓ ✓ ✓	✓ ✓ ✓		
Parenteral gold	Hypersensitivity, nephritis or nephritic syndrome		✓	✓	✓		2 months: weekly then: every 2nd dose	✓ ✓			✓ ✓	
Oral gold	Aplastic anemia during parenteral gold therapy Nephritis or nephritic syndrome		✓	✓	✓		3 months: 2-weekly 3 months: 4-weekly then 12-weekly	✓ ✓ ✓			✓ ✓ ✓	
(Hydroxy)chloroquine	Retinal disease Allergy to 4-aminoquinoline derivatives G6PD deficiency				✓	OPH	Regular visual acuity and retinal function tests				✓	OPH
D-Penicillamine	Allergy to penicillins Myasthenia gravis	Digoxin Antacids Iron	✓	✓	✓		2 months: weekly 5 months: 2-weekly then: 4-weekly	✓ ✓ ✓			✓ ✓ ✓	
Azathioprine		Allopurinol	✓	✓	✓		3 months: 2-weekly 3 months: 4-weekly then: 12-weekly	✓ ✓ ✓	✓ ✓ ✓		✓	
Cyclophosphamide	Severe bladder disease	Allopurinol	✓	✓	✓		3 months: 2-weekly 3 months: 4-weekly then: 8-weekly	✓ ✓ ✓	✓ ✓ ✓	✓ ✓ ✓	✓ ✓ ✓	
Cyclosporin A	Hypertension Renal failure	Erythromycine Calcium channel blockers Ketaconozole	✓	✓	✓	K^+ BP	every 2 weeks until dosage stable then: monthly	✓	✓	✓		K^+ BP

Fig. 14.9 Algorithm monitoring disease-modifying antirheumatic drug treatment. With permission from Wijnands & van Riel[75].

dosages up to 10mg are sufficient to treat most arthritic complaints. A higher dose may be needed when the patient has systemic manifestations such as vasculitis or serositis. Whether or not low-dose corticosteroid treatment has an impact on bone mineral content is still a matter for debate. Sambrook *et al.* evaluated the risk of osteoporosis, using low-dose prednisone (mean dose 8mg/day) over a mean period of 9 years[86]. Using dual photon absorptiometry they showed a reduced axial bone mass in the corticosteroid-treated group compared with patients not treated with corticosteroids, a finding which did not reach levels of statistical significance. In a study by Laan *et al.*[87], statistically significant vertebral bone loss detected by dual energy quantitative computed tomography (CT) was found in the first month of low-dose prednisone treatment (10mg/day) of patients with active RA.

In order to detect adverse events as early as possible regular monitoring should be carried out, including blood or urine glucose levels and, where high doses are given, blood pressure. Although no clear relationship between peptic ulcer disease and corticosteroid therapy has been established, prevention of peptic ulcer disease has to be considered in patients with concomitant NSAID treatment and other risk factors such as a history of peptic ulcer and advanced age[88]. If the anticipated duration of corticosteroid treatment is longer than 3 months and the expected daily dose higher than 7.5mg/day, bone densitometry is advised. Some measures recommended to retard bone loss may be effective, such as advice about nutrition and physical exercise and, in case of (suspected) deficiencies, supplementation with calcium salts and vitamin D. Treatment with bisphosphonates may also be beneficial[89–91]. Hormone (estrogen) substitution must be considered in women with established postmenopause-induced osteopenia.

THE RELATIONSHIP BETWEEN DOSE AND THE OCCURRENCE OF ADVERSE EFFECTS IN DISEASE-MODIFYING ANTIRHEUMATIC DRUGS

Drug	Adverse effect			
	Not influenced by dose	Influenced by dose	Not influenced by cumulative dose	Influenced by cumulative dose
Sulfasalazine	Leucopenia Cutaneous Hepatitis	GI, Headache Changes in mood Hemolysis		
Methotrexate	Pneumonitis Hepatocellular	Nausea and other GI effects Changes in transaminases Stomatitis	Pneumonitis	Liver fibrosis
Parenteral gold	Cutaneous Hematologic	Cutaneous (mild) Proteinuria (mild) Diarrhea		Chrysiasis
Oral gold	Cutaneous GI	Diarrhea		
(Hydroxy)-chloroquine	Keratopathy	Retinopathy GI Mucocutaneous	GI Cutaneous Keratopathy	Retinopathy
D-Penicillamine		Hematologic Renal		
Azathioprine	Nausea	Leukopenia Hepatotixity		
Cyclophos-phamide	Nausea Diarrhea	Alopecia Leukopenia		Hemorrhagic cystitis Malignancies Gonadal dysfunction

Fig. 14.10 The relationship between dose and the occurrence of adverse events in disease-modifying antirheumatic drugs. With permission from Wijnands & van Riel[75].

Intravenous (pulse) methylprednisolone therapy

Pulse methylprednisolone therapy is sometimes used to obtain prompt control of the inflammatory process. Usually 3 pulses are administrated on alternate days, with daily dose ranging from 200 to 1000mg. Minipulses of 100mg have also been shown to be effective in the treatment of RA flares[92]. A single dose can also be given and then repeated if necessary. The clinical response has a rapid onset and can have a prolonged duration, sometimes for 3–4 months.

Methylprednisolone pulses are usually well tolerated with a few minor and self-limiting side-effects such as flushing, psychological disturbance, palpitations and taste disturbance. Serious adverse reactions, such as cardiac arrest[93] and severe infection[94], have been reported in patients with failing cardiovascular or immune systems[95]. The methylprednisolone pulse should not be administered as a bolus, since sudden death has been attributed to rapid infusion[96].

Pulse therapy is free from the adverse effects associated with the long-term use of oral glucocorticoids. No prolonged suppressive effect has been reported on the hypothalamic–pituitary axis, and bone metabolism is not seriously affected in the short term.

Local corticosteroids

Intra-articular corticosteroids are frequently used to control local synovitis (see Chapters 12.2 & 3.7). This can produce prolonged relief of symptoms and signs of arthritis and markedly improved function. At present there is no scientific evidence to show that these injections can slow progression of erosive disease. Animal studies have suggested a negative effect of corticosteroids on cartilage[97]. Whether this is also true in humans is doubtful since corticosteroids ameliorate synovitis, which in itself is detrimental to cartilage (and bone). There is a dogma in clinical medicine that injections for a single joint should not exceed 2 or 3 per annum[98]. However, this is not well founded scientifically. The duration of action of intra-articular corticosteroid injection varies with the preparation used. Local corticosteroids are also frequently used for nonarticular manifestations of RA such as tenosynovitis, bursitis, carpal tunnel syndrome, etc.

NONPHARMACOLOGIC TREATMENT MODALITIES

Despite the success of pharmacologic treatments, many patients with RA requre other therapeutic modalities including synoviorthesis and surgical synovectomy. A multi-disciplinary approach encompassing physical therapy, occupational therapy and support from social workers and visiting nurses remain essential, especially for patients with moderate to severe chronic disease. Psychotherapy is sometimes necessary and patient education is vital. The following deals briefly with some of these therapies (discussed in greater detail in other chapters).

SYNOVIORTHESIS

There are two types of synoviorthesis: radiosynoviorthesis and chemical synoviorthesis (see Practical Problem 5.16, Recurrent knee synovitis in RA).

Radiosynoviorthesis – the intra-articular injection of radioisotopes – should be considered after several injections of (long-acting) corticosteroids have failed to relieve symptoms, especially when only a limited number of joints is involved. The injection can be performed under arthrographic control to avoid extra-articular leaks, especially for joints such as the hip or ankle which are difficult to inject. Strict inpatient immobilization for 3 days postinjection reduces spread of the radioisotope beyond the treated joint[99]. The choice of nuclide depends on the maximum tissue penetration of β-radiation in relation to the size of the joint. Erbium-169 is a β-emitting agent used for the treatment of rheumatoid digital joints (maximum tissue penetration 0.7mm). Rhenium-186 (maximum tissue penetration 3.1mm) is suitable for medium-sized joints such as the shoulder, elbow, wrist, hip and ankle. The small amount (about 10%) of γ radiation emitted by ^{186}Re, a predominantly β-emitter, can be used to detect any leakage. The use of radioactive colloidal gold, ^{198}Au (maximum tissue penetration 2.7mm), another β-emitter, is limited by its relatively high level of γ emission, causing undesirable irradiation of areas beyond the treated joint. Yttrium-90 silicate and ^{90}Y citrate have a greater maximum tissue penetration of β radiation (8.5mm) and are therefore used for larger joints (e.g. knee, ankle, hip)[100]. If the beneficial effect of radiosynoviorthesis is insufficient, the same joint can be treated again after 6 months[101]. However, repeat therapy with ^{90}Y in a previous nonresponder is associated with a high failure rate[102]. The total cumulative dose must not exceed approximately 15mCi (5.5×10^8Bq) for each joint. The injections do not jeopardize the outcome of later surgical treatment. The best results are obtained when synoviorthesis is used before the onset of joint destruction.

Complications, such as sepsis, subcutaneous sclerosis or radiation dermatitis, can be prevented if elementary precautions are taken during injection. Increased inflammation in the injected joint lasting several days and accompanied by fever, increased ESR and white blood cell count is very rare. In these cases an intra-articular corticosteroid injection may relieve symptoms. The major disadvantage of synoviorthesis is the extra-articular migration of the product, with the theoretical risk of chromosome damage. Because of this potential adverse reaction radiosynoviorthesis was initially restricted to patients beyond reproductive age. However, despite more than 30 years of experience, no long-term side effects have been reported and currently radiosynoviorthesis is done from about 18 years of age. There is very little experience in children, except in hemophiliac joint disease. Radiosynoviorthesis should not be performed during pregnancy or lactation.

In order to avoid the risks of irradiating the gonads, synoviorthesis has been carried out using chemicals, such as osmic acid (chemosynoviorthesis). This may be an alternative in young adults, especially for treatment of knee and hip synovitis[103,104]. It is not used in small joints because of its toxicity to skin and subcutaneous tissues. It can elicit an acute inflammatory reaction, despite the injection of a corticosteroid agent during treatment. Although this procedure is widely used in some countries, its efficacy has not been established.

SURGICAL SYNOVECTOMY

When intra-articular corticosteroids (and synoviorthesis) have failed to control local synovitis surgical removal of the synovium can be considered (see Chapter 3.12). There is a current preference for arthroscopic synovectomy, as opposed to open synovectomy, because of reduced morbidity, length of hospital stay and need for postoperative rehabilitation with a similar short-term reduction in pain and swelling[105].

Both synoviorthesis and surgical synovectomy can provide a prolonged remission of (local) synovitis, sometimes lasting several years. Whether or not they can retard eventual joint destruction is not clear. Most studies indicate progressive joint damage (especially osteoarthritis) after synovectomy[106].

REFERENCES

1. Edmonds JP, Scott DL, Furst DE, Brooks P, Paulus HE. Antirheumatic drugs: a proposed new classification. Arthritis Rheum. 1993;36:336–9.
2. Fries JF. The hierarchy of outcome assessment. J Rheumatol. 1993;20:546–7.
3. Felson DT, Anderson JJ, Boers M, *et al.* American College of Rheumatology preliminary definition of improvement in rheumatoid arthritis. Arthritis Rheum 1995;38:727–35.
4. van Gestel AM, Prevoo MLL, van 't Hof MA, van Rijswijk MH, van de Putte LBA, van Riel PLCM. Development and validation of the European League Against Rheumatism response criteria for rheumatoid arthritis. Arthritis Rheum. 1996;39:34–40.
5. Tugwell P, Bombardier C. A methodological framework for developing and selecting endpoints in clinical trials. J Rheumatol. 1982;9:758–62.
6. van der Heijde DMFM, van Riel PLCM, van Rijswijk MH, van de Putte LBA. Influence of prognostic features on the final outcome in rheumatoid arthritis: a review of literature. Semin Arthritis Rheum. 1988;17:284–92.
7. Emery P, Salmon M, Bradley H, *et al.* Genetically determined factors as predictors of radiological change in patients with early symmetrical arthritis. Br Med J. 1992;305:1387–9.
8. van der Heijde DMFM, van Riel PLCM, van Leeuwen MA, *et al.* Prognostic factors for radiographic damage and physical disability in early rheumatoid arthritis. A prospective follow-up study of 147 patients. Br J Rheumatol. 1992;31:519–25.
9. Tugwell P, Boers M, OMERACT Committee. Developing consensus on preliminary core efficacy endpoints for rheumatoid arthritis clinical trials. J Rheumatol. 1993;20:555–61.
10. van Riel PLCM. Provisional guidelines for measuring disease activity in RA clinical trials. Editorial. Br J Rheumatol. 1992;31:793–4.
11. Felson DT, Anderson JJ, Boers M, *et al.* The American College of Rheumatology preliminary core set of disease activity measures for rheumatoid arthritis clinical trials. Arthritis Rheum. 1993;36:729–40.
12. American College of Rheumatology Committee on Outcome Measures in Rheumatoid Arthritis Clinical Trials. Reduced joint counts in rheumatoid arthritis clinical trials. Editorial. Arthritis Rheum. 1994;37:463–4.
13. Smolen JS. Report on the EULAR Standing Committee on International Clinical Studies Including Therapeutic Trials. Rheumatol Eur. 1994;23:37–9.
14. Thompson PW, Kirwan JR. Joint counts: a review of old and new articular indices of joint inflammation. Br J Rheumatol. 1995;34:1003–8.
15. van der Heijde DMFM, van 't Hof MA, van Riel PLCM, van de Putte LBA. Validity of single variables and indices to measure disease activity in rheumatoid arthritis. J Rheumatol. 1993;20:538–41.
16. Anderson JJ, Chernoff MC. Sensitivity to change of rheumatoid arthritis clinical trial outcome measures. J Rheumatol. 1993;20:535–7.
17. Astbury C, Platt R, Dixon JS, Le Gallex P, Hill J, Bird HA. Optimizing the assessment of disease activity during treatment with anti-rheumatoid drugs. Br J Rheumatol. 1993;32:467–73.
18. Dixon JS. Hayes S, Constable PDL, Bird HA. What are the 'best' measurements for monitoring

patients during short-term second-line therapy? Br J Rheumatol. 1988;27:37–43.
19. Leeuwen van MA, Rijswijk van MH, Heijde van der DMFM, *et al.* The acute-phase response in relation to radiographic progression in early rheumatoid arthritis: a prospective study during the first three years of the disease. Br J Rheumatol. 1993;32:9–13.
20. Leeuwen van MA, Rijswijk van MH. Acute phase proteins in the monitoring of inflammatory disorders. Baillière's Clin Rheumatol. 1994;8:531–52.
21. Melzack R. The McGill pain questionnaire. Pain. 1975:1:277–99.
22. Meenan RF, Gertman PM, Mason JM. Measuring health status in arthritis: the arthritis impact measurement scales. Arthritis Rheum. 1980;23:146–52.
23. Anderson K, Bradley LA, McDaniel LK, *et al.* The assessment of pain in rheumatoid arthritis: disease differentiation and temporal stability of a behavioral observation method. J Rheumatol. 1987;14:700–4.
24. Buchbinder R, Bombardier C, Yeung M, Tugwell P. Which outcome measures should be used in rheumatoid arthritis clinical trials? Clinical and quality-of-life measures' responsiveness to treatment in a randomized controlled trial. Arthritis Rheum. 1995;38:1568–80.
25. Bosi Ferraz M, Quaresma MR, Aquino LRL, *et al.* Reliability of pain scales in the assessment of literate and illiterate patients in rheumatoid arthritis. J Rheumatol. 1990;17:1022–4.
26. Tugwell P, Boers M, Baker Ph, Wells G, Snider J. Endpoints in rheumatoid arthritis. J Rheumatol. 1994;21(Suppl 42):2–8.
27. Thompson PW. Functional outcome in rheumatoid arthritis. Br J Rheumatol. 1988:27(Suppl 1):37–43.
28. Ware JE, Donald-Sherbourne C. The MOS 36 item Short-Form Health Survey (SF-36): I. Conceptual framework and item selection. Med Care. 1992;6:473–83.
29. Bergner M, Bobbitt RA, Pollard WE, Martin DP, Gilson BS. The sickness impact profile: validation of a health status measure. Med Care. 1976;14:57–67.
30. Hunt SM, McKenna SP, McEwen J, Williams J, Papp E. The Nottingham Health Profile: subjective health status and medical consultations. Social Sci Med. 1981;15A:221–9.
31. Fries JF, Spitz P, Kraines RG, Holman HR. Measurement of patient outcome in arthritis. Arthritis Rheum. 1980;23:137–45.
32. Tugwell P, Bombardier C, Buchanan WW, Goldsmith CH, Grace E, Hanna B. The MACTAR patient preference disability questionnaire – an individualized functional priority approach for assessing improvement in physical disability in clinical trials in rheumatoid arthritis. J Rheumatol. 1987;14:446–51.
33. Jette AM. Functional status instrument: reliability of a chronic disease evaluation instrument. Arch Phys Med Rehabil. 1980;61:395–401.
34. Meenan RF, Anderson JJ, Kazis LE, *et al.* Outcome assessment in clinical trials: evidence for the sensitivity of a health status measure. Arthritis Rheum. 1984;27:1344–52.
35. Anderson JJ, Firschein HE, Meenan RF. Sensitivity of a health status measure to short-term clinical changes in arthritis. Arthritis Rheum. 1989;32:844–50.
36. Potts MK, Brandt KD. Evidence of the validity of the Arthritis Impact Measurement Scales. Arthritis Rheum. 1987;30:93–6.
37. Liang MH, Larson MG, Cullen KE, Schwartz JA. Comparative measurement efficiency and sensitivity of five health status instruments for arthritis research. Arthritis Rheum. 1985;28:542–7.
38. Sharp JT, Lidsky MD, Collins LC, Moreland J. Methods of scoring the progression of radiologic changes in rheumatoid arthritis. Arthritis Rheum. 1971;14:206–20.
39. Larsen A. How to apply Larsen Score in evaluating radiographs of rheumatoid arthritis in longterm studies? J Rheumatol. 1995;22:1974–5.
40. van der Heijde DM, van Riel PL, Nuver-Zwart HH, Gribnau FW, van de Putte LB. Effects of hydroxychloroquine and sulphasalazine on progression of joint damage in rheumatoid arthritis. Lancet. 1989;i:1036–8.
41. Sharp JT. Assessment of radiographic abnormalities in rheumatoid arthritis: what have we accomplished and where should we go from here? J Rheumatol. 1995;22:1787–91.
42. Pincus T, Callahan LF, Fuchs HA, Larsen A, Kaye J.Quantitative analysis of hand radiographs in rheumatoid arthritis: time course of radiographic changes, relation to joint examination measures, and comparison of different scoring methods. J Rheumatol. 1995;22:1983–9.
43. Weissmann BNW. Imaging techniques in RA. J Rheumatol. 1994;21(Suppl 42):14–19.
44. Gough AKS, Lilley J, Eyre S, Holder RL, Emery P. Generalised bone loss in patients with early rheumatoid arthritis. Lancet. 1994;334:23–7.
45. Deodhar AA, Brabyn J, Jones PW, Davis MJ, Woolf AD. Measurement of hand bone mineral content by dual energy X-ray absorptiometry: development of the method, and its application in normal volunteers and in patients with rheumatoid arthritis. Ann Rheum Dis. 1994;53:685–90.
46. Lansbury A. A method for summation of the systemic indices of rheumatoid activity. Am J Med Sci. 1956;232:300–10.
47. van der Putte LBA, Furst DE, van Riel PLCM, Williams X. Clinical assessments in rheumatoid arthritis: In Therapy of the systemic rheumatic disorders. Marcel Dekker, Inc. 1997.
48. Prevoo MLL, van 't Hof MA, Kuper HH, *et al.* Modified disease activity scores that include twenty-eight joint counts. Arthritis Rheum. 1995;38:44–8.
49. Fuchs HA. The use of the disease activity score in the analysis of clinical trials in rheumatoid arthritis. J Rheumatol. 1993;20:1863–6.
50. Mallya RK, Mace BEW. The assessment of disease activity in rheumatoid arthritis using a multivariate analysis. Rheumatol Rehab. 1981;20:14–17.
51. van Riel PLCM, Reekers P, van de Putte LBA, Gribnau FWJ. Association of HLA antigens, toxic reactions and therapeutic response to auranofin and aurothioglucose in patients with rheumatoid arthritis. Tissue Antigens. 1983;22:194–9.
52. Corkill M, Kirkham BW, Chikanza IC, Gibson T, Panayi GS. Intramuscular depot methylprednisolone induction of chrysotherapy in rheumatoid arthritis: a 24-week randomized controlled trial. Br J Rheumatol. 1990;29:274–9.
53. Davis MJ, Dawes PT, Fowler PD, *et al.* Comparison and evaluation of a disease activity index for use in patients with rheumatoid arthritis. Br J Rheumatol. 1990;29:111–15.
54. Pinals RS, Masi AT, Larsen RA. Preliminary criteria for remission in rheumatoid arthritis. Arthritis Rheum. 1981;24:1308–15.
55. Smythe HA, Helewa A, Goldsmith CH. 'Independent assessor' and 'pooled index' as techniques for measuring treatment effects in rheumatoid arthritis. J Rheumatol. 1977;4:144–52.
56. Paulus HE, Egger MJ, Ward JR, Williams HJ, CSSRD. Analysis of improvement in individual rheumatoid arthritis patients treated with disease-modifying antirheumatic drugs, based on the findings in patients treated with placebo. Arthritis Rheum. 1990;33:477–84.
57. Scott DL. A simple index to assess disease activity in RA. J Rheumatol. 1993;20:582–4.
58. Prevoo MLL, Gestel van AM, Hof van 't MA, *et al.* Remission in a prospective study of patients with rheumatoid arthritis. ARA preliminary remission criteria in relation to the disease activity score. Br J Rheumatol. 1996;35:1101–5.
59. Vliet Vlieland TPM, Zwinderman AH, Vandenbroucke JP *et al.* A randomized clinical trial of in-patient multidisciplinary treatment versus routine outpatient care in active rheumatoid arthritis. Br J Rheumatol. 1996;35:475–82.
60. DJ Hawley. Psycho-educational interventions in the treatment of rheumatoid arthritis. Ballière's Clin Rheumatol. 1995;9:803–23.
61. Ianuzzi L, Dawson N, Zein N, Kushner I. Does drug therapy slow radiographic deterioration in rheumatoid arthritis? N Eng J Med. 1983;309:1023–8.
62. van de Putte LBA, van Riel PLCM. Do disease modifying antirheumatic drugs actually modify disease course in rheumatoid arthritis? Clin Immunother. 1994;5:319–22.
63. Heijde DMFM van der, Leeuwen MA van, Riel PLCM van, *et al.* Biannual radiographic assessments of hands and feet in a three-year prospective followup of patients with early rheumatoid arthritis. Arthritis Rheum. 1992;35:26–34.
64. Heijde DM van der, Riel PL van, Nuver-Zwart IH, Gribnau FW, Putte LB van de. Effects of hydroxychloroquine and sulphasalazine on progression of joint damage in rheumatoid arthritis. Lancet. 1989;i:1036–8.
65. Pincus T, Callahan LF. Rheumatology function tests: grip strength, walking time, button test and questionnaires document and predict long term morbidity and mortality in rheumatoid arthritis. J Rheumatol. 1992;19:1051–7.
66. Felson DT, Anderson JJ, Meenan RF. Use of short term efficacy/toxicity tradeoffs to select second-line drugs in rheumatoid arthritis. Arthritis Rheum. 1992;35:1117–25.
67. Wijnands MJH, van 't Hof M, van Leeuwen MA *et al.* A prospective analysis of risk factors for the risk continuation of second-line antirheumatic drugs. Pharm World Sci. 1993;15:203–7.
68. Scott DL, Grindulis KA, Struthers GR, *et al.* Progression of radiological changes in rheumatoid arthritis. Ann Rheum Dis. 1984;43:8–17.
69. Scott DL, Dawes PT, Fowler PD, *et al.* Anti-rheumatic drugs and joint damage in rheumatoid arthritis. Q J Med. 1985;54:49–59.
70. Pullar T, Hunter JA, Capell HA. Effect of sulphasalazine on the radiological progression of rheumatoid arthritis. Ann Rheum Dis. 1987;46:398–402.
71. Stockman A, Emery P, Doyle T, *et al.* Relationship of progression of radiographic changes in hands and wrists, clinical features and HLA-DR antigens in rheumatoid arthritis. J Rheumatol. 1991;18:1001–7.
72. Leeuwen MA van, Rijswijk MH van, Heijde DMFM van der, *et al.* The acute-phase response in relation to radiographic progression in early rheumatoid arthritis: a prospective study during the first three years of the disease. Br J Rheumatol. 1993;32(suppl 3):9–13.
73. Jeurissen MEC, Boerbooms AMTh, Putte LBA van de, Doesburg WH, Lemmens AM. Influence of methotrexate and azathioprine on radiologic progression in rheumatoid arthritis. A randomized, double-blind study. Ann Intern Med. 1991;114:999–1004.
74. Heijde DMFM van der, Riel PLCM van, Nuver-Zwart HH, Putte LBA van de. Sulphasalazine versus hydroxychloroquine in rheumatoid arthritis: 3-year follow-up (letter). Lancet. 1990;539(i):33–5.
75. Wijnands MJH, van Riel PLCM. Management of adverse effects of disease-modifying antirheumatic drugs. Drug Safety. 1995;13:219–27.
76. Borigini MJ, Paulus HE. Combination therapy. Ballière's Clin Rheumatol. 1994;9:689–710.
77. Felson DT, Anderson JJ, Meenan RF. The efficacy and toxicity of combination therapy in rheumatoid arthritis: a meta-analysis. Arthritis Rheum. 1994;37:1487–91.
78. Tugwell P, Pincus T, Yocum D *et al.* Combination therapy with cyclosporine and methotrexate in severe rheumatoid arthritis. N Engl J Med. 1995;333:137–41.
79. O'Dell JR, Haire CE, Erikson N, *et al.* Treatment of rheumatoid arthritis with methotrexate alone, sulfasalazine and hydroxychloroquine, or a combination of all three medications. N Engl J Med. 1996;334:1287–91.
80. Kirwan JR, The Arthritis and Rheumatism Council Low-dose Glucocorticoid Study Group. The effect of glucocorticoids on joint destruction in rheumatoid arthritis. N Engl J Med. 1995;333:142–6.
81. Hench PS, Kendall EC, Slocumb CH, Polley HF. Effects of cortisone acetate and pituitary ACTH on rheumatoid arthritis, rheumatic fever and certain other conditions: a study in clinical physiology. Arch Intern Med. 1950;85:546–66.

82. Harris ED, Emkey RD, Nichols JE, Newberg A. Low dose prednisone therapy in rheumatoid arthritis: a double blind study. J Rheumatol. 1983;10:713–21.
83. Gestel AM van, Laan RFJM, Haagsma CJ, Putte LBA van de, Riel PLCM van. Oral steroids as bridge therapy in rheumatoid arthritis patients starting with parenteral gold. A randomized double-blind placebo-controlled trial. Br J Rheumatol. 1995;34:347–51
84. Million R, Poole P, Kellgren JH, Jayson MIV. Long-term study of management of rheumatoid arthritis. Lancet. 1984;i:812–16.
85. Joint Committee of the Medical Research Council and the Nuffield Foundation on Clinical Trials of Cortisone, ACTH, and other Therapeutic Measures in Chronic Rheumatic Diseases. A comparison of prednisolone with aspirin or other analgesics in the treatment of rheumatoid arthritis. Ann Rheum Dis. 1959;18:173–86.
86. Sambrook PN, Eisman JA, Yeates MG, *et al.* Osteoporosis in rheumatoid arthritis: safety of low dose corticosteroids. Ann Rheum Dis. 1986;45:950–3.
87. Laan RFJM, Riel PLCM van, Putte LBA van de, *et al.* Low-dose prednisone induces rapid reversible axial bone loss in patients with rheumatoid arthritis. A randomized, controlled study. Ann Intern Med. 1993;119:963–8.
88. Piper JM, Ray WA, Daugherty JR, Griffin MR. Corticosteroid use and peptic ulcer disease: role of nonsteroidal anti-inflammatory drugs. Ann Intern Med. 1991;114:735–40.
89. Harris ST, Watts NB, Jackson RD, *et al.* Four-year study of intermittent cyclic etidronate treatment of postmenopausal osteoporosis: three years of blinded therapy followed by one year of open therapy. Am J Med. 1993;95:557–67.
90. Adachi JD, Cranney A, Goldsmith CH, *et al.* Intermittent cyclic therapy with etidronate in the prevention of corticosteroid induced bone loss. J Rheumatol. 1994;21:1922–6.
91. Struys A, Snelder AA, Mulder H. Cyclical etidronate reverses bone loss of the spine and proximal femur in patients with established corticosteroid-induced osteoporosis. Am J Med. 1995;99:235–42.
92. Iglehart IW, Sutton JD, Bender JC, *et al.* Intravenous pulsed steroids in rheumatoid arthritis: a comparative dose study. J Rheumatol. 1990;17:159–62.
93. Moses RE, McCormick A, Nickey W. Fatal arrhythmia after pulse methylprednisolone therapy (letter). Ann Intern Med. 1981;95:781–2.
94. Garret R, Paulus H. Complications of intravenous methylprednisolone pulse therapy. Arthritis Rheum. 1980;23:677A.
95. Smith MD, Ahern MJ, Roberts-Thomson PJ. Pulse methylprednisolone therapy in rheumatoid arthritis: unproved therapy, unjustified therapy, or effective adjunctive treatment? Ann Rheum Dis. 1990;49:265–7.
96. McDougal BA, Whittier FC, Cross DE. Sudden death after bolus steroid therapy for acute rejection. Transplant Proc. 1976;8:493–6.
97. Gray RG, Gottlieb NL. Intra-articular corticosteroids. An updated assessment. Clin Orthop. 1983;177:235–63.
98. Barraclough D. The use of corticosteroid agents in connective tissue disorders. Med J Aust. 1986;144:427–32.
99. Jaworski R, McLean R, Choong K, Smart R, Edmonds J. Re-evaluating the need for hospitalization following synovectomy using yttrium-90 silicate. Br J Rheumatol. 1993;32:1012–17.
100. Boerbooms AMTh, Buijs WCAM, Danen M, Putte LBA van de,Vandenbroucke JP. Radiosynovectomy in chronic synovitis of the knee joint in patients with rheumatoid arthritis. Eur J Nucl Med. 1985;10:446–9.
101. Vella M, Zuckerman JD, Shortkroff S, Venkatesan P. Repeat radiation synovectomy with dysprosium 165-ferric hydroxide macro-aggregates in rheumatoid knees unresponsive to initial injection. Arthritis Rheum. 1988;31:789–92.
102. Stucki G, Bozzone P, Treuer E, Wassmer P, Felder M. Efficacy and safety of radiation synovectomy with yttrium-90: a retrospective long-term analysis of 164 applications in 82 patients. Br J Rheumatol. 1993;32:383–6.
103. Nissila M. Use of osmic acid in the topical treatment of exudative synovitis of the knee joint. Scand J Rheumatol. 1979;29(Suppl):3–44.
104. Menkes CJ. Is there a place for chemical and radiation synovectomy in rheumatic diseases? Rheumatol Rehabil. 1979;2:65–77.
105. Cohen S, Jones R. An evaluation of the efficacy of arthroscopic synovectomy of the knee in rheumatoid arthritis: 12–24 months results. J Rheumatol. 1987;14:452–5.
106. Ochi T, Iwase R, Kimura T, *et al.* Effect of early synovectomy on the course of rheumatoid arthritis. J Rheumatol. 1991;18:1794–808.

15

MANAGEMENT: END STAGE AND COMPLICATIONS

Johanna MW Hazes & Arnold Cats

- The primary goals of management of end-stage rheumatoid arthritis are to preserve and maximize function and prevent disability.
- Management decisions require distinguishing inflammatory from mechanical causes of joint disease.
- Aggressive physical, rehabilitative and occupational therapy are extremely important in management.
- Drug therapy including NSAIDs and SAARDs has a major role in the treatment of most patients with end-stage rheumatoid arthritis.
- Surgical treatment including synovectomy, tendon reconstruction, joint fusion and joint replacement can improve function and decrease pain in selected patients with end-stage rheumatoid arthritis (RA).
- Extra-articular complications including tendon ruptures, pressure ulcers, cervical spine instability, vasculitis and amyloidosis are important causes of morbidity.
- Reconstructive surgery is important in patients with disability from end-stage joint disease.

INTRODUCTION

The ability to manage the patient with end-stage RA has improved over the past several decades, not only because the therapeutic modalities have been improved considerably, but also because of changes in welfare. The outcome of RA in underdeveloped countries is still very poor[1]: in such countries incapacitated people who can no longer earn a livelihood have virtually no chance of survival. In developed countries, however, social improvements have contributed to the development of therapeutic facilities. Public assistance has become of major importance in the management of RA. Sickness and disability benefits enable the patient to maintain social and financial independence. Patients' associations have stimulated the evolution of welfare services. Furthermore the awareness which these patient groups have provoked has helped many patients to accept their disability. All these achievements have to be guarded as, with the constantly increasing health care costs, there is a tendency to economize on nonmedical care facilities.

The primary objective of the management of end-stage RA is to relieve pain and discomfort. The ultimate goal, however, is to prevent further damage to and loss of function of the locomotor apparatus, and to maintain patients' normal activities of daily life.

Several therapeutic modalities are of use in the management of RA at all stages of the disease. The principal elements of the management of end-stage RA are: education, balance between rest and exercise, physical therapy, occupational therapy, drug therapy and surgical intervention. The relative importance of each therapeutic modality varies with the stage of the disease (Fig. 15.1). Many other features of the disease itself (bad prognostic signs, extra-articular manifestations) or of the cultural and socioeconomic environment influence the choice of therapeutic intervention. The complexity of the disease process and the variable ways RA may affect the individual patient influences its management (Fig. 15.2).

THE ROLE OF THERAPEUTIC REGIMENS IN THE MANAGEMENT OF RHEUMATOID ARTHRITIS RELATED TO THE STAGE OF DISEASE

Therapeutic regimen	Early and established disease	End-stage disease
Conservative therapy		
Patient education	+++	+
Rest		
Systemic/therapeutic	+	+
Local/protective	++	++
Physical therapy		
Maintenance range of motion	++	+
Prevention of disuse atrophy of muscle, support of condition	+	++
Occupational therapy		
Joint protection	++	+
Adaptation	+	++
Drug therapy		
NSAIDs	++	++
Second-line drugs	++	+
Corticosteroids (systemic)	+	±
Intra-articular therapy	++	+
Surgical intervention		
Therapeutic (synovectomy)	+	–
Reconstructive	+	++
Joint replacement	–	+++

Fig. 15.1 The role of therapeutic regimens in the management of rheumatoid arthritis related to the stage of disease.

END-STAGE DISEASE

During the course of their disease the majority of RA patients will lose some functional capacity, but about half of the patients will develop a disabling, destructive joint disease. The path which eventually leads to widespread joint destruction will vary considerably. Patients may experience a slow or a rapid course of progressive RA, or their disease may be marked by exacerbations and remissions of variable duration.

FACTORS INFLUENCING MANAGEMENT OF RHEUMATOID ARTHRITIS

Patient	Disease
Age	Serologic phenomena
Sex	Radiologic lesions
Medical history	Activity
Family history	Extra-articular manifestations
Attitude/Schooling	Disease stage
Occupation	
Mental vulnerability	
Living conditions	
Marital status	

Fig. 15.2 Factors influencing the management of RA.

FEATURES OF AN EXACERBATION OF RHEUMATOID ARTHRITIS IN END-STAGE DISEASE

- Deterioration of general condition, fatigue, loss of appetite
- Increased synovial swelling and joint pain
- More intense morning stiffness
- Loss of function, progressive disability
- More nodules
- Changes in laboratory parameters: elevation of ESR, CRP and platelet count, diminished hemoglobin level

Fig. 15.3 Features of an exacerbation of RA in end-stage disease.

Even if widespread joint destruction already exists, RA patients may confront the physician with an unexpected deterioration of their functional ability or general condition. This may be attributed to an exacerbation of the arthritis, to mechanical problems caused by the extensive joint deformations or to systemic involvement of the disease. Differentiation between these three possibilities might be difficult because of the invariable presence of deformed and swollen joints. Hospital admission may be required for assessment and to exclude possible concurrent diseases.

EXACERBATION OF LONG-STANDING RHEUMATOID ARTHRITIS

Even destructive end-stage RA in remission may exacerbate, causing increased joint problems and a decline in functional ability. Increased synovial swelling and joint pain, together with changes in laboratory parameters such as erythrocyte sedimentation rate (ESR), C-reactive protein (CRP), hemoglobin level and platelet count, will provide clues as to the diagnosis (Fig. 15.3). The management of an exacerbation of long-standing RA is essentially the same as that of established RA, but in end-stage RA an individual approach to the problem is mandatory. The most important goal is to keep patients out of a nursing home and preserve their independence. The treatment program will therefore depend above all on the personal situation of the patient. The problems which the patients encounter are often multiple and complex and specialist care from various health care professionals is often required. An important feature of the multidisciplinary approach has to be based on team work. Specific treatment goals and strategies have to be coordinated by the health professionals. The effectiveness of multidisciplinary team care in improving disease activity and the quality of life has been established in an in-patient as well as in an out-patient setting[2,3]. Patients with long-standing, destructive disease and high level of disease activity may require hospitalization[4].

THE ROLE OF REST, PHYSICAL THERAPY AND OCCUPATIONAL THERAPY IN END-STAGE RHEUMATOID ARTHRITIS

When active inflammation of joints contributes to the patient's deterioration, limited bedrest and localized immobilization of the joints will be necessary to reduce the inflammatory process and consequently diminish pain, disability and further damage to joint and tendons. Along with rest (Fig. 15.4), the use of removable braces and specific splints (Fig. 15.5) is helpful in the treatment of active joint disease, even in already severely damaged joints. Resting in splints for an hour, three times a day, combined with goal-oriented exercise therapy, is a valuable procedure in preventing or abolishing nonfixed contractures. If a particular joint is inflamed out of proportion to others, then intra-articular injections with long-acting glucocorticosteroids might be beneficial, even if the joint is already destroyed to a large extent. It is important, however, to ensure the absence of an infection beforehand (see Chapter 5.16). The RA patient often cannot distinguish the increased joint symptoms from a 'flare' of the disease. Because of this confusion, the correct diagnosis is delayed with a resultant poor prognosis for both articular function and life. Almost half of all cases of polyarticular septic arthritis occur in patients with RA and one-third or more die during the infection[5]. An additional reason for intra-articular corticosteroid therapy is the possible small systemic effect of the drug. Injections of small joints in end-stage disease is not advocated because the results are poor: no significant functional improvement can be expected.

An exercise program plays an important role in end-stage RA. The aims of physical therapy are to loosen fixed positions of joints, to improve function of the damaged joints and to improve muscle

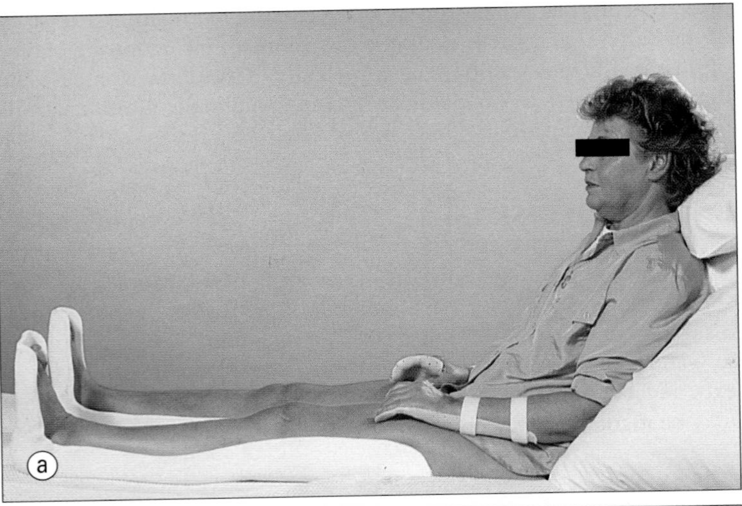

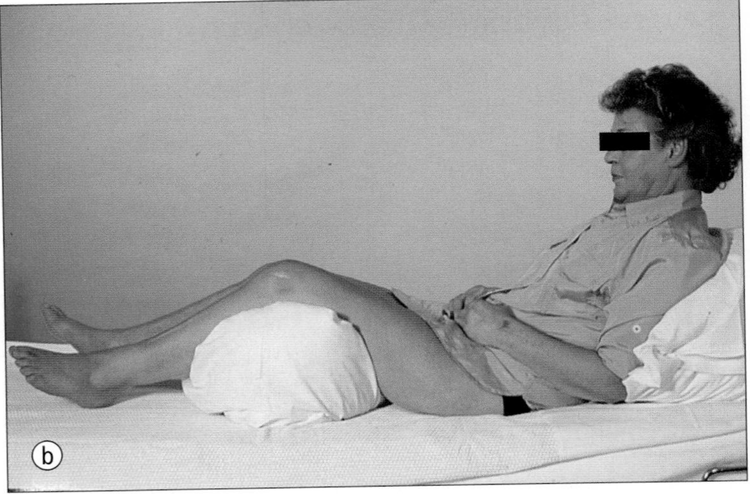

Fig. 15.4 Bed rests and splints in RA. Correct supine posture (a) and incorrect supine posture (b)

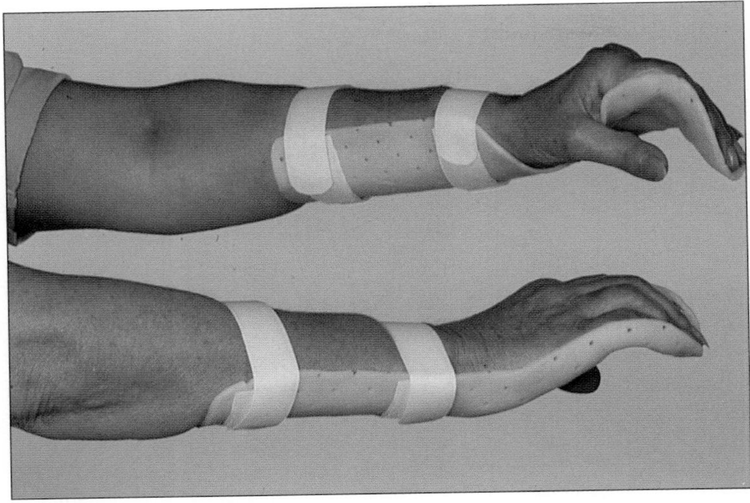

Fig. 15.5 Wrist and hand splint.

ELEMENTS OF PHYSICAL THERAPY PROGAM
Isometric and isokinetic exercises
Relaxation exercises
Preservation of range of joint motion
Physical conditioning excercises
Maintaining good posture

Fig. 15.6 Elements of a physical therapy program in end-stage RA.

strength and the general condition. Often the patient has to learn the proper use of walking aids. The main elements of a traditional physical therapy program are isometric muscle exercises, relaxation exercises, range of motion exercises, physical conditioning exercises and training to sustain a good posture (Fig. 15.6). In the past decade it has become clear that RA patients can participate in aerobic and weight-bearing exercises, including isokinetic exercises, without an increase in disease activity or detrimental effects in the short-term[6,7]. Dynamic exercises are more effective in improving muscle strength, aerobic condition, range of motion and physical capacity than are isometric exercises[7]. The knowledge of the effects of dynamic exercise in the long term is limited, but no harmful effects have been described so far[8]. The contribution of experienced therapists is essential as the physical therapy in very disabled patients demands special skills. Apart from their professional expertise, therapists must possess the talent to motivate patients and encourage them to keep up with a regular and sometimes strenuous program.

The occupational therapist has an important role in the management of end-stage RA. Aids and appliances, such as special grips, a raised toilet seat, special chairs and beds and other household adaptations, will improve the patients' abilities to perform the activities daily (see Chapter 3.11).

THE ROLE OF DRUG TREATMENT IN END-STAGE RHEUMATOID ARTHRITIS

Nonsteroidal anti-inflammatory drugs

Nonsteroidal anti-inflammatory drugs (NSAIDs) continue to play an important role in the treatment of long-standing RA. In consecutive groups of RA patients visiting an average rheumatology clinic, 75% of the long-standing RA patients (>25 years of disease) still used NSAIDs, a similar percentage to that found for patients with relatively recent RA. Because of their better tolerance, nonsalicylate NSAIDs have superseded the salicylates. After years of progressive disease RA patients probably continue to use the drug they tolerate best, even though the risk of side effects will increase considerably because of aging and concurrent diseases. Since the need for NSAIDs will not be diminished in patients with long-standing RA, the physician has to focus special attention on the adverse effects of these drugs (Fig. 15.7). Elderly women, a group particularly represented in end-stage RA, are especially at risk

RISK FACTORS ASSOCIATED WITH ADVERSE REACTIONS TO NSAIDs
Greater age
Female gender
History of gastric ulcers
Renal abnormalities
Hypovolemia, diuretics
Concomitant use of anticoagulants
Cardiovascular disease
Smoking

Fig. 15.7 Risk factors associated with adverse reactions to NSAIDs.

from gastropathy[9]. The risk of developing serious gastrointestinal bleeding is also increased because of the coexistence of arteriosclerotic vessels in the base of bleeding ulcers and inhibition of platelet aggregation mediated by NSAIDs. This group of patients may be receiving anticoagulant therapy, which adds to the bleeding risk. NSAID gastropathy may be asymptomatic and patients receiving these drugs must therefore be closely monitored for signs of gastric injury. Ulcers associated with NSAIDs usually heal rapidly when the NSAIDs are withdrawn. Fortunately, even with the continued use of NSAIDs, ulcers may heal spontaneously. This is accelerated by H2 blockers, omeprazole and prostaglandin analogs. In the case of large, troublesome ulcers omeprazole appears to be the best choice of therapy, especially when NSAIDs cannot be discontinued[10,11]. Elderly patients and patients with heart disease and previous peptic ulcer disease are generally accepted as high-risk patients[9–11] and should receive prophylactic therapy with a cytoprotective or a powerful acid-secretion reducing drug[10–13]. It remains to be seen if the cyclo-oxygenase-2 (COX-2) NSAIDs will obviate the problems of gastrointestinal side effects (see Chapter 3.5).

A second major problem of NSAID use in elderly end-stage RA patients is the adverse effect on renal function[14]; NSAIDs are particularly likely to decrease glomerular filtration in patients with hypovolemic states due to salt depletion or hypoalbuminemia and in those with preexisting renal impairment due to age, atherosclerosis, hypertensive renal disease or other intrinsic renal disease (see Chapter 5.16). All these conditions are commonly present in aged end-stage RA patients. An apparently 'normal' serum creatinine level is misleading in these RA patients because of a significant diminution of muscle mass[15]. Impairment of renal function is enhanced by the prostaglandin suppressing effect of NSAIDs in combination with the commonly prescribed medication of diuretics. It is advisable to measure the patients' creatinine clearance in order to assess renal function and monitor the renal side effects of NSAIDs and the other antirheumatic drugs. Choosing NSAIDs with a short half-life can minimize their complications by diminishing overdosing and shortening the duration of the adverse effects after stopping the drug.

Slow-acting antirheumatic drugs

Slow-acting antirheumatic drugs (SAARDs) are used in the management of RA to achieve remission of the disease and slow down the progression of joint erosions. Their place in the treatment strategy is primarily in the earlier years of the disease. It therefore seems illogical to treat end-stage RA patients with such drugs since the disease has already run its destructive course. However, according to many clinical trials, institution of a SAARD may be very helpful in controlling the inflammatory process and consequently in reducing further deterioration of functional capacity and general condition, even in advanced disease. There is some evidence now that consistent use of SAARDs is associated with better long-term functional outcomes[16]. Also, when a SAARD is stopped because of a remission of the disease the risk of an exacerbation is doubled[17].

When clinical and laboratory parameters show evidence of an exacerbation of the disease after 2–6 weeks of rigid conservative treatment consisting of rest, splinting, exercises and NSAIDs, a change in the SAARD therapy has to be considered. Although end-stage RA patients have already been on most of the conventional SAARDs, there will usually be a few drugs left with which to treat an eventual exacerbation of the disease. In addition, the use of combination therapy of SAARDs in refractory RA that has failed on one or more SAARDs seems to be promising and is increasingly used in current practice[18,19]. It is uncertain, however, which SAARDs would be available for the treatment of end-stage RA if combination SAARD therapy in early RA becomes common practice[20,21]. There are also insufficient data available about a beneficial effect of SAARDs that are administered for a second time after they had been stopped previously because of toxicity, inefficacy or temporary remission of the disease process. Reinstatement of intramuscular gold therapy is considerably less effective than the first course of gold therapy[22,23]. However, when recommenced, corticosteroids and

TREATMENT OF AN EXACERBATION OF INFLAMMATORY DESTRUCTIVE JOINT DISEASE
Limited bed rest
Splinting
Exercises
NSAIDs
Intra-articular corticosteroid therapy
SAARDs
If necessary: low dose prednisone

Fig. 15.8 Treatment of an exacerbation of inflammatory destructive joint disease.

NSAIDs appear to have a therapeutic effect similar to that of an earlier treatment period.

The efficacy of SAARDs in advanced RA can only be evaluated reliably after a 3–6 month period of a full dose regimen. As with NSAID therapy in elderly RA patients, the physician must be attentive to masked organ failure, in particular renal failure, which necessitates dose adjustment of the SAARD.

DIAGNOSTIC PROBLEMS: EXACERBATION VERSUS DESTRUCTION

There may be a considerable overlap between the clinical features of a flare-up of long-standing RA and the clinical and laboratory abnormalities found in patients with mechanical problems in end-stage disease. The latter condition may be accompanied by an active synovitis, most likely the result of release of degradation products from the damaged joints. As in crystal-induced synovitis, dissolution and absorption of osseous and cartilaginous debris may give rise to an inflammatory process, though crystals have never been shown in the joints of these patients. Treatment of this ‘overlap’ condition consists of rest and, if necessary, local corticosteroid injections. Systemic treatment with SAARDs is not indicated in these cases; generally NSAIDs suffice. With this treatment policy, clinical and laboratory abnormalities subside within a few weeks. Therefore it is advisable to start with a conservative regimen in end-stage RA patients with active joint disease rather than starting immediately with a (new) SAARD. When after a few weeks no improvement has been achieved, therapy with a new SAARD can still be instituted (Fig. 15.8).

THE ROLE OF SURGERY IN THE TREATMENT OF END-STAGE RHEUMATOID ARTHRITIS

Surgical procedures including tenosynovectomy, tendon reconstruction, joint synovectomy, peripheral nerve decompression, joint fusion, cervical spine fusion and joint replacement can benefit selected patients with advanced RA (see Fig. 15.1). Although patients with advanced RA have a substantial risks of local and systemic surgical complications, recent advances in preoperative preparation, surgical techniques, prevention of infection and thromboembolism and postoperative care have decreased these risks significantly. The development of joint replacement surgery is a major step forwards in the management of RA patients with destructive disease. No longer are RA patients with damaged joints necessarily confined to the wheelchair. Hip and knee replacements have become routine operations in RA patients and replacements of the shoulder, elbow, wrist and ankle are increasingly being used in the management of destructive disease (see Chapter 3.12). The potential local and systemic complications of joint replacements and the long-term problems of implant loosening and wear make it appropriate to exercise caution in proceding with these procedures[24]. However, delaying surgery as a patient develops progressive muscle atrophy and contractures can compromise the results of operative treatment and increase the risk of complications. The surgical treatment strategy must conform to the patient's complaints. Pain relief and functional improvement are legitimate indications for surgical treatment when conservative measures have failed. We should always try, however, to evaluate the intended operation beforehand, answering the questions of whether surgery will really improve daily functions and whether this improvement will be a lasting one (see Chapter 3.12) (Fig. 15.9).

In general, surgical procedures should be considered for patients with end-stage RA who have not had a satisfactory response to other treatments (Figure 15.10). Surgeons perform tenosynovectomies and joint synovectomies as isolated procedures, most frequently for treatment of symptomatic synovitis of the wrist and hand that fails to respond to other treatments; but, more commonly they combine synovectomies with other procedures including tendon reconstructions, removal of bony prominences that may abrade tendons, joint replacements and joint fusions. Tenosynovectomies and joint synovectomies can improve motion in some patients and removal of bony prominences combined with synovectomy may decrease the risk of tendon rupture. Many patients with tendon ruptures can benefit from tendon reconstructions or transfers. Fusions of wrist, finger, thumb, ankle and foot joints can decrease pain, realign the joints and provide stability. Fusions of the cervical spine may prevent development or progression of neurologic deficits. Joint replacement is indicated for severely damaged large joints including the hip, knee, shoulder and elbow that are painful at rest and at night in spite of adequate conservative therapy. As to function, the mobility of the joint will often not improve after insertion of the joint prosthesis, but if muscle

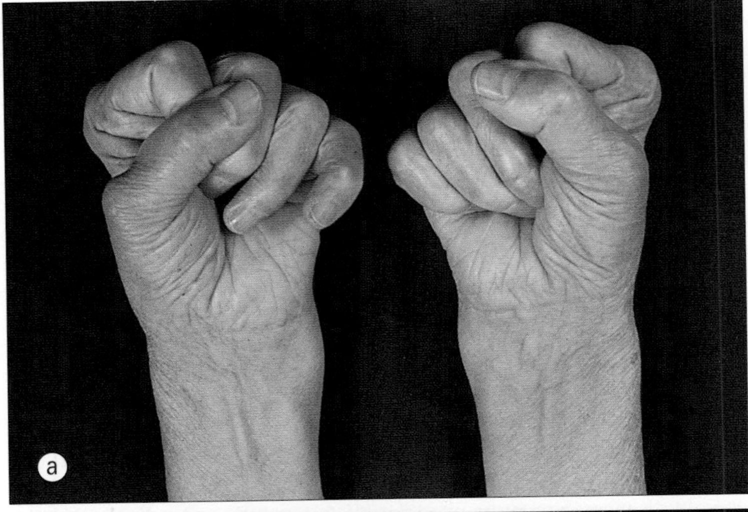

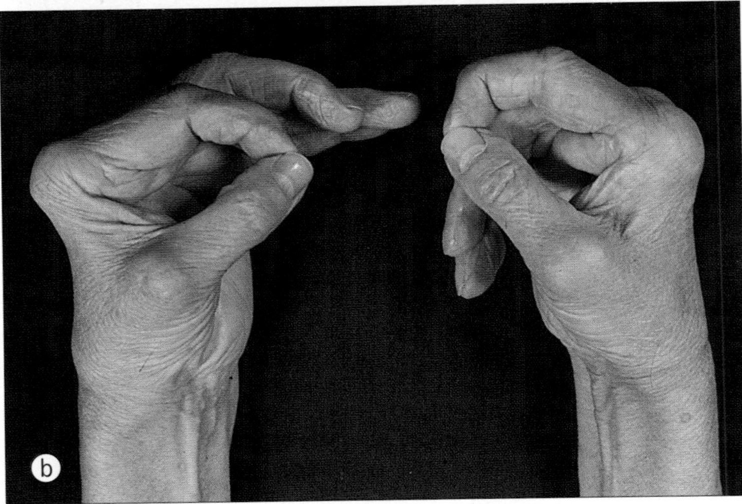

Fig. 15.9 Joint swelling, ulnar deviation, subluxation in metacarpophalangeal (MCP) joints. Grip function preserved (a). The same hands with sufficient pinch function (b).

SURGICAL TREATMENTS OF END-STAGE RHEUMATOID ARTHRITIS				
	Synovectomy	Arthrodesis	Joint replacement	Resection arthroplasty
Cervical spine		++		
Shoulder			+++	
Elbow	+		++	±
Wrist	+	++	±	
Thumb MCP & IP joint	+	++		
Finger MCP joint	+		+	
Finger IP joint	±	++	±	
Hip			+++	±
Knee			+++	
Talocrural joint		++	±	
Talocalcaneonavicular joints		++		
Big toe MTP joint		++		
Lateral toe MTP joint				+
Toe IP joint		+		±

Fig. 15.10 Surgical options available in end-stage RA. (IP, interphalangeal; MCP, metacarpophalangeal, MTP, metatarsophalangeal.)

strength is sufficient the joint can again exert its weight-bearing function, and joint replacement can correct skeletal deformities resulting from advanced RA. Ideally joint contractures can be improved by splints.

Since many patients with RA have involvement of multiple joints, optimal surgical treatment requires careful planning of the type and sequence of operative procedures and rehabilitation. The shoulder, elbow, wrist, hand, hip, knee, ankle and foot are all single elements of a functional chain which has to be looked upon as a whole[25]. For example, when a damaged hip has been replaced in order to reduce pain and improve mobility, the result in terms of functional improvement may be poor if problems of deformed ankles and feet have not been resolved. Sometimes it will be necessary first to perform a resection arthroplasty of the forefoot or an arthrodesis of the ankle to obtain the right functional result of the hip replacement. Also, in patients with destructive joint disease the replacement of one knee or hip often results in the replacement of both knees and hips (rule of four). Obviously, multiple surgery plays an important role in the management of end-stage disease. Fortunately, it may often be possible to resolve functional problems of several joints with conservative measures, such as shoe adaptation or functional aids. Sometimes joint replacement is not possible because of technical problems. In such cases excision arthroplasty or arthrodesis can provide acceptable pain relief (Fig. 15.10).

As to the surgical options for the shoulder and elbow, intractable pain is the most important indication for joint replacement[26,27]. Timing these operations may be very difficult, however, as bone and tendon condition may be very poor when the decision on surgical therapy has been made. The functional results of shoulder and elbow prostheses are not always favorable despite intensive postoperative physical therapy. Functional deterioration is the most important indication for surgical therapy of the hand in end-stage disease. Measurement of pinch and grip strength (see Fig. 15.9) is a simple and adequate method to assess hand function[28]. Severe malalignment of the MCP joints, inability to flex fingers or thumb and deformity of the thumb are important indicators of impaired hand function and are therefore potential objectives for surgical intervention[28]. For many patients arthrodeses of thumb or index finger produce better results in terms of function of the hand than do implants of finger prostheses.

The results of surgical treatment can be improved and the risks of surgical complications decreased by careful preoperative preparation and postoperative monitoring. Some patients will benefit from preoperative improvements in nutrition, joint range of motion and muscle strength. Preoperative adjustment of anti-inflammatory medications can decrease blood loss. Elimination of possible sources of infection including skin ulcers, the urinary tract and mouth before surgery helps decrease the risk of seeding the operative site. In some patients, especially those patients who undergo hip and knee replacement, thromboembolism prophylaxis is appropriate. Patients with joint replacements should be monitored indefinitely following surgery for radiographic evidence of periprosthetic osteolysis, which, when treated early, may halt progression to massive bone loss and implant failure. Any infections or skin ulcerations in these patients should be treated aggressively to decrease the risk of a bacteremia that leads to joint infection. Even those patients without signs of infection or skin ulceration must be carefully monitored for infection of their joint implants. Because joint infections in patients with end-stage RA may not cause striking clinical findings, physicians should consider joint aspiration in any patient with symptoms and signs that suggest the possibility of prosthetic joint infection. Early detection and aggressive treatment of a prosthetic joint infection may make it possible to save the implant or prevent the development of chronic osteomyelitis. In patients with multiple joint replacements, early treatment of an infected joint may prevent bacterial seeding of the other joints.

PROGRESSIVE MECHANICAL PROBLEMS IN END-STAGE RHEUMATOID ARTHRITIS

Pain and functional deterioration in end-stage RA patients are not always due to an exacerbation of the disease. Progressive joint destruction and secondary osteoarthritis will often lead to mechanically induced pain and functional deterioration. Treatment with SAARDs or NSAIDs will then make a limited contribution to the improvement of pain and functional status. The management of the progressively handicapped RA patient is complex. The patient needs an individual approach taking into account age, history, functional status, severity of pain, general condition, including concurrent diseases, psychologic and socioeconomic circumstances, and prognosis. The management team should include a rheumatologist, an orthopedic surgeon, a physical therapist, an occupational therapist and a social worker. The family doctor is also very important, being knowledgeable about the family situation.

It is clear that a program to restore functional ability may be very complex and will need the efforts of the whole management team, and indeed of the patients themselves who have to endure protracted hospital admissions, probably several operations with possible complications and then an intensive rehabilitation program.

When all possible medical, surgical and physical therapeutic treatments to restore patients' mobility and functional abilities have been exhausted, we are left with patients who have more or less severe handicaps. As patients' joint function cannot be improved anymore, there is a need to aim at maximal adaptation of the environment to patients' limitations. The occupational therapist and social worker will play an important role in this stage of the management. Many options are available to maintain the patients' independence, from simple aids that help to open a jar or pour tea to very complex constructional alterations of a house (see Chapter 3.11). Physical assistance may come from family, friends, neighbors and a community nurse. The success of this program is very much dependent on financial means and family circumstances.

It is obvious that great social and economic disparity between countries causes huge differences in therapeutic possibilities, in particular for incapacitated RA patients. This can not only result in an unsatisfactory living situation but also in early death[1]. It is known that patients with a bad functional status will develop more infections[29] and die earlier than patients who are functionally better off (see Chapter 5.14)[30].

MANAGEMENT OF EXTRA-ARTICULAR MANIFESTATIONS AND COMPLICATIONS

Being a systemic disease, RA not only affects the joints but may also cause a variety of systemic symptoms. It is often difficult to determine whether a specific symptom is attributable to an extra-articular manifestation, to a complication of RA, to a drug side effect or to a completely different illness. For example, neuropathy in a rheumatoid patient may be caused by an extra-articular manifestation (vasculitis of the vasa nervorum), by complications of RA, such as entrapment neuropathy (carpal tunnel syndrome) or polyneuropathy due to amyloidosis (see Chapter 8.27), by a drug side effect (chloroquine) or by a completely different disease, like diabetes mellitus or vitamin B deficiency. In the management of the extra-articular symptoms one has to be aware of all these various causes and a careful differential diagnosis is therefore demanded (Fig. 15.11).

EXTRA-ARTICULAR MANIFESTATIONS

Manifestations of vasculitis and systemic features are common in advanced disease and may even cause the predominant symptoms in patients with end-stage RA (see Chapter 5.4). In patients presenting with general malaise, excessive fatigue, diminished appetite, loss of weight or low-grade fever, the diagnosis of vasculitis has to be considered. Often, there are no signs of an active joint disease though other extra-articular features, such as nodules, episcleritis and pleural or pericardial effusions, are frequently present[31]. The laboratory results may record high ESRs often exceeding 90mm/h, anemia, a low serum albumin and sometimes elevated levels of liver enzymes. When neuropathy (either polyneuropathy or mononeuritis multiplex), palpable purpura, nail-fold lesions, digital gangrene, myopathy, skin ulcers that cannot be attributed to pressure (Fig. 15.12) or evidence of visceral ischemia are found, the suspicion of rheumatoid vasculitis is very high. A full thickness (skin and muscle) biopsy or a rectal biopsy must be performed in order to establish the diagnosis. In the biopsy a necrotizing arteritis of medium and large sized arteries similar to periarteritis nodosa can be found. The clinical syndrome accompanying this pathologic finding may vary considerably but can easily progress into life-threatening disease[32]. The overall mortality of patients with rheumatoid vasculitis is only slightly increased, however, when compared with RA controls which is probably due to the beneficial effect of prompt immunosuppressive and cytotoxic treatment of vasculitis patients with severe organ involvement[33]. Systemic necrotizing rheumatoid vasculitis is generally treated with a combination of high dose corticosteroids and cytotoxic drugs. A variety of treatments have been used, but the combinations of cyclophosphamide plus methylprednisolone, and azathioprine plus prednisone have been best

CLINICAL FEATURES DUE TO MANIFESTATIONS OF RHEUMATOID ARTHRITIS, ITS COMPLICATIONS OR TREATMENT, OR CONCURRENT DISEASE

Feature	Cause			
	Manifestation of RA	Complication of RA	Side effect of therapy	Concurrent disease
Neuropathy	Vasculitis	Local pressure Entrapment neuropathy Amyloid neuropathy	Chloroquine D-Penicillamine Gold	Diabetes mellitus complication of surgical procedures (hip/knee replacement)
Tendon rupture	Tenosynovitis	Irregular bone edge	Local corticosteroids	Trauma
Ulcers	Vasculitis	Pressure ulcers Perforated nodules Decubitus		Diabetes mellitus Corns, bunions Pyoderma gangrenosa
Anemia/leukopenia	Felty's syndrome	Gastric ulcers Vitamin deficiencies	NSAIDs SAARDs	Multiple myeloma Malignancy
Severe backache	Discitis	Osteoporosis	Corticosteroids	Menopause, aging
Pulmonary insufficiency	Pleuritis Pneumonitis	Cricoarytenoiditis	Methotrexate Gold D-Penicillamine	Congestive heart failure Sarcoidosis Malignancy Uremia/infection
Cardiac insufficiency	Pericarditis Carditis Valve disease Nodules	Conduction abnormalities	NSAIDs	Arteriosclerosis Viral disease Congenital abnormalities
Renal dysfunction	Vasculitis Proliferative glomerulonephritis	Amyloid	NSAIDs SAARDs	Nephrosclerosis Diabetes mellitus Intrinsic renal disease
Gastrointestinal symptoms	Vasculitis	Amyloid	NSAIDs SAARDs	Intestinal disease
Liver and spleen abnormalities	Felty's syndrome Sjögren's syndrome	Amyloid deposition	NSAIDs Azathioprine Methotrexate other SAARDs	Malignancy Viral infection and other causes
Headache	C1–C2 subluxation	Normal pressure hydrocephalus	NSAIDs	Arteriosclerosis Tumors
Eye involvement	Scleromalacia Scleritis (nodules, vasculitis)	Keratoconjunctivitis sicca	Chloroquine Corticosteroids	Eye diseases

Fig. 15.11 Clinical features due to manifestations of rheumatoid arthritis, its complications or treatment, or concurrent disease.

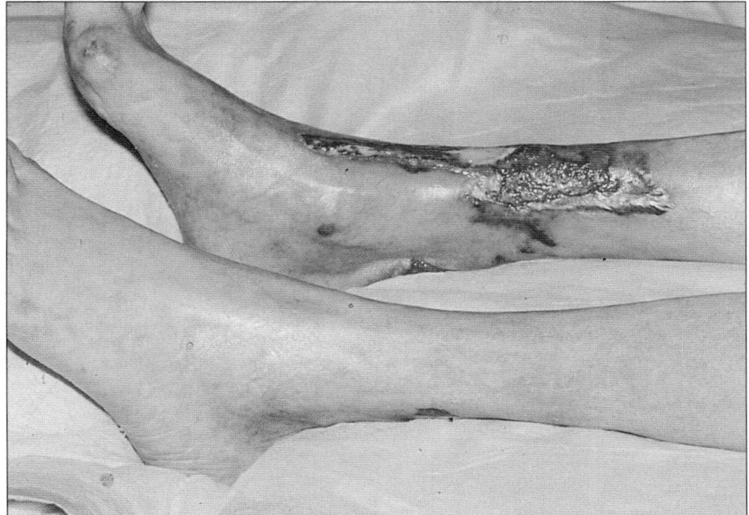

Fig. 15.12 Severe ulcers of the lower leg due to necrotizing vasculitis in RA.

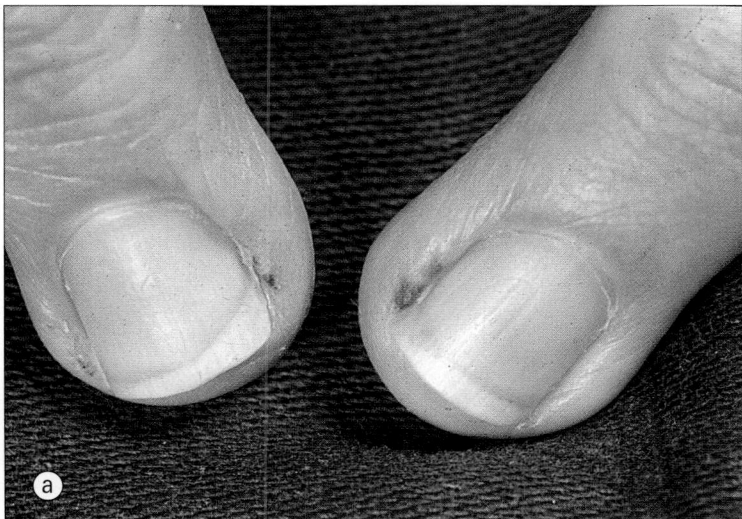

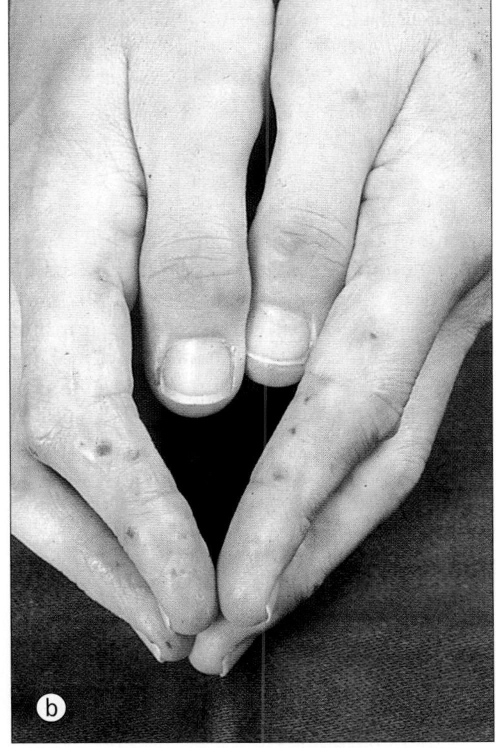

Fig. 15.13 Cutaneous vasculitis (a). Vasculitis lof the nailfolds (a) and thenar surfaces of the index fingers (b) in an RA patient with leuko-cytoclastic vasculitis (b).

documented and both have favorable results[34,35]. Rheumatoid vasculitis does not always cause severe systemic illness but comprises a broad spectrum of clinical and histologic features. Cutaneous vasculitis (leukocytoclastic vasculitis; Fig. 15.13) alone may not need immunosuppressive cytotoxic drugs, as conventional antirheumatic therapies appear to produce an equally good result[35].

Felty's syndrome

Felty's syndrome can be defined as seropositive RA with splenomegaly, and leukopenia, due to neutropenia. This syndrome has been shown to be associated with a number of extra-articular manifestations and recurrent infections. The extra-articular manifestations conform to those occurring in rheumatoid disease without neutropenia. The incidence of infections in Felty's syndrome is only increased if polymorphonuclear white cell counts fall below 100 cells/mm^3 [36]. Other factors influencing the incidence of infections are monocyte counts, complement activity, immune complex levels, skin ulcers and severity of physical handicap. A standard treatment for neutropenia in Felty's syndrome is not available. Splenectomy is still a controversial procedure. The results of various forms of drug treatment are not conclusive. There is no indication to administer potentially toxic drugs to patients with polymorphonuclear cell counts higher than 100 cells/mm^3; such treatment is only indicated when polymorphonuclear cells counts fall below this threshold[36].

Secondary Sjögren's syndrome

The prevalence of Sjögren's syndrome in RA varies between 11% and 62% depending on the definition used (see Chapter 7.32)[37]. Clinical features of this syndrome may become manifest at any time during the course of the disease. Keratoconjunctivitis sicca is the most common feature in RA patients with Sjögren's syndrome. Awareness of the benign course of secondary Sjögren's syndrome in RA may facilitate the patients' acceptance of this disorder. Artificial tears may ameliorate eye symptoms. Occlusion of the nasolacrimal ducts by electrocoagulation is rarely indicated. Topical antibiotics or antifungal treatment may be necessary in the case of secondary bacterial or fungal infections of the eye or mouth. In the case of xerostomia, meals should be taken with sufficient oral fluids. In between the meals ice cubes or water with some lemon juice will alleviate the discomfort of the xerostomia. Good dental care may prevent premature development of caries.

COMPLICATIONS OF RHEUMATOID ARTHRITIS

The most frequently occurring complications of RA are tendon ruptures and pressure ulcers. Potentially life-threatening complications are septic arthritis, instability of the cervical spine and amyloidosis. It is open to question whether osteoporosis has to be considered a manifestation or a complication of RA; it may be the result of ongoing disease activity, reduced mobility or treatment, in particular with corticosteroids[38,39]. The best treatment of osteoporosis is prevention by means of adequate antirheumatic therapy, exercise and sufficient daily intake of proteins, calcium and vitamin D. In overt osteoporosis treatment with bisphosphonates may be useful[40].

Tendon ruptures

Irregular bone edges resulting from the erosive process may erode tendons already weakened and attenuated by the action of proteinases produced by inflammatory cells. An active infiltrative tenosynovitis, though, may be enough by itself to cause tendon rupture. The dorsum of the wrist is the most vulnerable localization for rupture of the extensor tendons (Fig. 15.14). When the tenosynovitis does not respond to conservative treatment, dorsal tenosynovectomy, if necessary in combination with excision of the ulnar head, might prevent progressive damage to the extensor tendons. When one or more tendons have ruptured, prompt operative repair or tendon transfer is needed to restore hand function, often in combination with surgical

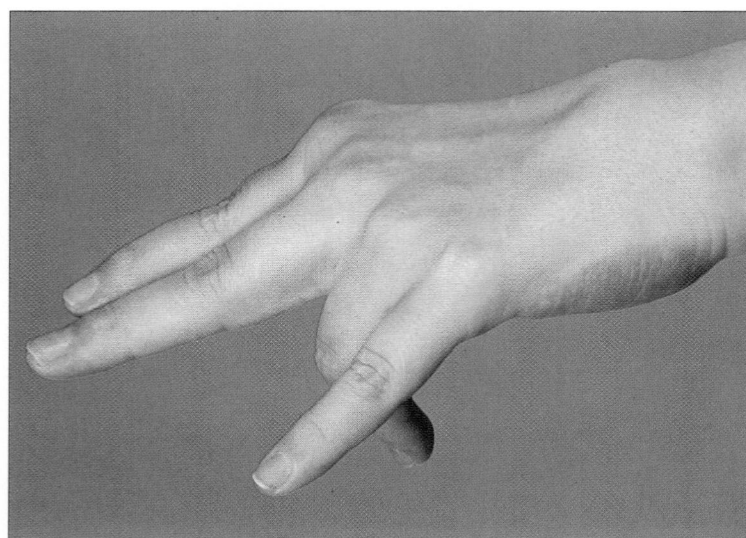

Fig. 15.14 Extensor tendon rupture of the fourth finger. Apart from repair of the tendon, tenosynovectomy, dorsal wrist synovectomy and ulnar head resection were also indicated.

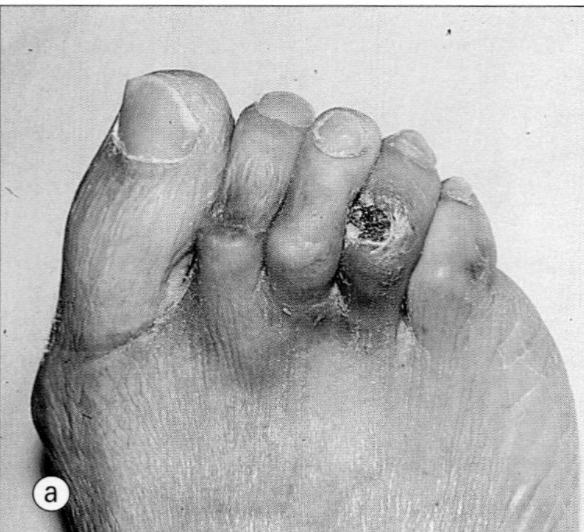

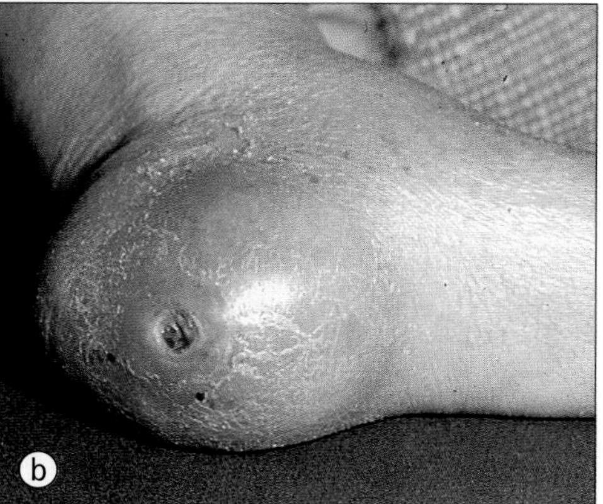

Fig. 15.15 Pressure ulcers. Ulceration over the surface of the PIP joints of the toe (a) and the olecranon bursa (b).

procedures to prevent rupture of the adjacent tendons (see Chapter 3.12). Not all tendon reconstructions are useful. The success of surgical repair is greatly dependent upon the size and the localization of the damaged tendon and the extent of joint deformation and destruction. For example, in patients with advanced ulnar deviation and subluxation in the MCP joints, repair of the ruptured extensor tendons of the third to fifth fingers hardly improves hand function. In ruptures of the flexor or extensor tendons of a distal interphalangeal (IP) joint (mallet finger) splinting will suffice. Ruptured thumb or index finger tendons should be repaired or reconstructed with tendon transfers as these digits are very important to hand function (tweezer and pinch grip)[28].

Pressure ulcers

In patients with advanced RA pressure ulcers are a common problem (see Chapter 5.16). In those immobile patients with severe joint deformations ulcers may develop at all sites exposed to pressure, e.g. above the IP joints of the toes, over bunions, ankles and elbows (Fig. 15.15). In patients confined to their bed ulcers may appear above the greater trochanter, in the lumbosacral region, on the buttocks or on the occiput and auricle. Sometimes these pressure ulcers may be preceded by the formation of small cutaneous nodules. The ulcers not only cause great inconvenience but also confer a considerable risk for bacterial arthritis, particularly in patients with prosthetic joints[41]. Eliminating the pressure, soaking the affected site in soda water or its equivalents and careful local therapy comprise the treatment of choice. Systemic antibiotic therapy is only indicated in case of bacteremia. It is sometimes difficult to determine whether pressure is the only cause of the ulcers, as vasculitic ulcers may appear at pressure sites. Irregular shaped purpuric lesions that proceed to nonhealing ulcers must be regarded as vasculitic lesions. In this case conservative treatment does not suffice and immunosuppressive therapy has to be added to the regime.

Entrapment neuropathy

Entrapment neuropathies in RA are caused by soft tissue swelling due to inflammation at a site where rigid structures constrain the peripheral nerve involved (see Chapter 4.16). The most common sites for pressure neuropathies are the carpal tunnel (median nerve), the elbow (ulnar nerve), popliteal space and fibular head (anterior tibial nerve) and tarsal tunnel (posterior tibial nerve). The main symptoms are dysesthesia and sensory loss in the area supplied by the entrapped nerve, sometimes accompanied by muscle weakness. Nerve conduction studies are helpful in the diagnostic process. The treatment aims to remove the pressure by reducing the inflammation by immobilization and local corticosteroid injection. The temporary use of a removable splint can be very helpful. If the inflammatory process is generalized, systemic therapy is needed. Surgical decompression is applied, particularly in median nerve compression, but for the other entrapment neuropathies a conservative approach is mostly pursued.

Instability of the cervical spine

In advanced RA the erosive process may lead to instability of the spine, in particular in the C1–C2 region (see Chapter 5.16). Nerve root compression due to the Cl–C2 subluxation may induce severe neck pain and occipital headache, whereas spinal cord compression causes neurologic symptoms such as sensory loss, paresis, disturbed bladder function and jerky legs. Surgical intervention is inevitable when neurologic abnormalities appear. Without surgical stabilization, the neurologic symptoms will progress with potentially devastating consequences including death[42]. It is possible, however, that after a few years the cervical segments below the ankylosed part become unstable. Occipital pain alone is not a firm indication for surgical fixation of the cervical spine. If a conservative approach with NSAIDs and immobilization with a neck collar ultimately does not suffice, surgical treatment for the intractable pain will be needed.

Amyloidosis

In advanced RA, amyloid deposits of the AA type may be found in various internal organs, but particularly in small vessels and parenchymal organs (see Chapter 8.27). The prevalence of amyloidosis in postmortem studies varies considerably, from 5–60%[43,44]. Approximately 10% of RA patients coming to autopsy have died from amyloidosis[45]. In the majority of patients the amyloidosis will not be recognized during life. Large deposits of amyloid in parenchymal organs may result in functional problems of specific organs. The kidney is almost invariably involved, with clinical symptoms of mild or severe progressive proteinuria, microscopic occult hematuria and mild or sometimes severe renal impairment. Gastrointestinal deposits of amyloid may cause gastrointestinal bleeding or malabsorption. Small vessel localization may lead to ischemic events and neuropathy. Restrictive heart disease and conduction disturbances may be the result of cardiac amyloid deposits.

In the case of the above-mentioned organ failures, particularly renal failure, amyloidosis should be considered. The most simple way to confirm the diagnosis is by performing a fine-needle biopsy of subcutaneous fat, or by a gingival or rectal biopsy (see Chapter 8.27). The sensitivity of rectal biopsy is somewhat higher, provided the sample contains submucosal tissue[46]. Renal or liver biopsy to establish the diagnosis is potentially hazardous because of the increased risk of hemorrhage. The histopathologic diagnosis is established by means of Congo red staining and the typical green and yellow birefringence under polarized light microscopy. Patients in whom the diagnosis of amyloidosis has been established have a poor prognosis. This is improving, however, due to the availability of better renal dialysis techniques and improved results of renal transplantation. There is no acceptable drug to dissolve the amyloid deposits already precipitated in the tissues. Together with the necessary symptomatic measures, adequate control of the activity of the inflammatory rheumatic process, with consequently less acute-phase protein formation and reduction of amyloid formation, is the most important step in the management of amyloidosis.

REFERENCES

1. Darmawan J. Rheumatic conditions in the Northern Part of central Java: an epidemiological survey. Doctoral Thesis, Erasmus University, Rotterdam.1988;97–102.
2. Vliet Vlieland TPM, Zwinderman AH, Vandenbroucke JP, Breedveld FC, Hazes JMW. A randomized clinical trial of in-patient multidisciplinary treatment versus routine out-patient care in active rheumatoid arthritis. Br J Rheumatol. 1996;35:475–82.
3. Ahlmén M, Sullivan M, Bjelle A. Team versus non-team out-patient care in rheumatoid arthritis. A comprehensive outcome evaluation including an overall health measure. Arthritis Rheum. 1988;31:471–9.
4. Vliet Vlieland TPM, Zwinderman AH, Vandenbroucke JP, Breedveld FC, Hazes JMW. In-patient treatment for active rheumatoid arthritis: clinical course and predictors of improvement. Br J Rheumatol. 1995;34:847–53.
5. Dubost, JJ Polyarticular septic arthritis. Medicine 1993:72:296.
6. Minor MA, Hewett JE, Webel RR, Anderson SK, Kay DR. Efficacy of physical conditioning exercise in patients with rheumatoid arthritis and osteoarthritis. Arthritis Rheum. 1989;32:1396–405.
7. Ende CHM van den, Hazes JMW, le Cessie S, *et al.* Comparison of high and low intensity training in well controlled rheumatoid arthritis. Results of a randomized clinical trial. Ann Rheum Dis. 1996;55:798–805.
8. Nordemar R, Ekblom B, Zachrisson L, Lundqvist K. Physical training in rheumatoid arthritis, a controlled long-term study I. Scand J Rheumatol. 1981;10:17–23.
9. Roth SH, Bennett RE. Nonsteroidal anti-inflammatory drug gastropathy. Arch Intern Med. 1987;147:2093–100.
10. Soll AH. Pathogenesis of peptic ulcer and implications for therapy. N Engl J Med. 1990;322:909–16.
11. Earnest DL. NSAID-induced gastric injury: It's pathogenesis and management. Arthritis Rheum. 1990;19(Suppl 2):6–10.
12. Raskin JB, White RH, Jackson JE, *et al.* Misoprostol dosage in the prevention of nonsteroidal anti-inflammatory drug-induced gastric and duodenal ulcers: a comparison of three regimens. Ann Intern Med. 1995;123:344–50.
13. Taha AS, Hudson N, Hawkey CJ, *et al.* Famotidine for the prevention of gastric and duodenal ulcers caused by nonsteroidal antiinflammatory drugs. N Engl J Med. 1996;334:1435–9.
14. Brooks PM, Day RO. Nonsteroidal antiinflammatory drugs: differences and similarities. N Engl J Med. 1991;324:1716–25.
15. Boers M, Dijkmans BAC, Breedveld FC, Mattie H. Errors in the prediction of creatinine clearance in patients with rheumatoid arthritis. Br J Rheumatol. 1988;27:233–5.
16. Fries JF, Williams CA, Morfeld D, Singh G, Sibley J. Reduction in long-term disability in patients with rheumatoid arthritis by disease-modifying antirheumatic drug-based treatment strategies. Arthritis Rheum. 1996;39:616–22.
17. Wolde S ten, Breedveld FC, Hermans J, *et al.* Randomised placebo-controlled study of stopping second-line drugs in rheumatoid arthritis. Lancet. 1996;347:347–52.
18. Tugwell p, Pincus T, Yocum D, *et al.* Combination therapy with cyclosporine and methotrexate in severe rheumatoid arthritis. N Engl J Med. 1995;333:137–42.

19. O'Dell JR, Haire CE, Erikson N, *et al.* Treatment of rheumatoid arthritis with methotrexate alone, sulfasalazine and hydroxychloroquine, or a combination of all three medications. N Engl J Med. 1996;334:1287–91.
20. Wilske KR, Healey LA. Remodeling the pyramid – a concept whose time has come. J Rheumatol. 1989;16:565–7.
21. McCarthy DJ. Suppress rheumatoid inflammation early and leave pyramids to the Egyptians. J Rheumatol. 1990;17:115–18.
22. Evers AE, Sundstrom WR. Second course gold therapy in the treatment of rheumatoid arthritis. Arthritis Rheum. 1983;26:1071–5.
23. Cats A. A multicentre controlled trial of the effects of different dosage of gold therapy, followed by a maintenance dosage. Agents Actions. 1976;6:355–63.
24. Hamalainen M, Hagena FW, Schwagerl W, Teigland J (volume editors). Revisional surgery in rheumatoid arthritis. Rheumatology: The interdisciplinary concept. Karger, Basel. 1990;13:1–265.
25. Hamalainen M, Hagena FW (volume editor). Rheumatoid arthritis. Surgery of the complex hand and foot. Rheumatology: An annual review. Karger, Basel. 1987;11:1–190.
26. Lettin AWF, Petersson C. (volume editors). Rheumatoid arthritis: Surgery of the shoulder. Rheumatology: The interdisciplinary concept. Karger, Basel. 1989;12:1–138.
27. Hagena FW (volume editor). Rheumatoid arthritis: Surgery of the elbow. Rheumatology: The interdisciplinary concept. Karger, Basel.1991;15:1–129.
28. Vliet Vlieland TPM, van der Wijk TP, Jolie IMM, Zwinderman AH, Hazes JMW. Determinants of hand function in patients with rheumatoid arthritis. J Rheumatol. 1996;23:835–40.
29. Albada-Kuipers GA, Linthorst J, Peeters EAJ, *et al.* Frequency of infection among patients with rheumatoid arthritis versus patients with osteoarthritis or soft tissue rheumatism. Arthritis Rheum. 1988;31;667–71.
30. Rasker JJ, Cosh JA. Cause and age at death in a prospective study of 100 patients with rheumatoid arthritis. Ann Rheum Dis. 1981;40:115–20.
31. Voskuyl AE, Zwinderman AH, Westedt ML, Vandenbroucke JP, Breedveld FC, Hazes JMW. Factors associated with the development of vasculitis in rheumatoid arthritis: results of a case-control study. Ann Rheum Dis. 1996;55:190–2.
32. Scott DGI, Bacon PA, Tribe CR. Systemic rheumatoid vasculitis: a clinical and laboratory study of 50 cases. Medicine. 1981;60:288–97.
33. Voskuyl AE, Zwinderman AH, Westedt ML, Vandenbroucke JP, Breedveld FC, Hazes JMW. The mortality of rheumatoid vasculitis compared to rheumatoid arthritis. Arthritis Rheum. 1996;395:266–71.
34. Scott DGI, Bacon PA. Intravenous cyclophosphamide plus methylprednisolone in treatment of systemic rheumatoid vasculitis. Am J Med. 1983;76:377–84.
35. Heurkens AHM, Westedt ML, Breedveld FC. Prednisone plus azathioprine treatment in patients with rheumatoid arthritis complicated by vasculitis. Arch Intern Med. 1991;151:224–54.
36. Breedveld FC, Fibbe WE, Hermans J, Cats A. Factors influencing the incidence of infections in Felty's syndrome. Arch Intern Med. 1987;147:915–20.
37. Andonopoulos AP, Drosos AA, Skopouli FN, Acriti NC, Moutsopoulos HM. Secondary Sjögren's syndrome in rheumatoid arthritis. J Rheumatol. 1987;14(6):1098–103.
38. Cough AKS, Liley, Eyre S, Holder RL, Emery P. Generalized bone loss in patients with early rheumatoid arhtritis. Lancet 1994;344:23–7.
39. Laan RFJM, van Riel PLCM, van de Putte LBA. Bone mass in patients with rheumatoid arthritis. Ann Rheum Dis. 1992;51:826–32.
40. Eggelmeijer F, Papapoulos SE, van Paassen HC, *et al.* Treatment with pamidronate increases bone mass in rheumatoid arthritis. Arthritis Rheum. 1996;39:396–402.
41. Kaandorp CJE, Schaardenburg van D, Krijnen P, Habbema JDF, Laar van de MAFJ. Risk factors for septic arthritis in patients with joint disease. Arthritis Rheum. 1995;38:1819–25.
42. Meyers KAE, Cats A, Kremer MHP, Luyendijk W, Onvlee GJ, Thomeer RTWM. Cervical myelopathies in rheumatoid arthritis. Clin Exp Rheumatol. 1984;2:239–45.
43. Saloman MI, Gallo G, Poon FP, Goldblat MV, Tehertkoff V. The kidney in RA. Nephron. 1974;12:297–310.
44. Boers M, Croonen AM, Dijkmans BAC, *et al.* Renal findings in rheumatoid arthritis. Clinical aspects of 132 autopsies. Ann Rheum Dis. 1987;46:658–63.
45. Laakso M, Mutru O, Ssomake H, Koota K. Mortality from amyloidosis and renal diseases in patients with rheumatoid arthritis. Ann Rheum Dis. 1986;45:663–7.
46. Breedveld FC, Markusse HM, Macfarlane JD. Subcutaneous fat biopsy in the diagnosis of amyloidosis secondary to chronic arthritis. Clin Exp Rheumatol. 1989;7:407–10.

RHEUMATOID ARTHRITIS 16

PRACTICAL PROBLEMS

RHEUMATOID FLARE

David L Scott

DEFINITION OF THE PROBLEM

Rheumatoid arthritis (RA) has a variable clinical course characterized by intermittent flares in disease activity. These flares comprise marked increases in the severity of the inflammatory synovitis together with systemic features of inflammation such as a very high acute phase response. There are variable constitutional symptoms.

THE TYPICAL CASE

A 49-year-old woman presented with RA 1 year previously. Her disease was mild and was controlled with the nonsteroidal anti-inflammatory drug (NSAID) ibuprofen 400mg q.i.d and intermittent analgesic (acetaminophen, 1 or 2 tablets p.r.n.). For the past month she had experienced increasing joint pain and swelling involving most of her peripheral joints and she was stiff for several hours each morning. She felt tired and unwell and had anorexia. Her peripheral joints were swollen and tender, she had large bilateral knee effusions and she walked slowly and with difficulty. Her hemoglobin was 9.6g/dl with a normochronic indices, platelet count 608 × 10^9/l, erythrocyte sedimentation rate (ESR) 98mm/h, C-reactive protein (CRP) 120g/dl, and rheumatoid factor titer (RA hemagglutination assay) 1:1024.

Medical treatment was changed to naproxen 500mg b.i.d. and dextropropoxyphene and acetaminophen (paracetamol) 2 tablets q.i.d. Intramuscular gold 50mg weekly was started together with a single intramuscular injection of methylprednisolone acetate 80mg. She was advised to rest at home for 1 week and was given advice on the nature of her medical treatment and the monitoring required. Her condition failed to settle and she was admitted to a specialized rheumatology unit, put on bed rest for a week and gradually improved. After discharge, the gold injections, naproxen and dextropropoxyphene and acetaminophen were continued without adverse effects. She had two more intramuscular methylprednisolone injections at monthly intervals. She continued an exercise program and planned rehabilitation.

DIAGNOSTIC PROBLEMS

The diagnosis of RA is usually well established and the flare in disease activity is self-evident, although intercurrent illnesses and sepsis can be difficult to differentiate. Rheumatoid disease follows a variable clinical course and disease activity waxes and wanes; it is sometimes difficult to ascertain whether current treatment has failed or a flare developed. A small group of RA patients (less than 10%) have progressive destructive

RHEUMATOID FLARE: THE KEY POINTS

- Characterized by marked activity of synovitis with variable systemic and constitutional symptoms
- Clinically many tender swollen joints (≥6), prolonged morning stiffness (>1 hour), and marked joint pain
- Elevated acute phase reactants with high ESR (>30mm/h or equivalent) and CRP
- A period of bed rest may help settle flares in some patients
- Principal drug treatment is to introduce a new or additional SAARD together with continuing NSAIDs and analgesia
- Short courses (1–3 months) of parenteral or oral corticosteroids are often needed
- Local intra-articular corticosteroids may benefit the worst-affected joints
- New therapeutic approaches, especially cytokine inhibition by antibodies to TNF-α, may be of considerable advantage, though they currently remain experimental

Fig. 16.1 Rheumatoid flare: the key points.

disease which is very difficult to control by most conventional therapies; it is as if they are in a continual state of flare. Discontinuing a slow-acting antirheumatic drug (SAARD) after a period of successful therapy, often due to an adverse effect, can precipitate a flare. In a few patients a flare can follow pregnancy, hinting at a hormonal etiology for at least some flares.

There are no absolute criteria for a disease flare; key points are given in Figure 16.1. Most will have active disease. Extra-articular features, such as an increased number of subcutaneous nodules, can accompany a flare. Although most flares are polyarticular, sometimes they are more restricted, involving a smaller number of joints, such as both knees. A related problem is when a flare occurs in late disease; there may be considerable joint destruction in long-standing RA and it can be problematic to differentiate a generalized disease flare from the pain and associated factors of end-stage joint failure. Another feature important to differentiate from a flare is the onset of extra-articular disease. Patients with systemic rheumatoid vasculitis usually develop this flare in their disease and many have inactive synovitis. Systemic vasculitis appears to be at the opposite end of the spectrum of disease pathogenesis from active synovitis and its treatment is somewhat different. However, in both circumstances serum acute-phase reactants are raised; constitutional symptoms such as fever, weight loss and malaise can occur.

THERAPEUTIC OPTIONS

Patients require a variety of antirheumatic drugs together with rest and subsequent rehabilitation. They normally need therapy with both a SAARD and a NSAID. There is insufficient evidence to demonstrate whether specific drugs in either category are especially effective for treating a disease flare. However, of the SAARDs, sodium aurothiomalate (injectable gold), methotrexate and cyclosporin should be preferred over penicillamine and sulfasalazine; auranofin (oral gold) and the antimalarials chloroquine and hydroxychloroquine seem less effective in such cases. Of the NSAIDs there is a broader choice of comparable drugs; diclofenac and naproxen are suitable examples and should be used together with an analgesic for pain control. Acetaminophen alone or in a compound formulation such as dextropropoxyphene or codeine and acetaminophen usually suffices.

In patients already taking a SAARD there is the question of maximizing therapy with one drug or starting a second SAARD. Most SAARDs are given at maximum dose from the initiation of therapy. But the dose of methotrexate can be increased to 20mg once a week (some rheumatologists give even higher dosages), intramuscular gold can be increased to weekly injections of 50mg, sulfasalazine to 3g daily and the dose of D-penicillamine up to 750mg daily, again with some rheumatologists giving even higher dosages. There is little evidence from randomized, controlled trials to support these increased dosages. There is debate about whether combining two or more SAARDs is of value in severe RA or an RA flare. Recent evidence favors this approach and the combination of methotrexate and cyclosporin has been shown to be more effective than methotrexate alone. More evaluation is needed before such combination therapy becomes part of routine clinical practice. But if a patient established on one SAARD has a flare it may be appropriate to start an additional SAARD concurrently.

The response to a SAARD such as injectable gold or methotrexate is not immediate, and it may take 6–8 weeks for an effect to be seen. Sometimes a response is delayed for 3 months or more. There is anecdotal evidence that some SAARDs have a more rapid onset of activity; this has been suggested for methotrexate, though the evidence is not strong. During this time, symptomatic treatment with NSAIDs and analgesics helps control the activity of the synovitis. It is often worthwhile changing the NSAID used at the onset of the flare, though there are no special advantages of one drug over another in this situation.

There is uncertainty about the relative benefits of hospitalization for RA. The balance of evidence suggests some time spent as an inpatient in a specialized unit helps control disease activity; with a very active arthritis, bed rest is advantageous. Supportive treatment in the form of physical therapy and occupational therapy is often used though there is also limited evidence for their effectiveness in a flare based on results of randomized, controlled trials

Local glucocorticosteroid injections into active joints are useful in controlling the extent of the synovitis and are frequently used. The place of systemic corticosteroids is more contentious. Short courses of oral prednisone or a depot intramuscular injection are often used in active disease when commencing therapy with a SAARD in an attempt to control symptoms before the SAARD has an appreciable effect. However, it is important to restrict these to short courses. The more prolonged use of oral corticosteroids has been shown to be advantageous in early disease and these agents may have a role in a flare in established disease, though most rheumatologists would exercise considerable caution in this situation. Pulse therapy with intravenous or intramuscular corticosteroids such as 0.5–1.0g methylprednisolone has a rapid onset of action but its advantage is often not maintained and its use remains dubious.

The rheumatoid flare has proved a good situation in which to test the value of cytokine inhibition in RA. This has been especially relevant in the use of monoclonal antibody therapy to inhibit tumor necrosis factor (TNF)-α, where there has been very impressive evidence of effectiveness with a rapid reduction in symptoms and the high levels of acute phase reactants such as CRP. Further work is needed to translate this approach into routine clinical practice, but it remains the most promising avenue for the control of flares in the foreseeable future.

Supportive measures such as patient education, the provision of simple aids, splinting of active joints and mobilizing physical therapy are all helpful adjuncts to medical treatment.

CONCLUSIONS

Rheumatoid patients with a flare in disease require assessment of disease severity, the introduction of, or change to a new SAARD, modification of treatment with NSAIDs and a period of rest. Education about their disease is important. Hospitalization and the use of glucocorticosteroids both have a role, although systemic corticosteroids should be restricted to short courses. Therapies to inhibit cytokine pathways by blocking specific cytokines, especially monoclonal antibody therapy to inhibit TNF-α, is an exciting area for future development.

REFERENCES

Elliott MJ, Maini RN, Feldmann M, *et al.* Randomised double-blind comparison of chimeric monoclonal antibody to tumour necrosis factor alpha (cA2) versus placebo in rheumatoid arthritis. Lancet. 1994;344:1105–10.

Hansen TM, Kryger P, Elling H, Haar D, *et al.* Double blind placebo controlled trial of pulse treatment with methylprednisolone combined with disease modifying drugs in rheumatoid arthritis. Br Med J. 1990;301:268–70.

Lansink M, de-Boer A, Dijkmans BA, Vandenbroucke JP, Hazes JM. The onset of rheumatoid arthritis in relation to pregnancy and childbirth. Clin Exp Rheumatol. 1993;11:171–4.

Murphy NG, Zurier RB. Treatment of rheumatoid arthritis. Curr Opin Rheumatol. 1991;3:441–8.

Tugwell P, Pincus T, Yocum D, *et al.* Combination therapy with cyclosporin and methotrexate in severe rheumatoid arthritis. N Engl J Med. 1995;333:137–41.

DEFINITION OF THE PROBLEM

If trauma can be shown to initiate or accelerate RA, the consequences for the patient would be considerable. Vigilance becomes salutary; if the noxious precipitant can be avoided, or thwarted, there should be fewer patients with RA or fewer in flare. But there is a downside; such cognizance is inherently inflammatory. After all, the patient suffering from RA learns he or she has been injured. 'Injury' implies more than proximate cause. To be injured is infuriating. It renders the pain more painful and the coping more challenging. Without injury, pain is one's fate to be managed, to be overcome. But the connotation of injury induces anger which can reduce the most rational of us even to animism. Otherwise, how is it that we can kick the door that just contused a finger? Injury connotes culpability which induces resentment and anger and the call for redress, if not revenge. Medicine is recruited by society – and the physician by the patient – to participate in each decision node of this syllogism. On what basis can we offer an opinion?

THE TYPICAL CASE

CA is a 23-year-old female college student who was injured in a head-on collision with an inebriated driver who lost control of his car. She suffered multiple fractures, a lacerated liver, a pneumothorax and a concussion and underwent hours of surgery followed by 3 weeks in an intensive care unit and 2 months of rehabilitation. Her recovery was miraculous. She returned to school, participating in a program of graduated exercises and progressing towards full health. Four months after the accident she noted the onset of polyarthritis which persisted and evolved into erosive seronegative RA. The consequences of the accident to the present were being fully indemnified by the insurer of the culpable driver. Her attorneys then advised her to claim that her RA was also a consequence of the accident. She was referred to a rheumatologist.

DIAGNOSTIC PROBLEMS

Neither the occurrence of trauma nor the outcome of RA are in question. The issue is how any confidence can be generated that this is more than coincidence. The clinical literature is a compendium of anecdote. Some of the more impressive anecdotes relate to psoriatic arthritis where discrete trauma to a joint is followed by psoriatic arthritis in that joint or post-traumatic reflex sympathetic dystrophy precedes psoriatic involvement in the same distribution. But these are anecdotes; they reflect the accrual bias of the publishing author. How many people with psoriasis who have traumatized a finger actually develop psoriatic arthritis in that finger? Precious few. Anecdotes of the coincidence of two events when one or both are common offer no substantive insight into pathogenesis.

However, there is some relevant science. Julkunen *et al.* in Helsinki determined the incidence of RA 2 years after 270 consecutive survivors of multiple trauma left the hospital. For comparison, 103 controls were randomly selected from the population at large and followed for two years. The principle results are presented in Figure 16.2. The study is easy to criticize. This case control study should be considered as hypothesis generating, not conclusive. However there exists no more compelling a data set.

What should the patient be advised? The only way to 'prove' causation in law is to overwhelm the 'finder of fact' (judge or jury) with pathos. Data alone will not suffice; any 'expert' who asserts causation based on the Helsinki data, let alone the compendium of anecdotes, will be challenged by another 'expert' capable of a potentially devastating critique. The pathos of the claimant is the most cogent argument. However, communicating the pathos, escalating the anger, dwelling on and recording the experience, living the incapacities are all necessary in order to sway the finder of the fact. All of these dynamics belie the wisdom of any rheumatologist experienced in managing the patient with RA. The process of tort is itself iatrogenic! Is the trade-off worthwhile, let alone reasonable?

And if the patient 'wins' – if the RA is adjudged a consequence of trauma – what is won? How much money is to be awarded for pain? for suffering? for incapacity? Pain cannot be measured, nor can suffering. So the patient–claimant is then faced with proving that she is as incapacitated as she claims. How is that determined? The opinion of a treating physician is seldom deemed valid. Rather, 'experts' are compensated to perform this task. Most rely on, or are constrained to rely on, a century-old tradition of 'impairment rating'; symptoms of incapacity are only valid if they correlate with the magnitude of pathoanatomic derangement. This tenet is so ingrained that most physicians are blind to the fact that it is a sophism. None the less, if the patient–claimant is not dramatically damaged by RA, it will be assumed that he/she is not as incapacitated as he/she claims.

Nothing is as debilitating as having to prove you are ill. No wonder it is far more likely that any patient/claimant will have escalating illness than that they will be awarded any substantial indemnity!

CONCLUSIONS

The wise treating physician will apprise his or her patient of the facts and fallacies of considering RA as a consequence of trauma. If they choose to pursue life in that algorithm, they need all the more support. Clinicians who are involved as the 'expert' who sits in judgment on a patient such as CA realize that they serve a master never envisioned by Maimonides.

As the 'expert' regarding the validity of the causal inference, physicians realize that the above 'typical case' took advantage of the only substantive data relating to traumatic causation in RA. More typical are the cases which try to argue that less dramatic trauma or even 'stress' was the culprit. Today such arguments are naught but fantasy. Nonetheless, they find a ready audience in the litigiousness which provides too ready a home for latter-day sophists.

INCIDENCE OF RA 2 YEARS AFTER MAJOR TRAUMA

RA	Trauma patients (%)	Controls (%)
Old cases	2.5	2.9
New cases	2.9	0

Fig. 16.2 Incidence of RA 2 years following major trauma. Data are taken from the Helsinki study performed by Julkunen *et al.*, 1974.

REFERENCES

Conca W, Laubenberger J, Krause T, Blumberg H, Peter HH. Posttraumatic reflex sympathetic dystrophy anteceding inverse psoriasis and psoriatic arthritis. J Rheumatol. 1995;24:783–5.

Hadler NM. Occupational musculoskeletal disorders. New York: Raven Press; 1993:1–272.

Julkunen H, Räsänen JA, Kataja J. Severe trauma as an etiologic factor in rheumatoid arthritis. Scand J Rheumatol. 1974;3:97–102.

DEFINITION OF THE PROBLEM

Destructive lesions of the cervical spine in RA are the result of chronic, nonspecific inflammation of the synovial tissue leading to the destruction of cartilage, bone and ligaments. Postmortem studies have frequently shown synovitis in the odontoid–atlas joints, in the uncovertebral joints (joints of Luschka) and in the interlaminar joints. The pathologic changes give rise to instability of the cervical spine. Abnormal mobility is most commonly found in the C1–C2 region, but may also occur at lower levels. Like arthritis of the peripheral joints, involvement of the cervical spine can cause pain and impaired mobility. The instability leads to nontraumatic dislocations that may occasionally cause neurologic disturbances.

THE TYPICAL CASE

A 63-year-old housewife with a 17-year history of seropositive RA was seen for evaluation of occipital headaches, heaviness of the arms and tingling and numbness in the hands. She had noted muscle weakness in the arms and intermittent, spontaneous jumping legs when recumbent. Micturition was not impaired. A global reduction in head movements of about 50% had been present for several years. Neurologic examination revealed a spastic paresis of both arms and the right leg with a positive Babinski's sign and impaired vibration sense in both lower arms, hands and legs. Radiographs of the cervical spine showed a subluxation of C1 on C2 of 15mm in flexion and 2mm in extension (Fig. 16.3). Magnetic resonance imaging (MRI) of the cervical spine revealed an anteroposterior slip of C1 on C2, obliteration of the subarachnoid space and compression of the cervical cord by the posterior arch of C1 (Fig. 16.4). Lying supine as much as possible during a week, followed by nearly 1 week's skull traction relieved the symptoms in the hands. She gained strength in her arms. Neurologic examination disclosed normal vibration sense in both legs and flexor plantar responses. At operation, fusion was performed of the occiput down to C4, using two autogenous bone grafts from the iliac crest fixed by steel wire (Fig. 16.5). After the operation, the patient received continuous skull traction applied through a Blackburn caliper and was nursed on a Stryker CircOlectric™ bed for a period of 3 months. After removal of the traction the patient was provided with a soft collar.

DIAGNOSTIC PROBLEMS

The prevalence of radiologically established instability of the atlantoaxial vertebrae in patients with RA has been estimated to be 6.4% in patients with clinical evidence of RA and 19% in RA patients admitted to a hospital. Other hospital studies have confirmed these figures, and percentages as high as 23–32% have been reported.

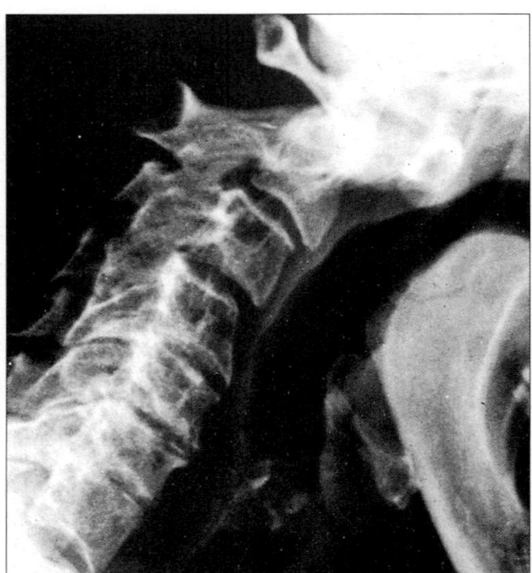

Fig. 16.3 Instability of the cervical spine. The slip of C1–C2 distance between atlas and ventral side odontoid process exceeds 15mm.

Motor power testing in these patients is often unreliable due to severe joint deformities and muscle wasting. It may be impossible to elicit reflexes. Sensory disturbances in the extremities are major pointers to a spinal cord lesion. Because the sensory loss in these patients may frequently be symmetric, other neurologic disorders such as carpal tunnel syndrome and polyneuropathy as a result of vasculitis or nutritional deficiency should be considered. It is striking that, just as in other cervical myelopathies and syringomyelia, the vibration sense is lost and the position sense retained in the majority of patients with rheumatoid cervical myelopathy. Painful arthritis of the knee(s) may mask jumping legs; the latter is a consequence of spinal automatism. Involvement of the cervical spine by the rheumatoid process is often accompanied by neck pain radiating to the occiput, even in the absence of spinal cord lesions. Occipital headache may occur in the absence of any visible radiologic spinal abnormality, but the reverse is also true: severe lesions can be seen in patients without any complaints.

However, severe neck pain, often radiating to the occiput, is one of the main features alerting the physician to the possibility of spinal cord damage. Clinical signs and symptoms as a result of vertebral artery dysfunction (vestibular features and diplopia) occur in only a minority of these patients. Additional alarm signs of spinal cord damage in RA are recognized (Fig. 16.6).

Collapse of the lateral mass of C1 may result in characteristic tilting of the head towards the affected side. A C1–C2 slip (or horizontal atlantoaxial dislocation) is the result of laxity or destruction by pannus of the transverse ligament of the atlas. This ligament connects the lateral masses of the atlas, keeping the odontoid process in close apposition to the anterior arch of the atlas. A C1–C2 subluxation can be visualized on a lateral radiograph of the upper cervical spine in maximal flexion (Fig. 16.7). The distance between the posterior rim of the anterior arch of the atlas and the anterior margin of the dens is abnormal if it exceeds 4mm. Destruction of the odontoid process by rheumatoid granulomatous inflammation may also produce a Cl–C2 slip.

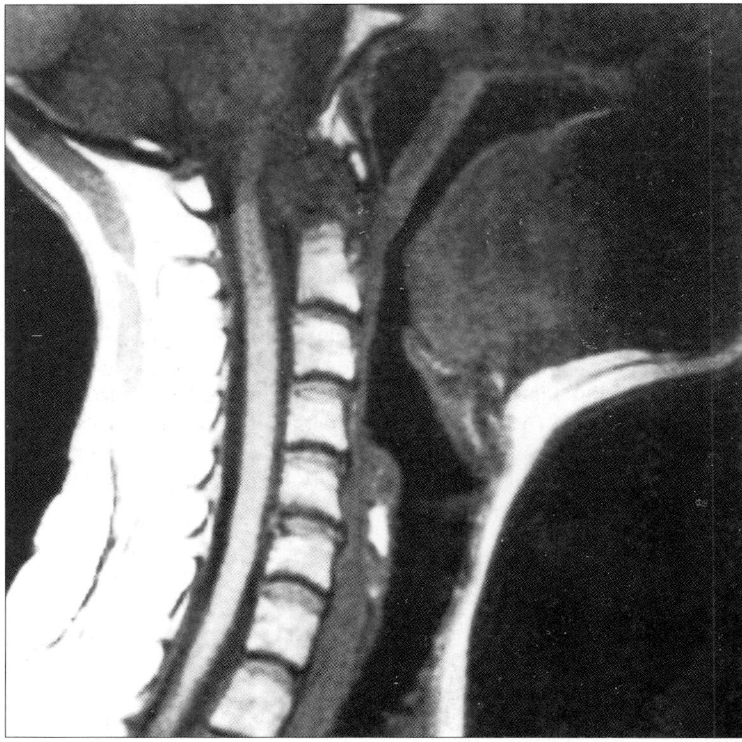

Fig. 16.4 MRI of the unstable cervical spine (Tl-weighted). There is compression of the cervical cord by pannus along the posterior margin of the . Courtesy of John L Sherman, Washington Imaging Center, Washington DC.

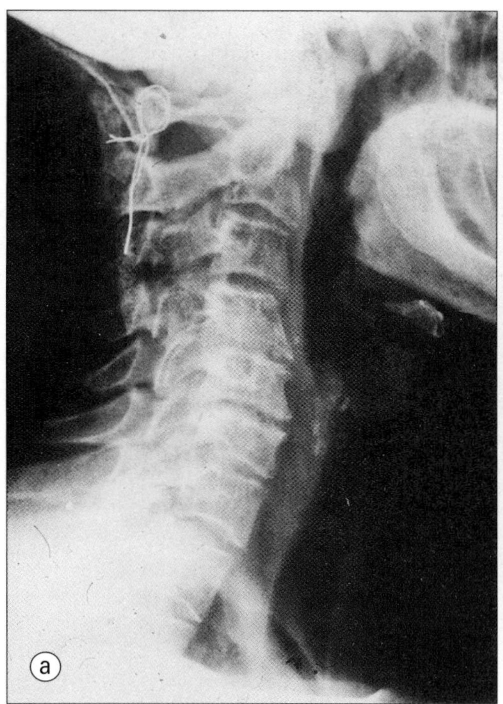

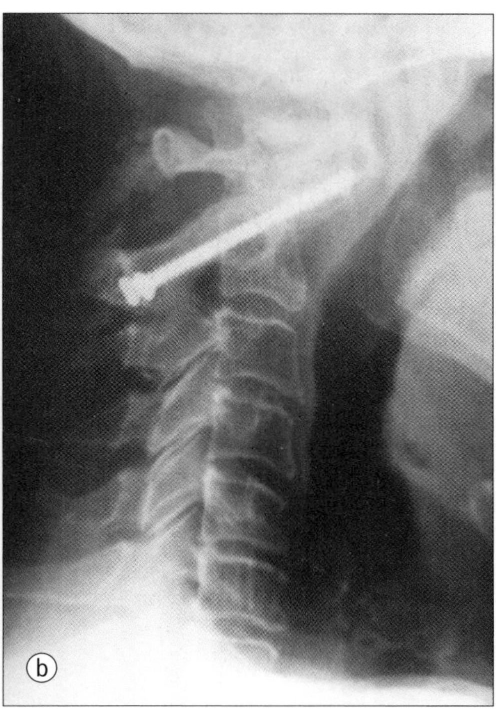

Fig. 16.5 Surgical procedures for C1–C2 instability. (a) Bone graft and wiring and (b) C1–C2 fusion with cannulated screws.

ALARM SIGNS OF SPINAL CORD DAMAGE IN RHEUMATOID ARTHRITIS
Severe neck pain, often radiating to the occiput
Diminished motor power in arms and legs
Tingling of the fingers and feet, or only numbness
A 'marble' sensation in the limbs and trunk
Jumping legs, as a consequence of spinal automatism
Disturbed bladder function, varying from incontinence to urinary retention

Fig. 16.6 Alarm signs of spinal cord damage in RA.

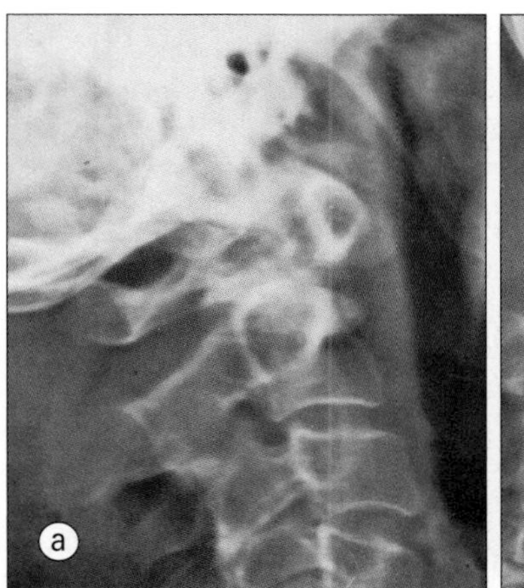

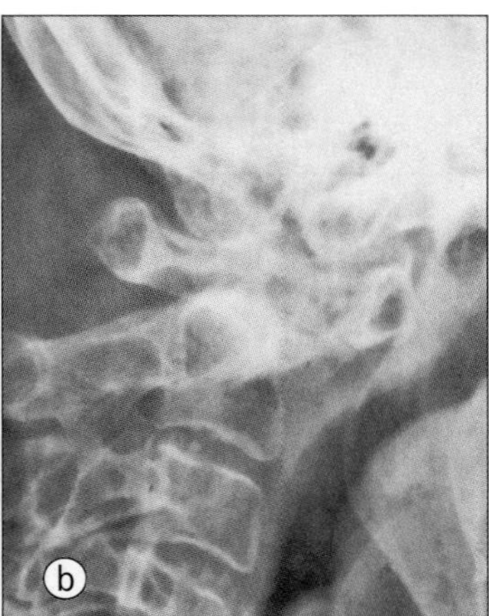

Fig. 16.7 Lateral views of the cervical spine. (a) Lateral view in extension: the distance between the dorsal side frontal bow C1 and ventral side of the odontoid process is 2mm. (b) Lateral view cervical spine in flexion: there is a slip of at least 8mm (distance between frontal bow C1 and odontoid process).

Vertical dislocations, also visible on lateral views, are caused by destruction or collapse of the lateral part of the atlas and axis. The odontoid process can then penetrate the foramen magnum, putting pressure on the brainstem, which may be fatal (basilar invagination). Destruction of the dens by the rheumatoid process may be lifesaving in both vertical and horizontal dislocations.

Myelography is a relatively difficult and hazardous procedure for establishing cord compression in patients with severe deformity; MRI thus appears to be a valuable addition in the assessment of spinal cord damage.

THERAPEUTIC OPTIONS

The presence of neurologic symptoms and signs and cord compression confirmed by MRI is a very strong indication for neurosurgery. A single horizontal or vertical spinal dislocation without significant neurologic features and no visible spinal cord damage on MRI requires no surgical intervention. Occipital headache often may be the only symptom present in these patients; for this a neck collar may suffice and, if necessary, NSAIDs and simple neck traction. This conservative approach is in contrast to that of others who advocate surgical treatment for intractable neck pain and instability without neurologic deficit. An operation is inevitable if a patient has cord compression and neurologic abnormalities. If an operation cannot be performed because of poor general health (involving too great an operative risk) or because of refusal, neurologic progression is to be expected and the 1-year prognosis is very poor (Fig 16.8). As most patients with this neurologic complication of RA are already severely crippled, ambulant postoperative treatment with halo traction and brace is not a practical alternative. Skull traction using a Blackburn caliper should be started a few days before operation. The aim of the operation is fusion of C1 and C2 spinous processes with the occiput and some lower vertebrae by means of transarticular facet screw fixation of C1–C2 and interspinous bone graft with cable fixation. Sometimes fusion with cannulated screws of C1–C2 may be sufficient (see Fig. 16.5b). There is a risk of vertebral artery injury during screw passage. Even in the presence of inflammatory tissue behind the odontoid peg, a posterior fusion is advocated because rheumatoid granulation tissue subsides with immobilization. Depending on the patient's condition, mobilization may start soon after the operation.

Recurrent subluxation has been observed after some years, often at subaxial levels. About 10% of patients in whom the diagnosis of C1–C2 slip has been established die either before surgery or shortly afterwards. Half the patients operated on have a life expectancy of approximately 5 years; in this latter group, death is not the direct result of cord compression.

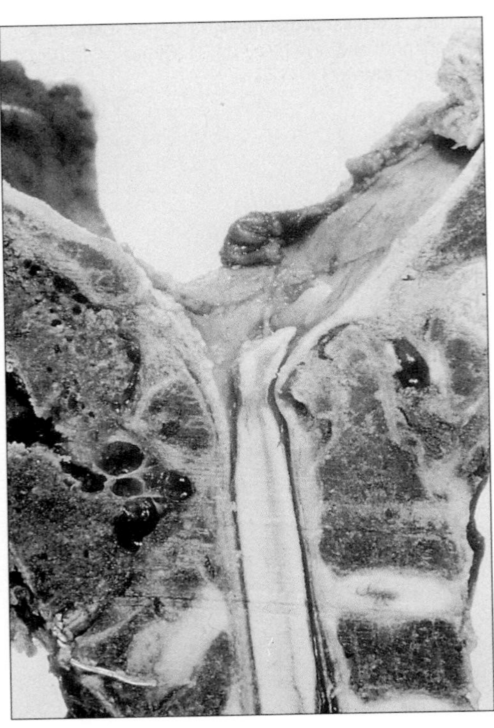

Fig. 16.8 Median saw cut of the cervical spine in RA. There is compression of medullary cord and forward dislocation of the atlas with respect to the axis.

CONCLUSIONS

Patients with RA are at risk of developing instability of the cervical spine. These patients should be carefully assessed because neurologic symptoms may develop. The preferred imaging modality for establishing the site of the cord compression is MRI. Surgical intervention is indicated in the presence of neurologic deficits and a neuroanatomic lesion.

REFERENCES

Agarwal AK, Peppelman WC Jr, Kraus DR, Eisenbeis CH Jr. The cervical spine in rheumatoid arthritis (editorial). Br Med J. 1993;306:79–80.

Breedveld FC, Algra PR, Vielvoye CJ, Cats A. Magnetic resonance imaging in the evaluation of patients with rheumatoid arthritis and subluxation of the cervical spine. Arthritis Rheum. 1987;26:624–9.

Dickman CA, Foley KT, Volker K, Sonntag VKH, Smith MM. Cannulated screws for odontoid screw fixation and atlantoaxial transarticular screw fixation. J Neurosurg. 1995;83:1095–100.

Horst-Bruinsma van der IE, Markusse HM, Macfarlane JD, Vielvoye CJ. Rheumatoid discitis with cord compression at the thoracic level. Br J Rheumatol. 1990;29:65–8.

Marks JS, Sharp J. Rheumatoid cervical myelopathy. Q J Med. 1980:199(NS):307–19.

CARPAL TUNNEL SYNDROME

Michael H Weisman

DEFINITION OF THE PROBLEM

Carpal tunnel syndrome (CTS) is an entrapment neuropathy caused by compression of the median nerve at the wrist in the carpal canal. Known causes include tenosynovitis associated with RA and other inflammatory disorders, acute trauma, pregnancy and repetitive use. Initially, the median nerve appears normal when examined microscopically, but as the process proceeds and becomes chronic, focal demyelination or wallerian degeneration may take place. In the late stages, frank axonal atrophy can occur both proximal and distal to the site of compression. Functional impairment of the thumb and hand can result from untreated disease.

THE TYPICAL CASE

A 74-year-old man was referred for evaluation of the abrupt onset of polyarthritis of his hands, wrists and shoulders. He had noted marked limitation in mobility of his wrists as well as his shoulders and had been entirely overcome by this illness such that he became almost nonfunctional. He was having difficulty even getting out of bed or a chair. On detailed questioning it became clear that he was waking in the middle of the night with quite severe pain in his hands, described as 'being like burning' and associated with a loss of feeling. He felt 'as if he has gloves on his hands' and could not feel fine objects. He found that rubbing his hands together and shaking them 'gets the circulation back' and improved the symptoms.

Sensory testing for light touch and pinprick was normal in both hands and wrists. Testing for thenar motor power was limited by pain in the thumb joints. Thenar muscle bulk appeared to be normal bilaterally. Phalen's sign was negative, although the patient was unable to complete the maneuver because of wrist pain. Tinel's sign was negative bilaterally.

DIAGNOSTIC PROBLEMS

The diagnosis of carpal tunnel syndrome is clinical and based upon the proper interpretation of symptoms and signs with confirmation by electrodiagnostic testing. The earliest signs of carpal tunnel syndrome are sensory; late findings are motor. Pain and paresthesias may occur in either the sensory distribution of the median nerve in the hand, thumb, index and long fingers, as well as the radial half of the ring finger or sometimes the whole hand. Forearm pain is not uncommon. Patients almost always experience the pain at night and give a typical history of awakening with their hands asleep, rubbing them together and shaking them to get the normal feeling back. When motor compromise occurs later, attention should be drawn to atrophy of the thenar eminence with selective weakness of abductor pollicis brevis and opponens pollicis.

The time-honored noninvasive tests are simple to do but are either nonspecific, in the case of Phalen's sign, or insensitive, for example Tinel's sign. Electromyography (EMG) and nerve conduction tests are more sensitive and have the virtue of providing quantification of the deficit, especially if there is motor involvement of the thumb. However, even these examinations are not 100% accurate.

It is not difficult to see why carpal tunnel syndrome occurs frequently in RA. Dramatic swelling of the hands is a common early finding in the disease; later, synovial hypertrophy and tenosynovial thickening are responsible for compressing the median nerve (Fig. 16.9). Not uncommonly older patients with seronegative arthritis present with swollen hands and paresthesias due to median nerve compression. In the early stages of seropositive RA, pain and stiffness in the joints may overshadow the sensory symptoms of carpal tunnel syndrome.

Several conditions that occur in patients with RA can mimic carpal tunnel syndrome (Fig. 16.10). Treatment for each of these conditions is highly specific, and distinction of one from another is required. Mononeuritis multiplex from vasculitis of the vaso nervorum can cause a mononeuropathy of the median nerve. The setting is usually (but not always) in long-standing RA and in patients seropositive for rheumatoid factor in high titer with evidence of other systemic manifestations. In the case of mononeuropathy, nerve conduction velocity will be slowed at different points, not just limited to the carpal canal.

Physical examination will usually distinguish between tendon rupture and weakness of the small abductor and opponens of the thumb associated with atrophy of the outer aspects of the thenar muscle bulk. A more difficult problem arises (discussed below) in differentiating extensor tendon rupture from radial nerve entrapment.

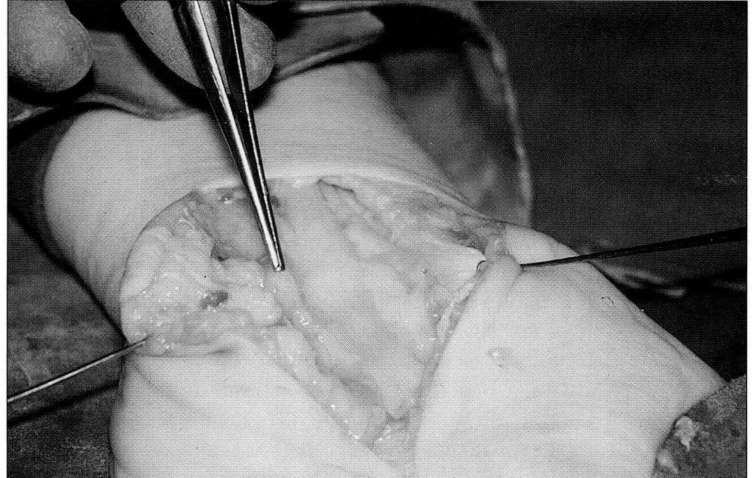

Fig. 16.9 Compression of the median nerve in carpal tunnel syndrome in RA. In this surgical decompression of the median nerve, the carpal tunnel is exposed from the palmar aspect and inflamed synovial tissue and the compressed median nerve are seen. Courtesy of Mr J Browett.

DIFFERENTIAL DIAGNOSIS OF CARPAL TUNNEL SYNDROME IN RHEUMATOID ARTHRITIS
Mononeuritis multiplex due to vasculitis
Tendon rupture
Cervical spine radiculopathy
Brachial plexus compression neuropathy
Ulnar nerve compression at the elbow
Posterior interosseous nerve syndrome

Fig. 16.10 Differential diagnosis of carpal tunnel syndrome in RA.

Cervical spine radiculopathy involving C6 may cause a sensory and motor neuropathy that could be confused with carpal tunnel syndrome. However, the sensory loss is in a C6 dermatome distribution with findings on the dorsal surface of the hand extending up the arm to the elbow. Diminished biceps and brachioradialis reflexes are usually associated with the weakness of the biceps and brachioradialis muscles.

The use of crutches by a RA patient can lead to radial nerve compression in the axilla and a brachial plexus compression neuropathy.

Ulnar nerve compression at the elbow, caused by rheumatoid inflammation and/or joint destruction, can produce ulnar nerve symptoms that range from minor irritating paraesthesias to weakness of the intrinsic muscles of the hand. Sensory loss involves the fifth finger and part of the fourth finger, the hypothenar eminence and part of the dorsum of the hand.

A posterior interosseous nerve syndrome, or compression of the pure motor branch of the radial nerve at several possible locations near the elbow, may be caused by rheumatoid disease and lead to some variability in physical findings. However, pain and paresthesias are always absent, pointing to the correct diagnosis. Inability to extend the four digits at the metacarpophalangeal (MCP) joints while maintaining wrist extension is the cardinal sign of this syndrome.

THERAPEUTIC OPTIONS

The first principle of treatment is to make an accurate diagnosis and differentiate CTS from other neuropathies.

In the recent-onset RA patient, treatment is usually not directed at the CTS *per se* but at the active synovitis. Once the swelling in the hands is reduced, the symptoms of median nerve compression will almost always abate. Treatments for RA such as NSAIDs, corticosteroids and the early introduction of disease-modifying agents should be sufficient. An important adjunct not only for the arthritis of the hands and wrists but also to control symptoms of carpal tunnel syndrome is the liberal use of resting hand and wrist splints in early-stage disease. Ideally, the splints should be custom-made for each patient from lightweight material and extend from the upper forearm to include the hand and all of the digits. They should be worn at night and as much as possible during the day.

The development of carpal tunnel syndrome symptoms in established RA under optimum treatment requires a different approach. When symptoms are minor and intermittent, empirical use of splints should be tried. If symptoms are not eliminated, then electrodiagnostic studies should be performed. If these reveal prolonged median nerve distal motor latency, or if there is evidence of denervation of the thumb muscles innervated by the median nerve, further conservative treatment is likely to fail, and the patient should be referred to an experienced hand surgeon for carpal tunnel release.

CONCLUSIONS

Carpal tunnel syndrome occurs frequently in RA and the diagnosis is based on the interpretation of clinical signs and symptoms. There is no convincing evidence that corticosteroid injections have a long-term benefit. Indications for tenosynovectomy are the same as in any other joint; they are synovitis and pain in one joint disproportionate to that in the rest of the joints in the body and producing significant important disability beyond that which can be controlled with systemic medications.

REFERENCES

Chamberlain MA, Corbett M. Carpal tunnel syndrome in early rheumatoid arthritis. Ann Rheum Dis. 1970;29:149–52.

Hadler N. The carpal tunnel syndrome. In: Medical management of the regional musculoskeletal diseases. Orlando: Grune & Stratton; 1984:143–55.

Katz JN, Stirrat CS. A self-administered hand diagram for the diagnosis of carpal tunnel syndrome. J Hand Surg (Am). 1990;15:360–3.

Katz JN. Carpal tunnel syndrome and other workplace-related upper extremity pain disorders. Postgrad Adv Rheumatol. 1991;16:4–9.

Kritchevsky M. Disease of peripheral and cranial nerves. In: Wiederholt W, ed. Neurology for non-neurologists. Philadelphia: Grune & Stratton; 1988:223–38.

DIAGNOSIS AND MANAGEMENT OF ACUTE SYNOVIAL RUPTURE OF THE KNEE

Allan St J Dixon

DEFINITION OF THE PROBLEM

Joints distended with synovial fluid under pressure may rupture, releasing the fluid into the surrounding tissue spaces. When the fluid contains mediators of inflammation, as in RA, it causes widespread inflammation and edema. Noninflammatory fluid, as in some forms of osteoarthritis (OA), causes little reaction other than transient swelling of the surrounding tissues.

THE TYPICAL CASE

A 42-year-old women recently developed RA and her right knee was swollen. She sat on a bench watching her son playing football. When the game was over she stood up but felt a sharp pain at the back of the knee. Later the calf began to swell painfully and she had difficulty in walking home. When examined, a deep vein thrombosis was suspected and she was sent to hospital where it was noted that the right calf was 2cm greater in girth than the left and that there was edema of the foot and calf (Fig. 16.11). A contrast arthrogram showed acute synovial rupture (Fig. 16.12).

DIAGNOSTIC PROBLEMS

The joint that most commonly ruptures in RA is the knee, usually via the interconnection with the semimembranosus–gastrocnemius bursa in the popliteal fossa. Vectors of the forces of contraction of the quadriceps muscle acting over the swollen knee are responsible for compressing the fluid; the pressure may rise to over 1000mmHg. The moment of the rupture may be felt as a sharp pain in the popliteal fossa or upper aspect of the calf: the subsequent swelling of the calf closely resembles that caused by deep crural vein thrombosis. The synovial membrane and capsule rupture where they are weakest. In long-standing RA the joint capsule thickens and scars, resisting rupture. Thus it is usually in early RA, when the muscles are still strong and the capsules of the joint and bursa thin, that acute synovial rupture is most likely to occur. The severity of the reaction also reflects the amount of fluid extravasated. Small leakages can be missed unless the calf muscles are inspected from behind and the girth of the calves routinely measured.

Typical features are early inflammatory arthritis, pain at the back of the knee on powered extension from the flexed position, and redness and tenderness maximal in the upper medial part of the posterior aspect of the calf. Sometimes the knee becomes less swollen as the calf swells. Pitting edema may spread both to the foot and above the knee. Fever and leukocytosis occur in some patients. Passive dorsiflexion of the ankle increases calf pain (positive Homan's sign). A palpable popliteal cyst is usually absent although ultrasonic scanning or MRI may reveal one. The prescence of fluid tracking along intermuscular fascial planes on T2-weighted MR images suggests rupture. Diagnosis is confirmed by a positive contrast arthrogram and, if necessary, a negative contrast venogram. The clinical resemblance to acute deep vein thrombosis in the calf is very strong. If in doubt, remember that, in the presence of arthritis of the knee, acute synovial rupture is much more common than deep vein thrombosis. Misdiagnosis can be hazardous as anticoagulation can turn the synovial fluid extravasation into a tense hematoma in the posterior muscular compartment of the calf, with the danger of muscle compression and necrosis.

The differential diagnosis includes rupture of the plantaris muscle, rupture of the medial head of the gastrocnemius (usually a football or skiing injury) and, rarely, a leaking popliteal artery aneurysm. During imaging, the patient lies supine on the radiography table, with a small cushion under the knee if full extension is too painful. Some fluid is aspirated by the lateral approach to ensure that the needle is in the synovial cavity. It is only necessary to remove about 5ml for diagnostic investigations unless the joint is very tense, when up to 20ml can be removed. The joint is injected with 20ml of a suitable contrast material, such as meglumine iothalamate, mixed with 5ml of 1% lidocaine (lignocaine). The patient gets down off the couch, walks a few steps and then climbs back on. This allows the contrast material to outline the complete distribution of the synovial fluid. The radiographs taken are anteroposterior with the knee extended, and lateral with the knee in 45° flexion, covering from the lower third of the femur to the lower third of the tibia. Repeat films after 10 and 20 minutes can follow the diffusion of the synovial fluid. A locally active corticosteroid, such as a suspension of of triamcinolone hexacetonide 20mg or methylprednisolone acetate, can be injected to control inflammation before the needle is withdrawn from the joint.

In acute synovial rupture, the contrast dye tracks down the back of the calf, most commonly along the course of the neurovascular bundle, and may outline the feathery appearance of the fibers of the soleus muscle. Occasionally a ruptured pre-existing enlarged popliteal cyst can be seen, and sometimes the upward spread of contrast into the lower thigh is visible.

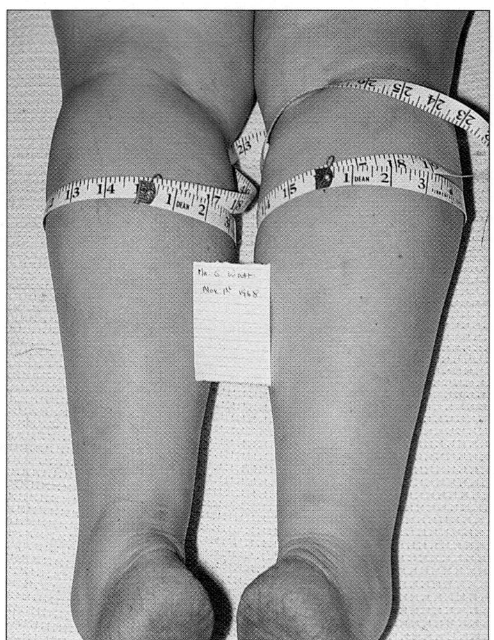

Fig. 16.11 Swelling of calf following acute synovial rupture of the knee in early inflammatory arthritis.

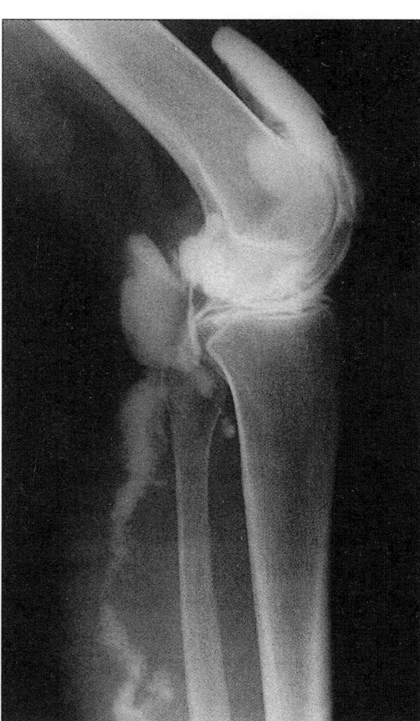

Fig. 16.12 Contrast arthrogram following acute synovial rupture of the knee.

THERAPEUTIC OPTIONS

Treatment is directed at decompressing the knee with bed rest, elevation of the limb and intra-articular corticosteroid injections as above (Fig. 16.13). These may need to be repeated after a week if the calf is still tense; diuretics are unnecessary and on no account should anticoagulants be given. If the calf muscle is very tense and painful, it may be helpful to needle it in several places under aseptic conditions. It will not be possible to aspirate fluid, but the puncture sites will continue to drain synovial fluid and edema as long as the calf is under pressure. If the synovial rupture has followed a persistent noninflammatory hydrarthrosis, decompression can be done by repeated aspiration of the knee. Follow up after a severe episode of synovial rupture has shown that some calf swelling persists for at least 3 years, presumably from residual stretching of the fascial envelopes of the calf.

REFERENCES

Dixon A St J, Emery P. Local injection therapy in rheumatic diseases, 4E. Basle: EULAR; 1992.

Dixon A St J, Grant G. Acute synovial rupture in rheumatoid arthritis. Lancet. 1964;i:742–4.

AN APPROACH TO DIAGNOSIS OF A SWOLLEN CALF IN RHEUMATOID ARTHRITIS

- There must have been previous swelling of the knee, which may have decreased as the calf swelling increased
- Other features are: onset after powered extension of the knee, relatively early arthritis, a popliteal cyst which is often not palpable, redness maximal in the upper posteromedial aspect of the calf, Homan's sign positive, edema may spread above the knee
- Complications include fever and leukocytosis and sometimes posterior compartment compression with danger of muscle necrosis
- An arthrogram is diagnostic
- Treatment is by decompression of the knee by aspiration, bed rest and injection of a locally active corticosteroid
- Recovery within a week is usual

Fig. 16.13 An approach to diagnosis of a swollen calf in RA.

LEG ULCERS

J Thomas Scott

DEFINITION OF THE PROBLEM

Approximately 5% of RA sufferers, especially women, develop leg ulcers. Ulcers tend to occur with severe rheumatoid disease, being usually situated between the ankle and the knee, less commonly over the feet.

THE TYPICAL CASE

JJ is a 55-year-old lady whose RA commenced at the age of 48 years. The disease ran a progressive course with erosions and the formation of nodules. Various anti-inflammatory drugs had been given with no obvious benefit, and 2 years ago her doctor commenced treatment with prednisone 10mg daily. Six months ago she knocked her ankle against a chair; subsequently, a small bruise over the lateral malleolus broke down into an ulcer. Two ulcers then developed over the other ankle. Examination showed that the fingers and toes were blue and cold with small infarcts at some of the nail edges. The peripheral pulses were easily palpable. There were signs of a peripheral sensory neuropathy. Serologic tests for rheumatoid factor were strongly positive.

She was admitted to the hospital and the legs were elevated to encourage healing of the ulcers, to which hydrocolloid dressings were applied, renewed at weekly intervals. The active RA with widespread vasculitis was treated with cyclophosphamide 100mg daily (monitored by serial blood counts); the prednisone dosage was unchanged. Careful attention was paid to physical therapy in the form of active exercises. Healing of the ulcers took place within 6 weeks, together with overall improvement in the condition of her RA.

DIAGNOSTIC PROBLEMS

Venous stasis and immobility of the ankle together with factors such as trauma, pressure, thinning of the skin due to corticosteroid therapy, and coexisting conditions such as diabetes and atheroma must be considered. Leg ulceration may be a feature of Felty's syndrome.

A most important cause, although evident in only a minority of patients, is systemic vasculitis with occlusion of small vessels. Small arteries are characteristically affected, but necrotizing vasculitis involving venules is also described. These patients are seropositive for IgM rheumatoid factor and often have nodules together with other features of vasculitis. The role of corticosteroids in the pathogenesis of necrotizing vasculitis remains uncertain. Ulceration of this type can be gross (Fig. 16.14).

Features of active vasculitis indicate that occlusion of small cutaneous vessels is responsible for ulceration. The foot pulses are easily palpable in such cases unless atheroma is present. It is possible that vasculitis is an underlying cause even when other clinical signs are lacking. In an immobile chair-bound patient, venous stasis is an important factor.

THERAPEUTIC OPTIONS

Treatment often involves long periods of hospitalization and recurrence rates are high. Management in the outpatient department and the community is also costly. Careful attention should therefore be paid to the prevention of ulceration by avoidance of trauma (including pressure from ill-fitting footwear) and prolonged sitting, and by active exercises.

With established ulceration the leg is kept in an elevated position as much as possible, foot and quadriceps exercises being encouraged. Traditional treatments, such as exposure, the use of irritant antiseptics

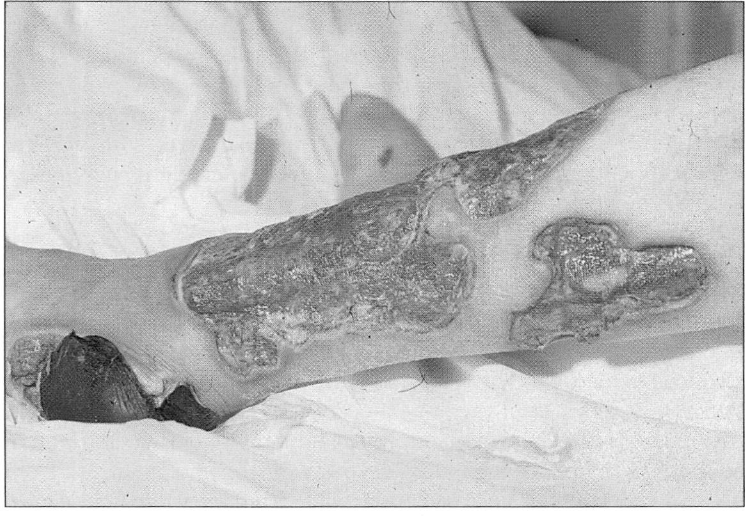

Fig. 16.14 Severe ulceration of the legs in a patient with RA and widespread polyarteritis. There is eschar formation over the heel.

such as peroxides and hypochlorites and the applications of dressings such as paraffin tulle gras that can adhere, are being replaced by newer nonirritant dressings. Disinfectant creams and local antibiotics are not usually required; normal saline is used for gentle cleaning. If swabbing reveals the presence of pathogenic bacteria, a course of systemic antibiotics can be considered.

Hydrocolloid dressings are nonadherent and protective, helping promote granulation and re-epithelialization. In addition, hydrocolloid paste can be applied to a depressed ulcer. The dressing can be reapplied at weekly intervals. These dressings are not suitable for very wet exudative lesions, for which calcium alginate may be preferred. The fibrous dressing absorbs fluid exudates by the formation of a hydrophilic gel. If a hard eschar has formed, a useful material is a hydrogel dressing, a thick liquid gel that promotes rapid debridement by facilitating rehydration and autolysis of dead tissue.

If the ulceration is part of a diffuse vasculitic syndrome, this should be treated with appropriate drug therapy.

CONCLUSIONS

Patients with severe RA are vulnerable to ulceration of the legs from various causes including immobility, dependency, trauma, vasculitis and corticosteroid-induced thinning of the skin.

Ulceration should be prevented by the avoidance of trauma (including pressure) and prolonged sitting and by leg exercises. Established ulceration should be managed by elevation of the limb and the use of modern nonirritant and nonadherent dressings. Diffuse vasculitis should be treated by systemic medication.

REFERENCES

Cullum N. Leg ulcer treatments: a critical review (part 2), Nurs Stand. 1994; 9:32–6.

Johnson A. Towards rapid tissue healing. Nurs Times. 1984;80:39–43.

Thurtle OA, Cawley MID. The frequency of leg ulceration in rheumatoid arthritis: a survey. J Rheumatol. 1983;10:507–9.

STRESS FRACTURES

J Thomas Scott

DEFINITION OF THE PROBLEM

Osteoporosis is common in patients with chronic RA. As a result they can develop stress fractures. Their constant pain, disability and rheumatoid deformities may obscure the diagnosis.

THE TYPICAL CASE

FF is a 68-year-old woman with a 21-year history of RA. Over recent years the disease has been active, causing progressive pain and deformity. She has become severely incapacitated, and can only shuffle from room to room in her house. She spends most of her time sitting in a chair or in bed. She has had numerous types of drug therapy over the years, including prednisone, which was commenced 3 years ago and which she has continued to take at doses of between 7mg and 12mg daily.

Two years ago she developed a fairly sudden increase of pain around her deformed, painful right ankle. A diagnosis of a rheumatoid flare was made, and the pain slowly subsided. Four months ago, while walking in her house, she stumbled slightly, afterwards beginning to complain of persistent pain in her right hip. Radiographs showed a fracture of the femoral neck with displacement, together with some collapse of several thoracic and lumbar vertebrae. Further investigations included some fresh radiographs of the ankles, and an old stress fracture of the right fibula was seen. Blood tests showed that she had a high acute-phase response and strongly positive rheumatoid factor, but renal and liver function tests were normal. Her calcium and phosphate levels were also normal, but there was a minimal elevation of alkaline phosphatase.

The femoral neck fracture was treated surgically by pinning. A bone biopsy was taken at the same time, and showed evidence of osteoporosis but no osteomalacia. She became relatively free from pain at the fracture sites, and further therapy was instituted, with cyclical etidronate 400mg daily for 2 weeks followed by calcium and vitamin D supplements for 13 weeks.

DIAGNOSTIC PROBLEMS

Patients with chronic RA develop demineralization of the entire skeleton. There may be several reasons for this (Fig. 16.15). Its severity is related to the degree of both their disease activity and disability. Reduced physical activity can lead to disuse osteoporosis which adds to the general effect of the RA process on the skeleton. The problem may be worsened by treatment, for example with corticosteroids. In addition, many patients are thin, elderly women, who are at risk from idiopathic postmenopausal osteoporosis. In a minority of cases, a combination of deprivation from sun, due to the disability, and/or a poor diet contributes to the development of osteomalacia.

Population-based observations have indicated a modest increase in the fracture incidence in patients with RA, with a relative risk of pelvic fractures of 2.6, and 1.5 for the proximal femur. Other common sites include the distal forearm, vertebrae and fibula.

In most patients, as in the case described, the osteopenia is entirely due to osteoporosis. However, a high index of suspicion of the possibility of osteomalacia must be maintained. Risk factors, such as diet and sun deprivation, should be thought of, and a search for Looser's zones, as well as biochemical evidence of the condition, should be carried out (see Chapter 8.41). The biochemistry may be misleading; RA and its treatment can cause mild elevations of alkaline phosphatase, and the tests may be only mildly deranged in cases of osteomalacia. A certain diagnosis may only be made with a bone biopsy.

It may also be difficult to exclude a pathologic fracture in patients with active RA, who are already ill, with a raised acute-phase response and in whom a scan will show hot spots around active joints. Clinical suspicion, careful radiologic examination with X-rays (Fig. 16.16) or MRI, a screen for myeloma-related gammopathy and, if need be, a biopsy of the fracture site can confirm the diagnosis.

Stress factors are particularly likely to occur at sites of abnormal mechanical stress caused by rheumatoid deformities. The lower end of the fibula may be stressed by a valgus ankle deformity causing impingement of the ankle on the malleolus. The resulting stress fracture can occur with normal activity, with an attendant increase in pain around an already painful ankle joint. The diagnosis is often missed. Clinical clues come from a careful history and examination. The pain may be localized and 'different' from that of the RA, and on examination a local area of bony tenderness is usually present. Running a pencil down

SOME CAUSES OF THIN BONES IN RHEUMATOID ARTHRITIS
Elderly and postmenopausal females
Persistent active disease
Disability, immobility and disuse osteoporosity
Corticosteroids
Smoking and alcohol
Prolonged low body weight
Osteomalacia secondary to sun deprivation and poor diet

Fig. 16.15 Some of the causes of thin bones in patients with RA.

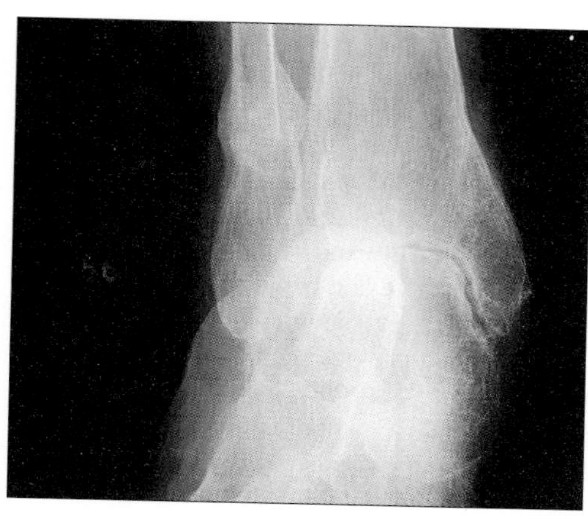

Fig. 16.16 Stress fractures of the fibula in RA. Radiography of the right ankle and foot shows severe osteoporosis, rheumatoid deformity with a valgus hindfoot and a healed stress fracture of the lower part of the fibula with extensive callous formation.

the fibula may result in a sudden shout of pain as the pencil pressure crosses the fracture point.

Vertebral collapse may occur with few symptoms in patients with RA, and even femoral neck fractures may be misdiagnosed as an exacerbation of hip arthritis.

THERAPEUTIC OPTIONS

It is a reasonable assumption that any postmenopausal woman with RA is at risk of developing osteoporosis and stress fractures. The position can be assessed quantitatively with dual-energy X-ray absorptiometry (DXA) or other techniques. It is difficult to restore lost bone, so prevention is of paramount importance.

Patients with RA can prevent osteoporosis by maintaining a good calcium intake, keeping as active as possible, avoiding smoking and excess alcohol, and not getting too thin. Milk, or calcium tablets, taken last thing at night may help counteract the normal nocturnal renal loss of calcium. Hormone replacement therapy (HRT) is known to delay postmenopausal loss of bone, and is best given within a few years of menopause. Therapy can be continued until the age of 60–65 years. Avoidance of corticosteroid therapy, particularly in higher doses, is also important. Care to prevent falls may reduce the incidence of fractures.

Therapy for established osteoporosis is not optional, and the same principles and problems apply to patients with RA as to those with idiopathic postmenopausal osteoporosis (see Chapters 8.39 and 8.40). Pain from stress fractures may respond well to calcitonin, and this agent, as well as the cyclical etidronate used in the case illustrated, may help maintain bone density. Analgesics should be used to help patients mobilize as quickly as possible, avoiding the many disadvantages of immobility in the RA subject with a thin skeleton.

CONCLUSIONS

Osteoporosis is present in many postmenopausal women with RA. There are many causes of this. Stress fractures commonly occur as a result of the thin bones, falls and abnormal biomechanics of the RA skeleton. Diagnosis is usually straightforward, but care must be taken to exclude osteomalacia or, more rarely, a pathologic fracture. Fractures may be relatively painless, or misdiagnosed as an exacerbation of RA.

Preventive measures should be instituted at or immediately after menopause.

REFERENCES

Hoogman JR, Melton LJ, Nelson AN, O'Fallon WM, Riggs BL. Fractures after rheumatoid arthritis. A population-based study. Arthritis Rheum. 1984;27:1352–61.

New treatments for osteoporosis (editorial). Lancet. 1990;335:1065–6.

Sambrook PN, Eisman JA, Champion DG, *et al.* Determinant of axial bone loss in rheumatoid arthritis. Arthritis Rheum. 1987;30:721–8.

Verstraeten A, Dequeker J. Vertebral and peripheral bone mineral content and fracture incidence in postmenopausal patients with rheumatoid arthritis: effect of low dose corticosteroids. Ann Rheum Dis. 1986;45:852–7.

DIAGNOSIS AND MANAGEMENT OF CORNEAL MELT

Beatrice E Frueh & Stuart I Brown

DEFINITION OF THE PROBLEM

Although not common, corneal melting can occur in patients with a long-standing history of RA as well as other collagen diseases, and it may have devastating consequences. The precise incidence of corneal melting in patients with RA is not known.

THE TYPICAL CASE

A 65-year-old woman with a 20-year history of severe RA complained of blurred vision, pain and redness of the left eye for 3 weeks. The current treatment for RA included ibuprofen and prednisone 7.5mg/day. The visual acuity was 20/20 in the right eye and 20/80 in the left eye. Slit-lamp examination of the left eye (Fig. 16.17) showed a peripheral corneal thinning from 4 to 9 o'clock and mild conjunctival injection adjacent to the ulcer. The adjacent sclera was not inflamed. Anterior chamber inflammation was absent. A Schirmer's test without anesthesia revealed borderline tear volume (7mm in the right eye and 5mm in the left eye after 5 min). A hydrophilic bandage contact lens was fitted to the left eye, followed by treatment with frequent application of artificial tears. Despite treatment, the thinning progressed and the conjunctiva and episclera became more inflamed (Fig. 16.18); 21 days after the initial presentation, a conjunctival

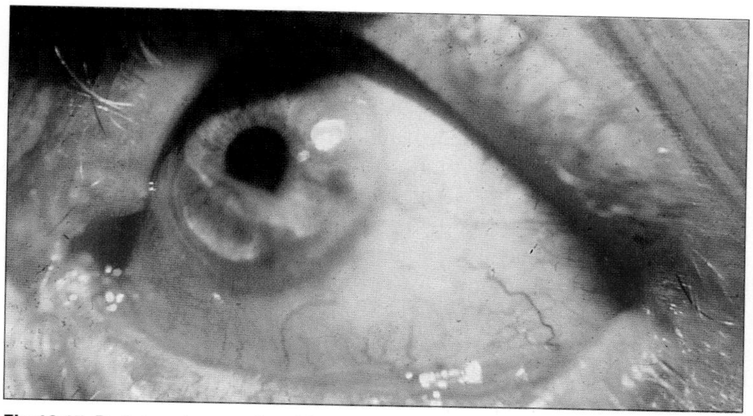

Fig 16.17 Peripheral corneal melting in a patient with RA. The melting extended from 4 to 9 o'clock at the initial presentation.

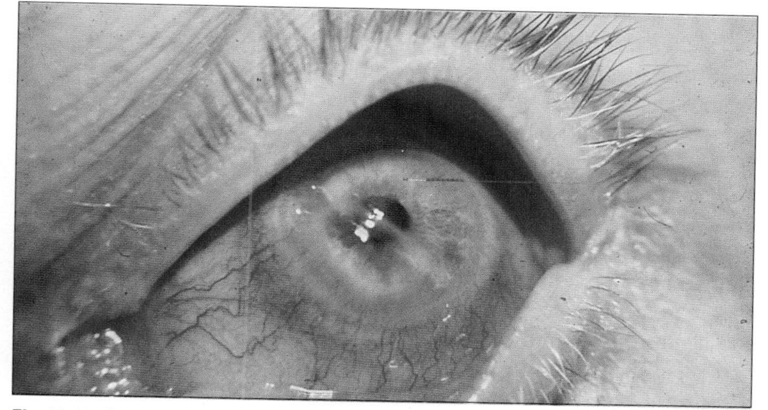

Fig 16.18 Ocular findings after 10 days' treatment of the patient in Figure 16.17. The conjunctiva and episclera are more inflamed and the corneal ulceration is deeper.

excision had to be performed. The epithelium recovered and the ulcer and the conjunctiva became free of inflammation. The visual acuity improved to 20/30 over the following 3 months.

DIAGNOSTIC PROBLEMS

Corneal thinning in patients with RA can present as:

- a marginal furrow with or without inflammatory signs in its base,
- a more inflamed necrotizing keratitis with infiltration (the base of the ulcer appears white from infiltration of inflammatory cells) without scleritis or
- a central ulceration.

Marginal furrows present as peripheral infiltrate and thinning, usually 1mm from the limbus, more often inferiorly. The epithelium is usually absent within the furrow and there is minimal vascularization present in the bed of the furrow. The conjunctiva is mildly inflamed initially and the eye is relatively indolent. If untreated, progression to perforation is not uncommon. A more inflamed peripheral ulcer with infiltration can result from the previous state or present *de novo*. The latter may be an active, rapid and painful necrotizing process. When scleritis is a prominent accompaniment, a lethal course due to systemic vasculitis is not infrequent. Previous cataract surgery can be the stimulus for developing a peripheral corneal and/or scleral ulceration in RA patients. Finally, central corneal melting is characterized by discrete noninflammatory ulcers that rapidly progress to perforation.

THERAPEUTIC OPTIONS

Corneal stromal melting in RA is a serious condition which has to be recognized early in the course in order to save the integrity of the eye. Because it can have minimal associated discomfort, patients with longstanding RA should be instructed to have routine examinations by an ophthalmologist and immediate examination for ocular discomfort, red eye or vision changes. Depending upon the clinical presentation of the melting process, different therapeutic approaches are possible (Fig. 16.19). Once an infectious etiology is ruled out, the treatment of the mildly inflamed peripheral corneal ulcers of RA should begin with simply fitting a bandage contact lens and with the application of artificial tears. If the ulceration continues to cause thinning or extend peripherally, excision of the conjunctiva adjacent to the ulcer should be performed and the bandage lens replaced postoperatively. If the conjunctival excision is unsuccessful and the cornea is thin, a peripheral lamellar graft may be performed. Finally, if the ulceration continues to progress and the previous treatments fail, immunotherapy may be considered. The latter is advised only when the ulcers are highly inflamed (with a white infiltrated base) and especially when associated with a scleritis. For these cases, a 1- or 2-day treatment with high-dose methylprednisone and cyclophosphamide (1–2mg/kg daily) should be tried first. Other possible immunosuppressive agents are azathioprine (1–2mg/kg daily) and methotrexate (5–15mg/week); the role of cyclosporin is at this time still under investigation. We reserve the use of topical corticosteroids after conjunctival resection for Mooren's-like ulcerations, i.e. for ulcers with a major infiltrative component, which begin at the limbus and progress centrally and circumferentially.

In case of perforation, tissue adhesive can be applied or a lamellar 'patch' graft can be performed. Postoperative melting of these grafts has been described. If not performed previously, conjunctival resection should then be performed at time of surgery. Central corneal melting in RA usually progresses rapidly, so that any central erosions should be quickly treated with a bandage contact lens, tissue adhesives or, if a perforation is already present, corneal transplantation.

CONCLUSIONS

Early and aggressive treatment of corneal melting in patients with RA is crucial and calls for a multidisciplinary approach involving both the rheumatologist and the ophthalmologist.

AN APPROACH TO THE MANAGEMENT OF CORNEAL MELT IN RHEUMATOID ARTHRITIS

- Peripheral corneal melt in rheumatoid arthritis: differentiate if it has or has not a prominent inflammatory component and if scleral involvement is present
- For mildly inflamed marginal furrows, first fit a bandage contact lens and use artificial tears; if progressive, excise adjacent conjunctiva
- If there are markedly inflamed and necrotic ulcers, conjunctival resection, fitting of a bandage lens and topical corticosteroids precede immunotherapy
- Concomitant scleritis is a bad prognostic sign, as it is often associated with systemic vasculitis
- In cases of scleral involvement, start immunosuppression

Fig 16.19 An approach to the management of corneal melt in RA.

REFERENCES

Brown SI, Grayson M. Marginal furrows. A characteristic corneal lesion of rheumatoid arthritis. Arch Ophthalmol. 1968;79:563–7.

Brown SI. Mooren's ulcer; treatment by conjunctival excision. Br J Ophthalmol. 1975;59:675–82.

Jayson MIV, Easty DL. Ulceration of the cornea in rheumatoid arthritis. Ann Rheum Dis. 1977;36:428–32.

THE RED EYE IN RHEUMATOID ARTHRITIS

Anthony J Bron

DEFINITION OF THE PROBLEM

There are several causes of red eye in patients with RA. Careful and prompt evaluation of the patient with a red eye is important to determine the exact cause of the problem and to plan effective therapy.

TYPICAL CASES

Case 1

LB is a 49-year-old woman with a 5-year history of RA. She complained of redness of the eyes for 7 months, with a stringy mucous discharge treated unsuccessfully as conjunctivitis. For a longer period she had been troubled by 'ocular fatigue', heaviness of the lids, a foreign body sensation and sensitivity to light. She had suffered a dry mouth for several years.

Examination showed mild redness of the globes and reduced tear stability, demonstrated by a premature break-up of the fluorescein-stained tear film (<10 seconds). Surface ocular damage was indicated by bilateral interpalpebral staining of the conjunctiva and cornea, using fluorescein and a blue light and viewing through a yellow barrier filter (the alternative, Rose Bengal, is more painful to use). The Schirmer test of tear flow showed wetting of less than 6mm on each side (0 and 2mm in her case) and this was not increased by nasal stimulation (this lack of reflex response is a distinguishing feature between Sjögren's and non-Sjögren's aqueous-deficient dry eye). LB was treated with two over-the-counter preparations, hydroxypropyl methylcellulose (HPMC) 2-hourly during the day, and liquid paraffin at night. This greatly improved her symptoms. However, she later developed a toxic reaction to the HPMC preservative, benzalkonium chloride, and switched successfully to a nonpreserved preparation, hydroxyethylcellulose. When her systemic and ocular condition later worsened, tear conservation was improved using spectacles with close-fittting side pieces to raise the periocular humidity (Everest Harris/Eagle Vision). Wettable sponge inserts permitted humidity to be increased on demand. The lacrimal canaliculi were also occluded on a semipermanent basis, with silicone punctal plugs.

Case 2

MR is a 63-year-old man with a 20-year history of R A. He is severely disabled due to deformities and widespread vasculitis. He presented recently with a deep, boring pain in the right eye and ocular redness without visual loss. He showed a patch of nodular scleritis on the right upper globe. His systemic prednisolone dosage was increased. On this regimen the scleritis diminished and the eye remained comfortable for 3 years. He then re-presented with further pain in the right eye. A large zone of avascular scleral necrosis had replaced the nodular scleritis, and the underlying ciliary body was exposed. A diagnosis of necrotizing scleritis was made. Immunosuppression was increased by the addition of cyclophosphamide to the regimen. Levels were adjusted over a period of time. At a later date, and under this regimen, a homologous scleral graft was performed.

DIAGNOSTIC PROBLEMS

Dry eye occurs in 11–13% of patients with RA as a part of secondary Sjögren's syndrome. Sjögren's syndrome is also associated with systemic lupus erythematosus (SLE), polyarteritis nodosa (PAN), Wegener's disease, relapsing polychondritis, primary biliary cirrhosis and mixed connective tissue disease. In the absence of overt systemic disease, the occurrence of dry eye and dry mouth in conjunction with antibodies such as anti-Ro and anti-La characterizes primary Sjögren's syndrome.

Sjögren's syndrome is an autoimmune exocrinopathy in which an inflammatory invasion of the lacrimal and salivary acini and ducts results in dry eyes and dry mouth. Dry eye is due to reduced lacrimal secretion. With continued evaporation, the tears become hyperosmolar and damage the exposed (and, rarely, the unexposed) conjunctiva and cornea. There may also be primary conjunctival damage.

Episcleritis and scleritis may be regarded as extra-articular manifestations of RA. If severe or poorly treated, scleritis can rapidly blind the patient. The least severe form of the disease is episcleritis, which can be simple or nodular (Fig. 16.21a) and affects the zone lying between the conjunctiva and sclera. The lesion may or may not be painful, but is usually tender. Simple episcleritis may be sectoral or diffuse. The mobility of nodular episcleritis over the underlying sclera distinguishes it from scleritis.

Scleritis is a manifestation of vasculitis. It is a serious, sight-threatening condition and implies a worsened prognosis for survival. It consists of an inflammation of the scleral wall. The inflammation, although most common in the anterior segment, can affect the whole eye, including the optic nerve. The most common presentation is redness of the eye without discharge, but it is always associated with pain or discomfort. Scleritis affects both eyes in 70% of patients and occurs in about 5% of all patients with RA.

SYSTEMIC ACCOMPANIMENTS OF RHEUMATOID EYE DISEASE		
	With episcleritis/scleritis (%)	Without episcleritis/scleritis (%)
Systemic complications	79	10
Rheumatoid nodules	71	26
Arteritis	71	12
Pericarditis/pleurisy	14	1

Fig 16.20 Systemic accompaniments of rheumatoid eye disease. From Jayson and Jones, 1971.

Anterior scleritis causes severe pain and a tender swelling of the scleral wall (Fig. 16.21a). It may be associated with sclerokeratitis (an involvement of the neighboring cornea) and may be necrotizing, particularly in patients with features of severe systemic vasculitis (Fig. 16.21b). Necrotizing scleritis causes a through-and-through scleral necrosis which may expose the underlying uvea (the ciliary body or choroid; (Fig. 16.21c), or so alter the scleral structure that it becomes almost transparent. In the absence of glaucoma, there is sufficient strength in the uvea to prevent ectasia. This condition should be distinguished from scleromalacia which results from arteriolar occlusion. There is progressive thinning of the anterior scleral wall in a quiet eye, leading to uveal ectasia (staphyloma).

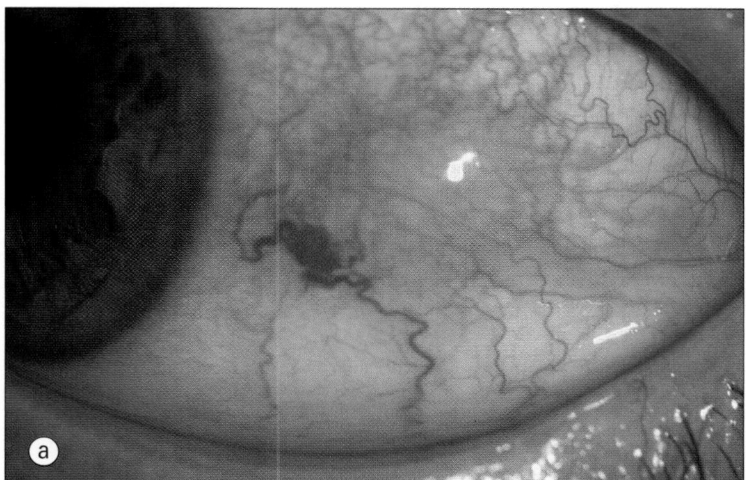

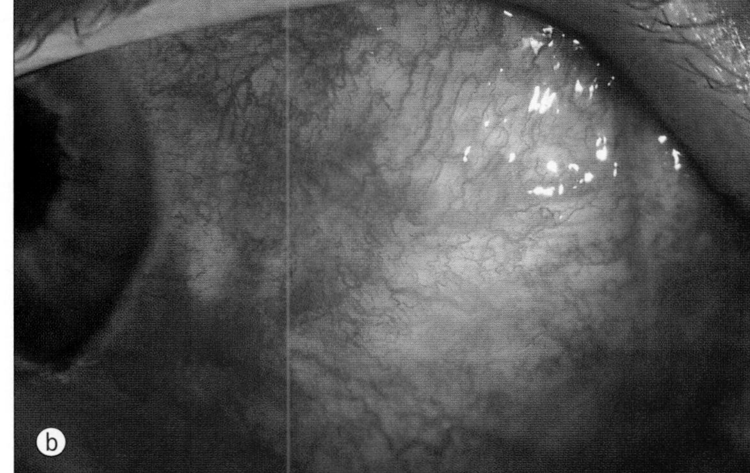

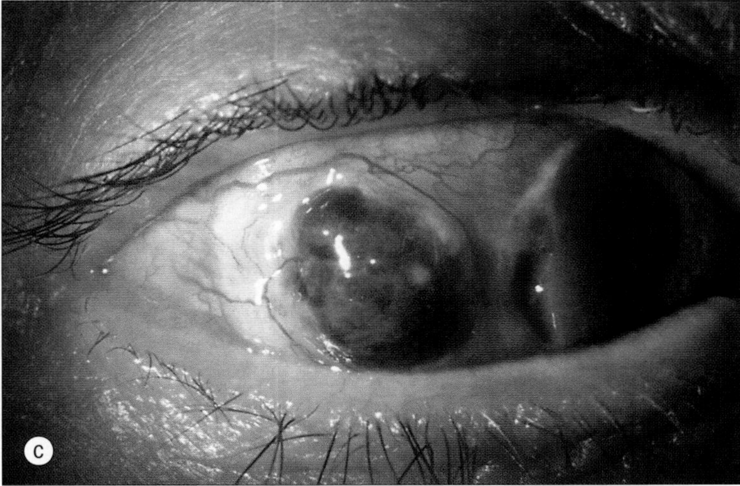

Fig 16.21 Scleritis in RA. (a) Nodular episcleritis. (b) Anterior scleritis. (c) Necrotizing scleritis may expose the underlying uvea. Here it is associated with marginal corneal melting.

Posterior scleritis is less common. It is usually associated with a diffuse anterior scleritis but may occur in isolation with minimal redness of the eye. It can cause exudative detachment of the retina, swelling of the optic nerve head, painful proptosis and angle closure glaucoma. Diagnosis is difficult because the affected sclera is obscured ophthalmoscopically, but ultrasound demonstrates thickening of the scleral wall. Corneal inflammation may accompany scleritis or episcleritis as a sclerokeratitis. Keratitis may also occur independently, with or without symptoms, with peripheral corneal infiltrates leading to corneal melting and ring-shaped, marginal guttering, often without significant inflammation.

THERAPEUTIC OPTIONS

Episcleritis may be relieved by topical corticosteroids or NSAIDs but is usually mild and self-limiting. Dry eyes in overt systemic disease such as Sjögren's syndrome, SLE and PAN are treated by tear substitutes and tear conservation. Newer approaches include local immune suppression, secretagogues and novel fluid delivery systems.

Anterior, diffuse and nodular scleritis and posterior scleritis in some patients respond to systemic NSAIDs. Flurbiprofen 100mg t.i.d. seems to be the most effective regimen. Severe cases require high-dose systemic corticosteroids (e.g. a starting dose of prednisone 80mg/day). If there is potential visual loss from perforation, keratitis or uveitis, or there is intense pain, pulsed methylprednisolone 1000mg i.v. repeated at 500mg on the 3rd or 4th day may be needed. Patients who are unresponsive may need systemic cyclophosphamide 2–3mg/kg by mouth daily in addition. Cyclosporin, azathioprine and methotrexate are less effective in this disease or should be used only if cyclophosphamide is contraindicated.

CONCLUSIONS

The most common cause of a red eye in RA is Sjögren's syndrome. The degree of redness is usually slight, but any patient with ocular symptoms should be tested for dry eye and dry mouth. A focal or diffuse redness of the globe should suggest episcleritis or scleritis. Both may cause pain. Pain-free redness is likely to be due to episcleritis while severe pain should suggest scleritis. Severe retrobulbar pain, not necessarily associated with redness of the eye, may be due to to posterior scleritis. Uveitis is not usually a feature of RA, but it may accompany scleritis, sclerokeratitis or keratitis. Poor or inadequate treatment can result in blindness. Expert ophthalmologic assistance should be sought if there is any doubt about the diagnosis.

REFERENCES

Foster CS, Forstot SL, Wilson LA. Mortality rate in rheumatoid arthritis patients developing necrotizing scleritis or peripheral ulcerative keratitis. Ophthalmology. 1984;91:1253–63.

Jayson MIV, Jones DEP. Scleritis and rheumatoid arthritis. Ann Rheum Dis. 1971;30:343–7.

Jones DT, Monroy D, Ji Z, Atherton SS, Pflugfelder SC. Sjögren's syndrome: cytokine and Epstein–Barr viral gene expression within the conjunctival epithelium. Invest Ophthalmol Vis Sci. 1994;35:3493–504.

McGavin DDM, Williamson J, Forrester JV, *et al.* Episcleritis and scleritis. A study of their clinical manifestations and association with rheumatoid arthritis. Br J Ophthalmol. 1976;60:192–226.

Watson PG, Hazleman BL. The sclera and systemic disorders. Philadephia: Saunders; 1976.

Williamson J. Incidence of eye disease in cases of connective tissue disease. Trans Ophthalmol Soc UK. 1974;94:742–52.

MANAGEMENT OF THE FRAIL ELDERLY RHEUMATOID PATIENT

Margaret Byron

DEFINITION OF THE PROBLEM

Demographic changes mean that the absolute and relative numbers of elderly people are growing, especially in the over 75 years age group. The frail elderly patient with RA can present particular management problems in addition to the ravages of long-standing RA and the secondary development of OA. These occur at impairment, disability and handicap levels (Fig. 16.22). The interaction of these factors makes development of a management plan very challenging. The psychosocial status of the patient, including family situation, ethnic and cultural background, religious beliefs and personality traits, is going to be of much more significance to the outcome than pills and potions. It is in this group that the multidisciplinary team approach is of paramount importance. The program should be goal-oriented with active participation of the patient and main care givers.

POTENTIAL PROBLEMS FACED BY THE ELDERLY PERSON WITH RA

Impairment (pathology, symptoms, signs)	Disability (functional limitation – task oriented)	Handicap (social context – role oriented)
Pain	Difficulty walking	Financial problems
Stiffness	Difficulty washing and dressing	Inadequate or inappropriate housing
Diminished renal function	Difficulty making snack/meal	Death of spouse/care-giver
Confounding illnesses	Difficulty keeping house	Isolation
Multiple drug therapy	Difficulty engaging in leisure activities	Social support limited (family scattered)
Predisposition to adverse drug reactions and interactions		Housebound
Diminishing vision and hearing		
Decline in cognitive function		
Incontinence		
Poor diet		
Poor skin		
Senile osteoporosis		
Depression		

Fig. 16.22 Potential problems faced by the elderly person with RA.

THE TYPICAL CASE

MN is a 77-year-old woman with a 31-year history of seropositive, erosive RA. Her arthritis has taken an undulating course with episodes of several years of good control. She has been treated with six second-line agents with variable response but all had eventually been stopped because of either lack of efficacy or side effects. Her medical history is complicated by bronchiectasis, a degree of cor pulmonale requiring diuretic therapy and a history of peptic ulceration. Over the past 10 years she has become increasingly disabled and dependent on her family for most of her care. She lives in public housing with her husband who has mild Parkinson's disease. Their daughter lives a few doors away and sees them daily.

This review was prompted by admission to hospital with an episode of pneumonia. She had become increasingly immobile over the preceeding 3 weeks, had been confined to bed and become incontinent of urine. Examination revealed a pyrexia with signs of consolidation at the right lung base and crepitant rales on the left. Her joints exhibited chronic rheumatoid deformities with marked limitation of movement at wrists, elbows, shoulders, knees, ankles and feet. Extra-articular features included nodules, leg ulcers and a penetrating ischial sore. She was pale and had poor muscle bulk generally (Fig. 16.23).

DIAGNOSTIC PROBLEMS

All acute problems precipitating loss of function must be diagnosed and treated appropriately. Sepsis in chest, urinary tract, joint or other site can cause a patient to become bedridden and, in the absence of localizing symptoms and signs, can require a careful search. Sudden worsening of cardiac or renal function or an acute metabolic

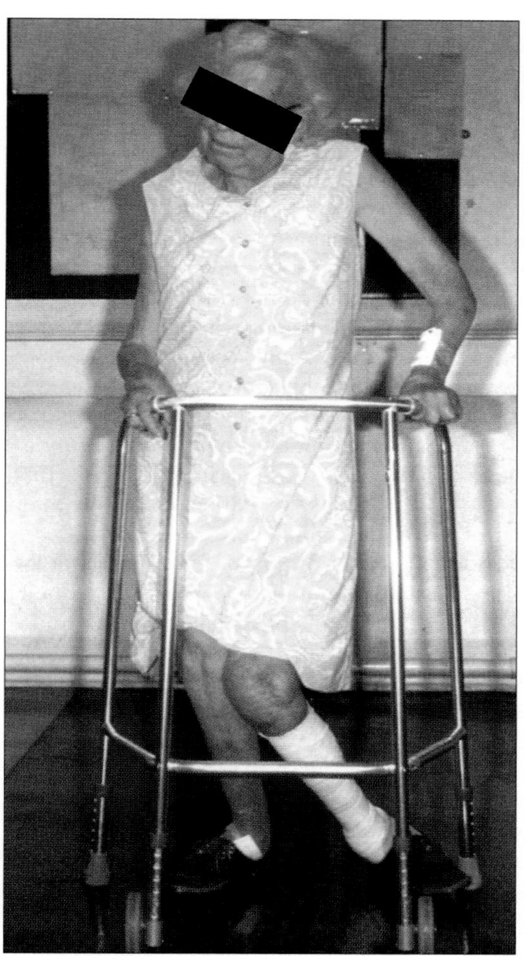

Fig. 16.23 Typical findings in a patient with long-standing rheumatoid arthritis. Note the multiple joint deformities, the poor muscle bulk and poor skin with ulceration on the left leg.

disturbance can also precipitate a crisis. Once the acute medical conditions are resolved or controlled, long-term management of the chronic disabling condition needs to be tackled.

THERAPEUTIC OPTIONS

The medical model of intervening at the pathologic or impairment level of disease with the aim of preventing or minimizing disability and handicap almost needs to be turned on its head in this age group. Coexisting medical conditions and multiple drug therapy should lead to caution in therapeutic enthusiasm. At this stage of arthritis disability is often established and the social situation may not be amenable to change. The first focus of management planning therefore should be at handicap level.

Handicap refers to the impact that impairments and disabilities have on a person's roles e.g. as parent, wage-earner, friend, spouse, etc. A given set of impairments does not lead to the same handicaps in every patient as the relationship is not necessarily linear nor hierarchical; each person is unique and requires a unique response. Setting the management plan within the framework of the patient's own expectations and wishes offers the best chance of a satisfactory outcome. In the illustrative case, medical and nursing team members felt that MN required 24 hour nursing care, best met within an institution. MN's main wish was to remain with her family, imposing a considerable burden of care on them. A case conference revealed that her family shared her wishes. The first goal therefore was to support MN at home. This required involvement of visiting nurses, voluntary services and the setting up of regular relief care at a primary care facility. Unfortunately the wishes of patients and care givers do not always coincide. In such cases sensitive negotiation of a compromise requires the skills of the whole multidisciplinary team to provide a realistic program of care.

A parallel step in management is a thorough assessment of impairment and disability so that interventions appropriate to the social context can be considered. Listing problems as in Figure 16.22 does provide a framework in which to work and examine the interactions. Relief of pain and stiffness can be achieved by a range of interventions: drugs, exercises, pacing, relaxation, transcutaneous electrical nerve stimulation (TENS), etc. Together with aids and equipment these can lead to improved function, enabling activities of daily living such as walking, dressing and preparing a snack. They may not prevent the patient from being housebound, however, and this mobility handicap may need to be approached in a different way – voluntary services visitor or transport, day centers, social clubs, etc. Although incontinence was identified as a problem for MN, a careful history revealed that it was due to immobility rather than a structural problem with the genitourinary tract. In view of her continuing immobility, skin breakdown and the burden on her family, catheterization was felt to be an appropriate intervention that was acceptable to patient and family.

After comprehensive assessment the next step is goal setting. The goals should be simple, realistic and measurable. Many elderly patients attempt to retain a measure of independence by rejecting help from all sources. The skill of the multidisciplinary team is to negotiate appropriate goals with the patient and main carers, with the aim of moving towards improved health status and function. For each goal, the actions required and the person who is to implement them must be identified together with some estimate of the time scale. One goal identified for MN was protection of skin and healing of the ischial sore. This required liaison with visiting nurses and provision of a specialist mattress and dressings, implemented by nursing staff. Appropriate seating was organized by the occupational therapist and dietary assessment by a dietitian. Nursing review was continuous with medical review after 3 months or at the nurse's request. The action plan included referral to the plastic surgeon if progress in the ischial lesion had not been made in the time agreed. Other goals could include specific tasks – preparing a snack; going to the toilet unaided – or may focus on the handicaps, e.g. advice on available services.

Periodic review is required in order to assess progress. Radical alteration of the goals is often required in this continuous process. Not all patients will accept what we have to offer and our main role is to provide the relevant information and the opportunity for intervention.

CONCLUSIONS

Management of the frail elderly patient with RA should focus primarily on the patient's and care-givers' expectations and wishes, within their social context. The impairment, disability and handicap framework is useful to sort out the multiple problems and their interactions. Goals should be negotiated with clear action plans and a time scale for review.

REFERENCES

Demlow LL, Liang MH, Eaton HM. Impact of chronic arthritis in the elderly. In: Kean WF, ed. Clinics in rheumatic diseases, 12. Arthritis in the elderly. Philadelphia: Saunders; 1986:329–35.

Ebrahim S. Measurement of impairment, disability and handicap. In: Hopkins A, Costain D, eds. Measuring the outcomes of medical care. London: Royal College of Physicians; 1990:27–41.

Gibson T, Grahame R. Rehabilitation of the elderly arthritic patient. In: Woolf D, ed. Clinics in rheumatic diseases, 7. Rehabilitation in the rheumatic diseases. Philadelphia: Saunders; 1981:485–95.

Rasker JJ, Cosh JA. Long term effects of treating rheumatoid arthritis. In: Scott DL, ed. Clinics in rheumatic diseases, 6. The course and outcome of rheumatoid arthritis. London: Baillière Tindall; 1992:141–160.

DEFINITION OF THE PROBLEM

In RA, the knee joint maintains a special place in the disease presentation and its potential for functional limitation and response to treatment. Clinically, while most other diarthrodial joints may be responsive to general disease control and intra-articular corticosteroid injection, the knee may be refractory to such treatment. Because of the large mass of synovial tissue present in the inflamed knee and/or its weight-bearing status, the knee may act as a sequestered site not amenable to treatment modalities successful elsewhere.

THE TYPICAL CASE

AW, a 40-year-old legal secretary with a 10-year history of seropositive RA, was seen for evaluation of progressive pain and swelling of the left knee. Despite combination therapy with low-dose prednisone and courses of multiple SAARDs (gold, hydroxychloroquine, D-penicillamine and methotrexate) she had continuous synovitis in multiple joints throughout the entire course of her disease. She indicated that the hydrocortisone injection given into the left knee 6 weeks earlier had produced relief that lasted only a day or two. Her current medications included prednisone 7.5mg each morning and methotrexate 22.5mg weekly.

On physical examination she was afebrile (37°C) and walked with obvious pain. The knees were warm, mildly tender to palpation and with bilateral (left greater than right) effusions (Fig. 16.24). Prominent wasting of the quadriceps muscles was noted. An aspiration of the left knee yielded 50ml of slightly cloudy fluid with a white cell count of 34,000 cells/mm^3 (75% neutrophils and 25% lymphocytes).

DIAGNOSTIC PROBLEMS

The main questions that must be answered in the rheumatoid patient with recurrent or persistent synovitis of a knee, despite maximal treatment efforts, are:

- is there a superimposed infection;
- does the knee complaint arise from the knee itself, or could its origin be from the ipsilateral hip or the back;
- is there a superimposed local or systemic disease process that is not being addressed by the treatment for RA; and
- is the recurrent or persistent knee synovitis due to refractory RA?

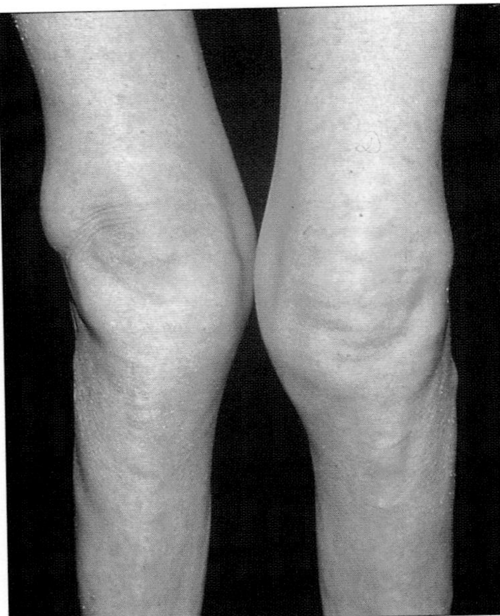

Fig. 16.24 Progressive pain and swelling of the left knee. Note the prominent wasting of muscles and effusion in the right knee also.

In any patient with RA, an infection should be strongly considered in a single disproportionately inflamed joint, especially when associated with a fever and/or ongoing immunosuppressive therapy. The potential sources of infection include: bacteremia, a surgical procedure or joint aspiration and/or injection, or contiguous osteomyelitis. The type of organism is ultimately definable by the culture of synovial fluid or tissue. However, the initial treatment decisions will be guided by the gram stain and the clinical presentation. Acute knee inflammation in an RA patient, associated with fever and chills, should raise the specter of *Staphylococcus aureus* or other pyogenic organisms. A subacute or chronic infectious disease would be a more typical presentation of infection with *Mycobacterium tuberculosis*. Superimposed Lyme disease should also be considered, especially in patients who live in or travel to highly endemic areas for the Lyme tick.

The RA patient may have synovitis of a knee joint, but, alternatively, the severity of the pain in that joint may be referrable to more proximal sites. Always examine the joints proximal and distal to the site of complaint.

The monoarticular knee inflammation may be related to inflammatory bowel disease, crystal-induced disease due to pseudogout or gout (an uncommon disorder in RA patients), a hemarthrosis due to trauma and/or anticoagulation, a mechanical derangement, such as a meniscal tear, ligamentous sprain or tear, patellofemoral dysfunction, secondary OA, osteonecrosis, a fracture due to osteoporosis, a primary or metastatic malignant process, hemangioma or pigmented villonodular synovitis and synovial chondromatosis. Often these diagnostic possibilities can be defined by a complete history, physical examination and an imaging study.

The possibility of refractory RA is strongly supported by the presence of generalized active joint and systemic disease. However, there is a subset of RA patients in whom recurrent or persistent knee synovitis is the sole site of disease activity. Often, the patient is already on a maximal treatment regimen, including an NSAID and SAARD, and, after infection has been ruled out with appropriate cultures, has already undergone one or more injections of a nonadsorbable intra-articular corticosteroid. Despite the injections, the synovitis either does not respond at all, responds only transiently (for 1–2 weeks) or worsens. After a maximum of 2–3 nonadsorbable corticosteroid instillations, over a period of 3–6 months, the physician should reassess the disease status and consider alternative treatment modalities, always with a high index of suspicion for an infection or alternative etiologies for the knee disease.

THERAPEUTIC OPTIONS

If the knee synovitis is clearly related to recurring or refractory RA, and infection, trauma or a superimposed systemic or local disorder is excluded, the following approach should be taken. First, the disease activity should be quantified employing clinical and laboratory measures. If the recurring knee synovitis is just one of many inflamed joints in the setting of poor general disease control, a reassessment of the treatment protocol is appropriate. This can take the form of the addition of, or switch to, an alternative SAARD, NSAID and/or a short course of oral corticosteroid. Certainly, if the knee synovitis is disproproportionate compared with all other joints, an intra-articular nonadsorbable corticosteroid injection is often quite helpful in improving local inflammation and its attendant functional limitation.

The usual clinical response to a nonabsorbable intra-articular corticosteroid injection (methylprednisolone 40mg or triamcinolone hexacetonide 20mg) is a rapid and marked initial and persistent improvement in knee inflammation. If the knee synovitis does not improve or if there is a recurrence of inflammation within 1–2 weeks, a second nonadsorbable corticosteroid injection is appropriate. One final injection may be considered in 1–2 weeks, but the likelihood of clinical response becomes less with each recurrence of synovitis. Overall, a greater likelihood of a clinical response is found in those patients in whom:

- a synovial effusion is present and inflammatory fluid can be aspirated,
- zero or minimal joint damage is present,
- 2–3 days of postinjection knee rest is instituted.

If after 2–3 corticosteroid injections and optimization of the treatment regimen, a significant knee synovitis remains or recurs, and infection and other potential causes are ruled out, an alternative treatment approach is needed. Knee ultrasound may be both diagnostically helpful and cost effective at this time in order to define abnormalities in the synovium, menisci and popliteal fossa. In this setting, arthroscopic synovectomy should be contemplated and is quite effective, in the vast majority of patients, in controlling the local inflammation and improving function. During the procedure, an assessment is made of the integrity of the cartilage, synovial fluid and tissue cultures taken and a synovial membrane histologic evaluation performed. In the rare patient who does not improve or improves only minimally after 'debulking' the knee synovial membrane via arthroscopic synovectomy, one final nonadsorbable intra-articular corticosteroid injection is commonly helpful.

Radiation synovectomy with yttrium-90 silicate colloid, rhenium-186 or dysprosium-165 hydroxide macroaggregate, if available, is an alternative modality prior to or after a failed response to arthroscopic synovectomy in order to decrease the overall mass of inflamed synovium. The typical RA patients in whom this procedure is considered are those in whom synovitis persists despite 6 months of systemic or local treatment and radiologic stages I or II are present. In patients who responded well to this treatment, synovial membrane histologic examination disclosed a reduction in inflammation and transitory synovial cell hyperplasia that ended in dense fibrosis. Postinjection immobilization and hospitalization is needed with all isotopes but is less with the shorter half-life dysprosium. Radionuclide-related cytogenetic damage, knee retention and extra-articular leakage are the same with all preparations.

A complete lack of response to synovectomy demands a total reassessment for alternative causes of synovitis, and may represent advanced cartilage and bone damage that could necessitate a total knee replacement.

If an infectious process can be defined, appropriate therapy is mandatory. If the offending organism is pyogenic, gram negative, mycobacterial or fungal, antimicrobial treatment should be guided by the clinical setting and culture results. Arthroscopic synovectomy is often indicated if initial antibiotic and joint aspirations are not rapidly successful in bringing about culture negativity and clinical improvement.

If Lyme disease has been diagnosed, supported by clinical and laboratory data, oral amoxicillin with probenecid or doxycycline should be instituted. Intravenous ceftriaxone is employed in the setting of persistent inflammation. In refractory cases, arthroscopic synovectomy is often curative.

CONCLUSIONS

Severe synovitis of the knee in RA may lead to the rapid development of functional limitation, quadriceps atrophy, altered gait pattern, and stress on other lower extremity joints and the back. The specific treatment for recurrent knee synovitis is dependent upon the etiology of the inflammation (Fig. 16.25).

RECURRENT RHEUMATOID KNEE SYNOVITIS: DIAGNOSTIC POSSIBILITIES AND TREATMENT

	Diagnostic possibilities	Treatment modalities
Refractory local rheumatoid synovitis		• Intra-articular nonabsorbable glucocorticosteroid injections and treatment of systemic disease • Arthroscopic synovectomy • Radiation synovectomy • Joint replacement, if extensive joint damage is present
Superimposed infection	• Pyogenic organisms – 80% *S. aureus* • Gram-negative organisms • Tuberculous • Fungal • Lyme	Antibiotic treatment guided by cultures; joint aspirations Surgical intervention for refractory infection, usually arthroscopic
Coexistent mechanical or bone disorders	• Meniscal or ligamentous sprain or tear • Patellofemoral dysfunction • Fracture • Osteonecrosis • OA • Loose bodies • Synovial chondromatosis • Hematoma: trauma, anticoagulation,hemophilia	Definition of the process by clinical physical diagnostic techniques Imaging study; treatment defined by the diagnosis
Coexistent inflammatory disorders	• Crystal-induced disorders • Pigmented villonodular synovitis • Inflammatory bowel disease	Synovial fluid analysis Imaging study; treatment of disease
Tumor	• Metastatic • Local • Hemangioma	History and physical examination Imaging study; treatment of disease

Fig. 16.25 Recurrent rheumatoid knee synovitis: diagnostic possibilities and treatment.

REFERENCES

Blyth T, Hunter JA, Stirling A. Pain relief in the rheumatoid knee after steroid injection. A single-blind comparison of hydrocortisone succinate, and triamcinolone acetonide or hexacetonide. Br J Rheumatol. 1994:33:461–3.

Edmonds J, Smart R, Laurent R, *et al.* A comparative study of the safety and efficacy of dysprosium-165 hydroxide macro-aggregate and yttrium-90 silicate colloid in radiation synovectomy – a multi centre double blind clinical trial. Australian Dysprosium Trial Group. Br J Rheumatol. 1994;33:947–53.

Menninger H, Reinhardt S, Sondgen W. Intra-articular treatment of rheumatoid knee-joint effusion with triamcinolone hexacetonide versus sodium morrhuate. A prospective study. Scand J Rheumatol. 1994;23:249–54.

DEFINITION OF THE PROBLEM

Foot pain in RA is one of the most common problems to present to rheumatologists and primary care physicians and occurs in 90% of patients. To deal with it effectively requires an accurate diagnosis of the problem and therefore an understanding of the anatomy and function of the foot.

Foot pain in RA is essentially articular or neurogenic in origin and the latter may be due to systemic disease, e.g. vasculitis, or to nerve traction or compression. Articular pain can occur at any stage of the disease, but neurogenic pain tends to present in people with severe and long-standing disease. Tarsal tunnel syndrome, for instance, is only seen in patients in classic/definite disease of more than 10 years' duration.

Other abnormalities that occur, but are not exclusive to RA, are peripheral neuropathies, which may be caused by small vessel vascular disease resulting in tissue damage and gangrene. These will not be mentioned specifically; it is sufficient to say that careful assessment of the foot is required to ascertain the nature of the underlying pathology.

THE TYPICAL CASE

JA is a 58-year-old woman with a 13-year history of classic RA. She has complained of metatarsalgia from the outset of her disease and 18 months afterwards was noted to have metatarsophalangeal (MTP) erosions in both feet.

She was treated with intramuscular gold and over the years had several courses of oral corticosteroids. She had a number of acute flares of her disease and was started with methotrexate with good effect.

Her foot pain continued and she was given a metatarsal dome for metatarsal pain and a medial arch support for developing pes planus. However, she could not tolerate these, as they increased the load on the lateral three MTP joints and caused pressure on the dorsal surfaces of the toes. Her first MTP joint was fused for a hallux valgus, but later she started to experience increased pain and dysesthesia in the medial and lateral aspects of the right foot and the lateral aspect of the left. She was noted to have a significant 30° subtalar valgus deformity. Nerve conduction studies confirmed:

- delayed right posterior tibial nerve conduction at the flexor retinaculum and
- a compressive neuropathy of the left lateral plantar nerve, as it passed under the medial arch.

Foot hygiene and tissue viability were discussed with the podiatrist and clinical nurse specialist. Bilateral medial wedge heel support insoles were provided to correct subtalar valgus deformities, which were the cause of the foot pronation in the apparent flat feet, thus diminishing further nerve injury. Her metatarsal domes were altered and depth shoes were supplied to allow sufficient room for her long-standing subluxed MTP joints and toes. Considerable relief resulted and, 6 months later, restoration of muscle bulk was noted in the right adductor hallucis muscle, in which reinnervation was confirmed on EMG.

DIAGNOSTIC PROBLEMS

Differentiating ankle and/or subtalar joint, hindfoot, midfoot and forefoot problems is essential for management. Although RA can involve any structure, the ankle and MTP joints are the most commonly affected.

Inflammation in the ankle causes alteration of gait with subsequent pain in the mid and forefoot. Subtalar valgus subluxation pronates the foot, which gives rise to an apparent flat foot. The posterior tibial nerve may be injured as it is stretched around the medial aspect of the ankle; this is more often the cause of a tarsal tunnel syndrome in RA, rather than true compression under the flexor retinaculum. It is therefore not really analogous to carpal tunnel syndrome and hindfoot correction with an appropriate insole in early RA may prevent its appearance later in the disease. Therefore, subtalar joint angle measurement (as shown in Fig 16.26) is useful with 20° or more of valgus on standing being significant in the definition of subluxation.

True pes planus is not peculiar to rheumatoid disease and most problems occur as a result of tibialis posterior tendon and talonavicular ligament injuries or overuse. The lateral plantar nerve may be compressed in the mid foot, as it passes under the arch between the quadratus plantae muscle and medial cuneiform bone, giving rise to pain in the lateral aspect of the foot and, if severe, sensory and motor changes.

Synovitis of the MTP joints often occurs early in the course of RA. With joint damage and instability, the ligamentous support of the forefoot weakens, resulting, in time, in MTP joint subluxation and valgus deformities of the toes. Bearing weight causes pain and the typical skin changes are found in the form of callouses under the metatarsal heads and on the dorsal aspect of the toes. Interphalangeal (IP) joint deformities and tendon changes result in further problems such as hammer toes, claw toes, etc., and this is further complicated by the effect of wearing badly fitting shoes. In addition, forefoot ischemia can cause irreversible changes.

As well as the above neurologic changes, which can decrease muscular control and disrupt musculoskeletal stability, trauma to the forefoot can result in the development of a Morton's neuroma in the plantar digital nerve, classically producing pain and paresthesia in the toes on walking.

THERAPEUTIC OPTIONS

The principle of treatment is to relieve pain and the load from damaged structures and protect the skin. The value of podiatry cannot be underestimated in the promotion of good foot hygiene and prevention of skin abnormalities, such as callouses, fissures, corns and nail and nailbed abnormalities, which cause considerable discomfort. Equally importantly, many people with RA cannot inspect their feet adequately and regular visits to a podiatrist will allow early detection and treatment of potentially disabling lesions, such as ulcers. A regular podiatry check for these people every 6–8 weeks is to be recommended.

The wearing of small medial wedge insoles early on in the course of the disease is a useful preventive measure and ensures a good foot posture in asymptomatic patients. For those requiring orthoses, this may involve the fitting of insoles, the provision of specialized footwear

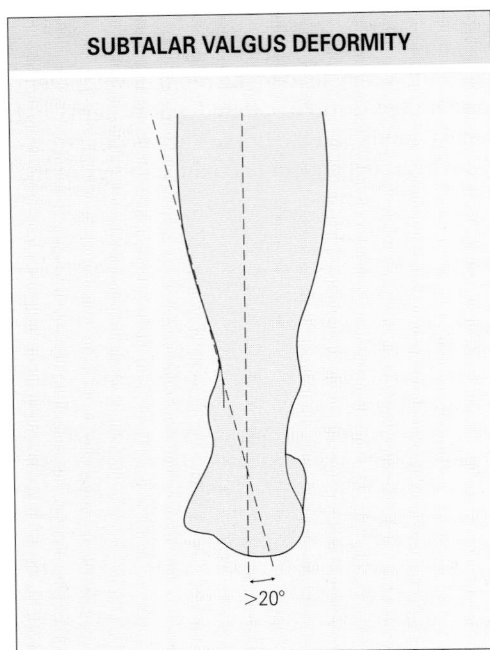

Fig. 16.26 Subtalar valgus deformity. This is the measurement at the ankle between a vertical line down from the middle of the popliteal fossa and a line between the ankle and the heel. The angle indicates the severity of subtalar valgus tilt. 20° or more with the patient standing is significant as a subtalar joint subluxation.

or a combination of both. The commercial availability of depth shoes and the use of new waterproof cosmetically acceptable materials have greatly increased treatment options. Depth shoes are enhanced footwear for people with deformed feet and are characterized by their lightweight, nonslip sole and wide opening to allow easy fitting. They are fairly cheap to produce and cater for most deformities. Importantly, they have sufficient space to fit appropriate insoles. Handmade shoes are available for patients with complex deformities, and consultation with a qualified orthotist will ensure provision of an appropriate item.

Insoles are directed to:

- wedge the heel medially or laterally to supinate or pronate the foot respectively,
- lift the arch to supinate the mid foot in pes planus and
- relieve the pain from MTP joint subluxation or from digital problems.

Injection of painful joints gives long-lasting relief only when the biomechanical issues have been addressed. Finally, surgery may be indicated to correct deformities, realign, excise or fuse joints or to decompress nerves and other structures.

CONCLUSIONS

Foot pain is thus a far more complex problem than it first appears. Accurate diagnosis is vital for effective treatment, which should address both the mechanical and pathologic problems of painful feet. Treatment is best prior to the onset of irreversible changes and prevention of deformity is a high priority in early disease. Cooperation with podiatrists and surgeons interested in foot problems is essential for good outcomes.

REFERENCES

Benjamin A, Hirschowitz D. Surgery of the rheumatoid foot. In: Helal B, Wilson D, eds. The foot. Edinburgh: Churchill Livingstone; 1988:535–41.

Francis BE. Chiropody in the foot. In: Helal B, Wilson D, eds. The foot. Edinburgh: Churchill Livingstone; 1988:1080–110.

Ward AB. Footwear and orthoses. In: Butler RC, Jayson MI, eds. Collected reports on the rheumatic diseases. Chesterfield: Arthritis & Rheumatism Council; 1995.

PREVENTING AND TREATING CONTRACTURES: JOINT PROTECTION AND SPLINTING

M Anne Chamberlain

DEFINITION OF THE PROBLEM

Joint protection is a method of preventing joint damage. This is sound in bioengineering terms although remains unproved. However, it has no side effects, few costs and is simple in concept even if in practice not easy to teach, enforce or sustain. It aims to decrease loads through synovial joints which are vulnerable to damage by virtue of inflammatory synovitis within them.

Joint protection seeks to:

- use regular exercise regimens to prevent contractures,
- avoid strain to any one joint and distribute strain over several joint systems,
- use simple working methods, aids and orthoses to achieve this, and
- adopt a positive and preventive lifestyle to further joint protection.

This may involve such strategies as respecting pain, or preventing large or uncoordinated loads passing through inflamed joints. The load should be carried near the body rather than farther away from it; it should be taken not through the joint, but, where possible, through a neighboring long bone. The load can also be distributed in time and tasks can be selected, delegated or not done.

Exercise should be sufficient to keep the muscles which pass across the involved joints in 'good trim', not contracted, having as far as possible normal bulk and normal fitness. Knowledge of joint protection is usually imparted to the patient as part of patient education training given by occupational therapists, nurse practitioners or members of voluntary organizations. It should normally be accompanied by information about pacing and energy conservation.

Where joints are deformed or likely to become so, particularly if they are unstable, subluxing or persistently contain effusions or are held in abnormal positions, they may need splinting.

THE TYPICAL CASE

AN is a 24-year-old woman who was first seen by the rheumatologist as a child with pauciarticular juvenile chronic arthritis (JCA). The brunt of her disease fell on the eyes (with unilateral treated uveitis). She was discharged well, with no residual disabilities, from the regional JCA clinic at the age of 18 years.

Recently AN attended the adult rheumatology clinic with acute inflammatory disease of the proximal interphalangeal (PIP) joints and MCP joints with impending swan neck deformities in several fingers. The right wrist was tender. There was an apparently fixed flexion deformity of the left elbow with a range of 30°–100° and limitation of left shoulder abduction to 90°. She experienced difficulty in driving due to neck involvement and had pain when using her typewriter. She found it tiring to run her household, look after her small child and do the cooking she enjoyed.

THERAPEUTIC OPTIONS

Such patients require comprehensive management. It is important not to 'run after' their disease, but to bring it under control promptly and keep it controlled to prevent unnecessary joint damage. Drug therapy, however, is not the only treatment: AN required functional assessment, advice from occupational and physical therapists and input from all who undertake patient education.

Her arthritis was treated with methotrexate, dosage rising as necessary from the 5mg/week regimen. She was referred to the occupational therapist who dealt with impending joint deformities by providing finger ring splints for the involved PIPs of the fingers (Fig. 16.27). These should be worn for as long as comfortable, in periods of 20–40

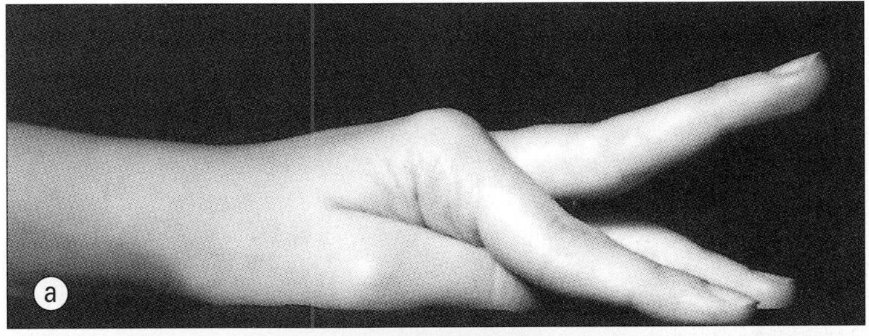

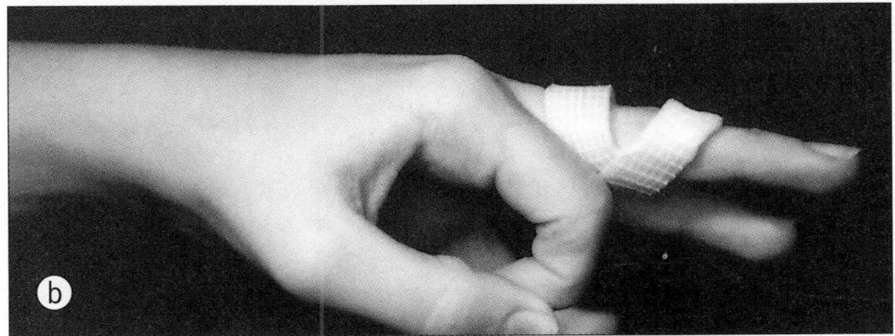

Fig. 16.27 Finger deformity in RA. (a) Hyperextension deformity of ring finger PIP. (b) Prevention of hyperextension at ring finger PIP by splintage (working or resting).

minutes during the day. AN was taught to stretch gently the intrinsic muscles and PIP joints.

The wrist was tender, grip painful and power grip reduced. A commercial working splint (Futuro) should be appropriate and should be worn when working. For some patients, it can be used at nights. Many patients are disconcerted by splints and stop wearing them, claiming they make the joint stiffer, though night resting splints are invaluable when many hand joints are involved (Fig. 16.28). It is important to reassure patients that splints do not produce joint damage.

Splintage is not appropriate for either elbow or shoulder. Preservation of function (particularly keyboard skills which may be lost if pronation is lost) and dressing and driving activities requires that the physical therapist teaches daily exercise to preserve range of movement at these joints. If daily home exercises fail to improve the range of movement it may be necessary to organize a period of more intensive exercise given by the physical therapist.

AN needed to be taught joint protection principles such as lifting both loads and her baby on her forearms and to rise (for example) by pressing her forearms on the arms of the chair, rather than by transmitting the weight of her arms through the finger joints. She was encouraged not to use a power grip (Fig. 16.29).

A small baby requires much handling and lifting. AN's central maternal role can be maintained by encouraging her to care for her baby while getting others, whether family members or paid help, to do household activities like shopping and cleaning. Disposable diapers, washers and driers and easy care clothes make doing the laundry much easier. Another person can do the shopping and put away food; the baby can be changed downstairs on a mat at convenient height to avoid repeated lifting. Ideally, the family should be taught the principles of joint protection to help them help the mother with RA.

AN will almost certainly have to 'pace' her domestic work and cooking and perhaps use simpler recipes. However, cooking not only provides her finger joints with desirable exercise; it is also an activity to enjoy doing with her child as she grows.

AN also wished to work part time. There are two components to the job – travel to and from work and the work itself. Commuting can be tiring: public transport is not friendly to those with poor grip and painful shoulders, so the whole journey may be tiring. A car with side or even panoramic mirrors is probably the aid most saving of energy and joints.

Work in a clerical capacity poses few problems, except for some keyboard operations which are not easy for those with PIP involvement. AN is able to manage at present but an assessment by the physical therapist and thence referral to the PACT (Placing, Assessment and Counseling Team of employment services) may be sought if the finger ring splints fail to hold the deformity or if the RA threatens her work. Numerous aids in the workplace are available through this route.

Splints are of four types: those for resting, those used during normal activities, those which are dynamic and those which can be re-set at increasingly improved angles. In inflammatory arthritis usually only resting and day splints are used in activities; dynamic splints are used mainly postoperatively. Splints selectively immobilize, stabilize or support joints, preventing subluxation where there is instability; they improve grip, e.g. when it is impaired by pain, allowing inflamed joints to rest and allowing (at the MCPs for example) patients to stretch contracted/shortened small muscles around the joint gently and effectively.

Splinting may be produced commercially or, preferably, by occupational therapists, particularly for children who grow quickly or when the problem is complex and requires frequent communication between the physician and the splint maker. Splint materials are numerous, some cheap, some remoldable, some more user-friendly, and familiarity with these by physicians is desirable. This author believes physicians should see all the splints that they have prescribed.

Most doctors neglect joint protection and splintage until too late. These should form part of routine practice within the management of early inflammatory arthritis, as principles of prevention rather than cure

CONCLUSIONS

Joint protection and splinting should be undertaken to suppress joint activity and prevent joint damage. Clinicians should view joint protection, exercise and function as essential to conserving normal function and preventing handicap.

REFERENCES

Brattstrom M. Joint protection and rehabilitation in chronic rheumatic disorders. London: Wolfe Medical Publications; 1987.

Lindroth Y, Bauman P, Brooks PM, Priestley D. A 5-year follow-up of a controlled trial of an arthritis education programme. Br J Rheumatol. 1995;34:647–52.

Lorig K, Fries JF. The arthritis handbook. New York: Addison-Wesley; 1993.

Melvin JL. Orthotic treatment of the hand. What's new? Bull Rheum Dis. 1995;44(4):5–8.

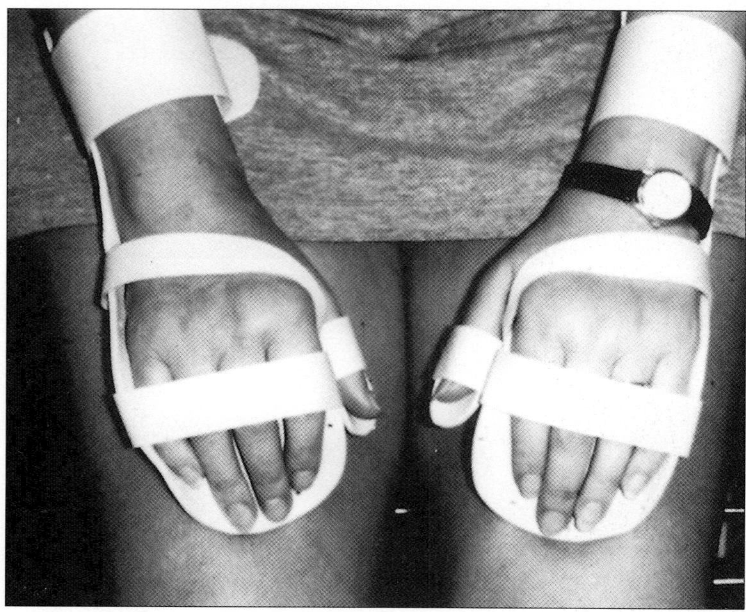

Fig. 16.28 Resting splints for inflamed wrists and hands.

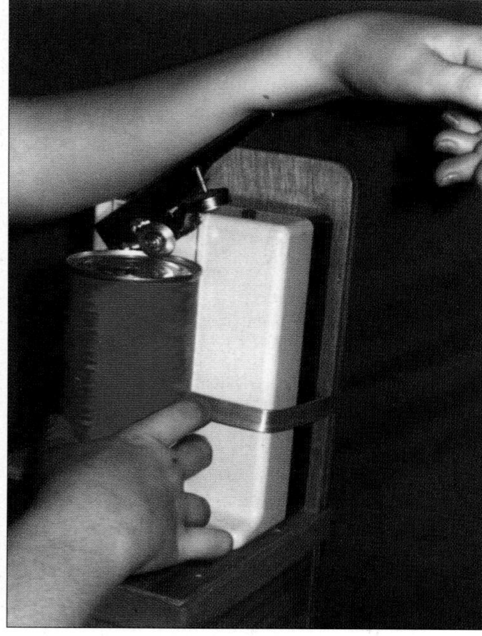

Fig. 16.29 To show joint protection – sparing of joints in this task which no longer requires power grip.

DEFINITION OF PROBLEM

Spontaneous tendon ruptures in the hand and wrist of patients with RA can occur at any time and at any age. Ruptures are caused by direct invasion of tenosynovium or attrition over roughened bone created by erosions or osteophytes. The patient is often unaware of the tendon rupture if hand function has been compromised for a long time. Clinical examination for tendon rupture is frequently complicated by joint deformities and other tendon problems and rarely by nerve lesions. The goals of treatment are to prevent further ruptures due to the same process and to restore hand function appropriate to the needs of the patient and the condition of the hand.

THE TYPICAL CASE

MS, a 74-year-old woman with RA of 29 years' duration, presented with a 3-week history of inability to flex the distal joint of her right thumb. She had not had an arthritic flare for several years and no specific physical activity preceded the loss. She did not seek medical advice initially because she attributed the loss to further general deterioration of her hand. Her main concern was loss of pinch strength and dexterity.

Physical examination of the right thumb revealed a hyperextended IP joint. The carpometacarpal (CMC) joint was slightly subluxed and had a mild flexion–adduction contracture. The MCP joint also had a mild extension contracture and slight subluxation. Osteoarthritic changes, including crepitus, were present in all thumb joints. There was no active synovitis or tenosynovitis in the hand and wrist.

Active IP joint flexion was absent in the thumb; however, passive flexion was nearly full. Combined passive extension of the wrist and the thumb MCP and CMC joints did not produce IP joint flexion (tenodesis test). All extensor tendons in the hand and wrist were intact. However, there was ulnar deviation of the fingers and subluxation of the extensor tendons at the MCP joints with an inability fully to extend the digits actively. The flexor digitorum superficialis and profundus tendons were intact in all fingers. There was mild wrist deformity and moderate limitation of motion. Nerve function was normal. Laboratory studies were unremarkable. Radiographs revealed diffuse, long-standing arthritic changes in the wrist and digits (Fig. 16.30).

A diagnosis of flexor pollicis longus tendon rupture was made. At surgery, a sharp osteophyte on the scaphoid was found projecting into the carpal tunnel which had caused an attrition rupture of the flexor pollicis longus tendon and partial erosion of the flexor digitorum profundus tendon to the index finger. The osteophyte was removed and a tendon transfer of the flexor digitorum superficialis of the ring finger was done.

DIAGNOSTIC PROBLEMS

The diagnosis of tendon rupture requires both an observant patient and an informed physician. Extensor tendon ruptures are usually caused by attrition and occur most frequently at the distal ulna or Lister's tubercle, which acts as a pulley for the extensor pollicis longus tendon. Chronic synovitis of the distal radioulnar joint causes erosions of the dorsal ulna leaving sharp spikes that erode through the joint capsule and extensor tendons. Typically, the extensor digiti quinti tendon ruptures first, followed by the extensor digitorum comminus tendons, beginning with the small finger and progressing radially as the remaining intact tendons shift ulnarwards. A rupture is often sudden and usually painless. Ruptures in patients accustomed to impaired hand function may go unrecognized, especially an isolated extensor digiti quinti tendon rupture which usually produces minimal loss. Extensor digiti quinti function is tested by holding the index, long and ring fingers in flexion to nullify the action of the extensor digitorum comminus and asking the patient to extend the small finger; an inability to extend the finger indicates a possible rupture. Radiographs may demonstrate dorsal subluxation and erosions of the ulnar head.

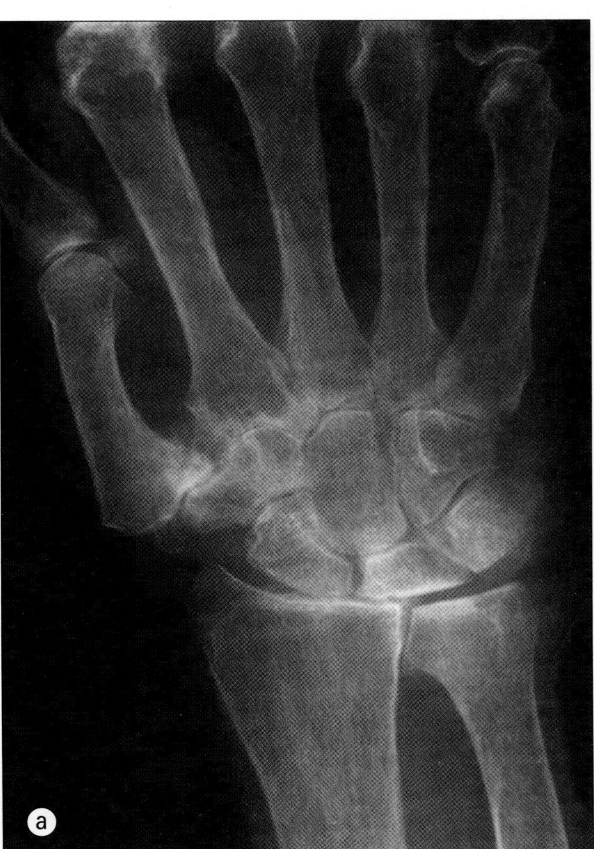

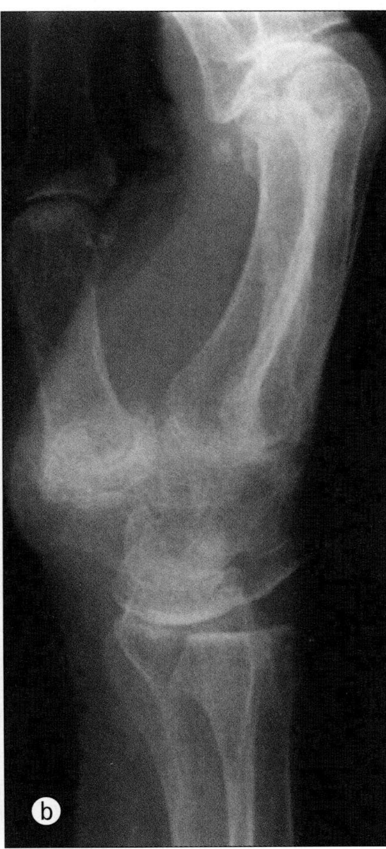

Fig. 16.30 Diffuse, long-standing arthritic changes are present in the wrist, including mild ulnar translation of the carpus. Osteophytes are present but the bony spike responsible for the rupture is not seen.

Although sudden loss of extension is usually the result of an attrition rupture, other conditions should be considered. Extensor tendon ruptures may also occur at the wrist due to invasive tenosynovitis. Metacarpophalangeal joint dislocation results in a flexed and ulnar deviated position of the finger. Lack of passive MCP joint extension and the presence of palpable or visible tendons make the differential diagnosis. Ulnar displacement of the extensor tendons at the metacarpal heads results in extensor lag of the MCP joints. Differentiation between tendon displacement and rupture can be difficult. If the patient is able to maintain MCP joint extension actively after the joint is extended passively the tendon is probably intact. The least common but most difficult condition that mimics tendon rupture is paralysis of the extensor digitorum comminus muscle from posterior interosseous nerve compression caused by elbow synovitis. There are several subtle findings between tendon rupture and muscle paralysis; however, the most reliable diagnostic test is the presence or absence of the tenodesis effect. With tendon rupture, wrist flexion has no effect on finger extension.

Flexor tendon ruptures are much less common than extensor tendon ruptures. Attrition ruptures occur in the carpal tunnel and are usually caused by an osteophyte on the scaphoid. The flexor pollicis longus tendon is affected first, followed by the index flexor digitorum profundus tendon. Clinical diagnosis of flexor pollicis longus tendon rupture is not difficult unless there is a fixed deformity of the IP joint. Although a carpal tunnel radiographic view would likely demonstrate an osteophyte projecting into the tunnel, wrist stiffness will nearly always preclude appropriate positioning for this view. Flexor tendon ruptures may also occur in the palm and digit from invasive tenosynovitis. Signs of flexor tenosynovitis in the hand and wrist include carpal tunnel syndrome, decreased dexterity, weakness, triggering, locking and pain. As tendon gliding becomes restricted, loss of active finger flexion ensues.

A discrepancy between active and passive finger flexion is characteristic of flexor tenosynovitis. An isolated flexor digitorum profundus rupture results in loss of active distal interphalangeal joint flexion, however, an isolated flexor digitorum superficialis rupture is difficult to detect in a rheumatoid patient. Joint stiffness makes flexor tenosynovitis and tendon ruptures more difficult to diagnose. A tendon nodule within the fibro-osseous canal of the finger can restrict tendon excursion and mimic a rupture.

Magnetic resonance imaging is highly sensitive to the full spectrum of tendon pathology, and has been shown to identify tendonitis and tendon rupture with greater accuracy than clinical examination (see Chapter 2.14). Tendon integrity can also be effectively evaluated with low-cost dedicated extremity MRI.

THERAPEUTIC OPTIONS

The factors responsible for a single tendon rupture maycause additional ruptures resulting in more significant functional loss. An isolated rupture of the extensor digitis quinti tendon may be the first sign of impending ruptures of the extensor digitorum comminus tendons. A flexor pollicis longus tendon rupture is often followed by ruptures of the flexor digitorum profundus tendons. Thus, even if the patient chooses to accept the present loss, surgical treatment is indicated to prevent further ruptures. An exception is an isolated rupture of the extensor pollicis longus tendon due to attrition at Lister's tubercle. The prognosis is better for restoration of function for attrition ruptures than for those caused by invasive tenosynovitis. Flexor tendon ruptures within the finger have a particularly poor prognosis. Thus, tenosynovectomy in the fingers should be considered for persistent tenosynovitis, especially if there is severely reduced active motion or if a rupture has already occurred in one finger. Because flexor tendon ruptures can occur in the wrist, palm or finger, surgical exploration is ultimately necessary to identify the site. Findings at surgery combined with the preoperative assessment of the patient's functional requirements will determine the appropriate surgical treatment.

CONCLUSIONS

Tendon ruptures in the hand and wrist are caused by attrition from roughened bone or by invasive tenosynovitis and may go unrecognized by the patient. Careful physical examination can usually differentiate tendon rupture from other causes of decreased function, including tendon subluxation, joint deformity and nerve compression. Surgical treatment is usually indicated to prevent further ruptures and to restore function. In some patients, tenosynovectomy may be indicated to decrease the risk of tendon rupture.

REFERENCES

Brown FE, Brown ML. Long-term results after tenosynovectomy to treat the rheumatoid hand. J Hand Surg. 1988;13A:704–8.
Ertel AN, Millender LH, Nalebuff EA, McKay D, Leslie BM. Flexor tendon ruptures in patients with rheumatoid arthritis. J Hand Surg. 1988;13A:860–6.
Leslie BM. Rheumatoid extensor tendon ruptures. Hand Clin. 1989;5:191–202.
Peterfy CG, Roberts T, Genant HK. Dedicated extremity MRI: an emerging technology. Radiol Clin North Am. 1997:
Rubens DJ, Blebea JS, Totterman SMS, Hooper MM. Rheumatoid arthritis: evaluation of wrist extensor tendons with clinical examination versus MR imaging – a preliminary report. Radiology. 1993;187:831–8.

AN INFECTED RHEUMATOID ARTHRITIS JOINT

Allen D Sawitzke & John R Ward

DEFINITION OF THE PROBLEM

While the exact frequency of bacterial joint infection in RA patients is unknown, these patients are at increased risk of joint infection. Usually, the patient is older and has long-standing seropositive disease. Almost half the patients are receiving systemic corticosteroids and essentially all are receiving NSAIDs, which may suppress signs of infection such as fever, pain and swelling. While usually a monoarticular disease involving large joints, septic arthritis in patients with RA may be polyarticular.

THE TYPICAL CASE

A 64-year-old woman with RA of 10 years' duration was receiving prednisone 5mg daily, sulindac 200mg b.i.d. and methotrexate 7.5mg weekly. She presented with a 36-hour history of redness, heat, increased swelling and pain in her left knee. There was no history of infection at other sites, fever or chills. On physical examination, she had mild synovitis of several joints and subcutaneous nodules over both extensor surfaces of the forearms. Her right knee was swollen, warm and had a palpable effusion (Fig. 16.31). While the joint was only moderately tender, there was marked pain on flexion and extension. There was no evidence of associated infection on physical examination and the skin was intact throughout. Her oral temperature was 37.3°C, the rheumatoid factor was 1:1280, ESR 56mm/h and blood leukocyte count 13,000/mm^3 with 80% neutrophils and 8% band forms. She was admitted to the hospital and blood cultures were obtained. The synovial fluid had 92,000 nucleated cells/mm^3 with 88% neutrophils. Examination for crystals was negative and no organisms were seen on the gram stain of centrifuged synovial fluid. Cultures were obtained for *Neisseria*, aerobic and anaerobic bacteria, mycobacteria and fungi. Radiographs of the right knee showed mild joint space narrowing. Because the gram stain of the synovial fluid was negative, and in view of the absence of an identifiable entry site, concomitant infection or features

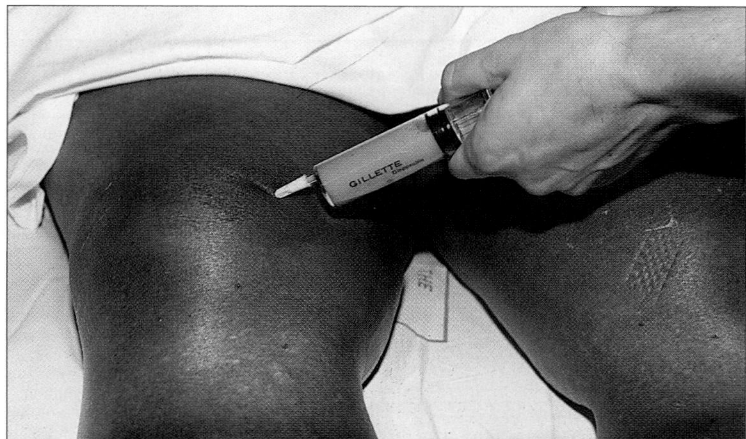

Fig. 16.31 An infected RA joint. A high degree of clinical suspicion of infection in patients with RA is essential. Pus may be present as in this case.

of bacterial sepsis, no antibiotic treatment was initiated.

The following day, re-aspiration of the left knee revealed similar findings as those on admission except that the gram stain revealed gram-positive cocci. Nafcillin, 2g i.v. q.i.d., was started. The next day, synovial fluid cultures grew *S. aureus*, which was sensitive to penicillin. Blood cultures yielded no growth. Antibiotic therapy was changed to penicillin G 1.2 million units i.v. q.i.d.

Daily joint aspirations were done and cultures became negative after 2 days. By day 7, the synovial fluid cell count had fallen to 20,000/mm^3 and the joint examination revealed only minimal effusion. The patient was then given penicillin V p.o. with serum bactericidal levels of greater than 1:16. The patient was discharged and continued taking oral penicillin for 3 weeks.

DIAGNOSTIC PROBLEMS

In the absence of trauma to or unusual use of a joint, a monoarticular flare in RA is unusual. Laboratory data, such as an elevated ESR, are not helpful. Mild blood leukocytosis is sometimes observed in RA and prednisone may increase the absolute number of mature granulocytes in the circulation. The degree of pain on motion in the knee observed in this patient would be unusual. While synovial fluid nucleated cell counts above 50,000/mm^3 can infrequently be seen in RA, a high proportion of neutrophils would be more consistent with a bacterial infection or crystal-induced disease.

Concomitant corticosteroids and NSAIDs can mask the early systemic and articular findings of joint infection. Care must be taken to exclude bacterial infection by repeated synovial fluid analysis, gram stain and cultures. Gout and pseudogout are uncommon in RA patients, such that even when crystals are observed, infection must be excluded. An entity termed 'pseudoseptic arthritis' occurs in RA patients who present with clinical and laboratory findings that are highly suggestive of bacterial infection. However, cultures are negative and attacks, lasting only 12–48 hours, do not require antibiotic treatment.

The usual approach to suspected bacterial infection of a joint in the patient with RA is to look for an associated infection such as urinary tract infection or a skin ulcer and to culture all suspected joints as indicated by clinical findings. Synovial fluid and blood cultures for *N. gonorrhoeae*, aerobic and anaerobic bacteria are taken. Cultures of asymptomatic sites, such as the mouth, cervix and rectum, and cultures for mycobacteria and fungi are considered. Synovial fluid analyses for total nucleated and differential cell counts, crystals and glucose content are obtained. A gram stain on the centrifuged fluid specimen is examined, and appropriate antibiotics are given immediately based on the most probable infecting organism.

THERAPEUTIC OPTIONS

When there is no evident entry site or concomitant systemic bacterial infection, and a gram stain of the synovial fluid is negative, antibiotic therapy is nevertheless implemented if the synovial fluid nucleated cell count is high and there are greater than 90% neutrophils. Since *S. aureus* is the most likely infecting organism, a penicillinase-resistant penicillin or first-generation cephalosporin (or vancomycin especially where methicillin resistance is frequent, or a fluoroquinolone and rifampin) is given parenterally and joint drainage is begun. If infection with a gram-negative bacillus is suspected, treatment with a ticarcillin–clavulanate combination or imipenem is initiated. Antibiotic therapy is then adjusted once culture results and sensitivities are known.

The best indicator of response to treatment is for a positive synovial fluid culture to revert to negative. This should occur within 24–72 hours. A reduction in arthritis, total nucleated cell count and neutrophil count may not be observed for at least 7 days.

Bacterial infection of joints most often results from hematogenous seeding of the synovium and spread to the joint space. If antibiotics are started at this stage, before extension to the joint space, synovial fluid cultures will be negative. Thus, the initial synovial fluid culture may yield no growth, and subsequent cultures ultimately become positive. The decision when to initiate antibiotic therapy is often difficult and must be decided for the individual patient. If the gram stain is positive, antibiotics should be initiated to cover the identified organism and selection of antibiotics reviewed after the organism is recovered on culture and sensitivities are determined. If initial gram stain and culture are negative, broad-spectrum antibiotics may be given pending final culture results. An alternative approach is to delay treatment pending isolation of the infecting organism from the synovial fluid or blood so that specific antibiotic treatment can be prescribed. Thus, the physician will be able selectively to administer antibacterial therapy and monitor the response by the absence of bacterial growth in synovial fluid cultures within 1–4 days of treatment. Long-term antibiotic treatment of an unidentified organism can be avoided by delaying treatment until culture results are positive. Also, patients with 'pseudoseptic arthritis' will be recognized by their spontaneous improvement without antibiotic therapy. Based on the available data, a delay of 2–5 days early in the course of bacterial infection of joints would not prevent successful results. In addition to appropriate antibacterial therapy, complete aspiration of the joint should be done whenever fluid reaccumulates. This can often be done successfully by needle aspiration but may require arthroscopic or open surgical drainage for joints in which needle aspiration is difficult, such as the hip, or when the fluid appears to be loculated. Range-of-motion exercises are implemented as tolerated by the patient.

CONCLUSIONS

Patients with RA have an increased susceptibility to bacterial infection of their joints. The typical signs of septic arthritis may not be present and the disease may be polyarticular (Fig. 16.32). Appropriate antibiotic therapy and complete joint drainage will generally produce excellent results. 'Pseudoseptic arthritis' can mimic a true bacterial infection and does not require antibacterial treatment.

DIAGNOSIS AND MANAGEMENT OF AN INFECTED JOINT IN RHEUMATOID ARTHRITIS

- Onset may be insidious
- May be polyarticular
- Confirm diagnosis by appropriate synovial fluid examination and cultures
- Monitor response to antibacterial therapy by repeated synovial fluid examination and cultures
- Adequately drain infected joint
- Start early range of motion
- Be aware of possible 'pseudoseptic arthritis'

Fig. 16.32 Diagnosis and management of an infected RA joint.

REFERENCES

Kaandorp CJ, Van Schaardenburg d, Krijnen P, Habbema JD, van de Laar MA. Risk factors for septic arthritis in patients with joint disease. A prospective study. Jan van Breemen Institute for Rheumatology and Rehabilitation, Amsterdam, The Netherlands. Arthritis Rheum 1995:Dec;38(12):1819–25.

Call PS, Ward JR, Samuelson CO Jr. Pseudoseptic arthritis in patients with rheumatoid arthritis. West J Med. 1985;143:471–3.

Goldenberg DL. Infectious arthritis complicating rheumatoid arthritis and other chronic rheumatic disorders. Arthritis Rheum. 1989;32:496–502.

DRUGS, PREGNANCY AND RHEUMATOID ARTHRITIS

Christopher Needs & Peter M Brooks

DEFINITION OF PROBLEM

Rheumatologists frequently encounter the management dilemma of rheumatic disease during pregnancy. Issues that need to be addressed include an awareness of the possible effects of medication on a developing fetus and advising patients of their potential impact should pregnancy occur. An appreciation of the effect of prescribed medication on fetal physiology is also important. The influence the rheumatic disease may have on pregnancy and vice versa needs to be considered, and the impact of the disease and treatment on female fertility is also important.

THE TYPICAL CASE

A 32-year-old nulliparous woman had a 2-year history of seropositive and erosive RA. At the onset of disease her hemoglobin was 9.8g/dl, ESR 68mm/h, rheumatoid factor 1:128 and antibodies to Ro(SS-A) and phospholipids were negative. Initial disease activity was such that weekly intramuscular Sodium Aurothiomalate (50mg) was introduced, with piroxicam 20mg/day. After 16 weeks of therapy, early morning stiffness was reduced to less than 5 minutes, and the patient remained on piroxicam in a reduced dose of 10mg daily. Radiologic evaluation 18 months later demonstrated several erosions in the right 3rd and 4th MTP joints. At this stage, she noted an increase in her morning stiffness, had some difficulty in walking and had pain in her wrists. At the time of consultation, she was 6 weeks pregnant while still receiving aurothiomalate 50mg each week and taking daily piroxicam. Investigations showed an ESR of 26mm/h, a hemoglobin of 12.2g/dl and a rheumatoid factor titre of 1:256.

This patient was already experiencing erosive disease affecting her feet and wrists and increasing difficulty could be anticipated in coping with a growing child if the disease was not suppressed.

After discussion with the patient, it was decided to give injections of gold aurothiomalate 20mg every 2 weeks during the pregnancy and to increase these injections to 50mg weekly for the first 6 weeks postpartum. Ibuprofen was provided as needed but was discontinued at 28 weeks as further analgesia was not required. Joint swelling began to recur 4 weeks postpartum and ibuprofen was reintroduced in a dose of 800mg q.i.d., timed to coincide with the beginning of breast-feeding (see below). Acetaminophen (paracetamol) was also required for pain relief during the immediate postpartum period.

MANAGEMENT PROBLEMS

About 70% of women with RA will have some amelioration of their disease during pregnancy. Even though improvement occurs, there are likely to be fluctuations during the pregnancy and thus there will be a need for continuing analgesia.

Unfortunately, the vast majority of women in whom disease stabilizes during pregnancy are likely to have a significant relapse in the postpartum period, usually in the first 8 weeks. Such recurrences are not influenced by breast-feeding or the return of menstruation. This makes it important to maintain suppression of disease activity as much as possible during pregnancy so that the risk of postpartum flare is reduced. It also means that almost all women with RA will at least need full-dose NSAID therapy in the postpartum period.

There is no evidence to suggest that RA alone will have an adverse effect on the outcome of pregnancy, although infants with mothers who have Sjögren's syndrome with antibodies to Ro(SS-A) are at increased risk of neonatal lupus syndrome (see Chapter 7.8).

PROBLEMS ASSOCIATED WITH NONSTEROIDAL ANTI-INFLAMMATORY DRUGS DURING PREGNANCY
Prolonged gestation
Prolonged labor
Increased risk of intracranial hemorrhage in premature infants and mothers receiving aspirin
Postpartum hemorrhage
Premature ductus arteriosus closure leading to pulmonary hypertension

Fig. 16.33 Problems associated with NSAIDs during pregnancy.

With NSAID therapy during the first 8 weeks of pregnancy there is a potential for teratogenicity, while in the last eight weeks there is the potential to influence fetal physiology. In general, no consistent teratogenic effects have been reported in humans taking NSAIDs. However, in animal models using higher than normal pharmacologic doses, various developmental abnormalities have been reported. The physiologic effects relate to the antagonism of the prostaglandins involved in the regulation of systemic and pulmonary blood vessels. Premature closure of the ductus arteriosus has been reported in both humans and animals taking NSAIDs prior to delivery. Thus, NSAID use in the third trimester should be restricted. Other considerations regarding NSAID use in pregnancy include the effect on platelet aggregation and uterine muscle tone at the time of birth (Fig. 16.33). From a practical point of view, it would seem reasonable to continue NSAIDs, if required, throughout the pregnancy but to restrict their use as much as possible in the last month of pregnancy and to use drugs that have a relatively short half-life.

In rats and rabbits, central nervous system malformations have been reported with gold aurothiomalate. Gold has been demonstrated to cross the placenta; indeed, therapeutic concentrations have been detected in umbilical blood samples of a developmentally normal infant at the time of delivery. There have been no adverse effects reported in a retrospective follow-up of seven pregnancies during which gold treatment was received. In these particular patients, at least one intramuscular gold injection had been given after the pregnancy commenced. In the patient described earlier, it would seem that the gold had controlled the RA to a certain extent but there was still some disease activity. There is no reason why gold should not be continued in a slightly lower dose throughout the pregnancy, but if the disease shows any increase in activity this would be a good argument for a return to full-dose treatment, at least during the last 6 months of pregnancy. All women of childbearing age who take methotrexate must be advised about adequate contraception. However, there is a suggestion that weekly low-dose methotrexate is not associated with fetal abnormalities when the drug is withdrawn on confirmation of pregnancy. Although spontaneous

FACTORS INFLUENCING DRUG CONCENTRATION IN BREAST-FED INFANTS
Maternal
Milk composition (fat, protein, water) and pH Mammary blood flow Maternal drug metabolism Time and frequency of feeding in relation to maternal dosing
Drug
Molecular weight p*Ka* Lipid solubility Pharmacokinetics Dose and dosage interval
Infant
Volume of milk consumed Absorptive capacity of infant Deconjugating ability of infant

Fig. 16.34 Factors influencing drug concentration in breast-fed infants.

ELIMINATION HALF-LIVES OF COMMONLY USED NONSTEROIDAL ANTI-INFLAMMATORY DRUGS	
Drug	Half life (hours)
Diclofenac	3
Diflunisal	10
Fenoprofen	2
Ibuprofen	2
Indomethacin	8
Ketoprofen	2
Naproxen	12
Piroxicam	26
Salicylate	4–15*
Sulindac	16
Tenoxicam	36
*Dose-dependant kinetics	

Fig. 16.35 Elimination half-lives of commonly used NSAIDs.

abortion may result from methotrexate use in rheumatic disease, birth defects have not been demonstrated in these fetuses.

Given the clinical setting of using NSAIDs in the postpartum period, only indomethacin has been reported to produce an adverse reaction during breast-feeding. As most medications will enter breast milk to some extent, the aim is to use medications which have minimal concentrations within breast milk. Basic drugs accumulate in milk compared with acidic compounds. Additional medication factors that need to be considered in deciding on appropriate agents to be used during lactation, include the propensity of the infant to release active medication from metabolites (Fig. 16.34). Glucuronide metabolites may be cleaved by the infant to release free drugs. The presence of active metabolites with a longer half-life than parent compounds may expose the infant to pharmacologic effects.

There are theoretical concerns with the use in the postpartum period of sulindac and phenylbutazone as well as diflunisal because of their long half-lives. Diclofenac has active metabolites that have a longer half-life than the parent compound, although clinical studies indicate that the amount of diclofenac present in breast milk is minimal.

When taking into account the above considerations, it would seem appropriate to use ibuprofen or ketoprofen (not in sustained-release form). The ideal situation would be to take the NSAID at the beginning of each breast-feed. Assuming that breast-feeding is not going to be repeated in under 4 hours and that each feeding lasts an average of 20 minutes, minimal infant exposure to the medication will be achieved.

No adverse effects have been reported in the breast-fed babies of mothers taking corticosteroids or sulfasalazine. Although there are theoretical risks with antimalarial drugs, babies are exposed to very small amounts in breast milk. Gold is excreted in breast milk with the infant being exposed to a greater concentration versus weight ratio of gold than the mother. There are no data on D-penicillamine excretion in breast milk, but it is likely to be low.

THERAPEUTIC OPTIONS

Rheumatoid arthritis is likely to flare in the postpartum period, and this should weigh heavily in deciding the management option during pregnancy itself. It may be safer in such women to reduce the dosage and frequency of gold administration during pregnancy in order to avoid a postpartum flare in disease activity, rather than discontinuing it altogether.

In order to reduce the physiologic impact of NSAIDs on the fetus, the use of medications with short half-lives is more appropriate. If an anti-inflammatory drug is required during the pregnancy, one of the short half-life propionic acid derivatives used intermittently should achieve the dual purpose of adequate pain relief with minimal effect on fetal pulmonary arterial musculature. Figure 16.35 lists the elimination half-lives of commonly available NSAIDs.

Likewise, in considering NSAIDs to be used in the postpartum period, short half-life agents are ideal. If used, infant exposure to medication is minimized when the dosing is timed to coincide with the beginning of breast-feeding. Given the average feeding time of 20 minutes with the medication having a half-life of 4–6 hours, minimum drug concentration would be present within the breast milk at 5–6 hours after the previous oral dose. Gold compounds have been detected in breast milk but cannot be absorbed by the infant. As such, exposure of the infant to gold compounds is minimal, and lactation itself is not a contraindication to the continued use of gold aurothiomalate.

CONCLUSIONS

Where possible, all medication should be withdrawn during pregnancy and avoided during the postpartum period. However, given adverse prognostic factors at the onset and the risk to the mother's and the child's physical and psychological well-being, a disease-suppressive agent is often required. This situation also reinforces the need to be vigilant with prescribed medications in all women of child-bearing age. Appropriate counseling as to the possible adverse effect of medication on the developing child is desirable.

REFERENCES

Kozlowski RD, Steinbrunner JV, Mackenzie AH, et al. Outcome of first trimester exposure to low dose methotrexate in eight patients with rheumatic disease. Am J Med. 1990;88:589–92.

Needs C, Brooks P. Anti-rheumatoid medication during pregnancy. Br J Rheumatol. 1984;24:282–90.

Ostensen M, Husby G. A prospective clinical study of pregnancy on rheumatoid arthritis and ankylosing spondylitis. Arthritis Rheum. 1983;26:1155–9.

Preston S, Needs C. Guidelines on the use of antirheumatic drugs in women during pregnancy and child-bearing age. Clin Rheumatol. 1990;4:687–98.

Tarp V, Graudal HA. Follow-up study of children exposed to gold *in vitro*. Arthritis Rheum. 1985:28;235–6.

HEPATIC AND PULMONARY COMPLICATIONS IN PATIENTS TAKING METHOTREXATE FOR RHEUMATOID ARTHRITIS

Daniel E Furst & Peter M Brooks

DEFINITION OF THE PROBLEM

Low-dose (7.5–50mg/week) methotrexate has been established as an effective therapy for inflammatory arthropathies and is now one of the most commonly used SAARDs. Patients with RA tolerate this drug for a longer time than other SAARDs, with up to 75% of patients still taking their treatment after 6 years.

THE TYPICAL CASE

RD is a 40-year-old woman with RA of 6 years' duration. Her past history includes alcohol abuse lasting for 10 years (although she has been abstinent by history for over 2 years) and type 2 (noninsulin-dependent) diabetes. Current treatment for her RA includes diclofenac 75mg b.i.d. and prednisone 5mg in the morning. Eighteen months ago she had an ESR of 42mm/h and swollen MCP and PIP joints and right knee and tender MTP joints, plus 2 hours of morning stiffness and fatigue within 1 hour of rising.

Methotrexate 15mg p.o. weekly was commenced and over the next 2 months the patient experienced a good response with joint swelling and tenderness reduced by 60%, morning stiffness reduced by 45 minutes and onset of fatigue delayed to 4 hours. The ESR decreased to 26mm/h. Six months prior to starting methotrexate, the patient's aspartate aminotransferase (AST) and alanine aminotransferase (ALT) were 45 and 48IU/l (upper limit of normal 40 and 42IU/l), respectively, and albumin was 4.2g/l. After 2 months on methotrexate, AST and ALT were 35 and 40IU/l and albumin was 4.6g/l. Over the ensuing year liver function tests were carried out at 4–8-week intervals and remained normal. Over the past 3 months her ALTs were noted to be 50, 60 and 198IU/l and ASTs were 60, 70 and 280IU/l. Albumin was 4.2, 3.9 and 3.8g/l.

Given the patient's previous history of alcohol abuse, the first concern was a recurrence of alcohol intake, but in addition the use of diclofenac may be suspected.

The patient was asked about alcohol intake (which she vociferously denied) and diclofenac was stopped for 4 weeks (some increase in disease activity was noted). Repeat ASTs on two occasions over 4 weeks were 152 and 120IU/l, ALTs were 160 and 180IU/l, albumins 3.5 and 3.4g/l.

No history of congestive heart failure was obtained, blood sugars were between 80 and 180mg/dl and the patient gave no history of appetite loss, weight loss, gastrointestinal symptoms or menstrual irregularity. Mammography 3 months previously was normal. Physical examination, including pelvic, was unremarkable. Glycosylated hemoglobin (HbA_{1C}) was 7.4%, hepatitis A, B and C screening was negative, there was no blood in the stool and the Pap smear was normal.

A liver biopsy was performed; this showed minimal periportal infiltration with lymphocytes plus some fatty degeneration but no fibrosis. Methotrexate was continued and hydroxychloroquine 400mg daily added after appropriate eye testing. Liver function tests were repeated and returned towards normal (ASTs and ALTs 40–60IU/l over the next 6 months) with albumin in the 3.6–4.0g/l range.

The patient's symptoms slowly improved over 6 months after starting a combination of methotrexate and hydroxychloroquine. The joint tenderness and swelling decreased to fewer than five joints, the ESR decreased to 18mm/h, morning stiffness decreased to less than 1 hour and the fatigue ceased being a significant problem. Prednisone was slowly decreased to 2mg/day. Although the patient developed two upper respiratory infections over this period, each cleared over 1 week, required no antibiotics and resulted in no interruption of methotrexate therapy.

Then the patient suddenly developed a persistent cough and a fever of 38°C. After 2 days she became quite short of breath and reported for review. Lung examination was unremarkable but the chest radiography showed patchy infiltrates in the right upper and left lower lobes; PaO_2 was 75mmHg and the PCO_2 30mmHg. Investigations for opportunistic infections such as *Pneumocystis carinii* were negative and it was decided to discontinue the methotrexate and provide supportive care with prednisone 60mg daily for 1 week. The prednisone was then rapidly tapered. The pulmonary lesion cleared promptly but it was considered unwise to restart the methotrexate.

DIAGNOSTIC PROBLEMS

A history of alcohol abuse increases the chance of serious liver damage from methotrexate and diclofenac, as any other NSAIDs, may have accounted for the transaminitis seen in this patient. Given the continued elevated liver function tests, despite withdrawal of diclofenac, a diagnosis of methotrexate-induced liver disease becomes more probable. Before proceeding to liver biopsy, a careful history and physical examination should to look for other causes of abnormal liver function such as congestive heart failure, diabetes or tumor as well as other forms of hepatitis. Since the liver function tests had been abnormal for more than 3 months in this patient and hepatitis screens were negative, liver biopsy would seem justified.

The American College of Rheumatology (ACR) has recently recommended baseline liver function tests and hepatitis B and C virus (HBV and HCV) serology for all RA patients commencing methotrexate to exclude pre-existing liver disease, together with baseline complete blood count and creatine phosphokinase (CPK).

Liver biopsies should be performed prior to commencing methotrexate therapy only for patients with a high risk of pre-existing pathology. In this case, the history of alcoholism is such a risk factor, but no baseline liver biopsy was done. Biopsies should then be considered in patients who have elevated AST levels in 5 of 9, or 6 of 12, liver function test determinations over a period of 1 year.

While the data for improvement of liver function tests with the addition of hydroxychloroquine to methotrexate are limited to cohort experience, and decreased liver function test results do not necessarily imply decreased risk of cirrhosis, the fact that albumin had stabilized in this patient was encouraging.

Low-dose methotrexate can result in a range of pulmonary pathologies, both infectious (especially opportunistic infections) and noninfectious. The literature has not always been clear in defining the particular methotrexate pulmonary problem, making incidence rates difficult to estimate. Rheumatoid arthritis may also be associated with interstitial lung disease, thus confounding the diagnosis.

Pulmonary infections, particularly with opportunistic organisms such as *P. carinii*, should be excluded; once this has been done, the diagnosis of methotrexate hypersensitivity or idiosyncratic drug reaction should be considered. Prevalence rates of between 0.3 and 12% have been reported, but the true risk is probably towards the lower end of the range. Risk factors for methotrexate pulmonary disease are poorly defined with disagreement between studies, but pre-existing lung disease, cigarette smoking and renal impairment have all been reported as possible predisposing factors.

CONCLUSIONS

Methotrexate is an extremely useful SAARD but toxicities do occur. Patients should be screened for pre-existing liver and renal disease prior to commencing therapy and monitored appropriately throughout. Minor toxic effects such as nausea, mucositis and weight loss may be prevented by initial dose reduction or by the addition of folic or folinic acid. The major difficulties come with liver disease and with pulmonary symptoms. These may be prevented in the main by strict adherence to the ACR's recommendations for monitoring liver function and by careful and prompt review of any pulmonary symptoms that develop in patients taking methotrexate.

REFERENCES

Barrera P, Laan RJFM, van Riel PLCM, *et al.* Methotrexate-related pulmonary complications in rheumatoid arthritis. Ann Rheum Dis. 1994;53:434–9.

Conaghan PG, Brooks PM, Quinn DI, Day RO. Hazards of low dose methotrexate. Aust N Z J Med. 1995;25:670–73.

Erickson AR, Reddy V, Vogel Gesang SA, West SG. Usefulness of the American College of Rheumatology guidelines for liver biopsy in methotrexate treated rheumatoid patients. Arthritis Rheum. 1995;38:1115–19.

Kremer JM, Alarcon GF, Lightfoot RW, *et al.* Methotrexate for rheumatoid arthritis. Arthritis Rheum. 1994;37:316–28.

Walker AM, Funch D, Dreyer NA, *et al.* Determinants of serious liver disease among patients receiving low dose methotrexate for rheumatoid arthritis. Arthritis Rheum. 1993;36:329–35.

Wilholm BE, Myrhed M, Ekman E. Trends and patterns in adverse drug reactions to non-steroidal anti-inflammatory drugs reported in Sweden. In: Rainsford KD, Velo GP, eds. Side effects of anti-inflammatory drugs, 1. Clinical and epidemiological aspects. Lancaster: MTP Press; 1987:55–70.

NONSTEROIDAL ANTI-INFLAMMATORY DRUGS AND PEPTIC ULCERATION

Neville Yeomans, Richard Day & Peter M Brooks

DEFINITION OF THE PROBLEM

Nonsteroidal anti-inflammatory drugs are among the most commonly prescribed medications, reflecting the high prevalence of chronic musculoskeletal disease in the community. However, there is now overwhelming evidence that NSAID use is associated with peptic ulceration (both gastric and duodenal ulcers), perforation and upper gastrointestinal hemorrhage (Fig. 16.36). Peptic ulcer complications in association with NSAID use are much more common in the elderly, but may be a result of the increased frequency of gastrointestinal adverse events with age rather than a specific effect of NSAIDs on the aged stomach. As NSAIDs are an important 'background' therapy for a whole range of rheumatic complaints, the question of arthritis treatment in the setting of peptic ulceration has frequently to be faced.

THE TYPICAL CASE

A 67-year-old woman with a 20-year history of erosive RA presented following a small hematemesis. Her hemoglobin had dropped from 11 to 8.5g/dl over a period of 2 days, and endoscopy revealed a chronic gastric ulcer with no evidence of malignancy. Arthritis treatment consisted of regular NSAIDs, prednisone 7.5mg daily and methotrexate 10mg once a week together with folic acid supplementation. Examination of her joints revealed active synovitis involving her MCP joints, wrists, shoulders and knees. Over the preceding 2 months her ESR had been elevated at 36mm/h. Initial treatment for the gastrointestinal bleeding involved bed rest, discontinuation of NSAIDs and increasing the prednisone to 10mg daily. Anti-ulcer therapy with a full-dose H_2-antagonist (ranitidine) was commenced and she was mobilized after 3 days. While ambulatory, she found she was restricted because of pain in her knees and her shoulders.

THERAPEUTIC OPTIONS

When peptic ulceration occurs, it is very important to treat both the ulceration and the RA (Fig. 16.37).

Treatment with NSAIDs should be discontinued, but this often leads to an exacerbation of synovitis, resulting in mobilization problems. As patients often have active synovitis, an attempt should be made to suppress symptoms in the following ways:

- local nonadsorbable corticosteroid injection can be given to painful joints, such as the knees and shoulders;
- oral prednisone dose may be increased slightly, i.e. to 15mg/day, but fairly rapid dose reduction (1mg/week) attempted to return to the dose required prior to ulceration;
- alternatively, methylprednisolone 100–200mg i.m. can be given;
- regular analgesia in the form of acetaminophen up to 4g daily should be provided; acetaminophen and codeine may also be required for short periods of time;
- liver function tests should be done, given the potential for increased hepatotoxicity in association with SAARD treatment, especially methotrexate.

Between 60 and 70% of NSAID-associated gastric ulcers will heal within 8 weeks even if NSAIDs are continued. This is substantially less than the mean healing rate in most studies of gastric ulceration not associated with NSAID use. One study randomized patients with

PEPTIC ULCER RISKS AND USE OF NONSTEROIDAL ANTI-INFLAMMATORY DRUGS		
	Relative risk of ulceration	95% confidence interval
Occurrence		
Gastric ulcer	5.0	1.4–26.9
Duodenal ulcer	1.1	0.4–3.7
Ulcer complication		
Bleeding:		
Gastric ulcer	2.8	1.5–5.4
Duodenal ulcer	2.7	1.3–5.8
Perforation:		
Peptic ulcer	7.3	4.4–11.8
Death		
Gastric ulcer	4.2	1.9–9.0
Duodenal ulcer	7.9	3.7–16.8

Fig 16.36 Peptic ulcer risks and use of NSAIDs. Data from Langman *et al.*, 1991.

AN APPROACH TO THE MANAGEMENT OF A PATIENT WITH A PEPTIC ULCER WHO IS DEPENDENT ON NSAIDS

- Try to stop/reduce dose of NSAID
- Provide symptomatic local pain relief
  Physical therapy
  Intra-articular corticosteroid
  Analgesic
- Increase or change suppressive therapy
  Increase oral corticosteroid
  Intramuscular depot corticosteroid
- Treat peptic ulcer
  H_2-antagonist
  Proton pump inhibitor
  Prostaglandin

Fig. 16.37 An approach to the management of a patient with a peptic ulcer who is dependent on NSAIDs.

gastric and duodenal ulcers into two groups, one continuing and one stopping NSAID therapy. Both groups continued ranitidine. After 4 weeks, regardless of ulcer type, of those who stopped the NSAID, 20% more healed than was the case in the group continuing with the NSAID. Prostaglandins have also been shown to accelerate ulcer healing, although the mean 8-week healing rate is still only about 70%. A significantly higher rate of healing (85%) at 8 weeks has been demonstrated with the proton-pump inhibitor (PPI) omeprazole. Thus if the NSAIDs have been stopped, as in this case, the ulcer could be healed with any one of the H_2-antagonists, a PPI or misoprostol. If NSAIDs need to be continued, the best option now is a PPI (e.g. omeprazole 20–40mg daily) for 8 weeks.

If the patient is known to be infected with *Helicobacter pylori*, it is probably advisable to treat this as well, e.g. with the combination of omeprazole 20mg, clarithromycin 250mg and metronidazole 400mg b.i.d. for 1–2 weeks. At present there is not sufficient information to recommend routine eradication of *H. pylori* in all patients who are to be given NSAIDs whether or not they have had ulcers. Once the ulcer has healed, the patient should be considered for prophylaxis if NSAIDs are still needed.

The epidemiology of NSAID-associated peptic ulceration is difficult to interpret because approximately 10% of the general population will experience frank peptic ulcer disease at some time. However, the best estimate of absolute risk of severe upper gastrointestinal adverse reactions seems to be approximately two cases of NSAID-induced reaction per 10,000 person-months of prescription. Using a variety of techniques, relative risks for perforated ulcer or hemorrhage as a result of NSAID therapy would seem to be of the order of 3:7. Given the relatively high rate of prescription of these drugs in the community, the most important way to reduce the number of NSAID-associated gastrointestinal problems is to reduce the overall prescribing of NSAIDs. However, since these agents do provide symptomatic relief for a variety of rheumatic complaints, the issue of ulcer prophylaxis is an important one. The histamine H_2-antagonists such as ranitidine appear to prevent duodenal but not gastric ulceration, whereas misoprostol prevents both and reduces most of the complications of peptic ulceration by about 50%. Two recent studies with a PPI (omeprazole) suggest that ulcer incidence is reduced by 70–80%.

Important in any discussion of ulcer prophylaxis is the subject of costs. Although the cost–benefit data are conflicting, it seems reasonable to provide prophylaxis with prostaglandins (misoprostol) or perhaps a PPI for NSAID-dependent patients over the age of 60 years who have a history of peptic ulcer disease or who are receiving corticosteroid therapy.

REFERENCES

Bjarnson I. Prophylaxis against non-steroidal induced upper gastrointestinal side effects. Ann Rhem Dis. 1991;50:207–9.

Ekström P, Carling L, Wetterhus S, Wingren PE. Omeprazole reduces the frequency of gastroduodenal lesions and dyspeptic symptoms during NSAID treatment. Gastroenterology. 1995;108:87A.

Kurata JH. Ulcer epidemiology: an overview and proposed research framework. Gastroenterology. 1989;96:569–80.

Lancaster-Smith MJ, Jaderberg ME, Jackson DA. Ranitidine in the treatment of NSAID-associated gastric and duodenal ulcers. Gut. 1991;32:252–5.

Langman MJS, Brooks P, Hawkey CJ, Silverstein F, Yeomans N. Non-steroidal anti-inflammatory drug associated ulcer: epidemiology, causation and treatment. J Gastroenterol Hepatol. 1991;6:442–9.

Langman MJS, Weil J, Lawson DH, *et al.* Risks of bleeding peptic ulcer associated with individual non-steroidal anti-inflammatory drugs. Lancet. 1994;343:1075–8.

Lichtenstein DR, Syngal S, Wolfe MM. Non-steroidal anti-inflammatory drugs and the gastrointestinal tract. Arthritis Rheum. 1995;38:5–18.

Silverstein FE, Graham DY, Senior JR *et al.* Misoprostal reduces serious gastrointestinal complications in patients with rheumatoid arthritis receiving non-steroidal and anti-inflammatory drugs: a randomised, double blind, placebo controlled trial. Ann Intern Med. 1995;123:241–9.

Walan A, Bader JP, Glassen M, Lamaers CB, Piper DW. Effect of omeprazole and ranitidine on ulcer healing and relapse rates in patients with benign gastric ulcer. N Engl J Med. 1989;320:69–7.

ANTIRHEUMATIC DRUGS AND RENAL DISEASE

Peter M Brooks, Richard Day & Elliott Savdie

DEFINITION OF THE PROBLEM

Many of the drugs used for rheumatic diseases, whether they are NSAIDs or drugs that affect the inflammatory process (SAARDs), can adversely affect renal function. Prescribing issues may arise when a patient with an underlying renal disease develops a musculoskeletal problem requiring antirheumatic drug therapy or when the antirheumatic drug therapy itself causes a renal adverse reaction.

THE TYPICAL CASE

A 64-year-old man with a long history of chronic renal failure following glomerulonephritis at the age of 20 years, who had been relatively stable from the point of view of his renal disease, presented with a serum creatinine of 0.2mmol/l (2.3mg/dl) and a creatinine clearance of 20ml/min. He had developed acute onset of an inflammatory arthritis, diagnosed as RA, with very severe pain, joint swelling and a positive rheumatoid factor.

The patient was treated with a small dose of prednisone (7.5mg daily) and intermittent acetaminophen to control his pain. Initially, he did reasonably well, but increasing synovitis and a persistently elevated ESR led to consideration of other specific antirheumatic therapy with a view to maintaining corticosteroid dose at less than 10mg daily. The patient had suffered from severe Stevens–Johnson syndrome when prescribed sulfa drugs some years previously and was not keen to start sulfasalazine. Methotrexate in a dose of 2.5mg was given and a methotrexate plasma level obtained 12 hours later. This was not significantly elevated and subsequent blood tests did not reveal any serious toxicity. The joint disease responded quite well to 2.5mg methotrexate once a week, with a fall in the ESR and a reduction in the number of swollen and tender joints. No decrease in renal function was noted.

REVERSIBLE EFFECTS OF NONSTEROIDAL ANTI-INFLAMMATORY DRUGS
Impairment of glomerular filtration
Renal vasoconstriction
Acute intestinal nephritis – heavy proteinuria (nephrotic) syndrome
Hyperkalemia
Increased reabsorption of sodium
Reduced effect of diuretics
Reduced effect of antihypertensive agents

Fig. 16.38 Reversible effects of NSAIDs.

THERAPEUTIC OPTIONS

The therapeutic issues are:

- whether NSAIDs can be used,
- what specific antirheumatic drugs may be used without compromising renal function and
- which monitoring procedure should be set in place and how frequently should monitoring be performed.

A number of renal adverse reactions are associated with NSAIDs (Fig. 16.38). Many of these adverse reactions are a direct effect of interference with prostaglandin production. Prostaglandins play an important role in autoregulation of renal blood flow and glomerular filtration. In chronic renal disease, prostaglandin mechanisms may be working to a maximum to maintain these functions, and any interference can precipitate a significant deterioration in renal function.

Although there have been some reports suggesting that some NSAIDs may have a differential effect on renal function, there is general agreement that no NSAID can be prescribed with absolute safety with respect to renal adverse effects. Some of the new NSAIDs which selectively inhibit cyclo-oxygenase (COX)-2 isoenzyme may be truly 'renal sparing' but clinical data are needed. If a patient with renal failure really does require an NSAID, then it might be reasonable to start the patient on sulindac because some studies suggest that, due to its particular metabolic profile (sulindac is converted into the active sulfide after absorption and deactivated in the renal cortex), it may have some 'renal sparing' effects. Even in this situation, it would probably be wise to try to control the pain with regular acetaminophen and other measures. If that is not possible, then small doses of sulindac should be introduced, with daily weight measurement, a check of serum creatinine and creatinine clearance after a week and advice to the patient to be careful regarding fluid intake. If a long half-life NSAID is used, then the serum creatinine and electrolytes should be checked after a further 2–3 weeks. Patients seem to be at particular risk of NSAID-induced adverse events if they are also elderly, hypovolemic or have cardiac or liver disease. This may be a particular problem when arthritic patients are undergoing surgery when still taking NSAIDs. Acute interstitial nephritis with heavy proteinuria is an unusual adverse effect of NSAIDs which seems to be particularly related to propionic acid drugs such a fenoprofen or naproxen. This adverse effect may be immunologic in origin.

In addition, NSAIDs can interfere with the action of a number of drugs that act on the kidneys. These include diuretics, particularly thiazides and aldosterone antagonists; NSAIDs tend to elevate blood pressure in hypertensive patients and may also impair the effectiveness of several antihypertensive drugs. Care should be taken when prescribing NSAIDs with digoxin or the aminoglycosides, particularly in patients with kidney impairment or hypovolemia, and with methotrexate and lithium. Although significant toxicity is recorded from interactions of NSAIDs and high-dose methotrexate, NSAIDs do not appear to interfere significantly with methotrexate in the standard weekly 'rheumatologic dose'. A few cases of toxicity have been reported with low-dose methotrexate, and renal function was reduced in the majority of these cases.

Specific antirheumatic drugs such as gold, D-penicillamine and cyclosporin are all well documented as being nephrotoxic. Gold can cause a membranous glomerulonephritis, D-penicillamine a membranous or crescentic glomerulonephritis, while cyclosporin may produce reversible renal dysfunction as a consequence of vasoconstriction, as well as a more chronic arteriolopathy with interstitial nephritis. Use of cyclosporin is also regularly associated with the development of hypertension. Cyclophosphamide may produce a hemorrhagic cystitis, although this can be reduced by the use of mesna, and chronic corticosteroid therapy and other immunosuppressive agents may increase the risk of renal infections.

CONCLUSIONS

Many drugs used to alter the course of RA or reduce symptoms of rheumatic diseases are nephrotoxic. Careful prescribing and regular monitoring of renal function are significant therapeutic issues in patients at risk of adverse renal events.

REFERENCES

Brooks PM, Day RO. Non-steroidal anti-inflammatory drugs – differences and similarities. N Engl J Med. 1991;324:1716–25.

Clive CM, Stoff J-S. Renal syndromes associated with non-steroidal anti-inflammatory drugs. N Engl J Med. 1984;310:563–72.

Johnson AG, Nguyen TV, Day RO. Do nonsteroidal anti-inflammatory drugs affect blood pressure? Ann Intern Med. 1994;121:289–300.

Pope JE, Anderson JJ, Felson DT. A meta analysis of the effects of nonsteroidal anti-inflammatory drugs on blood pressure. Arch Intern Med. 1993;153:477–84.

Schlondorff D. Renal complications of nonsteroidal anti-inflammatory drugs. Kidney Int. 1993;44:643–53.

Simon LS. Actions and toxic effects of the nonsteroidal anti-inflammatory drugs. Curr Opin Rheumatol. 1995;78:159–66.

MAINTAINING FITNESS IN RHEUMATOID ARTHRITIS

Christina H Stenström

DEFINITION OF THE PROBLEM

A progressive loss of functional capacity develops early in the course of RA and, despite drug therapy to suppress inflammatory activity, increases over the lifetime of the average patient. The functional limitation seems to be in part associated with decreased physical fitness as well as due to local factors in the joints leading to pain, stiffness and loss of movement. Other causes such as emotional, cognitive and behavioral factors also contribute to functional outcome. Exercises are frequently prescribed to maintain physical fitness and retain functional capacity.

THE TYPICAL CASE

ES is a 42-year-old woman with RA of about 1 year's duration. Knees, MTP and MCP joints, wrists and shoulders have been affected to a lesser or greater extent. She has been assigned to functional class II and stage II according to Steinbrocker *et al.* and her disease is under satisfactory control (ESR 22 mm/h, hemoglobin 13.5g/dl) with a combination of SAARDs and NSAIDs. Her main complaints arose from pain and fatigue, and she had difficulties in keeping up with her part-time job as an office worker as well as with household activities. She feared that her disease would progress and gradually exclude more and more physical activities as they caused pain and because she believed they would lead to a less favorable disease course. She needed to rest some 2–4 hours during the day on most days.

Examination revealed pain, and moderately limited active range of motion in all affected joints. Passive range of motion was close to normal in all limb joints except in individual MCP joints where moderate swelling persisted. No swelling was observed elsewhere, but she experienced significant joint tenderness and muscle soreness. Static muscle function was close to normal, while dynamic strength and

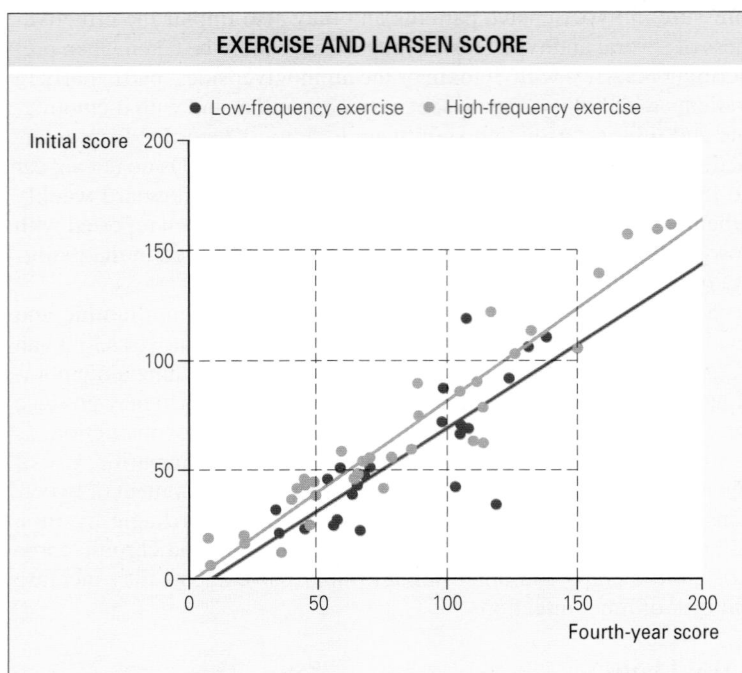

Fig. 16.39 Relationship between initial and 4th-year Larsen radiologic score for hands, wrists, shoulders, feet and knees in 36 RA patients exercising twice a week or more (upper regression line), and 23 RA patients exercising once a week or less (lower regression line). Adapted from CH Stenström, Radiologically observed progression of joint destruction and its relationship with demographic factors, disease severity, and exercise frequency in patients with rheumatoid arthritis. Phys Ther. 1994;74:32–9 with permission of the APTA.

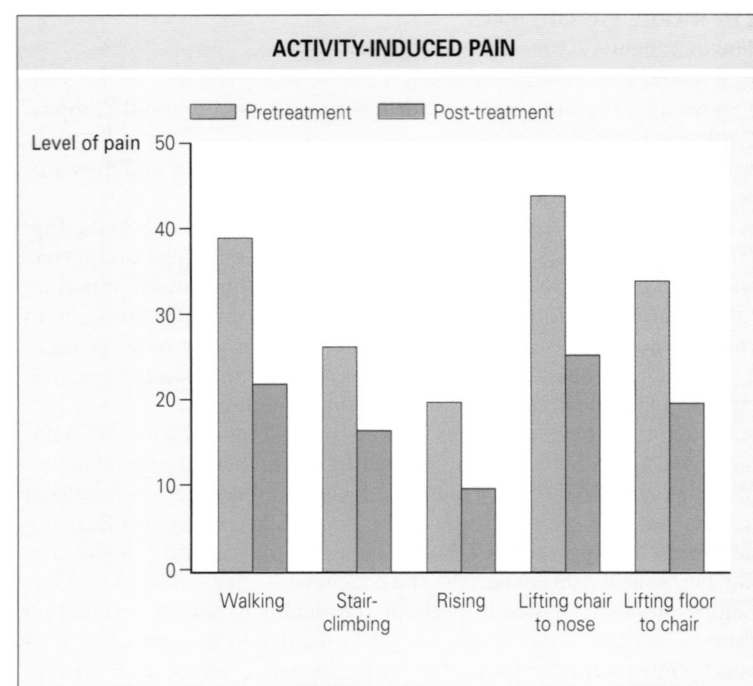

Fig. 16.40 Activity-induced pain (0–100) at five functional tasks before and after a 12-week home exercise program in 40 patients with RA. All reductions were statistically significant (*P* <0.01). Adapted from CH Stenström. Therapeutic exercise in rheumatoid arthritis. Arthritis Care Res.1994;7:190–7.

endurance were decreased, as were balance and co-ordination. The submaximal treadmill test of cardiovascular fitness was interrupted due to general pain and fatigue. The functional disability index of the Stanford health assessment questionnaire was 2, indicating that daily activities were carried out with much difficulty.

DIAGNOSTIC PROBLEMS

Through the years pain has frequently been considered as an indicator of inflammatory activity and thus as a limiting factor for exercise to maintain physical fitness. However, neurophysiologic as well as psychosocial theories offer additional explanations for pain that are also relevant for people with RA. In this particular case pain and fatigue do not seem indicative of active disease, but rather to be the result of limited knowledge about the disease, subsequent emotional and physical reactions and a reduction of physical activity.

THERAPEUTIC OPTIONS

Patients who fear the disease as well as its consequences and treatments, whether medication or exercise, need to be handled with care. Prescription of exercises is of no use unless the patient is well informed, secure and self-confident. Group education or self-help groups focusing on basic knowledge about the disease, treatment methods and self-care options, coping techniques and contact with people in similar situations usually form an excellent basis for motivating patients to undertake exercise.

The exercise goals, initially set by the patient and her physical therapist, are to achieve a reduction of exercise-induced pain, increase levels of physical activity, improve physical fitness and reduce fatigue. Treatment options are varied and include training in progressive muscle relaxation to reduce muscle tension and muscle soreness. Exercise in a hydrotherapy pool improves muscle function and cardiovascular fitness, and by reducing body weight improves exercise-induced pain. Gradual introduction of a self-administered program, such as aerobic walking or a dynamic home exercise program, is also helpful. Exercises may be performed individually or in a group, with or without sophisticated equipment, in a clinic or at home; the patient's preferences are more important than anything else to obtain compliance and to reach the goals. Although no negative side effects of exercise in persons with low to moderately active RA have been reported in the literature (e.g. Fig. 16.39), it seems wise to prepare the patient for a transient increase in pain associated with exercise, and to start out slowly with low exercise intensity and frequency. However, the exercise load may be gradually increased as the patient gains fitness with modifications to allow for acute flares. Signs of local and general disease activity, such as increased swelling and extreme fatigue, rather than increased pain alone, ought to determine the exercise load. Secure guidance and continuous supervision by a physical therapist improves compliance and outcome of exercise programs. In general, dynamic and/or aerobic exercise is recommended for functionally independent RA patients with low to moderate disease activity, whereas people with severe functional limitations and/or high disease activity would be instructed to exercise only with isometric muscle training and assisted range-of-motion exercises.

A number of studies have examined the possibility that exercise may suppress inflammatory disease activity. Although certain clinical features were noted to improve, the overall conclusion is that exercise has little effect on disease activity, as reflected by laboratory indices such as ESR. It thus seems exercise is often prescribed in order to increase physical fitness. However, it may also have an impact on cognitive and emotional factors that are equally important for the long-term preservation of functional capacity. In that respect it seems important to establish a rapport, set clear goals and offer feedback on progess to the patient engaged in the exercise program. This arrangement creates an excellent opportunity for learning how to cope with exercise-induced pain (Fig. 16.40) and, if performed in a group, enables the patient to derive benefit from good role models.

CONCLUSIONS

Exercise under secure guidance and continuous supervision, to maintain physical fitness as well as emotional and cognitive state, seems important for the retention of functional capacity in people with RA. Exercise-induced pain does not necessarily have to be an obstacle to exercise in people with low to moderately active disease, and adverse effects seem to be rare.

REFERENCES

Ekdahl C, Broman G. Muscle strength, endurance, and aerobic capacity in rheumatoid arthritis: a comparative study with healthy subjects. Ann Rheum Dis. 1992;51:35–40.

Gonzalez VM, Goeppinger J, Lorig K. Four psychosocial theories and their application to patient education and clinical practice. Arthritis Care Res. 1990;3:132–43.

Häkkinen A, Hannonen P, Häkkinen K. Muscle strength in healthy people and in patients suffering from recent-onset inflammatory arthritis. Br J Rheumatol. 1995;34:355–60.

Lorig K, Fries J. The arthritis helpbook. New York: Addison-Wesley; 1990.

Stenström CH. Therapeutic exercise in rheumatoid arthritis. Arthritis Care Res. 1994;7:190–7.

Stenström CH. Radiologically observed progression of joint destruction and its relationship with demographic factors, disease severity, and exercise frequency in patients with rheumatoid arthritis. Phys Ther. 1994;74:32–9.

PREDICTING OUTCOME IN EARLY RHEUMATOID ARTHRITIS

David L Scott

DEFINITION OF THE PROBLEM

Defining the outcome of RA means accurately describing of the ultimate effects of the disease process. Many factors are involved. Some are specific to the patients themselves, some reflect their personal circumstances and others result from the effects of treatment. While the chances of curing RA remain small, assessments of outcome focus on the amelioration of symptoms and prevention of disability over years and decades.

THE TYPICAL CASE

A 65-year-old retired man presented with a 4-month history of joint inflammation. The PIP, MCP and wrist joints of both hands were swollen; he had similar swelling in the MTP joints of both feet. He had marked joint pain and tenderness and over 60 minutes' morning stiffness. He felt unwell but there were no other medical problems and no extra-articular features of RA. He had always been previously fit and well. Investigations showed seropositivity for rheumatoid factor (titer 1:320), a high CRP level of 20mg/l, with normal hand and foot radiographs. Measurement of his functional ability showed marked impairment with a health assessment questionnaire (HAQ) score of 1.8. He is currently taking a NSAID (naproxen 500mg b.i.d.) and acetaminophen as needed.

DIAGNOSTIC PROBLEMS

The diagnosis of RA is not in doubt. But there are three key issues which are central to define the outcome of RA. These are:

- disease severity,
- optimum therapy and
- likely outcome.

Outcome is predicted by:

- demographic factors such as age, gender and disease duration;
- initial disability shown by functional impairment and joint damage;
- indicators of the type of RA, such as rheumatoid factor positivity; and
- clinical indicators of its severity, e.g. the number of swollen joints and the CRP.

Patients with the most severe RA have the worst outcome. This includes cases with a persistently high ESR, strongly positive tests for rheumatoid factor and severe extra-articular disease.

Age and gender influence outcome. Older women have a less favorable prognosis whereas younger men fare better. Formal educational level, which relates to social class, also predicts morbidity; lower educational attainments and lower social class are associated with a worse outcome. Poor initial function with high HAQ scores also indicates poor outcome.

Rheumatoid factor is an important indicator. Outcome is worst in seropositive rheumatoid patients and best in seronegative oligoarthritis of unknown etiology. Some types of rheumatoid factor may be predictive of severe RA; high level of IgA rheumatoid factor levels may indicate a more severe disease outcome. Patients with high ESRs or CRP levels have a worse outcome. The early appearance of radiologic erosions suggests more progressive disease. It is likely that a persistently elevated acute-phase response leads to a greater chance of subsequent erosive damage. Genetic markers do not have a role in routine clinical practice. Although RA is related to HLA-DR4 there is uncertainty about its value in predicting response. Some studies have shown little effect while others indicate a strong relationship.

Single measures of disease activity are weak predictors of outcome. A combination of measures improves prediction. In early RA the combination of the number of swollen joints, IgM rheumatoid factor and erosion score on plain radiology predict outcome well (Fig. 16.41).

In patients with early undifferentiated synovitis the subsequent development of destructive RA was predicted by:

- symmetric polyarthritis of peripheral joints,
- the presence of serum rheumatoid factor,
- prolonged morning stiffness,
- high ESR and
- old age.

CLINICALLY USEFUL PROGNOSTIC MARKERS IN EARLY RA		
Class of prognostic marker	Prognostic marker	Indicator of severity
General	Age	Older
	Sex	Female
	Social class	Poorer
Disease type	Distribution of joint involvement	Symmetric polyarthritis
	Rheumatoid factor	Positive
Disease severity	Number of swollen and tender joints	Many
	Pain	Severe
	ESR	High
	CRP	High
Destructive	Radiologic erosions	Present

Fig 16.41 Clinically useful prognostic markers in early RA.

In patients with definite early RA subsequent erosive damage was predicted by high disease activity, raised ESR and CRP levels, and rheumatoid factor positivity. The progression of radiographic damage could be correctly ascertained in over 80% of patients.

THERAPEUTIC OPTIONS

Treatment should improve the symptoms of RA and allow patients to maintain a normal lifestyle. Antirheumatic drugs may also control the disease process itself, reducing the inflammatory synovitis and consequent anatomic damage, together with improved and maintained function. Only second-line drugs (such as injectable gold and methotrexate) and corticosteroids can control the disease process in this way. Using second-line drugs in early disease, especially where there is a strong likelihood of progressive erosive RA, provides the greatest opportunity to control RA. Active RA with multiple swollen and tender joints or the early onset of erosions indicates a need for a SAARD. But the early use without adequate justification of drugs potentially toxic to many patients who may do well without them or who only have a transient synovitis is possibly unjustified. This is a difficult balance to achieve.

There is no agreement as to the best SAARD to use in early RA. In North America methotrexate is preferred whereas, in the UK, sulfasalazine is often used. Injectable gold and cyclosporin also have their adherents. Whichever drug is chosen 50% or more patients will discontinue therapy within the first year. There is some evidence that fewer patients withdraw from methotrexate. When one SAARD is discontinued and the disease is still active it is conventional to start a second drug.

The outcome of such sequential monotherapy is often disappointing. The alternative is to use several second-line drugs in combination, but this is controversial. It has been difficult to prove that a combination is more effective than its individual components used singly. Some studies suggest this is true, most notably the use of combination therapy with methotrexate and cyclosporin. There is also weak evidence to support the use of sulfasalazine with methotrexate. Finally there is some evidence that the use of corticosteroids in early RA may reduce the rate of subsequent joint damage.

The paradox between the successful results of short-term studies of antirheumatic therapy and the poor results in studies of long-term outcome is difficult to resolve. Prospective long-term clinical studies show that up to 80% of cases first seen as inpatients are moderately or severely impaired by 20 years whereas the average outpatient has a 30% chance of severe disability. Survival is reduced by 3–5 years. But there is some evidence that patients seen with early RA in specialist units may do better. For example, experience at one UK center after 15 years' follow up of early RA patients showed that only a minority of patients had severe disability and over 60% of survivors had normal function. Long-term studies inevitably reflect clinical practice of 10 or 20 years ago and modern approaches may be more effective. One example is the tendency for RA patients to be seen far earlier and for SAARDs to be used at an early stage. These changes in practice may mean the outcome is better than often suggested in long-term studies initiated in previous decades.

CONCLUSIONS

The best answer for patients with active RA is to start therapy with a SAARD as soon as the diagnosis is made, provided there are some indicators of severe disease. Thus the involvement of multiple joints, a high ESR or CRP, seropositivity for rheumatoid factor, poor function and early erosions all indicate the need for such therapy. I personally believe sulfasalazine is useful in slightly milder cases whereas injectable gold or cyclosporin is more useful in more severe cases with methotrexate as an alternative in both situations. I use combination therapy in a small number of cases where there has been only a partial response to the first-choice therapy. But my approach will change if new evidence becomes available about alternative therapeutic approaches.

REFERENCES

Corbett M, Dalton S, Young A, *et al.* Factors predicting death, survival and functional outcome in a prospective study of early rheumatoid disease over fifteen years. Br J Rheumatol. 1993;32:717–23.

Felson DT, Anderson JJ, Meenan RF. Use of short-term efficacy/toxicity tradeoffs to select second-line drugs in rheumatoid arthritis. A meta-analysis of published clinical trials. Arthritis Rheum. 1992;35:1117–25.

Kaarela K. Prognostic factors and diagnostic criteria in early rheumatoid arthritis. Scand J Rheumatol. 1985; 57(Suppl):1–54.

Scott DL, Huskisson EC. The course of rheumatoid arthritis. Baillière's Clin Rheumatol. 1992;6:1–21.

van der Heijde DM, van Leeuwen MA, van Riel PL, *et al.* Biannual radiographic assessments of hands and feet in a three year follow up of patients with early rheumatoid arthritis. Arthritis Rheum. 1992;35:26–34.

van Zeben D, Hazes JM, Zwinderman AH, *et al.* Factors predicting outcome of rheumatoid arthritis: results of a follow-up study. J Rheumatol. 1993;20:1288–96.

ARTHRITIS AND DRIVING

Jeremy G Jones

DEFINITION OF THE PROBLEM

Arthritis often impairs a person's ability to drive. Whether the problem relates to one part of the driving process (such as release of the emergency brake) or to several, the result is a loss of mobility. Arthritis also frequently limits a patient's ability to walk, so the mobility afforded by driving is precious. Indeed, whether such a person is able to drive can make the difference between work or unemployment, independence or dependence, or a social life or isolation.

THE TYPICAL CASE

RF, a 46-year-old woman, was well-to-do, outgoing and a keen bridge player. Recently widowed, she had a 15-year history of disabling RA. The visiting nurse reported that since her bereavement she had become housebound and was a virtual recluse in her custom-built bungalow in a somewhat isolated upscale suburb.

Evaluation in the clinic showed severe involvement of the hands, wrists, shoulders and feet, while other joints were mildly affected. Atlantoaxial subluxation caused pain on neck movement but there was no evidence of cord compression. The arthritis appeared well controlled with a NSAID and methotrexate. She claimed to have come to terms with her husband's death philosophically and denied that she was depressed.

Further questioning revealed that her husband had always driven the automobile and that without him she had lost her means of transport. The automobile remained in the garage even though she had an up-to-date driver's license. She said she had not driven the automobile because she didn't feel physically capable and added that she could not even unlock the door with the key.

She was referred to an occupational therapist with a special interest in driving problems. The initial interview revealed that RF had driven regularly until the onset of her arthritis 15 years previously. She

SOLUTIONS TO DRIVING DISABILITIES IN RHEUMATOID ARTHRITIS	
Disability problem	Solution
Securing/undoing seatbelt	Noninertia reel. Extend stem of seat belt attachment. Modify seat belt clip
Manipulating key	Build up key
Using handbrake	Convert to vertical lever for knock on/off action. Keep vehicle in gear when parked. Use accelerator/clutch for hill start. Use automatic vehicle
Opening and closing door	Keep door hinges and handles oiled. Modify buttons. Enlarge door handles
Adjusting mirror	Ask others to reposition mirror
Using gearstick	Increase length of gearstick. Modify hand piece. Use automatic vehicle. Modify automatic gear stick to 'push-down' type
Reaching seatbelt	Hook belt around seat lever. Prevent full recoil of seat belt
Steering/cornering	Use steering wheel cover to increase bulk of wheel. Learn 'threading' steering technique. Increase front tire pressure. Choose automobile with power steering
Reversing	Undo seat belt when reversing. Install wide rear-view mirror. Install near- and off-side mirrors. Reverse with mirrors
Seat comfort and position	Extend seat runners. Alter seat back position. Use wedge cushion and/or lumbar cushion
Vehicle entry and exit	Enter buttocks first rather than legs first. Extend seat runners
Using foot pedals	Modify pedals. Use automatic vehicle
Traffic sense and confidence	Practice with experienced driver in quiet streets. Limit driving to familiar streets. Take lessons with qualified driving instructor
Pain and fatigue on long drives	Make frequent stops on long trips. Make judicious use of NSAIDs and analgesics. Establish a relaxed driving position

Fig. 16.42 Solutions to driving disabilities in RA. Adapted by permission of Oxford University Press, from Jones *et al.*, 1991.

admitted she lacked confidence in her ability to drive again. The occupational therapist found that the automobile, with its power-assisted steering, automatic transmission and wide doors, met the patient's requirements. A static assessment found that RF was indeed unable to use the automobile key to open the door, getting in and out of the automobile posed no problems, reaching and manipulating the seat belt proved very difficult and the automobile seat was uncomfortable. A mobile assessment on a quiet road showed that she was unable to release the emergency brake, she had difficulty with manipulating the gear shift and her steering was erratic. Backing proved a problem because of her painful neck. It was also obvious that she was anxious while driving and that she lacked confidence.

The therapist felt that these difficulties could all be resolved. The simple expedient of increasing the bulk of the automobile key enabled RF to grip it and unlock the automobile door, and the addition of an extension to the stem of the seat belt and the trick of hooking the belt around the seat lever made seat belt use feasible. A wedge cushion produced a comfortable driving position. Increasing the length of the gear shift, introduction of a knock on/off vertical lever in place of the emergency brake button and the use of a steering wheel cover to increase the bulk of the wheel, resolved gear, brake and steering wheel difficulties.

The patient was instructed in the 'threading through' technique of steering (see below). She was also taught to back using her rear view mirror and two newly installed side mirrors. Like most people with arthritis, she quickly mastered these techniques and was soon able to steer and back accurately and comfortably. After her automobile had been adapted she had two more sessions on quiet roads with the occupational therapist. Her nervousness was rapidly disappearing, and after a few lessons with a driving instructor she became a capable, confident, safe driver.

Mrs F is now independent again with a full social life. She has renewed her interests in volunteer activities and is playing bridge with a vengeance. It is even rumored that she is more than just good friends with her handsome widower bridge partner. Her arthritis remains well controlled on methotrexate (ESR 18mm/h).

THERAPEUTIC OPTIONS

This rather whimsical tale illustrates how a nonmedical factor can be the major deleterious influence on the quality of life of a person with arthritis. Although arthritis and ESR may be under excellent control with methotrexate, the patient's horizons may be severely limited by loss of mobility. We are concerned here with driving, but the same principle applies to the use of public transport. The loss of the ability to negotiate the step up onto a bus can have devastating effects on a person's independence and mobility.

Driving is particularly important to people with arthritis because their walking ability is usually compromised. The ability to drive can determine whether a person with arthritis can continue to work, go shopping, go to the movies or meet friends. There is one other factor in this equation, and that is the provision of designated parking spaces for disabled drivers close to public facilities. The advantages of driving an automobile are negated if disabled people are forced to park half a mile from their destination.

In almost every case, an arthritic person's driving difficulties can be overcome by alterations to their driving technique and/or automobile.

Arthritis frequently makes steering and backing difficult and sometimes even dangerous. Beginner drivers are customarily taught to hold the steering wheel at 10 and 2 o'clock, which can be difficult for people with shoulder, wrist or elbow involvement. The 'threading through' technique, in which the steering wheel is held at its lowest pole with both hands and 'threaded through' from one hand to the other, usually overcomes this problem. In a similar way, the difficulty that people with neck and spinal involvement experience in looking behind them to back up can be avoided by using side mirrors in the manner of a truck driver. Both these techniques are easily learned and are very useful.

Simple modifications to the automobile, as listed in Figure 16.42, can enable most most driving problems caused by arthritis to be overcome. Most occupational therapists have on their books one or two sympathetic automobile mechanics who find such work satisfying. Often the modifications are so simple that they can be carried out by a friend or family member. Very few people with arthritis require referral to a specialized mobility unit with its sophisticated technology.

CONCLUSIONS

To drive safely a person needs confidence as well as a satisfactory technique and a suitable vehicle. Loss of confidence rather than physical disability is sometimes the reason people with arthritis do not drive. This can often be restored by a positive driving assessment from a sympathetic occupational therapist and a few driving lessons with an experienced instructor.

Every multidisciplinary rheumatology team should include a therapist with special knowledge about driving. This will keep people with arthritis on the road and will also encourage those with failing physical abilities to make good their loss of mobility by wise use of their automobile. Sometimes a dramatic improvement in quality of life can result.

REFERENCES

Bulstrode SJ. Car mirrors for drivers with restricted neck mobility. Int Disabil Stud. 1987;9:180–1.

Jones JG, McCann J, Lassere MN. Driving and arthritis. Br J Rheumatol. 1991;30:361–4.

Murray-Leslie C. Aids for disabled drivers. Br Med J. 1990;301:1206–9.

JUVENILE CHRONIC ARTHRITIS

17

HISTORY

Eric G L Bywaters

Definition

- A heterogeneous group of systemic inflammatory disorders affecting children below the age of 16 years.
- Major subsets defined on the basis of clinical features at onset have been described, which appear to differ in genetic associations and prognosis.

Clinical features

- Pauciarticular onset (≤ four joints involved) may be of several types – most common are early childhood with antinuclear antibodies (ANA) positivity and risk of ocular disease and late childhood with risk of spondyloarthropathy.
- Polyarticular onset are at greatest risk for chronic, severe arthritis.
- Systemic onset with fever, rash and arthritis may be associated with serious morbidity and mortality.

INTRODUCTION

The term juvenile chronic arthritis (JCA) as we now understand it represents a splendid epitome of the historical process as exemplified in medical thought (if such a pragmatic process can be thus dignified). This currently recognized disease-entity, defined by international criteria, came into being, like most such disease concepts, by first sightings, a sudden flurry of individual case records and a magisterial overview of a series of cases, followed by nosologic subdivisions on the clinical side, aided by application of newly developing medical science.

New entities are recognized in the hope of more specific etiology or treatment. Like any other disease concept, JCA started with a particular patient coming to consult a particular doctor. The doctor was gifted enough to be able to recognize a new experience for himself and then to ascertain that it was new to others. Finally, he had the impetus, the energy and the courage to announce this to the medical press (usually after he had seen and ascertained the second or third such case). His second case might be a coincidence; it was the third case that created the syndrome, and then there followed the differentiation from other similar entities.

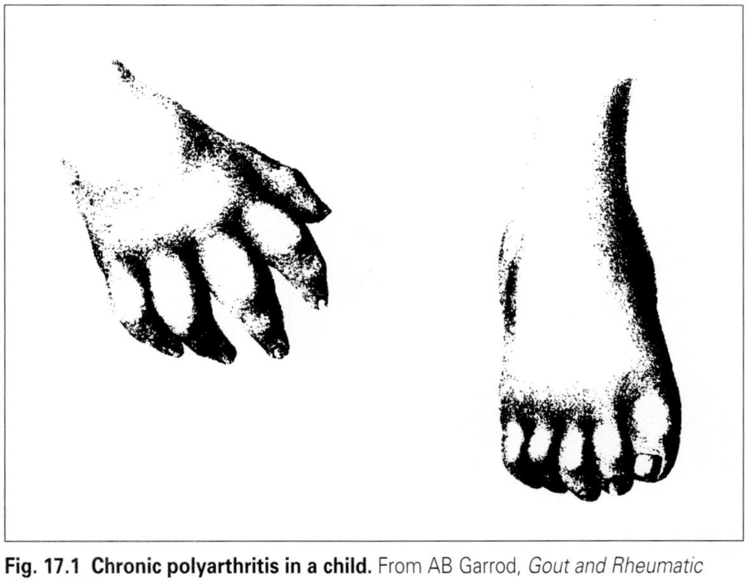

Fig. 17.1 Chronic polyarthritis in a child. From AB Garrod, *Gout and Rheumatic Gout*, 1876.

THE NINETEENTH CENTURY

This simple process started for JCA in 1864, but its history cannot be told without going further back, to the recognition of 'rheumatoid arthritis' (as Garrod named it in 1859) by Landré-Beauvais in 1800 as 'la goutte asthénique primitive'. Garrod differentiated this from gout and rheumatic fever. It was finally separated from osteoarthritis, clinically by Goldthwait (1904) and pathologically by Nichols and Richardson (1909). The recognition of rheumatoid arthritis (RA) in childhood in the latter part of the 19th century was not a major advance, since pediatric 'territorial rights' as they exist today had not been established.

Garrod for instance in his famous book *Gout and Rheumatic Gout* (third edition, 1876) refers to and pictures a patient with onset at the age of 3 years – 'rheumatoid arthritis may occur at any age' (Fig. 17.1). Most physicians and surgeons were generalists and for many years in the wake of rheumatic fever and tuberculosis, patients with JCA were referred primarily to cardiologists, prescribing bed rest and aspirin, and to orthopedic surgeons using splints in a disastrously wrong therapeutic regime. The patients ended up ankylosed. In the second half of the 19th century there were many case reports of such juvenile-onset RA (Fig.17.2). They were well detailed and referenced by Llewellyn Jones of Bath, UK, in 1909. Many of them were of French origin – Trousseau, Charcot, Laborde, Trastour,

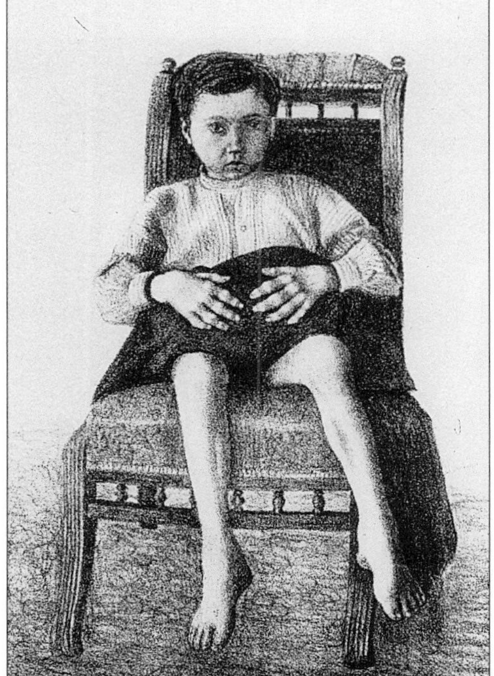

Fig. 17.2 Rheumatoid arthritis in an 8-year-old boy. Frontispiece from Hugh Lane, *Differentiation in the Rheumatic Diseases (so called)*. London: Churchill; 1892. Reproduced by permission of the Wellcome Institute Library, London.

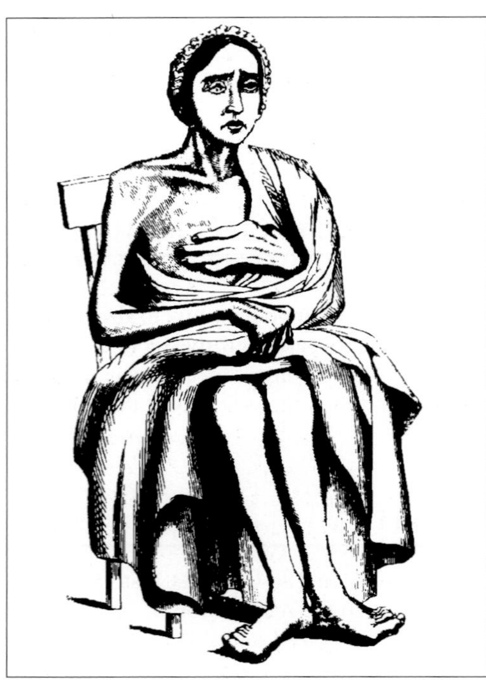

Fig. 17.3 A 27-year-old woman whose arthritis began at the age of 13 years. From Robert Adams, *Rheumatic Gout*, 1873.

Picot, Lacaze-Dori, Pelissie, etc., and Moncorvo. The latter, translated from the Portuguese by Dr Mauriac, was published in Paris in 1880 in 140 pages; it not only described fully his Brazilian case, with onset at 2.5 years, but provided 112 bibliographic references, including many by English and American authors [1].

But the most often quoted, perhaps the first and still the best of these earlier descriptions was that of Cornil (1864). Among others Cornil describes four cases in detail, one of which had developed at the age of 12 years a subacute and then chronic deforming polyarthritis and had died aged 29 years. Autopsy disclosed peritonitis, pleurisy and renal disease. Perhaps this was amyloidosis, which today affects about 6% of all JCA cases and a similar proportion in adult RA and ankylosing spondylitis. The majority of deaths then, as compared with now, were due to sepsis. Quite a large number of cases described at this time, and indeed since, are retrospective, that is adult chronic polyarthritis with onset in childhood (Fig. 17.3). The reverse, JCA with adult onset, was not described until 1956 [2]. The earlier stages of arthritis in this neglected field of pediatrics were usually mistaken for acute rheumatic fever, white swelling of joints if few in number, or confusedly named 'secondary chronic polyarthritis' (secondary to rheumatic fever) on the basis of a few cases of Jaccoud's syndrome.

The first overview of JCA was published in Paris in 1891 as a thesis; it is available xeroxed in the Heberden Library by courtesy of John Baum and the National Library of Congress [3]. Diamantberger there records two personal cases (Fig. 17.4) and 36 other published cases with a detailed bibliography. One of the two personal cases was from Bucharest and showed gross muscle wasting and exophthalmos. [Parenthetically, we have only found one such case out of several thousand of JCA at Taplow, but this patient had no other signs of Graves' disease. G.F. Still (see below) noted four cases with prominent eyes and illustrated one. There are also other such recordings by Rosenfeld (1917), Taylor and McKim (1899) and Reimold and Stoeber (1926). So far there is no explanation.]

This first survey of a rather limited field was overtaken 5 years later by a young registrar – George Frederic Still – at Great Ormond Street Hospital for Children in 1896. His personal history is given in detail by Eric Hamilton [4]. This famous Hospital was first founded in 1852 by Charles West – the first Children's Hospital in the UK and with 10 beds. Still was in a 2-year residency and was able to see 19 cases of JCA as well as three previously collected cases, enough to give a full description. His paper (to the Royal Medical and Chirurgical Society in London, 1896) was given by Archibald E. Garrod and is remarkable for its categorization of his cases into several nosologic groups, a process which has been going on ever since. He appeared to be a rather better pathologist than his mentor.

Why suddenly from the 1850s to the end of the century should so many case descriptions of this rare disease be published? I think partly because of the terrible state of society. The Industrial Revolution, starting in the mid 18th century, had produced not only urbanization, slums and appalling poverty, but also the painfully visible exploitation of children by factories, mines and shopkeepers, and also, as for centuries before, in the farms of the countryside. The response from the Victorian and Christian reformers, as Craig relentlessly describes [5], was the founding all over the UK and elsewhere in the industrialized world of charitably supported children's dispensaries, children's hospitals, schools, societies and homes, as well as much legislation for the protection of children. Such a comparatively rare disease as JCA (today affecting about 0.06% of the school population) would never have attracted notice amidst the pullulation and crowding of all those traditional diseases due to malnutrition, abuse, infection and neglect, unless there was a concentration of more chronic and less fatal cases in hospitals. The most severe of these was the white swelling of joints, the 'tumeur blanche' due to 'scrofula', or 'strumous disease', finally identified as due to *M. tuberculosis* in 1882 by Koch. New developments in hygiene and new knowledge of scurvy, and of the infectious diseases, including the dramatic decrease in smallpox due to vaccination, led to considerable positive advances in child health, but only to the better recognition of those still undefeatable chronic diseases.

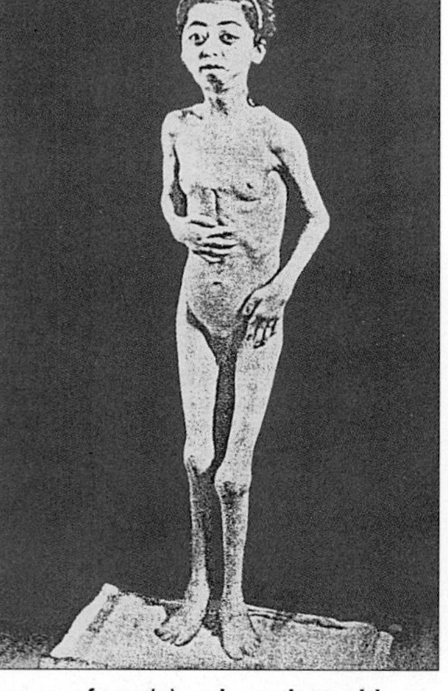

Fig. 17.4 A 9-year-old boy with onset at 5 years of age (a) and a patient with chronic generalized arthritis (b). Note exophthalmos and enlarged axillary lymph nodes in the latter. Reproduced from Diamantberger [3].

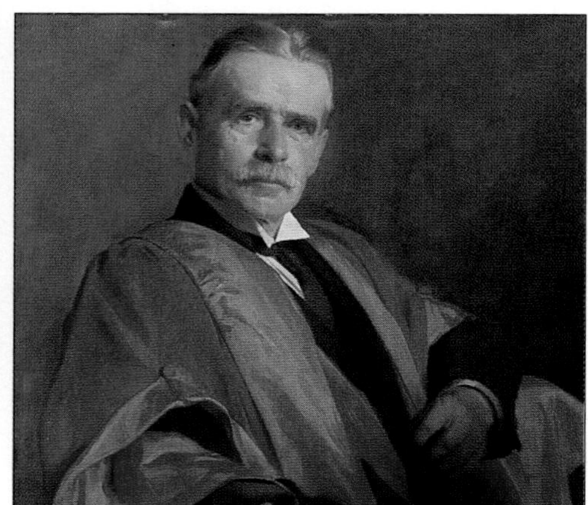

Fig. 17.5 George Frederic Still. Portrait by Sir Gerald Kelly. Reproduced with permission from King's College Hospital, through Dr Eric Hamilton.

1900–1940 THE NEW CENTURY

After the apotheosis of Sir Frederic Still as the first academic Professor of Paediatrics at King's College in London (Fig. 17.5), not only he but also most others lost interest in JCA in the face of more common and more soluble aspects of pediatric disease. Rheumatic fever, and the accompanying rheumatic heart disease which dominated cardiology, was still prevalent both in children and adults, but it was not until 1930 that improvements in the classification of streptococci allowed Collis, Schlesinger, Coburn and others to incriminate the beta-hemolytic streptococcus; the later discovery of Prontosil (1935) and sulfanilamide led to striking advances in prevention of second attacks, and this was furthered by the use of penicillin introduced during the Second World War. Tuberculosis was later attacked by bacille Calmette–Guérin (BCG) vaccination, tuberculin testing of cattle and pasteurization before its vanquishing by streptomycin, para-aminosalicylic acid (PAS) and isoniazid (INH) in 1944. But there was no such progress with regard to JCA, although occasional cases and small series were published between 1900 and 1940. Individual aspects began to be recorded in more detail: local growth defects affecting bones near inflamed joints, or general growth defects; the typical receding chin, which originally had been recorded by Diamantberger; eye involvement with band opacity described by Ohm in 1910; pericarditis previously mentioned by both Cornil and Diamantberger; lymph gland enlargement and splenomegaly sometimes wrongly linked with the names of Chauffard and Ramond (those authors described adults); the Wissler–Fanconi syndrome 'subsepsis allergica' in 1942; a rash which was first described by Boldero in 1930.

Amyloidosis then was due largely to tuberculosis and osteomyelitis, both in the UK and elsewhere, but JCA cases were recorded by Whitman and by Spitzy. No treatment of this was available until very recently.

One of the best historical surveys of JCA of this prewar period is that of Sury in 1952 [6]. He cites 107 references ranging from 1864 to 1951; of these the majority (one third) are from Scandinavian sources, the usual national language bias, followed by French (17%) and German (21%), mostly early references, and a very few from England and the USA, the latter more recent, on cortisone and rheumatoid factor. He records his early original series (and follow-up, really the most important aspect) of 158 cases.

1940–1990 JCA AND POSTWAR CHANGES

The study and care of JCA enjoyed a rebirth after the Second World War. Wars are a recurrent disgrace and hindrance to civilization, but they have often contributed to advances in health. With more closely defined priorities, our children's health improved in the Second World War on rationing with a better distribution of food and the unpremeditated destruction of old slums and subsequent rehousing. There was improved management of fractures, blood loss and infection. Penicillin and, later, streptomycin, PAS and INAH accelerated the fall in morbidity and mortality from those ancient infections of childhood. Rheumatic fever, highlighted during the Second World War by well-researched epidemics in all the Armed Forces, began to decline rapidly, until in 1956 the beds at Taplow, founded for research and care of rheumatism in children, were filled, not by rheumatic fever, as they had been from its inception 10 years earlier, but by children with chronic arthritis. The change in emphasis was furthered by the discoveries of 1948, the *annus mirabilis* of rheumatology (and notable in many other fields). The next year saw caronamide (and later probenecid) for gout, phenylbutazone as the first nonsteroidal anti-inflammatory drug (NSAID), the Rose–Waaler and lupus erythematosus (LE) cell tests, corticotrophin (ACTH) and cortisone, controlled clinical trials, and above all in the UK, the introduction of the National Health Service (NHS) as set out by Sir William Beveridge in his report of 1942, a service freely available to all, including those neglected patients with JCA.

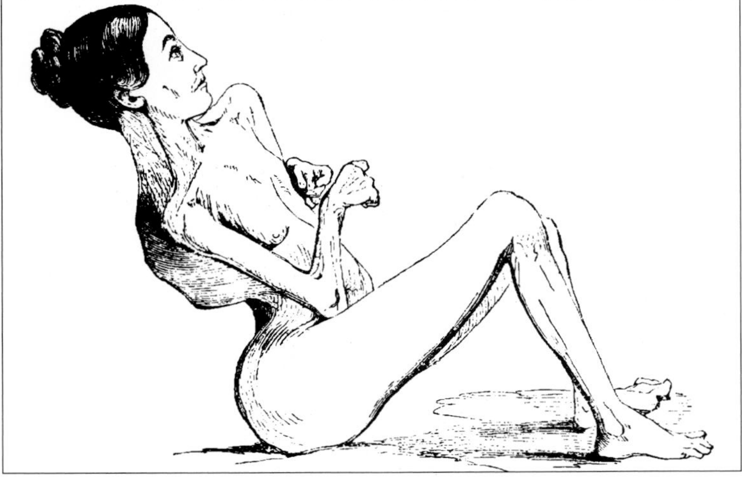

Fig. 17.6 A 20-year-old woman with chronic arthritis pictured after 7 years of disuse. Her arthritis began at the age of 6 years and progressively affected every joint in her body so that eventually she was unable to walk. Woodcut by Serny JB, in *Spinal Curvature, its Consequences and its Cure*. London: Sherwood; 1840.

Many children before that awakening must have been homebound in poor and rural areas, untreated because of poverty and ignorance, and because there was not known to be any useful treatment (Fig. 17.6). After 1948 interest in JCA became worldwide and was fostered by the concept of autoimmunity.

Perhaps the most important historic advance in this field has been the differentiation of at least nine varieties of JCA, promising clearer insight into etiology, prognosis and treatment. The process started with Still, who concluded that RA in children includes at least three distinct conditions, and more recent studies have strengthened this viewpoint. The entities differentiated today include:

- Spondylitis, starting in childhood, usually in pubescent males, may often present to the clinician with peripheral arthritis, and sometimes even without sacroiliac change, which may come on several years later [7]. This was recognized as early as 1965 [8]. The discovery of the role of HLA-B27 in ankylosing spondylitis, Reiter's syndrome and reactive arthritis (1974) made this early stage of the disease more easily identifiable – 'spondylitis *sine* spondylitis'.
- Psoriatic arthritis, ulcerative colitis and regional ileitis were recognized early on as occurring in children as well as in adults and again may present with arthritis alone.
- What we now call 'systemic onset JCA', which Still thought to be a new syndrome although he did not describe the specific rash, is now one of the most important subvarieties of JCA.
- Still also differentiated ordinary RA in children, which we now identify not only clinically but serologically using the Rose–Waaler factor.
- Separation of seropositive cases left the problem of the seronegatives. This was dealt with decisively by Schaller and Wedgewood in Seattle, who in 1969, studying children with iridocyclitis and few affected joints ('pauciarticular'), found that five out of eight cases had a positive antinuclear factor [7]. This was confirmed in a larger series at Taplow in 1972. This ANA-positive, early-onset pauciarticular set of children with chronic iridocyclitis is the only type not yet recognized to have an adult-onset disease counterpart. All other varieties of JCA have adult onset counterparts, including of course the syndrome of systemic-onset, described in adults [8].

These early-onset varieties pose interesting epidemiological questions, as do those inflammatory familial syndromes of fever, rash and arthritis [9] recently surveyed by Prieur [10]. Other congenital arthropathic syndromes [11] offer possible insight into the relationship between hereditary and environmental insults.

The historical evolution of the concept posed by G.F. Still is still continuing, but our future control is bound up with the etiology and management of the other common adult-onset chronic inflammatory diseases of joints, such as RA, ankylosing spondylitis, reactive arthritis and others.

The new freedom for youth in the 1950s and 1960s led to even greater differences between well and handicapped children, especially as Victorian rules persisited in many of the long-stay hospital units – six such recorded by Craig for heart cripples alone. At Taplow and elsewhere we endeavored to bring hospital care up to date by opening up the old-style hospital wards, subdividing them into play places, general open curtained wards and one-bed rooms. We instituted entertainment and talks by local groups – scouts, policemen, clowns – day trips in coaches and open visiting hours. We were even able to start a fund for travel fares for visits by parents (since we took children from all over the country and indeed from abroad). Schooling was mandatory from 1947, either at the bedside or in the adjacent purpose-built school. Central in the response to this challenge to integrate the handicapped children back into their own community when discharged were the tremendous efforts of our social workers, physiotherapists and occupational therapists to activate these patients' own local services. These children, sent back home with a letter to their general practitioner and the referring consultant, needed special help in education and transport: this was in the days when few families owned a car, people were means tested, unemployment was widespread and local authority hospitals were seldom concerned with the provision of jobs for and rehabilitation of the handicapped. These children needed regular hydrotherapy and resisted exercise, schooling or further education, and the provision of wheelchairs, kitchen appliances and other aids to self-help, self-pride and self determination.

There should be no gap of uncare left, as pediatrics tended to perpetuate, between the child and the adult he becomes.

Fortunately, in the UK, the NHS was inspired to provide such help and was conducive to the team approach as well as social help, which included physiotherapy, occupational therapy and arrangements for schooling, the orthopedic service and the eye surgeons. This combined effort was achieved with clinics and rounds shared between these professional experts and pediatricians and other members of the hospital team. Taplow was able to influence the development of such help in every county and country from where we had had patients, and from where we had seeded pediatric and rheumatologic centers through our training of registrars and fellows. There was a similar efflorescence of organized help for these needy children in many other European countries: in Poland on a limited scale with the Cheshire Homes; above all in Scandinavia (led by Edstrom, Bratstrom and others); Germany had Elizabeth Stoeber and her long recognized unit in Garmisch-Partenkirchen, struggles recounted well in the memoirs published on her retirement; and of course in the USA, where the Children's Home had been long established in the major cities, for example the Good Samaritan Hospital in Boston, La Rabida in Chicago and numerous others, well integrated by then with university clinics and teaching. Then there were the later polio palaces, built to deal with that last epidemic of 1953–4, and now devoted mainly to rehabilitation. Thus these two streams, scientific and academic progress and social improvement of handicapped children, ran together to form this recent surging advance in the care of chronic diseases of children, and particularly here of those with arthritis.

This culminated in the Park City Pediatric Rheumatology Conference of 1975, when the subspecialty was established. (Proceedings published as a Supplement to 'Arthritis & Rheumatism', 1977.)

THE HISTORY OF THE FUTURE

Where are we going today? Despite very considerable progress, particularly in care and treatment, and in the understanding and prevention of amyloidosis, we seem to be little further on in our understanding of JCA and RA than was Still in 1896 – there are too many 'promising leads'. Will the ultimate advance come from immunogenetic studies, as seems possible in ankylosing spondylitis (AS), or from born-again bacteria, from some dysregulation in the inflammatory process or from inbuilt designer-designed chaos in the immunoregulatory network? History awaits the joker in the pack!

CONCLUSIONS

All histories should look to the future and are often written for it. What otherwise is their use? As of 1992 we have a number of entities in JCA differentiated by clinical course, serological phenomena and genetic constitution, occurring in both children and adults alike, with so far one exception. The pediatric aspects are common to all children. But the prospects for etiological discovery are enormous and it seems just as, or even more, likely that studies of JCA will throw light on 'la goutte asthénique primitive' than vice-versa.

REFERENCES

1. Llewellyn RLJ. Arthritis Deformans. Bristol: Wright; 1909.
2. Bywaters EGL. Still's disease in the adult. Ann Rheum Dis. 1971;30:121–33.
3. Diamantberger MS. Du Rheumatisme noueux (polyarthrite deformante) chex less enfants. Paris: Lecrosner-Babe; 1891.
4. Hamilton, E. George Frederic Still. Ann Rheum Dis. 1986;45:1–5.
5. Craig WS. Child and adolescent life in health and disease.Edinburgh: Churchill Livingstone; 1940.
6. Sury B. Rheumatoid Arthritis in children. Munksgaard;1952.
7. Schaller J, Bitnum S, Wedgewood RS. Anklyosing spondylitis with childhood onset. J. Pediatr. 1969;74:505–16.
8. Bywaters EGL. Ankylosing spondylitis in childhood. Clin Rheum Dis. 1976;2:387–96.
9. Ansell BM, Bywaters EGL, Elderkin FM. Familial arthropathy with rash uveitis and mental retardation. Proc Roy Soc Med. 1975; 69:584–5.
10. Prieur AM, Lovell D. The chronic infantile neurologic cutaneous and articular syndrome. Paediatric Rheumatology Update. Edited by Woo P, White PA, Ansell M. Oxford: Oxford University Press. 1990;147–60.
11. Muckle TJ, Wells M. Urticaria - deafness and amyloidosis: a new heredo-familial syndrome. Quart J Med. 1963;31:235–48.

JUVENILE CHRONIC ARTHRITIS

18

CLINICAL FEATURES

Patience H White

Definition

- Most commonly diagnosed rheumatic disease in children, and an important cause of disability and blindness.
- The criteria for diagnosis include arthritis, age of onset under 16 years and the exclusion of other forms of juvenile arthritis.

Clinical features

- Three major onset subtypes can be identified after 6 months, which help in clarifying prognosis: pauciarticular onset, polyarticular onset and systemic onset.

INTRODUCTION

Juvenile chronic arthritis (JCA), known as juvenile rheumatoid arthritis (JRA) in the USA, is the most commonly diagnosed rheumatic disease in children and an important cause of disability and blindness. The criteria for diagnosis (Fig. 18.1) include age of onset under 16 years and the exclusion of other forms of juvenile arthritis[1,2]. After 6 months three major onset subtypes can be identified (Fig. 18.2) which

CRITERIA FOR DIAGNOSIS OF JRA/JCA

	Juvenile rheumatoid arthritis (American College of Rheumatology)	Juvenile chronic arthritis (European League Against Rheumatism)
Age of onset	<16 years	<16 years
Disease duration	>6 weeks	>3 months
Presence of arthritis	Joint swelling or effusion, or two of the following: painful or limited joint motion, tenderness, warmth	
Subtypes after 6 months of disease	Pauciarticular (<5 joints) Polyarticular (>4 joints) Systemic: arthritis, fever, rash	Pauciarticular (<5 joints) Polyarticular (>4 joints) IgM-RF negative Same
Other	Exclusion of other forms of juvenile arthritis	Polyarthritis IgM-RF positive Ankylosing spondylitis Psoriatic arthritis Exclusion of all other forms of juvenile arthritis

Fig. 18.1 Criteria for diagnosis of JRA/JCA.

CHARACTERIZATION OF JCA SUBTYPES

Subtype	% of JCA patients	F : M ratio	Age of onset	Joints affected	Iridocyclitis	Systemic complaints	Rheumatoid factors	Antinuclear antibodies	HLA associations: family history (fx)	Outcome: Remission at 5 years (%)	Outcome: Unremitting course (%)	Outcome: Articular erosions (%)	Outcome: Ultimate morbidity
Systemic onset	20	1.5:1	Throughout childhood (mean 4–6 years)	Any	Rare	High fever, rash, organomegaly polyserositis, leukocytosis, anemia, growth abnormalities	No	No	HLA-DR4	10–20	7	60	Mortality 1–2% Severe arthritis 40% worse outcome if < 5 years old at onset
Polyarticular rheumatoid factor negative	15	9:1	Throughout childhood (often early)	Any	Rare (10%)	Malaise, low grade fever, mild anemia growth abnormalities	No	25%	HLA-DRW8	10	7	48	Severe arthritis 10–15%
Polyarticular rheumatoid factor positive	10	4:1	Late childhood (teens)	Any	Rare	Malaise, weight loss, low grade fever, mild anemia, Sjögren's, Felty's, vasculitis	100%	50–70%	HLA-DR4 HLA-DW4 HLA-DW14	25	Majority	80	Severe arthritis 50% or more
Pauciarticular type I	25	4–7.5:1	Early childhood (<6 years old)	Large joints: knee, ankle, elbow	20% (95% if female ANA+ve with onset at 2 years old. 50% asymptomatic)	Rare growth abnormalities	5%	40–75%	HLA-DR5 HLA-DR8 HLA-DPW2	70	30 poly-arthritis	25	Ocular damage 40% blindness 10% polyarticular course more severe
Pauciarticular type II	15	1:6.9	Late childhood (>8 years old)	Lower extremities Large joints: sacroiliitis enthesitis (20% limited back motion)	10–20% acute	Rare (5–10%)	No	No	HLA-B27 (90% JAS) fx arthritis 60%	–	–	(100 sacroiliitis in JAS)	Subsequent spondyloarthropathy in 40% at follow-up 10 years later
Pauciarticular type III	15	4:1	Throughout childhood	Asymmetric large and small joints, dactylitis	10–20% chronic	Rare nail pits associated with subsequent psoriatic arthritis	No	17–50%	HLA-B27 associated sacroiliitis fx psoriasis 40%	–	majority poly-arthritis	–	Subsequent psoriasis

Fig. 18.2 The characterization of JCA subtypes.

help in clarifying prognosis.

- Pauciarticular onset (four or fewer joints involved) is the most common form, with 55–75% of cases presenting in this manner.
- Polyarticular onset (five or more joints affected) comprises 15–25% of the whole group.
- Systemic onset JCA comprises 10–20% of the whole group and is defined as arthritis associated with daily temperature spikes to 39.5°C for at least 2 weeks with or without a typical rash.

The true prevalence and incidence of JCA are still unknown[2,3]. Using the above mentioned criteria, the average mean incidence of JCA is 15.7/100,000 (range 9.2–25). The prevalence estimates range from 12–113/100,000 and it has been estimated that in the USA there are 31,775 active cases of JCA and 31,250 inactive cases of JCA. The female to male ratio is 2–3:1. There are a few studies suggesting the disease is less frequent among blacks and Chinese and more frequent in Native American Indian populations.

PAUCIARTICULAR ONSET JCA

This is the largest subtype of JCA. Three subtypes of pauciarticular onset JCA have been identified: those presenting with lower extremity arthritis before the age of 5 years; those presenting over the age of 9 years with or without sacroiliitis; and those who present at any age with asymmetric oligoarthritis and often develop psoriasis later in life. Other subtypes have not been well defined as yet; thus not all pauciarticular onset JCA can be assigned to one of the three subtypes discussed here. For example 30% of those presenting with pauci-articular JCA can go on to a more severe polyarticular course.

The majority of children with pauciarticular onset JCA present before the age of 5 years, with a peak onset between 1 and 3 years of age. Pauciarticular JCA occurs more frequently in females, with the ratio being 4–7.5:1. Commonly such children are brought to the physician because of a limp[4], complaints of pain are infrequent. Typically there are no constitutional signs or symptoms. The knee (Fig. 18.3) is the most commonly affected joint (47%) followed by the ankle and then either the small joints of the hand or the elbow. Involvement of other joints occurs but is less frequent. Arthritis limited to the hip is extremely rare in this subgroup, and if it is present the diagnosis should be questioned[5].

Antinuclear antibodies (ANA) are present in 40–75% of children with pauciarticular onset JCA and are largely associated with chronic anterior uveitis. The association with uveitis is particularly strong (95%) if the child with arthritis is female and below 2 years of age[6]. The child with uveitis is asymptomatic 50% of the time, thus making routine eye examination essential. On examination the iris may demonstrate irregularity due to posterior synechiae when a bright light is shone into the pupil (Fig. 18.4). This is a late finding, so a slit lamp examination is necessary for early detection of eye involvement. In most children the eye disease occurs within 7 years (median 2 years) of the onset of arthritis. It is generally a chronic condition with a remitting and relapsing course in 60% of patients, and it is bilateral in 66% of the cases[7]. The course of the eye disease is unrelated to the course of the arthritis and often persists after the arthritis has remitted.

A second subtype of pauciarticular JCA affects boys more than girls and presents most commonly after the age of 9 years. The lower extremity tends to be involved (especially the knee and ankle) but, in contrast to the younger onset pauciarticular group, the hip can also be affected[8]. Enthesitis or inflammation of the enthesis as it attaches to the periosteum, occurs frequently and is commonly seen as plantar fasciitis, or Achilles tendonitis. Many of these children develop sacroiliitis several

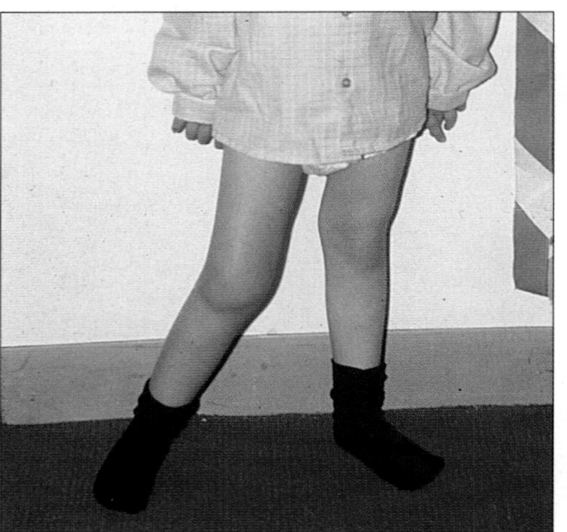

Fig. 18.3 A 6-year-old girl with pauciarticular onset JCA affecting her right knee. Her right leg is 3cm longer than her left leg.

Fig. 18.4 Iritis demonstrating cataract and irregular pupil secondary to posterior synechiae. Courtesy of JJ Kanski.

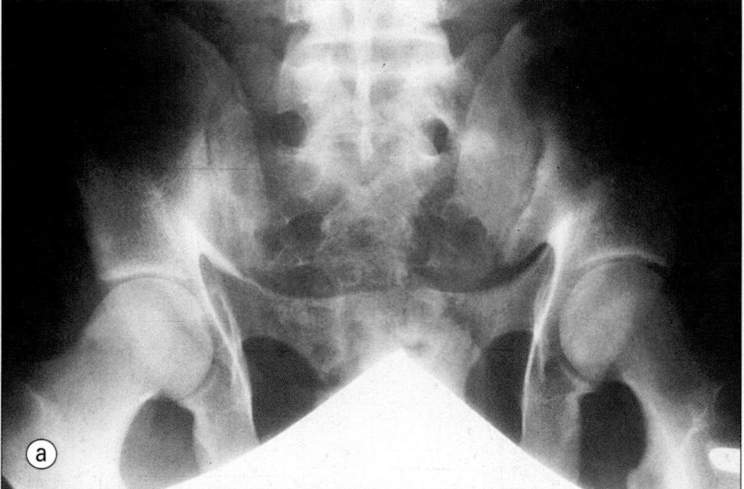

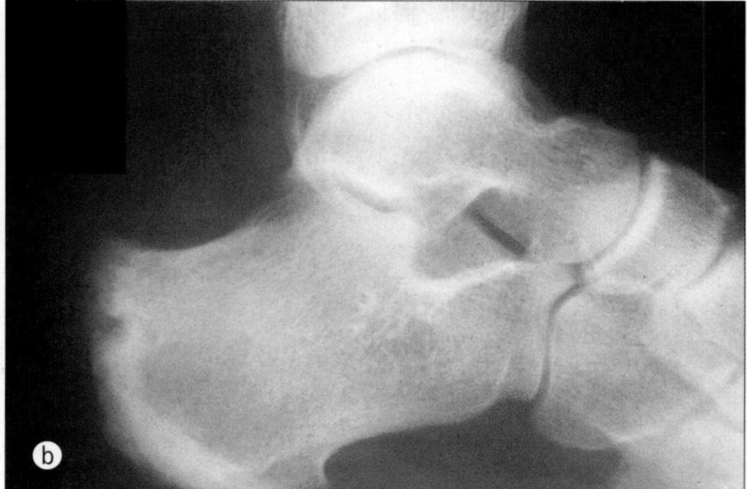

Fig. 18.5 A 19-year-old with bilateral heel pain since the age of 9 years. Sacroiliitis in the left sacroiliac joint (a). The patient was still without back symptoms. Erosion in the right heel was noted 10 years after onset of heel pain (b).

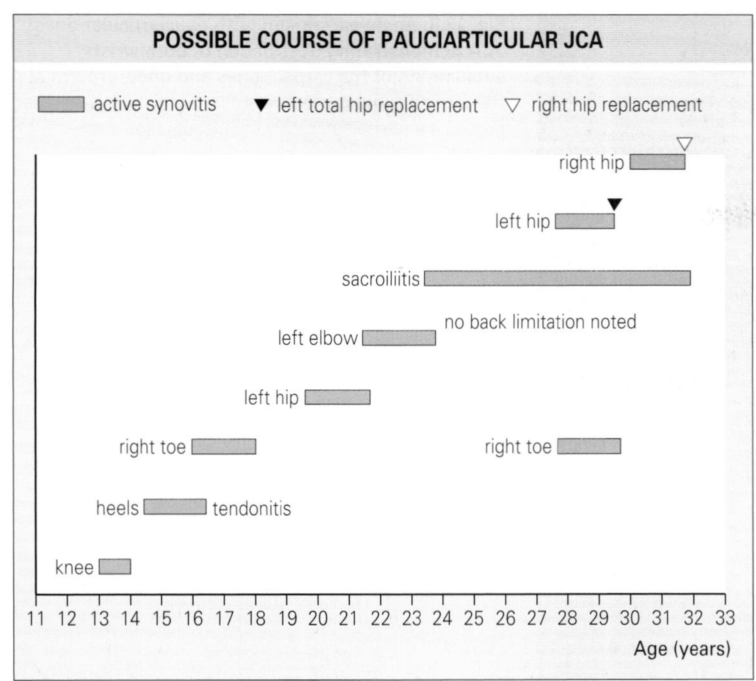

Fig. 18.6 Pauciarticular onset JCA with evolution into juvenile spondyloarthropathy.

years later (Fig. 18.5) and some will evolve into ankylosing spondylitis or other spondyloarthropathies (Fig. 18.6). Because back involvement and associated symptoms such as inflammatory bowel disease can occur many years after the onset of the arthritis, these patients are difficult to classify into particular spondyloarthropathy groups early in the course of disease. The Canadians have adopted a categorization called the seronegative enthesitis syndrome, or SEA[9]. These patients (usually boys) differ from those who can be classified from the outset as juvenile ankylosing spondylitis (JAS) in that they lack evidence of axial skeleton disease and less frequently inherit HLA-B27. The SEA group as well as the JAS group frequently have a family history of arthritis (65%), and sometimes there is a family history of ankylosing spondylitis (25%). The frequency with which SEA progresses to JAS or other spondyloarthropathies, such as those associated with psoriasis, inflammatory bowel disease or Reiter's syndrome, differs considerably from report to report[10]. Sheerin *et al.*[11] evaluated 36 HLA-B27-positive children and found that 8.9 years later 44% had developed a disorder associated with spondyloarthropathy; either JAS (6 cases), probable JAS (6 cases), inflammatory bowel disease with radiographic sacroiliitis (1 case), or psoriasis (2 cases) with sacroiliitis (1 case). In a 10-year follow-up of the originally described SEA group of 36 children, the 14 who had HLA-B27 had developed ankylosing spondylitis with definite sacroiliitis. Iritis, usually acute and symptomatic, occurs in 15–25% of this group. Another major problem can be severe hip disease requiring early total hip replacement (Fig. 18.7).

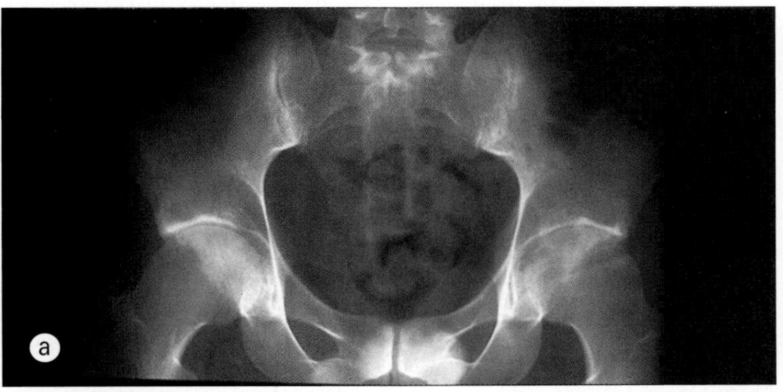

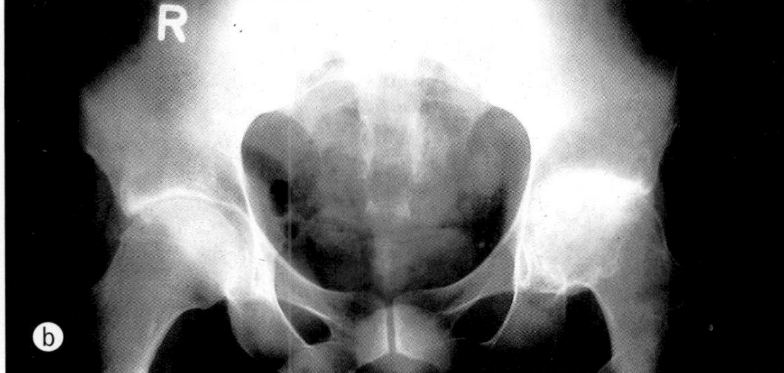

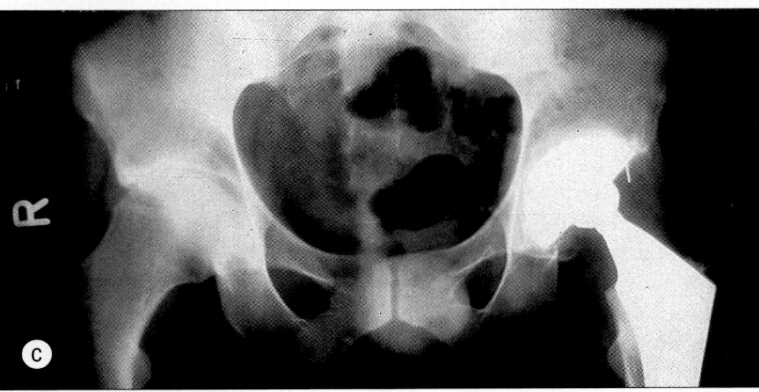

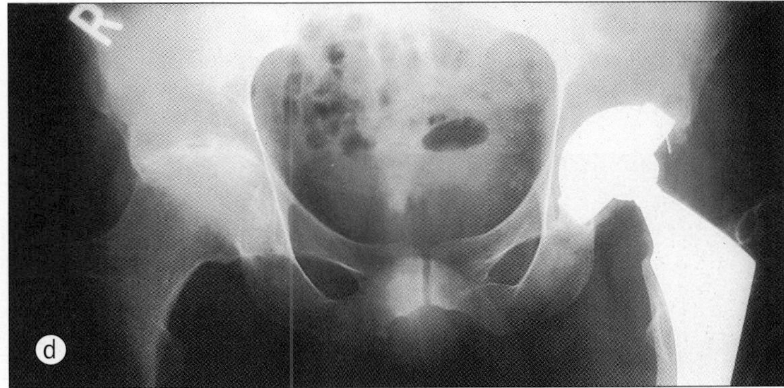

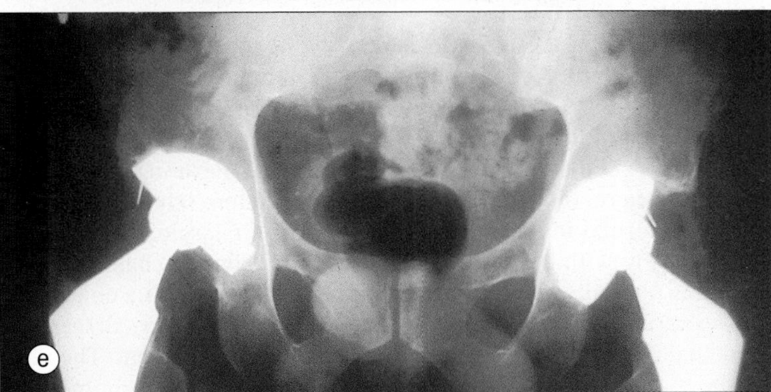

Fig. 18.7 A 21-year-old with evidence of sacroiliitis on the left. There is left hip joint space narrowing (a). Subsequently there was severe joint space narrowing 1 year later in the left hip (b); total hip replacement 6 months later (c); joint space narrowing of the right hip one year later (d); bilateral hip replacement (e).

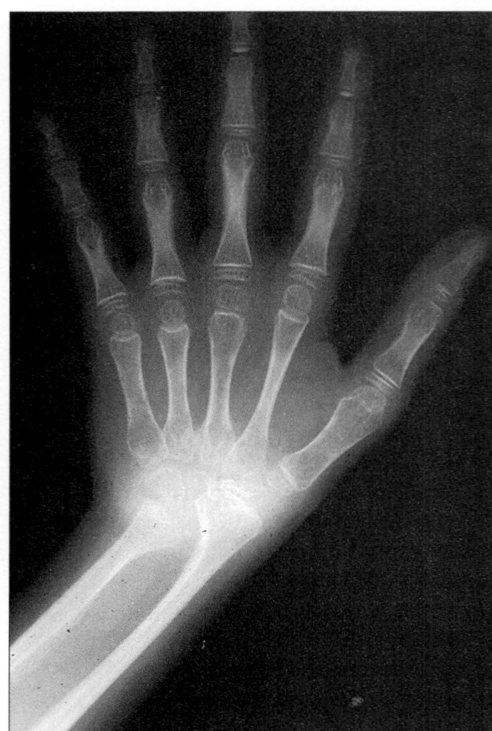

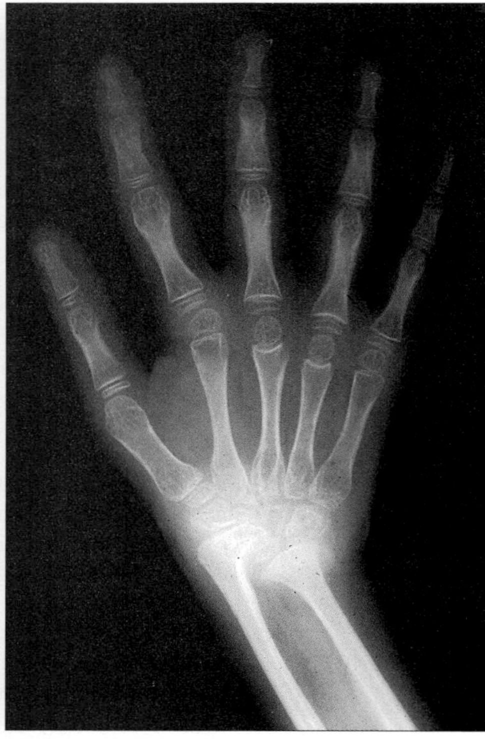

Fig. 18.8 An 8-year-old girl with pauciarticular onset JCA demonstrating destruction of both wrists, subluxation of the carpal bones and undergrowth of the ulnar styloids. There was a family history of psoriasis and she had a polyarticular course.

A third subtype of pauciarticular JCA comprises those children with dactylitis and asymmetric upper and lower extremity arthritis that can be locally very destructive. This subtype occurs slightly more frequently in girls, beginning around the age of 8 years. There is a family history of psoriasis in 40% of patients and psoriasis may develop many years later (Fig. 18.8)[12].

POLYARTICULAR ONSET JCA

Approximately 20% of children with JCA have polyarticular onset, with five or more joints involved in the first 6 months of disease. This subtype is divided into those who have persistent serum IgM rheumatoid factor (RF) and those who do not.

The RF-negative polyarticular onset JCA is often indistinguishable from the arthritis that follows systemic onset JCA[12]. These patients may have low grade fevers and mild hepatosplenomegaly. This form of the disease occurs throughout childhood. It comprises approximately 15% of the JCA cases. The joints tend to be symmetrically involved, with the knees, wrists and ankles being most commonly affected. In the hands the metacarpophalangeal (MCP) and proximal interphalangeal (PIP) joints are involved and there is flexor tenosynovitis. The neck is often involved and occasionally patients will present with torticollis. Hip and shoulder involvement occurs usually after at least 1 year of polyarthritis in those who present young and have persistently active disease. In the majority of patients the long-term prognosis is favorable.

The RF-positive polyarticular onset JCA is very similar to seropositive, adult onset rheumatoid arthritis (RA). Most patients are female and present between the ages of 12 and 16 years. This subtype comprises 10% of JCA cases. Symmetric small joint involvement is most typical including the MCP (Fig. 18.9), PIP and distal interphalangeal (DIP) joints as well as metatarsal phalangeal (MTP) joints. Large joints tend to be involved only in association with small joint involvement. Flexor tenosynovitis is common and often results in trigger fingers. Nodules similar to those seen in adult RA, and early development of erosions on radiographs, are significantly correlated with the presence of IgM RF. Systemic features are rare. IgM-RF-positive polyarticular onset JCA is frequently severe, unremitting and persists with active disease into adulthood. The complications of this form of arthritis include atlantoaxial subluxation with neurological impairment[12], aortic regurgitation[13], pulmonary fibrosis[14], vasculitis, sometimes associated with digital calcification[15], carpal tunnel syndrome, Sjögren's syndrome[16] and Felty's syndrome[17].

Fig. 18.9 An 11-year-old with seropositive JCA demonstrating erosions at several metacarpophalangeal joints and carpal bone fusion in the wrist.

SYSTEMIC ONSET JCA

This subtype is most often associated with the most serious short- and long-term morbidity as well as significant mortality. It makes up 20% of the total JCA population and is defined by its extra-articular features of fever and rash. The fevers typically rise to 39.5°C daily for at least 2 weeks before this diagnosis is considered. Fever usually occurs late in the afternoon or evening and the temperature returns to normal or below normal in the morning (Fig. 18.10). Classically the child appears toxic with the fever, can have accompanying shaking chills but looks normal when the fever abates. In 90% of cases a characteristic evanescent salmon colored eruption (Fig. 18.11) occurs on the trunk and thighs, most commonly when the fever is present. The rash can be brought out by scratching the skin (Koebner's phenomenon)

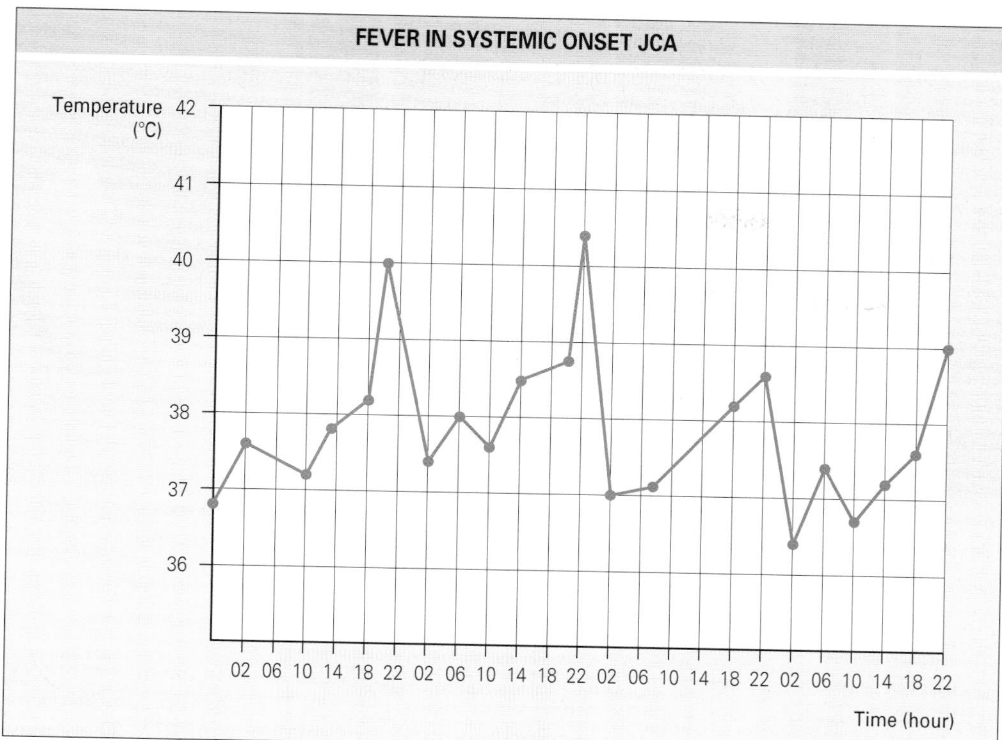

Fig. 18.10 Example of the typical fever curve seen in systemic onset JCA.

and occasionally is pruritic. Approximately 50–75% of patients will have generalized lymphadenopathy and hepatosplenomegaly. The lymph nodes are usually firm, movable and nontender and on biopsy show follicular hyperplasia and, rarely, necrotizing lymphadenitis. The child may complain of abdominal pain secondary to hepatomegaly and there can be a mild associated transaminitis[18]. Fulminant hepatic failure is rare but has been reported[19]. Polyserositis is common, with up to 36% of patients having documented pericarditis (Fig. 18.12)[20]. Most pericardial involvement is subclinical. Tamponade and myocarditis[21] can occur but are rare. Pulmonary disease is equally unusual and can manifest itself as pneumonitis, pleural effusion or pulmonary fibrosis[22]. Central nervous system involvement with coma and meningitis has been described but it is very unusual[23]. Approximately 75% of children with systemic onset JCA develop arthritis within 3–12 months of the onset of the fever. The wrists, knees and ankles are most commonly involved, with the cervical spine, hips, temporomandibular joints and hands also being affected. Cricoarytenoid arthritis resulting in laryngeal stricture occurs rarely.

The course of systemic onset JCA is variable. At least 50% of patients will recover completely, while the remainder will have a progressive polyarthritis. After 2–5 years, most of the systemic features usually disappear.

GROWTH ABNORMALITIES AND RADIOGRAPHIC FINDINGS

Growth abnormalities are a common finding in JCA and can be divided into two forms: local and systemic[24]. Local growth abnormalities affect 30% of children with polyarticular disease, 40% of those with systemic disease and over 50% of those with pauciarticular disease[25]. Local factors that influence bone growth include arterial blood supply, muscle

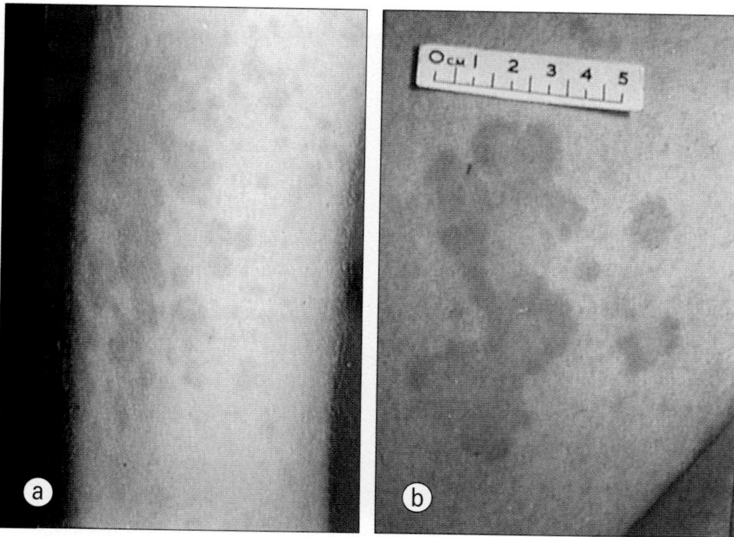

Fig. 18.11 The rash of systemic onset JCA. Larger lesions becoming confluent are shown (a). This must be differentiated from erythema marginatum, which is characteristic of the rash seen in rheumatic fever (b). By courtesy of B. Ansell.

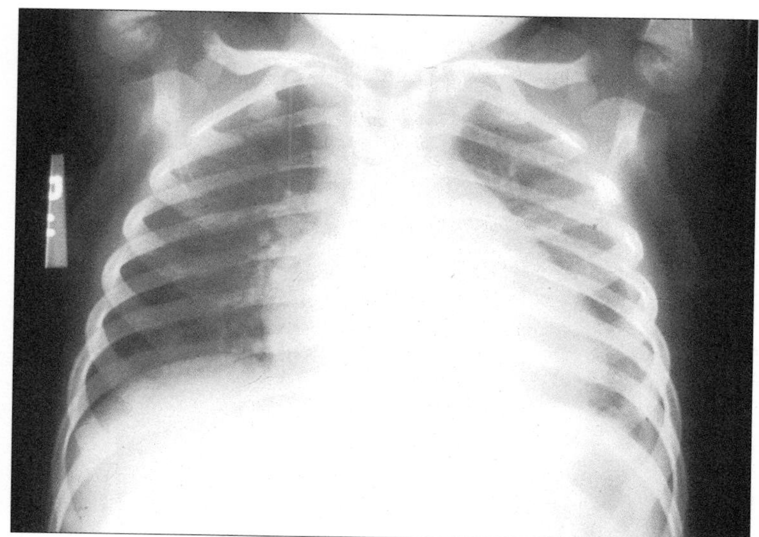

Fig. 18.12 A 3-year-old with systemic onset JCA with pericardial effusion.

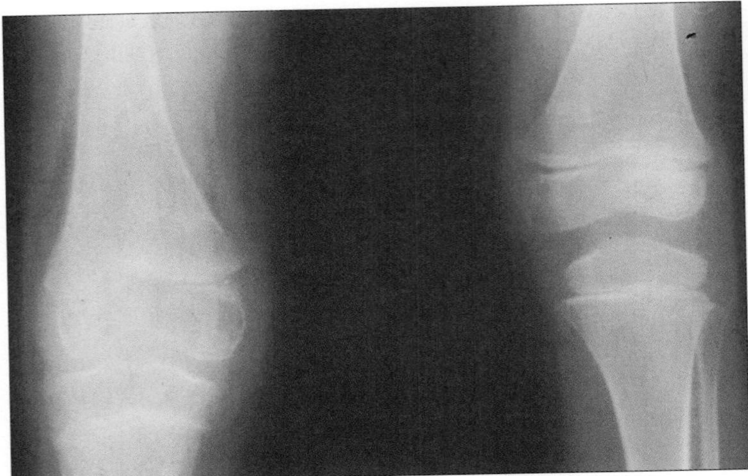

Fig. 18.13 Pauciarticular JCA involving the left knee with overgrowth of the leg and widening of the epiphysis.

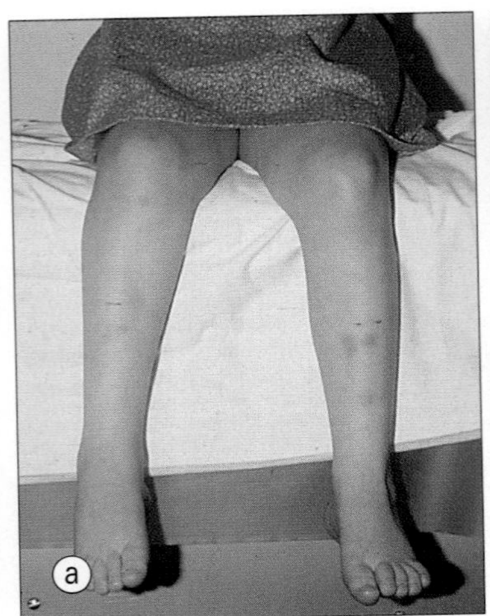

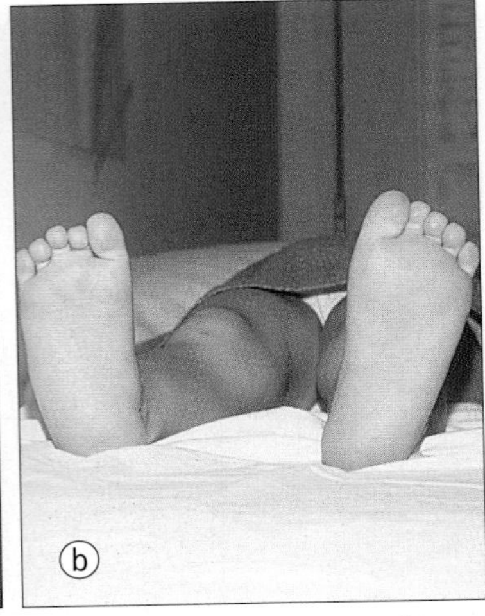

Fig. 18.14 Pauciarticular onset JCA in the right ankle. A shorter leg length from the knee to the ankle is demonstrated (a). The right foot is smaller, with underdevelopment of the right forefoot due to disuse (b).

spasm and use, capsular and ligamentous contracture or rupture, destructive synovitis eroding articular surfaces, and subluxed articular surfaces. Local growth disturbances can result in accelerated bone age. An example is the overgrowth commonly found in the knee. This results in leg length discrepancy, with the longer leg on the side of the involved knee, particularly if the disease begins before the age of 3 years (Fig. 18.13; also see Fig. 18.3). If the child is over 9 years of age, the local growth disturbance often results in early epiphyseal closure, causing a shortened leg on the side of the involved knee[26,27]. Another cause for undergrowth, or delayed bone and soft tissue maturity, is disuse (Fig. 18.14). This growth abnormality can be corrected with exercise. Leg length discrepancy should be diligently looked for as it can cause scoliosis[28,29].

The next most common joint to have growth abnormalities is the wrist. In contrast to the knee, many growth defects seen radiographically in the wrist are not observed clinically. The wrist can show increased bone age with early disease onset (Fig. 18.15) and carpal bone fusion with long-standing involvement. Growth defects are also seen in the ulna and the fourth and fifth metacarpal bones. The ulna, due to epiphyseal undergrowth, can be shorter than the radius, resulting in ulnar migration of the carpal bones, subluxation and severe deformity (Fig. 18.16). Brachydactyly can occur in the fingers or toes due to early epiphyseal closure (Fig. 18.15). The hip demonstrates some growth abnormalities in 35% of children with JCA. There may be lack of growth of the iliac bone and a coxa valga deformity, with either widening of the femoral neck and/or premature fusion leading to stunting of the femoral neck (Figs 18.17 & 18.18).

The cervical spine can develop growth abnormalities that result in apophyseal joint space narrowing and bony ankylosis (especially C2–C3) with a secondary decrease in the vertical and anteroposterior size of the adjacent vertebral bodies (Fig. 18.19). Similar findings are not seen in the dorsal lumbar spine, but compression fractures of the thoracic spine do occur particularly in those children taking corticosteroids. Micrognathia is observed clinically in 20% of children with JCA but noted radiographically in 40%. Mandibular hypoplasia may be due to inflammation in the temporomandibular joint or adjacent disease of the spine.

Generalized growth abnormalities have been observed in children with active disease and seem to be related to disease duration. Corticosteroid therapy also inhibits growth in height but not skeletal maturation (Fig. 18.20)[30]. The etiology of delayed growth and low weight is unclear. Studies suggest that severe weight loss or lack of weight gain may contribute to the lack of growth in height. Nutritional studies have suggested

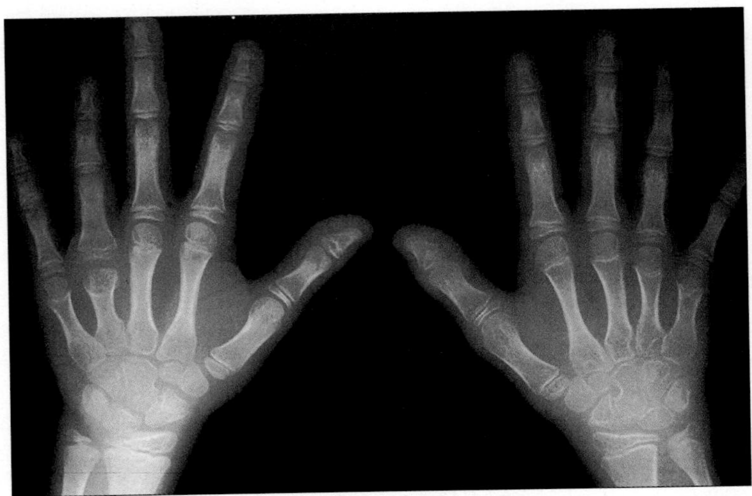

Fig. 18.15 An 8-year-old with pauciarticular JCA. Epiphyseal destruction and undergrowth of the third MCP joint of the left hand are seen as well as overgrowth of the carpal bones of the right wrist compared to the left wrist. Also note the widened appearance of the third phalanges due to periosteal new bone formation.

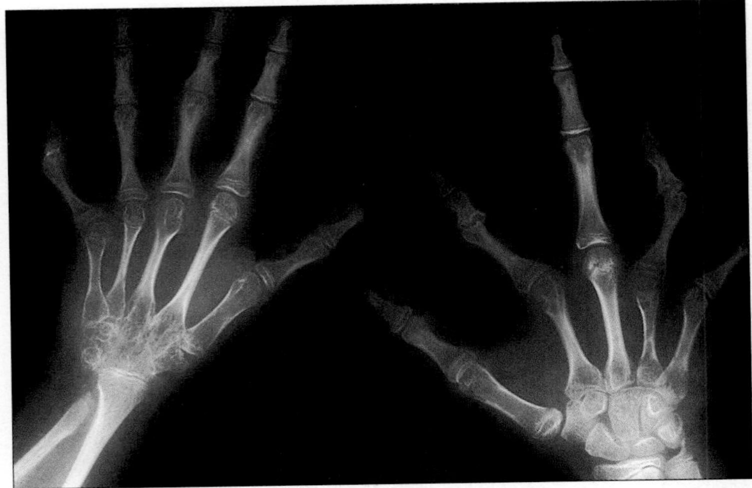

Fig. 18.16 A 12-year-old with seronegative polyarticular onset JCA since the age of 4 years. Note the asymmetry and obvious fusion and growth abnormalities of the right wrist compared to the left wrist.

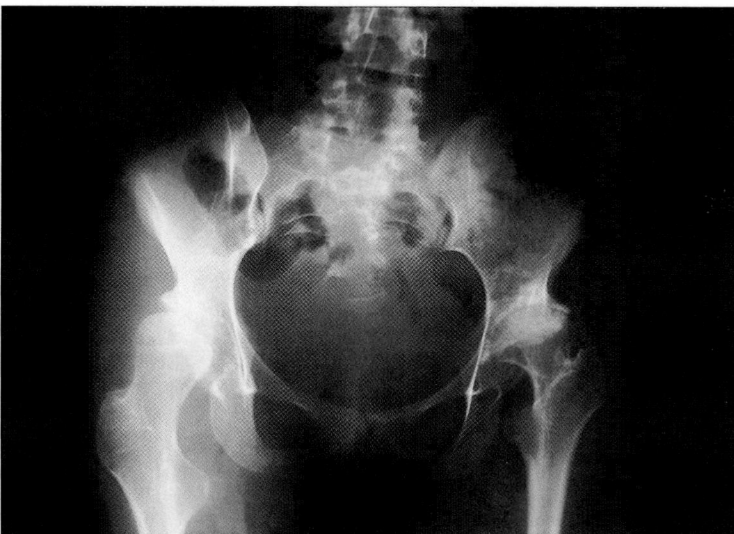

Fig. 18.17 A 12-year-old with JCA. Severe joint space narrowing and femoral head destruction are demonstrated as well as femoral neck anteversion and a shallow acetabulum on the opposite side.

that decreased caloric intake, increased metabolic needs beyond recommended daily requirements or lack of essential vitamins could result in decreased weight and height[31]. Although hormone levels are normal in children with JCA, a recent pilot study showed that giving growth hormone to children with JCA who had relatively inactive disease can increase growth velocity[32]. Osteoporosis is now being recognized in children with JCA, the etiology of which is multifactorial[33].

Radiographic changes in JCA are common. Early changes include soft tissue swelling around affected joints, and juxta-articular osteopenia and periosteal new bone formation (see Fig. 18.15) resulting in a widened midportion of the phalanges. Ballooning of the epiphysis also occurs (see Fig. 18.13). Erosions are a late finding because much of the cartilage in growing joints is not calcified; the visualization of erosions is possible only after the cartilage has calcified. Joint space narrowing is an early sign that cartilage has been eroded.

Cartilage that has been destroyed during the course of severe JCA can be replaced with fibrocartilage if the disease becomes quiescent (Fig. 18.21). Growth arrest lines may result from temporary loss of growth velocity and are frequently seen around the knee. Bony ankylosis, more common in children with arthritis than adults, is seen most frequently in the carpal and tarsal bones (see Fig. 18.16).

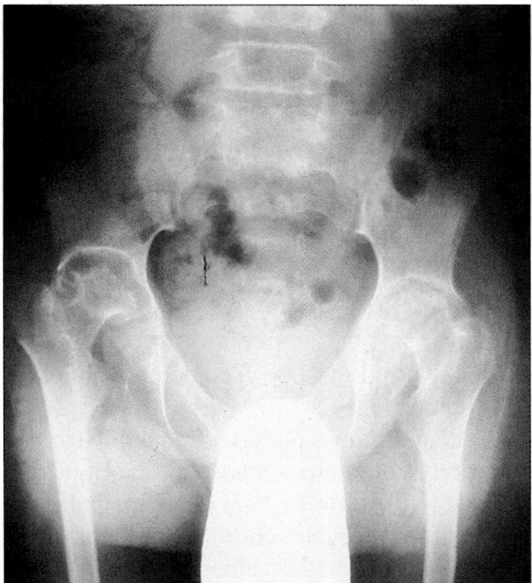

Fig. 18.18 Systemic onset JCA with polyarticular course. Severe hip destruction and protrusion.

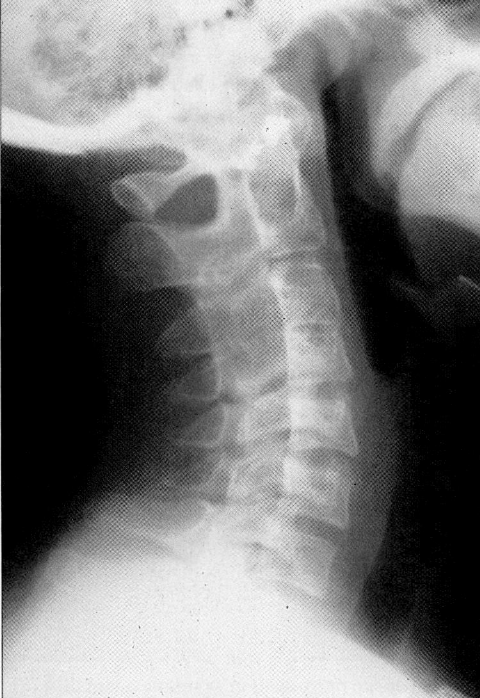

Fig. 18.19 Systemic onset JCA in a child who had a polyarticular course. Her neck shows apophyseal fusion of C2–C4 and undergrowth of adjacent vertebrae.

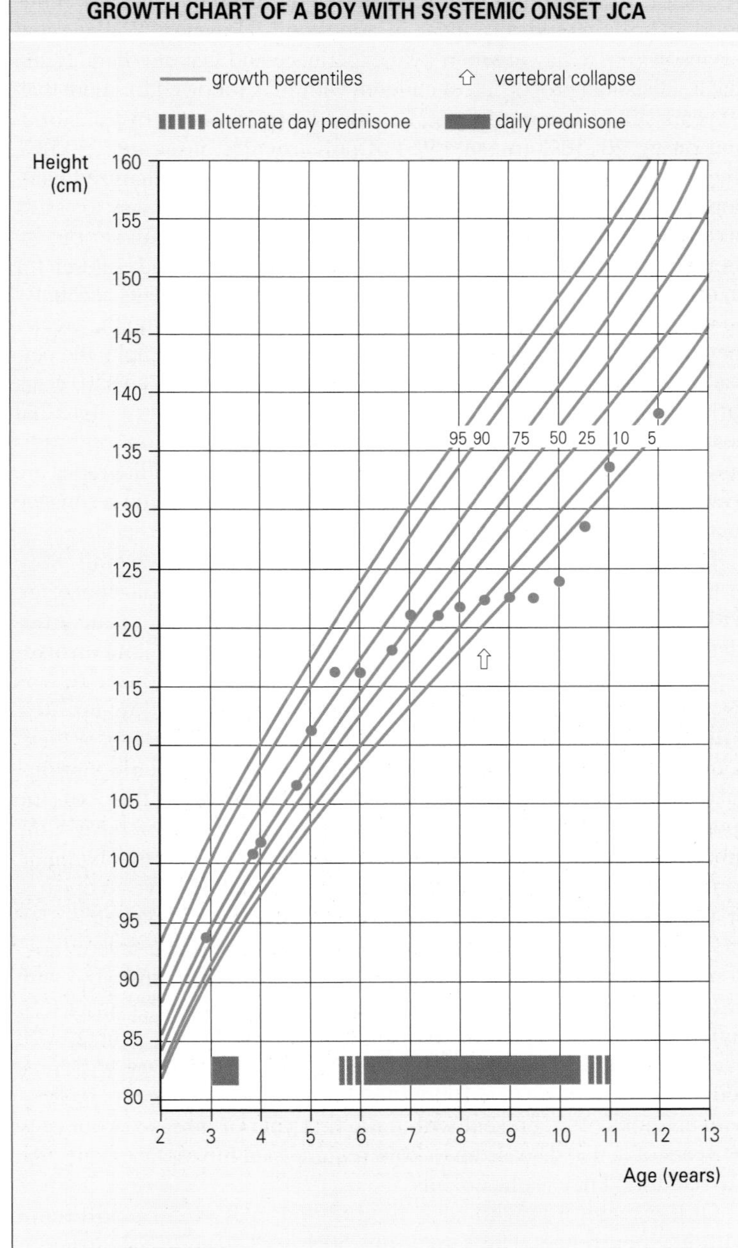

Fig. 18.20 Growth chart of a boy with systemic onset JCA.

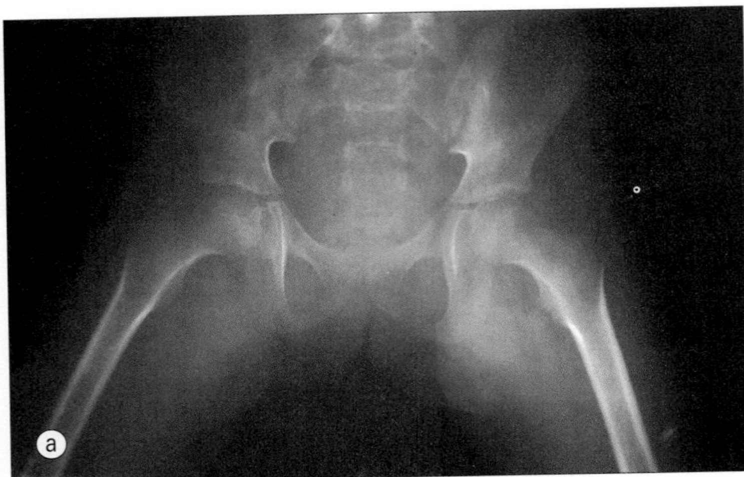

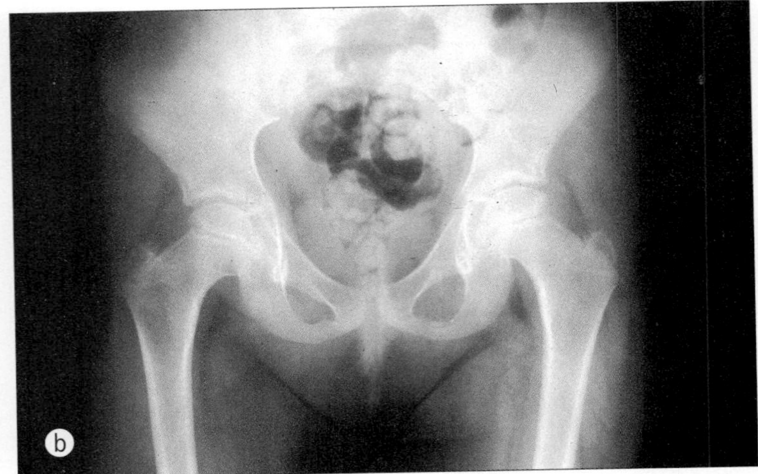

Fig. 18.21 Systemic onset JCA with polyarticular course. There is hip joint space narrowing bilaterally (a). There was recovery of joint space 2 years later (b) (standing view).

PROGNOSIS

The prognosis of JCA is variable depending on the subtype and course of disease[34–36]. A common misconception has been that most of childhood arthritis would disappear in adulthood. However, Wallace and Levinson[37], in reviewing their own experience and that of others, found that a substantial proportion of children with JCA followed for more than 10 years still had active disease, i.e. 30–70% (mean 44%) of pauciarticular onset, 40–50% (mean 45%) of polyarticular onset and 25–58% (mean 44%) of systemic onset. None of the studies they analyzed mentions resolution of the disease at or near puberty. The usual way to assess outcome in JCA has been by the functional classification set out by Steinbrocker *et al.*[38]. Wallace averaged studies that followed children for an average of 10 years and noted that one third of the patients at follow-up were in functional class III or IV. The longer the follow-up the greater the number who were in a worse functional state. For example, the percentage of patients in functional class III increased from 9% after 10 years to 17% at 15–20 years. Another way to look at outcome is to note that nearly 60% of all patients with JCA have bone erosion on joint radiographs after 10 years of disease[2]. Erosions detected by radiographs are a late finding in children with JCA, although using magnetic resonance imaging (MRI), erosions are seen more frequently, and earlier[39].

Prognoses in individual subtypes are fairly distinct. Overall, 80% of those with pauciarticular onset JCA who remain pauciarticular are without difficulty at a 15-year follow-up. Of those with a pauciarticular onset, 15% develop a polyarthritic course with severe joint involvement[40]. A major cause of morbidity in pauciarticular onset JCA is uveitis. Of such patients, 10% will be blind at 10-year follow-up, 50% will have decreased visual acuity and 25% will have cataracts or glaucoma[41]. The outcome for the child with later onset pauciarticular disease with enthesitis is quite variable due to the nature of the spondyloarthropathy that develops. As a group, only 12% have some functional limitation at 15 years, although 33% have hip involvement, some with only a small limitation of motion, and 25% have an episode of acute iritis. In the subtype with polyarticular onset and negative RF the prognosis is that of a mild disease: only 10–15% have severe functional limitation 10–15 years later. They often go into remission with little erosive disease residua. In contrast, those polyarticular onset JCA patients who have a positive RF will have a more severe course, with over 33% unable to live independently, and the majority will have active disease at a 15-year follow-up. Hip involvement occurs in 40%, with erosions often present within the first year of disease. After only 10 years of active disease up to 20% require total hip replacements and 7% had total knee replacements.

Of those children who have systemic onset JCA, 50% will remit without recurrence. The remaining 50% will have a polyarticular course with 33% having a severe destructive arthritis (Fig. 18.22) and local and generalized growth abnormalities. At risk for having a poor functional outcome are those whose disease onset is before age 5 years, with persistent disease activity for the first 5 years, accelerated radiologic changes, pericarditis and thrombocytosis[42]. Of children with systemic onset JCA, 4% die from infection or amyloidosis[43]. The incidence of amyloidosis is between 1% and 10% in all subtypes. In the past, diagnosis of amyloid depended on biopsy of an affected area such as the rectum, but a diagnostic technique with scintigraphy using radiolabeled serum amyloid P component which attaches to amyloid deposits is now available[44].

DIFFERENTIAL DIAGNOSIS OF JCA

JCA is a diagnosis of exclusion[45,46] and must be considered among the many causes of arthritis in children (Fig. 18.23). Making the diagnosis of arthritis in a child can be difficult because children frequently cannot describe their problems and rarely complain of pain. Instead they will tend not to use the area affected by the arthritis and develop abnormal growth and/or developmental patterns. Since children are constantly changing and progressing through well defined developmental milestones, the physician must be aware not only of disease entities commonly seen at particular ages but also of the age-related tasks a child should be performing. A functional abnormality may present as developmental delay, for instance inability to walk due to pauciarticular JCA.

Patterns of arthritis, such as monoarticular versus polyarticular,

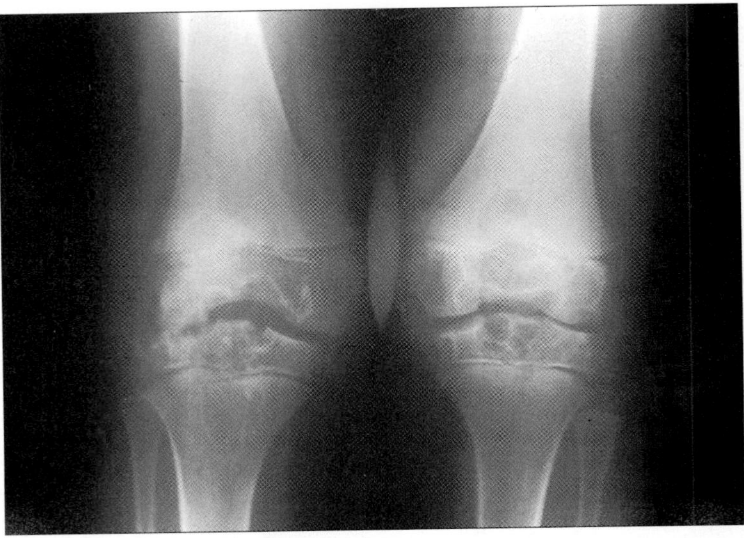

Fig. 18.22 Severe erosions and joint space narrowing in systemic onset JCA of 10 years' duration.

CONDITIONS THAT MIGHT BE CONFUSED WITH JCA

Type of condition	Example
Infections	Viral, fungal and mycoplasma Bacterial Aseptic arthritis associated with bacterial infections (osteomyelitis) Lyme disease Tuberculosis
Postinfectious	Rheumatic fever Poststreptococcal Postdysenteric arthritis
Noninflammatory	Hypermobility Trauma Reflex sympathetic dystrophy Foreign body synovitis Patellar femoral syndrome Toxic synovitis Osteochondroses Slipped capital femoral epiphysis Congenital and genetic disorders of bone and cartilage
Hematologic disorders	Sickle cell disease Hemophilia Christmas disease Von Willebrand's disease
Collagen vascular disorders	Systemic lupus erythematosus Ankylosing spondylitis Dermatomyositis Scleroderma Mixed connective tissue disease Behçet's syndrome Psoriatic arthritis Vasculitis Henoch–Schönlein purpura serum sickness Kawasaki disease
Miscellaneous	Immunologic abnormalities Sarcoidosis Hypertrophic osteoarthropathy Familial Mediterranean fever Idiopathic osteonecrosis and chondrolysis
Malignancy	Neuroblastoma Leukemia Localized bone tumor

Fig. 18.23 Conditions that might be confused with JCA.

migratory versus nonmigratory and the presence or absence of fever will help differentiate the causes of the arthritis. A child with JCA is likely to have a warm swollen joint that is nontender and generally does not look systemically ill. An exception is the systemic onset subtype. When evaluating a child with arthritis, infection must be excluded early through aspiration and culture of the affected joint. Most children with infectious arthritis appear systemically ill with fever and usually have a monoarthritis. There are notable exceptions, such as gonorrhea, which has an early migratory phase before settling in one joint. A diagnosis of bacterial septic arthritis can be especially difficult if it is partially treated with antibiotics. Lyme disease can masquerade as JCA, particularly since it tends to be migratory over several months to years, and a combination of clinical judgment and careful interpretation of serologic tests is needed in order to make the correct diagnosis. Hip disease is rare at the onset of JCA. Other causes of hip disease such as infection, toxic synovitis or congenital dislocation must be excluded. Children rarely complain of back pain without a mechanical cause[47] so processes such as spondylolysis, Scheuermann's disease, discitis and disc herniation must be excluded. Avulsion fractures can masquerade as enthesopathies associated with spondyloarthropathy. Another common nonrheumatic condition, the growing pains of childhood, should be considered in a child with bilateral lower extremity pain that is worse in the evening but leaves the child active during the day. Laboratory investigations are normal[48]. Fibrositis, a common diagnosis in adults, does occur in children and should be considered in the evaluation of the achy child[49].

Malignancy can masquerade as JCA for several months[50]. In a child with painful joints and fever, acute lymphoblastic leukemia and neuroblastoma are the most common malignancies seen. Often a clue to the diagnosis comes from noting thrombocytopenia and neutropenia which are not seen in systemic onset JCA. Another disease that can be difficult to differentiate from systemic onset JCA is rheumatic fever. Usually rheumatic fever has a sustained fever, the migratory arthritis is exquisitely painful in contrast to systemic JCA and the rash migrates. However, both diseases may have elevated antistreptolysin-O (ASO) titers.

A recent study of causes for joint complaints in children referred to a rheumatology clinic found that 65% had a recognizable form of inflammatory arthropathy, with only 23% having other connective tissue diseases. Henoch–Schönlein purpura, Kawasaki disease and systemic lupus erythematosus (SLE) were the other connective tissue diseases most commonly diagnosed[51]. Confirmation of SLE may take several years: a child can present with polyarthritis and a negative ANA but develop other signs of SLE months to years later and convert negative serologies to positive for ANA and anti-DNA antibodies[52].

Dermatomyositis and scleroderma can also present with arthritis, but the associated features of the disease result in a correct diagnosis. When a child has delayed growth and anemia, the diagnosis of inflammatory bowel disease should be considered even in the absence of diarrhea.

LABORATORY INVESTIGATIONS

As JCA is a diagnosis of exclusion, laboratory studies can be used only to support the clinical suspicion of JCA. Most of the laboratory abnormalities reflect the extent of the inflammatory response. Anemia is common in all forms of JCA and is more pronounced in the systemic onset subtype. Usually the anemia is secondary to chronic disease as reflected by low serum iron, low iron-binding capacity and normal hemosiderin stores. Serum ferritin may be elevated and mirrors systemic activity rather than iron stores. Treatment with corticosteroids and nonsteroidal anti-inflammatory drugs (NSAIDs) may cause intestinal blood loss; occasionally the anemia will respond to iron supplements. Anemia quickly resolves if the disease remits. Leukocytosis up to 15,000–25,000/mm^3 with a neutrophilic predominance is seen in 80% of those children with systemic onset JCA. Thrombocytosis is also seen in systemic and polyarticular onset JCA. Thrombocytopenia is rare, but if it is found a work-up for SLE or malignancy should be considered. Mild proteinuria, urinary red blood cells and white blood cells have been seen in 20–40% of children with JCA. These urinary abnormalities tend to occur early in the course of the disease. Mild glomerulitis has been diagnosed in 17 of 20 children on renal biopsy[53]. Abnormal renal tubular function has been noted[54]. Although NSAID-induced nephropathies are distinctly uncommon[55], some of the renal findings reported in JCA may be due to NSAIDs. However, few severe complications are observed in children taking NSAIDs[55]. The erythrocyte sedimentation rate (ESR) is usually elevated in all subtypes of JCA but most commonly is quite high in the systemic onset patients. The ESR often does not correlate well with the extent of clinical disease activity[56]. Serum immunoglobulins will often be elevated, as will the ASO titer, even though there is no evidence for a recent streptococcal infection. Occasionally IgA deficiency is seen in association with JCA[57]. IgM RFs are present in 15–20% of children with late onset polyarticular JCA. In those without IgM RF, IgG anti-IgG antibodies and hidden RF have been found in 40–60% of children with JCA[58]. Antinuclear antibodies occur in 40–60% of pauciarticular onset JCA, and this is associated with chronic uveitis. Usually homogeneous or speckled patterns are seen[59].

Radiographs may show no abnormalities early in the course of JCA, and a technetium bone scan may be more helpful. Looking at both immediate (15 minutes) and delayed (1–2 hours) radionucleotide studies helps identify arthritis (early increased tracer activity in soft tissue and joint) in contrast to other problems such as Legg–Perthes disease (reduced uptake in delayed study), reflex sympathetic dystrophy (decreased immediate scan) and malignancy[60].

Synovial fluid shows white blood cell counts ranging from 41,000 cells/mm^3 to 100,000 cells/mm^3, with between 18% and 88% polymorphonuclear neutrophils. The fluid may also show decreased glucose and glycosaminoglycans, and hyaluronic acid and chondroitin sulfate levels similar to those found in adult RA patients[61].

REFERENCES

1. Cassidy JT, Levinson JE, Bass JC,*et al.* A study of classification criteria for a diagnosis of juvenile rheumatoid arthritis. Arthritis Rheum. 1986;29:274–87.
2. Singsen BH. Rheumatic diseases of childhood. Rheum Dis Clin North Am. 1990;16:581–99.
3. Andersson Gäre BA, Fasth A. The natural history of juvenile chronic arthritis: a population based cohort study. II Outcome. J Rheumatol. 1995;22:308–19.
4. Sherry DD, Bohnsach J, Salmonsa K, Wallace LA Melins E. Painless juvenile rheumatoid arthritis. J Pediatr. 1990;116:921–3.
5. Ansell BM. Joint manifestations in children with juvenile chronic arthritis. Arthritis Rheum. 1977;20:204–6.
6. Chylack LT, Jr. The ocular manifestations of juvenile rheumatoid arthritis: pathology, fluorescein iris angiography and patient care patterns. In: Juvenile rheumatoid arthritis. Miller JJ, ed. Littleton: Massachussetts; 1979:149–63.
7. Kanski JJ, Shun-Shin GA. Systemic uveitis syndromes in childhood: analysis of 340 cases. Ophthalmology.1984;91:1247–51.
8. Rosenberg AM. Uveitis associated with juvenile rheumatoid arthritis. Semin Arthritis Rheum. 1987;16:158–73.
9. Rosenberg AM, Petty RE. A syndrome of seronegative entheropathy and arthropathy in children. Arthritis Rheum. 1982;25:1041–7.
10. Petty RE. HLA-B27 and rheumatic diseases of childhood. Perspect Pediatr Rheum. 1990;17 (Suppl.26):7–10.
11. Sheerin KA, Gianni EH, Brewer EJ, Jr, Banar KS. HLA-B27 associated arthropathy in childhood: long-term clinical and diagnostic outcome. Arthritis Rheum. 1988;31:1165–70.
12. Ansell BM. Juvenile chronic arthritis. Curr Orthop. 1986;1:81–9.
13. Leak AM, Miller Craig, MW, Ansell BM. Aortic regurgitation in seropositive JCA. Ann Rheum Dis. 1981;40:229–34.
14. Gordon JD, Snyder CH. Rheumatoid disease of the lung and observations in a child. Am J Dis Child. 1964;108:174–80.
15. Forsythe CC. Calcifications of the deposit arteries in a child with rheumatoid arthritis. Arch Dis Child. 1960;35:296–301.
16. Rosenberg AM, Dyck RK, George DH. Intravenous pulse methylprednisone for the treatment of a child with Sjögren's nephropathy. J Rheumatol. 1990;17:391–4.
17. Toomey K, Hepburn B. Felty syndrome in juvenile arthritis. J Pediatr. 1985;106:254–5.
18. Schaller J, Beakwith B, Wedgwood RJ. Hepatic involvement in juvenile rheumatoid arthritis. J Pediatr. 1970;77:203–10.
19. Boone JE. Hepatic disease and mortality in juvenile rheumatoid arthritis. Arthritis Rheum. 1977;20:257–9.
20. Bernstein B. Pericarditis in juvenile rheumatoid arthritis. Arthritis Rheum. 1977;20:241–2.
21. Miller JJ, French JW. Myocarditis in juvenile rheumatoid arthritis. Am J Dis Child. 1977;131:205–9.
22. Athreya B, Doughty RA, Bookspan M, *et al.* Pulmonary manifestation of juvenile rheumatoid arthritis: a report of eight cases and reviews. Clin Chest Med. 1980;1:361–4.
23. O'Connor D, Bernstein B, Hanson V, Kornreich H, King K. Disease of the central nervous system in juvenile rheumatoid arthritis. Arthritis Rheum. 1980;23:727–9.
24. White PH. Growth abnormalities in children with juvenile rheumatoid arthritis. Clin Orthop Rel Res. 1990;259:46–50.
25. Cassidy JT, Martel W. Juvenile rheumatoid arthritis: clinicoradiologic correlations. Arthritis Rheum. 1977;20:207–11.
26. Vostreg SM, Hollister JR. Muscle atrophy and leg length discrepancies in pauciarticular juvenile rheumatoid arthritis. Am J Dis Child. 1988;142:343–5.
27. Simon S, Whitten J, Shapiro F. Leg-length discrepancies in monoarticular and pauciarticular juvenile rheumatoid arthritis. J Bone J Surg. 1981;63A:209–15.
28. Moskowitz A. Scoliosis and JRA. Spine. 1990;15:46–9.
29. Papaioannov T, Stokes I, Keywright J. Scoliosis associated with leg length inequality. J Bone J Surg. 1982;64A:59–64.
30. Ansell BM, Bywaters EGL. Growth in Still's disease. Ann Rheum Dis. 1956;15:295–9.
31. Bacon M, White PH, Raiten DJ, *et al.* Nutritional status and growth in juvenile rheumatoid arthritis. Semin Arthritis Rheum. 1990;20:1–11.
32. Davies UM, Ansell BM, Woo P. Growth retardation in juvenile chronic arthritis: effect of treatment with biosynthetic human growth hormone. Arthritis Rheum. 1990;33:S14.
33. Cassidy JT, Langman CB, Allen SH, Hillman LS. Bone mineral metabolism in children with juvenile rheumatoid arthritis. Pediatr Clin North Am. 1995; 42:1017–34.
34. Ansell BM, Wood PHN. Prognosis in juvenile chronic arthritis. Clin Rheum Dis. 1976;2:397.
35. Dequeker J, Madjvadi A. Prognostic factors in juvenile chronic arthritis. J Rheumatol. 1982;9:909–15.
36. Hull RG. Outcome of juvenile rheumatoid arthritis. Br J Rheumatol. 1988;27:66–71.
37. Wallace CA, Levinson JE. JRA: outcome and treatment for the 1990s. Rheum Dis Clin North Am. 1991;17:891–906.
38. Steinbrocker O, Traeger CH, Batterman RC. Criteria for determination of progression of rheumatoid arthritis and of functional capacity of patients with the disease. JAMA. 1949;140:209.
39. Senac MO, Deutsch D, Bernstein BH, *et al.* MR imaging in juvenile rheumatoid arthritis. Am J Rheumatol. 1988;150:873–8.
40. Cush JS, Fink CW. Clinical outcome of pauciarticular onset juvenile arthritis. Arthritis Rheum. 1987;30(Suppl): S34.
41. Kanski JJ. Uveitis in juvenile chronic arthritis. Clin Rheumatol. 1990;8:499–503.
42. Schneider R, Lang BA, Reilly BJ, *et al.* Prognostic indicators of chronic destructive arthritis in systemic onset JRA. Arthritis Rheum. 1989;32:S83.
43. David J. Amyloidosis in juvenile chronic arthritis. Clin Exp Rheumatol. 1991;9:73–8.
44. Hawkins PN, Lavender JP, Myers MJ, Pepys MB. Diagnostic radionuclide imaging of amyloid: Biological targeting by circulating human serum amyloid P component. Lancet. 1988;1:1413–18.
45. Goldmuntz, EA, White PH. Diagnostic dilemmas in children with musculoskeletal complaints. Rheumatol Rev. 1991;1:13–21.
46. Brewer EJ. Pitfalls in the diagnosis of juvenile rheumatoid arthritis. Pediatr Clin North Am. 1986;33:1015–32.
47. King H. Prospective study of back pain. Pediatr Clin North Am. 1986; 33:1489–93.
48. Szer IS. Are those limb pains 'growing pains'? Contemp Pediatr. 1989;6:143–8.
49. Yunus M, Masi AT. Juvenile primary fibromyalgia syndrome. Arthritis Rheum. 1985;28:138–45.
50. Schaller J. arthritis are presenting manifestation of malignancy in children. J Pediatr. 1972;81:793.
51. Rosenberg AM. Ankylosis of a pediatric rheumatology clinic population. J Rheumatol. 1990;17:827–30.
52. Ragsdale CG, Petty RE, Cassidy JT, *et al.* The clinical progression of apparent juvenile rheumatoid arthritis to systemic lupus erythematosus. J Rheumatol. 1980;7:50–3.
53. Anttila R. Renal involvement in juvenile rheumatoid arthritis. Acta Paediatr Scan. 1972; 227 (Suppl):1–73.
54. Malleson PN, Lockitch G, Mackinnon M, Mahy M, Petty RE. Renal disease in chronic arthritis of childhood. Arthritis Rheum. 1990;33:1560–6.
55. Szer IS, Goldenstein-Schainberg C, Kurtin PS. Paucity of renal complications associated with non-steroidal anti-inflammatory drugs in children with chronic arthritis. J Pediatr. 1991;119:815–17.
56. Giannini EH, Brewer EJ. Poor correlation between the erythrocyte sedimentation rate and clinical activity in juvenile rheumatoid arthritis. Clin Exp Rheumatol. 1987;6:197–201.
57. Barkley DO, Hubermuth HJ, Howard H, Webster AD, Ansell BH. IgH deficiency in juvenile chronic polyarthritis. J Rheumatol. 1979;6:219–24.
58. Cassidy JT, Petty RE. Textbook of pediatric rheumatology, 3E. New York: Churchill Livingstone; 1995:168–76.
59. Szer W, Sierakowiska H, Szer IS. ANA profile in juvenile rheumatoid arthritis. J Rheumatol. 1991;18:401–8.
60. Conway JJ. Radionuclide bone imaging in pediatrics. Pediatr Clin North Am. 1977;24:701–12.
61. Spelling RF, Heisi N, Toledo OMS. Glycosaminoglycans in the synovial fluid of patients with juvenile rheumatoid arthritis. Clin Exp Rheumatol. 1991;9:195–8.

JUVENILE CHRONIC ARTHRITIS

19

SPECIAL PROBLEMS AND PRESENTATIONS IN CHILDREN

Barbara M Ansell

- Aches and pains in children are rarely due to serious diseases.
- Differential diagnosis of recognized forms of juvenile chronic arthritis includes:
  - bacterial and viral infections
  - reactive arthritis
  - connective tissue diseases (including vasculitides)
  - Familial Mediterranean fever
  - storage diseases.

INTRODUCTION

In children aches and pains are not uncommon, but rarely are they due to serious rheumatic illness. Successful management depends on the precision of diagnosis, which will be based largely on clinical features; the importance of an adequate history and examination cannot be overstressed. Older children will often give a very good account of their illness, while in infants and very young children, joint involvement may have to be inferred because of loss of function of a limb, a limp, general misery or an apathetic immobility. A careful history from the parents is essential, including details not only of the pain in the limb or limbs, but also at other sites such as the abdomen, associated features such as fever and rash, the state of the child's general health and any previous illness, particularly recent intercurrent infections, as well as the family history, which should include 'rheumatic symptoms' of all types. The child should be examined without clothing on and any physical abnormalities such as hepatosplenomegaly, lymphadenopathy, rash or heart murmurs noted. A relaxed child can usually be encouraged to point to the site of pain; this is helpful in differentiating between joint and limb pain, as is the history. An unwell child with fever, loss of weight or other constitutional signs should sound warning bells; a long history of pain with no abnormal signs and no deterioration in general health is unlikely to be the forerunner of a serious rheumatic illness.

In the differential diagnosis of acute polyarthritis with fever, it is important to consider pyogenic infection because of the need for urgent diagnosis and management with antibiotics; this can be mimicked by rheumatic fever as here the joints are frequently hot, exquisitely tender (Fig. 19.1) and may be associated with high sustained fever. The flitting nature of the arthropathy will only become obvious after 2 or 3 days, although the history of a preceding sore throat, particularly in the presence of a cardiac murmur, is suggestive of rheumatic fever.

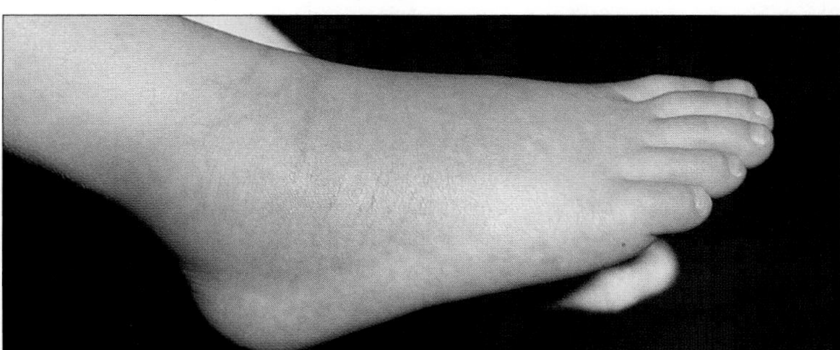

Fig. 19.1 Exquisitely painful acute arthritis of 3 days duration with persistent high fever in a 9 year old; there was a history of a sore throat 2 weeks previously. The differential diagnosis lay between septic arthritis and rheumatic fever. Blood cultures were negative and within 12 hours of this photograph this joint had subsided and a knee had become swollen. A mitral systolic murmur heard on day 3 of admission supported the diagnosis of rheumatic fever.

Viral infections are not uncommonly associated with limb pain, and frank arthritis develops in some, notably those associated with adenoviral infections, parvovirus, rubella, mumps and chicken pox as well as glandular fever and infectious hepatitis (see Chapter 6.6). Help in diagnosis may be obtained not only from a history of contact, but also from the character of the fever and rash. The fever, although intermittent, does not have the characteristic swings associated with systemic onset juvenile arthritis (Fig. 19.2), and yet it is not sustained, as in rheumatic fever, and the rash does not necessarily come at the height of the fever (Fig. 19.3). While the typical rash of systemic onset juvenile arthritis and the erythema marginatum of rheumatic fever can both

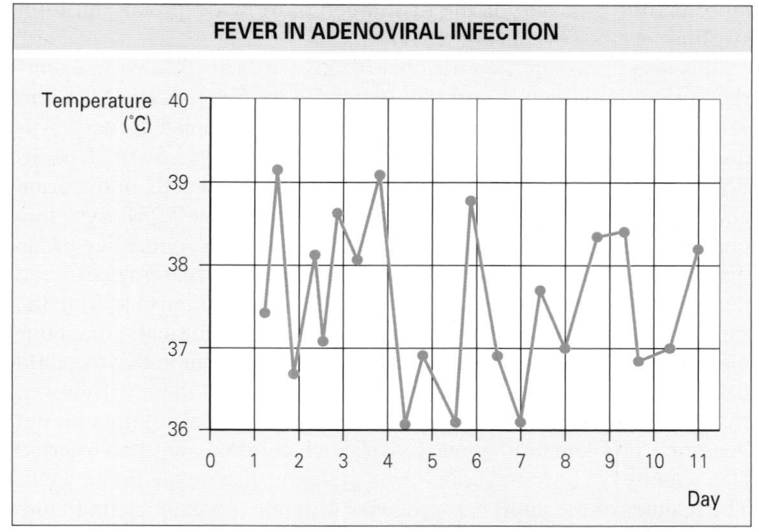

Fig. 19.2 Chart of the irregular fever seen in a child with an adenoviral infection.

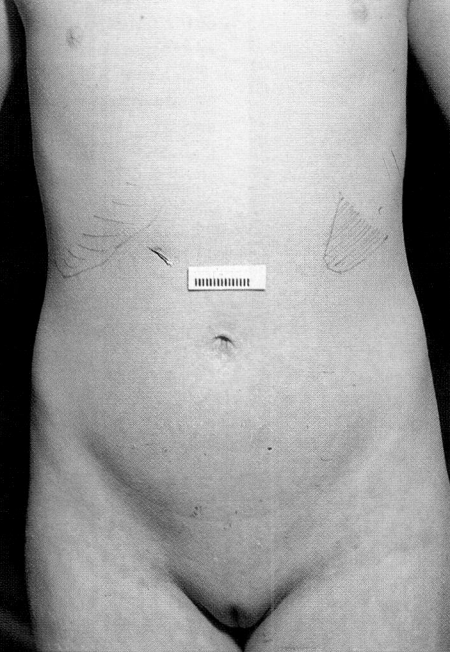

Fig. 19.3 Non-specific erythematosus rash in a girl with hepatosplenomegaly who presented as an acute arthropathy. She was later shown to have rising titers to the Epstein–Barr virus.

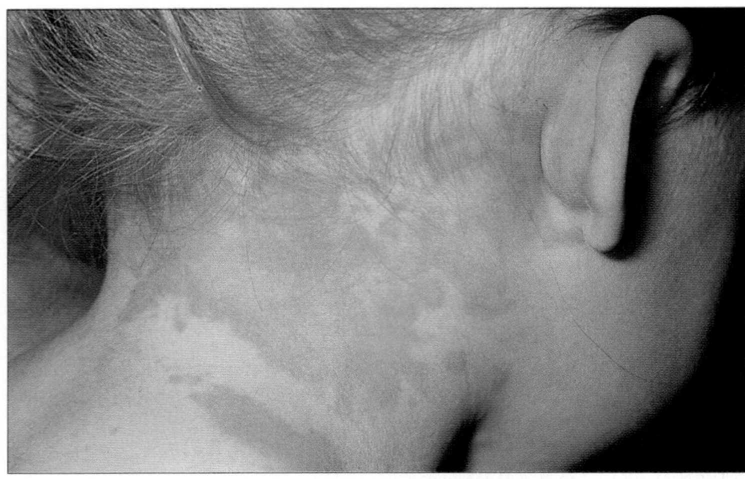

Fig. 19.4 Urticarial rash over the neck in a 6-year-old who had presented 5 days earlier with a sore throat which was treated with amoxycillin. This was a generalized urticarial rash associated with swelling and edema around the knees and fingers. Rapid resolution occurred on discontinuation of the amoxycillin.

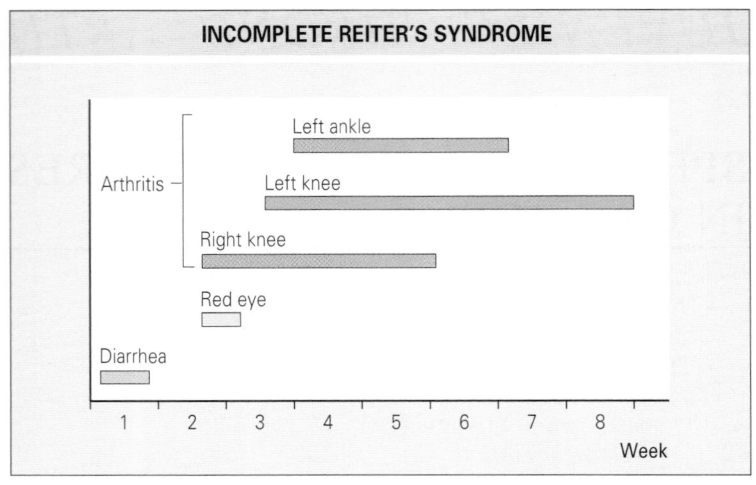

Fig. 19.5 Chart of incomplete Reiter's syndrome. This 6-year-old presented with swelling of both knees and a low grade fever. Only direct questioning produced the story of diarrhea 2 weeks previously and a red eye on day one of the arthritis.

occasionally have an urticarial element, urticaria from any cause can be associated with an arthritis. This is particularly difficult to differentiate if a child has recently had a sore throat and been treated with amoxycillin. Not only is the rash much more widespread, but joint swelling can be severe (Fig. 19.4).

It is also important to remember reactive arthritis following a diarrhea infection which is commonly caused by *Salmonella*, *Shigella*, *Yersinia* or *Campylobacter*; this tends to be an incomplete Reiter's syndrome (Fig. 19.5). The character of the rash is diagnostic in Henoch-Schönlein purpura, while other features include red cells in the urine and positive occult blood examinations (see Chapter 7.28). Systemic onset juvenile arthritis requires differentiation from connective tissue disorders such as systemic lupus erythematosus, dermatomyositis and the vasculitic syndromes. It will also need to be distinguished from the rare condition of CINCA (chronic infantile neurological, cutaneous and articular syndrome)[1]. Here the history is important in that the child usually presents with a rash in the neonatal period which is followed by the development of fever and hepatosplenomegaly; joints do not become a problem until about 1 year. Such children are often referred late, usually for a second opinion as 'systemic disease not doing well'. The features of the joints are somewhat different, for example in Figure 19.6 note the massive enlargement of the patella in a 6-year-old boy who has the very characteristic rash mimicking that of Still's disease, but which is itchy and tends to be continuous. Other clues to the CINCA syndrome include an anterior fontanelle that is persistently open for many years and a very prominent forehead, together with motor delay and ultimately central nervous system involvement.

Juvenile hyaline fibromatosis is associated with flexion contractures of the joints, causing generalized stiffness as well as skin lesions, fibrous nodules and gingival hypertrophy. The infantile form, with recurrent fevers, failure to thrive and joint contractures, can be mistaken for systemic onset disease, while milder forms which can present later with nodules and joint contractures, mimic polyarthritis[2]. Another very rare disorder which can mimic systemic disease is the hyper IgD syndrome with its recurrent febrile attacks and joint and skin lesions, but also abdominal distress and headaches[3].

It must also be remembered that ulcerative colitis and regional enteritis can present with fever, arthralgia or arthritis and anemia, but do not have a typical rash, although occasionally these diseases can be accompanied by erythema nodosum. If a child presents with apparent erythema nodosum, but which is in unusual sites, i.e. the back of the legs or thighs, consider whether this is a panniculitis, which can be associated with fever and limb pain (Fig. 19.7)[4].

Other problems in the differential diagnosis will be helped by the race

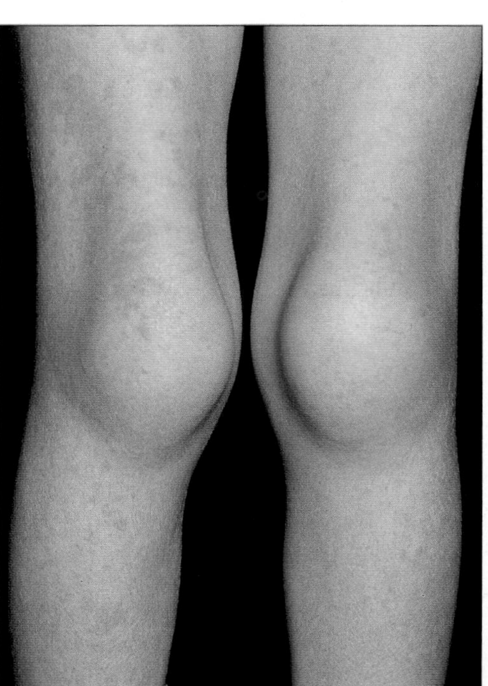

Fig. 19.6 Enlargement of the patellae in a boy who presented at birth with a rash followed by hepatosplenomegaly and later fever. Now at the age of 7 years there is still rash present down the legs and enormous patellae that prevent full extension of the knees, and difficulty in walking.

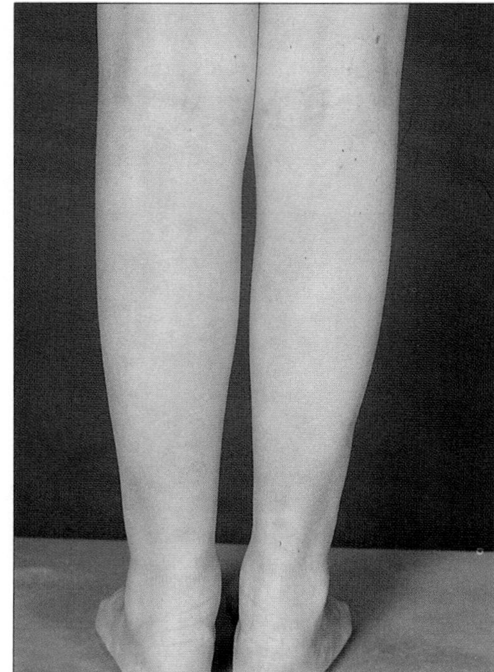

Fig. 19.7 Area of redness and induration together with slight swelling of the left ankle. A biopsy showed panniculitis.

of the child. For instance, familial Mediterranean fever, with its episodes of serious illness characterized by fever, abdominal pain, pericarditis, pleurisy and acute joints, can be seen in children of Mediterranean extraction (see Chapter 5.23), while sickle cell crises can present with acute swelling of the hands and feet in black babies (see Chapter 8.25).

Kawasaki syndrome, with its massive lymphadenopathy, conjunctivitis and arteritis, must always be considered in a young child presenting with fever[5,6] (see Chapter 7.27). In polychondritis the hot, red, tender ear cartilage is diagnostic. The presence of mouth ulcers will not only suggest regional enteritis, but also Behçet's syndrome; here acute iridocyclitis is common, as are small vasculitic lesions.

A polyarthritic onset of juvenile arthritis must be differentiated from a number of the conditions already referred to, such as inflammatory bowel disease, and will also need sorting according to the pattern of arthritis present: the age at onset, i.e. young (under 6 years) or older; sex; whether or not IgM rheumatoid factor is present and if there are associated features which might make the diagnosis that of psoriatic arthropathy or an HLA-B27 arthropathy.

Apparent joint swelling with loss of function can arise from other conditions. In the absence of an acute phase response, epiphyseal dysplasias must be considered. Multiple epiphyseal dysplasia is one of the more common skeletal dysplasias and is inherited as an autosomal dominant[7]. It presents in childhood with pain and stiffness in the affected limbs and is characterized by shortening and contractures and occasionally scoliosis[8]. Among the spondyloepiphyseal dysplasias it is the tarda form which gives rise to problems since it usually presents between 3 years and 10 years of age with pain in the knees and fingers, followed by deformity (Fig. 19.8). Because of the high heritable incidence it is not uncommon to have a family history of 'similar arthritis'. Such children are usually of short stature and radiographically there will be the characteristic beaking of the vertebra (Fig. 19.9). There is a progressive bony enlargement with deformity, particularly of the fingers and knees, and gradual loss of function of the knees and hips[9]. The condition is sometimes described as progressive pseudo juvenile rheumatoid arthritis[10].

Other skeletal anomalies include trichorhinophalangeal dysplasia, where the hypoplastic nares, short brittle hair, large ears and short stature allow differentiation when the child presents with bony enlargement of proximal interphalangeal joints[11].

Among the storage diseases (see Chapter 8.32) the two most likely to give rise to problems in diagnosis are Scheie's syndrome and Morquio–Brailsford syndrome (mucopolysaccharidosis type IV), in both of which the children have normal intelligence. In Scheie's syndrome the stature is well preserved but there is gradual progressive stiffening of the hands, elbows and knees without evidence of inflammation. In addition there may be clouding of the cornea. Carpal tunnel compression[12] can occur, while any of the mucopolysaccharidoses can present with a claw hand (Fig. 19.10) or carpal tunnel syndrome. In the Morquio–Brailsford syndrome symptoms do not usually begin until about the age of 3–4 years, with dwarfing, stiffening of the hands, valgus deformity of the knees and, ultimately, a waddling gait with kyphosis and protrusion of the sternum. Mucolipidosis type III, sometimes known

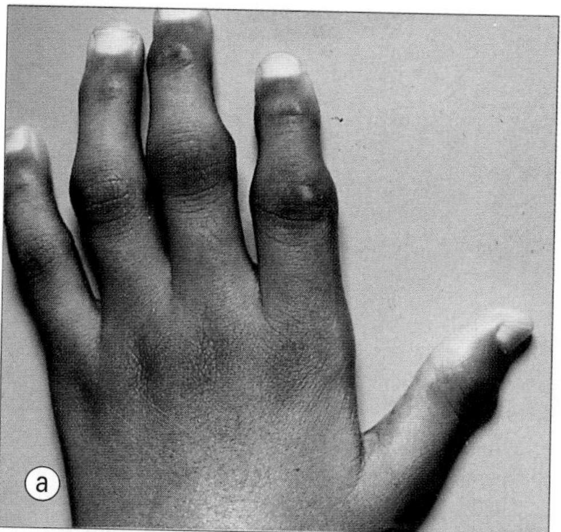

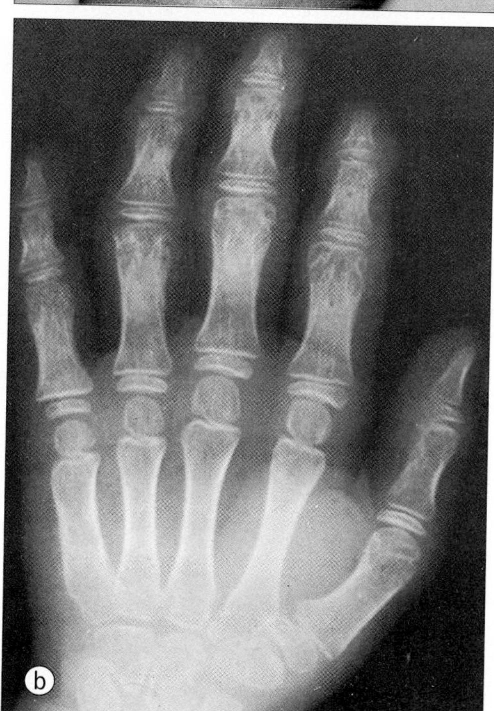

Fig. 19.8 Bony enlargement of proximal and distal interphalangeal joints in a child presenting with progressive loss of function in the hands and difficulty in walking (a). Radiograph showing bony change in proximal and middle phalanges consistent with an epiphyseal dysplasia (b).

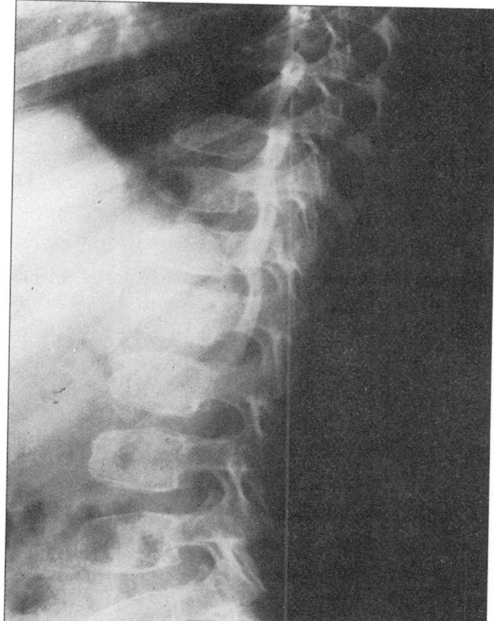

Fig. 19.9 Early spinal changes in a boy presenting with difficulty in gripping and failure to grow due to spondyloepiphyseal dysplasia tarda.

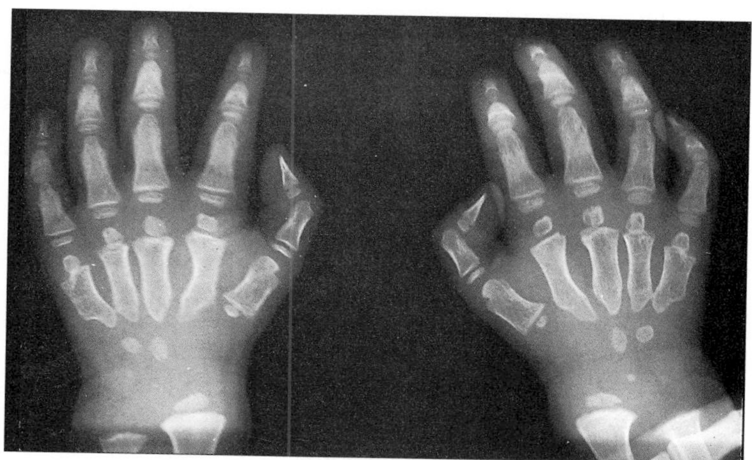

Fig. 19.10 Marked dysostosis of hands in a child with mucopolysaccharidosis of the Hurler type.

as pseudo-Hurler polydystrophy, is characterized by restriction of joint mobility, which does not become apparent until the second or third year of life; this also causes confusion.

In type 3 Gaucher's disease osteoarticular complaints are an important feature, with polyarthralgia affecting the large peripheral joints and ultimately secondary degenerative changes, particularly in the hips. Any child who presents with unusual deformities, evidence of multiple skeletal dysostosis and no inflammatory element must always be fully investigated in order to exclude those syndromes described here and many rarer ones.

An oddity which more closely mimics juvenile arthritis in its onset is acro-osteolysis, which usually affects the bones of the carpus and tarsus and which is associated with tender, swollen, limited wrists and ankles but no overt synovitis[13].

Acute leukemia may present with pain and swelling of joints, with the knees, shoulders and hands commonly affected and with limitation of movement. Bone lesions shown radiographically are helpful in distinguishing this condition. Silverstein and Kelly found 13.9% of acute leukemia patients had osteoarticular symptoms[14]. The other malignancy most commonly mimicking juvenile arthritis is that of neuroblastoma where limb pain with loss of weight and anemia occurs. The value of bone tenderness, on clinical examination, together with the illness and anemia of the child in sorting out both this and leukemia cannot be overstressed[15].

A long history of pain but with no abnormal signs or deterioration in general health is unlikely to be the forerunner of a serious rheumatic illness. However, such patients need careful appraisal, remembering the high frequency of recurrent limb pain in school children aged 6–13 years. This pain predominantly affects the legs and is often nocturnal. Emotional disturbances are common in such patients and their families. Hysteria is a curious pain disorder which can involve just one limb or joint[16]. Hysteric prolongation of symptoms originally part of an organic disease is particularly difficult to sort out but very important to recognize. Hypermobility of joints may occur as a feature of hereditary connective tissue disorders such as Marfan' and Ehlers–Danlos syndromes, but it is the 'benign hypermobility syndrome' that gives rise to most musculoskeletal complaints. The knees are the most common site, followed by the ankles. Discomfort tends to occur after exercise and is particularly common during periods of rapid growth. Adolescents who are good at sport can present with traumatic knee effusions and actual swelling of the ankles on one or both sides.

The persistence of pain and swelling in just one joint, i.e. monoarthritis, has similar exclusions to polyarthritis, but in addition a mechanical derangement also need to be sorted out. In particular it should be remembered that a partially treated bacterial infection can give rise to problems, as can bleeding into a joint as in hemophilia. Among synovial diseases haemangioma is the one most likely to give rise to recurrent blood stained effusions (Fig. 19.11).

In investigation of monoarticular arthritis it may be necessary to perform a biopsy, as the knee is the most common site of problems. In order to obtain appropriate samples, the biopsy should be performed arthroscopically by a surgeon used to dealing with children.

Other conditions to be thought of include Perthes disease, which not uncommonly presents as knee pain, often with quadriceps wasting in the young small child, while in adolescent females beware of slipping of the femoral epiphysis. Osteochondritis usually affects the knee, but it can also involve the elbow. Patella problems include recurrent subluxation, chondromalacia and infrapatella pain, which in a plumpish girl is common; the retropatella fat pad crosses on either side of the patella tendon and hangs partly into the joint where it is covered by synovial membrane. The fat pad is vulnerable to minor trauma, when it becomes edematous and inflamed, and closely simulates chondromalacia of the patella, although careful palpation will define the lesion. Localized bony lesions such as Osgood–Schlatter disease may need differentiation from enthesitis associated with HLA-B27 arthropathy, while osteoid osteoma, which tends to show a predilection for the trochanteric area, can mimic enthesitis or arthritis.

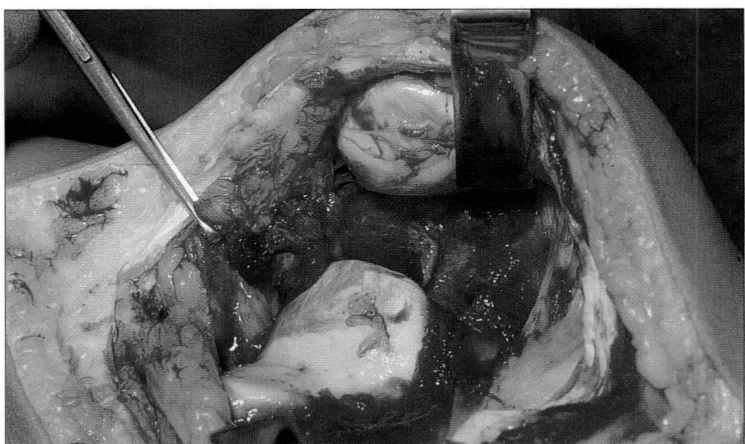

Fig. 19.11 The state of the synovium at synovectomy of a child who had recurrent bleeding into a knee associated with overgrowth of the leg over a 5 year period. Histologically the synovium looked like a pigmented villonodular synovitis, but at open surgery an angiomatous malformation was found which had caused the recurrent bleeding.

REFERENCES

1. Prieur AM, Lovell D. The chronic infantile neurological, cutaneous and articular syndrome (CINCA Europe IOMID USA). In: Paediatric Rheumatology Update. Oxford: Oxford University Press; 1990:147–60.
2. Glover MT, Lake BD, Harper J, Atherton DJ. Infantile systemic hyalinosis – a newly recognised disorder of collagen. Pediatrics. 1991;87:227–234.
3. Dreuth JP *et al.* Hyperimmunoglobulinaemia D and periodic fever syndrome. The clinical spectrum in a series of 50 patients. International Hyper IgD Study Group. Medicine (Baltimore). 1994;73:133–144.
4. Randle S, Richter MB, Palmer RG, Price A, Ansell BM. Panniculitis – a report of 4 cases and a literature review. Arch Dis Child. 1991;66:1057–60.
5. Kassiya T, Kawasaki T, Okuni M. *et al.* Report of Subcommittee on Standardisation of Diagnostic Criteria and Reporting of Coronary Artery Lesion in Kawasaki Disease. Tokyo: Japanese Ministry of Health and Welfare; 1984:1–10.
6. Dillon MJ. Kawasaki syndrome. In: The vasculitides – science and practice. Ansell BM, Bacon PA, Lie JT, Yazici H, eds. London: Chapman & Hall; 1996:384–91.
7. Amir D, Mogle P, Wenberg H. Multiple epiphyseal dysplasia in one family. A further review of seven generations. J Bone J Surg. 1985;67B:809–13.
8. Patroni NA, Kredich DW. Arthropathy in children with multiple epiphyseal dysplasia. J Rheumatol. 1985;12:145–9.
9. Wynne Davies R, Hall C, Ansell BM. Spondylo-epiphyseal dysplasia tarda with progressive arthropathy. J Bone J Surg. 1982;64B:442–5.
10. Spranger J, Albert C, Schilling F. *et al.* Progressive pseudo rheumatoid arthropathy of childhood – a hereditary disorder simulating juvenile rheumatoid arthritis. Eur J Paed. 1983;140:34–40.
11. Noltorp S, Kristofferson M, Mardahl N. Trichorhinophalanageal syndrome type 1. Symptoms and signs, radiology and genetics. Ann Rheum Dis. 1986;45:31–6.
12. Wrath JE, Alan SM. Carpal tunnel syndrome in the mucopolysaccharidoses and related disorders. Arch Dis Child. 1990;65:962–3.
13. Beals REI, Bird GB. Carpal and tarsal osteolysis: a case report and review of the literature. J Bone J Surg. 1975;57A:681–6.
14. Silverstein MN, Kelly PJ. Leukaemia and osteoarticular symptoms and signs. Ann Intern Med. 1963;59:637–45.
15. Schaller J. Arthritis as a presenting feature of malignancy. J Pediatr. 1972;81:793–9.
16. Nicol AR. Management of non-organic musculo-skeletal symptoms. In: Paediatric Rheumatology Update. Oxford: Oxford University Press; 1990:61–7.

ETIOLOGY AND PATHOGENESIS

Salvatore Albani

- Juvenile chronic arthritis has fundamental genetic, immunologic and clinical differences compared to rheumatoid arthritis.
- The etiopathogenesis is multifactorial.
- Strong, subset-specific genetic markers may affect immune responses.
- Multiple immune abnormalities are found.
- Aberrant immune responses to various infectious agents have been reported in the absence, however, of strong epidemiologic associations.
- Chronic inflammatory synovitis may be self-sustaining.

INTRODUCTION

Juvenile chronic arthritis (JCA), termed as juvenile rheumatoid arthritis (JRA) in North American literature, is an autoimmune disease characterized by chronic joint inflammation and accompanied by systemic symptoms. It is one of the major causes of chronic disability in childhood (see Chapter 5.18). Based on the number of joints involved, and on symptoms present during the first 6 months of disease, at least three different subtypes of JCA have been defined.

- The pauciarticular onset (divided into early and late onset, depending on the age of the patient) is characterized by involvement at onset of four or fewer joints, in general the large joints and in an asymmetric pattern. The early-onset form of this disease affects mainly girls; it is associated with uveitis and antinuclear antibodies (ANA) and the prognosis is usually good.
- The polyarticular form of JCA is the one most resembling adult rheumatoid arthritis (RA). It affects five or more joints, often in a symmetric fashion. It is often associated with HLA DRB1*0401, one of the genetic markers of RA, and it has a poor articular prognosis.
- Systemic-onset JCA often resembles an acute infection. A characteristic daily spiking fever, maculopapular, salmon pink rash, lymphadenomegaly, hepatosplenomegaly and serositis involving pleura and pericardium are features frequently seen in this form.

The heterogeneity of JCA is evident not only from a clinical standpoint, as the distinction in different subtypes implies, but also when an attempt is made to define its etiology and pathogenesis.

ETIOPATHOGENESIS OF JCA	
Genetic factors	Triggering factors
HLA TCR Immunoglobulins Peptide transporters	Various infectious agents acting on the same targets Single, still unidentified infectious agent Other environmental factors
Abnormal immune responses	
Autoimmunity? Hyperreactivity? Recruitment of inflammatory cells at the sites of inflammation Production of mediators of inflammation	
Chronic synovitis	
Self-sustaining? Continued antigenic challenge?	

Fig. 20.1 Etiopathogenesis of JCA.

Juvenile chronic arthritis is considered to be a disease of the immune system[1]. Abnormalities in the complex network that governs immune responses in patients with JCA may result in a loss of tolerance towards autoantigens that ultimately leads to chronic synovitis, accompanied by systemic symptoms of variable severity. Epidemiologic and immunologic data point towards a multifactorial process (genetic, immunologic and, perhaps, environmental) for the etiopathogenesis of JCA (Fig. 20.1).

GENETICS

HUMAN LEUKOCYTE ANTIGENS

The basis of immune distinction between self and nonself, as well as of the generation of antigen-specific immune responses, is the major histocompatibility complex (MHC) that in humans is called the human leukocyte antigens (HLA) (see Chapter 5.7). The HLA system comprises a family of polymorphic genes located on the short arm of

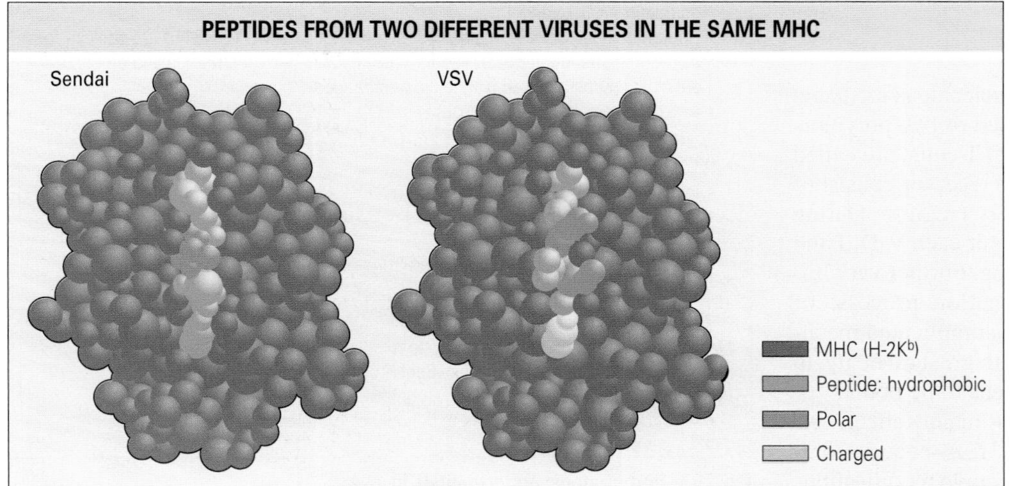

Fig. 20.2 Top view of the T-cell receptor binding site for two different MHC–peptide complexes. This complex represents the major ligand for the T-cell receptor. Its engagement leads to antigen recognition by the T-cell. Specifity of the interaction is based on tridimensional structure and charge. (VSV; vascular stomatitis virus.)

HLA RELATIONSHIPS IN CHILDREN WITH JCA		
Type of onset	Class I	Class II
Early onset oligoarthritis (ANA+, uveitis+)	A2 B44, 35, 16 Cw4	DR5 (1301) DRB1*0801 DPB1*0201 DQAI*0101
Polyarthritis (RF+)	B8, 15	DRB1*0401/0101
Systemic disease	B8, 35	DR4 DQA1*0101

Fig. 20.3 HLA relationships in children with JCA.

chromosome 6. The importance of these genes was first highlighted in the processes of transplant rejection. Later, the essential role that the HLA system plays in the generation and specificity of immune responses was defined at the molecular level[2].

The HLA system consists of two main groups of genes: the cluster called class I includes the A, B and C families of genes; the cluster called class II comprises the DR, DP and DQ gene families. The genes that encode for each of the HLA alleles are polymorphic and are transmitted to the progeny according to Mendelian laws. Therefore, the combination of the various maternal and paternal alleles is almost unique for each individual, and HLA haplotypes can be considered as a sort of a 'cellular ID'. The HLA molecules are polymeric transmembrane proteins, the function of which is to bind antigen and present it to specific T-cells. The specificity of the immune response is therefore based on a series of specific interactions that comprise:

- a certain HLA membrane phenotype;
- antigenic peptides derived from intracellular (with respect to HLA class I) or extracellular (for HLA class II) proteins (Fig. 20.2);
- a T-cell receptor specific for a given HLA–peptide complex (see also Chapter 5.7).

The most widely studied subtype of JCA is the early-onset pauciarticular form. Deoxyribonucleic acid (DNA) sequencing techniques have helped in defining association with specific alleles (Fig. 20.3). Unlike adult RA which has a strong association with HLA-DRB1*0401, JCA shows a pattern of polygenic inheritance[3–5]. The association among the various HLA alleles related to JCA is not based on linkage disequilibrium. Instead, the various alleles represent individual genetic risks, demonstrating the complexity and multiplicity of genetic interactions occurring in JCA. It is worth mentioning that autoimmune uveitis, which occurs predominantly with pauciarticular disease, is also associated with at least two HLA alleles that are frequently associated with the disease[3]. Moreover, patients with JCA do not have an increased frequency of HLA gene homozygosity, suggesting that, unlike what has been described in adult RA, a cumulative gene effect does not take place[4,5].

T-CELL RECEPTORS

Recognition of an antigen presented by the HLA molecule is mediated by the T-cell receptor (TCR). The TCR is composed of two polymorphic chains that, in the great majority of peripheral T-cells, are called α and/or β. The genes encoding for the α and/or β receptor consist of variable (V), diversity (D), joining (J) and constant (C) regions. During T-cell development, germline genes encoding one for each V, D, J and C region recombine by a mechanism called splicing. Further variability is given by addition, during the recombination process, of nucleotides that are not germline encoded. These complicated mechanisms have evolved in order to generate TCRs with great diversity, to accommodate the large number of potential antigens to be bound[6–7].

From a functional standpoint, diversity of the TCR mainly affects certain regions of the molecule that interact with the HLA–peptide complexes. These regions are hypervariable, and even simple modifications of their structure influences the binding ability of the TCR to the HLA–peptide complex and, ultimately, the generation of a specific cell-mediated immune response. The preferential usage of some of these combinations in JCA may, therefore, be related to recognition of a specific antigen (or autoantigen) that may be intimately related to disease pathogenesis. A recently identified subtype of the TCR Vβ6.1 allele has been associated with a subset of pauciarticular JCA that often evolves to the polyarticular form and has a reduced incidence of uveitis[3–5]. This TCR gene is genetically linked with HLA DQA1*0101, one of the alleles associated with pauciarticular JCA. However, the variant of the TCR Vβ6.1 gene associated with pauciarticular JCA is actually a 'null' gene, as it does not produce a functional protein. The significance of these findings therefore remains unclear[9]. An analysis using a semiquantitative polymerase chain reaction (PCR) of TCR gene usage in various tissues from patients with JCA has shown a preferential usage of certain Vβ families, such as Vβ2, 18 and 20. Presumably several different T-cell clones participate in the etiopathogenetic process of JCA[3,8–10].

PROTEASOMES, TRANSPORTERS AND OTHER HLA-LINKED GENES

Antigen processing and peptide transport may represent another possible pathway in the induction of abnormal cellular immune responses in JCA. Interestingly, in the human, rat and mouse systems, several genes clustered within the HLA class II region have been identified. Some of these genes (*tap*-1 and *tap*-2) encode for proteins that may be responsible for transport of endogenously derived peptides from the cytosol to the lumen of the endoplasmic reticulum. This pathway is used for presentation of intracellularly derived antigens to cytotoxic T-cells via HLA class I molecules. Other genes from the same cluster encode for proteins, Lmp-2 and Lmp-7, which are involved in the generation of endogenous immunogenic peptides by proteolysis.

The linkage of these genes to HLA and their functional association with antigen transport and presentation suggests a parallel evolution with HLA genes in establishing an effective immune response. These genes are also polymorphic. Allelic differences in these genes, in linkage combination with specific HLA genes, could therefore be responsible for the selection of a pathway of antigen processing and transport that may ultimately lead to the generation of peptides with an autoimmune potential. Indeed, several studies have shown that some association between HLA-associated autoimmune disease and polymorphisms of the proteasomes–transporters genes occurs[1,3]. Insulin-dependent diabetes mellitus, celiac disease and ankylosing spondylitis

IMMUNOLOGIC ABNORMALITIES IN JCA

Production of autoantibodies

- Antinuclear antibodies: mainly associated with early-onset pauciarticular JCA and with onset of uveitis
- Antihistone antibodies: associated with early-onset pauciarticular disease; good correlation with uveitis
- Rheumatoid factor: rare, mainly found in polyarticular HLA-DRB1*0401-positive form
- Anti-single-stranded DNA: present, cross-reactive between human and other species; no documented diagnostic or pathogenic significance
- Anti-double-stranded DNA: absent

Abnormalities in cytokine network

- Increased secretion of IL-1
- Reduced production of IL-2
- Increased secretion of IL-6
- TH1 pattern of lymphokine secretion from T-lymphocytes infiltrating the synovium

Abnormal immune responses to infectious agents

- Increased T- and B-cell responses to rubella or coxsackievirus antigens
- Molecular mimicry with Epstein–Barr virus proteins
- Retrovirus-mediated immune dysregulation
- Abnormal immune responses to heat-shock proteins, e.g. hsp60, dnaJ

Fig. 20.4 Immunologic abnormalities in JCA.

are among these. One variant of the *tap*-1 gene is represented with a significantly higher incidence in patients with the early-onset, oligoarticular form of JCA[11,12]. Thus, to a degree, mechanisms involved in the selection of 'arthritogenic' peptides to be presented to the immune system could be governed by genetic predisposition.

IMMUNOLOGIC ABNORMALITIES

Immunologic abnormalities in JCA include the production of autoantibodies, abnormalities in the cytokine network and immune responses to infectious agents (Fig. 20.4).

AUTOANTIBODIES

Antinuclear antibodies

Antinuclear antibodies (ANAs) are present in the sera of many patients with JCA and are associated with greatly increased risk of developing iridocyclitis. The ANAs are a heterogeneous family of autoantibodies that comprise various specificities. Previous studies have reported that reactivities to nuclear antigens such as double-stranded (ds) DNA, SS-A, SS-B and Sm are rare or absent in JCA. In contrast, antibodies to histones have been reported as significantly increased in JCA and often associated with iridocyclitis. Histones are components of the nucleosome, a highly organized structure with a core that consists of one H3H4 tetramer and two H2AH2B dimers surrounded by two turns of DNA. While the ultimate target of antihistone antibodies has yet to be defined, some studies have emphasized an increased titer of anti-H3 antibodies in JCA, and shown a definite correlation between the presence of such autoantibodies and the occurrence of iridocyclitis. Others have pointed out the role that conformational epitopes on the nucleosome structure may have in generation of antihistone antibodies. Elevated titers of anti-single-stranded DNA antibodies have been reported as well. Their lower affinity, in comparison with the anti-DNA antibodies of those from systemic lupus erythematosus (SLE) patients, may be a consequence of polyclonal B cell activation, which is one of the immune abnormalities found in JCA[13–18].

Rheumatoid factors

Rheumatoid factors (RFs) are autoantibodies directed against immunologically relevant determinants on the Fc fragment of the immunoglobulin class G molecules. They are found in approximately 70% of patients with adult RA. As with other autoantibodies, low-affinity rheumatoid factors can be found in the normal population and in other autoimmune diseases, such as JCA, that are correlated with B cell hyperactivation. One subgroup of patients with JCA, the HLA-DRB1*0401 subtype, is characterized by polyarticular erosive disease and a high prevalence of high-affinity rheumatoid factor. However, this latter group, due to the clinical picture, prognosis and HLA association, might more appropriately be classified as early-onset RA and not considered as a subtype of JCA.

Potential etiopathogenetic significance of autoantibodies in JCA

Immunoglobulins directed against autoantigens are a common feature of the normal B-cell repertoire. These 'natural' autoantibodies are often of low affinity for autoantigens and polyspecific (reacting with both self and exogenous antigens), and their interactions with autoantigens represents only an epiphenomenon of the diversity of the B cell repertoire. Elevated autoantibody titers in otherwise normal people, without pathologic implications, are often seen in situations with hyperactivation of the B cell compartment. Viral infections are good examples of such conditions. Autoimmune diseases, in contrast, are often associated with specific autoantibodies that may play a pathogenetic role in the disease.

This is the case, for instance, with the double-stranded anti-DNA antibodies found in SLE which have an important role in the generation of the immune damage. Autoantibodies produced in normal individuals, as well as in lymphoproliferative or transitory inflammatory conditions, are structurally and functionally dissimilar from those produced in autoimmune diseases, such as JCA. First of all, they differ genetically. Autoantibodies produced during lymphoproliferative disorders are generally encoded by a set of variable region genes that are germline. This means that these autoantibodies have not been developed by selective pressure, such as occurs following contact with environmental antigens. In contrast, genes encoding autoantibodies derived from patients with autoimmune diseases show a wide range of variable region usage, and the presence of somatic mutations in the autoantibodies derived from patients with autoimmune diseases indicates that a selection process has taken place.

The low affinity of 'natural' autoantibodies for autoantigen and the contrasting, high affinity of autoantibodies isolated from patients with autoimmune diseases underscore the role that autoantibodies have on physiologic mechanisms of defense against infection in normals, as well as on the pathogenesis of autoimmune disease. B cells that express autoantibodies on their surface are able to present antigens to T-cells, thereby contributing to the generation of a specific secondary immune response. In a physiologic situation, the production of low-affinity autoantibodies on the surface of B cells could act as a mechanism to enhance the local availability of an exogenous antigen in order to reach a threshold concentration for T-cell recognition. This amplification mechanism would therefore contribute to the generation of a specific T-cell response in the presence of very low concentrations of triggering antigen. In JCA, autoantibodies may be heterogeneous, have high affinity and are generally the products of somatic recombination, which is the outcome of T-helper cell-driven affinity maturation. Therefore, the production of autoantibodies in JCA appears to lack the regulatory self-limiting mechanism that governs autoantibody synthesis in normals. Considering the high efficiency of autoantibody-producing B cells in antigen presentation, one may speculate that autoantibodies can act as an amplification mechanism which increases the availability of a triggering antigen to specific T-cells, with generation of a noxious mechanism contributing to joint inflammation.

CYTOKINES

Cytokines are a family of cellular mediators produced in response to various stimuli. Three main categories of cytokines can be defined.

Proinflammatory cytokine family

This family comprises intercellular mediators that have a wide array of effects and targets. Two members of this family, interleukin-1 (IL-1) and tumor necrosis factor alpha (TNF-α), are particularly prominent in arthritis.

Interleukin-1 is mainly produced by activated macrophages in response to inflammatory stimuli. It has both systemic and localized effects on the immune system. In septic shock, IL-1 is considered as the endogenous pyrogen. At inflammatory sites, it induces T- and B cell activation and proliferation, and the release of proteolytic and chemotactic substances from macrophages; it has a stimulatory effect on osteoclasts with consequent bone resorption.

Also, TNF-α is a potent proinflammatory cytokine. As with most members of this family, it is produced mainly by cells that are involved in the nonspecific first line of immune response, such as activated macrophages. This type of potent inflammatory response is unbalanced in autoimmune arthritis and is probably involved in disease pathogenesis. TNF-α is a potent stimulator of T-cell activation. It upregulates expression of interferon-γ (IFN-γ) and IL-2 receptors on T-cells, induces B-cell activation and immunoglobulin production, and also has chemoattractant properties[19,20].

Immunomodulatory cytokines

This group includes mediators that play an essential role in qualitatively and quantitatively controlling the immune response[21]. Produced by T- and natural killer cells, IFN-γ is a powerful proinflammatory cytokine that has a potent stimulatory effect on most cells of the immune system. It plays a major role in controlling infections, particularly those of viral origin. It is also the cytokine associated in TH1-type responses. The immunomodulatory cytokine which is the natural antagonist of IFN-γ is IL-4, which is produced by CD4-positive T-cells and eosinophils and is a potent stimulator of B cell-mediated immune responses. Both IL-2 and IL-6 are intermediate mediators. They modulate immune responses by acting on other immune cells and stimulating production of other cytokines. Their effects are mainly stimulatory, and both have been implicated in the mechanisms of autoimmune inflammation. However, IL-2 production is downregulated in the synovium of JCA, pointing to a possible defect at the source, namely the T-cell. Conversely, IL-6 production is significantly elevated in JCA[22,23]. This cytokine plays several roles in the amplification and perpetuation of autoimmune inflammatory responses through its involvement in T- and B cell activation and in bone resorption. It has also been proposed as a principle responsible for rheumatoid cachexia.

The growth factors

Transforming growth factor β (TGF-β) is a pleuripotent cytokine made by a variety of cells, including macrophages and epithelial cells. It is a strong chemoattractant for inflammatory cells, and is important in the induction of wound healing and fibroblast proliferation. While stimulating some cells, it downregulates others. T-cell hyporesponsiveness in the synovium has been ascribed to TGF-β. Another cytokine of this group that has been implicated in the pathogenesis of articular inflammation is granulocyte–macrophage colony-stimulating factor (GM-CSF). This hematopoietic growth factor is produced by T-cells, macrophages and activated synoviocytes, and is a potent stimulus in inflammatory responses and in processes related to hyperplasia[21].

TH 1- AND TH 2-MEDIATED IMMUNE RESPONSES

The control of the balance of intracellular mediators of immune responses secreted by differing T-cell subsets is emerging as a major immunoregulatory mechanism. T-helper (TH) cells have been subdivided into TH1, secreting mainly INF-γ and IL-2, and TH2, secreting mainly IL-4, -5 and -10. These subdivisions, originally described in the mouse, are less well defined in humans but nevertheless may have important functional significance in the physiology of the immune response (see Chapter 5.13).

In general, TH1 cells are involved in responses to intracellular pathogens, while TH2 cells are elevated in allergic and parasitic diseases. An efficient immune response rests on a balance between the two networks. This balance is governed by, among other factors, inhibitory cytokines produced by non-T immune cells. Any alteration of this equilibrium would affect the quality of the immune response towards exogenous antigens and possibly a loss of tolerance toward autoantigens. Such a mechanism may occur in JCA, as well as in other autoimmune diseases. Cytokine patterns in the synovium of patients with RA differ significantly from those in patients with reactive arthritis, a disease in which inflammation is driven by the persistence of exogenous antigens. In RA a TH1 pattern has been described, whereas a TH2 pattern is more typical of patients with reactive arthritis. This difference may pinpoint the essential distinction between a chronic autoimmune inflammation that is self-sustained and an inflammatory process fueled by exogenous antigen. The latter process is more likely to be self-limiting, and the prevalence of inhibitory cytokines in reactive arthritis seems to support this idea[21,24].

ABNORMALITIES OF THE CYTOKINE NETWORK IN JCA

The autoimmune, self-sustaining inflammation that is one of the main features of JCA has prompted many studies of the role that proinflammatory cytokines may play in the process. Systemic-onset RA is the JCA subtype that has been most extensively studied.

Peripheral blood mononuclear cells from patients with systemic JCA contain detectable amounts of IL-6, and IL-6 serum levels are markedly elevated in comparison with controls. Interleukin-6 is correlated with disease activity, increases immediately before fever occurs and is associated with the extent of joint involvement. It may also contribute to thrombocytopoiesis, perhaps explaining the marked elevation in platelet number that occurs in patients with systemic JCA. Synovial fluid IL-6 concentrations are much higher than those in the blood. When compared with the other JCA subtypes, IL-6 levels in systemic-onset JCA are significantly higher[22,23]. This elevation does not correlate with the levels of IL-1β, as noted in the pauciarticular form of the disease. The massive IL-6 production in patients with systemic JCA may explain, at least in part, the occurrence of amyloidosis, one of the most dreaded complications of the disease.

Other proinflammatory cytokines are also markedly elevated in systemic JCA. Among them, IL-1β and TNF-α are of interest. Interleukin-1 is considered the endogenous pyrogen, and has important direct effects on the prostaglandin synthesis pathways. Elevated titers of TNFα can explain the occurrence of coagulopathies, including disseminated intravascular coagulation (DIC), may occur in systemic JCA. With respect to the pauci- and polyarticular forms of JCA, results from several studies show a pattern of inflammatory cytokines that are similar, although not so dramatic, as the ones described for systemic JCA.

One interesting therapeutic approach is based on a soluble IL-6 receptor that may act as a competitive inhibitor. As is the case for many experimental approaches that attempt to influence a chronic inflammatory process downstream of its origin, this system may be hampered by difficulties in maintaining effective serum concentrations of the inhibitor. An interesting alternative is offered by gene therapy. Injection into the inflamed joint of recombinant DNA constructs encoding for immunosuppressive agents, including biologics such as cytokines, may prove safe and effective.

INFECTIOUS AGENTS

The idea that microbial agents can be part of the etiopathogenesis of JCA continues to be a subject of great interest. Although a long list of candidates has been evaluated, to date no convincing evidence has been provided for a single infectious organism as an etiologic agent for JCA[25,26]. Attempts to identify viruses in synovium, by either direct visualization or immunologic techniques, have failed. Nevertheless, some interesting observations have been made.

Transient arthritis is a common complication of many viral infections, including mumps, varicella and rubella (see Chapter 6.6). In particular, rubella-specific immune responses have been measured in some children with polyarthritis and, in some instances, viable rubella virus has been recovered from peripheral blood mononuclear cells and synovial fluid cells from children with JCA[27,28]. Other viruses implicated, with similar rationale and degree of evidence, are parvoviruses and coxsackievirus. Both viruses can induce arthropathies, but available data do not demonstrate conclusively that they are etiologic agents for JCA. However, abnormal responses to such environmental agents may be part of the triggering events of the autoimmune process[29–31]. Epstein–Barr virus (EBV) has long been a suspect[32]. No direct correlation between EBV and the etiology of arthritis has been provided, but abnormal immune responses have been measured in children with pauciarticular JCA against epitopes shared between EBV antigens and disease-related HLA alleles[27]. Another family of viruses that some claim may play a role in the etiopathogenesis of RA is the retroviruses. These viruses permanently integrate into the host's genome and can express proteins that may, hypothetically, target or induce abnormal responses. According to some authors, retroviruses can also activate 'autogenes' that may trigger autoimmune disease.

Heat-shock proteins

A mechanism other than classic infection, but still involving human pathogens, that may contribute to the etiopathogenesis of JCA is represented by abnormal responses to a highly conserved, immunogenic family of bacterial proteins called heat-shock proteins (hsp). The initial enthusiasm over this family of proteins was fueled by the discovery that a *Mycobacterium tuberculosis* heat-shock protein, hsp65, is the triggering antigen of adjuvant arthritis in rats. In humans, hsp65, as well as other heat-shock proteins such as the *Escherichia coli* dnaJ, are probably implicated in the perpetuation of autoimmune inflammation rather than in its generation[33,34]. Bacterial heat-shock proteins are targets of specific humoral and cellular responses in patients with

JCA. Interestingly, the intensity of these responses correlates significantly with the degree of activity of the disease. These observations suggest that bacterial protein, once across the intestinal barrier, could, at inflammatory sites, activate T-cells that crossreact with proteins that are their human equivalents and overexpressed at these sites. This combination of exogenous activation increasing the availability of self-targets may fuel a reverberating circuit that is one of the components of the autoimmune inflammatory process.

SYNOVIAL MEMBRANE IN JUVENILE CHRONIC ARTHRITIS

The synovial histology of juvenile chronic arthritis (JCA) is very similar to adult rheumatoid arthritis (Fig. 20.5). In Wynne-Roberts' and Anderson's early biopsy studies of JCA synovium, eight out of fifteen patients had monoarticular disease[35]. Thus, these detailed histologic descriptions may not be fully representative of JCA (e.g,. all antinuclear antibodies were negative; only 13% had systemic disease). Macroscopically, the synovium in JCA appeared white–pink and had marked villous hypertrophy. Fibrin was widely distributed, and more abundant in recent onset disease. Intimal hyperplasia and marked hypertrophy were observed. Phagocytic synovial lining cells were common and often contained engulfed material. Fibroblasts were mildly increased in the subintimal synovium. There was a striking inflammatory infiltration of perivascular plasma cells and lymphocytes. The subintimal synovium was rich in plump macrophages, but polymorphonuclear cells were rare. Increased synovial vascularity was mainly arteriolar, at the expense of venules and capillaries. Mitotic figures were rare, not only among hyperplastic synoviocytes, but also among inflammatory cells[35]. Criteria for grading synovitis in pauciarticular JCA have been suggested[35]. 'Nonspecific synovitis' shows minimal round cell infiltration, increased vascularity, and synovial cell hyperplasia; 'active chronic synovitis' has moderate lymphocyte and/or plasma cell infiltration, with synovial cell hyperplasia that has progressed to the formation of villi. 'Probable rheumatoid synovitis' displays dense cellular infiltrate, with lymphocytes arranged in round clusters and marked synoviocyte hyperplasia.

ELECTRON MICROSCOPY IN JCA

Electron microscopic findings in JCA include increased separation between synovial cells. Most of the intimal hyperplasia is due to type A cells, with lesser numbers of type B and type C synoviocytes. As type C synoviocytes develop more phagocytic capabilities, they look progressively more like type B cells, with increasing types and numbers of lysosomes. Fibrocytes are not observed, but the numbers of mast cells are greatly increased. Synovial infiltrates are predominantly plasma cells, which are most prominent near blood vessels, fibroblasts, macrophages, and type A synoviocytes. By contrast, when JCA synovial tissues are disrupted and the cells eluted, immunoglobulin-bearing plasma cell precursors are found in very low concentrations, while rosette-forming T cells predominate[36]. Lymphocytes are the next most common cell type identified. These are found both near blood vessels and near type A and type B synoviocytes, throughout the two superficial layers. Larger lymphocytes appear to be metabolically active, but without mitoses. Markedly phagocytic macrophages are the third most common cell type 3. Endothelial cells and venules both display features of phagocytosis, with hyperplasia and hypertrophy[35]. These findings suggest an important pathogenic role for vascular cells, since they contain adhesion molecules that can react with cell surface ligands and mediate transport of inflammatory cells to the synovium.

ADHESION MOLECULES

Chronic inflammatory processes, such as those occurring in JCA, require continuous recruitment of inflammatory cells from the vascular compartment to tissues, such as the synovium, where inflammation takes place. This process is regulated by a family of molecules that are expressed on the membrane of inflammatory cells and mediate adhesion of these cells to the endothelium and recruitment to extravascular compartments. These molecules, which are often inducible, include the endothelial adhesion molecule 1 (E-selectin), intracellular adhesion molecules 1, 2 and 3 (ICAM-1, -2, -3), and vascular cell adhesion molecule 1 (VCAM-1). They play a role in the initial attachment of the cell to the endothelial wall. This attachment is stabilized by another family of molecules called integrins.

In the rheumatoid synovium a dynamic interplay exists in adhesion patterns among various inflammatory cells, the extracellular matrix and the resident cells (see Chapter 5.13). Any anomalous expression of adhesion molecules, or their ligands, could affect the normal pattern of cellular migration, and therefore attract in an abnormal fashion inflammatory cells to the site. Several reports have hinted that such anomalies may be present in arthritis. For instance, ICAM-3, an aberrant adhesion molecule and a costimulatory signal for both resting and activated lymphocytes, is overexpressed in rheumatoid synovium. In parallel, adhesion ligands such as endothelial leukocyte adhesion molecule (ELAM-1) and VCAM-1 are overexpressed on endothelial cells in RA patients. Together these data suggest that leukocyte trafficking and homing patterns are present in arthritis and may be part of the disease pathogenesis[37,38].

IMMUNOLOGICALLY ACTIVE CELLS IN THE JCA SYNOVIUM

Recent advances in immunopathology, monoclonal technology, and flow-cytometric analysis have permitted more precise assignment of phenotype and function of synovial cells in JCA. Macrophage-derived synoviocytes (type A cells) express MHC class II surface antigens, and also have Fc and C3 receptors, which suggests phagocytic and antigen-presenting capabilities[39]. Dendritic synoviocytes, derived from macrophages or type A synoviocytes, have a stellate morphology that gives them a unique appearance. They also express MHC class II surface antigens, but lack phagocytic activity. They may be important antigen-presenting cells during active synovitis. Fibroblast-like synoviocytes are nonphagocytic, but are able to release cytokines like IL-6 and GM-CSF. Studies of

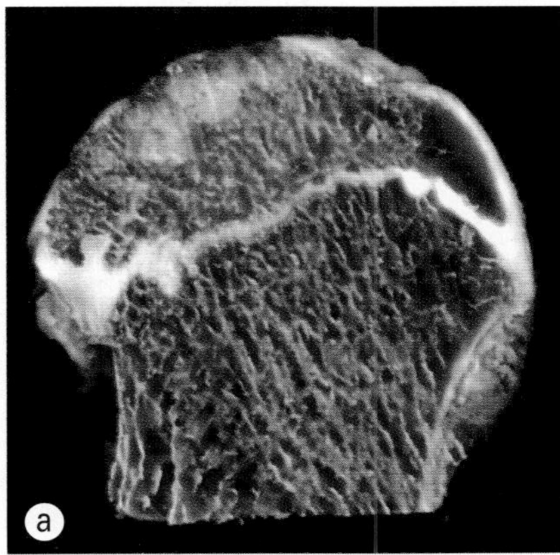

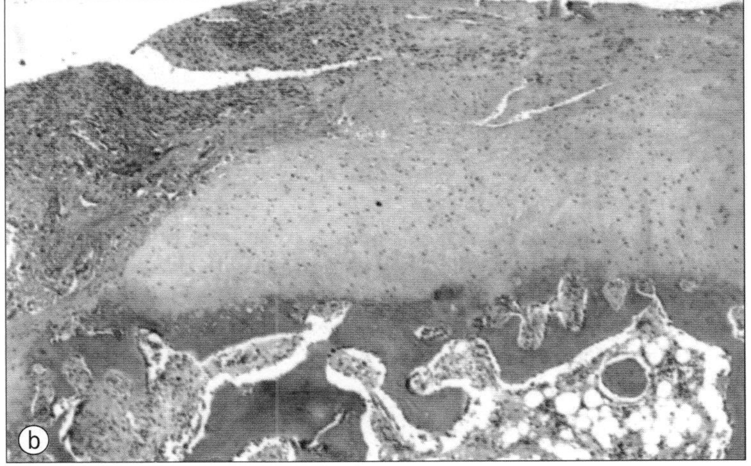

Fig. 20.5 (a) Photograph of a frontal section taken through the femoral head of a child with JCA. Extensive destruction of the articular cartilage has occurred, with associated erosion of the subchondral bone. (b) Photomicrograph of a section taken at the articular margin of the specimen demonstrated in (a) shows a destructive inflammatory pannus extending onto the articular surface. (Reproduced from Bullough PG. Orthopaedic Pathology, 3E. London: Mosby–Wolfe, 1997.)

proliferating adult rheumatoid synovium have shown that there is a direct 'traffic' of mononuclear cells which originate in the bone marrow and gain access to the synovium via subsynovial postcapillary venules. Their movement is facilitated by a cytokine-mediated chemotactic gradient and by adhesive vascular endothelial surface glycoproteins. Although great numbers of T and B cells are found in JCA synovia, 'lymphocentric' theories to explain the synovitis have recently been challenged[40]. CD4 (helper/inducer) T cells are predominant, and in close contact with dendritic-appearing, antigen-presenting cells, but CD8 (supressor/cytotoxic) cells are more commonly found among activated (MHC class II positive) T cells. The mechanism of T-cell recruitment and retention in the juvenile rheumatoid arthritis synovium is not clear. If cell recruitment were antigen driven, one would expect more oligoclonality within synovial infiltrates, while random chemotaxis (e.g., lymphocytes as bystanders) should result in more polyclonality. One study of 12 JCA synovial tissue samples has demonstrated identical T-cell receptor gene arrangements in two patients, suggesting some degree of oligoclonality[41]. Many of these cells also exhibit cell surface class II MHC antigens (activated stage), but not CD25 (the interleukin-2 receptor). Cytolytic natural killer (NK) activity was also noted, with 10–15% of the observed CD4 cells actually being NK cells, particularly in those children with polyarticular and/or destructive, rheumatoid factor (RF) negative JCA[41]. In another study of seropositive JCA patients, NK cell activity was found to be low[42]. Others have also found poor proliferative responses to mitogens in IgM RF1 JCA; this might relate to the high percentage of memory cells (CD41/CD291) in synovial fluid, which are normally poor responders, or to an abnormal mechanism of activation which permits expression of class II antigens but not IL-2R[43]. Several potential animal models of JCA have shown the importance of MHC-associated genetic susceptibility and a restricted repertoire of genes encoding for the variable region of the b chain[44]. It is possible that both specific MHC and T-cell receptors are needed for autoantigen presentation to activate the immune system. Additionally, T cells have at least two types of antigen receptors: those with α/β chains, and those with γ/δ chains. Normally, less than 15% of T cells exhibit the latter[45]. Reme et al. have recently studied JCA synovial fluids and tissues by double color flow-cytometry, using monoclonal antibodies specific for the two classes of T-cell receptors, and found increased numbers of the γ/δ subset among activated T-cell populations[46]. In another study of 24 children with JCA, activated γ/δ T cells were frequent in synovial fluids, but not in peripheral blood. Interestingly, γ/δ T cells are involved in responses to mycobacterial antigens[45]. Overall, as in adult RA, the synovial fluids and tissues in JCA contain large numbers of activated T cells, some showing oligoclonality. The CD8 subset is more common among activated cells, memory cells are more common than naive cells, and those with γ/δ receptors are over-represented.

REFERENCES

1. Sakkas, LI, Platsoucas CD. Immunopathogenesis of juvenile rheumatoid arthritis: role of T cells and MHC. Immunol Res. 1995;14:218–36.
2. Germain RN. MHC-dependent antigen processing and peptide presentation: providing ligands for T lymphocyte activation. Cell. 1994;76:287–99.
3. Grom AA, Giannini EH, Glass DN. Juvenile rheumatoid arthritis and the trimolecular complex (HLA, T cell receptor, and antigen). Arthritis Rheum. 1994;37:601–7.
4. Haas JP, Andreas A, Rutkowski B, *et al.* A model for the role of HLA-DQ molecules in the pathogenesis of juvenile chronic arthritis. Rheumatol Int. 1991;11:191–7.
5. Charmley P, Nepom BS, Concannon P. HLA and T cell receptor β-chain DNA polymorphisms identify a distinct subset of patients with pauciarticular-onset juvenile rheumatoid arthritis. Arthritis Rheum. 1994;37:695–701.
6. Von Boehmer H. Positive selection of lymphocytes. Cell. 1994;76:219–28.
7. Nossal G. Negative selection of lymphocytes. Cell. 1994;76:229–39.
8. Sioud M, *et al.* Limited heterogeneity of T cell receptor variable region gene usage in JRA. Eur J Immunol. 1992:2413–18.
9. Grom AA, *et al.* Dominant T cell receptor clones in JRA. Proc Natl Acad Sci, 1993: 11104–8.
10. Luyrink L, Gabriel CA, Thompson SD, *et al.* Reduced expression of a human Vβ6.1 T-cell receptor allele. Proc Natl Acad Sci USA. 1993;90:4369–73.
11. Stastny P, *et al.* Possible role of peptide transporter genes TAP1 and TAP2 in JRA. J Immunol. 1993: 1460.
12. Donn RP, Davies EJ, Holt PL, Thomson W, Ollier W. Increased frequency of TAP2B in early onset pauciarticular juvenile chronic arthritis. Ann Rheum Dis. 1991;53:261–4.
13. Monestier M, Losman J, Fasy T, *et al.* Anti-histone antibodies in antinuclear antibody positive juvenile arthritis. Arthritis Rheum. 1990;33:1836–40.
14. Albani S, Massa M, Viola S, Pellegrini G, Martini A. Antibodies against ssDNA of various species in children with diffuse connective tissue diseases. Autoimmunity. 1990;8(1):77.
15. Donn RP, Thomson W, Pepper L, *et al.* Antinuclear antibodies in early onset pauciarticular juvenile chronic arthritis (JCA) are associated with HLA-DQB1*0603: a possible JCA-associated human leucocyte antigen haplotype. Br J Rheumatol. 1995;34:461–5.
16. Burlingame RW, Rubin RL, Rosenberg, AM. Autoantibodies to chromatin components in juvenile rheumatoid arthritis. Arthritis Rheum. 1993;36:836–41.
17. Lawrence JM, Moore TL, Osborn TG, *et al.* Autoantibody studies in juvenile rheumatoid arthritis. Semin Arthritis Rheum. 1993;22:265–74.
18. Carson DA, Chen PP, Kipps TJ. New roles for rheumatoid factor. J Clin Invest. 1991;87:379–83.
19. Arend WP, Dayer JM. Inhibition of the production and effects of interleukin-1 and tumor necrosis factor alpha in rheumatoid arthritis. Arthritis Rheum. 1995;38:151–60.
20. McDowell TL, Symons JA, Ploski R, Forre O, Duff GW. A genetic association between juvenile rheumatoid arthritis and a novel interleukin-1 alpha polymorphism. Arthritis Rheum. 1995;38:221–8.
21. Mangge H, Kenzian H, Gallistl S, *et al.* Serum cytokines in juvenile rheumatoid arthritis: correlation with conventional inflammation parameters and clinical subtypes. Arthritis Rheum. 1995;38:211–20.
22. De Benedetti F, Massa M, Pignatti P, *et al.* Serum soluble interleukin 6 (IL-6) receptor and IL-6/soluble IL-6 receptor complex in systemic juvenile rheumatoid arthritis. J Clin Invest. 1994;93:2114–19.
23. De Benedetti F, Massa M, Robioni P, *et al.* Correlation of serum interleukin-6 levels with joint involvement and thrombocytosis in systemic juvenile rheumatoid arthritis. Arthritis Rheum. 1991;34:1158–63.
24. Liblan RS, Singer SM, McDevitt HO. TH1 and TH2 CD4$^+$ T cells in the pathogenesis of organ specific autoimmune disease. Immunol Today. 1995;16:34–8.
25. Schwartz B. Infectious agents, immunity and rheumatic diseases. Arthritis Rheum. 1990;33:457–65.
26. Albani S. Infection and molecular mimicry in autoimmune diseases of childhood. Clin Exp Rheumatol. 1994;12:535–41.
27. Ogra PI *et al.* Rubella-virus infection in JRA. Lancet. 1975:1157–61.
28. Chantler JK, *et al.* Persistent rubella virus infection associated with JCA. New Engl J Med. 1985;313:1117–23.
29. Sieper J, *et al.* Aetiological role of bacteria associated with reactive arthritis in JRA. Ann Rheum Dis. 1992: 1208–14.
30. Albani S, Keystone E, Martini A, Carson DA. Positive selection in autoimmunity: abnormal immune responses to a bacterial dnaJ antigenic determinant in patients with early rheumatoid arthritis. Nature Med. 1995;1:448–52.
31. Albani S, Carson D. A 'multistep molecular mimicry' hypothesis for the etiopathogenesis of rheumatoid arthritis. Immunol Today; in press.
32. Gear AJ, Venables PJW, Edwards JMB, Maini RN, Ansell BM. Rheumatoid arthritis, juvenile arthritis, iridocyclitis and the Epstein–Barr virus. Ann Rheum Dis. 1986;45:6–8.
33. Wauben MHM. (Altered) self peptides and the regulation of self reactivity in the peripheral T cell pool. Immunol Rev. 1996;149:55–73.
34. Houri JM, O'Sullivan FX. Animal models in rheumatoid arthritis. Curr Opin Rheumatol. 1995;7:201–5.
35. Wynne-Roberts CR, Anderson CH, Turano AM, Baron M. Light and electron microscopic findings of juvenile rheumatoid arthritis synovium. Comparison with normal juvenile synovium. Semin Arthritis Rheum. 1978;7:287–302.
36. Abrahamsen TG, Froland SS, Natvig JB, Pahle J. Lymphocytes eluted from synovial tissue of juvenile rheumatoid arthritis patients. Arthritis Rheum. 1977;20:772–7.
37. Morales-Ducret J, Wayner E, Elices MJ, *et al.* α_4/β_1 Integrin (VLA-4) ligands in arthritis: vascular cell adhesion molecule-1 expression in synovium and on fibroblast-like synoviocytes. J Immunol. 1992;149:1424–31.
38. Firestein GS. Mechanisms of tissue destruction and cellular activation in rheumatoid arthritis. Curr Opin Rheumatol. 1992;4:348–54.
39. Egeland T. Immunological aspects of the rheumatoid synovium. Scan J Rheumatol. 1987;66:S27–33.
40. Firestein GS, Zvaifler NJ. How important are T cells in chronic rheumatoid synovitis? Arthritis Rheum. 1990;33:768–73.
41. Pediatric rheumatology into the 90s: Proceedings of Park City III. March 2-6, 1990. J Rheumatol. 1992;19(S33):1–127.
42. Thoen J, Waalen K, Forre 0. Natural killer cells at inflammatory sites of patients with rheumatoid arthritis and IgM rheumatoid factor positive polyarticular JCA. Clin Rheumatol. 1987;6:215–25.
43. De Maria AF, Malnati MS, Poggi A. Clonal analysis of joint fluid T lymphocytes in patients with juvenile rheumatoid arthritis. J Rheumatol. 1990;17:1073–8.
44. David CS, Banerjee S. T-cell receptor genes and disease susceptibility. Arthritis Rheum. 1989;32:105–7.
45. Kjeldsen-Kragh J, Quayle A, Kalvenes C, et al. T gamma delta cells in juvenile rheumatoid arthritis and rheumatoid arthritis. Scand J Immunol. 1990;32:651–60.
46. Reme T, Portier M, Frayssinoux F, et al. T-cell receptor expression and activation of synovial lymphocyte subsets in patients with rheumatoid arthritis. Arthritis Rheum. 1990;**33**:485–92.

JUVENILE CHRONIC ARTHRITIS

21

MANAGEMENT

Anne-Marie F Prieur

Medical management
- The traditional pyramidal approach is the commonest way of treating children with JCA.
- Some drugs have specific side effects in children, such as corticosteroids on growth.

Surgical management
- Persisting joint inflammation can be treated either by synoviorthesis or with arthroscopic synovectomy.
- Reconstructive surgery can be used in older children and adolescents.
- Cervical spine involvement increases anesthesia risks because of limited mouth opening.

Rehabilitation
- Stretching and splinting reduce flexion contractures.
- Occupational therapy helps with activities of daily living.

INTRODUCTION

There is no single 'correct' way of managing children with juvenile chronic arthritis (JCA). As the etiology is unknown and the understanding of disease pathogenesis still limited, the therapeutic aims are to relieve pain, reduce general and local inflammation, prevent disability, maintain locomotor function and sustain satisfactory growth and development. Such a program cannot be achieved without an interdisciplinary team oriented towards child health care: consisting of a pediatric rheumatologist, orthopedic surgeon, ophthalmologist, dentist, family physician, nurses, physical therapist, dietitian, social worker, psychologist, parents, siblings and teachers. The management of JCA requires a thorough knowledge and understanding of the natural history of each of the subtypes – systemic, polyarticular and oligoarticular. It requires the use of various drugs, musculoskeletal rehabilitation, a surgical approach to prevent joint destruction in the early stages and restoration of joint function in the later stages, as well as psychosocial attention and appropriate education.

MEDICAL MANAGEMENT

The traditional pyramidal approach to treating JCA, which starts with drugs of minimal toxicity and progresses to the so-called second- and third-line agents, is the most common treatment. However, when there is unremitting progression of the disease and a severe prognosis is suspected, it may be necessary to 'invert the pyramid' and start with more aggressive therapy[1–2]. It must be borne in mind that some drugs have not been licensed for pediatric use and some formulations are unsuitable for very young children. Certain drugs have side effects specific to children. However, all drugs used to treat adults with rheumatoid arthritis (RA) can be given, as long as the risks are known and treatment is closely monitored.

FIRST-LINE THERAPY

NSAIDs

The class of drugs known as nonsteroidal anti-inflammatory drugs (NSAIDs) covers a wide variety of different agents (Fig. 21.1). Acetylsalicylic acid (ASA) was the first licensed drug for children of all ages. Other NSAIDs, such as propionic acid derivatives, phenylacetic acids, oxicams or indoleacatic acids, can be used in most countries. Legal recommendations are not universal, and some drugs which are available for pediatric use in some countries may not be elsewhere.

As well as anti-inflammatory activity, NSAIDs have analgesic and antipyretic properties. They mainly act by inhibiting cyclo-oxygenase (COX) and the generation of prostaglandins. Pharmacokinetic studies have shown only minor differences between adults and older children. The half-life is longer in synovial fluid than in plasma[3]. In contrast, noteworthy differences in pharmacokinetics have been found in infants[4]. Onset of effect of NSAIDs is usually rapid, but some have reported a delay of onset of several weeks[5]. These agents provide symptomatic relief and are used in most patients. They are not considered to be disease modifying.

Acetylsalicylic acid

Acetylsalicylic acid (ASA) is available in many different formulations. Recommendations vary according to the indication. Generally dosages are 60–80mg/kg/day divided into 3 or 4 doses for nonfebrile conditions and 100–120mg/kg/day given in divided doses every 4 hours (even during the night) in systemic disease. Blood salicylate levels must not exceed 150–200mg/l 2 hours after ASA administration; higher concentrations carry a risk of salicylate intoxication. Various factors can influence blood salicylate concentrations. A plateau concentration in blood is reached after about 10 days. At high doses even a minor change in dose can modify the blood salicylate level considerably. An increase in urinary pH, occurring, for example, with the use of aluminum- and magnesium hydroxide-containing antacids, increases ASA clearance. Urinary excretion increases 10-fold when the pH rises from 5.5 to 8[6]. Absorption is slowed when ASA is taken with food. The hypoalbuminemia associated with inflammatory diseases increases the volume of distribution. In combination with corticosteroids, blood salicylate levels are decreased by around 30%. Serum levels, however, only reflect the overall extracellular concentration of salicylate, not the bound fraction (especially that diffusing into the tissues). As a result, a low blood salicylate level does not neccessarily reflect low tissue concentrations. It is thus possible to obtain a satisfactory clinical effect

RECOMMENDED AND MAXIMUM DOSES OF NSAIDs IN CHILDREN

	NSAID	Recommended (mg/kg/day)	Maximum/ day (mg)
	Acetylsalicylic acid (ASA)	60–80 *or* 100–120	4000
Propionic acid derivatives	Naproxen	15–20	1500
	Ibuprofen	40–50	2400
	Ketoprofen	3–5	300
	Flurbiprofen	3–4	300
	Fenoprofen	40–50	3200
Indoleacetic acids	Sulindac	4–6	400
	Indomethacin	1.5–3	200
	Tolmetin	20–30	1800
Phenylacetic acids	Diclofenac	2–3	150
Oxicams	Piroxicam	0.2–0.3	20

Fig. 21.1 Recommended and maximum doses of NSAIDs in children.

despite apparently inadequate blood salicylate levels. In contrast, a blood salicylate level approaching 200–250mg/l may point to overdose and a risk of intoxication.

There are many side effects of ASA. The clinician must be alert to adverse events during long-term and high-dose ASA therapy in children. Parents must also be aware of the clinical signs of intolerance. Certain side effects are dose-dependent, including hearing loss and tinnitus, behavioral changes (irritability), tachypnea (not to be confused with tachypnea due to pericarditis), nausea and vomiting. The main side effects are:

- inhibition of platelet aggregation,
- gastrointestinal symptoms,
- nephrotoxicity and
- hepatotoxicity.

A bleeding tendency can result from the inhibition of platelet aggregation. This may be manifested as easy bruising while at play, epistaxis or, rarely, severe gastrointestinal bleeding. Gastrointestinal manifestations appear to occur less frequently than in adults. Occult bleeding is probably fairly common. Iron supplementation has been shown to increase low hemoglobin levels during ASA therapy of JCA[7]. Certain ASA preparations, especially enteric-coated forms and salicylates, reduce the risk of side effects. Cimetidine is recommended for gastrointestinal symptoms.

Renal toxicity is very rare, and consists of papillary and tubular necrosis. Regular monitoring for hepatotoxicity is necessary during ASA therapy in children with JCA. Liver damage can be reflected by a simple increase in serum transaminase activity, which is fairly common. A concomitant fall in the prothrombin time requires ASA withdrawal[8] to avoid the danger of complex manifestations with a hemorrhagic syndrome similar to disseminated intravascular coagulation (DIC), together with hepatic and neurologic signs characteristic of the 'macrophage activation syndrome' (MAS) (see below). These complications, which are not always associated with elevated blood salicylate levels, were recently reviewed[9].

Other NSAIDs

Figure 21.1 shows pediatric NSAID dosages.

The most frequent side effects are gastrointestinal (mainly abdominal pain), cutaneous (urticaria, rash and hypersensitivity[10]) and hematologic (anemia)[11]. Rare cases of renal damage and central nervous system manifestations (headache and dizziness) have been reported. Allergic reactions can also occur.

SECOND-LINE THERAPY

Patients who fail to respond to NSAIDs are candidates for slow–acting antirheumatic drugs (SAARDs) (Fig. 21.2). Their use in children must take into account age and clinical disease. Most of these should be avoided in systemic JCA because of the risk of reactions and poor efficacy[12]. They are primarily used in the treatment of children with polyarthritis. An improvement is usually observed during the first 6 months. There is no point continuing treatment if no result is obtained within this time.

Gold salts

No randomized, placebo-controlled studies have been carried out with intramuscular gold in JCA. In either prospective or retrospective open studies, mostly published in the 1980s, the rate of improvement varied from 20% to 80% and that of remission from 0% to 57%[13–18]. In some units the primary indication for gold is rheumatoid factor-positive JCA. Initial therapy is with weekly injections, with increasing dosages of 0.25mg/kg, 0.50mg/kg and 1mg/kg. If well tolerated, a dosage of 1mg/kg/week is continued for 4–6 months. Thereafter, if the drug is well tolerated and effective, dosage is changed to 1mg/kg biweekly or monthly. There is no definitive maximum duration of treatment and most authors agree that therapy should be continued several months after remission is obtained.

Oral gold, auranofin, has been used safely in children[19] at a dose of 0.10–0.20mg/kg/day. Because it is administered orally, it can be more

ANTIRHEUMATIC DRUGS IN CHILDREN		
Drug	**Dosage**	**Side effects**
Gold salts (intramuscular)	Progressive increase from 0.25mg/kg/week to 0.5mg/kg/week to 1.0mg/kg/week Monthly: 1.0mg/kg	Rash, cytopenia, proteinuria, bone marrow aplasia, MAS (with 2nd injection in systemic disease)
Auranofin (oral)	0.2mg/kg/day (max 9mg)	Diarrhea; as for gold salts but weaker
D-Penicillamine (oral)	Progressive increase from 5mg/kg/day to 10mg/kg/day to 15mg/kg/day	Rash, cytopenia, proteinuria, bronchiolitis obliterans, autoimmune – myasthenia gravis, SLE, Goodpasture's syndrome
Sulfasalazine (oral)	12.5–50mg/kg/day	Rash, cytopenia, increased transaminases, neurologic manifestations and MAS in systemic disease
Hydroxychloroquine (oral)	5–7mg/kg/day (max 200mg/day)	Retinopathy, cutaneous symptoms, neuropathies, cytopenia
Methotrexate (oral, i.m. or s.c.)	10–15mg/m²/week	Cytopenia, gastrointestinal (nausea), elevated transaminases, hepatotoxicity
i.m. = intramuscular; s.c. = subcutaneous.		

Fig. 21.2 Slow-acting antirheumatic drugs (SAARDs) used in children and their main side effects. Macrophage activation syndrome (MAS) may be particularly severe in some cases.

acceptable than intramuscular gold in young children. However, its efficacy seems to be weak and its place in treatment of childhood arthritis is now being questioned.

Adverse reactions to intramuscular gold are similar to those observed in adults, and include skin rashes and possibly severe dermatitis. Regular laboratory monitoring allows the detection of possible hematocytopenias and proteinuria. Usually, most of the side effects resolve when treatment is stopped. Severe complications, such as aplastic anemia[20] and gold-induced pneumonitis[21], are rare. In systemic JCA, MAS can be triggered with the second injection[9] (see below).

D-Penicillamine

Tolerance is similar to that in adults. However, one study in children claimed that up to 25% of children experienced side effects[16]. The spectrum of toxicity is similar to that of gold, but also includes autoimmune manifestations, e.g. systemic lupus erythematosus (SLE)-like syndrome, myasthenia gravis, myositis, Goodpasture's syndrome and bronchiolitis obliterans. Generally, these complications resolve when the drug is stopped. Monitoring must include regular clinical examination, blood cell counts and regular urinalysis.

Sulfasalazine

The first study of sulfasalazine in children, which showed very encouraging results[22], was contradicted by later studies[18]. Evidence for a differential effect according to the subtype of JCA has been suggested with a good response to patients with oligoarticular disease[23-26]. A majority of responders had disease classified among the group of spondyloarthropathies. The favorable effect was confirmed in juvenile cases[26] as well as in adults[27]. In contrast, sulfasalazine seems less effective in systemic disease[25] and life-threatening side effects have been observed[28]. Some authors consider this drug to be contraindicated in systemic disease.

The initial 12.5mg/kg/day dosage of sulfasalazine is progressively increased to 50mg/kg/day over 4 weeks. Monitoring includes biweekly blood counts and liver function studies; after 3 months these are carried out monthly. After a remission is obtained, the dose is decreased cautiously over 1 year.

In systemic disease, febrile and hepatic reactions have been reported[38,30]. In other cases, toxicity includes gastrointestinal manifestations, oral ulceration, dermatitis and cytopenias. Enteric-coated tablets may reduce gastrointestinal side effects. A desensitization program can be proposed for children with skin reactions[31].

Antimalarial drugs

Hydroxychloroquine has replaced chloroquine in rheumatologic practice. It seems to be used more often in Scandanavian countries[16,32]. The rate of improvement varies from 16% to 75% in open studies. In one controlled trial versus placebo, no significant improvement was obtained.

The recommended dose is 5–7mg/kg/day. Toxic reactions include gastrointestinal upset, dermatitis and bone marrow suppression. Retinal toxicity is the major concern with hydroxychloroquine. The drug may be progressively deposited in the cornea inducing asymptomatic alterations. Ophthalmologic examination every 4–6 months is necessary to test for changes in color vision and visual fields. Electroretinograms are the most sensitive indicator of hydroxychloroquine retinopathy.

Methotrexate

Methotrexate has been shown to be efficacious in JCA in an a number of studies[33–35]. A double-blind, placebo-controlled, multicenter study indicated a significant benefit at 10mg/m^2/week compared with 5mg/m^2/week or placebo[36]. Some studies have questioned whether the type of onset determines the response. Children with systemic onset may be less responsive[35,37], in contrast to the results of studies in adult-onset Still's disease[38,39]. Higher doses of methotrexate may be necessary in refractory cases[40,41]. No clinical characteristics seem to predict the remission of arthritis. In a study including 49 children, both responders and nonresponders had comparable duration of arthritis before starting the drug, age, maximum methotrexate dose, disease type at onset, presence of radiographic joint destruction, concomitant treatment and presence of autoantibodies[42]. In another study, no differences in methotrexate concentrations were observed between patients who responded to treatment and those who failed to respond[43]. In one report, radiologic progression of joint damage was reduced in children who responded to methotrexate[44], but this needs to be confirmed.

The currently recommended starting dose is 10–15mg/m^2/week orally. Higher doses can be administered safely up to 1mg/kg/week. The intramuscular or subcutaneous route can be used if gastrointestinal irritation occurs after a few months of oral administration. The total duration of treatment remains an open question. It seems that methotrexate may only have an effect while treatment continues as relapses are not unusual after discontinuation[45].

The pharmacokinetics of methotrexate seem to be age related. This may explain the observation that at least some children require higher doses than adults to obtain a sufficient therapeutic effect[46]. Interactions with other drugs, for example naproxen and other NSAIDs[47,48], suggest that close monitoring of patients is necessary. The bioavailability of oral methotrexate may be influenced by food, as bioavailability is greater in the fasting state[49].

The effect of methotrexate on liver function and histology remains a major concern. In adults, the development of hepatic disease, particularly fibrosis, seems to be related to predisposing factors such as alcoholism, malnutrition and viral hepatitis[50]. In children with JCA without these predisposing factors, the drug does not seem to cause major liver problems after at least 3 years' therapy[51,52], although some practitioners recommend regular liver biopsy. In 30% of children treated with methotrexate, a transient elevation of liver function tests may be observed, returning to normal when the dose is decreased briefly.

Other possible methotrexate adverse events include gastrointestinal, hematologic, renal, dermatologic, pulmonary and lymphoproliferative effects. Gastrointestinal upset with nausea is relatively common after a few months of oral administration[52]. This may be overcome by administering the drug intramuscularly or subcutaneously. The administration of folic acid (1mg/day) can also reduce the incidence of side effects[53]. Hematotoxic effects, including macrocytic anemia, leukopenia and thrombocytopenia, are rare. Renal insufficency may induce an increase in serum methotrexate levels and favor bone marrow depression. Skin problems are exceptional, although some patients may complain of hair-thinning. The risk of infection, particularly viral, has not been a major problem to date. However, any infectious event that occurs during methotrexate therapy should be promptly managed.

Lung toxicity has been reported in adults[54]. Pulmonary function evaluated in children over 3 years of treatment with methotrexate remained normal in one study[55]. The risk of methotrexate-induced nodules (with histologic characteristics of rheumatoid nodules) has been reported in adults. It seems to be extremely rare in children[56]. An increased risk of lymphoproliferative disease has been recognized in adults treated with low-dose methotrexate[57]. This complication, which must be borne in mind, has not yet been reported in children.

CORTICOSTEROIDS

Systemic corticosteroids

Among the available corticosteroid preparations (Fig. 21.3), the most frequently used in childhood rheumatic diseases is prednisone. The different enteric-coated and soluble tablets allow dosages to be easily adapted. The mineralocorticoid effect may differ between preparations. The daily dose must generally be divided in two in order to cover the whole day.

Several regimens are used. In severe systemic disease, prednisone (or its equivalent) 2mg/kg/day b.i.d. is necessary to control fever and pain. Once started, the dose should be reduced very slowly in order to avoid recurrence of symptoms, for example, decreasing the dose over 3–4 months to 1mg/kg/day and reaching 0.5mg/kg/day after 6–8 months. Then, the dose is gradually tapered to every other day to reach an alternate-day regimen whenever possible. Lower doses may be adequate in patients without systemic disease. In cases of severe eye involvement, alternate-day systemic corticosteroids may be prescribed. Intravenous pulse methylprednisolone therapy has been advocated by some[58,59].

The toxic effects of corticosteroids remain a major concern. For this reason these agents should only be used in well-defined indications. The child should be under the care of a physician who is experienced in managing rheumatic diseases to ensure that toxic effects are kept to a minimum (Fig. 21.4). Cushingoid features – moon face, buffalo hump, truncal obesity and striae – may develop very rapidly. These can be significantly reduced with a low carbohydrate diet. This diet is difficult to establish in children without the full cooperation of parents and regular support from a dietitian. Hypertension is rare in children, but blood pressure must be regularly checked.

Growth failure is a major complication of prolonged corticosteroid therapy in young children (see Chapter 5.24). In some with systemic disease, when daily corticosteroid intake is administered for years, growth arrest may lead to permanent severe short stature. The risk can be reduced if an alternate-day regimen can be achieved. Preliminary data from one study suggest that recombinant human growth hormone therapy improves growth velocity in children treated with corticosteroids[60]. After 5 years' follow up, children who received high-dose recombinant human growth hormone for 1 year maintained their achieved statural advantage[61]. This effect has been confirmed[62], providing the potential to reduce this significant adverse event of corticosteroid therapy in children.

Osteoporosis is one of the most troublesome consequences of long-term corticosteroid therapy. It can be complicated by osteonecrosis and vertebral collapse. It is particularly feared in severe JCA since osteoporosis can also occur independent of corticosteroid therapy. There is no preventive therapy. Recombinant human growth hormone stimulates osteoblastic as well as osteoclastic activity and does not reduce osteoporosis[60]. A good dietary intake of calcium and exercise may reduce osteoporosis. There is no definitive treatment of this complication, except stopping corticosteroids and reducing disease activity by other means. Glucose intolerance may be observed in children with a familial predisposition to diabetes. It rarely needs specific therapy. Adrenal insufficiency is also possible when corticosteroid therapy is stopped abruptly, although this is exceptional. More frequently, menstrual irregularities

COMPARISON OF SYSTEMIC CORTICOSTEROIDS				
Agent	Comparison of anti-inflammatory effect	Dose (mg) (equivalent)	Sodium-retaining capacity	Half-life (hr)
Cortisone	0.8	25	++	8–12
Hydrocortisone	1	20	++	8–12
Prednisone	4	5	+	12–36
Methylprednisolone	5	4	0	12–36
Triamcinolone	5	4	0	12–36
Dexamethasone	20–30	0.75	0	36–54
Betamethasone	20–30	0.6	0	36–54

Fig. 21.3 Various systemic corticosteroid preparations. Comparisons of anti-inflammatory effects, sodium-retaining capacity and half-life at dose equivalence.

occur in adolescents. Myopathy occurring as a consequence of corticosteroid therapy may be difficult to differentiate from muscle weakness secondary to the low physical activity in these disabled patients.

Skin anomalies are very common. Striae are the worst cutaneous manifestation since they last for life and are truly disfiguring in young girls. Acne and hirsutism disappear when treatment is stopped. In some children, the skin becomes thin and fragile with purpuric manifestations. Delayed healing may be a problem.

Potential gastrointestinal complaints require the use of antacid or cytoprotective agents. Pancreatitis is very rare. Prolonged corticosteroid treatment may induce postcapsular cataracts. Glaucoma may occur, particularly in children with uveitis, and must be looked for regularly. Neurologic effects can manifest as mood disturbances and insomnia. Headaches may rarely be a symptom of pseudotumor cerebri.

Corticosteroid therapy induces decreased resistance to infection. Viral infections, particularly varicella, can be life threatening. In case of exposure to varicella, specific varicella zoster immunoglobulins should be given.

Local corticosteroid therapy

Topical preparations may be applied locally to the joints and eyes. The use of intra-articular corticosteroids in children has completely transformed the prognosis of oligoarticular forms of JCA. Among the many available products, triamcinolone hexacetonide produces the most satisfactory results (Fig. 21.5). Multiple joint corticosteroid injection has been advocated for treating polyarticular JCA with a very significant reduction of joint manifestations after 1 year[63].

Uveitis, a very frequent complication of oligoarticular forms of JCA associated with antinuclear antibodies (ANA), is treated with corticosteroid-based eye drops and mydriatic agents. The ocular treatment must continue for weeks, often months. The ophthalmologist should closely monitor patients for response to treatment and detection of early relapse after the treatment has been stopped. Although there is a risk of corticosteroid-induced cataracts with local corticotherapy, the risk of uncontrolled uveitis is also high.

INTRAVENOUS IMMUNOGLOBULINS

The dramatic effect of intravenous immunoglobulins (IVIg) therapy in Kawasaki syndrome and in idiopathic thrombocytopenic purpura quickly led to its use in a large variety of diseases, particularly in the systemic forms of JCA. The numerous potential immune mechanisms of IVIg, for example blocking the Fc receptors of phagocytic cells, inhibiting the binding of complement components, modulating the cytokine network balance, modifying the structure and solubility of immune complexes, neutralizing autoantibody activity by idiotypic interaction and neutralizing a putative toxin or antigen as well as modifying lymphocyte reactivity[64], suggests a therapeutic role in controlling the immunoregulatory abnormalities in JCA[65].

Possible favorable effects have been reported[66–70]. An early publication described a significant effect on extra-articular manifestations in systemic JCA[66]. One trial with this therapeutic approach in 16 children, most of whom had systemic disease, produced ambiguous results[67]. Although injected doses and schedules of administration vary, differences between the studies do not appear spectacular. Following long-term follow up, results in patients who received long-term treatment over about 3 years did not seem to differ from those reported in patients who received only short-duration IVIg[67] (less than 3 months). These observations led to the design of a placebo-controlled trial which failed to demonstrate a benefit in children with systemic disease[68]. However, another recently published study of 27 patients followed up over a mean duration of 3 years reported some benefit on systemic features, although the effect on arthritis was not as clear[69]. These results could also describe the natural history of systemic disease. Most studies report that the tolerance of IVIg is generally good, although one study reported severe side effects in 3 patients, including SLE, systemic vasculitis and membranoproliferative glomerulonephritis[69]. Another recent trial with 25 children with poly-articular forms[70] concluded that a substantial improvement was observed in 65% of patients, but that the beneficial effects were short-lived after discontinuation. These ambiguous findings have been summarized in a recent editorial which concluded that IVIg should not be recommended in the treatment of JCA[71].

IMMUNOMODULATION – CYTOTOXIC DRUGS

The hyperimmune and autoimmune features of rheumatic diseases in children have prompted the use of immunosuppresive drugs. However, since these diseases are rarely life threatening, physicians must evaluate benefits versus potential harm. The disease course observed in

TOXIC EFFECTS OF CORTICOSTEROID THERAPY IN CHILDREN	
Endocrine, metabolic	Cushingoid features Growth failure Glucose intolerance Adrenal insufficiency Menstrual irregularities
Musculoskeletal	Osteoporosis Osteonecrosis Vertebral collapse Myopathy
Cutaneous	Striae Acne Hirsutism Thin, fragile skin Alopecia
Gastrointestinal	Gastritis Pancreatitis
Ocular	Cataracts Glaucoma
Neurologic	Mood disturbances Pseudotumor cerebri
Immunosuppression	Reduced resistance to infection

Fig 21.4 Main adverse reactions of systemic corticosteroid therapy in children.

some patients, with severe systemic complications or major joint destruction and functional disability, may necessitate the use of more aggressive treatment strategies.

ALKYLATING AGENTS

Chlorambucil

Chlorambucil was one of the first cytotoxic drugs studied in severe JCA. A significant effect on disease activity was clearly observed[72]. However, the major side effects of the drug, as well as the risks of infection due to its immunosuppressive activity, precludes its use in JCA. Sterility was confirmed by testicular biopsy in boys with nephrotic syndrome who were treated prepubertally with chlorambucil for more than 3 months[73]. Its use is now restricted to patients wwith JCA and secondary amyloidosis[74]. In this group, this therapy seems to be the only means of reducing the inflammatory activity of JCA[75]. The recommended dose is 0.1–0.12mg/kg/day.

Cyclophosphamide

Cyclophosphamide has not yet been fully evaluated in JCA. One study investigated its combination with other drugs (see below) [76]. The risk of inducing sterility[77] and malignancy[78] associated with the use of cyclophosphamide limits its use to more severe disease unresponsive to other drugs.

Azathioprine

The effects of azathioprine in JCA are controversial. Azathioprine is a purine analog that has been shown to be beneficial in the treatment of adult RA and in SLE. The effects of this drug in JCA are controversial. A mild benefit was reported in a retrospective study in systemic forms[12]. A placebo-controlled trial over 6 months in a group with severe JCA showed a significant improvement in patients' subjective evaluation but no difference in the objective measurements of disease activity[79]. Tolerance is generally good. The recommended doses are 2–2.5mg/kg/day with regular monitoring of the blood cell counts and liver function.

Cyclosporin

The immunosuppressive effect of this drug is related to its inhibition of T-cell activation. Its efficacy in JCA is controversial. In a retrospective study of 14 children with severe JCA, no significant improvement was observed with a dose ranging from 4 to 15mg/kg/day[80]. A recent study claimed a corticosteroid-sparing effect and safety in 45 patients with JCA treated with a mean dose of 3.5–4.6mg/kg/day. However, remission permitting cessation of treatment occurred in only 9 patients, whereas in 28 patients treatment was stopped because of disease flare, lack of improvement or side effects[81]. Toxic effects are common with increased serum creatinine, hypertension, hypertrichosis and gum hyperplasia. In order to assess carefully the value of cyclosporin in JCA, prospective, controlled studies should be undertaken in well-defined subgroups.

Tacrolimus (FK506)

A newer immunosuppressive agent used in transplantation inhibits T-cell activation and reduces the production of cytokines. A significant improvement was recently reported in a preliminary trial in 4 children with refractory JCA, and the drug was considered to be relatively safe[82].

Other immunomodulatory drugs have been tried. An open trial with γ-interferon in 9 children showed some improvement in extra-articular symptoms but no significant modification of joint manifestations[83]. Crude preparations of calf thymus[84] and thymopentin[85] were claimed to improve clinical symptoms in some cases of JCA.

INTRA-ARTICULAR LONG-ACTING CORTICOSTEROIDS

Product	Half-life (days)	Efficacy in JCA
Dexamethasone	8	±
Betamethasone	7–9	+
Cortivazol	40	+
Triamcinolone acetonide	14–20	++
Triamcinolone hexacetonide	26–60	++++

Fig. 21.5 Various preparation used for intra-articular injections and their effects.

COMBINATION THERAPY

The general feeling is that the current therapeutic drug strategies for JCA, particularly with disease-modifying antirheumatic drugs, lack real efficacy[86]. The complexity of the immune system dysregulation, with the imbalance of the cytokines implicated in the inflammatory reaction, suggests that single therapeutic agents will only provide transient or incomplete resolution of the disease[87].

In children, the combination of intravenous cyclophosphamide and methylprednisolone with oral methotrexate was reported to be of value in patients with severe systemic-onset JCA[76]. Further assessment is required to determine whether improvement can be sustained and these drugs are safe for long-term use. The uncertainty of long-term benefit is illustrated by the case history of a girl with systemic disease who was initially misdiagnosed as having malignant histiocytosis and treated with heavy cytotoxic chemotherapy, including corticosteroids, for 1 year with satisfactory results. After stopping therapy, however, she relapsed, allowing the correct diagnosis of JCA to be made. Thereafter, polyarthritis progressed for several years[88]. Although anecdotal, this observation draws attention to the difficulty of assuming that cytotoxic drugs are beneficial in the systemic forms of JCA.

MACROPHAGE ACTIVATION SYNDROME

Macrophage activation syndrome (Fig. 21.6) is not unusual in JCA, particularly in patients with systemic disease. It represents a life-threatening complication which appears to be triggered by a variety of events such as viral infection (e.g. varicella), and use of NSAIDs and disease-modifying drugs such as gold[9]. The syndrome is characterized by fever or hypothermia, hepatic and splenic enlargement, pancytopenia, decreased erythrocyte sedimentation rate (ESR), elevation of transaminases, hypertriglyceridemia and hypofibrinogenemia. The most characteristic diagnostic feature of MAS is the presence, although inconsistent, of well-differentiated macrophages that show hematophagocytosis in the bone marrow. It must be borne in mind that children with rheumatic diseases, particularly systemic JCA, are highly susceptible to this complication which appears to be more common than previously reported. The diagnosis must be promptly made as MAS represents a clinical emergency. High-dose corticosteroid therapy is generally effective. Cyclosporin induces rapid improvement in cases that respond incompletely to corticosteroids[29] and it should be preferentially employed to etoposide, an agent with potentially severe toxicity[89,90].

LOCAL INTRA-ARTICULAR INJECTION

Intra-articular therapy is indicated as soon as medical treatment fails to achieve complete control of synovitis and whenever functional impairment is progressive. In patients with oligoarthritis, intra-articular injections have radically transformed prognosis. It may prevent the need for escalation to potentially toxic drugs in young children. In polyarthritis, local therapy can improve the functional status in joints which are particularly liable to crippling damage. The control of synovitis can stabilize a joint, at least temporarily, and restore the functional status of a particularly important joint such as the hip. This may avoid the need to commence systemic corticosteroid therapy. It also allows the protection of a joint when general control of the disease is not achievable. Obviously, local therapy, even perfectly applied in severe cases, cannot prevent long-term joint destruction, but it may delay the process, thus ensuring an improved quality of life. The preservation of joint mobility, at least in part, spares bone development and limits muscle wasting, thus allowing these children to reach adolescence in better condition, when more sophisticated surgical procedures can be contemplated.

The most commonly used local drug is triamcinolone hexacetonide, a microcrystalized corticosteroid which, with a single injection, gives the longest period of improvement (see Fig. 21.5). This type of injection requires a clinician to have expertise in treating children's joints. The needle position must be precisely intra-articular, under the control of screening radiographs for deep joints, such as the hip, or other joints with difficult access such as the subtalar. In younger children, or when injections are planned at several sites, general anesthesia or sedation is necessary. There is no lower age limit for this type of treatment, as long as the precautions for use are observed. The injected dose is 40mg in large joints such as the knee; less is required for smaller joints. As much of the synovial fluid should be aspirated from the joint as possible before the drug is injected, without exerting pressure. Following the injection, the treated joint must be rested in a splint for 3 days. Two years after a single injection in the knee, the results achieved are very good to good in 40%, 60% and 80% of the systemic, polyarticular and oligoarticular forms, respectively. An improvement continues to be seen in 60% of treated hips 18 months after one injection.

Complications are rare. However, local injection can provoke severe cutaneous lesions such as skin atrophy (Fig. 21.7) or subcutaneous tissue fat necrosis (Fig. 21.8). Asymptomatic calcifications can also occur. The injection can be repeated if a there is a relapse more than 6 months later. An unsatisfactory result may be due to the presence of intra-articular rice bodies (Fig. 21.9). In this case an intra-articular drain with saline washout performed under general anesthesia can be helpful. The intra-articular injection is then performed 3 weeks later when the skin has healed.

Other products such as osmic acid are used in some centers, or can be proposed if intra-articular corticosteroids injections do not obtain a successful outcome. Radioactive synoviorthesis is contraindicated in children.

There do not appear to be any effects on the long-term growth or integrity of the joint after intra-articular injections, although subchondral fractures of the femoral head have been observed in some patients. The risk of cartilage damage may be increased after repeated intra-articular injections. Transient suppression of endogenous cortisol production immediately after the injection has been reported[91]. Because of the highly caustic nature of triamcinolone hexacetonide, its use is contraindicated in tendon sheaths, for which only hydrosoluble corticosteroids can be used, usually with only a mediocre result.

SURGICAL MANAGEMENT

Traditionally, surgical intervention has been regarded as a last resort, when medical and physical therapy have failed to prevent joint damage. During the past few decades, however, surgery has played an increasingly important role in the management of pediatric rheumatic diseases, from an early stage in the course of the disease, as part of the multidisciplinary approach[92].

Joint destruction results from synovitis, whatever the form of JCA. This process is more severe than in adults, since the destructive lesion involves not only the joint cartilage but the growing areas of bone as well. A combined approach of medical therapy and local injections may control the articular attack by the synovial pannus. However, complete recovery may not be achieved. There are two main objectives of surgery: the prevention of alteration of joint integrity in the early phases of the disease and the restoration of function in the later stages.

SYNOVECTOMY

When intra-articular injections have failed, or when the thickness of the pannus is such that chemical products are not effective, synovectomy should be considered. Synovectomy consists of the surgical ablation of the inflamed synovial membrane, either by a direct approach under an open arthrotomy or, more recently in children, by fragmentation using a rotorblade and aspiration of the synovium via arthroscopy[93]. Surgical synovectomy has been used for many years in JCA, particularly in Scandinavian countries[94,95]. Arthroscopic synovectomy performed on knees and shoulders in children significantly facilitates postoperative rehabilitation. Careful mobilization with a continuous passive motion machine is initiated immediately after synovectomy. Epidural analgesia is used to relieve pain and improve mobilization. At 2-year follow up, the results for knee joints are very good with reduced pain and improved mobility in 70%, and reduced synovial effusions in 50%, of treated children. In view of the difficulties of rehabilitation, surgical synovectomy is not performed in patients under 6 years of age.

Arthroscopic synovectomy carries some risks in children. The size of the arthroscope must be adapted to small joints. The inflamed synovium requires gentle excision in order to prevent bleeding and subsequent stiffness of the joint. Since only 70% of the tissue can be removed, and in order to suppress inflammatory activity, it is recommended that intra-articular triamcinolone hexacetonide be administered 3 weeks after surgery, when cutaneous healing has been achieved.

RECONSTRUCTIVE SURGERY

Despite adequate general and local therapy, severe JCA can lead to joint destruction, pain and functional impairment. At this stage of the disease process, numerous surgical procedures can be of benefit, including soft tissue release and lengthening to correct deformity, osteotomies, joint fusion and joint replacement. Surgery should not be delayed to the point that patients develop severe deformities or contractures that may compromise the success of the procedure. Unlike adults with arthritis, patients whose skeletal growth is not complete must be carefully evaluated for the immediate and potential effects of any surgical procedure on further development. For example, general joint replacements ideally would be delayed until the completion of skeletal growth. In addition, because many patients with JCA have significant bony abnormalities and may have very small bones, custom-made prostheses may be necessary to ensure optimum results. Very often, the patient has to undergo several interventions.

MACROPHAGE ACTIVATION SYNDROME	
Also known as	Hemophagocytosis Reye's syndrome Disseminated intravascular coagulation (DIC) Hepatitis
JCA forms at risk	Systemic
Clinical symptoms	Fever or hypothermia, anorexia Bleeding tendency, hepatosplenomegaly, icterus Neurologic symptoms Arthritis improvement Renal manifestations (rare)
Biological features	Anemia, decreased leukocyte count Normal or low platelet count Improved or normal ESR Hemophagocytosis in bone marrow (inconstant) Decreased coagulation factors (particularly VII, X) Decreased fibrinogen levels (usually high) Elevated transaminases Raised triglycerides Electrolytic disturbances Hypercytosis in cerebrospinal fluid (inconstant)
Main triggers	ASA, NSAIDs (particularly when combined) Injectable gold (second injection), sulfasalazine Viral infection (varicella + ASA)
Management	Admit immediately to hospital with access to intensive care unit Stop possible trigger Administer prednisone 2mg/kg/day or more Consider cyclosporin 3mg/kg/day Symptomatic therapy for visceral and/or biological anomalies

Fig. 21.6 Macrophage activation syndrome. Main manifestations and therapeutic indications.

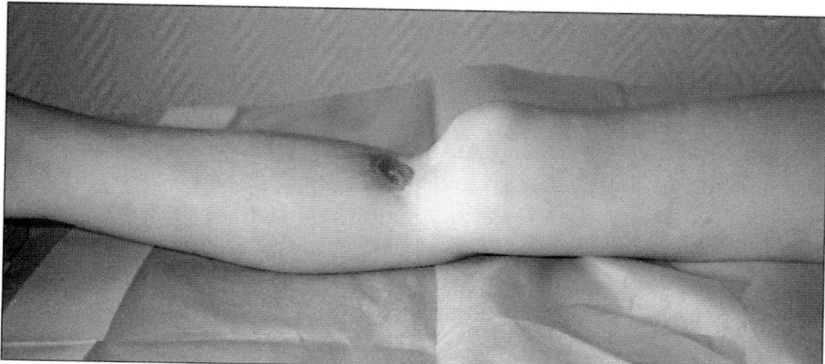

Fig. 21. 7 Severe skin atrophy after intra-articular injection of triamcinolone hexacetonide in oligoarticular disease. Courtesy of Professor Philippe Touzet.

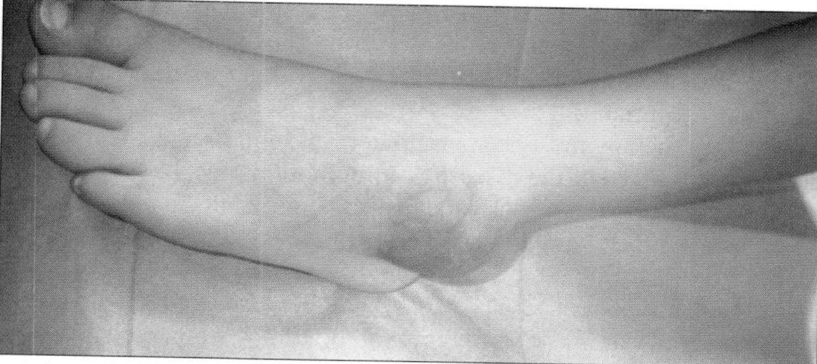

Fig. 21.8 Subcutaneous fat tissue necrosis in a boy with systemic disease after one injection of triamcinolone hexacetonide in the ankle. Courtesy of Professor Philippe Touzet.

Technical procedures differ according to the functional goal. In some joints, such as the wrist, ankle and cervical spine, stability is a priority. In such situations, arthrodesis may be considered. In other joints, such as the hip, shoulder, knee and elbow, joint mobility should be preserved as much as possible. Several surgical procedures are available depending on the underlying problems. However, it is rare to achieve a complete restoration of joint function, and only a few interventions lead to freedom from pain, improved motion and increased joint stability at the same time.

DEFORMITIES REQUIRING SURGICAL INTERVENTION

Subluxation and dislocation of joints

This deformity is the result of two mechanisms. Synovitis results in joint capsular distention leading to capsule destruction, fibrosis and instability. The destruction of the joint cartilage induces progressive subluxation, particularly in very mobile joints such as the wrist, shoulder and cervical spine. These subluxations can be prevented by physical therapy (splinting, traction, etc.). When the deformities no longer respond to physical therapy, they can be corrected by continuous traction with soft-tissue release. Soft-tissue release involves periarticular tendon lengthening and sometimes capsule incision[96], and is particularly indicated in the hip, knee and ankle. The joint can be further stabilized by various surgical procedures: muscle transfer (patellar subluxation), arthrodesis (e.g. in the cervical spine, wrist), prosthetic arthroplasties (hip, shoulder, etc.). Sometimes a simple epiphyseal resection may be necessary (e.g. of the ulnar or radial head).

Joint ankylosis

Spontaneous ankylosis (joint surface fusion) can be regarded as a natural cure for the condition. In some cases, this process can be improved by splinting the joint or surgically accelerated by arthrodesis in a good functional position. If the spontaneous ankylosis leads instead to joint deformity, the corrective approach varies according to the joint. When the foot deformity results in an equinovarus and/or adduction position, osteotomy and/or tarsectomy may be performed. If the mobility of the ankylosed joint needs to be restored, prosthetic arthroplasty can be considered.

Joint destruction

Ultimately, the disease process may result in a complete loss of architecture and function of the joint mechanism. The degree of erosive damage may necessitate preliminary bone reconstruction by means of grafting with autologous, heterologous or artificial bone, most often in the acetabulum or cervical spine. To date, total hip, knee, elbow and shoulder replacements have been performed in adolescents, often using specially designed or custom-made prostheses[97,98]. The strategy must be adapted to the individual case. For the lower limb, realignment and stabilization of the foot must precede hip and knee realignment by traction, followed by the various planned surgical procedures. On the contrary, for the upper limb, soft tissue release in the shoulder, for example, must precede corrective surgery of the elbow. Realignment arthrodesis of the wrist and arthroplasty or arthrodesis of the finger joints are performed last of all.

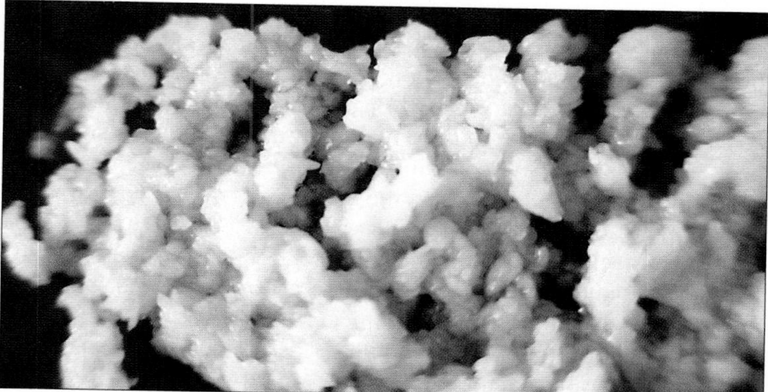

Fig. 21.9 Rice bodies obtained from draining the knee in a child with systemic disease. Courtesy of Professor Philippe Touzet.

Traditionally, surgery is planned for when the child has stopped growing. In a severely destroyed joint, when the growth cartilage plate has disappeared, however, the severity of the disability may require early consideration of surgery.

Local growth disturbance

Persisting inflammation in close proximity to an epiphyseal growth plate may cause either overgrowth of the affected limb or, less often, premature fusion of the growth cartilage. The latter is observed in the hind foot, resulting in a shorter length of the foot, or at a metacarpal bone (bradymetacarpus). In case of significant overgrowth, the surgical approach involves either a corrective osteotomy or epiphyseal stapling. Micrognathia may be improved with orthodontic surgery when dental development is complete.

ANESTHETIC RISKS

Anesthetic problems may result from intubation difficulties for several reasons. Cervical spine extension in children with JCA is often limited, temporomandibular joint involvement reduces mouth opening and long-standing disease is associated with mandibular hypoplasia, micrognathia, dental crowding and pharyngeal hypoplasia. Therefore, fiberoptic guidance for intubation may be required. Attention to medical therapy is mandatory, particularly in children using systemic corticosteroids or immunomodulatory drugs who require adjustment of their drugs. Postanaesthetic acute adrenal insufficiency, however, has not been reported in JCA patients.

REHABILITATION

The physical management of soft tissues and joints must be considered as soon as the diagnosis is made, even when only one joint is involved. The aim is to preserve functional capacity and the child's autonomy. It requires a great deal of energy and dedication to maintain a rehabilitation program over months and years. The physical therapist is a privileged member of the therapeutic team because of contact with the child and family several times a week. The need to establish both a good rapport with the child and parents and easy access is essential.

Physical therapy must be appropriate to the child's age, the involved joint and the stage of the disease[99]. Joint motion must be preserved at all costs. The use of hot packs and heated pools results in muscle relaxation and reduced pain and stiffness. It may precede joint mobilization. In the morning, a hot bath is highly recommended. Cold packs may also be of benefit.

Actively or passively stretching the joint allows anatomically correct movements to be maintained. However, the latter must remain painless. Splinting of joints at rest reduces flexion contractures. Nighttime traction of the lower limbs with a small abduction wedge pillow between the legs maintains a correct alignment of the lower limbs and avoids hip adduction. Lying in the prone position reduces hip flexion contractures. Hand splinting may be necessary, either during the night to avoid wrist deformity or when the child is writing or playing to improve hand strength and position. Dynamic splinting can also be recommended for finger deformity. Each joint requires specific attention[99].

Occupational therapy aims to maintain functional skills and independence[100]. Therapeutic sessions must not exceed the child's concentration span and the activities must be appropriate to the developmental level. The child must be instructed as to how to cope with the obstacles encountered in daily life. Booklets that describe difficulties encountered by a child with JCA are available and should be provided. The need for various technical aids, such as tricycles, walking aids, equipment for school, should be assessed by the occupational therapist and given as required.

THERAPEUTIC STRATEGIES

The three main forms of JCA cover a wide range of pathophysiologic conditions that differ both in terms of their response to various treatments and the side effects with which they are associated. The main therapeutic indications are summarized in Figure 21.10.

SYSTEMIC DISEASE

Systemic forms of JCA are associated with high fevers, they affect very young children and can spare the joints at onset. Characteristically there is some difficulty in controlling clinical symptoms (with the exception of relief obtained by corticosteroid therapy) and a high risk of therapeutic side effects. The following therapeutic approach may be indicated:

- NSAID therapy, starting in hospital,
- corticosteroid therapy,
- second-line therapy,
- IVIg,
- immunomodulators.

The most commonly used NSAID in this setting is high-dose ASA 100mg/kg/day in 6 divided doses (even at night). Doses of 110–120mg/kg can be reached gradually as long as it is tolerated, but the total daily dose must not exceed 4g. Pain relief is usually rapid, but fever abates more slowly. There are no noteworthy effects on laboratory parameters. This treatment can be continued at home for several months if it is effective and well tolerated. It is very important for parents to be warned of potential side effects, and they must be able to call a doctor immediately if problems arise. Up to 50% of children less than 5 years old initially respond to this treatment. Other NSAIDs can be used to treat older children. Indomethacin, although not used in all countries until the age of 15 years, is effective and shows acceptable tolerance in the older child. In principle, two NSAIDs should not be combined because of the increased risk of MAS[9]. However, in cases of morning stiffness taking aspirin only, indomethacin 1–2mg/kg/day, taken in the evening, can improve the patient's comfort.

Corticosteroid therapy – prednisone 2mg/kg/day orally or the equivalent – is indicated if NSAIDs are ineffective after appropriate treatment (at least 1 month) or if intolerance or pericarditis occur. Once started, corticosteroids are continued for several months as attempts to reduce the dose rapidly or switch to alternate-day dosing are doomed to failure. A NSAID can be added to the corticosteroid regimen. It should be remembered that blood salicylate levels are reduced by 30% during corticosteroid therapy. Corticosteroids have a spectacular effect on all clinical and biological manifestations, but this benefit is only obtained at high doses which also carry a risk of severe adverse effects. The effect is purely suppressive and in no way appears to prevent progression to severe arthritis. The effect of intravenous methylprednisolone pulses is generally rapid, but rarely long lasting.

Second-line therapies are rarely effective in systemic forms of disease[12], and may even be dangerous (especially gold)[47,50]. Serious adverse events have been reported with sulfasalazine[28]. The effect of methotrexate is controversial in this setting, but is probably less marked than in some other forms of JCA[35]. Intravenous immunoglobulins are less efficient than in Kawasaki syndrome. This therapy is not recommended for systemic disease because of its questionable efficacy and high cost. There is no formal evidence that heavy immunosuppressive treatments are effective in the systemic forms, but multicenter trials are warranted, despite the risk of side effects.

POLYARTICULAR DISEASE

Polyarticular disease encompasses several clinical entities. A subset with rheumatoid factor (RF^+) (10% of all polyarticular disease) is generally distinguished from other forms (RF^-).

NSAIDs are the first-line treatment of choice; as polyarticular disease mainly affects older children, there is a fairly wide choice of agents.

Second-line therapies are indicated early in the RF^+ subset, given its rapid progression; the indications are similar to those for adults. The response in RF– forms varies according to the degree of clinical and biological inflammation. It appears that a subset of 'dry' juvenile arthritis (without effusions) is particularly resistant to all available drugs. Methotrexate is indicated, mainly in RF^+ disease.

Systemic corticosteroid therapy is rarely indicated in these patients. However, corticosteroids at daily doses of less than 5mg/day, or alternate-day corticosteroid therapy, may improve these patients' comfort. Intra-articular injections can improve the function of a severely affected joint.

Immunomodulators may be used in some patients with severe disease refractory to second-line therapies, particularly in the RF^+ group and in other patients.

OLIGOARTICULAR DISEASE

Routine use of NSAIDs is for more of an analgesic than an anti-inflammatory effect. As these forms of JCA are generally associated with little pain, NSAIDs may be discontinued if the patients gain no benefit.

Local treatments have completely changed the prognosis in these disorders. Intra-articular triamcinolone is injected in a joint inflamed for 6–8 weeks. In very small children, it is important to treat the inflamed knee early to avoid the risk of flexion contracture with posterior subluxation of the tibia, which can occur rapidly. Local treatment gives very good results with larger joints, but is less effective with smaller and more complex joints such as those of the feet and hands.

Ophthalmologic involvement correlates with circulating ANA. The presence of ANA calls for routine ophthalmologic examination for iridocyclitis every 3–4 months for several years. Iridocyclitis occurs in about 30% and 50% of cases within 5 and 10 years, respectively, even in the absence of articular progression[101]. Ocular involvement is persistent and thus calls for local treatment with corticosteroid eye drops and mydriatic agents for months or even years. The failure to provide appropriate treatment can lead to cataracts and band keratopathy. Alternate-day systemic corticosteroids can be used in some cases if local treatment fails to control ocular inflammation.

Second-line therapies are not indicated for oligoarticular disease as affected patients show a poor response. However, methotrexate appears to be useful in patients with disease of oligoarticular onset which spreads and persists in multiple joints[37].

THERAPEUTIC STRATEGIES IN FORMS OF JCA				
Agent	Systemic	Polyarticular	Oligoarticular	Spondyloarthropathy
ASA	100–120mg/kg/day	Rarely used	60–80mg/kg/day	Rarely used
Other NSAIDs	In older patients, indomethacin 2.5mg/kg/day	Yes	According to licensed dosages in young children	Yes, active on pain (Amor criteria)[112]
Systemic corticosteroids	Prednisone 2mg/kg/day if NSAIDs fail or are not tolerated	Rarely used 5mg/day to improve comfort	Alternate-day regimen if needed for eye inflammation	Used in exceptional circumstances
Gold	Risk of MAS (2nd injection)	Used in all forms, especially RF+	Not indicated	Rarely used
D-Penicillamine	Poor efficacy? Risk of side effects	Used in all forms, especially RF+	Not indicated	Rarely used
Sulfasalazine	Risk of MAS	Probable efficacy	Not indicated	Efficacy confirmed
Antimalarials	Poor efficacy	Used in all forms, especially RF+	Not indicated	Rarely used
Methotrexate	Higher doses probably needed	Used in all forms, especially RF+	Indicated in 'extended' forms	Probable efficacy
Immunomodulators	Efficacy not documented	Used in refractory cases	Not indicated	Not indicated
Intra-articular corticosteroids	In particularly crippling joints	In particularly crippling joints	Very good efficacy	Very good efficacy

MAS = Macrophage activation syndrome.

Fig. 21.10 Main therapeutic indications in the various forms of JCA.

SPONDYLOARTHROPATHIES

Undifferentiated forms of arthritis account for 80% of pediatric cases according to the ESSG (European Spondyloarthropathy Study Group) and Amor criteria[102].

Useful pain control can often be achieved with NSAIDs. Among the second-line therapies, sulfasalazine appears ro be drug of choice[26]. Local (intra-articular) treatment with corticosteroids is indicated when arthritis is persistent and problematic. Treatment of enthesopathies is difficult, and is based on local infiltration with cortisteroids along with physical therapy or, if needed, orthopedic procedures.

CONCLUSIONS

Although progress continues and new and improved therapeutic measures are emerging, clinicians yearn for more effective and proved treatments. Advances in basic sciences and immunogenetics will contribute to the understanding of JCA and related diseases and new therapeutic strategies will become available in the future. The development of worldwide, multicenter collaborative research represents a means of ensuring continued progress in the management of children with JCA.

REFERENCES

1. Malleson PN, Petty RE. Remodelling the pyramid. A pediatric perspective. J Rheumatol. 1990;17:867–8.
2. Wallace CA, Levinson JE. Juvenile rheumatoid arthritis: outcome and treatment for the 1990's. Rheum Dis Clin North Am. 1991;17:891–905.
3. Hallé F, Marfil F, Sioufi A, *et al.* Pharmacokinetics of pirprofen in children with juvenile chronic arthritis. Eur J Drug Metab Pharmacokinet. 1991;16:29–34.
4. Rey E, Pariente-Khayat A, Gouyet L, *et al.* Stereoselective disposition of ibuprofen enantiomeres in infants. Br J Clin Pharmacol. 1994;38:373–5.
5. Lovell DJ, Giannini EH, Brewer EJ Jr. Time course of response to nonsteroidal anti-inflammatory drugs in juvenile rheumatoid arthritis. Arthritis Rheum. 1984;27:1433–7.
6. Dromgoole SH, Furst DE, Paulus HE. Rational approaches to the use of salicylate in the treatment of rheumatoid arthritis. Semin Arthritis Rheum. 1981;11:257–83.
7. Koeper MA, Sempel DA, Dallman JR. Anemia in patients with juvenile rheumatoid arthritis. J Pediatr. 1978;92:930–2.
8. Athreya BH, Moser G, Cecil HS, Myers AR. Aspirin induced hepatotoxicity in juvenile rheumatoid arthritis. A prospective study. Arthritis Rheum. 1975;18:347–52.
9. Prieur AM, Stephan JL. Macrophage activation syndrome in pediatric rheumatic diseases. Rev Rheumatol. 1994;61B:385–8.
10. Levy ML, Barron KS, Eichenfield A, Honig PJ. Naproxene induced pseudoporphyria. J Pediatr. 1990;117:660–4.
11. Barron KS, Person DR, Brewer EJ. The toxicity of nonsteroidal anti-inflammatory drugs in juvenile rheumatoid arthritis. J Rheumatol. 1982;9:149–55.
12. Manners PJ, Ansell BM. Slow acting anti rheumatic drugs in systemic onset juvenile chronic arthritis. Pediatrics. 1986;77:99–103.
13. Brewer EJ, Giannini EH, Barkley E. Gold in the management of juvenile rheumatoid arthritis. Arthritis Rheum. 1980;23:404–10.
14. Ansell BM, Hall MA, Ribero S. A comparative study of gold and penicillamine in seropositive juvenile chronic arthritis (juvenile rheumatoid arthritis). Ann Rheum Dis. 1981;40:522A.
15. Svantesson H. Gold in rheumatoid arthritis therapy today. Paediatr Scand J Rheumatol. 1983;51:125–6.
16. Kvien TK, Hoyerall HM, Sandstad B. Slow acting antirheumatic drug in patients with juvenile rheumatoid arthritis. Evaluation in a randomized, parallel 50 week clinical trial. J Rheumatol. 1985;12:533–9.
17. Malleson PN, Grondin C, Petty RE. Outcome of gold therapy in juvenile rheumatoid arthritis. Arthritis Rheum. 1987;30:528–32.
18. Grondin C, Malleson P, Petty RE. Slow acting anti rheumatic drugs in chronic arthritis of childhood. Semin Arthritis Rheum. 1988;18:38–47.
19. Giannini EH, Barron KS, Spencer CH, *et al.* Auranofin therapy in juvenile rheumatoid arthritis: result of the five-year open label extension trial. J Rheumatol. 1991;18:1240–2.
20. Alvaro Garcia JM, Castaneda-Sanz S, Arranz R, *et al.* Antithymocyte globulin in the treatment of gold-induced severe aplastic anemia. J Rheumatol. 1988;15:43–5.
21. Pegg SJ, Lang BA, Mikhail EL, Hughes DH. Fatal bronchiolitis obliterans in a patient with juvenile rheumatoid arthritis receiving chrysotherapy. J Rheumatol. 1994;21:349–51.
22. Ozdogan H, Turunc M, Deringol B, Yurdakul S, Yacizi H. Sulphasalazine in the treatment of juvenile rheumatoid arthritis: a preliminary open trial. J Rheumatol. 1986;314:1269–70.
23. Joos E, Veys EM. Sulfasalazine treatment in juvenile chronic arthritis: an open study. J Rheumatol. 1991;18:880–4.
24. Gedalia A, Barash J, Press J, Buskila D. Sulphasalazine in the treatment of pauciarticular onset juvenile chronic arthritis. Clin Rheumatol. 1993;12:511–14.
25. Ansell BM, Hall MA, Loftus JK, *et al.* A multicenter pilot study of sulphasalazine in juvenile chronic arthritis. Clin Exp Rheumatol. 1991;9:201–3.
26. Job-Deslandre C, Menkes CJ. Treatment of juvenile spondylarthropathies with sulphasalazine. Rev Rheum. 1993;60:489–91.
27. Dougados M, Maetzel A, Mijiyawa H, Amor B. Evaluation of sulphasalazine in the treatment of spondylarthropathies. Ann Rheum Dis. 1992;51:955–8.
28. Hertzberger-Ten Cate R, Cats A. Toxicity of sulfasalazine in juvenile chronic arthritis. Clin Exp Rheumatol. 1991;9:85–8.
29. Van Rossum MAJ, Fiselier Th, Franssen M, *et al.* Sulfasalazine in the treatment of juvenile chronic arthritis. Arthritis Rheumatol. 1996;39(Suppl).
30. Mouy R, Stephan JL, Pillet P, *et al.* Efficacy of cyclosporin A in the treatment of macrophage activation syndrome in juvenile arthritis. Report of five cases. J Pediatr. 1996; 129: 750-4.
31. Kummerle-Deschner J, Dannecker G. Sulphasalazine desensitization in a paediatric patient with juvenile chronic arthritis. Acta Paediatr. 1995;84:952–4.
32. Laaksonen AL, Koskiahde V, Juva K. Dosage of antimalarial drugs for children with juvenile rheumatoid arthritis and systemic lupus erythematosus. A clinical study with determination of serum concentrations of chloroquine and hydroxychloroquine. Scand J Rheumatol. 1974;3:103–8.

33. Truckenbrodt H, Hafner R. Methotrexate therapy in juvenile rheumatoid arthritis: a retrospective study. Arthritis Rheum. 1986;29:801–7.
34. Rose CD, Singsen BH, Eichenfeld AH, Goldsmith DP, Athreya BH. Safety and efficacy of methotrexate therapy for juvenile rheumatoid arthritis. J Pediatr. 1990;117:653–9.
35. Speckmaier M, Findeisen J, Woo P, Ansell BM. Low-dose methotrexate in systemic onset juvenile chronic arthritis. Clin Exp Rheumatol. 1989;7:647–50.
36. Giannini EH, Brewer EJ, Kuzmina N, *et al.* Methotrexate in resistant juvenile rheumatoid arthritis. Results of the USA–USSR double-blind, placebo-controlled trial. The Pediatric Rheumatology Collaborative Study Group and the Cooperative Children's Study Group. N Engl J Med. 1992;326:1043–9.
37. Hallé F, Prieur AM. Evaluation of methotrexate in the treatment of juvenile chronic arthritis according to the subtype. Clin Exp Rheumatol. 1991;9:297–302.
38. Kraus A, Alargon-Segovia D. Fever in adult onset Still's disease. Response to methotrexate. J Rheumatol. 1991;18:918–20.
39. Aydintug AO, D'Cruz D, Cervera R, Khamashta MA, Hughes GR. Low dose methotrexate treatment in adult Still's disease. J Rheumatol. 1992;19:431–5.
40. Wallace CA, Sherry DD. Preliminary report of higher dose methotrexate treatment in juvenile rheumatoid arthritis. J Rheumatol. 1992;19:1604–7.
41. Reiff A, Shaham B, Wood BP, *et al.* High dose methotrexate in the treatment of refractory juvenile rheumatoid arthritis. Clin Exp Rheumatol. 1995;13:113–18.
42. Wallace CA, Sherry DD, Mellins ED, *et al.* Predicting remission in juvenile rheumatoid arthritis with methotrexate treatment. J Rheumatol. 1993;20:118–22
43. Ravelli A, Di Fuccia G, Molinaro, *et al.* Plasma levels after oral methotrexate in children with juvenile rheumatoid arthritis. J Rheumatol. 1993;20:1573–7.
44. Harel L, Wagner-Weiner L, Poznanski AK, *et al.* Effects of methotrexate on radiologic progression in juvenile rheumatoid arthritis. Arthritis Rheum. 1993;36:1370–4.
45. Ravelli A, Viola S, Ramenghi B, *et al.* Frequency of relapse after discontinuation of methotrexate therapy for clinical remission in juvenile rheumatoid arthritis. J Rheumatol. 1995;22:1574–6.
46. Albertioni F, Flato B, Seideman P, *et al.* Methotrexate in juvenile rheumatoid arthritis. Evidence of age dependent pharmacokinetics. Eur J Pharmacol. 1995;47:507–11.
47. Wallace CA, Smith AL, Sherry DD. Pilot investigation of naproxen/methotrexate interaction in patients with juvenile rheumatoid arthritis. J Rheumatol. 1993;20:1764–8.
48. Dupuis LL, Koren G, Shore A, Silverman ED, Laxer RM. Methotrexate nonsteroidal antiinflammatory drug interaction in children with arthritis. J Rheumatol. 1990;17:1469–73.
49. Dupuis LL, Koren G, Silverman ED, Laxer RM. Influence of food on the bioavailability of oral methotrexate in children. J Rheumatol. 1995;22:1570–3.
50. Kremer JM. Liver biopsies in patients with rheumatoid arthritis receiving methotrexate: where are we going? (editorial). J Rheumatol. 1992;19:189–91.
51. Kugathasan S, Newman AJ, Dahms BB, Boyle JT. Liver biopsy findings in patients with juvenile rheumatoid arthritis receiving long term weekly methotrexate therapy. J Pediatr. 1996;128:149–51.
52. Graham LD, Myones BL, Rivas CR, Rivas-Chalon RF, Pachman LM. Morbidity associated with long-term methotrexate therapy in juvenile rheumatoid arthritis. J Pediatr. 1992;120:287–95.
53. Morgan SL, Baggott JE, Vaughn WH, *et al.* The effect of folic acid supplementation on the toxicity of low dose methotrexate in patients with rheumatoid arthritis. Arthritis Rheum. 1990;33:9–18.
54. St Clair EN, Rice JR, Snyderman R. Pneumonitis complicating low-dose methotrexate therapy in rheumatoid arthritis. Arch Int Med. 1985;145:2033–5.
55. Pelucchi A, Lomater C, Gerloni V, *et al.* Lung function and diffusing capacity for carbon monoxide in patients with juvenile chronic arthritis: effect of disease activity and low dose methotrexate therapy. Clin Exp Rheumatol. 1994;12:675–9.
56. Muzaffer MA, Schneider R, Cameron BJ, Silverman ED, Laxer RM. Accelerated nodulosis during methotrexate therapy for juvenile rheumatoid arthritis. J Pediatr. 1996;128:698–700.
57. Zimmer-Galler I, Ue JT. Choroidal infiltrates as the initial manifestations of lymphoma in rheumatoid arthritis after treatment with low-dose methotrexate. Mayo Clin Proc. 1994;69:258–61.
58. Miller JJ III. Prolonged use of large intravenous steroid pulses in the rheumatic diseases of children. Pediatrics. 1979;65:989–94.
59. Job-Deslandre C, Menkes CJ. Administration of methylprednisolone pulse in chronic arthritis in children. Clin Exp Rheumatol. 1991;9(Suppl 6):915–18.
60. Davies UM, Rooney M, Preece MA, Ansell BM, Woo P. Treatment of growth retardation in juvenile chronic arthritis with recombinant human growth hormone. J Rheumatol. 1994;21:153–8.
61. Rooney M, Davies UM, Ansell BM, Woo PM. The recombinant growth hormone (rGH) in juvenile chronic arthritis (JCA) five years on. Clin Exp Rheumatol. 1993;13(Suppl):63.
62. Touati G, Prieur AM, Ruiz JC, *et al.* Recombinant human growth hormone (rhGH) treatment in children affected with long term corticosteroid treated juvenile chronic arthritis. Effects on growth and metabolic parameters. Clin Exp Rheumatol. 1996;14:464.
63. Pugh MT, Grosse R, Southwood TR. Multiple joint corticosteroid injections in polyarticular juvenile chronic arthritis: a single-blind one year follow up study. Arthritis Rheum. 1995;38(Suppl).
64. Hurez V, Kaveri SV, Kazatchkine MD. Normal polyspecific immunoglobublin (IVIg) in the treatment of autoimmune diseases. J Autoimmun. 1993;6:675–81.
65. Lang BA, Shore A. A review of the current concepts on the pathogenesis of juvenile rheumatoid arthritis. J Rheumatol. 1990;17(Suppl 1):15–23.
66. Silverman ED, Laxer RM, Greenwald M, *et al.* Intravenous gamma globulin therapy in systemic juvenile rheumatoid arthritis. Arthritis Rheum. 1990;33:1015–22.
67. Prieur AM, Adleff A, Debré M, Boulate P, Griscelli C. High dose immunoglobulin therapy in severe juvenile chronic arthritis. Clin Exp Rheumatol. 1990;8:603–9.
68. Silverman ED, Cawkwell GD, Lovell DJ, *et al.* Intravenous immunoglobulin in the treatment of systemic juvenile rheumatoid arthritis. A randomized placebo controlled trial. J Rheumatol. 1994;21:2353–8.
69. Uziel Y, Laxer RM, Schneider R, Silverman ED. IVIG therapy in systemic onset JRA. A follow study. J Rheumatol. 1996;23:910–18.
70. Giannini EH and the Pediatric Rheumatology Collaborative Study Group. IVIG in the treatment of polyarticular JRA: a phase I/II study. J Rheumatol. 1996;23:919–24.
71. Prieur AM. IVIG in Still's disease: Still controversial, still unproven (editorial). J Rheumatol. 1996;23:797–800.
72. Prieur AM, Balafrej M, Griscelli C, Mozziconacci P. Résultats et risques à long terme du traitement par chlorambucil dans le traitement des arthrites chroniques juvéniles. A propos de 40 cas. Rev Rhum Mal Ostéoart. 1979;46:85–90.
73. Guesry P, Lenoir G, Broyer M. Action à long terme des immunosuppresseurs sur la fonction de reproduction. Arch Fr Pédiatr. 1977;34:792–8.
74. Deschênes G, Prieur AM, Hayem F, Broyer M, Gubler MC. Renal amyloidosis in juvenile chronic arthritis: evolution after chlorambucil treatment. Pediatr Nephrol. 1990;4:463–9.
75. David J. Amyloidosis in juvenile chronic arthritis. Clin Exp Rheumatol. 1991;9:73–8.
76. Shaikov AV, Maximov AA, Speransky AI, *et al.* Repetitive use of pulse therapy with methylprednisolone and cyclophosphamide in addition to oral methotrexate in children with systemic juvenile rheumatoid arthritis. Preliminary results of a long term study. J Rheumatol. 1992;19:612–16.
77. Trompeter RS, Evans PR, Barratt TH. Gonadal function in boys with steroid responsive nephrotic syndrome treated with cyclophosphamide. Lancet. 1981;i:1177–9.
78. Hofeman GS, Gerr GS, Leavitt RY, *et al.* Wegener granulomatosis: an analysis of 158 patients. Ann Int Med. 1992;116:488–98.
79. Kvien TK, Hoyeraal HM, Sandstad B. Azathioprine versus placebo in patients with juvenile chronic arthritis. J Rheumatol. 1986;13:113–23.
80. Ostensen M, Hoyeraal HM, Kass E. Tolerance of cyclosporine A in children with refractory juvenile arthritis. J Rheumatol. 1988;15:1536–8.
81. Fantini F, Gerloni V, Gattinara H, *et al.* Corticosteroid sparing effect and safety profile of cyclosporin A in the treatment of juvenile chronic arthritis. Arthritis Rheum. 1996;39(Suppl).
82. Goel A, Londino AV. FK506 treatment in severe resistant juvenile rheumatoid arthritis. Arthritis Rheum. 1996;39(Suppl).
83. Pernice W, Schuchmann L, Dippel J, *et al.* Therapy for systemic juvenile rheumatoid arthritis with gamma-interferon: a pilot study of nine patients. Arthritis Rheum. 1998;32:643–6.
84. Pernice W, Stahn R, Fabricius HA, Klingshirn R. Steroid economising effects of calf thymus extracts in three patients with juvenile chronic arthritis. Klin Woch. 1983;61:429–31.
85. Bardare M, Corona F, Ogliari MT, Cohen E. Thymopentin in the treatment of juvenile chronic arthritis. Clin Exp Rheumatol. 1990;8:89–93.
86. Rooney M. Is there a disease-modifying drug for juvenile chronic arthritis? Br J Rheumatol. 1992;31:635–41.
87. Kahn MF. Aggressive therapy for rheumatoid arthritis. Clin Exp Rheumatol. 1995;13(Suppl 12):31–4.
88. Heaton DC, Moller PW. Still's disease associated with Coxsackie infection and haemophagocytic syndrome. Ann Rheum Dis. 1985;44:341–4.
89. Stephan JL, Zeller J, Hubert PH, *et al.* Macrophage activation syndrome in rheumatic disease in childhood: a report of four new cases. Clin Exp Rheumatol. 1993;11:451–6.
90. Fishman D, Rooney M, Woo P. Successful management of reactive haemophagocytic syndrome in systemic onset juvenile arthritis. Br J Rheumatol. 1995;34:388.
91. Huppertz HI, Pfüller H. Transient suppression of cortisol production after intraarticular steroid therapy for chronic arthritis in children. Arthritis Rheum. 1996;39(Suppl).
92. Touzet P, Prieur AM, Wouters K. Arthritis in children and adolescents. The surgical management of juvenile chronic arthritis. Baillière's Clin Paediatr. 1993;1:875–95.
93. Hope PG. Arthroscopy in children. J Roy Soc Med. 1991;84:29–31.
94. Kvien TK, Pahle JA, Hoyeraal HM, Sandstad B. Comparison of synovectomy and no synovectomy in patients with juvenile rheumatoid arthritis. Scand J Rheumatol. 1987;16:81–91.
95. Ovregard T, Hoyeraal HM, Pahle JA, Larsen S. A three year retrospective study of synovectomies in children. Clin Orthop. 1990;259:76–82.
96. Moreno Alvarez MJ, Espada G, Maldonado Cocco JA, Gagliardi SA. Longterm followup of hip and knee soft tissue release in juvenile chronic arthritis. J Rheumatol. 1992;19:1608–10.
97. Wiit JD, Swann M, Ansell BM. Total hip replacement for juvenile chronic arthritis. J Bone J Surg. 1991;73B:770–3.
98. Boublik M, Tsahakis PJ, Scott RD. Cementless total knee arthroplasty in juvenile onset rheumatoid arthritis. Clin Orthop. 1993;286:88–93.
99. Emery HM. Arthritis in children and adolescent. The rehabilitation of the child with juvenile chronic arthritis. Baillière's Clin Paediatr. 1993;1:803–23.
100. Lawton S. In: Woo P, White P, Ansell BM, eds. Paediatric rheumatology update. Occupational therapy. Oxford: 1990;99–105.
101. Peralta JL, Prieur AM. Arthrite chronique juvénile avec présence d'anticorps antinucléaires sériques. Arch Fr Pédiatr. 1990;47:497–502.
102. Prieur AM, Listrat V, Dougados M, Amor B. Critères de classification des spondylarthropathies chez les enfants. Arch Fr Pédiatr. 1993;50:379–85.

ADULT STILL'S DISEASE

John M Esdaile

Definition

- An acute febrile syndrome in young adults.
- Typically affects multiple organs.
- Although the diagnosis is one of exclusion, a striking constellation of clinical and laboratory abnormalities is present.

Clinical features

- High spiking fever, arthralgia or arthritis, sore throat, transient maculopapular rash, lymphadenopathy, hepatosplenomegaly, serositis.
- Morbidity arises predominantly from chronic arthritis in addition to constitutional symptoms.

HISTORY

In 1971, Bywaters described 14 adult patients with features similar to the systemic form of juvenile rheumatoid arthritis (formerly, Still's disease)[1,2]. Subsequently, more than 300 cases have been reported[3–5].

EPIDEMIOLOGY

This rare disease is found worldwide[3–4]. It is predominantly a disorder of young adults aged 16–35 years[5] (Fig. 22.1). The incidence in the Brittany and Loire regions of France has been estimated at 0.16 per 100,000 [6]. This is likely to be a minimum estimate.

A familial tendency has not been reported. Inconsistent results have been found with HLA typing. Separate studies have reported an association with HLA-DR2, -DR4 and -DR7[5,7,8] and an increased frequency of HLA-B35 has been found in both children and adults with the disease[5].

CLINICAL FEATURES

Adult Still's disease affects multiple organs (Fig. 22.2)[3,5]. It is important to note that the full constellation of clinical features may not be present at onset and that evolution to a 'typical' case of adult Still's disease may take a number of weeks, or, rarely, even months (see Fig. 22.3)[8,9].

EPIDEMIOLOGY OF ADULT STILL'S DISEASE	
Peak age (years)	16–35
Sex distribution (F:M)	1:1
Prevalence and incidence	Unknown
Geographic distribution	Worldwide

Fig. 22.1 Epidemiology of adult Still's disease.

FEVER

Adult Still's disease commonly presents with a high fever (>39°C), spiking once a day, usually in the evening or night, with return of the temperature to below normal. Occasionally, two fever spikes a day are seen, and in 20% of patients the temperature does not return to a normal level[5].

MUCOCUTANEOUS LESIONS

The 'Still's rash' is salmon pink, macular or maculopapular (see Fig. 22.4). It is frequently evanescent and is most likely to be observed with the fever spike (hence the need to evaluate the patient in the evening). The rash is most commonly found on the trunk and proximal extremities, but in up to 15% of those affected it may be found on the face[5]. In over one third the rash is mildly pruritic and thereby may be mistaken for drug allergy[5]. It may appear in areas of mechanical irritation, for example those caused by clothing. In one third of patients it can be precipitated by rubbing (Koebner's phenomenon) or, less commonly, by a hot bath[5]. The typical Still's rash has only rarely been observed in other diseases. These include ulcerative colitis, vasculitis and leukemia.

CLINICAL MANIFESTATIONS OF ADULT STILL'S DISEASE		
	Number	%
Female	145/283	51
Childhood episode (≤15 years)	38/236	16
Onset 16–35 years	178/233	76
Arthralgia	282/283	100
Arthritis	249/265	94
Fever ≥39°C	258/266	97
≥39.5°C	54/62	87
Sore throat	57/62	92
JRA rash	248/281	88
Myalgia	52/62	84
Weight loss ≥10%	41/54	76
Lymphadenopathy	167/264	63
Splenomegaly	138/265	52
Abdominal pain	30/62	48
Hepatomegaly	108/258	42
Pleuritis	79/259	31
Pericarditis	75/254	30
Pneumonitis	17/62	27
Alopecia	15/62	24

Fig. 22.2 Clinical manifestations of adult Still's disease. Data from Pouchot *et al.*[5] including patients reviewed by Ohta *et al.*[3]. For fever ≥39.5°C, sore throat, myalgia, weight loss, abdominal pain, pneumonitis and alopecia the data are from Pouchot *et al.*[5] only, as these clinical manifestations were likely to be under-reported in early studies.

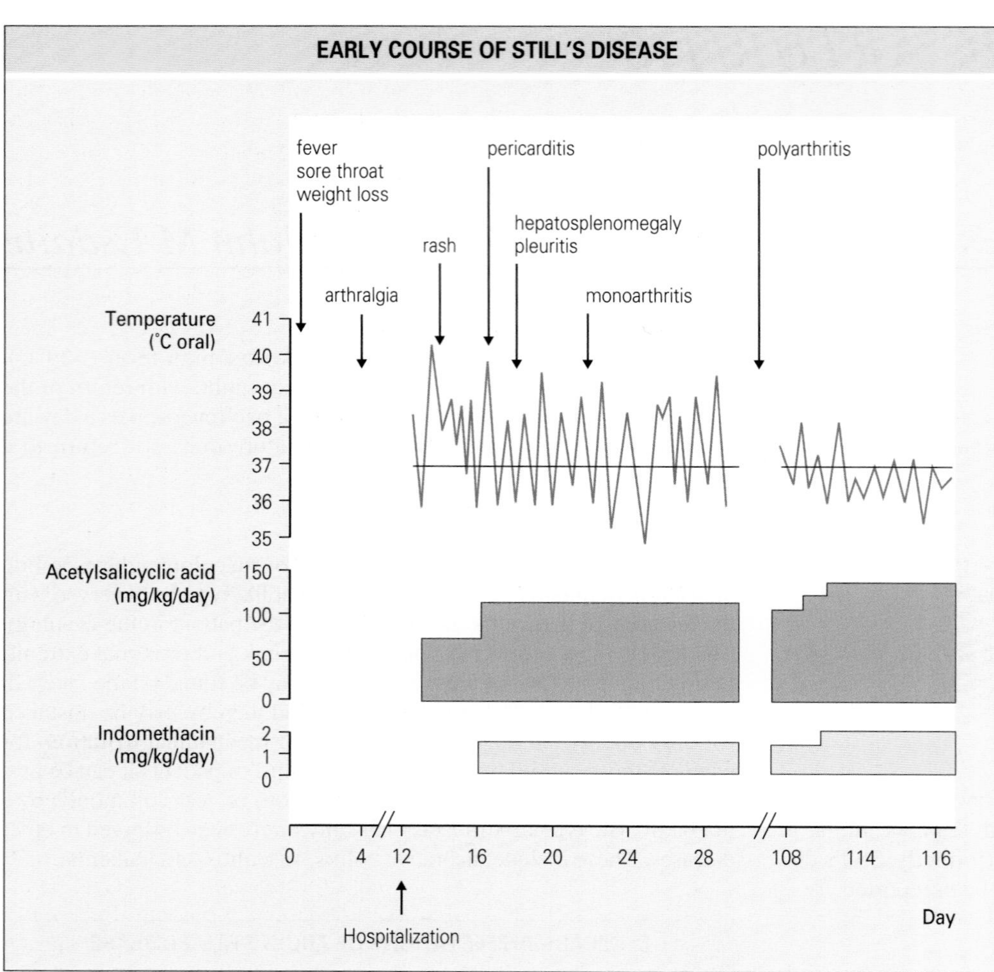

Fig. 22.3 Early course of Still's disease. The fever pattern and early evolution of the clinical manifestations in relation to therapy of a typical case of adult Still's disease in a 20-year-old male. The patient was hospitalized on day 12 of the illness. On admission the hemoglobin was 10.6g/dl, the WBC 25,600/mm^3 and the ESR 32mm/h (corrected Wintrobe). Adapted from Esdaile *et al.*[10].

Mild diffuse hair loss is noted in 24% of patients: increased hair on the pillow-case or hair brush is reported. An aseptic non-exudative pharyngitis is extremely common at presentation. Rarely, it can interfere with eating[5,11].

JOINTS AND MUSCLE

Arthralgia is universal and usually increases in intensity, sometimes markedly, with the fever spike. While articular involvement is common (Fig. 22.5), at least 5% of patients never demonstrate an arthritis, and at presentation the arthritis may be transient, confined to only a few joints, or be mild and overshadowed by the other dramatic clinical manifestations of the disease (Fig. 22.3)[2,5,9,11]. By 6 months, the majority of patients have polyarticular disease[5].

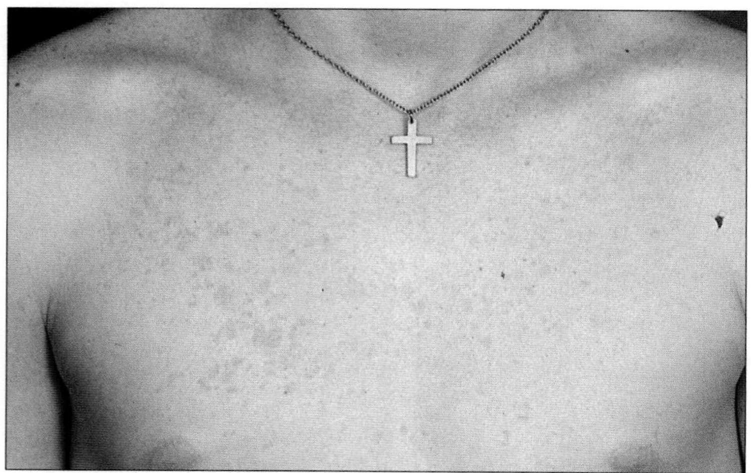

Fig. 22.4 Still's rash. The faint salmon-colored rash of Still's disease. More erythematous eruptions may also be seen. Although the rash is most common on the trunk and upper extremities, it may also be seen on the face.

While the joints affected resemble those of many other polyarticular inflammatory joint diseases, the involvement of the distal interphalangeal joints of the hand in 18% of cases is notable (Fig. 22.5). With the exception of psoriatic arthritis, this joint is spared in many of the common articular disorders of young adults.

JOINTS AFFECTED BY ADULT STILL'S DISEASE

Joint affected	Patients (%)
Knee	84
Wrist	74
Ankle	57
Elbow	50
Proximal interphalangeal – hands	47
Shoulder	43
Metacarpophalangeal	34
Metatarsophalangeal	19
Distal interphalangeal – hands	18
Hip	14
Neck	11
Temporomandibular joint	8
Interphalangeal – feet	3

Fig. 22.5 Joints affected by adult Still's disease. (From 90 patients described in Pouchot *et al.*[5], Cush *et al.*[12] and Del Paine and Leek[13].)

Myalgia can be severe and debilitating and may require drug therapy for relief. Like the arthralgia it can increase markedly in severity with the fever spike. Proximal muscle weakness is rare. Transient minimal elevation of muscle enzyme tests may occur[4,5].

LYMPHADENOPATHY, SPLENOMEGALY, HEPATOMEGALY AND ABDOMINAL PAIN

Lymph nodes are mobile and slightly tender. The cervical region is most commonly affected. Splenomegaly and hepatomegaly are common (see Fig. 22.2) but usually mild.

Although abdominal pain has been described in only 12% of cases worldwide, it has been present in approximately 50% of patients in some series[5,12,14]. In general it is mild, but severe cases can simulate a 'surgical abdomen'. It is important to recognize this as a clinical feature of the underlying disorder in order to avoid unnecessary surgical exploration.

PLEUROPULMONARY AND CARDIAC MANIFESTATIONS

Pleuritic pain, sometimes incapacitating, is universal with pleural or pericardial effusions. Pleural and pericardial involvement may be less common in Japanese patients[4]. Aseptic pneumonitis, often transient and affecting either upper or lower lung regions, is not uncommon. Rare manifestations include acute respiratory distress syndrome, chronic restrictive lung disease, pericardial tamponade and myocarditis[5].

RARE MANIFESTATIONS AND ASSOCIATED DISORDERS

Other manifestations include sicca syndrome, aseptic meningitis, transient cranial nerve palsies, peripheral neuropathy, retinal exudates, iritis, panophthalmitis, Brown's syndrome and inflammatory orbital pseudotumor[4,5,11]. Adult Still's disease has been associated with interstitial nephritis[3], subacute glomerulitis[14] and thrombotic thrombocytopenic purpura[5].

DISEASE COURSE

Self-limited, intermittent and chronic disease courses have been described. Self-limited, or monocyclic, disease refers to a single episode of illness. The episode usually lasts less than 1 year and is followed by persistent good health. Intermittent, or polycyclic, disease remits completely but is then characterized by one or more exacerbations of disease activity. The timing of these flare-ups cannot be predicted. The flare-ups most commonly include fever, Still's rash, arthritis and serositis. They tend to be less severe and of shorter duration than the initial episode[5,12,15].

A chronic disease course refers to persistently active disease, usually due to chronic destructive arthritis. Nonetheless, the majority of patients improve and up to 25% enter a remission at least temporarily, although this frequently takes years to occur[2,4,5,8,12,15].

The different definitions used to characterize the disease course, as well as the different methods of selecting patients for inclusion in a study and the different observation periods used, permit only general statements about the relative frequency of self-limited, intermittent and chronic disease courses[5]. Approximately 30–50% of patients have a chronic disease course[2–5,8]. Of the remainder, self-limited disease occurs with a frequency approximately equal to that of intermittent disease.

Predictors of disease course

Probably as a result of the rarity of adult Still's disease and the limited time since its recognition as a distinct disorder, studies of prognosis have been uncommon. Of the several studies of prognosis, three have identified as a marker of a poor outcome the presence of polyarthritis early in the disease course[5,8,12] and two have found the same to be true of proximal joint arthritis (involvement of one or more shoulders or hips)[5,8]. These markers appear to predict both a chronic disease course and a prolonged time to clinical remission[5]. In addition, a prior episode in childhood, hip involvement and the requirement for over 2 years' treatment with systemic corticosteroids have been associated with poorer long-term function[12]. A recent study[5] has also reported that the absence of a Still's rash in the initial illness denotes a better outcome.

Other clinical markers and routine laboratory tests do not predict the course of adult Still's disease. Autoantibodies such as rheumatoid factor and antinuclear antibodies are rarely present in adult Still's disease and when present are customarily transient. Nonetheless, a tendency towards a more prolonged active disease course has been noted when either are detected[5]. These antibodies may be markers for a more severe inflammatory state. HLA-B35 has been associated with a greater likelihood of a self-limited disease course[16], and HLA-DR6 with proximal joint arthritis and greater disability[17]. Neither result has been confirmed[5].

FUNCTIONAL AND OCCUPATIONAL OUTCOMES

As with the assessment of disease course, assessment of outcome is affected by issues relating to patient selection, the length of follow-up and the small number of patients in many studies. Similar results have been interpreted by some as supporting a good prognosis and by others as indicating a less favorable one. This discrepancy probably arises because adult Still's disease was initially believed to be predominantly a benign, self-limited disease. This is clearly not the case. Nonetheless, in studies with follow-up from 4.5–20 years 81–85% of patients are in American Rheumatism Association Functional Class I or II[5].

Standardized health status measures have recently been used to assess outcome. Cush *et al.*[12] used the Stanford Health Assessment Questionnaire to measure physical disability. With a mean follow-up of 12 years, patients with adult Still's disease were less disabled than patients with rheumatoid arthritis of similar duration. Sampalis *et al.*[16] compared Still's patients after a mean of 10 years disease to age- and sex-matched healthy controls. Psychologic disability and social functioning in Still's disease was similar to that in the controls. Scores for physical disability and pain were significantly elevated compared to healthy controls but less than those reported for systemic lupus erythematosus (SLE) and rheumatoid arthritis (RA)[18].

Adult Still's disease patients completed their education and obtained jobs of similar occupational prestige and income as age- and sex-matched controls[18]. Pessimistic views of adult Still's disease based on the frequency of chronic disease can be tempered by the data suggesting that patients appear to overcome much of the disability of their disease and play an active role in society.

SURVIVAL

Twenty-seven deaths have been reported as a result of adult Still's disease[4,5]. The most common causes were infection, amyloidosis and liver failure. Adult respiratory distress syndrome, heart failure, status epilepticus, diffuse intravascular coagulation and thrombotic thrombocytopenic purpura were other causes[4,5].

INVESTIGATIONS

BASIC LABORATORY TESTS

The laboratory test results largely reflect the systemic inflammatory nature of the disease process in adult Still's disease (see Fig. 22.6). An elevated sedimentation rate is universal. The platelet count is high in over 50% of patients and hypoalbuminemia is present in 81%; 68% have a significant anemia, which is almost always an anemia of chronic disease. Coomb's tests are negative, as are tests for hemolysis[3]. Although intravascular coagulation has been noted in childhood Still's disease, this is a rare manifestation in adults[5,8,11]. In at least some cases the disseminated intravascular coagulation reflects the underlying disease process[5,8].

The most striking abnormality is a marked leukocytosis (see Fig. 22.6). Over 75% of patients have a peripheral white blood cell (WBC) count $\geq$ 15,000/mm^3. The increase in cells is predominantly due to an increase in mature and juvenile neutrophils[5]. Less than 2% of cases present with a diminished WBC count[3].

LABORATORY TESTS IN ADULT STILL'S DISEASE		
	Number	%
Elevated ESR	265/267	99
WBC ≥10,000/mm³ ≥15,000/mm³	228/248 50/62	92 81
Neutrophils ≥80%	55/62	88
Serum albumin <3.5g/dl	143/177	81
Elevated hepatic enyzmes*	169/232	73
Anemia (hemoglobin ≤10g/dl)	159/233	68
Platelets ≥400,000/mm³	37/60	62
Negative antinuclear antibody test	256/278	92
Negative rheumatoid factor	259/280	93
* Any elevated liver function test.		

Fig. 22.6 Laboratory tests in adult Still's disease. From Pouchot *et al.*[5], including patients reviewed by Ohta *et al.*[3]. For WBC ≥ 15,000/mm³, neutrophils ≥ 80%, and elevated platelet count, the data are from Pouchot *et al.*[5].

Elevation of one or more liver function tests, particularly the transaminases, is seen in two thirds of patients. While these results may reflect preceding treatment with hepatotoxic drugs, especially nonsteroidal anti-inflammatory agents, in many cases they result from the underlying disease process[7,10,16].

Recent reports have noted a striking elevation of serum ferritin in patients with active adult Still's disease in comparison to other inflammatory disorders and inactive Still's disease[4,19,20].

Tests for rheumatoid factor, antinuclear antibodies and other autoantibodies are generally negative[5,8]. Occasionally positive tests are seen for rheumatoid factor and antinuclear antibodies, which are present in low-titer and generally transient. While they may be a marker of severe disease[5], they may also represent repeated testing on previously test-negative patients (Fig. 22.6).

In the blood, immunoglobulins may be elevated, complement levels are normal or elevated and circulating immune complexes have been detected in up to one-third of patients[4]. The true frequency of abnormality of these tests is uncertain because the vast majority of patients have not had them performed, or at least the results have not been reported.

SYNOVIAL AND SEROSAL FLUIDS

Synovial fluids are inflammatory. In two recent studies[5,11] the mean synovial fluid WBC counts were 11,200 cells/mm³ (n=15, range 1,800–40,700 cells/mm³) and 15,250 cells/mm³ (n=25, range 1560–48,200 cells/mm³). Two additional patients had normal synovial fluids. The proportions of polymorphonuclear leukocytes were 70% (range 10–95%) and 86% (range 33–100%), respectively. Synovial fluid complement levels were normal[11].

Pleural and pericardial fluids have demonstrated sterile inflammatory exudates[5].

RADIOGRAPHY

The radiographic findings at presentation are nonspecific. Radiographs of affected joints may be normal or demonstrate soft-tissue swelling or periarticular osteopenia. With time, cartilage narrowing or erosion may be detected in the majority[5].

A characteristic late radiographic finding was noted by Medsger and Christy[21] (Fig. 22.7). They described selective nonerosive narrowing of carpometacarpal and intercarpal joint spaces of the wrist, which went on to bony ankylosis. The changes were most marked about the capitate. Bjorkengren *et al.*[22] suggested that pericapitate and intercarpal bony fusion, as opposed to merely cartilage loss, are the specific radiographic findings. These were increased six fold and 11 fold, respectively, in adult Still's disease compared to appropriately matched patients with adult RA. In contrast, radiocarpal involvement was eight times more common in RA.

Radiographic intertarsal and tarsometatarsal changes occur, albeit less frequently than wrist involvement. There are insufficient data to determine how characteristic tarsal involvement is for adult Still's disease[5]. Other uncommon features include ankylosis of the cervical spine apophyseal joints, and distal interphalangeal joint changes that clinically result in Heberden's nodes[5].

Destruction of one or both hip joints, and to a lesser extent of the knee joints, occurs, sometimes rapidly, in from 5% to over 33% of patients[5,8,11,12,23]. Unlike wrist or ankle involvement, which often results in fusion and only limited disability, the hip or knee disease is disabling and often requires total joint replacement.

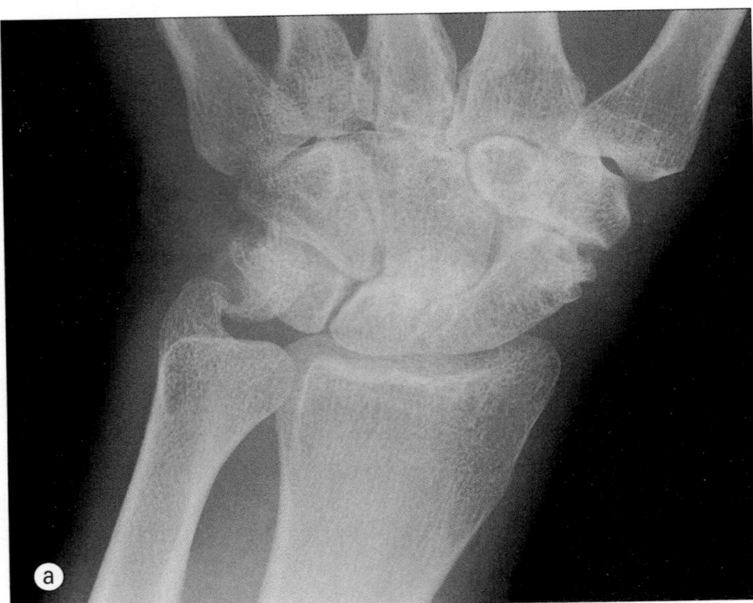

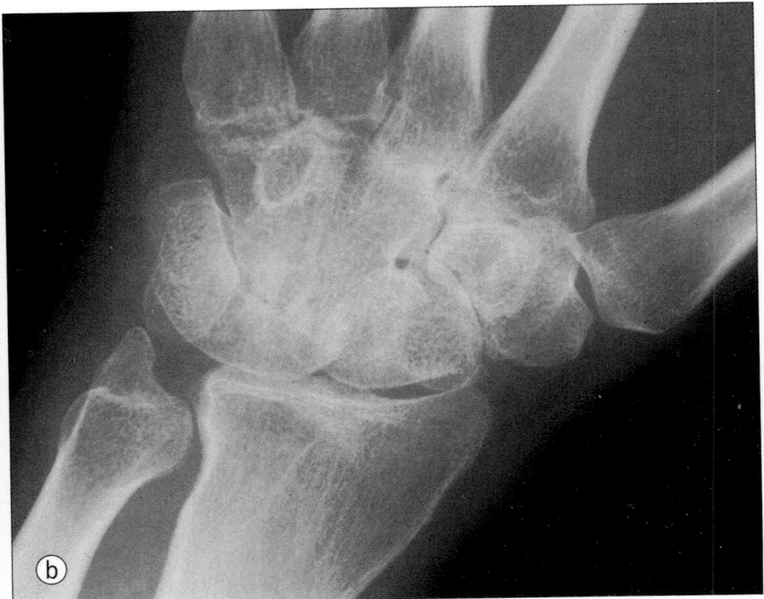

Fig. 22.7 Radiographic findings in the wrist. There is soft-tissue swelling at the wrist (a). There is pericapitate cartilage loss as well as cartilage loss between the lunate and scaphoid and the scaphoid and trapezium. The radiocarpal and radioulnar jonits are normal. More advanced changes (b). There is soft-tissue swelling and the bones are demineralized. The joint space loss is more marked than in (a) and bony fusion has occurred. There is relative sparing of the radiocarpal joint but erosive disease is present in the radioulnar joint, and the radial styloid is demineralized.

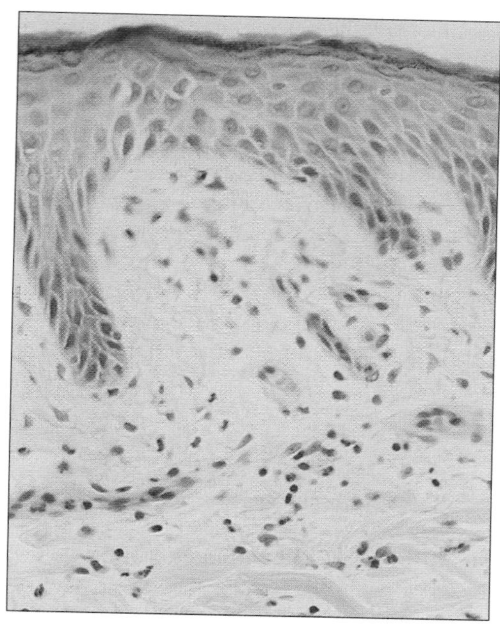

Fig. 22.8 Histopathology of Still's rash. Sparse perivascular infiltrate of lymphocytes and neutrophils in the superficial dermis with dermal edema. (Hematoxylin and eosin stain, original magnification x 25.) Courtesy of A. Kevin Watters MD.

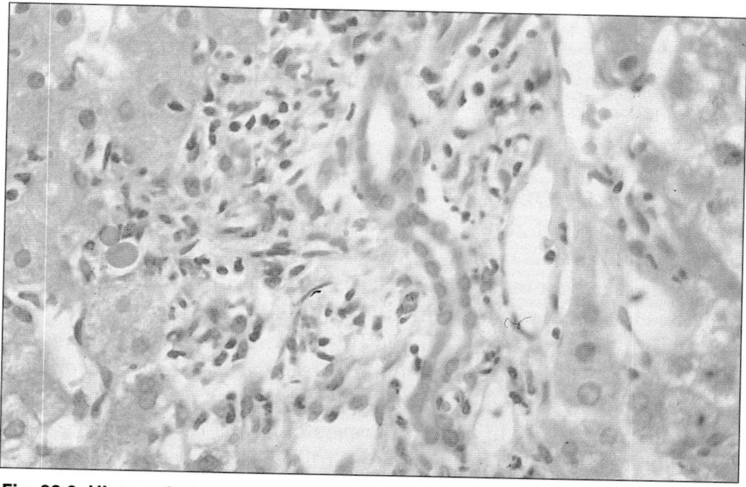

Fig. 22.9 Histopathology of Still's liver involvement. Pericholangitis in a patient with adult Still's disease not receiving anti-inflammatory drugs. The portal triad has a mixed inflammatory infiltrate consisting of polymorphonuclear leukocytes and occasional eosinophils. (Hematoxylin and eosin stain, original magnification x 250.) Courtesy of John Lough MD.

BIOPSY

The findings on biopsy of affected tissues and organs in adult Still's disease are entirely nonspecific. Thus, the place of biopsy is to exclude an alternative diagnosis that cannot be excluded clinically or by simpler investigations. Awareness of the clinical features of adult Still's disease will diminish the frequency of unnecessary tissue biopsy[9].

The most commonly performed and least invasive biopsy is skin biopsy. Histologically, the eruption consists of mild perivascular inflammation of the superficial dermis with sparse numbers of lymphocytes and neutrophils. Dermal edema is present (Fig. 22.8)[5,10]. Direct immunofluorescent study is usually negative for immunoglobulins and complement[5,11,15]. Skin biopsy may be performed to exclude vasculitis or Sweet's syndrome.

In patients who have not been treated with nonsteroidal anti-inflammatory drugs (NSAIDs), liver biopsy has demonstrated mononuclear sinusoidal and portal tract infiltrates with mild Kuppfer cell hyperplasia, even in patients with normal liver function tests (Fig. 22.9). Less frequently, focal hepatitis with feathery degeneration and necrosis of liver parenchymal cells may be seen[5,10,11]. These findings are identical to the description of salicylate hepatitis and it has been suggested that NSAIDs may unmask the underlying liver disease of adult Still's disease[8,10–12]. Massive hepatic necrosis occurs and has been fatal[5,10,17]. Liver biopsy is usually performed to exclude a granulomatous disorder such as sarcodosis.

Lymph node biopsy demonstrates infiltrates of plasma cells and polymorphonuclear leukocytes as well as signs of reactive hyperplasia[5,11]. Necrotizing lymphadenitis is a rare finding[1]. The major indication for lymph node biopsy is to exclude lymphoma[11]. Histopathology of splenic tissue is either normal or reveals histiocytic and sinus hyperplasia[5,11].

Muscle biopsies are usually normal. Occasional biopsies have demonstrated mild mononuclear infiltrates without evidence of significant necrosis. Inflammatory myositis is not a notable feature of adult Still's disease[5,11,14].

Biopsies of other tissues such as pleura and pericardium have demonstrated nonspecific inflammatory changes.

DIFFERENTIAL DIAGNOSIS

Diagnostic or classification criteria have been proposed by a number of authors[11,12,19,21,24]. The most commonly used currently are those of Cush *et al.*[12] (Fig. 22.10). Even a 'typical' patient may take weeks or months to satisfy the criteria (Fig. 22.3).

In a disease such as adult Still's, which lacks a diagnostic or confirmatory test, the diagnosis is one of exclusion and the differential diagnosis might be lengthy. Often the diagnosis will be suspected early on, and the alternative diagnoses (Fig. 22.11) can be excluded by blood cultures, serologic tests, skin tests and an occasional biopsy to exclude a specific entity. Patience and a trial of therapy are sometimes required.

CRITERIA FOR THE DIAGNOSIS OF ADULT STILL'S DISEASE
A diagnosis of adult Still's disease requires the presence of all of the following:
Fever ≥39°C
Arthralgia or arthritis
Rheumatoid factor <1:80
Antinuclear antibody <1:100
In addition to any two of the following:
White blood cell count ≥15,000 cells/mm³
Still's rash
Pleuritis or pericarditis
Hepatomegaly or splenomegaly or generalized lymphadenopathy

Fig. 22.10 Criteria for the diagnosis of adult Still's disease. Adapted from Cush *et al.*[12].

DIFFERENTIAL DIAGNOSIS OF ADULT STILL'S DISEASE	
Granulomatous disorders	Sarcoidosis, idiopathic granulomatous hepatitis, Crohn's disease
Vasculitis	Serum sickness, polyarteritis nodosa, Wegener's granulomatosis, thrombotic thrombocytopenic purpura, Takayasu's arteritis
Infection	Viral infection, such as hepatitis B, rubella, parvovirus, Coxsackie, Epstein–Barr virus, cytomegalovirus or HIV Subacute bacterial endocarditis, chronic meningococcemia, tuberculosis, Lyme disease, syphilis, rheumatic fever
Malignancy	Leukemia, lymphoma, angioblastic lymphadenopathy
Connective tissue disease	Systemic lupus erythematosus, mixed connective tissue disease

Fig. 22.11 Differential diagnosis of adult Still's disease.

ETIOLOGY AND PATHOGENESIS

Almost a century ago, George Still noted that the etiology of the disease he had described was 'very uncertain'. Uncertainty remains, but progress has been made.

INFECTIOUS ETIOLOGY

The constellation of abrupt onset, sore throat, high fever, evanescent rash, generalized adenopathy, splenomegaly and leukocytosis suggests an infectious trigger in the pathogenesis of adult Still's disease. A viral agent has been that most commonly proposed.

Rubella virus has been isolated from the urine of one patient. In two cases of systemic onset juvenile chronic arthritis (JCA), rubella virus has been identified in lymphoid tissue in one and synovial fluid in the other[5]. Serologic changes consistent with rubella have been detected in several patients with adult Still's disease, but these changes may have been nonspecific[5]. A study of five cases early in the disease detected abnormalities consistent with echovirus 7 infection in one case and with rubella infection in two others[25]. Isolated case reports have noted an association of adult Still's with Epstein–Barr virus, cytomegalovirus, mumps virus, para-influenza virus, parvovirus B19, *Yersinia enterocolitica* and *Mycoplasma pneumonia*[4,5,26].

IMMUNE COMPLEXES

Elkon *et al.*[15] have suggested that Still's disease may be a vasculitis mediated by non-necrotizing immune complexes. Circulating immune complexes have been detected in only the minority of patients, and immune reactants have only rarely been detected in biopsy tissue. Nonetheless, this hypothesis requires further study. Levels of circulating immune complexes may decline rapidly and go undetected. Nor is it incompatible with the hypothesis that an infectious agent is the trigger.

GENETIC PREDISPOSITION

As for other rheumatic diseases, an association has been sought between adult Still's disease and HLA loci. No consistent results have been obtained (Fig. 22.12). This may result from the absence of an association or from heterogeneity in the disease. Larger studies will be required to determine whether HLA associations exist within distinct subsets of adult Still's disease.

PREGNANCY AND HORMONAL INFLUENCES

Unlike adult RA and SLE, where hormonal influences have been considered potentially important, both sexes are affected with equal frequency in adult Still's disease. An exception is Japan, where women predominate[4]. Pregnancy does not appear to be a risk factor for the development of Still's disease and does not increase the risk of relapse to any extent, if at all. Also, fetal outcomes are normal in Still's disease[5,27,28].

RELATIVE RISKS FOR SELECTED HLA ANTIGENS IN ADULT STILL'S DISEASE COMPARED TO CONTROLS

Study	Elkon *et al.*[15]	Miller *et al.*[7]	Wouters[9]	Pouchot *et al.*[5]
Number of subjects	9	30(B locus) 28(DR locus)	42	55(B locus) 57(DR locus)
HLA-B35	3.8	1.1	0.1*	2.9*
HLA-DR1	2.4	1.3	0.0*	0.6
HLA-DR2	0.5	0.7	0.8	2.1*
HLA-DR4	1.6	0.4	2.2*	0.9
HLA-DR6	0.4	–	0.6	0.5
HLA-DR7	0.8	2.6*	0.7	1.2

* Significantly different from expected relative risk of 1.0

Fig. 22.12 Relative risks for selected HLA antigens in adult Still's disease compared to controls. (Data provided by Dr Jacques Pouchot.)

OTHER RISK FACTORS

A case-control study of risk factors for adult Still's disease revealed no association with smoking, alcohol consumption, diet, use of oral contraceptives, exposure to toxic substances, vaccination, blood transfusion or surgery including tonsillectomy, adenoidectomy or appendectomy. Physical and emotional stress in the year preceding the onset of Still's disease was more common than expected[27]. Allergy, possibly an allergic response to an infectious agent, has been raised as a possible cause[6,27]. These results are unconfirmed and require caution in interpretation.

MANAGEMENT

INTRODUCTION

The management of adult Still's disease is first directed at the acute systemic features of the disease. In chronic disease the arthritis is the major concern, although chronic or recurrent systemic disease occurs[2,5,12,24], especially in Japanese patients[4]. With increased knowledge of predictors for a chronic disease course, more aggressive early treatment may be warranted for those with a poorer prognosis.

Adult Still's disease predominantly affects young adults, aged 16–35 years. This is a time when those affected are attempting to make their own way as independent adults: a sudden incapacitating disease of unknown etiology can be particularly devastating. Fortunately, it is also a time when one is still resilient[5,18]. Physicians who are knowledgeable about what is understood about the prognosis and therapeutic choices, who can obtain the necessary help from allied health professionals such as physical therapists, occupational therapists and psychologists, and who can intervene to obtain appropriate support from family members, teachers or employers, will make a major difference to the well-being of their patients.

ACUTE DISEASE

Nonsteroidal anti-inflammatory drugs

Some authors favor an early use of systemic corticosteroids both as a rapid way of controlling the acute manifestations of the disease and as a means of avoiding potentially hepatotoxic NSAIDs[4,24]. Nonetheless, 20–25% of all patients do respond to NSAIDs, and an initial therapeutic trial with these agents is appropriate[2,3,5,11,12]. Those who respond frequently fall into the good prognosis group with self-limited or intermittent disease[5].

Enteric-coated aspirin has been the main NSAID used. The dose required is frequently much higher than that required for other aspirin-responsive rheumatic diseases in this age group (Fig. 22.3). An advantage of aspirin is that salicylate levels can be obtained. The desired objective is a serum level of 15–25mg/dl. The aspirin dose should be titrated cautiously to obtain this level. Why much higher doses are needed to obtain a standard anti-inflammatory level of aspirin is unknown.

Often a second NSAID may need to be added to aspirin. A number of studies found high-dose indomethacin (100–200mg/day) to be of benefit[2,9,11,14]. Other NSAIDs have been used instead of indomethacin. Response to single agent or combination NSAID treatment may be slow (Fig. 22.3).

The major concerns with NSAID therapy are hepatotoxicity and intravascular coagulation[5,8,11]. Abnormal liver function tests prior to therapy with NSAIDs do not preclude the use of these agents[5]. However, in that liver abnormality[8,10,11] and posssibly intravascular coagulopathy[8] are likely to be an integral part of the disease, frequent monitoring of liver function and clotting tests are mandatory, even after discharge from hospital, while the disease remains active.

For the acute disease, NSAIDs should be continued for 1–3 months after the disease has remitted.

Systemic corticosteroids

These agents usually provide prompt control of the acute disease. Doses of 0.5mg/kg/day to more than 1.0mg/kg/day of prednisone have been required initially[5,8,11,12,24]. Alternative day therapy has occasionally been used successfully[2,15], presumably in those with milder disease. One reason for delay in initiating corticosteroids is the well known long-term side effects of these agents[2,11,12,14–16] (see Chapter 3.6).

If a trial of NSAIDs is instituted, approximately two thirds of patients will require systemic corticosteroids in addition to the NSAIDs[5]. During tapering of the dose of corticosteroids, close monitoring of the patient is necessary, since disease exacerbations are common as the dose is reduced. Pulse methylprednisolone may be a reasonable treatment in those requiring high doses of prednisone chronically (≥ 1mg/kg/day) or in those with acute life-threatening disease[29,30].

Absolute indications for systemic corticosteroids include myocarditis, pericardial tamponade, intravascular coagulation, rising liver function tests while receiving NSAIDs and other potentially life-threatening manifestations of Still's disease. Financial considerations, such as the need for a wage earner to return to work because of the lack of disability insurance, would be another reasonable indication for initiating corticosteroid therapy early.

Relapse

Once the acute disease has remitted and a patient is off all treatment, a relapse of adult Still's disease occurs in 50% of cases. The timing of the relapse is unpredictable. The relapse tends to be milder and briefer than the initial episode and usually responds to a similar, or even less aggressive, therapeutic regimen[5,12,15].

CHRONIC DISEASE

In the literature, chronic disease has been defined as persistent disease activity 12 months after diagnosis[5,16]. Most commonly, chronic polyarthritis, frequently uncontrolled by low-dose corticosteroids (e.g. prednisone 5–20mg daily), dominates. In Caucasians chronic systemic features such as fever, rash, reticuloendothelial enlargement and serositis are less frequent than arthritis[4,5].

Second-line drugs such as intramuscular (i.m.) gold, D-penicillamine, sulfasalazine (salazopyrin) and hydroxychloroquine have been used, mainly to control articular symptoms[5]. Intramuscular gold has been used most often. Uncontrolled results suggest that up to 40% of patients may improve coincidentally with use of this agent. Immunosuppressive agents including azathioprine, cyclophosphamide and intravenous bolus cyclophosphamide have been used. Recently, low-dose methotrexate has been reported to have a corticosteroid-sparing effect[31,32]. Methotrexate has also been thought to control the systemic disease[33]. High-dose intravenous immunoglobulin infusions have been used as an experimental therapy[34].

The absence of controlled studies and the limited number of even uncontrolled long-term studies justify a conservative approach, while

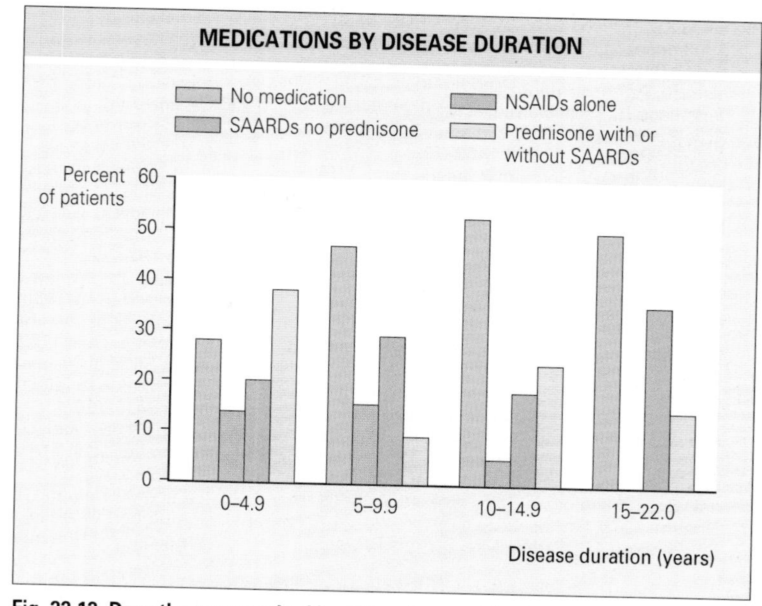

Fig. 22.13 Drug therapy required by 104 patients with adult Still's disease based on time from diagnosis. Courtesy of Sampalis *et al.*[18].

increased knowledge of predictors for chronic disease, such as root joint involvement or polyarthritis, may indicate an aggressive approach in those with these markers.

For those with persistent systemic disease without major articular involvement, hydroxychloroquine can be used early in the disease course. For those who continue to require systemic corticosteroids and hydroxychloroquine, the latter agent might be replaced with low-dose (5–15mg) once weekly methotrexate.

In patients with persistent polyarthritis, with or without root joint arthritis, a trial of i.m. gold, hydroxychloroquine or sulfasalazine could be instituted early on. Methotrexate would be reserved for those who fail on one or more of these agents, at least until more information is available on its use. Similarly, azathioprine should be reserved for those who fail on all these agents. Because of its toxicity, cyclophosphamide should be used only in the most exceptional cases, and consideration might be given to using a pulse regimen.

Patients with adult Still's disease do remit even years after disease onset[5]. Only half of the patients with adult Still's disease require pharmacologic treatment after 10 years or more of disease (Fig. 22.13)[18]. The role of treatment in disease remission is not clear, although it seems reasonable to believe that it may have helped. For those patients who remit a year or more after diagnosis, it is probably justified to continue treatment indefinitely with the safer agents (e.g. hydroxychloroquine, sulfasalazine, i.m. gold).

REFERENCES

1. Bywaters EGL. Still's disease in the adult. Ann Rheum Dis. 1971;30:121–32.
2. Larson EB. Adult Still's disease. Evolution of a clinical syndrome and diagnosis, treatment, and follow-up of 17 patients. Medicine (Baltimore). 1984;63:82–91.
3. Ohta A, Yamaguchi M, Kaneoka H, Nagayoshi T, Hiida M. Adult Still's disease: review of 228 cases from the literature. J Rheumatol. 1987;14:1139–46.
4. Ohta A, Yamaguchi M, Tsunematsu T, *et al.* Adult Still's disease: a multicenter survey of Japanese patients. J Rheumatol. 1990;17:1058–63.
5. Pouchot J, Sampalis JS, Beaudet F, *et al.* Adult Still's disease: manifestations, disease course and outcome in 62 patients. Medicine (Baltimore). 1991;70:118–36.
6. Magadur-Joly G, Billaud E, Barrier JH, *et al.* Epidemiology of adult Still's disease: estimate of the incidence by a retrospective study in west France. Ann Rheum Dis. 1995;54:587–90.
7. Miller ML, Aaron S, Jackson J, *et al.* HLA gene frequencies in children and adults with systemic onset juvenile rheumatoid arthritis. Arthritis Rheum. 1985;28:146–50.
8. Wouters JMGW, van de Putte LBA. Adult-onset Still's disease; clinical and laboratory features, treatment and progress of 45 cases. Q J Med.1986;61:1055–65.
9. Esdaile JM, Tannenbaum H, Hawkins D. Adult Still's disease. Am J Med. 1980;68:825–30.
10. Esdaile JM, Tannenbaum H, Lough J, Hawkins D. Hepatic abnormalities in adult onset Still's disease. J Rheumatol. 1979;6:673–9.
11. Reginato AJ, Schumacher HR, Baker Jr DG, O'Connor CR, Ferreiros J. Adult onset Still's disease: experience in 23 patients and literature review with emphasis on organ failure. Semin Arthritis Rheum. 1987;17:39–57.
12. Cush JJ, Medsger Jr TA, Christy WC, Herbert DC, Cooperstein LA. Adult-onset Still's disease: clinical course and outcome. Arthritis Rheum. 1987;30:186–94.
13. Del Paine DW, Leek JC. Still's arthritis in adults: disease or syndrome? J Rheumatol. 1983;10:758–62.
14. Bujak JS, Aptekar RG, Decker JL, Wolff SM. Juvenile rheumatoid arthritis presenting in the adult as fever of unknown origin. Medicine (Baltimore). 1973;52:431–44.

15. Elkon KB, Hughes GRV, Bywaters EGL, *et al.* Adult-onset Still's disease. Twenty-year follow-up and further studies of patients with active disease. Arthritis Rheum.1982;25:647–54.
16. Terkeltaub R, Esdaile JM, Décary F, *et al.* HLA–Bw35 and prognosis in adult Still's disease. Arthritis Rheum. 1981;24:1469–72.
17. Wouters JMGW, Reekers P, van de Putte LBA. Adult-onset Still's disease: disease course and HLA associations. Arthritis Rheum. 1986;29:415–18.
18. Sampalis JS, Esdaile JM, Medsger Jr TA, *et al.* A controlled study of the long-term prognosis of adult Still's disease. Am J Med. 1995;98:384–8.
19. Yamaguchi M, Ohta A, Tsunematsu T, *et al.* Preliminary criteria for classification of adult Still's disease. J Rheumatol. 1992;19:424–30.
20. Van Reeth C, Le Moel G, Lasne Y, Revenant M-C, Agneray J, Kahn M-F, Bourgeois P. Serum ferritin and isoferritins are tools for diagnosis of active adult Still's disease. J Rheumatol. 1994;21:890–5.
21. Medsger Jr TA, Christy WC. Carpal arthritis with ankylosis in late onset Still's disease. Arthritis Rheum. 1976;19:232–42.
22. Bjorkengren AG, Pathria MN, Sartoris DJ, *et al.* Carpal alterations in adult-onset Still's disease, juvenile chronic arthritis and adult-onset rheumatoid arthritis: a comparative study. Radiology. 1987;165:545–8.
23. Cabane J, Michon A, Ziza J-M *et al.* Comparison of long term evolution of adult onset and juvenile onset Still's disease, both followed up for more than 10 years. Ann Rheum Dis. 1990;49:283–5.
24. Kahn M-F, Delaire M. Maladie de Still de l'adulte. In: Maladies Systémiques. Kahn M-F, Peltier AP, eds. Paris: Flammarion, Médecine/Sciences; 1985:197–201.
25. Wouters JMGW, van der Veen J, van de Putte LBA, de Rooij DJRAM. Adult onset Still's disease and viral infections. Ann Rheum Dis. 1988;47:764–7.
26. Pouchot J, Ouakil H, Debin ML, Vinceneux P. Adult Still's disease associated with acute human parvovirus B19 infection (letter). Lancet. 1993;341:1280–1.
27. Sampalis JS, Medsger TA, Fries JF, *et al.* Risk factors for adult Still's disease. J Rheumatol. 1996;23:2049–54 .
28. Le Loët X, Daragon A, Duval C, Thonime E, Lauret P, Humbert G. Adult onset Still's disease and pregnancy. J Rheumatol. 1993;20:1158–61.
29. Kharaishi M, Fam AG. Treatment of fulminant adult Still's disease with intravenous pulse methylprednisolone therapy. J Rheumatol. 1991;18:1088–90.
30. Bisagni-Faure A, Job-Deslandre C, Menkès CJ. Treatment of Still's disease with bolus methylprednisolone. Rev Rhum Mal Osteoartic. 1992;59:228–32.
31. Bourgeois P, Palazzo E, Belmatoug N, Kahn M-F. Low dose methotrexate in adult Still's disease: second-line treatment or steroid-sparing? Arthritis Rheum. 1989;32(suppl. 60) (abstract).
32. Aydintug AO, D'Cruz D, Cervera R, Khamashta MA, Hughes GRV. Low dose methotrexate treatment in adult Still's disease. J Rheumatol. 1992;19:431–5.
33. Kraus A, Alarcón-Segovia D. Fever in adult onset Still's disease. Response to methotrexate. J Rheumatol. 1991;18:918–20.
34. Permal S, Wechsler B, Cabane J, Perrot S, Blum L, Imbert JC. Traitement de la maladie de Still de l'adulte par immunoglobulines intraveineuses. Rev Med Intern. 1995;16:250–4.

FAMILIAL MEDITERRANEAN FEVER

Mordechai Pras & Daniel L Kastner

Definition

- A genetic disorder restricted mainly to certain ethnic groups of Mediterranean and Middle Eastern origin.
- Onset usually in childhood or early adolescence.
- The FMF gene has been localized to the short arm of chromosome 16, but the metabolic deviation underlying the disorder has so far not been elucidated.

Clinical features

- Characterized by two independent phenotypic features: brief attacks of fever recurring at irregular intervals accompanied by peritonitis, arthritis or pleuritis and insidious development of systemic AA amyloidosis presenting clinically as nephropathy; and leading, in untreated patients, to terminal renal failure.
- In almost all patients, chronic colchicine treatment prevents both clinical attacks and amyloidosis.

HISTORY

Though certainly not a new disease, familial Mediterranean fever (FMF)[1] was recognized only 50 years ago[2,3]. The affected population, which lived in geographic isolation, came into contact with modern clinical science mainly after the Second World War. A small number of FMF cases are 'hidden', and discussed under a variety of names in publications from the early 1900s. In 1945 Siegal called attention to the recurrent abdominal attacks of these patients[2]. Many cases of 'periodic disease' are recognizable as typical cases of FMF[3]. In the early 1950s Mamou, Cattan and other French authors drew upon their experience with Jewish patients of North African origin and published excellent descriptions of the clinical features of FMF[4,5]. In 1954, Heller and coworkers defined the clinical features and diagnostic criteria of the disease, and named it 'familial Mediterranean fever'. They established its genetic nature, mode of inheritance and ethnic restriction, determined the fatal significance of the amyloidosis and described the articular syndrome characteristic of FMF[1,6–10]. The 4000 patients from the Tel-Hashomer hospital were mostly immigrants and their offspring from Mediterranean and Middle Eastern countries. Only symptomatic treatment was available until 1972, when Goldfinger suggested daily colchicine treatment, which prevents attacks in most patients and the development of amyloidosis probably in all of them. Large series of FMF patients have been subsequently reported among Armenians in California[11], Turks in Anatolia[12] and Arabs in the Middle East.

EPIDEMIOLOGY

FMF is ethnically restricted. The highest gene frequencies, 1:14 and 1:16, occur in the Sephardi Jews and in Armenians, while in Arabs and the Ashkenazi Jews it occurs less frequently. In contrast, FMF appears practically absent among northern Europeans, Serbians, blacks, Chinese and Indians. 'Sephardi' means Spanish and denotes the Jewish communities who lived for thousands of years around or near the shores of the Mediterranean; 'Ashkenazi' Jews derive from Eastern Europe. Though statistics are not available, among Anatolian Turks the FMF gene seems to be relatively frequent, and less so in Arabs of the Middle East. Sporadic cases have been reported from several countries. As a consequence of the mass migrations of the 20th century, cases of FMF may now be found all over the world.

A genetic analysis of 229 complete pedigrees indicated an autosomal recessive inheritance[7]. However, in one Jewish family of Georgian origin and in one Ashkenazi family, the mode of inheritance apparently conformed to dominant transmission, affecting members in four consecutive generations[13].

CLINICAL FEATURES

The febrile, painful attacks which are the hallmark of the disease are characterized by marked elevation of body temperature, acute inflammation of the peritoneum, synovia or pleura. The attacks are of short duration and patients are entirely normal between attacks.

The repetitive occurrence of the attacks at irregular intervals and in unpredictable sequence is typical of the disease. Periods of febrile attacks weekly can be followed by remissions of weeks, months or even years with no apparent cause. During the illness the patient will probably encounter several forms of attack, but the monotonous recurrence of one type over many years is not uncommon.

ABDOMINAL ATTACK

Abdominal attack is the most frequent type, experienced by 90% of the patients, in 68% of whom it is the presenting sign. Its dramatic manifestation draws attention and initiates extensive diagnostic efforts. Onset of fever up to 39–40°C is sudden, often with chills and pain spreading over the entire abdomen. As the attack gains intensity, guarding, rebound tenderness, board-like rigidity, distention and absence of peristalsis appear. Multiple small fluid levels in small bowel radiographs suggest an acute abdominal catastrophe. After 6–12 hours, signs and symptoms begin to recede, the fever drops to subfebrile levels and, within 24–72 hours, the attack is usually over, leaving the patient as well as before.

In patients operated on during attacks, the only findings have been hyperemia and a small amount of cloudy exudate rich in polymorphonuclear cells. Organization of the exudate may result in fibrous adhesions, which in rare cases may give rise to mechanical ileus. This may be responsible for chronic abdominal symptoms in some patients and ascites in others. It is probably the cause of sterility in some affected women.

PLEURAL ATTACK

Pleural attack has been experienced by 45% of our patients, and in 5% it was the presenting sign. It resembles the peritoneal attack in its abrupt onset, high fever, rapid resolution and unpredictable recurrence. The pleuritic attack may be limited to one side of the chest or might shift to the abdomen. Breathing is painful and breath sounds are diminished on the affected side. There may be radiologic evidence of a small exudate in the costophrenic angle, which is difficult to aspirate and which resolves within 48 hours. No sequelae have been noted.

ARTICULAR ATTACK

Arthritis is the second most common form of attack. It was experienced by 75% of our Sephardi patients and was the presenting symptom in 16% of them. Joint symptoms may recur for years as the only feature of the disease, until eventually other forms of attack appear[14].

The arthritic symptoms of FMF form a characteristic clinical picture. As a rule, one large joint is involved at a time, mostly in the lower extremities. Arthritic attacks may present in two forms: a short, acute or subacute form, and a chronic one. In the short attacks the onset is abrupt, fever ranges from 39–40°C lasting 24 hours and the single joint affected is tender and swollen and held immobile because of the severe pain. Redness and local heat are frequently less marked than expected in a process so acute. The signs and symptoms usually peak in 1–2 days and then gradually subside, leaving no residue. The attacks can sometimes be precipitated by trauma or effort, such as prolonged walking. Synovial effusion is often demonstrable. The synovial fluid is sterile and varies in appearance from cloudy to purulent, depending upon the acuteness and severity of the synovitis. A short attack can resolve within 3–5 days, but more commonly this takes a week and sometimes nearly a month[1].

About 6% of the patients experience protracted attacks, which are defined as persisting for more than a month. Usually the knees or hips are involved, but sometimes other joints (Fig. 23.1), such as the ankle and, rarely, the temporomandibular or the sternoclavicular joints, are affected. Rather than recovering after several days, the joint remains markedly swollen and painful, presenting a picture of chronic monoarthritis. Although spontaneous pain decreases, passive and active movements are resisted since they induce marked aggravation of pain. Atrophy of adjacent muscles appears rapidly, often within 2 weeks, and progresses proportionally to the duration of the attack, becoming extreme in the most protracted. Marked disuse osteoporosis can develop in adjacent bones leading to spontaneous fractures in rare cases. In extreme cases, the affected knee joint resembles a fluid bag (Fig. 23.2). Surprisingly, in most cases no functional impairment results. During such protracted joint attacks, short attacks involving other joints, the abdomen or chest may occur[14].

In some protracted cases, especially in the hips, damage to the joints can be so severe as to cause permanent deformity, which ultimately may require joint replacement[14]. Many knees affected by protracted arthritis regain completely normal function. Among Armenians living in California articular involvement is less common[11].

DERMAL ATTACKS

Attacks of erysipelas-like erythema is one of the most characteristic manifestations of FMF, reported in 3% to 46% of patients, sometimes combined with arthritis. Rather sharply bordered red patches, which are hot, tender and swollen, appear on the skin of the lower extremities. Usually located between the knee and ankle, or on the dorsum of the foot or ankle region, the dermatitis is often accompanied by abrupt elevation of body temperature and lasts about 24–48 hours. Biopsies of the affected skin show edema and hyperemia of the dermis, and cellular infiltration predominantly by polymorphonuclear cells.

OTHER MANIFESTATIONS

Vasculitis is more common among FMF patients than in the general population. Henoch-Schönlein purpura develops in about 5% of children with FMF. Periarteritis nodosa (PAN) has also been reported in several FMF patients[15]. Among FMF patients PAN tends to occur at a younger age, and perirenal hematoma is a more frequent complication[16]. Abdominal pain and fever are seen both in FMF attacks and in PAN; the presence of hypertension and nephritis and the persistence of symptoms favor the possibility of PAN. Hematuria, sometimes only microscopic, has been observed in some patients during and between attacks of FMF.

Various types of glomerulonephritis have also been reported in FMF, but data are insufficient to state whether these disorders are more common in FMF than in the general population[17].

Muscle pain occurs in about 20% of FMF patients. Usually the pain is not severe, appears in the lower extremities after physical exertion, lasts from a few hours to 1–2 days and subsides with rest or NSAIDs. In 12 FMF patients a syndrome of protracted, severe, debilitating myalgia accompanied by fever, abdominal pain, high ESR, leukocytosis and hyperglobulinemia. In patients that were treated by NSAIDs the attacks lasted 6–8 weeks, but all symptoms subsided promptly after a high dose of prednisone[18]. Since colchicine is known to induce neuropathy and myopathy in rare cases, especially in transplanted patients treated with cyclosporine, it is important to differentiate colchicine-induced myopathy from an attack of protracted febrile myalgia.

Among 160 patients with protracted arthritis we found a small group of 11 patients, in whom the HLA-B27 was negative, who fulfilled the criteria for seronegative spondyloarthropathy. Most of these patients responded to therapy with NSAIDs, but some of them required the addition of disease modifying anti-rheumatic drugs (DMARDs).

AMYLOIDOSIS

Amyloid nephropathy becomes first evident clinically with the appearance of proteinuria. The role of amyloidosis in the natural history of the disease was studied in an untreated group of 470 FMF patients, and some typical features were described[1]. Its clinical presentation occurs at an early age: 90% of the patients who died from amyloidosis were under the age of 40 years. Subsequent evaluation showed a lower incidence of amyloidosis in some Jewish ethnic groups and in Armenians[19]. The onset of the clinical signs of amyloidosis is not related to the frequency or intensity of the febrile attacks.

The amyloidotic nephropathy passes through several stages (Fig. 23.3). A preclinical stage exists which is diagnosable only by repeated rectal and renal biopsies, or occasionally found in a Congo red stain of a surgical specimen. Amyloidosis becomes clinically overt upon the appearance of proteinuria. This may be mild and intermittent at first, but later sustained and increasing to nephrotic proportions, progressing to uremia and renal death. Persistent proteinuria in an otherwise typical

PROTRACTED ARTHRITIS IN FMF PATIENTS

Joint	Number of patients
Knee	36
Hip	25
Ankle	7
Wrist	5
Shoulder	3
Sacroiliac	2
Sternoclavicular	2
Metatarsophalangeal	2
Elbow	1
Temporomandibular	1
Total	84

Fig. 23.1 Protracted arthritis in FMF patients. Adapted from Sneh *et al.* 14.

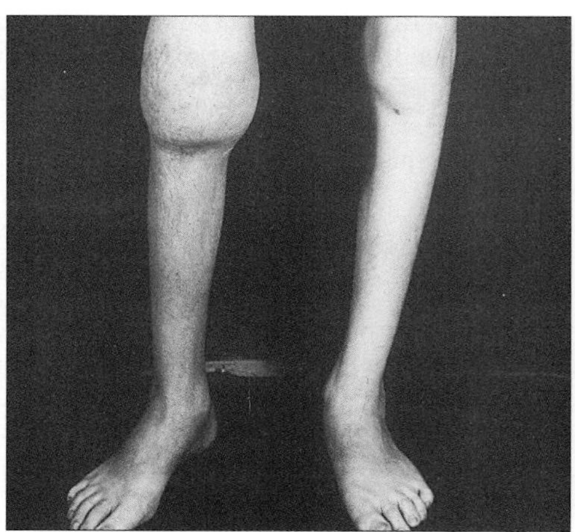

Fig. 23.2 Protracted arthritis of the right knee in a 19-year-old male, 7 months after its onset. Resolution started after 2 more months and was complete within a year (precolchicine era).

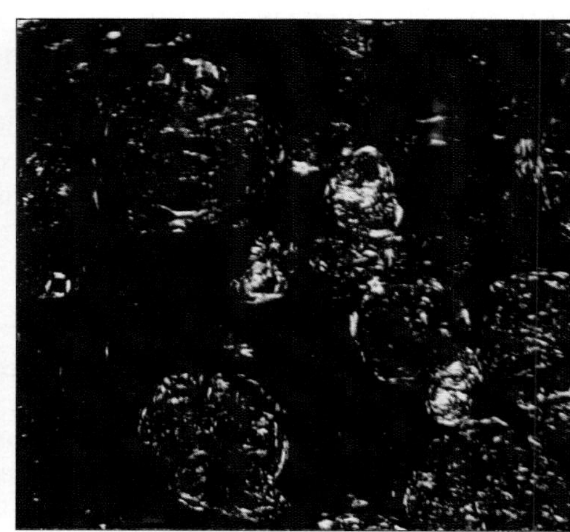

Fig. 23.3 Endstage amyloid nephropathy. Heavy AA amyloid deposits in glomeruli and blood vessels. (Polarizing microscopy of Congo red stained slide, magnification × 100.)

FMF patient has proved to be a sure indication of renal amyloidosis.

Clinical evidence of extrarenal amyloidosis is rare in early stages of the disease but may develop in end stage renal disease patients whose lives have been prolonged by chronic dialysis and renal transplantation. Adrenal insufficiency is not apparent despite the severe involvement observed at autopsy. Amyloid cardiopathy and cardiac valvular disease, hepatic amyloid, and amyloid goiter have been reported in FMF patients. The most frequent extrarenal form of amyloidosis occurs in the small bowel and leads to malabsorption.

In some patients amyloidosis occurs before the appearance of the febrile attacks, and in a few it is the only manifestation of the disease.

Amyloidosis is prevalent mainly in Jewish patients of North African origin and in Anatolian Turks. It occurs in Arabs and Ashkenazi Jews and rarely in Armenians. In the precolchicine era, only 2.5% of North African Jewish patients survived and reached the age of 40 years without demonstrating clinical signs of amyloidosis[19]. Environmental factors may also play a role in susceptibility to amyloidosis, since Armenians in Armenia reportedly have much higher rates of amyloidosis than Armenian–Americans.

INVESTIGATIONS

Laboratory findings are meager and nonspecific. Erythrocyte sedimentation rate is accelerated, and acute phase proteins such as serum amyloid A (SAA), C-reactive protein (CRP), α_2-globulin and fibrinogen are increased, particularly during attacks but also in between[1,20].

Examination of fluid from the peritoneal, pleural and synovial cavities during attacks yields a cloudy exudate, rich in fibrin and leukocytes and sterile in culture. At the height of the abdominal attack, multiple small fluid levels may be seen on radiologic examination of the abdomen. During pleural attacks there may be evidence of a small exudate on the affected side, which resolves within 48 hours.

The radiographic findings in chronic joint attacks, though not specific, are more pronounced and characteristic. During the chronic inflammation, osteoporosis around the affected joint appears out of proportion to that expected from disuse. In some of the affected hips typical osteonecrosis of the femoral head is seen, and in others there is sclerosis and narrowing of the joint space (Figs 23.4 & 23.5).

Histologic examination of the synovia during acute attacks shows acute inflammation, with enlarged synovial lining cells and infiltration of subjacent fibrous tissue by polymorphonuclear cells. In protracted attacks chronic synovitis with nodular perivascular aggregation of lymphocytes is seen. In patients with joint involvement there are no LE cells, antinuclear factor or rheumatoid factor, and there is no elevation of antistreptolysin-O titers.

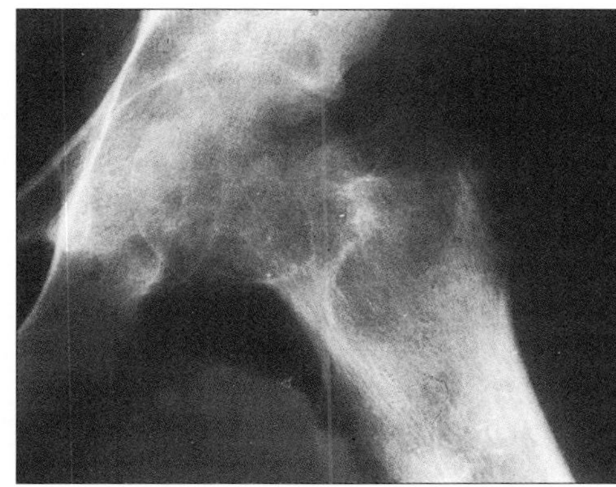

Fig. 23.4 Radiograph of protracted arthritis of right hip in a 22-year-old male. Lytic lesions, osteonecrosis and narrowing of the joint space can be seen.

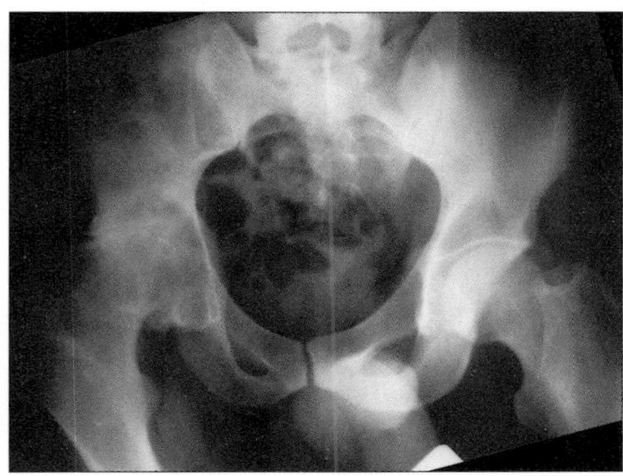

Fig. 23.5 Radiograph of protracted arthritis of right hip in a 36-year-old male, showing sclerosis and narrowing of the joint space.

TEL-HASHOMER CRITERIA FOR THE DIAGNOSIS OF FMF
Major criteria 1. Recurrent febrile episodes accompanied by peritonitis, synovitis or pleuritis. 2. Amyloidosis of the AA-type without predisposing disease. 3. Favorable response to continuous colchicine treatment.
Minor criteria 1. Recurrent febrile episodes. 2. Erysipelas-like erythema. 3. FMF in a first degree relative.
Definitive diagnosis: 2 major or 1 major and 2 minor. Probable diagnosis: 1 major and 1 minor.

Fig. 23.6 Tel-Hashomer criteria for the diagnosis of FMF.

DIFFERENTIAL DIAGNOSIS

The diagnosis of FMF must be made on clinical grounds, since there is no specific test available. Although the infusion of metaraminol reportedly induced mild attacks in FMF patients but not in controls, there are serious concerns about the safety of this test, and it is therefore not recommended. The combination in an otherwise healthy child, or young adult, of irregularly recurrent, short, febrile episodes; abdominal, arthritic or pleuritic symptoms; a favorable response to colchicine; and AA amyloidosis in the absence of another disease are the main features on which the diagnosis should be based.

Other hereditary causes of intermittent fever and abdominal pain include the hyperimmunoglobulinemia D syndrome and familial Hibernian fever. The hyper-IgD syndrome can be distinguished by the frequent occurrence of a characteristic skin rash, the presence of lymphadenopathy, and elevated serum IgD levels. It is apparently inherited as an autosomal recessive gene, and thus far has been reported primarily in Western European populations. Familial Hibernian fever differs from FMF in that it is inherited as a dominant trait, has only been described among the Irish and symptoms respond to corticosteroids but not to colchicine.

A syndrome of recurrent high fever lasting 4–8 days was described in children, often accompanied by pharyngitis and cervical lymphadenopathy. The febrile attacks that recur every 2–9 weeks did not respond to antibiotics, NSAIDs or colchicine, but did resolve with prednisone[21].

Diagnostic criteria for FMF have been developed (Fig. 23.6). Either two of the major criteria, or of one major and two minor criteria, is enough to establish a definite diagnosis of FMF, while that of one major and one minor is considered a probable diagnosis. Ethnic origin (Sephardi Jewish, Armenian or Anatolian Turk) and elevated ESR and acute reactive proteins cannot serve as criteria, but can add support to the diagnosis.

PATHOPHYSIOLOGIC MECHANISMS

Amyloidosis in FMF is of the AA type[20]. Its structure does not differ from the AA fibrils of reactive amyloidosis of, for example, rheumatoid arthritis, tuberculosis, Hodgkin's disease or hypernephroma. FMF amyloidosis is the only preventable form of systemic amyloidosis (see Chapter 8.27).

The special attention accorded to SAA is due to the fact that its N-terminal fragment is AA protein, which is the protein part of the amyloid AA fibril. Serum amyloid A is greatly increased in amyloidotic FMF patients and in all FMF patients during acute attacks[20]. The high levels decrease gradually in the days following an attack. However, even during remission, SAA levels in FMF patients are usually two or three times the normal value. Since SAA is a universal acute phase protein, it is elevated in other inflammatory febrile diseases and therefore cannot be considered a diagnostic measure of FMF.

A C5a inhibitor deficiency in joint and peritoneal fluids from FMF patients may play a role in the febrile attacks. An unconfirmed abnormality in catecholamine metabolism (high levels of dopamine β-hydroxylase in untreated patients) was suggested as a pathogenetic mechanism.

GENETIC STUDIES

FMF is caused by a single autosomal recessive gene that has been mapped to a small interval on the short arm of chromosome 16 between the gene causing adult-onset polycystic kidney disease and the gene of Rubinstein–Taybi syndrome[22]. The function of its encoded protein and the pathogenesis of the inflammatory attacks of the disease remain to be elucidated. The same locus is implicated in Jews, Arabs, Armenians and Turks. Identical twins are concordant for FMF, although there are differences in the type and severity of attacks. Because of the recessive mode of inheritance, a history of consanguinity is often elicited, especially in families from the Middle East.

MANAGEMENT

Daily prophylactic colchicine treatment for FMF was first suggested by Goldfinger in 1972[23] and its efficacy in preventing attacks shown by double blind studies[24]. Since the dose is not weight dependent, treatment is started with 1mg/day colchicine, regardless of age or severity of attacks. If necessary this dose is increased to 1.5mg/day and later to 2mg/day, until remission from attacks is achieved. Doses larger than 1mg have to be divided in two. If 2mg/day does not produce remission, further elevation of the dose does not improve responsiveness. Omission of the daily dose may be followed promptly by an attack.

Of these patients, 65% enjoy complete remission of attacks if they adhere to their daily dose of colchicine. Partial remission, defined as either a significant decrease in the frequency and severity of all forms of attack or remission of one form (usually abdominal) but not of another (usually arthritic), is experienced by an additional 30%, but protracted arthritis is a rarity among treated patients in partial remission. In 5% of the treated patients the attack rate remains unchanged. These patients are maintained on 2mg/day to prevent amyloidosis.

Continuous prophylactic colchicine treatment in FMF patients prevents the development of nephropathic amyloidosis[25]. None of our patients who started treatment without proteinuria have developed amyloidosis (22 years of follow up) while an involuntary 'control group' of noncompliant patients showed a 30% incidence – the same rate of amyloidosis as expected in the natural history of the disease.

The side effects of colchicine are mild in the main. Diarrhea and nausea are the most common and usually prove transient and easily controllable. Desensitization by progressively increasing doses of colchicine makes possible continuation of the drug in cases of angioneurotic edema, epistaxis and leukopenia. Intravenous (i.v.) injections of colchicine to FMF patients should be restricted to patients who cannot ingest food, such as those undergoing surgery. Fatal toxicity has been reported in FMF patients who have been treated with high doses of i.v. colchicine in the setting of an acute FMF attack.

Hundreds of children have taken the drug daily for more than 10 years, and in none of them, including children in their first decade of life, has colchicine caused any deviation from normal in physical examination, routine laboratory tests, linear growth or sexual development.

In our first series of 91 pregnancies in colchicine-treated FMF patients, two cases of trisomy 21 occurred. No further cases were found in a subsequent 110 closely monitored pregnancies under colchicine treatment, or in a total of 420 amniocenteses of colchicine-treated FMF patients in Israel. We also encountered two babies with Down's syndrome that were born to colchicine-treated FMF fathers. Routine amniocentesis is recommended to exclude chromosomal aberrations possibly related to colchicine.

Many FMF patients, who in the precolchicine era deteriorated to terminal renal failure due to amyloidosis, were treated by dialysis or transplanted. It seems that patients with renal amyloidosis of FMF fare better with transplantation than with dialysis treatment. A daily dose of 1.5–2.0mg colchicine protects the engrafted kidney by delaying the development of amyloidosis.

Prevention of amyloidosis requires strict adherence to daily prophylactic colchicine treatment. This is also vital in patients who have not experienced attacks for months or even years. There are cases on record in which lapses of treatment, or noncompliance in adhering to the drug for relatively short periods of time, brought about clinically manifest amyloidosis.

REFERENCES

1. Sohar MJ, Gafni J, Pras M, Heller H. Familial Mediterranean fever. A survey of 470 cases and review of the literature. Am J Med. 1967;43:227–53.
2. Siegal S. Benign paroxysmal peritonitis. Ann Intern Med. 1945;2:1–21.
3. Reimann HA. Periodic disease. Probable syndrome including periodic fever, benign paroxysmal peritonitis, cyclic neutropenia, and intermittent arthralgia. JAMA. 1948;136;239–44.
4. Mamou H, Cattan R. La maladie periodique (sur 14 cas personnels dont 8 compliques de nephropathies). Sem Hop Paris. 1952;28:1062–70.
5. Siguier F, Zara M, Funck-Bretano JL, Lagrue G. Maladies periodiques a formes degradees evoluant chez plusieurs members d'une meme famille. Bull Mem Soc Med Hop Paris. 1954;69:679–84.
6. Heller H, Sohar E, Sherf L. Familial Mediterranean fever. Arch Intern Med. 1958;102:50–71.
7. Sohar E, Pras M, Heller J, Heller H. Genetics of familial Mediterranean fever. Arch Intern Med. 1961;107:529–38.
8. Heller H, Sohar E, Gafni J, Heller H. Amyloidosis in familial Mediterranean fever. Arch Intern Med.1961;107:539–50.
9. Gafni J, Ravid M, Sohar E. The role of amyloidosis in familial Mediterranean fever. A population study. Isr J Med Sci. 1968;4:995–9.
10. Heller H, Gafni J, Michaeli D, *et al.* The arthritis of familial Mediterranean fever (FMF). Arthritis Rheum. 1966;9:1–17.
11. Rogers DB, Shoat M, Peterson GM, *et al.* Familial Mediterranean fever in Armenians Am J Med Genet. 1989;34:168–72.
12. Ozdemir AI, Cavit S. Familial Mediterranean fever among the Turkish people. Am J Gastroenterol. 1969;51:311–6.
13. Yuval Y, Hemo-Zisser M, Zemer D, Sohar E, Pras M. Dominant inheritance in two families with familial Mediterranean fever. Am J Med Genet. 1995;57:455–7.
14. Sneh E, Pras M, Michaeli D, Shahi N, Gafni J. Protracted arthritis in familial Mediterranean fever. Rheumatol Rehabil. 1977;16:102–6.
15. Glikson M, Galun E, Schlezinger M,*et al.* Polyarteritis nodosa and familial Mediterranean fever. A report of two cases and review of the literature. J Rheumatol. 1989;16:536–9.
16. Sachs D, Langevitz P, Morag B, Pras M. Polyarteritis nodosa in familial Mediterranean fever. Br J Rheumatol. 1987:26:139–41.
17. Said R, Hamzeh Y, Said S, Tarawneh M, Al-Khateeb M. Spectrum of renal involvment in familial Mediterranean fever. Kidney Int. 1992;41:414–19.
18. Langevitz P, Zemer D, Linveh A, Shemer J, Pras M. Protracted febrile myalgia in patients with familial Mediterranean fever. J Rheumatol. 1994;21:1708–9.
19. Pras M, Bronshpigel N, Zemer D, Gafni J. Variable incidence of amyloidosis in familial Mediterranean fever among different ethnic groups. Johns Hopkins Med J. 1982;150:22–6.
20. Knecht A, De Beer FC, Pras M. Serum amyloid A protein in familial Mediterranean fever. Ann Intern Med. 1985;102:71–2.
21. Marcshall GS, Edwards KM, Butler J, Lawton AR. Periodic fever, pharyngitis and aphthous stomatitis. J Paediatr. 1987;110:43–6.
22. Pras E, Aksentijevich I, Gruberg L, *et al.* Mapping of a gene causing familial Mediterranean fever to the short arm of chromosome 16. N Engl J Med. 1992;326:1509–13.
23. Goldfinger SE. Colchicine therapy for familial Mediterranean fever. N Engl J Med. 1974;291:934–7.
24. Zemer D, Revach M, Pras M, *et al.* A controlled of trial of colchicine in preventing attacks of familial Mediterranean fever. N Engl J Med.1974;291:932–4.
25. Zemer D, Pras M, Sohar E, Modan B, Cabili S, Gafni J. Colchicine in the prevention and treatment of the amyloidosis of familial Mediterranean fever. N Engl J Med. 1986;314:1001–5.

JUVENILE CHRONIC ARTHRITIS

24

PRACTICAL PROBLEMS

NONORGANIC MUSCULOSKELETAL PAINS IN CHILDREN

Peter Hollingworth

DEFINITION OF THE PROBLEM

Musculoskeletal pains without apparent cause are reported in 4–15% of children in the community and up to 25% of children attending a pediatric rheumatology clinic.

Many will improve without a diagnosis being made. In some, a change in the line of questioning, a more pertinent examination or the appropriate test reveals the diagnosis, often minor and responding to simple measures or reassurance, but occasionally a serious non-rheumatologic disorder. In others, the diagnosis becomes apparent only after extended follow up.

A substantial minority remain in whom nonorganic factors are suspected. Nonorganic symptoms are a common cause of confusion in children suffering or recovering from recognized rheumatic diseases.

SOME DISORDERS THAT CAUSE DIAGNOSTIC DIFFICULTIES
Infection post-immunization
Human parvovirus
Adenovirus
Rubella
Mycoplasma
Borrelia
Orthopedic causes
Overuse syndromes
Neurologic disease
Hypermobility
Synovitis, enthesitis, arthritis (SEA) syndrome
Osteoid osteoma
Immunodeficiency
Malignancy, e.g. preleukemic leukemia
Cold sensitivity
Sarcoidosis
Inherited epiphyseal dysplasias
Storage diseases
Hemoglobinopathies
Inherited connective tissue diseases
Autoimmune connective tissue diseases
Regional osteoporosis
Osteochondritis

Fig. 24.1 Disorders to consider if an organic cause is suspected in children with nonorganic musculoskeletal pains.

In some, the problem can be recognized: attention seeking, school phobia, 'growing pains', fibromyalgia, reflex sympathetic dystrophy or conversion hysteria. Others will defy such specific diagnoses, while seeming to lie within their ambit.

THE TYPICAL CASE

JK, a 12-year-old girl, was brought by her mother for evaluation of joint pain and stiffness that had resulted in increasing absenteeism from school. Over the past several months the child had complained of diffuse joint pains. The symptoms were most notable in the morning, causing her to remain in bed until midday and stay home from school for 1–2 days each week. On physical examination, the girl was afebrile and in the 90th percentile of height and weight. The musculoskeletal examination was entirely normal. Laboratory studies revealed a white blood cell (WBC) count of 6.7×10^9/l with normal differential, hemoglobin of 13.5g/dl and a Westergren erythrocyte sedimentation rate (ESR) of 10mm/h.

DIAGNOSTIC PROBLEMS

Figure 24.1 lists some of the disorders to be considered if an organic cause is still suspected even though the examination and the usual screening tests are normal. Hypermobility warrants special mention: peripubertal girls are particularly affected, presenting with usually lower-limb joint pains after exercise (see Chapters 4.18 and 8.51).

Musculoskeletal symptoms in children felt to have a predominantly nonorganic cause can be due to:

- attention seeking,
- growing pains, recurrent limb pains,
- conversion hysteria,
- school phobia and
- fibromyalgia, reflex sympathetic dystrophy and related disorders.

Attention seeking

Young children soon learn that complaints of pain receive particular notice and may copy family members with rheumatic complaints.

'Growing pains'; recurrent limb pains

Growing pains and recurrent limb pains seem to be a distinct entity. The child wakes at night crying from pain in the legs, the calves, shins or thighs, but settles when they are rubbed. This happens repeatedly over several months. In one third, the upper limbs or trunk are also affected. Symptoms by day are uncommon and there is never a limp. Four percent of children are affected, girls and boys equally, chiefly aged 6–13 years. Recurrent abdominal pain or headaches are common at the same time or later, and the parents often give a similar history from their childhood. Stress factors such as bullying, lack of friends or domestic difficulties are usual.

Conversion hysteria

Musculoskeletal complaints are a common manifestation of conversion hysteria which often follows a minor illness. The symptoms and signs are typically manifestly bizarre, grossly exaggerated and wholly inappropriate to an organic disorder. Tertiary referrals have often undergone extensive investigations. Trick maneuvers often reveal the nonorganic nature of the signs. An interest in amateur dramatics should raise suspicion. Frequently, overt psychopathology is strikingly absent as the purpose is to communicate the child's distress in a coded form.

School phobia

The child with school phobia complains of vague limb pains on the morning of, or night before, school and consequently has a poor attendance record. However, the pains usually resolve after the school bus has left and rarely occur at weekends or on holiday.

Fibromyalgia, reflex sympathetic dystrophy and related disorders

Fibromyalgia, reflex sympathetic dystrophy and related disorders are believed to represent a continuum as they share a similar epidemiology, certain features and patterns of psychopathology. Typically, the child is a pubescent girl. Half or more have pain in multiple sites and in the remainder it is localized. In 10% the pattern switches from one to the other. The majority of either group respectively fulfil criteria for fibromyalgia or reflex sympathetic dystrophy in adults. The remainder seem to fit in a continuum between the two. In many, the onset follows a minor illness or injury. Headaches and abdominal pains are common and these children feel globally less well than children with proven arthritis. While their pain and disability is often incapacitating and unresponsive to the usual measures, they commonly remain incongruously cheerful.

Signs of note include hyperesthesia on stroking the affected part and, in reflex sympathetic dystrophy, the *tache cérébrale*: a stroke with a blunt object causes a weal in 20 seconds, persisting for 5 minutes in the affected limb only. This sign of autonomic dysfunction is also seen in known central nervous system disease. The radionuclide bone scan is often abnormal in those with localized pain, some not fulfilling criteria for reflex sympathetic dystrophy.

Two patterns of family dynamics are recognized. In one, the family is cohesive, stable and intolerant of separation. In the other it is chaotic and unsupportive with high levels of conflict. In both, the closeness between mother and child appears to be inappropriate, with the parent speaking for the child, and overt nonverbal messages passing between them. If a hospital admission is suggested, the mother typically becomes unduly distressed and it transpires the child has never spent a night away from home.

Other stress factors may be identified or suspected, such as domestic strife, unrealistic academic expectations or sexual abuse. Frank depression is rare. The majority respond to physical therapy, sometimes with psychotherapy, within a year, though relapses are common.

THERAPEUTIC OPTIONS

Organic disease needs to be excluded but without over- or repeated investigation as this implies that an organic cause is still suspected. The problem should be approached with delicacy, sensitivity and tact. The clinician should avoid saying that there is nothing wrong or that it is psychosomatic, so suggesting to the child, the parents and nonmedical colleagues that it is 'all in the mind'. It is unhelpful to deliberate whether the problem is predominantly psychologic or organic. It is important to recognize that treatment must be multifaceted. The child and parents should know that the symptoms are being taken seriously and are not being dismissed because they are believed to arise from nonorganic pain.

Secondary problems, such as flexion contractures, which may occur in conversion hysteria require treatment. There may also be a social handicap, such as transport to school, that needs to be managed. The child should be approached optimistically and reassured that, with treatment, he or she will improve. It is important to look for psychologic stresses and address them. Liaison with nonmedical colleagues is helpful. In conversion hysteria a conjoint family assessment and active psychotherapeutic management are necessary.

Whatever the diagnosis, rest or immobilization worsens the problem. A cornerstone of treatment is a program of graded physical activity supervised by the physical therapist. This rehabilitates underused joints and provides a face-saving way through to recovery. Early intervention may relieve the immediate morbidity, such as loss of schooling, and could prevent persisting symptoms.

CONCLUSION

Non-organic causes must be considered in a child with limb pain when the cause is not obvious. Diagnosis and management require particular skills and sensitivity. Serious and protracted disability commonly results without appropriate intervention.

REFERENCES

Cincuttini F, Littlejohn GO. Female adolescent rheumatological presentations: the importance of chronic pain syndromes. Aust Paediat J. 1989;25:21–4.

Malleson PN, Al-Matar M, Petty RE. Idiopathic musculoskeletal pain syndromes in children. J Rheumatol. 1992;19:1786–9.

Sherry DD, McGuire T, Mellins E, *et al.* Psychosomatic musculoskeletal pain in childhood: clinical and psychological analysis of 100 children. Pediatrics. 1991;88;1093–9.

TOXIC SYNOVITIS OF THE HIP

Charlotte Grondin

DEFINITION OF THE PROBLEM

Toxic synovitis of the hip is the most common cause of hip pain in children aged 18 months to 13 years. The peak incidence is between 4 and 7 years of age; boys are affected more than girls. This is a benign self-limiting condition of acute onset, which is often preceded by a respiratory tract infection within the previous 2 weeks. The acute illness lasts 5–35 days with an average duration of 16 days. Bilateral involvement and recurrences may be seen. The etiology remains unknown. The infrequent long-term sequelae include a moderate overgrowth of the femoral head and a persistent widening of the joint space.

THE TYPICAL CASE

A 4-year-old boy was first seen in the clinic with a 2-day history of limping and pain in the right knee and hip. There was no history of trauma or previous hip problems. He had had an upper respiratory tract infection 1 week before, with a fever of 38°C for 24 hours. Upon examination, he appeared well and was afebrile. There was some guarding on movement of the right hip, which had painful mild restriction of abduction and internal rotation; the spine, pelvis and abdomen were normal, as were the other joints. Complete blood count (CBC) and urinalysis were normal. The ESR was increased to 25mm/h. A throat swab for *S. pyogenes* was negative. Radiographs of the pelvis and both hips

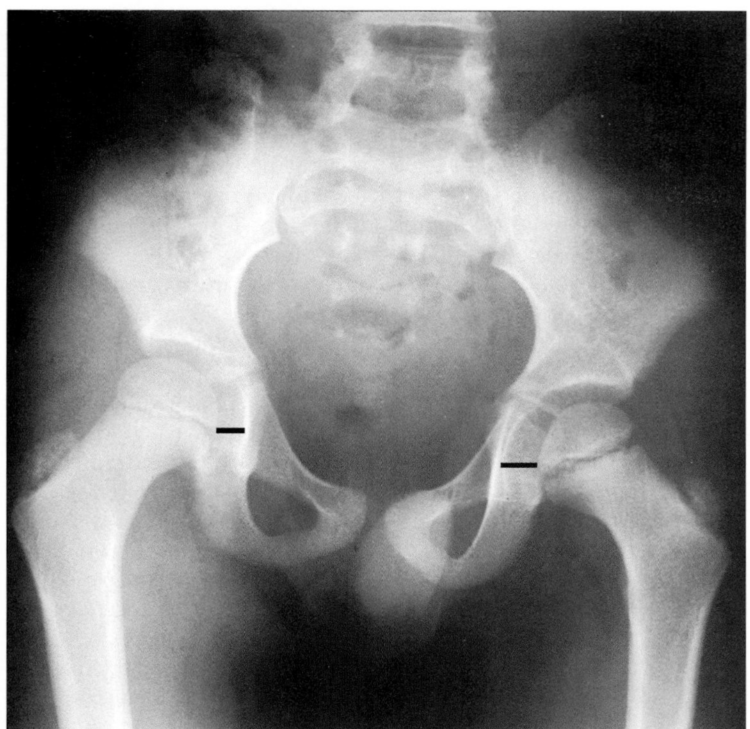

Fig 24.2 Widening of the medial joint space in toxic synovitis of the left hip.

were normal. A presumptive diagnosis of toxic synovitis of the hip was made. The child was treated with acetaminophen (paracetamol) and bed rest at home, and the parents were instructed to return if the condition worsened or if fever recurred. At the follow up visit, 1 week later, the child had fully recovered.

DIAGNOSTIC PROBLEMS

Limping associated with painful limitation of the hip is the predominant complaint in toxic synovitis of the hip as well as in other conditions, such as septic arthritis, osteomyelitis, Legg–Perthes disease, slipped capital femoral epiphysis, neoplasia, osteoid osteoma, juvenile chronic arthritis (JCA) and, less commonly, sickle cell disease and hemophilia. The initial diagnostic steps include a history and physical examination, CBC, differential leukocyte count, ESR, urinalysis and a throat swab for *S. pyogenes*. The results of these tests are normal in most cases of toxic synovitis of the hip. Radiographs of the pelvis and both hips, anteroposterior and frog views, are also usually normal, though joint-space widening has been described (Fig. 24.2). The subsequent course of the disease will confirm the diagnosis of toxic synovitis of the hip.

Toxic synovitis of the hip may present with low-grade fever, a slightly increased leukocyte count, and a moderately increased ESR. If the effusion in the hip joint is important, the child may be irritable and have moderate limitation of hip movement. In the presence of persistent fever, blood and urine cultures should be performed and the child hospitalized. Hip joint aspiration should be performed to rule out septic arthritis, especially if clinical signs worsen or if a high spiking fever is associated with severe hip pain and limitation at the initial presentation. Unless the systemic features subside within a few days after admission, technetium and gallium scintigraphy should be performed to exclude osteomyelitis and septic arthritis. A bloody joint effusion suggests hemophilia, which should be confirmed by the appropriate coagulation tests.

Legg–Perthes disease predominantly affects boys in the age group 3–12 years and is bilateral in 10% of cases (see Chapter 8.48). In earlier retrospective reports, toxic synovitis of the hip was associated with the risk of subsequent Legg–Perthes' disease in 1–20% of the cases, whereas Landin *et al.* reported in their prospective study a risk of 3.7%. On the initial radiographs, one should look for early signs of Legg–Perthes disease, which include subchondral translucency of the femoral epiphysis and smaller epiphysis on the affected side. In children with toxic synovitis of the hip, early recurrences of symptoms or prolonged bed rest to regain a normal painless hip movement have been associated with subsequent Legg–Perthes disease. These children should therefore be followed more closely and bone scintigraphy and/or magnetic resonance imaging (MRI) should be done in doubtful cases.

Slipped capital femoral epiphysis should be suspected in the obese or the tall slim young patient. The clinical course is prolonged if not treated, and initial radiographs show widening of the epiphyseal line and irregular demineralization of the adjacent area.

Hip pain and limping may be the presenting complaints of neuroblastomas in younger children. In leukemia and other solid tumors, the pain may be out of proportion to the physical findings. Neoplasms should be suspected if there are systemic signs associated with severe anemia, leukopenia or thrombocytopenia, and/or blast cells on the peripheral blood smear. Radiographs may be normal or show pathologic fractures, lytic lesions or a periosteal reaction. Bone scintigraphy may be useful to demonstrate metastases.

Osteoid osteomas occur mainly in the proximal half of the femur and may simulate synovitis when near the hip joints. However, at presentation, the symptoms have usually been present for a long time, and the pain is worse at night and is relieved with aspirin. Physical findings may already include thigh atrophy and leg-length inequality. On radiographs, a central nidus circumscribed by a thin translucent peripheral rim, which in turn is surrounded by a zone of dense bone sclerosis, is typical of osteoid osteoma. If radiographs are normal, radioisotope bone scan and computed tomography (CT) scan should be performed to demonstrate the lesion.

Juvenile chronic arthritis rarely presents with hip monoarthritis and therefore remains a diagnosis of exclusion. Older boys who are HLA-B27 positive, rheumatoid factor negative, and have enthesitis and a family history positive for uveitis, psoriasis, inflammatory bowel disease (IBD) or spondyloarthropathy (SEA syndrome) form a subset of pauciarticular JCA which may present with arthritis predominating in the lower extremities. In this subgroup, IBD must be considered, once septic arthritis has been excluded, especially if there is a persistent fever associated with hip synovitis.

THERAPEUTIC OPTIONS

Most cases of toxic synovitis of the hip are managed at home with bed rest and acetaminophen. Mobilization is allowed when the child is pain free and the hip has recovered a full range of movement. However, complete prevention of weight bearing on the involved hip is often difficult to achieve. Admission to the hospital must be considered in a child with borderline clinical features suggesting septic arthritis. Skin traction with the hip flexed at 45° and nonsteroidal anti-inflammatory drugs (NSAIDs) may relieve severe hip pain. Follow up visits, until the child has recovered, are necessary to confirm the initial diagnosis.

CONCLUSIONS

Toxic synovitis of the hip is the most common cause of hip pain in children. This benign, acute, self-limiting condition may mimic more serious problems that may require further investigation. Bed rest and acetaminophen remain the treatment of choice.

REFERENCES

Aston JW. Pediatric update No. 16: the orthopaedic presentation of neuroblastoma. Orthop Rev. 1990;19:929–32.

Choban S, Killian JT. Evaluation of acute gait abnormalities in preschool children. J Pediatr Orthop. 1990;10:74–8.

Haueisen DC, Weiner DS, Weiner SD. The characterization of 'transient synovitis of the hip' in children. J Pediatr Orthop. 1986;6:11–17.

Kallio P, Ryoppy S, Kunnamo I. Transient synovitis and Perthes' disease. Is there an aetiological connection? J Bone Jt Surg. 1986;68B:808–11.

Landin LA, Danielsson LG, Wattsgard C. Transient synovitis of the hip. Its incidence, epidemiology and relation to Perthes' disease. J Bone Jt Surg. 1987;69B:238–42.

Petty RE, Malleson P: Spondylarthropathies of childhood. Pediatr Clin North Am. 1986;33:1079–96.

DEFINITION OF THE PROBLEM

Parents of children with JCA commonly ask how much exercise they should allow, often fearing that the child will damage his or her joints. In brief, the advice is for as much exercise as can be encouraged, but with certain provisos, depending on the age of the child and the severity and extent of the arthritis.

THE TYPICAL CASE

FM is a 7-year-old boy with pauciarticular JCA. He was first seen 2 years ago with acute swelling of both knees, left ankle and right elbow. Over the past 6 months he has been treated with aspirin (75mg/kg/day) and oral methotrexate (10mg/m^2/week) with good results. On physical examination, there was mild tenderness and swelling evident in the right elbow; the knees and ankles were entirely normal. The boy and his father asked for advice as to whether he would be able to play on the school basketball team this season.

THERAPEUTIC OPTIONS

Inactivity is deleterious and liable to be enforced by parents whose response is to overprotect and infantilize their child. A striking feature of JCA is the propensity to periarticular fibrosis with the early development of flexion contractures, restricted joint movement and muscle wasting. Regular exercise is the cornerstone of prevention (Fig. 24.3): even a child with severe systemic disease should be encouraged to walk every day.

Lack of weight bearing is thought to contribute to the growth abnormalities of the hips seen when JCA starts before the age of 5 years. A thick anteverted vertical femoral neck bears an enlarged femoral head subluxing laterally out of a shallow acetabulum. While hyperemia is thought to contribute to these changes, they also develop in symptomless hips of children unable to walk owing to knee disease. The dysplasia is believed to predispose to the development of destructive changes.

AN APPROACH TO EXERCISE IN JUVENILE CHRONIC ARTHRITIS

Exercise helps prevent impairment of joint function from:
- Flexion contractures
- Joint restriction
- Muscle wasting
- Growth defects
- Cartilage loss

Participation in games and sports can help emotional difficulties:
- Feeling different
- Social isolation
- Poor self-image

Encourage swimming and cycling

Avoid:
- Body-contact sports
- Repeated impact loading in lower-limb joint disease
- Rugby with neck involvement
- Jumps or point work in ballet
- Riding with hip disease

Formal physical therapy is essential:
- Supervised by the parents
- Seen as a routine
- A general exercise regime

Balance exercise with appropriate rest

Make exercise possible:
- Encourage the child
- Counsel parents
- Liaise with the school, community and other health workers
- Clubs for the disabled
- State aid for transport
- Treat joints preventing exercise

Fig. 24.3 An approach to exercise in JCA.

Limited joint motion contributes to cartilage loss in hips and knees. Restoration of mobility, notably of the hips following soft tissue release, can be accompanied by radiographic improvement, with widening of the joint space and smoothing of the articular surface from 'healing' by fibrocartilage.

Exercise cannot damage the articular surface but inflamed joints and weak muscles predispose to injury which takes longer to heal than in healthy joints. Accordingly, until synovitis is settled and the muscles are strengthened, repeated impact loading should be avoided with lower limb joint disease, as should body-contact sports, jumps and point work in ballet, rugby with neck disease, and horse-riding with hip disease.

Swimming and cycling should be encouraged. The former is the one sport in which arthritic children can excel. Many public swimming pools are fitted with hoists and have sessions for disabled people. While expensive low-resistance bicycles are available, a 'normal' geared cycle is as effective and more acceptable.

Above all, these children want to be normal and like other children. Social isolation is a common difficulty and often does not correlate with the severity of the disease, with some of the most mildly affected children being the most severely isolated. This can stem from withdrawal because of a poor self-image, impaired mobility (both locomotor and transport) and parental overprotection. Factors such as these may leave the child with emotional problems more disabling than any physical handicap. These difficulties may be minimized by encouraging participation in physical activities in school and in clubs, some designated for handicapped children. To facilitate this, overprotective parents need counseling and financial assistance may be needed for transport.

Formal physical therapy is necessary as an adjunct to exercise as play, as the child tends to overprotect the very joints that should be exercised. Range of motion and muscle strengthening exercises are initiated by the physical therapist and taught to the parents, who supervise them at home, once or twice daily. Physical therapy must be as much a routine as cleaning teeth, with the aim of the child becoming self-sufficient. Morning exercises are easier after a hot bath. The regimen should be general, but concentrating on the affected joints because new joint involvement will be detected early and because asymmetric exercises result in unequal muscle pull; for example, with knee arthritis, the glutei and calf muscles are secondarily affected.

Children unable to participate in games at school should do their exercises instead. When starting, exercises need to be graded: for the severely ill child, from passive to active to resisted. Hydrotherapy is used for hip spasm or to enable a chairbound child to walk again.

CONCLUSIONS

Exercise has to be balanced with a period of rest, particularly during active disease. Predominant hip or knee synovitis or contracture, preventing participation in games, may warrant a corticosteroid injection or soft tissue release. Liaison with the physical education teacher and the physical therapist is essential. Information booklets are available for parents and teachers who deal with these children.

REFERENCES

Arthritis and Rheumatism Council. When a young person has arthritis: a guide for teachers. Arthritis and Rheumatism Council.

Bernstein B, Forrester D, Singsen B, *et al.* Hip restoration in juvenile arthritis. Arthritis Rheum. 1977;20:1099–104.

Gallino L, Pountain G, Mitchell N, Ansell BM. Development aspects of the hip in juvenile chronic arthritis. Scand J Rheumatol. 1984;13:310–18.

Wilkinson VA. Juvenile chronic arthritis: facing the reality. Int Rehabil Med. 1981;3:11–17.

PREVENTION AND TREATMENT OF GROWTH ABNORMALITIES INDUCED BY CORTICOSTEROIDS IN JUVENILE CHRONIC ARTHRITIS

Barbara M Ansell

DEFINITION OF THE PROBLEM

Failure of overall growth as a result of chronic disease, possibly associated with a poor nutritional status, is aggravated by daily corticosteroid therapy, particularly when given in divided dose. The younger the child in whom corticosteroid therapy is used the more likelihood there is of growth failure. It is appropriate, however, to use corticosteroid therapy in the seriously ill child with systemic JCA complicated by pericarditis, myocarditis or hepatotoxicity, and in those with polyarthritis who are failing to improve on a full regimen and, very occasionally, in a child with serious eye disease.

THE TYPICAL CASE

MF developed a systemic onset of JCA just before her fourth birthday. Initially managed with aspirin she had a serious relapse after 14 months for which long-term corticosteroids were required because of recurrent pericarditis associated with high fevers and severe anemia (hemoglobin 5–6g/dl). She continued with this severe systemic disease for almost 5 years, during which time she developed a progressively severe arthritis. Once the systemic features subsided she was treated with sodium aurothiomalate. Satisfactory transfer to alternate-day prednisone was not achieved until more than 5 years of daily corticosteroid therapy (Fig. 24.4). During this time she had a fall off in growth rate from above the 50th percentile to below the third, with resumption of some growth on transfer to alternate-day corticosteroid therapy just prior to the puberty growth spurt. Her height was further affected by contractures of both hips and valgus deformity of the knees which were treated by bilateral soft tissue release operations at the hips just before her 14th birthday, followed by supracondylar osteotomies; she is now a fully functional adult but is below the 3rd percentile in height.

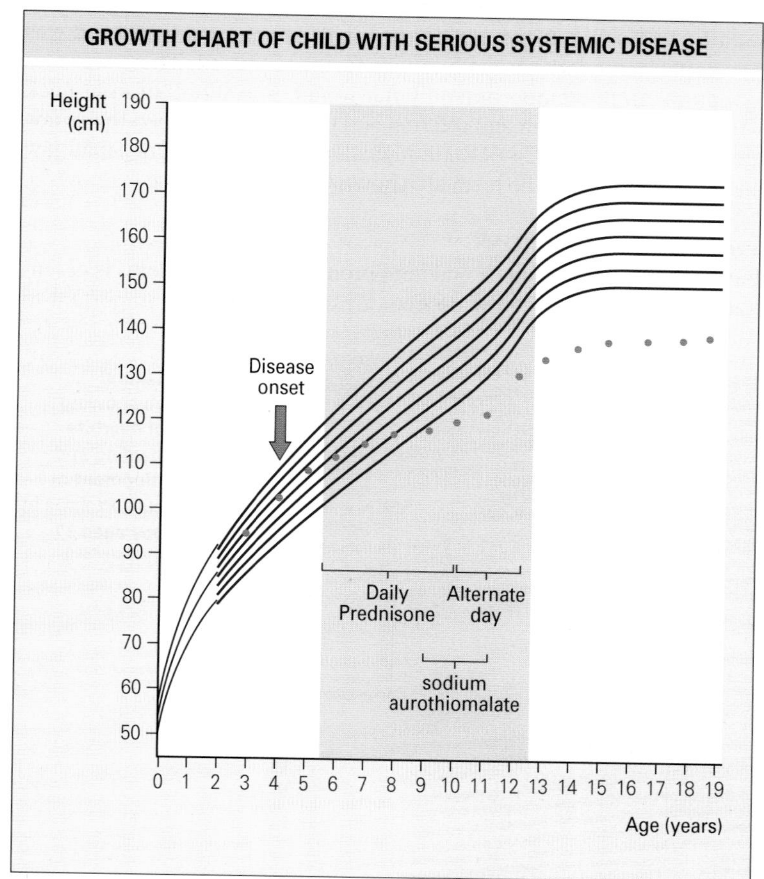

Fig 24.4 Growth chart of child with serious systemic disease. Note the fall off in height and subsequent resumption of growth on alternate-day therapy.

DIAGNOSTIC PROBLEMS

In order to assess growth rate, regular standing measurements of height should be plotted on an appropriate chart, while the weight should also be measured regularly and plotted. This will allow impairment of the growth rate in height or weight to be spotted early.

THERAPEUTIC OPTIONS

Children with systemic onset disease may have a low calorie intake for their age and weight. It is therefore important, particularly when a child is febrile, to make sure that he or she receives adequate nutrition, if necessary supplementing fruit drinks, soups, etc., with glucose and other high-calorie foods. From time to time overnight tube feeding may even be considered.

Even when corticosteroids are deemed essential, if at all possible oral therapy should be given as a single morning dose; at 1–2mg/kg body weight per 24 hours. Ideally this should be at two different levels on alternate days, to make the change to an alternate-day regimen easier. A full-dose of NSAID should also be given to keep corticosteroids at the lowest possible dosage. Severe systemic disease may also be treated by pulses of intravenous methylprednisolone, but this is not a very satisfactory regimen for continuous use in the young child. It may, however, be very valuable when there is an acute exacerbation, e.g. after an intercurrent infection, to give one or two pulses at 48- or 72-hour intervals to tide the child over and allow the dose of oral prednisone to remain unchanged.

When systemic features persist, consideration of the use of intravenous gammaglobulin will be required. If the arthritis is becoming severe, it would be wise to consider the adding of methotrexate. This, if effective, will allow reduction of corticosteroid dosage and hopefully transfer to an alternate-day regime. As yet the role of cyclosporine early in the course of systemic disease in reducing the need for prolonged corticosteroid therapy has not been established.

For children who are given corticosteroid therapy primarily for general deterioration in health and extension of joint involvement, an alternate-day regimen should be used from the outset, even though it may take several weeks for the effects to be noted. If the hypothalmic–pituitary–adrenal axis is suppressed at the time of the puberty growth spurt, this will not take place (Fig. 24.5). Therefore every effort should be made to ensure the child is on a good alternate-day regimen at approximately 0.5mg/kg well before this is likely to occur.

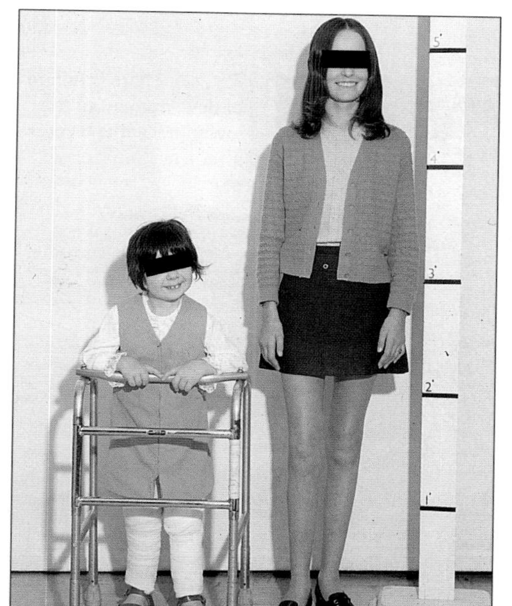

Fig 24.5 These girls are both 14 years of age. The one on the left had a systemic onset Still's disease at 1 year of age and was treated with daily divided corticosteroid therapy, which was only relatively recently changed to alternate-day therapy. The one on the right also had a systemic onset of JCA, but not until the age of 7 years. She has been treated with NSAIDs and short courses of alternate-day corticosteroid therapy and is on the normal centile for her age.

In a comparative study of children with serious disease requiring prednisone over a 1 year period, using lumbar densitometry, deflazacort (an oxazolone derivative of prednisone) has been shown to have a sparing effect with regard to the development of osteoporosis in a dosage range of 6mg of deflazacort to 5mg of prednisone and was just as effective in controlling disease activity. This improved rate of mineralization has continued in the second year of therapy. In our studies we also noted loss of the cushingoid state. Preliminary results on its use as the first corticosteroid suggest that growth can be better maintained with this preparation than with an equivalent dose of prednisone.

The possible use of recombinant human growth hormone to give an improved growth rate in these children has been under study using two different dosage levels, 12IU per week or 24IU per week given in divided doses on 6 of 7 days. While both dosage levels undoubtedly gave some overall improvement in growth rate, in those patients in whom corticosteroids had to be increased because of the severity of the disease process, this dose of human growth hormone was not sufficient to allow growth to proceed. Thus the use of human growth hormone cannot be relied on to overcome moderately high doses of corticosteroids.

CONCLUSIONS

Corticosteroid-induced growth failure can be minimized by the use of an alternate-day regimen. It may well be that deflazacort will prove a more acceptable corticosteroid for young patients with JCA. Other appropriate medication may allow reduction of the corticosteroid dosage. Human growth hormone could have a role in improving growth rate in some patients on relatively low corticosteroid dosage.

REFERENCES

David J, Loftus J, Hesp R, Ansell BM, Woo P. Spinal and somatic growth in patients with juvenile chronic arthritis treated for 1 or 2 years with deflazacort. Clin Exp Rheumatol. 1992;10:621–4.

Davies UM, Rooney M, Reeve J, *et al.* Growth retardation in juvenile chronic arthritis: effect of treatment with biosynthetic human growth hormone. J Rheumatol. 1994;21:153–8.

Gattorno M, Faraci M, Picco P, Buoncompagni A, Pistoia V. Early treatment of systemic onset juvenile chronic arthritis with low-dose cyclosporin A. Letter. Clin Exp Rheumatol. 1995;13:409–10.

Kotaniemi A, Savolainen A, Kautiainen H, Kroger H. Estimation of central osteopenia in children with chronic polyarthritis treated with glucocorticoids. Pediatrics. 1993;91:1127–30.

Reiff A, Shaham B, Wood BP, *et al.* High dose methotrexate in the treatment of refractory juvenile arthritis. Clin Exp Rheumatol. 1995;13:113–18.

Varonos S, Ansell BM, Reeve J. Vertebral collapse in juvenile chronic arthritis: its relationship with glucocorticoid therapy. Calcif Tissue Int. 1987;41:75–8.

PREVENTION AND MANAGEMENT OF DEVELOPMENTAL ABNORMALITIES OF THE LOWER JAW IN JUVENILE CHRONIC ARTHRITIS

Barbara M Ansell

DEFINITION OF THE PROBLEM

Micrognathia (bird-like face profile) is seen in children with a young onset of polyarthritis, either *de novo* or following a systemic onset. Temporomandibular joint involvement itself is relatively common, possibly as high as 50%, although it is difficult to obtain exact figures. It is associated with neck involvement, particularly loss of extension and failure of growth in the cervical spine, although the exact relationship is uncertain. Initially condylar growth is deficient, followed after some years by condylar erosions. Computed tomography of the temporomandibular joints allows division of lesions into mild, moderate and severe, and allows for better planning of orthodontic treatment. A dysplastic mandible causes alteration in dental function and occlusion as well as masseter muscle weakness.

THE TYPICAL CASE

A 3-year-old boy presented with a systemic onset disease. He had a high fever, with rash intermittently for about a year, followed by the development of widespread polyarthritis. He was treated predominantly with NSAIDs, with two short periods on prednisone at a maximum dose of 15mg on alternate days. In the eleventh month of the disease he developed a progressive arthritis with particular problems in the neck, wrists, hips and knees. Although he had no complaint of pain in the temporomandibular joints, he started to lose function. By 5-year follow up he had marked loss of movement in the cervical spine and radiologically was showing early fusion of apophyseal joints and was developing an overbite; his bite was further reduced. There were no symptoms in the temporomandibular joints. The short, straight neck which lacked extension and rotation and the underdeveloped lower jaw are obvious in Figure 24.6. Radiologically the neck problem, small jaw and overcrowding of the teeth are shown from another case (Fig. 24.7).

THERAPEUTIC OPTIONS

Early identification of neck and temporomandibular problems is essential. In trying to reduce the degree of micrognathia it is important to

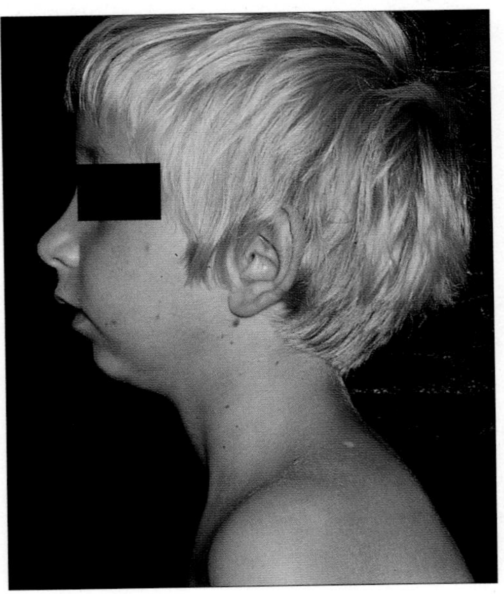

Fig 24.6 There is failure of development of the lower jaw some 5 years after a systemic onset of disease. The neck is short and slightly flexed.

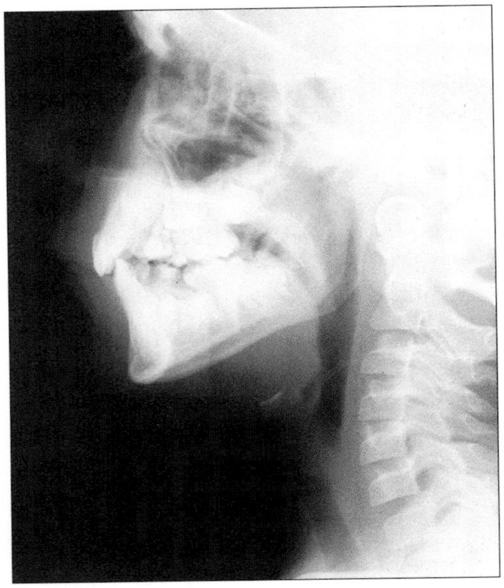

Fig 24.7 Lateral radiograph showing severity of overbite, dental crowding and poor development of the cervical vertebrae in another boy aged 11 years. Courtesy Dr J. Sills.

maintain mobility, not only in the temporomandibular joints but also in the cervical spine by a very active program of physical therapy. Exercise of the temporomandibular joints by opening and closing the mouth, rotation and blowing into a bag is important. It is also necessary to look at the way collars are used; except in the very rare patient who has atlantoaxial subluxation, there is little place for the old-fashioned collar with a chin piece. For acute pain in the neck, a small collar can be equally effective provided attention is paid to good posture when sitting at a desk or table, or when lying down. Any collar should always be removed for eating. Although severe pain in the temporomandibular joints limiting movement is very rare, when it does occur it can be effectively treated by a local injection of corticosteroid. However, this will require an experienced orthodontist. Prior to the recognition of the need for maintenance of movement of the neck and temporomandibular joints, ankylosis did occasionally occur, but now is rare except in the juvenile spondyloarthropathy subgroup. Here asymmetric involvement of the temporomandibular articulator may cause pain, loss of function in the joint and unilateral abnormality of growth.

It is important that an orthodontist monitors any child in whom there is evidence of poor growth with dental occlusion becoming altered. Using panoramic radiographs the state of the secondary dentition can be confirmed as well as the state of the condylar heads, which can become flattened and notched early and eroded later. When there is malocclusion during growth, particularly before and around puberty, a functional appliance as described by Frankel (1969), which aims at forcing the mandible to assume a measured forward position with the upper and lower teeth held slightly apart, appears to be helpful in altering the growth pattern of the mandible. Braces may be required for minor cosmetic realignment. Facial asymmetry will require more active orthodontic treatment carried out over a prolonged period. Numerous techniques have been described for surgical revision of the withdrawn mandible and augmentation of the chin. These include bilateral sagittal split osteotomies of the mandible and sliding anterior horizontal osteotomy of the chin. In the past alloplastic materials, particularly silicone, were considered a possible method but are no longer used.

CONCLUSIONS

The realization of the importance of maintaining neck and jaw mobility would appear to have reduced the frequency with which micrognathia is now seen. It does, however, still occur in children who have very severe disease, early neck involvement and overall stunting of growth. It is important that temporomandibular joint function is noted at each assessment and the bite checked. Any suggestion of dental problems should call for immediate consultation with a pediatric orthodontist.

REFERENCES

Frankel R. The treatment of class II division 1 malocclusion and functional correctors 1. Am J Orthod. 1969;44:265–75.

Krieberg S, Bakke M, Kirkeby S, *et al.* Facial growth and oral function in a case of juvenile rheumatoid arthritis. Eur J Orthod. 1990;12:119–34.

Larheim TA, Haanaes HR, Rudel AF. Mandibular growth, temporo-mandibular joint changes and dental occlusion in juvenile rheumatoid arthritis. Scand J Rheumatol. 1981;10:225–33.

Mayro RF, DeLozier JB, Whitaker LA. Facial reconstruction consideration in rheumatic diseases. Rheum Dis Clin North Am. 1991;17:943–69.

Myall RWT, West RA, Horwitz H, Schaller JG. Jaw deformity caused by juvenile rheumatoid arthritis and its correction. Arthritis Rheum. 1988;31:1305–10.

Ronchezel MV, Hilario MOE, Goldenberg J, *et al.* Temporomandibular joint and mandibular growth alterations in patients with JRA. J Rheumatol. 1995;22:1956–61.

AMYLOIDOSIS

Barbara M Ansell

DEFINITION OF THE PROBLEM

In reactive amyloidosis, which is a complication of chronic inflammatory disorders, fibrillar proteins are deposited together with glycosaminoglycans, serum amyloid P (SAP) component and fibrinonectin which interfere with cellular function. The spleen is always involved and the kidneys, liver, adrenal glands and gastrointestinal tract are frequently affected.

THE TYPICAL CASE

SF, a 9-year-old girl with a systemic onset of JCA was treated with intramuscular sodium aurothiomalate for progressive arthritis. After 4 months proteinuria was noted so the aurothiomalate was stopped. Her ESR was then 54mm/h, C-reactive protein (CRP) 24mg/dl, hemoglobin 11g/dl, WBC 13,000 mm^3 and platelets 800,000 mm^3. Intermittent proteinuria continued over the next 8 months; a rectal biopsy was performed but showed no evidence of amyloidosis. Over the next 2 years, although the systemic features declined and despite the introduction of 10mg of prednisone on alternate days, her arthritis continued to be extremely active. Her ESR rose to 117mm/h with the hemoglobin falling to 8.6g/dl; CRP remained at 23mg/dl and proteinuria now became persistent, the 24-hour excretion being in the order of 1g. The rise in ESR with reduction of the hemoglobin and persistently high CRP, together with a fall in serum albumin, all suggested a diagnosis of amyloidosis, so a renal biopsy was undertaken which confirmed the diagnosis of amyloidosis which had been suspected for the preceding 12 months.

DIAGNOSTIC PROBLEMS

Proteinuria during the course of aurothiomalate therapy can occur and initially this was assumed to be the case. However, despite discontinuation, occasional intermittent proteinuria without red cells, white cells or infection in the urine continued; at this stage a rectal biopsy was negative for amyloidosis. With the persistence of proteinuria varying between 1 and 2 g per 24 hours, combined with a rising ESR, falling hemoglobin and persistently high CRP, together with a fall in serum albumin, a renal biopsy was undertaken which showed deposition of amyloid. Particularly in the early stages of amyloidosis deposition is patchy; rectal biopsy is usually performed first as this is a relatively safe procedure; renal biopsy is not without risk in this condition and some patients have had serious bleeding following the procedure.

A positive tissue biopsy shows an amorphous eosinophilic material under the light microscope which, when stained with Congo Red and under polarized light, has a characteristic apple green birefringence (Fig. 24.8). The diagnostic technique described by Hawkins *et al.* (1988) relies on the specific binding of the normal circulating protein SAP to amyloid

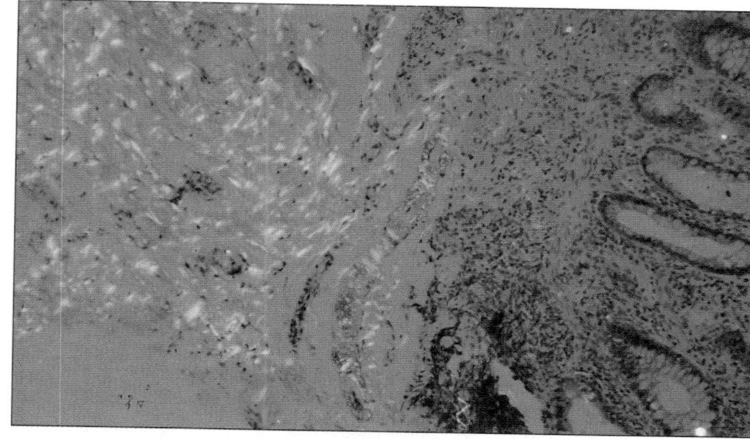

Fig 24.8 Rectal biopsy positive for amyloidosis. The tissue has been stained with Congo Red and examined by polarized light. Note the apple green birefringence present.

tissue, so that purified human SAP labeled with ^{123}I is given. A rapid plasma clearance is seen when there are large amyloid deposits and increased whole body retention observed (Fig. 24.9). Regional views obtained 24 hours after injection allow a much better assessment of the organs involved and of the severity of the deposition. This is now used for diagnostic purposes, although occasionally it may be considered necessary to confirm it by an appropriate biopsy; it also allows monitoring of the progress of the amyloid deposition by regular sequential scans.

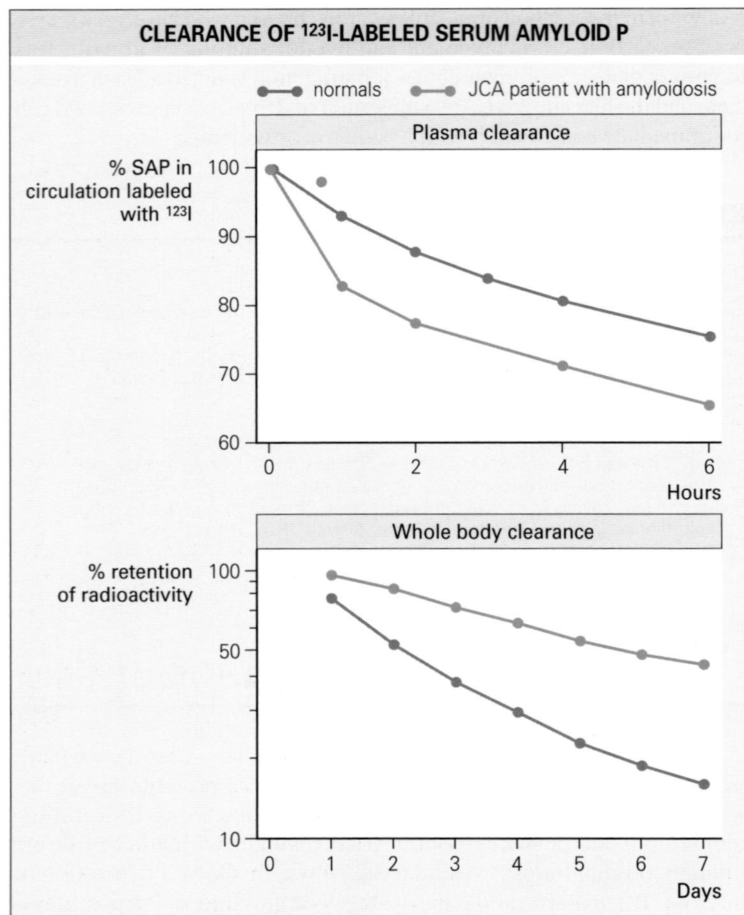

Fig 24.9 Clearance profiles after intravenous injection with serum amyloid P labeled with ^{123}I from plasma and whole body, showing mean values for 10 normal volunteers and patients. In amyloidosis deviation from normal values is due to sequestration of tracer within amyloid deposits. Courtesy of Dr P Hawkins.

THERAPEUTIC OPTIONS

The aim of treatment is to reduce the overall disease activity and thereby reduce the acute phase response. Initially high-dose corticosteroids were tried, and while patients were temporarily improved, this therapy proved impractical because of the side effects at the dosage required to suppress the acute phase response. For this reason various other drugs were studied; it would appear that cytotoxic therapy in the form of chlorambucil is an effective means of reducing the acute phase response (Fig. 24.10) and improving life expectancy. Initially chlorambucil was selected rather than cyclophosphamide as it was felt to have fewer side effects and would also allow easier monitoring of the urinary state. It has the same disadvantage as cyclophosphamide of impairing ovarian function in some female patients and testicular function appears to have been affected in all the boys so treated; therefore when adolescents are started on therapy, the possibility of banking semen will need to be considered.

In the course of management it is important to recognize intercurrent infections which need prompt and adequate treatment. Extrarenal uremia can occur in association with anything which has caused diarrhea and vomiting: on such an occasion it is very important to watch the fluid balance as these compromised patients may rapidly go into extrarenal uremia. Hypertension should be treated promptly with appropriate antihypertensive therapy. Nephrosis may call for an increased protein intake and a reduction in sodium; very rarely albumin infusions may be helpful in tiding a patient over. Should renal failure occur, provided the overall disease is well controlled, renal transplantation will need consideration.

CONCLUSIONS

In the assessment of JCA, any patient with persistent activity of the disease who develops proteinuria, a rising ESR with a falling hemoglobin and serum albumin, should be considered for serum amyloid P protein scan. To date it is the most sensitive method for demonstrating deposition of amyloid. When a diagnosis of amyloidosis is made, every effort should be undertaken to control the disease activity. At the present time, the most effective slow-acting agent appears to be chlorambucil.

REFERENCES

David J, Vouyiouka O, Ansell BM, Hall A, Woo P. Amyloidosis in juvenile chronic arthritis: a morbidity and mortality study. Clin Exp Rheumatol. 1993;11:85–90.

Hawkins PN, Lavender JP, Pepys MB. Evaluation of systemic amyloidosis by scintigraphy with ^{123}I-labelled serum amyloid P component. N Engl J Med. 1990;323:508–13.

Hawkins PN, Myers MJ, Epentos AA, Caspi D, Pepys MB. Specific localization and imaging of amyloid deposits *in vivo* using ^{123}I-labelled serum amyloid P component. J Exp Med. 1988;167:903–13.

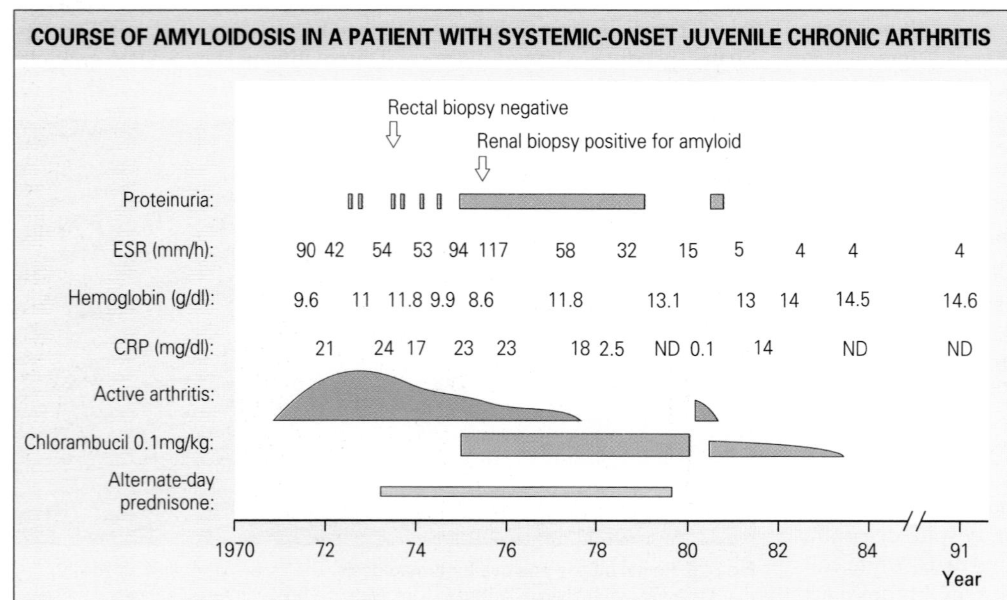

Fig 24.10 This chart shows the course of the patient's disease and response to chlorambucil. Note the marked improvement in the arthritis, rise in hemoglobin and fall in ESR. When therapy stopped there was a flare in the arthritis and recurrence of proteinuria, which rapidly responded to a lower dose of chlorambucil.

Barbara M Ansell

DEFINITION OF THE PROBLEM

Total replacement arthroplasty in a growing child is an operation not to be undertaken lightly. It should be reserved for those cases when the hips or knees severely limit the child's physical capacity, which in the majority of cases will be associated with severe pain. A secondary consideration is whether the joint is causing deterioration in other joints.

THE TYPICAL CASE

A 7-month-old girl was noticed by her mother to have swelling of both knees and to dislike her knees, ankles or wrists being moved. On examination she was found to have widespread polyarthritis with an ESR of 60mm/hour, hemoglobin of 11g/dl and white blood cell count of 14,000/mm^3, 80% polymorphs, and platelets 560,000/mm^3; she thus represents a polyarthritic onset of JCA at a young age. She was treated initially with NSAIDs, but had marked pain and misery which prevented adequate splinting and physiotherapy. Alternate-day steroid therapy (prednisone 7.5mg) was therefore introduced in an attempt to reduce her pain and allow appropriate physical management. At the age of 18 months corticosteroid injections in both knees were performed. After these she was able to stand and take a few tottering steps when her hand was held, but she did not really walk independently until she was nearly 3 years old. By this time intramuscular gold had been commenced; this did not appear to benefit her, so it was stopped after 2 years and penicillamine introduced. This was continued for 5 years but her arthritis persisted, with varying degrees of activity but causing very widespread joint involvement so that all her major joints were involved, including the neck, hands and feet. Despite physiotherapy she was never able to walk freely without an aid. From the age of 12 to 14 years her hip function steadily deteriorated clinically and radiologically.

She now has serious flexion contractures of the hips and is unable to take more than a few steps even with gutter crutches (Fig. 24.11). At school and at home she has become completely wheelchair-bound, and she is in pain when she attempts to move the hips. In addition to the lower limb joint deformities, she has a straight neck and foreshortened lower jaw.

THERAPEUTIC OPTIONS

Children suffer the effect not only of chronic inflammation on the growing skeleton, but also that of immobility, which further alters and delays development of joints, particularly the hips. In addition, those children who are seriously ill, usually with systemic disease, will have had their growth further altered by the use of systemic corticosteroid therapy, with its attendant side effects of impaired height, growth rate, osteoporosis and tendency to osteonecrosis. Such patients will have severe multiple joint involvement and particular problems with anesthesia. Another group in which prosthetic replacement, particularly of the hips and knees, is common is the small group of seropositive juvenile arthritics. In childhood-onset systemic lupus erythematosus, osteonecrosis without other abnormalities of joints, usually affecting the hips, may require surgery.

Any implant must be small enough to fit the stunted skeleton and this may mean a custom-made prosthesis. Thus before surgery is considered, a radiographic measurement must be made to determine the size of the prosthesis required. This will require a posteroanterior and a lateral radiograph, the latter particularly for the size of the bone shaft, while for the hips a CT scan is essential to look for the degree of anteversion.

Although skeletal immaturity is a relative contraindication, hip joints considered for replacement have usually become totally destroyed and may be subluxed. The surgeon undertaking such prosthetic work in children must be prepared for considerable bleeding, the anteverted femoral neck and a femoral shaft which is greater in its coronal diameter. The remnants of the femoral head often have to be removed piecemeal with bone nibblers. An initial report on such young patients brought out the value of the operation, but the longer term follow-up showed that by 10 years a significant proportion are failing, usually due to loosening of the prosthesis; other problems include late infection. In the past, prostheses were all cemented; nowadays, custom-made cementless prostheses (Fig. 24.12) are available, and it is hoped that this will overcome the problem of late loosening.

The aim of total knee replacement is a stable, painless joint allowing mainly flexion and extension, with some small degree of rotatory movement. Because growth of the femur continues at the lower end

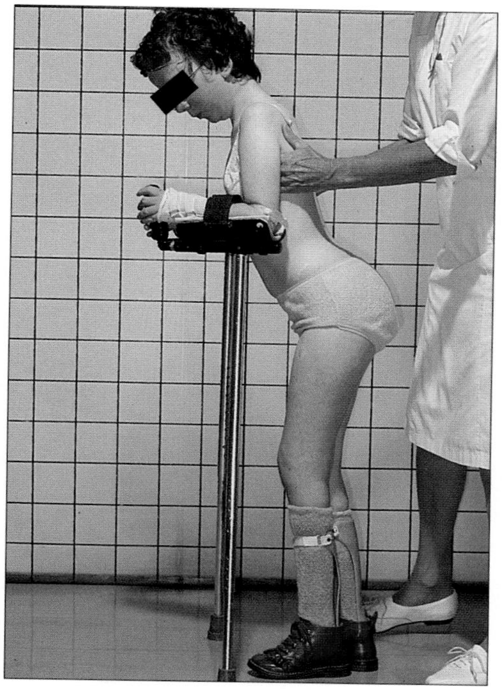

Fig. 24.11 Polyarthritic onset of JCA at the age of 7 months. Despite gold, first followed by penicillamine, this 14-year-old girl continued to have active disease with severe damage to multiple joints. The hips became gradually destroyed, causing severe flexion contractures. She was just able to take a few steps with two crutches, but in the last 3 months she had been wheelchair-bound. Note the short neck and poor development of the lower jaw.

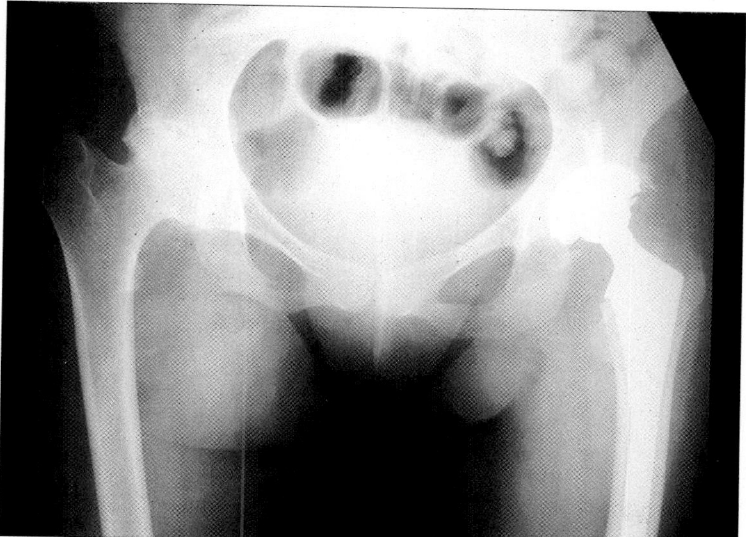

Fig. 24.12 Prosthesis in JCA. This 16-year-old girl had a systemic onset of disease at the age of 6 years, with the later development of bilateral hip disease. The radiograph shows the preoperative state of her right hip, with a short femoral neck, some persistence of anteversion and the destroyed joint. The left hip has been replaced by a custom-made cementless prosthesis. Courtesy of Mr M Swann, Slough.

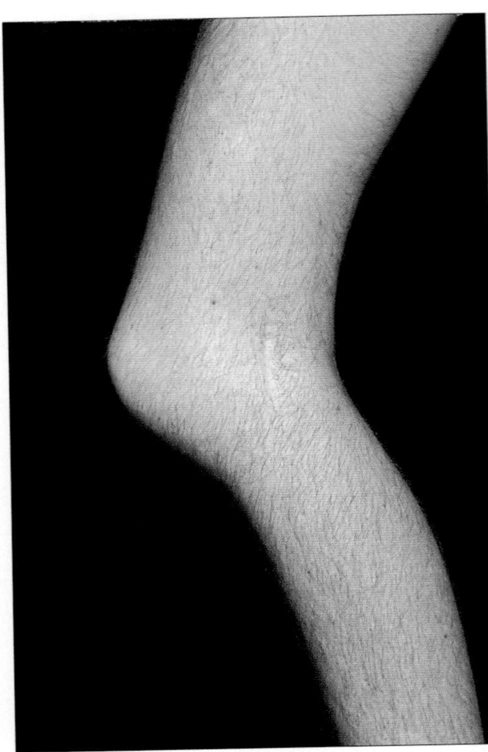

Fig. 24.13 Posterior subluxation of one knee in a seronegative 13-year-old boy with JCA and considerably stunted growth. The scar of a previous soft tissue release is obvious.

until the epiphysis closes, which would be well after damage occurs in the articular surface of the epiphysis, knee surgery tends to be done at a somewhat later age. Such a knee may have already undergone a soft tissue release, or lateral release of the patella. In the seronegative group of JCA patients, the knee may well show posterior subluxation of the tibia (Fig. 24.13), an altered shape and position of the patella, and occasionally evidence of an old supracondylar fracture, a common occurrence in JCA. The older seropositive JCA patient's knee resembles that of adult rheumatoid arthritis.

The newer prostheses, either unconstrained or partially constrained, should be used; while the femoral prosthesis can be press-fit type and uncemented, the tibial prosthesis is probably better cemented to prevent settling. Hyman and Gregg suggest a CT-scan-generated styroform model of the knee to practice cut preoperatively. This may improve surgeons' ability to correct angular deformities and flexion contracture by appropriate removal of bone with femoral or tibial cuts. Again, custom-made prostheses may be required.

Most of the work on prostheses in patients under 16 years has been confined to hips and knees, although other joints are now under consideration. Thus the Swanson arthroplasty of the wrists has been performed in eight patients. Mr W. Souter (Edinburgh) has successfully used his own elbow prosthesis in some young patients, including some over the age of 16 years. To date, shoulder arthroplasty has been tried in only a few cases and then usually with a custom-made prosthesis.

Before considering any arthroplasty, careful assessment of all joints must be made. If surgery is to be on the lower limbs, are the upper extremities satisfactory for walkers or crutches required for postoperative rehabilitation? The need for rehabilitation both pre- and postoperatively should be stressed, and any new apparatus (such as a passive motion machine) likely to be used should be introduced early. Family support is essential and sometimes psychological counseling will be required. What is likely to be achieved must be indicated at the outset.

CONCLUSIONS

This type of surgery should only be undertaken where preoperative assessment can be made and the whole team is used to dealing with such young patients. In particular, the surgeon should have had experience in managing such children and the physician should be able to discuss the problems with the surgeon and the family. For those youngsters who have lost function and are becoming chair bound because of severe hip or knee destruction, total replacement arthroplasty is now a possibility, but special-sized prostheses may need to be prepared; whenever possible, these should be of the type that do not require cement. Even when disease onset is at 10 years and over and the hip is reasonably developed before damage starts, there is a tendency to severe protrusio, so that technically the operation can still be very difficult.

REFERENCES

Evans DM, Ansell BM, Hall A. The wrist in juvenile arthritis. J Hand Surg. 1991;16B:293–30.

Hyman BS, Gregg JR. Arthroplasty of the hip and knee in juvenile rheumatoid arthritis. Rheum Dis Clin N Am. 1991;17:971–83.

Ruddelston C, Ansell BM, Arden GP, Swann M. Total hip replacement in children with juvenile chronic arthritis. J Bone Joint Surg. 1986;68B:218–22.

Smith B. Anaesthesia in paediatric rheumatology. In: Woo P, White P, Ansell BM, eds. Paediatric rheumatology update. Oxford: Oxford University Press; 1990:124–30.

Swann M. The surgery of juvenile chronic arthritis. Clin Orthop. 1990;259:70.

Witt JD, Swann M, Ansell BM. Total hip replacement for juvenile chronic arthritis. J Bone Joint Surg. 1991;73B:770–3.

ERYTHEMA NODOSUM

Josh Dixey

Definition

- An acutely tender and nodular skin eruption with marked erythema and bruising as a consequence of inflammation of subcutaneous fat.
- Can be triggered by infection, drugs, sarcoidosis and, rarely, neoplasia.

Clinical features

- Cutaneous nodules, 1–10cm in diameter, occur on extensor aspects of the legs. The eruption lasts for 6–8 weeks.
- Associated with fever, polyarthralgia, ankle synovitis and hilar lymphadenopathy.
- The erythrocyte sedimentation rate is usually elevated.
- The overall prognosis is good.

HISTORY

Erythema nodosum (EN) was first described by Robert Willan in 1798[1]. It was not until the early 20th century that the association between EN and infection, particularly tuberculosis and streptococcal pharyngitis, was recognized. In 1941, King[2] observed on chest radiography a high incidence of bilateral hilar lymphadenopathy in patients with EN and soon the strong association between EN and sarcoidosis was recognized[3]. More recently, with the falling incidence of tuberculosis (TB) in industrialized societies, many different micro-organisms have been found to trigger EN, including typical and atypical bacteria, and fungi. Similarly, the number and variety of drugs which have been found to trigger EN continues to expand.

EPIDEMIOLOGY

There are few data available to provide an accurate estimate of the incidence and prevalence of EN (Fig. 25.1). With a strong association between EN and infection, demographic factors are obviously important, since varying patterns of infection occur in different populations. Collecting data is further complicated by the fact that EN cases often present to different specialists – rheumatologists, chest physicians, dermatologists or primary care physicians – which can create biases in epidemiologic studies. In an English rural population, the prevalence has been estimated at 2.4 per 100,000[4]. In the 1950s, 62 cases were seen over a period of 7 years in an area of south-east England (population 275,000) [5].

The rash is more common in women (estimates vary between 2.5:1.0 and 4:1; F:M) and occurs in young people (25–40 years old). EN is seen in childhood but is uncommon in the elderly.

EPIDEMIOLOGY OF ERYTHEMA NODOSUM	
Peak age (years)	25–40
Sex distribution (F:M)	4:1
Annual incidence (per 100,000)	2–3
Genetic association	HLA-B8

Fig. 25.1 Epidemiology of erythema nodosum.

There is increased incidence of the HLA antigen phenotype HLA-B8 in cases of EN associated with both sarcoidosis and nonsarcoidosis triggers[6]. In sarcoidosis, the presence of the HLA-B8 antigen is associated with EN and arthritis and an overall good prognosis. However, unlike the HLA status in autoimmune diseases, there is no linkage disequilibrium between HLA-B8 and HLA-A1 in EN[6]. It is tempting to speculate that there may be a linkage between HLA-B8 and -DR3, leading to abnormal processing of foreign antigen and EN. Unfortunately, there is as yet no information about HLA-DR status and EN.

CLINICAL FEATURES

Erythema nodosum is an acute lesion. The nodules are exquisitely tender and are normally situated on the anterior aspect of the lower leg, less commonly on the thighs and occasionally on the forearms. At first, the nodule is a light red color with surrounding erythema, with a diameter of 0.2–2.0cm but sometimes as large as 10cm (Fig. 25.2). As the lesion ages, the color deepens and becomes a livid dark red and local bruising is apparent (Fig. 25.3). In black skin, EN appears as hyperpigmented lesions (see Fig. 25.4). In convalescence, when the nodule is no longer palpable, the pain disappears and there remains a yellowish hue before there is complete resolution. The nodules do not ulcerate and they heal without scarring.

Once seen, the diagnosis of EN is relatively straightforward. The majority (70%)[7] will be febrile and systemically unwell in the early stages, with a temperature pattern resembling rheumatic fever. Often, the taking of a careful history will reveal the cause, and questions should be asked about triggering infection (especially sore throat) and drug therapy. Careful examination may also identify the cause; for instance, up to 50% of those presenting with sarcoidosis and EN will have superficial and palpable lymph nodes suitable for biopsy, and other cutaneous manifestations of sarcoidosis may also be found[7].

The acute illness of EN normally resolves within 6–8 weeks and is self-limiting. Recurrence is unusual and suggestive of lymphoma.

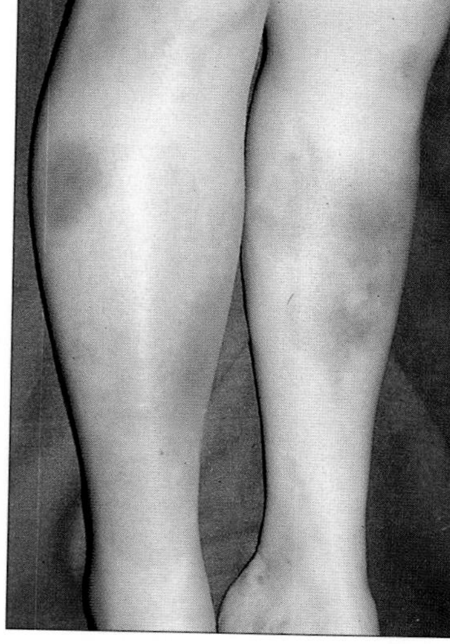

Fig. 25.2 Erythema nodosum: early lesions with prominent bruising. Courtesy of Dr R Butler.

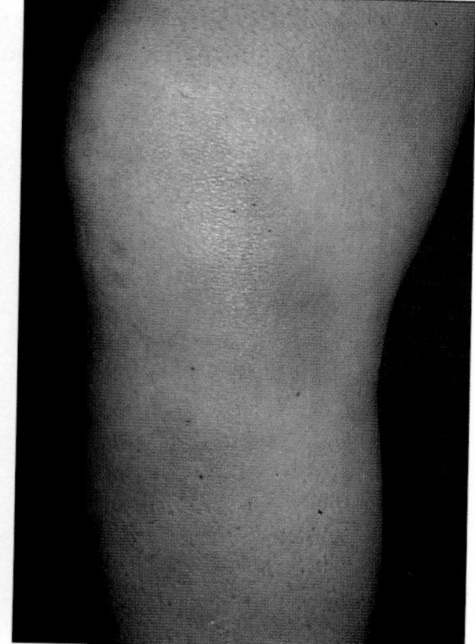

Fig. 25.3 Erythema nodosum. Bruising is apparent.

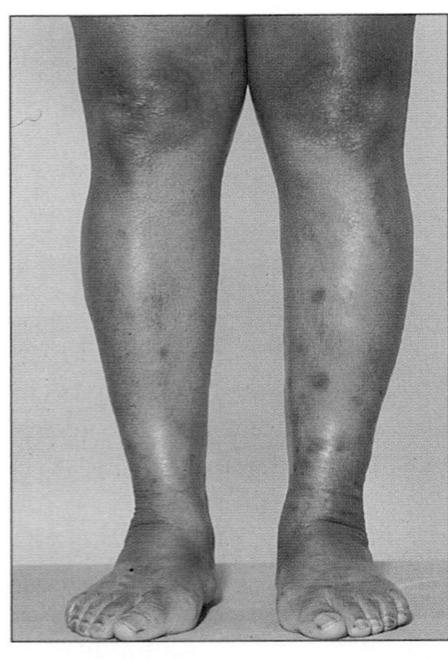
Fig. 25.4 Erythema nodosum in black skin: hyperpigmented lesions.

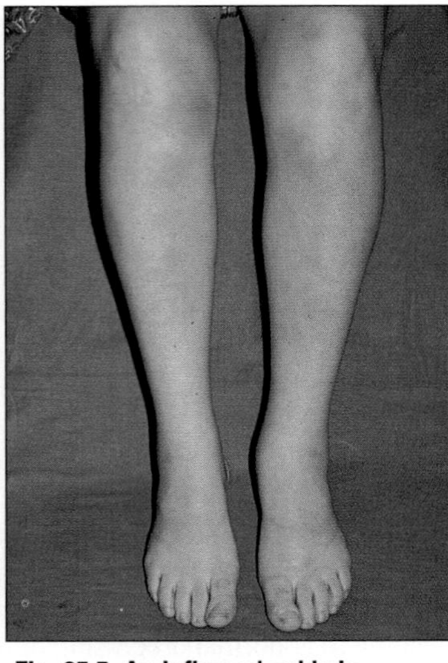
Fig. 25.5 An inflamed ankle in erythema nodosum.

Because of the presence of local pain, EN is often referred to the rheumatologist. Fifty percent of cases, or more, will have an arthropathy. When joint symptoms appear, the joint pain tends to precede the skin eruption. A flitting polyarthritis with fever starting 2–4 weeks before the onset of rash has been described[8]. More commonly, the patient with EN complains of joint stiffness and polyarthralgia at the onset. In order of relative frequency, ankles (Fig. 25.5), knees, wrists, fingers, shoulders, elbows and hips[8] are painful. Joint tenderness is the predominant feature, but effusion and soft tissue swelling occur in ankles and knees. Synovial fluid is relatively acellular and the sparsity of inflammatory cells can help to distinguish the arthritis of EN from other causes of acute joint inflammation.

The synovitis usually resolves with the skin lesions; joint pain and stiffness may persist for up to 6 months but will eventually resolve. The acute arthropathy of EN is readily distinguishable from the persistent arthropathy of chronic sarcoidosis.

INVESTIGATIONS

In 75% of those with EN, the erythrocyte sedimentation rate is raised to 50mm/h or more and will fall to normal once the rash has resolved. Further investigations are required to establish the cause, as the diagnosis of the skin lesions is usually apparent. The chest radiograph is abnormal in the majority, with bilateral hilar lymphadenopathy found in approximately 50%. In a series of 170 patients reported by James[9], 140 had radiographic abnormalities: bilateral hilar lymphadenopathy (124 patients), bilateral hilar lymphadenopathy with pulmonary mottling (8) and right paratracheal lymphadenopathy (5). The combination of EN and bilateral hilar lymphadenopathy is a form of acute sarcoidosis that has an excellent prognosis, as there is a complete resolution of the adenopathy within 12 months in 90% of cases and only a few will progress to a more chronic sarcoidosis. Histologic examination of palpable lymph nodes, when present, will often confirm the diagnosis. Measurement of serum angiotensin converting enzyme is not discriminatory in establishing the diagnosis of sarcoidosis in the presence of EN and hilar lymphadenopathy. The Kveim test is more specific but concern has been expressed about the safety of the use of the antigen made from a spleen extract from patients with sarcoidosis.

In EN triggered by streptococcal infection, there is usually a history of sore throat preceding the eruption, and significant infection is confirmed by a rise in antistreptolysin-O titer. Although uncommon in industrialized societies, active TB should be considered, especially in children under 5 years old. In children[10] and adults with active TB, the Mantoux test will be strongly positive. In contrast, the Mantoux is usually negative when EN and hilar lymphadenopathy are the manifestations of acute sarcoidosis. With the increasing prevalence of mycobacterial infection in human immunodeficiency virus (HIV) infection, when EN develops in an HIV positive patient a careful search should be made for TB and here a Mantoux test will be very informative[11].

In those with hilar lymphadenopathy, follow-up chest radiography is mandatory to ensure resolution. If the lymph nodes fail to diminish in size or enlarge, a lymphoproliferative disorder should be considered, although, fortunately, EN as a manifestation of neoplasia is unusual.

DIFFERENTIAL DIAGNOSIS

The early lesion of EN is commonly mistaken for insect bites by those who have not seen the skin disorder before. Otherwise, EN is distinct and normally is easily distinguished from other causes of subcutaneous fat inflammation. Erythema nodosum does not ulcerate and heals without a scar, properties that should distinguish the lesion clinically from vasculitic lesions such as nodular vasculitis and polyarteritis nodosa. Weber–Christian disease, a widespread vasculitic disease of subcutaneous fat, differs from EN in that punched out lesions of fat necrosis, situated predominantly over the buttocks, occur with scarring. Widespread fat necrosis of skin is occasionally seen in acute pancreatitis, in which case the symptoms of pancreatitis itself should provide the diagnosis. A biopsy of the lesion should be diagnostic.

STRUCTURE AND FUNCTION

In normal skin, the subcutaneous fat cells are stored within lobules parceled by septa of connective tissue. The diagnostic lesion of EN is

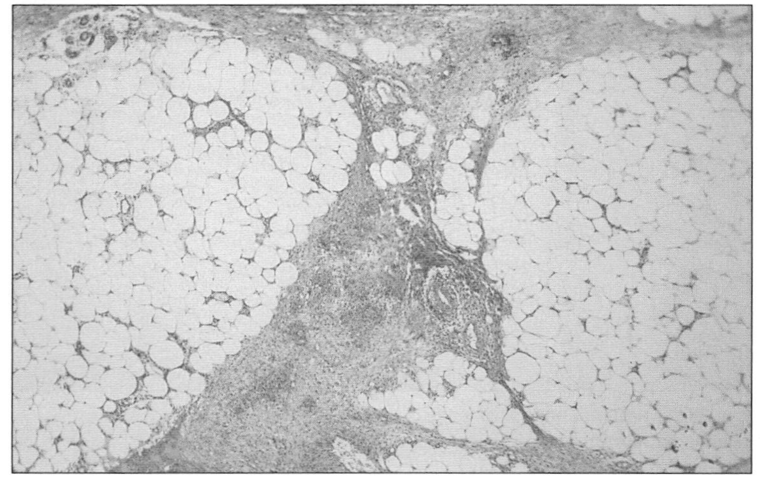

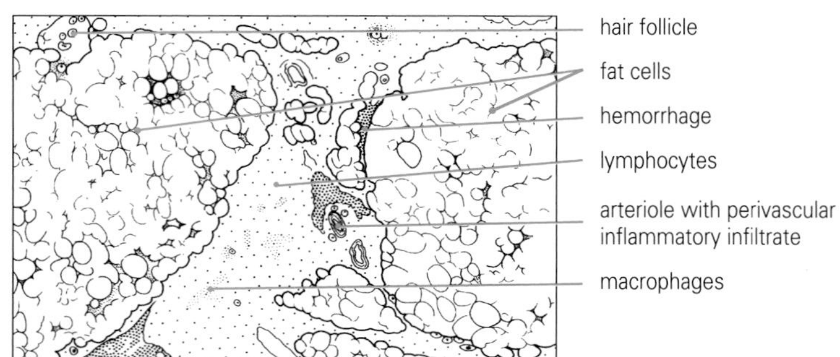

Fig. 25.6 Erythema nodosum: early lesion showing marked inflammation of the septum and focal hemorrhage. Courtesy of Dr PH McKee.

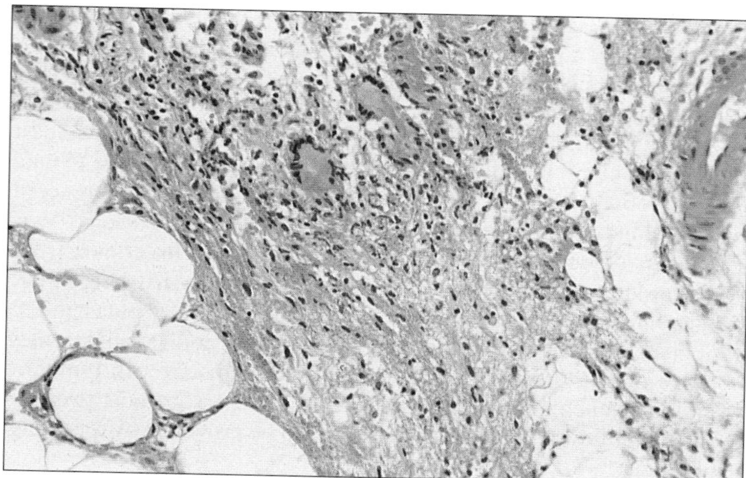

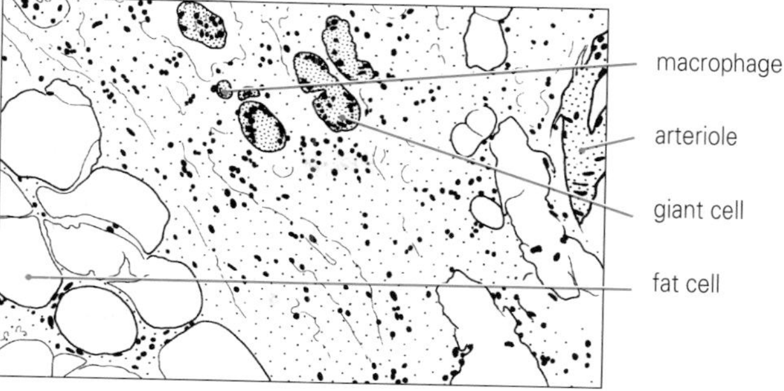

Fig. 25.7 Erythema nodosum: late lesion showing giant cells and granuloma formation. Courtesy of Dr PH McKee.

an inflammatory response around the septa, a septal panniculitis. In the early lesion (Fig. 25.6), an infiltrate of lymphocytes and the occasional macrophage is seen in the septal areas. If a more widespread and lobular panniculitis is observed, this is suggestive of nodular vasculitis or other vasculitic process.

The characteristic sheen of EN results from capillary leak and bleeding and this appearance can be compared with a bruise. Therefore, hemorrhage is a prominent microscopic feature. In approximately 30% of cases a venulitis is seen, but arterial inflammation or fat necrosis is not a feature. The dermis overlying the abnormal fat cells is inflamed also.

In the later lesion (Fig. 25.7), macrophages coalesce to form giant cells and, with further organization, septal granulomas form. Healing is brought about by fibrosis but, in contrast to nodular vasculitis, there is no scarring.

ETIOLOGY

INFECTION

The list of microorganisms capable of triggering EN is extensive (Fig. 25.8). Typical and atypical bacteria are well represented, as are fungal infections, but viral triggers are unusual and EN following protozoal infection has not been described. The relative frequency with which individual microorganisms trigger EN varies according to the pattern of infections within populations. For example, as seen with reactive arthritis, the incidence of *Yersinia* infections triggering EN is higher in Scandinavia[12] than in the UK, and the relative frequencies are likely to be different in the developing world (though no information on the latter is available). EN should not be confused with the erythema nodosum leprosum that occurs in the lepromatous phase of leprosy and is distinctly different, with widespread hemorrhagic and ulcerating skin nodules forming and plentiful acid-fast bacilli seen on microscopy. As in reactive arthritis, host factors are probably more important than the initial infectious trigger in establishing disease. Recurrent EN following infections by two different microorganisms has been described[13]. Similarly, in an epidemic of histoplasmosis[14] in North America, 4% of the 435 documented cases also developed EN – the patients with EN could not be distinguished serologically, but the prognosis appeared better than it was for the majority who were infected with *Histoplasma* but did not have EN.

INFECTIOUS TRIGGERS OF ERYTHEMA NODOSUM
Bacteria
Streptoccocal pharyngitis
Salmonella enteritis
Yersinia enteritis
Psittacosis
Chlamydia pneumoniae (strain TWAR) infection
Mycoplasma pneumonia
Meningococcal infection
Gonorrhea
Syphilis
Lymphogranuloma venereum
Tularemia
Cat scratch disease
Leprosy
Tuberculosis
Fungi
Histoplasmosis
Coccidioidomycosis
Blastomycosis
Trichophyton verrucosum
Viruses
Cytomegalovirus
Hepatitis B
Epstein–Barr

Fig. 25.8 Infectious triggers of erythema nodosum.

DRUGS

Proving a causal relationship between drug therapy and EN is difficult, especially in the case of antibiotics when the infection for which they are prescribed may also trigger EN. But antibiotics, especially sulfonamides, are the drugs most frequently implicated. The oral contraceptive is another culprit. Again proving the causal link is difficult, given the frequency of this form of birth control among women at risk for EN. Many other drugs (Fig. 25.9) have also been implicated, and it is therefore reasonable to conclude that EN is, on occasions, an adverse drug reaction.

SARCOIDOSIS

Of patients in whom EN is a cutaneous manifestation of sarcoidosis, the majority will have hilar lymphadenopathy visible on chest radiography (see Investigations) and the overall prognosis is excellent compared with that of other presentations of sarcoidosis, such as parenchymal lung disease or lupus pernio. Tuberculosis presenting with this combination of clinical features is most unusual, but this diagnosis should be considered in children and in populations in which the

DRUG TRIGGERS OF ERYTHEMA NODOSUM
Sulfonamides
Penicillins
Oral contraceptives
Gold salts
Prazosin
Aspirin
Phenazone
Bromides

Fig. 25.9 Drug triggers of erythema nodosum.

incidence of TB is high. As there is a direct association of EN with infection, the association here can only strengthen the argument that sarcoidosis is caused by a microorganism, albeit unidentified as yet.

CANCER

There are a few reports of EN as the presenting feature of Hodgkin's and non-Hodgkin's lymphomas, but EN as a paraneoplastic phenomenon is rare. The finding of right paratracheal hilar lymphadenopathy on chest radiography should heighten suspicion, but sarcoidosis is still the likely diagnosis. Recurrent EN in a patient with chronic ill health should also raise the possibility of lymphoma. Erythema nodosum as a pointer of lymphoma relapse has been described[15].

SPONDYLOARTHROPATHY

Erythema nodosum is an unusual complication of spondyloarthritis and has been described in Behçet's syndrome and with chronic inflammatory bowel disease. In Behçet's syndrome, classic EN occurs but other skin lesions do arise which might be mistaken for EN despite being a manifestation of phlebitis or vasculitis[16] – skin biopsy should be diagnostic here. With inflammatory bowel disease, EN reflects heightened disease activity and is often combined with arthritis and uveitis. Erythema nodosum is a complication in 3% of those with chronic inflammatory bowel disease and is more common in Crohn's disease than in ulcerative colitis. As might be expected from this association with spondyloarthritis, EN is more common in chronic inflammatory bowel disease complicated by arthritis than in chronic bowel disease alone.

PATHOGENESIS

Erythema nodosum is a form of cell-mediated hypersensitivity. Cellular hypersensitivity results from an exaggerated interaction between antigen and cell-mediated immune mechanisms and is best exemplified by the formation of granulomata in tuberculosis. The evidence that EN is brought about by this mechanism comes from study of the histology. The early lesion of EN is characterized by an inflammatory infiltrate of lymphocytes and macrophages into the septal region of the fat panniculus, followed later by the formation of giant cells and granuloma. The presence of granuloma provides an important clue to etiology. Granuloma formation is a host tissue response to foreign antigen or immune complex and is most often seen in chronic infections. In sarcoidosis, the 'foreign antigen' has not been identified. In EN, serum immune complexes[17] and local vascular deposits of immunoglobulins and complement have been demonstrated, which indicates that the local inflammatory response is at least initiated by circulating factors. However, there is no evidence to date that microbial antigen is found locally when EN has been triggered by infection.

Further evidence of cell-mediated hypersensitivity comes from positive skin testing to bacterial antigens in EN. For instance, in EN triggered by TB, the Mantoux test is strongly positive whereas, in EN with bilateral hilar lymphadenopathy, it is negative at first and becomes positive during the convalescent phase of the disease. In lymphogranuloma venereum, EN appears when the Frei test is most strongly positive[18]. Furthermore, a relapse of EN can be provoked by repeating the Frei test[18].

MANAGEMENT

Erythema nodosum is an acute self-limiting disease. Therefore, once the diagnosis has been recognized, the management is straightforward.

In the acute phase of the disease, when the skin lesions are very tender and joints painful, the patient should and will want to rest. In most cases, there is a reasonable symptomatic response to nonsteroidal anti-inflammatory drug (NSAID) therapy taken with simple analgesics. The lesions are likely to be very painful for at least 2 weeks, and this should be pointed out to the patient.

If the acute pain persists or fails to respond symptomatically to the drug regimen described above, then a short course of systemic corticosteroids is indicated and will often produce good relief from symptoms. An alternative to corticosteroids is a course of oral potassium iodide (900mg daily in divided doses). Potassium iodide is described[19] as bringing about a rapid resolution of symptoms in the majority of patients with EN. Some success has also been attributed to the use of local heparinoid ointments. Hydroxychloroquine is another option for those with chronic EN[20].

The skin lesions of EN will normally resolve within 6–8 weeks, but the joint pain may take longer (up to 6 months) to resolve and here NSAIDs are normally sufficient to control pain.

REFERENCES

1. Willan R. On cutaneous diseases, vol 1. London: J Johnson; 1808:483.
2. King DS. Sarcoid disease as revealed by the chest roentgenogram. Am J Roentgenol. 1941;45:505–12.
3. Löfgren S. Primary pulmonary sarcoidosis. Part 1. Early signs and symptoms. Acta Med Scand. 1953;145:424–31.
4. Ryan TJ, Wilkinson DS. Cutaneous vasculitis 'angiitis'. In: Rook A, Wilkinson DS, Ebling FJG, Champion RH, Burton JL, eds. Textbook of dermatology. 4th ed. Oxford: Blackwell Scientific Publications; 1986:1121–87.
5. Vesey CMR, Wilkinson DS. Erythema nodosum. A study of seventy cases. Br J Dermatol. 1959;71:139–55.
6. Guyatt GH, Bensen WG, Stolmon LP, Fagnilli L, Singal DP. HLA-B8 and erythema nodosum. Can Med Assoc J. 1982;127:1005–6.
7. James GD, Thomson AD, Willcox A. Erythema nodosum as a manifestation of sarcoidosis. Lancet. 1956;ii:218–21.
8 Truelove LH. Articular manifestations of erythema nodosum. Ann Rheum Dis. 1960;19:174–80.
9. James GD. Erythema nodosum. Br Med J. 1961;1:853–7.
10. Various. Aetiology of erythema nodosum in children. Lancet. 1961;ii:14–16.
11. Feqeux S, Maslo C, De Truchis P, Matheron S, Couland JP. Erythema nodosum in HIV-infected patients. J Am Acad Dermatol. 1991;25:113.
12. Niemi K, Hannuksela M, Salo OP. Skin lesions in human yersiniosis. Br J Dermatol. 1976;94:155–60.
13. Hudson M, Smith CC. Erythema nodosum after two separate infective stimuli. Is the host more important than the stimulus? J Infect. 1989;19:185–6.
14. Ozols II, Wheat J. Erythema nodosum in an epidemic of histoplasmosis in Indianapolis. Arch Dermatol. 1981;117:709–12
15. Taillan B, Ferrari E, Fuzibet JG, Vinti H, Pesce A, Dujardin P. Erythema nodosum and Hodgkin's disease. Clin Rheumatol. 1990;9:397–8.
16. Chun SI, Su WPD, Lee S, Rogers RS. Erythema nodosum-like lesions in Behçet's syndrome: a histopathological study of 30 cases. J Cutan Pathol. 1989;16:259–65.
17. Niemi KM, Forstrom L, Hannuksela M, Mustakallio KK, Salo OP. Nodules on legs. Acta Dermatov (Stockh). 1977;57:145–54.
18. Hellerström S. Erythema nodosum. Acta Derm Venereol. 1966;46:469–72.
19. Schulz EJ, Whiting DA. Treatment of erythema nodosum and nodular vasculitis with potassium iodide. Br J Dermatol. 1976;94:75–8.
20. Alloway JA, Franks LK. Hydroxychloroquine in the treatment of chronic erythema nodosum. Br J Dermatol. 1995;132:661–73.

SARCOIDOSIS WITH SKELETAL INVOLVEMENT *Donald N Mitchell*

Definition

- A noncaseating granulomatous disease process affecting bone, synovial tissues, and muscle.

Clinical features

- Acute and chronic forms of polyarthritis, particularly involving the knees and ankles.
- Cystic bone lesions may produce dactylitis, or rare involvement of the skull, vertebrae, ribs or pelvis.
- Nonmusculoskeletal features are common and include bilateral hilar adenopathy, pulmonary infiltrates, skin lesions such as erythema nodosum, lupus pernio and uveitis.

ACUTE POLYARTHRITIS

In sarcoidosis the most common form of joint involvement is the febrile arthropathy which is often associated with bilateral hilar lymph node enlargement (BHL) and erythema nodosum (EN). The larger joints, especially the ankles and knees, are most frequently affected, although the shoulders, hips, wrists, elbows and the small joints of the hands and feet may also be involved[1,2]. In a study by the British Thoracic and Tuberculosis Association[3], arthropathy without EN was more frequent in men, occurring in 4%, as compared to 1% of women. In most patients, there are flitting pains, especially in knees and ankles, without objective signs. Pain and stiffness in the joint may be the only evidence, but in the more severely affected there may be considerable periarticular swelling and tenderness with effusions into the affected joints (Fig. 26.1). In these patients, tenderness and limitation of movement are found. Joints are usually affected symmetrically, although various joints may be affected consecutively. Painful swelling of the ankles (or other joints) may occur with or without EN. Joint symptoms may precede EN and may persist after its resolution, nor is their severity related to its extent. The arthropathy may resolve within a few weeks, but may persist for several months[2]. Biopsy of the synovial membrane has shown only an infiltration of mononuclear cells around small blood vessels extending into the synovium[4] or normal synovium[5]. Recurrence of acute polyarthritis during the course of sarcoidosis is uncommon and may be associated with generalized lymphadenopathy and granulomatous skin lesions[6,7] or with recurrent BHL and EN[8]. Glennas *et al.*[9] found that the number of new cases of acute sarcoid arthritis (SA) in the city of Oslo was 2.9/100,000. All presented with bilateral ankle involvement and BHL and more than half also had EN. The mean duration of the arthritis was 11 weeks, the EN was mild and transient and the intrathoracic manifestations resolved spontaneously within 2 years.

CHRONIC POLYARTHRITIS

Most, although not all, cases of chronic polyarthritis without involvement of the adjacent bone have been in black patients (Fig. 26.2). Sokoloff and Bunim reported five cases of sarcoidosis, all in young black men[10]. All had clinical and histologic evidence of sarcoidosis in several other organs. In three, the joints were affected early in the clinical course and, in two, about 2 years after other symptoms. In three, the joint symptoms had persisted for up to 8 years and both small and large joints were involved. In four patients, epithelioid and giant cell granulomas were

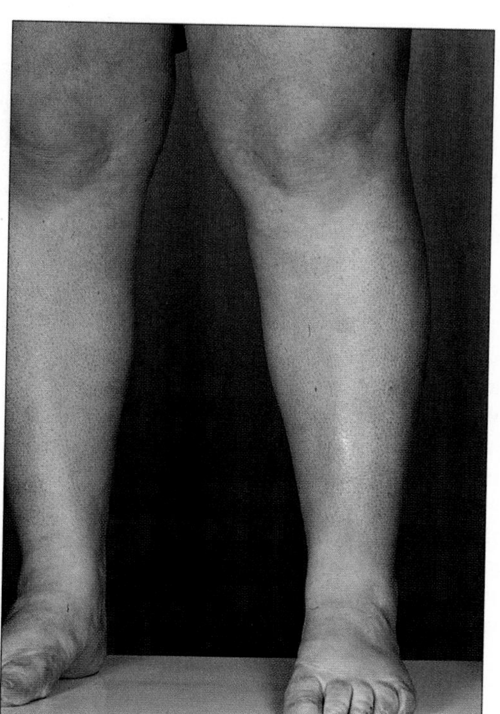

Fig. 26.1 Erythema nodosum. This patient presented with an arthropathy of knee joints associated with BHL. Symptoms (extreme lassitude, with pain and stiffness of large joints) were unusually persistent, and failed to resolve spontaneously or respond to treatment with nonsteroidal anti-inflammatory drugs. This picture was taken after 3 weeks' treatment with prednisolone.

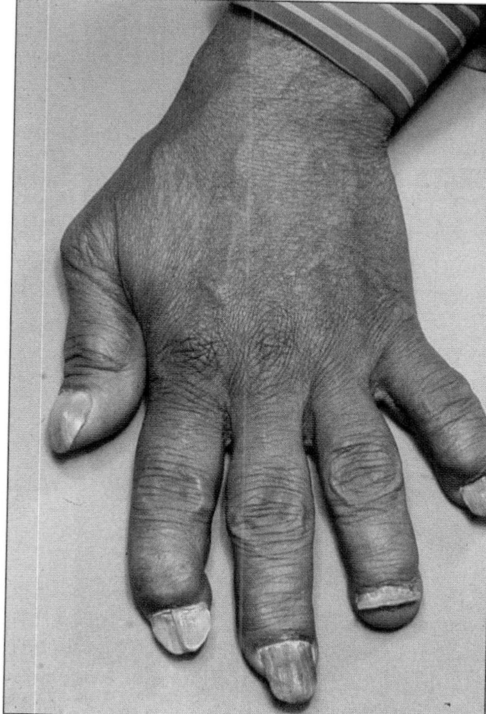

Fig. 26.2 Chronic polyarthritis. This patient with long-standing pulmonary sarcoidosis and granulomatous skin lesions developed polyarthritis of the interphalangeal joints.

obtained by biopsy of the synovium of the knee or elbow and in the fifth, who had five brief episodes of polyarthritis in 3 years, biopsy of synovial tissue from the wrist showed nonspecific changes. Although there was no radiographic evidence of the destruction of bone near the involved joints, one of these patients had associated lupus pernio and one showed cystic changes in the metatarsal bones of the feet. Serologic tests for rheumatoid factor (RF) were negative and no lupus erythematosus cells were found. Bianchi and Keech studied 12 black sarcoidosis patients with chronic joint changes[11]. Biopsy of joint synovia was undertaken in six; five showed synovitis with hypertrophy of the lining cells but epithelioid and giant cell granulomas were also present. Spilberg *et al.* studied seven patients with sarcoidosis in whom arthropathy had appeared at 7 months or up to 6 years after presentation[12]. Tenosynovitis of the wrists was present in two of the patients and, in both, biopsy of the tendon sheath yielded epithelioid and giant cell granulomas. In a review of 154 South African patients with sarcoidosis, Benatar found deforming arthritis in the hands of two of 30 black patients and none among 27 white and 102 patients of mixed race[13].

Migratory polyarthalgia or polyarthritis resembling acute rheumatic fever may be an initial feature and may precede other manifestations of sarcoidosis by several months. Polyarthritis is occasionally present in young children in whom other clinical manifestations are usually present. Most reported cases have been in patients under 5 years of age and have had granulomatous skin eruptions, uveitis, salivary gland involvement or splenomegaly[14–19]. Pulmonary involvement has infrequently been reported. The joints most commonly affected are ankles, knees, wrists and elbows; the metacarpophalangeal and interphalangeal joints are less commonly affected. Although the clinical picture of the joint changes may resemble Still's disease, the diagnosis of sarcoidosis is established by biopsy, either from other sites, from the synovium of the large joints or, most commonly, from tendon sheaths. Palmer and Schumacher investigated polyarthritic episodes in seven patients with chronic sarcoidosis[20]. Needle synovial biopsies at between 10 days and 7 weeks after the onset of joint symptoms showed that noncaseating granulomas are not necessarily a readily detectable feature of the episodic polyarthritis which may evolve in the course of chronic sarcoidosis. The synovial fluid from the involved joints is usually of a non- or mildly inflammatory type, although the onset of the arthropathy may be acute and dramatic. There is a preponderance of mononuclear cells in the synovial fluid. The diffuse synovial infiltrate consists principally of histocytic cells and lymphocytes and may be representative of the change that precedes epithelioid transformation and granuloma formation. Although some inflammatory cell infiltrate is common, it is less marked than that seen in chronic rheumatoid disease, so that adequate biopsies might help separate this from sarcoidosis even in the absence of granulomas.

ASSOCIATION WITH RA AND OTHER CONNECTIVE TISSUE DISORDERS

Some 40% of patients with RA develop lung function abnormalities consistent with a restrictive defect of lung function and some 6% have an abnormal chest radiograph with shadowing in one or both lung fields[21–24]. A review of the world literature shows only eight patients reported in whom sarcoidosis has developed after the onset of RA, and that there are few reports of patients with sarcoidosis who subsequently developed RA[25–28], although Menard *et al.*[29] have reported the association of histologically confirmed pulmonary sarcoidosis with RA proven by means of synovial biopsy. Fallahi *et al.* addressed the difficulty in differential diagnosis and emphasized the need for vigilance among patients with RA who develop extra-articular disease, such as uveal tract involvement, cranial neuropathies or clinically progressive lung disease[25]. Kucera reported two patients with RA who developed sarcoidosis[30]. Both were shown to have the HLA antigen DR4, which is known to be associated with RA[31], and both had Sjögren's syndrome. These findings raise the possibility that sarcoidosis may have an increased propensity to develop in patients with RA when Sjögren's syndrome was present in association with HLA-DR4.

Reports of sarcoidosis coexisting with connective tissue diseases are rare. Wiesenhutter and Sharma found that an extensive review of the literature disclosed only one case of sarcoidosis coexisting with progressive systemic sclerosis (PSS) and two cases coexisting with systemic lupus erythematosus (SLE)[32]. They reported a further three cases of sarcoidosis coexisting with PSS and one case coexisting with SLE, and reviewed the relationships between autoimmune disorders and sarcoidosis.

BONE CYSTS AND SARCOID DACTYLITIS

Among patients with early acute or subacute sarcoidosis, bone changes which cause no symptoms may be found in a small proportion (approximately 5%) on routine radiography of the hands and feet. Löfgren described 212 patients with BHL, of whom more than half had EN; in 30 of these, the hands and feet were examined radiographically and two were found to have skeletal lesions (Fig. 26.3)[33]. Series which include a high proportion of white patients presenting with recent BHL contain fewer patients with bone lesions than those which include a high proportion of black patients or those referred from dermatology clinics. Neville *et al.* reported that, of 567 patients attending a sarcoidosis clinic in London, 26 had changes in the bones of the hands or feet, one in the temporal bone, one in the hard palate and three in the nasal bones in association with nasal mucosal involvement[34]. Granulomatous skin lesions were present in 19 (66%) of those with bone changes, and took the form of lupus pernio in 14 (Fig. 26.4). Erythema nodosum had occurred in only one of 26 with bone involvement, as compared with 33% of the whole series. Thus, bony lesions of clinical significance are most often found among patients with chronic sarcoidosis and are often associated with lupus pernio and/or other granulomatous skin lesions. Leibowitz *et al.* reported six cases of sarcoid dactylitis in black South African patients and drew attention to the fact that in three of these six patients, dactylitis was the presenting feature of sarcoidosis and appeared without evidence of chronic fibrotic sarcoidosis elsewhere[35]. The significance of this localized presentation is that it is easily confused with tuberculoid leprosy and may therefore be misdiagnosed. It is rare for the long bones to show evidence of involvement by sarcoidosis. Zickel *et al.*[36] have reported the case of a patient seen initially because of pathologic fractures with nonunion. Despite extensive investigation the diagnosis of sarcoidosis was not firmly established until many years after the initial fracture. When there is osseous involvement the most common radiographic finding is diffuse rarefaction with reduction of the thickness of medullary trabeculae and cortical atrophy; when bone is involved the mortality rate is of the order of 21%, some four times greater than the overall mortality rate associated with sarcoidosis[37]. There are few reports of pathologic fracture through bone in patients with known sarcoidosis[34,38,39]. The results of treatment have been poor despite bone grafts, splinting or internal fixation and fractures often progress to nonunion.

The most common symptom of sarcoid dactylitis is swelling of the soft tissues over the affected digits, associated with tenderness and with painful stiffness of the adjacent joints: the overlying skin may be erythematous (Fig. 26.5). When the terminal phalanges are involved, the nails may show thickening, ridging distortion and dystrophy (Fig. 26.6). In severe cases, the affected bones may be completely resorbed, leading to virtual disappearance of the phalanges and marked deformity, sometimes complicated by pathologic fractures. Benatar has shown that these changes are more frequent in black patients and are rare in white patients with sarcoidosis[40,41]. Jüngling described three types of changes in phalanges[42]. In type I, the phalanx is diffusely expanded, the compact bone is thinned and the bone appears to consist of a number of cyst-like spaces of various sizes. In type II, the changes include round or oval punched-out areas. In type III, the radiograph of the affected bone shows a fine lattice-like structure. With

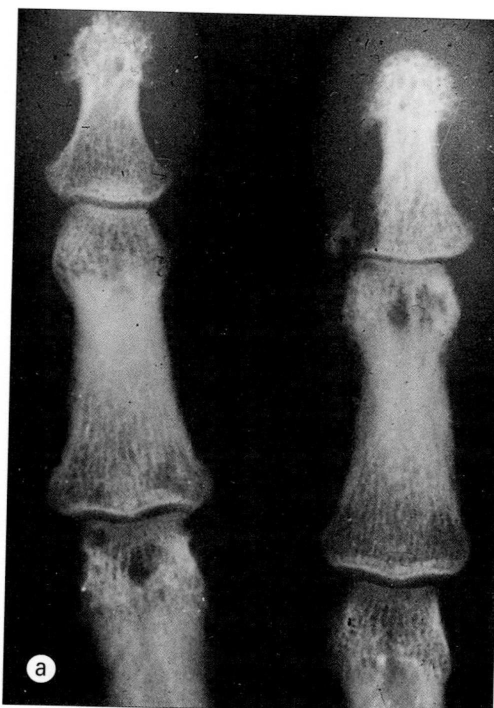

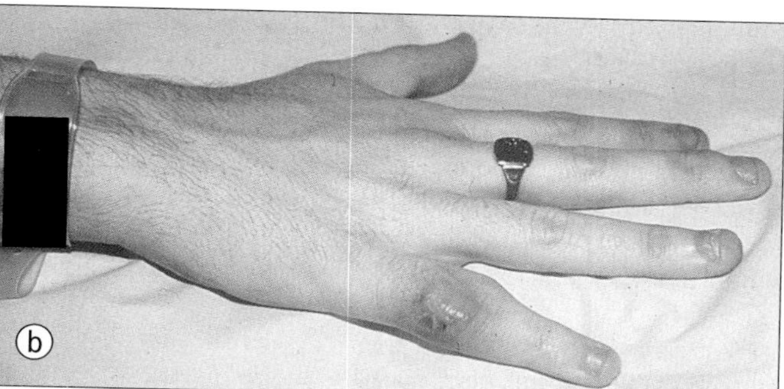

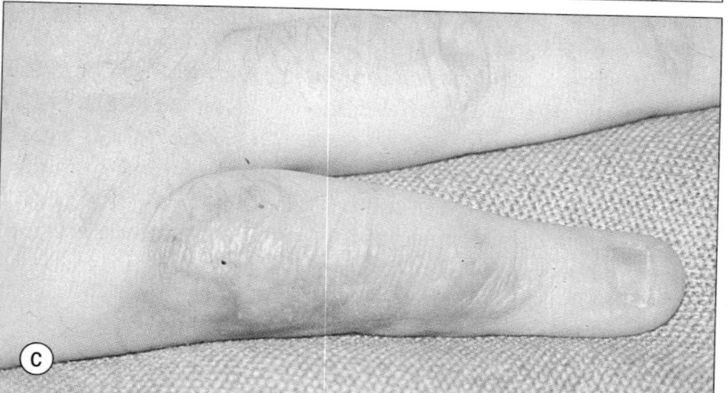

Fig. 26.3 Bone cysts and sarcoid dactylitis. Macroradiograph of small bones of the hand showing bone cysts in an asymptomatic patient with bilateral hilar lymphadenopathy (a). Dactylitis, with a small underlying bone cyst, in a patient with long-standing sarcoidosis (b). Resolution of the dactylitis after treatment with oral prednisolone (c).

all patterns of bone change, periosteal reaction is rare, sclerosis occurring only perifocally as part of the healing process; joints are involved only when adjacent bone is destroyed. The process is indolent and there is no sequestration, the possibility of healing being limited only by the degree of bone destruction and deformity. Schaumann gave a detailed account of the pathology of the changes in the small bones of the hands and feet[43,44]. Tuberculoid follicles surrounded by lymphocytes replaced the marrow between normal trabeculae; in the parts showing rarefaction, the trabeculae were resorbed leaving a space filled with tuberculoid granulation tissue. In the compact bone, there was irregular resorption with enlargement of Haversian canals containing granulomas. In a few places near the ends of the phalanx, granulomatous tissue extended into the tissues around the bone, infiltrating the tendon sheaths but leaving the tendons intact.

JOINT CHANGES ACCOMPANYING BONE INVOLVEMENT

When the small bones of the hands and feet are severely affected, the intervening joints are frequently involved. In these circumstances, confusion with primary diseases of joints is unlikely, especially when,

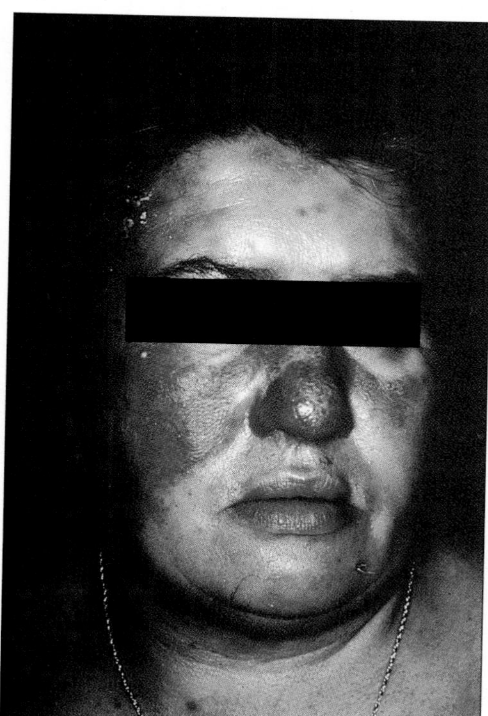

Fig. 26.4 Lupus pernio. Violaceous nodular and plaque eruption on the nose, cheeks and forehead in a patient with long-standing sarcoidosis.

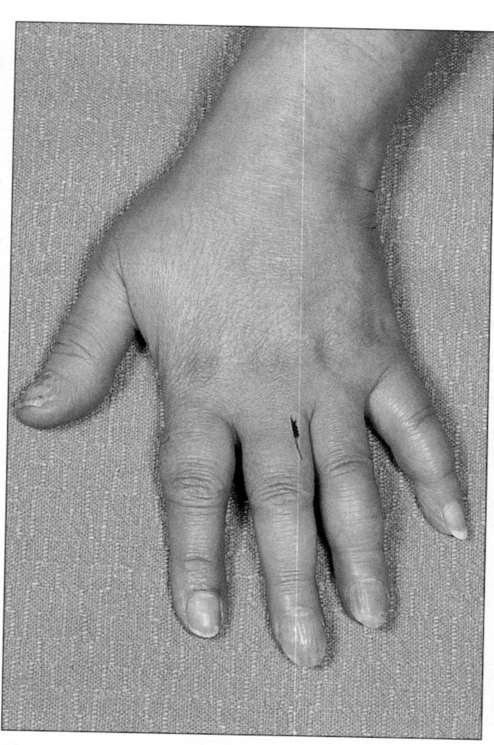

Fig. 26.5 Sarcoid dactylitis. Soft tissue swelling of the digits is seen in this patient with long-standing scaroidosis.

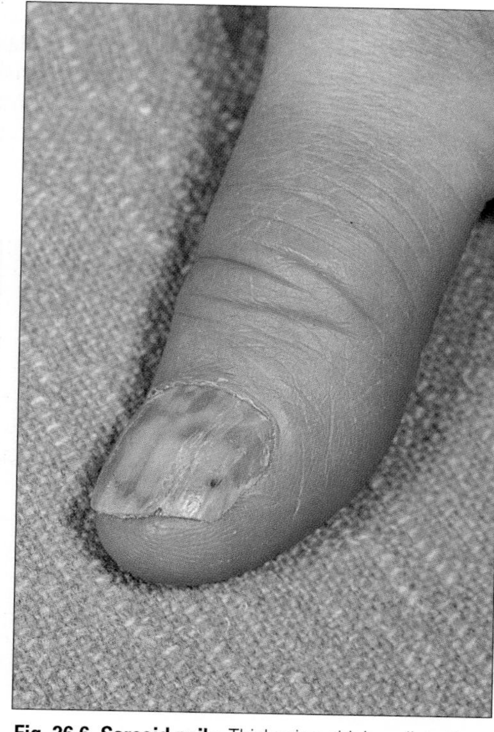

Fig. 26.6 Sarcoid nails. Thickening, ridging, distortion and dystrophy of nails in a patient with sarcoidosis.

as is the rule, there are changes of lupus pernio in the overlying skin. Very occasionally, the bone changes may present an atypical appearance and if, in such cases, there are no skin changes, the clinical picture may resemble that of RA. Synovitis of the tendon sheaths may occur in association with lupus pernio, and it is probable that granulomatous changes in the tendon sheaths and in the joint synovia, adjacent to affected bones, contribute to the soft tissue swelling that occurs in some cases of sarcoidosis of the bones of the hands[45].

NASAL BONES

The nasal bones may be involved in patients with lupus pernio affecting the nose[39] or in those with intranasal sarcoidosis (Fig. 26.7)[46]. To help guide treatment Krespi *et al.*[47] have developed a new staging system dividing sinonasal sarcoidosis into three categories according to the extent and reversibility of disease. Patients in stage 1 have limited, reversible involvement with hypertrophic turbinates, nucosal edema, and partial nasal airways obstruction: the paranasal sinuses are not involved. Patients in stage 2 have moderate but still potentially reversible disease with crusting, epistaxis, limited synechiae, vestibular granulomas or limited single sinus involvement or mucoperiosteal thickening. Stage 3 categorizes patients with irreversible disease that progresses to ulcerations, extensive intranasal synechiae, nasal stenosis, cartilage destruction, saddle nose deformity, nasal cutaneous fistulization or extensive multiple sinus involvement.

SKULL

Sarcoidosis of the skull is a rare manifestation of sarcoidosis, only 11 cases having been reported over the past 40 years[48–50]. Radiographically, the lesions in the skull appear as multiple areas of bone translucency with well-demarcated margins and no surrounding sclerotic or reactive changes. The diameter of the lesions varies from 0.1cm to 4.0cm. In contrast to metastatic neoplasms, the calvarial tables are intact and the serum alkaline phosphatase is usually normal despite the massive bone destruction. Although reactive sclerosis is usually absent, some irregular peripheral sclerosis has occasionally been found[51] and Silver *et al.* reported a case in which widespread changes in bones, including the skull, were radiographically dense[52]. Most reported cases have been discovered incidentally but there may be tenderness over the vertex of the skull. Headache may be a feature and lead to radiography of the skull. This was a presenting symptom in a 46-year-old woman whose case was reported by Perrin-Fayolle *et al.*[51]. In a few other cases, local soft tissue swellings or headache have drawn attention to cranial lesions in patients with sarcoidosis[53,54]. Partial or complete resolution of the lesions may occur spontaneously and the role of adrenocortical steroids in the treatment of calvarial sarcoidosis is therefore difficult to assess[55].

VERTEBRAE

In a small number of patients with sarcoidosis, a complaint of back pain has led to the detection of vertebral involvement. In most patients, the changes have been lytic or destructive with collapse or wedging of the vertebral bodies[56–58]. Disc spaces adjacent to affected vertebrae may be narrowed[57–59]. In some patients, the condition of the affected vertebrae may improve[60] or resolve spontaneously[61]. Responses to corticosteroid treatment have appeared favorable[62] or doubtful[56].

RIBS

Involvement of ribs in connection with vertebral sarcoidosis has been reported by Young and Laman[63], Baldwin *et al.*[59], Stump *et al.*[57] and Cutler *et al.*[58], and was detected by radioisotope survey in a case of bone sarcoidosis reported by Silver *et al.*[52]. Radiographically there may be localized rarefactions or densities. Young and Laman found thickening of bone trabeculae, replacement of marrow by connective tissue, and well-defined granulomas following biopsy of a rib showing increased density[63]. Similarly, Baldwin *et al.*, following open biopsy of a rib which showed erosion of its lower border, found edematous periosteum and a soft rib, each structure showing many noncaseating granulomas[59].

PELVIC BONES

Bonakdapour *et al.*[64], Lin *et al.*[65] and Silver *et al.*[52] have each reported involvement of the pelvic bones; all were in black patients with widespread clinical involvement by sarcoidosis. Radiographically, there may be areas of rarefaction or of increased bone density. Bonakdapour *et al.* performed biopsy of the iliac crest in one patient and found thick cancellous bone with paucity of osteoblastic and osteoclastic activity[64]. Noncaseating granulomas were present throughout the hemopoietic and fatty bone marrow. Silver *et al.* found that their patient had complained of low back pain for some 20 years following the diagnosis of sarcoidosis[52]. Radiographically, there were dense areas in both iliac bones; biopsy of the iliac crest showed epithelioid and giant cell granulomas. Treatment with prednisolone gave relief of pain but no radiographic improvement was noted. The patient reported by Lin *et al.* showed diffuse osteosclerotic changes in the pelvis and sacrum[65]. Biopsy of the iliac crest again yielded sarcoid granulomas.

HEEL PAIN

Gumpel *et al.* noted heel pain in two of 50 patients presenting with sarcoid arthritis[66]. Subsequently, Shaw *et al.* reported seven patients with sarcoidosis in whom heel pain was a significant feature of their illness[67]. All had polyarticular involvement and hilar adenopathy. Ott and van Linthoudi reported a patient who presented with arthralgia and hilar lymphadenopathy in whom heel pain persisted after spontaneous improvement of other associated symptoms and suggested that such

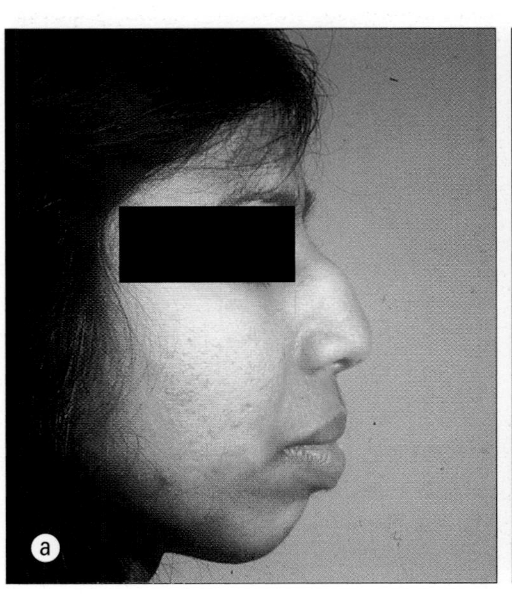

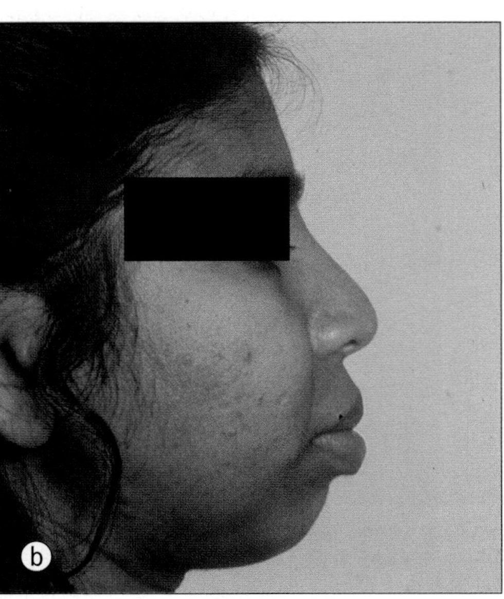

Fig. 26.7 Sarcoidosis involving the nasal bones. Stage 1 nasal involvement in this patient with BHL and lupus pernio (a).The same patient is shown after treatment with oral prednisolone for one year(b).

patients could develop a true spondyloarthropathy[68]. Certainly bilateral heel pain can be a presenting symptom of sarcoidosis and may accompany or precede sarcoid arthritis. Blacksin *et al.*[69] report the use of magnetic resonance imaging (MRI) performed to evaluate possible rupture of the posterior tibial tendon and Archilles tendinitis. MRI showed no evidence of tendinopathy or rupture but did demonstrate multiple foci of abnormal bone marrow signal throughout the bones of the foot. Biopsy of the calcaneal lesion seen on MRI showed noncaseating granulomas within the calcaneus.

MYOPATHY

First described by Myers *et al.*[70], sarcoid myopathy is rare. Symptomatic patients typically have a chronic, slowly progressive muscle disease that closely resembles chronic polymyositis or muscular dystrophy. Other symptomatic forms include palpable muscle nodules and acute myositis.

Asymptomatic muscle involvement is thought to occur in 50–80% of cases[71]. Wolfe *et al.* reported four patients with muscle weakness and reviewed the clinical features of 75 previously reported cases of sarcoid myopathy[72]. Asymptomatic muscle granulomas may occur in the course of sarcoidosis and random muscle biopsy has provided one method of tissue diagnosis in sarcoidosis[73]. The least common form of symptomatic sarcoid muscle disease is the palpable nodule, which may cause pain, stiffness and cramps.

An acute myositis may occur, but is rare; in such cases, creatine kinase (CK) has been found to be elevated[74]. It is the least frequent form of sarcoid muscle involvement; only some 18 cases have been reported in the English language literature. Most present with fevers and myalgias over a period of weeks or months and may simulate the presentation of acute polymyositis: the majority of patients so affected are female and black. All show predominant proximal muscle weakness, most commonly of hips and shoulders. Ost *et al.*[75] have reported a single case of acute sarcoid myositis affecting the respiratory muscles, responsive to prednisolone with resolution of symptoms and improvement of pulmonary function tests. Al-Saffar *et al.*[76] have reported acute sarcoid myositis in a West Indian woman with pulmonary sarcoidosis who showed markedly elevated CK levels associated with eosinophilia for which no other cause could be found. She was treated with prednisolone and showed marked improvement in muscle strength with rapid return of the eosinophilia and CK levels to normal. Chronic myopathy is frequently seen and is a slowly progressive, often symmetric disease, involving the proximal muscles of the extremities, trunk and neck, often with muscle wasting. Distal muscle involvement may be secondary to peripheral neuropathy. Chronic myopathy usually occurs in older patients, predominantly postmenopausal women. Muscle enzymes are often increased and electromyogram (EMG) shows a myopathic pattern. Pseudohypertrophy is occasionally seen[77–79].

The response of acute myopathy to treatment with corticosteroids is good and the course usually benign, but in chronic myopathy it is unpredictable, with a variable but chronic course with remissions and exacerbations needing continued suppression and adjustments of corticosteroid dose[72].

The association of myasthenia gravis (MG) with sarcoidosis is rare. Sarcoidosis has developed during remission of MG in some and during a resurgence of sarcoidosis in others. Regression of MG and sarcoidosis after thymectomy has also been reported. Takanana *et al.*[80] have described such an association in which, as one would expect, MG became less severe after thymectomy, but sarcoidosis did not.

CLINICAL INVESTIGATIONS

Apart from the clinical, radiographic and biopsy findings (including technetium-99m pyrophosphate or gallium-67 scans where appropriate), the diagnosis of sarcoidosis will often be supported by evidence of the presence of sarcoid granulomas in a number of other organs or tissues. Although the number of patients who present with a normal chest radiograph varies with the nature and source of their referral, it is of the order of 5–10%[81]. Computed tomography (CT) may in some cases show quite marked mediastinal nodal involvement and/or unexpected parenchymal disease, even in the presence of a virtually normal chest radiograph (Fig. 26.8). Moreover, CT changes may match pulmonary function abnormalities more closely than the chest radiograph[82]. Accordingly, if a patient with a normal or near normal chest radiograph shows significant impairment of standard lung function tests, it may well be profitable to proceed to CT, which may assist in a more critical assessment.

In the majority of patients, hilar node enlargement is bilateral, but apparently unilateral and usually right-sided hilar adenopathy and/or unilateral paratracheal adenopathy is present in some 4% of patients[83–85]. It is important that this possibility be appreciated because of the increasing recognition of the prevalence of sarcoidosis among the Asian population of the UK, in whom it is especially important to exclude the possibility that mediastinal lymphadenopathy may be attributable to tuberculosis. Transbronchial biopsy of the radiologically

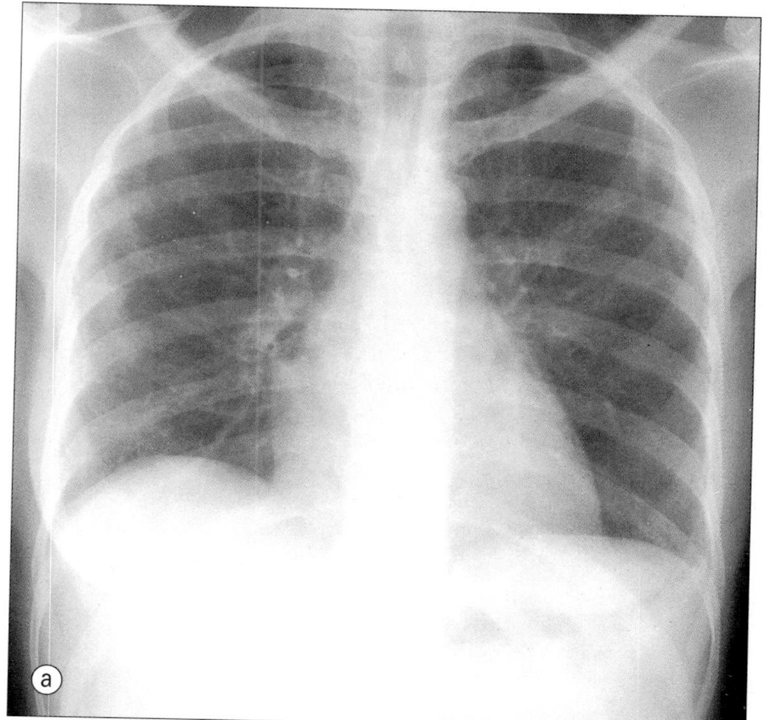

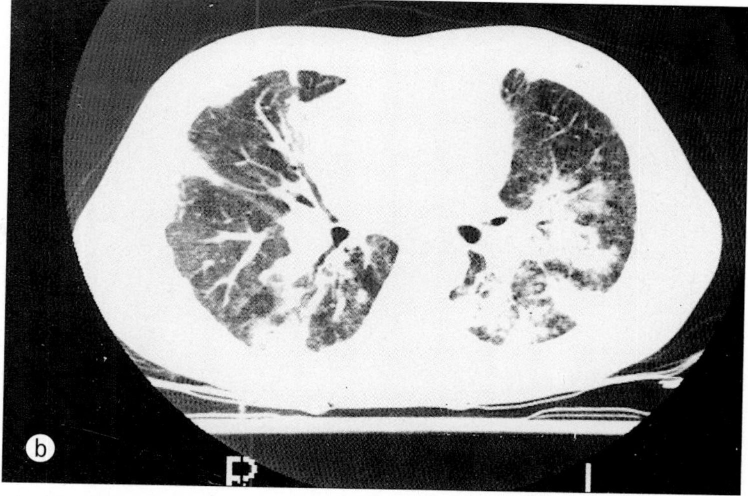

Fig. 26.8 Pulmonary sarcoidosis. Radiograph of patient with pulmonary sarcoidosis showing minimal changes (a). CT scan of the chest done at the same time shows extensive changes (b).

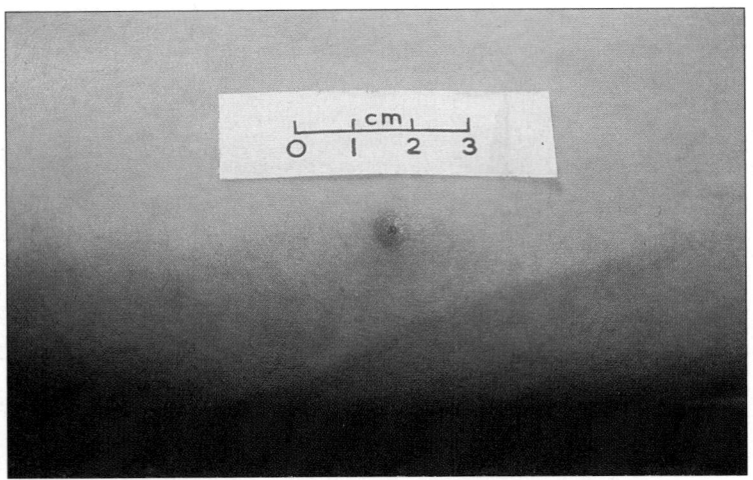

Fig. 26.9 Classical Kveim papule. The histology of the lesion showed noncaseating epithelioid and giant cell granulomas.

normal lung will yield the presence of epithelioid and giant cell granulomas in some 60% of such patients[86].

Alternatively, and provided the diagnosis of sarcoidosis remains highly probable on clinical grounds so as to justify the delay of 4–6 weeks incurred between its insertion and biopsy of the resultant test site, a Kveim test will provide histologic support for the diagnosis in a substantial proportion (50–70%) of such cases (Fig. 26.9). The rates of Kveim reactivity fall off with increasing duration of disease[87]. In appropriate circumstances of doubt as to the diagnosis, recourse may be made to mediastinal lymph node biopsy via mediastinoscopy or mediastinotomy. The essential histologic features of sarcoidosis are well-circumscribed epithelioid cell tubercles with a variable amount of lymphocytic infiltration peripherally. The tubercles show no caseation, although there may be some central eosinophilic necrosis with or without disruption of the reticulin pattern (Fig. 26.10). The latter finding may correlate with the acute symptomatic onset of sarcoidosis[88].

It is noteworthy that Kunkel *et al.* found positive latex fixation tests for rheumatoid factor (RF) in six of 61 patients with sarcoidosis, although the Rose-Waaler test was negative in all[89]. Similarly, Oreskes and Siltzbach found that 38% of 64 patients with sarcoidosis had positive tanned red cell tests for RF, compared with 8% of a control group; 3% had positive Rose-Waaler tests; positive tests were found twice as often in women as in men and were more frequent in those with active disease and with persistent lung changes[90]. Antinuclear factor with a speckled pattern of immunofluorescence may be found in low titer in the serum of a few patients with sarcoidosis[11], but no more frequently than among control subjects[91].

Gallium citrate scanning may reveal a characteristic pattern of uptake and thereby assist in providing support for a diagnosis of sarcoidosis (Fig. 26.11). It is important to note however that ^{67}Ga is also taken up by other inflammatory and malignant diseases, including tuberculosis and lymphomas. Moreover the pattern of gallium uptake may change rapidly, with different regions of the lung being involved with varying intensity patterns.

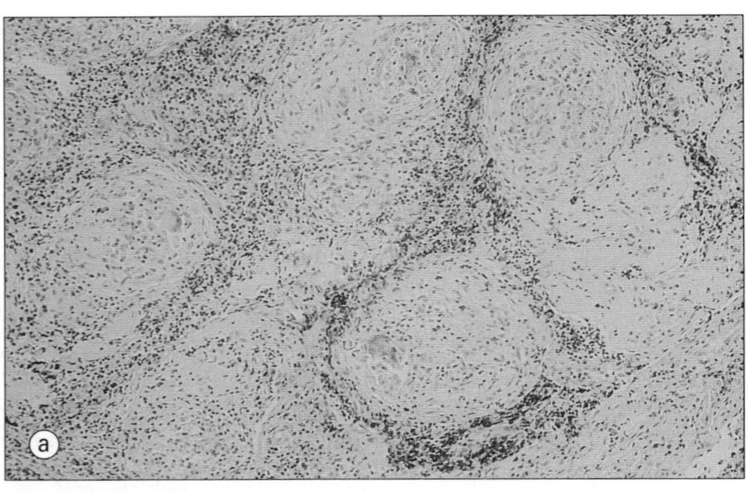

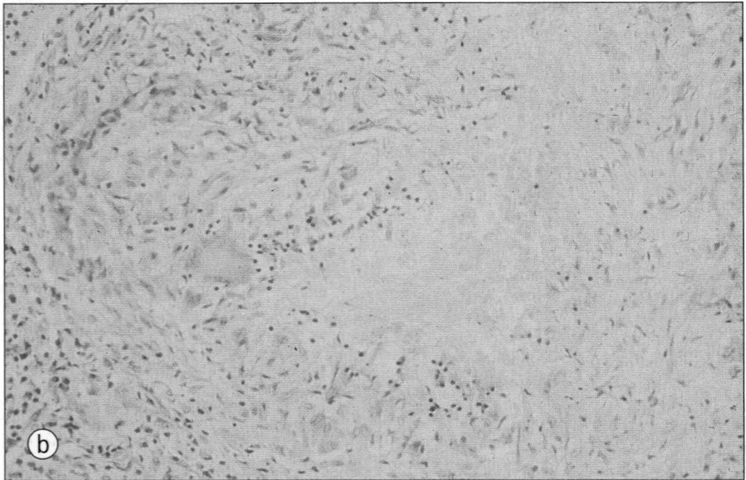

Fig. 26.10 Changes to reticulin pattern. Histology of the lymph node from a patient with sarcoidosis, showing noncaseating epithelioid and giant cell granulomas (a). Histology from a patient with sarcoidosis, showing noncaseating epithelioid and giant cell granulomas with central eosinophilic necrosis of collagen, correlating here with acute symptomatic onset of sarcoidosis (b). There was subsequent natural resolution without treatment in this case.

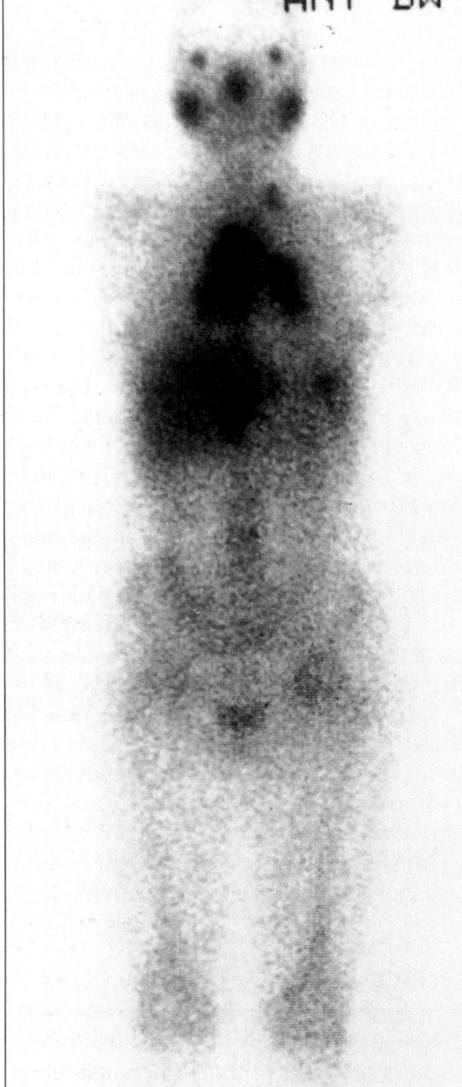

Fig. 26.11 Abnormal gallium scan in sarcoidosis. The scan shows uptake in lacrimal, parotid and salivary glands as well as in mediastinum and lungs.

In the majority of patients, however, the combination of the clinical, radiologic, physiologic and laboratory findings, including serum angiotensin-1-converting enzyme (ACE), are sufficient to reach a definite or highly probable diagnosis of sarcoidosis. In all doubtful cases and in cases where treatment is likely to be needed, support for the diagnosis from tissue biopsy or by Kveim testing is, wherever possible, essential.

MANAGEMENT

Most patients with acute musculoskeletal manifestations of sarcoidosis respond well to nonsteroidal anti-inflammatory drugs (NSAIDs), such as indomethacin. The chronic, persistent form of arthritis often accompanies an aggressive course of sarcoidosis in which major organs are affected and corticosteroids are required. Oral prednisone in doses of 40–60mg daily is recommended, with gradual tapering of the dose to an acceptable maintenance level that controls the disease. Reparative changes are sometimes observed in affected bones following prolonged suppression of sarcoidosis with corticosteroids, but it is often difficult to be certain as to whether a similar degree of resolution might not have accrued during the natural evolution of the disease. Case reports have appeared on the efficacy of immune modulating drugs, such as chlorambucil or cyclosporin A in sarcoidosis; however these agents should be reserved for patients with progressive, severe disease that is unresponsive to corticosteroid therapy.

REFERENCES

1. Williams MJ. Sarcoidosis presenting with polyarthritis. Ann Rheum Dis. 1961;20:138–43.
2. Gumpel JM, Johns CJ, Shulman LE. The joint disease of sarcoidosis. Ann Rheum Dis. 1967;26:194–205.
3. British Thoracic and Tuberculosis Association. Geographical variations in the incidence of sarcoidosis in Great Britain: a comparative study of four areas. Tubercle. 1966;50:211–32.
4. Ferguson EH, Paris J. Sarcoidosis: study of 29 cases, with review of splenic, hepatic, mucous membrane, retinal and joint manifestations. Arch Intern Med. 1958;101:1065–84.
5. Siltzbach LE, Duberstein JL. Arthritis in sarcoidosis. Clin Orthop. 1968;57:31–50.
6. Moreau MR. Formes articulaires de la maladie de Besnier–Boeck–Schaumann. Bull Acad Nat Med [Paris]. 1949;133:89–91.
7. Ridley CM. Sarcoidosis with unusual arthritis. Proc R Soc Med. 1957;59:609–10.
8. MacFarlane JT. Recurrent erythema nodosum and pulmonary sarcoidosis. Postgrad Med J. 1981;57:525–7.
9. Glennas A, Kvien K, Melby K, *et al.* Acute sarcoid arthritis: occurrences, seasonal onset, clinical features and outcome. Br J Rheum. 1995;34:45–50.
10. Sokoloff L, Bunin JJ. Clinical and pathological studies of joint involvement in sarcoidosis. N Engl J Med. 1959;260:841–7.
11. Bianchi FA, Keech MK. Sarcoidosis with arthritis. Ann Rheum Dis. 1964;23:463–79.
12. Spilberg I, Siltzbach LE, McEwen C. The arthritis of sarcoidosis. Arthritis Rheum. 1969;12:126–37.
13. Benatar SR. Sarcoidosis in South Africa. S Afr Med J. 1978;52:602–6.
14. Burman MS, Mayer L. Arthroscopic examination of knee joint: report of cases observed in course of arthroscopic examination, including instances of sarcoid and multiple polypoid fibromatosis. Arch Surg. 1936;32:846–74.
15. Zweifel E. Gleichzeitiges Vorkommen eines, Boeckschen Sarkoids mit einer primaren chronischen Polyarthritis (beginnendes Sjögren-Syndrom). Helv Paediatr Acta. 1946;1:475–84.
16. Castelanos A, Galan E. Sarcoidosis: report of a case in child simulating Still's disease. Am J Dis Child. 1946;71:513–29.
17. Schweizner VG, Kanaar P. Sarcoidosis with polyarthritis in a child. Arch Dis Child. 1967;42:671–4.
18. Toomey F, Bautista A. Rare manifestations of sarcoidosis in children. Radiology. 1970;94:569–73.
19. North AF Jr, Fink CW, Gibson WM, *et al.* Sarcoid arthritis in children. Am J Med. 1970;48:499–555.
20. Palmer DG, Schumacher HR. Synovitis with non-specific histological changes in synovium in chronic sarcoidosis. Ann Rheum Dis. 1984;43:778–82.
21. Patterson CD, Harville WE, Pierce JA. Rheumatoid lung disease. Ann Intern Med. 1965;62:689–97.
22. Frank ST, Weg JG, Harkleroad LE, Fitch RF. Pulmonary dysfunction in rheumatoid arthritis. Chest. 1973;63:27–34.
23. Laitinen O, Nissila M, Salorinne Y. Pulmonary involvement in patients with rheumatoid arthritis. Scand J Resp Dis. 1975;56:297–304.
24. Cervantes-Perez P, Toro-Perez AH, Rodriguez Jurado P. Pulmonary involvement in rheumatoid arthritis. JAMA. 1980;243:1715–19.
25. Fallahi S, Collins RD, Miller RK, Hala JT. Coexistence of rheumatoid arthritis and sarcoidosis: difficulties encountered in the differential diagnosis of common manifestations. J Rheum. 1984;11:506–29.
26. Davis MW, Crotty RQ. Sarcoidosis associated with polyarthritis. Ann Intern Med. 1952;36:1098–106.
27. Putkonen T, Virkkunen M, Wager O. Joint involvement in sarcoidosis with special reference to the coexistence of sarcoidosis and rheumatoid arthritis. Acta Rheum Scand. 1965;11:53–61.
28. Tane N, Hayashi M, Sakoda A, Mayeda A, Uda H. Extra-articular sarcoid lesions in a case treated as rheumatoid arthritis – a case report. Ryumachi. 1980;20:358–67.
29. Menard O, Petit N, Gillet P, Laucher A, Martinet Y. Association of histologically proven rheumatoid arthritis with pulmonary sarcoidosis. Eur Respir J. 1995;8:472–3.
30. Kucera RF. A possible association of rheumatoid arthritis and sarcoidosis. Chest. 1989;95:604–6.
31. Carpenter B. The major histocompatibility gene complex. In: Petersdorf RG, Adams RD, Braunwald E, *et al.*, eds. Harrison's principles of internal medicine, 10E. New York: McGraw-Hill;1983:330–1.
32. Wiesenhutter CW, Sharma OP. Is sarcoidosis an autoimmune disease? Report of four cases and review of the literature. Semin Arthritis Rheum. 1979;9:124–40.
33. Löfgren S. Primary pulmonary sarcoidosis. Acta Med Scand. 1953;145:424–31, 465–74.
34. Neville E, Carstairs LS, James DG. Sarcoidosis of bone. Q J Med. 1977;46:215–27.
35. Leibowitz MR, Essop AR, Shamroth D, Blumsohn D, Smith EH. Sarcoid dactylitis in black South African patients. Semin Arthritis Rheum. 1985;14:232–7.
36. Zickel RE, Bernstein RS, Ryan SF Carney WP. Pathological ununited fractures of the long bones in a patient who had sarcoidosis. J Bone J Surg. 1995;77:440–3.
37. Redman DS, McCarty RE, Jimenez JE. Sarcoidosis in the long bones of a child. A case report and review of the literature. J.Bone Joint Surg. 1983;65A:1010–14.
38. Adelaeer RS. Sarcoidosis of the upper extremity: case presentation and literature review. J Hand Surg. 1983;8:492–6.
39. Watson RC, Cahen I. Pathological fracture in long bone sarcoidosis. Report of a case. J Bone J Surg. 1973;55A:613–17.
40. Benatar SR. Sarcoidosis in South Africa. S Afr Med J. 1978;52:602–6.
41. Benatar SR. A comparative study of sarcoidosis in white, black and coloured South Africans. In: Jones-Williams W, Davies BH, eds. Proceedings of the Eighth International Conference on Sarcoidosis, Cardiff (1978). Cardiff: Alpha Omega; 1980:508–13.
42. Jüngling O. Uber Ostitis tuberculosa multiplex crystoides, zugleich ein Beitrag zur Lehre von der Tuberkuliden des Knochens. Beitr Klin Chirug. 1928;143:401–75.
43. Schaumann J. Etudes histologiques et bactériologique sur les manifestations médallaires du lymphogranulome bénin. Ann Dermatol Syphiligr. 1919;7:385–98.
44. Schaumann J. Benign lymphogranuloma and its cutaneous manifestations. Br J Dermatol Syph. 1924;36:515–44.
45. Neville E, Mills RJS, Jash DG. Sarcoidosis of the upper respiratory tract and its association with lupus pernio. Thorax. 1976;31:660–4.
46. Wilson R, Sweatman M, Mitchell DN. Upper respiratory tract involvement in sarcoidosis and its management. Eur Respir J. 1988;1:269–72.
47. Krespi YP, Kuriloff DB, Aner M. Sarcoidosis of the sinonasal tract: A new staging system. Otolaryngol Head Neck Surg. 1995;112:221–7.
48. Tierstein AS, Wolf BS, Siltzbach LE. Sarcoidosis of the skull. N Eng J Med. 1961;265:65–8.
49. Zimmerman R, Leeds NE. Calvarial and vertebral sarcoidosis. Radiology. 1976;119:384.
50. Landsberger D, Ravé D, Friedman G. The skull in chronic sarcoidosis. Postgrad Med J. 1988;64:875–7.
51. Perrin-Fayolle M, Bouvier M, Queneau P, Deplante JP. Lacunes craiennes au cours d'une

sarcoidose gangliopulmonare. Lyon Med. 1971;225:945–53.
52. Silver HM, Shirkhoda A, Simon DB. Symptomatic osseous sarcoidosis with findings on bone scan. Chest. 1978;73:238–41.
53. Nou E. Sarcoidosis with skull lesions. Acta Tuberc Scand. 1965;47:147–52.
54. Rohatgi PK. Radioisotope scanning in osseous sarcoidosis. Am J Radiol. 1980;134:189–91.
55. Cinti DC, Hawkins HB, Slavin JD. Radioisotope bone scanning in a case of sarcoidosis. Clin Nucl Med. 1986;10:192–4.
56. Bloch S, Morison IJ, Seedat YK. Unusual skeletal manifestations in a case of sarcoidoisis. Clin Radiol. 1968;19:226–8.
57. Stump D, Spock A, Grossman H. Vertebral sarcoidosis in adolescents. Radiology. 1976;121:153–5.
58. Cutler SS, Sankaranarayanan G. Vertebral sarcoidosis. JAMA. 1978;24:557–8.
59. Baldwin DM, Roberts JG, Croft HE. Vertebral sarcoidosis. J Bone J Surg. 1974;56:629–32.
60. Brody PA, Pripstein S, Strange G, Kohout ND. Vertebral sarcoidosis. Am J Roentgenol. 1976;126:900–2.
61. Berk RN, Brewer TD. Vertebral sarcoidosis. Radiology. 1964;82:660–3.
62. Goobar JE, Gilmer WS Jr, Carroll DS, Clark GM. Vertebral sarcoidosis. JAMA. 1961;178:1162–3.
63. Young DA, Laman ML. Radiodense skeletal lesions in Boeck's sarcoid. Am J Roentgenol. 1972;114:533–8.
64. Bonakdapour A, Levy W, Aegertev EE. Osteosclerotic changes in sarcodosis. Am J Roentgenol. 1971;113:646–9.
65. Lin SR, Levy W, Go EB, Lee I, Wong WK. Unusual osteosclerotic changes in sarcoidosis, simulating osteoblastic metastases. Radiology. 1973;106:311–12.
66. Gumpel JM, Johns CJ, Sculman, LE. The joint disease of sarcoidosis. 1967;26:194–205.
67. Shaw RA, Holt PA, Stevens MB. Heel pain in sarcoidosis. Ann Intern Med. 1988;109:675–7.
68. Ott H, van Linthoudi D. Heel pain in sarcoidosis – is sarcoid a cause of spondarthropathy? Br J Rheumatol. 1987;26:468.
69. Blacksin M, Acello AN, Kowalec J, Lyons MM. Osseous sarcoidosis of the foot: detection by MR imaging. Am J Roentgenol. 1994;163:1444–5.
70. Myers GB, Gottlieb AM, Mottiman PE. Joint and muscle manifestations in sarcoid. Am J Med. 1952;12:161–9.
71. Silverstein A, Siltzbach LE. Muscle involvement in sarcoidosis. Arch Neurol. 1969;21:235–41.
72. Wolfe SM, Pinals RS, Aelion JA, Goodman RE. Myopathy in sarcoidosis: clinical and pathologic study of four cases and review of the literature. Semin Arthritis Rheum. 1987;16:300–6.
73. Phillips RW, Phillips AM. The diagnosis of Boeck's sarcoid by skeletal muscle biopsy. Arch Intern Med. 1956;98:732–6.
74. Alpert JN, Groff AE, Bastian FO. Acute polymyositis caused by sarcoid: report of a case and review of the literature. Mt Sinai J Med. 1979;46:486–8.
75. Ost D, Yeldani A, Cudgell D. Acute sarcoid myositis with respiratory muscle involvement. Chest. 1995;107:879–82.
76. Al-Saffar ZS, Kelsey CR, Kennet RP, Webbey M. Myositis and eosinophilia in a patient with sarcoidosis. Postgrad Med J. 1994;70:833–5
77. Douglas AC, MacLeod JG, Matthews JO. Symptomatic sarcoidosis of skeletal muscle. J Neurol Neurosurg Psychiatry. 1973;36:1034–40.
78. Dyken PR. Sarcoidosis of skeletal muscle. Neurology. 1962;12:643–51.
79. Delaney P. Neurologic manifestations of sarcoidosis. Ann Intern Med. 1977;87:336–45.
80. Takanami I, Imanura T, Kodaira S. Myasthenia gravis complicated by sarcoidosis. J Thorac Cardiovasc Surg. 1995;109:183–4.
81. Dunbar RD. Sarcoidosis and its radiologic manifestations. CRC Crit Rev Diagnostic Imaging. 1978;11:185–221.
82. Putman CE, Rothman SL, Littner MR. Computerized tomography in pulmonary sarcoidosis. Comput Tomog. 1977;1:197–209.
83. Kirks DR, McCormick VD, Greenspan RH. Pulmonary sarcoidosis: roentgenologic analysis of 150 patients. Am J Roentgenol. 1973;117:778–86.
84. Kent DC. Recurrent unilateral hilar adenopathy in sarcoidosis. Am Rev Resp Dis. 1965;91:272–6.
85. Mikhail JR, Mitchell DN, Sutherland I, McNicol MW. Sarcoidosis presenting in a district general hospital. In: Jones-Williams W, Davies BH, eds. Proceedings of the Eighth International Conference on Sarcoidosis (1978). Cardiff: Alpha Omega; 1980:532–42.
86. Mitchell DN, Emerson CJ, Collins JV. Transbronchial lung biopsy (TBB) in 433 patients. In: Nakhosteen JA, Maasen W, eds. Bronchology. The Hague: Martinus Nijhoff; 1981:333–7.
87. Munro C, Mitchell D. The Kveim test: still useful, still a puzzle. Thorax. 1987;44:371–2.
88. Carlens E, Hanngren A, Ivemark B. The concomitance of feverish onset of sarcoidosis and necrosis formation in the lymph nodes. In: Iwai K, Hosoda Y, eds. Proceedings of the VI International Conference on Sarcoidosis (1972). Tokyo: University of Tokyo Press; 1974:409–12.
89. Kunkel HG, Simon HJ, Fudenberg H. Observations concerning positive serologic reactions for rheumatoid factor in certain patients with sarcoidosis and other hyperglobulinaemic states. Arthritis Rheum. 1958;1:289–96.
90. Oreskes I, Siltzbach LE. Changes in rheumatoid factor activity during the course of sarcoidosis. Am J Med. 1968;44:60–7.
91. Turner-Warwick M. Autoantibodies in allergic respiratory disease. In: Brent L, Holborow, J, eds. Progress in immunology, 11, vol 4. Amsterdam: Elsevier; 1974:238.

27

RELAPSING POLYCHONDRITIS

Harvinder S Luthra

Definition
- A rare autoimmune disease of unknown etiology with episodic but potentially progressive inflammatory manifestations.
- Cartilaginous structures throughout the body are primarily involved, including the ears, nose, eyes, laryngobronchial and costal cartilage and joints, in a heterogeneous pattern and sequence.
- May be associated with other autoimmune diseases.

Clinical features
- Chondritis of the auricular, nasal, laryngotracheal, costal and articular cartilage.
- Ocular and inner ear inflammation.
- An associated systemic vasculitis, or glomerulonephritis may contribute significant morbidity and premature mortality.
- Extremely varied in its manifestations, course and response to therapy.

HISTORY

Relapsing polychondritis is a rare disease of unknown etiology. The first clinical description of it is attributed to Jaksch-Wartenhorst[1], who called it 'polychondropathia' and considered it to be a degenerative disorder. Pearson *et al.*[2] reported in the English literature the case of a 32-year-old brewer with fever, asymmetric polyarthritis, pain in and swelling of his external ears, and collapse of his nose bridge. This patient went on to develop external auditory canal stenosis and diminished hearing. A biopsy of the nasal septum showed a hyperplastic mucous membrane and absence of any cartilage. Pearson *et al.* first coined the term 'relapsing polychondritis', which is the currently accepted name. More than 450 cases have been reported[2–6] so far and, as expected, the clinical spectrum has widened considerably.

EPIDEMIOLOGY

Relapsing polychondritis (RP) is a rare disease, as demonstrated by the estimated annual incidence rate of 3.5/million in Rochester, Minnesota (personal observations). The peak age at onset is between 40 and 50 years, but cases in children and in the very elderly (over the age of 80 years) have been observed. It occurs with equal frequency in both sexes and all racial groups. Over 30% of the cases are associated with an existing autoimmune or hematologic disease (Fig. 27.1), the chondritis usually occurring after the onset of the other condition. One transplacental case has been observed, but there are no documented reports of familial RP. A recent study from France reported an increase of HLA DR4 (56.1%) in patients with RP compared with controls (25.5%). However when these investigators performed oligonucleotide-based genotyping, no significant subtype was found to be increased[7]. The life expectancy of RP patients is reduced, with an estimated 5-year survival of 74% in one large series. In the subgroup of patients with systemic vasculitis, the estimated survival is similar to that of patients with polyarteritis – 45% at 5 years. Infection and respiratory involvement are frequent and contribute to reduced survival[6].

CONDITIONS ASSOCIATED WITH RELAPSING POLYCHONDRITIS	
Systemic vasculitis syndromes	Behçet's syndrome
Rheumatoid arthritis	Primary biliary cirrhosis
Systemic lupus erythematosus	Retroperitoneal fibrosis
Sjögren's syndrome	Dermatitis herpetiformis
Overlapping connective tissue	Dysmyelopoietic syndromes
Mixed cryoglobulinemia	Hodgkin's disease
Churg–Strauss vasculitis	Hydralazine-induced cases
Löffler's syndrome	Hypogammaglobulinemia
Ankylosing spondylitis	Thymoma with myasthenia gravis
Psoriatic arthritis	Weber–Christian disease
Reiter's syndrome	Diabetes mellitus
Inflammatory bowel disease	Psoriasis vulgaris

Fig. 27.1 Conditions associated with relapsing polychondritis.

CLINICAL FEATURES

OTORHINOLARYNGEAL DISEASE

The classic clinical manifestation of RP is acute unilateral or bilateral auricular chondritis. The onset is characteristic with redness or violaceous discoloration, warmth and swelling involving the cartilaginous portion of the pinna, sparing the lobe (Fig. 27.2a). The episode lasts days to weeks and resolves with or without treatment. Over time and with repeated attacks, the pinna loses its firmness and becomes soft and flops over (Fig. 27.2b) or assumes a knobby, cauliflower appearance. In our series of 112 patients at the Mayo Medical School this was the presenting feature in 39%, ultimately developing in up to 85% of the patients. Damage to the nasal bridge causes the saddle nose deformity (see Fig. 27.3). Swelling of the external auditory canal causes conductive deafness. Vasculitis of the internal auditory artery, or its cochlear or vestibular branch, results in auditory and/or vestibular impairment leading to varying degrees of vertigo and/or neurosensory hearing loss. This may occur in up to 30% of the patients (see Fig. 27.4).

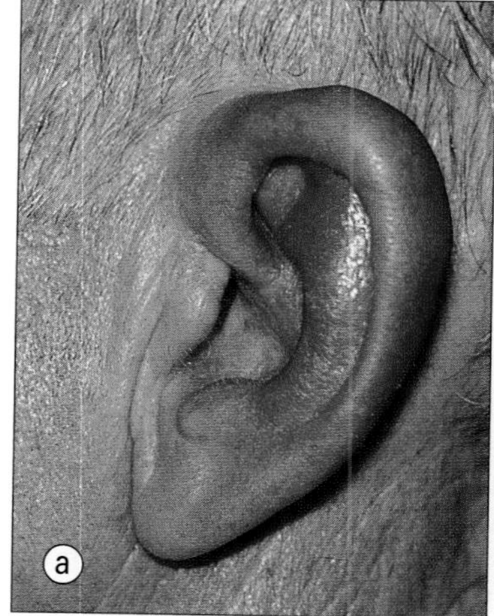

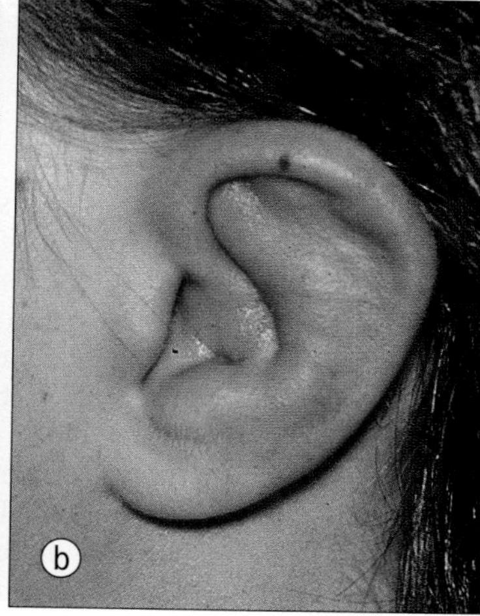

Fig. 27.2 Otorhinolaryngeal disease in relapsing polychondritis. The pinna of the ear becomes inflamed: note the sparing of the noncartilaginous portion of the ear (a). Recurrent attacks cause loss of cartilage, with the ear flopping over (b).

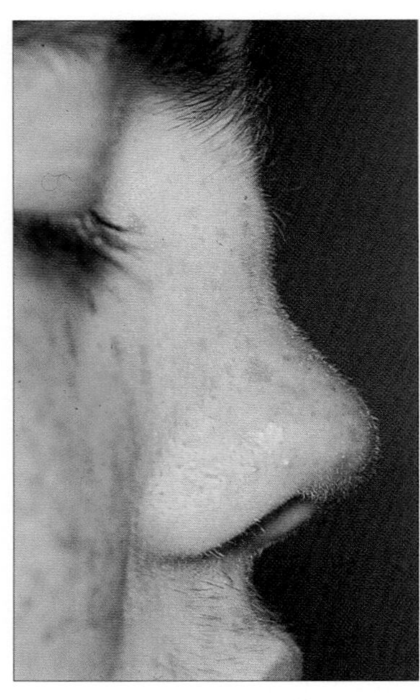

Fig. 27.3 Otorhinolaryngeal disease in relapsing polychondritis. The saddle nose deformity is caused by damage to the nasal bridge.

CLINICAL MANIFESTATIONS OF RELAPSING POLYCHONDRITIS		
	Frequency %	
	At diagnosis	Total
Auricular chondritis	39	85
Saddle nose deformity	18	29
Hearing loss	9	30
Arthritis	36	52
Costochondral symptoms	2	2
Nasal cartilage changes	24	54
Ocular symptoms	19	51
Scleritis/episcleritis	19	47
Laryngotracheal–bronchial symptoms	26	48
Laryngotracheal stricture	15	23
Systemic vasculitis	3	10
Valvular dysfunction	0	6
Cutaneous symptoms	7	28

Fig. 27.4 Clinical manifestations of relapsing polychondritis. Modified from Izaak *et al.* [9].

RESPIRATORY DISEASE

Respiratory symptoms are common and can be potentially lethal. At onset, 25% of patients present with these, although ultimately 50% develop them. Tenderness of the thyroid cartilage and the anterior trachea, hoarseness, persistent cough, choking spells, and wheezing and dyspnea on exertion can occur. Inflammation of the tracheobronchial tree leads to varying degrees of localized (Fig. 27.5) or diffuse obstruction, and damage to the cartilaginous rings can cause a dynamic obstruction leading to respiratory difficulty in inspiration and during anesthesia. Strictures usually form in the subglottic region, causing increased susceptibility to secondary infections. The reported mortality from respiratory complications varies from 10 to 50% – the lower figure is probably more realistic.

MUSCULOSKELETAL SYMPTOMS

The arthritis of RP is episodic, seronegative, asymmetric oligo- or polyarticular. It can occur before, during or after the diagnosis is established, and is the presenting feature in 30% of cases, ultimately developing in 75%. The episodes may last weeks to months, but the arthritis is nondeforming and nonerosive. Its activity does not correlate with the activity of RP. The joints most commonly involved are the ankles, followed by the wrists, proximal interphalangeal and metacarpophalangeal joints, elbows and metatarsophalangeal joints. The hips, knees and sacroiliac joints are involved less frequently, and inflammation of the costochondral cartilages may lead to a pectus deformity. Since RP can be accompanied by another connective tissue disease, the patient may have the musculoskeletal manifestations of the associated disease[8].

CARDIOVASCULAR DISEASE

The cardiovascular system is involved in less than 10% of cases. The spectrum of vasculitis is broad, with small-vessel disease presenting as cutaneous leukocytoclastic vasculitis and large-vessel disease presenting as Takayasu's arteritis. Aneurysms of the thoracic and abdominal aorta can occur. Aortitis causes thinning of the media and leads to dilatation of the root of the aorta and leakage of the aortic valve. Systemic polyarteritis nodosa has been observed in 9% of the cases; the underlying disease dictates the prognosis. Aortic and mitral valves can be sites of inflammation, with incompetence of the valve developing because of aortic root dilation, valvulitis or papillary muscle dysfunction. Conduction abnormalities causing arrhythmias, heart block and supraventricular tachycardia, due to myocarditis and involvement of the conduction system, occur rarely. Myocarditis and pericarditis are infrequent. Recurrent aneurysms and valvular function abnormalities can occur in spite of treatment[9].

OCULAR SYMPTOMS

The eye is a frequent site of involvement. Initially, 19% of the patients have eye symptoms but eventually about 50% are affected. The extraocular involvement includes periorbital edema, tarsitis, chemosis and proptosis. Extraocular muscle palsy can occur. Episcleritis, local or diffuse, and scleritis, both anterior and posterior, can occur at onset or during the course of this disease. Keratitis, thinning of the cornea and corneal melt have been reported but are rare. Iridocyclitis, chorioretinitis, retinal hemorrhages and retinal vasculitis have been observed[9].

RENAL DISEASE

In RP, although up to 26% of patients may have abnormal urinalysis, creatinine is elevated in only 10%[10]. A few patients have had renal biopsies showing segmental proliferative glomerulonephritis with crescent formation. Immunoglobulins (IgG, or IgM) and C3 component of complement, deposited in a granular pattern or as subendothelial and mesangial deposits, have been observed on electron microscopy. Renal involvement by the associated autoimmune disease, for example systemic vasculitis, Wegener's granulomatosis or systemic lupus erythematosus, has also been observed.

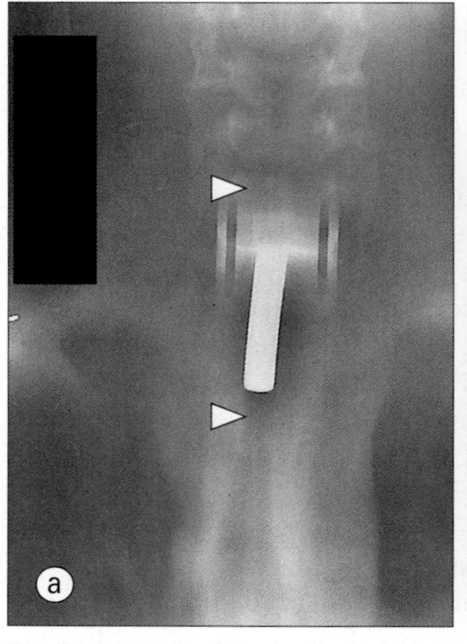

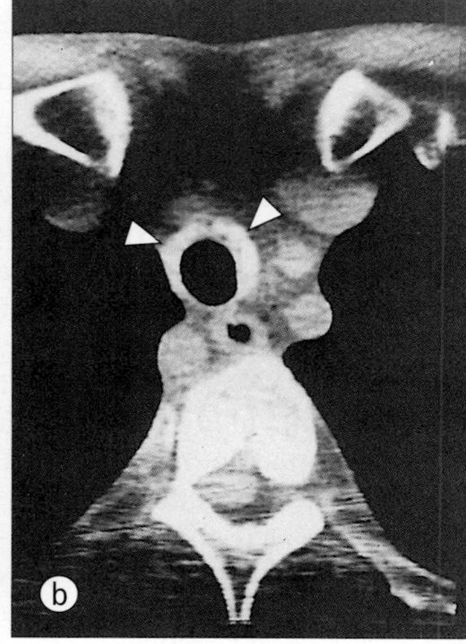

Fig. 27.5 Localized tracheobronchial obstruction due to relapsing polychondritis. The radiograph shows narrowing in both the larynx above the tracheostomy tube and the tracheal stenosis below (a). CT scan of the trachea shows the thickening of the tracheal wall due to inflammatory changes (b).

DERMATOLOGIC DISEASE
The skin manifestations are variable. The presence of palpable purpura, urticaria and angioedema has been observed. Livedo reticularis, migratory superficial thrombophlebitis, erythema nodosum, erythema multiforme and panniculitis are rare but known.

NEUROLOGIC DISEASE
Vasculitis involving the central and peripheral nervous system is seen in some patients who develop cranial neuropathies, headaches, encephalopathy, hemiplegia and ataxia. Transverse myelitis, mononeuritis multiplex and temporal artery nongranulomatous vasculitis have been observed.

HEMATOLOGIC DISEASE
Several cases of RP associated with the myelodysplastic syndrome have recently been described[11].

FEVER
Fever has been observed in 22% of the patients at presentation and up to 44% during the course of the illness. The pattern is variable and a few patients have presented as fever of unknown origin.

DIAGNOSIS AND INVESTIGATIONS

Although the diagnosis of RP is relatively easy, many conditions can mimic the initial changes, or an associated disease may confuse the clinical picture. McAdam *et al.*[5] used the following criteria, requiring three or more of the clinical features to confirm the diagnosis:

- bilateral auricular chondritis,
- nonerosive, seronegative inflammatory polyarthritis,
- nasal chondritis,
- ocular inflammation (conjunctivitis, keratitis, scleritis and/or episcleritis, uveitis),
- respiratory tract chondritis (laryngeal and/or tracheal cartilages),
- cochlear and/or vestibular dysfunction (neurosensory hearing loss, tinnitus and/or vertigo),
- cartilage biopsy confirmation of a compatible histologic picture.

Biopsy of auricular chondritis is performed to confirm the diagnosis of polychondritis (Fig. 27.6). In patients where the presentation is very characteristic, such as simultaneous chondritis in both auricles or chondritis in multiple sites, a biopsy is frequently not necessary. In others, if there is early disease or another underlying disease, it may be required.

All patients should be evaluated for laryngotracheal disease because of the potential for serious airway involvement. Pulmonary function tests, such as inspiratory and expiratory flow-volume curves[12], as well as a radiologic assessment by tomography or computed tomography (CT), scanning each are necessary, as either test alone may not reveal the full functional impact on the airway[13]. Combinations of intra- and extrathoracic airway involvement with expiratory and inspiratory obstruction occur. Laryngotracheal biopsy should be considered with caution as it may be hazardous, leading to acute respiratory distress in cases with stenotic or collapsing airways.

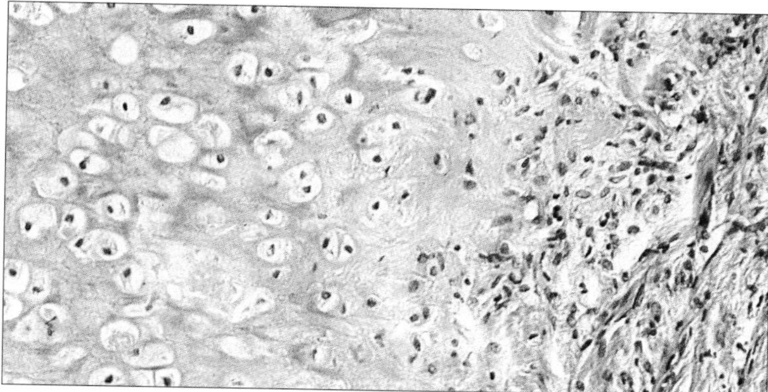

Fig. 27.6 Biopsy of auricular chondritis. Biopsy of the ear shows perichondritis with presence of mononuclear cells and occasional polymorphonuclear leukocytes at the fibrochondral junction. (Hematoxylin and eosin stain, original magnification× 200.) Courtesy of Dr Lester E. Wold.

The usual findings on CT of the trachea include wall thickening by edema or granulation tissue, collapse of the lumen by edema or granulation tissue, fibrosis and calcification of the tracheal wall. An examination by cine CT of the respiratory cycle may demonstrate flaccidity of the airway with dynamic collapse during breathing.

Renal status should always be investigated to exclude the possibility of an accompanying glomerulonephritis[10]. Echocardiography may be indicated to evaluate large vessel involvement. Nonspecific parameters of inflammation are often observed, including an elevated erythrocyte sedimentation rate (ESR), anemia of chronic disease, leukocytosis, thrombocytosis and hypergammaglobulinemia. If macrocytic anemia is present, the possibility of a rare associated early myelodysplastic syndrome should be considered.

Positive serologic tests, such as rheumatoid factor and antinuclear antibodies, are observed in the setting of RP associated with rheumatoid arthritis or other connective tissue disease. Complement levels are usually normal in RP. The arthropathy of polychondritis is radiographically characterized by a nonerosive process resulting in juxta-articular osteoporosis and uniform joint-space narrowing. The anti-neutrophil cytoplasmic antibody (ANCA) has not been reported with RP; however, because Wegener's granulomatosis or renal 'microscopic' polyarteritis nodosa is occasionally accompanied by RP, it is possible that an ANCA may be observed in some cases. Anti-type II collagen antibody tests are not routinely available and, when they are undertaken, antibodies are not observed in all cases. Their utility in the diagnosis or monitoring of RP, remains to be established. Urinary glycosaminoglycans may be elevated in RP but their usefulness in monitoring the disease activity has also not been clarified. Recently, a serum 148kDa noncollagenous cartilage matrix protein was identified in patients with rheumatoid arthritis and RP[14]. Currently, however, no reliable laboratory marker for ongoing cartilage damage is clinically available.

DIFFERENTIAL DIAGNOSIS

Although the clinical manifestations of this disease are characteristic, there are circumstances when the diagnosis may be difficult. The pinna of the ear is readily exposed to injury by trauma, chemicals, frostbite and so on. The trachea is similarly liable to be injured during prolonged endotracheal intubation. Acute streptococcal infection, fungal infection, syphilis and leprosy all may lead to perichondritis that may be easily mistaken for RP. Although the sparing of the ear lobe is characteristic, sometimes the only way to make a definite diagnosis is to perform a biopsy. Nasal damage can occur due to several different conditions, including local infections from fungi, tuberculosis, syphilis and leprosy, or granulomatous lesions, such as Wegener's granulomatosis, lymphomatoid granulomatosis and lethal midline granuloma. Eye involvement by RP or the associated disease can be difficult to separate. Necrotizing scleritis and keratitis can occur with rheumatoid arthritis, Wegener's granulomatosis, polyarteritis nodosa, Behçet's syndrome or Cogan's syndrome. Other features of these associated diseases aid differential diagnosis. Systemic vasculitis with pulmonary, renal, central nervous system (CNS) and other organ involvement can occur. Involvement of the root of the aorta by other diseases should be considered, especially Ehlers–Danlos syndrome, Marfan's syndrome, idiopathic medial cystic necrosis or associated ankylosing spondylitis.

STRUCTURE AND PATHOGENESIS

Cartilage is an avascular structure made up of chondrocytes, type II collagen, proteoglycan aggregates and noncollagenous matrix proteins. It is immunologically protected and thus tolerance does not develop to these antigens. This is also the reason that it is likely to be a target for an autoimmune response. Because of the association of RP with autoimmune disease, the finding of immune-mediated changes in sites of damage and humoral and cell-mediated immunity to cartilage components, and the recent observation of similar changes in rats, this disease should be classified as an autoimmune disorder.

Over the past 10 years there have been several reports of collagen-induced and, more recently, proteoglycan-induced arthritis. It is clear that both of these cartilage antigens can function as autoantigens and can lead to disease. That this may be involved in the pathogenesis of RP is suggested by several lines of evidence. The pathology of the lesion shows collections of lymphocytes and few plasma cells. The presence of immunoglobulins and C3 component of complement locally at the fibrocartilaginous junction suggests local complement activation[15]. Antibodies to type II collagen have been reported to correlate with the activity of the disease[16], and cell-mediated immunity to cartilage antigens has been observed in patients with RP[17]. Recently, two groups of investigators have observed chondritis in rats immunized with native type II collagen, and fawn-hooded rats develop it spontaneously[18,19]. In addition, doubly transgenic mice for human HLA-DQ6 and HLA-DQ8 have recently been observed to develop chondritis and arthritis which appear similar to human disease. This model may shed further light on the pathogenetic mechanisms involved[20]. These observations reconfirm that autoimmune mechanisms are probably important in the pathogenesis of RP. The role of enzymatic destruction is probably just as important and local release of proteinases and oxygen metabolites contribute to the damage. Whether the immune damage initiates the process that is perpetuated by the enzymatic damage, or whether enzymatic damage exposes the privileged antigens that can activate the immune system, thus allowing the disease to appear, is not known.

MANAGEMENT

The initial management of acute RP is well established. In situations of mild auricular and/or nasal chondritis or arthritis, initial treatment is with nonsteroidal anti-inflammatory drugs and low-dose prednisone. For cases with serious manifestations such as laryngotracheal or ocular symptoms, inner ear inflammation, severe auricular or nasal chondritis, systemic vasculitis, aortitis or glomerulonephritis, prednisone at a dose of 1mg/kg is indicated. In most instances, the acute inflammation responds well and the corticosteroids can be gradually tapered off. However, if relapses occur with dose reduction, patients require maintenance doses of prednisone to control the disease. Strategies for refractory disease or frequent relapses during tapering are less certain.

As RP is so rare controlled therapeutic trials have not been carried out. The literature is replete with successful anecdotes of therapies ranging from dapsone and colchicine to immunosuppressants. Generally, the former two agents may be useful in milder disease as corticosteroid-sparing agents, whereas immunosuppressants are reserved for those with manifestations refractory to moderate-to-high-dose steroids. Plasmapheresis, azathioprine, cyclophosphamide, chlorambucil and cyclosporin have all been reported to be beneficial, but patients may not reliably respond to any of these therapies. Treatment is monitored by clinical response.

The ESR may be useful in some cases. Urinary glycosaminoglycans, serum anticollagen antibodies and antibodies to 148kDa non-collagenous cartilage matrix protein have all been proposed as potential laboratory markers for disease activity, but their roles in monitoring RP have not been satisfactorily established.

In the situation of an initial presentation with unilateral auricular chondritis alone, the differential diagnosis and initial treatment must include the possibility of a bacterial external otitis, cellulitis and/or perichondritis. A biopsy with culture may be necessary in this setting, as well as concurrent treatment with an antibiotic until culture results are known.

Laryngotracheal involvement presents special management issues in following the activity of the disease and dealing with the consequences of a structurally impaired airway. Indirect laryngoscopy and serial CT scanning of the trachea can be used to monitor disease activity, although experience with this radiographic procedure in RP is limited. Once airway damage has occurred, tracheostomy is necessary to treat a symptomatic subglottic stenosis. If diffuse airway involvement with flaccid collapse has occurred, effective therapies are limited. Recurrent pulmonary infections require antibiotic and respiratory care treatment. Experience with successful tracheal stents is limited. Nasal continuous positive airway pressure can be tried at night to assist the patient in keeping the airway open while recumbent and asleep. Surgical correction of subglottic stenosis and collapsed nasal cartilage can be performed once the disease is quiescent.

Heart valve replacement and aortic graft surgery have been successful. Due to the nature of the disease, surgical failure has been observed: continued annular inflammation leading to perivalvular leaks, as well as recurrent aortitis adjacent to grafts.

REFERENCES

1. Jaksch-Wartenhorst R. Polychondropathia. Wien Arch F Inn Med.1923;6:93–100.
2. Pearson CM, Kline HM, Newcomer VD. Relapsing polychondritis. N Engl J Med. 1960;263:51–8.
3. Bean WB, Drevets CC, Chapman JS. Chronic atrophic polychondritis. Medicine. 1958;37:353–63.
4. Kaye RL, Sones DA. Relapsing polychondritis: clinical and pathologic features in fourteen cases. Ann Intern Med. 1964;60:653–64.
5. McAdam LP, O'Hanlon MA, Bluestone R, Pearson CM. Relapsing polychondritis: prospective study of 23 patients and a review of the literature. Medicine. 1976;55:193–215.
6. Michet CJ Jr, McKenna CH, Luthra HS, O'Fallon WW. Relapsing polychondritis; survival and predictive role of early disease manifestations. Ann Intern Med. 1986;104:74–8.
7. Lang B, Rothenfusser A, Lanchbury JS, *et al.* Susceptibility to relapsing polychondritis is associated with HLA-DR4. Arthritis Rheum. 1993;36:660–4.
8. O'Hanlon M, McAdam LP, Bluestone R, Pearson CM. The arthropathy of relapsing polychondritis. Arthritis Rheum. 1976;19:191–4.
9. Isaak BL, Liesegang TJ, Michet CJ Jr. Ocular and systemic findings in relapsing polychondritis. Ophthalmology. 1986;93:681–9.
10. Chang-Miller A, Okamura M, Torres VE, *et al.* Renal involvement in relapsing polychondritis. Medicine. 1987;66:202–17.
11. Diebold L, Rauh G, Jager, Lohrs U. Bone marrow pathology in relapsing polychondritis: high frequency of myelodysplastic syndromes. Br J Haematol. 1995;89:820–30.
12. Krell WS, Staats BA, Hyatt RE. Pulmonary function in relapsing polychondritis. Am Rev Respir Dis. 1986;133:1120–3.
13. Booth A, Dieppe PA, Goddard PL, Watt I. The radiological manifestations of relapsing polychondritis. Clin Radiol. 1989;40:147–9.
14. Saxne T, Heinegard, D. Involvement of nonarticular cartilage, as demonstrated by release of a cartilage-specific protein, in rheumatoid arthritis. Arthritis Rheum 1989;32:1080–6.
15. Homma S, Matsumoto T, Abe H, Fukuda Y Nagano M, Suzuki M. Relapsing polychondritis: pathological and immunological findings in an autopsy case. Acta Pathol Jpn. 1984;34:1137–46.
16. Foidart J, Abe S, Martin GR, *et al.* Antibodies to type II collagen in relapsing polychondritis. N Engl J Med. 1978;299:1203–7.
17. Herman JH, Dennis MV. Immunopathologic studies in relapsing polychondritis. J Clin Invest.1973;52:549–58.
18. Cremer MA, Pitcock JA, Stuart JM, Kang AH, Townes AS. Auricular chondritis in rats. J Exp Med. 1981;154:535–40.
19. Prieur DJ, Young DM, Counts DF. Auricular chondritis in fawn-hooded rats: a spontaneous disorder resembling that induced by immunization with type II collagen. Am J Pathol. 1984;116:69–76.
20. Bradley DS, Das P, Griffiths MM, Luthra HS, David CS. Double transgenic HLA-DQ6/8 mice provide a new model of polychondritis following type II collagen immunization. Arthritis Rheum. 1996;39:S229.

CANCER AND MISCELLANEOUS ARTHROPATHIES

Nathan J Zvaifler

- Joint systems may accompany many kinds of cancer. Different mechanisms operate in cancer related rheumatic complaints, including local invasion, metastic disease and several paraneoplastic syndromes
- Intermittant and relapsing arthritides are rare or uncommon disorders, usually with episodic polyarticular joint pain and swelling, which although exceedingly chronic, produce little or no permanent joint abnormalities
- Musculoskeletal symptoms are recognized complications of disorders of hemoglobin production, leukemias, lymphomas and plasma cell myelomas. Angioimmunoblastic lymphadenopathy (AILD) shares a number of features with several connective tissue diseases
- Multicentric reticular histiocytosis is a rare disease of soft tissues and joints associated with the accumulation of lipid-la den histiocytes and multi-nucleated giant cells

CANCER-ASSOCIATED RHEUMATIC SYNDROMES
Arthropathies
Local articular involvement by cancer
Rheumatoid and rheumatoid–like arthritis
Cancer polyarthritis
Hypertrophic osteoarthropathy
Polymyalgia rheumatica
Palmar fasciitis and arthritis
Relapsing polychondritis
Other arthropathies
Muscular disorders
Dermatomyositis and polymyositis
Localized nodular myositis
Necrotizing myopathy
Scleroderma, panniculitis and fasciitis syndromes
Systemic sclerosis
Eosinophilic fasciitis
Erythema nodosum
Panniculitis–arthritis
Vasculitides
Miscellaneous rheumatic disorders
Reflex sympathetic dystrophy
Sjögren's syndrome
Antiphospholipid antibody syndrome

Fig. 28.1 Classification of rheumatic syndromes reported to be associated with neoplasia. Adapted from Naschetz *et al.*[1].

CANCER-RELATED ARTHROPATHIES

Malignancies of various kinds are occasionally associated with connective tissue diseases, particularly dermatomyositis, Sjögren's syndrome and perhaps rheumatoid arthritis (RA). In some instances the coexistent cancer may be coincidental but in others there is a real but unexplained associations (Fig. 28.1). Primary malignancies can also give rise to musculoskeletal complaints as a result of direct invasion of bone and joints by tumor metastasis, or indirectly as paraneoplastic syndromes. The latter are frequently a source of confusion because of their polyarticular nature[1–3].

METASTATIC DISEASE

In elderly patients with pain in or around a joint, the possibility of metastatic malignancy, particularly from carcinoma of the lung or breast, should be considered. Typically the process is monoarticular, involving large joints, such as the knee or hip, but rarely an asymmetric polyarthritis may reflect a disseminated carcinoma[4]. Symptoms are the result of a reactive synovitis secondary to invasion of the synovium or periarticular bone. Swelling and pain in the small joints due to phalangeal metastasis have been confused with a primary rheumatic condition[5] and children with neuroblastoma can have fever and joint symptoms mimicking the Still's form of juvenile arthritis.

PARANEOPLASTIC SYNDROMES

Carcinomatous polyarthritis

Occult malignancy, particularly of the breast in women and the lung in men, is a rare cause of polyarthritis[1–3]. Its prevalence is unknown. The arthritis differs from typical RA. In general, the patients are older and symptoms usually appear abruptly, with asymmetric involvement tending to spare the small joints of the hands and wrist[6]. Most patients have an elevated erythrocyte sedimentation rate, negative blood rheumatoid factor serology and a mildly inflammatory synovial fluid. Joint radiographs tend to be normal.

Carcinomatous polyarthritis may antecede or follow the clinical appearance of the underlying neoplasm[1–2]. The most convincing demonstration that this is a real entity is the occasional disappearance of joint symptoms following resection of the cancer and reappearance of arthritis with recurrence of the tumor[3]. Good responses to nonsteroidal anti-inflammatory drugs (NSAIDs) have been reported.

Pancreatic panniculitis and arthritis

Patients with pancreatic neoplasms, pseudocysts, or acute and chronic pancreatitis may develop a liquifying panniculitis that gives rise to skin lesions and polyarthritis[7]. The former consists of tender, red, subcutaneous nodules that appear on the buttocks, thighs, upper arms, thorax and scalp. The most typical location is on the dorsum of the leg. Unlike the lesions of erythema nodosum, these nodules generally are movable when they first appear. Subsequently, they may become fluctuant and drain sterile material containing globules of fat[8].

Hypertrophic osteoarthropathy

The combination of clubbing of the fingers plus pain, swelling, tenderness and stiffness of peripheral joints, especially the wrists, ankles and fingers, is called hypertrophic osteoarthropathy. Carcinoma of the lung is by far the most common etiology, although metastatic malignancies and diseases involving the pleura (e.g. pleural mesothelioma) can produce similar symptoms. Hypertrophic osteoarthropathy is discussed in detail in Chapter 8.46.

INTERMITTENT AND RELAPSING ARTHRITIDES

Included under this heading are a disparate group of disorders that share certain attributes:

- The conditions are rare or very uncommon;
- They are associated with episodic attacks of joint pain and swelling, which are usually polyarticular;

- The interval between attacks is highly variable but during this time the joints appear normal;
- Despite a remarkable chronicity, permanent joint abnormalities or deformities are exceedingly infrequent.

Several members of this group, such as familial Mediterranean fever (see Chapter 5.24), relapsing polychondritis (see Chapter 5.27), and Behçet's syndrome (see Chapter 7.26), are detailed in other chapters; the remainder are included here for completeness.

PALINDROMIC RHEUMATISM

Palindromic rheumatism is characterized by recurrent attacks of painful swelling of the joints associated with articular and periarticular inflammation. The attacks are abrupt in onset and short lived, frequently lasting only hours and rarely more than a few days. The pattern is peculiar to individual patients, and the intervals between attacks vary from days to weeks to months[9]. Once established, the pattern remains relatively unchanged for the duration of the illness, which may go on for decades. Any joint can be affected, and there is an unusual accompaniment of a periarticular swelling of the heels, finger pads or palms that resembles angioedema. Despite the chronicity, the joints are not damaged. Both sexes are affected equally and the joint symptoms usually begin in the third to sixth decade[9–11]. During attacks the blood acute-phase reactants may be elevated, but they are normal in between. Rheumatoid factor is sometimes positive, most often in subjects who will subsequently develop RA. In one third to one half of patients, the disease becomes less episodic and progresses into typical RA. The remainder continue unchanged. Treatment with NSAIDs is of questionable benefit. The use of glucocorticosteroids or NSAIDs is seldom successful, although prophylactic colchicine treatment may be helpful. Some patients are reported to improve with chrysotherapy.

INTERMITTENT HYDROARTHROSIS

This condition consists of recurrent attacks of unilateral, relatively painless, noninflammatory joint effusions (usually in women, in the knees) that occur with a predictable periodicity. The disease appears once or twice monthly, often in association with the menses. Fluid accumulates rapidly and is resorbed over a period of several days. Laboratory studies are unremarkable, and synovial fluid obtained from the affected joint appears benign. No cause has been found, but an allergic diathesis is suspected. There is no satisfactory treatment.

WHIPPLE'S DISEASE

Whipple's disease (WD) occurs predominantly in white middle-aged men who reside in the US or Northern Europe[12–18]. In some instances there has been definite geographic clustering of cases. A retrospective analysis of the prevalence of HLA antigens suggests WD may be associated with a two- to three-fold increase in HLA-B27, even in the absence of concomitant spondylitis[15].

WD can involve many organs, but an almost invariable symptom is malabsorption because of widespread infiltration of the lamina propria and submucosa of the small intestine by macrophages containing periodic acid-shiff (PAS) staining material, and obstruction of mesenteric lymphatics. Gastrointestinal symptoms are often striking and include diarrhea, steatorrhea, weight loss, abdominal bloating and pain. Peripheral edema, generalized lymphadenopathy and skin hyperpigmentation are characteristic findings. Constitutional symptoms (fever, sweats, malaise), central and peripheral neurologic features (confusion, memory loss, bizarre behavior, myoclonus, supranuclear ophthalmoplegia and focal cranial nerve lesions), and cardiac (pericarditis and endocarditis as manifested by heart valve disease) and pulmonary involvement (chronic unexplained cough, pleuritis and pneumonitis) are frequent accompaniments (Fig. 28.2). Arthritis occurs in at least 60% of patients with WD and, most importantly, it may precede the onset of bowel symptoms by many years or even decades. Rheumatoid arthritis, ankylosing spondylitis or intermittent (palindromic) arthritis are common misdiagnoses during this prodromal period. Typically the arthritis is episodic, migratory, symmetric and polyarticular, lasting a few hours to days and clears without residua[12–14]. The knees, ankles and wrists are most commonly involved, although any joint may be affected, and inflammation in the small joints of the hands and feet have been reported. Attacks of arthritis are accompanied by joint effusions, pain, limitation of motion and evidence of inflammation in the affected joints in some, but not all, patients. Despite a prolonged history of arthritis, joint radiographs seldom show abnormalities, although in at least two instances erosive changes and ankylosis were noted in the hands and wrists. Infiltration of the skin with PAS-staining macrophages has been confused with rheumatoid subcutaneous nodules.

Axial arthritis (both isolated sacroiliitis and spondylitis) can occur alone or in combination with peripheral arthritis [15]. Overall, however, spine involvement is less common than peripheral joint disease. Unexplained is the observation that, although the frequency of HLA-B27 is two to three times greater in WD than predicted, it does not appear to have a direct association with either sacroiliitis or spondylitis.

Synovial fluid findings are variable. White blood cell counts range from 5000–30,000/mm^3 in inflamed joints with a preponderance of polymorphonuclear leukocytes. Mononuclear cells may be seen in the interval between acute attacks. In synovial biopsies, both PAS-positive macrophages and rod-shaped bacilli have been identified.

The diagnosis of WD is established by histologic examination of involved tissues. The procedure of choice is peroral small intestinal biopsy, since the proximal small intestine is involved in the vast majority of patients. The process can be patchy, however, and more than one biopsy may be required. Diagnosis depends on the demonstration of both foamy, PAS-positive macrophages and the typical Whipple's bacillus. The causative organism has not been cultured, but a unique actinomycetes' species (*Tropheryma Whippelii*) has been detected by amplifying RNA from patient materials by polymerase chain reaction (PCR)[16]. The relationship of this new organism to disease pathogenesis is still not understood[17].

Joint symptoms do not respond to anti-inflammatory agents or second-line drugs, but antibiotics effective against gram-positive organisms can induce dramatic improvement. A variety of regimens have been advocated; the most recent are trimethoprim–sulfamethoxazole or chloramphenicol. These agents are favored because they readily penetrate the blood–brain barrier and may have the potential to eliminate occult central nervous system (CNS) involvement. Generally, diarrhea and other findings of malabsorption are the first to improve with antibiotic treatment, often within several weeks. Organisms will disappear from the intestinal mucosa after 2–4 months, and this is considered a useful guideline for discontinuing antibiotics. The joints are somewhat slower to respond, often requiring weeks to months. Neurologic symptoms are the least responsive to antibiotic therapy. The development

CLINICAL MANIFESTATIONS OF WHIPPLE'S DISEASE

Symptoms and features	Percentage of patients
Gastrointestinal	
Weight loss	95
Diarrhea	75
Abdominal pain	60
Articular	
Peripheral joints	60
Axial joints	10–30
Fever	40
Lymphadenopathy	50
Peripheral edema	30
Skin hyperpigmentation	50
Cardiac	
Clinical	50
Postmortem	80
Pulmonary	30
Neurologic	10
Ocular	10

Fig. 28.2 Clinical manifestations of Whipple's disease. Percentages are approximate. Adapted from Weiner and Utsinger[12] and Dobbins[19].

of new CNS symptoms, or the recurrence of previously noted neurologic complaints, may herald relapses even in the absence of the return of intestinal symptoms[18].

BYPASS ARTHROPATHY

Recurrent episodes of polyathralgia, nondeforming arthritis, myalgia and stiffness lasting a few days to several weeks may complicate the intestinal bypass operations that in the past were done for the treatment of morbid obesity (see Chapter 6.24)[20–22]. Depending on the type, length and location of the blind loop produced (jejunocecal or jejunoileal), an arthritis–dermatitis syndrome develops in up to 40% of patients, often many months or years after the surgical procedure. Symptoms appear to be related to bacterial overgrowth in the blind loop. The subsequent release of bacterial antigens into the circulation gives rise to circulating immune complexes that deposit in target organs, such as the joints and skin[23]. In support of this explanation is the rapid improvement that follows when the blind loop is taken down, or after appropriate antibiotic treatment[24].

The episodic arthritis can involve any peripheral joint. Both sacroiliitis and spondylitis have also been reported. Joint tenderness is often disproportionate to the physical findings. In two thirds or more of patients a characteristic skin rash precedes or accompanies the musculoskeletal symptoms. Exquisitely painful red macules progress to papules and then pustules on the extremities and upper trunk (Fig. 28.3). Additional immune complex-related findings include pericarditis, pleuritis, mild glomerulonephritis and Raynaud's phenomenon. Rheumatoid factors and antinuclear antibodies are seldom present, and radiographic changes are rare in the joints. Immune complexes have been detected in blood and joint effusions. The synovial fluid is usually inflammatory, but leukocyte counts are very variable. Skin biopsies show vasculitis and epidermal necrosis as well as immune deposits at the dermal–epidermal junction of involved skin.

NSAIDs, corticosteroids and dapsone (50–100mg daily) are all reported to relieve symptoms in individual patients. Oral antibiotics help by reducing bacterial overgrowth in the isolated loop of bowel, but re-establishment of the normal intestinal anatomy is the only curative procedure[25]. Gastric stapling has superseded intestinal bypass operations for treating morbid obesity, but there are still large numbers of people who possess intact anastomoses and who are at risk for the development of this condition.

HEMATOLOGIC DISEASES

LEUKEMIA

Joint pain and true arthritis develop in only a small percentage of adults with either acute or chronic leukemia, but are common symptoms in children with acute lymphoblastic leukemia (ALL) (up to 60% of cases)[29, 30]. The arthritis of ALL tends to be asymmetric, additive, polyarticular and may antedate the appearance in the blood of abnormal cells. Occasionally, there is bilateral involvement of both small and large joints, mimicking RA. Knees, ankles and shoulders are most commonly affected, presumably due to leukemic infiltration of the synovium or periosteal elevation of the intra- and periarticular bone. In children, the association of arthritis and fever can mimic Still's disease or acute rheumatic fever. To add to the confusion, autoantibodies develop in some patients with ALL, including rheumatoid factor and antinuclear antibodies. Clues to the diagnosis include nocturnal bone pain, hematologic abnormalities and radiographs that show growth arrest lines or other recognized radiologic features of leukemia (Fig. 28.4). Joint symptoms usually respond to aspirin or NSAIDs. Occasionally the use of prednisone to treat the arthritis masks the underlying ALL.

In adults with leukemia, crystal-induced joint inflammation (both monosodium urate and calcium pyrophosphate) has been reported, but this is probably coincidental.

Hairy cell leukemia is a rare neoplasm of unknown origin. In most patients the disease appears to represent the clonal expansion of cells committed to the B-lymphocyte lineage, but the expression of T-cell markers and interleukin-2 (IL-2) surface receptors on the abnormal cells, plus functions usually associated with monocytes and histiocytes, all add to the confusion. Both polyarthritis and polyarteritis nodosa have been described in patients with hairy cell leukemia[31]. The former may antedate the diagnosis of leukemia, whereas vasculitis generally appears late in the course of the disease, usually after splenectomy done for treatment. The vasculitis is postulated to result from viral infection transmitted by blood transfusion, but there is no evidence to support this contention.

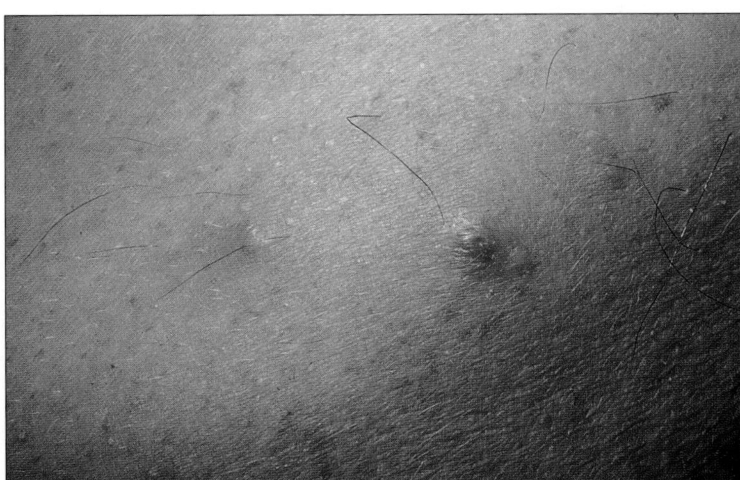

Fig. 28.3 Typical vesiculopustular skin lesion on the leg of a patient with bypass arthropathy.

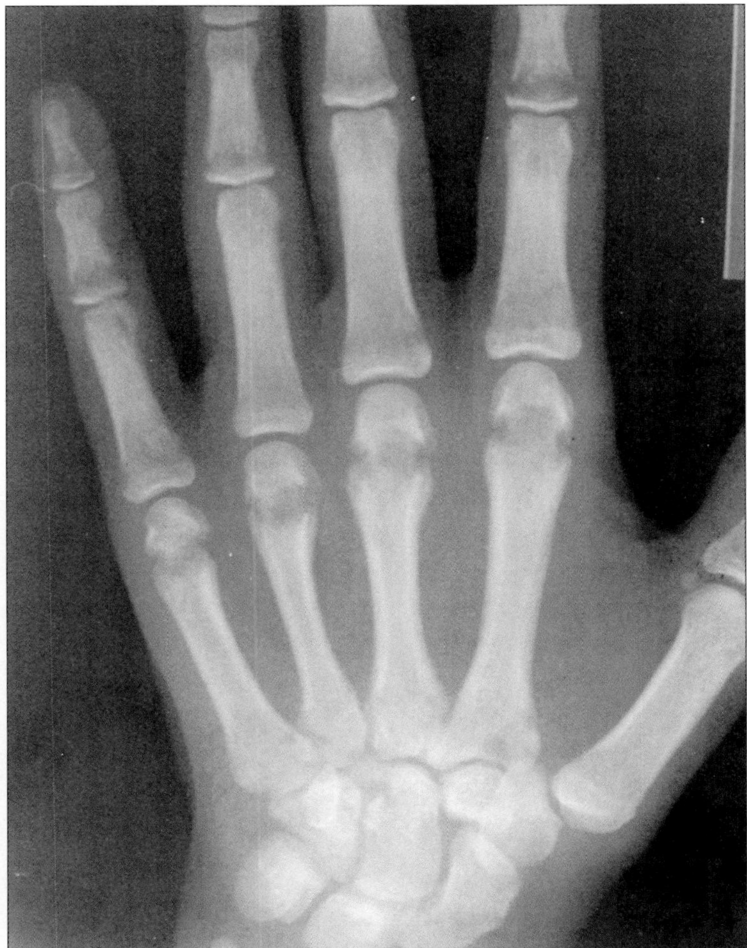

Fig. 28.4 Radiograph of the hand in a child with luekemia showing extensive metaphyseal destruction and periosteal new bone formation.

LYMPHOMA

Skeletal involvement is a recognized accompaniment of lymphomas[29,30]. At autopsy, perhaps half the patients with Hodgkin's disease show bony lesions, but as a rule these are asymptomatic. In the rare instance in which articular symptoms are present, these are usually related to involvement of periarticular bone. In the setting of aggressive chemotherapy or radiation therapy, given without concomitant allopurinol treatment, a rapid breakdown of rapidly dividing cells can result in a remarkable hyperuricemia and secondary gout can be a consequence. An uncommon but confusing finding can be positive tests for rheumatoid factor or antinuclear antibody or lupus erythematosus cells in the blood of lymphoma patients.

Leukocytoclastic vasculitis is a recognized complication of Hodgkin's disease, other lymphomas and leukemias. A relationship with circulating immune complexes containing antigens from the neoplasm has been proposed as the mechanism.

ANGIOIMMUNOBLASTIC LYMPHADENOPATHY

Angioimmunoblastic lymphadenopathy (AILD) is a lymphoproliferative disorder with well-established clinical and histologic features[32–34]. It shares a number of similarities with connective tissue diseases, including Sjögren's syndrome, RA and systemic lupus erythematosus, with which it has been associated. Characteristic signs and symptoms of AILD include enlarged lymph nodes, hepatosplenomegaly, fever, weight loss, urticaria or maculopapular skin rash. Hemolytic anemia and hypergammaglobulinemia are common accompaniments. An infrequent complaint is arthritis, usually described as symmetric, peripheral and nonerosive. The polyarthritis is inflammatory with joint fluid leukocytosis; white blood cells up to 20,000/mm^3 with 70–85% neutrophils have been reported. The cause of angioimmunoblastic lymphadenopathy is not known. Diagnosis is based on the classic appearance of the biopsy, which shows replacement of normal lymph-node architecture by proliferation of small blood vessels and a polymorphous infiltrate including plasma cells, immunoblasts and eosinophils. The results of treatment are variable. A proportion of patients respond poorly despite corticosteroid and cytotoxic therapy. About a third progress to malignant lymphoma. The remainder appear to have a self-limited disease.

PLASMA CELL MYELOMA

Pain in the bones of the back or chest wall is a characteristic of multiple myeloma. Symptoms are gradual in onset and exacerbated by motion. Spontaneous fractures, however, can cause sudden disability. Classic radiographs of plasma cell myeloma show well-circumscribed lytic lesions in vertebrae, ribs, sternum, skull, pelvis or proximal long bones, but often only decreased bone density is seen. Because plasma cell myeloma has its onset in the later decades of life, differentiation from senile osteoporosis may be difficult. The demonstration of a monoclonal immunoglobulin spike on serum electrophoresis, or an excessive immunoglobulin light chain excretion in the urine, or a bone marrow aspiration demonstrating an increased number of plasma cells, will usually clarify the issue.

Osteosclerotic myeloma is a rare form of the disease, characterized by a typical radiographic appearance and an indolent disease course. A severe progressive sensory motor polyneuropathy is a common accompaniment. Less frequent is an unusual multisystemic syndrome characterized by polyneuropathy, organ enlargement (especially hepatosplenomegaly), endocrine dysfunction, M protein and skin alterations, including thickening and abnormal pigmentation that can be confused with scleroderma; this is described by the acronym POEMS[35]. Characteristic radiographic features include single or multiple osteosclerotic bone lesions and a peculiar variety of bone proliferation.

A regular accompaniment of myelomatosis is amyloid deposition. When this occurs around joints, it can give rise to a carpal tunnel (medium nerve compression) syndrome, or rarely a confusing symmetric polyarthritis, particularly of the hands, wrists and shoulders[36]. Amyloid deposits in the skin can be confused with rheumatoid nodules, and accumulation around the shoulder joints gives rise to a striking appearance described as the 'shoulder pad sign'[37]. Biopsy of the synovium or a demonstration of crystal violet-positive amyloid deposits in the sediment of an otherwise bland-appearing synovial fluid suggest the diagnosis.

MULTICENTRIC RETICULOHISTIOCYTOSIS

Multicentric reticulohistiocytosis (lipoid dermatoarthritis) is a rare disease that affects the joints and skin by virtue of the accumulation of lipid-laden histiocytes and multinucleated giant cells[38–40]. The disease usually begins insidiously as a symmetric polyarthritis. Women are affected three times more often than men and are generally in the fifth or sixth decades when the process starts. Skin nodules usually follow months to years (average 3 years) later, but they can precede or occur simultaneously with the arthritis (Fig. 28.5). Small and large peripheral joints and the cervical spine are the targets of what is often a severe, destructive, inflammatory arthritis sometimes confused with RA. Predominant involvement of the distal interphalangeal joints, however, can be a distinguishing

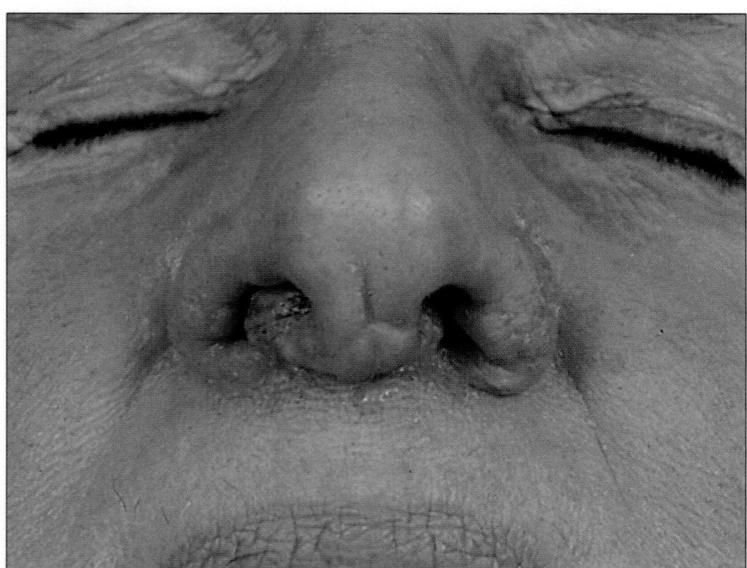

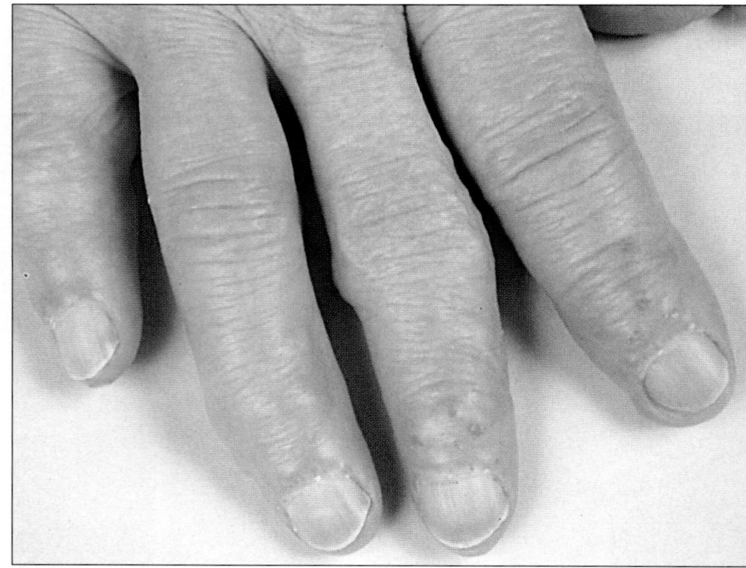

Fig. 28.5 Multicentric reticulohistiocytosis. Small tumorous swellings around the nose and xanthomata around the eyes (left). The typical nail bed tumors and interphalangeal joint arthropathy are also shown (right).

feature[38]. Rheumatoid factor tests are negative. Joint-fluid analysis is quite variable; most often the effusions are inflammatory with either polymorphonuclear or mononuclear cell predominance. The diagnosis of the joint disease is usually suggested by radiographs (Fig. 28.6), which show disproportionate bone destruction, as compared to articular cartilage loss, and remarkably mild osteopenia around the affected joints[40]. Soft tissue swellings, which represent the reddish brown or yellow skin nodules, can often be seen on the radiograph. Striking resorption of subchondral bone can develop over a fairly short period of time and lead to arthritis mutilans ('opera-glass' hands).

The skin lesions, which vary in number from a few to hundreds, tend to wax and wain independent of the symmetric polyarthritis. They are most numerous over the dorsum of the hands, the face and behind the ears. A frequent coexistence of xanthelasma may increase confusion about the diagnosis. A confluence of nodules about the nail folds is characteristic. Lesions on the buccal mucosa, the nasal septum or the lips are present in about half of the patients with skin nodules. A coalescence of large numbers of skin lesions on the face and about the eyes can be confused with leprosy or even give an acromegalic appearance.

The cause of multicentric reticulohistiocytosis is not understood; neither is the finding that almost 50% of patients have a positive tuberculin skin test. The vivid staining of the cytoplasm of the histiocytes and multinucleated giant cells with the PAS reagent is reminiscent of a lipid storage disease, but the actual infiltrate has not been characterized biochemically. Because it is such a rare disease, and severe cases are probably more often recognized and reported, the natural history of multicentric reticulohistiocytosis is incompletely described. A significant proportion of patients (30–50%) progress to severe joint destruction in the first decade of disease, but mild disease is well recognized, as are spontaneous remissions. The latter make evaluation of treatment difficult. Both corticosteroids and cytotoxic drugs have been claimed to be effective[41]. Control of the joint inflammation with NSAIDs or small (5.0–7.5mg) daily doses of prednisone, combined with physical therapy to minimize the effects of contracture and joint destruction, constitutes initial treatment. Alkylating agents (cyclophosphamide 1.25–2.5mg/kg/day or chlorambucil 0.1mg/kg/day orally) alone or in combination with methotrexate can induce remissions of multicentric reticulohistiocytosis[41,42]. Occasionally, cosmetic surgery may be required for the removal of masses of nodules.

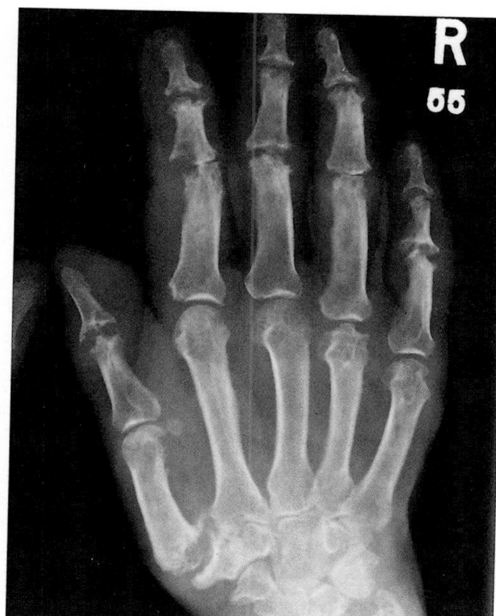

Fig. 28.6 Multicentric reticulohistiocytosis. Hand radiograph showing well-defined erosions at many joints with normal bone density and normal, or apparently widened, joint spaces. Soft tissue swelling is present.

REFERENCES

1. Naschetz, J, Rosner, I, Rozenbaum, *et al.* Cancer associated rheumatic disorders: clues to occult neoplasia. Sem Arthritis Rheum. 1995;24:231–41.
2. Mills JA. Spectrum of organ systems that respond to cancer: The joints and connective tissue. Ann NY Acad Sci. 1974;230:443–7.
3. Mackenzie AH, Scherbel AL. Connective tissue syndromes associated with carcinoma. Geriatrics. 1963;18:745–53.
4. Murray GC, Persellin RH. Metastatic carcinoma presenting as monoarticular arthritis: A case report and review of the literature. Arthritis Rheum. 1980;23:95–100.
5. Vaezy A, Budson DC. Phalangeal metastases from bronchogenic carcinoma. JAMA. 1978;239:226–7.
6. Caldwell DS. Musculoskeletal syndromes associated with malignancy. Semin Arthritis Rheum. 1981;10:198–223.
7. Simkin PA, Brunzell JD, Wisner D, Fiechtner JJ, Carlin JS, Willkens RF. Free fatty acids in the pancreatitic arthritis syndrome. Arthritis Rheum. 1983;26:127–32.
8. Virshup AM, Sliwinski AJ. Polyarthritis and subcutaneous nodules associated with carcinoma of the pancreas. Arthritis Rheum. 1973;16:388–92.
9. Hench PS, Rosenberg EF. Palindromic rheumatism: A 'new', oft recurring disease of joints (arthritis, periarthritis, paraarthritis) apparently producing no articular residues: Report of 34 cases; its relation to 'angioneural arthrosis', 'allergic rheumatism'. Arch Intern Med.1944;73:293–321.
10. Schumacher HR. Palindromic onset of rheumatoid arthritis: Clinical, synovial fluid, and biopsy studies. Arthritis Rheum. 1982;25:361–9.
11. Wajed MA, Brown DL, Currey HLF. Palindromic rheumatism: Clinical and serum complement study. Ann Rheum Dis. 1977;36:56–61.
12. Weiner SR, Utsinger P. Whipple's disease. Semin Arthritis Rheum. 1986;15:157–67.
13. Dobbins WO III. Whipple's disease: An historic perspective. Q J Med. 1985;56:523–31.
14. Rubinow A, Kanoso JJ, Goldenberg DL, *et al.* Arthritis in Whipple's disease. Isr J Med Sci. 1981;17:445–50.
15. Kahn MA. Axial arthropathy in Whipple's disease. J Rheumatol. 1982;9:928–9.
16. Relman D, Schmidt T, MacDermott RP, *et al.* Identification of the uncultured bacillus of Whipple's disease. N Engl J Med.1992;327:293–301.
17. Keren, DF. Whipple's disease: the agent defined – its pathogenesis remains obscure. Medicine. 1993;72:335–58.
18. Knox DL, Bayless TN, Pittman FE. Neurologic diseases in patients treated with Whipple's disease. Medicine. 1976;55:467–76.
19. Dobbins WO III.HLA antigens in Whipple's disease. Arthritis Rheum. 1987;30:102–5.
20. Shagrin JW, Frame B, Duncan H. Polyarthritis in obese patients with intestinal bypass. Ann Intern Med. 1971;75:377–80.
21. Stein HB, Schlappner OL, Boyko W, *et al.* The intestinal bypass arthritis–dermatitis syndrome. Arthritis Rheum. 1981;24:684–90.
22. Clegg DO, Samuelson CO, Williams HJ, *et al.* Articular complications of jejunoileal bypass

surgery. J Rheumatol. 1980;7:65–70.
23. Wands JP, Lamont JT, Mann E, *et al.* Arthritis associated with intestinal bypass procedure for morbid obesity. N Engl J Med. 1976;294:121–4.
24. Leff RD, Aldo-Benson MA, Madura JA. The effect of revision of the intestinal bypass on post intestinal bypass arthritis. Arthritis Rheum. 1983;26:678–81.
25. Schumacher HR. Rheumatological manifestations of sickle cell disease and other hereditary haemoglobinopathies. Clin Rheum Dis. 1975;1:37–53.
26. de Ceulaer K, Forbes M, Roper D, *et al.* Non-gouty arthritis in sickle cell disease: Report of 37 consecutive cases. Ann Rheum Dis. 1984;43:599–603.
27. Ebong WW, Kolawole TM. Aseptic necrosis of the femoral head in sickle cell disease. Br J Rheumatol. 1986;25:34–9.
28. Reynolds MD. Gout and hyperuricemia associated with sickle cell anemia. Semin Arthritis Rheum. 1983;12:404–13.
29. Spillberg I, Meyer GJ. The arthritis of leukemia. Arthritis Rheum. 1975;15:630–5.
30. Evans, TI, Nercessian, BM, Sanders, KM. Leukemic arthritis. Semin Arthritis Rheum. 1994;24:48-56.
31. Elkon KB, Hughes GRV, Catovsky D. Hairy cell leukemia with polyarteritis nodosa. Lancet. 1979;ii:280–2.
32. Davies PG, Fordham JN. Arthritis and angioimmunoblastic lymphadenopathy. Ann Rheum Dis. 1983;42:516–18.
33. Cullen MH, Stansfeld AG, Oliver RT, *et al.* Angioimmunoblastic lymphadenopathy: Report of 10 cases and a review of literature. Q J Med. 1979;48:151–77.
34. Frizzera G, Moran ZM, Rappaport H. Angioimmunoblastic lymphadenopathy. Diagnosis and clinical course. Am J Med. 1975;59:1–18.
35. Bardwick PA, Zvaifler NJ, Gill GN, Newman D, Greenway GD, Resnick DL. Plasma cell dyscrasia with polyneuropathy, organomegaly, endocrinopathy, M protein, and skin changes: The POEMS syndrome. Report on two cases and a review of the literature. Medicine. 1980;59:311–22.
36. Gordon DA, Pruzanski W, Ogryzlo MA, *et al.* Amyloid arthritis simulating rheumatoid disease in five patients with multiple myeloma. Am J Med. 1974;55:142–54.
37. Hickling P, Wilkins M, Newman GR, *et al.* A study of amyloid arthropathy in multiple myeloma. Q J Med. 1981;50:417–33.
38. Barrow MB, Holubar K. Multicentric reticulohistiocytosis: A review of 33 patients. Medicine. 1969;48:287–305.
39. Heathcote JG, Guenther LC, Wallas AC. Multicentric reticulohistiocytosis: A report of a case and a review of the pathology. Pathology. 1985;17:601–8.
40. Gold RH, Metzger AL, Mirra JM. Multicentric reticulohistiocytosis. An erosive polyarthritis with distinctive clinical, roentgenographic, and pathologic features. Am J Roentgenol Radium Ther Nucl Med. 1975;124:610–24.
41. Ginsburg WW, O'Duffy JD, Morris JL, Huston KA. Multicentric reticulohistiocytosis: Response to alkylating agents in six patients. Ann Intern Med. 1989;111:384–8.
42. Liang GC, Granston AS. Complete remission of multicentric reticulohistiocytosis with combination therapy of steroid, cyclophosphamide, and low-dose pulse methotrexate: case report, review of the literature, and proposal for treatment. Arthritis Rheum. 1996;39:171–4.
43. Adebajo A. Rheumatic manifestations of tropical diseases. Curr Opin Rheumatol. 1996;8:85–9.

29

SYNOVIAL TUMORS

F Richard Convery, Roger Lyon & Carlos Lavernia

Definitions

- Synovial tumors are uncommon and usually benign.
- The most frequent benign articular tumors are pigmented villonodular synovitis and synovial osteochondromatosis.
- Synovial sarcomas are very rare.

Clinical features

Pigmented villonodular synovitis appears in three forms:

- Pigmented villonodular tenosynovitis (giant cell tumor of the tendon sheath), a localized lesion, usually of the fingers.
- Diffuse intra-articular PVNS, which can cause effusions and localized bone destruction in weight-bearing joints.
- Localized pedunculated villonodular synovitis.

Synovial osteochondromatosis:

- Cartilage formation within the synovium of any articular structure.
- Ossification of portions of the lesions gives a characteristic radiographic appearance, which underestimates the extent of the disease.

Synovial sarcomas:

- Misnomer because most arise from periarticular structures.
- Symptoms result from local growth or metastasis.
- Soft tissue tumors with a poor prognosis.
- Proper diagnosis and classification requires biopsy of the lesion.

PIGMENTED VILLONODULAR SYNOVITIS

Pigmented villonodular synovitis (PVNS) is a slowly progressive benign proliferation of synovial tissue that presents in three different clinical forms – an isolated discrete tenosynovitis; a diffuse villonodular synovitis; and a rare pedunculated lesion. The etiology is unknown, the nomenclature is uncertain and the results of treatment less than completely satisfactory.

EPIDEMIOLOGY

All three forms of the disease may occur at almost any age. The youngest reported patient in an epidemiologic study was 11 years and the oldest 84 years[1]. The most frequent age of initial onset is in the third decade[1,2]. However, in a Mayo Clinic series of pigmented villonodular tenosynovitis (PVTS) the peak incidence was approximately 20 years older[3]; 45% of the patients had associated degenerative joint disease. The younger ages in the first two series cited above were determined at the time of initial diagnosis, which may not have been the case in the Mayo Clinic series.

Pigmented villonodular synovitis is slightly more common in women. Myers *et al.* tabulated the literature to 1980 and reported a 56% incidence in females[1], which is somewhat less than the 47/33 female/male ratio reported by Byers *et al.*[2] and the much higher female predilection reported by the Mayo Clinic (79/38 [3] and 59/40 [4]).

The frequency of the disease is difficult to determine because of the small numbers of patients involved and the comparisons made. Clark reviewed the records of 2000 patients seen for joint complaints at the Massachusetts General Hospital, and found 18 documented cases, an incidence of approximately one in 100 patients with joint complaints[5].

The incidence of one localized pedunculated villonodular (LPVS) lesion per 250 meniscectomies[6] and one per 650 arthroscopies for both localized and diffuse lesions has been cited[7].

A comprehensive epidemiologic study in a large, well-defined community was performed to provide 'a global perspective'[1]. In this series, heavily weighted with cases of giant cell tumor of tendon sheath (PVTS), that is 80 patients with PVTS and only 16 with PVNS, the overall incidence in all age groups was 9.2 cases per million population.

CLINICAL FEATURES

Giant cell tumor of tendon sheath (PVTS), is the most common expression of what is believed to be a disease spectrum of three basic types of clinical presentation[1]. This isolated discrete lesion is usually painless, slowly progressive and may cause erosions of adjacent bone[3,8–10]. Rarely does PVTS cause any dysfunction, but slow enlargement over a long period of time usually results in surgical excision, primarily for diagnostic reasons. The hand, especially the fingers, is by far the most common site; rarely, the lesion occurs elsewhere, such as the foot, wrist, toe or ankle.

After ganglions, PVTS is the next most common tumor seen in the hand. It is grossly identical to localized PVNS and is histologically identical to diffuse pigmented villonodular synovitis. The label benign synovioma is histologically accurate since the tumor does not metastasize[8,11]. Typically PVTS presents in adulthood, most commonly in the third, fourth and fifth decades of life, and in most series it is more prevalent in women.

The second presentation is as diffuse intra-articular PVNS. This form of the disease has attracted the most attention, and serves as the prototype for etiologic investigation. The knee is the most frequent joint involved by PVNS, followed by the hip and ankle[1,4,12]. Infrequently, the diffuse form will present in the hand, shoulder, wrist and, surprisingly, in the vertebral column[13], where the lytic destruction of bone simulates a much more ominous diagnosis. The onset is nonspecific, although, as in many chronic diseases of the extremities, the patient may well implicate a traumatic incident. The progression is slow with initially intermittent and later steady joint swelling and pain. A joint effusion is usually present (see Fig. 29.1). Unlike the localized form of the disease, which may simulate a meniscal lesion, diffuse PVNS more closely resembles the chronic synovitis of rheumatoid arthritis (RA).

The third and least common presentation is a localized pedunculated nodule within the joint (LPVS). The knee is the joint most usually involved. The lesion is initially thought to be a torn meniscus or a loose body, since the patient presents with mechanical symptoms of locking and clicking. Radiographs are normal and the diagnosis is most often determined at the time of arthrotomy.

INVESTIGATIONS

Two comprehensive literature reviews and extensively illustrated reports that emphasize the radiologic features of diffuse PVNS have been published[14,15]. Soft tissue swelling without calcification, a significant differential feature with respect to synovial osteochondromatosis, is the most common radiologic finding. Hemosiderin deposition may produce a subtle homogeneous increase in soft tissue density, a finding most easily demonstrated with knee involvement. Osteophytes and juxta-articular osteoporosis, important findings in the differential diagnosis of degenerative joint disease and RA, respectively, are characteristically absent.

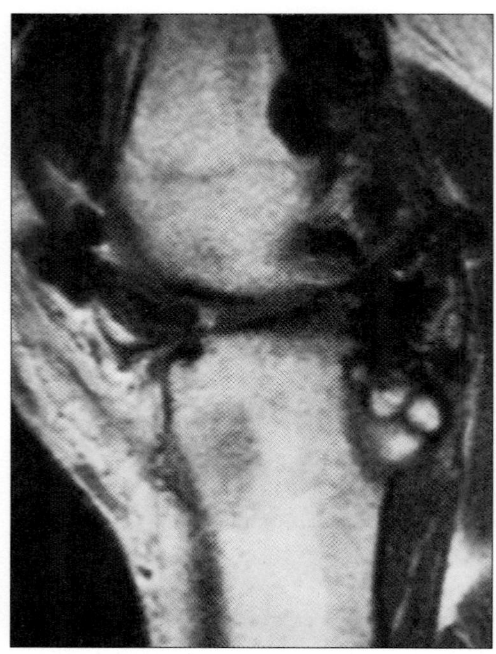

Fig. 29.1 Pigmented villonodular synovitis. Sagittal T2-weighted MRI of the knee shows diffusely thickened synovium darkened by hemosiderin deposition from recurrent hemarthrosis.

Osseous involvement, as by subchondral cysts and pressure erosions, is more usually seen in joints other than the knee, where soft tissue findings predominate. Hip involvement, although much less frequent than that of the knee, seems to be particularly associated with bone destruction[4,8,16–18], perhaps because of the tight unyielding capsule of the hip, as compared to the voluminous expansive capsule of the knee joint. An alternative explanation is that the osseous involvement is not the result of pressure, but more likely direct invasion of proliferating pannus via vascular foramina[19]. This also might explain the massive destruction reported in the cervical spine[11], wrist[7] and ankle[14]. Prior to 1960, when McMaster reported six cases of bone involvement, three each in the knee and the hip, bone destruction in association with knee involvement was not known[19].

The amount of hemosiderin in PVNS is usually greatly in excess of that seen in RA, and the MRI appearance reflects this, with PVNS appearing diffusely black on T1– and Tx–weighted MRI as in Figure 29.1 and RA typically high on T2– and intermediate on T1–weighted images.

ETIOLOGY

The etiology of PVNS is unknown. The three different forms of clinical presentation are, however, thought to be a continuum of the same disease caused by a single unknown entity[1–3,22–23]. The absence of a known cause is reflected in the variable terminology. A partial list of synonyms for PVNS includes synovial xanthoma, synovial fibroendothelioma, synovial endothelioma, benign fibrous histiocytoma, xanthomatous giant cell tumor and giant cell tumor of tendon sheath.

Prior to 1941, the various forms of the disease were thought to be different entities of neoplastic origin. In an effort to emphasize the inflammatory reaction of the proliferative process and to group the three seemingly disparate forms into a single non-neoplastic group, Jaffe *et al.* introduced the comprehensive term 'pigmented villonodular synovitis'[20] and, for the most part, this terminology has been accepted. Various etiologic theories have been proposed, based primarily on which of the several cell types present in the lesion is emphasized. Microscopically, a proliferation of synovial cells, foam cells (hemosiderin-laden histiocytes) and multinucleated giant cells are seen intermixed with fibrous tissue. The case for a neoplastic etiology is suggested by the presence of multinucleated giant cells, a high rate of recurrence following surgical excision and a more ominous histologic pattern seen in tissue examined after recurrence. The presence of bone erosions, seen most frequently in the hip[4,16–19], has been interpreted as a malignant etiology. However, the relative infrequency of bone erosions and the absence of metastases argues against a neoplastic etiology. Granowitz *et al.* failed to discover a single reported case of malignant degeneration or distant metastasis[23].

The benign clinical course, as well as the histologic appearance, suggested to Jaffe *et al.* that PVNS is not a neoplasm, but represents an inflammatory response to an unknown inciting agent[21], and this is still the prevailing view[9,21,23].

The presence of hemosiderin-laden histiocytes in the PVNS lesion has stimulated efforts to reproduce the disease[24,25]. Young and Hudacek[26], who believed that trauma was a significant factor in the etiology, repeatedly injected autologous blood into canine knee joints for up to 13 months. After 8 months of injections, they reported the production of brownish-stained hypertrophic synovium that was villous and contained firm brown nodules. Histologic examination of the joints of the dogs sacrificed after 8 months or longer demonstrated hyperplastic villi, often a marked fibroblastic response, scattered multinucleated giant cells and collections of lipid-laden macrophages. Hemosiderin was found in the synovial cells and deeper tissues and there were many hemosiderin-laden macrophages in the subsynovial tissues. The gross and histologic pictures were similar to PVNS. There was no control, such as saline injection. McCollum *et al.*[25] showed that repeated saline injection, as well as blood, produced synovial proliferation that seemed to meet the histologic criteria for PVNS. Hoagland also injected blood and saline into the joints of immature puppies[27]. The injections were done six times a week for 12–18 weeks. The joints that received blood had a thickened yellow-to-brown pigmented synovium with pannus over the anterior tibial plateau. Microscopically there was hyperplasia of the synovial surface cells, an increase in synovial fibrous tissue and hemosiderin deposition. Multinucleated giant cells and foam cells were not observed and the synovial changes seen were interpreted as similar to previous studies of experimental hemarthrosis and human hemophilia rather than to PVNS.

PATHOLOGY

In 1941, Jaffe *et al.*[20] published the landmark paper that united the three forms of PVNS and emphasized the inflammatory nature of the lesion. Grossly, the synovium in PVNS is hypertrophic and a red–brown to mottled orange–yellow color (Fig. 29.2). Villous projection of synovium and soft nodules are present. Microscopically there is a marked synovial cell hyperplasia with surface proliferation and subsynovial round cells. Along with the proliferation of synovial

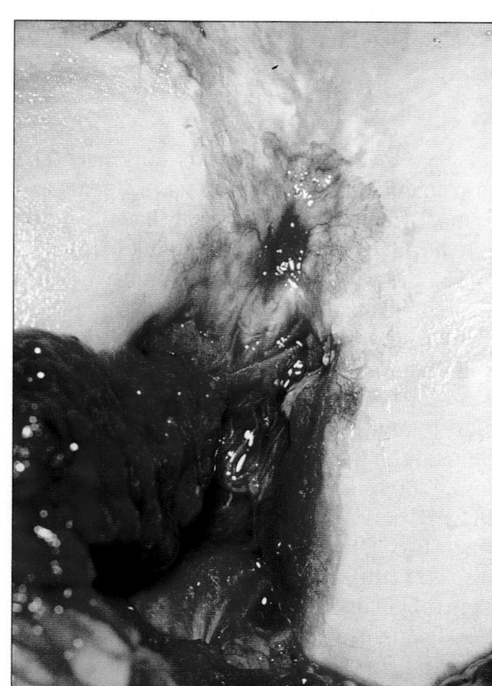

Fig. 29.2 Pigmented villonodular synovitis. Dark brown synovial hypertrophy surrounding the anterior cruciate ligament in the femoral notch. Creeping pannus formation in the inferior trochlea and on the femoral condyle.

cells, there are collections of giant cells, with the nuclei tending to collect in the center of the cell, hemosiderin-laden macrophages and fibroblasts. Hemosiderin can also be found between cells, in the synovial lining cells and in the round cells. Lipid-filled histiocytes (foam cells) are often prominent. To some investigators, this feature has suggested a disorder of lipid metabolism as the inciting agent, with the inflammation a secondary response.

The microscopic differential diagnosis includes synovial hemochromatosis, synovial hemosiderosis and the synovitis of hemophilia (see Chapters 8.24 and 8.26). The collection of foam cells and giant cells are unique to PVNS. It is important to point out that all brown synovium is not PVNS[28].

The histologic appearance seen in the localized form of the disease and in localized giant cell tenosynovitis is identical to that of diffuse PVNS, with the exception that in each of these localized forms the predominant synovial villi are absent.

MANAGEMENT

The treatment of PVNS is surgical and is frequently complicated by recurrence. Because surgical excision is often unsatisfactory, newer treatment techniques are under investigation. The disease is relatively rare, however, making controlled studies impossible. Reported series are small in numbers, usually include various joints and all three forms of the disease are combined. Moreover patients with recurrence, as well as those at initial presentation, are usually included. For these reasons, it is difficult to interpret most clinical studies.

Diffuse lesions of the knee, although treated by wide synovectomy, still have high range from 20–50%[29]. The usual explanation for recurrence is the technical inability to completely excise all the pathologic tissue without injury to the knee. There is no series to document the consensus that, as in RA, the results of synovectomy in PVNS are proportional to the degree of joint damage at the time of surgery, so that, with greater joint destruction, results are less satisfactory. In one series, routine manipulation for 2 weeks postoperatively seemed to improve the overall results. There were no unsatisfactory ratings in the knees that had been manipulated, mostly because of a better range of motion[29].

In the past, high recurrence rates after surgical synovectomy have led to the use of radiotherapy, either in combination with synovectomy[30,31] or alone[32]. Reluctance to employ radiation therapy in young patients with a benign disease, and the fear of creating joint stiffness, have limited this application. Intra-articular radionuclides are being investigated. Eight patients who received one or two intra-articular injections of yttrium-90 silicate have been reported[33]. Six experienced recurrence of PVNS after surgical synovectomy. At a mean follow-up of 32 months, four of the eight patients showed improvement of the synovitis as determined by clinical examination, a decrease in technetium-99m uptake and arthroscopic biopsy. More recently, a group from Boston has reported their experience with dysprosium-65 ferric hydroxide macroaggregate[34]. Intra-articular radiation was combined with surgical synovectomy. The 24 patients were treated and divided into two groups, depending upon the time elapsed since surgical synovectomy. Those patients irradiated 6 months or longer after synovectomy all had a poor result. When irradiation was done within 6 months of surgical treatment, 81% had a good result, with no recurrence up to 6 years later.

Surgical excision of the localized form (PVNS) in the knee is usually more successful[22,23,29], although in one series there were two recurrences following surgical excision in 13 patients[2]. Interestingly, these same authors reported the highest recurrence rate (46%) in their group of patients with diffuse lesions. Localized lesions in the knee have in the past been excised via open arthrotomy. Arthroscopic resection is now much more commonly employed[12,13,35]. In view of the high recurrence rate following open synovectomy, it seems unlikely that arthroscopic synovectomy alone will be routinely successful for diffuse lesions.

Since the diffuse form of PVNS in the hip joint is usually associated with significant bone destruction, and synovectomy of the hip joint in RA is usually not successsful, prosthetic replacement is the consensus recommendation for hip joint involvement. The method of fixation and design of the implant have and will be determined by the prevailing concepts at the time of treatment[4,17,18]. In a series of 99 patients with PVNS of large joints, only 25 joints (20 hips) had associated bone destruction. There were no recurrences in those patients who had a prosthetic joint replacement as their initial procedure, combined with a complete synovectomy[4].

Pigmented villonodular tenosynovitis which occurs most commonly in the hand, especially the fingers, is isolated, accessible and should be easily excised. Modern surgical techniques, such as tourniquet hemostasis and operating microscopes, as well as knowledge of the high rates of recurrence in this form of the disease[2,3,6,23], should improve the results in the future.

SYNOVIAL OSTEOCHONDROMATOSIS

Synovial osteochondromatosis is an uncommon condition characterized by cartilage formation within the synovium. It has also been termed synovial chondromatosis, synovial chondromata, joint chondroma, diffuse chondromatosis of the joint capsule and enchondroma of the joint capsule[36–39].

Synovial osteochondromatosis can be divided into two types: primary and secondary. Primary osteochondromatosis is thought to reflect a metaplasia of fibroblasts within the synovium that develop into cartilage-making cells. The exact mechanism that causes these changes is not known. Possibilities include residual pleuripotential cells, (embryologic in nature), neoplasia, trauma and infection[37,38,40–42].

Secondary synovial osteochondromatosis can result from osteoarthritis, as well as trauma. The radiologic appearance of secondary synovial osteochondromatosis is identical to that of primary disease. Histologically, however, intrasynovial cartilage nodules are not common and the appearance of the chondrocytes within the loose bodies is quite different. In secondary disease, cartilage nests are almost always absent and the cells appear mature.

CLINICAL FEATURES

Primary synovial osteochondromatosis usually presents with monoarticular pain and swelling, as well as limitation of motion. Locking of the joint will be present in some cases, but is relatively uncommon.

Synovial osteochondromatosis can occur in any synovial tissue, including bursae and tendon sheaths, but it is by far most usual within joint cavities[38,40,43,44]. The knee is the most commonly affected joint, in more than 50% of cases, followed by the hip[44] and elbow[38–40,45–49]. Synovial osteochondromatosis has also been described in the spine[50], shoulder[51], temporomandibular joint[52] and hand[53–55], as well as in the proximal tibiofibular joint[56]. The average age at presentation is around 50 years. In some series, osteochondromatosis is most common in the third, fourth and fifth decades (range to 67 years); men appear to be more commonly affected than women[37], although other authors report just the opposite[39]. There are case reports of children with synovial chondromatosis in the area of the knee[43,57].

INVESTIGATIONS

Several radiologic imaging modalities have been utilized, including bone scans, computer tomography and MRI[58,59]. Synovial osteochondromas with negative bone scans have been noted[37,44,58]. Thus, MRI is likely to play an increasingly important role[59].

DIFFERENTIAL DIAGNOSIS

In primary synovial osteochondromatosis, laboratory values are usually normal, but they are helpful in excluding other diagnoses. Routine radiographs usually demonstrate well-calcified loose bodies within a synovial or bursal cavity (Figs. 29.3a, b). Radiologic evaluation, however, markedly underestimates the extent of the disease, since the bulk of the nodules are not radiopaque (Figs 29.3c, d). Additionally, cases with negative radiographs have been reported[44]. On arthrotomy or arthroscopy, the soft tissues of the joints are markedly thickened and the joint cavity is filled with a large number of small, very irregular, cartilaginous nodules. It is characteristic to find some secondary osteoarthritic changes on the side of the joint surface and this is most common in long-standing cases, particularly in weight-bearing joints.

The differential diagnosis includes osteoarthritis, RA, osteochondral fractures, tumoral calcinosis and calcium pyrophosphate disease[60,61].

ETIOLOGY

The cause of this disease has been studied by many authors[39,45,62], but there is no consensus as to its origins and no convincing experimental models are available.

PATHOGENESIS

Histologically the synovium appears to be very vascular and thickened with numerous villous projections. Focal collections of lymphocytes, as well as multiple hypertrophic foci of cartilage nodules, are seen within the synovium. It is possible to trace the transition of spindle-shaped fibroblasts into cartilage-forming tissue. The cartilage cells seen in these foci appear as rapidly reproducing cells with some cellular atypia, but they are easily distinguished from malignant cells on other grounds[38]. The three stages of synovial osteochondromatosis described by Milgram[36] are frequently seen in primary disease: stage I – intrasynovial bodies; stage II – cartilaginous bodies partially attached to the synovium; and stage III – loose bodies floating within the joint space. In most cases, all three stages coexist.

MANAGEMENT

The treatment of synovial osteochondromatosis is controversial. Some authors advocate observation while others postulate that the disease will progress to osteoarthritis and should be aggressively treated with removal of the loose bodies and complete synovectomy. This is the accepted procedure, although Maurice *et al.* have stated that synovial osteochondromatosis does not necessarily lead to osteoarthritic changes and have presented 53 cases, some with follow up of 7 years, to support this view[47].

Arthroscopic treatment for synovial osteochondromatosis of the knee may represent a more conservative approach. In a recent report, excellent results were obtained by removal of the loose bodies from the knee joints of 39 patients without synovectomy[63].

SYNOVIAL SARCOMA

Synovial sarcoma is a soft tissue tumor that occurs most commonly around the large joints of both the upper and lower extremities. The tumor is thought to originate from tendon sheaths, bursae and joint capsules. It is among the most common soft tissue sarcomas and, like the others, has a poor prognosis. Surgical resection remains the mainstay of therapy.

HISTORY

Historically, synovial sarcoma has been grouped together with several other tumors including epithelioid, clear cell and chorioid sarcomas.

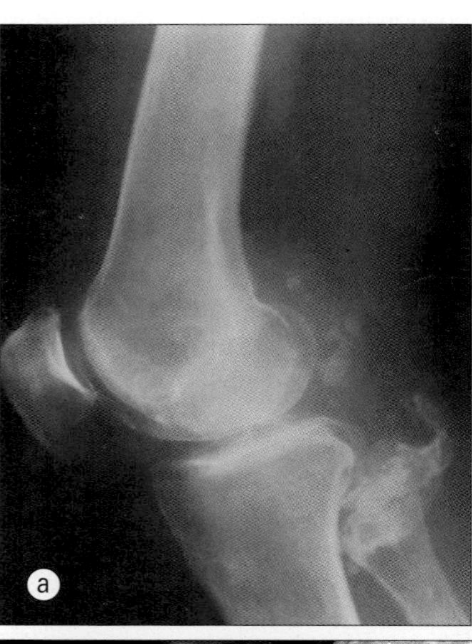

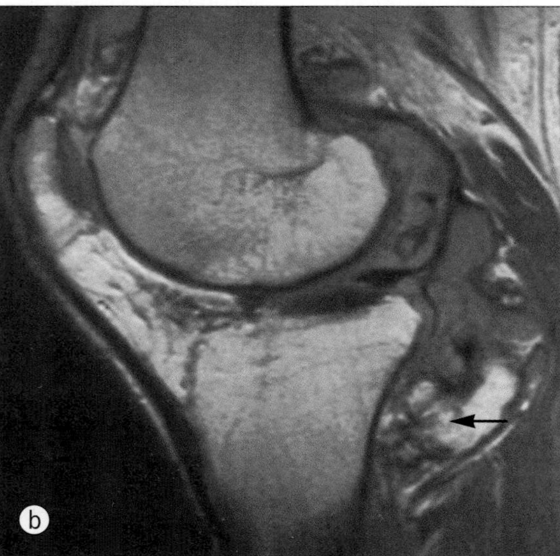

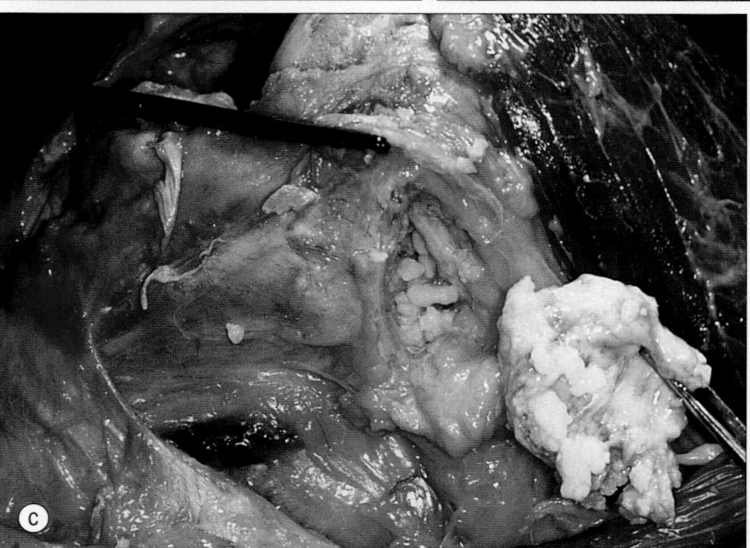

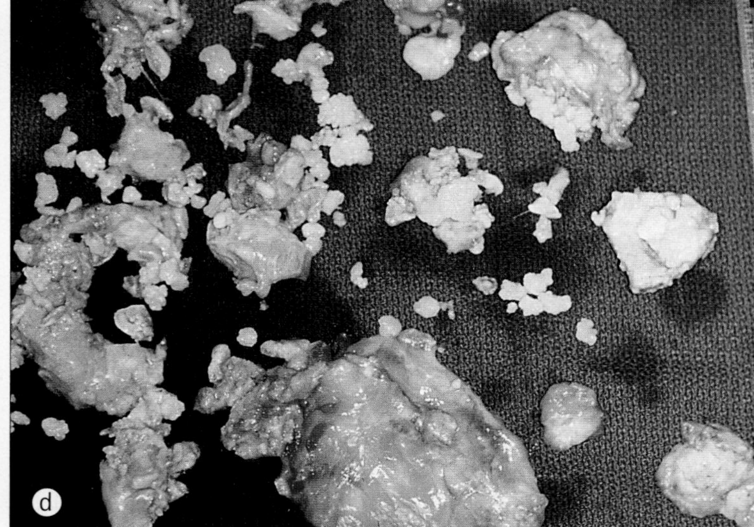

Fig. 29.3 Synovial osteochondromatosis. Radiograph shows numerous ossific bodies within the knee joint (a). T1-weighted MRI of the same knee shows extensive synovial thickening associated with the ossifications; note the high-signal marrow fat within some of the ossific bodies (arrow) (b). The synovial mass of embedded and free-floating cartilaginous loose bodies is excised from another patient (c). The volume of tissue removed (d) is much greater than demonstrated by the radiograph.

However synovial sarcoma is a clinically and microscopically distinct entity. First described in 1893, this lesion has been variously described as adenosarcoma, perithelial sarcoma, synovial sarcoendothelioma, sarcomesothelioma and mesothelioma of joints[9]. In 1927, Smith used the term 'synovioma'[64] and, in 1936, Knox proposed the term 'synovial sarcoma'[65].

EPIDEMIOLOGY

Synovial sarcoma most commonly occurs in adolescents and young adults aged 15–40 years. Scattered cases in children as young as 1 or 2 years old are reported, as well as cases in the seventh and eighth decades of life. Occurrences in males slightly outnumber those in females. There appears to be no predilection as to race.

CLINICAL FEATURES

Most synovial sarcomas occur in the extremities near the large joints. Rarely are they found within the joint cavity. In general, they are associated with tendons, tendon sheaths and bursal structures. They do arise less commonly from fascial structures, ligaments, aponeuroses and interosseous membranes. Approximately 60% of synovial sarcomas occur in the lower extremities, and another 25% in the upper extremities. The knee is by far the most involved site, in more than one third of all cases. Then, in decreasing order of occurrence, are the foot and ankle, elbow, upper arm and shoulder regions. Synovial sarcoma is the most common noncutaneous primary malignant tumor of the foot. The remaining 10–15% of synovial sarcomas are found in the head, neck and trunk regions. In the head and neck, these tumors arise in the paravertebral connective tissue spaces and present as solitary peripharyngeal masses near the carotid bifurcation. Similar lesions can also occur in the trunk and are usually deep seated, in the lower half of the abdomen and specifically involve the abdominal wall.

Synovial sarcomas usually present as large, deep-seated, rapidly growing masses in and about the thigh, buttocks and shoulder or upper arm. Occasionally they are painful and cause limitation of motion because of their location near joints. A lesser percentage appear as small, superficial, indolent lumps located about the hands or feet. In some of these cases, the tumor is soft and slow growing, and thought to be benign by the patient and physician. They are often excised routinely and only after histologic examination of sections is the physician aware of the actual diagnosis.

Lesions about the head and neck cause difficulties with breathing and swallowing, and can cause voice changes. Other clinical complaints are related to the specific location of the tumor and the structures which are compromised.

The duration of symptoms prior to medical attention varies considerably, ranging from 2 to 4 years, but sometimes lasts as long as 20 years. Initial diagnoses of synovitis, tendonitis, bursitis or ganglions are common.

INVESTIGATIONS

Plain radiographs remain an essential first step in the evaluation of synovial sarcoma. The characteristic, but not diagnostic, radiographic appearance of a synovial sarcoma is that of a round or oval soft tissue mass of moderate density, located near a large joint. Approximately one-third of all cases have spotty opacities of localized calcification within the lesion (Fig. 29.4). There is occasional periosteal reaction and rare bone invasion (Fig. 29.5a). In one study, soft tissue swelling only was present in 20% of cases, calcification in 20% and adjacent bone involvement in 11%. The plain radiographs were interpreted as normal in 49% of the cases[66].

Radionuclide bone scans can be helpful in determining the extent of the tumor by showing increased uptake in adjacent bone, occult bony involvement and assessing the vascularity of the lesion and the surrounding reactive zone[67].

Angiographic studies of synovial sarcoma usually show a neovascular reaction in the early arterial phase, and a prominent tumor blush in the late venous phase (Fig. 29.5b). When regional lymph nodes are involved, they are evident on the early arterial phase. If synovial sarcoma is suspected, visualization of the regional lymph nodes is recommended.

Computer tomography can help delineate the extent of the tumor and the presence of calcification or ossification, but MRI is rapidly becoming the procedure of choice for characterization of soft tissue

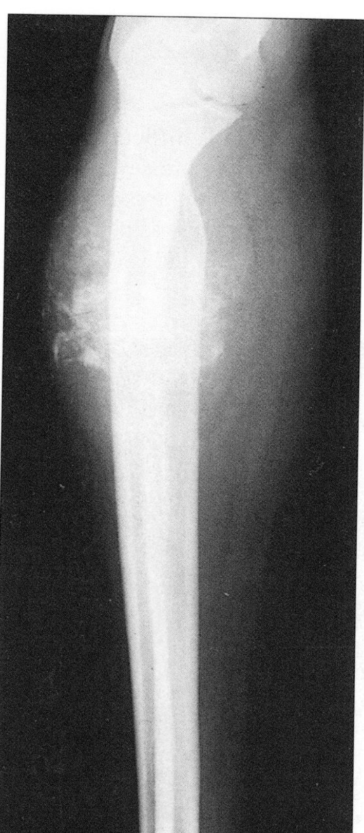

Fig. 29.4 Synovial sarcoma of the forearm: radiograph demonstrating soft tissue calcification.

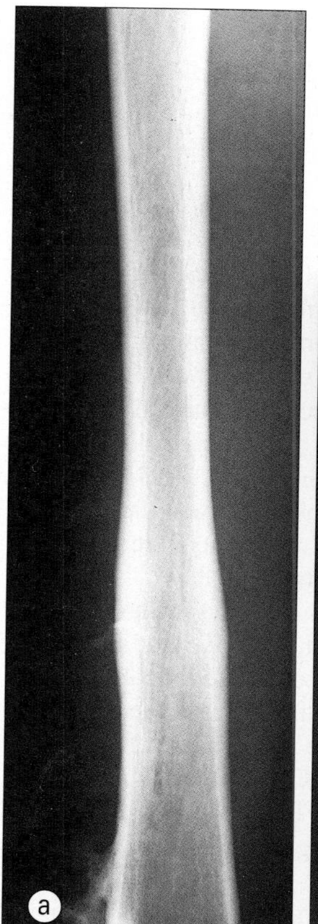

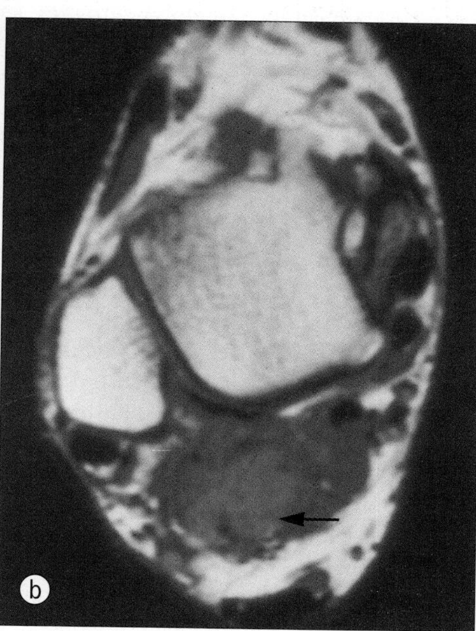

Fig. 29.5 Synovial sarcoma. Plain radiograph of a synovial sarcoma, demonstrating minimal osseous involvement and periosteal reaction (a). Transverse T1-weighted MRI shows a large soft-tissue mass (arrow) adjacent to but outside the ankle joint. The MRI appearance of this lesion is nonspecific, but its anatomic extent is clearly delineated allowing accurate presurgical staging (b).

tumors[68]. Such studies are able to localize lesions in reference to major structures, including nerves, vessels and bone. Also, MRI can aid in staging the lesion in terms of extra- or intracompartmental extent and in identifying the reactive zone of the sarcoma.

The definitive step in the work-up of a suspected sarcoma is a biopsy, because none of the radiographic studies are absolutely diagnostic. There are several reasonable options for obtaining tissue for histologic examination. An incisional biopsy remains the standard for biopsy of soft tissue lesions in general, and synovial sarcoma specifically. When this is done and an adequate specimen is obtained, the diagnosis is rarely in doubt. To obtain an adequate specimen, the tissue should come from a fleshy area of the lesion, including the edge along the pseudocapsule or surrounding tissue, and measure at least $1cm^3$. In many cases, a specimen is sent intraoperatively for frozen section to confirm that an adequate sample has been obtained for diagnosis. Occasionally, for small superficial lesions (under 5cm), an excisional biopsy is performed[69]. This is not the optimal approach because rarely are sufficient margins obtained[70]

A closed biopsy of a suspected synovial sarcoma is an accepted method of obtaining a tissue diagnosis[71,72]. Although less accurate than an open biopsy, needle biopsy has the advantage of being simple and having minimal risk of contaminating normal tissue planes. It is best reserved for large, deep-seated lesions, where open biopsy is difficult and would involve extensive dissection with associated contamination of several compartments.

DIFFERENTIAL DIAGNOSIS

If a lesion has the typical biphasic histologic appearance and is located in an extremity near a large joint in a young adult, then synovial sarcoma is a reliable diagnosis. In less clear cases, differentiation of synovial sarcoma from other neoplasms can be difficult.

Epithelioid sarcoma has a multinodular histologic pattern with central necrosis, eosinophilic tumor cells and no clear biphasic component. These tumors occur mainly in the hand or forearm and frequently have ulceration of the overlying skin.

Clear cell sarcoma is a rare tumor composed of fusiform and polygonal cells with abundant, finely vacuolated cytoplasm and large round pale-staining nuclei with prominent nucleoli. The cells are arranged into a nest-like pattern, have abundant glycogen and stain for S-100 protein and melanin, but not for cytokeratin.

Fibrosarcoma can resemble the monophasic spindle-cell type of synovial sarcoma. However, unlike synovial sarcoma, fibrosarcoma lacks mast cells, areas of calcification and cytokeratin. Fibrosarcoma has a classic herringbone pattern of the cells.

PATHOLOGY

The gross appearance of slowly growing lesions tends to be sharply circumscribed, round or multilobular, and may be surrounded by a pseudocapsule. Occasionally, cyst formation is a prominent feature. Most are attached to tendon sheaths, to the exterior wall of the joint capsule or to tendons themselves. On cut section, synovial sarcomas range in color from yellow to grayish-white, are usually solid and calcification is found only occasionally. Lesions of up to 15.3cm have been reported. Poorly differentiated and rapidly growing lesions are more often soft gelatinous masses which, on cut section, are yellow or light brown, with multiple areas of small hemorrhage.

The histologic differentiation of synovial sarcoma from other soft tissue sarcomas can occasionally be difficult. Unlike other sarcomas, they comprised two distinct cell types that characteristically form a biphasic pattern: the fibrosarcoma-like spindle cell and the epithelial cell. The spindle cells which are usually the predominant feature are mostly plump, of uniform appearance, with scant cytoplasm and oval, darkly stained nuclei. These cells tend to lie in a nondescript manner, but occasionally are organized in a swirling arrangement similar to fibrosarcoma.

The epithelial cells are always a less prominent feature of synovial sarcoma than the spindle-cell component. The epithelial cells tend to have large, round or oval, vesicular nuclei and abundant pale-staining cytoplasm with distinct cellular borders. There are no set patterns for these cells, but they tend to be oriented about slits or spaces that have the appearance of epithelial-lined clefts. In the clefts are glandular or homogeneous eosinophilic secretions representing mucoproteins that stain red with periodic acid–Schiff (PAS).

Two histologic types of synovial sarcoma are generally recognized depending on the relative prominence of the spindle and epithelial cell components, that is monophasic or biphasic. The histologic pattern varies widely between types and likely represents a continuous morphologic spectrum from a monophasic fibrous type, through a biphasic type, to a rare monophasic epithelial type. Although more difficult to characterize there is also a poorly differentiated type.

Classic biphasic type

Synovial sarcomas are most easily recognized when they are biphasic (Fig. 29.6). The spindle cell component is usually the most prominent with these cells forming solid, compact masses in an irregular nodular arrangement. Mitotic figures occur in both cell types, with only the poorly differentiated forms having more than two mitotic figures per high-power field. The epithelial cell component has typical cuboidal to tall columnar cells arranged in solid cords, whorls or nests, or surround clefts or irregular cyst-like spaces. Silver stains are helpful for locating the sometimes sparse epithelioid areas devoid of reticulum fibers in contrast to the positively staining spindle-cell areas.

Calcification is a characteristic feature in about 30% of cases and ranges in amount from a few small areas to extensive calcifications occupying a large portion of the tumor. Usually the calcifications are more pronounced at the periphery of the lesion.

Other cellular elements found in synovial sarcoma include mast cells, especially in the spindle cell component, and rarely giant cells. Vascular elements can be a dominant feature and vascular invasion, which is not uncommon, is an unfavorable prognostic sign.

Monophasic spindle-cell type

In this form of synovial sarcoma, the epithelioid formation is rare or lacking. Its existence has been confirmed by immunostaining of the spindle cells for keratin and a specific epithelial membrane antigen, and the presence of characteristic ultrastructural features, such as occasional intercellular spaces with filopodia.

Monophasic epithelial type

This rarely recognized form of synovial sarcoma is difficult to diagnose, because without a biphasic component there are several other neoplasms that have an almost identical microscopic appearance. In making the diagnosis, other factors are important, such as patient age, tumor location, presence of mast cells, calcifications and PAS-positive

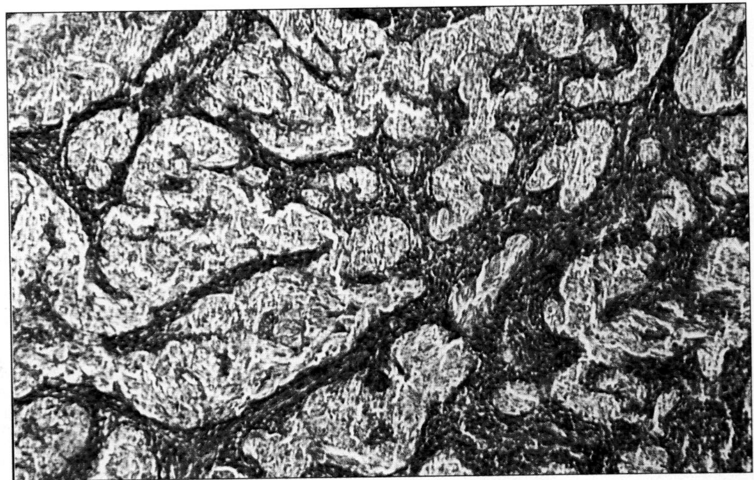

Fig. 29.6 Photomicrograph of a synovial sarcoma: demonstrating the characteristic biphasic pattern.

material within the cells or intercellular spaces. This diagnosis can only be made with confidence if some portion of the primary or recurrent neoplasm has a biphasic component.

Poorly differentiated type

There are no sharp criteria for distinguishing between well- and poorly differentiated synovial sarcoma. Histologically the cells appear intermediate between epithelial and spindle cells with little evidence of differentiation. Areas with more or less cellular differentiation often coexist within the same lesion. This type of synovial sarcoma accounts for about 20% of cases, and behaves more aggressively and metastasizes more frequently.

PATHOGENESIS

Although thorough studies of the natural history of synovial sarcoma are not available, it is clear that the outcome is usually very poor. In general the patient only comes to medical attention months to years after first noting symptoms. Metastases occur frequently and are occasionally present at the initial presentation. The most common sites of metastases are the lungs (80%), lymph nodes (20%) and bone marrow (20%). Metastases as late as 25 years after initial presentation have been reported, as has 10 years of survival after the first evidence of metastases.

The 5-year survival rates for synovial sarcoma range from 36 to 55%[66–73]. Ten-year survivals are from 11 to 38%[66–73]. Favorable clinical factors include a tumor size smaller than 5cm, localized disease at presentation, younger age patient and a distal lower extremity lesion. Several studies have attempted to relate histologic features to overall prognosis in synovial sarcoma. Although there is no consensus on the prognostic significance of microscopic type, a study by Cagle *et al.* showed that patients with biphasic lesions, with greater than 50% glandularity and mitotic rates of less than 15 per 10 × high-power field, had a longer disease-free interval and significantly improved survival than patients with other histologic subtypes[74]. Extensive calcification and ossification within the lesion also seem to predict a better survival.

MANAGEMENT

Surgery remains the mainstay of treatment. Simple local excision without ancillary therapy is clearly inadequate, as earlier studies using this treatment reported recurrence rates as high as 70%. Wide surgical excision through seemingly normal tissue is usually definitive if done for a small peripheral intracompartmental lesion (under 5cm) with favorable histologic features. If recurrence occurs, a wide amputation is necessary.

For larger intracompartmental (over 5cm) lesions with unfavorable histologic features, a radical local resection gives the best overall survival rates[75]. Because of the proximity of these lesions to large joints, they are usually extracompartmental and essentially unresectable with clear wide margins. In such cases, either a wide excision based on imaging studies or an amputation with a bone level 10cm above the lesion is required.

The effect of radiation therapy on synovial sarcoma specifically has not been well studied. However, from more general studies of other soft tissue sarcomas[76,77], several conclusions have been drawn: first, that radiation therapy alone cannot control the tumor; second, that preoperative radiation therapy of over 40Gy (4000rads) decreases the rate of local recurrence and can help in determining the radiosensitivity of the lesion; and, finally, postoperative radiation therapy with 50–70Gy (5000–7000rads) leads to significantly improved survival and relapse-free survival rates in patients who have undergone incomplete (non-radical but at least marginal) surgical resection.

Similar studies concerning the effects of adjuvant chemotherapy on soft tissue sarcomas[78,79] suggest that, although its beneficial effects are not proved, preoperative chemotherapy significantly improves overall survival, continuous disease-free survival and distant metastases-free survival in patients judged to have clinical response to chemotherapy and subsequently undergoing local surgery and radiation therapy.

It is encouraging that more recent studies have demonstrated improved survival rates using a combination of surgery, chemotherapy and radiation therapy. Hopefully the next generation of studies will specifically address synovial sarcomas and resolve the issues of appropriate timing and amount of these three modalities.

REFERENCES

1. Myers BW, Masi AT, Feigenbaum SL. Pigmented villonodular synovitis and tenosynovitis: a clinical epidemiologic study of 166 cases and literature review. Medicine. 1980;59:223–38.
2. Byers BD, Cotton RE, Deacon OW, *et al.* The diagnosis and treatment of pigmented villonodular synovitis. J Bone J Surg. 1968;50B:290–305.
3. Jones FE, Soule, EN, Coventry MD. Fibrous xanthoma of synovium (giant cell tumor of tendon sheath, pigmented nodular synovitis). J Bone J Surg. 1969;51A:76–86.
4. Schwartz HS, Unni KK, Pritchard DJ. Pigmented villonodular synovitis, a retrospective review of affected joints. Clin Orthop. 1989;247:243–55.
5. Clark WS. Case records of the Massachusetts General Hospital. N Engl J Med. 1976;245:59–63.
6. Dandy DJ, Rao NS. Benign synovioma causing internal derangement of the knee. J Bone J Surg. 1990;72B:641–2.
7. Bequin J, Locker B, Vielpeau L, Souquières G. Arthroscopy. J Arthroscopy Rel Surg. 1989;5:62–4.
8. Phaen GS, McCormack LJ, Gazule WS. Giant cell tumor of tendon sheath. Clin Orthop. 1959;15:140–51.
9. Schajowicz F, Blumenfeld I. Pigmented villonodular synovitis of the wrist with penetration into bone. J Bone J Surg. 1968;50B:312–17.
10. Scott PM. Bone lesions in pigmented villonodular synovitis. J Bone J Surg. 1968;50B:306–11.
11. Lichtenstein L. Diseases of bone and joints, 2E. St Louis: Mosby; 1975:296–300.
12. Flandry F, Hughston JC. Current concepts review, pigmented villonodular synovitis. J Bone J Surg. 1987;69A:942–9.
13. Karnezis TA, McMillan RD, Ciric I. Pigmented villondular synovitis in a vertebra. J Bone J Surg. 1990;72A:927–30.
14. Goldman AB, DiCarlo EF. Pigmented villonodular synovitis, diagnosis and differential diagnosis. Radiol Clin North Am. 1988;26:1327–47.
15. Flandy F, McCann SB, Hughston SG, Kurtz DM. Roentgenographic findings in pigmented villonodular synovitis of the knee. Clin Orthop. 1989;247:208–19.
16. Jaffe HL. Discussion. Pigmented villonodular synovitis with invasion of bone. J Bone J Surg. 1960;42A:1183.
17. Chung SMK, Jones JM. Diffuse pigmented villonodular synovitis of the hip joint. Review of the literature and report of four cases. J Bone J Surg. 1965;47A:293–303.
18. Danzig LA, Gershuni DH, Resnick D. Diagnosis and treatment of diffuse pigmented villonodular synovitis of the hip. Clin Orthop. 1982;168:42–7.
19. McMaster PE. Pigmented villonodular synovitis with invasion of bone. J Bone J Surg. 1960;42A:1170–83.
20. Jaffe HL, Lichtenstein L, Sutro CJ. Pigmented villonodular synovitis, bursitis and tenosynovitis. Arch Pathol. 1941;31:731.
21. Jaffe HL. Pigmented villonodular synovitis, bursitis and tenosynovitis. In: Jaffe HL, ed. Tumors and tumorous conditions of the bones and joints. Philadelphia: Lea & Febiger; 1958:532–57.
22. Rao AS, Vigorita VS. Pigmented villonodular synovitis (giant cell tumor of tendon sheath and synovial membrane). J Bone J Surg. 1984;66A:76–94.
23. Granowitz SD, D'Antonio J, Mankin HL. The pathogenesis and long-term end results of pigmented villonodular synovitis. Clin Orthop. 1976;114:335–51.
24. Key JA. Experimental arthritis, the reaction of joints to mild irritants. J Bone J Surg. 1929;11:705–38.
25. McCollum DE, Musser AW, Rhangos WC. Experimental villonodular synovitis. South Med J. 1966;59:966–70.
26. Young JM, Hudacek AB. Experimental production of pigmented villonodular synovitis in dogs. Am J Pathol. 1954;30:799–812.

27. Hoagland FT. Experimental hemarthrosis, the response of canine knees to injection of autologous blood. J Bone J Surg. 1967;49A:285–98.
28. Collins DH. Haemosiderosis and haemochromatosis of synovial tissue. J Bone J Surg. 1951;33B:436–41.
29. Johansson JE, Ajjoub S, Coughlin LP, Wener JA, Cruess RL. Pigmented villonodular synovitis of joints. Clin Orthop. 1982;163:159–66.
30. Shafer SJ, Larmon WA. Pigmented villonodular synovitis, a report of seven cases. Surg Gynecol Obstet. 1951;92:574–80.
31. Friedman M, Schwartz EE. Irradiation treatment of pigmented villonodular synovitis. Bull Hosp Jt Dis. 1957;18:19–32.
32. Greenfield MM, Wallace KM. Pigmented villonodular synovitis. Radiology. 1950;54;350–6.
33. Franssen MJAM, Boerbooms AMTH, Karthaus RP, Buijs, WCAM, van de Putte LBA. Treatment of pigmented villonodular synovitis of the knee with ^{90}Y silicate: prospective evaluation by arthroscopy, histology and ^{99m}Tc pertechnetate uptake measurements. Ann Rheum Dis. 1989;48:1007–13.
34. Tsahakis PS, Shortkrott S, Boyd AD, Wilson MG, Zuckerman JD, Sledge CB. Role of radiation synovectomy in the treatment of pigmented villonodular synovitis of the knee. In: AAOS (American Academy of Orthopaedic Surgeons) annual meeting, Anaheim 1991. AAOS;65.
35. Lopez-Vazquez, E, Lopez-Peris, JI, Via-Donat E, Martinez-Garcia JB, Bru-Pomer, A. Localized pigmented villonodular synovitis of the knee: diagnosis and arthroscopic resection. J Arthroscopy Rel Surg. 1988;4:121–3.
36. Milgram JW. Synovial osteochondromatosis. J Bone J Surg. 1977;59A:790–801.
37. Ginai A. Case report 607. Skeletal Radiol. 1990;19iii:110–16.
38. Dahlin DC. Bone tumors, 4E. Springfield: Thomas; 1986:462–5.
39. Jones HT. Loose body formation in synovial osteochondromatosis with special reference to etiology and pathology. J Bone J Surg. 1924;6:407–58.
40. McCarthie FN, Dorfman HD. Primary chondromatosis. Clin Orthop. 1982;168:178–86.
41. Ryan LM, Cheung HS, Schwab JP, Johnson RP. Predominance of type II collagen and synovial chondromatosis. Clin Orthop. 1982;168:173–7.
42. Jeffries TE. Synovial chondromatosis. J Bone J Surg. 1967;49B:530–4.
43. Carey LS. Synovial chondromatosis of the knee in childhood, report of two cases. J Bone J Surg. 1983;65B:444–7.
44. Wilson WJ, Parr TJ. Synovial chondromatosis. Orthopedics. 1988;11:1179–83.
45. Milgram JW. The development of loose bodies. Clin Orthop. 1977;124:292–303.
46. Milgram JW. The classification of loose bodies in human joints. Clin Orthop. 1977;124:282–91.
47. Maurice H, Crone M, Watte I. Synovial chondromatosis. J Bone J Surg. 1988;6:807–11.
48. Milgram JW, Hadesman WM. Synovial osteochondromatosis in the subacromial bursa. Clin Orthop. 1988;236:154–9.
49. Patzak HJ. Chondromatosis of the elbow. Unfallchirurgie. 1990;16ii:107–9.
50. Cosci MF, Edmonson AS, Pitcock JA. Paravertebral synovial osteochondromatosis. Spine. 1986;11:82–7.
51. Richman JD, Rose DJ. The role of arthroscopy in the management of synovial chondromatosis of the shoulder. Clin Orthop. 1990;257:91–3.
52. Gusenbauer AW, White GC. Synovial osteochondromatosis of the TMJ: case report and review of the literature. J Can Dent Assoc. 1989;55:897–9.
53. Harvey N, Negrine J. Synovial chondromatosis in the DIP. J Hand Surg. 1990;15:102–5.
54. Nather N, Chong PY. A rare case of carpal tunnel syndrome due to synovial osteochondroma. J Hand Surg [Br]. 1986;11:478–80.
55. Minissinger B, Millender LH. Tenosynovial osteochondroma of the hand. Clin Orthop. 1985;96:248–52.
56. Weiss C, Averabuch PF, Steiner GC, Rusoff GH. Synovial osteochondromatosis and instability of the proximal tibial fibular joint. Clin Orthop. 1975;108:187–90.
57. Jacob RA, Campbell WP, Niemann KW. Synovial chondrometaplasia, case report. Clin Orthop. 1975;109:152–4.
58. Shih SH. Synovial osteochondroma of the knee in ^{99m}TcHMDP bone imaging. Clin Nuc Med. 1988;27:615–18.
59. Sundaram M, McGuire MH, Shields JB. Magnetic resonance imaging of lesions of synovial origins. Skeletal Radiol. 1986;15:110–16.
60. Komatasu T, Oshida M, Saski K. Massive deposition of calcium pyrophosphate dihydrate crystals in the knee. J Bone Joint Surg. 1990;72A:931–4.
61. Sim FH, Dahlin CD, Ivins SC. Extra-articular synovial chondromatosis. J Bone J Surg. 1977;59A:492–6.
62. Kay PR, Freemont HA, Davis DRA. The etiology of multiple loose bodies, snowstorm knee. J Bone J Surg. 1989;71:501–4.
63. Dorfmann H, Debie JP, Boyer T. Arthroscopic treatment of synovial chondromatosis of the knee. Arthroscopy. 1989;5:48–52.
64. Smith LW. Synovial sarcoma. Am J Pathol. 1927;3:355–64.
65. Knox LC. Synovial sarcoma: report of 3 cases. Am J Cancer. 1936;28:461–80.
66. Wright PH, Sim EH, Soule EG, Taylor WF. Synovial sarcoma. J Bone J Surg. 1982;64A:112–22.
67. Enneking WF, Chew FS, Springfield DS, Hudson TM, Spanier SS. The role of radionuclide bone-scanning in determining the resectability of soft-tissue sarcomas. J Bone J Surg. 1981;63A:249–57.
68. Wetzel LH, Levine E. Soft-tissue tumors of the foot: value of MR imaging for specific diagnosis. AJR. 1990;155:1025–30.
69. Rydholm A, Rooser B, Persson BM. Primary myectomy for sarcoma. J Bone J Surg. 1986;68A:586–9.
70. Mankin HJ, Lange TA, Spanier SS. The hazards of biopsy in patients with malignant primary bone and soft-tissue tumors. J Bone J Surg. 1982;64A:1121–7.
71. Moore TM, Meyers MH, Patzakis MJ, Terry R, Harvey JP. Closed biopsy of musculoskeletal lesions. J Bone J Surg. 1979;61A:375–9.
72. Dollahite HA, Tatum L, Moinuddin SM, Carnesale PG. Aspiration biopsy of primary neoplasms of bone. J Bone J Surg. 1989;71A:1166–9.
73. Ryan JR, Baker LH, Benjamin RS. The natural history of metastatic synovial sarcoma. Clin Orthop Rel Res. 1982;164:257–60.
74. Cagle LA, Mirra JM, Storm K, Roe DJ, Eilber FR. Histologic features relating to prognosis in synovial sarcoma. Cancer. 1987;59:1810–14.
75. Simon MA, Enniking WF. The management of soft-tissue sarcomas of the extremities. J Bone J Surg. 1986;6:317–27.
76. Suite HD, Proppe KH, Mankin HJ, Wood WC. Preoperative radiation therapy for sarcoma of soft tissue. Cancer. 1981;47:2269–74.
77. Leibel SA, Tranbaugh RF, Wara WM, Beckstead JH, Bovill EG, Phillips TL. Soft tissue sarcomas of the extremities: survival and patterns of failure with conservative surgery and postoperative irradiation compared to surgery alone. Cancer. 1982;50:1076–83.
78. Simon MA, Nachman J. Current concepts review: the clinical utility of preoperative therapy for sarcomas. J Bone J Surg. 1986;68A:1458–63.
79. Pezzi CM, Pollock RE, Evans HL, *et al.* Preoperative chemotherapy for soft-tissue sarcomas of the extremities. Ann Surg. 1990;211:476–81.

FOREIGN BODY SYNOVITIS

Nathan J Zvaifler

Foreign body synovitis

Definition

- Penetration of the joint capsule by a foreign material can produce a chronic, inflammatory, noninfectious synovitis.
- Plant thorns, wood, silica, glass and sea urchin spines have all been implicated.

Clinical features

- Chronic monoarticular arthritis.
- Fingers, wrists and knees are most often involved.
- Initial injury is frequently overlooked. Acute inflammation subsides and may remain quiescent for a long interval before the development of a persistent synovitis.

Silicone synovitis

Definition

- Silicone synovitis is a reaction to particulate material at the site of silicone joint replacement arthroplasty.

Clinical features

- Pain, stiffness and swelling at the site of an implant arthroplasty.
- Swelling of regional lymph nodes may occur.

FOREIGN BODY SYNOVITIS

HISTORY

For more than 50 years it has been recognized that the introduction of foreign material into a joint, tendon sheath or the soft tissue surrounding a joint can induce a chronic, inflammatory monoarticular synovitis or tenosynovitis. In earlier times this was believed due to the introduction of an infectious agent, but subsequently the joint inflammation was shown to represent a nonspecific, foreign body reaction. Coincident with an increased recognition of this rare cause of monoarticular arthritis is an appreciation of the many materials that can evoke this response (Fig. 30.1).

EPIDEMIOLOGY

Although any joint can be affected by foreign body synovitis, the fingers, wrists and knees are most usually involved. A variety of materials have been implicated but the most commonly described include plant thorns, wood splinters, sea urchin spines and inert foreign bodies such as silica and glass[1,2]. In England, the blackthorn, a perennial shrub of the West Midlands is the most common offender, whereas in the southwestern United States, date palm and sentinel palm thorns are often implicated. Children, construction workers and professional and home gardeners are most likely to develop a foreign body synovitis. Swimmers and surfers are at risk for penetrating injuries from the spines of sea urchins.

CLINICAL FEATURES

The clinical picture is one of localized pain in and around a joint that occurs soon after the initial injury, followed by a relatively quiescent period lasting a few days and even occasionally weeks or months[1,2]. By then the initial injury has been forgotten by the patient. After the latent period a persistent monoarticular synovitis develops accompanied by an elevated erythrocyte sedimentation rate, but minimal systemic symptoms. An exception is the foreign body synovitis caused by a sea urchin spine which may have, in addition, fever and myalgia, enlargement of regional lymph nodes and even synovitis beyond the affected joint[3].

DIAGNOSIS AND INVESTIGATIONS

Diagnosis of a foreign body synovitis depends on recognition of the antecedent injury, which is easily overlooked, and exclusion of other causes of chronic inflammatory monoarthritis. Joint aspiration usually yields a cloudy synovial fluid with white blood counts ranging from 5,000–50,000/mm^3 with polymorphonuclear leukocytes as the predominant cell. Bacterial and fungal cultures are negative, although occasionally an infectious agent can be introduced along with the foreign body. The results of imaging studies depend on the etiologic agent[4]. Vegetable particles, such as plant thorns, are not radiodense and thus radiographs of the joint show only soft tissue swelling, generally without associated bone change. Glass and silica are likewise not usually detected, but nonmetallic particles can be demonstrated in the skin by ultrasonography[5]. Sea urchin spines are an exception; because they are composed of calcium carbonate, they are readily seen on routine radiographs. Although there is little published information, magnetic resonance images likely will reveal the responsible agent. The correct diagnosis almost invariably depends upon an excisional biopsy with appropriate pathologic and bacteriologic studies. Synovial lining cells are often increased in number and the subintimal area contains

REPORTED CAUSES OF FOREIGN BODY SYNOVITIS

Plant thorns	Miscellaneous	Detritus from joint prosthesis
Date palm	Sea urchin spine	Cement
Sentinel palm	Wood splinter	Methylmethacrylate
Blackthorn	Fish bone	Silicone
Rose	Stone	Metallic fragments
Cactus	Gravel	
Citrus	Sea shell fragments	
Hawthorn	Glass	
Mesquite	Rubber	
Ulex europaeus (tojo)	Fiberglass	
	Plastic	
	Starch granules	

Fig. 30.1 Reported causes of foreign body synovitis.

monocytes and foreign body giant cells and/or a granulomatous reaction in the histologic examination, but provocative vegetable tissue can only be identified with the aid of a polarizing microscope. Characteristically, plant thorn fragments appear as intensely birefringent multiple cell walls separated by thin fibrous septae (Fig. 30.2). In the past the diagnosis of the foreign body synovitis required an arthrotomy. Currently arthroscopic observation of the synovium and biopsy are usually sufficient.

MANAGEMENT

Treatment usually begins with nonsteroidal anti-inflammatory drugs (NSAIDs) and antibiotics which most often prove to be inadequate. When the proper diagnosis is recognized then removal of the foreign body and observation are indicated. Sometimes this is all that is needed, but often an extensive synovectomy is required to eliminate the problem.

SILICONE SYNOVITIS

HISTORY

Silicone synovitis is a foreign body reaction to particulate material (silicone elastomer, dimethylpolysiloxane) characterized by pain, stiffness and swelling at the site of silicone joint replacement arthroplasty. Flexible silicone implants for finger joint resection arthroplasty were introduced in the 1960s. Over the ensuing decade a significant incidence of implant failure was recognized. Accordingly the conventional 'soft' silicone elastomer was replaced by a prosthesis with improved resistance and a 400% greater increase in strength. Whereas the conventional implants tended to disintegrate at the site of failure with little soft tissue reaction, the high performance elastomer remained in place subject to compression, shearing and abrasion, resulting in microparticle formation. Thus implant failure was replaced by silicone synovitis[6]. The highest incidence of synovitis is observed with carpal–metatarsal and head-of-the-radius implants. These are the implants subjected to the most constant compression and repeated abrasion against bone surfaces during normal activity.

DIAGNOSIS AND MANAGEMENT

Silicone synovitis is diagnosed when a previously asymptomatic patient develops localized pain and swelling at the site of an implant arthroplasty. The diagnosis can be confirmed by evidence of foreign body giant cells and silicone particles in biopsy specimens or radiologic evidence of intramedullary bone destruction, with endosteal scalloping and widening, secondary to bone erosion, especially in bones adjacent to the implant. Swelling of regional lymph nodes with the presence of typical multinucleated giant cells and refractile particles is a recognized complication. Treatment requires removal of the prosthesis.

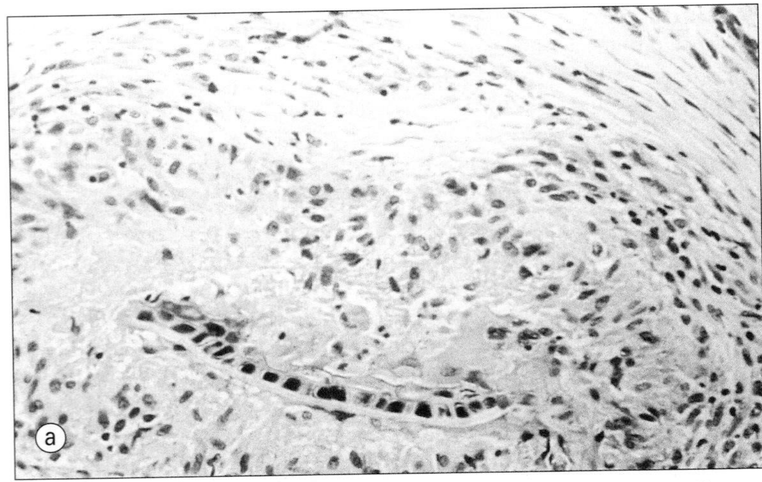

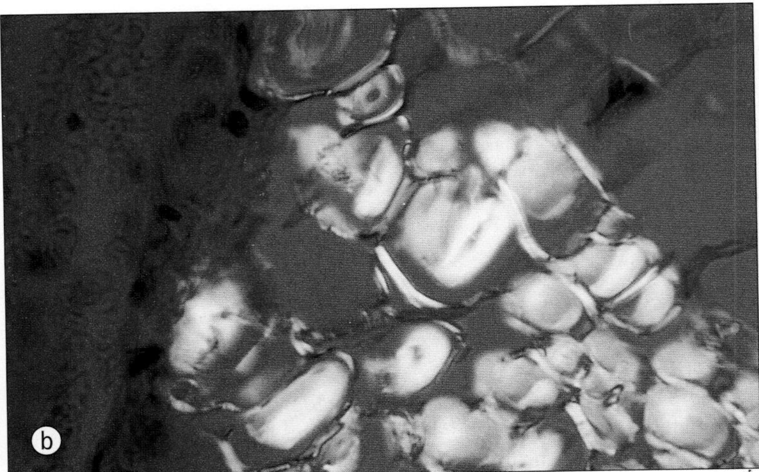

Fig. 30.2 Plant thorn fragment. Example of a plant thorn fragment, surrounded by mononuclear cells and a giant cell in synovium from the knee (a). (Original magnification × 300.) Birefringent cells and septum of a fragment of an *Ulex europaeus* thorn in the synovium from a proximal interphalangeal joint (b). (Original magnification × 300.) Reproduced with permission from Reginato *et al.*[1].

REFERENCES

1. Reginato AJ, Frerreiro JL, O'Connor CR, *et al.* Clinical and pathologic studies of 26 patients with penetrating foreign body injury to the joints, bursa and tendon sheaths. Arthritis Rheum. 1990;33:1753–62.
2. Olenginski TP, Bush DC, Harrington TM. Plant thorn synovitis. An uncommon cause of monoarthritis. Semin Arthritis Rheum. 1991;21:40–46.
3. Cracchiolo A III, Goldberg L. Local and systemic reactions to puncture injuries by the sea urchin spine and the date palm thorn. Arthritis Rheum. 1977;20:1206–12.
4. Bauer AR, Yutani D. Computer tomography localization of wooden foreign bodies in children's extremities. Arch Surg. 1983;118:1084–6.
5. Little CL, Parker MG, Callowich MC, *et al.* The ultrasonic detection of soft tissue foreign bodies. Invest Radiol. 1986;21:275–7.
6. Khoo CT. Silicone synovitis (review article) the current role of silicone elastomer implants in joint reconstruction. J Hand Surg. 1993;18B:679–86.

INDEX

INDEX

A

Introductory note:

- Page numbers in bold refer to major discussions; page numbers followed by (P) refer to Practical Problems; page numbers followed by (i) refer to illustrations; page numbers preceded by A refer to the Appendix; *vs* denotes differential diagnosis or comparisons.
- Page references to sections 1–5 refer to Volume 1. Page references to sections 6–8 refer to Volume 2. **You are in Volume 1**.
- This index is in letter-by-letter order, whereby hyphens and spaces within index headings are ignored in the alpahabetization. Terms in brackets are excluded from the initial alphabetization.
- Cross-reference terms in italics are either general cross-references, or refer to subentry terms within the main entry.

Index abbreviations:

RA (rheumatoid arthritis) • AIDS (acquired immunodeficiency syndrome) • SAARDs (slow acting anti-rheumatic drugs) • SLE (systemic lupus erythematosus)
OA (osteoarthritis) • HIV (human immunodeficiency virus) • NSAIDs (nonsteroidal anti-inflammatory drugs) • HLA (human leukocyte antigen)
AS (ankylosing spondylitis) • JCA (juvenile chronic arthritis) • SPA (spondyloarthropathies) • ReA (reactive arthritis)

A

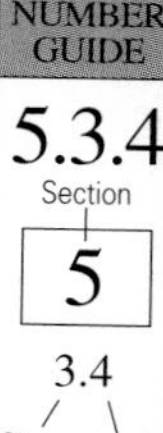

INDEX

A

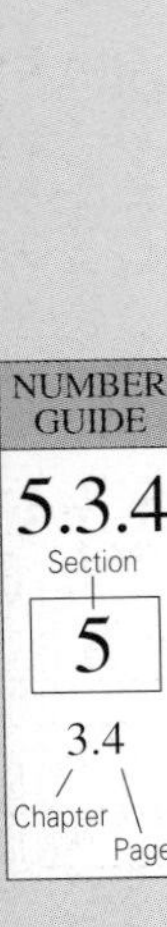

INDEX

A

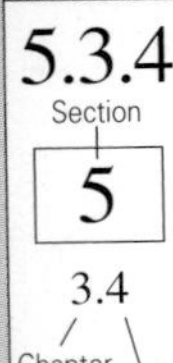

B

C

Page numbers in bold print refer to main subject entries. Page numbers followed by (P) refer to Practical Problems; (i) refers to illustrations. Page numbers preceded by A refer to the Appendix .

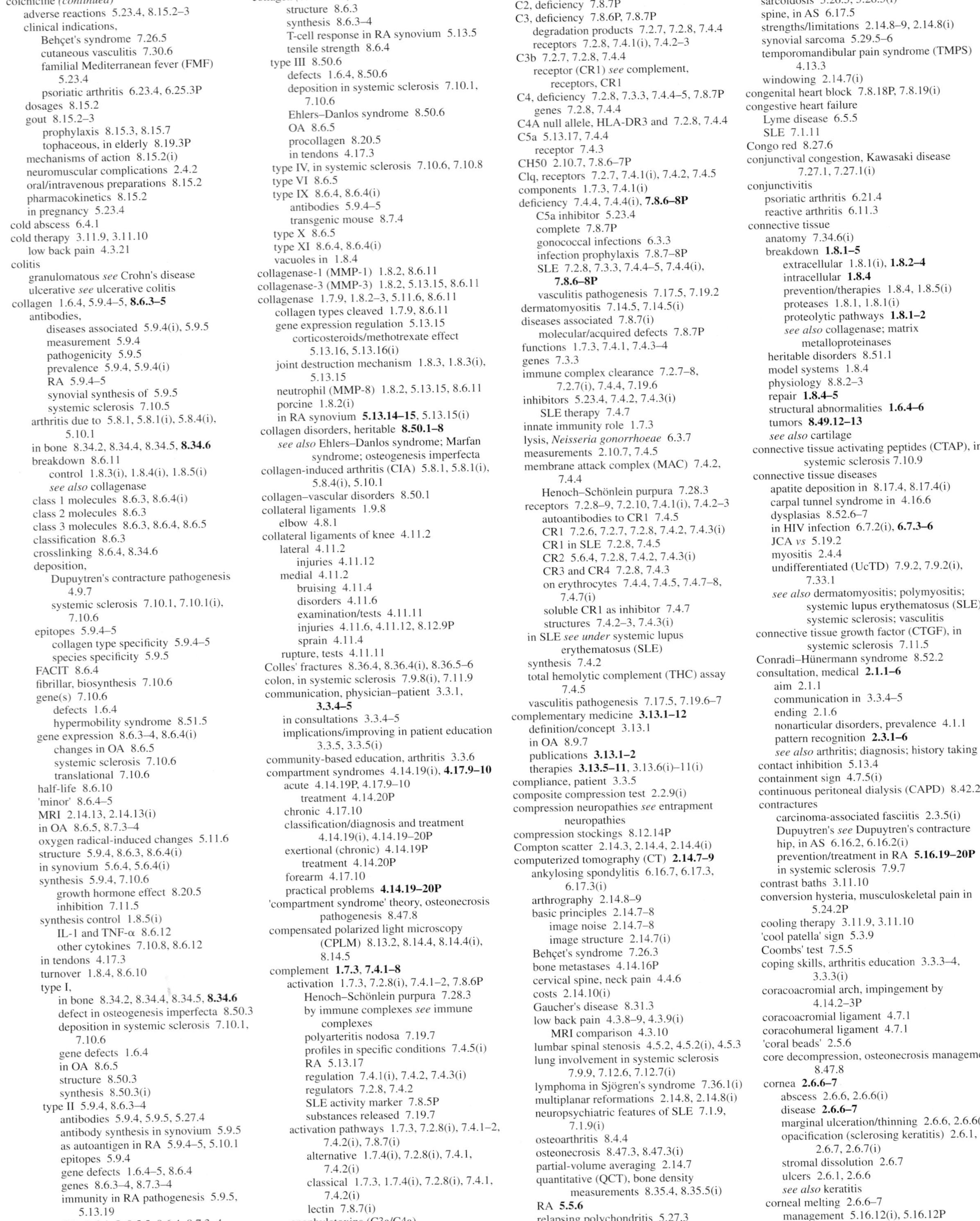

D

E

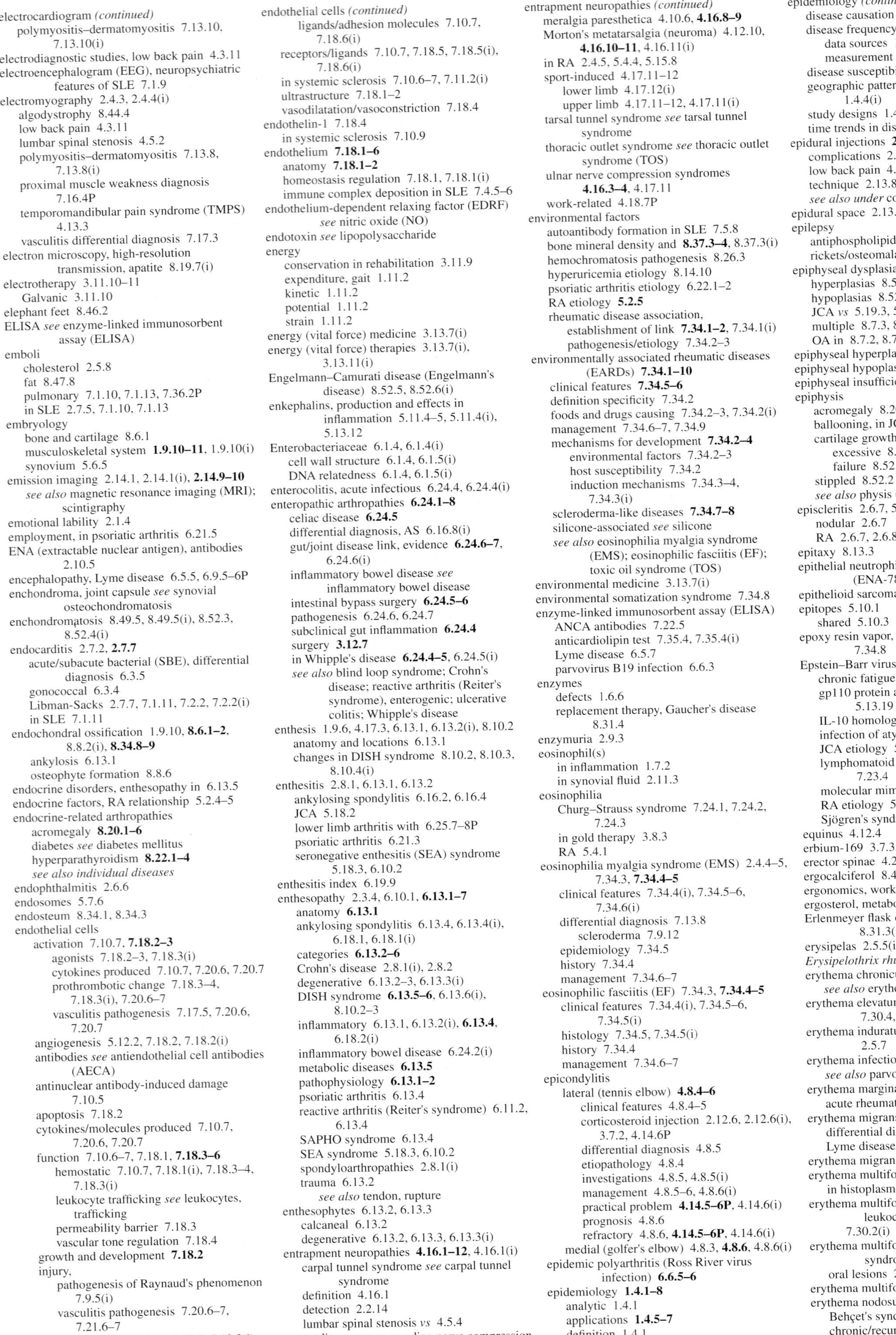

F

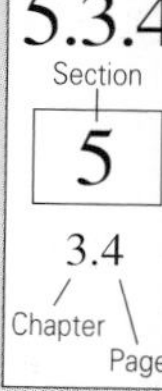

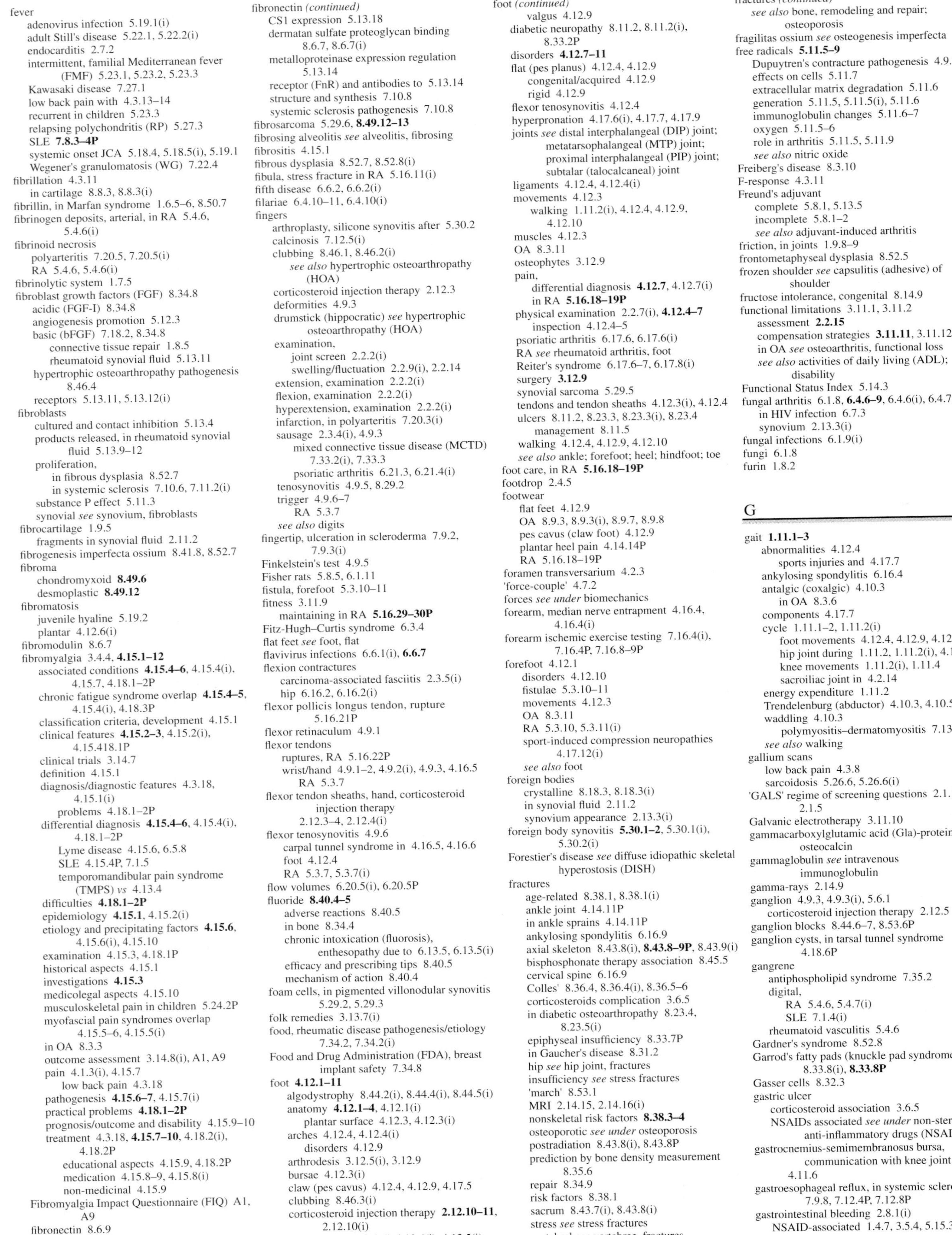

G

NUMBER GUIDE

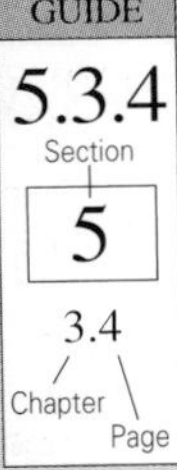

NUMBER GUIDE
5.3.4
Section 5
3.4
Chapter Page

J

K

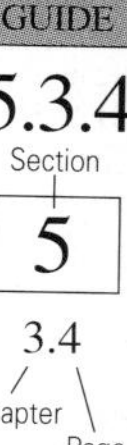

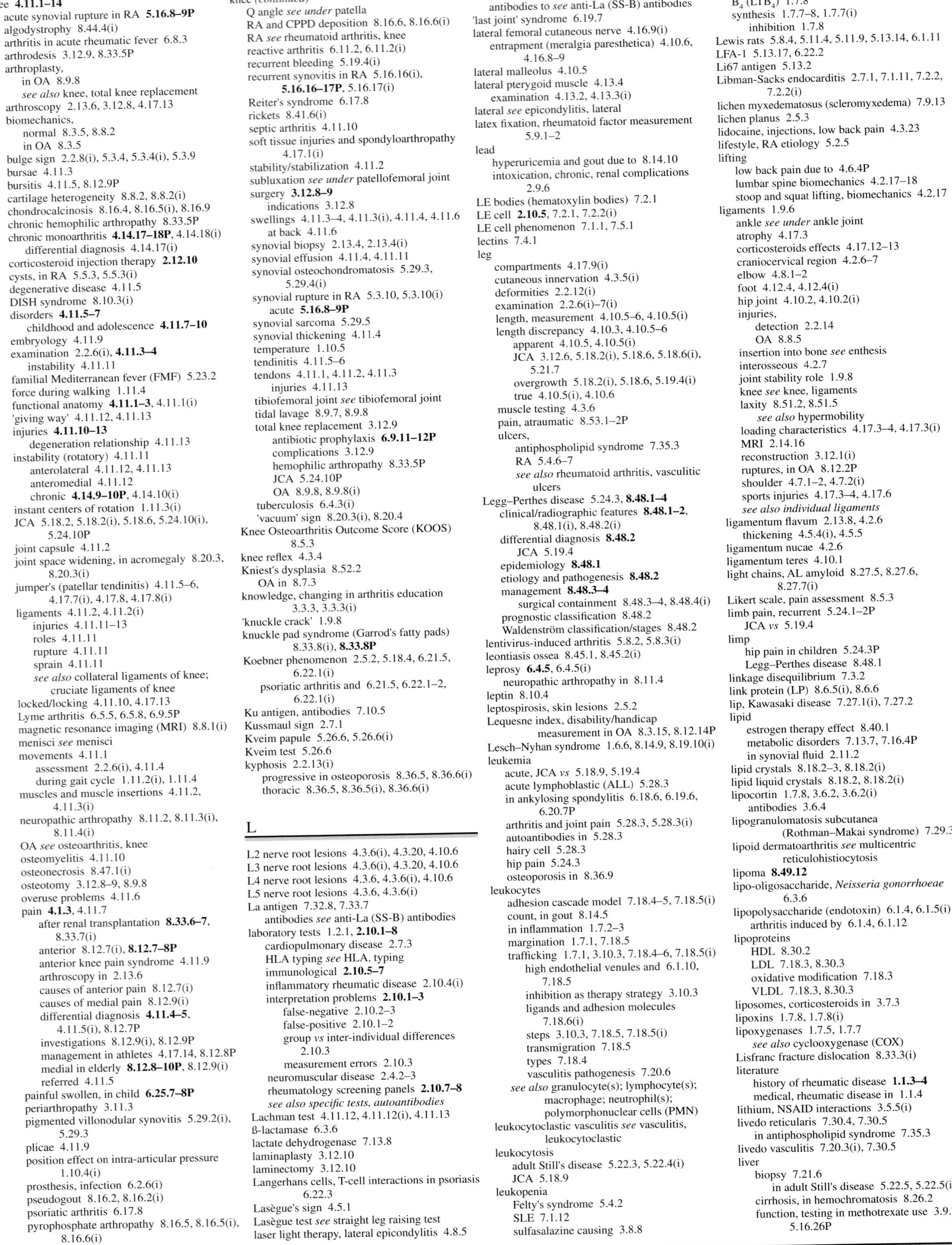

L

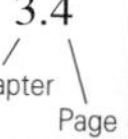

M

O

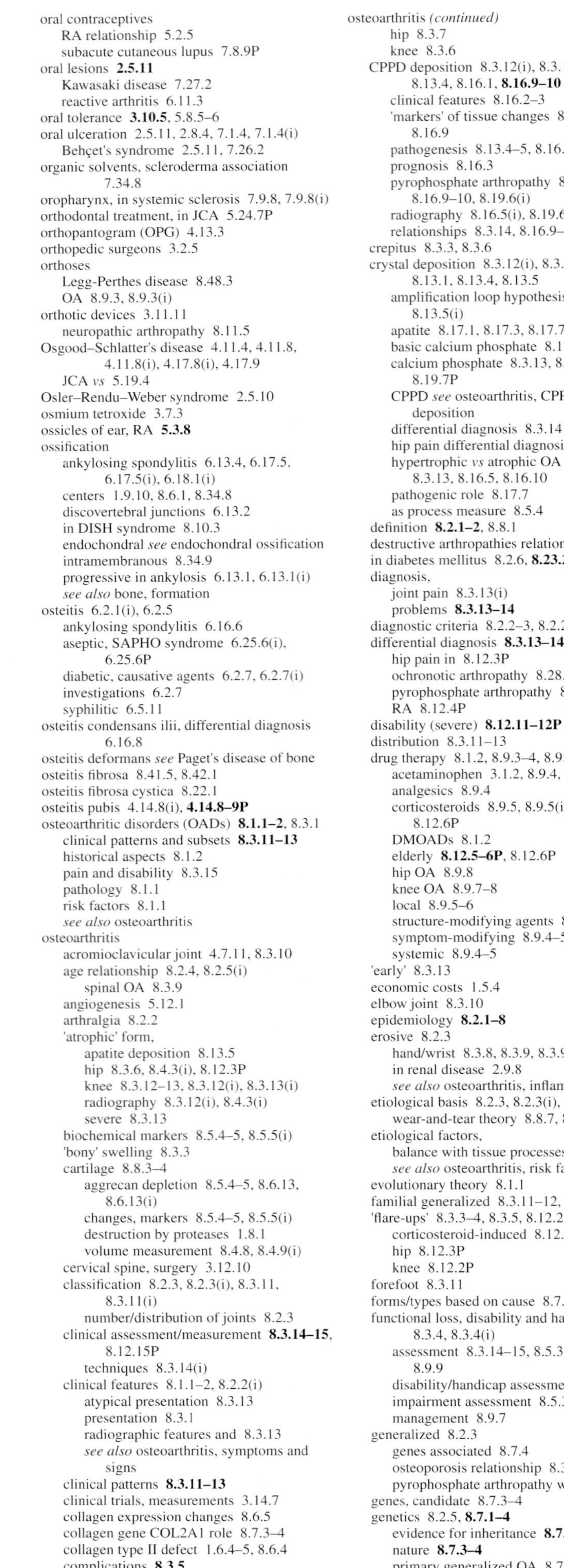

NUMBER GUIDE

5.3.4

Section 5

3.4 Chapter / Page

NUMBER GUIDE
5.3.4
Section
5
3.4
Chapter
Page

P

NUMBER GUIDE
5.3.4
Section 5
3.4
Chapter / Page

INDEX

P

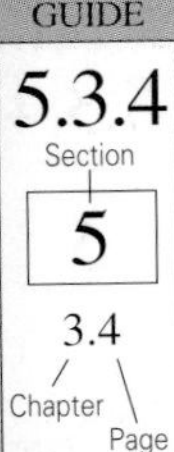

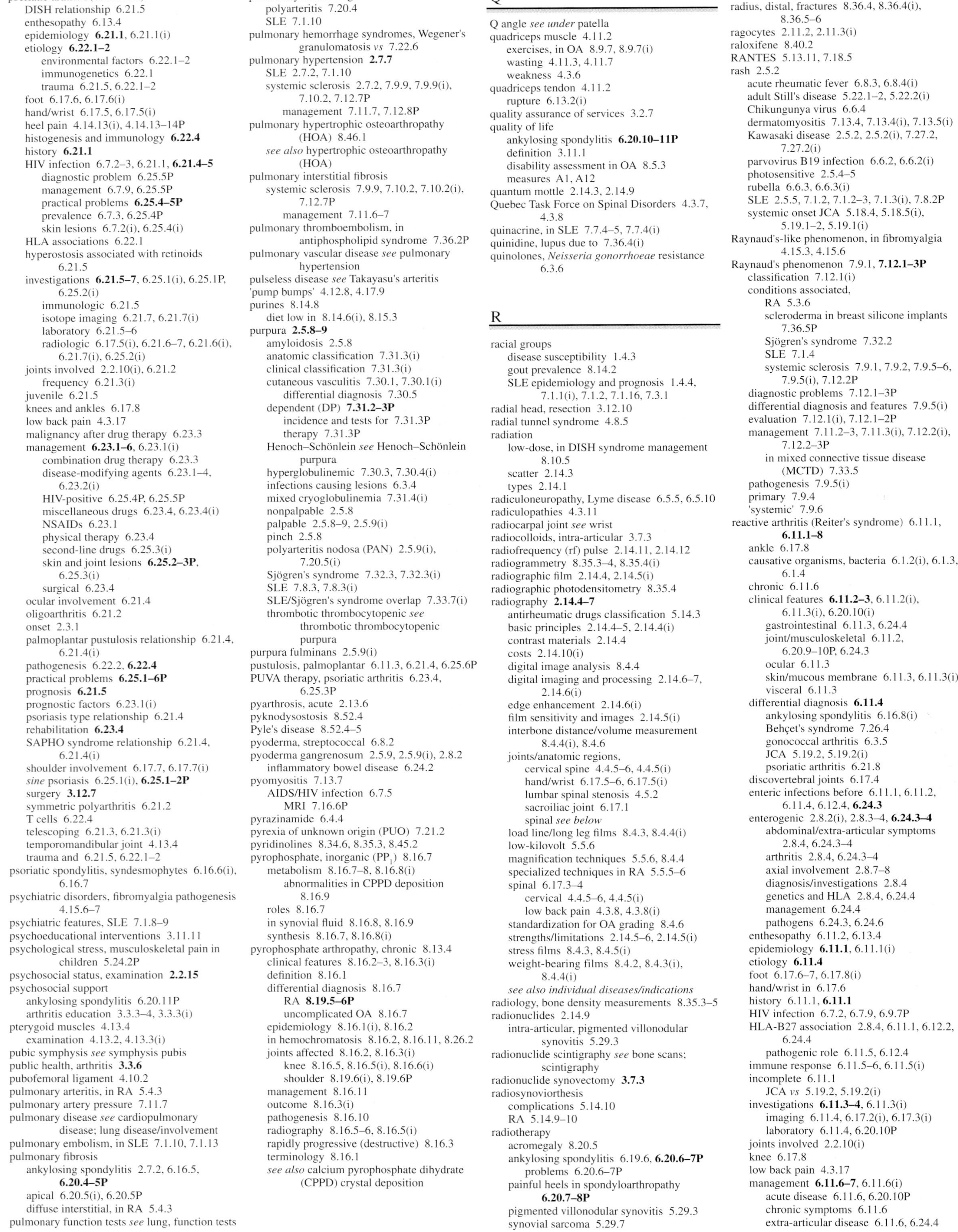

Q

R

NUMBER GUIDE
5.3.4
Section
5
3.4
Chapter / Page

NUMBER GUIDE
5.3.4
Section 5
3.4
Chapter Page

INDEX

S

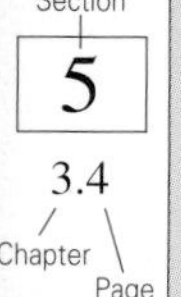

Page numbers in bold print refer to main subject entries. Page numbers followed by (P) refer to Practical Problems; (i) refers to illustrations. Page numbers preceded by A refer to the Appendix.
Volume 1: Sections 1–5; Volume 2: Sections 6–8. You are in Volume 1

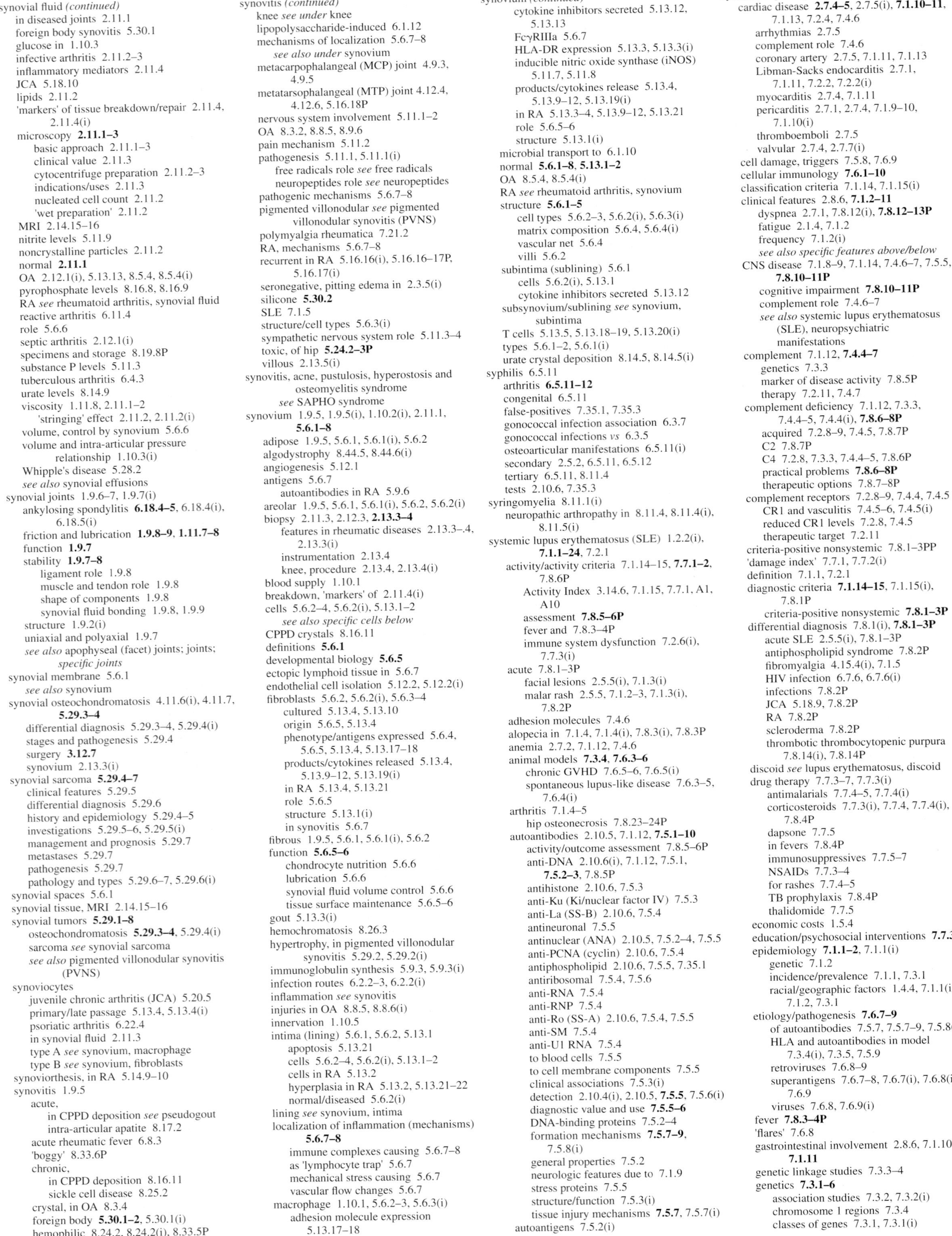

U

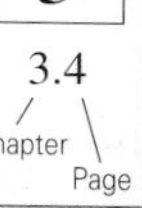

V

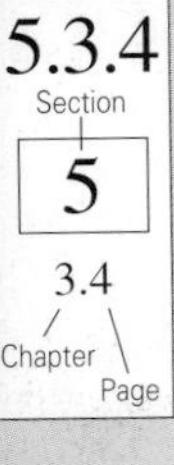

W

X

Y

Z

NUMBER GUIDE

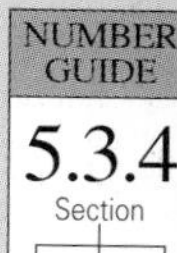